Pain Relief and Anesthesia in Obstetrics

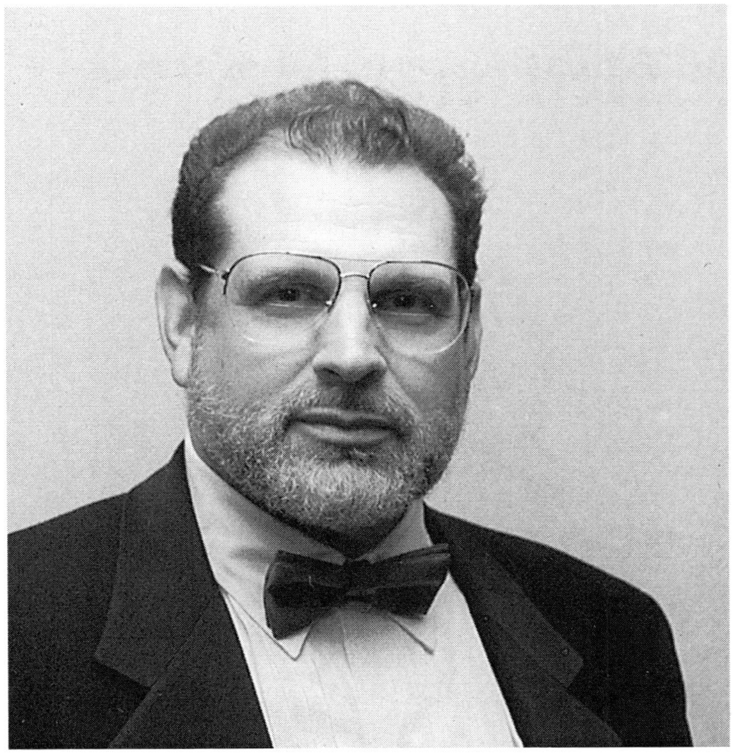

GERARD W. OSTHEIMER
1940–1995

The anesthesia community was stunned by the announcement of the untimely death on October 1 of Gerard W. Ostheimer. The House of Regional Anesthesia has lost another giant. Gerry was regarded as a true friend, a respected colleague and an expert advisor to a worldwide community of regional and obstetrical anesthesiologists, whom he guided in his own professional way as a clinician, mentor, teacher, leader and compassionate human being, whose heart was always woven of human joys and cares.

I was very proud that Gerry supported the idea to write our book Pain Relief and Anesthesia in Obstetrics. Without Gerry's help, this dream would never have been realized. This title is, therefore, dedicated to the memory of my dear friend Gerard W. Ostheimer, who shall be painfully missed by all who knew him.

André Van Zundert
1995

For Churchill Livingstone
Commissioning Editor: Geoffrey Nuttall
Copy Editor: Helen McDonald
Indexer: Monica Trigg
Production: Mark Sanderson, Nora Cameron
Design Direction: Erik Bigland

Pain Relief and Anesthesia in Obstetrics

Edited by

André Van Zundert MD PhD

Department of Anesthesiology, Intensive Care and Pain Therapy, Catharina Hospital, Eindhoven, The Netherlands;
Secretary-General, European Society of Regional Anaesthesia

The Late Gerard W. Ostheimer MD

Formerly Professor of Anaesthesia, Harvard Medical School;
Vice Chairman, Department of Anaesthesia, Brigham and Women's Hospital, Boston, Massachusetts, USA

Line drawings by
Emily Harris

CHURCHILL
LIVINGSTONE

NEW YORK EDINBURGH LONDON MADRID MELBOURNE SAN FRANCISCO AND
TOKYO 1996

CHURCHILL LIVINGSTONE
Medical Division of Pearson Professional Limited

Distributed in the United States of America by Churchill Livingstone Inc., 650 Avenue of the Americas, New York, N.Y. 10011, and by associated companies, branches and representatives throughout the world.

First published 1996

ISBN 0 443 04474 0

British Library Cataloguing in Publication Data
A catalogue record for this book is available from the British Library.

Library of Congress Cataloging in Publication Data
A catalog record for this book is available from the Library of Congress.

The publisher's policy is to use **paper manufactured from sustainable forests**

Printed in Singapore

Contents

SECTION 7
Controversies

Contributors

Ezzat I. Abouleish MB ChB DA DM MD
Professor of Anesthesiology, Professor of Obstetrics and Gynecology, Director of Obstetric Anesthesia, Medical School, University of Texas at Houston, Texas, USA

S. Alahuhta MD
Department of Obstetrics and Gynecology, University of Oulu, Oulu, Finland

Claudine Amiel-Tison MD
Associate Professor of Pediatrics, Baudelocque Maternity Hospital, Paris, France

Katherine Amundson MD
Anesthesiologist, Mercy Medical Center, Baltimore, Maryland, USA

John E. Arnold MD
Anesthesia Service Medical Group Inc.; Staff Anesthesiologist, Sharp Memorial Hospital, San Diego, California, USA

Albert Aynsley-Green MA DPhil MB BS FRCP FRCP(Edin)
Nuffield Professor of Child Health, Institute of Child Health, London, UK

Angela M. Bader MD
Assistant Professor of Anaesthesia, Harvard Medical School; Staff Anesthesiologist, Brigham and Women's Hospital, Boston, Massachusetts, USA

William H. Barth Jr. MD
Chief of Obstetrics, Wilford Hall Medical Center, San Antonio, Texas; Assistant Professor, Department of Obstetrics and Gynecology, Uniformed Services, University of the Health Sciences, Bethesda, Maryland, USA

Gerard M. Bassell MB BS
Professor of Anesthesiology, Obstetrics and Gynecology, University of Kansas School of Medicine; Medical Director, Surgicare of Wichita, Kansas, USA

P. Belfrage MD
Department of Anesthesiology and Intensive Care, Karolinska Hospital, Stockholm, Sweden

Sergio D. Belzarena MD
Chairman, Department of Anesthesiology, Santa Casa de Misericordia, Livramento RS, Brazil

Dan Benhamou MD
Associate Professor, Department of Anesthesia and Intensive Care, Hôpital Antoine Béclère, Clamart, Université Paris-Sud, Paris, France

Frederick M. Bennett PhD
Co-Director, Center for Analysis of Heart Rate Dynamics, Department of Anesthesia, Beth Israel Hospital, Boston Massachusetts, USA

David J. Birnbach MD
Director of Obstetric Anesthesia, St Luke's-Roosevelt Hospital Center; Assistant Professor of Anesthesiology and Obstetrics and Gynecology, Columbia University College of Physicians and Surgeons, New York, USA

Norman H. Blass MD
Professor of Anesthesia and Obstetrics, University of Texas Medical Branch, Galveston, Texas, USA

The Late John J. Bonica MD DSc DMedSc(Hon) FRCAnaes(Hon)
Formerly Professor and Chairman Emeritus, Department of Anesthesiology; Founder and Honorary President, International Association for the Study of Pain; Director Emeritus, Multidisciplinary Pain Center, University of Washington, Seattle, Washington, USA

A. I. J. Brain MA LMSSA FFARCSI
Honorary Consultant Anaesthetist, Northwick Park Hospital, Harrow,; Honorary Consultant Anaesthetist, Royal Berkshire Hospital, Reading; Honorary Research Fellow, Institute of Laryngology, University of London, UK

Philip R. Bromage MB BS FRCA FRCP(C)
Post-retirement Professor, McGill University Department of Anaesthesia, Montreal, Canada

Peter Brownridge MB ChB FRCA FANZCA
Director of Obstetric Anaesthesia and Senior Lecturer, Department of Anaesthesia and Intensive Care, Flinders Medical Centre, Adelaide, South Australia, Australia

Bernard Bruguerolle MD PhD
Professor and Head of Experimental and Clinical Pharmacology, Faculty of Medicine of Marseille, Marseille, France

Corey A. Burchman AB MD
Staff Anesthesiologist, York Hospital, York, Pennsylvania, USA

Randall L. Busch MD MS
Director, Center for Pain Management, Department of Anesthesiology, Mercy Medical Center, Dubuque, Iowa, USA

William Camann MD
Assistant Professor of Anaesthesia, Harvard Medical School, Staff Anesthesiologist, Brigham and Women's Hospital, Boston, Massachusetts, USA

Enrico Mario Camporesi MD
Professor and Chairman, Department of Anesthesia, SUNY Health Science Center, Syracuse, New York, USA

Harvey Carp PhD MD
Associate Professor of Anesthesiology and Obstetrics and Gynecology, Oregon Health Sciences University, Portland, Oregon, USA

Len E. S. Carrie MB ChB FRCA
Consultant Anaesthetist, The John Radcliffe Maternity Hospital and Nuffield Department of Anaesthetics, Oxford; Clinical Lecturer, University of Oxford, Oxford, UK

José Carlos A. Carvalho MD PhD
Supervisor Obstetric Anesthesia, University of São Paulo, São Paulo, Brazil

I. Castelletti MD
Primario Anestesia e Rianimazione, Ospedale Santa Anna, Turin, Italy

Paula D. M. Chantigian MD FACOG
Obstetrician Gynecologist, Rochester, Minnesota, USA

Robert C. Chantigian MD
Assistant Professor, Department of Anesthesiology, Mayo Clinic, Rochester, Minnesota, USA

David H. Chestnut MD
Professor and Chairman, Department of Anesthesiology, University of Alabama, Birmingham, Alabama, USA

Paul Clyburn MB BS MRCP(UK) FRCA
Consultant Obstetric Anaesthetist, University Hospital of Wales, Cardiff, UK

Jacqueline Conard PhD
Maître de Conferences des Universités; Practicien Hospitalier - Laboratoire Central d'Hematologie, Hotel Dieu, Paris, France

Kenneth A. Conklin MD PhD
Associate Professor, Director of Obstetric Anesthesia, Department of Anesthesiology, University of California, Los Angeles School of Medicine, Los Angeles, California, USA

Stephen B. Corn MD
Instructor, Department of Anaesthesia, Harvard Medical School; Anesthesiologist, Brigham amd Women's Hospital; Anesthesiologist, Children's Hospital, Boston, Massachusetts, USA

Michael J. Cousins MB BS MD(Syd) FANZCA FRCA
Professor and Head, Anaesthesia and Pain Management, Sydney University, Royal North Shore Hospital, Sydney, Australia

The Late Benjamin G. Covino PhD MD
Formerly Professor and Chairman, Department of Anaesthesia, Brigham and Women's Hospital, Harvard Medical School, Boston, Massachusetts, USA

P. G. W. Cramp MRCP FRCA
Consultant Anaesthetist, Bradford Hospitals NHS Trust, Bradford, UK

Yves Darbois MD
Professeur des Universités, Centre Hôpitalier Universitaire Pitié-Salpétrière, Université Pierre et Marie Curie, Paris, France

Sanjay Datta MD FFARCs(Eng)
Director of Obstetric Anaesthesia, Brigham and Women's Hospital; Professor of Anaesthesia, Harvard Medical School, Boston, Massachusetts, USA

P. Defoort MD ScD(Biomed)
Consultant, Department of Gynecology, University Hospital, Gent, Belgium

José A. De Andrés
Medica Anestesiologa, Eratamiento del dolar, Valencia, Spain

André M. De Wolf MD
Associate Professor of Anesthesiology, University of Pittsburgh School of Medicine, Pittsburgh, Pennsylvania, USA

Marie Dreyfus MD
Associate Professor, Department of Hematology, Hôpital Bicêtre, Le Kremlin Bicêtre, France

David Ecker MD
Associate Professor, Department of Obstetrics and Gynecology, Brigham and Women's Hospital, Boston, Massachusetts, USA

Francesco Emma MD
Division of General Pediatrics, Child Development Unit, The Children's Hospital, Harvard Medical School, Boston, Massachusetts, USA

Gilbert F. Fanciullo MD MS
Instructor, Harvard Medical School; Staff Anesthesiologist, Pain Management Center, Department of Anesthesia, Brigham and Women's Hospital, Boston, Massachusetts, USA

Bruce B. Feinberg MD
Associate Professor, Maternal-Fetal Medicine, Department of Obstetrics and Gynecology, Harvard Medical School, Brigham and Women's Hospital, Boston, Massachusetts, USA

F. Michael Ferrante MD
Assistant Professor of Anaesthesia, Harvard Medical School, Director Pain Management Center, Department of Anesthesia, Brigham and Women's Hospital, Boston, Massachusetts, USA

Mieczyslaw Finster MD
Professor of Anesthesiology, Obstetrics and Gynecology, College of Physicians and Surgeons, Columbia University, New York, USA

Kenneth J. Freese MD
Clinical Associate Professor of Anesthesiology, State University of New York at Stony Brook, New York; Chairman, Department of Anesthesiology, Nassau County Medical Center, New York, USA

David R. Gambling MB BS DRCOG FRCPC
Director, Obstetric Anesthesia Research; Assistant Professor, Department of Anesthesiology and Pain Management, University of Texas Southwestern Medical Center at Dallas, Texas, USA

James Gardiner MB FFARCSI FRCA
Director of Anaesthesia, Rotunda Hospital, Dublin, Eire

Stephen P. Gatt MRCS MD FFARACS FANZCA FFA Int Cr
Director of Anaesthesia, Royal Hospital for Women, Paddington; Senior Lecturer in Anaesthesia, University of New South Wales, Kensington, Sydney, Australia

Elisabeth Giaufré MD
Department of Anesthesiology, Fondation Hôpital Saint-Joseph, Marseille, France

Mathieu J. M. Gielen MD PhD
Associate Professor, Institute for Anaesthesiology, University of Nijmegen, The Netherlands

Evelina Gollo MD
Servizio Di Anesthesia e Rianimazione, Ospedale S Anna, Torino, Italy

Bernard Gonik MD
Professor and Vice Chairman, Department of Obstetrics and Gynecology, Wayne State University School of Medicine; Chief, Department of Obstetrics and Gynecology, Grace Hospital, Detroit, Michigan, USA

Inmaculada Guasp MD
Instructor in Anesthesia, New York University School of Medicine, New York, USA

Simon Halevy MD
Professor of Anesthesiology, State University of New York; Director of Anesthesia Research, Nassau County Medical Center, East Meadow, New York, USA

Jamil Hamza MD
Assistant Professor in Anesthesiology, Départemant d'Anesthésie-Réanimation, Hôpital St Vincent de Paul, Paris, France

Michael Harmer MB BS FRCA
Consultant Anaesthetist, University Hospital of Wales, Cardiff, UK

Martha A. Hauch MD
Instructor, Department of Anaesthesia, Harvard Medical School, Boston; Staff Anaesthesiologist, Brigham and Women's Hospital, Boston, Massachusetts, USA

J. M. Hawdon MA MB BS MRCP
Lecturer in Neonatology, Institute of Child Health, University of Liverpool, Liverpool, UK

Joy L. Hawkins MD
Associate Professor of Anesthesiology, University of Colorado Health Sciences Center, Denver, Colorado, USA

Michelle A. Hayes FRCA
Research Fellow in Intensive Care, St Bartholomew's Hospitals at Smithfield and Homerton, London, UK

Michel Henry PhD MD
Hôpital de la Pitié, Paris, France

Arno I. Hollmén MD PhD
Professor, Department of Anaesthesiology, University of Oulu, Oulu, Finland

Laurel A. Hortvet MD
Staff Anesthesiologist, Hartford Hospital, Hartford, Connecticut, USA

McCallum R. Hoyt MD
Assistant Professor, Department of Anesthesiology, Case Western Reserve University; Chief, Division of Obstetric Anesthesia, University Hospitals of Cleveland, Cleveland, Ohio, USA

T. Huckaby MD
Director of Anesthesiology, Arnold Palmer Hospital for Women and Children, Orlando, Florida, USA

N. Hughes FFARCSIRI DABA FACPM
Consultant Anaesthetist, St James' Hospital, Dublin, Ireland

Catherine O. Hunt MD
Staff Anesthesiologist, Beverly Hospital, Beverly, Massachusetts, USA

Ronald J. Hurley MD
Assistant Professor of Anesthesia, Harvard Medical School; Associate Director of Obstetric Anesthesia, Brigham and Women's Hospital, Boston, Massachusetts, USA

Lars Irestedt MD PhD
Associate Professor, Department of Anaesthesiology and Intensive Care, Karolinska Hospital, Stockholm, Sweden

Ronaldo R. Joco MD
Senior Resident in Anesthesiology, Albert Einstein College of Medicine, Bronx, New York, USA

Calvin Johnson MD
Assistant Professor of Anesthesia, Wayne State University; Chief of Anesthesia, Hutzel Hospital, Detroit, Michigan, USA

M. D. Johnson BS MT MD
Chairman, Department of Anesthesiology, Melrose Wakefield Hospital, Melrose, Massachusetts, USA

Pentti Jouppila MD PhD
Associate Professor, Department of Obstetrics and Gynaecology, University of Oulu, Oulu, Finland

R. Jouppila MD
Department of Obstetrics and Gynaecology, University of Oulu, Oulu, Finland

Thomas H. Joyce III MD
Professor of Anesthesiology, University of Cincinnati, Cincinnati, Ohio, USA

Patricio J. Kelly MD DM DA
Chairman, Department of Anaesthesia, British Hospital of Buenos Aires, Buenos Aires, Argentina

R. M. Knapp MD
Staff Anesthesiologist, Jordan Hospital, Plymouth, Massachusetts, USA

Betty Lou Koffel MD
Associate Professor, Department of Anesthesiology, Boston City Hospital, Boston, Massachusetts, USA

John Kolbe MB BS FRACP
Senior Lecturer in Medicine, University of Auckland, Respiratory Physician, Green Lane Hospital, Auckland, New Zealand

Hector Lacassie MD
Associate Professor of Anesthesiology, University of Chile School of Medicine, Santiago, Chile

Ian A. Laing MA MD FRCP(Edin)
Clinical Director, Neonatal Unit, Simpson Memorial Maternity Pavilion, Edinburgh, UK

Donald H. Lambert PhD MD
Anaesthesiologist, Brigham and Women's Hospital; Associate Professor of Anaesthesia, Harvard Medical School, Boston, Massachusetts, USA

Daniel P. Landry MD
Instructor in Anesthesia, Harvard Medical School, Beth Israel Hospital, Boston, Massachusetts, USA

Robert F. LaPorta PhD MD
Anesthesiologist, Department of Anesthesia, North Shore University Hospital, New York, USA

K. A. Leavitt MD
Assistant Professor of Anesthesiology, George Washington University Hospital, Washington DC, USA

Barbara L. Leighton MD
Associate Professor of Anesthesiology, Jefferson Medical College, Thomas Jefferson University, Philadelphia, Pennsylvania, USA

Catherine K. Lineberger MD
Assistant Professor of Anesthesiology, Duke University Medical Center, Durham, North Carolina, USA

Barbara Lynn Loferski BA MD
Instructor in Anesthesia, Harvard Medical School; Staff Anesthesiologist, Brigham and Women's Hospital, Boston, Massachusetts, USA

Steven A. Lussos MD
Staff Anesthesiologist, Fairfax Hospital, Falls Church, VA, USA

Willem Luyendijk MD PhD
Emeritus Professor of Surgical Neurology, State University Leiden, The Netherlands

Eileen Lynch MD AB
Instructor in Anaesthesia, Harvard Medical School, Staff Anesthesiologist, Brigham and Women's Hospital, Boston, Massachusetts, USA

John H. McClure BSc MB ChB FRCA
Consultant Anaesthetist, Royal Infirmary, Edinburgh; Honorary Senior Lecturer, University of Edinburgh, UK

Robert S. F. McKay MD
Clinical Associate Professor of Anesthesiology, University of Kansas-Wichita; Director of Obstetric Anesthesia, HCA/Wesley Medical Center, Wichita, Kansas, USA

S. A. Macklin MB BS FRCA
Senior Registrar, Department of Anaesthesia, Guy's Hospital, London, UK

Graham H. McMorland MB ChB FRCPC
Professor Emeritus, Department of Anaesthesia, University of British Columbia, Vancouver, Canada

T. Philip Malan Jr PhD MD
Assistant Professor, Department of Anesthesiology, University of Arizona, Tucson, Arizona, USA

Andrew M. Malinow MD
Director, Obstetric Anesthesia and Associate Professor of Anesthesiology, Obstetrics and Gynecology, University of Maryland School of Medicine, Baltimore, Maryland, USA

Virgil Manica MD
Instructor in Anesthesia, Department of Anesthesia, New England Medical Center, Massachusetts, USA

Elsa Margaria MD
Professoressa, Primario Anestesia e Rianimazione, Ospedale S. Anna, Turin, Italy

Ramon F. Martin MD PhD
Assistant Professor of Anesthesia, Harvard Medical School, Staff Anesthesiologist, Department of Anesthesia, Brigham and Women's Hospital, Boston, Massachusetts, USA

Gertie F. Marx MD
Professor of Anesthesiology, Albert Einstein College of Medicine, Bronx, New York, USA

Kenneth Mintz MD
Chairman, Department of Anesthesia, Lourdes Hospital, Binghamton, New York; Clinical Instructor, Department of Anesthesia, State University of New York Health Science Center at Syracuse, Syracuse, New York, USA

Beth H. Minzter MD MS
Instructor, Department of Anaesthesia, Harvard Medical School; Staff Anesthesiologist, Pain Management Center, Department of Anesthesia, Brigham and Women's Hospital, Boston, Massachusetts, USA

Daniel C. Moore MD FFARCS
Department of Anesthesiology (Emeritus), The Mason Clinic, Seattle, Washington, USA

James Moore MD FRCA FFARCS(I)
Chief of Anaesthesia, King Fahad Armed Forces Hospital, Jeddah, Saudi Arabia

Barbara Morgan MB ChB FRCA
Senior Lecturer in Obstetrics and Anaesthesia, Institute of Obstetrics and Gynaecology; Consultant Anaesthetist, Queen Charlotte's Hospital, London, UK

Lachlan M. M. Morrison MB ChB BSc FFARCSI
Consultant Anaesthetist, St John's Hospital, Livingston, West Lothian, UK

Rhonda M. Mullins MD
Assistant Professor, Department of Anesthesiology, University of Texas Health Science Center, San Antonio, Texas, USA

Julius Neumark MD FACA
Chairman, Department of Anaesthesiology, Donauspital-SMZO, Vienna, Austria

Hans Nolte MD(D) MD(DK) PhD(Priv Doz)
Professor and Head, Department of Anaesthesia, Academic Hospital, Minden, Germany

Mark C. Norris MD
Professor of Anesthesia, Jefferson Medical College, Thomas Jefferson University, Philadelphia, Pennsylvania, USA

B. O'Kelly MD
Department of Anesthesia and Intensive Care, Hôpital Antoine Béclère, Clamart, Université Paris-Sud, Paris, France

Nancy E. Oriol MD
Assistant Professor, Harvard Medical School; Director, Obstetric Anesthesia, Beth Israel Hospital, Boston, Massachusetts, USA

The Late Gerard W. Ostheimer MD
Formerly Professor of Anaesthesia, Harvard Medical School; Vice Chairman, Department of Anesthesia, Brigham and Women's Hospital, Boston, Massachusetts, USA

Geraldine O'Sullivan MD FRCA
Consultant Anaesthetist, St Thomas' Hospital, London, UK

L. M. Padilla MD
Department of Anesthesiology, New York University School of Medicine, New York, USA

Michael J. Paech MB BS DRCOG FRCAnaes FANZCA
Staff Anaesthetist and Acting Head of Department, Department of Anaesthesia, King Edward Memorial Hospital, Perth, Western Australia, Australia

James F. Pearson MD FRCOG
Reader in Obstetrics and Gynaecology, University of Wales College of Medicine, Cardiff, UK

Hilda Pedersen MB ChB FFARCS
Professor of Clinical Anesthesiology, College of Physicians and Surgeons, Columbia University, New York, USA

Michael D. Popitz MD
Instructor, Department of Anaesthesia, Harvard Medical School; Anesthesiologist, Department of Anesthesia, Beth Israel Hospital, Boston, Massachusetts, USA

Marcia A. Procopio BS MD
Attending Anesthesiologist, Assistant Professor of Anesthesia, Dartmouth Hitchcock Hospital, Lebanon

Narinder Rawal MB BS MD PhD
Associate Professor, Department of Anesthesiology, Örebro Medical Center Hospital, Sweden; Visiting Professor, Department of Anesthesiology, University of Texas Medical School, Houston, Texas, USA

Felicity Reynolds MB BS MD FRCA
Professor of Obstetric Anaesthesia, St Thomas' Hospital, London, UK

Jorge Riquelme MD
President, CLASA; Director, LASRA; Director of Anesthesiology, Chilean Air Force Hospital, Santiago, Chile

Carlo Romanini MD
Professor and Chairman, Department of Obstetrics and Gynecology, University of Rome, 'Tor Vergata', Italy

Michael Rosen CBE FRCA FRCOG
Professor in Anaesthetics, University of Wales College of Medicine, Cardiff, UK

A. Runyon-Hass MD
608 Jackson Boulevard, Nashville, Tennessee, USA

David Sage MB ChB Dip. Obstet. FANZCA
Chairman, Department of Anaesthesia, Green Lane/National Women's Hospital, Auckland, New Zealand

Meyer Michel Samama MD
Professor of Hematology, Director of Central Laboratory of Hematology, Hôtel-Dieu Hospital, Paris, France

Alan C. Santos MD
Associate Attending Anesthesiologist, Bronx Municipal Hospital, Eastchester Road and Pelham Parkway, Bronx, New York, USA

John W. Scanlon MD
Director of Neonatology, Columbia Hospital for Women; Professor of Pediatrics, Georgetown University, Washington DC, USA

Dan Schneeweiss MD
Private Practice, Yakima, Washington, USA

Steven S. Schwalbe MD
Assistant Professor of Anesthesiology, Director of Obstetric Anesthesia, Albert Einstein College of Medicine and Montefiore Medical Center, Bronx, New York, USA

D. Bruce Scott MD FRCPE FRCA
Consultant and Senior Lecturer (ret), Royal Infirmary, University of Edinburgh, Edinburgh, UK

Jeanne Seebacher MD
MGU-PH d'Anesthesie Reanimation responsable d'Anesthesie en obstetrique, Département d'Anesthésie-Réanimation, Centre Hôpitalier Universitaire Pitié-Salpétrière, Paris, France

M. J. Segal MD
Assistant Professor of Anesthesia, Tulane University School of Medicine, New Orleans, Louisiana, USA

Ferne B. Sevarino MD CM
Associate Professor of Anesthesiology, Yale University School of Medicine, New Haven, USA

D. Sfoggia MD
Hôpital Pitié Salpétrière, Paris, France

Farrokh Shahrivar MD
Associate Clinical Professor of Pediatrics, College of Physicians and Surgeons, Columbia University; Director, Neonatology Division, St Luke's-Roosevelt Hospital Center, New York, USA

Cathy Shea MSc
Marketing Manager, Becton Dickinson Co, Franklin Lakes, New Jersey, USA

Donald M. Sherline MD
Brooks Professor and Chairman, Department of Obstetrics and Gynecology, Medical College of Georgia, Augusta, Georgia, USA

The Late Sol M. Shnider MD BSc(Med) FRCA(Hon)
Formerly Professor and Vice Chairman, Department of Anesthesia; Professor of Obstetrics, Gynecology and Reproductive Sciences, University of California, San Francisco, California, USA

Raymond S. Sinatra PhD MD
Associate Professor of Anesthesiology; Director, Post Surgical Pain Service, Yale University School of Medicine, New Haven, Connecticut, USA

Elizabeth B. Skerman RNC
Clinical Specialist in Inpatient Obstetrics, University Hospital, Louisiana State University Medical Center, Shreveport, Louisiana, USA

Jonathan H. Skerman BDSc MScD DSc
Professor of Anesthesiology, Professor of Obstetrics and Gynecology, Vice Chairman for Administration and Research, Department of Anesthesiology, School of Medicine in Shreveport, Louisiana State University Medical Center, Shreveport, Louisiana, USA

Ross Francis Smith MB BS FANZCA
Visiting Medical Officer, Prince of Wales Hospital, Mater Misericordiae Hospital and St Margaret's Maternity Hospital, Sydney, New South Wales, Australia

Maurits A.G. Soetens MD
Anaesthesiologist, Lecturer Katholieke Universiteit Leuven; Head, Department of Anaesthesiology and Reanimation, St Elisabethziekenhuis, Turnhout, Belgium

Donna E. Stewart MD DPsych FRCP(C)
Professor of Psychiatry, Obstetrics & Gynecology and Anesthesia, University of Toronto; Chief of Psychiatric Consultation-Liaison Service, St Michael's Hospital, Toronto, Ontario, Canada

T. H. Taylor MB BS FRCA
Consultant Anaesthetist, Royal London Hospital, London, UK

Gil Tchernia MD
Professor and Head of Department of Hematology, Hôpital Bicêtre, Le Kremlin Bicêtre, France

Gérard Tertian MD
Associate Professor, Department of Hematology, Hôpital Bicêtre, Le Kremlin Bicêtre, France

Michel Thiery MD PhD FRCOG
Emeritus Professor and Head of Department of Obstetrics, University of Gent, Belgium

Trevor A. Thomas MB ChB FRCA
Senior Consultant Anaesthetist, St Michael's Hospital (Maternity) Bristol; Consultant Anaesthetist, Bristol Royal Infirmary; Clinical Lecturer, University of Bristol, Bristol, UK

John Thorburn MB ChB FRCA FRCP(Glas)
Consultant Anaesthetist, The Queen Mother's Hospital and Western Infirmary, Glasgow, UK

M. Thornhill MD
Assistant Chief of Anesthesia, Holy Name Hospital, Teaneck, New Jersey, USA

Silvia Treves MD
Staff Anesthesiologist, Ospedale Ostetrico-Ginecologico, Santa Anna, Turin, Italy

E. Z. Tronick PhD
Chief, Child Development Unit, Children's Hospital, Boston; Associate Professor of Pediatrics, Harvard Medical School, Massachusetts, USA

The Late Leo Vaes MD
Formerly Head, Department of Anesthesiology and Intensive Care, St Elisabethziekenhuif, Turnhout, Belgium

Herbert Valensise MD
Assistant Professor, Department of Obstetrics and Gynecology, University of Rome, 'Tor Vergata', Italy

Albert Van Steenberge MD
Professor of Anesthesiology, University of Brussels, Belgium

André Van Zundert PhD MD
Department of Anesthesiology, Intensive Care and Pain Therapy, Catharina Hospital, Eindhoven, The Netherlands; Secretary–General, European Society of Regional Anaesthesia

Jasmine Vartikar MD
Department of Anesthesia, Norwood Hospital, Norwood, Massachusetts, USA

D. Vauthier-Brouzes MD
Department of Obstetrics and Gynecology, Hôpital Pitié Salpetrière, Paris, France

P. H. Vehring MD
Department of Anesthesiology, University Hospital, Leiden, The Netherlands

Donald H. Wallace MD FFARCS(Eng.)
Associate Professor of Anesthesiology, Department of Anesthesiology and Pain Management, University of Texas Southwestern Medical Center at Dallas, Dallas, Texas, USA

Martin P. Ward Platt MD MRCP
Consultant Paediatrician (Neonatal Medicine), Department of Child Health, Princess Mary Maternity Hospital, Newcastle Upon Tyne, UK

David Watson BSc MB FRCA
Consultant and Senior Lecturer, Department of Anaesthesia and Intensive Care Medicine, St Bartholomew's Hospitals, London, UK

Moira D. Westmore MB BS FFARACS FANZCA MBA
Head, Department of Anaesthesia, King Edward Memorial Hospital for Women, Subiaco, Perth, Australia

J. A. W. Wildsmith MD FRCA
Professor of Anaesthesia, University Department of Anaesthesia, Ninewells Hospital and Medical School, Dundee, UK

W. Desmond R. Writer MB FRCA FRCPC
Professor, Department of Anaesthesia, Dalhousie University, Halifax, Nova Scotia; Staff Anaesthetist, Grace Maternity Hospital, Halifax, Nova Scotia, Canada

E. Yau MD FRCA
Department of Anaesthesia and Intensive Care Medicine, St Bartholomew's Hospital, London, UK

Paul C. Youngstrom MD CM
Ohio Permanente Medical Group, Kaiser Health Plan of Ohio; Assistant Professor of Anesthesiology and Reproductive Biology, Case Western Reserve University, Cleveland, Ohio, USA

Esther M. Yun MD
Department of Anesthesiology, State University of New York at Stony Brook, New York, USA

Preface

The editors are pleased to introduce you to *Pain Relief and Anesthesia in Obstetrics*. Distinguished authors from all over the world were prepared to focus on one or more different subjects and provide a collection of highly readable chapters. Their invaluable efforts are greatly appreciated and have contributed to a large extent to the success of this project. We have tried to give a broad view on obstetrics-related anesthesia problems. For that reason, leading experts in anesthesiology, obstetrics and pediatrics from the five continents were invited to give their own perspective on a topic, so that we sometimes have the same material dealt with by more than one person. This might lead to some inevitable overlap, but at the same time it stresses that there is not always a uniform way of practicing obstetric anesthesia and it may suggest alternatives in the treatment of our patients. Scientific input is increased by the opinion of experts in the field, allowing greater in-depth coverage of specific areas which practitioners can apply to their own practice.

Being editors of such a major textbook, with more than 100 contributors, was not an easy task. In 1989, our plan was to produce a small book dedicated to Dr Albert van Steenberge, the initiator of the use of low dose-low concentration epidural technique for vaginal deliveries. The project evolved into a major textbook. The unfortunate death of Dr B. G. Covino also influenced the publication of the book, as Dr Ostheimer had to take over as interim Chairman of the Department of Anesthesiology at the Brigham and Women's Hospital in Boston.

The goals of pain relief during anesthesia for obstetrics are to provide effective and safe pain relief during the first, second and third stages of labor and delivery without interfering with the progress of labor and delivery, to minimize the side effects for the mother and the fetus and, finally to improve maternal satisfaction. Pain relief during labor and delivery, as well as intraoperative and post-operative pain relief are presented in depth, along with all of the possible problems and complications of pregnancy.

The winding river of obstetric anesthesia takes many turns before reaching the ocean. We are confident that *Pain Relief and Anesthesia in Obstetrics* will prove a major source of innovative ideas and effective solutions for your practice and look forward to receiving your ideas and comments on how to improve possible future editions of this book.

André Van Zundert, M.D., Ph.D.,
Gerard W. Ostheimer, M.D.

Acknowledgements

We chose Churchill Livingstone as our publisher in this massive undertaking because of their pre-eminence in the field of anesthesiology publishing. We have been ably assisted throughout our project by Lowri Daniels, the MacDonnald Group, Elspeth Masson and Nora Cameron. Without the yeoman work of my secretary, Alyce Russo, we would still be copy editing articles and processing page proofs. Sometimes one finds gold in one's own back yard and such has been the case with our discovery of Emily Harris, a medical illustrator working in our own department. She has contributed her talents to many of the illustrations in the text. Without Alyce and Emily I do not know how we could possibly have finished this project. To my colleague and co-editor André Van Zundert, he has become a friend that I respect, admire and thank for approaching me with the idea to work with him on this tremendous project.

Gerard W. Ostheimer, M.D.

1. Introduction

G. F. Marx   P. R. Bromage

The world has become small! In 1846 it took two months for the letter describing the successful ether anesthesia at the Massachusetts General Hospital to reach London from Boston. Currently, transatlantic information transfer takes but two days by air express and mere minutes by FAX. Despite this ability to exchange ideas so rapidly, anesthetic practices in various countries are not uniform. There are differences between the United States and the European nations in concepts, equipment, and in both the choice and dosage of drugs. Katz et al,[1] studying the effects of suxamethonium (succinylcholine) and tubocurarine in comparable patients in London and in New York City, found the magnitude of action of tubocurarine and the duration of action of both relaxants to be less in the British than in the American patients. This Anglo-American disparity was explained by a combination of three factors: a difference in the response of patients to relaxants, a difference in clinical practice, and differing concentrations in the preparation of the agents. In contrast, the original dosage recommendations for midazolam, which were based on European evaluations, were found to be too high for many patients in the USA.[2]

Similar factors apply to obstetric anesthesia. For instance, self-administered nitrous oxide analgesia, an old stand-by in Great Britain and Ireland, is rarely employed in North America; thus, Entonox, the mixture of N_2O and O_2, is not manufactured there. Important differences also exist in obstetric practice. For example, exteriorization of the uterus for repair at cesarean delivery has become routine practice in many obstetric units throughout the USA since the mid-70s, whereas exteriorization is only rarely performed, and then for specific diagnostic purposes, in Britain and many parts of Europe. Consequently, differences in nociceptive afferent input confound attempts at statistical comparisons between regional anesthetic requirements for cesarean delivery on both sides of the Atlantic. Governmental regulations also play a role in creating international differences. Some local anesthetics, because of regulatory requirements, have been withheld for many years in the USA; two examples are EMLA cream for topical anesthesia or carbonated lidocaine, with its enhanced onset, for regional blockade. On the other hand, 2-chloroprocaine, widely used in the USA because of its prompt action, is not available in many European countries. Pain responses also vary with differing cultural backgrounds from country to country, so that the apparent need for labor analgesia is not geographically consistent.

A textbook on obstetric analgesia–anesthesia providing information on the practices of more than one country is a useful new approach to our management of mother and baby and to an unveiling of the hidden variables that handicap meta-analysis of obstetric anesthetic outcomes on both sides of the Atlantic. While many chapters describe European and USA approaches, others are even more detailed. Pregnancy-induced hypertension is discussed by experts from three countries (UK, USA, Australia), whereas the intricacies of two important entities – the organization of an obstetric anesthesia service and the financial considerations of obstetric anesthesia – are each reviewed by representatives of ten nations. Such diversification will benefit health care providers worldwide and will make the book a valuable addition to all medical libraries.

REFERENCES

1. Katz R L, Norman J, Seed R F, Conrad L 1969 A comparison of the effects of suxamethonium and tubocurarine in patients in London and New York. Br J Anaesth 41: 1041–1047
2. Midazolam. The Medical Letter on Drugs and Therapeutics 1986; 28: 73–74

2. History of pain relief in childbirth

L. M. M. Morrison J. A. W. Wildsmith G. W. Ostheimer

ANCIENT METHODS

Those techniques that produce obstetric analgesia and anesthesia are similar to those that are used for surgical anesthesia, but the history of their application in labor is clearly different. Folklore, superstition and opposition from the church as well as members of the medical profession have all played a part in delaying the development of various techniques for pain relief.

The concept of pain relief during childbirth is a relatively recent one. Unfortunately for women, the biblical reference (Genesis 3, v. 16) in which God says to Eve in the Garden of Eden 'I shall greatly multiply thy sorrow and thy conception. In sorrow thou shalt bring forth many children' was construed to imply that childbirth must be painful and that any attempt to abolish that pain was to thwart God's will. This interpretation was used as an argument against relief of pain during childbirth as recently as the late nineteenth century. There are many references in the Bible that suggest an appreciation of the pain involved in labor. For example, King David remarked 'Fear took hold upon them there and pain, as of a woman in travail', and in Jeremiah it is said 'For I have heard a voice as of a woman in travail'. However, there are few references to relief for that pain. There is an obscure mention of Rachel requesting mandrake, but this may have been for use as a love potion rather than as an aid to labor. In Exodus the king of Egypt mentioned the birthing stools that were used by Hebrew women.

Some ancient tribes used mechanical aids to gravity to assist parturition, but more often these resembled crude methods of torture. In Pago Pago the strong men in the tribe were employed to assist with the birth by pressing their heels into the lower ribs of laboring women during the contractions. The later discovery by Aburel and Cleland that uterine pain pathways entered the cord at the 11th and 12th thoracic segments may have provided a pseudoscientific basis for this practice.

Other ancient civilizations may have been more sympathetic to the plight of women in labor. The ancient Chinese employed opioids and soporific potions for relief of pain in labor, while Helen of Troy learned how to prepare herbal remedies that banished sorrow from the memory. The Greeks may have attempted the use of anesthetic agents to relieve pain of childbirth for Hippocrates, the father of medicine, remarked 'Divinum est opus sedare dolorem.' (divine is the work to subdue pain.). In medieval times alcohol was used in childbirth, and in Salem, Massachusetts, an early form of mesmerism was employed. However, more than a few 'witches' were burned at the stake for attempting to relieve the pain of labor.

INHALATION METHODS: VAGINAL DELIVERY

Morton first publicly demonstrated the use of ether anesthesia at the Massachusetts General Hospital on 16 October 1846. This event was witnessed by Henry J. Bigelow, who then wrote a letter to Francis Boot, an American physician practicing in London. Two months later, on 21 December 1846, Robert Liston successfully amputated the lower limb of Frederick Churchill under ether anesthesia.

As soon as James Young Simpson, the professor of midwifery in Edinburgh, heard of this success, he immediately traveled to London during the Christmas holiday to obtain first-hand information from Liston himself. On his return to Edinburgh, he became the first person to document the use of ether anesthesia in obstetric practice. On 19 January 1847 he used it to aid delivery of a dead fetus after internal podalic version in obstructed labor had failed. Credit for the first documented use of ether for analgesia in a naturally progressing labor must go to Nathan Colley Keep, a Boston dentist, who either gave the drug or supervised its administration by Henry Wadsworth Longfellow to Fanny Longfellow on 7 April 1847. He wrote that, 'consciousness was unimpaired and labor was not retarded'. He had synchronized the administration of ether with the contractions. The obstetrician in attendance was Walter Channing, one of the founders of the Boston Lying-In Hospital and the first Dean of Harvard Medical School. He subsequently published a treatise on etherization in childbirth, describing its use in 581 cases.[1] Two paragraphs from his introduction are timeless since they state what we believe about obstetric anesthesia to this day.

> My great, I had almost said my sole, object in this circular—in short, in my whole efforts—was to ascertain here at home, in the birthplace of etherization, what had been the precise results of many experiments, made by many physicians, of the employment of the remedy of pain. My object was to learn if this use of it had been *safe*—safe both to *mother* and *child*; and thus, as far as such results might reach, to contribute something towards settling the most important point concerning its further use, namely, that of its safety.

Subsequently, Simpson published his paper describing the use of ether in obstetrics but he was searching for another anesthetic that did not have the disadvantages of ether: 'The disagreeable and very persistent smell, its occasional tendency to irritation during its first inspirations and the large quantity occasionally required to be used'. Simpson's attention was drawn to chloroform by David Waldie, a Liverpool chemist, in October 1847. Waldie recommended chloric ether because of its 'volatility, agreeable flavour and medicinal properties' and promised to send some to Simpson. Simpson obtained a sample in Edinburgh and, on 4 November 1847, arranged for a dinner party where all present inhaled chloroform vapor. The next day Simpson administered chloroform to a patient in labor and he presented his findings to the Medico-Chirurgical Society of Edinburgh later that month. In his publication in the *Lancet* he noted the advantages of chloroform over ether. He describes placing the patient 'under the influence of chloroform by moistening with half a teaspoonful of the liquid a pocket handkerchief rolled up in a funnel shape and with the broad or open end of the funnel placed over her mouth and nostrils'. The patient wakened later, describing that 'sleep had stopped the pains'.[2]

Simpson's example was followed in the USA by Gardner of New York, who used chloroform in obstetrics in February 1848. Obstetric anesthesia quickly became popular in America, aided by Channing's book *A Treatise on Etherisation in Childbirth*. At the American Medical Association meeting in 1848, the Committee on Obstetrics reported the use of ether and chloroform in 2000 patients with no deaths and few if any untoward results. One year later, the same committee recommended the use of anesthesia in obstetrics, preferably with chloroform, believing it to be justified for relieving pain in labor. They reported that 'in all difficult and instrumental labors their application could not be rightfully withheld'.

However, controversy continued over the next 6 years, with Simpson defending the concept of pain relief in labor against both medical and religious objections. Wakley, the influential editor of the *Lancet*, felt that there was no justification for the use of chloroform in a normal labor. Many obstetricians regarded the mother's reaction to labor pain as a valuable guide and argued that it would be dangerous to abolish it, Pickford concluding 'Pain is mother's safety and its absence her destruction'. Others felt that the pain was trivial and transient and there were fears over the safety of the anesthetic. Simpson opposed those who argued against pain relief, accusing them of impeding progress, and compared their resistance to that displayed 50 years earlier to the introduction of vaccination. Religious and moral objections were based on the reference from Genesis noted above, and also the observation that the effects of anesthesia in labor were similar to alcohol intoxication. The turning point in the controversy occurred when chloroform was recommended to Queen Victoria by her obstetrician, Sir James Clark, for the delivery of Prince Leopold, and it was administered by Dr John Snow on 7 April 1853. Queen Victoria later wrote 'Dr Snow administered the blessed chloroform and the effect was soothing, quieting and delightful beyond measure'. Snow's technique was similar to that used by Nathan Cooley Keep[3] and involved having the parturient inhale chloroform (instead of ether) from a handkerchief intermittently with each contraction. By 1862 anesthesia in midwifery was in general use and the only remaining argument was whether ether or chloroform was the safer drug. In America, ether was preferred to chloroform and, although the latter was initially more popular in Britain, grave doubts began to be expressed about its safety.

The Royal Medical and Chirurgical Society recommended the use of the ACE mixture (alcohol one part, chloroform two parts, ether three parts), devised by George Harley and Thomas Nunneley. However, concern slowly grew over the use of chloroform, leading to the comment in the British Medical Journal in November 1872: 'In the face of the great mortality from chloroform and the almost deathless record of ether, it has become our duty to interpose to call the urgent attention of professional men throughout the country to the claims which ether has upon their confidence and to urge that the anesthetic which was introduced by Simpson should have a fair trial'. Further evidence in support of ether was cited by Jeffries, a visiting surgeon from Boston, who remarked 'I believe that there are others like myself who do not desire to run the risk of killing a patient with chloroform and who perhaps would gladly avail themselves of ether were they rendered as familiar with its administration and harmlessness as we are in America'. Jeffries' use of ether bore similarities to Simpson's recipe for success described in his original paper published in the *Lancet*. A survey of the London hospitals in the *British Medical Journal* from 1875 revealed that three-quarters of respondents had abandoned the use of chloroform except for specific indications, including midwifery. In this context, chloroform was felt to be highly suitable because it was given in small intermittent doses and the risk of overdose causing cardiac syncope was negligible. It was not generally realized, however, that the main value of chloroform used in this manner in labor was as an analgesic and not an anesthetic, and it fell into disrepute.

Chloroform was reevaluated in America by Waters in 1951, who concluded that it was safe to use provided that small increments could be delivered carefully. The Tecota chloroform inhaler was developed to achieve this, although it is no longer used in routine practice.

Humphry Davy was the first to describe the analgesic properties of nitrous oxide, but it was Horace Wells who illustrated its value as an anesthetic when he inhaled it for his own dental extraction. Wells had first seen it demonstrated in Hartford, Connecticut, by the showman, Gardner Quincy Colton, and realized its potential practical application. When Wells attempted to demonstrate the use of nitrous oxide for a dental extraction before a group of students from the Harvard Medical School it was a fiasco, and both the drug and Wells' reputation fell into disrepute. He eventually committed suicide by inhaling ether and cutting his thigh (and probably his femoral artery) while imprisoned for throwing acid into a prostitute's face. Eighteen years later Colton revived the use of nitrous oxide in America and in 1863 instructed T W Evans, an American practicing in Paris, on its use. Evans demonstrated nitrous oxide at the National Hospital in 1868, and this led to its renewed popularity in Britain. In the same year Edmund Andrews wrote 'I have for some time been experimenting to see whether by the addition of free oxygen to the nitrous oxide a mixture would not be obtained by which a patient might be anesthetised for an indefinite period without danger of asphyxia'. Andrews named this combination of gases 'the oxygen mixture'. Joseph T Clover, who had been present at the demonstrations given by Evans, perceived the possibility of modifying his own chloroform apparatus to deliver a mixture of nitrous oxide and ether, which he called gas ether. B W Richardson was less impressed by Evans' demonstration and maintained that 'no substance had been more deservedly given up as unfit and unsafe for use'.

In 1880 Stanislav Klikovich[4] was the first clinician to use a mixture of 80% nitrous oxide and 20% oxygen to provide analgesia in labor. He observed that this mixture was an effective analgesic throughout labor and safe for both mother and child, although the apparatus was expensive and difficult to transport. A number of other European physicians tried the technique employed by Klikovich, but it failed to become established and it was not until 1911 that A E Guedel devised the first machine for self-administration of nitrous oxide and air in labor. In his paper he says that 'the patient soon learns that her relief depends upon the result of a race between the action of the gas and the approaching pain with the gas winning always if given an equal start'. However, Guedel's method was abandoned because of resultant maternal cyanosis.

After attending a meeting to discuss the use of nitrous oxide and oxygen in obstetrics in 1933, R Minnitt perceived that the disadvantages related to the use of nitrous oxide might be overcome by substituting air for oxygen. He later developed a piece of apparatus that became the accepted method for patient self-administration in Britain in the early part of this century. At the same time in America there was an increasing suspicion that when nitrous oxide was used part of its action was dependent on the patient's hypoxia. Courville, a neurologist, in 1936 described the neuropathologic lesions found in patients who died from asphyxia during nitrous oxide anesthesia.[6] In the same year Eastman further demonstrated, by examination of umbilical blood samples that were withdrawn during nitrous oxide anesthesia, that the fetus was affected by hypoxia. In 1949, Seward in a paper from the *Proceedings of the Royal Society of Medicine* described how he used a new machine from Denmark, which he adjusted to give 25% oxygen and 75% nitrous oxide. Incorporated into this machine was a safety valve that cut off the supply of nitrous oxide if the supply of oxygen failed.

The problem of asphyxia was solved in later designs of the Minnitt apparatus by mixing nitrous oxide with oxygen, but it was never really successful because it was superseded by the Lucy Baldwin modification of the Walton 5 dental anesthetic machine introduced in 1958. This allowed the woman to self-administer varying concentrations of nitrous oxide in a minimum of 30% oxygen. If there were any sign of fetal distress the gas–oxygen mixture was discontinued.

In 1961, Tunstall, following up on a technique described by Barach and Rovenstine in the USA, used a mixture of 50% nitrous oxide and 50% oxygen in one cylinder with the advantage of delivering nitrous oxide to the patient in a safe concentration of oxygen. Developed by the British Oxygen Company and called Entonox, the cylinder had a two-stage demand valve and midwives were allowed to administer it without supervision because there was no reduction in maternal oxygen saturation. With the development of Entonox and the demand valve apparatus in 1963 the Minnitt and Lucy Baldwin machines became obsolete. Nitrous oxide delivered in this form is still a first-line method of pain relief in labor. Recent modifications include the use of a mouthpiece instead of the traditional face mask advocated by Dolan and Rosen in 1975, and Arthurs and Rosen in 1981 suggested that the efficacy of the method could be improved by supplying the mother with a continuous flow of Entonox via a nasal catheter as well as inhaling it with the contractions.

Nitrous oxide was not the only inhalation agent to be used to ameliorate labor in the middle part of the twentieth century. Ethylene–oxygen was developed by Luckhardt and first used as an analgesic agent in obstetrics in the USA in 1923. Cyclopropane, discovered in 1882, had its anesthetic properties described by Lucas and Henderson in 1928. These agents enjoyed success especially in the USA because they provided better analgesia at lower concentrations than nitrous oxide, therefore allowing a greater proportion of oxygen in an effective mixture and so preventing fetal asphyxia. In 1924 Heaney reported that ethylene–oxygen provided satisfactory analgesia after two breaths, while with nitrous oxide four were required. Knight and Urner reported in 1936 on the administration of cyclopropane by means of a patient-operated apparatus. Analgesia with cyclopropane and ethylene–oxygen, although popular in many centers, had the drawbacks of expensive, complicated apparatus and the necessity of the constant presence of a physician fully acquainted with their use. Both agents produced rapid unconsciousness and the patient could not be encouraged to bear down with her contractions as effectively as with nitrous oxide. Such difficulties prevented more widespread use of these agents.

Divinyl ether was first used by Wesley Bourne in obstetrics in 1936 after it had been introduced by Gelfan and Bell in 1933. It was more powerful and rapid in its anesthetic action than ether and less irritating. Ethyl chloride was first employed clinically by Heyfelder in 1848. For many years, it was used as a topical anesthetic and played only a minor role in pain relief in childbirth for a time because its extreme potency made it dangerous in inexperienced hands.

In 1944 Spitzer pointed out that 'all general anesthetics weaken uterine contractions and retractions' and that they all have fetal effects that early studies failed to recognize.[7] There had been concern at an early stage about the effects of anesthetics on the fetus. In 1853 Snow noted that mothers who had chloroform anesthesia produced children who did not kick and scream as much and he documented placental transfer of the inhaled anesthetic agent when he detected the odor of chloroform on the breaths of these infants. He concluded that the fetus was affected by chloroform. Interestingly, in 1848, Channing concluded that ether did not cross the placenta because there was no odor from the cut end of the umbilical cord. In 1850 Harvey gave many examples to support the theory of placental transport, but it was not until 1877 that the controversy was clarified when Zweifel demonstrated that chloroform could be detected chemically in the umbilical blood and urine of the newborn.[8]

The fetal effects were difficult to quantify, but in 1953 Virginia Apgar published her description of a method to establish a simple clear classification or 'grading' of newborn infants which can be used as a basis for discussion and comparison of the results of obstetric practices, types of maternal pain relief and the effects of resuscitation'.[9] Initially the Apgar score was used to assess the effects of inhalation anesthetics on the newborn, and it then became apparent that potent drugs such as cyclopropane increased the incidence of neonatal depression if given for more than 5 mins before delivery. There was no such increase if less potent agents such as nitrous oxide or ethylene were used or if potent agents were administered in much lower analgesic concentrations.

Between 1943 and 1984 both trichloroethylene (Trilene) and, to a lesser extent, methoxyflurane (Penthrane) were also used successfully. Trilene was introduced into anesthesia by Striker and Jackson in 1935 and was used for the first time in obstetrics in 1943, Freedman's inhaler allowing the administration of an analgesic concentration. However, this method was found to be unreliable, and some mothers received an apparent overdose. The Medical Research Council defined the standards that inhalation apparatus had to achieve in the UK in 1952. Epstein and MacIntosh designed their Emotril inhaler in 1949 and the Tecota inhaler was developed in 1952. Both of these instruments were draw-over temperature-compensated vaporizers, and their output was unaffected by the patient's respiration.

Methoxyflurane was introduced by Artusio in 1960 and was widely used for obstetric analgesia in the USA. However, methoxyflurane did not become popular elsewhere, and anxiety about its adverse effects on renal function led eventually to its withdrawal in 1984. More general concerns about the depressant effect of all volatile agents on the fetus, and the gradual development and spread of better techniques of pain relief in labor, led to a decline in their use.

The first forceps delivery under general anesthesia was performed in Boston by Walter Channing on 5 May 1847. On 16 September 1847 the first instance of in-patient obstetric anesthesia was recorded by Dr Charles G Putnam. Ether was administered to Catherine Fisher for a forceps delivery at the Boston Lying-In Hospital. She was the first woman in that institution or any other American maternity hospital to receive an *anesthetic* for childbirth.

The first recorded cesarean delivery from a living woman occurred in 1500 when Jacob Nufer, a Swiss sow gelder, performed the surgery on his own wife. Supposedly, she and the child survived; however, there is some dispute since no published record appeared until 1582. In Great Britain, in 1737, Robert Smith of Edinburgh performed a cesarean delivery but the mother died some hours later. During the remainder of the eighteenth century, there were scattered reports of cesarean deliveries, but in no instance did the mother survive, although a few children did. In 1793, James Barlow performed a cesarean delivery on Jane Foster, who survived, although the baby was born dead. In *Barlow's Essays on Surgery and Midwifery*, he noted that, while the operation was performed almost 50 years before ether or chloroform was introduced as anesthetic agents, 'the poor woman scarcely complained during the operation, so great was her fortitude. Soon after she was put to bed she slept without any medicine and passed a good night.'

The first cesarean delivery performed under general anesthesia with ether or chloroform is not recorded. In these early operations, sometimes the mother or baby or both died – usually because of the prolonged labor or infection.

PARENTERAL TECHNIQUES

Parallel to the evolution of inhalation methods of pain relief in childbirth was the development of parenteral techniques. These were pioneered by Alexander Wood, who tried to improve the analgesic effect of morphine, isolated from crude opium by Sertürner in 1806, by injecting it close to the site of pain in a patient with neuralgia. He had modified the Ferguson syringe by adding graduations and using a finer, sharper needle so that he was able to bring 'some narcotic to bear more directly than I had hitherto been able to accomplish on the affected nerve'. In his description[10] of this technique in the *British Medical Journal* of 1858 he wrote:

> I believe the remedy I have been speaking of acts in two ways. First the injection into the cellular tissue in the neighbourhood of the nerve, the needle being charged with narcotic solution, affects the nerve. In the second place I believe it acts by being passed into a part which rapidly absorbs the medicine and sends it through the system thus producing an almost instantaneous effect. In this little instrument we possess the means of bringing the patient almost directly under the influence of opium.

It was Hunter who later concluded that the effect obtained was the same irrespective of whether the injection was local or distant from the nerve. Administration of morphine to control the pain of labor by hypodermic injection was suggested by Kormann in Germany in 1860, but problems associated with its use had already been recognized. In 1834 Ramsbotham wrote that children born to opium-addicted mothers were dull and sleepy in the first few hours of life. Morphine was not used very much for over 100 years after its discovery because, in the words of Snyder, 'respiratory injury of the child was the chief hazard in the use of morphine for obstetric analgesia'.

Green, in America, and Nussbaum, in Europe, in 1864 were the first to report the combination of morphine and inhalation anesthesia for general surgery. They showed that an injection of morphine appeared to intensify and prolong chloroform anesthesia and there was a long period of post-operative tranquility. Subsequently, it was Claude Bernard who did the definitive investigations on this combination, which he termed 'mixed anaesthesia'.

In 1870 Guilbert was one of the first people to test the combination of chloroform and morphine in obstetric practice. He described how he obtained 'two distinct states, one analgesia and two anaesthesia'. He wrote that the 'analgesic state will be of great service in cases of difficult labour'. For parturition, Guilbert used:

> a subcutaneous injection of about one centigram of hydrochloride of morphine into the forearm at the moment when uterine contractions begin to become unbearable . . . a quarter of an hour after the injection I begin chloroform inhalation . . . at a time when the woman announces the beginning of another contraction. After ten or so inspirations the woman ceases to feel acute pain although the contraction continues. I suspend the inhalation before the end of the contraction and continue in this manner throughout labour allowing chloroform to be inhaled only during contraction.

Scopolamine was introduced with the express aim of reducing the dose of morphine required during labor to try to avoid the problems associated with it. After Schneiderlin described the narcotic effect that was produced by a combination of morphine and scopolamine in 1899, it was successfully used during surgery by Korff and Bloss, and Von Steinbuchel became the first to use the technique in labor in 1902.[11] It became known as 'twilight sleep' from the German word 'Dämmerschlaf' used to describe the state of impaired consciousness induced by this combination. It was realized that scopolamine did not increase the pain threshold but appeared to act by a psychological effect, inducing amnesia, but not unconsciousness, of the events surrounding labor. Subsequent studies painted a mixed picture of the success of twilight sleep. Hocheisen concluded that the mixture caused protraction of birth and fetal asphyxia, but Gauss spent much time developing a technique that in his hands gave satisfactory results in 70–90% of his patients. Around 1912 a popular magazine promoted the use of twilight sleep for pain relief in labor and it was widely read by women in the USA. This created awareness among women that it was possible for them to have pain relief and forced obstetricians and anesthesiologists to consider this problem more urgently. The combination of analgesia, sedation and amnesia made morphine and scopolamine a popular method for some time, but twilight sleep eventually fell into disrepute because of the high incidence of asphyxia neonatorum, inadequate pain relief and the adverse effect on uterine contractions. Excessive restlessness was also described in many patients. In 1928 Van Hoosen and in 1942 Kirschbaum advocated the use of scopolamine alone, suggesting that it was the only drug that would not depress intrauterine fetal respiratory effort. It was hoped that papaveretum would be a suitable alternative to morphine without its adverse effects, and this was first tried by Jaeger in 1910, but it did not fulfill these expectations.

One of the few legacies from this period was the introduction of meperidine in obstetric analgesia. It was synthesized in Germany in 1939 by Schaumann and Eisleb in their search for an analgesic with spasmolytic atropine-like qualities. Its combined analgesic, antispasmodic and sedative actions suggested that it might be a very useful drug for producing obstetric analgesia. The belief that it was less of a respiratory depressant than morphine led to the expectation that it would be less harmful to the baby. It was first used in labor in Germany by Benthin in 1940, then by Gilbert and Dixon in America in 1943 and by Spitzer in Britain the following year. However, it became clear that its use in labor could also result in depression of the infant at birth, and Shnider and Moya in 1964 concluded that even small doses of meperidine given intramuscularly to the mother could significantly depress the newborn infant, with the time interval between administration and delivery being the most important determinant of the degree of neonatal depression produced. In 1970 Scott used a technique of self-administering meperidine intravenously in labor with a clamp that closed automatically if the patient fell asleep under the influence of the drug. He believed that the unnecessary peaks and troughs of the intramuscular method of administration were abolished, and reported that 89% of his patients regarded the method as good or very good. He felt that the technique 'carried the prospect of bringing narcotic analgesia up to the level of efficiency of conduction block'. In 1984 Crawford wrote of the technique that 'It is salutory to record that in our experience mothers who are provided with this apparatus will be found not infrequently to have self-administered three to four hundred milligrams of pethidine during a labour of average duration: evidence surely of the relatively inadequacy of our established regimes'.

Many newer opioids have been tried in labor, but meperidine remains the parenteral analgesic of choice in spite of its well-established side-effects resulting from the ease of transfer across the placenta demonstrated by Apgar. For example in 1966, Filler and Filler suggested that pentazocine would be a suitable alternative that would produce effective analgesia of rapid onset and short duration. Clinical trials have failed to reveal any difference between meperidine and pentazocine with respect to neonatal depression when used in equianalgesic doses, although Refstead and Lindback in 1980 found that the respiratory depression with pentazocine was finite, whereas with meperidine it was cumulative. In 1973 Monkovich reported the synthesis of butorphanol, but again equipotent doses in labor were no better than meperidine, as Maduska demonstrated in 1978. Meptazinol and nalbuphine have also been used in labor with no real advantage to parturient or her fetus/newborn.

With the development of major tranquilizers in the 1950s, trials of meperidine with the phenothiazines took place with the so-called meperidine ataractic combinations during labor. It was hoped that the potentiating effect of the phenothiazine would allow a reduction in the dose of meperidine. Chlorpromazine was used by Hershenson in 1954 after he had observed that when it was used as an antiemetic during labor it produced hypnotic effects. However, later reports began to indicate that it produced undesirable effects, such as maternal indifference to cooperation and hypotension. Promazine was promoted as a superior alternative to chlopromazine by Kuntze.

There was also a vogue for combining meperidine with narcotic antagonists in the hope of producing equivalent pain relief without respiratory depression, but Telford and Keats in 1961 failed to show any advantage with this combination.

Sedatives were first used in 1869 when Oscar Liebreich used chloral hydrate in Berlin. However, chloral hydrate alone does not provide good pain relief and it was therefore used in combination with opioid analgesics. Barbiturates eventually superseded chloral hydrate. The first of these compounds was named barbitone and was synthesized by Fischer and Von Mering of Munich in 1903. Barbiturates were not used in labor until 1923 by Cleisz. They remained popular for a number of years and the main drugs used were pernocton (1927), sodium amytal (1929) and pentobarbital sodium (1931). It was hoped that these drugs would have less depressant effect on the fetal respiratory centre than opioids. They were frequently used in combination with morphine and/or scopolamine. In doses sufficient to allow adequate analgesia fetal depression occurred and, even in low doses, violent maternal restlessness had been documented, requiring forcible restraint.

RECTAL PREPARATIONS

Besides using ether as an inhalation agent, Pirogoff in Russia and Dupuy in France instilled the liquid rectally as early as 1847. It was not until 1913, however, that Gwathmey[12] rediscovered that ether absorbed into the alimentary tract produced an analgesic effect; it was first applied in obstetrics in 1933. The so-called Gwathmey[12] analgesia consisted of a combination of morphine and magnesium sulfate injected hypodermically, and colonic ether in a mixture with olive oil, alcohol and quinine. Gwathmey and his co-workers stated that their object was to 'ameliorate pain by a harmless, inexpensive method, which could be used by a physician without special training in the home or hospital and which would employ drugs in common use'. They relied on the synergistic action of these agents for their major effect. The rectal ether oil method became widespread and was modified by McCormick, who devised apparatus to facilitate its administration in 1931. Quinine was initially included as an oxytocic but it was later abandoned and the morphine–magnesium sulfate combination was thought to be responsible for too many narcotized babies. The original formula was modified many times and the most popular formulation included the substitution of oral barbiturates for intramuscular injection.

Paraldehyde was introduced as a hypnotic by Cervello in 1882, and its rectal instillation in oil was suggested by Rosenfield and Davidoff of Boston and Colven and Bartholomew of Atlanta in 1932. By combining paraldehyde with barbiturates these workers reported successful analgesia and amnesia in labor. The method was modified by Kane and Roth, who replaced the oil with benzyl alcohol. They subsequently advocated the initial administration of the paraldehyde by mouth for a quicker onset of action, despite its noxious odor. Kotz and Katzman supported the use of this method along with supplements of morphine when the mother became restless and claimed that it was a satisfactory method even though labor did not occur spontaneously and outlet forceps were necessary. They also claimed that the mother suffered no ill-effects and the only effect on the baby might be difficulty in clearing its airway. Other rectal preparations were used. For example, Willstatter and Duisberg introduced a type of basic anesthesia with rectal administration of tribromomethylalcohol (Avertin), which proved to be popular for a time after 1926. But Butzengiger wrote of this technique: 'I should like to emphasize the fact that each session of anaesthesia actually is not a harmless incident and that it must be managed with the greatest caution'.

Gwathmey also suggested the rectal administration of Evipal, a barbiturate compound, but its effects were highly variable. Irving made a critical comparison of all the different methods of pain relief in labor in 1934. He rated them according to degree of amnesia, lack of effect on the infant and freedom from excitement. He found that pentobarbital with scopolamine with or without rectal ether for controlling restlessness was the best method. He was against using morphine at all because of its marked effect in delaying the initial respiration of the infant. He was also one of the earliest workers to express concern about the potential of agents to impair the reflex responses that prevented patients who were vomiting from aspirating during labor. For this reason, he was not in favor of giving barbiturates to patients who had recently eaten.

There was an increasing realization among many workers of the importance of the effect of commonly used analgesics on respiration. Waters concluded that opioids, barbiturates and other nonvolatile agents in sufficient doses all caused depression of the respiratory center of both mother and baby, and the better the pain relief the worse this became. Rosenfield and Snyder, and Henderson, demonstrated that the effect on the child of a hypnotic given to the mother is directly proportional to the amount given and the duration of its action. These workers advocated that anyone administering analgesia in labor must perfect the art of resuscitation and tracheal intubation. Cole pointed out that 'all sedative drugs increase the incidence of asphyxia' and the danger to the fetus is 'in direct proportion to the amount used'. Rosenfield and Snyder also demonstrated that the nonvolatile anesthetics depressed fetal respiratory movement at doses well below those required to anesthetize the mother.

Other agents investigated included glutethimide used by Abbas in 1957, which was reported to reduce meperidine requirements. Diazepam was used by Bepko in 1965 after a suggestion that 'it cut through the anxiety-tension-pain cycle during labor without harmful effects on mother or baby'. Ketamine was used in 1974 by Akamatsu, who described the dream-like state that frequently accompanied the analgesic effect of this agent.

LOCAL ANESTHETIC TECHNIQUES

With the development of the glass syringe and the hypodermic needle, substances began to be injected for pain relief and surgery. In 1853, Alexander Wood of Edinburgh, who refined a syringe for injections, began to administer drugs into the area of nerve trunks to alleviate neuralgia. Subsequently, he has been referred to as the 'father-in-law of nerve block'. The industrial revolution brought an explosion of developments in the field of surgery, including steam sterilization of dressings and the use of surgical rubber gloves. It also brought about the production of numerous pharmaceuticals. Of these, cocaine was the key in the development of local anesthesia.

Albert Niemann successfully isolated the alkaloid from the leaves of the *Erythoxylon coca* plant in 1860. Thomas Moreno y Maiz experimented with frogs to determine the anesthetic properties of cocaine in 1868. Sigmund Freud suggested to Carl Koller that he evaluate its effect on the nervous system. Freud hoped that cocaine would prove useful in curing a friend of his addiction to morphine. Koller, an ophthalmologist, used cocaine in animal experiments and then experimented with it on himself and colleagues in 1884. After demonstrating that the anesthetic properties of cocaine were sufficient to produce anesthesia of the eye, he began to use it topically for eye surgery. Koller wrote a paper on the subject and gave it to a friend to present at a meeting of the Congress of Ophthalmology in Heidelburg.

The news of the anesthetic properties of cocaine reached the USA, and its use in ophthalmology spread rapidly. Regional anesthesia using cocaine was preferable to inhalation anesthesia because the pain relief was similar; less time was needed to establish the anesthetic effect; engorgement of the ocular vessels produced by ether was avoided and there was decreased vomiting by the patient. Burke performed the first nerve block later in 1884, and, by the end of 1885, Halsted and Hall had used cocaine to block most peripheral nerves.

However, the use of cocaine for other surgery was limited by the drug's toxicity and and its limited duration of anesthetic effect. In 1885, Corning improved the duration of cocaine anesthesia by using a constricting bandage to decrease circulation to the anesthetized limb. Braun in 1903 used epinephrine in place of the elastic bandages for this same purpose. Braun also demonstrated that epinephrine would act to decrease the rate of absorption of cocaine and therefore limit its toxic effects while increasing the duration of the anesthetic effect.

J. Leonard Corning, a prominent neurologist, attended one of Halsted's demonstrations in New York and later became the first to inject cocaine around the spinal cord in order to anesthetize the lower half of the body.[13] He wrote:

> I reasoned that it was highly probable that if the anaesthetic was placed between the spinous processes of the vertebra it would be rapidly transported by the blood to the substance of the cord and would give rise to anaesthesia of the sensory and perhaps also of the motor tracts of the same.

He foresaw that this method might be used as a substitute for etherization in genitourinary and other branches of surgery. Because he injected a very substantial dose of cocaine (120 mg in a period of 5 mins) into the thoracic region of the patient with no untoward effects, it is thought that he obtained an epidural block and not true spinal anesthesia.

Quincke, a German, first described the correct paramedian approach for performing a lumbar dural puncture for the purpose of draining off cerebrospinal fluid in the treatment of hydrocephalus in 1891, using a device originally designed by Wynter for draining edema fluid in dropsy. Ziemsson suggested replacing the cerebrospinal fluid with a therapeutic fluid.

In 1899, August Bier attempted 'to render large areas of the body insensible to pain by introducing cocaine into the spinal cord'. He was also the first to describe to post-dural puncture headache. Bier and his associate, Hildebrandt, experimented on each other to perfect a technique of administering spinal anesthesia. Their experiments, and the unfortunate spinal headaches that ensued, led Bier to conclude that the loss of cerebrospinal fluid should be avoided during lumbar dural puncture and that the spinal needle should be of a small gauge.

Tuffier, a Parisian, popularized cocainization of the spinal cord and this encouraged Oskar Kreis to use spinal anesthesia for operative vaginal delivery in 1900, in Basle, Switzerland.[14] He injected cocaine into the subarachnoid space of several women and claimed that it alleviated pain with little impairment of muscular power of uterine contractility. He said that the patients described the contractions merely as sensations of abdominal pressure but, unfortunately, the majority experienced side-effects of nausea, vomiting and headache. One would suspect he would have used it for cesarean delivery although no record has been found.

The first cesarean delivery in the UK utilizing cocaine spinal anesthesia was performed at the Manchester Maternity Hospital in May, 1901, and reported by Sinclair in 1902 in great detail. At the same time in the USA, Marx used spinal anesthesia to 'still the agonising and maniacal shrieks of these poor women'. With the introduction of stovaine synthesized by Fourneau in 1903 and procaine by Einhorn in 1904 the technique was revived. However, the use of spinal anesthesia in labor was not without its drawbacks. In 1915, in experiments on cats, Smith showed that the fall in blood pressure which had been noted as one of the principal dangers of spinal anesthesia was due to paralysis of the vasomotor fibers regulating the tone of blood vessels in the splanchnic area. In 1937 Cosgrove and colleagues summarized the experiences of the use of spinal anesthesia in labor. They concluded that spinal anesthesia had no place in the first stage of labor unless operative delivery was required. The statistical evidence suggested that it was the most dangerous anesthetic technique and cases of peripheral vascular collapse and respiratory paralysis due to phrenic and intercostal nerve block were described. Attempts to limit the site of action of the local anesthetic were carried out in the 1920s and 1930s by Pitkin and Sise, who varied the baricity of the solution by adding glucose. This technique had been described by Barker 20 years previously. Parmley and Adriani utilized this process and developed the technique of saddle block anesthesia using hyperbaric nupercaine, which they applied to relieve the pain in childbirth in 1946. Lemmon noted that the two most common problems with spinal anesthesia using procaine were 'failure to take' and 'wearing off too soon'. He found that by leaving the needle in the subarachnoid space he could continue to administer the drug until an effect was obtained and to give further doses when the effect began to wear off. To achieve this he used a malleable spinal needle and a specially designed mattress. In 1940 he presented these findings in a paper entitled 'A method for continuous spinal anesthesia'.[15] In 1945, Tuohy modified Lemmon's technique using a ureteral catheter introduced into the subarachnoid space via a needle with a Huber point.

In 1943 Greenhill hoped that 'perhaps the tendency of confining anesthetics to the lower region of the body, the use of smaller doses, the employment of continuous spinal anesthesia and hyperbaric solutions which are more controllable will prove safer'.

In the early days of the use of cocaine as a local anesthetic, a wide number of applications were found for it. However, concern began to grow about its safety as a number of deaths associated with its use were reported. In 1894 Schleich in Germany developed the technique of infiltration anesthesia using a weaker solution of cocaine, as had been suggested by Paul Reclus, in order to reduce the incidence of toxicity. In 1910 Stiassney applied topical cocaine to the vulva and vagina to attempt to reduce the pain of labor and then, in 1927, Gellhorn infiltrated the perineum with local anesthetic solution.

An interesting application for infiltration anesthesia was tried by Rose in 1929. He applied the concept of referred pain described by MacKenzie and reasoned that:

> In labour the contraction of the uterus sets up repeated stimuli which cause the cord centres supplying the uterus to become hyperirritable. The normal skin impulses entering these irritable centres are recorded by the brain as pain arising in those skin areas.

By accurately determining and infiltrating these areas in the skin with procaine he attempted to reduce the pain of labor in 100 cases and only obtained poor results in six. He concluded that 'intradermal infiltration of definite areas of the abdomen produces decided relief and absence of pain during the first stage of labour'. Greenhill reported on the safety of local infiltration anesthesia as a technique for pain relief during labor and delivery in 1943.

Pudendal nerve block was first described by Muller in 1908, and both transperineal and transvaginal routes have been described. The chief application of this procedure is in instrumental delivery, but it is also used in combination with other blocks. In 1953, Jeffcoate asserted in the *British Medical Journal* that the greatest danger of forceps delivery was in the attendant general anesthesia (as it was given at that time) and he recommended the use of pudendal block as a safer alternative. The usefulness of this technique is not in dispute, but doubts have been expressed as to its mode of action. It has been suggested that the analgesia produced by this method is simply due to perineal infiltration and not to pudendal nerve block.

Paracervical nerve block was described by Gellert in 1926 as a method of providing effective pain relief. It was popular in Europe, but Rosenfield reviewed the literature about the use of this technique in 1945 and found an ill-explained depression of fetal heart rate in 4% of cases. Freeman revived its use in the USA in 1956, and Baggish recommended an indwelling catheter to provide continuous analgesia in 1964. The risk of infection prevented this method from becoming popular. In addition, alterations in the fetal heart rate and a high incidence of fetal distress secondary to the uptake of local anesthetic and uterine hypertonus has led to the decreasing use and outright abandonment of paracervical block in many centers throughout the world.

EPIDURAL TECHNIQUE

In 1901, Cathelin, a urologist, and Sicard, a neuroradiologist, independently published papers within 1 week of each other about the injection of cocaine into the epidural space through the caudal canal via the sacral hiatus. Sicard[16] confirmed that:

> Unfortunately there is no doubt that the subarachnoid injection of cocaine may present certain difficulties, consequently we have sought another procedure, one which is completely harmless and which allows us to reach, by means of a liquid injection, the nerve trunks at the sites of their exit from the spinal cord. The extradural space located between the dura mater and the bony canal presents itself for this purpose.

Despite differences of opinion about the nomenclature and injection technique used, Sicard and Cathelin agreed in seeing little practical surgical application for the procedure in man. However, they suggested that it might be of use in sciatica, cancer, hemorrhoids, fissures, tabes and possibly the relief of labor pains.

It was von Stoeckel, a gynecologist,[17] who applied the above technique to childbirth using procaine in 1909. He hypothesized that if the pain of labor was largely uterine in origin then this technique could be useful and he coined the term 'sacral anesthesia'. He was so impressed with the success of this method of pain relief that he abandoned the technique of twilight sleep that he had been using until that time. He achieved pain relief for an average of $1–1\frac{1}{2}$ h, but he cautioned that the greater the analgesic effect, the greater the risk of impairing the force of labor.

LUMBAR EPIDURAL ANESTHESIA

The introduction of the modern technique of lumbar epidural anesthesia was preceded by important scientific studies. Although the first suggestion that pain was mediated by specific pathways was made in 1846, part of the reason for inadequacy of analgesia by all methods of local anesthesia was lack of understanding of the anatomy and physiology relating to the pathways of pain in childbirth. Until this time pain in labor was considered to be the result of neuralgia of lumboabdominal nerves and compression of uterosacral plexus.

Aburel, a Romanian working in Paris, distinguished between pain in the first stage 'avant la periode d'expulsion' and 'la periode d'expulsion'. He believed that pain in the first stage was caused by distension of either the body or the cervix of the uterus. He thought that this pain was of visceral origin and was referred to those somatic areas supplied by the segments of the spinal cord (thoracic 11 and 12) into which the afferent uterine fibers entered. He considered pain in the second stage to be caused by distension of the perineum transmitted via pudendal nerves to the second, third and fourth sacral segments. By careful dissection studies in 1930, Aburel traced the afferent fibers carrying pain impulses from the uterus to a plexus lying in the angle between the aorta and the vertebral column. He demonstrated that by blocking this plexus the pain of early labor was relieved without interfering with uterine contraction. Aburel's theory of the pain pathways of labor continues to be accepted today. In 1931[18] he presented his paper 'Continuous local analgesia in obstetrics', in which he described his technique of continuous caudal and lumboaortic plexus block for pain relief in childbirth. His technique of catheter insertion is similar to that used in the present day. He wrote 'It becomes possible to obtain prolonged local anesthesia in obstetrics. This approach should no longer be considered experimental but as an everyday procedure'.

The technique of paravertebral block was described as long ago as 1906 by Sellheim. Although Cleland began his investigation into this area in Montreal in 1927, he did not report his findings until 1933. Like Aburel, he independently identified the pathways of pain in labor. In his paper[19] 'Paravertebral anaesthesia in obstetrics, experimental and clinical basis', he concluded:

> Pain in labor still remains a necessary concomitant of normal delivery. There seems to be two valid reasons for this. First, the disadvantages of general anesthesia and/or narcosis are enhanced in obstetrics by the peculiarly long period of administration, producing toxic effects on the child, the mother or the uterus itself which contraindicate adequate dosage. Second, the lack of definite knowledge concerning the paths of afferent nerves of the uterus to the cord has prevented the scientific application of regional anesthesia' and that 'regional anesthesia . . . should find its ideal application in obstetrics . . . spinal anesthesia not only lacks the safety of other forms of regional block but also impairs the expulsive power of the uterus, whereas caudal block does not relieve the pain of uterine contraction.

His studies culminated in the demonstration that 'the pain of uterine contraction may be abolished without affecting the contractions by paravertebral block of only two adjacent nerves'.

As early as 1901, Tuffier had attempted epidural analgesia by the lumbar approach, but technical difficulties discouraged further interest in this procedure for many years. In 1921, Pages, a Spanish military surgeon, and Siccard and Forrester independently described their use of the lumbar epidural approach. Pages called it 'metameric anesthesia', and his method of detecting the space demanded a high level of manual dexterity which, along with his untimely death, limited the spread of this technique. He had written 'last November whilst giving a spinal anesthetic it occurred to me to block the nerves between the intervertebral spaces and the meninges rather than pierce the dura'. Dogliotti, an Italian, rediscovered the method in 1931 using the now standard 'loss of resistance' technique and he named it 'segmental peridural spinal anesthesia'. Dogliotti's method was easier than the paravertebral techniques as only one skin puncture was required.

In the USA, the lumbar approach to the epidural space for analgesia in labour was first used by Graffagnino and Seyler in 1938. Hingson and Edwards had previously experimented with the lumbar epidural space but had abandoned the procedure because of the theoretical risk of injection into the subarachnoid space. From the evidence in the thesis of one of his pupils, Atanasiu, in 1938, it was clear that Aburel had also begun to use lumbar epidural blocks.

The main problem with all the techniques of local anesthesia at this time was the short duration of action of the drugs used. In 1923, Meeker predicted that there would be a wider field of use 'when a means has been devised to prolong the action of an epidural injection'. This means was provided by Hingson and Edwards in 1942, when they developed a method of supplying continuous caudal analgesia for the relief of pain in childbirth using a semiflexible malleable steel needle.[20] This was an adaptation of Lemmon's spinal catheter technique. They wrote that:

> We consider this form of anesthesia to be an improvement over the conventional type of peridural anesthetic administered by a single injection. In this latter procedure the limit of satisfactory anesthesia is from 45 minutes to two and a half hours. While with caudal administration the anesthesia can be safely prolonged indefinitely.

In the same year, Manalan used a ureteral silk catheter for caudal block in obstetrics, but he did not use a continuous technique of injection. Block and Rochberg in 1943 devised a continuous gravity drip into the caudal epidural space to 'decrease the attendant risks of large rapidly injected doses of the anesthetic agent'. Nicodemus observed a marked reduction in stillbirth and asphyxia neonatorum following continuous caudal anesthesia, in contrast to results after sedation with barbiturates or rectal ether followed by delivery under nitrous oxide or ethylene. However, its critics were quick to point out the 'definite though slight risk of death and chance of producing minor or major complication'. An editorial in *Anesthesiology* in 1945 expressed the view that 'the merits of continuous caudal anesthesia during parturition are not conclusively proved' and 'before the final definitive place it should occupy in relieving pains of labor and delivery is established it must be reviewed critically'. In addition, there was a 15% failure rate owing to variations in the anatomy of the caudal canal and problems finding it in pregnant women.

Caudal anesthesia did not relieve the pain of uterine contraction unless, as suggested by Schlimpert, large doses were used. This approach produced the added problems of toxic effects and retardation of labor, as also occurred with spinal anesthesia.

In 1944 Hingson and Southworth published their first paper concerning lumbar epidural anesthesia using a Barker spinal needle and a ureteral catheter similar to that used by Aburel in 1931 for continuous analgesia. In 1949 Curbelo adapted the equipment first described by Tuohy in 1945 and used it with a ureteral catheter for continuous epidural anesthesia in surgery. In the same year Flowers and colleagues recommended using continuous lumbar epidural with a catheter in labor and directing its effect by changes in posture. However, they initially recommended its use only in patients in whom the caudal approach was unsuitable or unsuccessful. Cleland promoted the same technique and took it further in 1952 when he suggested a two-catheter method called segmental peridural block.

The development of local anesthesia received a setback in the 1950s because of the article by Kennedy[21] entitled 'The grave spinal cord paralysis caused by spinal anesthesia', which asserted that 'paralysis below the waist is too large a price for a patient to pay in order that the surgeon should have a fine relaxed field of operation'. However, in the USA, Mendelson differentiated between the effects produced by aspirating solid and liquid gastric contents and furthered the case for the use of regional anesthesia in labor. He wrote in 1946: 'The aspiration of stomach contents into the lung is preventable. The dangers of this complication as an obstetric hazard may be avoided by... wider use of local anesthesia where indicated and feasible'.

The introduction of lidocaine by Torsten Gordh in 1949 helped to promote the use of local anesthesia. Lidocaine was more chemically stable, three times as active, less toxic and longer acting than procaine. Bupivacaine was introduced by Widman in 1963, had a long duration of action which allowed repeated injections to be given with a smaller risk of cumulative toxicity, and became the major factor in promoting the use of continuous epidural techniques in labor.

Bromage in 1961, produced a simple diagram of the dual afferent pathways of labor and helped to popularize lumbar epidural analgesia/anesthesia. He wrote:

> In childbirth this sort of analgesic capability opened the door to revolutionary changes in obstetric methods. No longer were centrally depressant analgesics and anesthetics required, labor could be pain free from start to finish without the need for any pharmacological depression of the fetus, and with judicious use of elective induction, 'daylight obstetrics' became a practical possibility.

In spite of these advances the use of epidural anesthesia in labor was slow to be accepted for general use. Eisen reported a series of 9532 lumbar epidural anesthetics in 1960 in Toronto, and Hellman followed this with a study of 16 000 from the same unit in 1965. However, these authors appeared to apply the technique late in labor to avoid the hazard of a general anesthetic. The popularity of epidural anesthesia was enhanced by headlines in the press proclaiming 'painless childbirth at last' after the Fourth World Congress of Anesthesiologists in London in 1968. There had been a growing concern about general anesthesia in labor. In the UK from 1952 to 1954 deaths from aspiration of vomit accounted for 32 out of 49 anesthetic maternal deaths, and Marston, who compiled the section about anesthetic fatalities in the report of the newly commissioned confidential enquiry into maternal deaths, pointed out that there were particular hazards with general anesthesia in labor. However, in addition to a lack of anesthesiologists adequately trained in the technique of giving epidural anesthesia in the UK, midwives were unhappy about the technique. They were concerned that epidural analgesia required closer observation and so increased their workload, that the progress of labor was more difficult to assess, that they would lose some of their responsibilities in caring for the laboring woman and that they would not obtain sufficient experience in using more conventional methods of pain relief during their training. Obstetricians also provided some resistance in that some of them contended that existing methods of pain relief were adequate. According to a study by Beasley in 1967 using parenteral opioids in the first stage of labor, it was found that in spite of an intensive program to improve patient satisfaction with the pain relief provided in childbirth 'that there remained 40% of women whose childbirth was painful'.[22] Other obstetricians maintained a lingering suspicion that epidural anesthesia might be responsible for some neonatal neurologic damage, while others were concerned that their junior staff would be subjected to a greater workload because of an increased number of forceps deliveries.

Neurobehavioral assessments of the newborn have demonstrated little, if any, effect of local anesthetics administered by spinal or epidural anesthesia. Present-day concerns have shifted to the avoidance of hypotension, even for a brief period of time, to avoid any effect on the newborn.

Any concerns that epidural anesthesia might be detrimental to the fetal circulation were removed in 1978 when Jouppila[23] used a radioactive clearance technique to measure the placental blood flow and demonstrated that epidural analgesia resulted in no change or an improvement in the intervillous blood flow.

More recently, researchers have looked at other ways of relieving labor pain via the epidural space. It was suspected that segmentally applied epidural anesthesia had undesirable effects, including reducing the efficiency of uterine contractions, weakening the abdominal musculature and inhibiting the pushing reflex in the second stage, resulting in an increased number of outlet extractions. In 1980 Booker injected small doses of morphine into the epidural space, but 52% of the mothers had only partial pain relief or no pain relief at all. The authors concluded, however, that the striking success with some patients and the potential advantages over more traditional methods merited further study.

Initially epidural anesthetics were given primarily for medical indications, and Doughty in 1971 found that this resulted in a frequency of use in 15% of mothers; however, when epidural on request was allowed the frequency increased to 30%. In order to accommodate the supply for this demand an increase in consultant anesthesiologists committed to obstetrics and an increase in 24-h coverage was required and introduced.

A questionable use of local anesthesia was promoted by Allen in 1945 and by Johnston and Gilbert in 1946. These workers advocated the intravenous administration of procaine by infusion using two different dosage regimens, a lower concentration to produce analgesia by a so-called peripheral effect in the earlier part of labor and a higher dose producing anesthesia with partial loss of consciousness by a central effect in the second stage of labor. In Allen's series there were apparently no serious complications in either mother or child. However, tetany and convulsions could occur when the dosage was increased. This technique is apparently still utilized in some developing countries.

PSYCHOLOGICAL METHODS

Charles Meigs, an early opponent of Simpson, asserted in 1848 that he had 'no doubt of some physiological and therefore needful and useful connection of the pain and powers of parturition'.[24] Although the necessity for providing relief of pain in childbirth by pharmacologic means has been assiduously sought by modern practitioners, during the last five decades a movement advocating the so-called 'natural childbirth' has grown. The first modern proponent of this school of thought was Dick-Read in 1933.[25] He believed that the pain of childbirth was engendered mainly by fear and anxiety and that if the woman could be taught to relax through understanding the events of labor then that pain could be eliminated. Followers of Dick-Read devised a series of lectures and exercises which became known as preparation for natural childbirth. Unfortunately, this method did not encourage the concurrent use of drug treatment when necessary and women who went on to require drug treatment for pain or operative delivery for complications felt a sense of failure and could possibly become psychologically scarred. Astbury later wrote that 'those whose expectations of labor are violated by the actual labor experience report more severe pain'.

Velvowski, in 1947, described conditioned reflex training for childbirth, which became known as psychoprophylaxis. This training involved a series of lectures describing the physiology of normal labor and exercises to practice during pregnancy which were used as a form of distraction therapy during labor itself. However, the patient is told that labor may be abnormally painful and other analgesia may be required. Lamaze and Leboyer adopted and refined these techniques. More recent scientific analyses of these techniques by Scott and Rose in 1976 revealed that Lamaze-treated patients required opioids or epidural analgesia less frequently than controls. However, this does not imply that these women experience less pain than the controls but that the obstetricians withhold analgesia more often in these patients whether or not at the request of the mothers. It was concluded that the Lamaze technique was not harmful to the mother or infant.[26]

In 1981 Melzack, who described the gate theory of pain, said pain was 'a complex perceptual experience that is profoundly influenced by psychologic variables, such as fear, attention and suggestion as well as by injurious or potentially harmful stimuli' and that therefore 'clinical pain is often substantially reduced by psychologic procedures'.[27] When he applied the McGill pain questionnaire to women, labor pain ranked among the most intense pains recorded. The primiparous woman who had received prepared childbirth training had lower pain scores but the effects were small. Most women who received prepared childbirth training requested epidural anesthesia. Melzack concluded that 'Prepared childbirth and obstetric anesthesia are compatible complementary procedures aimed at assisting women in childbirth to suffer less fear, anxiety and pain.' Buckston hoped that 'In the future a gradual process of distillation and refinement will place in its proper perspective this concentration on the psychological needs of the parturient woman' and that it would 'merge imperceptibly with the overall concept of good prenatal and intrapartum obstetric care'.

Hypnosis, which has been used since ancient times, was placed on a scientific footing by Mesmer, a medical graduate from Vienna, in the late eighteenth century. As Goldsmith wrote: 'His theories bridged the gap between ancient superstition and modern psychotherapy.' Elliotson and Esdaile, two Edinburgh graduates at the beginning of the nineteenth century, developed the use of hypnotism as a form of analgesia/anesthesia during surgical procedures. The use of hypnotism in obstetrics was promoted because it avoided neonatal respiratory depression and the patient could remain awake and cooperative during labor. However, only 25% of mothers can be hypnotized to a level producing effective analgesia; it is a time-consuming process and requires the personal attention of the hypnotist for the best result. In addition Wahl, in 1962, advised caution in the use of hypnotism in labor because it might lead to subtle psychological problems in the future, particularly among women who expressly wished to avoid the experience of labor.

OTHER TECHNIQUES

Heyns, in 1959, found unexpectedly that parturients experimentally paralyzed with succinylcholine exhibited 'rapid dilation of the cervical os' and this reduced the duration of labor. From this finding he developed the abdominal decompression technique to try to relax the anterior abdominal muscles by the external application of negative pressure so that the uterus could move forward freely during contractions. There was dispute about the efficacy of this technique. In 1964 Quinn published the largest series with 593 patients. He obtained excellent or good pain relief in 86% and confirmed that the duration of labor was shortened. However, Castellanos and Newman disputed the value of this technique. The use of acupuncture was tried in labor because of claims that it provided 'hypoanalgesia' in 70% of surgical procedures in which it was used in China. In 1974 Wallis employed a trained Chinese acupuncturist to evaluate its use in 21 volunteers and found that none of them obtained successful analgesia. She concluded that hypnosis might be an important element in successful acupuncture. In 1975 Abouleish tested acupuncture in labor in 10 patients: only one patient had adequate pain relief, while in three it was partial. He concluded that the analgesia obtained was incomplete, unpredictable and inconsistent compared with regional techniques.

The clinical application of the gate theory of pain to explain the sensation of pain led to the development of transcutaneous electrical nerve stimulation (TENS). Among the first workers to apply TENS in labor were Shealy and Maurer,[28] in 1974, who with later groups found it to be of most value in backache occurring during labor. Augustinsson found that 88% of women derived some benefit from TENS. However, Nesheim in 1981 found no difference compared with placebo for degree of pain relief or the need for analgesic supplements. Bundsen also in 1981 suggested that the infants of TENS-treated mothers tended to have better Apgar scores and these women had a reduced requirement for nitrous oxide supplements but it could not be used optimally as it interfered with electronic fetal heart rate monitoring, although Harrison in 1986 did not find that this was a problem. In the same study, Harrison, finding a highly significant difference in favorable comments by mother and midwife after delivery comparing TENS and placebo concluded that 'such evident consumer satisfaction suggests that TENS has a part to play in analgesia in labour particularly where labour is likely to be short'.

Persianinov, a Russian, developed a variation of electrical stimulation that involved applying electrodes to the region of the forehead and mastoid processes in 1975. He claimed that 'It has been successfully used for preparing the pregnant woman for labor'.[29]

Burt and Korn in 1964 promoted the little-heard-of technique of audioanalgesia as distraction therapy during labor after hearing of its effectiveness in dentistry. The patient is subjected to white sound via earphones and a control box is used to increase the volume as the pain increases. They claimed good results in two-thirds of cases and a reduction in meperidine requirements was noted.

Our attitudes towards pain relief continue to change. Initial progress was retarded by the overenthusiastic use of drugs in labor. In 1936 Galloway described how 'five different drugs are given . . . within a few hours by mouth, by hypodermic, and by rectum, combining narcotics, a hypnotic and a uterine stimulant. Then during delivery gas is used'.[30] However, it has been shown in recent years that pain is not only not a necessary accompaniment of childbirth but that in some instances may be harmful. Recent work in animals has shown that maternal stress is hazardous to the fetus and that maternal sedation can have a beneficial effect on the fetus. Women receiving an epidural anesthetic during labor have a lower incidence of metabolic acidosis. In tandem with both the humanitarian ideal of eliminating pain in childbirth and the improvement in physiological well-being produced is the recognition of the sense of deprivation of the normal experience of childbirth felt by mothers who have excessive and perhaps unnecessary interference. Billewiez and Driemel in 1976 comparing mothers who were given epidural anesthesia with those who were not $1\frac{1}{2}$ years after delivery and found that more than half of the mothers who did not wish an epidural in future labor had had a completely pain-free labor and one of these women stated that 'Painless labor is unemotional. I would like to feel the whole experience of having a baby'.

The future direction of intrapartum analgesic and anesthetic care would appear to be in the direction of a balance between the physiological, psychological and emotional needs of the mother and child. In the words of Simpson: 'I esteem it the office of the physician not only to restore health but to mitigate pain and dolours'.

REFERENCES

1. Channing W 1848 A treatise on etherization in childbirth, illustrated by five hundred and eighty one cases. William D Ticknor, Boston
2. Simpson J Y 1847 On a new anaesthetic agent more efficient than sulphuric ether. Lancet 2: 549–550 (November 20)
3. Keep N C 1847 Inhalation of ethereal vapor for mitigating human suffering in surgical operations and acute diseases. Boston Med. Surg. Journal 36: 199–201
4. Klikovich S 1881 Nitrous oxide and experiences with its therapeutic administration. A M Kotomin St Petersburg
5. Guedel A E 1911 Nitrous oxide–air anaesthesia self administered in obstetrics. A preliminary report. Indianapolis Med Journal (October)
6. Courville C B 1936 Asphyxia as a consequence of nitrous oxide anaesthesia. Medicine 15: 129–145
7. Spitzer W 1944 Obstetric analgesia with pethidine. BMJ 179–181 (February 4)
8. Zweifel P 1877 Der Übergang von Chloroform und Salicylsaure in die Placenta Nebst Bemerkungen uber den Icterus Neonatorum. Arch Gynakol 12: 235–257
9. Apgar V 1953 A proposal for a new method of evaluation of the newborn infant. Anesth Analg 32: 260–267
10 Wood A 1858 Treatment of neuralgic pains by narcotic injections. BMJ 2 (August 28)
11. Von Steinbuchel 1902 Vorlaufige Mittheilung über die Anwendung von Skopolamin–Morphium–Injectionem in der Geburtshilfe. Zentralbl F Gynak 26: 1304
12. Gwathmey J T 1930 Obstetrical analgesia: a further study, based on more than twenty thousand cases. Surg Gynec and Obst 51: 190–195
13. Corning J L 1885 Spinal anesthesia and local medication of the cord. New York Med Journal 42: 483–485
14. Kreis O 1900 Über Medullarnarkose bei Gebarenden. Zentralbl F Gynakol 24: 724
15. Lemmon, W T 1940 A method for continuous spinal anaesthesia: a preliminary report. Ann Surg 111: 141–144

16. Sicard M A 1901 Les injections medicamenteuses extradurales par voie sacro-coccygienne. Compt Rend Soc de Biol 53: 396–398
17. Stoeckel W 1909 Über sakrale Anaesthesie. Zentralbl F Gynaekol 33: 1
18. Aburel E 1931 L'anaesthesie localé continué (prolongée) en obstetrique. Bulletin de la Societe D'Obstetrique et Gynaecologie de Paris 20: 35–37
19. Cleland J G P 1933 Paravertebral anaesthesia in obstetrics: experimental and clinical basis. Surg Gynecol and Obst 57: 51–62
20. Hingson R A, Edwards W B 1943 Comprehensive review of continuous caudal analgesia for anesthetists. Anesthesiology 4: 181–196
21. Kennedy F G, Effron A S, Perry G 1950 The grave spinal cord paralyses caused by spinal anesthesia. Surg Gynecol and Obstet 91: 385–398
22. Beazley J M, Leaver E P, Morewood J H M, Bircumshaw J 1967 Relief of pain in labour. Lancet i: 1033–1035
23. Jouppila R, Jouppila P, Hollmen A, Kuikka J 1978 Effect of segmental extradural analgesia on placental blood flow during normal labour. Br Journal of Anaesthesia 50: 563–566
24. Meigs C D 1848 Letter to Prof W Channing, dated 26 April, 1848. In: Channing W (ed) A treatise on etherization in childbirth. William D Ticknor, Boston p 14
25. Dick-Read G 1944 Childbirth without fear. Harper, New York
26. Scott J R, Rose N B 1976 Effect of psychoprophylaxis on labor and delivery in primaparas. New England Journal of Medicine 294: 1205–1207
27. Melzack R 1984 The myth of painless childbirth. Pain 19: 321–337
28. Shealy C N, Maurer D 1974 Transcutaneous nerve stimulation for control of pain. Surg Neurol 2: 45–47
29. Persianinov L S 1975 The use of electro-analgesia in obstetrics and gynaecology. Acta Obstet Gynecol Scand 54: 373–384
30. Galloway, Grier, Blessing 1936 Pentobarbital–sodium and scopolamine hydrobromide. JAMA 107: 1707

SECTION 1

Maternal–fetal–neonatal considerations

3. The nature of pain in parturition

J. J. Bonica

A thorough understanding of all aspects of the nature of pain of childbirth is a *sine qua non* for optimal obstetric anesthesiologic care. Effective relief of the pain of childbirth has long been and today remains an important health and sociologic issue worldwide. The importance stems from several interrelated reasons. For one thing, contrary to the claims of proponents of 'natural childbirth' and 'psychoprophylaxis' that this physiologic process should be painless, it has long been appreciated that labor and vaginal delivery are painful events for most women. For another, misconceptions exist among the public, some physicians, nurses, midwives and other health professionals about its nature, function and effects and about methods for its control. Many believe that pain has an important biologic function and should not be relieved, while others believe that pharmacologic methods of pain relief have deleterious effects on the mother and fetus and should be avoided.

As emphasized later, while pain has the important biologic function of indicating to the gravida that labor is imminent, it should be effectively relieved once it has served this function because persistent, severe pain has harmful effects on the mother and might also have harmful effects on the fetus and newborn. Although *improperly* administered analgesia/anesthesia can entail the risk of complications, and can contribute to maternal and perinatal morbidity and even mortality, there is now an impressive body of evidence that *properly administered*, it does *not* contribute to maternal and perinatal morbidity or mortality but may help to reduce them, especially in high-risk pregnancies. Finally, many gravidae in developed countries have been informed of the benefits of modern pharmacologic analgesia by the news media and other sources, and many expect effective pain relief during childbirth.

*In this chapter I present a comprehensive overview of all aspects of the pain of childbirth. The material is presented in three major sections:

1. a brief overview of the current concepts of acute pain in general including its neurophysiologic and biochemical substrates, its modulation and its function;
2. the nature of the pain of childbirth, including discussion of the incidence, intensity and quality of labor pain; detailed description of the intrinsic mechanisms and other factors that influence it; the peripheral pathways and the central nociceptive mechanisms; and
3. the effects of parturitional pain and their modification by properly administered analgesia/anesthesia.

This chapter represents an updated summary of the subject as I presented it previously[1] and as described in two recent review articles[2,3] and chapters recently published in major textbooks on pain.[4,5]

CURRENT CONCEPTS OF PAIN

The study of the nature of pain has consumed the interest and efforts of many philosophers and scientists for centuries. Aristotle considered pain a state of feeling, the experience antithetic to pleasure and the epitome of unpleasantness.[6] Although during the ensuing two millenia many philosophers/scientists attempted to provide more precise and diverse hypotheses, the Aristotelian concept remained predominant until the early part of the nineteenth century when physiology emerged as an experimental science and the study of pain in the modern sense was initiated. Toward the end of the century there emerged two opposing 'theories' of pain:[6] the specificity theory, which stated that pain is a pure (primary) sensation with its own specific receptor organs and conducting pathways that transmit nociceptive information to the brain with little modification; and the intensive theory, which stated that pain results from intense stimulation of any nerve and central summation of impulses provoked by the stimuli. These two opposing theories embraced by physiologists were in opposition with the Aristotelian

* The information in this chapter is contained in Chapter 9 of *Principles and Practice of Obstetric Analgesia and Anesthesia*, 2nd edn, edited by J. J. Bonica and J. McDonald 1994 (in press). Lea & Febiger, Pennsylvania.

concept that pain was an affective quality which at this time was being supported by most philosophers and psychologists (see ref. 6 for detailed description of these theories). During the first five decades of the present century, most of the research on pain was done to support one of the these theories, but by mid-century the specificity theory prevailed.

To take into account the influence of psychologic and environmental factors and integrate them into the specificity theory, some authorities, but particularly Wolff and associates,[7–9] suggested that the total pain experience is composed of pain perception and the associated sensations, emotional reactions, affective (feeling) states and the psychophysiologic reactions consequent thereto. They further contended that the reaction is independent of the original sensation or perception and can be dissociated from it, and that the perception is the same for all individuals and is measurable. However, it is doubtful there is such a thing as a pure sensation separate and distinct from the influence of reaction.[10] Beecher[10] believed that processing of the psychic reaction to the original stimulus probably begins before awareness of the sensation has been achieved. Moreover, the essential part of pain is awareness and no other sensation or perception can be called 'pain' unless it is experienced as such.[10] Therefore, although the original stimulus may be the same for all individuals, it probably loses that sameness as a result of modifying neuronal and emotional influences. Consequently, the reactions to pain vary not only among individuals, but in the same individual at different times. The pattern of reactions depends in part on what the sensation means to the individual in light of his past life experiences, as well as his attitude, judgment, mood, and emotional status at the time pain is perceived, and its symbolic meaning to him.[11] The presence or absence of anxiety, fear and apprehension and the significance, seriousness and importance assigned to the cause of pain are also very important in determining the individual's reaction to his/her pain.[10]

While these modifications of the specificity theory were definitely an improvement, the concept of pain perception assumes a one-to-one relationship between the intensity of the stimulus and the pain perception and relegates the reaction to pain as a secondary response consequent to the sensation achieved in a straight-through push-button or alarm system fashion. Moreover, these modifications did not explain many phenomena associated with pain nor did they provide correct explanation of how these emotional and psychologic reactions influenced nociception and pain. After carefully assessing the advantages and limitations of the various theories, Melzack and Wall[12] in 1965 proposed the now well known 'gate control' theory which two years later was modified by Melzack and Casey.[13] This theory is appealing because it helps to explain certain peculiar phenomena of pain and also because it suggested a possible explanation of how emotions and other cerebral processes can influence the pain experience. Pain, they said, is not due to neural activity which resides exclusively in a 'pain pathway' as implied by the simple straight-through neural system of the specificity theory, but rather it is a result of activity in several interacting neural systems each with its own specialized function. The publication of this theory, together with a number of other factors, generated much new research, and consequently we have acquired a great deal of new information during the past quarter-century. The new data emphasize that the acute pain experience provoked by injury or disease is the net effect of many interacting physiologic and psychologic mechanisms which involve the activity of most parts of the nervous system concerned with sensory, motivational and cognitive processes and psychodynamic mechanisms.

In this chapter only a brief review of some of the new facts will be given under the following headings:

1. neurophysiology and biochemistry of acute pain including the peripheral system; central mechanisms and spinal cord; ascending afferent systems, brain stem and cerebral cortex;
2. modulating systems; and
3. psychologic aspects.

Comprehensive reviews of many of these aspects appear in recently published books and articles.[14–17]

Neurophysiology and biochemistry of acute pain

Peripheral system

The peripheral system consists of afferent neurons of spinal and cranial nerves; their distal axonal branches, which end as, or into, receptors in body tissues; their cell bodies in sensory ganglia; and their proximal axonal branches, which make contact with second-order neurons in the neuraxis (Fig. 3.1A). Many recent electrophysiologic studies have shown an impressive degree of specialization among receptor–afferent units.[14–17] Several types of receptors have been identified: mechanoreceptors, thermoreceptors and nociceptors or pain receptors. Nociceptors are characterized by high threshold, small receptive fields, persistent discharge for a suprathreshold stimulus and are terminals of small A delta and C afferent fibers. Some A delta afferents are activated only by very strong mechanical stimulation, and thus are known as mechanical nociceptors (high-threshold mechanoreceptors or HTMs). Other A delta afferents respond well to both noxious heat stimuli (>45°C) and to intense mechanical stimuli and are thus known as myelinated mechano-thermal nociceptors (MMTNs). Most (95% in human skin) C afferent fibers are activated by intense mechanical (>1 g), thermal (maximal firing range 45–53°C) and chemical stimuli and are therefore known as polymodal nociceptors (CPNs).

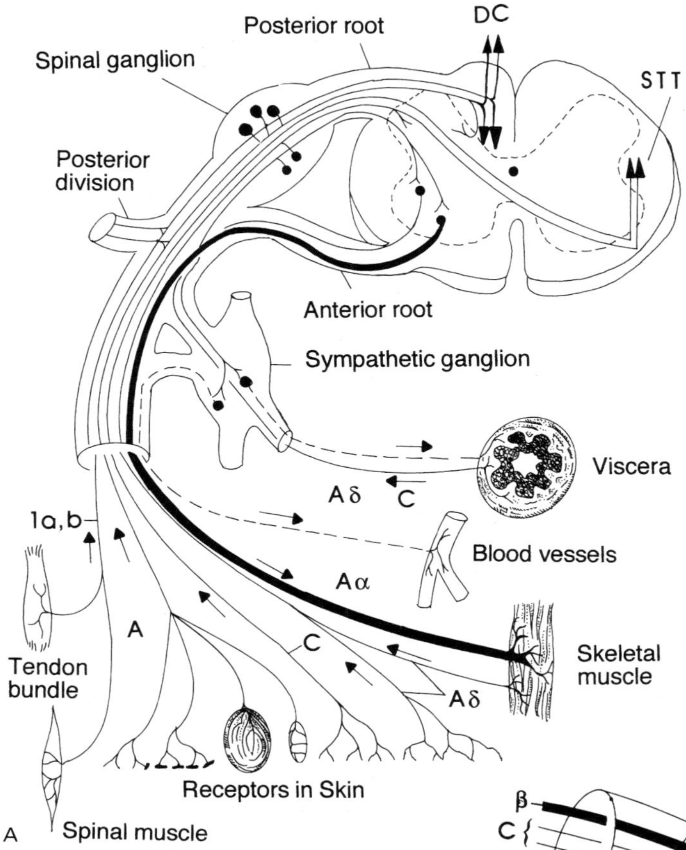

A

Fig. 3.1 A very simplified schema of the components of a peripheral nerve (A) and a cross-section of the input of the dorsal horn of the spinal cord as well as the interneurons and axonal terminals of the descending control systems. Many of the small, thinly myelinated A delta and unmyelinated C fibers transmit innocuous mechanical and thermal information, but a significant number transmit nociceptive impulses. These A delta and C fibers supply skin, deep somatic structures and viscera. They synapse primarily in laminae I, IIo, and V, although they make synaptic contact through interneurons with cells in other laminae. Cutaneous nociceptive afferents project to laminae I, IIo and V, whereas visceral and muscle nociceptive afferents project to laminae I and V but not to lamina II. Note the convergence of cutaneous and visceral afferents on viscerosomatic neurons in laminae I and V [C cells, which are wide dynamic range (WDR) neurons], the axons of which pass to the anterolateral fasciculus (ALF) of the opposite side and project to the brain. Similarly, A delta and C muscle nociceptive afferents and cutaneous afferents also converge on neurons in laminae I and V, including some with long ascending axons that form part of the ALF. Although most of the axons ascend in the contralateral ALF, some ascend ipsilaterally. The collaterals from A beta fibers, which course along the medial side of the dorsal horn, take a retroflex course at the level of lamina V, ascend dorsally, and then branch out to make contact with interneurons and output neurons. In this way they modulate dorsal horn output. Note the interneurons in laminae II and III and an 'antenna' cell in lamina IV (cells B) that may project rostrally as dorsal column post-synaptic fibers or as spinocervical fibers. Raphespinal and reticulospinal fibers (from n. reticularis magnocellularis) descend in the lateral fasciculus to make contact with cells in laminae I, II and V and deeper laminae to exert modulating influences on dorsal horn function (see Fig. 3.4). S-stalk cell, I-islet cell. The dorsolateral horn funiculus (DLF) contains descending axons of cells in the brain stem that are inhibitory (off-cells) of perhaps facilitatory (on-cells). (From Bonica J J 1990 The management of pain, 2nd edn. Lea & Febiger, Philadelphia, 1990. (A) Fig. 3–2, p 30; (B) Fig. 3–26, p 51.)

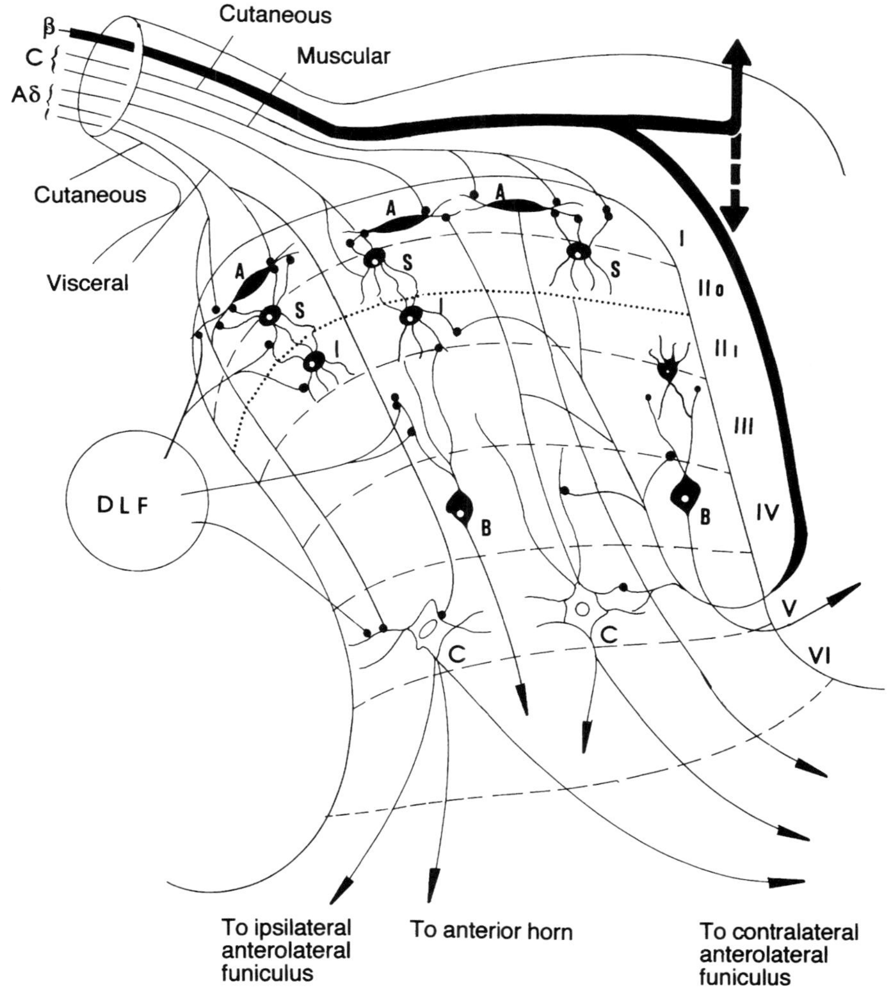

B

Studies have also indicated that repeated thermal stimulation produces sensitization or lowering of the threshold of the nociceptors.[18,19] Sensitization is also produced by biochemical agents liberated with tissue damage or inflammation. Data from single- and multiple-fiber studies in animals and in man support earlier observations that these A delta and C fibers are essential for pain sensation.[17,20] These nociceptor-afferent fibers supply not only the skin and subcutaneous tissue, but also the muscle, fascia, periosteum and other deep structures (Fig. 3.1). Viscera are also supplied by afferent fibers, which under certain circumstances [inflammation, spasm of hollow viscera, contraction of hollow viscera under isometric conditions (contraction against obstruction), sudden abnormal distension, stretching or tearing of these structures] act as nociceptive afferents.[16]

From the peripheral spinal nerves, the sensory information from below the head is transmitted to dorsal horn cells of the spinal cord while the sensory information from the head is carried via the cranial nerves to the nucleus caudalis of the trigeminal nuclear complex, also called the 'medullary dorsal horn'. It is then transmitted to higher parts of the neuraxis via ascending neural systems. In contrast to the idea of the straight-through transmission without modification, it is now clear that there is a great degree of modulation all along the course of transmission of impulses: at the first synapse in the spinal dorsal horn or medullary horn and at every level of the neuraxis.[12,13,17,21–23] Within the somatosensory system there are mechanisms that permit distinction between mechanical, thermal, and chemical events in spatial, temporal and intensity domains.

Spinal and medullary dorsal horn

On reaching the dorsal horn of the spinal cord or the nucleus caudalis, some primary peripheral nociceptive afferents terminate and make direct or indirect contact with cells in the superficial part of these structures (laminae I and IIo) and send collaterals that terminate in deeper laminae (V), while others terminate more medially (laminae VII and VIII)[15,16] (Fig. 3.1B). Some of the cells in laminae I and II of the dorsal horn are known as nociceptive-specific (NS) neurons because they receive input exclusively from high-threshold peripheral afferents. Those in lamina V (and perhaps IV and VI) are known as 'wide dynamic range' (WDR) neurons because they receive input from low-threshold fibers concerned with touch sensation and also from nociceptive afferents so that they are able to respond with increasingly higher frequency of impulse discharge to touch, pressure and noxious stimuli. The convergence of visceral high-threshold afferents and low-threshold afferents from the skin, supplied by the same spinal cord segments on lamina V neurons, are said to provide the neural basis for the phenomenon of referred pain associated with visceral deep and somatic disorders.[16]

In addition to making synaptic contact and receiving input from primary nociceptive afferents, these dorsal horn neurons also receive input from the large myelinated peripheral afferents, from short-axon interneurons of the substantia gelatinosa and from the terminals of supraspinal descending neural control systems. Thus, it is obvious that the dorsal horn and nucleus caudalis, which were traditionally considered simple relay stations, are very complex structures containing a large number and many varieties of neurons and synaptic arrangements that permit not only reception and transmission, but a high degree of sensory processing, including local abstraction, integration, selection and appropriate dispersion of sensory impulses. This complex form of local processing is achieved through the phenomena of central convergence, central summation, excitation and inhibition coming from the periphery, from local and segmental interneurons, and from the brain and brainstem. These processes involve the liberation of putative excitatory neurotransmitters, including substance P and somatostatin, and the liberation of the endogenous opioid peptide enkephalin and other inhibitory neurotransmitters including norepinephrine and 5-hydroxytryptamine. These very complex interactions determine the modulation, transmission and dispersion of nociceptive information.

After being subjected to these modulating influences in the dorsal horn, some of the nociceptive impulses pass through internuncial neurons to the anterior and anterolateral horn cells, where they stimulate somatomotor neurons that supply skeletal muscles and sympathetic neurons that supply blood vessels, viscera and sweat glands. These are involved in segmental reflex (autonomic) responses, which are described later. Other nociceptive impulses are transmitted to neurons, the axons of which make up the spinothalamic tract and other ascending systems and are thus conveyed to the brainstem and the brain to provoke suprasegmental reflex responses and cortical responses.

Ascending pathways

It has long been known that the spinothalamic tract transmits pain messages from below the head and that the trigeminothalamic tract transmits impulses from the head.[17,24] However, evidence acquired during the past two decades indicates that this system also transmits other sensory information and is composed of two parts that have different anatomic, physiologic and functional characteristics: the neospinothalamic tract and the paleospinothalamic tracts (Fig. 3.2). More recent evidence also suggests that several other ascending systems participate in transmission of pain signals; on the basis of their anatomic and functional characteristics, these and

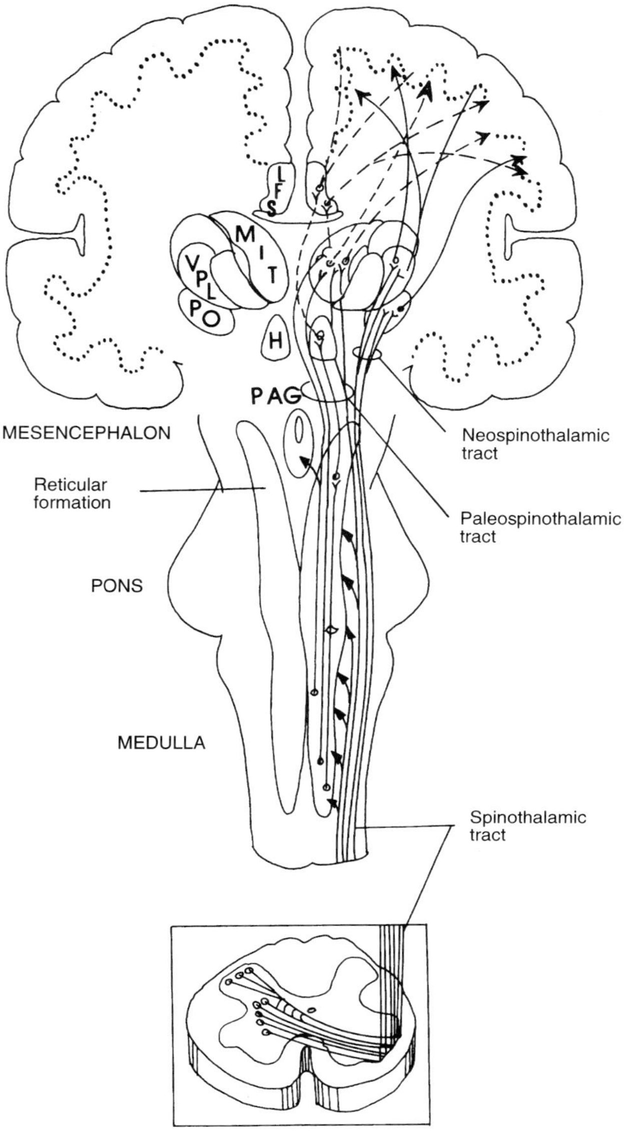

Fig. 3.2 Simple diagram of the course and termination of the spinothalamic tract. Most of the fibers cross to the opposite side and ascend to the brainstem and brain, although some ascend ipsilaterally. The neospinothalamic (nSTT) part of the tract has cell bodies located primarily in laminae I and V of the dorsal horn, whereas the paleospinothalamic tract (pSTT) has its cell bodies in deeper laminae. The nSTT fibers ascend in a more superficial part of the tract and project without interruption to the caudal part of the ventroposterolateral thalamic nucleus (VPLc), the oral part of this nucleus (VPLo), the medial part of the posterior thalamus (POm). In these structures they synapse with a third relay of neurons, which project to the somatosensory cortex (SI, SII and retroinsular cortex) (solid lines). Some of the fibers of the pSTT pass directly to the medial/intralaminar thalamic nuclei (MIT), and others project to the nuclei and the reticular formation of the brainstem and thence to the periaqueductal gray (PAG), hypothalamus (H), nucleus submedius and MIT. In these structures these axons synapse with neurons that connect with the limbic forebrain structure (LFS) via complex circuits and also send diffuse projection to various parts of the brain (dashed lines). See text section on limbic system for details. (From Bonica J J 1990 The management of pain, 2nd edn. Lea & Febiger, Philadelphia, Fig. 3–29, p 54.)

the spinothalamic tracts have been grouped into two major systems: the lateral system and the medial system[25] (Fig. 3.3).

The lateral system. The lateral system includes the neospinothalamic and neotrigeminothalamic tracts, the spinocervical tract and the dorsal column post-synaptic system.[16] This group is composed of long, thick fibers that conduct rapidly, have a discrete somatotopic organization and make connection with the ventrobasal thalamus and posterior thalamic nuclei where they synapse with another relay of fibers that project to the somatosensory cortex. The evidence suggests that the lateral system is concerned with rapid transmission of phasic discriminative information about the onset of injury, its precise location, its intensity and duration, and can quickly bring about responses that prevent further damage.

The medial system. The medial system is composed of the paleospinothalamic, paleotrigeminothalamic, spinoreticular and propriospinal systems.[16,25] The paleospinothalamic, paleotrigeminothalamic and spinoreticular fibers consist of a few long and many short, thin fibers that are not somatically organized and which pass medially to project to the reticular formation, the periaqueductal gray matter (PAG), the hypothalamus and the medial and intrathalamic nuclei where they synapse with neurons that connect with the limbic forebrain structures and with diffuse projections to many other parts of the brain. The multisynaptic propriospinal system also consists of very short, thin fibers that ascend through the cord in the gray matter (in contrast to the ventrolateral tracts, which lie in the white matter) and project to unknown destinations in the brain. Because of the thinness of the fibers, their multisynaptic nature and the lack of somatotopic organization, impulses passing through this system are said to transmit tonic information about the state of the organism. As previously mentioned, these impulses also provoke the suprasegmental reflex responses, the powerful motivational drive and the unpleasant effect characteristic of pain, and some stimulate cells in the PAG and thus activate descending control systems.

Brainstem

The reticular formation serves an integrative function and from the midbrain level an ascending activating system of fibers maintains both tonic and phasic stimulation of an overlying diffuse thalamic projection system, which in turn modulates the level of arousal of widespread areas of cerebral cortex, particularly the association cortex.[16,17,26–31] The *hypothalamus* integrates and regulates autonomic nervous system functions and the neuroendocrine response to stress, and organizes visceral and somatic reaction patterns.[16,28,29] *The limbic system* does not have primary control of behavioral processes, but rather has a complex modulatory suppressor influence upon attention,

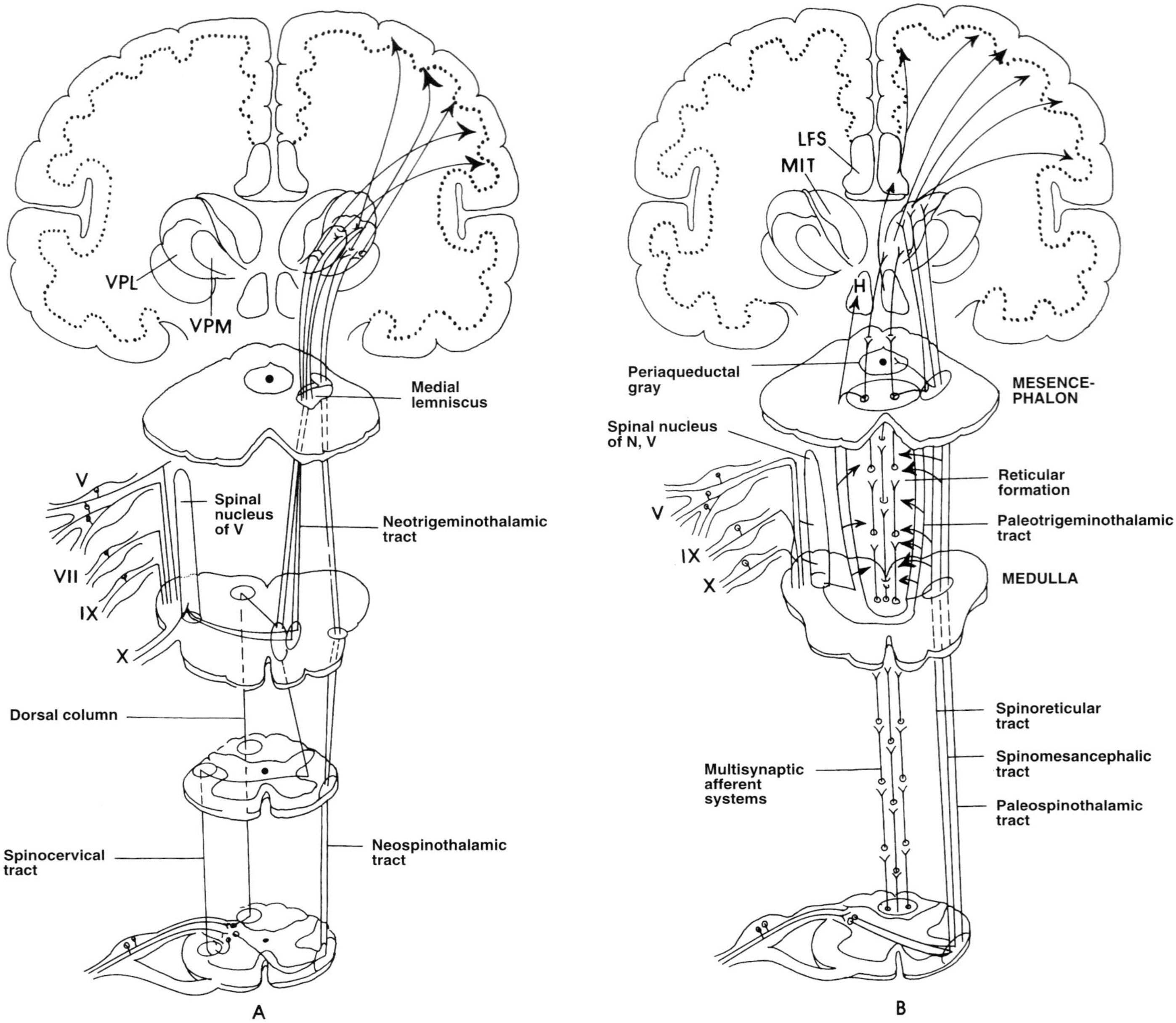

Fig. 3.3 Diagrams illustrating the origin, course and projection of the lateral system (A) and the medial system (B). See text for details. (From Bonica J J 1990 The management of pain, 2nd edn. Lea & Febiger, Philadelphia, Fig. 3–66, p 89.)

mood and motivation, as well as upon processes underlying the performance of certain types of behavior.[16,30,31]

Cerebral cortex

The somatosensory cortex serves a discriminative function and may regulate subcortical activity related to pain through highly complex reflexes, but is not essential to pain perception.[12,13,16,32] The frontal cortex probably plays a significant role in mediating between cognitive activities and motivational and affective features of pain since it receives information via intracortical fiber systems from virtually all sensory and associated cortical areas and projects strongly to reticular and limbic structures.[13–16] These make possible mobilization of all sorts of associations based upon past experience, judgments and emotions, and is involved in the evaluation of the sensation. It appears essential in maintaining a negative effect and aversive motivational dimension of pain. Neocortical processes subserve cognitive and psychologic factors, including early experience, prior conditioning anxiety, attention, suggestion, cultural background and evaluation of the meaning of the pain-producing situation. Through the neocortical processes and corticofugal impulses these factors may affect sensory, affective and motivational dimensions of pain or they may modify primarily the affective and motivational and leave the sensory discriminative dimensions relatively undisturbed.[13–16]

Modulation of nociception and pain

One of the most exciting areas in recent research concerns the various neural, biochemical and psychophysiologic mechanisms that participate in the modulation of nociceptive information from tissues to the brain.[21–24] In the peripheral system, injury or inflammation causes the liberation of pain-producing substances and/or damages nerves and thus lowers the threshold of the nociceptive afferent units so that innocuous stimulation (light touch) produces pain. On the other hand, innocuous stimulation of the skin by rubbing, by application of cold or by transcutaneous electrical stimulation in some way impairs the transmission of nociceptive impulses from the periphery to the dorsal horn. Nociceptive transmission in the dorsal horn is affected by the activity and interactions of local interneurons and supraspinal descending systems (Fig. 3.4).

In 1969 Reynolds[33] reported that electrical stimulation of the lateral periaqueductal gray (PAG) and periventricular gray (PVG) matter of the midbrain produced a profound analgesia without apparently interfering with motor function or with the animal's response to other sensory stimuli. A series of brilliant experiments by Liebeskind and co-workers[34–36] and many others[37] (see also ref. 21 for all references) done during the ensuing decade have shown that: (a) this phenomenon, known as stimulation-produced analgesia (SPA), often outlasts stimulation by many seconds or minutes; (b) SPA inhibits the activity of dorsal horn neurons involved in nociception but not those concerned with other sensations; (c) the effects of SPA are partly or wholly diminished by administration of naloxone, a morphine antagonist; and (d) injection of very small amounts of morphine directly into PAG produces analgesia, indicating that a major effect of morphine is to activate descending inhibitory neurons in

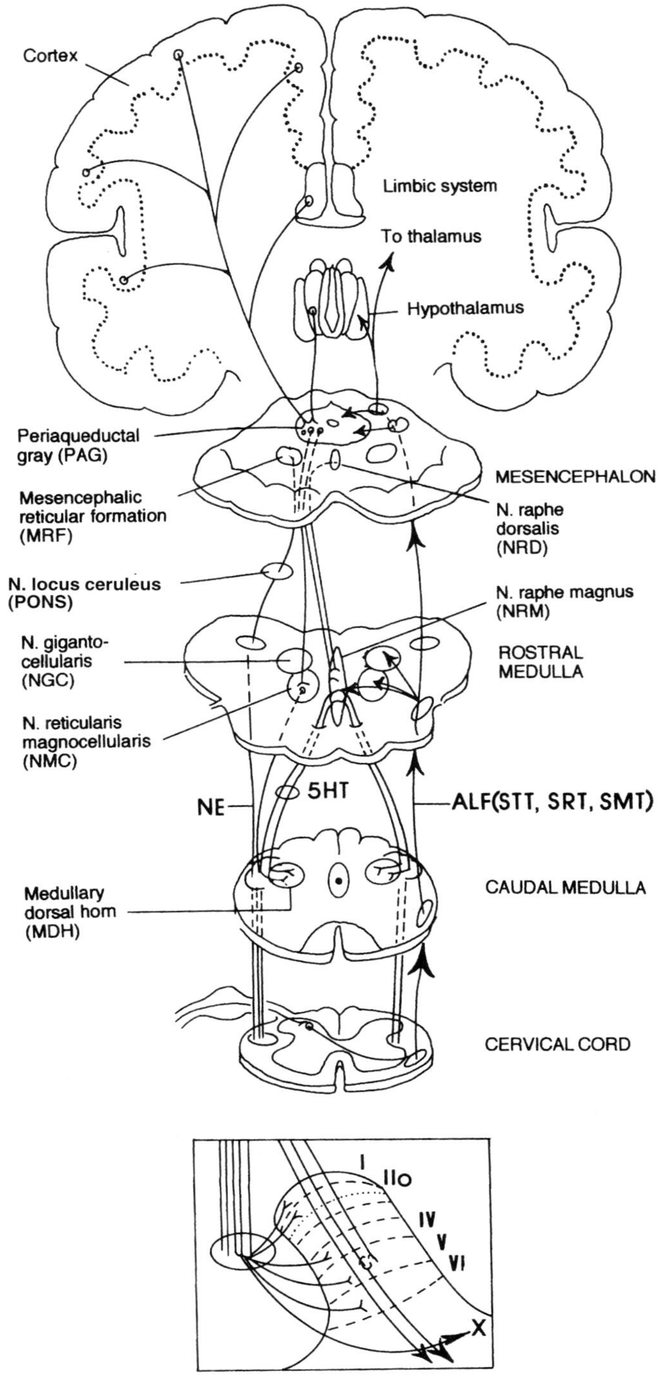

Fig. 3.4 Schema of the most extensively studied and probably the most important descending control system, composed of four tiered parts. The ascending anterolateral fasciculus (ALF), composed of the spinothalamic, spinoreticular and spinomesencephalic tracts, has important inputs into the nucleus raphe magnus (NRM), nucleus magnocellularis (NMC), nucleus reticularis gigantocellularis (NGC) and the periaqueductal gray (PAG) via the nucleus cuneiformis. The ALF also has input to the medullary/pontine reticular formation, the nucleus raphe dorsalis (NRD) and the mesencephalic reticular formation (MRF). The PAG receives important input from such rostral structures as the frontal and insular cortex and other parts of the cerebrum involved in cognition, and from the limbic system, the thalamus and, most importantly, the hypothalamus, which sends beta-endorphin axons to the PAG. The locus ceruleus in the pons is a major source of noradrenergic input to the PAG and dorsal horn (tract labeled NE). These mesencephalic structures (PAG, NRD, MRF) contain enkephalin (ENK), dynorphin (DYN), serotonin (5HT) and neurotensin (NT) neurons, but only the last two send axons that project to NRM and NGC. Here they make synapse with neurons that are primarily serotonergic, whose axons project to the medullary dorsal horn and descend in the dorsolateral funiculus to send terminals to all laminae of the spinal gray (the densest populations are found in laminae I, IIo and V of the dorsal horn and the motor neuron pools of lamina IX). The projection from NRM is bilateral, whereas the projection from NGC is ipsilateral. Noradrenergic fibers descend and project to the medullary dorsal horn and then descend in the dorsolateral funiculus of the spinal cord to send terminals to laminae I, IIo, IV–VI and X. (From Bonica J J 1990 The management of pain, 2nd edn. Lea & Febiger, Philadelphia, Fig. 4–9, p 108.)

the brainstem. The anatomic and biochemical characteristics of this descending pathway have been elucidated[22,23] (see ref. 21 for all references) (Fig. 3.4).

These studies were paralleled by the discovery of opioid receptors on nerve cells, which led to the quest for and identification of endogenously produced substances which were named endorphins (endogenous morphine-like substances) and enkephalins (opioid substances in the brain). As a result of these and other studies, it was found that SPA produced impulses that descend in the dorsolateral funiculus and make contact with and stimulate a variety of short-axon interneurons in the substantia gelatinosa at every level of the spinal cord. Some of these interneurons contain enkephalin, which inhibits transmission of nociceptive information by preventing the release of substance P, the neurotransmitter that permits the transfer of nociceptive impulses from one nerve to another. This descending modulating system has input from the brain, limbic system and other structures which are known to be involved in the psychologic dimensions of pain.

More recent studies have suggested there are other descending inhibitory systems that do not involve opioids[38,39] (see ref. 21 for all references). The data acquired to date make it perfectly clear that there are a number of mechanisms of pain inhibition, some involving spinal mechanisms; others involving supraspinal mechanisms; some involving opioids and some not; and some involving centrifugal control on spinal nociceptive systems and some not. In addition to drastically changing our conceptualization of pain mechanisms, the new data have had a major impact on the development of new modalities for relief of pain.

Even more recent electrophysiologic experiments in animals revealed that stimulation of the rostral ventromedial medulla (RVM) can also exert facilitatory effects on spinal nociceptive neurons. Fields et al[40] used a tail-flick reflex (TF) response in lightly anesthetized rats to study the characteristics of cells in the RVM and found a class of TF-related bulbospinal neurons in this region that they called 'on-cells'. Pharmacologic evidence supports the thesis that on-cells have an enhancing effect on nociception. The activity of these on-cells is completely suppressed by morphine given in doses sufficient to block TF – a response that is due to stimulation of 'off-cells'. When the 'spontaneous' activity of on-cells and off-cells is studied simultaneously, they are found to have a reciprocal period of activity. When on-cells are active, TF response latency is short and the threshold is lower, whereas when off-cells are active TF response latency is longer. Given the extensive independent support for the role of RVM neurons and modulation of spinal nociception, these observations that TF response latency is inversely related to on-cell firing and is directly related to off-cell firing are consistent with bidirectional modulation or control of nociception by these two populations of RVM neurons: on-cells that enhance nociceptive transmission and off-cells that suppress it.

Psychologic and emotional factors

During the past quarter-century many new scientific data have been acquired which impressively emphasize the importance of motivational, affective, cognitive, emotional and other psychological factors on the individual's total pain experience.[41–46] Moreover, these data have put in sharper focus the influence of perceptual factors, learning, personality, ethnic and cultural factors, and the environment, and have helped to clarify the psychodynamics of anxiety: anticipation of pain, the meaning or significance of the pain-producing sensation, attention, motivation, suggestion and placebos – factors well known to influence the pain experience. Early experience, perceptual factors, personality, ethnic and cultural patterns play varying roles in the individuals's pain behavior. In some cultures tolerating pain without expression of suffering is required, while in others overt expression of suffering is encouraged.

Anxiety is a particularly powerful factor in reducing pain tolerance or, in other words, producing greater pain behavior.[45,46] Conversely, pain tolerance can be increased by reducing anxiety with information or attention to another task. *Attention*, the selective orientation of the receptor system to one source or pattern of stimulation to the exclusion of others, can either enhance or diminish the painful experience. It is, of course, well known that athletes injured during play and soldiers injured in battle often do not experience pain at the moment of injury. In contrast, the same individuals often manifest overt pain behavior consequent to minimal noxious stimulation induced by hypodermic needles in the emergency room. Under such conditions, attention and anxiety both decrease tolerance to pain.

Motivation is another psychodynamic mechanism which can have marked influence on the physiologic, behavioral and affective aspects of pain experience.[10,44] In some instances motivation is so strong as to permit the individual to sustain severe injury without any of the pain responses. In such cases, psychophysiologic mechanisms probably inhibit transmission of impulses in the dorsal horn as well as other parts of the nervous system. In others the mechanism is not sufficient to block reflex responses but is sufficient to suppress overt pain behavior.

How do these psychologic factors influence pain? In view of the recent data, it is not taking an unreasonable degree of scientific license to suggest that various emotional, motivational and affective factors can stimulate parts of the brain which, when activated, exert powerful inhibition. These send descending impulses which have the capability of preventing transmission of noxious impulses in the dorsal horn and at different levels of the neuraxis. On the other hand, under appropriate conditions psychologic factors through action of the limbic system and descending pathways can stimulate 'on-cells' and thus enhance transmission of noxious impulses to the brain with consequent greater pain experience.

Biology and pathophysiology of acute pain

Transient acute pain, as occurs when an individual touches a hot stove or steps on a sharp object, promptly alerts the individual and causes him or her to immediately withdraw the limb and thus avoid further damage. Acute pain associated with severe injuries involving deep somatic structures, such as fractures or sprains, imposes limitation of action and therefore tends to prevent further damage or aggravation of pathophysiology. The biologic function of acute pain under these circumstances is widely accepted and appreciated. Similarly, acute pain of visceral disease has the biologic function of warning the individual that something is wrong: it prompts him or her to consult a physician, and it is used by the physician as an aid in making the diagnosis. Moreover, acute pain caused by injury or disease is often associated with certain segmental and suprasegmental reflex responses that help the organism maintain homeostasis (see below).

Although the biologic function of acute pain is widely and universally accepted, what is not generally realized or appreciated, even by some physicians, is that some types of pain, such as that which occurs after an operation, have no biologic function, but instead produce abnormal physiologic and psychologic reactions that often cause complications. Similar deleterious effects result if the severe pain of injury or of such diseases as myocardial infarction and acute pancreatitis is not effectively relieved after it has served its biologic function. Indeed, as will be duly emphasized later, even severe pain associated with certain physiologic processes such as parturition, if allowed to persist, will produce deleterious effects. These detrimental effects are consequent to progression of the segmental and suprasegmental reflex responses and cortical responses to an abnormal state. In order to fully appreciate this thesis, a brief discussion of the responses to tissue injury is presented.

Responses to tissue injury

Tissue destruction, whether from crush injury, fracture, operation, internal disease or the injury inherent in parturition, results in local biochemical changes and autonomic reflex responses that are intended to maintain body integrity (see refs. 47 and 48 for comprehensive reviews). The local biochemical changes produced by liberation of intracellular chemical substances into the extracellular fluids surrounding nerve endings to induce local pain, tenderness, and hyperalgesia have been discussed earlier. In addition to sensitizing the nerve endings, these algogenic substances also act indirectly by altering the microenvironment consisting of smooth muscles, capillaries and efferent sympathetic fibers. The nociceptors, thus activated, transduce the noxious stimuli into impulses that are transmitted to the neuraxis. As previously mentioned, upon reaching the spinal or medullary dorsal horn, these impulses are promptly subjected to peripheral local segmental and supraspinal descending modulating influences which, together with other factors, determine their further transmission throughout the neuraxis. Some stimulate somatomotor and sympathetic preganglionic fibers of the same and adjacent segments to produce segmental (spinal) reflex responses. Other nociceptive impulses stimulate dorsal horn neurons, the axons of which make up ascending afferent systems and thus provoke suprasegmental reflex responses and cortical responses (Fig. 3.5).

Segmental (spinal) reflexes

Segmental (spinal) reflexes may, and often do, enhance nociception and produce alteration of ventilation, circulation and gastrointestinal and urinary function. Thus stimulation of somatomotor cells results in increased skeletal muscle tension or spasm, which decreases chest wall compliance and initiates positive feedback loops that generate nociceptive impulses from the muscle.[47,48]

Stimulation of sympathetic preganglionic neurons in the anterolateral horn of the spinal cord causes an increase in heart rate, stroke volume and, consequently, cardiac work and myocardial oxygen consumption. Moreover, severe pain may cause cardiac arrhythmias, which may become serious. In addition, sympathetic hyperactivity causes decrease of gastrointestinal tone that may progress to ileus and a decrease in urinary function that reduces urinary output. Because these responses to noxious stimuli occur in animals which have undergone vagotomy and C1 spinal section, they are produced by truly spinal segmental reflexes.

Suprasegmental reflex responses

Suprasegmental reflex responses result from nociceptive-induced stimulation of medullary centers of ventilation and circulation, of hypothalamic (predominantly sympathetic) centers of neuroendocrine function, and of some limbic structures.[47] These responses consist of hyperventilation, increased hypothalamic neural sympathetic tone and increased secretion of catecholamines and other endocrine secretions. The increased neural sympathetic tone and catecholamine secretion add to the effects of spinal reflexes and further increase cardiac output, peripheral resistance, blood pressure, cardiac workload and

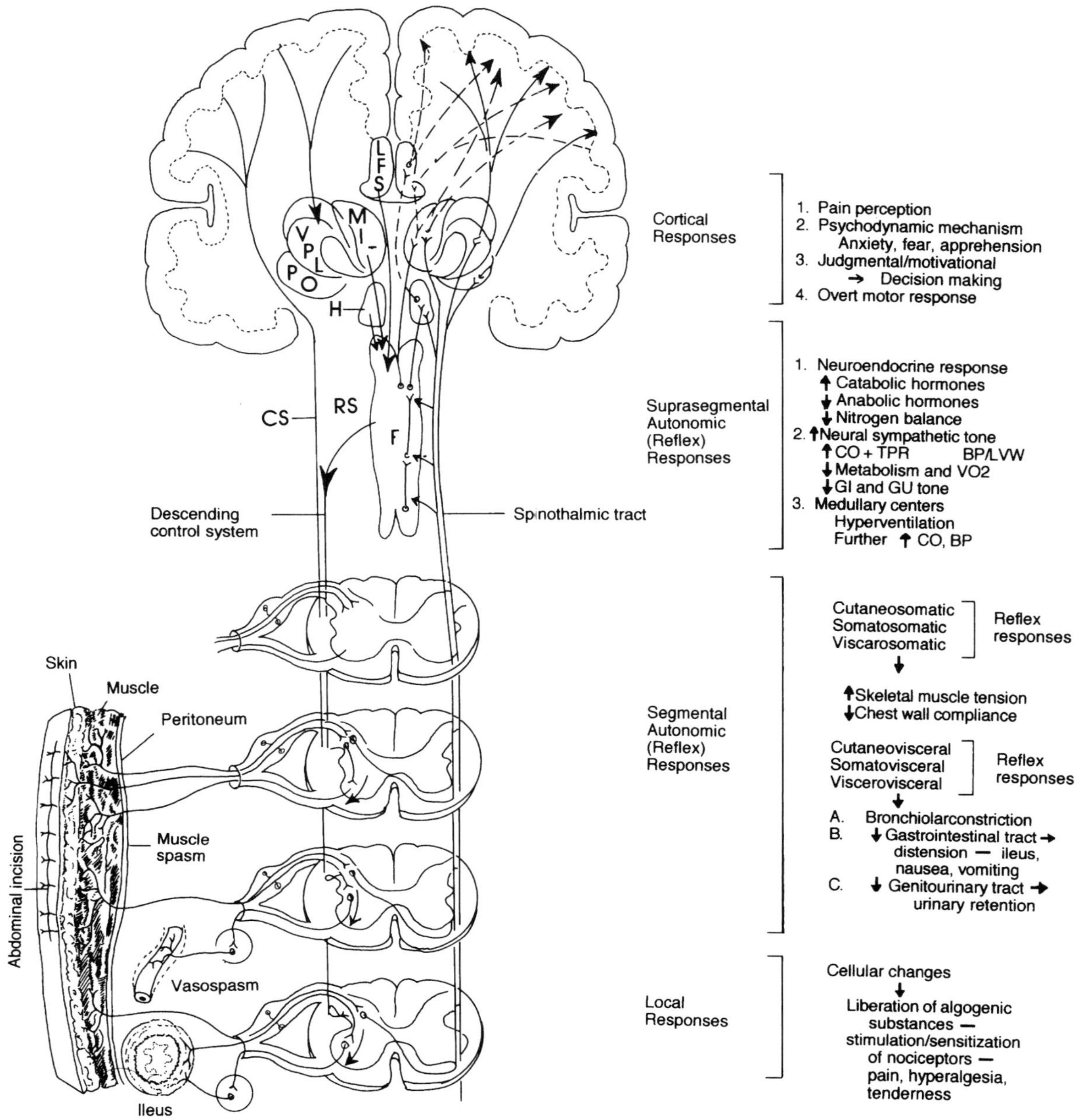

Fig. 3.5 Schematic depiction of the responses to noxious stimuli induced by trauma during intra-abdominal surgery. LFS, limbic forebrain structure; MIT, medial and intralaminar thalamic nuclei; VPL, ventroposterolateral nucleus; PO, posterior group of thalamic nuclei; H, hypothalamus; CS, central gray substance; RS, rubrospinal tract; and RF, reticular formation). (Modified from Bonica, J J 1979 Introduction to recent advances in the management of acute and chronic pain. Hosp Pract (Special Report), January, pp 4–10.)

myocardial oxygen consumption.[48] In addition to catecholamine release there is an increased secretion of cortisol, ACTH, glucagon, cAMP, antidiuretic hormone (ADH), growth hormone (GH), renin and other catabolically acting hormones, with a concomitant decrease in the anabolically acting hormones insulin and testosterone.[47–50] This type of endocrine secretion, characteristic of the stress response, produces widespread metabolic effects, including increased blood glucose, free fatty acids, blood lactate and ketones, as well as generalized increased metabolism and oxygen consumption. The endocrine and metabolic changes result in substrate utilization from storage to central organs and injured tissue and lead to a catabolic state with a negative nitrogen balance. The degree and duration of these endocrine and metabolic changes are related to degree and duration of tissue damage, and many of these biochemical changes last for days.[50]

Cortical responses

The intense anxiety and fear that invariably develop in patients who experience severe acute pain consequent to an unexpected severe injury or acute myocardial infarction greatly enhance the hypothalamic responses characteristic of stress through cortical stimulation. Indeed, cortisol and catecholamine responses to anxiety may exceed the hypothalamic responses provoked directly by nociceptive impulses reaching the hypothalamus.[47] Moreover, anxiety causes cortically mediated increased blood viscosity, clotting time, fibrinolysis and platelet aggregation (see ref. 47 for references). Recent advances in medicine and surgery and anesthesia, together with much new information about the metabolic and biochemical responses to injury, now suggest that these reflex responses might have become maladaptive because the persistent pain and associated reflex responses may cause a variety of complications. In the next section I will present impressive evidence that blocking the afferent and efferent pathways involved in these responses prove beneficial.

THE NATURE OF PARTURITIONAL PAIN

Magnitude of the problem

Mention has been made of the misconceptions and confusion about the nature of the pain of childbirth and its treatment. This has been and continues to be a result of inadequate dissemination of information to the public about advances in knowledge and current therapeutic procedures. Many proponents of natural childbirth have compounded the problem by insisting that pain need not occur during normal labor and that when it occurs it is the product of modern cultural and environmental factors. The origin of this notion is not known, but in 1914 Behan[51] stated in his classic book that 'like menstruation, childbirth naturally should be a painless process. It is only as culture advances that the labor becomes painful, for in women of primitive races pain is absent. Savages of a low degree of civilization are generally little troubled by parturiency.' Nineteen years later the same argument was put forth by Dick-Read,[52] who for the ensuing 25 years traveled worldwide espousing this thesis, strongly condemning pharmacologic analgesia, and encouraging the use of his method of 'natural childbirth'. In 1950, in the USSR, Velvovski et al[53] began to use the technique of 'psychoprophylaxis', which they had developed and which was a modification of the Dick-Read method. Psychoprophylaxis was subsequently embraced by Lamaze[54] of France, who did much to popularize it in Europe and the Western hemisphere. The claim by these clinicians and their followers that childbirth among primitive peoples is painless has been disputed by many studies.[55–59]

Ford,[55] who studied this and other problems of reproduction in 64 primitive societies, wrote that 'the popular impression of childbirth in primitive society as painless and easy is definitely contradicted by our cases. As a matter of fact, it is often prolonged and painful.' After studying 80 primitive groups, Freedman and Ferguson[56] reported that the pain response in these groups during childbirth was similar to that observed in American and European parturients. Similar views have been expressed by others who studied the problem of labor pain in primitive societies.[57] I observed over 24 parturients in primitive societies in Australia and Africa, most of whom manifested severe pain behavior (unpublished data). Mention of the prevalence of pain during childbirth and its importance is found in the writings of the ancient Babylonians, Egyptians, Chinese, Hebrews and Greeks, and in the writings of many subsequent cultures and civilizations.[58] Finally, a recent study by Lefebre and Carli[59] of parturition of 88 individuals of 29 species of captive and wild non-human primates revealed that 69 (78%) manifested moderate to very severe pain characterized by straining, stretching, arching, grimacing, writhing, shaking, doubling-up, restlessness and vocalizations. This article provides impressive evidence that, while the behavior of the monkeys varied upon the circumstances of the environment, the process of parturition in these animals provoked what in humans we call pain of varying degrees.

Incidence, intensity and quality of parturitional pain

Although it is a common observation in obstetrics that parturients vary in the amount of suffering associated with labor and vaginal delivery, few well-designed studies on the prevalence, intensity and quality of labor pain have been performed. Lundh[60] published a survey of several Swedish investigations, which included both primiparae and multiparae; these revealed that the prevalence of intolerable severe pain ranged from 35 to 58%, with the remainder having moderate pain. Bundsen[61] found that 77% of primiparae reported that their pain during childbirth was severe or intolerable. In a study of 78 Swedish randomly selected primiparae, Nettelbladt et al[62] found that 35% reported intolerable pain, 37% had severe pain and 28% had moderate pain during labor and delivery. Records on 2700 parturients observed (and many interviewed) by Bonica while visiting or working (demonstrating obstetric anesthetic techniques) in 121 obstetric centers (with some having 100–150 deliveries daily) in 35 countries on six continents indicated that the frequency and intensity of labor pain was as follows: 15% had little or no pain, 35% had moderate pain, 30% had severe pain and 20% had extremely severe pain. The data are similar to those noted among over 8000 American parturients to whom I have administered or directly supervised anesthetic care during a period of 40 years (J Bonica, unpublished data).

Part 2. What Does Your Pain Feel Like?

Some of the words below describe your present pain. Circle ONLY those words that best describe it. Leave out any category that is not suitable. Use only a single word in each appropriate category--the one that applies best.

1	2	3	4	5
Flickering Quivering Pulsing Throbbing Beating Pounding	Jumping Flashing Shooting	Pricking Boring Drilling Stabbing Lacerating	Sharp Cutting Lacerating	Pinching Pressing Growing Cramping Crushing
6	**7**	**8**	**9**	**10**
Tagging Pulling Wrenching	Hot Burning Scalding Searing	Tingling Itchy Smarting Stinging	Dull Sore Hurting Aching Heavy	Tender Taut Rasping Splitting
11	**12**	**13**	**14**	**15**
Tiring Exhausting	Sickening Suffocating	Fearful Frightful Terrifying	Punishing Gruelling Cruel Vicious Killing	Wretched Blinding
16	**17**	**18**	**19**	**20**
Annoying Troublesome Miserable Intense Unbearable	Spreading Radiating Penetrating Piercing	Tight Numb Drawing Squeezing Tearing	Cool Cold Freezing	Nagging Nauseating Agonizing Dreadful Torturing

Part 4. How Strong is Your Pain?

People agree that the following 6 words represent pain of increasing intensity. They are:

1	2	3	4	5
Mild	Discomforting	Distressing	Horrible	Excruciating

To answer each question below, write the number of the most appropriate word in the space next to the question.

1. Which word describes your pain right now? ______________
2. Which word describes it at its worst? ______________
3. Which word describes it where it is least? ______________
4. Which word describes the worst toothache you ever had? ______________
5. Which word describes the worst headache you ever had? ______________
6. Which word describes the worst stomach ache you ever had? ______________

Fig. 3.6 The McGill Pain Questionnaire. (From Melzack R 1975 The McGill Pain Questionnaire: Major properties and scoring methods. Pain 1: 277, Fig. 2, pp 280–81.)

Obviously, these surveys and observations were based on simple numeric or verbal descriptions of pain, and thus lack quantification. One of the first attempts to quantify the intensity of labor pain was made by Javert and Hardy,[63] who used the Hardy–Wolff–Goodell dolorimeter to induce experimental pain and asked the parturients to compare it to the pain of their labor. The method entails the application of thermal heat, measured in millicalories (mc), to 3.5 cm of skin for 3 s. The stimulus is increased in intensity stepwise until perceptible pain (pain threshold) and eventually the greatest perceivable pain (ceiling or maximum pain) are induced. They used a pain scale that ranged from 1 pain unit ('dol'), assigned to pain threshold, to $10\frac{1}{2}$ dol, denoting maximum pain, which was produced by a stimulus of sufficient intensity to produce a third-degree burn. They studied 26 primiparae and six multiparae during the course of normal labor and delivery and found that the intensity of pain in the early part (latent phase) of the first stage was 2–3 dol (very mild), increasing progressively to 3–4 dol at about 4 cm cervical dilatation, 5–7 dol at 6–8 cm and 8–9 dol at full dilatation, and ranging from $9–10\frac{1}{2}$ dol (maximum pain) as the head of the baby dilated and stretched the perineum during the second stage of labor.

The incidence, intensity, quality and other aspects of labor pain have been elucidated more precisely by Melzack and associates,[64–67] who have carried out a series of studies using the McGill Pain Questionnaire (MPQ),[68] the most extensively tested multidimensional scale of pain measurements available. The MPQ consists of 20 sets of words describing the sensory, affective and evaluative dimension of the pain experience. The first 10 sets represent sensory quality, the next five are affective, 16 are evaluative and the last four are miscellaneous words (Fig. 3.6). Two major indices can be obtained from the questionnaire. First is a pain rating index (PRI), which is the sum of the rank values of the words chosen based on the position of the words in each category of subclass. The second is an index of present pain intensity (PPI), a measure of the overall pain intensity on a scale of 0–5 with 0 representing no pain, 1 mild, 2 discomforting, 3 distressing, 4 horrible and 5 excruciating pain.

In their first study[64] labor pain was measured with the MPQ in 87 primiparae and 54 multiparae, all of whom had cervical dilatation of at least 2–3 cm and contractions at intervals of 5 mins or less. Of the 141 parturients, 61 primiparae and 31 multiparae had received prepared childbirth training in specialized training units in hospitals or private clinics, while 26 primparae and 24 multiparae had received no training. Although the MPQ was completed between contractions, the patients were asked to measure the amount of pain they felt during contractions. They found that the mean total pain rating index (PRI) was 34 for primiparae and 30 for multiparae, thus confirming the widely held view that labor is significantly

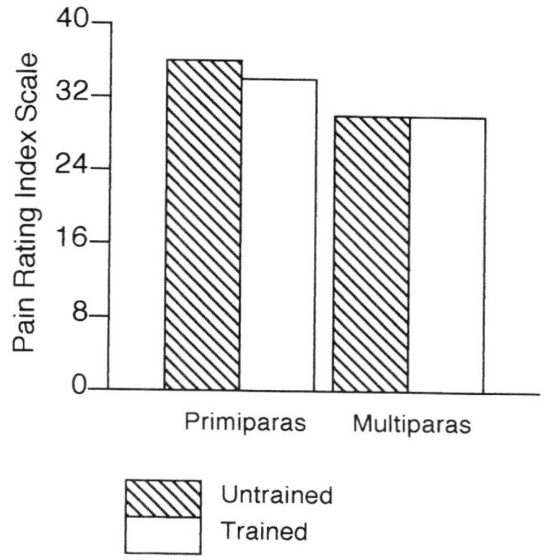

Fig. 3.7 The mean PRI scores of pain by untrained and trained primiparas (a) and multiparas (b). Untrained primiaras had a PRI score of 37, while the trained primiparas had a score of 33, but both untrained and trained multiparas had a similar score of 30. [Modified from (a) Melzack R 1984 The myth of painless childbirth (The John J. Bonica Lecture). Pain 19: 321, Fig. 4, p 327. (b) Melzack R et al 1981 Labour is still painful after prepared childbirth training. Can Med Assoc J 125: 357, Fig. 2.A, p 360.]

more painful for the first birth than for later births (Fig. 3.7). Significant differences were also found between primiparae and multiparae for each of the four classes of words describing their pain. The *sensory* qualities of the pain were described as sharp, cramping, aching, throbbing, stabbing, hot, shooting or heavy; the *affective* qualities were described as tiring by half and exhausting by more than a third. The *evaluative* word 'intense' was chosen by 52% and the *miscellaneous* word 'tight' by 44%. Subsequently, Melzack[69] compared the mean total PRI scores for several pain syndromes obtained in earlier studies[68,70] with those of labor and noted that the scores for labor pain were some 8–10 points higher than those associated with back pain, cancer pain, phantom limb pain or post-herpetic neuralgia and even greater than acute pain that occurs after accidents (Fig. 3.8).

As might be expected, although the average intensity of labor pain was extremely high, a wide range in pain scores was observed, which Melzack[69] divided into six groups within the range of the PRI scores recorded (ranging from 2 to 62) (Fig. 3.9). Assigning verbal descriptors of pain intensity to these data suggests that about 10% of primiparae and about 24% of multiparae experienced mild to moderate pain, about 30% of both groups rated their pain as severe, about 38% of primiparae and 35% of multiparae felt very severe pain, and 23% of primiparae and 11% of multiparae experienced horrible or excruciating pain. The mean PRI scores of 61 primiparae who received prepared childbirth training was 33 and, for the 26 primiparae who received no training, it was 37. On the other hand, no significant difference was noted in any of the PRI

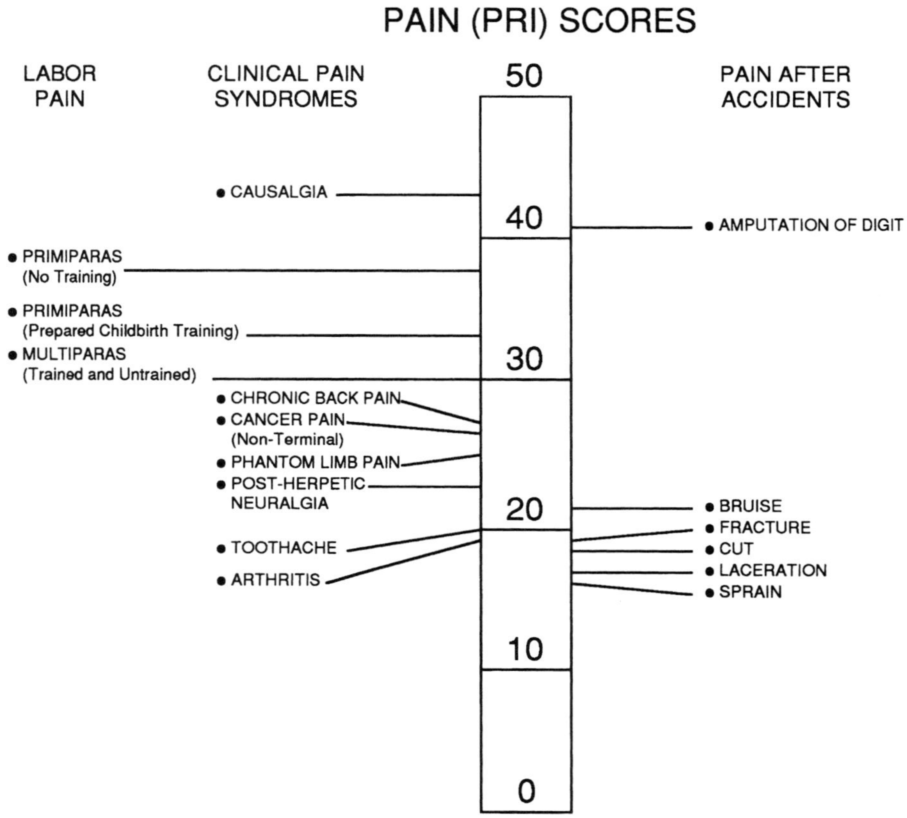

Fig. 3.8 Comparison of pain scores using the McGill Pain Questionnaire obtained from women during labor and from patients in general hospital clinics and an emergency department. The pain rating index (PRI) represents the sum of the rank values for all words chosen from 20 sets of pain descriptions. (From Melzack R 1984 The myth of painless childbirth (The John J. Bonica Lecture). Pain 19: 321, Fig. 2, p 325.)

measures of the 30 multiparae who had received training and 24 who received no training. Of the 28 parturients who were given successful epidural analgesia, the PRI score decreased from a mean of 28 before the block to a mean of 8 and 7.6 at 30 and 60 mins, respectively, after induction of analgesia. These scores were based on the use of such words as numbness, pressing and tingling.

In the second study[65] 79 parturients (42 primiparae and 37 multiparae) were given several successive questionnaires at hourly intervals until they entered the delivery room, or had an epidural block, or asked the experimenter to stop. Figure 3.10 shows the average pain curves for trained and untrained women. Although these curves indicate a gradual rising pain intensity, graphs of pain scores obtained from individual parturients revealed a high level of variability as labor progressed. Instead of the idealized rising curve usually seen in obstetric textbooks which reflects the group scores shown in Figure 3.8, they noted a remarkable variety of patterns. Some parturients showed the expected rising curve while others showed rises and falls in pain level. Some women had extremely high levels of pain early in labor, while others, up to the time of delivery, showed fairly low, constant pain scores.

In both studies Melzack and associates[64,65] noted that the high level of individual variability was also reflected in the spatial distribution of the pain. Some women had widespread pain of a large part of the abdomen and back, while others had discrete painful areas. Spatial variability prompted Melzack and Schaffelberg[67] to carry out another study involving 46 parturients (29 primiparae and 17 multiparae) to define more precisely the location of the pain during contractions and between contractions. All 46 women had abdominal pain and 44 (96%) rated the contraction pain as the worst. In contrast, 34 parturients (74% of the subjects) had low back pain with 19 having the pain only during contractions, while 15 (33% of the whole group) had continuous low back pain which was rated worse than the abdominal and back pain associated with contractions. The parturients found this type of pain as intense and difficult to bear and described it as 'unrelenting' and 'exhausting'. The mechanisms of back pain are discussed in the next section.

Gaston-Johansson et al[71] carried out a study similar to that of Melzack et al in 138 Swedish women (50 primiparae, 88 multiparae) using the Johansson Pain-O-Meter individual and visual analog scale (VAS) when the

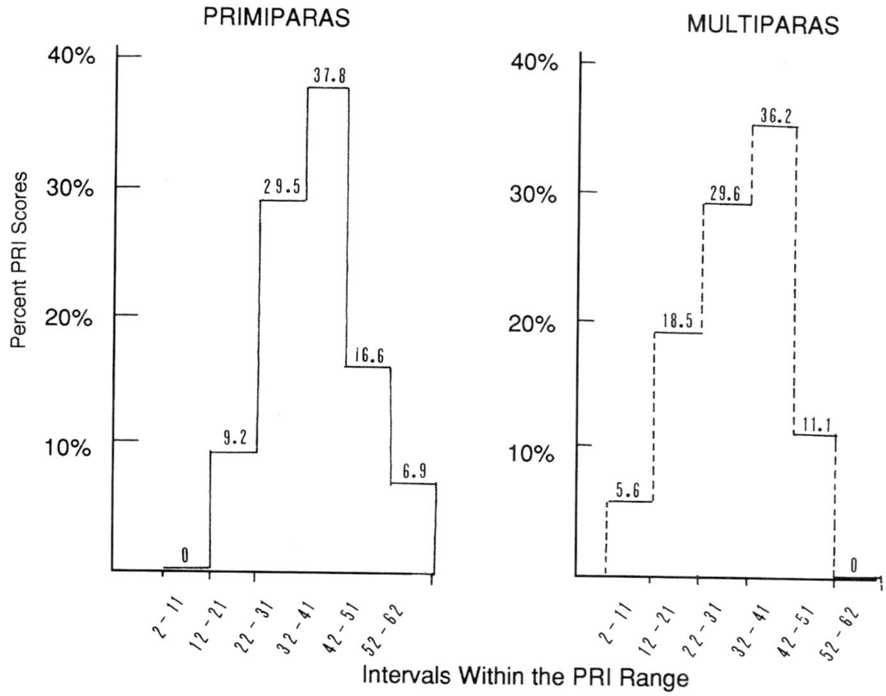

Fig. 3.9 Distribution of PRI scores for primiparas and multiparas in six intervals of the total PRI range. (From Melzack R 1984 The myths of painless childbirth (The John J. Bonica Lecture). Pain 19: 321, Fig. 3, p 326.)

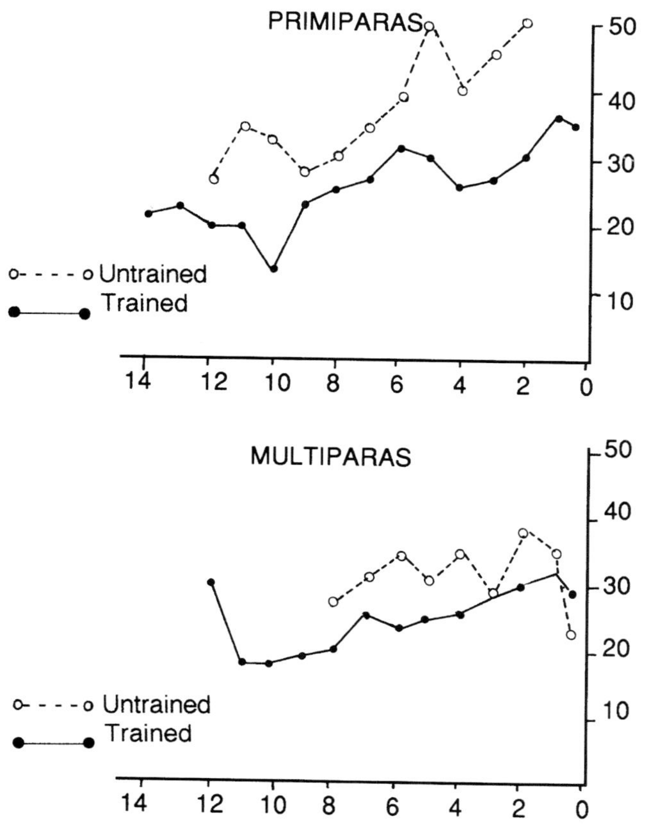

Fig. 3.10 Average pain rating index (PRI) scores reported by primiparas and multiparas at successive hours prior to delivery. Pain scores, shown separately for trained and untrained women, were assigned to the nearest hour for purposes of calculation. (From Melzack R 1984 The myths of painless childbirth (The John J. Bonica Lecture). Pain 19: 321, Fig. 5, p 328.)

cervix was dilated 2–4 cm (stage I), 5–7 cm (stage II) and 8–10 cm (stage III). The Pain-O-Meter is made of a hard plastic and is 8 inches long by 2 inches wide and 1 inch thick with one side having 11 affective and 12 sensory pain word descriptors and the other side having the VAS scale. Two major indices obtained from the sensory and affective components of pain are: (a) the number of words chosen (NWC); and (b) the pain rating index rank (PRIR), based on accumulation of numerical values assigned to the chosen words. Among the 138 women, 80% of the primiparae and 20% of the multiparae had received prepared childbirth training. Moreover, 72% of primiparae and 27% of multiparae received meperidine, epidural anesthesia was administered to 30 and 7% respectively, and nitrous oxide oxygen was administered to 70% and 57% respectively. The intensity scores for the sensory component of pain were 6.11 during stage I, while pain intensity scores for the affective component reached the highest peak during stage III of labor and delivery (4.23 in I, 4.32 in II and 5.60 in III). Primiparae reported more intense sensory pain in stages I (7.36) and III (7.24) and more intense affective pain in all three stages of labor than multiparae (5.80, 4.70, 7.80), even though they consumed significantly more pain medication than did the multiparae. It is of interest to note that subjects who had participated in prepared childbirth training reported a significantly higher in-labor pain scores during stage I and stage III than those who did not participate. The authors commented that prepared childbirth, while providing much information, may lead to unrealistic expectations about in-labor pain. In another study, Fridh and Gaston-Johansson[72] found that neither primiparae had realistic expectation of in-labor pain and experienced much more pain than they had anticipated. The findings reported in this study are in agreement with earlier reports by Javert and Hardy,[63] Cogan et al[73] and Scott-Palmer and Skevington.[74]

Mechanisms of the pain of parturition

To provide optimal pain relief with regional analgesia, it is essential for the obstetric team to understand the peripheral mechanisms and pathways of the pain of parturition and the factors that influence its intensity, duration and quality. Most of these factors vary during the different phases and stages of labor and are therapeutically significant, so they are considered separately.

Pain of the first stage of labor

During the first stage, labor pain initially is entirely in the uterus and its adnexa during contractions. Earlier, it was proposed that labor pain was caused by the following:

1. pressure on nerve endings between the muscle fibers of the body and fundus of the uterus;[75]
2. contraction of the ischemic myometrium and cervix consequent to expulsion of blood from the uterus during the contraction[76] or as a result of vasoconstriction consequent to sympathetic hyperactivity;[52]
3. inflammatory changes of uterine muscles;[75]
4. contraction of the cervix and lower uterine segment consequent to fear-induced hyperactivity of the sympathetic nervous system;[52] and
5. dilatation of the cervix and lower uterine segment.[76]

Most data support the concept that the pain of the first stage of labor is predominantly a result of dilatation of the cervix (CX) and lower uterine segment (LUS) and of the consequent distension, stretching and tearing of these structures during contractions. Contractions of the uterus under isometric conditions – that is, against the obstruction presented by the cervix and perineum – also probably contribute to the pain of uterine contractions.

These hypotheses are based on the following considerations:

1. Stretching of smooth muscle of a hollow viscus is an adequate stimulus for visceral pain.[77]
2. The degree of CX and LUS dilation is correlated with the rapidity with which it occurs on the one hand and with the intensity of the pain on the other.[1]
3. The time of onset of uterine contractions is related to the time of onset of the pain. This lag, which is longest in the early stages of labor and lessens as labor progresses, occurs because uterine contractions need time to increase the amniotic fluid pressure to 15 mmHg above tonus (Fig. 3.11). This has been determined to be the minimum pressure required to initiate dilatation of the CX and LUS.[78]

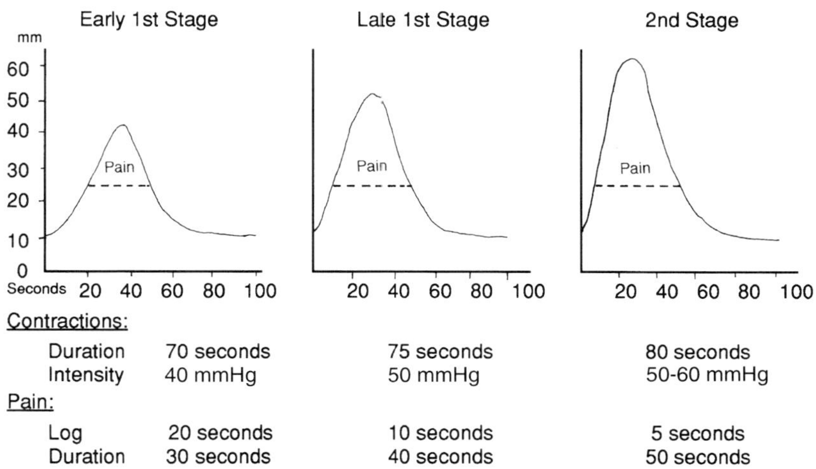

Fig. 3.11 Relation between duration of uterine contraction and duration of pain associated with the contraction. Since intensity of contraction must reach 25 mmHg before pain is provoked, there is a lag of 20 s during early phase of first stage when the build-up of the contraction is slower. As labor progresses the contraction reaches its peak more rapidly and the lag is shortened. (From Bonica J J 1967 Principles and practice of obstetric analgesia and anesthesia. F A Davis, Philadelphia, Fig. 5–5, p 104.)

4. In the parturient undergoing cesarean delivery with abdominal field block, the exposed but unanesthetized uterus can be incised and gently palpated without discomfort to the conscious parturient,[63,76] while forceful palpation and stretching of the CX and LUS produce pain similar in quality and location to that experienced during labor.[78]

5. When the cervix is suddenly and widely dilated in parturients or in gynecologic patients, they feel pain similar in quality, distribution and intensity to that experienced during uterine contractions.[63,76,79]

The evidence that contractions of the body of the uterus contribute to the pain of labor is somewhat puzzling. Braxton–Hicks contractions of prelabor are frequently painless, even though they can attain the intensity of labor contractions, and this detracts from this hypothesis. Moreover, during the immediate post-partum period, the intensity of uterine contractions of the empty uterus might be two to three times higher than the contractions of active labor but post-partum uterine contractions are associated either with much less intense pain or with no pain at all. On the other hand, strong contractions are associated with severe pain in most parturients with mechanical distortion caused by abnormal fetal positions and in those in whom the cervix dilates slowly. Because in such situations the uterine muscle is contracting under isometric conditions (i.e. its exit, the cervix and perineum, present an obstruction), the strong contractions are probably also a source of pain.

The validity of various other hypotheses is also disputed. The suggestion that pain is a result of ischemia during uterine contractions is disputed by monkey studies that showed that, although placental (intervillous) perfusion decreased to nearly 50% of control values, myometrial blood flow increased significantly during contractions[80] and increased to an even greater degree during a sustained (8-min) contraction.[81] Moreover, no evidence of an inflammatory process in the uterine muscles has been found.[1,3] Dick-Read's[52] hypothesis that contraction of the cervix brought about by fear-induced hyperactivity of the sympathetic nervous system as the cause of pain is unwarranted in view of the fact that the cervix is composed mostly of connective tissue, with little muscle and elastic tissue.[82] Moreover, during uncomplicated childbirth, the LUS and CX manifest only a small contractile force, which becomes even weaker as labor progresses.[78]

Second and third stages of labor

Once the cervix is fully dilated, the amount of nociceptive stimulation arising in this structure decreases, but the contractions of the body of the uterus and distension of the lower uterine segment continue to cause pain in the same areas of reference as in the first stage of labor. In addition, the progressively greater pressure of the presenting part on pain-sensitive structures in the pelvis and distension of the outlet and perineum become new sources of pain. Progressively greater distension causes intense stretching and actual tearing of fascia and subcutaneous tissues and pressure on the skeletal muscles of the perineum.

Other factors that influence the pain of childbirth

In addition to the role played by such intrinsic factors as the intensity, duration and pattern of contractions and related physiologic and biochemical mechanisms, the amount or degree of pain and suffering associated with childbirth is influenced by physical, physiologic, psychologic, emotional and motivational factors.[60–62,64–66,74,83–87] Although different investigators found differences in the role played by each of the various factors mentioned below, there is consensus that many of these play an important role in determining the incidence, intensity and quality of pain in the general parturient population.

Physical factors

Physical factors that influence the incidence, severity and duration of the pain of childbirth include the age, parity and physical condition of the parturient, the condition of the cervix at the onset of labor and the relationship of the size of the infant to the size of the birth canal. Many of these factors are interrelated. Generally, an uninformed unmarried teenage gravida may experience more anxiety-induced pain. Moreover, older (>40 years) primiparae experience a longer, more painful labor than young primiparae. The cervix of the multipara begins to soften even before the onset of labor and is less sensitive than that of the primipara. In general, the intensity of uterine contractions in early labor tends to be higher in primiparae than in multiparae, whereas in the later phase of labor the reverse is true.[64–66,71]

In the presence of dystocia caused by a contracted pelvis, a large baby or abnormal presentation, the parturient experiences more pain than under normal conditions. Melzack et al[65] found that the heavier the primipara per unit of height, the higher the pain scores. The same variable contributed to the pain scores of multiparae and, in addition, heavier mothers and those with heavier babies had higher pain scores. There are also a number of reports cited by Kohenen[86] that women who labor and deliver in the vertical position (sitting, standing or squatting), experience less pain and have a shorter second stage of labor. However, in a recent study by Melzack and Belanger (personal communication, 1990) in which they used part of the McGill Pain Questionnaire and visual analog scale to measure pain intensity, they found that in the latent and early first stage of labor parturients had less pain in the vertical position, but in the late stage and second stage they experienced less pain in the lateral supine position. This confirms results reported by others.

Melzack and associates[64,66] found that high pain scores were associated with menstrual difficulties. They also noted that menstrual pain felt in the back, but not in the front, was correlated with increasing levels of pain in the abdomen and back during contractions and with continuous low back pain previously mentioned. Similar relationships between menstrual pain and higher pain scores were reported by Fridh and Gaston-Johansson,[72] who noted that primiparae had more pain in late first stage, whereas multiparae had more pain in the early first stage. Marx[87] has presented strong evidence that women who have dysmenorrhea produce excessive amounts of prostaglandins which trigger uterine contractions and that drugs that inhibit prostaglandin synthesis also diminish menstrual pain. Melzack[69] has suggested that because of the positive correlation between menstrual pain and the pain during childbirth, it is conceivable that parturients who suffer severe labor pain may also produce excessive prostaglandins during labor.

Fatigue, loss of sleep and general debility influence a parturient's tolerance of the painful experience and increase the pain behavior. This is particularly significant in parturients with prolonged labor.

Physiologic and biochemical factors

A number of studies have demonstrated a progressive increase in plasma beta-endorphin, beta-lipotropin and ACTH levels, all of which are derived from a common precursor.[88–93] These values have been found to peak at delivery or in the immediate post-partum period at 4–10 times the prelabor and nonpregnant values. These findings have led to the speculation that plasma beta-endorphin might have an intrinsic analgesic role during parturition.[93] The fact that plasma beta-endorphin levels that are considerably higher than those observed in these studies do not appear to cross the blood–brain barrier or have analgesic effects on nonpregnant humans[94] has questioned the efficacy of beta-endorphin as an analgesic during parturition.

On the other hand, other opioid systems may play a role in increasing the pain tolerance threshold. This suggestion is based on the findings of Gintzler,[95] who in 1980 noted in rats that pain threshold rises at the end of pregnancy, peaks around delivery and returns to normal nonpregnant levels within 12 h of delivery. This 'pregnancy-induced analgesia' or more properly 'hypalgesia' is blocked by the opioid antagonists naloxone and naltrexone. This phenomenon has been observed using several noxious modalities including response threshold to electric foot shock and tail withdrawal latencies.[96,97] Similar increases in pain threshold have been noted in studies involving humans during late pregnancy in which responses to radiant heat to dermatomes C1 or S1 or intense pressure applied to the forearm were used as aversive (noxious) stimuli[98,99] Gintzler et al[97] have identified the pregnancy-induced hypalgesia as resulting from the action of spinal dynorphin/kappa opioid receptor systems. These data suggest that in parturients who experience low levels of pain the activation of this system may be sufficient to lower the intensity and perhaps modify the quality of the pain of parturition.

Related to this issue are the recent studies carried out by Kristal and associates,[100–103] which show that ingestion of amniotic fluid or the placenta by rats enhanced several types of opioid-mediated analgesia: that induced by morphine, by foot shock, by vaginal/cervical stimulation and that of late pregnancy, but not analgesia produced by aspirin injection. In the absence of opioid-mediated analgesia, however, ingestion of placenta and amniotic fluid does not produce the enhancing effects. Opioid antagonists such as naloxone and naltrexone not only block the opioid-mediated analgesia, but also render placental ingestion and amniotic fluid ingestion ineffective. Kristal and associates[101–103] have named the active substance in placenta and amniotic fluid, placental opioid-enhancing factor or POEF. They have also shown that POEF enhances the central effects of opioid analgesia but not its peripheral effects, perhaps by stimulating 'off-cells' in the periaqueductal gray.

Because most nonaquatic, nonhuman mammalian mothers engage in ingestion of the afterbirth (termed *placentophagia*) or at least lick amniotic fluid from themselves or the newborn infant, and in view of the measurable increase in pain threshold produced by elevated endogenous opioids present prior to delivery, Kristal and associates[103] have explored the possibility in rats that a significant benefit of parturitional placentophagia is an enhancement of the pregnancy-mediated analgesia during labor and delivery. Their studies have revealed that 1 ml of placenta or 0.25 ml of amniotic fluid, which is the amount available during the delivery of one rat pup, is the optimum dose for enhancement of morphine-induced analgesia. Moreover, the enhancement produced by 0.25 ml of amniotic fluid by orogastric tube is detectable within 5 min and lasts for about 30 min, the approximate duration of the interpup interval during delivery. Since amniotic fluid is available to the mother before the emergence of the first neonate and the placenta is not available until after delivery of each pup, amniotic fluid is probably the more important substance in enhancement of pregnancy-mediated analgesia.

The importance of these findings is twofold. First it demonstrates that nonaquatic, nonhuman mammalian mothers have two factors which tend to diminish nociception and pain behavior: pregnancy-induced hypalgesia and the hypalgesic effect of amniotic fluid and placenta. Secondly, it may be possible to isolate the active substance in human placenta and on the basis of the findings to develop new and different analgesic agents.

Psychologic factors

Psychologic factors that can and frequently do affect the incidence and intensity of parturition pain include the mentation, attitude and mood of the parturient at the time of labor, and other emotional factors. Fear, apprehension and anxiety probably enhance pain perception and pain behavior.[85,104–108] One of the most frequent causes of fear and anxiety is ignorance of or misinformation about the process of pregnancy and parturition, and what the onset of labor signifies. An uninformed parturient, especially a primipara, can be disturbed by fear of the unknown, death, suffering, mutilation, possible complications and concern for her condition or that of her fetus.[71,85,107] Parturients who have had an unplanned or illegitimate pregnancy or have an ambivalent or negative reaction to gestation report more pain than those who do not.[62,77]

The relationship between the parturient and her spouse plays an important role in the degree of pain she experiences. Melzack[69] reported that the affective pain scores were higher when the husband was in the labor room than when he was absent. He suggested that this may reflect genuinely higher affective pain scores or may be due to a deliberate choice of descriptors in the attempt to impress the husband or express anger at him, but in any case the finding was not spurious. Wallach[108] found a similar effect in an independent study. In contrast, Nettelbladt et al[62], Norr et al[84] and Fridh et al[85] found that positive feelings of the expectant father toward the pregnancy seemed to be an important factor in decreasing the mother's feelings of apprehension during pregnancy. When fathers were more supportive of their mates during pregnancy and labor, women experienced less pain during parturition. Fridh et al[85] emphasized the need to include supportive fathers in prenatal training.

In contrast, other emotional factors such as intensive motivation and cultural influences can affect modulation of sensory transmissions and certainly can influence the affective and behavioral dimensions of pain. Moreover, cognitive intervention such as giving the parturient preparatory information about labor, thus reducing uncertainty while focusing attention or producing distraction and dissociation from pain (all parts of an 'educated' childbirth program) reduces pain behavior. In a study of 134 low-risk parturients at term, Lowe[109] found that confidence in ability to handle labor was the most significant predictor of all components of pain during active labor. The greater the confidence the parturient had, the lesser the pain and vice versa.

Cultural and ethnic factors

Racial, cultural and ethnic factors have long been considered to be important in influencing pain tolerance and pain behavior. Persons of Italian and other Latin cultures or of Jewish of Mediterranean background are said to express pain in an emotive fashion and to exaggerate their verbal report, whereas those of Anglo-Saxon origin (e.g. English, third-generation Americans, Irish), as well as Scandinavians, Asians, American Indians and Eskimos, are said to be more stoic and to manifest less pain behavior.[110] Experimental data and clinical observations, however, suggest that, although racial, cultural and ethnic differences do exist, they appear to be differences in expressiveness consequent to underlying attitudes toward the pain rather than differences in the sensory experience or pain perception.

True[111] reported that Mohave Indian women experienced a great deal of pain during childbirth but avoided expressing their suffering for fear of ridicule. In an experimental study, Meehan et al[112] found no significant differences between pain tolerance of American Indians, Eskimos and Whites. In a study of Turkomenian women, Preissman and Ogoulbostan-Essenova[113] noted that they behaved calmly during childbirth and manifested no pain behavior, but inquiry revealed that the process was very painful. Nettelbladt et al,[62] in a study of 78 women, noted that 56% of parturients who reported intolerable pain were not rated by the midwives as having very painful deliveries. This discrepancy probably occurred because the parturients manifested less overt pain behavior than they actually felt, which is a characteristic of Scandinavian culture. Winsberg and Greenlick[114] examined pain behavior in Black and White parturients who were matched on such parameters as age, social class and education and found no differences in pain responses or estimated degrees of pain.

The thesis that cultural and racial differences can have some influence on pain behavior but probably not on the pain felt by parturients is supported by my own studies (unpublished data) of 2700 parturients in other countries and of 8000 parturients in the USA (see above: Incidence and intensity of labor pain). In Western and Eastern Europe, Latin America, Africa, Asia–Australia, the Near East and North America parturients who were not 'educated' and who were psychologically unprepared for childbirth manifested a similar incidence of pain behavior, although the patterns of behavior varied. During the contractions some women moaned, others screamed, others writhed and had facial expression of suffering with little or no verbal expression, while still others used incantations (said to be specific for labor pain in that particular country). Contrary to traditional belief, Asian women (including Japanese, Chinese, Malaysians, Indians, Cambodians and Thais) did not remain stoic but manifested as much pain behavior as American and European parturients. Moreover, the large Oriental population of Seattle and the recent influx of refugees from Indochina afforded the opportunity to observe and interview several hundred parturients from various countries in South-East Asia. These studies revealed that the frequency and intensity of labor pain and the request for analgesia was the same as for Occidental parturients living in Asia, and the pain behavior was similar to that observed among parturients in their native countries (J Bonica, unpublished data).

The influence of education and psychologic conditioning inherent in psychoprophylaxis and natural childbirth in modifying pain behavior without significantly affecting pain sensation is now widely appreciated. During 5- to 10-day visits to obstetric centers that practice psychoprophylaxis or natural childbirth in the Soviet Union, France, Germany, Italy, The Netherlands, Sweden and the USA, made over a 5-month period in 1959, Bonica observed about 700 parturients (and interviewed many) who had received training in one of these methods, and over 85% of them manifested little or no pain behavior during labor and delivery. When questioned the next day, however, most of them indicated that the process had been painful but many quickly added that they were pleased to cooperate with their instructor and obstetric team. Especially impressive was the marked change in behavior of Italian parturients in a large obstetric center in Turin noted during two visits made 5 years apart. During the first visit, in 1954, the labor ward was a scene of cacophony caused by the screaming, pleading and praying of the nearly 50 laboring women in the same ward. In contrast, 5 years later, one heard only an occasional moan from a similar number of parturients who had undergone an intensive course of psychoprophylaxis. Most went through the entire labor and delivery with minimal pain behavior but later stated that they had had moderate to severe pain.

Summary

It is obvious that the pain-associated responses to noxious stimulation provoked by uterine contractions and other tissue-damaging factors during labor and vaginal delivery are the net effects of highly complex interactions of various neural systems, modulating influences and psychologic and cultural factors. Through the interaction of the afferent system and neocortical processes, the parturient receives perceptual and discriminate information that is analyzed and that usually activates motivational cognitive processes. These, in turn, act on motor system and initiate psychodynamic mechanisms of anxiety and apprehension that produce the complex physiologic, behavioral and affective responses that characterize acute pain.

Neural pathways of parturitional pain

Although the extrinsic nerve supply to the uterus was well described during the seventeenth and eighteenth centuries, it was not until 1893 that Henry Head[115] published the first description of the specific nociceptive pathways of the uterus and cervix. Based on his studies of the segments of hyperalgesia associated with various uterine disorders, as well as of hyperalgesia during the second stage of labor, Head[115] concluded that the sensory nerve supply of the uterus always involved the T11, often the T12, and not infrequently the T10 and L1 and sometimes L2 segments, and that the cervix was supplied by the S2, S3 and S4. During the ensuing four decades, much confusing and conflicting evidence and difference of opinion existed in textbooks concerning this issue. It remained for John Cleland[116] to clarify the issue by extensive animal experiments and studies on parturients. Cleland used the visceromotor reflex to determine the critical sensory pathways from the uterus and subsequently carried out paravertebral somatic nerve block in parturients to eliminate the pain of the first stage of labor. Based on these studies, Cleland concluded that in humans the sensory supply of the uterus is through the T11 and T12 spinal segments and that pain caused by stretch of the birth canal was transmitted through 'undetermined sacral segments'. This finding was interpreted to mean that the cervix and vagina are supplied by the sacral segments. As a result of these two studies it became widely taught that nociceptive impulses from the body of the uterus are transmitted through the T11 and T12 nerves, and that pain from the LUS and CX is transmitted through the pelvic nerves to the S2, S3 and S4 spinal segments.

Because my clinical observations were at variance with this concept, in collaboration with my colleagues Akamatsu, Kohl and others, I carried out a study that involved 240 parturients and 35 gynecologic patients investigated over a period of 22 years.[117] The study entailed the use of discrete blocks of various nociceptive pathways by paravertebral block, segmental epidural block, caudal block and trans-sacral block of various segments. Their results demonstrated conclusively that the upper part of the CX and the LUS are *not* supplied by sensory fibers that accompany the pelvic nerves (nervi erigentes), as stated in almost every modern anatomy and obstetric textbook. Rather, these structures are supplied by afferents that, like those that supply the body of the uterus, accompany the sympathetic nerves in the following sequence: the uterine and cervical plexus; the pelvic (inferior hypogastric) plexus; the middle hypogastric plexus or nerve; and the superior hypogastric and aortic plexuses. The nociceptive afferents then pass to the lumbar sympathetic chain and course cephalad through the lower thoracic sympathetic chain, which they leave by way of the rami communicantes associated with the T10,

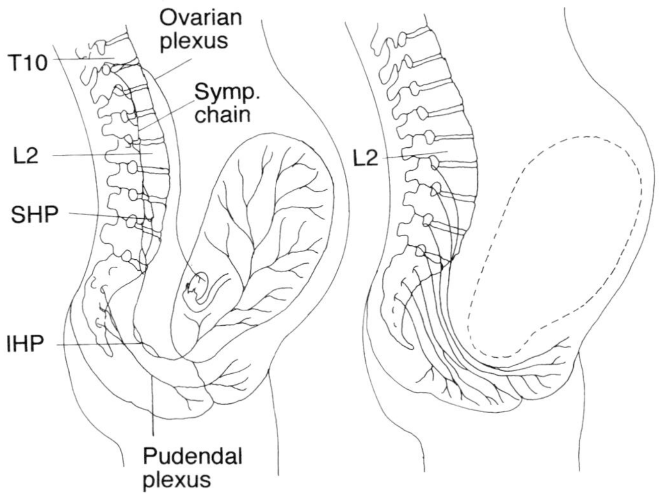

Fig. 3.12 Schematic depiction of the peripheral nociceptive pathways involved in the pain of childbirth. (a) The uterus, including the cervix and lower uterine segments, is supplied by afferents that pass from the uterus to the spinal cord by accompanying sympathetic nerves through the inferior hypogastric plexus (IHP), the hypogastric nerve, the superior hypogastric plexus (SHP), the lumbar and lower thoracic sympathetic chain and the nerves at T10, T11, T12 and L1. (b) The nerves involved in transmission of nociceptive impulses are provoked by noxious stimulation of pelvic structures. See text for details. (From Bonica J J 1990 The management of pain, 2nd edn. Lea & Febiger, Philadelphia, Fig. 66–22, p 1327.)

T11, T12 and L1 spinal nerves. Finally they pass through the posterior roots of these nerves to make synaptic contact with interneurons in the dorsal horn (Figs 3.12 and 3.13).

These findings have been recently confirmed in animal experiments carried out by a number of investigators.[118–122] Berkeley and associates[118–120] have carried out a series of systematic comprehensive experiments using in vitro and in vivo electrophysiologic studies and behavioral studies of the nerve supply of the uterus and other pelvic organs. These investigators used mechanical and chemical stimuli of the uterine cavity including the cervix and vagina. The results can be summarized as follows:

1. Afferent fibers in the hypogastric nerve have receptive fields confined to the uterus and cervix with most fibers located in the lower portion of the cervix and they respond primarily to noxious stimuli. Effective mechanical stimuli include steady pressure, stretching, squeezing and probing in intensities greater than 5 g, which produced transient ischemia around the probe.[118–119] Using in vitro preparations the fibers responded to injection into the uterine artery of high doses of algesic substances such as bradykinin, 5-hydroxytryptamine and potassium chloride, and they also responded to high doses of carbon dioxide in saline and sodium cyanide (NaCN) but rarely to lower doses. Afferent fibers in the hypogastric nerve also responded to uterine contractions.

2. Afferent fibers in the pelvic nerve (nervi erigentes) have receptive fields located mostly in the upper part of the vaginal canal near, but not including, the cervix. Effective stimuli that activated these fibers were much less intense, rarely producing ischemia, and these fibers responded to much lower doses of algesic substances.

3. Gentle distension of the vaginal canal of anesthetized rats showed response of sensory fibers in the pelvic nerve and the responses increased as distension increased into the noxious range. Berkeley and Wood[119] also examined the relation between this neural response and sensation caused by vaginal distension in rats that had previously been trained to perform an operant escape response to terminate noxious somatic stimulus (tail pinch). At gentle levels of distension rats oriented towards the stimulus, but failed to make the escape responses, but as the levels of stimulation were gradually increased into the noxious range the probability of the rats making an escape response gradually increased to 100%. Although this would suggest that both pain and nonpainful stimulation arising from mechanical stimulation of the vaginal canal are subserved at least in part by activity in afferent fibers of pelvic nerve, this apparently is not the case because bilateral pelvic neurectomies had no significant effect on the animal's response to noxious stimulation of the vagina.[119,120]

The above findings led Berkeley and associates[118–120] to conclude that afferent fibers in the hypogastric nerves are concerned with the transmission of nociceptive information. In contrast, the uterine pelvic nerve afferent fibers are capable of conveying information regarding more physiologic innocuous events that are likely to subserve a wide range of reproductive functions. These afferent fibers differ considerably from, but must somehow be coordinated with, those of the hypogastric nerve fibers during the lifetime course of reproductive events.

Patterns of pain of parturition

Typical of pain arising from viscera, the pain of the first stage of labor is referred to the dermatomes supplied by the same spinal cord segments that receive nociceptive input from the uterus and cervix. During the latent (very early) phase of the first stage the pain is felt as an ache or moderate cramp and is limited to the T11 and T12 dermatomes (Fig. 3.14A). As labor progresses to the active phase of the first stage (usually 3–4 cm cervical dilation) and the uterine contractions become more intense, the pain in the T11 and T12 dermatomes becomes more severe, is described as sharp and cramping, and spreads to the two adjacent (T10 and L1) dermatomes (Fig. 3.14B).

The distribution of the T10, T11, T12 and L1 dermatomes in the back overlies the lower three lumbar vertebrae and the upper half of the sacrum. This distribution of pain during the first stage of labor has been misinterpreted by some as being transmitted by the lower

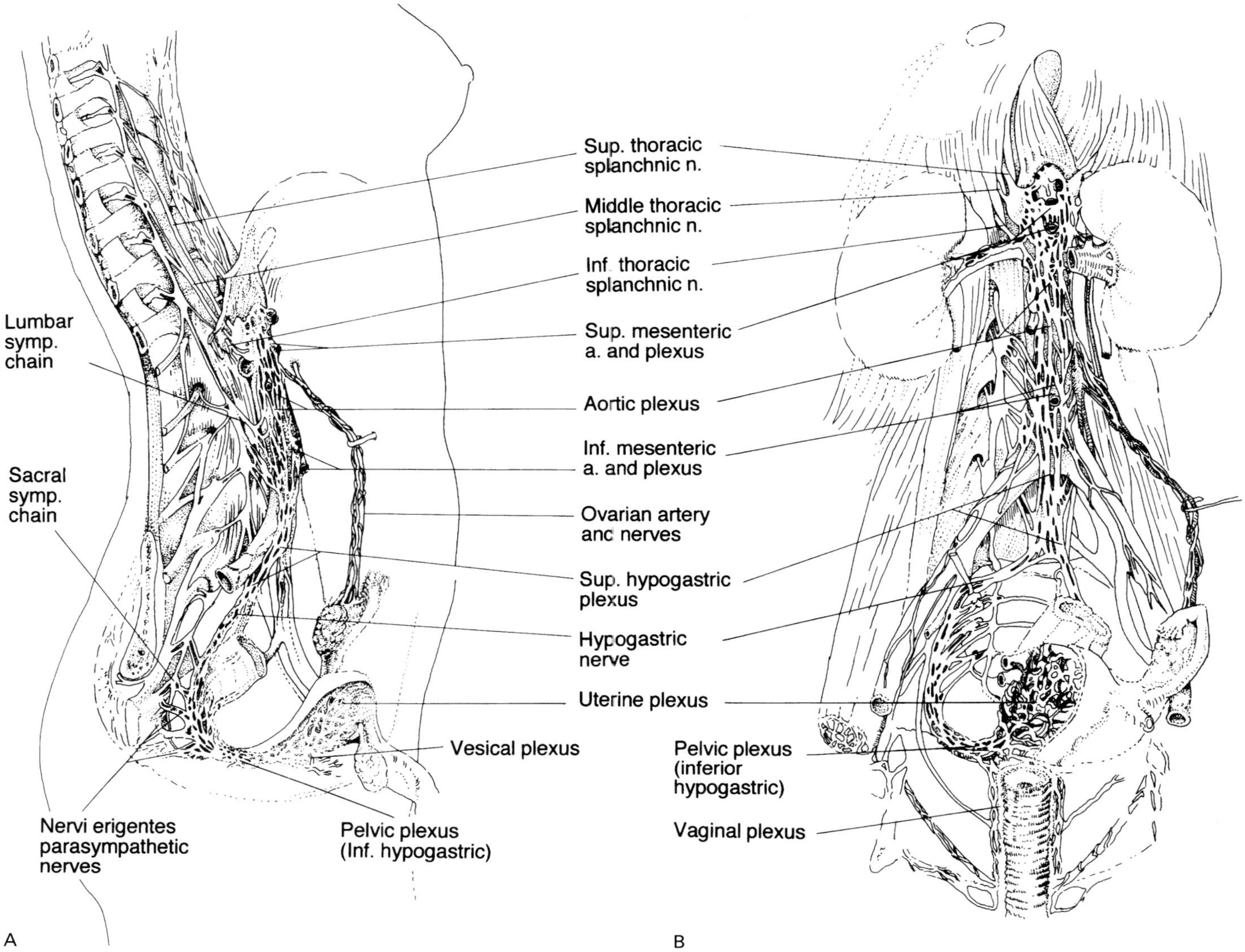

Fig. 3.13 Gross anatomy of the nerve supply to the uterus. (A) Lateral view. (B) Anterior view. The uterus is shown in the nonpregnant state to permit the various nerves that supply it to be depicted. Note that the uterine and cervical plexuses are derived from the pelvic plexus, which contains parasympathetic and sympathetic efferents. The parasympathetic efferents have their cell bodies in the middle three sacral segments, and the parasympathetic afferents pass through these segments and progress cephalad through the neuraxis. The sympathetic efferents and afferents pass through the hypogastric nerve, which in turn is a continuation of the superior hypogastric and aortic plexuses. Note that fibers from the last two plexuses pass on to the lumbar sympathetic chain, the afferents of which mediate nociceptive impulses and accompany the sympathetic fibers through these structures. From the lumbar and lower thoracic sympathetic chain the nociceptive afferents pass to the T10, T11, T12 and L1 spinal nerves and reach the spinal cord via their posterior roots and rootlets. (Modified from Bonica J J 1967 Principles and practice of obstetric analgesia and anesthesia. F A Davis, Philadelphia, pp 110–111.)

lumbar and sacral spinal segments. Proof that the low back pain is the result of nociceptive transmission in the T10–L1 segments is derived from the fact that epidural block limited to these four segments produces relief of the low back pain until descent of the presenting part causes pressure on the pelvic structures that are supplied by lower lumbar and the sacral segments (see below). As previously mentioned, often the pain is not referred to the entire dermatome, but can be more severe in one or more patches of varying size within a territory of one or more dermatomes. However, one can demonstrate hyperalgesia in the entire extent of the involved dermatomes.

In the late first stage and second stages of labor the pain is felt most sharply in the perineum, in the lower part of the sacrum, anus and frequently in the thighs (Fig. 3.14B and C). Like other pain caused by stimulation of superficial somatic structures, the perineal pain is sharp and well localized, predominantly in the region supplied by the pudendal nerves, and can be eliminated by block of these nerves. Moreover, in the late part of the first stage and during the second stage a number of parturients develop aching, burning or cramping discomfort in the thigh and less frequently in the legs (Fig. 3.14C and D). This is presumably a result of stimulation of pain-sensitive structures in the pelvic cavity, including the following: (a) traction on the pelvic parietal peritoneum and on the structures it envelops, including the uterine ligaments; (b) stretching and tension of the bladder, urethra and rectum; (c) stretching and tension of ligaments, fascia and muscles in the pelvic cavity; and (d) undue pressure on one or more roots of the lumbosacral plexus. These factors usually produce mild pain referred to the lower lumbar and sacral segments; (Fig. 3.12A) but, if the fetus is in an abnormal position, with undue pressure by the presenting part, the referred pain can become moderate or severe (Fig. 3.14C and D).

The transmission of the nociceptive information that arises from these various structures to the dorsal horn and then to other parts of the spinal cord and to the ascending systems to the brain is presumably similar to that of other

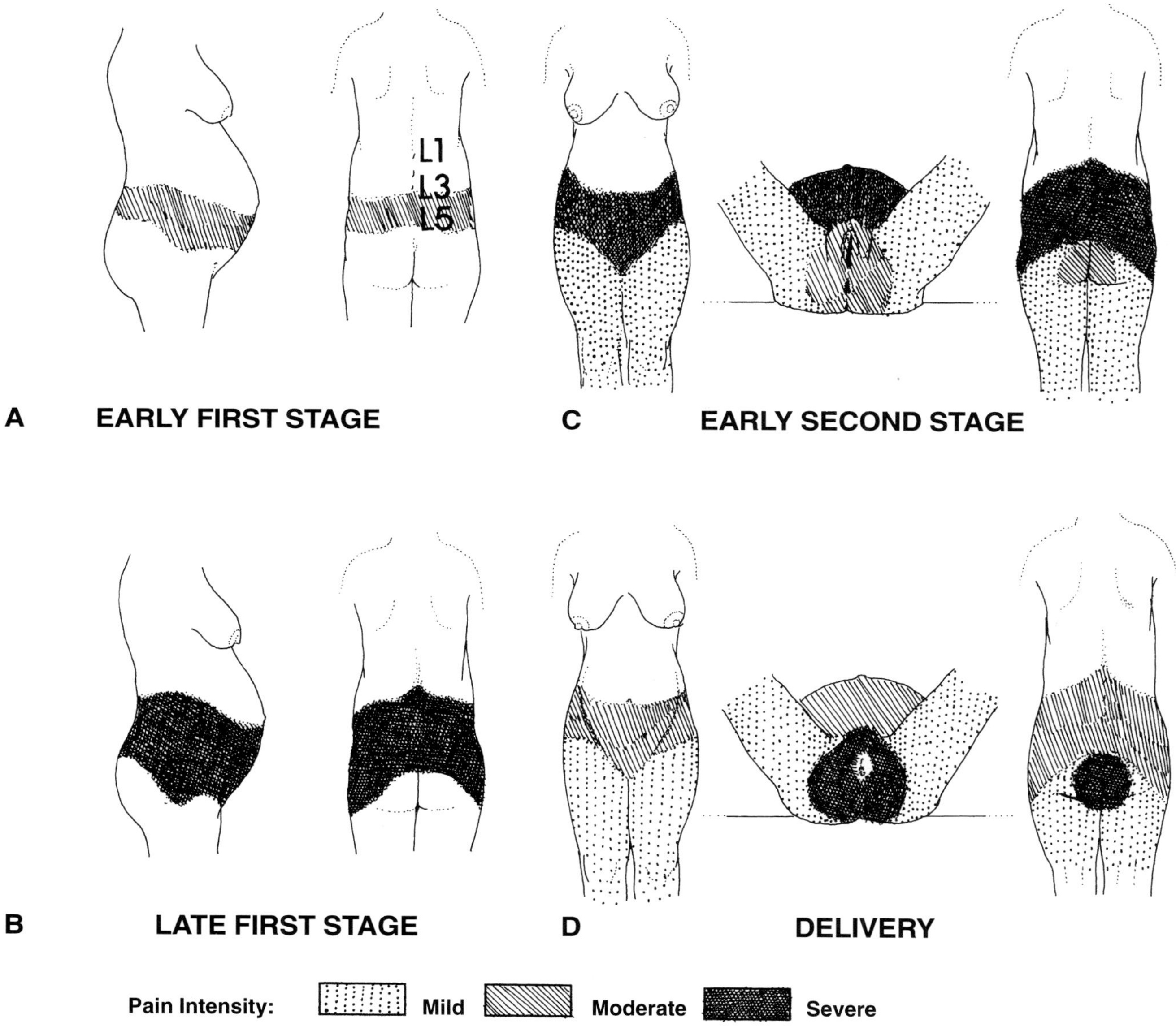

Fig. 3.14 The intensity and distribution of parturition pain during the various phases of labor and delivery. (A) In the early first stage the pain is referred to the T11 and T12 dermatomes. (B) In the late first stage, however, the severe pain is also referred to the T10 and L1 dermatomes. (C) In the early second stage uterine contractions remain intense and produce severe pain in the T10 to L1 dermatomes. At the same time the presenting part exerts pressure on pelvic structures and thus causes moderate pain in the very low back and perineum and often produces mild pain in the thighs and legs. (D) Intensity and distribution of pain during the later phase of the second stage and during actual delivery. The perineal component is the primary cause of pain whereas uterine contractions produce moderate pain. (From Bonica J J 1980 Obstetric analgesia and anesthesia, 2nd edn. University of Washington Press, Seattle, pp 46–47.)

types of acute pain. Since this was discussed in the first section of this chapter, nothing more will be said except to re-emphasize that the tissue damage in the cervix and perineum causes the responses to injury mentioned in the section on pathophysiology of the pain of parturition.

EFFECTS OF PARTURITIONAL PAIN AND THEIR MODIFICATION WITH ANALGESIA

This last section is devoted to discussion of the effects of parturitional pain on the mother, fetus and newborn and how these can be modified and in many instances, completely eliminated. In addition, I will stress the effects of labor pain on uterine contraction and on the fetus and newborn.

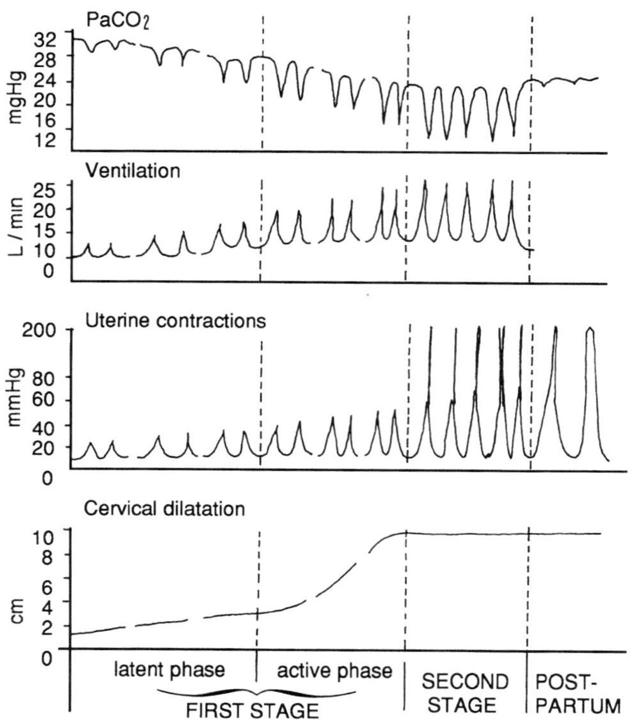

Fig. 3.15 Schematic representations of ventilatory changes during labor in an unpremedicated gravida. Note the correlation of the stages of labor as reflected by the Friedman's curve (bottom tracing), the frequency and intensity of uterine contractions, minute ventilation and arterial carbon dioxide tension (top tracing). Early in labor uterine contractions are slight and are associated with mild pain, causing only small increases in minute ventilation and decreases in the $Pa\text{CO}_2$. As labor progresses, however, the greater intensity of contractions causes greater changes in ventilation and $Pa\text{CO}_2$. During the active phase, contractions with an increased intrauterine pressure of 40–60 mmHg cause severe pain, which acts as an intense stimulus to ventilation with a consequent reduction of the $Pa\text{CO}_2$ to 18–22 mmHg. During the second stage the reflex bearing-down efforts further increase intrauterine pressure and distend the perineum, producing consequent additional pain that prompts the parturient to ventilate at a rate almost twice that of early labor and causing a commensurate reduction in the $Pa\text{CO}_2$. (Modified from Bonica J J 1973 Maternal respiratory changes during pregnancy and parturition. In Marx G F (ed) Parturition and Perinatology. Clinical Anesthesia Series, Vol 10, No 2, F A Davis, Philadelphia.)

Effects of childbirth pain

Changes in ventilation

In Chapter 5 the remarkable changes in ventilation are described in detail. Because the pain of childbirth is a powerful respiratory stimulus, it causes marked increases in tidal volume and minute ventilation and even greater increases in alveolar ventilation, causing a fall of $Pa\text{CO}_2$ from a normal pregnant level of 32 mmHg (4.27 kPa) to a value of 16–20 mmHg (2.13–2.67 kPa), with some as low as 10–15 mmHg (1.33–2.00 kPa), and a concomitant increase in pH to 7.55–7.60 (Fig. 3.15). With the onset of the relaxation phase, pain no longer stimulates respiration, so that hypocapnia causes a transient period of hypoventilation that decreases the maternal $Pa\text{O}_2$ by 10–50%, with a mean of 25–30%. In parturients who received an opioid the depressant effects of the respiratory alkalosis are enhanced by the action of the opioid. When the maternal $Pa\text{O}_2$ falls below 70 mmHg (9.33 kPa) it has a significant effect on the fetus, consisting of a decrease in the fetal $Pa\text{O}_2$ and late decelerations (Fig. 3.16).

Effects of Analgesia. Partial relief of pain with opioids decreases hyperventilation somewhat so that the $Pa\text{CO}_2$ is in the 22–25 mmHg (3–3.3 kPa) range and oxygenation improves.[123] However, between contractions the respiratory alkalosis combined with the depressant effects of the opioid may cause hypoventilation and hypoxemia

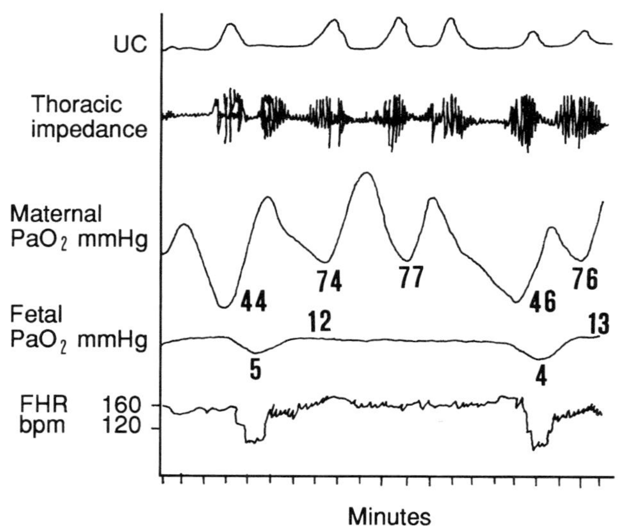

Fig. 3.16 Continuous recording of uterine contractions (UC), maternal thoracic impedance, maternal transcutaneous oxygen tension ($Pa\text{O}_2$), fetal oxygen tension and fetal heart rate (FHR) in a primipara 120 mins before spontaneous delivery of an infant with an Apgar of 7. Marked hyperventilation during uterine contraction was followed by hypoventilation or apnea between contractions. With the parturient breathing air during and after the first and fourth periods of hyperventilation, the maternal $Pa\text{O}_2$ fell to 44 and 46 mmHg, with a consequent decrease in fetal $Pa\text{O}_2$ and variable decelerations, which reflected fetal hypoxia. (Modified from Huch A, Huch R, Schneider H, Rooth G 1977 Continuous transcutaneous monitoring of foetal oxygen tension during labour. J Obstet Gynecol 84 (suppl 1): 1

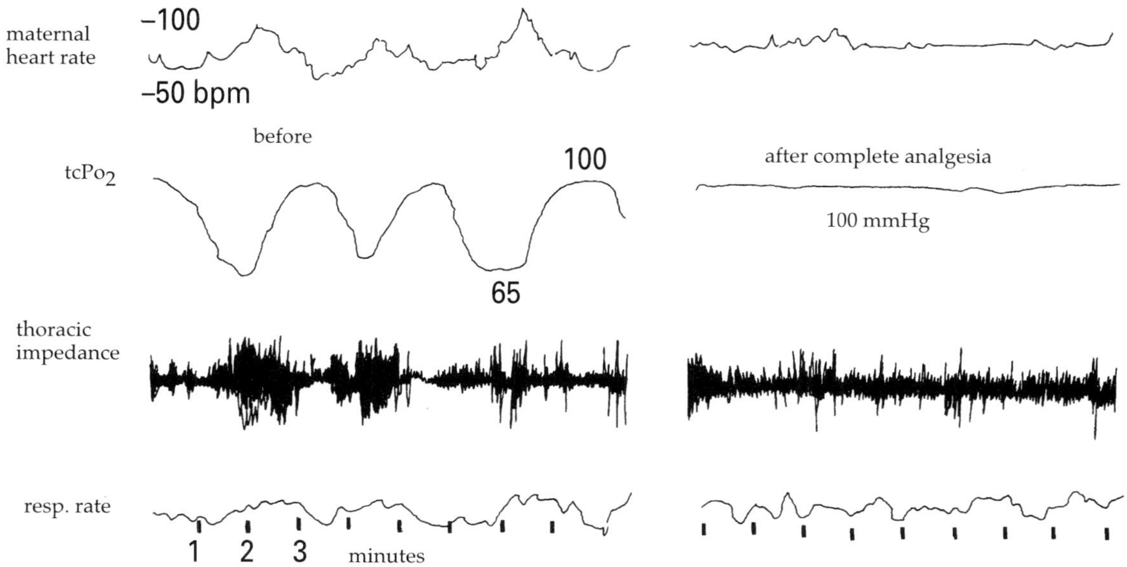

Fig. 3.17 Continuous recording of maternal heart rate, transcutaneous (tc) Po_2, thoracic impedance, uterine pressure (labor intensity) and respiratory rate after the parturient was given 100 mg of meperidine i.m. With each uterine contraction marked hyperventilation caused the tcPo_2 to increase to 110 mmHg but then to fall to low levels as a result of the marked respiratory alkalosis and of the respiratory depressant effect of the meperidine. The large decreases in tcPo_2 were avoided by giving the parturient breathing instructions during the relaxation period. (From Peabody J L 1979 Transcutaneous oxygen measurement to evaluate drug effect. Clin Perinatol 6: 109

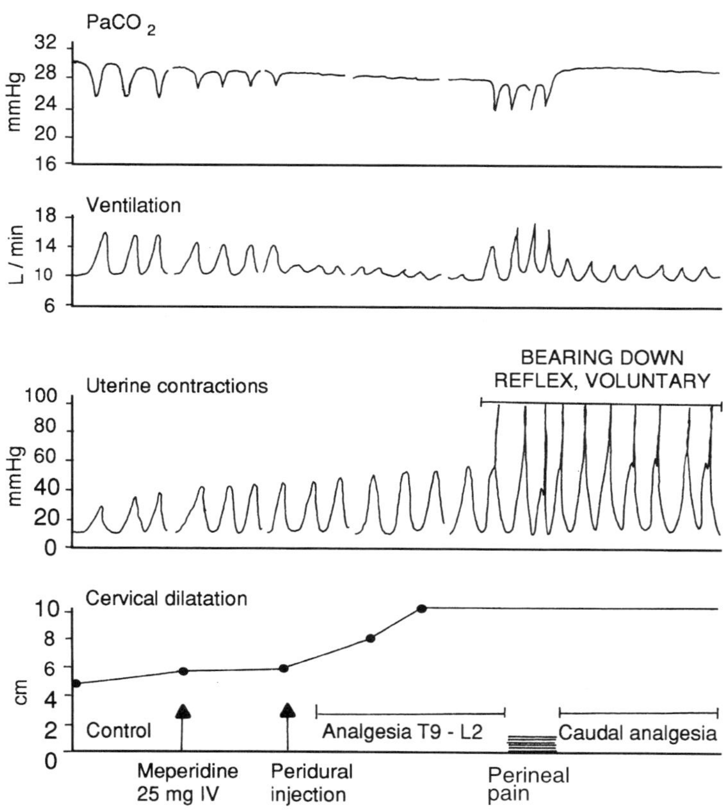

Fig. 3.18 Schematic representation of the effects of analgesia on ventilation based on measurements in a primipara. At 5 cm cervical dilation 25 mg of meperidine i.v. resulted in partial relief of pain and consequently produced smaller changes in ventilation and $Paco_2$. Subsequent induction of segmental epidural analgesia produced complete pain relief, which eliminated maternal hyperventilation and $Paco_2$ changes without affecting uterine contractions. During the second stage the onset of perinatal pain and initiation of reflex bearing-down efforts caused a concomitant increase in ventilation and a slight decrease in the $Paco_2$, which were eliminated with the induction of low caudal (S1–S5) analgesia. (From Bonica J J 1980 Obstetric analgesia and anesthesia, 2nd edn. University of Washington Press, Seattle, p 114.)

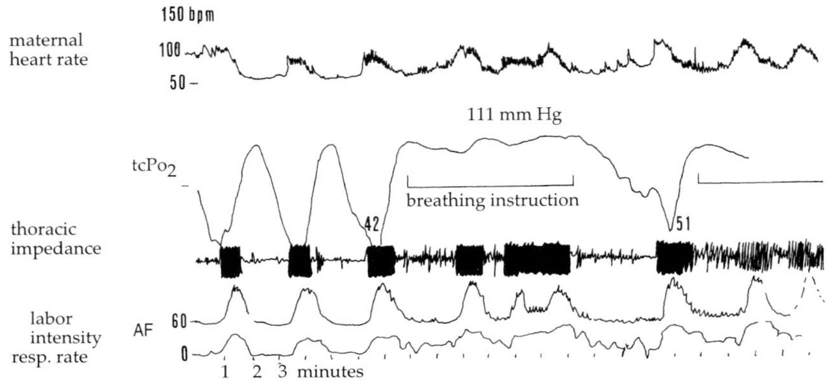

Fig. 3.19 Polygraph recording of maternal heart rate, transcutaneous oxygen tension ($tcPo_2$), thoracic impedance and respiratory rate during labor. Before the induction of epidural analgesia the pain of uterine contractions caused marked hyperventilation and a consequent increase in $tcPo_2$ to 100 mmHg (13.3 kPa, which fell to 65–70 mmHg (8.7–9.3 kPa) between contractions. After complete epidural analgesia all curves were more regular, and the $tcPo_2$ was maintained at a stable 100 mmHg. (From Peabody J L 1979 Transcutaneous oxygen measurement to evaluate drug effect. Clin Perinatol 6: 109.)

(Fig. 3.17). Complete pain relief achieved with epidural analgesia prevents the transient period of hyperventilation during a contraction and prevents hypoventilation during relaxation, so that the $Paco_2$ remains in the range 28–32 mmHg (3.73–4.27 kPa) and the Pao_2 increases to about 100 mmHg (13.3 kPa) (Figs 3.18 and 3.19).

Neuroendocrine effects

Animal studies have shown that acute pain caused by noxious stimulation produces a significant (20–40%) increase in catecholamine levels, particularly norepinephrine, with a consequent 35–70% decrease in uterine blood flow[124,125] (Figs 3.20 and 3.21). Human studies have shown that severe pain and anxiety during active labor cause a 300–600% increase in the epinephrine (E) level, a 200–400% increase in the norepinephrine (NE) level, a 200–300% increase in the cortisol level and significant increases in corticosteroid and ACTH levels during the course of labor; these reach peak values at or after delivery.[126–128] Lederman et al[126,127] noted that, during the period of active labor, the E level increased by nearly 300%, the NE level by 150% and the cortisol level by 200%. They noted that the higher epinephrine levels were significantly associated with uterine contractile activity at the onset of active labor (3 cm cervical dilation) and with longer labor during the active phase (3–10 cm cervical dilation). Increased epinephrine and cortisol levels were correlated significantly with anxiety and pain.

Ohno et al[129] carried out a comprehensive study of catecholamines and cyclic nucleotides during labor and following delivery and noted a nearly twofold increase in the dopamine level, a threefold increase in the E level and a twofold increase in the NE as well as a small increase in the cAMP level. They noted a positive correlation between

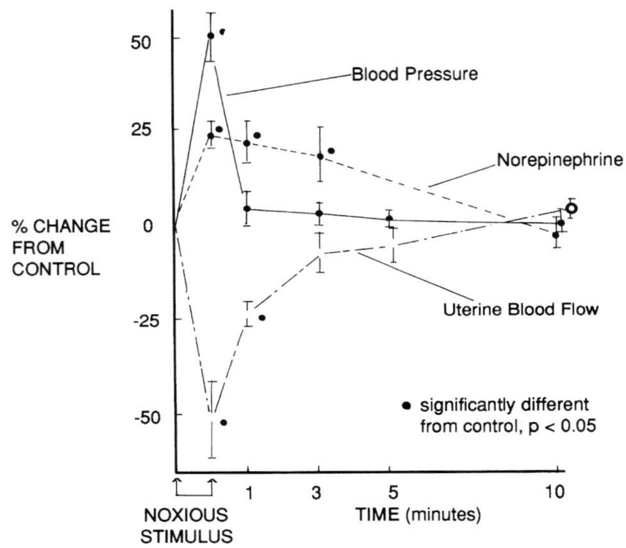

Fig. 3.20 Effects of noxius stimulus on maternal arterial blood pressure, norepinephrine blood level and uterine blood flow. The stress was induced by application of an electric current onto the skin of an ewe at term. The increase in arterial pressure is transient but the decay in norepinephrine level is more protracted, and is reflected by a mirror-image decrease in uterine blood flow. (From Shnider S M, Wright R G, Levinson G et al 1979 Uterine blood flow and plasma norepinephrine changes during maternal stress in the pregnant ewe. Anesthesiology 50: 524.)

E on the one hand and heart rate and systolic blood pressure on the other, as well as a correlation between NE and cAMP during labor. The greater increase in E than in NE was contrasted with the findings of a previous study, which showed that NE was much greater than E during physical exercise. This led them to conclude that elevated sympathoadrenal activity during labor is a result of pain and anxiety rather than of physical effort. Other data, however, show that, although pain is a major factor in the

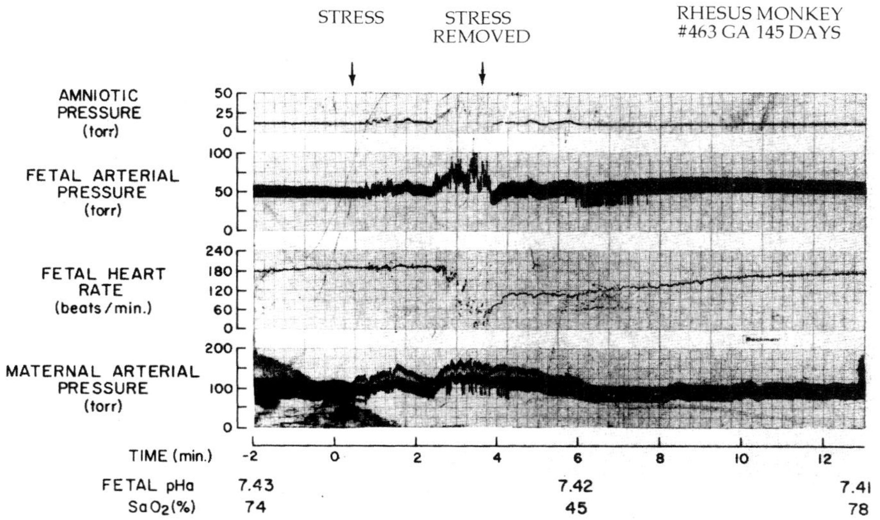

Fig. 3.21 Effects of pain-induced stress on maternal arterial pressure, intrauterine pressure and fetal heart rate in a pregnant monkey. Note the adverse effect of the stress on fetal heart rate and oxygenation. (Modified from and courtesy of Morishima, H D, Pedersen H, Finster M 1978 Am J Obstet Gynecol 131: 286.)

elevation of catecholamine levels, physical effort during the second stage does contribute to the increase in catecholamine levels.

Effect of analgesia. Recent studies have provided impressive evidence that epidural analgesia, by blocking nociceptive input and sympathetic efferents, reduces the release of catecholamines, beta-endorphins, ACTH and cortisol.[130–137] This neuroendocrine lowering effect is primarily a result of relief of pain during labor and was demonstrated by Abboud et al,[138] who noted that spinal anesthesia at the T4 dermatomal level decreased catecholamine levels in women in labor, but did not do so in women who were not in labor. This selectivity suggests that the mechanism by which catecholamine release is decreased is relief of maternal pain.

Epidural analgesia during labor and delivery does not decrease catecholamine and beta-endorphin release in the fetus and newborn,[92,131,135–138] and norepinephrine predominates over epinephrine.[138] This response indicates that, even during completely uncomplicated deliveries with adequate maternal analgesia, the infant is considerably distressed by the process of birth by vaginal delivery. A number of studies have suggested that catecholamines have an important role for neonatal adaptation to the extrauterine environment, including surfactant synthesis and release, lung liquid resorption, nonshivering thermogenesis, glucose homeostasis, cardiovascular changes and water metabolism.[138]

Cardiovascular changes

During labor cardiac output progressively increases to a value that is about 40–50% higher than the prelabor value during the late first and second stages, and some parturients have an increase of nearly 100% with a further increase of 20–30% during each painful uterine contraction[139–143] (Fig. 3.22). Available data suggest that 40–50% of the increase during the contraction is caused

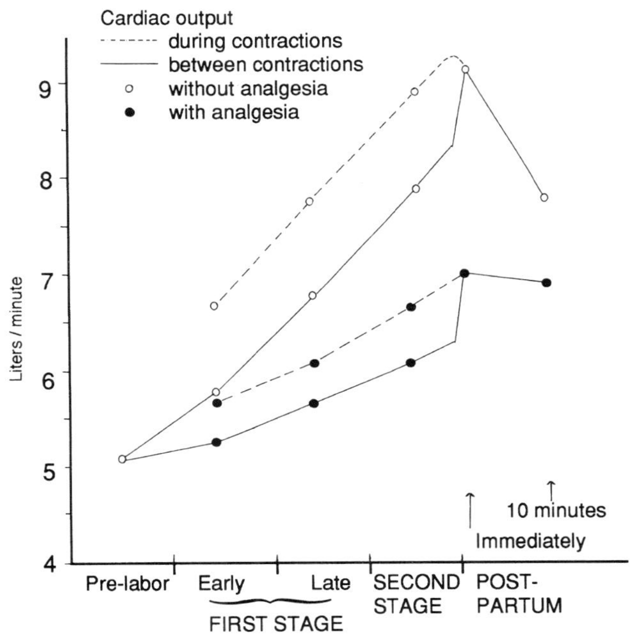

Fig. 3.22 Cardiac output during various phases of labor between contraction and during contractions. In a group of patients laboring without analgesia, the progressive increases between contractions and the further increases during each contraction were much greater than corresponding changes in a group of patients who received continuous epidural analgesia. (From Bonica J J 1967 Principles and practice of obstetric analgesia and anesthesia. F A Davis, Philadelphia, p 383.)

by the extrusion of 250–300 ml of blood from the uterus and by increased venous return from the pelvis and lower limbs into the maternal central circulation.[139,142] The rest is caused by an increase in sympathetic activity provoked by pain, anxiety, apprehension and the physical effort of labor, which contribute to the progressive rise in cardiac output as labor advances.[140,141] Uterine contractions in the absence of analgesia also cause increases of 20–30 mmHg (2.6–6.4 kPa) in the systolic and diastolic blood pressures. The increases in cardiac output and systolic blood pressure lead to a significant increase in left ventricular work that is tolerated by healthy parturients but can prove deleterious if the parturients have heart disease, pregnancy-induced hypertension (preeclampsia), essential hypertension, pulmonary hypertension or severe anemia.

Effect of analgesia. By decreasing the pain-induced sympathetic hyperactivity and neuroendocrine response, epidural analgesia eliminates that portion of the increase in cardiac output and blood pressure caused by pain. Figures 3.23 and 3.24 show that epidural analgesia decreases the progressive increase in cardiac output and its further increase during uterine contractions to about 50% of that without analgesia. A similar decrease in periodic increase in blood pressure is depicted in Figure 3.24. Several studies have proven the value of epidural analgesia in dampening the increase in cardiac output, cardiac work and blood pressure in laboring parturients with heart disease, pregnancy-induced hypertension (preeclampsia) and pulmonary hypertension, provided of course that maternal hypotension is avoided.[143,144]

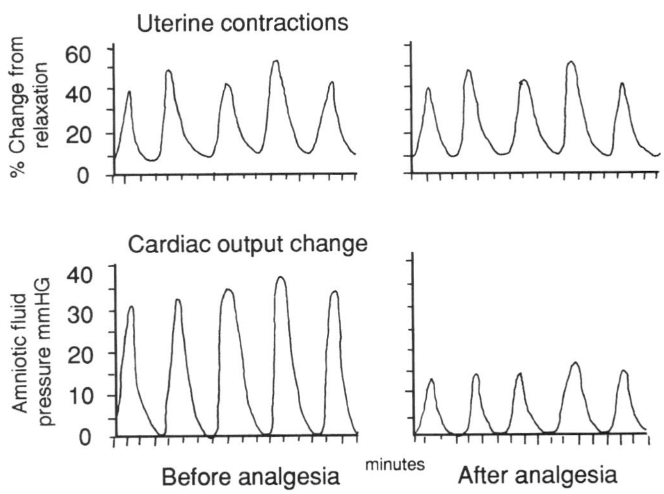

Fig. 3.23 Increases in cardiac output during each uterine contraction before and after induction of continuous epidural analgesia in a primipara. With pain relief the increase in cardiac output during contractions was about 50% of at before induction of analgesia. (From Bonica J J 1984 Labour pain. In Wall P D, Melzack R (eds) Textbook of pain. Churchill Livingstone, Edinburgh, pp 327–392.)

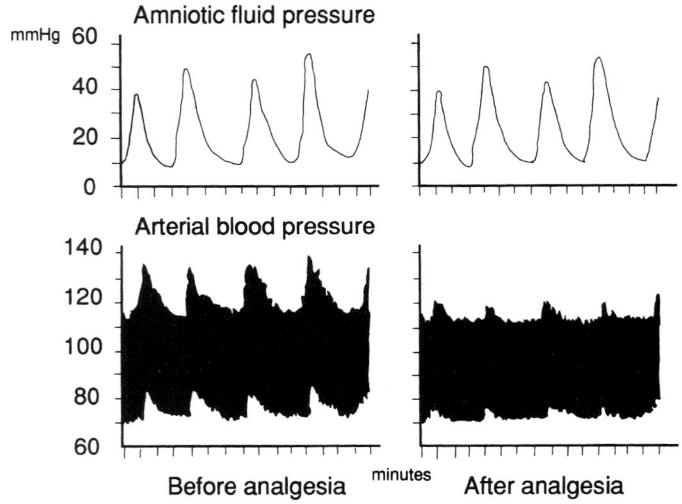

Fig. 3.24 Fluctuations in blood pressure produced by uterine contractions before and after induction of continuous epidural analgesia. Like the cardiac output changes (Fig. 3.23), complete relief of pain resulted in decreasing the contraction-induced fluctuations to nearly 50% of the values measured before analgesia. (From Bonica J J 1984 Labour pain. In Wall P D, Melzack R (eds) Textbook of pain. Churchill Livingstone, Edinburgh, pp 327–392.)

Metabolic effects

During the first and second stages of labor free fatty acids and lactate levels increase significantly, apparently as a result of the pain-induced release of catecholamines and the consequent sympathetic-induced lipolytic metabolism.[133] This assumption is based on the fact that, with complete blockade of nociceptive (afferent) and efferent pathways achieved with epidural or other forms of regional analgesia, only slight increases in maternal free fatty acid and lactate levels and acidosis are seen. During the second stage of labor maternal acidosis is a result of the pain and physical exertion inherent in the active bearing-down (pushing) effort during contractions.

Increased sympathetic activity caused by labor pain and anxiety also increases metabolism and oxygen consumption and decreases gastrointestinal and urinary bladder motility. The increased oxygen consumption, plus that inherent in the work of labor, together with the loss of bicarbonate from the kidney as compensation for the pain-induced respiratory alkalosis and often reduced carbohydrate intake, produce a progressive metabolic acidosis that is transferred to the fetus. The maternal pyruvate level increases, along with an even greater increase in the lactate level and a progressive accumulation of excess lactate, which is reflected by a progressive increase in base excess.[145–147]

Effects of analgesia. The relief of pain and associated anxiety with continuous epidural analgesia decreases the total work of labor, maternal metabolism and oxygen consumption. Buchan[133] showed that, during labor, epidural analgesia reduced internal stress by abolishing pain, thus eliminating the progressive increase in the 11-hydroxycorticosteroid levels normally seen throughout labor. Consequently, epidural analgesia significantly reduces maternal and fetal metabolic acidosis. The superiority of epidural analgesia over opioids and other systemic drugs in decreasing maternal work, oxygen consumption and maternal and fetal metabolic acidosis has been impressively demonstrated by a number of investigators[130,145–152] (Figs 3.17, 3.18 and 3.22). Because active pushing during the second stage of labor contributes to metabolic acidosis, epidural analgesia does not completely eliminate metabolic and fetal acidosis. Figure 3.25 demonstrates that epidural analgesia and elimination of the bearing-down effort (pushing) during the second stage almost eliminates maternal metabolic acidosis. Moreover, under these conditions it decreases but does eliminate the degree of fetal acidosis. Undoubtedly, this is a result of the physical stress on the fetus inherent in the process of birth.

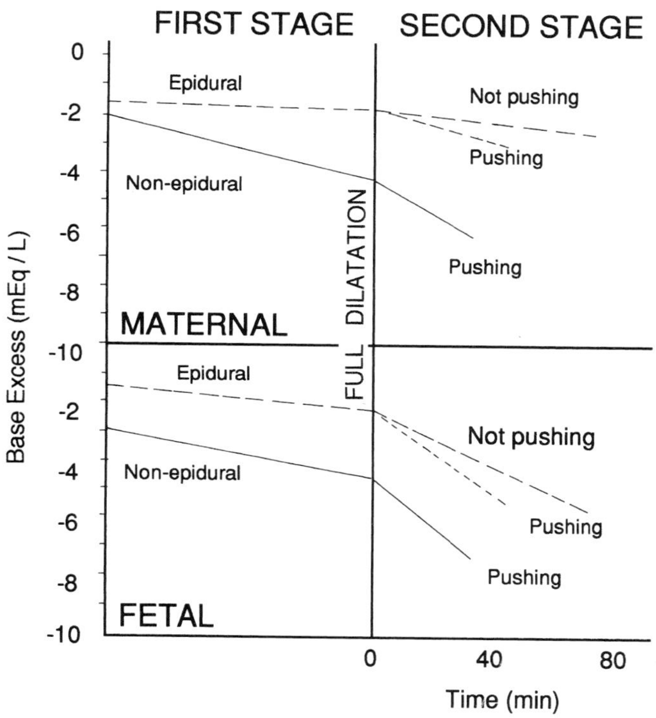

Fig. 3.25 Mean changes in extent of maternal (above) and fetal (below) metabolic acidosis during the first and second stages of labor in a group of parturients managed without lumbar epidural analgesia and in two similar groups managed with epidural analgesia, one of which retained the bearing-down reflex and the other did not. The parturients were delivered by outlet forceps. Significant metabolic acidosis was experienced by those in the nonepidural group of parturients, whereas those given epidural analgesia experienced little or no changes in their acid–base status. Fetuses born of mothers managed without epidural also developed metabolic acidosis during the first stage, and to an even greater degree during the second stage. In contrast, fetuses of mothers given epidural had no change in acid–base status during the first stage but showed a time-dependent increase in metabolic acidosis during the second stage. From Bonica J J 1980 Obstetric analgesia and anesthesia, 2nd edn. University of Washington Press, Seattle, p 115.)

Changes in gastrointestinal function

The pain of labor affects the function of the gastrointestinal tract. Gastrin release is stimulated during painful labor and results in an increase in gastric acid secretion.[153] Moreover, the pain and associated anxiety and emotional stress produce segmental and suprasegmental reflex inhibition of gastrointestinal motility and function, and consequently a significant delay in gastric emptying. These reflex effects of nociception are aggravated by the recumbent position and by the use of opioids and other depressant drugs.[153–155] The combined effect of pain and depressant drugs can cause food and fluids other than water to be retained for as long as 36 h or more, and during this period swallowed air and gastric juices accumulate progressively, with the pH of the stomach contents decreasing below the critical value of 2.5 in most parturients. Delayed gastric emptying of acidic gastric contents increases the risk of regurgitation and pulmonary aspiration, especially during the induction of general anesthesia.

Effect of analgesia. Epidural analgesia, by completely blocking the nociceptive input, obviates the reflex inhibition of gastrointestinal function and, unlike opioids, has no effect on gastrointestinal function. Consequently the parturient does not incur the delay in gastric emptying and other changes mentioned above in gastrointestinal function.[155]

Psychologic effects

Severe labor pain can produce serious long-term emotional disturbances that might impair the parturient's mental health, negatively influence her relationship with her baby during the first few crucial days and cause fears of future pregnancies that could affect her sexual relationship with her husband.[62–65,148–151] Kartchner,[156] Rogers,[157] Melzack et al,[64,65,69] Gaston-Johansson and associates[71,72] and others[74,158] reported that a significant number of women who had participated in natural childbirth developed or had aggravation of prelabor depression and other deleterious emotional reactions in the postpartum period, consequent to the pain experienced during their childbirth without analgesia. Cheetam and Rzadkowolski[157] reported that nearly two-thirds of parturients experienced some type of emotional upset characterized predominantly by a decrease in mental acuity and in social interests, and an increase in their feelings of dysphoria, depression and anxiety. They pointed out that psychologic aspects of labor are accentuated by the well-cited triad of 'fear–tension–pain', which might in turn decrease uterine activity and thus prolong labor. In addition, Melzack et al[69] noted that some women might experience an added burden of guilt, anger and failure when they anticipate 'natural, painless childbirth' and are then confronted with such severe pain that they require epidural analgesia. Stewart[159] reported that some women who failed to achieve 'painless' childbirth and experienced such severe pain as to require epidural analgesia subsequently became miserable, depressed, and even suicidal, and lost interest in sex. In some cases, the husbands of women who anticipated 'natural' childbirth had to undergo psychotherapy for serious reactions after seeing their wives experience such severe pain that they developed feelings of guilt and subsequent impotence and phobias. Melzack[69] also mentioned other reports of similar reactions by parturients who failed to achieve painless childbirth.

Effects of analgesia. *Properly administered* epidural analgesia will relieve most of the pain and thus obviate many of the psychologic and emotional reactions to the severe pain mentioned above. Melzack[69] summarized the data from the studies mentioned earlier in this chapter in a review article titled 'The myth of painless childbirth'. As previously mentioned, epidural analgesia decreased the PRI scores from a mean of 28 before the block to a mean of about 8 at 30 and 60 mins after induction of analgesia, and these scores were based on the use of such words as numbness, pressing and tingling. Based on his studies and data from other sources, Melzack[69] pleaded for a well-developed and well-balanced approach, whereby all prospective parturients are given education and training for childbirth and, if they experience more than mild pain, have skilfully administered epidural analgesia, because these are compatible and complementary procedures that allow the recognition of the individuality of each woman.

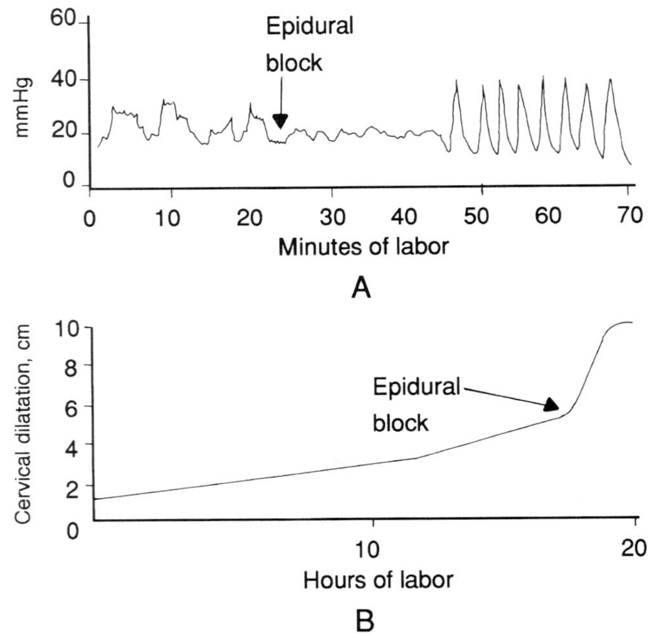

Fig. 3.26 Effect of epidural block on incoordinate uterine contractile pattern. (a) Intrauterine pressure tracings. Note the temporary decrease in uterine contractions and the subsequent normalization of the previously irregular contractions. (b) Cervimetric curve showing the rapid cervical dilation that followed start of the epidural block. (From Bonica J J 1969 Principles and practice of obstetric analgesia and anesthesia, Vol 2. F A Davis, Philadelphia, p 1200.)

Effects on uterine activity and labor

Through increased secretion of catecholamines and cortisol, pain and emotional stress can either increase or decrease uterine contractility and thus influence the duration of labor. Norepinephrine increases uterine activity, whereas epinephrine and cortisol decrease it.[126,127] Morishima et al1[24,160] reported that, in pregnant baboons and rhesus monkeys, nociceptive stimulation increased uterine activity about 60–65%, and was associated with a decrease in fetal heart rate and oxygenation. In contrast, severe pain and anxiety in some parturients cause such an increase in epinephrine and cortisol levels that uterine activity was consequently decreased and labor was prolonged.[126,127] In a small number of parturients, pain and anxiety produce 'incoordinate uterine contractions' manifested by a decrease in intensity coupled with an increase in frequency and uterine tonus.[161]

Effects of analgesia. By decreasing the sympathetic-induced hyperactivity, sedation and complete analgesia can reduce or eliminate uterine hyperactivity or hypoactivity and can change incoordinate uterine contractions to a normal labor pattern[161,162] (Fig. 3.26). Equally important is the efficacy of analgesia in reducing placental hypoperfusion and any existing deterioration in uterine blood flow, thus decreasing or even eliminating any impairment of blood gas transfer that might be a result of increased catecholamines or uterine hyperactivity.[122]

Effects on the fetus

During labor the intermittent reduction of intervillous blood flow during the peak of a contraction leads to a temporary decrease in placental gas exchange. This impairment is often further increased by pain-induced severe hyperventilation, which causes severe respiratory alkalosis (see above) and results in the following: (a) shift (to the left) in the maternal oxygen dissociation curve, which diminishes the transfer of oxygen from mother to fetus; (b) maternal hypoxemia during uterine relaxation; and (c) a reduction in uterine blood flow, which is provoked by an increase in norepinephrine and cortisol release (Fig. 3.20). These deleterious effects on the fetus have been demonstrated in several species of animals and in humans.[118,119,130,132,160] Figure 3.16 depicts the deleterious effects on fetal heart rate that are caused by marked hyperventilation during a contraction and by hypoventilation between contractions. Lederman et al[127] also noted that parturients who were anxious and had pain had a higher incidence of abnormal fetal heart rate patterns, and that their infants had lower 1- and 5-min Apgar scores.

Under the conditions of normal labor, such series of transient and intermittent impairments of blood gas exchange are tolerated by the normal fetus because oxygen is stored in the fetal circulation and intervillous space, and is sufficient to maintain adequate fetal oxygenation during the brief period of placental hypoperfusion. Moreover, the fetus can compensate by increasing the proportion of cardiac output that is distributed to the myocardium and brain.[163,164] If the above factors are combined with an excessive increase in uterine activity, however, fetal hypoxia, hypercapnia and acidosis develop that might still be tolerated by the normal fetus, although its ability to withstand oxygen deprivation is limited. If the fetus is already at risk because of obstetric or maternal complications (e.g. preeclampsia, heart disease, diabetes), the pain-induced reductions of oxygen and carbon dioxide transfer can be the critical factors that produce perinatal morbidity, and could even contribute to mortality.[124,125,160] The maternal metabolic acidosis is transferred to the fetus, making it more vulnerable to the effects of intrauterine asphyxia caused by cord compression, prolapse or other obstetric complications.[160,165]

Effects of analgesia. These benefits of pain relief, best achieved with epidural analgesia, are likely to be of value to many infants, but they are especially important to the fetus at risk.[1,130,145–152,155,166,167] It has been found to be the best method of analgesia for breech delivery and for multiple pregnancies.[1,155,166,167] It has been shown that epidural analgesia, through its vasomotor blocking effect, increases intervillous blood flow in parturients with severe preeclampsia and probably also in those with hypertension, diabetes and other conditions that decrease placental blood flow and function.[1,155,166,167] Janisch et al[168] found that continuous epidural analgesia administered to preeclamptics during their last few weeks of gestation produced a 100% increase in placental blood flow. Jouppila et al[169] studied the influence of lumbar epidural analgesia that was limited to a few segments and the effect of a more extensive type of lumbar epidural block on parturients with severe preeclampsia. They found that the limited block increased intervillous blood flow by 34%, whereas the more extensive block increased it by a mean of 77%. They attributed this effect to the relief of severe vasoconstriction by the vasomotor block. Maternal hypotension must be strictly avoided by appropriate prophylactic measures (e.g. intravenous infusion of fluids, lateral displacement of the uterus) to achieve these benefits.

REFERENCES

1. Bonica J J 1967 and 1969 Principles and practice of obstetric analgesia and anesthesia, Vols 1 and 2. F A Davis, Philadelphia
2. Bonica J J 1975 The nature of pain of parturition. Clin Obstet Gynecol 2: 499
3. Bonica J J 1986 Pain of parturition. Clin Anesthesiol 4: 1
4. Bonica J J, Chadwick H S 1989 Labour pain. In: Wall P D, Melzack R (eds) Textbook of pain, 2nd edn. Churchill Livingstone, New York, pp 482–499
5. Bonica J J 1990 The pain of childbirth. In: Bonica J J The management of pain, 2nd edn. Lea & Febiger, Philadelphia, pp 1313–1343
6. Bonica J J 1990 History of pain concepts and therapies. In: Bonica, J J: The management of pain, 2nd edn. Lea & Febiger, Philadelphia, pp 2–17
7. Wolff H G , Wolf S 1948 Pain. Charles C Thomas, Springfield, I L
8. Hardy J C, Wolff H G, Goodell H 1952 Pain sensations and reactions. Williams & Wilkins, Baltimore
9. Hardy J C 1956 The nature of pain. J Chron Dis 4: 22
10. Beecher H K 1959 Measurement of subjective responses. Oxford University Press, New York
11. Szasz T S 1957 Pain and pleasure. Basic Books, New York
12. Melzack R, Wall P D 1965 Pain mechanisms: a new theory. Science 150: 971
13. Melzack R, Casey K L 1967 Sensory, motivational, and central control determinants of pain: a new conceptual model. In: Kenshalo D (ed) International symposium on the skin senses. Charles C Thomas, Springfield, I L
14. Bonica J J 1983 Presidential address. In: Bonica J J, Lindblom U, Iggo, A (eds) Advances in pain Research and therapy, Vol 5. Raven Press, New York
15. Wall P D Melzack R (eds) Textbook of pain, 2nd edn. Churchill Livingstone, New York
16. Bonica J J 1990 Anatomic and physiologic basis of nociception and pain. In: Bonica, J J (ed) The management of pain, 2nd edn. Lea & Febiger, Philadelphia, pp 28–94
17. Dubner R, Bennett G J 1983 Spinal and trigeminal mechanisms of nociception. Ann Rev Neurosci 6: 381
18. Perl E R 1984 Pain and nociception. In: Handbook of physiology. Section I, The Nervous System, Vol 3. American Physiologic Society, Bethesda, pp 915–975
19. Lynn B 1984 The detection of injury and tissue damage. In: Wall P D, Melzack R (eds) Textbook of pain. Churchill Livingstone, New York, pp 19–31
20. Hallim R G, Torebjork H E, Wiesenfeld Z 1981 Nociceptors and warm receptors innervated by C fibers in human skin. J Neurol Neurosurg Psychiat 44: 313
21. Bonica J J 1990 Biochemistry and modulation of nociception and pain. In: Bonica J J (ed) The management of pain, 2nd edn. Lea & Febiger, Philadelphia, pp 95–121
22. Fields H L, Basbaum A I 1978 Brain stem control of spinal pain transmission neurons. Annu Rev Physiol 40: 193
23. Basbaum A I, Fields H L 1984 Endogenous pain control systems: brain stem spinal pathways and endorphin circuitry. Annu Rev Neurosci 7: 309
24. Willis W D 1985 The pain System: The neural basis of nociceptive transmission in the mammalian nervous system. Karger, Basle
25. Dennis S G, Melzack R 1977 Pain signalling systems in dorsal and ventral spinal cord. Pain 4: 97
26. Casey K L 1980 Reticular formation and pain: toward a unifying concept. In: Bonica J J (ed) Pain. Raven Press, New York, pp 93–105
27. Brodal A 1957 The reticular formation of the brain stem. Anatomical aspects and functional correlations. Charles C Thomas, Springfield, I L
28. Jänig W 1983 The autonomic nervous system. In Schmidt R F, Thews G (eds) Human physiology. Springer, New York, pp 111–144
29. Haymaker W, Anderson E, Nauta W J H (eds) 1969 The hypothalamus. Charles C Thomas, Springfield, I L
30. Isaacson, R L: The limbic system. Plenum Press, New York, 1974
31. MacLean P D 1958 Contrasting functions of limbic and

neocortical systems of the brain and their relevance to psychophysiological aspects of medicine. Am J Med 25: 611
32. Kenshalo Jr, D R Isensee O Responses of primate S1 cortical, neurons to noxious stimuli. J Neurophysiol 50: 1479
33. Reynolds D V 1969 Surgery in the rat during electrical analgesia induced by focal brain stimulation. Science 164: 444
34. Mayer D J et al 1971 Analgesia from electrical stimulation in the brain stem of the rat. Science 174: 1351
35. Liebeskind J C 1976 Pain modulation by central nervous system stimulation. In: Bonica J J, Albe-Fessard D (eds) Advances in pain research and therapy, Vol 1. Raven Press, New York, pp 445–453
36. Liebeskind J C, Paul L A 1977 Psychological and physiological mechanisms of pain. Annu Rev Psychol 28: 41–60
37. Besson J M R 1980 Supraspinal modulation of the segmental transmission of pain. In: Kosterlitz H W, Terenius L Y (eds) Pain and Society. Verlag Chemie, Weinheim, 1980, pp 161–181
38. Lewis J W et al 1984 Neural, neurochemical, and hormonal bases of stress-induced analgesia. In: Bonica J J, Kruger L, Liebeskind J C (eds) Advances in pain research and therapy, Vol 6. Raven Press, New York, pp 277–288
39. Mayer D J, Watkins L R 1984 Multiple endogenous opiate and nonopiate analgesia systems. In: Bonica J J, Kruger L, Liebeskind J C (eds) Advances in pain research and therapy, Vol 6. Raven Press, New York, pp 253–276
40. Fields H L et al 1983 The activity of neurons in the rostral medulla of the rat during withdrawal from noxious heat. J Neurosci 3: 2545
41. Merskey H, Spear F G 1967 Pain: psychological and psychiatric aspects. Bailliere, Tindall & Cassell, London,
42. Fordyce W E 1976 Behavioral methods of chronic pain and illness. Mosby, St Louis
43. Sternbach R A 1978 The psychology of pain. Raven Press, New York
44. Pilowsky I 1980 Abnormal illness behavior and sociocultural aspects of pain. In: Kosterlitz H W, Terenius L Y (eds) Pain and society, Verlag Chemie, Weinheim, pp 445–460
45. Chapman C R, Turner J A 1990 Psychologic and psychosocial aspects of acute pain. In: Bonica J J (ed) The management of pain, 2nd edn. Lea & Febiger, Philadelphia, pp 122–132
46. Chapman C R 1985 Psychological factors in postoperative pain and their treatment. In: Smith G, Covino B (eds) Acute pain, Vol 1. Butterworths International Medical Review, London
47. Bonica J J 1990 General considerations of acute pain. In: Bonica J J (ed) The management of pain, 2nd edn. Lea & Febiger, Philadelphia, pp 159–179
48. Kehlet H 1978 Influence of epidural analgesia on the endocrine-metabolic response to surgery. Acta Anesthesiol Scand 70: 39
49. Kehlet H 1986 Pain relief and modification of the stress response. In: Cousins M J, Philips G D (eds) Acute pain management. Churchill Livingstone, New York, pp 49–75
50. Wilmore D W et al 1976 Stress in surgical patients as a neurophysiologic reflex response. Surg Gynecol Obstet 142: 257
51. Behan R J 1914 Pain. Appleton, New York
52. Dick-Read G 1953 Childbirth without fear. Harper, New York
53. Velvovski I Z, Chougom E A, Plotitcher V A 1950 The psychoprophylactic and psychotherapeutic method in painless childbirth. Pediatriya, Akusherstvo ta Ginekologiya 1: 32–41
54. Lamaze F 1956 Qu'est-ce que l'accouchement sans douleur par la methode psychoprophylactique? Ses principes, sa realisation, ses resultats. Savour et Connaitre, Paris
55. Ford C S 1945 A comparative study of human reproduction. Yale University Publications in Anthropology. Yale University Press, New Haven
56. Freedman L Z, Ferguson V S 1950 The question of 'painless childbirth' in primitive cultures. Am J Orthopsychiatry. 20: 363–379
57. Jochelson W 1910 The Yukaghir and the Youkaghirized Tungus: Vol XIII of the Memoirs of American Museum of Natural History which constitutes at the same time Vol IX, Part I, of the Jesup North Pacific expedition. Am Museum of Natural History, New York
58. Lévi-Strauss C 1956 Sorciers et psychanalyse. LeCourier de l'Unesco, Geneva, pp 808–810
59. Lefebvre L, Carli G 1985 Parturition pain in non-human primates: pain and auditory concealment. Pain 21: 315
60. Lundh W 1974 Modraundervisning, Forlossningstraning eller foraldrakunskap? Ph.D. Dissertation, Pedagogiska Institutionen, Stockholms Universitet
61. Bundsen P 1975 Subjectiva resultat av smartlindring under forlossning-En enkatundersokning. Lakartidningen 3: 129–136
62. Nettelbladt P, Fagerstrom C F, Uddenberg N 1976 The significance of reported childbirth pain. J Psychol Res 20: 215–221
63. Javert C T, Hardy J D 1950 Measurement of pain intensity in labour and its physiologic, neurologic and pharmacologic implications. Am J Obstet Gynecol 60: 552–563
64. Melzack R, Taenzer P, Feldman P, Kinch R A 1981 Labour is still painful after prepared childbirth training. Can Med Assoc J 125: 357–363
65. Melzack R, Kinch R A, Dobkin P, Lebrun M, Taenzer P 1984 Severity of labour pain: influence of physical as well as psychological variables. Can Med Assoc J 130: 579
66. Melzack R, Schaffelberg D 1987 Low-back pain during labor. Am J Obstet Gynecol 156: 901
67. Melzack R, Belanger E 1989 Labour pain: correlations with menstrual pain and acute low-back pain before and during pregnancy. Pain 36: 225
68. Melzack R 1975 The McGill Pain Questionnaire: major properties and scoring methods. Pain 1: 277–299
69. Melzack R 1984 The myth of painless childbirth. The John J Bonica Lecture. Pain 19: 321
70. Melzack R, Wall P D, Ty T C 1982 Acute pain in an emergency clinic: latency of onset and descriptor patterns related to different injuries. Pain 14: 33
71. Gaston-Johansson F, Fridh G, Turner-Norvell K 1988 Progression of labor pain in primiparas and multiparas. Nurs Res 37: 86
72. Fridh G, Gaston-Johansson F 1988 Expectations of labor pain held by primiparas and multiparas. Unpublished
73. Cogan R, Henneborn W, Klopper F 1976 Predictors of pain during prepared childbirth. J Psychosom Res 20: 523
74. Scott-Palmer J, Skevington S M 1981 Pain during childbirth and menstruation: a study of locus of control. J Psychosom Res 25: 151
75. Reynolds S R M 1949 Physiology of the uterus, 2nd edn. Paul B Hoeber, New York
76. Moir C 1939 The nature of the pain of labor. Br J Obstet Gynaecol 46: 409–424
77. Hurst A F 1911 The sensibility of the alimentary canal. Oxford University Press, Oxford
78. Caldeyro-Barcia R, Poseiro J J 1960 Physiology of the uterine contraction. Clin Obstet Gynaecol 3: 386–408
79. Paul W M, Glickman B I, Cushner I M, Reynolds S R M 1956 Clinical tone and pain threshold. Am J Obstet Gynecol 7: 510
80. Lees M H, Hill J D, Ochsne A J, Thomas C L, Novy M J 1971 Maternal placental and myometrial blood flow of the rhesus monkey during uterine contractions. Am J Obstet Gynecol 110: 68–81
81. Novey M J 1972 The effect of sustained uterine contractions on myometrial and placental blood flow in the rhesus monkey. In: Longo L D, Bartels H (eds) Respiratory gas exchange and blood flow in the placenta. Department of Health, Education and Welfare, Bethesda, Publ No (NIH) 7–361, pp 143–152
82. Danforth D N 1954 Distribution and functional significance of the cervical musculature. Am J Obstet Gynecol 68: 1261–1271
83. Eustace D 1978 Cognitive, attitudinal, and socioeconomic factors influencing parent's choice of childbirth procedure. Dissertation Abstracts International 39: 1474B
84. Norr L, et al 1977 Explaining pain and enjoyment in childbirth. J Health Soc Behav 18: 260
85. Fridh G, et al 1988 Factors associated with more intense labor pain. Res Nurs Health 11: 117
86. Kohnen N 1986 'Natural' childbirth among the kankanaly-Igorot. Bull N Y Acad Med 62: 768
87. Marx J L 1979 Dysmenorrhea: basic research leads to a rational therapy. Science 205: 175
88. Csontos K, Rust M, Hollt V 1980 The role of endorphins during parturition. National Institute of Drug Abuse Research, Monograph Series, Rockville M D pp 264–271
89. Goland, R S, Wardlaw S L, Stark R I, Frantz A G 1981 Human

plasma beta-endorphin during pregnancy, labour and delivery. J Clin Endocrinol Metabol 52: 74–78
90. Abbound T K, et al 1983 Effects of epidural anesthesia during labor on maternal plasma beta endorphin levels. Anesthesiology 59: 1
91. Fettes I, et al 1984 Plasma levels of immunoreactive beta-endorphin and adrenocorticotropic hormone during labor and delivery. Obstet Gynecol 64: 359
92. Goebelsmann U et al 1984 Beta-endorphin in pregnancy. Eur J Obstet Gynecol Reprod Biol. 17: 77
93. Facchinetti F et al 1982 Opioid plasma levels during labour. Gynecol Obstet Invest 13: 155
94. Foley K M et al 1979 B-endorphin: analgesic and hormonal effects in humans. Proc Natl Acad Sci USA 76: 5377
95. Gintzler A R 1980 Endorphin-mediated increases in pain threshold during pregnancy. Science 210: 913
96. Gintzler A R, Peters L C, Komisaruk, B R 1983 Attenuation of pregnancy-induced analgesia by hypogastric neurectomy in rats. Brain Res 277: 186
97. Sander H W, Portoghese P S, Gintzler A R 1988 Spinal k-opiate receptor involvement in the analgesia of pregnancy: effects of intrathecal norbinaltorphimine, a k-selective antagonist. Brain Res 474: 343
98. Cogan R, Spinnato, J A 1986 Pain and discomfort thresholds in late pregnancy. Pain 27: 63
99. Rust M et al 1983 Verminderte Schmerzempfindung wahrend Schwangerschaft und Geburt. Arch Gynecol 235: 676
100. Kristal M B, Thompson A C, Grishkat H L 1985 Placenta ingestion enhances opiate analgesia in rats. Physiol Behav 35: 481
101. Kristal M B et al 1988 Modification of periparturitional pain threshold by ingestion of amniotic fluid in the rat. Soc Neurosci Abstr 14 (Part 2): 1158
102. Kristal M B, Tarapacki J A, Barton D 1990 Amniotic fluid ingestion enhances opioid-mediated but not nonopioid-mediated analgesia. Physiol Behav 47: 79
103. Kristal M B et al 1990 Amniotic-fluid ingestion by parturient rats enhances pregnancy-mediated analgesia. Life Sci 46: 693
104. Reading A E, Cox D N 1985 Psychosocial predictors of labor pain. Pain 22: 309
105. Brown W A, Manning T, Grodin, J 1972 The relationship of antenatal and perinatal psychologic variables to the use of drugs in labor. Psychosom Med 34: 119
106. Zuckerman M et al 1963 Psychological correlates of somatic complaints in pregnancy and difficulty in childbirth. J Consult Psychol 27: 324
107. Deutsch H 1955 Psychology of pregnancy, labour and puerperium. In: Greenhill J P (ed) Obstetrics, 11th edn. W B Saunders, Philadelphia, pp 349–360
108. Wallach H 1982 Psychological and physiological childbirth-related variables affecting pain of labour. Unpublished Master's Thesis, Lakehead University
109. Lowe N K 1989 Explaining the pain of active labor: the importance of maternal confidence. Res Nurs Health 12: 237
110. Wolff B B, Langley S 1975 Cultural factors and the response to pain: a review. In: Weisenberg M (ed) Pain: clinical and experimental perspectives. C V Mosby, St Louis, pp 144–151
111. True R M 1954 Obstetrical hypnoanalgesia. Am J Obstet Gynecol 67: 373–376
112. Meehan J P, Stoll A M, Hardy J D 1954 Cutaneous pain threshold in Native Alaskan Indians and Eskimos. J Appl Physiol 6: 397–400
113. Preissman A B, Ogoulbostan-Essenova E 1956 Some details of psychoprophylactic preparation for childbirth in the Turkomenian. Proceedings of the S.S.R. Kiev Congress 90: 66–67
114. Winsberg B, Greenlick M 1967 Pain response in Negro and white obstetrical patients. J Health Soc Behav 8: 222–228
115. Head H 1893 On disturbances of sensation with special reference to the pain of visceral disease. Brain 16: 1–132
116. Cleland J G P 1933 Paravertebral anaesthesia in obstetrics. Surg Gynaecol Obstet 57: 51–62
117. Bonica J J 1974 Current role of nerve blocks in diagnosis and therapy of pain. In: Bonica J J (ed) Advances in Neurology, Vol 4. Raven Press, New York, pp 445–454
118. Berkley K J, Robbins A, Sato Y 1988 Afferent fibers supplying the uterus in the rat. J Neurophysiol 59: 142
119. Berkely K J, Wood E 1989 Responses to varying intensities of vaginal distension in the awake rat. Soc Neurosci Abstr 15: 979
120. Berkely, K J 1990 The role of various peripheral afferent fibers in pain sensation produced by distension of the vaginal canal in rats. Abstract of the 6th World Congress on Pain
121. Peters L C, Kristal M B, Komisaruk B R 1987 Sensory innervation of the external and internal genitalia of the female rat. Brain Res 408: 199
122. Kawatani, M et al 1988 An analysis of the afferent and efferent pathways to the uterus of the cat using axonal tracing techniques. Soc Neurosci Abstr 12: 1055
123. Bonica, J J 1973 Maternal respiratory changes during pregnancy and parturition. In: Marx G F (ed) Parturition and perinatology. Clinical Anesthesia Series, Vol 10, No 2. F A Davis, Philadelphia, pp 9–21
124. Morishima H O, Pedersen H, Finster M 1978 The influence of maternal psychological stress on the fetus. Am J Obstet Gynecol 134: 286–290
125. Shnider S M, Wright R G, Levinson G 1979 Uterine blood flow and plasma norepinephrine changes during maternal stress in the pregnant ewe. Anesthesiology 50: 524–527
126. Lederman R P, McCan D S, Work B, Huber M J 1977 Endogenous plasma epinephrine and norepinephrine in last-trimester pregnancy and labour. Am J Obstet Gynecol 129: 5–8
127. Lederman R P, Lederman E, Work Jr B A et al 1978 The relationship of maternal anxiety, plasma catecholamines, and plasma cortisol to progress in labor. Am J Obstet Gynecol 132: 495–500
128. Falconer A D, Powles, A B 1982 Plasma noradrenalin levels during labour. Anesthesiology 37: 416
129. Ohno H, et al 1986 Maternal plasma concentrations of catecholamines and cyclic nucleotides during labor and following delivery. Res Commun Chem Pathol Pharmacol 51: 183
130. Joupplila R, Hollmen, A 1976 The effect of segmental epidural analgesia on maternal and foetal acid-base balance, lactate, serum potassium and creatine phosphokinase during labour. Acta Anaesthesiol Scand 20: 259–268
131. Abbound, T K, et al 1983 Effects of epidural anesthesia during labor on maternal plasma beta-endorphin levels. Anesthesiology 59: 1
132. Motoyama E K, et al 1967 The effects of changes in maternal pH and $P\text{CO}_2$ on the $P\text{O}_2$ of fetal lambs. Anesthesiology 28: 891–903
133. Buchan P C 1980 Emotional stress in childbirth and its modification by variations in obstetric management – epidural analgesia and stress in labor. Acta Obstet Gynecol Scand 59: 319
134. Shnider S M, et al 1983 Maternal catecholamines decrease during labor after lumbar epidural anesthesia. Am J Obstet Gynecol 147: 13
135. Raisanen I, et al 1986 Beta-endorphin in maternal and unbilical cord plasma at elective cesarean section and in spontaneous labor. Obstet Gynecol 67: 384
136. Westgren M, Lindahl S G E, Norden N E 1986 Maternal and fetal endocrine stress response at vaginal delivery with and without an epidural block. J Perinat Med 14: 235
137. Neumark J, Hammerle A F, Biegelmayer C 1985 Effects of epidural analgesia on plasma catecholamines and cortisol in parturition. Acta Anaesthesiol Scand 29: 555
138. Abboud T K, et al 1982 Effects of spinal anesthesia on maternal circulating catecholamines. Am J Obstet Gynecol 142: 252
139. Adams J Q, Alexander A M 1958 Alterations in cardiovascular physiology during labor. Obstet Gynecol 12: 542
140. Hansen J M, Ueland K 1966 The influence of caudal analgesia on cardiovascular dynamics during normal labor and delivery. Acta Anaesthesiol Scand 23 (suppl 10): 449
141. Lees M M, Scott D B, Kerr M G: Haemodynamic changes associated with labour. Br J Obstet Gynecol 77: 29
142. Hendricks C H, Quilligan E J 1956 Cardiac output during labour. Am J Obstet Gynecol 71: 953–972
143. Bonica J J, Ueland K 1969 Heart disease. In: Bonica J J (ed) Principles and practice of obstetric analgesia and anesthesia, Vol 2. F A Davis, Philadelphia, pp 941–977

144. Sorenson M B, et al 1982 The use of epidural analgesia for delivery in a patient with pulmonary hypertension. Acta Anaesthesiol Scand 26: 180
145. Pearson J F, Davies P 1973 The effect of continuous lumbar epidural analgesia on maternal acid–base balance and arterial lactate concentration during the second stage of labour. Br J Obstet Gynecol 80: 225–229
146. Marx G F, et al 1969 Effect of pain relief on arterial blood gas values during labor. NY J Med 69: 819
147. Marx G F, and Greene N M 1964 Maternal lactate, pyruvate and excess lactate production during labour and delivery. Am J Obstet Gynecol 90: 786
148. Pearson J F, Davies P 1974 The effect of continuous lumbar epidural analgesia upon fetal acid–base status during the first stage of labour. Br J Obstet Gynecol 81: 971
149. Pearson J F, Davies P 1974 The effect of continuous lumbar epidural analgesia upon fetal acid–base status of maternal arterial blood during the first stage of labour. Br J Obstet Gynaecol 81: 975
150. Thalme B, Belfrage P, Raabe N 1974 Lumbar epidural analgesia in labour. Acta Obstet Gynaecol Scand 53: 27–35
151. Thalme B, Raabe N, Belfrage P 1974 Lumbar epidural analgesia in labour. Acta Obstet Gynaecol Scand 53: 113–119
152. Zador G, et al 1974 Low dose intermittent epidural anaesthesia with lidocaine for vaginal delivery. Acta Obstet Gynaecol Scand 34 (suppl): 17–30
153. Hayes J R, et al 1972 Stimulation of gastrin release by catecholamines. Lancet 1: 1
154. Nimmo W S, Wilson J, Prescott L F 1975 Narcotic analgesics and delayed gastric emptying during labour. Lancet 1: 890
155. Crawford J S 1984 Principles and practice of obstetric anesthesia, 5th edn. Blackwell Scientific Publications, Oxford
156. Kartchner F D 1950 A study of the emotional reactions during labour. Am J Obstet Gynecol 60: 19–29
157. Rogers F S 1956 Dangers of the Read method in patients with major personality problems. Am J Obstet Gynecol 71: 1236–1241
158. Cheetam R W, Rzadkowolski A 1980 Psychiatric aspects of labour and the puerperium. S Afr Med J 58: 814
159. Stewart D E 1982 Psychiatric symptoms following attempted natural childbirth. Can Med Assoc J 127: 713
160. Morishima H O, Pedersen H, Finster M 1980 Effects of pain on mother, labour and fetus. In: Marx G F, Bassell G M (eds) Obstetric analgesia and anaesthesia. Elsevier, Amsterdam, pp 197–210
161. Bonica J J, Hunter Jr C A 1969 Management in Dysfunction of the forces of labor. In: Bonica J J (ed) Principles and practices of obstetric analgesia and anesthesia, Vol 2. F A Davis, Philadelphia, pp 1188–1208
162. Moir D, Willocks J 1967 Management of incoordinate uterine action under continuous epidural analgesia. Br Med J 3: 396–400
163. Assali N S, Holm I W, Sehgal N 1962 Hemodynamic changes in foetal lamb in utero in response to asphyxia, hypoxia and hypercapnia. Circ Res 11: 423
164. Cohn H E, Sacks E J, Heymann M A, Rudolph A M 1974 Cardiovascular responses to hypoxemia and acidemia in foetal lambs. Am J Obstet Gynecol 120: 817–824
165. Beard R W, Morris E D, Clayton S G pH of foetal capillary blood as an indication of the conditions of foetus. Br J Obstet Gynaecol 74: 812
166. Shnider S M, Levinson G 1984 Anesthesia for obstetrics. Williams & Wilkins, Baltimore
167. Albright G A 1986 Anesthesia and obstetrics: maternal, fetal and neonatal aspects, 2nd edn. Butterworths, Boston
168. Janisch H, Leodolter S, Neumark J et al 1978 Der Einfluss der kontinuierlichen Epiduralanaesthesia auf die uteroplazentare Durchblutung. Z Gerburtshilfe Perinatol 182: 343–346
169. Jouppila P, Jouppila R, Hollmén A, Koivula A 1982 Lumbar epidural analgesia to improve intervillous blood flow during labour in severe pre-eclampsia. Obstet Gynecol 59: 158–161

4. Adverse effects of labor pain on the fetus

S. M. Shnider

INTRODUCTION

Up until the last two decades the administration of analgesic drugs during labor and delivery was viewed as potentially dangerous to both the mother and the fetus. Apnea of the newborn infant secondary to use of these agents at high doses, frequently observed during the 1930s and 1940s, was considered a major cause of brain injury at birth. In contrast to this view that these agents are excessively dangerous, many animal and human clinical studies suggest that, skillfully administered, they instead offer the possibility of fetal and neonatal benefits even in the circumstance of asphyxia of the fetus. These agents may act therapeutically by increasing the oxygen supply to the fetus by diminishing maternal sympathetic nervous system activity, decreasing uterine blood vessel tone, and improving uterine blood flow.

In addition, during labor, particularly towards the end of first stage and in second stage as pain becomes severe, maternal minute ventilation may be increased by as much as 300% compared with the nonpregnant state, with the development of marked maternal hypocarbia ($Pa\text{CO}_2$) of 20 mmHg or less and alkalemia (pH greater than 7.55).[1] This marked respiratory alkalosis may cause hypoventilation between painful contractions, resulting in maternal and fetal hypoxemia[2] (Fig. 4.1). It has been demonstrated that effective epidural anesthesia alone can markedly diminish this hyperventilation,[3] resulting in normal maternal oxygenation,[4,5] which indicates that hyperventilation is in part due to the pain of labor.[3,6]

HISTORICAL PERSPECTIVES

On October 16, 1846, William T. J. Morton demonstrated the use of ether for pain relief during surgery. Within a few years, ether[7] and chloroform were introduced to provide analgesia and anesthesia for many other procedures, including 'painless deliveries'. Other pharmacologic agents soon became available to aid in controlling labor pain: morphine and scopolamine in 1902 to produce 'twilight sleep'[8] and the barbiturates in 1924 to produce sedation.[9] Though viewed with skepticism and worry by some, these drugs eventually gained wide acceptance because they greatly allayed the anxiety and pain of women in labor and provided the physician with a considerable measure of control over the progress of labor.

At the time these drugs were introduced into obstetrics, they were poorly understood and little investigated. Furthermore, when administered to parturients they presented special hazards because, until the 1950s, obstetric anesthesia was administered by individuals with no special training in anesthesiology.[10] The early enthusiastic reception that these drugs received was often associated with their use at excessive doses,[11] with inadequate patient surveillance,[10,12] a lack of individualization of treatment, and a haphazard mixing of drugs. For example, in 1936 a program of pain relief was suggested in which 'five different drugs are given . . . within a few hours, by mouth, by hypodermic and by rectum, combining narcotics, a hypnotic and a uterine stimulant, then during delivery gas is used'.[13] With respect to excessive drug dose, the highly respected obstetrician, Mengert,[14] described the administration of morphine at doses in excess of 30 mg in 20% and of 65 mg or more in 1% of 293 deliveries in primigravid patients in 1942.

Reports appearing as early as 1928 showed that gaseous anesthetics improperly used could result in reduced fetal oxygenation.[15] It was also noted that the use of other sedative, analgesic, and anesthetic drugs at high doses could result in prolongation of labor.[10,16,17]

There really was never any doubt that the use of sedative, analgesic and anesthetic drugs at *high* doses depress the central nervous system.[10] Pediatricians had long noted that the neonates of women heavily dosed with these drugs were usually somnolent, flaccid, and pale. Their respirations were shallow and these babies rarely objected to handling. Their cry was weak and their primary reflexes suppressed. They were usually indifferent to drinking fluids and their nursing was inadequate.[13] It was Taylor et al[18] who correctly noted that anesthesia-

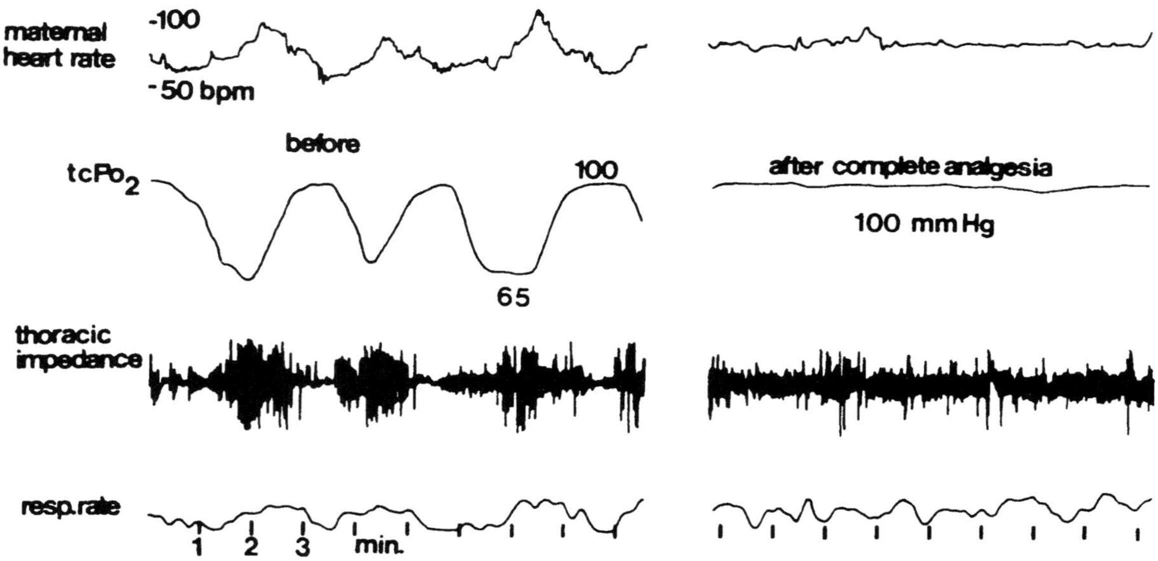

Fig. 4.1 Maternal hyperventilation during painful uterine contractions resulting in hypoventilation between contractions with a corresponding fall in transcutaneous oxygen tension ($TcPo_2$) to 65–70 mmHg. After effective epidural analgesia $TcPo_2$ is maintained at a stable 100 mmHg. (Reprinted by permission from Huch R, Huch A, Lübbers D W 1981 Transcutaneous PO2. Thieme Stratton, New York, p 139.)

induced nervous system depression was accompanied by maternal respiratory depression, which resulted in lowered oxygen content of arterial blood in newborn infants of anesthetized mothers, and that these depressed values persisted for a considerable time. Some reported that respiratory depression in the neonate was associated with atelectasis and increased risk of pneumonia.[19,20]

Physicians in the 1930s began to write extensively about the dangers of the use of central nervous system depressants in obstetrics,[16, 21–23] and in 1948 Mengert stated that 'the relief of the pain of labor is numerically and relatively the biggest single cause of asphyxia of the newborn'.[24]

Through all these years of criticism of the obstetric use of sedative, analgesic and anesthetic drugs, there always remained a number of investigators who still concluded that sedative and anesthetic agents, when used under properly controlled conditions, were compatible with a favorable delivery outcome.[13,16, 25–27] Hershenson,[27] in an early textbook devoted solely to obstetric anesthesia, concluded that infants delivered under heavy sedation suffer no remote effects. Bowes[28] summarized information available by stating that 'the medication used for analgesia and anesthesia . . . appear to be well tolerated by the fetus, and though there may be transient narcosis, there are probably few long-term untoward effects'.

Eastman et al[29] later demonstrated that use of analgesic agents at moderate doses did not affect the oxygen content of umbilical vein blood taken at birth. They also pointed out that numerous maternal and fetal factors other than drug use, such as maternal hypotension, prolonged second stage of labor, and compression of the umbilical cord, also could cause fetal asphyxia demonstrable from changes in cord blood acid–base status.

It has been well documented that the Apgar score may be lowered by the use of central nervous system depressants at high doses during labor and delivery;[30–32] however, when these same drugs are prescribed in amounts that fall within traditional or recommended doses, no lowering of Apgar score results.[33]

ADVERSE FETAL EFFECTS OF MATERNAL STRESS

As early as 1941, Sontag[34] reported that maternal emotional agitation induced by sound caused decreases in the fetal heart rate. Since then, an increasing body of literature has accumulated indicating that maternal anxiety can indeed produce adverse effects on the fetus. For example, in 1970, the Taylor Manifest Anxiety Scale was used to rate 150 healthy, married primigravidas.[35] The mothers who were prone to anxiety during pregnancy gave birth to smaller babies than women not prone to anxiety.

I believe it is worth remembering that the anxiety state can be of at least two types: the acute response evoked by single repeated stressful experiences, for instance labor pains; and prolonged anxiety, which recurs at sustained intensities at periodic intervals during all of pregnancy. Both types activate the sympathetic nervous system, reducing uterine circulation and fetal oxygenation.

Animal studies

Adrenergic stimulation can constrict uterine vessels and reduce uterine blood flow.[36–43] High blood epinephrine levels achieved by unintentional intravascular injection produce alpha effects with consequent uterine artery vasoconstriction, increased uterine activity, and decreased uterine blood flow. In ewes given 0.10–1.00 μg/kg/min epinephrine, uterine blood flow was reduced by 55–75%.[40] Exogenous norepinephrine infusion[44] or electrical stimulation of the major sympathetic branch of the hypogastric plexus[39] also significantly reduces uterine blood flow in the pregnant ewe.

It now appears that maternal stress, anxiety, and pain may adversely affect the fetus. The result of such stress may be an increase in the rate of spontaneous abortion,[45–48] premature delivery or fetal growth retardation,[49–52] or perinatal death.[53–55] The cause of the fetal compromise induced by maternal anxiety probably involves a number of factors, including abnormal metabolism of adrenal corticoid and other steroid hormones, or of protein hormones from the central nervous system. Increased maternal secretion of catecholamines with a consequent decrease in uteroplacental blood flow must also be a factor.

For example, in order to observe the influence of maternal epinephrine on fetal outcome, two groups of 10 rats each received epinephrine during different periods of gestation (duration of total gestation = 21 days).[56] A third group served as controls. In the group receiving the drug during the first 6 days, six failed to produce any living offspring. In addition, neonatal weight was significantly lower in this group. A sample of the offspring of rats receiving epinephrine on the seventh to twelfth days of gestation revealed significant behavioral differences compared with control group offspring. The etiologic factor thought to be responsible for these findings was intrauterine fetal hypoxia secondary to placental vasoconstriction produced by epinephrine.

Administration of catecholamines (epinephrine and norepinephrine) to the pregnant rhesus monkey produces varying degrees of fetal asphyxia under controlled conditions.[57] In fact, these agents infused in sufficient doses for a given period likely diminish uterine blood flow to the point of asphyxiating the fetus. Uterine blood flow was not measured, but vasoconstriction, resulting in reduced intervillous space perfusion, was the prime factor implicated in reducing fetal oxygenation. By contrast, direct administration of catecholamines to the fetus, as with nicotine, produced only insignificant effects on fetal oxygenation.

Again using both a sheep[58] and a primate study model[59] with catheters implanted in maternal and fetal arteries and the amniotic cavity, with ECG leads attached to the fetus, environmental influences were studied during labor or just before its onset. It was noted that when the mother was exposed to an anxiety-inducing environment, such as appearance of strangers in the operating room, loud ringing of a telephone or some decrease of anesthesia while the mother was on the operating table, the fetus invariably became asphyxiated.

In the pregnant rhesus monkey, progression of fetal asphyxia could be prevented by sending visitors out of the room, cutting down the noise level, or covering the mother's eyes so that she could not see what was happening. Another method was to give the mother more sedation; fetal oxygen tension and other indicators of fetal well-being, such as blood pressure and heart rate, then returned toward their original levels.

Myers et al[60] and Morishima et al[61] also examined this problem in a more systematic way and subjected pregnant rhesus monkeys to measured amounts of psychologic stress. After anesthetizing term pregnant animals and placing catheters in maternal and fetal circulations, the investigators subjected them, after full recovery from anesthesia, to various psychologically stressful stimuli. Some of these stimuli were incidental to handling of the animals, and others were planned. Planned stimuli included suddenly lighting up a darkened room in which a monkey was resting, making auditory or physical 'threats' to the mother, clapping of the hands, etc. All episodes were timed to last 60 or 150 s. These experiments showed that 50 s after the beginning of the stress stimulation, fetal bradycardia and hypotension developed, and arterial blood P_{O_2} values fell. When the episode ended, the vital signs and P_{O_2} values returned to prestimulation levels. These studies again indirectly point to uterine vasoconstriction and reduced blood flow, associated with increased sympathetic nervous system activity, as the mechanism that induces the change in vital signs and fetal asphyxia.

Morishima et al[61] studied the effects of maternal agitation, induced by exposure to bright lights, upon fetal well-being in pregnant rhesus monkeys at 139–148 days of gestation. Fetuses were classified as 'healthy' or 'asphyxiated' according to their initial acid–base state. Following variable periods of maternal excitement, a decrease in heart rate and arterial oxygenation was seen in all fetuses. Recovery occurred more rapidly in the healthy group, after maternal sedation was achieved, either by removing the stimulus or by additional administration of pentobarbital, 5–20 mg intravenously. The beneficial effects of maternal sedation on the fetus were thus demonstrated. In this study the pregnant monkey was deliberately exposed to stress by means of bright light shining in her face. Prior to the application of this stimulus, the animal was quiescent and in most cases (13 out of 19) the fetus was in good condition, with a pH above 7.30. In the period of agitation, significant elevation in maternal arterial blood pressure and heart rate occurred, probably through an increase in sympathetic activity. The tachycardia was accompanied by arrhythmias in the majority of mothers. Uterine activity also increased in most instances. Fetal bradycardia and decreased arterial oxygenation were noted in both healthy and asphyxiated fetuses (Fig. 4.2). All fetuses recovered (although more slowly in the asphyxiated group), probably because maternal agitation was terminated shortly after fetal distress became manifest. Fetal deterioration associated with maternal agitation undoubtedly resulted from an increase in uterine activity and an impairment of uteroplacental circulation, but uterine blood flow was not measured in these studies.

Uterine blood flow studies and maternal stress in animals

In the late 1970s our laboratory studied uterine blood flow and plasma norepinephrine changes during maternal stress in the pregnant ewe. We tested the effects of brief episodes (15–60 s) of maternal stress in 18 awake pregnant ewes.[58] Maternal agitation and struggling occurred either following nonpainful stimuli such as loud noises or sudden movements of personnel (10 animals) or following the brief application to the ewe's skin of a uniform electrical stimulus of 30 v with a frequency of 167 Hz for 30–60 s (eight animals). Stimulation of either type produced a 45–50% increase in mean maternal arterial blood pressure and a concomitant 32–52% decrease in uterine blood flow ($P<0.05$) (Fig. 4.3). The decreases in uterine blood flow were brief, lasting less than 3 min, and were not associated with fetal asphyxia. Maternal plasma norepinephrine levels were measured following electrically-induced maternal stress and were increased by 23%. We concluded that maternal stress may decrease uterine blood flow secondary to release of endogenous catecholamines. Morishima et al[62] later studied pregnant baboons and also demonstrated that maternal pain or fear resulted in decreased uterine blood flow.

Human studies of anxiety and exercise and catecholamine secretion

Dimsdale & Moss[63] devised a technique to monitor plasma catecholamines in a minimally obtrusive fashion in subjects going about their working activities. Nine young physicians were studied as they went about their normal hospital chores. Subjects were either house staff or junior faculty and in good general health. A heparin sodium-impregnated catheter was inserted in a peripheral vein and attached to a small (10×9 cm) portable blood-withdrawal pump. Blood was collected in tubes that had been heparinized.

Vigorous physical activity, in this case, was climbing stairs for 1 min: the pump was started, and subjects proceeded with an additional 3 min of continuous climbing (usually amounting to a total of 20 flights). For measurement of significant emotional stress, the investigators obtained a sample during the first 3 min of the subjects' presentations at various medical conferences

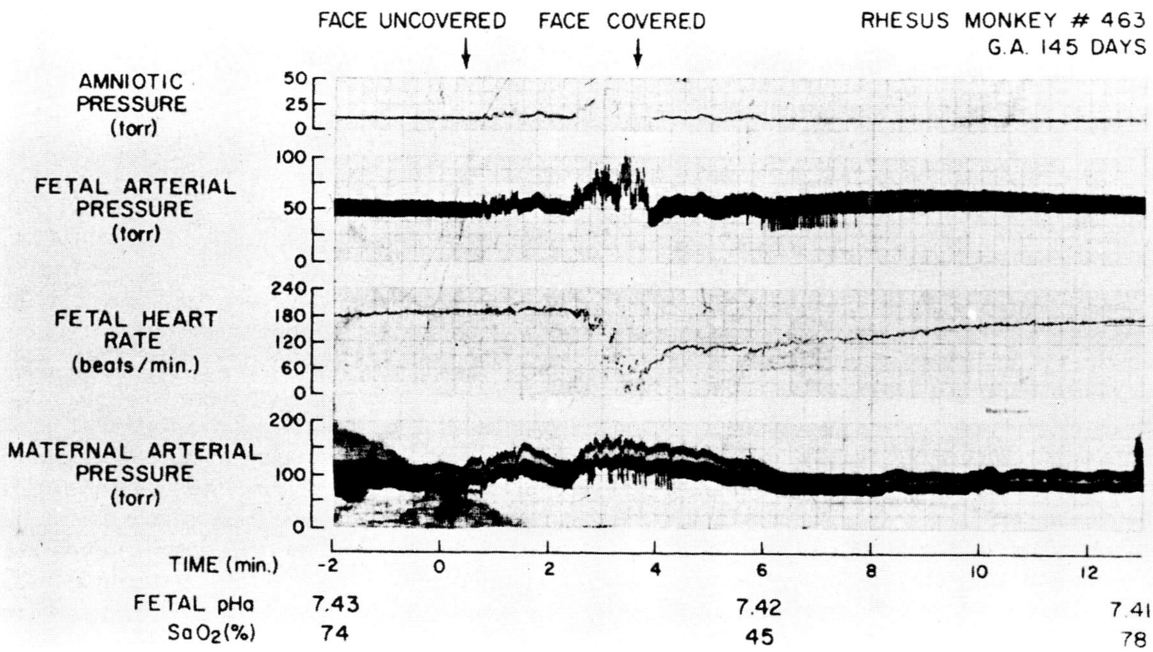

Fig. 4.2 Record of intra-amniotic pressure, fetal arterial blood pressure and heart rate, and maternal arterial pressure (expt no. 436). Note that maternal agitation did not cease until after intravenous administration of pentobarbital. (Reprinted by permission from Morishima H O, Pedersen H, Finster M 1978 The influence of maternal psychological stress on the fetus. Am J Obstet Gynecol 131: 286–290.)

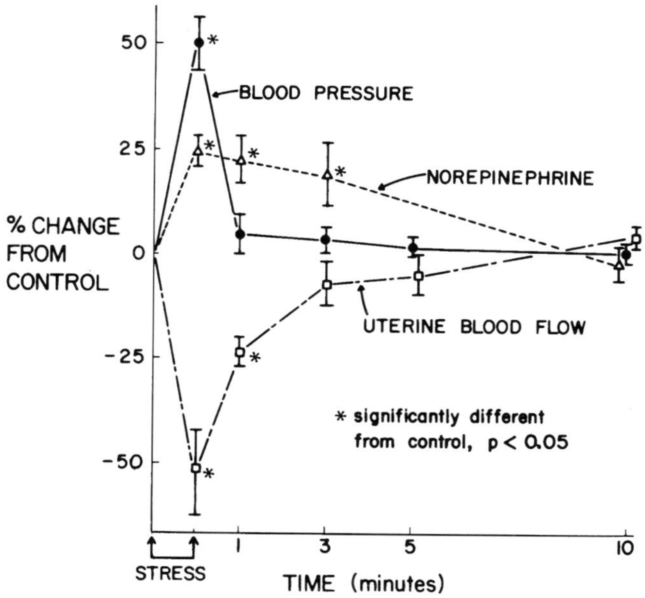

Fig. 4.3 Effect of electrically-induced stress (30–60 s) on maternal arterial blood pressure, plasma norepinephrine levels, and uterine blood flow. All values subsequent to control are given as mean percentage change with standard error. (Reprinted by permission from Shnider S M, Wright R G, Levinson G, Roizen M F, Wallis K L, Rolbin S H, Craft J B 1979 Uterine blood flow and plasma norepinephrine changes during maternal stress in the pregnant ewe. Anesthesiology 50: 524–527.)

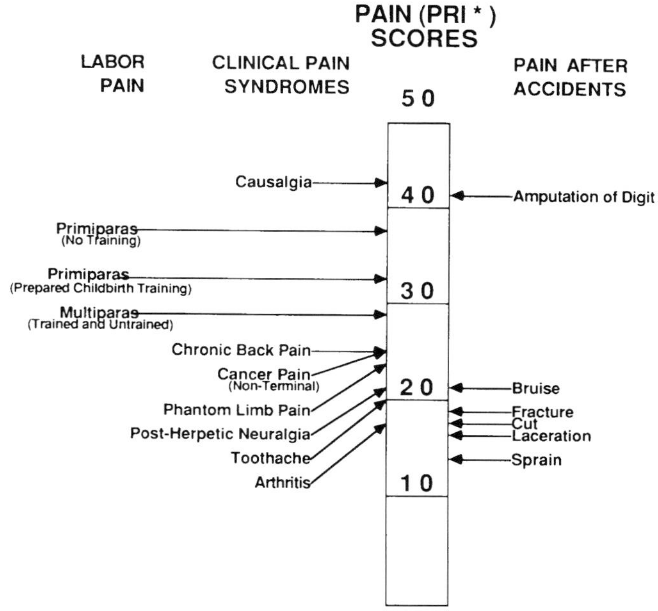

Fig. 4.4 This figure represents a comparison of pain scores using the McGill Pain Questionnaire. It compares labor pain and pain of other patients in a general hospital pain clinic. McGill Pain Questionnaire Pain Rating Index. [Modified from Melzack R 1987 The myth of painless childbirth (The John J. Bonica Lecture). In: Shnider S M, Levinson G (eds) Anesthesia for obstetrics, 2nd edn. Williams & Wilkins, Baltimore, p 79.]

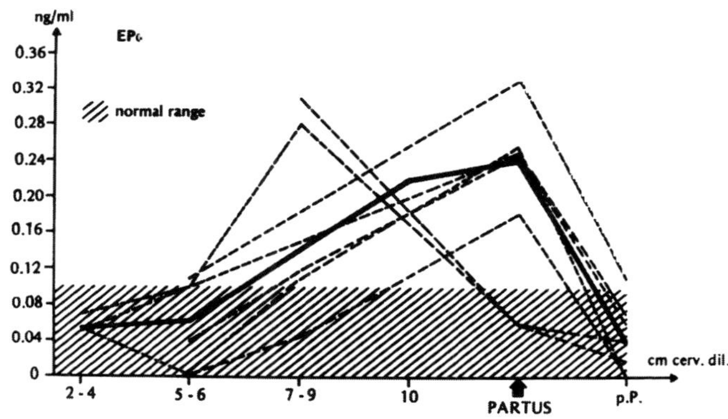

Fig. 4.5 Rising epinephrine plasma levels during various stages of labor. (Reprinted by permission from Neumark J, Hammerle A F, Kemeter P 1980 The influence of epidural block on cortisol, catecholamines and cardiotocography. Abstract No 1250, Seventh World Congress of Anesthesiology, Hamburg, September 14–21, 1980, Excerpta Medica International Congress, Series No. 533.)

(e.g. formal case conferences and death and complications conferences).

Each subject was tested serially and the investigators were able to use each person as his or her own control. The investigators found that there was disparity between plasma norepinephrine and epinephrine levels in different situations. During public speaking, epinephrine levels increased twofold, whereas during physical exercise norepinephrine levels increased threefold. It appeared that, while exercise induced a response of the sympathetic nervous system, psychologic stress induced primarily an adrenal response.

Human labor pain and endogenous catecholamines

Very few doubt that the experience of childbirth can be extremely painful. A comparison of pain scores in a Canadian review revealed that the degree of pain accompanying labor ranged between that of cancer pain and amputation of a digit (Fig. 4.4). It is well documented that during normal labor there is a steady increase in plasma catecholamines and cortisol levels.[64] The highest levels of epinephrine are found at delivery (Fig. 4.5). When the authors compared eight women who received meperidine with eight who received epidural anesthesia, the levels in the epidural group were significantly lower than in the meperidine group.

In another study plasma epinephrine and norepinephrine concentrations during labor and immediately after delivery were compared with those of the third trimester in 21 uncomplicated pregnancies of married primigravid women, 20–32 years old.[65] Third-trimester catecholamine concentrations were similar to those of normal, nonpregnant subjects; samples were obtained under identical conditions. Compared with third-trimester levels, significant elevations of plasma epinephrine and norepinephrine were found in three phases of labor (at 3–5 cm and 9–10 cm of cervical dilatation and immediately after delivery). Epinephrine values returned to normal within 3–21 min after delivery; norepinephrine values remained high or continued to rise in this time interval. Maternal analgesia and anesthesia influenced plasma catecholamine levels. Patients given regional anesthesia during labor tended to have lower levels of plasma epinephrine following the block. These investigators,[65] however, studied only two patients given epidural anesthesia during labor and six given spinal anesthesia for delivery. With this small population, statistically significant differences could not be demonstrated, nor did these investigators relate catecholamine levels to the clinical and biochemical conditions of the newborn.

The same investigators also found that parturients who are the most anxious have higher levels of epinephrine and decreased uterine activity during labor and also have longer labors compared with the calmer low-epinephrine group of women.[66]

Occasionally, dysfunctional labor associated with incoordinate uterine activity is improved dramatically by lumbar epidural anesthesia.[67] I would speculate that a relative increase in the proportion of plasma epinephrine (a predominantly β-adrenergic agonist) is responsible.

To determine whether epidural anesthesia during labor affects maternal circulating catecholamines, we took blood samples from 15 patients at the peak of and immediately after two consecutive painful contractions.[68] A lumbar epidural local anesthetic without epinephrine was then administered. After the onset of pain relief four blood samples were again drawn. All samples were analyzed by a radioenzymatic assay for epinephrine and norepinephrine concentrations. Before anesthesia, the mean (± SEM) plasma epinephrine level was 280 ± 49 pg/ml and the mean norepinephrine level was 866 ± 122 pg/ml. After anesthesia, epinephrine levels decreased by 56% ($P<0.01$). Although norepinephrine levels decreased by approximately 19%, this reduction was not statistically significant. At the height of a contraction, catecholamine levels did not differ significantly from those occurring between contractions. Lumbar epidural anesthesia during labor reduced maternal epinephrine levels, probably by eliminating the psychological and physical stress associated with painful uterine contractions or by denervating the adrenal medulla. Whatever the mechanism, reducing pain and activity of the sympathetic nervous system increases uterine blood flow.

In human studies, using the radioactive xenon technique to measure intervillous blood flow, Finnish investigators confirmed that the reduction in circulating catecholamines produced by uncomplicated lumbar epidural anesthesia has salutary effects on the progress of labor and uterine blood flow. Lumbar epidural anesthesia properly administered to healthy[69] and severely toxemic[70] parturients significantly improved uteroplacental blood flow during labor (Fig. 4.6).

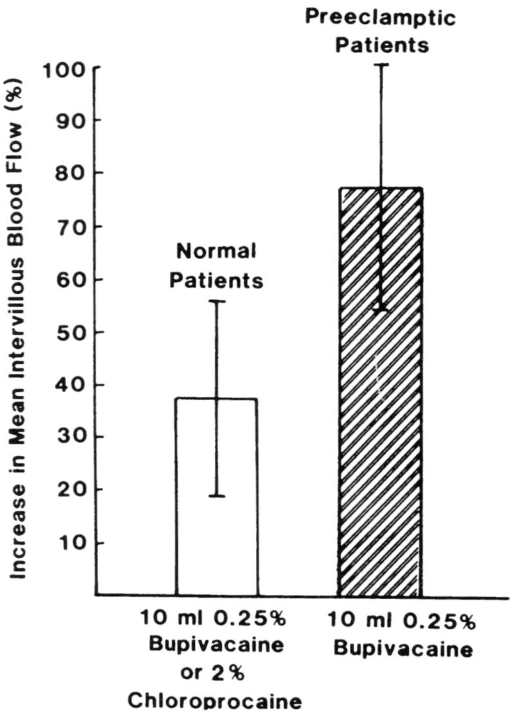

Fig. 4.6 Percent increase in mean intervillous blood flow values (± SE) after epidural anesthesia for labor in normal and preeclamptic patients. In: Shnider S M, Levinson G (eds) 1987 Anesthesia for obstetrics, 2nd edn. Williams & Wilkins, Baltimore, p 30. (Redrawn by permission from Hollmén A, Jouppila R, Jouppila P, Kolvula A, Vierola H 1982 Effect of extradural analgesia using bupivacaine and 2-chloroprocaine on intervillous blood flow during normal labor. Br J Anaesth 54: 837–842; and Jouppila P, Jouppila R, Hollmén A, Kolvula A 1982 Lumbar epidural analgesia to improve intervillous blood flow during labor in severe preeclampsia. Obstet Gynecol 59: 158–161.)

Lederman et al[71] have demonstrated that the incidence of abnormal fetal heart rate patterns is higher for very anxious patients with high epinephrine levels and their babies tend to have lower Apgar scores at 1 and 5 min.

CONCLUSION

It can be concluded, therefore, that maternal pain and hyperexcitability represent hazards to the fetus. Evidence suggests that obstetric anesthesia actually benefits the fetus. In pregnant sheep, stress results in maternal hypertension and increased plasma norepinephrine, which is associated with a precipitous decrease in uterine blood flow. In pregnant rhesus monkeys, psychologic stress results in fetal bradycardia and asphyxia, whereas alleviation of stress with a barbiturate causes an immediate and significant improvement in heart rate and oxygenation. Studies of women in labor also indicate that lumbar epidural anesthesia decreases plasma catecholamines and improves uterine blood flow. This is not meant to imply that *all* parturients should have regional anesthesia. Some well-prepared parturients with supportive attendants and/or sympathetic husbands will probably have lower levels of pain, anxiety, and plasma catecholamines than the average parturient. However, when nonpharmacologic techniques have not been effective, skillful anesthesia, coupled with reassurance and emotional support, may make birth less stressful not only for the mother but also for the fetus.

REFERENCES

1. Bonica J J 1973 Maternal respiratory changes during pregnancy and parturition. In: Marx G (ed) Parturition and Perinatology, Clinical Anesthesia Series (Vol 10, No 2). F A Davis, Philadelphia, p 9
2. Huch A, Huch R, Schneider H et al 1977 Continuous transcutaneous monitoring of fetal oxygen tension during labour. Br J Obstet Gynaecol (suppl) 84: 1–39
3. Fisher A, Prys-Roberts C 1968 Maternal pulmonary gas exchange. A study during normal labor and extradural blockade. Anaesthesia 23: 350–356
4. Curtis J, Shnider SM, Saitto C et al 1980 The effect of painful uterine contractions, position and epidural anesthesia on maternal transcutaneous oxygen tension ($TcPO_2$). Anesthesiology 53: S315
5. Peabody J L 1979 Transcutaneous oxygen measurement to evaluate drug effects. Clin Perinatol 6: 109–121
6. Bonica J J (ed) 1972 Obstetric analgesia and anesthesia, Springer, Berlin, p 5
7. Channing W 1848 Etherization in Childbirth. Wm D Lichnow, Boston, MA
8. von Steinbuckel R 1902 Vorlaufige Mittheilung über die Anwendung von Skopalamin-morphium Injektionen in der Geburtshilfe. Zentralbl Gynaekol 26: 1304
9. Cleisz L 1924 L'Anesthésie obstetricale par injection intraveineuse de somnifère. Presse Med 32: 1001
10. Waters R M, Harris J W 1940 Factors influencing the safety of pain relief in labor. Am J Surg 48: 127
11. Montgomery T L 1940 The use of analgesics in labor. Anesth Analg 19: 341
12. Shields L V, Taylor E S 1957 Serial oxygen saturation studies of newborn infants following obstetrical complications, difficult deliveries, and caesarean section. Am J Obstet Gynecol 73: 1011–1021
13. Galloway C E, Grier R M, Blessing R 1936 Pentobarbital-sodium and scopolamine hydrobromide: three years' experience with these drugs in obstetrics at the Evanston Hospital. J Am Med Assoc 107: 1707–1710
14. Mengert W F 1942 Morphine sulfate as an obstetric analgesic. Am J Obstet Gynecol 44: 888–896
15. Davis C H 1928 The evaluation of methods in obstetric analgesia and anesthesia with special reference to gas-oxygen. Anesth Analg 7: 176
16. Irving F C, Berman S, Nelson H B 1934 The barbiturates and other hypnotics in labor. Surg Gynecol Obstet 58: 1–11
17. Friedman E A (ed) 1967 Labor: clinical evaluation and management. Appleton Century Crofts, New York
18. Taylor E S, Govan C D, Scott W C 1951 Oxygen saturation of the blood of the newborn as affected by maternal anesthetic agents. Am J Obstet Gynecol 61: 840–854
19. Cruickshank J N 1930 Child life investigations, the causes of neonatal death. Medical Research Council Special Report, Series No 145. HMSO, London
20. Henderson J L 1943 Infection in the newborn. Edinburgh Med J 50: 535–553
21. Eastman N J 1936 Fetal blood studies. V. The role of anesthesia in the production of asphyxia neonatorum. Am J Obstet Gynecol 31: 563–572
22. Rosenfeld M, Snyder F F 1939 The factor of anesthesia in the pathogenesis of asphyxia neonatorum. Am J Obstet Gynecol 38: 424–430
23. Cole W C C, Kimball D C, Daniels L E 1939 Etiologic factors in neonatal asphyxia. J Am Med Assoc 113: 2038–2045
24. Mengert W F 1948 Fetal and neonatal mortality: causes and prevention. Am J Obstet Gynecol 55: 660–668
25. Embree E D 1939 A discussion of obstetrical anesthesia and analgesia based on 6000 cases. Anesth Analg 18: 329
26. Snyder F F (ed) 1949 Obstetric analgesia and anesthesia. W B Saunders, Philadelphia, p 206
27. Hershenson B B (ed) 1955 Obstetrical anesthesia: its principles and practice. Charles C Thomas, Springfield, Il
28. Bowes W A 1970 I. Obstetrical medication and infant outcome: a review of the literature. Monogr Soc Res Child Dev 35: 3
29. Eastman N J, Kohl S G, Maisel J E et al 1962 The obstetrical background of 753 cases of cerebral palsy. Obstet Gynecol Surv 17: 459–500
30. Moya F, Thorndike V 1963 The effects of drugs used in labor on the fetus and newborn. Clin Pharmacol Ther 4: 628–653
31. Batt B 1968 Are large doses of intravenous barbiturates justified for use as premedication in labor? Am J Obstet Gynecol 102: 591–596
32. Flowers C E 1960 The effect of analgesia and anesthesia on the fetus. Clin Obstet Gynecol 3: 890
33. Bonica J J 1967 Principles and practice of obstetric analgesia and anesthesia. F A Davis, Philadelphia
34. Sontag L W 1941 The significance of fetal environmental differences. Am J Obstet Gynecol 42: 996–1003
35. Shaw J A, Wheeler P, Morgan D W 1970 Mother–infant relationship and weight gain in the first months of life. J Am Acad Child Psychiatr 9: 428–443
36. Ahlquist R P, Woodbury R A 1947 Influence of drugs and uterine activity upon uterine blood flow. Fed Proc 6: 305
37. Berry Jr F A 1967 Vasopressors in pregnancy. Va Med Mon 94: 697–701
38. Greiss Jr F C 1967 A clinical concept of uterine blood flow during pregnancy. Obstet Gynecol 30: 595–603
39. Greiss Jr F C, Gobble Jr F L 1967 Effect of sympathetic nerve stimulation on the uterine vascular bed. Am J Obstet Gynecol 97: 962–967
40. Greiss Jr F C, Pick Jr J R 1964 The uterine vascular bed: adrenergic receptors. Obstet Gynecol 23: 209–213
41. Greiss Jr F C 1963 The uterine vascular bed: effect of adrenergic stimulation. Obstet Gynecol 21: 295–301
42. Martin Jr C B, Gingerick B 1976 Uteroplacental physiology. J Obstet Gynecol Nurs 5 (suppl): 16–25
43. Nimwegn D V, Dyer D C 1974 The action of vasopressor on isolated uterine arteries. Am J Obstet Gynecol 118: 1099–1103
44. Barton M D, Kilam A P, Meschia G 1974 Response of ovine uterine blood flow to epinephrine and norepinephrine. Proc Soc Exp Biol Med 145: 996–1003
45. Javert C T 1954 Repeated abortion. Obstet Gynecol 3: 420–433
46. Berle B B, Javert C T 1954 Stress and habitual abortion: their relationship and the effect of therapy. Obstet Gynecol 3: 298–306
47. James W H 1963 The problem of spontaneous abortion. X. The efficacy of psychotherapy. Am J Obstet Gynecol 85: 38–40
48. Tupper C, Weil R J 1962 The problem of spontaneous abortion. IX. The treatment of habitual aborters by psychotherapy. Am J Obstet Gynecol 83: 421–424
49. Shaw J A, Wheeler P, Morgan D W 1970 Mother–infant relationship and weight gain in the first months of life. J Am Acad Child Psychiatr 9: 428–424
50. Sontag L W 1940 Effect of fetal activity on the nutritional state of the infant at birth. Am J Dis Child 60: 621–630
51. Smith D J, Jaffe J M, Heseltine G F D 1974 Modification of prenatal stress effect in rats by adrenalectomy, dexamethasone and chlorpromazine. Fed Proc 33: 223
52. Myers R E 1972 The pathology of the rhesus monkey placenta. Acta Endocrinol 166 (suppl): 221–257
53. Hockman C H 1961 Prenatal maternal stress in the rat: its effect on emotional behavior in the offspring. J Comp Psychol 54: 679–684

54. Caldwell D F 1962 Stillbirths from adrenal demedullated mice subjected to chronic stress throughout gestation. J Embryol Exp Morphol 10: 471–475
55. James W H 1969 The effect of maternal psychological stress on the fetus. Br J Psychiatr 115: 811–825
56. Crist T, Hulka J F 1970 Influence of maternal epinephrine on behavior of offspring. Am J Obstet Gynecol 106: 687–691
57. Adamsons K, Mueller-Heubach E, Myers R E 1971 Production of fetal asphyxia in the rhesus monkey by administration of catecholamines to the mother. Am J Obstet Gynecol 109: 248–262
58. Shnider S M, Wright R G, Levinson G et al 1979 Uterine blood flow and plasma norepinephrine changes during maternal stress in the pregnant ewe. Anesthesiology 50: 524–527
59. Myers R E, Myers S E 1979 Use of sedative, analgesic and anesthetic drugs during labor and delivery: bane or boon? Am J Obstet Gynecol 133: 83–104
60. Myers R E 1975 Maternal psychological stress and fetal asphyxia: a study in the monkey. Am J Obstet Gynecol 122: 47–59
61. Morishima H O, Pedersen H, Finster M 1978 The influence of maternal psychological stress on the fetus. Am J Obstet Gynecol 131: 286–290
62. Morishima H O, Yeh N M, James L S 1979 Reduced uterine blood flow and fetal hypoxemia with acute maternal stress: experimental observation in the pregnant baboon. Am J Obstet Gynecol 134: 270–275
63. Dimsdale J E, Moss J E 1980 Plasma catecholamines in stress and exercise. JAMA 243: 340–342
64. Neumark J, Hammerle A F, Kemeter P 1980 The influence of epidural block on cortisol, catecholamines and cardiotocography. Abstract No 1250, Seventh World Congress of Anesthesiology, Hamburg, September 14–21, 1980, Excerpta Medica International Congress, Series No. 533
65. Lederman R P, McCann D S, Work B et al 1977 Endogenous plasma epinephrine and norepinephrine in last-trimester pregnancy and labor. Am J Obstet Gynecol 129: 5–8
66. Lederman R P, Lederman L, Work Jr B A et al 1978 The relationship of maternal anxiety, plasma catecholamines, and plasma cortisol to progress in labor. Am J Obstet Gynecol 132: 495–500
67. Bonica J J, Hunter Jr C A 1967 Management in dysfunction of the forces of labor. In: Bonica J J (ed) Principles and practice of obstetric analgesia and anesthesia. F A Davis, Philadelphia, p 1188
68. Shnider S M, Abboud T K, Artal R et al 1983 Maternal catecholamines decrease during labor after lumbar epidural anesthesia. Am J Obstet Gynecol 147: 13–15
69. Hollmén A I, Jouppila R, Jouppila P et al 1982 Effect of extradural analgesia using bupivacaine and 2-chloroprocaine on intervillous blood flow during normal labour. Br J Anaesth 54: 837–841
70. Jouppila P, Jouppila R, Hollmén A et al 1982 Lumbar epidural analgesia to improve intervillous blood flow during labor in severe preeclampsia. Obstet Gynecol 59: 158–161
71. Lederman E, Lederman R P, Work Jr B A et al 1981 Maternal psychological and physiologic correlates of fetal-newborn health status. Am J Obstet Gynecol 139: 956–958

5. *Maternal physiologic considerations during pregnancy and delivery

K. A. Conklin

Anemia. Hyperventilation. Hypervolemia. Hypercoagulability. These terms are frequently used to describe maternal physiology. However, since they describe abnormal or pathologic conditions, their use implies that a woman's physiology during gestation constitutes an abnormal state. Despite the fact that many physiologic parameters of a pregnant woman differ from those of a nonpregnant woman, the physiologic adaptions are *normal*, and, at least teleologically, important for maternal and fetal well-being. Thus, the above descriptive terms are inappropriate when applied to normal pregnancy.

This chapter will describe the physiologic distinctness of the pregnant patient, emphasizing those areas with relevance to obstetric anesthesia. Since changes in respiratory, cardiovascular and gastrointestinal physiology have the greatest impact upon management, these systems will be presented in detail. Changes in other systems, when relevant to obstetric anesthesia, will be discussed within the context of anesthetic implications.

BODY COMPOSITION AND METABOLISM

Weight gain (Table 5.1) during pregnancy averages 11 kg, and is accounted for by a gain of 1 kg during the first trimester and 5 kg during each of the second and third trimesters.[1] The uterus and its contents account for approximately half of the parturient's weight gain at term, with the uterus, weighing 1 kg, containing approximately 1000 ml of amniotic fluid along with the fetus and placenta for a combined weight of about 4 kg. Blood volume increases by 1500–2000 ml, with the balance of maternal weight gain being the deposition of extrauterine fat and protein.

Table 5.1 Weight gain at term

Uterus	1 kg
Amniotic fluid	1 kg
Fetus and placenta	4 kg
Maternal blood	2 kg
Maternal tissue mass	3 kg
Total weight gain	11 kg

Basal metabolic rate (Fig. 5.1) is slightly depressed during early pregnancy, but rises after 12–16 weeks of gestation to a level at term that is 15% above the nonpregnant level.[2] Women who have the lowest nonpregnant basal metabolic rates tend to have the greatest pregnancy gains in this parameter.[3]

Resting oxygen consumption (Fig. 5.1) increases progressively throughout gestation to a level at term that is 35% above the nonpregnant level.[4–8] The increased metabolic demand is due primarily to the metabolic needs of the products of gestation, plus a small contribution from increased maternal cardiac and respiratory work. Subjects with low weight gain during gestation and obese patients on calorie-restricted diets exhibit smaller increases in oxygen consumption.[9] During the first and second stages of labor oxygen consumption is elevated by approximately 40% and 75%, respectively, over the resting level.[10,11] The increased metabolic demand of

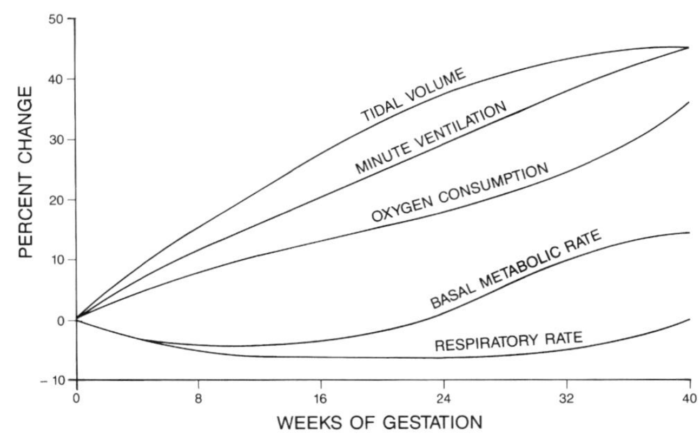

Fig. 5.1 Metabolic and ventilatory parameters during pregnancy. The curves are derived from data in the following references cited in the text: 2, 4–8, 23, 24, 28, 29.

*Previously published in part in Conklin K A 1991 Seminars in Anesthesia 10: 221–234.

labor is due to elevated respiratory work, which results from increased minute ventilation, uterine activity and, during the second stage, pushing.

RESPIRATORY PHYSIOLOGY

Anatomy

Airways

Capillary engorgement of the nasal and oropharyngeal mucosa and larynx, which is due to elevated levels of estrogens and progesterone, begins early in the first trimester.[12] Involvement of the false vocal cords and the arytenoid region of the larynx frequently results in voice changes.[13] Nasal mucosal engorgement commonly makes nose breathing difficult, and may result in nosebleeds.[13] Below the larynx the larger airways apparently dilate, as indicated by the increase in airway conductance.[14] This may be attributed to direct dilation by progesterone, cortisone and related substances or relaxin;[14] or possibly enhanced beta-adrenergic activity induced by progesterone.[15]

Thorax

The circumference of the thoracic cage increases by 5–7 cm during pregnancy,[13] with increases in both the anteroposterior and transverse diameters.[12,16] Flaring of the ribs occurs, with an increase in the subcostal angle from 68.5° at the beginning of the second trimester (which is equivalent to the subcostal angle 7 weeks post partum) to 103.5° at term.[16] These changes are accompanied by a decrease of up to 4 cm in the vertical diameter of the chest because the diaphragm is elevated from upward pressure exerted by the gravid uterus.[16]

Lung radiograph

The chest radiograph shows no characteristic changes of the lung parenchyma or pulmonary vasculature due to pregnancy per se, which indicates that the same criteria for interpretation should be applied for pregnant and nonpregnant women.[17]

Mechanics (Table 5.2)

Mechanism of lung expansion

Inspiration results from expansion of the thoracic cage and contraction (descent) of the diaphragm. Compared with the nonpregnant woman, the term pregnant woman at end expiration has an expanded thoracic cage and an elevated diaphragm.[12,13,16] Thus, breathing in the parturient is primarily by diaphragmatic excursion since, during inspiration, expansion of the thorax is limited, whereas descent of the diaphragm, movement of which is unimpaired in pregnancy,[16] is increased.[18,19]

Table 5.2 Changes in respiratory physiology at term* (From Conklin K A 1991 Semin Anesth 10: 221–234)

Parameter	Change†
Mechanics	
Diaphragm excursion	Increased
Chest wall excursion	Decreased
Total pulmonary resistance	−50%
Lung compliance	No change
FEV_1‡	No change
FEV_1/FVC§	No change
Flow–volume loop	No change
Lung volumes	
Inspiratory reserve volume	+ 5%
Tidal volume	+ 45%
Expiratory reserve volume	−25%
Residual volume	−15%
Lung capacities	
Inspiratory capacity	+ 15%
Functional residual capacity	−20%
Vital capacity	No change
Total lung capacity	−5%
Dead space	+ 45%
Respiratory rate	No change
Ventilation	
Minute ventilation	+ 45%
Alveolar ventilation	+ 45%
Closing capacity	No change
Diffusion capacity	Decreased

* Values are derived from data in the following references cited in the text: 4, 7, 8, 14–18, 20–30.
† Changes relative to values for nonpregnant individuals.
‡ Forced expiratory volume in 1 second.
§ Forced vital capacity.

Airway function

Reduction of the resting lung volume normally increases airway resistance because of lesser outward traction on the airways which reduces the size of their lumen. However, pregnant women exhibit a decrease in total pulmonary resistance (by 50%), or an increase of its reciprocal, airway conductance, despite a reduction in resting lung volume.[14,20,21] These findings are consistent with dilatation of the large airways, which compensates for the lower resting lung volume, as well as the increase in airway resistance that results from the decrease in arterial partial pressure of carbon dioxide (Pa_{CO_2}) during pregnancy.[15] Unimpaired function of the large airways during pregnancy is also shown by the lack of change in the forced expiratory volume in 1 second and the ratio of this parameter to forced vital capacity,[4,15,21–25] as well as the unaltered flow–volume loop.[25]

Small airway function is unaltered during pregnancy, as shown by the absence of change in closing capacity,[26,27] the lung volume at which small airway closure begins, and by the flow characteristics manifested in the flow–volume loop, which are similar in pregnant and nonpregnant subjects.[25]

Lung volumes and capacities (Fig. 5.2 and Table 5.2)

Tidal volume increases by approximately 20% during the first trimester of pregnancy.[4,8,23,28] This change is accounted for by a reduction in the inspiratory reserve volume since it occurs without a change in functional residual capacity or inspiratory capacity. Tidal volume increases throughout the remainder of gestation to a level at term that is 45% above the nonpregnant level.[4,7,8,28,29] The change during late pregnancy is accounted for by a progressive decline in functional residual capacity, since it occurs while inspiratory reserve volume increases and total lung capacity remains essentially unchanged.

A significant reduction in functional residual capacity is observed by the fifth to sixth month of gestation, and at term it has decreased to 80% of the nonpregnant level.[4,7,14,23,27] The decrease in functional residual capacity is attributable to elevation of the relaxed diaphragm.[7] This results from a less negative intrathoracic pressure, caused by alteration of the balance between the elastic recoil of the lungs and the chest wall, and an increase in intra-abdominal pressure, caused by the enlarged uterus entering the abdominal cavity. The change in functional residual capacity, at term gestation, is accounted for by a 25% reduction in expiratory reserve volume[4,7,14,21,23,25,30] and a 15% reduction in residual volume.[4,23,24] When the term parturient assumes the supine position, functional residual capacity falls to 70% of its volume measured with the patient sitting.[27,30]

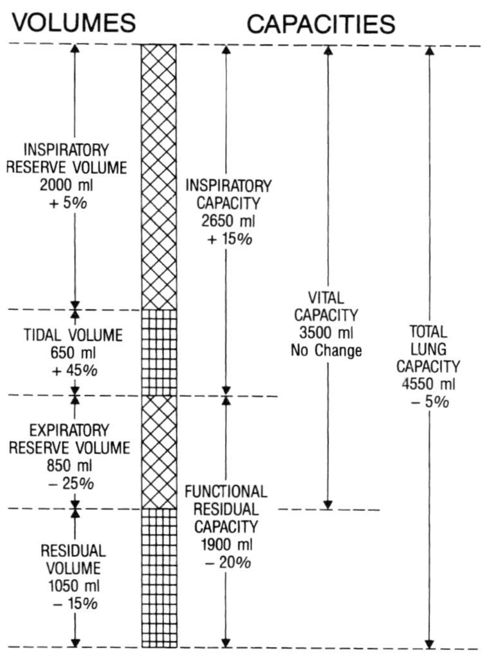

Fig. 5.2 Lung volumes and capacities at term gestation in absolute volumes and as the percentage change from nonpregnant values. The curves are derived from data in the following references cited in the text: 4, 7, 8, 16, 21, 23–25, 27–29, 30.

Inspiratory capacity increases during the third trimester to a level at term that is approximately 15% above that of nonpregnant individuals.[7,14,23,24] This change, which is due to an increase in inspiratory reserve volume, compensates for the reduction in expiratory reserve volume, so that vital capacity is unchanged,[4,7,14,16,21,23–26,30] and, in part, for the reduction of functional residual capacity, so that total lung capacity is only minimally reduced.[4,7,14,23,25,26]

Ventilation (Fig. 5.1 and Table 5.2)

Pregnancy is associated with an elevation of minute ventilation to a level at term that is 45% above that of nonpregnant individuals.[4,7,8,23,24,28,29] Since respiratory rate changes little during pregnancy, although it decreases slightly during mid-gestation,[4,8,23,24,28,29] the increase in minute ventilation parallels that of tidal volume.

Dead space increases by 40%–50% during gestation,[28,29] a change that is observed as early as the third month of gestation.[28] This is attributable to dilatation of the conducting airways, as evidenced by the decrease in airway resistance during gestation.[14,20,21] Since the ratio of dead space to tidal volume does not change during pregnancy,[28] the increase in alveolar ventilation (45%) is equivalent to the increase in minute ventilation.

Increased ventilation is accounted for by two factors. First, the increase in carbon dioxide production during pregnancy[8,29] necessitates an increase in alveolar ventilation to maintain the $Pa\text{CO}_2$. Ventilation is also affected by the hormonal changes of pregnancy. Progesterone increases the slope of the ventilatory response curve to arterial carbon dioxide, indicating an elevated sensitivity of the central respiratory center to carbon dioxide.[31] This hormone may also act as a primary respiratory center stimulant.[32] During pregnancy, as well as during the luteal phase of the menstrual cycle, the decrease in $Pa\text{CO}_2$ is closely related to the progesterone level in arterial blood.[33] Estrogens appear to have an additive effect to that of progesterone, and probably contribute to the increase in minute ventilation during gestation.[34] Since the elevation of minute ventilation[4,8,23,24,28] and fall in the $Pa\text{CO}_2$[28,35] precede the increase in carbon dioxide production,[8] the early changes in minute ventilation are attributable to the hormonal changes of pregnancy, whereas the later changes are due to both factors.

Gas exchange, blood gases and acid–base status

Diffusion capacity (Table 5.2)

The diffusion capacity of the lungs is the measure of gas

transferred per mmHg of partial pressure difference, which is proportional to the alveolar capillary surface area and the permeability of the respiratory membrane. During the first trimester, diffusion capacity has been reported to be significantly elevated over that of the nonpregnant state,[36] although a more limited study found first-trimester and nonpregnant values to be the same.[24] During the second and third trimesters, diffusion capacity is below that measured 2.5–5 months post-partum or in nonpregnant controls,[24,36,37] although pregnant subjects do have an appropriate increase in diffusion capacity with exercise.[37] The mechanism for the change in diffusion capacity is unclear since it does not correlate with pulmonary capillary blood volume, which is unchanged during gestation,[24] or with changes in hemoglobin concentration or hormone concentrations;[24,36] and it cannot be explained solely by alteration of alveolar volume, which decreases during gestation.[36]

Blood and alveolar gases (Fig. 5.3 and Table 5.3)

The $Pa\text{CO}_2$ decreases to a level of 28–32 mmHg by the end of the first trimester[28,35] and remains at that level until term gestation.[28,33,35,38–40] End-tidal carbon dioxide ($ETCO_2$) also decreases,[41] as expected, and, although there is a significant difference between $ETCO_2$ and $Pa\text{CO}_2$ in nonpregnant subjects, the partial pressures are essentially equivalent in pregnant individuals in early pregnancy,[42] at term[43,44] and in the early post-partum period.[45] The change in the relationship of $ETCO_2$ to $Pa\text{CO}_2$ can be attributed to a reduction of alveolar dead space (un- or under-perfused alveoli) which results from the marked increase of output during pregnancy (see below).

The decline in the $Pa\text{CO}_2$ results in an increase in the arterial partial pressure of oxygen ($Pa\text{O}_2$) because of the inverse relationship between the partial pressures of these two alveolar gases. For pregnant subjects in the upright position, reports have documented an increase in the $Pa\text{O}_2$ to 106–108 mmHg in the first trimester, 103–107 mmHg in the second trimester and 101–104 mmHg at term gestation, all of which are increased significantly compared with values for nonpregnant subjects.[28,35,40] The increase is also due, in part, to the decrease of physiologic shunt[28] and the reduced arteriovenous oxygen difference,[5,46] with an increase in the latter parameter in the last trimester accounting for the decline of the $Pa\text{O}_2$ in late pregnancy. The decrease in the arteriovenous oxygen difference during early pregnancy is due to an increase in cardiac output that is proportionately greater than the increase in oxygen consumption. This results in an increase in the mixed venous oxygen content since tissues extract a smaller proportion of the oxygen contained in blood when flow increases. When venous blood with a higher oxygen content passes through the

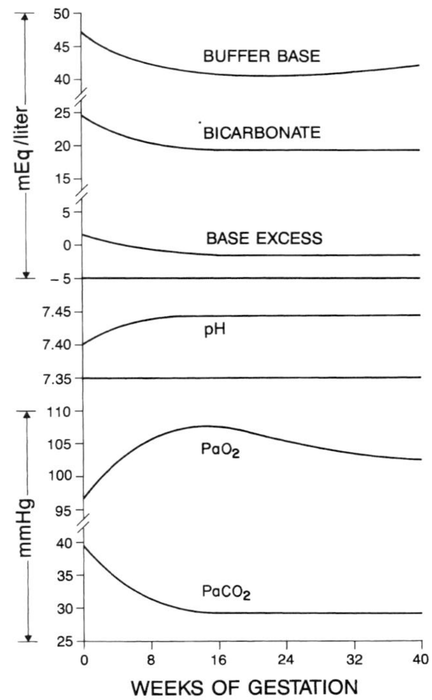

Fig. 5.3 Blood gas and acid–base values during pregnancy. The curves are derived from data in the following references cited in the text: 28, 33, 35, 38–41, 49–54.

Table 5.3 Blood gases and acid–base status at term* (From Conklin K A 1991 Semin Anesth 10: 221–234)

Arterial $P\text{O}_2$	103 mmHg
Arterial $P\text{CO}_2$	30 mmHg
Arterial pH	7.44
Base excess	−1.5 meq./l
Serum bicarbonate	19 meq./l
Total buffer base	42 meq./l

* Values are derived from data in the following references cited in the text: 28, 33, 35, 38–40, 49–51, 53, 54.

physiologic shunt in the lungs, it causes a smaller decrease of the arterial oxygen content and $Pa\text{O}_2$. In late pregnancy, the mixed venous oxygen content decreases because oxygen consumption continues to rise while cardiac output changes minimally.

The elevated $Pa\text{O}_2$ of pregnant subjects in erect posture suggests that, although functional residual capacity decreases during gestation,[4,7,14,23,27] it remains greater than closing capacity (the lung volume at which dependent lung zones cease to ventilate because of airway closure, causing an increase in physiologic shunt during normal tidal ventilation). This is supported by the observations that physiologic shunt does not increase and the alveolar to arterial oxygen gradient is unchanged during pregnancy,[28] and confirmed by measurements of functional residual capacity and closing capacity in pregnant subjects.[26,27]

When the $P\text{a}O_2$ is determined with pregnant patients in the supine position after mid-gestation, values are frequently below 100 mmHg.[38,39] Two factors contribute to the decreased $P\text{a}O_2$. First, functional residual capacity decreases in the supine position whereas closing capacity does not change, and Russell and Chambers[27] observed that closing capacity exceeds functional residual capacity in more than 50% of supine pregnant subjects during the second half of gestation, although Craig and Toole[26] found the prevalence to be only 8%. The second factor is reduced cardiac output, secondary to aortocaval compression (see below), which results in decreased mixed venous oxygen content. Several studies have documented these effects by demonstrating an increase in the $P\text{a}O_2$ and a decrease in the alveolar to arterial oxygen gradient in moving from the supine to the erect position,[40,47] and improved oxygen saturation in the lateral compared with the supine position.[48] Although an elevated $P\text{a}O_2$ was observed in supine pregnant subjects in one of the above-cited studies,[35] they were supine for only a short period of time before arterial sampling. Thus, there may have been insufficient time for airway closure or aortocaval compression to affect the $P\text{a}O_2$.

Acid–base status (Fig. 5.3 and Table 5.3)

The respiratory alkalosis of pregnancy is compensated for by an increase in renal excretion of bicarbonate. This is reflected by a decrease in serum bicarbonate to 18–21 meq./1,[35,38,49,50] a reduction of base excess by 2–3 meq./1[28,35,49,50] and a lowering of total buffer base, which includes protein and hemoglobin in addition to bicarbonate, by approximately 5 meq./1.[51] However, metabolic compensation does not fully compensate for the respiratory alkalosis. This has been shown by several investigators who have compared venous,[52] capillary[49,53,54] and arterial[28] blood pH in pregnant and nonpregnant individuals, documenting a pH increase of 0.02–0.06 units during gestation. Enhanced renal excretion of bicarbonate is attributable primarily to respiratory changes, although it may be due, in part, to reduced renal bicarbonate reabsorption resulting from hypervolemia and the increased levels of parathyroid hormone during pregnancy.[54]

Respiratory changes during labor

When parturients do not receive analgesia or anesthesia, minute ventilation, compared with that before labor begins, increases during contractions by 75–150% in the first stage of labor and by 150–350% during the second stage of labor.[10,55–57] The hyperventilation of labor is associated with significant hypocapnia. In patients who receive opioid analgesia, $P\text{a}CO_2$ values measured during contractions are 21–28 mmHg in the active phase of the first stage of labor and 16–24 mmHg during the second stage of labor and at the time of delivery.[56,58–61] Somewhat higher values are found between contractions.[58] When parturients do not receive analgesia during labor, $P\text{a}CO_2$ levels as low as 10–15 mmHg may be observed.[57]

The metabolic cost of hyperventilation is substantial. In pregnant subjects, a doubling of ventilation results in an increase of oxygen consumption by approximately 50% due to the elevated work of breathing, a cost substantially greater than that of nonpregnant subjects.[62] During labor, not only is ventilation commonly in excess of 100% above that before labor, but uterine activity further increases the metabolic demand. Thus, it is not surprising that the maternal aerobic requirement for oxygen exceeds oxygen consumption during parturition, which is confirmed by the progressive increase in blood lactate concentration (an index of anaerobic metabolism) during labor.[11,60,61,63,64]

Epidural anesthesia has a substantial effect on the respiratory changes induced by labor. When effective pain relief is accomplished during the first stage of labor, minute ventilation,[10,55,56] oxygen consumption[10,55] and the $P\text{a}CO_2$[56,59–61] remain at (or return to) values similar to those measured before labor begins. Additionally, the blood lactate concentration does not change,[60,61,63] which suggests that the aerobic oxygen requirement is being met. However, during the second stage of labor and at the time of delivery, even with epidural anesthesia, minute ventilation,[10] oxygen consumption[10] and the lactate concentration[61,63] increase, and the $P\text{a}CO_2$ decreases.[61] These effects are due to the elevated metabolic requirements of pushing, the increase in uterine activity that occurs as labor progresses and the stress and/or excitement of the delivery process, which increases muscular activity.

CARDIOVASCULAR PHYSIOLOGY

Examination of the heart

During the later stages of gestation the enlarging uterus alters the position of the heart, shifting it to the left and anteriorly and rotating it to a more transverse position.[12] This results in a shift of the apical impulse, which is more prominent during pregnancy, cephalad to the fourth intercostal space and laterally to, or beyond, the mid-clavicular line.

Beginning early in the second trimester, auscultation reveals accentuation of both components of the first heart sound with exaggerated splitting.[65] Phonocardiographic examination reveals that, although both the mitral and tricuspid elements move closer to the Q-wave, the mitral element moves more, thus increasing the time interval of the split. The second heart sound is little affected by pregnancy, although, during the last trimester, the interval between the aortic and pulmonic components tends to vary less than normal with respiration.[65] The third heart sound becomes loud and easily heard by mid-gestation.[65] Rarely, during early pregnancy, a fourth heart sound can be identified by phonocardiography (16% of patients) or auscultation (4% of patients), although it always disappears by term gestation in normal individuals.[65] An early to mid-systolic murmur, of grade I or II and heard best at the left sternal border, is commonly heard in pregnant individuals.[65] This appears to be secondary to tricuspid regurgitation resulting from dilation of the tricuspid annulus.[66]

The electrocardiogram during gestation reveals sinus tachycardia and a shortening of the uncorrected QT interval, reflecting the change in heart rate.[67] There is also shortening of the PR interval.[67] Depressed S–T segments and isoelectric or low voltage T-waves in the left-sided precordial and limb leads are observed in pregnant subjects more frequently than in nonpregnant individuals.[68] A Q-wave and negative T-wave may be observed in lead III during pregnancy.[69] The QRS axis exhibits a small rightward deviation during the first trimester,[67] but, during the third trimester, both rightward[70] and leftward[67] deviation have been reported. The T-wave axis exhibits a leftward deviation during pregnancy.[67] None of the electrocardiographic changes during pregnancy are clinically significant.

The radiographic appearance of the heart during pregnancy shows no characteristic changes, and it has been suggested that the same criteria for interpretation be utilized for pregnant and nonpregnant individuals.[17]

Echocardiographic measurements reveal progressive myocardial hypertrophy during pregnancy, with left ventricular enlargement being evident by mid-pregnancy and returning to the nonpregnant state by 4–6 weeks post-partum.[71,72]

Hemodynamics

Central hemodynamics (Fig. 5.4 and Table 5.4)

Measurements made by thermodilution,[73] echocardiography,[71,72,74–77] dye dilution[78,79] and cardiac catheterization using the Fick method[80] demonstrate that cardiac output increases substantially during gestation. Although there are discrepancies, most studies have yielded similar results when performed with the pregnant subjects in the resting state. Measurements were made with the subjects in the lateral position (during the second half of gestation), and an appropriate control (a matched group of nonpregnant subjects or the pregnant individuals studied several weeks post-partum) was utilized for comparison.

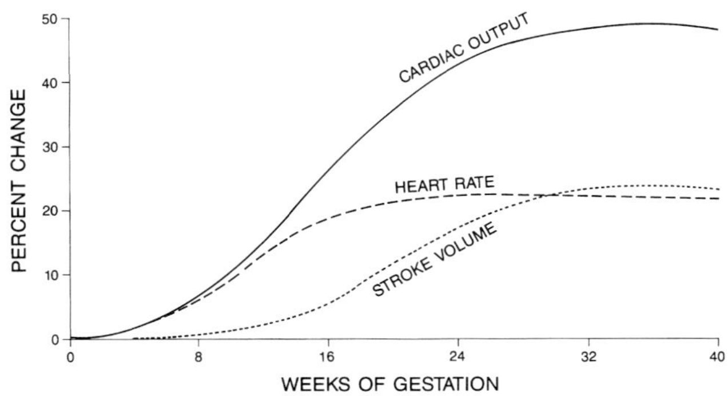

Fig. 5.4 Hemodynamic parameters during pregnancy. The curves are derived from data in the following references cited in the text: 71–80.

Table 5.4 Hemodynamic changes at term* (From Conklin K A 1991 Semin Anesth 10: 221–234)

Parameter	Change†
Cardiac output	+ 50%
Stroke volume	+ 25%
Heart rate	+ 20%
Left ventricular end-diastolic volume	Increased
Left ventricular end-systolic volume	No change
Ejection fraction	Increased
Left ventricular stroke work index	No change
Pulmonary capillary wedge pressure	No change
Central venous pressure	No change
Systemic vascular resistance	− 20%

* Values are derived from data in the following references cited in the text: 71–80.
† Changes relative to values for nonpregnant individuals.

Cardiac output is significantly elevated by 8–10 weeks of gestation and reaches a value that is 20% above the nonpregnant level by the end of the first trimester.[76,78,80] At the end of the second trimester cardiac output is elevated by nearly 50% and it remains essentially at that level until term.[71–79]

The rise in cardiac output during early pregnancy is attributable primarily to an increase in heart rate, which is elevated as early as 8 weeks of gestation and reaches a value that is 15% above the nonpregnant level by the end of the first trimester.[76,78] Stroke volume changes minimally during this time period.[71,72,76,78] During the second and third trimesters the further rise in cardiac output is due primarily to a progressive increase of stroke volume to a level at term that is approximately 25% above that of nonpregnant individuals.[71,72,74,76,77] Heart rate increases minimally during the last two trimesters of pregnancy.[72,76,77]

The elevation of stroke volume is accounted for by an increase in left ventricular end diastolic volume that occurs without a change in end-systolic volume.[71,74,76,77] Thus, ejection fraction increases.[74,76,77] This occurs without a change in myocardial contractility, since left ventricular stroke work index, measured by invasive means, is unaffected by pregnancy.[73] These results confirm observations using noninvasive techniques.[72] Additionally, elevation of end-diastolic volume occurs without a change in pulmonary capillary wedge pressure.[73] The lack of change of pulmonary artery diastolic pressure[46] is further evidence that left ventricular filling pressure during pregnancy is within the normal range for nonpregnant individuals. The apparent discrepancy between the filling pressure and end-diastolic volume is explained by ventricular dilatation, with the dilated left ventricle accommodating a greater volume without an increase in pressure. Right ventricular filling pressure (central venous pressure) is also unchanged during gestation.[73]

Regional blood flow

The elevation of cardiac output during the latter part of pregnancy amounts to at least 2000 ml/min.[72–75,79] The uterus, kidneys and extremities are the primary recipients of this increased blood flow.

The greatest proportionate increase in blood flow is that to the uterus. The relationship of factors that determine uterine blood flow (UBF) are as follows:

$$\text{UBF} = \text{UPP}/R = (\text{UAP}-\text{UVP})/(R_i+R_e)$$

In this relationship uterine perfusion pressure (UPP) equals uterine arterial pressure (UAP) minus uterine venous pressure (UVP), R_i is intrinsic vascular resistance (uterine vascular tone) and R_e is extrinsic vascular resistance (intrauterine pressure).[81] The pressure–flow relationship is nearly linear (as measured in sheep), with the pressure intercept at about 25 mmHg.[82] Under normal circumstances vascular resistance is at its minimum and uterine blood flow is maximal. Since vasodilation cannot occur by physiologic means, i.e. the uteroplacental vascular bed lacks an autoregulatory mechanism, uterine blood flow will not be maintained when perfusion pressure decreases due to reduction of uterine arterial pressure or elevation of uterine venous pressure.[83] From the above relationship, it also follows that an increase in intrinsic or extrinsic vascular resistance causes a decrease in uterine blood flow. For example, catecholamines cause uteroplacental vasoconstriction, and exposure of the uterine vasculature to these agents can result in a marked reduction of uterine blood flow.[84–86] An increase in extrinsic vascular resistance, as occurs during uterine contractions, similarly reduces uterine blood flow,[87–89] although an increase in uterine venous pressure[90] and a decrease in uterine arterial pressure[87] during contractions also contributes to the effect.

Assali et al,[91] using an electromagnetic flowmeter during therapeutic abortions, have made the only direct measurements of uterine blood flow in humans. They reported that uterine blood flow increased from 50 to 185 ml/min from weeks 10 to 28 of gestation. However, these measurements may not reflect actual uterine blood flow since determinations were made during administration of general or spinal anesthesia, either of which may reduce uterine blood flow by elevating catecholamines (general anesthesia) or causing maternal hypotension (spinal anesthesia).[92] Additionally, these patients may have been in the supine position, which can also reduce uterine blood flow after mid-gestation (see below). At term gestation, uterine blood flow has been estimated to be 500 ml/min utilizing the Fick principle with nitrous oxide,[93,94] although these determinations were also performed during administration of anesthesia, and most likely with patients in the supine position. More recently, measurements of uterine blood flow using intravenously injected ^{133}Xe in awake patients at term have obtained values of approximately 150 ml/min/100 g for intervillous blood flow and 8.5 ml/min/100 g for myometrial blood flow.[95–98] Since the weight of the uterus is approximately 1000 g and the estimated blood volume of the placenta is 500 ml,[99] blood flow determined by this technique would yield values of approximately 750 ml/min for intervillous blood flow, 85 ml/min for myometrial blood flow and 800–850 ml/min for total uterine blood flow.

Renal plasma flow increases during the first trimester, reaches a level by mid-pregnancy that is approximately 80% above the nonpregnant level, and is followed by a moderate decline as term gestation approaches.[100–103] Elevated renal plasma flow is associated with a 50% increase in the glomerular filtration rate,[100–103] a 50% increase in creatinine clearance,[102] and a reduction in the plasma creatinine concentration to a level of approximately 0.6 mg/100 ml.[102]

Skin perfusion, estimated by finger pulse volume, does not change until about 16 weeks of gestation, after which there is a slow rise until 20 weeks followed by a sharp increase between 20 and 30 weeks to a level at term that is 3–4 times the nonpregnant level.[104] Measurements by venous occlusion plethysmography yield similar results for hand perfusion, which, although less than nonpregnant values until 14 weeks, increase to a level at term that is 3–4 times higher.[105] Foot perfusion is reduced until 26 weeks of gestation, after which it increases to approximately twice the nonpregnant level at term.[105] An increase in skin temperature parallels the increase in perfusion.[106] Peripheral vasodilation provides a means to dissipate the additional heat production that accompanies the enhanced metabolism of pregnancy.

Other blood flow measurements have revealed no change in cerebral[107] or hepatic[108] perfusion during gestation.

Peripheral circulation

Serial blood pressure measurements by brachial sphygmomanometry reveal that systolic and diastolic arterial pressures decrease during gestation.[109–111] In the sitting or standing position, diastolic blood pressure decreases significantly by 8 weeks of gestation,[110] reaches its lowest level of approximately 15 mmHg below that of nonpregnant subjects between 20 and 30 weeks and returns nearly to the nonpregnant level at term.[109–111] In the lateral position, diastolic blood pressure is approximately 10 mmHg lower than in the sitting position.[109]

The decline in systolic blood pressure parallels that of diastolic blood pressure, although the magnitude depends upon how the study is performed. In patients who remain normotensive throughout pregnancy,[109] systolic blood pressure is approximately 20 mmHg below that of nonpregnant individuals by 17–20 weeks, and, although it increases throughout gestation as does diastolic blood pressure, it remains approximately 10 mmHg below the nonpregnant level at term. These investigators also observed that systolic blood pressure, like diastolic blood pressure, was 10 mmHg (or more) lower in the lateral position than in the sitting position. In contrast, when individuals that become hypertensive during gestation are included in the study population, the maximum decline in systolic blood pressure is less than 10 mmHg, and it returns to the nonpregnant level at term.[110,111] These results suggest that hypertensive disorders of pregnancy involve primarily systolic blood pressure, since diastolic blood pressures were similar in the three studies despite the differences in experimental design.

Age and parity also affect blood pressure during gestation, as does the technique of measurement. Blood pressure increases with advancing age, with diastolic blood pressure exhibiting a steady rise with increasing age whereas systolic blood pressure does not begin to increase until age 35.[112] For a given age, nulliparas have a higher mean blood pressure than parous individuals.[112] When measured intra-arterially, systolic blood pressure was found to be 7 mmHg lower and diastolic blood pressure 13 mmHg lower than values obtained using a sphygmomanometer.[113]

Changes in the peripheral vasculature are reflected in the decrease of systemic vascular resistance (Table 5.4). Bader et al[46] measured this parameter between the 14th and 40th weeks of gestation and found the value in early pregnancy to be approximately 25% below that at term, although at term, it is still 20–25% below that measured 2 weeks[75] or 11–13 weeks post-partum.[73] This change is due primarily to the low resistance of the uteroplacental vascular bed, although enhanced renal blood flow[100–103] and blood flow to the extremities[105] suggest a significant contribution from the kidneys, skeletal muscle and skin. The etiology of these changes is both anatomic, i.e. the addition of a low-resistance vascular bed (the intervillous space) during pregnancy, and hormonal. Prostacyclin production increases during gestation,[114,115] causing peripheral vasodilation. It also increases uterine blood flow in sheep,[116] although its effect on uterine blood flow in humans has been questioned.[117] Estrogens also cause a substantial increase in uterine blood flow[118] and produce peripheral vasodilation.[119,120] Progesterone may also exert a vasodilative effect.[120] The increase in systemic vascular resistance during the third trimester can be explained by compression of the aorta by the gravid uterus.

The changes in systemic vascular resistance, which reflects arteriolar tone, are consistent with the observed variation in diastolic blood pressure,[109–111] the value of which is dependent primarily upon systemic vascular resistance. Systolic blood pressure is determined by stroke volume and the distensibility of the larger arterial vessels, with a smaller influence from systemic vascular resistance. Since stroke volume increases during gestation, the decrease in systolic blood pressure must be due to enhanced arterial distensibility. This explanation is consistent with the observations that systolic blood pressure is lower during early gestation[109–111] when stroke volume has changed minimally,[71,72,76,78] but that it increases during late gestation[109–111] in parallel with the increase in stroke volume.[71,72,74,76,77]

Aortocaval compression

Angiographic studies reveal that the aorta and inferior vena cava are compressed by the gravid uterus when a pregnant woman, after mid-gestation, assumes the supine position. Kerr and co-workers[121,122] studied 10 patients between 38 and 40 weeks of gestation and two patients at 32 weeks with polyhydramnios. Ten of 12 individuals exhibited complete obstruction of the inferior vena cava at the level of the bifurcation, with venous return to the heart occurring primarily via the vertebral venous plexus and paraspinal veins, which empty into the azygos vein. Caval obstruction is also bypassed by the ovarian plexuses, which drain the uteroplacental vascular bed and enter the inferior vena cava proximal to the site of caval compression.[123] Partial obstruction of the aorta, at the level of the lumbar lordosis (L3–L5), has also been demonstrated in patients studied between week 27 of pregnancy and term gestation.[87,124] The higher pressure in the aorta, compared with the vena cava, prevents total occlusion in normotensive individuals, with the degree of occlusion increasing during arterial hypotension.[87]

However, collateral circulation via the azygos and ovarian veins does not compensate for obstruction of the inferior vena cava when a pregnant patient assumes the supine position. This is illustrated by venous pressure measurements. Femoral venous pressure, in the supine position, increases to 50% above nonpregnant or post-partum levels by 13–16 weeks of gestation,[125] which suggests that the hemodynamic consequences of aortocaval compression begin early in pregnancy. It progressively rises from there to a value at term that is approximately 2.5 times the nonpregnant level,[125,126] which corresponds to the pressure measured in the inferior vena cava below the level of compression by the uterus.[122,127] Although moving from the supine to the lateral position at term gestation results in a fall in femoral[126] and inferior vena cava[127] pressures, they remain approximately 100% above those of nonpregnant and post-partum subjects. These observations are consistent with angiographic studies,[121] and demonstrate that compression of the vena cava by the gravid uterus is not completely relieved in the lateral position.

The term pregnant woman in the lateral position exhibits a right ventricular filling pressure (central venous pressure) that is similar of that of a nonpregnant individual.[73] These data suggest that venous return in this position is maintained by collateral circulation, despite partial caval obstruction.[121] In the supine position, however, right atrial pressure falls substantially,[122,128] demonstrating that collaterals cannot compensate for complete, or nearly complete, caval obstruction. The fall in the cardiac filling pressure in moving from the lateral to the supine position results in a decrease in stroke volume of approximately 25%.[74,79,128–131] Since heart rate changes little with this maneuver,[79,122,129–131] cardiac output decreases to the same magnitude as does stroke volume.[74,79,122,128–133] These positional changes in stroke volume and cardiac output are evident by 20–28 weeks of gestation.[79] Additionally, a 15° tilt to the left also improves cardiac output compared with that in the supine position,[134] and once the fetal head is engaged in the pelvis the effect of the supine position on stroke volume and cardiac output is much reduced.[122,128]

In the pregnant patient at term, moving from the lateral to the supine position is associated with significant changes in regional blood pressure and blood flow. In the upper extremities, systolic, diastolic and mean blood pressures are substantially elevated in most patients[72,110,129] although blood flow exhibits little change.[135,136] The change in blood pressure is associated with a marked increase in systemic vascular resistance,[129] which can be attributed to compression of the aorta by the gravid uterus, and enhanced sympathetic nervous system outflow. In approximately 5% of individuals, however, a substantial drop in blood pressure occurs ('supine hypotensive syndrome'), which is associated with bradycardia (usually following a transient tachycardia) and maternal symptoms of hypotension including pallor, sweating and possibly syncope.[48,126,128,137] This is attributable to a profound drop in venous return for which the cardiovascular system cannot compensate.

When the pregnant patient assumes the supine position, blood flow decreases below the site at which the aorta is compressed, as shown by a decline of 20% in uterine blood flow[96] and of 40–50% in flow to the lower extremities.[135,136] Angiographic studies also document these changes, and confirm that perfusion of the uterus is affected to a lesser degree than that of the lower extremity and pelvic circuits.[123] The difference between the changes in blood flow to the uterus and the lower extremities is attributable to differences in venous outflow. Venous drainage of the uteroplacental vascular bed occurs, in part, via the ovarian plexuses, which enter the inferior vena cava proximal to the site of caval compression. Thus uterine blood flow decreases primarily as a result of compression of the aorta and reduction of uterine arterial pressure, with only a moderate obstruction of venous outflow and increase in uterine venous pressure. In contrast, venous drainage of the lower extremities is via the common iliac veins, which join to form the inferior vena cava distal to the site of caval obstruction. Therefore, lower extremity blood flow decreases due to the decrease in arterial pressure as well as a marked increase in venous pressure.[125,126]

Hemodynamics during parturition

Cardiac output, during labor and in the absence of uterine contractions, increases over prelabor values by 10% in the early first stage, 25% in the late first stage and 30–50% in the second stage.[138–140] Since heart changes are minimal, these elevations are due to increases in stroke volume. There is also a rise in systolic and diastolic blood pressures during the late first stage and the second stage of labor. These effects can be attributed to sympathetic nervous system activity, which increases during the active phase of the first stage and the second stage of labor and peaks at the time of delivery,[141–146] and results in elevation of systemic vascular resistance, myocardial contractility and central venous pressure.[139,140] This mechanism explains why epidural analgesia/anesthesia which reduces the maternal sympathetic nervous system response to the stress,[143–146] reduces cardiac output during labor.[139]

Uterine contractions cause a further increase of 15–30% in cardiac output and stroke volume[130,138–140,147,148] and a rise in mean arterial pressure of approximately 10%.[90,138,140,148] During contractions, augmentation of stroke volume can be attributed to a significant elevation of central venous pressure,[90,138,140] which results from further elevation of maternal sympathetic nervous system activity and from displacement of 300–500 ml of blood from the intervillous space.[90,148] The mechanism responsible for the latter effect has been illustrated by radiographic techniques. During a uterine contraction, complete (or nearly complete) occlusion of the abdominal aorta occurs, which prevents blood from entering the intervillous space.[87,124,149] Uterine venous outflow, however, is less impeded because of drainage via the ovarian plexuses,[123] and, as intrauterine pressure rises, blood is forced from the intervillous space into the central venous circulation. These changes also markedly impair uterine blood flow, due primarily to enhanced compression of the aorta during contractions, although maternal stress also contributes to the effect.[150,151] However, the effect of stress on uterine blood flow is relieved when maternal blood levels of catecholamines are reduced by administration of epidural analgesia/anesthesia.[152,153]

Immediately post-partum, cardiac output and stroke volume increase to 80% above prelabor values, while heart rate does not change.[139] During the next hour, cardiac output decreases to approximately 30% above prelabor levels, with a lesser decline in stroke volume and a moderate decrease in heart rate.[139,140] Central venous pressure, compared with values measured during labor, is elevated by 50% throughout this period[140] and accounts for the increase in stroke volume. The sustained elevation of central venous pressure can be explained by relief of aortocaval compression which improves venous return, transcapillary refill in the lower extremities which results from reduced venous pressure and a reduction of vascular capacitance (at least 500 ml owing to loss of the intervillous space) that exceeds the volume of blood lost at the time of delivery ('autotransfusion'). These changes result in a hypervolemic state compared with the predelivery condition.

Hematology

Red blood cell, plasma and blood volumes (Fig. 5.5 and Table 5.5)

Measurement of plasma and total blood volume must be made with patients in the lateral position since determina-

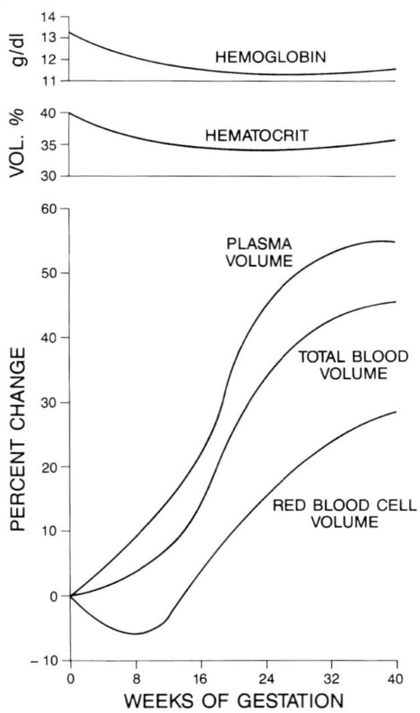

Fig. 5.5 Hemoglobin concentration, hematocrit, blood volume, plasma volume and red blood cell volume during pregnancy. The curves are derived from data in the following references cited in the text: 7, 76,

Table 5.5 Hematologic changes at term* (From Conklin K A 1991 Semin Anesth 10: 221–234)

Blood volume	+ 45%†
Plasma volume	+ 55%†
Red blood cell volume	+ 30%†
Hematocrit	35.5
Hemoglobin	11.6g/dl

* Values are derived from data in the following references cited in the text: 7, 76, 78, 155–167.
† Changes relative to values for nonpregnant individuals.

tions performed in the supine position in individuals beyond 30–32 weeks of gestation will underestimate these parameters.[154] Inaccurate measurements in the supine position of near-term subjects results from loss of plasma volume to the extravascular compartment of the lower extremities, because of the increased venous pressure, and from incomplete mixing of the marker (dye or isotopically labeled compound) within the plasma volume.

An increase in plasma volume is evident by 6 weeks of pregnancy,[155] reaching a value by the end of the first trimester that is 15% above the nonpregnant level.[155–159] Subsequently there is a steep increase until 28–30 weeks of gestation, followed by a more gradual rise to a volume at term that is 55% above the nonpregnant level.[155–161] In contrast, red blood cell mass decreases during the first 8 weeks of gestation,[155,158] but increases thereafter to a level at term that is nearly 30% above the nonpregnant level.[155,158,159,161,162] At term, these changes result in a 45% increase in total blood volume,[7,161–163] and a reduction in the hemoglobin concentration and hematocrit to values of 11.6 g/100 ml and 35.5 vol % respectively. However, the decline in the latter two parameters is greater during the second trimester (15%) than at term (10%)[7,78,158–162,164–167] because red cell mass increases to a proportionately greater degree than does plasma volume during the last trimester.[155] The changes in hemoglobin concentration and hematocrit occur even when iron is administered during gestation,[158,159,162,166] although the decreases are greater in individuals who do not receive this therapy.[158]

The changes in red blood cell, plasma and blood volume tend to show considerable variability between individuals, although the same changes tend to be repeated in successive pregnancies in any given individual.[155,162] Additionally, these volumes increase to a greater degree with twin pregnancies than with single pregnancies.[161,162] The changes are also positively correlated with the size of the fetus in single pregnancies.[157]

Estrogens and progesterone appear to be responsible for the increase in plasma volume during pregnancy. Estrogens increase plasma renin activity,[168] which enhances hepatic angiotensinogen production. This results in an elevation of the blood level of angiotensin, which stimulates adrenal aldosterone production.[169] The actual control may be by the fetus since the estrogen precursor, dehydroepiandosterone, is produced by the fetal adrenal glands.[170] Progesterone also enhances aldosterone production[171] by inhibiting its sodium-retaining action on the renal tubules,[172] which results in sodium diuresis, relative hypovolemia, decreased renal blood flow and elevated renin secretion. Placental lactogen also increases aldosterone production.[173] The hyperaldosteronism of pregnancy results in retention of 500–900 meq. of sodium and an increase of 6000–8000 ml of total body water, of which 70% is extracellular.[174]

Elevated red blood cell volume can be attributed to an increase in the serum erythropoietin concentration during pregnancy, with the absence of increased activity until 8–12 weeks of gestation explaining the early delay in enhanced erythrocyte production.[175,176] Erythropoiesis may also be stimulated by prolactin, progesterone and placental lactogen.[170,173]

The clinical significance of hemodilution during pregnancy is open to conjecture. However, since increased blood viscosity is associated with thrombosis, Koller[177] suggests that hemodilution and decreased viscosity of maternal blood decreases the risk of intervillous thrombosis and infarction, occurrences that are frequent even in normal pregnancy.[178] Thus, adequate hemodilution may be essential for preservation of the patency of the uteroplacental vascular bed. This contention is supported by the observation that large placental infarcts, leading to intrauterine growth retardation and fetal death, are positively correlated with the maternal hemoglobin concentration and hematocrit.[179] It could also be argued that fetal well-being is jeopardized in an abnormal fetus who is unable to secrete adequate estrogen precursors, thus impairing plasma volume expansion.

Plasma proteins and colloid osmotic pressure (Table 5.6)

The total serum protein concentration decreases by approximately 10% during the first trimester, from a nonpregnant value of 7.3 g/100 ml to 6.6 g/100 ml, and subsequently changes little, reaching a value at term of 6.5 g/100 ml.[164,180–184] The change is due primarily to a decline in the albumin concentration, which decreases from 4.4 to 3.9 g/100 ml in the first trimester and progressively declines throughout the remainder of pregnancy to a level (3.4 g/100 ml) at term that is 20–25% below that of nonpregnant individuals.[160,164,180–185] Although the concentration of globulins declines by 10% during the first trimester, the level rises subsequently to a value at term that is 5–10% above the nonpregnant level.[164,181–185] These changes result in a progressive decrease in the albumin to globulin ratio from approximately 1.5 in nonpregnant individuals to 1.1 at term. Maternal colloid osmotic pressure decreases in parallel with the decline in serum albumin concentration, from nonpregnant values of 25–26 mmHg to approximately 22 mmHg at term.[164,186–188]

Table 5.6 Plasma proteins and colloid osmotic pressure*

	Nonpregnant	Term
Albumin	4.4 g%	3.4 g%
Globulin	2.9 g%	3.1 g%
A/G ratio†	1.5	1.1
Total protein	7.3 g%	6.5 g%
COP‡	26 mmHg	22 mmHg

* Values are derived from data in the following references cited in the text: 160, 164, 180–188.
† Albumin to globulin ratio.
‡ Colloid osmotic pressure.

Coagulation (Table 5.7)

Significant changes in the concentration of most coagulation factors occur during pregnancy. The fibrinogen (factor I) concentration increases early in pregnancy, reaching a level by the end of the first trimester that is 20–30% above the nonpregnant value.[184,189–192] The fibrinogen concentration at term is approximately 100% higher than that of nonpregnant individuals,[184,189–193] with the concentration of some subjects reaching 600 mg/100 ml.[190,194] The concentrations of factor VII (proconvertin),[195,196] factor VIII (antihemophilic factor)[190,192,195] and factor IX (Christmas factor)[197] also increase by at least 100% during gestation, whereas that of factors X (Stuart–Power factor)[190,195,196] and XII (Hageman factor)[190] increases by approximately 30%. The concentrations of prothrombin (factor II)[194–196] and factor V (proaccelerin)[192,194,195] do not change during

Table 5.7 Coagulation at term*

Parameter	Change†
Factor I (fibrinogen)	+ 100%
Factor II (prothrombin)	No change
Factor V (proaccelerin)	No change
Factor VII (proconvertin)	+ 100%
Factor VIII (antihemophilic factor)	+ 150%
Factor IX (Christmas factor)	+ 100%
Factor X (Stuart–Power factor)	+ 30%
Factor XI (thromboplastin antecedent)	+ 40%
Factor XII (Hageman factor)	+ 30%
Factor XIII (fibrin-stabilizing factor)	− 50%
Platlet count	− 5%
Prothrombin time	Shortened (20%)
Partial thromboplastin time	Shortened (20%)
Bleeding time	Shortened (10%)
Fibrin degradation products	+ 100%

* Values are derived from data in the following references cited in the text: 165, 184, 189–201, 204, 205.
† Changes relative to values for nonpregnant individuals.

pregnancy, and there is a 40–50% decrease in the concentrations of factors XI (plasma thromboplastin antecedent)[190] and XIII (fibrin-stabilizing factor).[198] These changes result in a shortening, by approximately 20%, of the prothrombin time and the partial thromboplastin time.[194]

Most investigators have observed a moderate decline of the platelet count during gestation, with the reduction at term amounting to approximately 15%.[165,190,194,199–201] Since the mean platelet volume rises constantly and significantly throughout pregnancy, the decline in platelet count is attributable to increased platelet consumption.[201] Pregnancy does not affect platelet adhesiveness[192] or ADP- and epinephrine-induced aggregation.[199] Bleeding time, however, is reported to be reduced by 10% in pregnant patients at term.[199]

Elevated intravascular fibrin deposition, presumably involving the uteroplacental circulation, is evident by the second month of gestation and progressively increases until term.[189] Although the fibrinolytic system appears to be depressed, as shown by the decrease in plasminogen activator,[190–192,202] the increase in fibrinolytic inhibitors[202] and the prolonged euglobulin lysis time,[203] fibrinolysis overall is increased.[189] This is evidenced by the elevation of fibrin degradation products throughout pregnancy,[204,205] and possibly explained by the marked increase in the plasminogen concentration.[190–192,202]

Plasma cholinesterase

The concentration of plasma cholinesterase falls abruptly during pregnancy to approximately 80% of the nonpregnant level by the end of the first trimester.[206–209] A further decline, to 70–75% of control values, occurs by mid-gestation, and it remains at that level until term.[206–209]

Hematologic changes during parturition and the puerperium

Blood loss at the time of vaginal delivery averages 450 ml, which amounts to 25–30% of the blood volume expansion of pregnancy.[163,210] Loss of another third (approximately 600 ml) of the volume expansion occurs during the first 24 h post-partum,[163,211] which is followed by little change in blood volume for the next 3–6 days.[163,210,211] Subsequently, plasma volume continues to fall while red blood cell volume remains constant, which results in hemoconcentration, as reflected by the increasing hematocrit.[155] Blood volume returns to normal by 6–9 weeks post-partum.[155]

During cesarean delivery, blood loss is approximately 900 ml,[163,210] and appears to be independent of the type of anesthesia used since the change in post-delivery hematocrit is the same with regional anesthesia as with general anesthesia utilizing nitrous oxide/oxygen or nitrous oxide/oxygen/halothane (0.3–1.0% before delivery).[212] By 1 week post-partum, the blood volume changes following vaginal delivery and cesarean delivery are equivalent, although the hematocrit of patients delivered by cesarean delivery is less because of their greater blood loss at the time of delivery.[163,210]

Total protein and albumin concentrations decline following delivery, remain below those of term pregnant patients until 2–3 days post-partum and, although subsequent increases occur, are still below values for nonpregnant subjects at 6–12 weeks post-partum.[180,182,184] Globulins are moderately elevated during the first week post-partum compared with term pregnant subjects,[182,184] and the albumin to globulin ratio during this time period falls to values below that of term gestation.[182] These changes in protein concentrations are associated with a marked drop in colloid osmotic pressure following delivery,[186] with return to the nonpregnant level by 6 weeks post-partum.[164]

Placental separation during delivery is associated with activation of the clotting mechanism, reflected by a reduction in clotting time and a decrease in plasma fibrinogen.[213] Within an hour after delivery, fibrinolytic activity returns to nonpregnant levels and the concentration of fibrin/fibrinogen degradation products increases[213] and remains elevated during the first week post-partum.[214] In the early puerperium, the fibrinogen concentration rises to a level above that measured at term, remaining elevated for approximately 1 week before it declines to the nonpregnant level 1 month following delivery.[184,189,213] The platelet count also rises within 3–5 days after delivery.[213]

Plasma cholinesterase activity falls during the early puerperium to a level that is approximately 15% below that measured at term, and 30–35% below the nonpregnant level.[207–209]

GASTROINTESTINAL PHYSIOLOGY

Pregnant patients, at term gestation, are generally considered to be at greater risk of aspiration pneumonitis than are nonpregnant individuals. Factors that may alter the risk during pregnancy include changes in gastrointestinal anatomy, motility or secretions. However, measurements of gastric volume, gastric acidity and barrier pressure, i.e. the difference between intragastric pressure and the tone of the lower esophageal high-pressure zone (sphincter), provide a more objective assessment of risk.

Anatomy

The stomach and intestines during pregnancy are displaced cephalad into the left dome of the diaphragm by the enlarging uterus, and the axis of the stomach is rotated to the right approximately 45° and shifted from a vertical to a horizontal position.[215] This changes the angle of the gastroesophageal junction and may cause pocketing of the gastric contents.

Gastrointestinal motility

Esophageal peristalsis in pregnant individuals has a lower wave speed and lower amplitude compared with nonpregnant women.[216] Davison et al,[217] using a dye dilution technique, found gastric emptying to be significantly prolonged in individuals whose pregnancy was at least 34 weeks. They also found that pregnant individuals with symptomatic gastroesophageal reflux exhibited a greater delay in gastric emptying. O'Sullivan et al,[218] however, using an epigastric impedance technique, found gastric emptying to be similar in nonpregnant and term pregnant women. Assessments by absorption of paracetamol following oral administration[219] and applied potential tomography[220] also show that gastric emptying is the same in nonpregnant women as it is in first, second and third trimester, and term pregnant. Thus most data provide evidence that gastric emptying is unaltered during pregnancy.

Small intestinal transit time is prolonged during the first half of gestation.[221] Transit time from ingestion of a test meal to its delivery to the cecum is also significantly prolonged in individuals during the third trimester.[222]

Gastric secretions

Murray et al,[223] observed that the basal gastric acid secretion rate and the histamine-induced maximal secretory capacity were reduced between the 10th and 30th weeks of gestation. These results explain earlier results that demonstrate that pregnant women exhibit a relative hypochlorhydria, which is most marked during early to mid-gestation.[224] Consistent with these findings are those which show that the plasma level of gastrin, which stimulates gastric acid secretion, is depressed during early pregnancy but increases toward the nonpregnant level during the last trimester,[225] although this study also reported that the basal and pentagastrin-stimulated acid secretory rates were the same at 12, 24 and 36 weeks of gestation and between 1 and 4 weeks post-partum. Additionally, the plasma pepsin level, which is an indirect measure of the rate of gastric secretions, is depressed through the seventh month of gestation and returns to the nonpregnant level during the eight month.[226]

Gastric volume and pH (Table 5.8)

The use of gastric volume and acidity as a measure of patient risk of aspiration pneumonitis has limitations. Most authors have utilized a pH of ≤ 2.5 and a volume of ≥ 25 ml as the definition of 'at risk'. However, these criteria for the volume[227] and pH[228] of gastric contents that are necessary to produce pneumonitis were derived from animal experiments. The authors who originally proposed the criteria even stated that they had been arbitrarily defined.[227] Additionally, there is an important interaction between volume and pH of aspirates, i.e. the lower the pH the lower the volume required to produce severe pulmonary damage and death.[229] Finally, most authors have determined volume by means of gastric aspiration via a nasogastric tube, which is a technique that does not reliably remove all stomach contents and may be less efficient in pregnant patients because of pocketing of gastric contents.

Table 5.8 Volume and pH of gastric contents* (From Conklin K A 1991 Semin Anesth 10: 221–234)

Patients†	Volume ⩾ 25 ml	pH ⩽ 2.5	'At risk'‡
Nonpregnant	44%	87%	42%
Early gestation (15 weeks)	51%	69%	37%
Term gestation	59%	71%	49%
In labor	69% (>40 ml)	36%	23%

* Values are derived from data in the following references cited in the text: 227, 230–242, 255–259.
† None received opioids, anticholinergic agents, antacids, histamine-2 antagonists or metoclopramide.
‡ Volume ≥ 25 ml and pH ≤ 2.5.

Despite the limitations of using gastric volume and acidity measurement to determine the risk of aspiration pneumonitis, these parameters, when measured by uniform techniques, do provide a means for comparing the relative risk of pregnant and nonpregnant subjects. This, of course, assumes that nasogastric aspiration is equally effective in obtaining gastric contents from both groups of subjects. Additionally, since individuals may respond differently to medication that alters gastric volume or acidity, e.g. antacids, opioids, anticholinergics, histamine-2 antagonists and agents such as metoclopramide, data for comparative purposes should be derived only from unmedicated subjects.

Several investigators have reported such results for nonpregnant individuals undergoing elective surgery[230–237] and pregnant patients undergoing elective cesarean delivery[227,238–242] with all measurements being made shortly after induction of general anesthesia. Combining the results of these studies, 87% of the 166 nonpregnant patients studied had a gastric pH of ≤ 2.5. In 71% of 79 parturients the findings were similar,[238–242] with a lower proportion of low pH values, possibly because of the relative hypochlorhydria of pregnancy.[223,224] 44% of 55 nonpregnant subjects[235–237] and 59% of 54 parturients[240–242] had a gastric volume of ≥ 25 ml. The percentages of patients 'at risk', i.e. having a pH of 2.5 or less and a volume of 25 ml or greater, were 42% of 55 nonpregnant subjects[235–237] and 49% of 78 parturients.[227,240–242] Therefore, based on criteria of gastric volume and acidity, pregnant patients who have been without oral intake in preparation for elective cesarean delivery appear to be at little, if any, greater risk for aspiration pneumonitis than are nonpregnant individuals for elective surgery.

During early gestation (mean of 15 weeks), 69% of patients have a pH of 2.5 or less, 51% have a volume of 25 ml or greater and 37% are 'at risk' by the above criteria.[237] Although the overall 'at risk' proportion was low for the pregnant patients, it was similar to that of the nonpregnant individuals who were investigated in this study.

Barrier pressure

Pyrosis (heartburn) occurs in 50–80% of pregnant women,[243–245] although the prevalence may vary significantly between races.[243] Gastroesophageal reflux, the cause of pyrosis, occurs when there is a reduction in the barrier pressure, due to either an elevation of intragastric pressure or a reduction in tone of the lower esophageal high-pressure zone.

Intragastric pressure of women during the last trimester and at term is substantially elevated compared to that of nonpregnant subjects,[216,243,244,246–249] with no difference between pregnant patients with and without pyrosis.[246–249] In pregnant patients without pyrosis, the tone of the high-pressure zone also rises,[243,244,247–249] in response to the increase in intragastric pressure, and the barrier pressure is equivalent to[247,249] or greater than[244,248] that of nonpregnant subjects. In contrast, pregnant women with pyrosis have a decrease,[244,246,248,249] no change[244] or only a small increase[247] in the tone of the high-pressure zone, and these women exhibit a decrease in the barrier pressure.[244,246–249] This is attributed to displacement of the intra-abdominal segment of the esophagus into the thorax, which prevents the usual increase in lower esophageal tone that accompanies a rise in intragastric pressure.[243,244] Thus, compared with asymptomatic pregnant women, those with pyrosis are at an increased risk of regurgitation and pulmonary aspiration of gastric contents during administration of obstetric anesthesia.

Women with pyrosis during early gestation (8–20 weeks) also have a reduction in barrier pressure, which is reported to be due to an increase in intragastric pressure without a change in tone of the high-pressure zone.[250] Some authors have found a reduction in the barrier pressure even in asymptomatic women between 12 and 20 weeks of gestation, although these subjects exhibited a reduction of lower esophageal tone.[251] It has been proposed that progesterone reduces the tone of the high-pressure zone,[252] which would account for these results. However, if progesterone exerts this effect, other factors, e.g. the increase in intragastric pressure during late pregnancy, counteract the effect and account for the increase in tone at term gestation.[243,244,247–249]

Effects of labor on gastrointestinal function

Roberts and Shirley[227] observed that, during labor, gastric volume decreases slowly; the minimum gastric volume is attained between 12 and 20 h after a meal; and, after 20 h following a meal, gastric volume increases. Other investigators, by measuring the rate of gastric emptying following a test meal[217,218,253] or the rate of acetaminophen absorption after oral administration,[254] have confirmed that labor delays gastric emptying in term pregnant subjects.

Several investigators have evaluated gastric volume and acidity of parturients who have not received medication that would alter gastric contents. Taylor and Pryse-Davies[225] found that 69% of 52 patients in labor had gastric volumes greater than 40 ml, which contrasts with only 59% of patients at term but not in labor who have volumes ≥25 ml[240–242] (Table 5.8). Others have also found that the mean gastric volume increases during labor.[227,256,257] However, only 36% of 74 patients in labor were reported to have a gastric pH ≤2.5,[255,258] and only 23% of 35 patients met the criteria of being 'at risk'[227,259] (Table 5.8). Therefore, these data suggest that, compared with individuals at term but not in labor, patients in labor have delayed gastric emptying and elevated gastric volume, but their gastric pH is higher and the proportion of individuals 'at risk' is lower.

Effect of analgesia during labor on gastrointestinal physiology

O'Sullivan and Bullingham[260] measured gastric pH changes following sodium citrate administration during labor and observed that epidural anesthesia delayed the return to basal pH. They suggested that this represents delayed gastric emptying, although other explanations, such as an alteration of gastric secretion during epidural anesthesia, could also explain the results. In contrast, Holdsworth[257] found a lower mean gastric volume in laboring patients with epidural anesthesia than in those without.

Administration of intramuscular opioids during labor results in a substantial delay of gastric emptying as shown by delayed acetaminophen absorption,[254,256] prolonged retention of a test meal[218,253] and a delay in the return to basal gastric pH following antacid administration.[260] These results are consistent with those that demonstrate that parturients who receive intramuscular opioids have a substantial increase in mean gastric volume compared with those who receive no analgesia.[257,261,262] Opioids also decrease the barrier pressure by reducing the tone of the lower esophageal high-pressure zone.[263,264] Thus, opioids that are administered during labor enhance a patient's risk of aspiration pneumonitis.

It is also common practice to utilize epidural opioids for analgesia during labor with or without local anesthetics.

However, epidural fentanyl used for analgesia during labor[265] or following cesarean delivery[266] does delay gastric emptying. Thus, this form of obstetric analgesia also increases the parturient's risk of aspiration pneumonitis.

Post-partum changes in gastrointestinal physiology

Gastric pH, gastric volume and the proportion 'at risk' are the same in nonpregnant individuals undergoing elective surgery as in patients who have been without oral intake for 1–42 h post-partum.[230,267] However, gastric volume is greater from 1 to 8 h and from 24 to 42 h post-partum than it is from 9 to 23 h post-partum.[230]

ANESTHETIC IMPLICATIONS

Patient positioning

Aortocaval compression by the term gravid uterus may result in 'supine hypotensive syndrome' when a pregnant patient assumes the supine position, although this is an infrequent occurrence.[48,126,137] However, uterine blood flow is significantly reduced in all term pregnant women when they assume the supine position.[96] Although this decrease is tolerated by the healthy fetus, further impairment of uterine blood flow compromises fetal well-being. For example, the added reduction of uterine blood flow caused by uterine contractions[87–89] and elevation of sympathetic nervous system activity[150,151] results in an increase in late decelerations,[268] reduced fetal scalp capillary blood pH,[268–270] a drop in fetal transcutaneous Po_2[271] and lower neonatal Apgar scores[270] when parturients labor in the supine position as compared with other positions. Similarly, neonatal acidosis is greater[272,273] and Apgar scores are lower[272] when patients, during cesarean delivery, are placed in the supine position as compared with the lateral tilted position. Since neonatal depression correlates with prolonged uterine incision to delivery intervals,[274,275] uterine blood flow is, most likely, impaired during this period of time and adds to the adverse effect of the supine position.

During administration of anesthesia, as well as at other times, measures should be taken to minimize aortocaval compression. Effective maneuvers include positioning the patient in the lateral position, elevating the right hip with a wedge or utilizing a device that manually displaces the uterus to the left, although mechanical devices appear to be less effective than other means since they do not relieve the aortic component of vascular compression.[276] Since adverse effects of supine positioning are evident early in pregnancy, i.e. elevated femoral venous pressure by 13–16 weeks[125] and depressed stroke volume and cardiac output by 20–28 weeks,[79] the above measures should be utilized for pregnant patients before they reach term gestation.

'Full-stomach' considerations

Evidence suggests that gastric volume and acidity of pregnant patients,[227,238–242] even those in labor,[227,255,258,259] does not place them at greater risk of aspiration pneumonitis than nonpregnant individuals[230–237] (Table 5.8). Thus, there is controversy as to the need to administer an antacid, e.g. sodium citrate,[242] to elevate gastric pH; a histamine-2 receptor antagonist, e.g. cimetidine or ranitidine,[239,241] to reduce gastric acid secretions; or an agent, such as metoclopramide,[240] to enhance gastric emptying and elevate lower esophageal tone. However, since 50–80% of pregnant patients, i.e. those with pyrosis,[243–245] are predisposed to pulmonary aspiration of gastric contents because of their reduced barrier pressure,[244,246–249] justification can be made to reduce gastric volume and acidity by pharmacologic or chemical means.

Prudent management dictates the use of endotracheal intubation to secure the airway whenever general anesthesia is utilized for obstetric procedures. This should be accomplished following the rapid-sequence administration of an intravenous induction agent and succinylcholine during induction of anesthesia, accompanied by the Sellick maneuver.[277] Many authors also suggest the use of a small dose of nondepolarizing muscle relaxant, prior to administration of succinylcholine, to prevent the rise of intragastric pressure caused by fasciculations.[278] However, barrier pressure increases when succinylcholine-induced fasciculations occur since the lower esophageal pressure rises more than the intragastric pressure.[279] Additionally, precurarization delays the onset, reduces the intensity and shortens the duration of a succinylcholine-induced block,[280,281] which could cause either a delay or failure when attempting endotracheal intubation. Therefore, it is best to avoid the practice of precurarization in pregnant patients.

General anesthesia (Table 5.9)

Endotracheal intubation

Pregnant patients, beginning early in the first trimester, experience capillary engorgement of the nasal and oropharyngeal mucosa and larynx.[12] Thus, the internal diameter of the trachea is reduced and the endotracheal tubes used for pregnant women should be smaller than those used for nonpregnant women. Since mucosal engorgement predisposes to nasopharyngeal trauma in pregnant women,[13] nasotracheal intubation should be avoided.

Maternal oxygenation and ventilation

Moving from the upright to the supine position results in a greater decrease of the Pao_2 in pregnant than in non-

Table 5.9 Anesthetic implications of maternal physiology: general anesthesia (From Conklin K A 1991 Semin Anesth 10: 221–234)

Endotracheal intubation
Smaller endotracheal tube required (e.g. 6–8 mm)
Greater risk of trauma with nasotracheal intubation
Maternal oxygenation
Greater increase of physiologic shunt when supine
More rapid denitrogenation
More rapid fall in Pa_{O_2} during apnea (139 mmHg/min)
Maternal ventilation
Higher minute ventilation required (121 ml/kg/min)
Inhalation anesthesia
More rapid rate of induction
Reduced minimum alveolar concentration (30%)
Muscle relaxants
Reduced sensitivity to succinylcholine (?)
Elevated sensitivity to nondepolarizing relaxants

pregnant women.[47] This is due to a decline of functional residual capacity to a volume that is below closing capacity in many pregnant individuals.[26,27] It is evident during preparation for general anesthesia since, following 5 min of acute oxygenation or denitrogenation, the Pa_{O_2} of parturients was 473 mmHg compared with 507 mmHg in nonpregnant women.[282] The decrease in functional residual capacity also reduces the parturient's oxygen reserve during periods of apnea. Thus, during induction of general anesthesia, the Pa_{O_2} falls more rapidly in pregnant women (139 mmHg/min) than it does in nonpregnant women (58 mmHg/min),[282] although the elevation of oxygen consumption during pregnancy[4–8] also contributes to the more rapid decline. The reduction of functional residual capacity and elevation of minute ventilation result in more rapid denitrogenation during pregnancy.

Optimal minute ventilation during general anesthesia, i.e. that required to maintain a normal Pa_{CO_2} for the parturient (approximately 30 mmHg), is 121 ml/kg/min, a value much greater than that (77 ml/kg/min) required to maintain a comparable Pa_{CO_2} in nonpregnant women.[284] This is attributable to the elevation of carbon dioxide production during pregnancy. Maternal hyperventilation, however, should be avoided because it reduces uterine blood flow and results in fetal hypoxia and acidosis and low neonatal Apgar scores.[285–288] The reduction of uterine blood flow is due to a decrease of cardiac output, resulting from positive-pressure ventilation, which increases intrathoracic pressure and reduces venous return,[289] and to the increase of uterine vascular resistance that occurs when the Pa_{CO_2} falls below 30 mmHg.[290] Hypocapnia, and its associated respiratory alkalosis, also contributes to deterioration of the fetus by reducing umbilical blood flow and increasing the affinity of maternal hemoglobin for oxygen.[285]

Inhalation anesthesia

The rate of induction of anesthesia, i.e. the rate of rise of the alveolar anesthetic concentration relative to that of the inspired gas, increases during pregnancy.[291] This is due to the decrease of functional residual capacity and the increase of minute ventilation, both of which enhance lung washout during induction. Although cardiac output is also elevated in the parturient, which would tend to slow the rate of induction, the overall effect of the combined cardiorespiratory changes is an enhanced rate of rise of the alveolar anesthetic concentration.

The anesthetic requirement (minimum alveolar concentration) during pregnancy, as determined in animals, is reduced by 20–40%.[292,293] The mechanism for this change is uncertain, although several factors may be responsible. Progesterone levels increase substantially during pregnancy, and this hormone has been shown to have sedative activity[294] and, in very high doses, to produce unconsciousness in humans.[295] Increased central nervous system serotoninergic activity during gestation may also play a role.[296] Activation of the endorphin system could contribute to the decreased anesthetic requirement, although conflicting data have been reported with respect to changes in plasma levels of beta-endorphin during gestation. Some investigators have found levels to be elevated during the later part of gestation[297] and at term,[297–299] whereas others report no change from nonpregnant values during pregnancy[300] or at term.[301] Beta-endorphin does rise during general anesthesia for cesarean delivery[302] although it is likely to be elevated in nonpregnant individuals undergoing anesthesia since stress is an effective stimulus. In support of a role for beta-endorphin is the finding that the placenta has precursors from which beta-endorphin-like material is released.[303] Also, beta-endorphin in the brain increases throughout gestation in the pregnant rat,[304] and administration of an opioid antagonist abolishes the progressive rise in pain threshold that occurs in these animals during gestation.[305]

Muscle relaxants

The duration of action of succinylcholine in nonpregnant subjects varies inversely with the concentration of plasma cholinesterase.[306,307] However, despite a reduction in the plasma cholinesterase concentration in pregnant patients at term,[206–209,308,309] the time to 10%, 25%, 50% and 90% twitch height recovery and the 25–75% recovery time following succinylcholine administration does not differ significantly between nonpregnant controls and genotypically normal parturients receiving the same (mg/kg or mg/m^2) relaxant dose.[308,309] The results even suggest that recovery time may be faster in the pregnant individuals.[308,309] These findings may be explained by the increased volume of distribution for succinylcholine in pregnant patients,[309] largely due to the marked elevation of plasma volume, which would result in a lower initial concentration of the relaxant and a shorter time period before the threshold for recovery is reached. It has also been suggested that modified pharmacodynamics account for these observations,[310] i.e. the pregnant woman may be less sensitive than the nonpregnant woman to similar plasma concentrations of succinylcholine.

Patients who are 1–2 days post-partum exhibit a prolonged recovery from succinylcholine compared with term pregnant and nonpregnant subjects receiving the same relaxant dose,[309] and require a significantly reduced dose compared with nonpregnant subjects for 80% depression of control twitch height.[311] These results can be explained by a further decline of the plasma cholinesterase concentration[206–209,308,309] and the reduction of plasma volume (i.e. volume of distribution) which occurs in the post-partum period.

The pharmacology of nondepolarizing muscle relaxants is also affected by pregnancy. In rabbits, the ED_{50} for vecuronium is reduced by more than 50% during pregnancy.[312] Enhanced sensitivity during the puerperium is also suggested by the prolonged duration of action of vecuronium in patients undergoing post-partum tubal ligation compared with nonpregnant women having gynecologic procedures.[313] Although altered pharmacokinetics could explain these results, this is unlikely since parturients, unlike nonpregnant individuals, exhibit a reduced elimination half-life for vecuronium,[314] as well as for pancuronium.[314,315]

Magnesium, which is used for seizure prophylaxis in preeclamptic patients and for tocolysis, interacts with depolarizing and nondepolarizing muscle relaxants. The neuromuscular blocking effects of magnesium and succinylcholine have been described as additive,[316] although the interaction may represent potentiation.[317] The effect of concurrent administration of these agents is evident in the management of preeclamptic patients given a loading dose and supplemental doses of magnesium,[318] although administration of a single 60 mg/kg dose of magnesium does not alter the clinical effect of succinylcholine.[319] Laboratory[320,321] and clinical studies[316,317] demonstrate that magnesium enhances the effects of nondepolarizing muscle relaxants.

Regional analgesia and anesthesia (Table 5.10)

Cerebrospinal fluid and epidural pressures

Cerebrospinal fluid pressure at term gestation, between contractions and with the patient in the lateral position, is within the range of normal for nonpregnant individuals.[322–324] Thus, the rate of flow of cerebrospinal fluid during lumbar dural puncture should be similar in pregnant and nonpregnant women. However, cerebrospinal fluid pressure increases significantly during contractions, and to even a greater degree with bearing down.[322–324]

Table 5.10 Anesthetic implications of maternal physiology: regional anesthesia (From Conklin K A 1991 Semin Anesth 10: 221–234)

Technical consideration
Reduced sensitivity of 'hanging drop' technique
Dose of local anesthetic
Reduced subarachnoid dose requirement (25%)
Epidural dose requirement
Large dose: no change
Small dose: reduced requirement (30%)
Hydration
Increased fluid requirement to prevent hypotension

The epidural pressure is increased significantly in pregnant patients. In the lateral position, the pressure in the lumbar epidural space is negative in more than 90% of nonpregnant individuals,[325] whereas the pressure is positive in all pregnant patients studied at term gestation.[325–327] During labor, between contractions, the epidural pressure increases as labor progresses, although contractions cause a further increase and pushing a still greater increase.[326,327] Elevation of the epidural pressure in the parturient may reduce the sensitivity of the 'hanging drop' technique for identification of the epidural space. In the post-partum period, the epidural pressure returns to normal by 6–12 h after delivery.[327]

Elevation of the epidural pressure during pregnancy can be attributed to compression of the inferior vena cava by the gravid uterus. This increases the venous pressure below the obstruction[122,125–127] and causes diversion of venous return via the vertebral plexus within the epidural space, which distends these veins.[121,122] Hehre et al[328] confirmed this mechanism experimentally (in dogs) by obstructing the inferior vena cava with a balloon-tipped catheter. Increasing the degree of aortocaval compression by turning the parturient from the lateral to the supine position results in an increase in the epidural pressure.[326,327] Patients in the lateral tilt position have epidural pressures between those of the lateral and supine positions, suggesting some relief of aortocaval compression. However, the higher epidural pressure in pregnant women than in nonpregnant subjects in the lateral position is further evidence that this position does not fully relieve the effects of the gravid uterus on venous return. These results are consistent with radiographic studies[121] and venous pressure measurements,[126,127] which show only partial relief of aortocaval compression in the lateral position.

The increase in the epidural pressure during uterine contractions[326,327] can be explained by an increase in abdominal muscle tone in response to pain, since epidural anesthesia abolishes the increase.[327] Pushing, with its attendant increase in intra-abdominal pressure, appears to elevate the epidural pressure[326,327] by a similar means. The increase in cerebrospinal fluid pressure during contractions and pushing[322–324] can also be explained by the same mechanism, with the increase in pressure being attributed to enhanced diversion of venous return via the vertebral plexus of veins when intra-abdominal pressure rises.

Complications of epidural catheter placement

Despite distension of the epidural veins of pregnant women, the prevalence (6–12%) of venous cannulation with an epidural catheter in these patients does not differ from that (10%) in nonpregnant individuals.[229–334] However, whereas injection of 10 ml of air or fluid does not change the prevalence of venous cannulation in nonpregnant patients, it results in a substantial reduction in the frequency of this complication (to 2–3%) in parturients.[332–334]

Changes in the epidural space during pregnancy do not affect the occurrence of paresthesias during passage of epidural catheters, since the prevalence is between 25% and 50% in pregnant and nonpregnant[333] subjects alike.[329,332] The wide variation between the results of these studies may be due to differences in catheter design.[330] The incidence of paresthesias in pregnant and nonpregnant subjects is reduced by the prior injection of 10 ml of air or local anesthetic solution.[332,334]

Local anesthetic dose requirements for spinal anesthesia

Pregnant women, at term gestation, require less local anesthetic for spinal anesthesia than do nonpregnant women. Barclay et al[335] and Marx and Orkin[336] observed that 4 and 5 mg of tetracaine resulted in an upper level of anesthesia that was 3–5 spinal segments higher in pregnant patients, which corresponds to a 20–33% reduction of the segmental dose requirement (mg of drug per spinal segment). Datta et al[337] observed a 17% decrease in the segmental dose requirement in patients receiving spinal anesthesia for cesarean delivery. Dose requirements return to that of nonpregnant women shortly after delivery, as shown by the elevated segmental dose requirement within 8–24 h post-partum,[338] the reduced spread of a fixed dose of bupivacaine in patients 2–51 h post-partum as compared with patients for cesarean delivery[339] and the significant increase in the post-partum dose requirement to achieve a certain level of anesthesia in individuals studied at term and again at 36–48 h post-partum.[340]

Several factors account for the reduced dose requirement for spinal anesthesia in pregnant patients. First, distension of the epidural veins, secondary to aortocaval compression, results in reduction of cerebrospinal fluid volume. This is because the epidural space is effectively a rigid tube containing two distensible tubes, the dural sac and the veins,[328] with the boundaries of the rigid tube being formed superiorly by the dura, which adheres firmly to the periosteum around the foramen magnum; inferiorly by the sacrococcygeal membrane; anteriorly by the posterior longitudinal ligament; posteriorly by the lamina of the vertebrae and ligamentum flavum; and laterally by the intervertebral foramina, which provide a means for entry or exit of nerves and blood vessels, and the pedicles of the vertebrae.[341] Thus, when the volume within the veins increases, as occurs with compression of the vena cava,[121,122,328] there is an obligatory loss of cerebrospinal fluid. This mechanism has been illustrated by Barclay et al,[335] who demonstrated, in nonpregnant subjects, that acute compression of the inferior vena cava resulted in enhanced spread of tetracaine, which was injected into the subarachnoid space.

A second factor that may contribute to the reduced dose requirement for spinal anesthesia during pregnancy is enhanced neural sensitivity to local anesthetics, an effect that has been demonstrated in humans[342] and rabbits.[343,344] This may account for the observation that pregnant women exhibit a more rapid onset and a longer duration of anesthesia than nonpregnant women who receive the same dose of local anesthetic.[336] Progesterone probably contributes to this effect, since ovariectomized rabbits injected with the hormone also exhibit enhanced neural sensitivity.[345] Other contributing factors may be the reduced cerebrospinal fluid protein concentration during pregnancy,[346] which would increase local anesthetic effectiveness by reducing protein binding, and the elevated cerebrospinal fluid pH,[347] which would increase the proportion of unionized local anesthetic, thus facilitating movement across neural membranes.

Local anesthetic dose requirements for epidural analgesia and anesthesia

Several factors could alter the spread of local anesthetic in the epidural space during gestation. Acute occlusion of the vena cava with distension of the epidural veins has been shown to produce enhanced spread of contrast media in the epidural space (of dogs), with the Valsalva maneuver producing even a more extensive spread.[328] Elevated epidural pressures in nonpregnant (elderly) individuals are also associated with increased spread.[325] Extending these results to pregnant individuals, vena cava compression by the gravid uterus, which distends the epidural veins[121,122,328] and elevates the epidural pressure,[325–327] might be expected to produce the same effect. However, whether acute vena cava occlusion (in dogs) has the same effect as continuous compression in pregnant women is unclear, and uterine contractions, which increase the epidural pressure and venous distension,[326,327] have no apparent effect on the spread of local anesthetic in the epidural space.[348] Enhanced neural sensitivity[342–344] would be expected to facilitate spread, although the increased blood flow and surface area of the epidural veins could enhance local anesthetic absorption and reduce the spread. Finally, a change in the patency of the intervertebral foramina, through which local anesthetic could leave the epidural space, may alter the spread during pregnancy.

Clinically, administration of a large dose of local anesthetic, i.e. that used for cesarean delivery or major abdominal surgery, produces the same spread of epidural anesthesia in term pregnant and nonpregnant patients.[349,350] In contrast, parturients receiving a small epidural 'labor' dose (140 mg) of lidocaine,[351] or a similar dose of bupivacaine,[349] exhibit a 20–40% decrease of the segmental dose requirement compared with nonpregnant subjects. Bromage[352] also reported enhanced spread (approximately a 30% reduction of the segmental dose requirement) in pregnant subjects, although the local anesthetic dose that these individuals received is unclear. However, since the dosage he used varied from 7 to 25 ml of 2% lidocaine or mepivacaine for surgical procedures in nonpregnant subjects and for obstetric procedures, it is likely that most (or all) of the obstetric data are from the use of small doses for labor. Thus, these results appear to support those of others,[349,351] which demonstrate enhanced spread in pregnant subjects when small doses are administered.

During the first trimester of pregnancy, individuals who receive a large dose of local anesthetic (400 mg of lidocaine) have a reduced (21%) segmental dose requirement compared with nonpregnant subjects,[353] thus exhibiting a different response to epidural administration of local anesthetics than women at term gestation.[349,350]

Considerations for selection of local anesthetic doses

The spread of subarachnoid bupivacaine administered for cesarean delivery is unaffected by the parturient's age, height, weight or body mass index (weight/height in m^2).[354–356] Vertebral column length, which does not correlate with height,[357] also appears to be without affect on the spread of local anesthetic in the subarachnoid space,[354] although a weakly significant correlation was reported in one study.[356] Thus, it appears to be appropriate to use a standardized dose of local anesthetic (i.e. 'one dose fits all') when performing spinal anesthesia for cesarean delivery, except in the very short (<5 ft/150 cm) or very tall (>6 ft/180 cm).

In contrast to the management of spinal anesthesia, patient variables should be considered when selecting the local anesthetic dose for epidural analgesia and anesthesia for obstetric patients. Although age[358,359] and height[358–361] are not correlated with the spread of local anesthetic in the epidural space, spread is positively correlated with body weight and body mass index[358,359] and inversely correlated with vertebral column length.[361]

Hydration requirements for regional anesthesia

The sympathetic nervous system has a minor role in the maintenance of hemodynamic stability in nonpregnant individuals who are normovolemic and at rest. During pregnancy, under similar conditions, the contribution of the sympathetic nervous system to the maintenance of vasomotor tone increases progressively and reaches a peak near term.[340,362–365] The effect is predominantly on the capacitance system of the lower extremities,[364,365] which counteracts the adverse effects that uterine compression of the vena cava has on venous return. Thus, pharmacologic sympathectomy by ganglionic blockade or high spinal anesthesia, in the absence of an acute volume loading, produces a minimal change of blood pressure in nonpregnant individuals (approximately a 10% decrease), whereas individuals with normal-term pregnancies experience nearly a 50% decrease in blood pressure.[340] The response to sympathectomy returns to that of nonpregnant individuals by 36–48 h post-partum.[340] Therefore, fluid administration is mandatory if hemodynamic stability is to be maintained in pregnant patients receiving regional anesthesia.

Infusion of 500–1000 ml of balanced electrolyte solution prior to cesarean delivery is insufficient to maintain blood pressure when spinal or epidural anesthesia is administered, since 45–85% of parturients receiving this volume experience a decrease in systolic blood pressure of at least 20%, or to a value less than 100 mmHg.[366–369] 25–50% of these individuals will have a fall in systolic blood pressure of more than 30% or to a value less than 90 mmHg.[366,367,370,371] Hemodynamic stability can be provided by administering 1000 ml (15 ml/kg) of a colloid solution[367,372] or 2000 ml (30 ml/kg) of a crystalloid solution.[366,373]

Effects of regional anesthesia on respiratory function

The diaphragm and the fifth to ninth external intercostal muscles are the principal muscles of inspiration,[374] although, during pregnancy, inspiration is almost exclusively the role of the diaphragm.[18,19] Expiration is essentially a passive function. The abdominal muscles have no function in inspiration or normal ventilation, but are the most important muscles of forced expiration and coughing.[375]

In pregnant[376] and nonpregnant[375,377–379] subjects, paralysis of the intercostal muscles during administration of high spinal or epidural anesthesia has no effect on resting minute ventilation or arterial blood gases. Paralysis of the abdominal muscles in nonpregnant individuals results in a reduction of the peak expiratory flow rate[375,379] and a marked decrease in the ability to increase intra-abdominal and intrathoracic pressures during vigorous coughing.[380] Pregnant subjects[381,382] experience a much greater reduction of the peak expiratory flow rate during regional anesthesia than do nonpregnant subjects,[375] which suggests that the ability to cough effectively may be impaired to a greater degree during pregnancy. Therefore, although patients receiving regional anesthesia for cesarean delivery maintain their laryngeal reflexes, they are at an increased risk for pulmonary aspiration of gastric contents because of their inability to cough effectively. These results provide support for the contention that pharmacologic and chemical means should be used to reduce gastric volume and acidity of pregnant patients undergoing operative procedures.

Blood replacement

At the time of delivery, loss of the volume of blood contained within the placenta does not result in maternal hypovolemia since its loss is accompanied by an equivalent reduction in the size of the maternal vascular compartment (loss of the intervillous space). Therefore, when assessing blood loss for the purpose of volume replacement, the initial 500 ml (at least), i.e. the volume of the intervillous space, should not be considered. Decisions concerning blood administration should also take into consideration the post-partum changes in the maternal vascular compartment, which decreases in size from approximately 85 ml/kg at term gestation[163] to 65–70 ml/kg in the nonpregnant state. Following the acute reduction, by at least 500 ml at the time of delivery, maternal vascular capacitance decreases by another 500–600 ml during the first 24 hs post-partum,[163,211] with a further reduction of 500–1000 ml in the subsequent weeks.[155] Since the latter reductions in size of the vascular compartment are accounted for by a reduction of plasma volume without a substantial loss of red blood cell volume, a significant degree of hemoconcentration occurs in the post-partum period.[155] Thus, it is appropriate to withhold administration of red blood cells from parturients who sustain but acutely tolerate a substantial blood loss during delivery, and to administer only crystalloid or colloid solutions to maintain hemodynamic stability in anticipation of the patient's hemoconcentration during the puerperium.

REFERENCES

1. Chesley L C 1944 Weight changes and water balance in normal and toxic pregnancy. Am J Obstet Gynecol 48: 565–593
2. Watrous J, Blakely S B 1952 Usefulness of the basal metabolic rate in pregnancy. Am J Obstet Gynecol 64: 1310–1315
3. Sontag L W, Reynolds E L, Torbet V 1944 The relation of basal metabolic gain during pregnancy to nonpregnant basal metabolism. Am J Obstet Gynecol 48: 315–320
4. Cugell D W, Frank NR, Gaensler E A, Badger, T L 1953 Pulmonary function in pregnancy. I. Serial observations in normal women. Am Rev Tuberculosis 67: 568–597
5. Ueland K, Novy M J, Metcalfe J 1973 Cardiorespiratory responses to pregnancy and exercise in normal women and patients with heart disease. Am J Obstet Gynecol 115: 4–10
6. Pernoll M L, Metcalfe J, Schlenker T L, Welch J E, Matsumoto J A 1975 Oxygen consumption at rest and during exercise in pregnancy. Resp Physiol 25: 285–293
7. Knuttgen H G, Emerson Jr K 1974 Physiological response to pregnancy at rest and during exercise. J Appl Physiol 36: 549–553
8. Plass E D, Oberst F W 1938 Respiration and pulmonary ventilation in normal nonpregnant, pregnant and puerperal women. With an interpretation of the acid–base balance during normal pregnancy. Am J Obstet Gynecol 35: 441–452
9. Emerson Jr K, Saxena B N, Poindexter E L 1972 Caloric cost of normal pregnancy. Obstet Gynecol 40: 786–794
10. Hägerdal M, Morgan C W, Sumner A E, Gutsche BB 1983 Minute ventilation and oxygen consumption during labor with epidural analgesia. Anesthesiology 59: 425–427
11. Gemzell C A, Robbe H, Stern B, Ström G 1957 Observations on circulatory changes and muscular work in normal labour. Acta Obstet Gynecol Scand 36: 75–92
12. Bonica J J 1967 Physiology of pregnancy, principles and practice of obstetric analgesia and anesthesia, Vol 1. FA Davis, Philadelphia pp 13–39
13. Leontic E A 1977 Respiratory disease in pregnancy. Med Clin N Am 61: 111–128
14. Gee J B L, Packer B S, Millen J E, Robin E D 1967 Pulmonary mechanics during pregnancy. J Clin Invest 46: 945–952
15. Milne J A, Mills R J, Howie A D, Pack A I 1977 Large airways function during normal pregnancy. Br J Obstet Gynaecol 84: 448–451
16. Thomson K J, Cohen M E 1938 Studies on the circulation in pregnancy. II. Vital capacity observations in normal pregnant women. Surg Gynecol Obstet 66: 591–603
17. Turner A F 1975 The chest radiograph in pregnancy. Clin Obstet Gynecol 18: 65–74
18. McGinty A P 1938 The comparative effects of pregnancy and phrenic nerve interruption on the diaphragm and their relation to pulmonary tuberculosis. Am J Obstet Gynecol 35: 237–248
19. Grenville-Mathers R, Trenchard H J 1953 The diaphragm in the puerperium. J Obstet Gynaecol Br Emp 60: 825–833
20. Garrard G S, Littler W A, Redman C W G 1978 Closing volume during normal pregnancy. Thorax 33: 488–492
21. Rubin A, Russo N, Goucher D 1956 The effect of pregnancy upon pulmonary function in normal women. Am J Obstet Gynecol 72: 963–969
22. Sims C D, Chamberlain G V P, de Swiet M 1976 Lung function tests in bronchial asthma during and after pregnancy. Br J Obstet Gynaecol 83: 434–437
23. Alaily A B, Carrol K B 1978 Pulmonary ventilation in pregnancy. Br J Obstet Gynaecol 85: 518–524
24. Gazioglu K, Kaltreider N L, Rosen M, Yu P N 1970 Pulmonary function during pregnancy in normal women and in patients with cardiopulmonary disease. Thorax 25: 445–450
25. Baldwin G R, Moorthi D S, Whelton J A, MacDonnel K F 1977 New lung functions and pregnancy. Am J Obstet Gynecol 127: 235–239
26. Craig D B, Toole M A 1975 Airway closure in pregnancy. Can Anaesth Soc J 22: 665–672
27. Russell I F, Chambers W A 1981 Closing volume in normal pregnancy. Br J Anaesth 53: 1043–1047
28. Templeton A, Kelman G R 1976 Maternal blood-gases (PAo_2-Pao_2), physiological shunt and V_D/V_T in normal pregnancy. Br J Anaesth 48: 1001–1004
29. Pernoll M L, Metcalfe J, Kovach P A, Wachtel R, Dunham M J 1975 Ventilation during rest and exercise in pregnancy and postpartum. Resp Physiol 25: 295–310

30. Holdcroft A, Bevan D R, O'Sullivan J C, Sykes M K 1977 Airway closure and pregnancy. Anaesthesia 32: 517–523
31. Lyons H A, Antonio R 1959 The sensitivity of the respiratory center in pregnancy and after the administration of progesterone. Trans Assoc Am Physicians 72: 173–180
32. Skatrud J B, Dempsey J A, Kaiser D G 1978 Ventilatory response to medroxyprogesterone acetate in normal subjects: time course and mechanism. J Appl Physiol 44: 939–944
33. Machida H 1981 Influence of progesterone on arterial blood and CSF acid–base balance in women. J Appl Physiol 51: 1433–1436
34. Novy M J, Edwards M J 1967 Respiratory problems in pregnancy. Am J Obstet Gynecol 99: 1024–1045
35. Andersen G J, James G B, Mathers N P, Smith E L, Walker J 1969 The maternal oxygen tension and acid–base status during pregnancy. J Obstet Gynaecol Br Cwlth 76: 16–19
36. Milne J A, Mills R J, Coutts J R T, MacNaughton M C, Moran F, Pack A I 1977 The effect of human pregnancy on the pulmonary transfer factor for carbon monoxide as measured by the single-breath method. Clin Sci Mol Med 53: 271–276
37. Bedell G N, Adams R W 1962 Pulmonary diffusing capacity during rest and exercise. A study of normal persons and persons with atrial septal defect, pregnancy, and pulmonary disease. J Clin Invest 41: 1908–1914
38. Lucius H, Gahlenbeck H, Kleine H O, Fabel H, Bartels H 1970 Respiratory functions, buffer system, and electrolyte concentrations of blood during human pregnancy. Resp Physiol 9: 311–317
39. Blechner J N, Cotter J R, Stenger V G, Hinkley C M, Prystowsky H 1968 Oxygen, carbon dioxide, and hydrogen ion concentrations in arterial blood during pregnancy. Am J Obstet Gynecol 100: 1–6
40. Awe R J, Nicotra M B, Newsom T D, Viles R 1979 Arterial oxygenation and alveolar–arterial gradients in term pregnancy. Obstet Gynecol 53: 182–186
41. Boutourline-Young H, Boutourline-Young E 1956 Alveolar carbon dioxide levels in pregnant, parturient and lactating subjects. J Obstet Gynaecol Br Emp 63: 509–528
42. Shankar K B, Moseley H, Vemula V, Ramasamy M, Kumar Y 1989 Arterial to end-tidal carbon dioxide tension difference during anaesthesia in early pregnancy. Can J Anaesth 36: 124–127
43. Burger G A, Datta S, Chantigian R A, Warren T M, Naulty J S, Raemer D, Weiss J B, Ostheimer G W 1983 Optimal ventilation in general anesthesia for cesarean delivery. Anesthesiology 59: A420
44. Shankar K B, Moseley H, Kumar Y, Vemula V 1986 Arterial to end tidal carbon dioxide tension difference during caesarean section anaesthesia. Anaesthesia 41: 698–702
45. Shankar K B, Moseley H, Kumar Y, Vemula V, Krishnan A 1987 Arterial to end-tidal carbon dioxide tension difference during anaesthesia for tubal ligation. Anaesthesia 42: 482–486
46. Bader R A, Bader M E, Rose D J, Braunwald E 1955 Hemodynamics at rest and during exercise in normal pregnancy as studied by cardiac catheterization. J Clin Invest 34: 1524–1536
47. Ang C K, Tan T H, Walters W A W, Wood C 1969 Postural influence on maternal capillary oxygen and carbon dioxide tension. Br Med J 4: 201–203
48. Calvin S, Jones O W III, Knieriem K, Weinstein L 1988 Oxygen saturation in the supine hypotensive syndrome. Obstet Gynecol 71: 872–877
49. MacRae D J, Palavradji D 1967 Maternal acid–base changes in pregnancy. J Obstet Gynaecol Br Cwlth 74: 11–16
50. Dayal P, Murata Y, Takamura H 1972 Antepartum and postpartum acid–base changes in maternal blood in normal and complicated pregnancies. J Obstet Gynaecol Brit Cwlth 79: 612–624
51. Oard H C, Peters J P 1929 The concentration of acid and base in the serum in normal pregnancy. J Biol Chem 81: 9–27
52. Seeds A E, Battaglia F C, Hellegers A E 1964 Effects of pregnancy on the pH, PCO_2, and bicarbonate concentrations of peripheral venous blood. Am J Obstet Gynecol 88: 1086–1089
53. Sjöstedt S 1962 Acid–base balance of arterial blood during pregnancy, at delivery, and in the puerperium. Am J Obstet Gynecol 84: 775–779
54. Lim V S, Katz A I, Lindheimer M D 1976 Acid–base regulation in pregnancy. Am J Physiol 231: 1764–1770
55. Sangoul F, Fox G S, Houle G L 1975 Effect of regional analgesia on maternal oxygen consumption during the first stage of labor. Am J Obstet Gynecol 121: 1080–1083
56. Fisher A, Prys-Roberts C 1968 Maternal pulmonary gas exchange. A study during normal labour and extradural blockade. Anaesthesia 23: 350–356
57. Bonica J J 1970 Obstetric analgesia and anesthesia. Recent trends and advances. NY State J Med 70: 2079–2084
58. Andersen G J, Walker J 1970 The effect of labour on the maternal blood-gas and acid–base status. J Obstet Gynaecol Br Cwlth 77: 289–293
59. Pearson J F, Davies P 1974 The effect of continuous lumbar epidural analgesia upon fetal acid–base status during the first stage of labour. J Obstet Gynaecol Br Cwlth 81: 971–974
60. Pearson J F, Davies P 1973 The effect of continuous lumbar epidural analgesia on the acid–base status of maternal arterial blood during the first stage of labour. J Obstet Gynaecol Br Cwlth 80: 218–224
61. Jouppila R, Hollmén A 1976 The effect of segmental epidural analgesia on maternal and foetal acid–base balance, lactate, serum potassium and creatine phosphokinase during labour. Acta Anaesth Scand 20: 259–268
62. Bader R A, Bader M E, Rose D J 1959 The oxygen cost of breathing in dyspnoeic subjects as studied in normal pregnant women. Clin Sci 18: 223–235
63. Thalme B, Raabe N, Belfrage P 1974 Lumbar epidural analgesia in labour. II. Effects on glucose, lactate, sodium, chloride, total protein, haematocrit and haemoglobin in maternal, fetal and neonatal blood. Acta Obstet Gynecol Scand 53: 113–119
64. Marx G F, Greene N M 1964 Maternal lactate, pyruvate, and excess lactate production during labor and delivery. Am J Obstet Gynecol 90: 786–793
65. Cutforth R, MacDonald C B 1966 Heart sounds and murmurs in pregnancy. Am Heart J 71: 741–747
66. Limacher M C, Ware J A, O'Meara M E, Fernandez G C, Young J B 1985 Tricuspid regurgitation during pregnancy: two-dimensional and pulsed doppler echocardiographic observations. Am J Cardiol 55: 1059–1062
67. Carruth J E, Mirvis S B, Brogan D R, Wenger N K 1981 The electrocardiogram in normal pregnancy. Am Heart J 102: 1075–1078
68. Oram S, Holt M 1961 Innocent depression of the S–T segment and flattening of the T-wave during pregnancy. J Obstet Gynaecol Br Cwlth 68: 765–770
69. Hollander A G, Crawford J H 1943 Roentgenologic and electrocardiographic changes in the normal heart during pregnancy. Am Heart J 26: 364–376
70. Schwartz D B, Schamroth L 1979 The effect of pregnancy on the frontal plane QRS axis. J Electrocardiol 12: 279–281
71. Laird-Meeter K, Van de Ley G, Bom T H, Wladimiroff J W, Roelandt J 1979 Cardiocirculatory adjustments during pregnancy – an echocardiographic study. Clin Cardiol 2: 328–332
72. Katz R, Karliner J S, Resnik R 1978 Effects of a natural volume overload state (pregnancy) on left ventricular performance in normal human subjects. Circulation 58: 434–441
73. Clark S L, Cotton D B, Lee W et al 1989 Central hemodynamic assessment of normal term pregnancy. Am J Obstet Gynecol 161: 1439–1442
74. Rubler S, Damani P M, Pinto E R 1977 Cardiac size and performance during pregnancy estimated with echocardiography. Am J Cardiol 40: 534–540
75. Robson S C, Boys R J, Hunter S, Dunlop W 1989 Maternal hemodynamics after normal delivery and delivery complicated by postpartum hemorrhage. Obstet Gynecol 74: 234–239
76. Robson S C, Hunter S, Boys R J, Dunlop W 1989 Serial study of factors influencing changes in cardiac output during human pregnancy. Am J Physiol 256: H1060–H1065
77. Robson S C, Hunter S, Moore M, Dunlop W 1987 Haemodynamic changes during the puerperium: a Doppler and M-mode echocardiographic study. Br J Obstet Gynaecol 94: 1028–1039
78. Walters W A W, MacGregor W G, Hills M 1966 Cardiac output at rest during pregnancy and the puerperium. Clin Sci 30: 1–11
79. Ueland K, Novy M J, Peterson E N, Metcalfe J 1969 Maternal

cardiovascular dynamics. IV. The influence of gestational age on the maternal cardiovascular response to posture and exercise. Am J Obstet Gynecol 104: 856–864
80. Hamilton H F H 1949 The cardiac output in normal pregnancy. As determined by the Cournand right heart catheterization technique. J Obstet Gynaecol Br Emp 56: 548–552
81. Greiss Jr F C 1966 Pressure-flow relationship in the gravid uterine vascular bed. Am J Obstet Gynecol 96: 41–47
82. Ladner C, Brinkman III C R, Weston P, Assali N S 1970 Dynamics of uterine circulation in pregnant and nonpregnant sheep. Am J Physiol 218: 257–263
83. Berman Jr W, Goodlin R C, Heymann M A, Rudolph A M 1976 Relationships between pressure and flow in the umbilical and uterine circulations of the sheep. Circ Res 38: 262–266
84. Tabsh K, Nuwayhid B, Erkkola R et al 1981 Hemodynamic responses of the pelvic vascular bed to vasoactive stimuli in pregnant sheep. Biol Neonate 39: 52–60
85. Rosenfeld C R, West J 1977 Circulatory response to systemic infusion of norepinephrine in the pregnant ewe. Am J Obstet Gynecol 127: 376–383
86. Rosenfeld C R, Barton M D, Meschia G 1976 Effects of epinephrine on distribution of blood flow in the pregnant ewe. Am J Obstet Gynecol 124: 156–163
87. Bieniarz J, Crottogini J J, Curuchet E, Romero-Salinas G, Yoshida T, Poseiro J J, Caldeyro-Barcia R 1968 Aortocaval compression by the uterus in late human pregnancy. II. An arteriographic study. Am J Obstet Gynecol 100: 203–217
88. Borell U, Fernström I, Ohlson L, Wiqvist N 1965 Influence of uterine contractions on the uteroplacental blood flow at term. Am J Obstet Gynecol 93: 44–57
89. Brotanek V, Hendricks C H, Yoshida T 1969 Changes in uterine blood flow during uterine contractions. Am J Obstet Gynecol 103: 1108–1116
90. Hendricks C H 1958 The hemodynamics of a uterine contraction. Am J Obstet Gynecol 76: 969–982
91. Assali N S, Rauramo L, Peltonen T 1960 Measurement of uterine blood flow and uterine metabolism. VIII. Uterine and fetal blood flow and oxygen consumption in early human pregnancy. Am J Obstet Gynecol 79: 86–98
92. Conklin K A 1990 Effects of obstetric analgesia and anesthesia on uterine activity and uteroplacental blood flow. In: Carsten M E, Miller J D (eds) Uterine function: molecular and cellular aspects. Plenum Publishing, New York, pp 539–575
93. Metcalfe J, Romney S L, Ramsey L H, Reid D E, Burwell C S 1955 Estimation of uterine blood flow in normal human pregnancy at term. J Clin Invest 34: 1632–1638
94. Assali N S, Douglass Jr R A, Baird W W, Nicholson D B, Syuemoto R 1953 Measurement of uterine blood flow and uterine metabolism. IV. Results in normal pregnancy. Am J Obstet Gynecol 66: 248–253
95. Rekonen A, Luotola H, Pitkänen M, Kuikka J, Pyörälä T 1976 Measurement of intervillous and myometrial blood flow by an intravenous ^{133}Xe method. Br J Obstet Gynaecol 83: 723–728
96. Kauppila A, Koskinen M, Puolakka J, Tuimala R, Kuikka J 1980 Decreased intervillous and unchanged myometrial blood flow in supine recumbency. Obstet Gynecol 55: 203–205
97. Jouppila P, Kuikka J, Jouppila R, Hollmén A 1979 Effect of induction of general anesthesia for cesarean section on intervillous blood flow. Acta Obstet Gynecol Scand 58: 249–253
98. Jouppila R, Jouppila P, Kuikka J, Hollmén A 1978 Placental blood flow during caesarean section under lumbar extradural analgesia. Br J Anaesth 50: 275–279
99. Pritchard J A, MacDonald P C, Gant N F 1985 Maternal adaptation to pregnancy. Williams Obstetrics, 17th edn. Appleton Century Crofts, Norwalk pp 181–210
100. Dignam W J, Titus P, Assali N S 1958 Renal function in human pregnancy. I. Changes in glomerular filtration rate and renal plasma flow. Proc Soc Exp Biol Med 97: 512–514
101. Dunlop W 1981 Serial changes in renal haemodynamics during normal human pregnancy. Br J Obstet Gynaecol 88: 1–9
102. Ezimokhai M, Davison J M, Philips P R, Dunlop W 1981 Non-postural serial changes in renal function during the third trimester of normal human pregnancy. Br J Obstet Gynaecol 88: 465–471
103. Dunlop W 1976 Investigations into the influence of posture on renal plasma flow and glomerular filtration rate during late pregnancy. Br J Obstet Gynaecol 83: 17–23
104. Katz M, Sokal M M 1980 Skin perfusion in pregnancy. Am J Obstet Gynecol 137: 30–33
105. Ginsburg J, Duncan S L B 1967 Peripheral blood flow in normal pregnancy. Cardiovasc Res 1: 132–137
106. Burt C C 1949 Peripheral skin temperature in normal pregnancy. Lancet 2: 787–790
107. McCall M L 1953 Cerebral circulation and metabolism in toxemia of pregnancy. Observations on the effects of veratrum viride and apresoline (1-hydrazinophthalazine). Am J Obstet Gynecol 66: 1015–1030
108. Munnell E W, Taylor Jr H C 1947 Liver blood flow in pregnancy–hepatic vein catheterization. J Clin Invest 26: 952–956
109. Gallery E D M, Hunyor S N, Ross M, Györy A Z 1977 Predicting the development of pregnancy-associated hypertension. The place of standardised blood-pressure measurement. Lancet 1: 1273–1275
110. Wilson M, Morganti A A, Zervoudakis I et al 1980 Blood pressure, the renin–aldosterone system and sex steroids throughout normal pregnancy. Am J Med 68: 97–104
111. MacGillivray I, Rose G A, Rowe B 1969 Blood pressure survey in pregnancy. Clin Sci 37: 395–407
112. Christianson R E 1976 Studies on blood pressure during pregnancy. I. Influence of parity and age. Am J Obstet Gynecol 125: 509–513
113. Ginsburg J, Duncan S 1969 Direct and indirect blood pressure measurement in pregnancy. J Obstet Gynaecol Br Cwlth 76: 705–710
114. Lewis P J, Boylan P, Friedman L A, Hensby C N, Downing I 1980 Prostacyclin in pregnancy. Br Med J 280: 1581–1582
115. Goodman R P, Killam A P, Brash A R, Branch R A 1982 Prostacyclin production during pregnancy: comparison of production during normal pregnancy and pregnancy complicated by hypertension. Am J Obstet Gynecol 142: 817–822
116. Clark K E, Austin J E, Seeds A E 1982 Effect of bisenoic prostaglandins and arachidonic acid on the uterine vasculature of pregnant sheep. Am J Obstet Gynecol 142: 261–268
117. Ylikorkala O, Jouppila P, Kirkinen P, Viinikka L 1983 Maternal prostacyclin, thromboxane, and placental blood flow. Am J Obstet Gynecol 145: 730–732
118. Greiss Jr F C, Anderson S G 1970 Effect of ovarian hormones on the uterine vascular bed. Am J Obstet Gynecol 107: 829–836
119. Goodrich S M, Wood J E 1966 The effect of estradiol-17-beta on peripheral venous distensibility and velocity of venous blood flow. Am J Obstet Gynecol 96: 407–412
120. Goodrich S M, Wood J E 1964 Peripheral venous distensibility and velocity of venous blood flow during pregnancy or during oral contraceptive therapy. Am J Obstet Gynecol 90: 740–744
121. Kerr M G, Scott D B, Samuel E 1964 Studies of the inferior vena cava in late pregnancy. Br Med J 1: 532–533
122. Kerr M G 1965 The mechanical effects of the gravid uterus in late pregnancy. J Obstet Gynaecol Br Cwlth 72: 513–529
123. Bieniarz J, Yoshida T, Romero-Salinas G, Curuchet E, Caldeyro-Barcia R, Crottogini J J 1969 Aortocaval compression by the uterus in late human pregnancy. IV. Circulatory homeostasis by preferential perfusion of the placenta. Am J Obstet Gynecol 103: 19–31
124. Abitbol M M 1976 Aortic compression by pregnant uterus. NY State J Med 76: 1470–1475
125. McLennan C E 1943 Antecubital and femoral venous pressure in normal and toxemic pregnancy. Am J Obstet Gynecol 45: 568–591
126. Howard B K, Goodson J H, Mengert W F 1953 Supine hypotensive syndrome in late pregnancy. Obstet Gynecol 1: 371–377
127. Scott D B, Kerr M G 1963 Inferior vena caval pressure in late pregnancy. J Obstet Gynaecol Br Cwlth 70: 1044–1049
128. Lees M M, Scott D B, Kerr M G, Taylor S H 1967 The circulatory effects of recumbent postural change in late pregnancy. Clin Sci 32: 453–465
129. Milsom I, Forssman L 1984 Factors influencing aortocaval

compression in late pregnancy. Am J Obstet Gynecol 148: 764–771
130. Ueland K, Hansen J M 1969 Maternal cardiovascular dynamics. II. Posture and uterine contractions. Am J Obstet Gynecol 103: 1–7
131. Ueland K, Gills R E, Hansen J M 1968 Maternal cardiovascular dynamics. I. Cesarean section under subarachnoid block anesthesia. Am J Obstet Gynecol 100: 42–54
132. Vorys N, Ullery J C, Hanusek G E 1961 The cardiac output changes in various positions in pregnancy. Am J Obstet Gynecol 82: 1312–1321
133. Lees M M, Taylor S H, Scott D B, Kerr M G 1967 A study of cardiac output at rest throughout pregnancy. J Obstet Gynaecol Br Cwlth 74: 319–328
134. Newman B, Derrington C, Dore C 1983 Cardiac output and the recumbent position in late pregnancy. Anaesthesia 38: 332–335
135. Weaver J B, Pearson J F, Rosen M 1975 Posture and epidural block in pregnant women at term. Effects on arterial blood pressure and limb blood flow. Anaesthesia 30: 752–756
136. Drummond G B, Scott S E M, Lees M M, Scott D B 1974 Effects of posture on limb blood flow in late pregnancy. Br Med J 4: 587–588
137. Holmes F 1960 Incidence of the supine hypotensive syndrome in late pregnancy. A clinical study in 500 subjects. J Obstet Gynaecol Br Emp 67: 254–258
138. Hansen J M, Ueland K 1966 The influence of caudal analgesia on cardiovascular dynamics during normal labor and delivery. Acta Anaesth Scand 23: suppl 449–452
139. Ueland K, Hansen J M 1969 Maternal cardiovascular dynamics. III. Labor and delivery under local and caudal analgesia. Am J Obstet Gynecol 103: 8–18
140. Kjeldsen J 1979 Hemodynamic investigations during labour and delivery. Acta Obstet Gynecol Scand 89 (suppl): 1–252
141. Lederman R P, Lederman E, Work Jr B, McCann D S 1985 Anxiety and epinephrine in multiparous women in labor: relationship to duration of labor and fetal heart rate pattern. Am J Obstet Gynecol 153: 870–877
142. Lederman R P, Lederman E, Work Jr B A, McCann D S 1978 The relationship of maternal anxiety, plasma catecholamines, and plasma cortisol to progress in labor. Am J Obstet Gynecol 132: 495–500
143. Lederman R P, McCann D S, Work Jr B, Huber M J 1977 Endogenous plasma epinephrine and norepinephrine in last-trimester pregnancy and labor. Am J Obstet Gynecol 129: 5–8
144. Grenman S, Erkkola R, Kanto J, Scheinin M, Viinamäki O, Lindberg R 1986 Epidural and paracervical blockades in obstetrics. Catecholamines, arginine vasopressin and analgesic effect. Acta Obstet Gynecol Scand 65: 699–704
145. Falconer A D, Powles A B 1982 Plasma noradrenaline levels during labour. Influence of elective lumbar epidural blockade. Anaesthesia 37: 416–420
146. Jouppila R, Puolakka J, Kauppila A, Vuori J 1984 Maternal and umbilical cord plasma noradrenaline concentrations during labour with and without segmental extradural analgesia, and during caesarean section. Br J Anaesth 56: 251–255
147. Hendricks C H, Quilligan E J 1956 Cardiac output during labor. Am J Obstet Gynecol 71: 953–972
148. Adams J Q, Alexander Jr A M 1958 Alterations in cardiovascular physiology during labor. Obstet Gynecol 12: 542–549
149. Borell U, Fernström I, Ohlson L, Wiqvist N 1964 Effect of uterine contractions on the human uteroplacental blood circulation. An arteriographic study. Am J Obstet Gynecol 89: 881–890
150. Morishima H O, Yeh M N, James L S 1979 Reduced uterine blood flow and fetal hypoxemia with acute maternal stress: experimental observation in the pregnant baboon. Am J Obstet Gynecol 134: 270–275
151. Shnider S M, Wright R G, Levinson G, Roizen M F, Wallis K L, Rolbin S H, Craft J B 1979 Uterine blood flow and plasma norepinephrine changes during maternal stress in the pregnant ewe. Anesthesiology 50: 524–527
152. Hollmén A I, Jouppila R, Jouppila P, Koivula A, Vierola H 1982 Effect of extradural analgesia using bupivacaine and 2-chloroprocaine on intervillous blood flow during normal labour. Br J Anaesth 54: 837–842
153. Brotanek V, Vasicka A, Santiago A, D'Arc Brotanek J 1973 The influence of epidural anesthesia on uterine blood flow. Obstet Gynecol 42: 276–282
154. Chesley L C, Duffus G M 1971 Posture and apparent plasma volume in late pregnancy. J Obstet Gynaecol Br Cwlth 78: 406–412
155. Lund C J, Donovan J C 1967 Blood volume during pregnancy. Significance of plasma and red cell volumes. Am J Obstet Gynecol 98: 393–403
156. Pirani B B K, Campbell D M, MacGillivray I 1973 Plasma volume in normal first pregnancy. J Obstet Gynaecol Br Cwlth 80: 884–887
157. Hytten F E, Paintin D B 1963 Increase in plasma volume during normal pregnancy. J Obstet Gynaecol Br Cwlth 70: 402–407
158. Taylor D J, Lind T 1979 Red cell mass during and after normal pregnancy. Br J Obstet Gynaecol 86: 364–370
159. Flanagan B, Muldowney F P, Cannon P J 1966 The relationships of circulating red cell mass, basal oxygen consumption and lean body mass during normal human pregnancy. Clin Sci 30: 439–451
160. Hønger P E 1967 Intravascular mass of albumin in pre-eclampsia and normal pregnancy. Scand J Clin Lab Invest 19: 283–287
161. Rovinsky J J, Jaffin H 1965 Cardiovascular hemodynamics in pregnancy. I. Blood and plasma volumes in multiple pregnancy. Am J Obstet Gynecol 93: 1–15
162. Pritchard J A 1965 Changes in the blood volume during pregnancy and delivery. Anesthesiology 26: 393–399
163. Ueland K 1976 Maternal cardiovascular dynamics. VII. Intrapartum blood volume changes. Am J Obstet Gynecol 126: 671–677
164. Robertson E G, Cheyne G A 1972 Plasma biochemistry in relation to oedema of pregnancy. J Obstet Gynaecol Br Cwlth 79: 769–779
165. Sill P R, Lind T, Walker W 1985 Platelet values during normal pregnancy. Br J Obstet Gynaecol 92: 480–483
166. Efrati P, Presentey B, Margalith M, Rozenszajn L 1964 Leukocytes of normal pregnant women. Obstet Gynecol 23: 429–432
167. Rath C E, Caton W, Reid D E, Finch C A Conroy L 1950 Hematological changes and iron metabolism of normal pregnancy. Surg Gynecol Obstet 90: 320–326
168. Tapia H R, Johnson C E, Strong C G 1973 Effect of oral contraceptive therapy on the renin-angiotensin system in normotensive and hypertensive women. Obstet Gynecol 41: 643–649
169. Watanabe M, Meeker C I Gray M J, Sims E A H, Solomon S 1963 Secretion rate of aldosterone in normal pregnancy. J Clin Invest 42: 1619–1631
170. Longo L D, Hardesty J S 1984 Maternal blood volume measurement, hypothesis of control, and clinical considerations. Rev Perinat Med 5: 35–59
171. Laidlaw J C, Ruse J L, Gornall A G 1962 The influence of estrogen and progesterone on aldosterone excretion. J Clin Endocrinol Metab 22: 161–171
172. Landau R L, Lugibihl K 1958 Inhibition of the sodium-retaining influence of aldosterone by progesterone. J Clin Endocrinol Metab 18: 1237–1245
173 Jepson J H 1968 Endocrine control of maternal and fetal erythropoiesis. Can Med Assoc J 98: 844–847
174. Lindheimer M D, Katz A I 1973 Sodium and diuretics in pregnancy. New Eng J Med 288: 891–894
175. Cotes P M, Canning C E, Lind T 1983 Changes in serum immunoreactive erythropoietin during the menstrual cycle and normal pregnancy. Br J Obstet Gynaecol 90: 304–311
176. Živný J, Kobilková J, Neuwirt J, Andrasová V 1982 Regulation of erythropoiesis in fetus and mother during normal pregnancy. Obstet Gynecol 60: 77–81
177. Koller O 1982 The clinical significance of hemodilution during pregnancy. Obstet Gynecol Survey 37: 649–652
178. Rolschau J 1978 Infarctions and intervillous thrombosis in placenta, and their association with intrauterine growth retardation. Acta Obstet Gynecol Scand 72 (suppl): 22–27

179. Naeye R L 1977 Placental infarction leading to fetal or neonatal death. A prospective study. Obstet Gynecol 50: 583–588
180. Hoch H, Marrack J R 1948 The composition of the blood of women during pregnancy and after delivery. J Obstet Gynaecol Br Emp 55: 1–16
181. Rinehart R E 1945 Serum protein in normal and toxemic pregnancy. Am J Obstet Gynecol 50: 48–56
182. Coryell M N, Beach E F, Robinson A R, Macy G, Mack H C 1950 Metabolism of women during the reproductive cycle. XVII. Changes in electrophoretic patterns of plasma proteins throughout the cycle and following delivery. J Clin Invest 29: 1559–1567
183. Hamilton H G, Higgins R S 1949 A correlated study of serum protein, erythrocyte count, leucocyte count, hemoglobin and hematocrit in normal pregnancy. Am J Obstet Gynecol 58: 345–353
184. de Alvarez R R, Afonso J F, Sherrard D J 1961 Serum protein fractionation in normal pregnancy. Am J Obstet Gynecol 82: 1096–1111
185. Mendenhal H W 1970 Serum protein concentrations in pregnancy. I. Concentrations in maternal serum. Am J Obstet Gynecol 106: 388–399
186. Cotton D B, Gonik B, Spillman T, Dorman K F 1984 Intrapartum to postpartum changes in colloid osmotic pressure. Am J Obstet Gynecol 149: 174–177
187. Wu P Y K, Udani V, Chan L, Miller F C, Henneman C E 1983 Colloid osmotic pressure: variations in normal pregnancy. J Perinat Med 11: 193–199
188. Jones M M, Longmire S, Cotton D B, Dorman K F, Skjonsby B S, Joyce T H III 1986 Influence of crystalloid versus colloid infusion on peripartum colloid osmotic pressure changes. Obstet Gynecol 68: 659–661
189. Fletcher A P, Alkjaersig N K, Burstein R 1979 The influence of pregnancy upon blood coagulation and plasma fibrinolytic enzyme function. Am J Obstet Gynecol 134: 743–751
190. Hellgren M, Blombäck M 1981 Studies on blood coagulation and fibrinolysis in pregnancy, during delivery and in the puerperium. I. Normal conditions. Gynecol Obstet Invest 12: 141–154
191. Bonnar J, McNicol G P, Douglas A S 1969 Fibrinolytic enzyme system and pregnancy. Br Med J 3: 387–389
192. Nilsson I M, Kullander S 1967 Coagulation and fibrinolytic studies during pregnancy. Acta Obstet Gynecol Scand 46: 273–285
193. Ratnoff O D, Colopy J E, Pritchard J A 1954 The blood-clotting mechanism during normal parturition. J Lab Clin Med 44: 408–415
194. Talbert L M, Langdell R D 1964 Normal values of certain factors in the blood clotting mechanism in pregnancy. Am J Obstet Gynecol 90: 44–50
195. Kasper C K, Hoag M S, Aggeler P M, Stone S 1964 Blood clotting factors in pregnancy: factor VIII concentrations in normal and AHF-deficient women. Obstet Gynecol 24: 242–247
196. Pechet L, Alexander B 1961 Increased clotting factors in pregnancy. New Engl J Med 265: 1093–1097
197. Ratnoff O D, Holland T R 1959 Coagulation components in normal and abnormal pregnancies. Ann NY Acad Sci 75: 626–633
198. Coopland A, Alkjaersig N, Fletcher A P 1969 Reduction in plasma factor XIII (fibrin stabilizing factor) concentration during pregnancy. J Lab Clin Med 73: 144–153
199. Sagi A, Creter D, Goldman J, Djaldetti M 1981 Platelet functions before, during and after labor. Acta Haematol 65: 67–70
200. Pitkin R M, Witte D L 1979 Platelet and leukocyte counts in pregnancy. J Am Med Assoc 242: 2696–2698
201. Fay R A, Hughes A O, Farron N T 1983 Platelets in pregnancy: hyperdestruction in pregnancy. Obstet Gynecol 61: 238–240
202. Hedner U, Åstedt B 1971 Studies on fibrinolytic inhibitors during pregnancy. Acta Obstet Gynecol Scand 50: 99–103
203. Shaper A G, Evans C M, MacIntosh D M, Kyobe J 1965 Fibrinolysis and plasminogen levels in pregnancy and the puerperium. Lancet 2: 706–708
204. Hahn L 1974 On fibrinolysis and coagulation during parturition and menstruation. With special reference to fibrinogen–fibrin degradation products. Acta Obstet Gynecol Scand 28 (suppl): 7–40
205. Woodfield D G, Cole S K, Allan A G E, Cash J D 1968 Serum fibrin degradation products throughout normal pregnancy. Br Med J 4: 665–668
206. Robertson G S 1966 Serum cholinesterase deficiency. II. Pregnancy. Br J Anaesth 38: 361–369
207. Shnider S M 1965 Serum cholinesterase activity during pregnancy, labor and the puerperum. Anesthesiology 26: 335–339
208. Hazel B, Monier D 1971 Human serum cholinesterase: variations during pregnancy and post-partum. Can Anaesth Soc J 18: 272–277
209. Evans R T, Wroe J M 1980 Plasma cholinesterase changes during pregnancy. Their interpretation as a cause of suxamethonium-induced apnoea. Anaesthesia 35: 651–654
210. Pritchard J A, Baldwin R M, Dickey J C, Wiggins K M 1962 Blood volume changes in pregnancy and the puerperium. II. Red blood cell loss and changes in apparent blood volume during and the following vaginal delivery, cesarean section, and cesarean section plus total hysterectomy. Am J Obstet Gynecol 84: 1271–1282
211. McLennan C E, Lowenstein J M 1959 Blood volume changes immediately after delivery. Stanford Med Bull 17: 152–156
212. Hood D D, Holubec D M 1990 Elective repeat cesarean section. Effect of anesthesia type in blood loss. J Reprod Med 35: 368–372
213. Bonnar J, McNicol G P, Douglas A S 1970 Coagulation and fibrinolytic mechanisms during and after normal childbirth. Br Med J 2: 200–203
214. Bonnar J, Davidson J F, Pidgeon C F, McNicol G P, Douglas A S 1969 Fibrin degradation products in normal and abnormal pregnancy and parturition. Br Med J 3: 137–140
215. Williams N H 1941 Variable significance of heartburn. Am J Obstet Gynecol 42: 814–820
216. Ulmsten U, Sundström G 1978 Esophageal manometry in pregnant and nonpregnant women. Am J Obstet Gynecol 132: 260–264
217. Davison J S, Davison M C, Hay D M 1970 Gastric emptying time in late pregnancy and labour. J Obstet Gynaecol Br Cwlth 77: 37–41
218. O'Sullivan G M, Sutton A J, Thompson S A, Carrie L E, Bullingham RE 1987 Noninvasive measurement of gastric emptying in obstetric patients. Anesth Analg 66: 505–511
219. Macfie A G, Magides A D, Richmond M N, Reilly C S 1991 Gastric emptying in pregnancy. Br J Anaesth 67: 54–57
220. Sandhar B K, Elliott R H, Windram I, Rowbotham D J 1992 Peripartum changes in gastric emptying. Anaesthesia 47: 196–198
221. Parry E, Shields R, Turnbull A C 1970 Transit time in the small intestine in pregnancy. J Obstet Gynaecol Br Cwlth 77: 900–901
222. Wald A, Van Thiel D H, Hoechstetter L, Gavaler J S, Egler K M, Verm R, Scott L, Lester R 1982 Effect of pregnancy on gastrointestinal transit. Dig Dis Sci 27: 1015–1018
223. Murray F A, Erskine J P, Fielding J 1957 Gastric secretion in pregnancy. J Obstet Gynaecol Br Emp 64: 373–381
224. Arzt F 1930 Further observations on the gastric juice in pregnancy. Am J Obstet Gynecol 20: 382–385
225. Van Thiel D H, Gavaler J S, Joshi S N, Sara R K, Stremple J 1977 Heartburn of pregnancy. Gastroenterology 72: 666–668
226. Gryboski W A, Spiro H M 1956 The effect of pregnancy on gastric secretion. New Engl J Med 255: 1131–1134
227. Roberts R B, Shirley M A 1974 Reducing the risk of acid aspiration during cesarean section. Anesth Analg 53: 859–868
228. Teabeaut II J R, 1952 Aspiration of gastric contents. An experimental study. Am J Pathol 28: 51–67
229. James C F, Modell J H, Gibbs C P, Kuck E J, Ruiz B C 1984 Pulmonary aspiration – effects of volume and pH in the rat. Anesth Analg 63: 665–668
230. James C F, Gibbs C P, Banner T 1984 Postpartum perioperative risk of aspiration pneumonia. Anesthesiology 61: 756–759
231. Ong B Y, Palahniuk R J, Cumming M 1978 Gastric volume and pH in out-patients. Can Anaesth Soc J 25: 36–39
232. Morison D H, Dunn G L, Fargas-Babjak A M, Moudgil G C,

Smedstad K, Woo J 1982 A double-blind comparison of cimetidine and ranitidine as prophylaxis against gastric aspiration syndrome. Anesth Analg 61: 988–992
233. Rao T L K, Madhavareddy S, Chinthagada M, El-Etr A A 1984 Metoclopramide and cimetidine to reduce gastric fluid pH and volume. Anesth Analg 63: 1014–1016
234. Barnes P J, Havill J H 1980 Preoperative cimetidine – effects on gastric fluid. Anaesth Intens Care 8: 464–468
235. Manchikanti L, Grow J B, Colliver J A, Hadley C H, Hohlbein L J 1985 Bicitra (sodium citrate) and metoclopramide in outpatient anesthesia for prophylaxis against aspiration pneumonitis. Anesthesiology 63: 378–384
236. Detmer M D, Pandit S K, Cohen P J 1979 Prophylactic single-dose oral antacid therapy in the preoperative period – comparison of cimetidine and Maalox. Anesthesiology 51: 270–273
237. Wyner J, Cohen S E 1982 Gastric volume in early pregnancy: effect of metoclopramide. Anesthesiology 57: 209–212
238. Baraka A, Saab M, Salem M R, Winnie A P 1977 Control of gastric acidity by glycopyrrolate premedication in the parturient. Anesth Analg 56: 642–645
239. McCaughey W, Howe J P, Moore J, Dundee J W 1981 Cimetidine in elective caesarean section. Effect on gastric acidity. Anaesthesia 36: 167–172
240. Cohen S E, Jasson J, Talafre M L, Chauvelot-Moachon L, Barrier G 1984 Does metoclopramide decrease the volume of gastric contents in patients undergoing cesarean section? Anesthesiology 61: 604–607
241. Boschi S, Di Marco M G, Pigna A, Rossi R 1984 The effect of ranitidine on gastric pH and volume in patients undergoing cesarean section: possible relationship to Mendelson's syndrome. Curr Ther Res 35: 654–662
242. Dewan D M, Floyd H M, Thistlewood J M, Bogard T D, Spielman F J 1985 Sodium citrate pretreatment in elective cesarean section patients. Anesth Analg 64: 34–37
243. Bassey O O 1977 Pregnancy heartburn in Nigerians and Caucasians with theories about aetiology based on manometric recordings from the oesophagus and stomach. Br J Obstet Gynaecol 84: 439–443
244. Nagler R, Spiro H M 1961 Heartburn in late pregnancy. Manometric studies of esophageal motor function. J Clin Invest 40: 954–970
245. Atlay R D, Gillison E W, Horton A L 1973 A fresh look at pregnancy heartburn. J Obstet Gynaecol Br Cwlth 80: 63–66
246. Brock-Utne J G, Downing J W, Dimopoulos G E, Rubin J, Moshal MG 1980 Effect of domperidone on lower esophageal sphincter tone in late pregnancy. Anesthesiology 52: 321–323
247. Brock-Utne J G, Dow T G B, Welman S, Dimopoulos G E, Moshal M G 1978 The effect of metoclopramide on the lower oesophageal sphincter in late pregnancy. Anaesth Intens Care 6: 26–29
248. Lind J F, Smith A M, McIver D K, Coopland A T, Crispin J S 1968 Heartburn in pregnancy – a manometric study. Can Med Assoc J 98: 571–574
249. Dow T G B, Brock-Utne J G, Rubin J, Welman S, Dimopoulos G E, Moshal M G 1978 The effect of atropine on the lower esophageal sphincter in late pregnancy. Obstet Gynecol 51: 426–430
250. Brock-Utne J G, Dow T G B, Dimopoulos G E, Welman S, Downing J W, Moshal M G 1981 Gastric and lower oesophageal sphincter (LOS) pressures in early pregnancy. Br J Anaesth 53: 381–384
251. Bainbridge E T, Nicholas S D, Newton J R, Temple J G 1984 Gastro-oesophageal reflux in pregnancy. Altered function of the barrier to reflux in asymptomatic women during early pregnancy. Scand J Gastroenterol 19: 85–89
252. Van Thiel D H, Gavaler J S, Stremple J 1976 Lower esophageal sphincter pressure in women using sequential oral contraceptives. Gastroenterology 71: 232–234
253. La Salvia L A, Steffen E A 1950 Delayed gastric emptying time in labor. Am J Obstet Gynecol 59: 1075–1081
254. Murphy D F, Nally B, Gardiner J, Unwin A 1984 Effect of metoclopramide on gastric emptying before elective and emergency caesarean section. Br J Anaesth 56: 1113–1116
255. Taylor G, Pryse-Davies J 1966 The prophylactic use of antacids in the prevention of the acid-pulmonary-aspiration syndrome (Mendelson's syndrome). Lancet 1: 288–291
256. Wilson J 1978 Gastric emptying in labour: some recent findings and their clinical significance. J Int Med Res 6 (suppl 1): 54–60
257. Holdsworth J D 1978 Relationship between stomach contents and analgesia in labour. Br J Anaesth 50: 1145–1148
258. Lahiri S K, Thomas T A, Hodgson R M H 1973 Single-dose antacid therapy for the prevention of Mendelson's syndrome. Br J Anaesth 45: 1143–1146
259. Wheatley R G, Kallus F T, Reynolds R C, Giesecke Jr A H 1979 Milk of magnesia is an effective preinduction antacid in obstetric anesthesia. Anesthesiology 50: 514–519
260. O'Sullivan G M, Bullingham R E 1985 Noninvasive assessment by radiotelemetry of antacid effect during labor. Anesth Anal 64: 95–100
261. Johnston J R, McCaughey W, Moore J, Dundee J W 1982 A field trial of cimetidine as the sole oral antacid in obstetric anesthesia. Anaesthesia 37: 33–38
262. Johnston J R, Moore J, McCaughey W, Dundee J W, Howard P J, Toner W, McClean E 1983 Use of cimetidine as an oral antacid in obstetric anethesia. Anesth Analg 62: 720–726
263. Hey V M F, Ostick D G, Mazumder J K, Lord W D 1981 Pethidine, metoclopramide and the gastro-oesophageal sphincter. A study in healthy volunteers. Anaesthesia 36: 173–176
264. Hall A W, Moossa A R, Clark J, Cooley G R, Skinner D B 1975 The effects of premedication drugs on the lower oesophageal high pressure zone and reflux status of Rhesus monkeys and man. Gut 16: 347–352
265. Wright P M C, Allen R W, Moore J, Donelly J P 1992 Gastric emptying during lumbar extradural analgesia in labour: effect of fentanyl supplementation. Br J Anaesth 68: 248–251
266. Geddes S M, Thorburn J, Logan R W 1991 Gastric emptying following caesarean section and the effect of epidural fentanyl. Anaesthesia 46: 1016–1018
267. Blouw R, Scatliff J, Craig D B, Palahniuk R J 1976 Gastric volume and pH in postpartum patients. Anesthesiology 45: 456–457
268. Abitbol M M 1985 Supine position in labor and associated fetal heart rate changes. Obstet Gynecol 65: 481–486
269. Humphrey M D, Chang A, Wood E C, Morgan S, Hounslow D 1974 A decrease in fetal pH during the second stage of labour, when conducted in the dorsal position. J Obstet Gynaecol Br Cwlth 81: 600–602
270. Humphrey M, Hounslow D, Morgan S, Wood C 1973 The influence of maternal posture at birth on the fetus. J Obstet Gynaecol Br Cwlth 80: 1075–1080
271. Huch A, Huch R, Schneider H, Rooth G 1977 Continuous transcutaneous monitoring of fetal oxygen tension during labour. Br J Obstet Gynaecol 84 (suppl 1): 1–39
272. Crawford J S, Burton M, Davies P 1972 Time and lateral tilt at caesarean section. Br J Anaesth 44: 477–484
273. Datta S, Alper M H, Ostheimer G W, Brown Jr W U, Weiss J B 1979 Effects of maternal position on epidural anesthesia for cesarean section, acid–base status, and bupivacaine concentrations at delivery. Anesthesiology 50: 205–209
274. Crawford J S, James F M III, Davies P, Crawley M 1976 A further study of general anaesthesia for caesarean section. Br J Anaesth 48: 661–667
275. Datta S, Ostheimer G W, Weiss J B, Brown W U Jr, Alper M H 1981 Neonatal effect of prolonged anesthetic induction for cesarean section. Obstet Gynecol 58: 331–335
276. Eckstein K L, Marx G F 1974 Aortocaval compression and uterine displacement. Anesthesiology 40: 92–96
277. Sellick B A 1961 Cricoid pressure to control regurgitation of stomach contents during induction of anesthesia. Lancet 2: 404–406
278. Muravchick S, Burkett L, Gold M I 1981 Succinylcholine-induced fasciculations and intragastric pressure during induction of anesthesia. Anesthesiology 55: 180–183
279. Smith G, Dalling R, Williams T I R 1978 Gastro-oesophageal pressure gradient changes produced by induction of anaesthesia and suxamethonium. Br J Anaesth 50: 1137–1143
280. Freund F G, Rubin A P 1972 The need for additional

succinylcholine after d-tubocurarine. Anesthesiology 36: 185–187
281. Walts L F, Dillon J B 1969 Clinical studies of the interaction between d-tubocurarine and succinylcholine. Anesthesiology 31: 39–44
282. Archer G W Jr, Marx G F 1974 Arterial oxygen tension during apnoea in parturient women. Br J Anaesth 46: 358–360
283. Norris M C, Kirkland, M R, Torjman M C, Goldberg M E 1989 Denitrogenation in pregnancy. Can J Anaesth 36: 523–525
284. Rampton A J, Mallaiah S, Garrett C P O 1988 Increased ventilation requirements during obstetric general anaesthesia. Br J Anaesth 61: 730–737
285. Cook P T 1984 The influence on foetal outcome of maternal carbon dioxide tension at caesarean section under general anaesthesia. Anaesth Intens Care 12: 296–302
286. Peng A T C, Blancato L S, Motoyama E K 1972 Effect of maternal hypocapnia v. eucapnia on the foetus during caesarean section. Br J Anaesth 44: 1173–1178
287. Low J A, Boston R W, Cervenko F W 1970 Effect of low maternal carbon dioxide tension on placental gas exchange. Am J Obstet Gynecol 106: 1032–1043
288. Moya F, Morishima H O, Schnider S M, James L S 1965 Influence of maternal hyperventilation on the newborn infant. Am J Obstet Gynecol 91: 76–84
289. Scott D B, Lees M M, Davie I T, Slawson K B, Kerr M G 1969 Observations on cardiorespiratory function during caesarean section. Br J Anaesth 41: 489–495
290. Fuller E O, Galletti P M, Chou H Y, Peirce E C II 1972 Effect of P_{CO_2} on the vascular resistance of the pregnant sheep uterus. Physiologist 15: 140
291. Moya F, Smith B E 1965 Uptake, distribution and placental transport of drugs and anesthetics. Anesthesiology 26: 465–476
292. Palahniuk R J, Shnider S M, Eger II E I 1974 Pregnancy decreases the requirement for inhaled anesthetic agents. Anesthesiology 41: 82–83
293. Strout C D, Nahrwold M L 1981 Halothane requirement during pregnancy and lactation in rats. Anesthesiology 55: 322–323
294. Selye H 1941 Studies concerning the anesthetic action of steroid hormones. J Pharmacol Exp Ther 73: 127–141
295. Merryman W, Boiman R, Barnes L, Rothchild I 1954 Progesterone 'anesthesia' in human subjects. J Clin Endocrinol Metab 14: 1567–1569
296. Spielman F J, Mueller R A, Corke B C 1985 Cerebrospinal fluid concentration of 5-hydroxyindoleactic acid in pregnancy. Anesthesiolgy 62: 193–195
297. Genazzani A R, Facchinetti F, Parrini D 1981 Beta-lipotrophin and beta-endorphine plasma levels during pregnancy. Clin Endocrinol 14: 409–418
298. Budiamal L R, Muetterties C L, Seltzer J L, Jacoby J, Vogel W H 1981 Beta-endorphin in pregnant women at term. Anesthesiology 55: A322
299. Abboud T K, Sarkis F, Hung T T et al 1983 Effects of epidural anesthesia during labor on maternal plasma beta-endorphin levels. Anesthesiology 59: 1–5
300. Goland R S, Wardlaw S L, Stark R I, Frantz A G 1981 Human plasma beta-endorphin during pregnancy, labor, and delivery. J Clin Endocrinol Metab 52: 74–78
301. Steinbrook R A, Carr D B, Datta S, Naulty J S, Lee C, Fisher J 1982 Dissociation of plasma and cerebrospinal fluid beta-endorphin-like immunoactivity levels during pregnancy and parturition. Anesth Analg 61: 893–897
302. Datta S, Carr D B, Lambert D H et al 1983 Anesthesia for cesarean delivery: relationship of maternal and fetal plasma beta-endorphin concentrations to different types of anesthesia. Anesthesiology 59: A418
303. Houck J C, Kimball C, Chang C, Pedigo N W, Yamamura H I 1980 Placental beta-endorphin-like peptides. Science 207: 78–80
304. Wardlaw S L, Frantz A G 1983 Brain beta-endorphin during pregnancy, parturition, and the postpartum period. Endocrinology 113: 1664–1668
305. Gintzler A R 1980 Endorphin-mediated increases in pain threshold during pregnancy. Science 210: 193–195
306. Viby-Mogensen J 1980 Correlation of succinylcholine duration of action with plasma cholinesterase activity in subjects with the genotypically normal enzyme. Anesthesiology 53: 517–520
307. Baraka A, Wakid N, Noueihed R, Karam H, Bolotova N 1986 Pseudocholinesterase activity and atracurium v. suxamethonium block. Br J Anaesth 58: 91S–95S
308. Blitt C D, Petty W C, Alberternst E E, Wright B J 1977 Correlation of plasma cholinesterase activity and duration of action of succinylcholine during pregnancy. Anesth Analg 56: 78–83
309. Leighton B L, Cheek T G, Gross J B, Apfelbaum J L, Shantz B B, Gutsche B B, Rosenberg H 1986 Succinylcholine pharmacodynamics in peripartum patients. Anesthesiology 64: 202–205
310. Ramzan I M 1986 Succinylcholine in peripartum patients. Anesthesiology 65: 441–442
311. Ganga C C, Heyduk J V, Marx G F, Sklar G S 1982 A comparison of the response to suxamethonium in post-partum and gynaecological patients. Anaesthesia 37: 903–906
312. Rodrigue R, Durant N N, Nguyen N, Katz L, Conklin K A 1986 Comparison of vecuronium-induced neuromuscular blockade in pregnant and nonpregnant female rabbits. Anesthesiology 65: A401
313. Camp C E, Tessem J, Adenwala J, Joyce T H III 1987 Vecuronium and prolonged neuromuscular blockade in postpartum patients. Anesthesiology 67: 1006–1008
314. Dailey P A, Fisher D M, Shnider S M et al 1984 Pharmacokinetics, placental transfer, and neonatal effects of vecuronium and pancuronium administered during cesarean section. Anesthesiology 60: 569–574
315. Duvaldestin P, Demetriou M, Henzel D, Desmonts J M 1978 The placental transfer of pancuronium and its pharmacokinetics during caesarian section. Acta Anaesth Scand 22: 327–333
316. Giesecke A H Jr, Morris R E, Dalton M D, Stephen C R 1968 Of magnesium, muscle relaxants, toxemic parturients, and cats. Anesth Anal 47: 689–695
317. Ghoneim M M, Long J P 1970 The interaction between magnesium and other neuromuscular blocking agents. Anesthesiology 32: 23–27
318. Morris R, Giesecke Jr A H 1968 Potentiation of muscle relaxants by magnesium sulfate therapy in toxemia of pregnancy. S Med J 61: 25–28
319. James M F M, Cork R C, Dennett J E 1986 Succinylcholine pretreatment with magnesium sulfate. Anesth Analg 65: 373–376
320. Tran B, Nguyen N, Chung H, Murad S, Lee C 1984 Interaction between magnesium and vecuronium in rabbits. Anesthesiology 61: A403
321. Lee C, Nguyen N B, Tran B K, Katz R 1982 Quantification of magnesium–pancuronium interaction in the diaphragm and the tibialis anterior. Anesthesiology 57: A392
322. Hopkins E L, Hendricks C H, Cibils L A 1965 Cerebrospinal fluid pressure in labor. Am J Obstet Gynecol 93: 907–916
323. Marx G F, Zemaitis M T, Orkin L R 1961 Cerebrospinal fluid pressures during labor and obstetrical anesthesia. Anesthesiology 22: 348–354
324. Marx G F, Oka Y, Orkin L R 1962 Cerebrospinal fluid pressures during labor. Am J Obstet Gynecol 84: 213–219
325. Usubiaga J E, Wikinski J A, Usubiaga L E 1967 Epidural pressure and its relation to spread of anesthetic solutions in epidural space. Anesth Analg 46: 440–446
326. Galbert M W, Marx G F 1974 Extradural pressures in the parturient patient. Anesthesiology 40: 499–502
327. Messih M N A 1981 Epidural space pressures during pregnancy. Anaesthesia 36: 775–782
328. Hehre F W, Yules R B, Hipona F A 1966 Continuous lumbar peridural anesthesia in obstetrics. III. Attempts to produce spread of contrast media by acute vena cava obstruction in dogs. Anesth Analg 45: 551–556
329. Rolbin S H, Relle A, Hew E M 1985 Hyperventilation does not affect the incidence of paresthesiae and blood vessel cannulation during epidural catheter insertion. Can Anaesth Soc J 32: 568

330. Rolbin S H, Hew E, Ogilvie G 1987 A comparison of two types of epidural catheters. Can J Anaesth 34: 459–461
331. Rolbin S H, Halpern S H, Braude B M, Kapala D, Unger R, Radhakrisnan S 1990 Fluid through the epidural needle does not reduce complications of epidural catheter insertion. Can J Anaesth 37: 337–340
332. Philip B K 1985 Effect of epidural air injection on catheter complications. Reg Anesth 10: 21–23
333. Verniquet A J W 1980 Vessel puncture with epidural catheters. Experience in obstetric patients. Anaesthesia 35: 660–662
334. Halpern S, Onayemi A, Swartz J, Rosaeg O 1987 Does an epidural test dose prevent complications of epidural catheter insertion? Anesth Analg 66: S77
335. Barclay D L, Renegar O J, Nelson Jr E W 1968 The influence of inferior vena cava compression on the level of spinal anesthesia. Am J Obstet Gynecol 101: 792–800
336. Marx G F, Orkin L R 1969 Anesthetic considerations: the mother. In: Adriani J (ed) Physiology of obstetric anesthesia. Charles C Thomas, Springfield pp 83–114
337. Datta S, Hurley R J, Naulty J S et al 1986 Plasma and cerebrospinal fluid progesterone concentrations in pregnant and nonpregnant women. Anesth Analg 65: 950–954
338. Abouleish E I 1986 Postpartum tubal ligation requires more bupivacaine for spinal anesthesia than does cesarean section. Anesth Analg 65: 897–900
339. DeSimone C A, Norris M C, Leighton B L, Epstein R H, Palmer C 1989 Spinal anesthesia for cesarean section and post partum tubal ligation. Anesthesiology 71: A837
340. Assali N S, Prystowsky H 1950 Studies on autonomic blockade. I. Comparison between the effects of tetraethylammonium chloride (TEAC) and high selective spinal anesthesia on blood pressure of normal and toxemic pregnancy. J Clin Invest 29: 1354–1366
341. Cheng P A 1963 The anatomical and clinical aspects of epidural anesthesia. Anesth Analg 42: 398–406
342. Butterworth IV J F, Walker F O, Lysak S Z 1990 Pregnancy increases median nerve susceptibility to lidocaine. Anesthesiology 72: 962–965
343. Datta S, Lambert D H, Gregus J, Gissen A J, Covino B G 1983 Differential sensitivities of mammalian nerve fibers during pregnancy. Anesth Analg 62: 1070–1072
344. Flanagan H L, Datta S, Lambert D H, Gissen A J, Covino B G 1987 Effect of pregnancy on bupivacaine-induced conduction blockade in the isolated rabbit vagus nerve. Anesth Analg 66: 123–126
345. Flanagan H L, Datta S, Moller R A, Covino B G 1988 Effect of exogenously administered progesterone on susceptibility of rabbit vagus nerves to bupivacaine. Anesthesiology 69: A676
346. Sheth A P, Dautenhahn D L, Fagraeus L 1985 Decreased CSF protein during pregnancy as a mechanism facilitating the spread of spinal anesthesia. Anesth Analg 64: 280
347. Dautenhahn D L, Fagraeus L 1984 Acid–base changes of spinal fluid during pregnancy. Anesth Analg 63: 204
348. Sivakumaran C, Ramanathan S, Chalon J, Turndorf H 1982 Uterine contractions and the spread of local anesthetics in the epidural space. Anesth Analg 61: 127–129
349. Sharrock N E, Greenidge J 1979 Epidural dose responses in pregnant and non pregnant patients. Anesthesiology 51: S298
350. Grundy E M, Zamora A M, Winnie A P 1978 Comparison of spread of epidural anesthesia in pregnant and nonpregnant women. Anesth Analg 57: 544–546
351. Kalas D B, Senfield R M, Hehre F W 1966 Continuous lumbar peridural anesthesia in obstetrics. IV. Comparison of the number of segments blocked in pregnant and nonpregnant subjects. Anesth Analg 45: 848–851
352. Bromage P R 1962 Spread of analgesic solutions in the epidural space and their site of action: a statistical study. Br J Anaesth 34: 161–178
353. Fagraeus L, Urban B J, Bromage P R 1983 Spread of epidural analgesia in early pregnancy. Anesthesiology 58: 184–187
354. Norris M C 1990 Patient variables and the subarachnoid spread of hyperbaric bupivacaine in the term parturient. Anesthesiology 72: 478–482
355. Norris M C 1988 Height, weight, and the spread of subarachnoid hyperbaric bupivacaine in the term parturient. Anesth Analg 67: 555–558
356. Hartwell B L, Hauch M A, Aglio L S, Datta S, Ostheimer G W 1989 Vertebral column length and the spread of hyperbaric subarachnoid bupivacaine in the term parturient. Society of Obstetrical Anesthesia and Perinatology, Seattle
357. Chen B J, Kwan W F, Virtusio L 1990 Comparison of body height and vertebral column length in the term pregnant women. Anesth Analg 70: S55
358. Hodgkinson R, Husain F J 1981 Obesity, gravity, and spread of epidural anesthesia. Anesth Analg 60: 421–424
359. Hodgkinson R, Husain F J 1980 Obesity and the cephalad spread of analgesia following epidural administration of bupivacaine for cesarean section. Anesth Analg 59: 89–92
360. Gambling D R, McMorland G H, Mayson K, Moore R 1989 Predictability of spread of epidural anesthesia for cesarean section using incremental doses of lidocaine hydrocarbonate with epinephrine. Reg Anesth 14: 133–137
361. Santos D J, Juneja M, Denson D D, Nicholson C, Bridenbaugh P O 1987 Is there a correlation between vertebral length and volume of local anesthetic required to produce epidural anesthesia? Reg Anesth 12: 39
362. Assali N S, Prystowsky H 1950 Studies on autonomic blockade. II. Observations on the nature of blood pressure fall with high selective spinal anesthesia in pregnant women. J Clin Invest 29: 1367–1375
363. Tabsh K, Rudelstorfer R, Nuwayhid B, Assali NS 1986 Circulatory responses to hypovolemia in the pregnant and nonpregnant sheep after pharmacologic sympathectomy. Am J Obstet Gynecol 154: 411–419
364. Edouard D, Pannier B, London G, Safar M 1990 Differential influence of pregnancy on limbs venous tone in humans. Anesthesiology 73: A955
365. Goodlin R C 1986 Venous reactivity and pregnancy abnormalities. Acta Obstet Gynecol Scand 65: 345–348
366. Gibbs C P, Spohr L, Petrakis J, Paulus D, Schultetus R 1981 Prevention of hypotension with hydration. Anesthesiology 55: A308
367. Hallworth D, Jellicoe J A, Wilkes R G 1982 Hypotension during epidural anaesthesia for caesarean section. A comparison of intravenous loading with crystalloid and colloid solutions. Anaesthesia 37: 53–56
368. Clark R B, Thompson D S, Thompson C H 1976 Prevention of spinal hypotension associated with cesarean section. Anesthesiology 45: 670–674
369. Downing J W, Houlton P C, Barclay A 1979 Extradural analgesia for caesarean section: a comparison with general anaesthesia. Br J Anaesth 51: 367–374
370. Fox G S, Smith J B, Namba Y, Johnson R C 1979 Anesthesia for cesarean section: further studies. Am J Obstet Gynecol 133: 15–19
371. James F M III, Crawford J S, Hopkinson R, Davies P, Naiem H 1977 A comparison of general anesthesia and lumbar epidural analgesia for elective cesarean section. Anesth Analg 56: 228–235
372. Mathru M, Rao T L K, Kartha R K, Shanmugham M, Jacobs H K 1980 Intravenous albumin administration for prevention of spinal hypotension during cesarean section. Anesth Analg 59: 655–658
373. Lewis M, Thomas P, Wilkes R G 1983 Hypotension during epidural analgesia for caesarean section. Arterial and central venous pressure changes after acute intravenous loading with two litres of Hartmann's solution. Anaesthesia 38: 250–253
374. Campbell E J M 1955 An electromyographic examination of the role of the intercostal muscles in breathing in man. J Physiol 129: 12–26
375. Moir D D 1963 Ventilatory function during epidural analgesia. Br J Anaesth 35: 3–7
376. Moya F, Smith B 1962 Spinal anesthesia for cesarean section. Clinical and biochemical studies of effects on maternal physiology. J Am Med Assoc 179: 609–614
377. Askrog V F, Smith T C, Eckenhoff J E 1964 Changes in pulmonary ventilation during spinal anesthesia. Surg Gynecol Obstet 119: 563–567

378. de Jong R H 1965 Arterial carbon dioxide and oxygen tensions during spinal block. J Am Med Assoc 191: 698–702
379. Pitkänen M T 1987 Body mass and spread of spinal anesthesia with bupivacaine. Anesth Analg 66: 127–131
380. Egbert L D, Tamersoy K, Deas T C 1961 Pulmonary function during spinal anesthesia: the mechanism of cough depression. Anesthesiology 22: 882–885
381. Gamil M 1989 Serial peak expiratory flow rates in mothers during caesarean section under extradural anaesthesia. Br J Anaesth 62: 415–418
382. Norris M C, Torjman M, Leighton B L, DeSimone C A 1990 Respiratory and motor function during bupivacaine spinal anesthesia for cesarean section. Anesth Analg 70: S283

6. Maternal assessment

Part A USA view *E. M. Yun*
Part B European view *M. A. G. Soetens*

PART A
USA VIEW
E. M. Yun

There are many differences in the anesthetic care of parturients and nonpregnant patients, including their preoperative evaluation. Although preoperative assessment is a crucial part of anesthetic management, many obstetric patients are not interviewed by an anesthesiologist until just prior to the administration of an anesthetic, whether during active labor or in emergency situations, such as a 'stat' cesarean delivery or hemorrhage from a retained placenta. However, it is in the early preoperative period that the parturient can be best informed of her options for anesthesia, while she is relatively calm and is in less discomfort than during the painful active stages of labor or in emergency situations. Owing to the nature of the progress of labor, it is difficult to ensure that every patient will be evaluated by an anesthesiologist except immediately prior to the administration of anesthesia. It would be prudent, however, to make this effort, especially in a 'high-risk' obstetric population who may require a surgical procedure.

It is helpful to divide obstetric patients into two groups for preoperative evaluation: those desiring labor analgesia and those patients with systemic disease that may influence the anesthetic management or will increase the likelihood of cesarean delivery. Good communication with the obstetric team is important. On occasion, a patient may require additional medical evaluation and intervention to place her in the best possible condition for the delivery of her baby. Therefore, early evaluation of the parturient and good communication between the care givers are essential for the high-risk group.

PREOPERATIVE EVALUATION FOR LABOR ANALGESIA

The goals for the preoperative evaluation are twofold: to inform the patient of the risks and benefits of anesthesia and to obtain a history that will aid in the delivery of a safe and pleasant anesthetic. As with any preoperative evaluation, the review of any available medical record is helpful prior to the interview. The interview itself consists of a history with a review of systems including any medical therapy that the patient is receiving and a physical examination. It is also during this time that the patient can be informed about the various anesthetic techniques available, along with the risks and the benefits of each, the procedures and events expected and, lastly, she can give informed consent if she desires an anesthetic.

History

A full record of the patient's current and past medical history must be obtained including any prior anesthetic experiences, surgery, allergies, medications, as well as height and weight. There are many physiologic changes during pregnancy that can exacerbate the parturient's systemic disease and influence the anesthetic management. Therefore, a careful review of systems is crucial.

A suggested review of systems of particular interest in obstetric patients:

- Cardiovascular: mitral valve prolapse, palpitations, increase in blood pressure, generalized edema;
- Respiratory: asthma, cigarette use;
- Hepatic: history of hepatitis, alcohol use;
- Neurologic: seizure, headache;
- Gastrointestinal: gastroesophageal reflux, hiatal hernia, peptic ulcer disease;
- Hematologic: easy bruising, bleeding tendency;
- Endocrine: diabetes, thyroid disease;
- Musculoskeletal: scoliosis, history of back pain, rheumatoid arthritis;

- Reproductive: previous obstetric complications, pregnancies, parity, gestational age.

All parturients are considered to have a 'full stomach', but it is important to note their last oral intake. Current drug therapy must also be carefully reviewed and any potential adverse drug interaction with anesthetics must be considered.

Physical examination

Routine auscultation of the heart and lungs should be performed and special attention should be given to any area of concern elicited by the history. Baseline BP and HR should be noted, as well as the patient's size and the anatomy of the back, examining for excessive lordosis and obesity.

Perhaps one of the most critical, if not the most crucial, part of the physical examination is the assessment of the airway. Any laboring patient is at risk of an emergency procedure, such as cesarean delivery, at any time. Parturients are considered to have a 'full stomach' and are at increased risk for regurgitation and aspiration. In addition to the airway being edematous with friable mucous membranes, the patient has increased breast size, all of which contribute to problems during airway management. If the patient has already had an epidural anesthetic for labor, this is not as concerning; however, if regional anesthesia is not an option, the operating room table is not the place to discover a difficult airway when two lives are in danger. For these reasons, the airway must always be routinely examined. The combination of the Mallampati airway classification, the measurement of the distance from thyroid cartilage to tip of the mandible, and the ability to extend the neck gives a good assessment of the airway and the possibility of a difficult intubation. If a difficult laryngoscopy is anticipated, the patient should be strongly advised to have an early epidural placement to decrease the likelihood of requiring a general anesthetic for an emergency procedure.

Laboratory information

Elaborate laboratory studies are not cost-effective and are not warranted, since the majority of parturients are young and healthy. However, depending on the patient, the complexity of the medical history, as well as the planned procedure, appropriate studies should be performed. Of particular interest in the labor and delivery suite, where regional anesthesia is the technique of choice, are the coagulation studies. Currently there is a great deal of controversy concerning the best test for assessing the patient's coagulation status. Each institution may have its own guidelines to follow prior to the administration of a regional technique. The overall clinical status of the patient, the risks and benefits of a regional technique, along with the patient's history of bleeding and easy bruisability, should govern the choice of anesthetic technique.

Initiation of epidural anesthetic

A thorough explanation of the procedure is helpful for the patient's understanding as well as her ability to cooperate during the placement of an epidural anesthetic. The patient can be placed in the lateral or the sitting position, but the importance of flexing the head, bending the knees up to the chest and curving the lower back out like a letter 'C' should be emphasized. A step-by-step description is given, such as cleaning the back with a cold antiseptic solution, a sharp needle stick to inject local anesthetic to numb the skin, pressure sensation of the epidural needle insertion which may be followed by a possible transient paresthesia during the insertion of the epidural catheter. The needle is removed while the catheter is left in place and then taped to the back. Common side-effects and complications should be explained. Hypotension can occur even after a prior fluid bolus necessitating frequent BP measurements and treatment with additional fluid and or vasopressor. A possible headache from an unintentional dural puncture may occur, and is very 'operator dependent'. Symptoms of local anesthetic toxicity from an unintentional intravenous injection through an epidural vein include tinnitus and circumoral numbness. Postpartum backache is perhaps one of the most common complaints in the obstetric patient; however, this can occur whether or not regional anesthesia is used. Patients should be aware that not all the sensations of labor will disappear with an epidural anesthetic. It is normal to feel the pressure of contractions along with rectal and vaginal pressure towards the second stage of labor and delivery.

Rare complications such as an epidural hematoma and epidural abscess are surgical emergencies and should be explained to any patient with a possibility of high risk for such an event. The possibility of replacing the epidural catheter due to an unintentional intravascular catheter insertion, unilateral block, malfunctioning catheter, accidental displacement of the catheter, as well as a rare event such as subdural or subarachnoid injection of local anesthetic resulting in a high spread of anesthesia should also be mentioned.

All questions regarding anesthesia should be answered and any misconceptions should be dispelled. One of the most frequently asked question is whether epidural analgesia slows the progress of labor. Despite a large number of studies, there is no single accepted viewpoint. Most believe that there is a transient slowing in the progress of labor. This is less of a concern for patients in active labor and can be offset by the use of oxytocic stimulation of the uterus.

The risks of an epidural anesthetic should be weighed against its many advantages. It provides good to excellent pain relief without maternal or fetal depression. The parturient is awake and participating in the labor and delivery of her baby with decreased risk of aspiration. A proper analgesic level will decrease catecholamine release and decrease maternal hyperventilation. A well-functioning labor epidural anesthetic can be used for instrumentations such as vacuum extraction, forceps delivery, episiotomy repair, removal of retained placenta and, most importantly cesarean delivery avoiding the use of general anesthesia.

Finally, informed consent should be obtained early in the process when the laboring parturient is in less pain and discomfort.

HIGH-RISK CONSULTATION

Advances in medical and obstetric care have allowed an increasing number of women with significant medical histories to conceive and deliver babies. This has also increased the number of high-risk patients in the obstetric population. This group includes those patients with underlying systemic disease, conditions associated with pregnancy that require special attention such as difficult airway, or a prior unpleasant experience of anesthesia. Some of the medical problems include cardiac disease, asthma, diabetes, renal disease, morbid obesity, hematologic and neurologic disorders, scoliosis with a Harrington rod placement, and even rare problems such as patients with heart or lung transplants. Problems associated with pregnancy may include hypertensive disorders, peripartum hemorrhage and conditions involving the fetus.

The obstetrician should refer these patients to the anesthesiologist during the patient's routine prenatal care visit. A full history and physical examination should be performed and an anesthetic plan developed and discussed with the patient. Early evaluation would allow for proper work-up and management of the patient to place her in an optimal condition for labor and delivery.

It is helpful to have a list of high-risk patients that is updated on a regular basis for the obstetric anesthesia team. The list may include a brief history of the patient, estimated date of birth and anesthetic plans and concerns. The consultation form can be filed so that it is easily accessible when the patient is admitted to the labor and delivery suite.

Whether the patient is seen for a routine labor epidural analgesia or for a high-risk consultation, it is crucial to convey any pertinent history of the patient and plans for her anesthetic management to the rest of the anesthesia team since emergency situations can arise at any time.

PART B
EUROPEAN VIEW
M. Soetens

The routine preoperative anesthetic evaluation is considered to be an essential part of any anesthetic procedure. However, many parturients are not seen except immediately before entry into the operating room or when they are already in labor. In 1968, an obstetric anesthesia service was started in the author's hospital, mainly utilizing the lumbar epidural technique. After 2 years of practice we felt the need to institute an outpatient consultation service for pregnant women. Others feel the same need.[1] Usually, this prepartum consultation takes place either in a prenatal clinic outside the hospital or in the hospital itself.

Ideally, every parturient should be seen by an anesthesiologist at a prepartum consultation before labor. As with any other anesthetic procedure an epidural anesthetic can lead to complications such as total spinal anesthesia or possible toxic reactions after unintentional intravenous injection of local anesthetic. Any labor may end at any time with a cesarean delivery.

Because it is not appropriate to do a prepartum consultation with the parturient in painful labor or in the middle of the night, we like to see the parturient prior to admission. It would be better to arrange the prepartum consultation close to the delivery date, but this would mean that a number of preterm labors would be missed. Therefore, we try to see the patients during the last 3–4 weeks before the expected delivery date.

The prepartum consultation for labor and delivery, with the anesthesiologist, fulfills a variety of functions concerned with the administration of regional analgesia or anesthesia and, occasionally, general anesthesia. Although it has some analogy with a routine preoperative evaluation, the prepartum consultation obviously has its own distinguishing characteristics.

The first function of the prepartum consultation is to inform the parturient fully about the risks and benefits of the various anesthetic techniques and to reduce her anxiety.

Therefore, 3–4 weeks before the expected delivery date, the parturients, along with their partners attend one of our weekly sessions in stress-free surroundings. An anesthesiologist, who performs lumbar epidural anesthesia for obstetrics, gives information about the aims of this type of anesthesia as well as technical details.

Preposterous and unfounded rumors regarding epidural analgesia abound: 'it causes deformed babies and eye problems in the baby'; 'the mother gets alopecia'; the performance of a future section is impossible'. All these misconceptions must be dispelled.

It is advisable to explain, step by step, the performance of the epidural technique. The first subject is the placement of an intravenous line through which an infusion can be started. The benefits of an intravenous line are three fold: comfort – different drugs can be injected through one needle puncture; safety – it provides fast access to administer drugs during unexpected complications; nutrition value – fluids with electrolytes and calories can be given. We explain that the best position for the patient during lumbar epidural puncture is the lateral position with flexed head, curved back and bended knees while remaining motionless. We disinfect the back with a cold moistened tampon and warn the patient not to touch her back to prevent infection. In order to allay the common apprehension of the actual introduction of the needle into the back we explain that the skinprick and the placement of the epidural needle is less painful than the puncture and the intravenous placement of a catheter in an arm vein. We show an epidural catheter to the group so that they can see it and understand how the local anesthetic can reach the epidural space through the hollow plastic tube. We explain that sometimes one can feel pressure in the back or tingling in one leg or in the buttocks while the epidural needle is being inserted or, thereafter, with the plastic catheter; these feelings must be reported to the anesthesiologist because they give him important information about the correct positioning of the needle or the catheter. Finally we discuss how the catheter is taped onto the back and how it is brought over the left shoulder and how the syringe is fixed to the gown in order to make manipulation easier for giving top-ups.

We give a short physiologic explanation about segmental pain relief: during the first stage of labor, the block stays in the lumbar region of the back while during late first stage, representing perineal and rectal involvement, the pain stimuli reach the sacral region. The parturient can then easily understand why at the onset of the analgesia she is laid for 10 min in Trendelenburg position and then before expulsion is sat upright for the last top-up.

Parturients who have not been seen for a prepartum consultation may be refused routine regional analgesia except upon the personal request of their obstetrician, who must indicate a medical reason, e.g. a prolonged labor. Our reasons for refusal are that a frightened woman in labor with painful contractions can neither judge objectively nor accept a technique that she would otherwise, or in a normal situation, reject. On the other hand, the parturient who was seen at a prepartum consultation is not committed to take an epidural analgesia if she decides to endure the pain of her contractions. Nor is attendance at the prepartum consultation a 100% guarantee of epidural analgesia if, for instance, she enters the hospital fully dilated and with bearing-down reflexes. A parturient who refuses epidural analgesia should not be coerced to accept it because her refusal per se is an absolute contraindication.

One should explain that the patient cannot choose the anesthesiologist to give her the epidural catheter and to follow her entire labor and delivery; indeed there is a great chance she will be attended by more than one anesthesiologist during the progress of the labor and the delivery because the continuity by the department of anesthesia is assured by a team of anesthesiologists who work on a rotation system.

The best moment for the epidural catheter to be placed is as soon as the parturient experiences painful contractions regularly every 5 min. It is more convenient for the anesthesiologist to perform the epidural technique early, and it is safer for the parturient if surroundings are quiet and the parturient is in full control of herself than under time pressure with an anxious, moving and uncooperative parturient.

Shortcomings should be stressed. These may be due to the epidural catheter technique. For example, a catheter can come out of the epidural space or become obstructed by a blood clot – these problems are solved by replacement of the catheter; a kinked catheter can be withdrawn a short distance and retaped. Shortcomings can be due to the parturient or to the anesthesiologist. For example: anatomic problems, such as difficult identification of the epidural space in a morbidly obese parturient; difficult access to the epidural space after operations such as herniated disk, spinal fusion, Harrington rod fixation or spinal deformity; unilateral analgesia or root segment analgesia due to a malpositioned catheter; analgesia established too late if labor progresses too fast; post dural puncture headache because of a dural puncture with loss of cerebrospinal fluid through a patent hole in the dura; or a massive injection from a misplaced or secondarily migrated catheter into either the subdural or subarachnoid space causing extended segmental anesthesia or into the bloodstream causing drowsiness and possible eventual progression to convulsions and cardiovascular depression. This review of untowards effects at the prepartum consultation appeases the parturient. The blood pressure is routinely measured every 5 min after the injection of local anesthetic and for at least 15 min in order to discover and treat hypotension quickly. Hypotension can be caused by vasodilation of the blood vessels in the anesthetized part and/or by compression of the inferior vena cava and abdominal aorta, which may be prevented by lying the parturient on her left side, producing left uterine displacement, and administering intravenous fluids. The parturient will perceive numbness increasing to a temporary feeling of paresis in the leg muscles and abdominal muscles; therefore, parturients are encouraged to follow prepartum physiotherapy lessons and exercises to learn how to push down effectively during the expulsion process. Occasionally unilateral or bilateral blurred vision occurs because of high spreading of the local anesthetic (Horner's syndrome). It is abolished by application of one eyedrop of phenylephrine 5%. The possibility of a relative overdose and excessively high segmental blockade with undue vasomotor and temporary muscular paralysis is mentioned. Post-partum backache has a prevalence of 30–40% regardless of whether regional or general anesthesia is used: its occurrence is related to ligamentous strain from lordosis during pregnancy. Shivering after induction of the block usually stops spontaneously within 10–15 min and is of no serious concern. Bladder dysfunction during epidural analgesia may cause retention and catheterization is performed if necessary.

Rare complications should be explained with emphasis that these are extremely rare events. With an epidural hematoma there is a chance of paralysis if it goes unrecognized and untreated for more than 6 h; therefore, parturients with preeclamptic toxemia undergo laboratory tests to evaluate clotting abnormalities before the epidural catheter is introduced. An epidural abscess, if not urgently treated at an early stage, can give rise to paraplegia; therefore the procedure for placing an epidural catheter is sterile, i.e. the lumbar region is prepared and draped.

There are also many advantages of lumbar epidural analgesia. For the mother, epidural analgesia can provide complete pain relief for labor and delivery and brings about maternal relaxation without the need for various depressant drugs for mother and child; being awake, the parturient can participate in the labor and delivery and the risk of pulmonary aspiration of gastric contents is minimized; it prevents maternal hyperventilation, which may occur during painful contractions and may be harmful to the fetus. For the obstetrician, it provides ideal conditions for vaginal delivery, episiotomy, forceps and vacuum extraction and twin delivery and, in addition, the analgesia can be rapidly extended for cesarean delivery. The epidural technique incurs no neonatal depression and its use can be considered in the case of preeclampsia–eclampsia.

The presence of an anesthesiologist in the labor and delivery room is advantageous in emergencies – the life of one parturient who had an amniotic fluid embolism with severe shock was saved. We describe how, after delivery, the newborn is scored on a 10-point scale at 1 and 5 min, which gives an indication of any need for resuscitation. All tools and drugs are always at hand to resuscitate the newborn with no waste of time; of course, if a problem is anticipated the pediatrician should also be present. Besides the resuscitation score, the newborn is examined for anomalies such as esophageal atresia or intestinal obstructions by passing a gastric tube through the mouth into the stomach and inspecting the volume aspirated; in addition the anus is inspected to exclude imperforation.

At the end of the group session, the parents can ask questions, which should be answered avoiding difficult medical and technical language. The whole session lasts 30–45 min depending on the activity and curiosity of the group. The group size is 10–15 mothers with their partners.

Another function of a prepartum consultation is to acquire information about the medical history and the physical and mental condition of the parturient. After the group session, each parturient can be seen privately but usually in the presence of her partner. Parturients can ask more questions if they wish for more details or explanations for any reason. Parturients who have had a previous epidural analgesia do not attend the group session but should have, like the others, a private prepartum consultation.

During the prepartum consultation the patient is interviewed and a record sheet is completed. This completed record should be kept at the desk of the obstetric department and should be available on admission.

During the progress of the pregnancy, the obstetrician will have explained to the parturient the different types of local or regional analgesia available to relieve or attenuate pain from contractions and he will have informed her of the 24-h epidural service, assuring her that there will be an anesthesiologist in the hospital to administer her epidural analgesia. If she is interested she fills in and signs an anesthesia questionnaire which she brings along to the prepartum consultation.

At the beginning of the prepartum consultation the anesthesiologist checks the completed items of the questionnaire, noting the relevant data on the record sheet: allergy to drugs; current and recent medications; previous operations; specific diseases such as cardiac disease, lung (asthma) or liver disease (icterus), tendency to bleed or other diseases, e.g. a parturient with multiple sclerosis should be informed about possible exacerbation during pregnancy and the post-partum period. We feel that there is no reason to refuse an epidural analgesia for such a parturient who asks for one after an explanation. Up to the present we have refused an epidural analgesia to only two groups of parturients. One patient had Lobstein's disease (fragilitas ossium) and we felt that the risk of breaking up a piece of bone during the epidural technique was too high. The second group are the morbidly obese in whom the vertebral column cannot even be identified.

The anesthesiologist fills in his or her own name on the record form and starts the routine clinical examination: systolic and diastolic pressure, heart and lung auscultation. Special attention is paid to the back: previous and recent complaints about backache radiating to the legs or buttocks are noted because post-partum back problems are often ascribed to lumbar epidural analgesia by the parturient as well as by some physicians, even when the parturient has the same complaints before pregnancy or labor and delivery. Excessive lordosis or obesity is noted since they might hamper either the identification of the site to introduce the epidural needle or the degree of bending of the back. A laminectomy scar, spinal fusion or a Harrington rod placement is quoted as 'serious' because they can make the access to the lumbar epidural space difficult. The parturient should be informed of problems such as the possibility of an unintentional dural puncture or analgesia zones with residual pain area(s) along with the possibility of solving the problem by the introduction of a second catheter caudally. In these cases it is important to view the earlier radiographs either during the prepartum consultation or at the latest on her admission to the hospital. One should note the weight and the height of the parturient and inquire about any unpleasant experiences with previous anesthetics such as poor analgesia, difficult insertion or post-partum backache and/or other remarks from previous epidural complications. At the end of the prepartum consultation, the classic ASA score is given together with a psychologic score. The psychologic score is divided in three grades: grade 1 is a normal apprehensive parturient; grade 2 is a parturient who easily exaggerates minor discomfort; and grade 3 is one with a pathological psychiatric disease.

When there are attendant obstetric problems such as preeclampsia–eclampsia or other cardiac, pulmonary, endocrine, psychiatric or other important disorders, the obstetrician receives separately, in a sealed envelope, a description of the disorder with the relevant laboratory tests. The obstetrician regularly checks levels of hemoglobin, hematocrit, glucose and electrolytes and informs the anesthesiologist accordingly.

Thus, at the prepartum consultation every parturient has a completed and signed anesthesia questionnaire and some bring a written note about a known disorder, laboratory tests or back radiographs. The gathering of all this relevant information before the hospital admission of the parturient is always useful, and especially so when the parturient's own obstetrician is absent and a locum attends the labor and performs the delivery. With a 24 h anesthesia service, the parturient will practically never have a preassigned anesthesiologist and, if the labor is long-lasting, several may attend in succession.

Obtaining an informed consent is a third function of the prepartum consultation. We introduced a consent form into our prepartum consultation after our experiences with one particular patient. A 26-year old primigravida weighing 71 kg was seen during the prepartum consultation. The history was negative except for limitation of salt, mefruside tablets and ritodrine hydrochloride. Blood pressure was 100/60. All these data were noted on the record sheet. One week later she delivered a girl weighing 2650 g with 1- and 5-min Apgar scores of 9 and 10 respectively. In the post-partum period, the bladder was catheterized on several occasions because she was unable to void. A diagnosis of hemorrhagic cystitis was made by the urologist. Six weeks later the patient was discharged from the hospital. She could spontaneously void but still complained of dysuria and low back pain. She consulted various neurologists and urologists, of whom one stated that the lumbar epidural analgesia was the cause of her voiding problem. A pacemaker for her bladder sphincter was implanted and, after threatening to sue the anesthesia department to pay for the operation, she proceeded against the anesthesiologist who had performed the lumbar epidural technique. After his refusal, a suit was taken out against the anesthesiologist and the whole story was uncovered: 11 years previously she had had a hip operation for recuring hip luxation; 1 year later she was treated for pathologic obesity (96 kg). Seven years later she suffered psychic depression lasting 1 year while she lost 20 kg in weight. In the meantime she underwent an operation for coccygodynia and was admitted to a psychiatric institution because of anorexia nervosa. Three years before her delivery she underwent a laparoscopy for an ovarian biopsy with a fractional curettage; at that time she complained of dysuria with urinary retention and regular bladder catheterization. Because of her recurrent psychiatric problems, the psychiatrist noted in her record at the time 'this is a very negative and rationalizing woman'.

So, even with all our precautions, some women purposely do not reveal their previous problems or operations. Because of this case we added to our questionnaire a written consent signed by the parturient before the prepartum consultation in order to obtain all pertinent information. This consent form is signed by the parturient after the anesthesiologist has conducted an informed consent discussion for the anesthetic.

Ideally, all parturients should give informed consent. In the USA, consent forms can be attacked in litigation if the plaintiff can prove she signed the consent form before she had met the anesthesiologist although medicolegal cases are rarely, if ever won or lost solely on the issue of informed consent.

We believe that better-informed anesthesiologists and parturients as well as their partners contribute to safety and comfort and that these prepartum consultations should be continued and extended to all parturients as far as possible in every obstetric department where obstetric anesthesia is performed on a 24 h basis. Referral to the anesthesia department by the obstetrician should be routine so that all parturients have the opportunity to speak to the anesthesia staff if they have questions about anesthesia. Additionally, the anesthesiologists will have all the relevant information about the parturient.

REFERENCE

1. Hew-Wing P, Rolbin S, Hew E 1989 Outpatients anaesthetic consultations for pregnant patients. Can J Anaesth 36: 102

7. Fetal assessment

Part A Fetal well-being during pregnancy
C. Romanini H. Valensise
Part B Fetal well-being during labor *H. Valensise C. Romanini*
Part C Fetal and neonatal hemodynamic adaptations at birth *J. Hamza*

PART A
FETAL WELL-BEING DURING PREGNANCY
C. Romanini H. Valensise

FETAL HEART RATE

The recording of the fetal heart rate allows several parameters of fetal well-being during pregnancy to be monitored:

1. basal fetal heart rate;
2. heart rate variability;
3. recurrent variations (accelerations and decelerations).

Basal fetal heart rate

The basal fetal heart rate is normally in the range 120–160 beats per minute (bpm) (Fig. 7.1). Higher or lower rates constitute tachycardia or bradycardia respectively. The basal fetal heart rate gradually decreases and ultimately reaches neonatal values (about 120 bpm). An essential characteristic of the basal heart rate is its irregularity, as it can be seen from the tracing in Figure 7.1. This 'relative instability' is caused by conflicting autonomic nervous system effects on the heart rate: increased sympathetic tone causes acceleration and increased vagal tone causes deceleration.

Fetal tachycardia must be considered a defensive precaution. The causes can be either maternal or fetal. On a cardiotocographic tracing it is important to evaluate the amplitude of tachycardia, but it is also important to evaluate the occurrence and persistence of other adverse

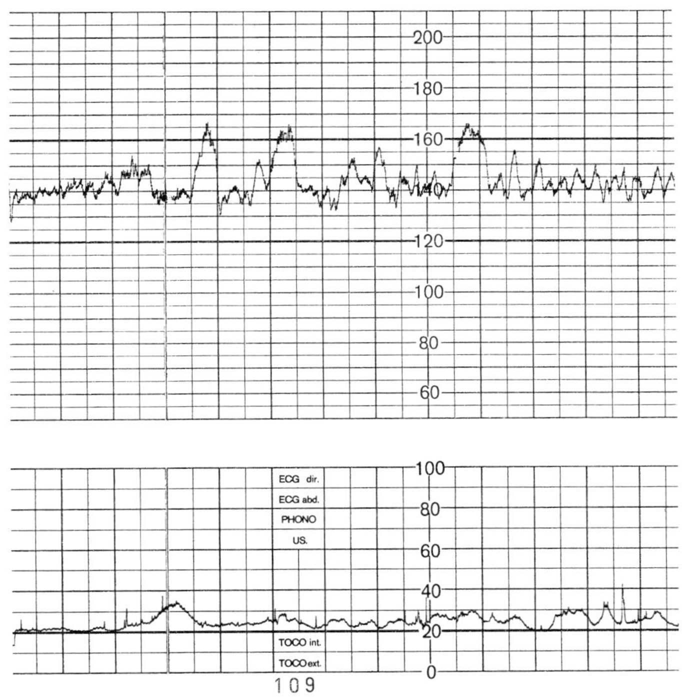

Fig. 7.1 Normal fetal heart rate tracing with basal heart rate of 140, normal variability (> 10 bpm) and frequent heart rate accelerations.

prognostic signs, such as a reduction in the variability, the absence of accelerations or the occurrence of decelerations (Figs 7.2 and 7.3). Maternal pyrexia and the administration of beta-mimetic drugs are often associated with a cardiotocographic tracing with normal characteristics (variability > 10 bpm, presence of accelerations) even if the fetal heart rate is increased by about 20–25 bpm. In these cases the fetal prognosis is good: the heart rate shows adaptation to the pharmacologic or metabolic conditions of the intrauterine environment.

With regard to bradycardia, it is important to consider the time at which it begins. It should be remembered[2] that throughout pregnancy there is a progressive reduction in the basal rate from 160–170 bpm (at a gestational age of 16–18 weeks) to 120–125 bpm in late pregnancy and at

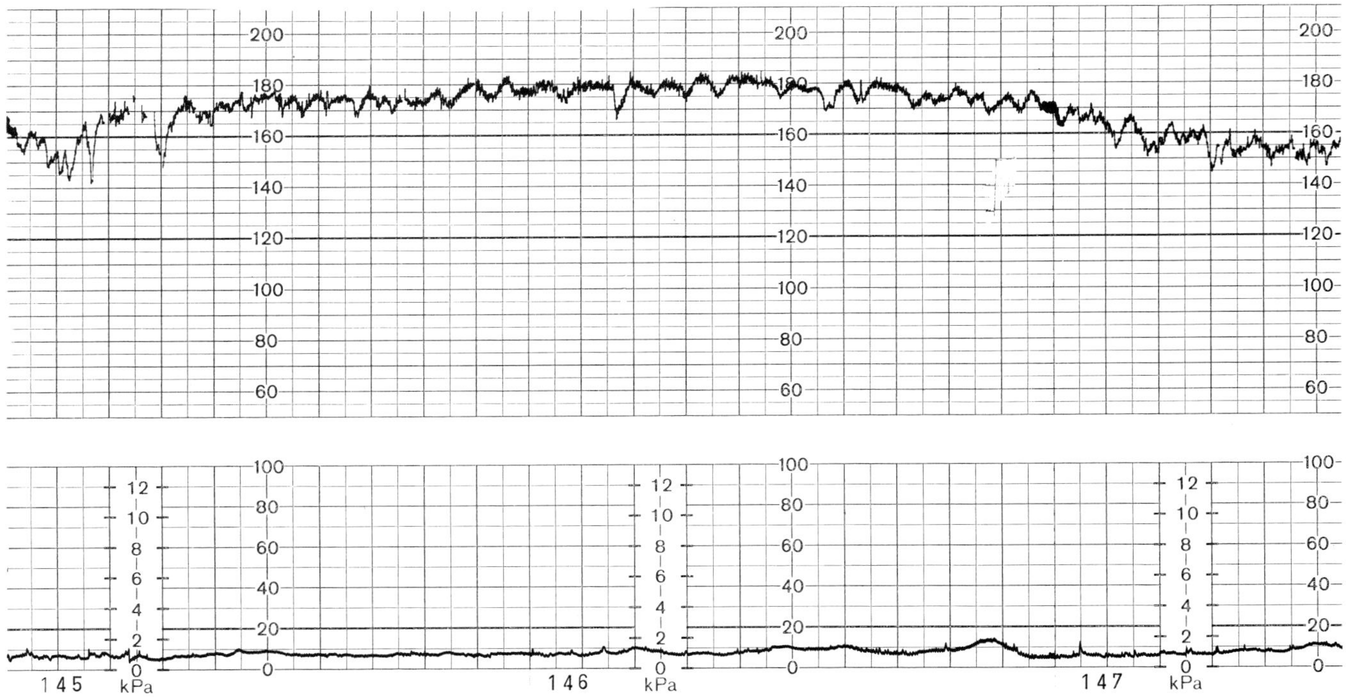

Fig. 7.2 Transient episode of fetal tachycardia during pregnancy lasting 17 min between two episodes of normal fetal heart rate. Maternal supine hypotension was the main cause of the fetal heart rate variation.

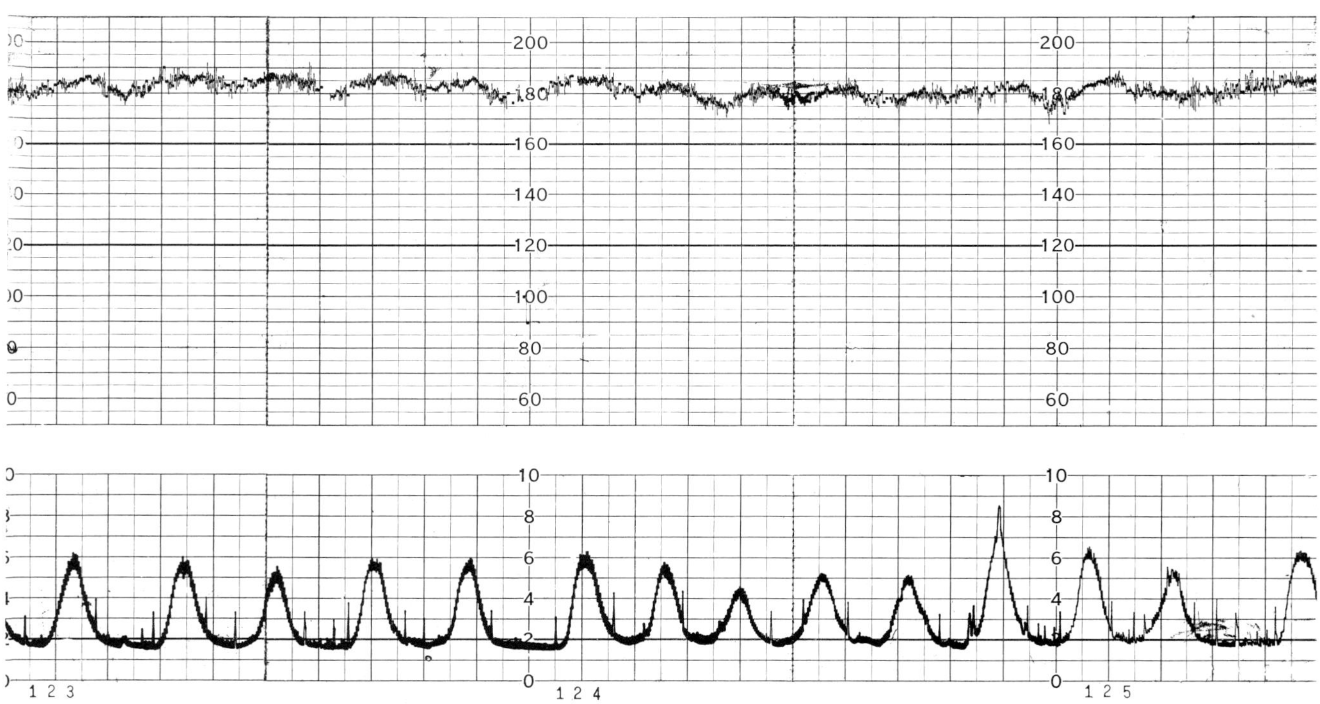

Fig. 7.3 Persistent fetal tachycardia in labor with reduced variability and absence of fetal heart rate accelerations. A Cesarean delivery was performed at 39 weeks and healthy 1980-g male fetus was delivered.

birth. A persistent bradycardia below 110 bpm at a gestational age of 30–32 weeks in a nonstress situation can indicate an anomaly and must be thoroughly investigated; however, a persistent bradycardia of 110–120 bpm in a term fetus can be considered physiologic (Fig. 7.4). In both cases other parameters should be considered (variability, accelerations, decelerations) to determine whether the bradycardia is abnormal. An important sign of a

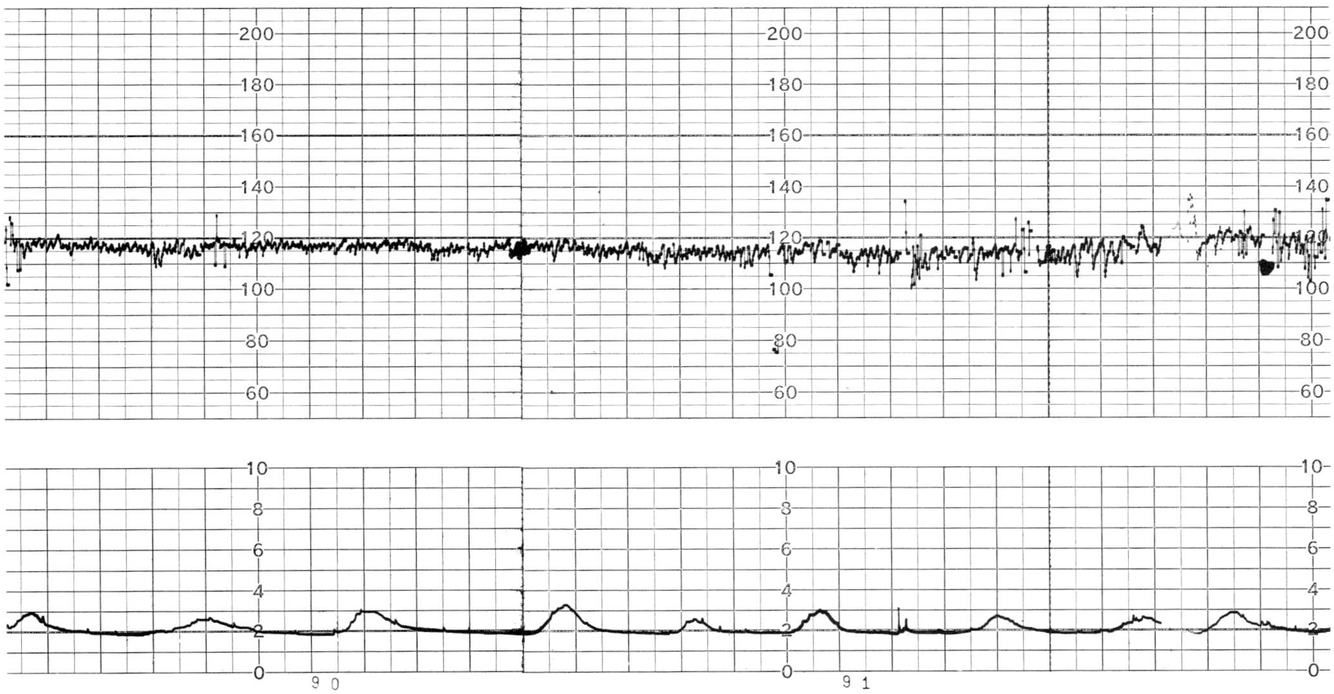

Fig. 7.4 Persistent fetal bradycardia with heart rate of 110–115 bpm in a term fetus. Although the recording shows no acceleration and 30 min of reduced variability, the fetus was delivered vaginally in excellent condition.

hypoxic event is bradycardia that occurs after a heart rate tracing within the normal range; it generally occurs when the mother receives drugs or during labor if there is a prolapse or continuing compression of the umbilical cord (Fig. 7.5). If bradycardia is preceded in the tracing by other signs of fetal distress, such as tachycardia, reduced variability and repeated variations, it may indicate ischemia of the fetal myocardium.

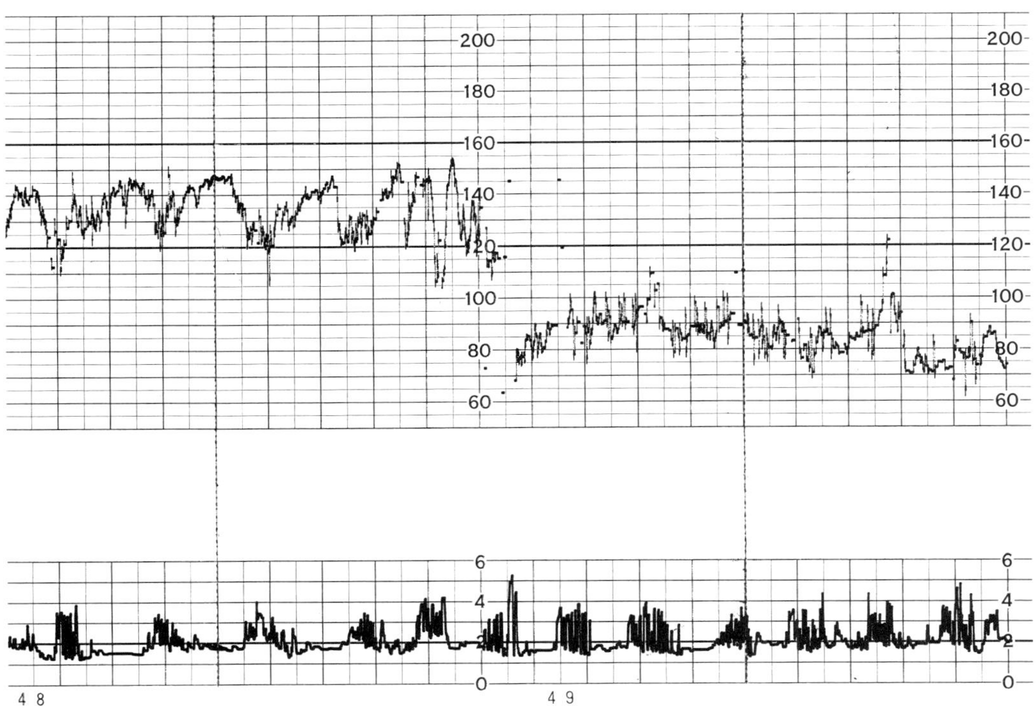

Fig. 7.5 Episode of 9 minutes bradycardia with fetal heart rate of 80–85 bpm after a normal heart rate due to prolapse of the umbilical cord.

Heart rate variability

Fetal heart rate variability is the expression of the spontaneous activity that the autonomous fetal nevous system exercises on fetal rate.[3] It can be defined as:

- 'Short-term variability', beat-to-beat variability or microvariations. This is the variation in heart rate between one beat and the next. It can be calculated only if the fetal heart rate is measured by abdominal or direct electrocardiographic techniques.
- 'Long-term variability' or macrovariations. This is the heart rate variation over an arbitrarily defined time period (usually 1 min).
- Number of passages to zero. This is the number of cycles in relation to a reference line that crosses the basal rate. Some authors consider this to be long-term variability.
- Range. This measures heart rate variation in periods of 1 min and allows a numeric evaluation of long-term variability.

Good fetal oxygenation results in a normal variability range between 10 and 25 bpm. In a cardiotocographic tracing there can be periods of normal variability (10–25 bpm) and periods of reduced variability (<10 bpm). Both types of variation are physiologic and linked to the different 'states' of fetus during recording. A quiet behavioral state in the fetus, with an absence of active movements, is characterized by a reduced variability that can last 35 or 40 min.[4,5] Fetal well-being is characterized by alternating episodes of quiet and active behavioral states. Cardiotocographic recording during the active state shows standard variability, accelerations and active fetal movements. A phase of reduced variability followed by a tracing that demonstrates fetal well-being is considered normal. If a period of reduced variability is observed, monitoring should be continued until the fetus enters an active phase. The presence of these physiologic modifications in variability is correlated with the gestational age: there are generally no modifications until a gestational age of 28 or 30 weeks. Before this time cardiotocographic recording can present an 'immature' aspect without the clear distinction between quiet and active fetal behavioral states.

The persistence of reduced variability on cardiotocographic tracing (<10 or 5 bpm) and the absence of accelerations and active fetal movements for periods >40–60 min should be of concern as they could be the first sign of hypoxic fetal distress.[6] In some cases, the fall in heart rate variation is associated with other signs of fetal hypoxia such as tachycardia, whether moderate or severe, and the occurrence of periodic variable or late decelerations.

Recurrent variations

Acceleration

Heart rate acceleration is technically defined as 'a transient abrupt rise in fetal heart rate of at least 15 beats/min above the baseline, of at least 15 seconds' duration, returning towards the baseline after reaching a peak'. The acceleration is caused by the sympathetic autonomous nervous system which, by intensifying its activity, causes the initial rise in heart rate. The return towards the baseline is associated with a decline in the sympathetic activity and a rise in vagal activity. Accelerations can be divided into periodic and sporadic: the former are related to uterine activity, the latter to active fetal movements. Fetal heart rate acceleration is a sign of fetal well-being[7]:

> The fetus that can execute a vigorous movement needing a heart rate acceleration can be considered as having a good functional reserve. A chronically reduced reserve might prevent the fetus from making this type of movement which requires the acceleration of fetal heart rate.

The presence of accelerations on the cardiotocographic tracing is a sign of good fetal 'reactivity', whether during pregnancy or labor. On the other hand, accelerations that precede or follow the variable deceleration (pre-and post-deceleration) are the hemodynamic result of transient fetal hypotension.

Precocious (early) deceleration

This type of deceleration shows a uniform trend, related to uterine contraction (Figs 7.6 and 7.7). There is no time interval between deceleration and contraction. It is caused

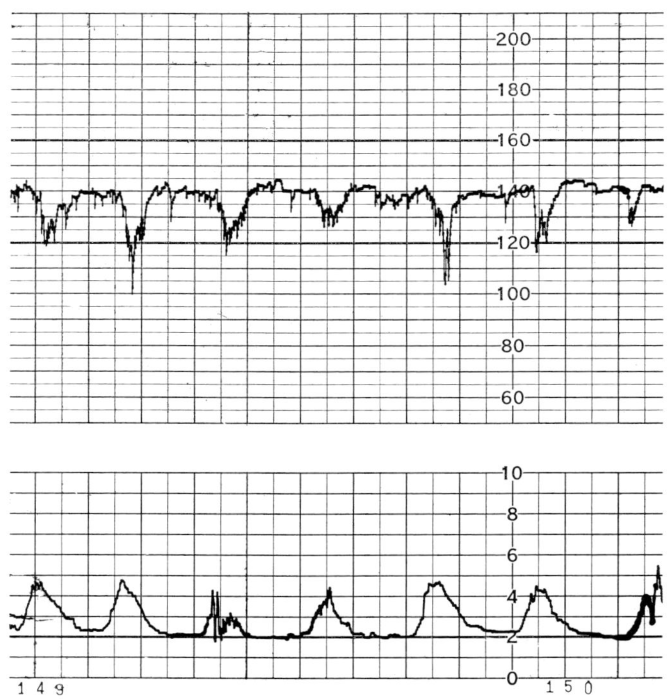

Fig. 7.6 Early decelerations of fetal heart rate.

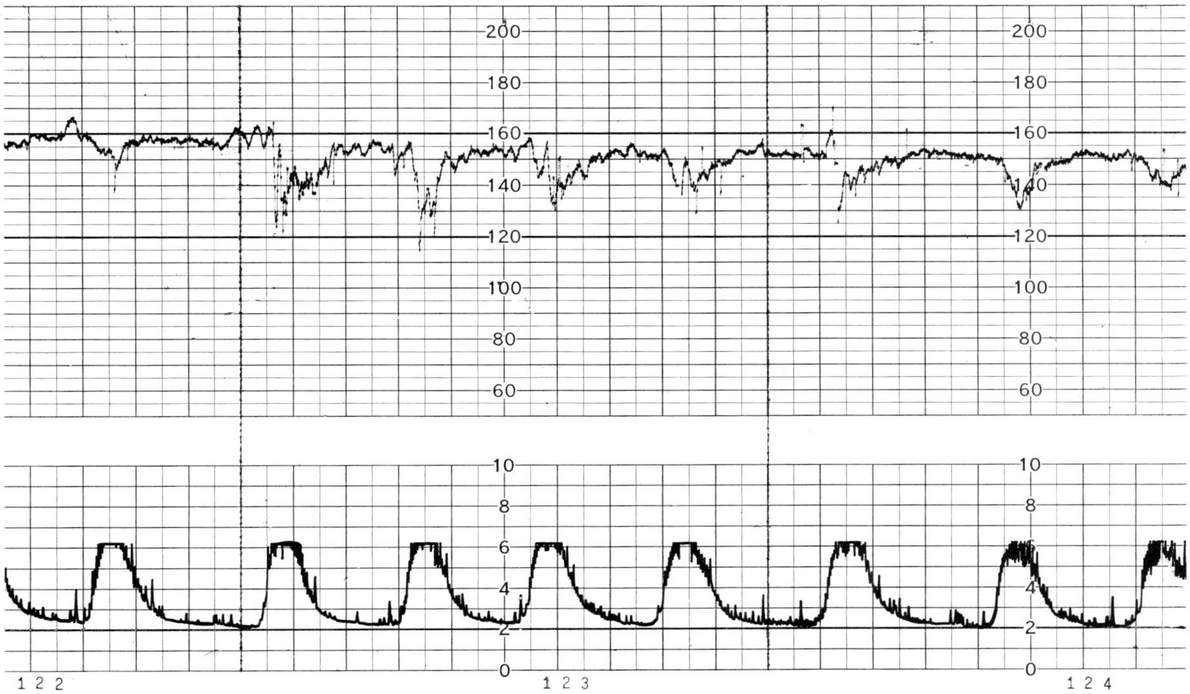

Fig. 7.7 Early decelerations of fetal heart rate.

by compression of the fetal head and of maternal tissue. It reduces the heart rate directly through activation of parasympathetic pontine–mesencephalic centers, or through activation of baroreceptors stimulated by circulatory pressure changes.

It is evidence of the integrity of the fetal nervous system, which is capable of responding to different stimuli. In the presence of significant brain damage, there will be no precocious deceleration. It appears more frequently during the dilating phase of labor when the fetal head is compressed on the pelvic floor; it can occur in cases of fetal pelvic disproportion because of compression of the fetal structures. It is not associated with adverse neonatal outcome. It is not an expression of a reduction in fetal oxygenation and it is not due to a change in placental or umbilical flow.

Late deceleration

The cardiotocographic pattern of late deceleration can vary but usually it is uniform and similar to an upside-down bell (Fig. 7.8). Its amplitude is normally 10–15 bpm, but its clinical significance differs from greater decelerations of the same type. To classify a deceleration as late it is essential to consider its temporal relationship with uterine contraction: late decelerations begin 20–30 s after the beginning of a contraction. This behavior of heart rate is easily understandable if pressure during uterine contraction is considered. The pressure increase causes a reduction first in myometrial blood flow and then in the intervillous space. At the peak of the contraction the flow is totally abolished and flow begins slowly as the uterine contraction attenuates and intrauterine pressure is reduced. The mechanism responsible for the late deceleration is the reduction in intervillous space perfusion during a contraction. The reduced perfusion causes a reduction in gas exchange with the fetus and subsequent fetal hypoxia.[9,10] For the ‘retarded’ temporal relationship between contraction and deceleration to be understood it has to be remembered that fetal oxygenation during the first half of a contraction depends on blood that perfused the intervillus space before the contraction.

Thus, both normally and in placental insufficiency, there will be no modification of fetal heart rate during the ascending phase of a contraction. During the descending phase of a contraction, fetal oxygenation is correlated with the amount of blood that reached the intervillous space during the ascending phase. The reduction in the oxygen concentration in fetal blood stimulates chemoreceptors, which act reflexly to decrease heart rate. Fetal hypoxia occurs during the descending phase of a contraction and the reduction in the fetal heart rate begins after the peak of the contraction. After the contraction, fetal oxygenation depends on the amount of maternal blood that reached the intervillous space during the descending phase of the contraction. Late deceleration is never a normal event, and is often a sign of fetal impairment. It is often associated with other modifications of fetal heart rate such as a reduction in variability, bradycardia or tachycardia. Events of this type should not be ignored especially if they

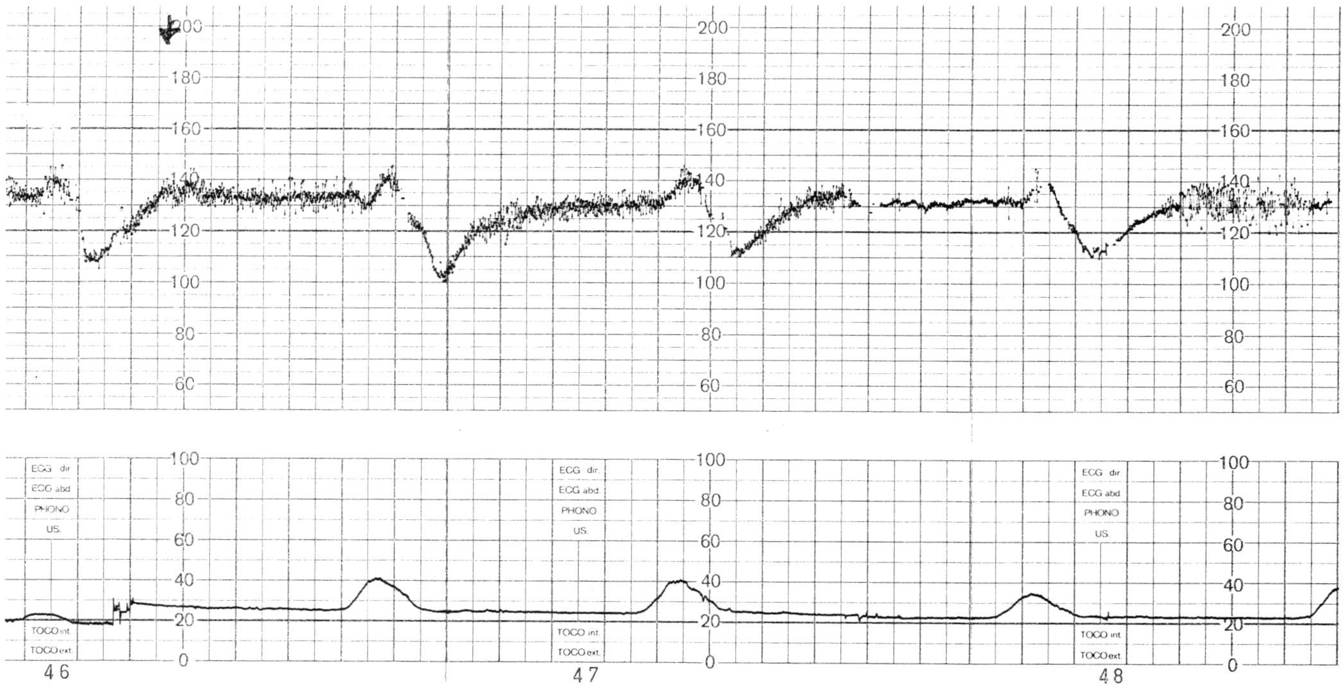

Fig. 7.8 Late decelerations of fetal heart rate.

are recurrent and are associated with other adverse cardiotocographic signs. The cause of deceleration is always uteroplacental hypoperfusion which can be divided into factors linked to a serious maternal pathology (diabetes, hypertension, preeclampsia) and factors that modify uteroplacental flow causing a persisting (myomas) or temporary compression (aortocaval compression). Uterine hyperactivity, hypertonia and tachycardia alone or in association with other factors cannot explain the presence of repetitive late decelerations.

Variable deceleration

Fetal heart rate deceleration that has no constant temporal relation with uterine contractile activity is defined as 'variable' (Figs 7.9 and 7.10) because of its abnormal pattern (as a U, V, W or other irregular form). The shape is a manifestation of reflex changes in fetal heart rate secondary to abrupt circulatory modifications. These modifications cause an acceleration that precedes a deceleration. In fact, variable deceleration is an expression of reduced perfusion of the fetal circulation correlated with a reduction in blood flow through the umbilical cord. The early phase of cord compression blocks the flow through the umbilical vein, which carries oxygenated blood from the placenta to the fetus. When this happens, the blood flow is reduced while the flow in the umbilical arteries is still unrestricted. This causes fetal hypotension, which induces an increase in the fetal heart rate. This is followed by compression of the two umbilical arteries: the blood flowing from the fetus to the placenta is forced into the fetal circulation, creating a state of fetal hypertension that causes an abrupt reduction in fetal heart rate, and the descending phase of deceleration occurs. As soon as cord compression is lessened, flow in the umbilical arteries resumes, while the umbilical vein, because of its wall characteristics, remains closed. From a hemodynamic point of view, fetal hypertension declines and there is an immediate return to the baseline. The phase explains the ascending phase of deceleration seen on the cardiotocographic tracing. Nevertheless, the temporary closure of the umbilical vein causes a state of fetal hypotension. As a consequence, futher sympathetic stimulation is accompained by an acceleration, called a post-deceleration acceleration. The duration of a deceleration depends on the duration of umbilical cord compression. The shape of the deceleration can vary from an simple V to more complex shapes.[12] Pathogenetic elements occur in addition to cord compression, for example:

1. loss of the acceleration that precedes and follows the deceleration;
2. a secondary prolonged acceleration (overshoot);
3. loss of variability during overall deceleration;
4. a 'two-phase' deceleration in which the first ascending phase does not reach the baseline but is interrupted by a reduction of the new rate;
5. an ascending phase of deceleration that gradually returns towards the baseline;
6. suspension of the ascending phase of the

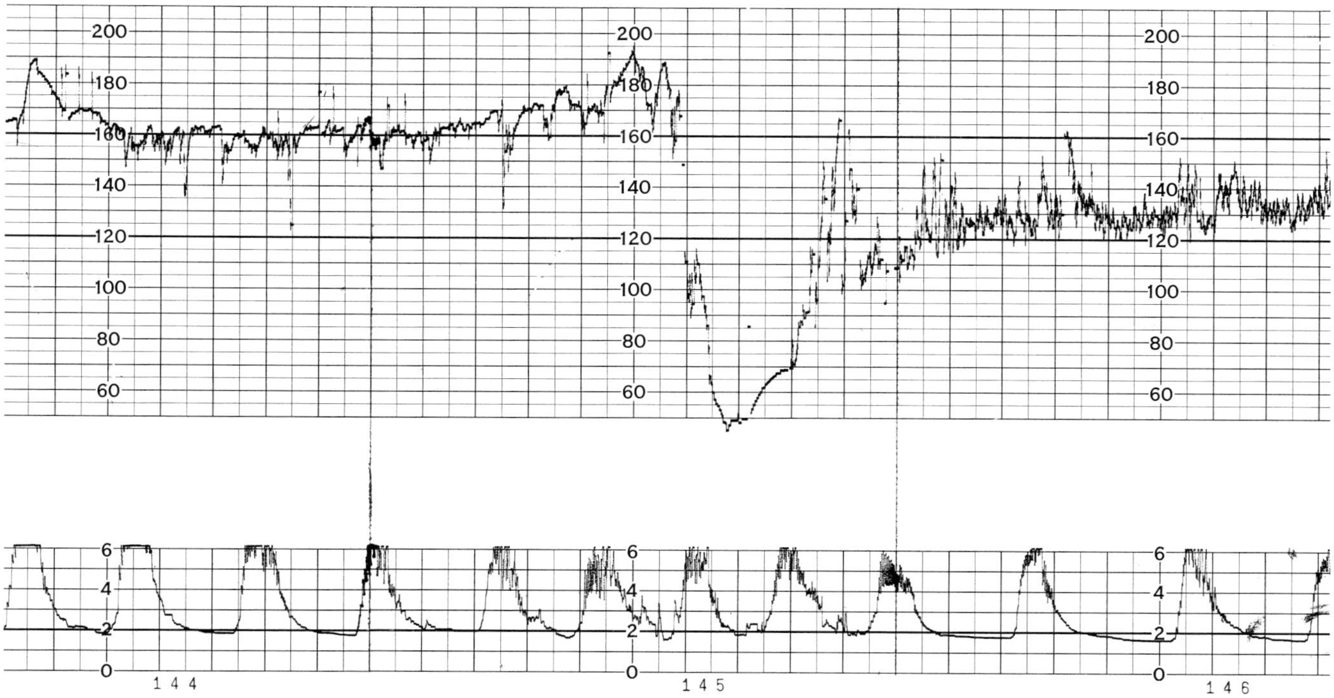

Fig. 7.9 Isolated variable deceleration of fetal heart rate.

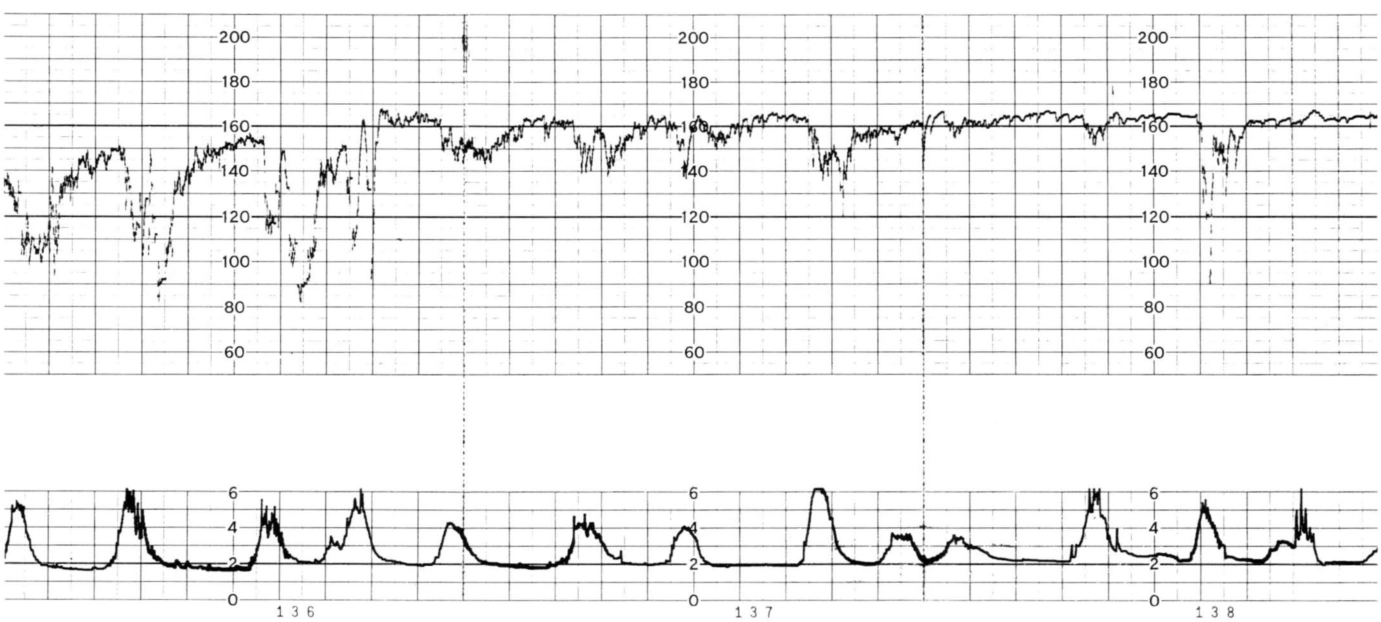

Fig. 7.10 Cluster of variable decelerations of fetal heart rate.

deceleration and return towards a baseline below or beyond the starting-line.

Abnormalities within a variable deceleration can weaken the prognostic value and are adverse elements to be considered together with the deceleration's duration and amplitude. Loss of variability during deceleration, absence of the secondary acceleration (post-deceleration) and 'two-phase' deceleration seem to be the main predictors of subsequent fetal distress. Disappearance of the initial acceleration (predeceleration), although the most common atypical deceleration, is not associated with adverse fetal outcome at birth.

CARDIOTOCOGRAPHY DURING PREGNANCY

In the late 1950s, Caldeyro-Barcia et al,[13] pioneers of electronic fetal monitoring in labor, applied an electrode to the fetal scalp after rupture of the membranes. In 1968 Hammacher[14] studied the cardiotocographic signal. He used an external transducer applied to the maternal abdomen that revealed fetal heart rate with a non-invasive procedure when the parturient was not in labor. During the following years, the Doppler effect was used for heart rate monitoring: this technique has contributed to broaden biophysical monitoring during both pregnancy and labor. The aim of cardiotocography is to monitor fetal well-being and to prevent intrauterine death. Fetal heart rate variations have been ascertained to be a fetal response to stress; some particular changes indicate that the fetus is unable to react adequately.

In the 1970s cardiotocographic monitoring, both the contraction stress test (CST) and the nonstress test (NST) broadly replaced biochemical monitoring (estriol and human placental lactogen, hPL) as a means of predicting risk linked to uteroplacental insufficiency. Kubli et al[15] and Pose et al[16] were the first to described the CST, that is cardiotocographic evaluation of fetal response to contractile activity. Spontaneous uterine contractions occur in 12–32% of pregnant women; oxytocin is used to induce contractions in the remainder.

The oxytocin challenge test (OCT), introduced by Ray et al[17] and later modified by Schifrin et al[18] is the most common type of CST. Oxytocin, 5 IV in 500 ml of isotonic saline solution is administered at the rate of 0.5 mU/min, increasing by 2 mU every 2 min until adequate contractile activity is achieved (three contractions in 10 min). Cardiotocographic tracings obtained by CST are classified as positive, negative, questionable or unsatisfactory. Positive tests show repeated, uniform late decelerations. Negative tests show a stable heart rate without periodic decelerations. In questionable tests either nonrepetitive late decelerations or fetal bradycardia due to excessive uterine activity are found. In unsatisfactory tests either the fetal heart is not perfectly recorded or these is no contractile activity after 2 h from the beginning of the test.

A positive test is evidence of reduced uteroplacental reserves and is often followed either by an immediate cesarean delivery or by induction.[19,20,21] In a study by Schulman et al[22] the number of cesarean deliveries increased approximately twofold after questionable or positive oxytocin tests. A negative CST is normally repeated after a week unless other circumstances do not require a closer check. The questionable test is repeated within 24–72 h.

Exogenous oxytocin has not been demonstrated to have severe clinical and neurologic effects on the fetus. The oxytocin test, as a collateral effect, produces uterine hypertonus in 0–18% of women, with a mean around 7%; moreover, spontaneous labor can occur after a CST within 24 h. Indications for CST include an increased risk of uteroplacental deficiency, e.g. post-maturity, diabetes or hypertension, or suspected intrauterine fetal growth retardation. CST is used as a diagnostic test following a nonreactive NST or persisting anomalous levels of hPL or estriol. Contraindications to the use of CST include the risk factors of preterm labor, such as multiple pregnancies, previous uterine operation and cervical incompetence.

The CST was widely used in the past but has gradually been replaced by Doppler velocimetry and ultrasonic biometry and is now rarely performed. Currently a greater importance seems to be placed on fetal heart rate recording under basal conditions (NST). The occurrence of late or variable decelerations after the induction of contractile activity (evaluation of 'placental reserve') is no longer considered to be a useful indicator of fetal distress. The NST reveals well-being or precocious signs through the study of heart rate variability and the occurrence of repetitive and recurring accelerations.[23] The NST is simple, not at all invasive, inexpensive and more widely used than the CST. Moreover, it can be carried out by nonqualified staff. In many obstetric departments, NST has totally replaced CST as a means of diagnosing utero-placental insufficiency.

The NST is classified as reactive or nonreactive. It is considered reactive if during a 20 min period there occur one,[24] two or more accelerations of at least 15 beats and of 15 s duration associated with active fetal movements. If these criteria are not met, the NST is continued for a futher 20 min with acoustic stimulation of the fetus. If there are still no signs of fetal activity on the tracing, the test is considered to be nonreactive.[25] The number of tracings that cannot be correctly classified is about 5%, but it depends on the gestational age at which the test is carried out and on the duration of the recording: the percentage of nonreactive tests falls as the period of observation increases. A study of 1101 nonreactive NSTs[26] performed on 343 high-risk women showed that 24% of tests were nonreactive for the first 20 min. After 40 min 5% and after 80 min only 2% of the tests were still nonreactive. In addition, no correlation between the time required to obtain a reactive test and neonatal outcome was found. Nevertheless, the cost and the time and staff required, and the acceptability could discourage the extensive use of the NST.

Some clinicians[27] consider more than one factor to define a normal or pathologic tracing, evaluating the baseline, the beat-to-beat variability and the presence of accelerations associated with either fetal active movements or spontaneous contractions. It is unanimously accepted[28,29] that a NST tracing is normal if the basal heart rate is between the range of 120–150 bpm, if the beat-to-beat variability is >5 bpm and if there are accelerations in response to fetal active movements and no variable or late decelerations are revealed.[30] In addition, an NST classification can be based on other biophysical parameters, such as the number of fetal movements, the presence of respiratory movements and the amniotic fluid volume. Some authors[31,32,33] give a score to each of these parameters, identifying in this way a biophysical profile of the fetus. Nevertheless, this methodology has been discussed because variables that differ from a pathogenetic point of view might have the same score, preventing clinicians from distinguishing between well fetuses and those already compromised. The diagnostic accuracy of the NST and surveillance techniques has been evaluated.[34] As far as perinatal mortality is concerned, the cardiotocographic tests are characterized by high specificity (ability to identify true negatives) but low sensitivity (ability to identify true positives). Thus they cannot be totally trusted with regard to perinatal and neurologic morbidity. This being the case, the predictive value of cardiotocography in pregnancy is reduced.

FETAL BEHAVIORAL STATES

The prevention of slight or severe neonatal neurologic handicaps depends on the obstetrician's ability to prevent intrapartum acute and prolonged fetal distress. Unfortunately, the correlation between fetal distress by cardiotocography and amniotic fluid characteristics is not as linear as would be wished. In particular, it has been noted that not all fetuses that show signs of severe fetal distress are afflicted by handicaps, and in those in whom labor and delivery is optimum some neurologic disability may occur later.[35] It must be remembered that low-risk prenatal conditions can also cause outcomes associated with asphyxia, especially intrauterine growth retardation, prematurity or birth weight less than the 10th percentile. Nevertheless, the number of affected fetuses in the group characterized by normal weight and gestation is higher than expected.[36] The attention of researchers has thus shifted towards the evaluation of fetal well-being during pregnancy by biophysical means. Given the validity of NST in fetal well-being evaluation, and also its relative weakness in predicting fetal outcome, biophysical methodologies have turned towards combination of cardiotocography and observations of fetal somatic motor and eye activity obtained by real-time sonography.

Fetal neurologic integrity has been evaluated by measuring spontaneous heart rate changes; in fact, when recorded for prolonged periods of time, it is possible to determine a continuous alternation between 'active' and 'quiet' states in normal oxygenated near-term fetuses. More recent studies have followed the direction of an integrated evaluation of some fetal variables as a direct expression of the spontaneous activity of the central nervous system.[37] By integrating cardiotocographic and the sonographic recordings, it is possible to determine and identify a series of fetal 'behavioral states'.[38] This means that neonatal neurologic condition can be assessed by combining polygraphy and spontaneous behavior methodologies, in order to detect the slightest sign of neurologic impairment that may escape a test of neonatal well-being.[39,40,41] Thus, fetal central nervous system activity can be evaluated by controlling different variables and observing not single modifications but the capacity of the fetal CNS to integrate variations in different variables in a coordinated and synchronous way.

Four behavioral states have been indentified; they are designated 1F, 2F, 3F and 4F according to the cardiotocographic tracing variations and the association of this variable with the other two essential ones: eye movements and spontaneous body movements.[38] From a 36–38 weeks' gestation onwards the fetus shows all four alternative states in different but stable proportions. The 1F state, corresponding to 'quiet sleep', occurs 25.3% of the time and the 2F state, corresponding to 'active sleep', occurs about 60% of the time. The 3F and 4F states are relatively rare and jointly represent 10–12%. Other fetal variables have been described but, because they do not vary regularly, they cannot be considered as indicators of fetal well-being. These parameters are: regular breathing movements in 1F, more frequent in 2F, rare in 3F and irregular in 4F; vesical emptying that occurs within 30 min after the passage from a 1F state to a 2F state; and regular mouth movements in 1F. It is possible to detect a progressive increase in amount of time spent in the 1F state from 5% at 30 weeks' gestation to 14.6 ± 3.7% at 36 weeks of gestation and 22.16 ± 7.8% near term. In the same way, the proportion of time in the 2F state increases from 34.8 ± 13.9% at a gestational age of 30 weeks to 62.5 ± 14.6% at 40 weeks of gestation. The total time at 30 weeks of gestation is 40.5 ± 14.4%; the percentage gradually increases to 68.43 ± 15.3% at 36 weeks and reaches 78.07 ± 13.0% near term. Analysing these trends reveals the development and neurologic coordination of the fetus at different gestational ages. It can be seen that the tendency is towards a progressive increase in behavioral states between 34 and 36 weeks of gestation and a plateau after 38 weeks.[42] In early gestation, the behavioral states occur less often, separated by periods of 'noncoincidence' in which single variables do not vary in a synchronous way, and are therefore completely controlled by fetal central inhibitory mechanisms. In the same way an increase in the representation of the two most common states (1F and 2F) is due to progressive fetal maturation and an increase in central coordinative capacity. It is particularly interesting to measure the progression of the 1F state, which represents the development of central inhibitory activities with a positive neuronal control of peripheral somatic motor and visual activity and of heart rate regulation. The drawing of reference normality curves allows us to compare any particular pregnancy with other abnormal pregnancies. In the clinical situation of intrauterine growth retardation, modifications of behavioral states are particularly evident and affect both the percentage of representation of the single states, and above all the percentage of time in which the three variables do not coincide ('noncoincidence'). In particular, the 2F state, corresponding to 'active sleep', decreases to 35–45% and the 1F state to 15–17%. In more severe cases the 3F and 4F states totally disappear. The percentage of noncoincidence is the parameter that is mostly modified; from normal values of 10% it increases to values of 35–40%. At the same time the 'interruptions' of single states increase considerably.[43] These results indicate that in conditions of fetal compensation or intrauterine growth retardation, a central 'uneasiness' can be expressed by the fetus through the absence of coincidence in the variations of single variables. This could reflect the correct availability of essential substrates.[44] At the same time the results demonstrate that in these conditions it could be unreliable to determine fetal health state merely on the basis of the presence/absence of the single variables (body movements, eye movements); in the initial compensation phase, and when there are no decelerations, fetal body movements are still present, but the absence of coincidence between body movements and the variations of the other fetal variables makes it possible to recognize an abnormal situation.

DOPPLER SYSTEMS

Monitoring during pregnancy has been radically modified by the development of Doppler ultrasonographic systems: these systems, either a simple continuous Doppler instrument or more complicated instruments such as pulsed Doppler or color Doppler, have made it possible to assess vascular adaptation of the maternal uteroplacental environment or fetal umbilical, splanchnic and cerebral adaptation which distinguishes normal conditions from conditions in which fetal peripheral resistance tends to increase or distant diastolic flow velocity tends to decrease.

Doppler principles

Doppler shift (fd) can be used to determine blood flow velocity by means of ultrasound frequency measurement. fd is expressed by the formula:

$$\text{fd} = \frac{2f \times V \times \cos\theta}{c}$$

where f represents the frequency of ultrasound discharge, c the constant of diffusion of ultrasound in the medium, V is the velocity of the moving object and $\cos\theta$ is the cosine of the angle between the incident beam and the direction of the moving surface. This value ranges from a maximum of 1 when the angle of incidence is 0° and therefore the probe is parallel to the flow direction to a minimum value of 0 when the ultrasound probe angle of incidence is 90° in relation to the vessel's direction. Doppler shift is supposed to be a function of flow velocity at a certain angle of incidence.

When the Doppler principle is applied to arterial vascular structures, a Doppler velocity waveform is visualized on a system of Cartesian axes where the abscissa represents time and the ordinate the Doppler shift, fd. The Doppler wave presents peak systolic and end-diastolic velocity. The waveform is determined by various factors, such as:

- the heart contractile force;
- the vessel compliance;
- the vessel diameter;
- the distance of the examined point from the heart;
- the flow intensity;
- the peripheral vascular resistance.

Experimental and clinical studies have demonstrated that the Doppler velocity waveform is influenced by peripheral vascular resistance; Doppler ultrasonographic equipment is currently used in obstetrics to detect this resistance. Some indices have been elaborated in order to estimate flow velocity waveform. The most frequently used are:

- A/B ratio, i.e. systolic:diastolic ratio;
- Resistance index (RI), the systolic–diastolic difference divided by diastolic velocity;
- Pulsatility index (PI), is calculated by dividing the systolic–diastolic velocity difference by the mean velocity.

Doppler velocimetry of maternal vessels

The uterine artery (Fig. 7.11) originates from the internal iliac artery. Along the uterine wall it gives off branches that penetrate the thickness of myometrium (arcuate arteries), anastomosing on the anterior or posterior uterine wall. Radial arteries, which originate from the arcuate arteries, pass to the uterine cavity and become spiral arteries after penetrating the mucosa. During pregnancy the spiral arteries experience a trophoblastic invasion that causes destruction of the elastic lamina and leads to a low-resistance vascular system in which maternal arteries are linked to fetal intervillous spaces. When the fetal vascular system is compromised, the persistence of the spiral arteries prevents a reduction in uteroplacental resistance. Doppler velocimetry makes it possible to study the uterine artery and spiral and subplacental arteries.[45,46–47,48] As outlined

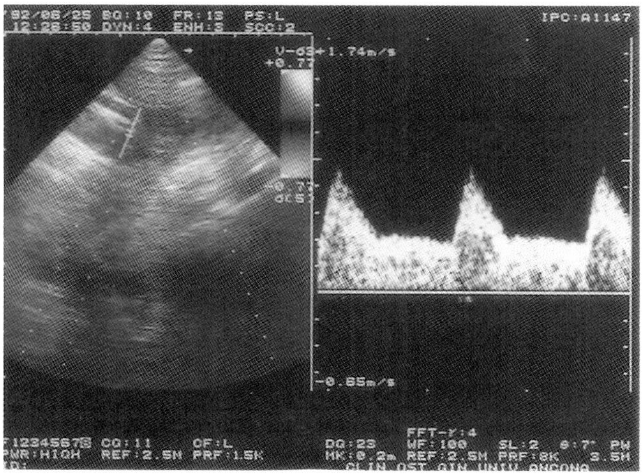

Fig. 7.11 Doppler evaluation of uterine vessel waveform with increased resistance index.

above, a technique to determine the degree of vasodilation of the uteroplacental bed can be extremely useful. Gestational hypertension seems to adapt to this pathogenetic mechanism and to cause severe maternal or fetal complications. For this reason some authors have proposed Doppler analysis of uterine arteries as a method of screening for gestational hypertension. The accuracy of this method in predicting gestational hypertension and fetal growth retardation method has recently been reported to be 76%.[49]

Doppler velocimetry of fetal vessels (Fig. 7.12)

In an optimally oxygenated fetus arterial flow is greatest to the organs that most need oxygen. The fetal circulation is characterized by a cardiac anatomy that conveys the most oxygenated blood, coming from the ductus venosus and from the left hepatic vein, through the foramen ovale to the superior portions of the body. This circulation provides oxygen and glucose to the heart and the central nervous system. In chronic hypoxic stress conditions there is a rearrangement of fetal hemodynamics. From a pathophysiologic point of view, the most interesting model of fetal chronic asphyxia is asymmetric fetal growth retardation; sonograpy reveals a discrepancy between cerebral growth and abdominal growth. Hemodynamic measurements demonstrate an increase in vascular resistance in the peripheral, aortic, renal and umbilical areas associated with a significant reduction in cerebral resistance.[50–54] A large number of studies have confirmed that a reduction in diastolic flow in the fetal umbilical arteries is associated with intrauterine growth retardation.[55,56] The absence of diastolic flow or the presence of a reversed flow in this area indicates an adverse prognosis. The presence of a reversed flow is often related to adverse cardiotocographic signs; neonatal prognosis is worsened by the occurrence of complications (intracranial hemorrhages) and neonatal death may occur. In asymmetric growth retardation, aortic resistance increases with a subsequent reduction in peripheral tissue flow. Also, the degree of aortic constriction is variable to the extent that there may be absence of distant diastolic flow with or without reversed flow. The increase in resistance mostly affects the fetal liver and gastrointesinal tract. A higher incidence of necrotizing enterocolitis has been reported in fetuses with asymmetric growth retardation; this could be due to a chronic intestinal hypoxia. At a cerebral level, chronic hypoxia causes a reduction in circulating PO_2 and a vasodilation that involves all Willis polygon cerebral zones. The initial aim of cerebral vasodilation is to maintain the correct cerebral metabolic equilibrium. The mechanisms that cause the flow redistribution are not yet completely understood; it is accepted that PO_2 and the acid–basic equilibrium have an essential role in determining brain-sparing effect. Many studies have been carried out to evaluate whether Doppler methodology may be trusted in predicting this type of growth retardation and fetal well-being with different but encouraging results as regards patients at risk.[57–60]

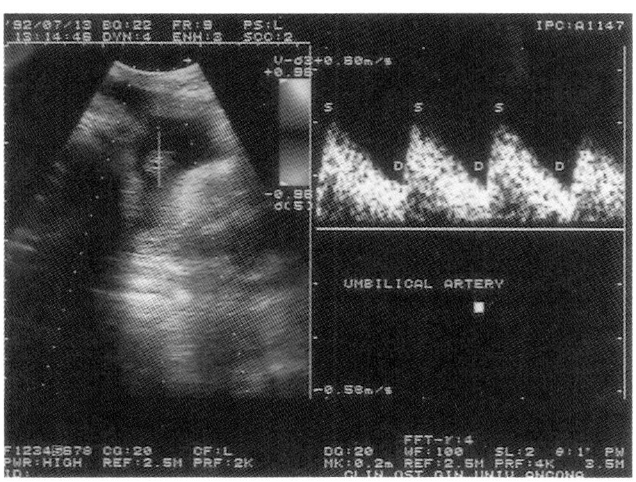

Fig. 7.12 Doppler evaluation of normal umbilical artery: systolic (S) and diastolic (D) peaks of Doppler waveforms are demonstrated.

COMPUTERIZED CARDIOTOCOGRAPHY

Computerized systems for fetal heart rate analysis have recently become commercially available. The reduction in intra-observer and inter-observer variability demonstrated in several reports[61,62] is the principal aim of these devices.

Of these systems, 'System 8000' is based on the studies carried out by Dawes and his associates over the last 15 years.[63–66] The fetal heart rate is calculated by means of an ultrasound probe. Analysis is performed on a personal computer connected directly to the cardiotocograph. A computerized system makes it possible to assess

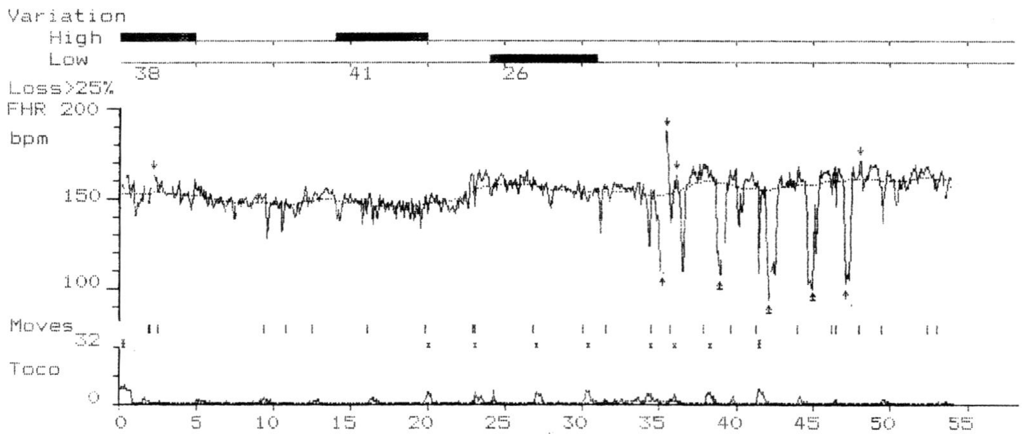

Fig. 7.13 Printout of computerized fetal heart rate using 'System 8000'. An abnormal heart rate tracing is shown with three deep decelerations. The numerical analysis of the heart rate is shown.

analytically and objectively a series of observations that up until now have been interpreted by the operator alone (Fig. 7.13). With this system a baseline is drawn on the fetal heart rate (FHR) cardiotocographic tracing; accelerations and decelerations are then recognized. Variability or FHR interval (in minutes) is calculated minute by minute of the tracing. Episodes of high FHR variability are identified when for 5 out of 6 successive minutes the range of pulse intervals is >32 min. When this criterion is not met, a new analysis is performed (threshold 24 min) and episodes of high variation are identified when pulse intervals are >24 min. Episodes of low FHR variability are identified when 5 out of 6 successive minutes have a range of pulse intervals <30 min. Again when this criterion is not met, a new analysis is performed (interval <22 min). In borderline cases a third analysis is performed: the baseline is reset and small decelerations are investigated (<5 bpm). No other parameters are recalculated. Short-term variability is measured as variation lasting 1/16 min calculated for every minute throughout the tracing. Together with FHR variation maternally perceived fetal movements are recorded as frequency per hour. The mean number of movements per minute within episodes of high or low variation is also noted. At the end of every recording the following parameters can be obtained:

- signal loss (%);
- basal fetal heart rate;
- fetal movements per minute in high variability;
- fetal movements per minute in low variability;
- accelerations;
- decelerations >20 bpm;
- duration of high variability;
- duration of low variability;
- variation overall (mean range);
- short-term variation.

Some of these parameters (short-term variation, high/low ratio, movements during periods of low variability have been shown to be reliable indexes of fetal well-being as they vary early in fetuses with intrauterine growth retardation and in those who will progress to acute fetal distress. The most significant aspect is the automated analysis of periods of high and low variability, their duration, the coincidence between periods of high and low variability and fetal movements revealed by maternal observation. It identifies variations of movement distribution revealed by study of fetal behavior. In a preliminary study performed on a sample group of patients with an intrauterine growth-retarded fetus compared with controls of the same gestational age, we could verify that in normal fetuses movements occur mostly during periods of high FHR variability periods while, on the other hand, in growth-retarded fetuses movements occur during periods of both high and low variability. This is evidence of the difficulty in controlling spontaneous movements in relation to other variables such as fetal heart rate.

REFERENCES

1. Hon E H (ed) 1986 An atlas of fetal heart rate patterns. Hardy Press, New Haven, Ct
2. Pillai M, James D 1990 The development of fetal heart rate patterns during normal pregnancy. Obstet Gynecol 76: 812–816
3. Martin Jr C B Physiology and clinical use of fetal heart rate variability Clin Perinatol 9: 339–352
4. Hoppenbrowers T, Combs D, Ugartchea J C et al 1981 Fetal heart rates during maternal wakefulness and sleep Obstet Gynecol 57: 301–304
5. Timor Trish I E, Dierker J, Zador I et al 1978 Fetal movements associated with fetal heart rate accelerations. Am J Obstet Gynecol. 131: 276–280
6. Henson G, Dawes G S Redman C W G 1984 Characterization of the reduced heart rate variation in growth-retarded fetuses. Br J Obstet Gynaecol 91: 751–755
7. Lee C Y Di Loreto P C, O'Lane J M 1975 A study of fetal heart rate acceleration patterns. Obstet Gynecol 45: 142–146

8. Cibils L A 1975 Clinical significance of fetal heart rate patterns during labor. II. Late decelerations. Am J Obstet Gynecol 124: 437–477
9. Harris J L, Krueger T R, Parer J T 1982 Mechanism of late decelerations of the fetal heart rate during hypoxia. Am J Obstet Gynecol 144: 491–496
10. Itskovitz J, Goetzman B W Abraham M, Rudolph A M 1982 The mechanism of late deceleration of the heart rate and its relationship to oxygenation in normoxemic and chronically hypoxemic fetal lambs. Am J Obstet Gynecol 142: 66–73
11. James L S, Yeh M N, Morishima H O et al 1976 Umbilical vein occlusion and transient acceleration of the fetal heart rate. Am J Obstet Gynecol 126: 276–279
12. Krebs H K, Petres R E, Dunn L J 1983 Intrapartum fetal heart rate monitoring. VII. Atypical variable decelerations. Am J Obstet Gynecol 145: 297–301
13. Caldeyro Barcia R, Mendez Bauer C, Poseiro J J et al 1966 Control of human fetal heart rate during labor. In: Cassels D E (ed) The heart and circulation in the newborn and infant. Grune & Stratton, New York) pp 13–27
14. Hammacher K 1968 The clinical significance of cardiotocography. In: Huntingford P J, Hunter E S, Saling E (eds) Perinatal medicine Academic Press, New York, pp 80–93
15. Kubli F, Boos R, Ruttgers H et al 1977 Antepartum fetal heart rate monitoring. In Current status of fetal heart rate monitoring and ultrasound in obstetrics. Beard R W, Campbell S (eds) Royal College of Obstetricians and Gynaecologists, London, pp 28–45
16. Pose S V, Castillo J B Mora Rojas E O et al 1969 Test of fetal tolerance to induce uterine contractions for the diagnosis of chronic distress, perinatal factors affecting human development. Pan American Health Organization, Scientific Publication No 185, place, pp 96–104
17. Ray M, Freeman R, Pine S, Hesselgesser R 1972 Clinical experience with the oxytocin challenge test. Am J Obstet Gynecol 114: 1–9
18. Schifrin B S, Lapidus M, Doctor G, Leviton A 1975 Contraction stress test for antepartum fetal evaluation Obstet Gynecol 45: 433–436
19. Freeman R K 1975 The use of oxytocin challenge test for antepartum clinical evaluation of uteroplacental respiratory function Am J Obstet Gynecol 121: 481–489
20. Farahani G, Vasudeva K, Petris R, Fenton A N 1976 Oxytocin challenge test in high risk pregnancy. Obstet Gynecol 47: 159–168
21. Baskett T F, Sandy E A 1977 The oxytocin challenge test and antepartum fetal assessment. Br J Obstet Gynaecol 84: 39–43
22. Schulman H, Lin C, Saldana L, Randolph G 1977 Quantitative analysis in the oxytocin challenge test Am J Obstet Gynecol 129: 239–245
23. Flynn A M, Kelly J 1977 Evaluation of fetal well being by antepartum fetal heart monitoring Br Med J 1: 936–939
24. Mendenhall H W, O'Leary J A, Phillips K O 1980 The non stress test: the value of a single acceleration in evaluating the fetus at risk. Am J Obstet Gynecol 136: 87–92
25. Brown R, Patrick J 1981 The non stress test: how long is enough? Am J Obstet Gynecol 141: 646–651
26. Phelan J 1981 The non stress test: a review of 3000 tests. Am J Obstet Gynecol 139: 7–12
27. Visser G H A, Huisjes H J 1977 Diagnostic value of the unstressed antepartum cardiotocogram Br J Obstet Gynaecol 84: 321
28. Keegan K A, Paul R H 1980 Antepartum fetal heart rate testing. IV. The non stress test as a primary approach. Am J Obstet Gynecol 136: 75–80
29. Brown V A, Sawers R S, Parson R J et al 1982 The value of antenatal cardiotocography in the management of high risk pregnancy: a randomized controlled trial Br J Obstet Gynaecol 89: 716–722
30. Sadovsky E, Navot D, Yaffe A 1981 Antenatal evaluation of fetal heart rate accelerations associated with fetal movements. Int J Gynaecol Obstet 19: 441–445
31. Manning F A, Morrison I, Lange I R, Harman C 1982 Antepartum determination of fetal health: composite biophysical scoring. Clin Perinatol 9: 285–296
32. Manning F A 1985 Assessment of fetal condition and risk: analysis of single and combined biophysical variable monitoring. Semin Perinatol 9: 4–16
33. Baskett T F, Gray J H, Prewett S J et al 1984 Antepartum fetal assessment using a fetal biophysical score. Am J Obstet Gynecol 148: 630–633
34. Thacker S B, Berkelman L Assessing the diagnostic accuracy and efficacy of selected antepartum fetal surveillance techniques. Obstet Gynecol Survey 41(3): 121–141
35. Huisjes H J, Towen B C L, Hoekstra J T et al 1980 Obstetrical neonatal neurological relationship. A replication study. Eur J Obstet Gynecol Reprod Biol 10: 247–256
36. Nelson K B, Ellenberg J H 1983 Antecedents of cerebral palsy. New Engl J Med 315: 81–86
37. Terao T, Kawashima Y, Noto H, Inatomo Y, Tzan Yu Lin Y, Sumimoto K, Maeda M 1984 Neurological control of fetal heart rate in 20 cases of anencephalic fetuses. Am J Obstet Gynecol 149: 201–207
38. Nijhuis J G, Martin C, Prechtl H F R 1984 Behavioural states of the human fetus. In: Prechtl HFR (ed) Continuity of neural functions from prenatal to postnatal life. Lavenham Press, Suffolk, pp 65–78
39. Prechtl H F R 1974 The behavioral states of the newborn infant (a review). Brain Res 76: 185–212.
40. Prechtl H F R 1982 Assessment methods for the newborn infant, a critical evaluation. In: Stratton P (ed) Psychobiology of the human newborn, John Wiley, Chichester, pp 21–52
41. Prechtl H F R 1984 Continuity and change in early human development. In: Prechtl H F R (ed) Continuity of neural functions from prenatal to postnatal life. Lavenham Press, Suffolk, pp 1–16
42. Romanini C, Valensise H 1990 Fetal Behavior and fetal health. In: Papini M, Pasquinello A, Gidoni E A (eds) Development, Handicap, rehabilitation: practice and theory, Elsevier, Amsterdam, pp 9–14
43. Valensise H, Ciotti G, Giobbi D, et al 1988 Behavior of fetuses from hypertensive mothers. Clin Exp Hypertens–Hypertens pregnancy B7: 227–233
44. Romanini C, Valensise H, Ciotti G, et al 1989 Tryptophan availability and fetal behavioural states. Fetal Ther 4 (suppl 1) 68–72
45. Campbell S, Griffin D R, Pearce J M, Diaz-Recanses J, Cohen-Overbeek T E, Wilson K, Teague M J New doppler technique for assessing uteroplacental blood flow. Lancet i: 675–677
46. Trudinger B J, Giles W B, Cook C M Flow velocity waveforms in the maternal uteroplacental and fetal umbilical placental circulation. Am J Obstet Gynecol 152: 155–163
47. Schulman H, Fleischer A, Farmakides G, Bracero L, Rochelson B, Grunfeld L 1986 Development of uterine compliance in pregnancy as detected by doppler ultrasound. Am J Obstet Gynecol 155: 1031–1036
48. Schulman H, Ducey J Farmakides G, Guzman E, Winter D, Penny B, Chi-Lee Y 1987 Uterine artery Doppler velocimetry: the significance of divergent systolic diastolic ratios. Am J Obstet Gynecol 157: 1539–1542
49. Arduini D, Rizzo G. Romanini C, Mancuso S 1987 Uteroplacental blood flow velocity waveforms as predictors of pregnancy induced hypertension. Eur J Obstet Gynecol Reprod Biol 26: 335–339
50. Stuart B, Drumm J, Fitzgerald D E, Duignan N M 1980 Fetal blood velocity waveform in normal pregnancy. Br J Obstet Gynaecol 87: 780–785
51. Lingman G, Marsal K 1986 Fetal central blood circulation in the third trimester of normal pregnancy – a longtudinal study. I. Aortic and umbilical blood flow. Early Hum Dev 13: 137–150
52. Lingman G, Marsal K 1986 Fetal central blood circulation in the third trimester of normal pregnancy-a longitudinal study. II. Aortic blood velocity waveform. Early Hum Dev 13: 151–159
53. Woo J, Liang S T, Roxy L S, Fung Yee Chan S 1987 Middle cerebral artery Doppler flow velocity waveforms. Obstet Gynecol 70: 613
54. Wladimiroff J W, Tonge H M, Stewart P A 1986 Doppler ultrasound assessment of cerebral blood flow in the human fetus. Br J Obstet Gynaecol 93: 471–475
55. Bekedam D J, Visser G H, van der Zee A G, Snijders R J, Poelmann Weesjes G 1990 Abnormal velocity waveforms of the umbilical artery in growth retarded fetuses: relationship to antepartum late heart rate decelerations and outcome. Early Hum Dev 24: 79–89

56. Wladimiroff J W, Wijngaard J A, Degani S, Noordam M J, Eyck J V, Tonge M D 1987 Cerebral and umbilical arterial blood flow velocity waveforms in normal and growth-retarded pregnancies. Obstet Gynecol 69: 705–709
57. Arduini D, Rizzo G, Romanini C, Mancuso S 1987 Fetal blood flow velocity waveforms as a predictor of growth retardation. Obstet Gynecol 70: 7–10
58. Pattinson R, Dawes G, Jennings J Redman C 1991 Umbilical artery resistance index as a screening test for fetal well-being. I. Prospective revealed evaluation. Obstet Gynecol 78: 353–358
59. Hofmeyr G J, Pattinson R, Buckley D, Jennings J, Redman C W 1991 Umbilical artery resistence index as a screening test for fetal well-being. II. Randomized feasibility study. Obstet Gynecol 78: 359–362
60. Arduini D, Rizzo G, Soliani A, Romanini C 1991 Doppler velocimetry versus nonstress test in the antepartum monitoring of low-risk pregnancies. J Ultrasound Med 10: 331–335
61. Flynn A M, Kelly J, Mathews K et al 1982 Predictive value of and observer variability in several ways of reporting antepartum cardiotocographs. Br J Obstet Gynaecol 89: 434–440
62. Nielsen P V, Stigsby B, Nickelsen C, Nim J 1987 Intra and inter observer variability in the assessment of antepartum cardiotocograms. Acta Obstet Gynecol Scand 66: 421–424
63. Dawes G S, Houghton C R S, Redman C W G 1982 Baseline in human fetal heart-rate records. Br J Obstet Gynaecol 89: 270–275
64. Dawes G S, Houghton C R S, Redman C W G, Visser G H A 1982 Pattern of normal human fetal heart-rate. Br J Obstet Gynaecol 89: 279–284
65. Dawes G S, Redman C W G, Smith J H 1985 Improvements in the registration and analysis of fetal heart rate records at the bedside. Br J Obstet Gynaecol 92: 317–325
66. Dawes G S Moulden M, Redman C W G 1990 Limitation of antenatal fetal heart rate monitors. Am J Obstet Gynecol 162: 170–173

PART B
FETAL WELL-BEING DURING LABOR

H. Valensise C. Romanini

INDICATORS OF FETAL DISTRESS

Fetal heart rate

Based on the characteristics of the fetal heart rate recordings, two fetal conditions during labor can be easily distinguished by examining the FHR variations. The first condition is characterized by a regular FHR, a basal level within the norm, frequent accelerations and an absence of decelerations. These characteristics are usually associated with optimal oxygenation and with a high Apgar score at birth.[1]

The cardiotocographic tracing associated with poor fetal condition is characterized by tachycardia, reduced variability and repeated late decelerations. If persistent, such characteristics are associated with a high risk of intrauterine or neonatal mortality or late neonatal morbidity. Similarly, bradycardia occurring rapidly, and which is prolonged and associated with reduced heart rate variability, may be an indicator of severe fetal distress preceding fetal death[2] if the labor has not yet reached second stage. The evaluation of tracings intermediate between normal and indicative of severe fetal distress depends on four factors:

- episodic and repeated occurrence of the event;
- degree of growth and intrauterine fetal development;
- the duration of labor;
- the presence of other maternal pathology.

The presence of meconium in amniotic fluid may also be significant.[3]

Various reports[4,5] that have attempted to correlate of cardiotocography during labor with fetal well-being or distress have not always taken these factors into account, therefore it is not always possible to obtain correlations. In addition, because of differences in obstetric management between centers with different indications for performing a cesarean delivery or using forceps or vacuum extraction, the cardiotocographic tracing may be useful in deciding when intervention is necessary. However, it is more useful as a means of distinguishing between dangerous situations and those that require more careful evaluation.

Fetal pH

The determination of fetal acidosis by withdrawing a small amount of blood from the fetal scalp was widely used until the early 1980s.[6] The popularity of the technique has declined since the development and widespread use of cardiotocographic instruments, but it remains of some value in determining fetal condition in some borderline situations. The fetal pH is considered normal if >7.25; pH between 7.20 and 7.25 indicates a state of preacidosis; and values <7.20 indicate acidosis.

Comparison of cardiotocograph tracings and fetal pH shows:[7,8]

- pH >7.25 when there is a normal tracing with the previously described characteristics;
- significant but small variations in the fetal pH are associated with slight bradycardia and good variability or slight tachycardia and good variability;
- progressive reduction in fetal pH value when repeated, longer and more serious decelerations occur.

Decelerations in order of seriousness may be classified as follows: early, variable, variable with worsening signs and late decelerations. The reduction in the fetal pH value as fetal condition progressively worsens is significant. This is principally due to the change in fetal metabolism that begins at the moment of deceleration. Late decelerations are associated with a change to anaerobic metabolism because of the prolonged hypoxia that occurs and thus the production of lactic acid. The slow rise in the heart rate at the end of a contraction is due to the restoration of aerobic metabolism.

Variable decelerations and early decelerations are usually not correlated with the vascular mechanisms responsible or with the mechanisms involved in changing from aerobic to anaerobic metabolism. In such cases, therefore, the fetal pH variation is not so frequent. This association between heart rate and pH variation may be found only in the presence of serious repeated variable decelerations or other signs of worsening fetal health.

CLINICAL RELEVANCE OF FHR DURING LABOR

The value of fetal heart rate recording during trial of labor is controversial.[9–12] Neonatal mortality and morbidity results obtained during randomized trials have caused doctors to question the utility of heart rate recording during trial of labor as compared with intermittent auscultation with a stethoscope. However, data correlating fetal monitoring with a reduction in intrapartum mortality favor its use. Furthermore, a correlation between prolonged and serious acidosis and the absence of intensive prenatal control during labor has been reported.[13] The presence of acidosis is significantly correlated with a high incidence of long-term neurologic damage compared with subjects who have not suffered from acidosis. Those who oppose monitoring FHR during labor maintain that its use has not significantly reduced the incidence of cerebral palsy in the past few years.

The use of the cardiotocography during labor has led to an increased number of cesarean deliveries with a consequent increase in maternal morbidity, and it has also led to an increase in the number of legal and medical controversies in which the cardiotocographic tracing is a decisive element. Opponents of cardiotocography during labor mistakenly believe that the recording of the variation in the heart rate in relation to uterine contractile activity may be an indication of the normality or otherwise of fetal and neonatal psychoneurologic development. The normal development of the neonatal brain is not dependent on the heart rate trend during trial of labor.[14] This was verified by neurophysiologists and pediatricians by comparing term neonates with premature neonates who had reached the same gestational age in extrauterine conditions.

The development of the neonatal brain and the occurrence of cerebral palsy are slightly correlated with fetal hypoxia developed during labor, although other factors during pregnancy also affect the central nervous system and play an important role. It is, however, possible that fetal hypoxia may cause permanent neurologic damage.

Currently most pregnant women reaching the trial of labor stage have received comprehensive prenatal care, in particular, monitoring of fetal growth and maternal pathology during pregnancy. This has resulted in a low-risk population reaching trial of labor: thus acute fetal distress in combination with a chronic condition (slowing of growth, hypertension) is thus rarer and more difficult to verify. Monitoring of FHR during labor is therefore a very valuable tool when used in the physiopathologic circumstances for which it was devised.

EPIDEMIOLOGY OF MENTAL RETARDATION

Mental development was previously measured using the intelligence quotient (IQ). This test has well-known limitations: it has some cultural influences and it does not evaluate important aspects of cognitive functions. However, it has the advantage of being a numeric indicator. Mental retardation is defined as severe if the IQ is < 50 and slight if it is between 50 and 70. Studies[15–17] in industrialized populations have found similar prevalence of severe mental retardation in different samples, the prevalence in schoolchildren being 3–4 per 1000. The prevalence of slight mental retardation is more variable: 1–3% of schoolchildren. In severe mental retardation, clinical signs of cerebral damage such as motor handicap and convulsions are present, while these are not present in individuals with slight mental retardation. Slight mental retardation seems to be more common in the lower social classes although class differences in the prevalence of severe mental retardation do not seem to exist. Previously these two forms of mental retardation were considered to have a different etiology; socioeconomic in the former and biologic in the latter. This view has changed and a high percentage cases of slight mental retardation are reported to be due to biologic damage. The main causes of mental retardation are: chromosome anomalies (36%), complex malformation syndromes (20%), congenital metabolic errors (7%), perinatal causes (asphyxia, trauma) (8%), prenatal causes (intrauterine growth retardation, IUGR) (8%), infections (6%) and other causes (unknown) (15%). In many cases it is difficult to assign a definite etiology, but it should be noted that trisomy 21 is the major cause of mental retardation, and in various studies accounts for a one-third to one-half of all individuals with mental retardation. Taken together, perinatal events would seem to account for >10–15% of cases of severe mental retardation, i.e. 3–4 per 10 000 schoolchildren.

CORRELATION BETWEEN OBSTETRIC EVENTS AND NEUROLOGIC OUTCOMES

Some factors must be considered when attempting to link obstetric events and neonatal neurologic problems. If these factors are unknown it is difficult to evaluate individual cases.

The factors are:

- gestational age at birth;
- fetal growth;
- maternal risk factors;
- history and trend of labor;
- fetal health indicators during labor and at birth;
- duration and degree of the hypoxic event;
- neurologic follow-up;
- socioeconomic conditions.

It is very difficult to relate fetal history with neurologic outcome in fetuses of different gestational ages and with different degrees of intrauterine growth. Even lesions which can be identified at the cerebral structure level can vary in location, distribution and morphology. Intraventricular hemorrhage is more frequent in the premature neonate up to 37 weeks of gestation associated with secondary leukomalacia; it can cause cerebral palsy, mental retardation, hydrocephalus and sensory disturbances, and it very often has a post-natal origin. On the other hand, in a term fetus of normal weight the most frequent histopathologic lesion is cerebral cortical necrosis or encephalic trunk necrosis, which are often the result of perinatal damage. The symptoms may vary from cerebral palsy in the most serious cases to every degree of behavioral, sensory and learning problems. These two different physiopathologic models must be kept separate when statistical data are being analyzed.

One must be similarly cautious when evaluating the effect of obstetric variables during pregnancy and labor. A clear correlation exists between long-term neurologic anomalies and severe prematurity. Delivery between 24 and 29 weeks of gestation[18–20] is associated with a high mortality rate which decreases as the gestational age increases. Prematurity and associated neonatal respiratory difficulties must be taken into consideration when identifying the causes of a handicap. Motor handicap occurs in 10% of neonates delivered at 24–28 weeks' gestation, while mental retardation occurs in 12% of surviving infants at the same age. There is a progressive reduction in mortality with increasing gestational age associated with an increase in the risk of mental retardation in the survivors. In neonates delivered at 27–31 weeks, a decrease in mortality is accompanied by an increase in neurologic morbidity. If prematurity is associated with reduced intrauterine growth, the prevalence of neuromotor handicaps in the surviving neonates is high but variable: between 30 and 45%. It is often difficult to separate the roles of prematurity and IUGR in determining handicap, but together they play a decisive role. It is important to remember that mental retardation does not affect only high-risk pregnancies, such as premature fetuses or fetuses with slow intrauterine growth. In fact most neonates with cerebral palsy or permanent neurologic syndromes are born to low-risk subjects. Data gathered by Nelson and Ellenberg[21, 22] show that, out of the 54 000 births examined, 58% of the affected neonates were born after 37 weeks and weighed >2500 g.

Various risk indices have been described in order to reduce to a minimum the incidence of neurologically handicapped neonates. These include the concept of 'obstetric optimality' described by the school of Groningen,[23–25] in which 76 obstetric risk indicators are scored in an attempt to identify an ideal pregnancy. This score is correlated with a similar post-natal neurologic evaluation of the neonate. However, in some almost ideal pregnancies achieving very high scores and, therefore, of low perinatal obstetric risk, neonates subjected to examination and a neurologic follow-up were found to be abnormal or suspect.

When evaluating obstetric risk conditions for post-natal neuromotor or sensory handicap the existence of adverse obstetric factors cannot be ignored, but it is almost impossible to eliminate the risk totally, even in ideal obstetric conditions.[26–28]. These considerations are even more important if observation of the relationship between obstetric events and long-term outcomes is restricted to the length and mode of labor. Generally, hypoxic stress during trial of labor is considered to be responsible for long-term neurologic sequelae. Although the severity and correlation with the duration of hypoxia are crucial, the development of poor fetal oxygenation and the change to anaerobic metabolism with cerebral damage is not linear. This is the finding of a series of studies that have evaluated the ability of indicators of fetal/neonatal stress/well-being to predict neurologic normality. For example, the 1-min Apgar score[21] was described as normal in 55% of neonates that later developed cerebral palsy. In neonates with a normal Apgar score at 5 min this percentage rises to 73%. However, as an indicator of early neonatal mortality, the Apgar score maintains its value, with a mortality rate of 17% if < 4 at 1 min, 44% if < 4 at 5 min, and 88% if < 4 at 10 min.

FHR and acid–base balance (pH) are important indicators of fetal health and good predictors of long-term neurologic outcome. Both measures together are a more reliable indicator of fetal well-being than heart rate alone. Numerous clinical trials have shown no difference in long-term outcome between neonates that showed signs of fetal hypoxia and controls, and thus some authors have suggested not monitoring labor by cardiotocography.

In contrast, Low[29] reported 60 neonates with metabolic acidosis during trial of labor who, during follow-up at 6 and 12 months, showed a high percentage of motor and cognitive defects (13% major defects, 16% minor defects). In 90% of the neonates with no handicap intensive monitoring was carried out during the 5 h before delivery; in 80% of the neonates with minor handicap, the intensive monitoring before delivery lasted 2.5 h. In 63% of those with major handicap no monitoring of the FHR was performed, while only in 37% of the pregnancies was intensive monitoring carried out during the last hour before delivery. Acidosis of duration > 60 min can be directly correlated with a progressive increase in neuromotor and cognitive risk: a briefer period of acidosis can be associated with a successful neonatal outcome.

Thus, fetuses at risk may be identified only by means of a combination of historic and current, biophysical and biochemical, data. Nevertheless, long-term outcome seems to be more closely linked to the sensitivity of an individual fetus to potentially damaging intrauterine events.

These findings have stimulated further perinatal research in order to broaden our knowledge of the development of the fetal nervous system during pregnancy with the aim of determining indicators of normality and abnormality during the period preceding labor, so reducing the importance of the trial of labor in the genesis of long-term perinatal damage.

REFERENCES

1. Cibils L A 1980 Clinical significance of fetal heart rate patterns during labor. Am J Obstet Gynecol 136: 392–397
2. Herbert C M, Boehm F H 1981 Prolonged end-stage fetal heart rate deceleration: a reanalysis. Obstet Gynecol 57: 589
3. Kariniemi V, Harrela M 1990 Significance of meconium staining of the amniotic fluid. J Perinat Med 18: 345–349
4. Mac Donald D, Grant A, Seridan Pereira M et al 1985 The Dublin randomized trial of intrapartum fetal heart rate monitoring. Am. J Obstet Gynecol 152: 524–539
5. Leveno K J, Cunningham R G C, Nelson S et al 1986 A prospective comparison of selective and universal electronic fetal monitoring in 34,995 pregnancies. New Eng J Med 315: 615–619
6. Fleisher A, Schulman H, Jagani N, Mitchell J, Randolph G 1982 The development of fetal acidosis in the presence of an abnormal fetal heart rate tracing. Am J Obstet Gynecol 144: 55–59
7. Fee S C, Malee K, Deddish R, Minogue J P, Socol M L 1990 Severe acidosis and subsequent neurologic status. Am J Obstet Gynecol 162: 802–806
8. Nickelsen C, Weber T 1991 The current status of intrapartum continuous fetal tissue pH measurements. J Perinat Med 19: 87–92
9. Haverkamp A D, Orleanes M, Langendoerfer S et al 1979 A controlled trial of the differential effects of intrapartum fetal monitoring. Am J Obstet Gynecol 134: 399–412
10. Wood C, Renou P, Oats J et all 1981 A controlled trial of fetal heart rate monitoring in a low risk obstetrics population. Am J Obstet Gynecol 141: 527–534
11. Ducey J, Guzman E, Schulman H, Farmakedis G, Karmin I 1990 Value of a screening fetal heart rate tracing in the latent phase of labor. J Reprod Med 35: 899–900
12. Sandmire H F 1990 Whither electronic fetal monitoring? Obstet Gynecol 76: 1130
13. Low J A, Galbralth R S, Muir D W, Killen H L, Pater E A, Karchmar E J 1983 Intrapartum fetal hypoxia. A study of long-term morbidity. Am J Obstet Gynecol 145: 129
14. Blair E, Stanley F J 1988 Intrapartum asphyxia: a rare cause of cerebral palsy. J Pediatr 112, 515–519
15. Hagberg B, Hagberg G, Olow I 1984 The changing panorama of cerebral palsy in Sweden. IV. Epidemiological trends 1959–78. Acta Pediatr Scand 73: 433–440
16. Keegan K A, Waffarn F, Quilligan E J 1985 Obstetric characteristics and fetal heart rate patterns of infants who convulse during the newborn period. Am J Obstet Gynecol 153: 732–737
17. Grant A, O'Brien N, Joy M T 1989 Cerebral palsy among children born during the Dublin randomised trial of intrapartum monitoring. Lancet 2: 1233
18. Shennan A T, Milligan J E 1980 The growth and development of infants weighing 1,000–2,000 grams at birth and delivered in a perinatal unit. Am J Obstet Gynecol 136: 273–237
19. Kitchen W H, Yui V G H, Orgik A A, et al 1982 Infants born before 29 weeks' gestation: survival and morbidity at 2 years of age. Br J Obstet Gynaecol 89: 887–890
20. Milligan J E, Sheenan A T, Hoskins E M 1984 Perinatal intensive care: where and how to draw the line. Am J Obstet Gynecol 149: 499
21. Nelson K B, Ellenberg J H 1984 Obstetric complications as a risk factors for cerebral palsy or seizure disorders. J Am Med Assoc 251: 1843–1848
22. Nelson K B, Ellenberg J H 1986 Antecedents of cerebral palsy. New Engl J Med 315: 81–86
23. Towen B C Variability and stereotype in neurological development. 1982 In: Kong E (ed) Zerebrale Bewegungs-storungen. Aktuelle Fragen der Klinik und Forschung. (Karger), Basle, pp 70–77
24. Towen B C 1979 Developmental neurology. In: Clifford Rose F (ed) Paediatric neurology. Blackwell Scientific Publications, Oxford, pp 86–97
25. Huisjes H J, Towen B C L, Hoekstra J T et all 1980 Obstetrical neonatal neurological relationship. A replication study Eur J Obstet Gynecol Reprod Biol 10: 4,247
26. Niswander K, Henson G, Elbourne D et all 1984 Adverse outcome of pregnancy and the quality of obstetric care. Lancet 2 827–831
27. Murphy K W, Johnson P, Moorcraft J, Pattinson R et all 1990 Birth asphyxia and the intrapartum cardiotocograph. Br J Obstet Gynaecol 97: 470–479
28. Melone P J, Ernest J M, O'Shea Jr M D, Klinepeter K L 1991 Appropriateness of intrapartum fetal heart rate management and risk of cerebral palsy. Am J Obstet Gynecol 165: 272–276
29. Low J A, Galbraith R S, Muir D W, Killen H L, Pater E A, Karchmar E J 1988 Motor and cognitive defects after intrapartum asphyxia in the mature fetus. Am J Obstet Gynecol 158: 356–361

PART C

FETAL AND NEONATAL HEMODYNAMIC ADAPTATIONS AT BIRTH

J. Hamza

The transitional circulation occurs between the fetal hemodynamic state and the neonatal circulation. It is important for the obstetric anesthesiologist to understand these hemodynamic changes since certain neonatal problems may induce a persistence of this transitional circulation after birth, particularly after fetal asphyxia.

FETAL CIRCULATION

Fetal hemodynamics

The umbilical vein carries blood from the placenta to the fetus. The liver is the first organ to receive blood flow, but more than 50% of this blood flow bypasses the liver and flows into the ductus venosus, which empties into the inferior vena cava.[1]

Umbilical venous blood has a relatively low oxygen saturation (65%): this is explained by the reduced affinity of fetal hemoglobin for 2,3-diphosphoglycerate (2,3-DPG), which results in a leftward shift of the oxygen dissociation curve.[2] These properties of fetal hemoglobin explain why, despite this low $Sa\text{O}_2$, sufficient oxygen is brought to the fetal tissues.

In the full-term fetal lamb, blood received through the right atrium is distributed as follows:

1. One-third of the blood flows through the foramen ovale to the left atrium and is distributed to the left ventricle and then to the ascending aorta; vital organs, such as the myocardium and brain, receive relatively more oxygenated blood (oxygen saturation, 65%) than other non-essential organs.[3,4]
2. Two-thirds of the blood is mixed in the right atrium with the desaturated superior vena caval blood and is distributed to the right ventricle and into the main pulmonary artery. As pulmonary vascular resistance is high and placental resistance is low, only 10% of the blood in the main pulmonary artery is distributed to the pulmonary vascular bed, whereas the remaining 90% is shunted to the descending aorta through the ductus arteriosus. Blood is then distributed to the abdominal viscera and returns to the placenta through the two umbilical arteries.

Therefore, the outflow from the left ventricle is important for myocardial and cerebral perfusion, whereas the outflow from the right ventricle is essential for abdominal, placental and lower extremity perfusion. As they face the same placental resistance, the two fetal ventricles work in parallel and not in series: the right and left ventricular systolic pressures are equal. The ventricular output is approximately 200 ml/kg/min,[5] but the contribution of each ventricle is different: the left ventricle contributes to only one-third of the total cardiac output whereas the right ventricle contributes the remaining two-thirds.

Although their outputs are different, right and left ventricular size and function are similar throughout gestation, as demonstrated by echocardiography.[6]

Because of the parallel arrangement of the two ventricles, fetal aortic blood flow is not altered by complete obstruction of right or left circulation: the ductus arteriosus and the foramen ovale allow blood flow to bypass these obstructions.

Determinants of fetal cardiac output

The main determinants of fetal cardiac output are preload, myocardial contractility, afterload and heart rate.

Preload

In fetal lambs, left ventricular end-diastolic pressure is 3–5 mmHg above intra-amniotic pressures. Although the Frank–Starling mechanism appears to function within the normal range of pressures, there is no significant increase in combined ventricular output when ventricular end-diastolic filling pressures are increased above the normal range by infusing saline rapidly.[7] Nevertheless, ventricular output decreases significantly if the filling pressures falls below the lower limit of the normal range.

Contractility

Fetal ventricular tissue contains more noncontractile elements and fewer sarcomeres than adult ventricular tissue. Fetal lamb myocardium is less able to increase its contractility and is less compliant (limited increase in sarcomere length with higher filling pressures) than the adult sheep myocardium.[8] These two properties of fetal myocardium limit its ability to increase cardiac output when filling pressures are increased.

Afterload

As the placental resistance is low and placental blood flow is high, fetal afterload is normally relatively low. However, increased afterload induces an important fall in combined ventricular output, mainly due to a drop in right ventricular output.[9]

Heart rate

Heart rate is considered the main determinant of fetal cardiac output. Between 100 and 250 beats per minute in

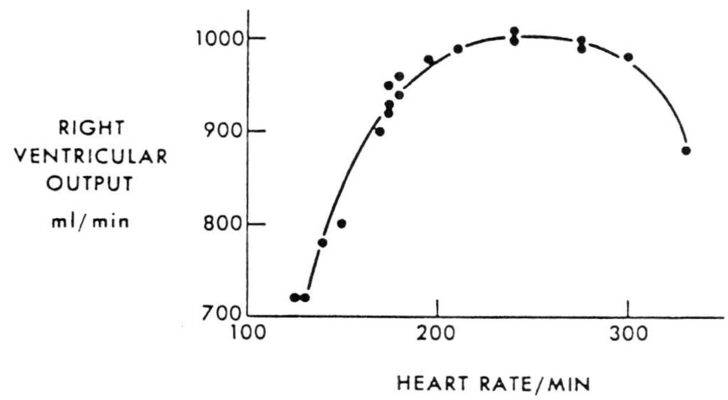

Fig. 7.14 The relationship between right ventricular output and heart rate in one fetus is shown. A marked rise in output occurs as the rate rises from 125 to 200 bpm. Above a rate of 300 bpm output falls.

the fetal lambs, heart rate is linearly related to left and right ventricular output[10] (Fig. 7.14). Relatively small reductions in heart rate reduce right ventricular output dramatically, whereas only very rapid atrial pacing (>315 bpm) may induce a rapid fall in right ventricular output. In addition, all the reflexes that cause severe bradycardia in the fetus may reduce cardiac output to a dangerously low level.

Fetal pulmonary circulation

Fetal pulmonary vascular resistance is very high and this limits the pulmonary blood flow to 7% of the combined ventricular output,[3] which is sufficient to meet the requirements of fetal lung growth.

Pulmonary vascular resistance in the fetus is thought to be controlled by numerous factors (catecholamines, acetylcholine, bradykinin, histamine), but hypoxia and acidosis appear to be the main pulmonary vasoconstrictors. The degree of hypoxemia required to induce vasoconstriction decreases with advancing gestational age.[11] In full-term fetal animals, mild hypoxemia induces an important increase in pulmonary vascular resistance. Pulmonary vasoconstriction is observed in the lung receiving hypoxemic blood but not in the other lung, which is perfused with normoxemic blood: this vascular response is therefore due to the direct effect of local hypoxemia.[12] A similar age-related responsiveness of the pulmonary vascular vessels to acidemia has been shown in other studies.[13,14]

The role of prostaglandins is not yet clearly understood. Nevertheless, prostacyclin (PGI_2), which is released by fetal lung distension, induces a pulmonary vasodilation when given to fetal lambs.[15]

Fetal response to stress

The redistribution of blood flow in response to hypoxia has been documented in fetal lambs: heart, brain, adrenal glands and placenta are well perfused while blood flow is reduced to other organs (gut, kidneys, lungs). Similarly, in human fetuses, blood flow to brain, heart and adrenal glands is 3–4 times higher during asphyxia than under normal conditions.[16]

TRANSITIONAL CIRCULATION

Many important changes are necessary to establish the adult pathway of circulation at birth.

Changes of systemic and pulmonary vascular resistances

Systemic blood pressure increases just after umbilical cord clamping because of the sudden rise in systemic vascular resistance. Simultaneously, pulmonary blood flow increases just after the first breath because of the reduction in pulmonary vascular resistance. The decrease in pulmonary vascular resistance is mainly caused by the increase in alveolar and pulmonary venous oxygen tension, whereas physical expansion of the lung has a lesser effect.

Closure of the ductus arteriosus

Closure of the ductus arteriosus is a two-stage process after birth. Functional closure, which occurs during the first 15 hs after birth, is reversible, particularly if hypoxemia or acidosis occurs. Anatomic closure, which occurs between the second and third week after birth, is mainly caused by the permanent increase in aortic $P\text{O}_2$. Although oxygen has a dose-dependent effect,[17] the ability of the ductus to contract in response to oxygen depends on gestational age. In contrast to full-term lambs, immature lambs have no ductal constriction in response to high oxygen concentrations.[17]

Some prostaglandins (PGE_1, PGE_2, and PGI_2) may induce or maintain ductal dilation particularly in immature fetal lamb. However, the vasoconstricting effects of indomethacin, a prostaglandin synthetase inhibitor, are less effective in closing an immature ductus than one in a mature fetus.

Whatever the gestational age, the ductus may reopen after birth in response to hypoxemia or acidemia and blood may flow through it (from right to left), leading to futher hypoxemia.

Closure of the foramen ovale

The decreased pulmonary vascular resistance and the increased pulmonary blood flow of the neonate induce simultaneously a fall in right atrial pressure and a rise in left artrial pressure. These events facilitate the functional, and later the anatomic, closure of the foramen ovale.

As in the case of the ductus arteriosus, right-to-left shunting may occur through the foramen ovale after birth.

NEONATAL CIRCULATION

The normal neonatal circulation

During the first hours of life, the increase in systemic vascular resistance and the decrease in pulmonary vascular resistance causes more than 30% of the left ventricular output to flow from left-to-right through the ductus arteriosus. Cardiac output decreases from 500 ml/kg/min to 425 ml/kg/min when the newborn's ventricles begin to work in series.[18] Right ventricular output increases by 25% from 340 ml/kg/min to 425 ml/kg/min, while left ventricular output increases by 150% from 170 ml/kg/min to 425 ml/kg/min. Cardiac output is higher in neonates delivered vaginally than in those born by cesarean delivery.[19,20]

Neonatal blood pressure at birth depends on gestational age and increases gradually with post-natal age.[21]

Determinants of neonatal cardiac output

Preload

In newborn lambs, increasing left ventricular end-diastolic pressure (LVEDP) to 10 mmHg increases stroke volume and stroke work, but stroke work decreases when LVEDP is increased above 15 mmHg. Thus, the Frank–Starling mechanism is intact when preload is in the normal range.[22]

Heart rate

The neonatal heart rate is subject to important spontaneous changes. In a study of full-term human newborns continuously monitored for 1 day,[23] the mean heart rate was higher (145 ± 15 bpm range 78–222) during the awake state than during sleep (123 ± 12 bpm, range 72–210).

Contractility

Although left ventricular contractility increases in lambs at birth,[24] the major noncontractile tissue present in the newborn's myocardium may explain the lower compliance of the neonatal left ventricle when compared with the right ventricle.[8]

Afterload

Afterload changes in the newborn are not well understood. Nevertheless, a 73% increase in the systemic vascular resistance index was noted between the first and third weeks after birth in one study in neonatal lambs.[21]

The newborn pulmonary circulation

During the first minutes after birth, the pulmonary vessels dilate in response to the higher ambient oxygen concentration.[1] Pulmonary vascular resistance rapidly decreases to 20% of its fetal level, and pulmonary blood flow increases from 35 ml/kg/min to 160–200 ml/kg/min.

Immediately after birth, pulmonary arterial pressure remains approximately equal to aortic systolic pressure because the ductus arteriosus transmits the aortic pressure to the pulmonary artery. In the newborn lamb, mean pulmonary arterial pressure is 55 mmHg at birth and decreases to 38 mmHg during the first day, and to 18 mmHg several days after birth.[25]

The neonatal pulmonary vascular bed is highly reactive to vasoactive substances. The full-term newborn has a greater vasoconstrictor response to hypoxemia and acidemia[1] than the premature baby because the medial smooth muscle layer is thicker in the former.[26]

The persistent pulmonary hypertension resulting from the occasional persistence of high pulmonary vascular resistance after birth allows pulmonary arterial blood to shunt from right to left across the ductus arteriosus and/or the foramen ovale, leading to severe neonatal hypoxemia.

CONCLUSION

The newborn's circulation is characterized by continuous changes in cardiovascular anatomy and physiology from the fetal to the neonatal state. Some changes are reversible, such as closure of the ductus arteriosus or the reduction of pulmonary vascular tone. When subjected to hypoxemia, acidemia or hypervolemia, the newborn's circulation may revert to the fetal state, which may endanger the newborn. Therefore, it is important that the obstetric anesthesiologist be fully aware of these problems so that they may be avoided or treated rapidly if they occur.

REFERENCES

1. Rudolph A M 1970 The changes in the circulation after birth: their importance in congenital heart disease. Circulation 41: 343–359
2. Lister G, Moreau G, Moss M et al 1984 Effects of alterations of oxygen transport on the neonate. Semin Perinatol 8: 192–204
3. Rudolph A M, Heymann M A 1970 Circulatory changes during growth in the fetal lamb. Circ Res 26: 289–299
4. Rudolph A M, Heyman M A 1974 Fetal and neonatal circulation and respiration. Annu Rev Physiol 36: 187–207
5. Assali N S, Rauramo L, Peltonen T 1960 Measurement of uterine blood flow and uterine metabolism. VIII. Uterine and fetal blood flow and oxygen consumption in early human pregnancy. Am J Obstet Gynecol 79: 86–98
6. St. John-Sutton M G, Gewitz M H, Shah B et al 1984 Quantitative assessment of growth and function of the cardiac chambers in the normal human fetus: a prospective longitudinal echocardiographic study. Circulation 69: 645–654
7. Heymann M A, Rudolph A M 1973 Effects of increasing preload on right ventricular output in fetal lambs in utero. Circulation 48 (suppl 4): 37

8. Friedman W F 1973 The instrinsic physiologic properties of the developing heart. In: Friedman W F, Lesch M, Sonnenblick E H (eds) Neonatal heart disease. Grune & Stratton, Orlando, F L, pp 21–49
9. Reller M D, Morton M J, Reid D L, Thornburg K L 1987 Fetal lamb ventricles respond differently to filling and arterial pressures and to in utero ventilation. Pediatr Res 22: 621–626
10. Rudolph A M, Heymann M A 1976 Cardiac output in the fetal lamb: the effects of spontaneous and induced changes of heart rate on right and left ventricular output. Am J Obstet Gynecol 124: 183–192
11. Lewis A B, Heymann M A, Rudolph A M 1976 Gestational changes in pulmonary vascular responses in fetal lambs in utero. Circ Res 39: 536–541
12. Campbell A G M, Cockburn F, Dawes G S et al 1976 Pulmonary vasoconstriction in asphyxia during cross-circulation between twin foetal lambs. J Physiol 192: 111–121
13. Rudolph A M, Yuan S 1966 Response of the pulmonary vasculature to hypoxia and H^+ ion concentration changes. J Clin Invest 45: 399–411
14. Cohn H E, Sacks E J, Heymann M A et al 1974 Cardiovascular responses to hypoxemia and acidemia in fetal lambs. Am J Obstet Gynecol 120: 817–824
15. Cassin S, Winikor I, Tod M et al 1981 Effects of prostacyclin on the fetal pulmonary circulation. Pediatr Pharmacol 1: 197–207
16. Rudolph A M, Heymann M A, Teramo K A W et al 1971 Studies on the circulation of the previable human fetus. Pediatr Res 5: 452–465
17. McMurphy D M, Heyman M A, Rudolph A M et al 1972 Developmental changes in constriction of the ductus arteriosus: responses to oxygen and vasoactive agents in the isolated ductus arteriosus of the fetal lamb. Pediatr Res 6: 231–238
18. Klopfenstein H S, Rudolph A M 1978 Postnatal changes in the circulation and responses to volume loading in sheep. Circ Res 42: 839–845
19. Adams F H 1983 Fetal and neonatal circulations. In Adams F H Emmanouilides G C (eds) Heart disease in infants, children, and adolescents. Williams & Wilkins, Baltimore, pp 11–17
20. Gessner I, Krovetz L H, Benson R W et al 1965 Hemodynamic adaptations in the newborn infant. Pediatrics 36: 752–762
21. Bucci G, Scalamandre A, Savignoni P G et al 1972 The systemic systolic blood pressure of newborns with low weight: a multiple regression analysis. Acta Paediatr Scand 229 (suppl): 1–26
22. Romero T E, Friedman W F 1979 Limited Left ventricular response to volume overload in the neonatal period: a comparative study with the adult animal. Pediatr Res 13: 910–915
23. Montague T J, Taylor P G, Stokton R et al 1982 The spectrum of cardiac rate and rhythm in normal newborns. Pediatr Cardiol 2: 33–38
24. Reimenschneider T A, Brenner R A, Mason D T 1981 Maturational changes in myocardial contractile state of newborn lambs. Pediatr Res 15: 349–356
25. Rudolph A M 1974 Congenital diseases of the heart. Year Book Medical Publishers, Chicago, pp 29–48
26. Naeye R L 1961 Arterial changes during the perinatal period. Arch Pathol Lab Med 71: 121–128

8. Neonatal assessment

Part A Neonatal evaluation *R. C. Chantigian P. Chantigian*

Part B Direct and indirect effects of obstetric anesthesia on infant functional development *F. Emma E. Z. Tronick*

Part C The Neurologic and Adaptive Capacity Scoring System (NACS): 10 years later *C. Amiel-Tison S. M. Shnider*

PART A NEONATAL EVALUATION

R. C. Chantigian P. Chantigian

There are many ways to evaluate the neonate at birth. Early in the systematic evaluation of the neonate, breathing time (time to the beginning of spontaneous respiration) was used. In 1952, the Apgar score[1] was introduced and continues to be widely used. Because extrinsic uterine events can affect uteroplacental blood flow, umbilical blood gas data at the time of delivery have been utilized. To detect more subtle changes in the neonate's adaptation to extrauterine life, neurobehavioral tests were developed. This section presents an overview of these methods of neonatal evaluation.

RESPIRATORY TIMES

Breathing time is defined as the time from delivery of the head to the first breath (normally within 30 s of delivery). Time to sustained respiration (TSR) occurs when breathing becomes sustained (normally by 90 s after delivery). Crying time is the time until the establishment of a satisfactory cry.

Apgar[1] pointed out some problems with breathing and crying times. She noted that breathing time can be difficult to interpret when the mother has received excessive amounts of depressant drugs in the antepartum period, as the neonate may take a breath and then become apneic for several minutes. Crying time may also be difficult to interpret, as a satisfactory cry may not be established in a particular neonate by the time the infant leaves the delivery room. Because of the difficulty in interpreting the meaning of these times, they are not widely used today but are presented for historical interest.

APGAR SCORE

Since Apgar[1] introduced her scoring system in 1952, the Apgar score has become the most frequently used method for evaluating the well-being of the neonate and the effects of maternally administered medications. Although subjective, her scoring system proved to be rapid and reproducible. A summary of her scoring system of five evaluations (heart rate, respiratory effort, reflex irritability, muscle tone and color) is presented in Table 8.1. Each evaluation is given a score (0, 1 or 2) and the scores are totaled (0 to 10) to obtain the Apgar score.

The five evaluations used are essentially a set of vital signs that can be used to describe the healthy neonate's condition and can serve as a guide to success during neonatal resuscitation. Care of the neonate, however, begins at the time of delivery and not after a score is performed. Scoring is performed on all neonates at 1 and 5 min after birth, and, if the neonate is depressed, also at 10, 15 and 20 min. Table 8.2 shows typical percentages of neonatal scores.

Of the five scores, Apgar[3] stated that heart rate and

Table 8.1 The Apgar Score (Modified from Apgar[1])

Score	0	1	2
Heart rate	Absent	< 100	> 100
Respiratory effort	Apneic	Irregular, shallow	Good, crying
Reflex irritability	No response	Grimace	Cough, sneeze
Muscle tone	Flaccid	Some flexion	Active motion
Color	Blue, pale	Pink body, extremities blue	Entirely pink

Table 8.2 Normal distribution of Apgar scores (From Drage and Berendes[2] with permission)

Score	1 min(%)	5 min(%)
0–3 (severely depressed)	6.7	1.8
4–6 (moderately depressed)	14.5	3.5
7–10 (normal)	78.9	94.8

respiratory effort are much more important than reflex irritability and muscle tone. Color has the least significance. As a result, some researchers use an Apgar minus color (A–C) score.[4]

The scoring is easy to perform, however given the same neonate different scores may be given by different examiners.[5–7] This makes interpretation of the results more difficult.

The 1-min score is thought to be a reflection of the acid–base status of the neonate. However, this correlation is not strong.[4] In 1982, Sykes et al[8] showed that only 21% of neonates with a 1-min Apgar score of <7 had severe acidosis (umbilical artery pH $\leqslant$7.10 and base deficit $\geqslant$13 mmol/l), whereas 73% of neonates with severe acidosis had a 1-min Apgar score of $\geqslant$7. In premature infants, this correlation is particularly poor. In 1984, Goldenberg et al[9] showed that 'the more premature the infant, the more likely the Apgar score was low in the presence of a pH $\geqslant$7.25'. This may be related to the premature infant not being strong enough to elicit the responses recorded on the Apgar score.

The 5-min score is thought to be a predictor of both survival and neurologic abnormalities.[5] In 1966, Drage and Berendes[2] showed that a 5-min Apgar score of 0 or 1 was associated with a 49% incidence of neonatal death. They also reported a correlation between the 5-min Apgar scores and neurologic abnormalities in infants at 1 year of age. Infants with a 5-min Apgar score of 0–3 had a higher incidence of neurologic abnormalities than those infants with a score of 7–10 (7.4% versus 1.7%). Thus, over 90% of surviving infants with low Apgar scores (0–3) were neurologically normal at 1 year of age! In 1975, Niswander et al[10] failed to show a correlation between Apgar score and neurologic abnormalities in 4-year-olds. Perhaps this is due to the enormous growth of nervous tissue that occurs after birth. In 1983, Paneth and Stark[11] noted that the majority of infants with cerebral palsy had no evidence of depression at birth (73% of the subjects had a 5-min Apgar score of $\geqslant$7).

Thus, the Apgar score has encouraged us to look more objectively at the neonate in a quick, systematic, and inexpensive manner. The value of the Apgar score to predict neonatal acidosis and neurologic abnormalities is poor. By itself, a low score indicates neonatal depression. However, the reason for a low score may include inaccurate scoring, prematurity, drug effects, congenital abnormalities, endotracheal intubation, nasopharyngeal suctioning and/or asphyxia. Recently, it has been suggested that the Apgar score should be abandoned because of its misuse and inaccuracies.[12] Many,[13] including this author (and the editors), still believe that its use is important, if for no other reason than to give a common reference for evaluating how the neonate is adapting to extrauterine life.

UMBILICAL BLOOD GAS DATA

To appreciate placental perfusion, umbilical blood gas studies are often performed. Chronic fetal asphyxia is associated with neonatal metabolic acidosis (i.e. low pH, normal or high $P\text{CO}_2$, and high base deficit), whereas brief asphyxia is associated with the more common respiratory acidosis (i.e. low pH, high $P\text{CO}_2$, and normal base deficit).[14,15] Umbilical cord blood gas analysis can be performed to determine how well the fetus adapted to the intrauterine environment (Table 8.3).

NEUROBEHAVIORAL TESTS

One problem with the Apgar score is that only the most severe neonatal depression from excessive or poorly timed maternal medications can be detected by the score at birth. To better evaluate the more subtle effects of maternally administered drugs, neurobehavioral tests were developed. Neurobehavioral assessment is not a standard part of the neonatal examination but has been used to assess the neonate's response to its environment. Although there are several neurobehavioral tests, three are most commonly used: Brazelton's Neonatal Behavior Assessment Scale,[17] Scanlon's Early Neonatal Neurobehavioral Scale[18] and the Neonatal Neurologic and Adaptive Capacity Score of Amiel-Tison et al.[19]

Brazelton[17] states: 'The neonate and his behavior cannot be assumed to be purely of genetic origin. Intrauterine influences are powerful and have already influenced the physiologic and behavioral reactions of the baby at birth.' Because intrauterine influences such as nutrition, infection, hormones and medications may affect the fetus, a behavioral scale to evaluate the neonate was proposed.

The baby's state of consciousness (deep sleep, light sleep, drowsy, alert, active, crying) is probably the most

Table 8.3 Normal-term neonate blood gas data (± 1SD) (From Yeomans et al[16] with permission)

	Umbilical vein	Umbilical artery
$P\text{O}_2$ (mmHg)	29.2 ± 5.9	18.0 ± 6.2
$P\text{CO}_2$ (mmHg)	38.2 ± 5.6	49.2 ± 8.4
pH	7.35 ± 0.05	7.28 ± 0.05
Bicarbonate (mEq/L)	20.4 ± 2.1	22.3 ± 2.5

important element of the behavioral examination, since the neonate's responses to external stimuli depend on his or her state of consciousness. The Neonatal Behavioral Assessment Scale includes 27 behavioral items (nine point scale) and 20 elicited responses (three-point scale). The midpoint of the scale is the norm. Brazelton[17] states: 'This mean is related to the expected behavior for an 'average' 7 + pound, full-term (40-week gestation), normal Caucasian infant, whose mother has had not more than 100 mg of barbiturates and 50 mg of other sedative drugs prior to delivery, whose Apgar scores were no less than 7 at 1, 8 at 5 and 8 at 15 minutes after delivery, who needed no special care after delivery, and who had an apparently normal intrauterine experience.' The score is based on the neonate's best performance. Tests repeated on several days in the neonatal period are more valuable than one examination. Because many infants are uncoordinated during the first 48 h after delivery, the behavior on the third day is the expected norm.

A period of 3–4 weeks of training is needed in order to become adequately trained in performing the Brazelton examination. About 45 min is required to perform each test.[20] As a result of the amount of training needed and the time required to perform this test, the Brazelton examination is not as widely used today as the other tests discussed below. It is, however, considered the 'gold standard' for neurobehavioral evaluations, particularly in the research setting.

Scanlon et al,[18] in 1974, developed a neurobehavioral examination called the Early Neonatal Neurobehavioral Scale (ENNS) in an attempt to simplify neurobehavioral testing and to assess the neonatal effects of epidural anesthesia. The main advantages of this examination are that it is simple and rapid to perform (it takes only 5–10 min) and personnel can be trained to 85% reliability in only 2–3 days.

The examination begins with the evaluation of the neonate's state of consciousness (four awake and two sleep states). It is then followed by specific tests. Tests 1–9 are scored on a 0, 1, 2, 3 scale. Test 10 is scored as abnormal, borderline, normal, or superior. Again, an important aspect of the ENNS is the assessment of state and its changes during the examination.

In regard to statistical analysis for the ENNS, it should be noted that none of the items is a continuous scale. For several scores (tone in particular), both extremely high and low scores may be abnormal; a summation of 'total score' can therefore be misleading. Statistical techniques should attempt to measure differences in median scores. Several nonparametric tests are useful, such as chi-square and the Fisher exact test. *F*-testing and matched-pair median subtest covariance analysis are also appropriate.[19]

Amiel-Tison et al,[19] in 1982, introduced another neurobehavioral test called the Neonatal Neurologic and Adaptive Capacity Score (NACS), also called the ABS score. This examination takes less time than the ENNS (4.4 min versus 7.2 min), places greater emphasis on motor tone and avoids the use of noxious stimuli. It is divided into five sections and includes 20 criteria. Each criterion is scored 0, 1 or 2. The scores of each criterion can be added together to give a maximum score of 40. A score of 35–40 denotes a vigorous neonate.

These neurobehavioral assessments were designed only to evaluate the neonate in the first few hours to days after delivery. If abnormal behavior is identified in the early neonatal period, it may influence the interaction between the care giver and the infant, which in turn may set the stage for abnormal interactions throughout childhood.

The Apgar score, which looked at dramatic depressive effects of drugs on the neonate for the first few minutes after delivery, has proved to be of little predictive value for long-term neurologic behavior. Will the neurobehavioral evaluations, which look at more subtle effects of drugs on the neonate over a few days, be of better predictive value? The answer to that question is still unanswered, as there are few long-term evaluations of infants originally tested with a neurobehavioral assessment.

REFERENCES

1. Apgar V 1953 A proposal for a new method of evaluation of the newborn infant. Anesth Analg 32: 260
2. Drage J S, Berendes H 1966 Apgar scores and outcome of the newborn. Pediatr Clin N Am 13: 635
3. Apgar V, Holaday D A, James S et al 1958 Evaluation of the newborn infant—second report. J Am Med Assoc 168: 1985
4. Marx G F, Mahajan S, Miclat M N 1977 Correlation of biochemical data with Apgar scores at birth and at one minute. Br J Anaesth 49: 831
5. Apgar V 1966 The newborn (Apgar) scoring system – reflections and advise. Pediatr Clin N Am 13: 645
6. Clark D A, Hakanson D O 1988 The inaccuracy of Apgar scoring. J Perinatol 8: 203
7. Schifrin B S 1989 Polemics in perinatology – the Apgar score – what should we call it? J Perinatol 9: 331
8. Sykes G S, Hohnson P, Ashworth F et al 1982 Do Apgar scores indicate asphyxia? Lancet 1: 494
9. Goldenberg R L, Huddleston J F, Nelson K G 1984 Apgar scores and umbilical arterial pH in preterm newborn infants. Am J Obstet Gynecol 149: 651
10. Niswander K R, Gordon M, Drage J S 1975 The effect of intrauterine hypoxia on the child surviving to 4 years. Am J Obstet Gynecol 121: 892
11. Paneth N, Stark R I 1983 Cerebral palsy and mental retardation in relation to indicators of perinatal asphyxia. An epidemiologic overview. Am J Obstet Gynecol 147: 960
12. Anon 1989 Is the Apgar score outmoded? Lancet 1: 591
13. Editorial Board 1989 Point-counterpoint – the Apgar score . . . revisited. J Perinatol 9: 338
14. James L S, Weisbrot I M, Prince C E et al 1958 The acid-base status of human infants in relation to birth asphyxia and the onset of respiration. J Pediatr 52: 379
15. Wilbe J L, Petrie R H, Koons A et al 1982 The clinical use of umbilical cord acid–base determinations in perinatal surveillance and management. Clin Perinatol 9: 387
16. Yeomans E R, Hauth J C, Gilstrap L C III et al 1985 Umbilical cord pH, PCO_2, and bicarbonate following uncomplicated term vaginal deliveries. Obstet Gynecol 151: 798
17. Brazelton T B 1973 Neonatal behavioral assessment scale. Clinics

in Developmental Medicine, No. 50. Spastics Int Med Publ., London
18. Scanlon J W, Brown W U Jr, Weiss J B et al 1974 Neurobehavioral responses of newborn infants after maternal epidural anesthesia. Anesthesiology 40: 121
19. Amiel-Tison C, Barrier G, Shnider S M et al 1982 A new neurologic and adaptive capacity scoring system for evaluation obstetric medications in full term newborns. Anesthesiology 56: 340
20. Ostheimer G W 1981 Neurobehavioral effects of local anesthesia and fetal resuscitation. Reg Anesth 6: 136

PART B
DIRECT AND INDIRECT EFFECTS OF OBSTETRIC ANESTHESIA ON INFANT FUNCTIONAL DEVELOPMENT

F. Emma E. Z. Tronick

INTRODUCTION

More than 50 studies have been published that show that deficient neonatal behavior performance is related to obstetric medication.[1] However, these effects are not simply the result of the direct effects of the medications but are rather the result of direct and indirect effects acting in concert.

Some of the earliest studies that found major effects of obstetric medication on neonatal behavior assessed larger doses and different drugs from those used today. For example, Hughes et al[2] found an association between large doses of meperidine, phenobarbital and morphine and drowsiness and cortical depression in neonates. Brazelton[3] found that high doses of barbiturate and general anesthesia impaired feeding patterns and delayed weight gain. These early studies led to a significant revision in the use of obstetric medication, resulting in a decrease in the use of opioids, sedatives and general anesthesia and an increase in the use of local or regional anesthesia. Nervertheless, the findings serve as a constant reminder of the powerful effects that medication can have on early behavior. Even today, this is still the situation for those clinical conditions that require the use of unusual amounts or kinds of medication. In these conditions we may once again see not only the direct effects of the drugs but also behavioral effects resulting from the synergistic action of the drug and the clinical condition. Similar concerns must be kept in mind when new medications with unknown behavioral effects are administered.

RECENT RESEARCH

More recent research has focused on behavioral effects of revised obstetric practices. Overall, the results appear mixed, ranging from no effects of medication to 'long-term' effects. However, many of these studies suffer from significant problems, making it difficult to draw conclusions. First, unmedicated control samples have been rare and no study to our knowledge has utilized randomized assignment. Many studies group different types and routes of analgesia and anesthesia into weighted clinical categories that disregard principles of perinatal pharmacology. Other studies focus on single agents and disregard other obstetric medication utilized in the sample. Additionally, important drug-related parameters, such as dose and background variables known to affect behavior

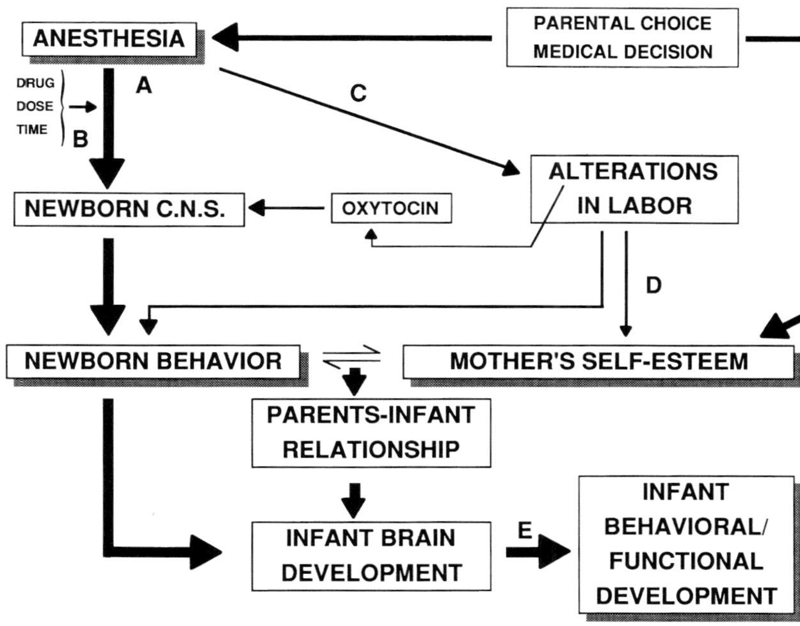

Fig. 8.1 A proposed model of factors and processes related to epidural anesthesia that can influence newborn behavioral outcome.

have been ignored. Even more glaring is the lack of attention paid to many factors that synergistically interact with the effect of the drug (such as birth weight, nutritional status and fetal acidosis). Finally, along with the direct effect of the drug on the central nervous system, there are also indirect effects of anesthesia that can stress the fetus and/or the mother (such as maternal hypotension, prolonged labor, increased use of forceps, etc.). These effects, labeled 'indirect' because they are affecting one system that in turn affects the infant, nonetheless are critical and a potentially common pathway leading to compromised brain development and behavior. To understand all these implications, we propose a model of factors and processes related to epidural anesthesia which can influence the newborn behavioral outcome (see Fig. 8.1).

To analyze the effects of drugs on neonatal behavior, one group of studies[4–9] have either compared epidural anesthesia groups with non-medicated controls or examined the dose–behavior relationship. These studies have utilized the Brazelton Neonatal Behavioral Assessment Scale (NBAS).[10] This scale was designed to measure the behavioral capacities and individual differences of infants during the first month of life. It is based on the concept that the neonate is a complex and competent organism, adapted to interact with the environment in such a way as to elicit responses necessary for future growth and development. Thus, this scale goes beyond traditional examinations in its assessment of a range of behaviors that may affect the development of the infant–caregiver relationship. It has been demonstrated to be sensitive to slight but significant variations in behavior.

These studies have found that anesthetics affect the following neonatal behaviors: habituation, motor maturity, orientation and alertness, range and regulation of states of consciousness and autonomic regulation. In contrast to the findings from the NBAS, none of the studies using the Scanlon Early Neonatal Neurobehavioral Scale[10] or the Neurologic and Adaptive Capacity Scoring System[11] have demonstrated adverse effects due to bupivacaine, one of the most commonly used drugs. While these findings clearly establish that there are drug-related effects on newborn behavior, as well as the greater sensitivity of the NBAS for detecting drug-induced behavioral changes, they also indicate that the effects are relatively minor.[12]

Direct effects of the drug are expected to be related to the choice of the drug, the dosage and the time of administration. Some differences between drugs have been observed. For example, infant behavior appears to be less influenced by anesthesia with bupivacaine than with chloroprocaine, as measured by the NBAS.[13]

Studies have attempted to relate infant behavior to the amount of bupivacaine exposure and/or to umbilical cord blood concentration at birth. Rosenblatt et al[14] demonstrated a significant dose-related impairment in most of the NBAS criteria (visual orientation, alertness, motor organization, state control and response to stress), with the exception of the muscle tone, which appeared to be improved.*

**Editor's note*: This study has been severely criticized for its lack of appropriate controls and absence of obstetric and anesthetic information.

Similarly, Sepkoski et al found a dose effect on the mean orientation and the motor cluster scores of the NBAS.[9] Using a lower dose of bupivacaine, other authors have not found dose-related effects.[6] Once again, these effects are relatively minor when found, but the findings on specificity and dose relation speak to the reality of these effects.

Epidural anesthesia may increase the length of the first and second stage of labor depending on when it is administered. Therefore, oxytocin may be given to stimulate contractions. Depression of neonatal behavior has been reported when epidural anesthesia is administered along with oxytocin, even when the length of labor is statistically controlled.[6] Because of its very short half-life ($T^1/_2$ <15 min), the added effect of oxytocin is unlikely to be a direct effect, but rather an indirect effect by increasing the frequency and the forcefulness of the contractions. Sepkoski et al[9] reported that both oxytocin administration and the use of forceps have additive effects with bupivacaine on neonatal behavior, but only forceps had an independent effect on the motor cluster. Recently, Hoult et al[17] have reported a fivefold increase in instrumental delivery and a threefold increase in fetal head malposition, regardless of the reason for anesthesia (elective choice or medical indication). However, the summation of several studies supports the increase in instrumental deliveries, especially in the primigravidas, while not supporting the increased incidence of fetal malposition.

Compared with the medications used two decades ago, modern anesthetic agents are much safer for obstetric analgesia and anesthesia and affect infant behavior in more limited ways. These limited effects may lead to developmental compromise and are the result of the effects of these medications on the *mother's functioning and her interaction with her infant*. And as the neurologist Prechtl[18] has emphasized, the mother-infant relationship is a critical influence on the infant's brain development.

The use of obstetric anesthesia may be associated with a disruption of maternal functioning. The pain relief provided by obstetric analgesia and anesthesia has to be evaluated in the context of an accumulation of possible indirect negative effects due to prolonged and more difficult labor that not only increases the mother's fatigue but also increases her sense of failure. Shea and Tronick[19] found that self-esteem after delivery affected both the infant's behavior and the sensitivity of the mother to the infant at 6 weeks of age. Maternal self-esteem was affected by the health and behavior of the newborn and by paternal and familial support. Other studies have demonstrated that maternal self-esteem is affected by delivery variables including medication, type of delivery and maternal health and separation from the infant. The mother's personality and her personal decision in receiving analgesia or anesthesia, may be factors determining the final psychological maternal effect.

Finally, although minor, differences in neonatal behavior at one month of age have also been reported, especially when the velocity of neurobehavioral recovery is analyzed.[9,20] These differences cannot be attributed to a direct effect of the drug as a strict pharmacokinetics model would predict. More likely, they are the result of the cumulative effect in the post-natal period of the parental perception and the infant's behavior. The parents' perception of their baby may indeed account for later interactional problems. Murray et al[6] found that a group of mothers receiving epidural anesthesia perceived their infants' behavior to be inferior to that of a non-medicated group at 1 month of age, even though objective assessments indicated no difference in infant performance. It is quite likely that the mother's perception may have been accurate earlier on when the infant's behavior may have been compromised by medication. Again, other factors (such as family history, parental personality, economic stress and even doctor–patient relations) can modify parental self-esteem and perceptions and, ultimately, parent–infant relationship.

SUMMARY

Drug effects operate through multiple pathways and Figure 8.1 shows only a simplified model. Many methodological problems still prevent the drawing of definitive conclusions. Although analgesia and anesthesia in obstetrics have become increasingly common and have been proved to be efficient in relieving maternal pain without major effects on the newborn, we believe that obstetricians and anesthesiologists must be aware of the possible negative effects of these procedures on both the mother and the infant. The key to this awareness is to move beyond the pharmacokinetic model of direct drug effects and realize that (1) development, including the structuring of the brain, is affected by many factors but most critically by the quality of the parent–infant interaction, and (2) an accumulation of several small synergistically acting negative effects that compromise newborn and maternal behavior can have significant and cascading effects on the infant's development. Thus the decision to administer pain relief should be taken on a case-to-case basis, after discussion with the parents, to prevent possible post-partum adverse effects. The decision to use new medications with unknown behavioral effects should be made carefully.

Finally, many of these possible effects of obstetric analgesia and anaesthesia can be abrogated by having the care giver encourage a positive maternal–familial–infant interaction from birth.

REFERENCES

1. Sepkoski C 1985 Maternal obstetric medication and newborn behavior. In: Scanlon J W (ed) Perinatal anesthesia. Blackwell Scientific Publications, London, p 131–173

2. Hughes J G, Hill F S, Green C R et al 1950 Electroencephalography of the newborn. 5. Brain potentials of babies born of mothers given meperidine hydrochloride (demerol hydrochloride), vinbarbital sodium (delvinal sodium) or morphine. Am J Dis Child 79: 996–1007
3. Brazelton T B 1961 Psychophysiologic reactions in the neonate. 2. The effects of maternal medication on the neonate and his behavior. J Pediatr 58: 513–518
4. Alexandrowicz M K, Alexandrowicz D R 1974 Obstetrical pain relieving drugs as predictors of infant behavior variability. Child Dev 45: 935–945.
5. Kuhnert B R, Harrison M J, Linn P L et al 1984 Effects of maternal epidural anesthesia on neonatal behavior. Anesth Analg 63: 301–308
6. Murray A D, Dolby R M, Nation R L et al 1981 Effects of peridural anesthesia on newborns and their mothers. Child Dev 52: 71– 82
7. Sepkoski C 1984 The cumulative effects of bupivacaine epidural anesthesia and obstetric variables on neonatal behavior. Dissertation, University of Florida, Gainesville.
8. Tronick E, Wise S, Als H et al 1976 Regional obstetric anesthesia and newborn behavior: effect over the first ten days of life.Pediatrics 58: 94–100
9. Sepkoski C M, Lester B M, Ostheimer G W, Brazelton T B et al 1992 The effects of maternal anesthesia on neonatal behaviour during the first month. Developmental Medicine and Child Neurology 34: 1072–1080
10. Scanlon J W, Brown W U, Weiss J B et al 1974 Neurobehavioral responses of newborn infants after maternal anesthesia. Anesthesiology 40: 121–128
11. Amiel-Tison C, Barrier G, Shnider S M et al 1982 A new neurologic and adaptive capacity scoring system for evaluating obstetric medications in full-term newborns. Anesthesiology 56: 340–350
12. Tronick E Z 1982 A critique of the Neonatal Neurologic and Adaptive Capacity Score (N.A.C.S.). Anesthesiology 5: 2–3
13. Kuhnert B R, Kennard M J, Linn P L 1988 Neonatal neurobehavior after epidural anesthesia for cesarean section: a comparison of bupivacaine and chloroprocaine. Anesth Analg 67: 64–68
14. Rosenblatt D B, Belsey E M, Lieberman B A et al 1981 The influence of maternal analgesia on neonatal behavior. 2. Epidural bupivacaine. Br J Obstet Gynaecol 88: 407–413
15. Chantigian R C 1992 Pain relief and vaginal delivery. In: Ostheimer G W (ed) Manual of Obstetric Anesthesia, 2nd end. Churchill Livingstone, New York, p 63
16. Scanlon J W, Ostheimer G W, Lùrie A O et al 1976 Neurobehavioral responses to drug concentrations in newborns after maternal epidural anesthesia with bupivacaine. Anesthesiology 45: 400
17. Hoult I J, MacLennan A H, Carrie L E S 1977 Lumbar epidural analgesia in labor: relation to fetal malposition and instrumental delivery. Br Med J 6052: 14–16
18. Prechtl H R 1981 Maturation and development: Biological and psychological perspectives. Clinics in Developmental Medicine No 77/78. Spastics International Medical Publications. London: William Heinemann Medical Books, J B Lippincott, Philadelphia
19. Shea E, Tronick E Z 1988 The Maternal Self-Report Inventory: a research and clinical instrument for assessing maternal self-esteem. In: Fitzgerald H E, Lester B M, Yogman M W (eds) Theory and research in behavioral pediatrics, vol 4. Plenum, New York, p 101–141
20. Muhlen-Schulte L, Wade K 1988 Intervention in childbirth neonatal responsiveness. Community Health Studies 12: 6981

PART C
THE NEUROLOGIC AND ADAPTIVE CAPACITY SCORING SYSTEM: 10 YEARS LATER

C. Amiel-Tison S. M. Shnider

PRELIMINARY REMARKS

It is difficult to correlate abnormal or suboptimal neonatal neurologic signs with various obstetric factors, and particularly difficult to distinguish between signs related to fetal asphyxia, mechanical compression of the fetal head during labor and delivery and/or medications administered during labor and delivery. Clinical signs of brain dysfunction are not specific: some degree of brain edema is often present in the first days of life. Many abnormalities are transient, without any late sequelae. The French obstetrician Pajot[1] was puzzled, 100 years ago, by the difficulty in relating clinical neurologic signs to, for example, subarachnoid hemorrhage in the newborn. He wrote in 1882: 'Les symptômes de ces sortes d'épanchements sont assez obscurs, en ce sens qu'on les observe aussi dans les cas où cette altération n'existe pas'. Loosely translated, Pajot noted that the 'typical' signs and symptoms of subarachnoid hemorrhage are often present in neonates in which such bleeding is absent. He thus described the nonspecificity of neurologic signs during the neonatal period while implying a large cohort of 'false positives'.

For the sick neonate, the neurologic examination must be detailed, repeated and interpreted as part of a general examination. The neurologic signs and symptoms may be classified at the end of the first week of life into one of three grades depending upon the severity. Signs and symptoms commonly cluster in a few typical patterns, which are easily recognizable.[2,3] We have found that grading this continuum of signs and symptoms is necessary and potentially useful for prognosis at birth and prevention of most neurologic morbidity. We have found that no single, specific type of neurologic, psychologic or behavioral handicap characterizes the outcome following a difficult birth. Any type of motor handicap, seizure disorder, mental retardation or behavioral problem, ranging in severity from coma to very mild dysfunction, can be the consequence of a difficult birth.[4] However, there is a good correlation between the neonatal gradation of cerebral dysfunction at birth and late outcome, a correlation suggesting the validity of gradation, as recently reviewed.[5]

To describe a normal newborn infant has proved to be a much easier task, even though there are not enough data in the world literature to demonstrate definitively that a normal neurologic or neurobehavioral assessment within the first week of life is a guarantee of a normal outcome.

However, our experience and preliminary data suggest that such a statement is valid.[6] A normal central nervous system (CNS) in the neonate born *at term* can be verified very rapidly by routine systematic examination. A normal head circumference, a lively look, a vigorous cry, efficient sucking and swallowing, grasping and an active response to forward traction can provide an evaluation of alertness, primary reflexes and muscle tone within 30 s. This is universally accepted clinical experience, with very few contradictions.

In parallel with the advances in clinical neurology, the field of developmental psychology has been very productive in the last 20 years, accumulating data on the neurobehavior and sensory function of the neonate.[7,8] However, the increasing sophistication of this research creates a wider and wider gap between our knowledge and the practical applications. And thus, for the time being, defining a 'normal' neonate becomes an exceedingly ambitious task. Moreover, it is not yet clearly understood how much of the neonate's response is mediated by the brainstem and how much by the cerebral cortex.[9,10] We believe that many of the claims of neonatal neuropsychologists regarding evaluating cognitive functions by sophisticated testing are not yet absolutely convincing.

Nevertheless, in order to evaluate the effects of labor and drugs, several basic questions have to be answered for everyday practice: Is CNS function grossly satisfactory? Are feeding and sleep within normal limits? Is communication with the caregiver possible? If abnormalities are present at the first examination, how quickly, if at all, will the recovery occur and what is the possible mechanism involved in each case to explain suboptimal response?

To answer these questions accurately, one would have to design large prospective and randomized studies comparing, for instance, different anesthetic or obstetric interventions in similar populations and then attempt to determine the possible precise mechanism of any dysfunction. This is indeed a major undertaking, which will seldom be practical and acceptable to committees concerned with human research.

For the sake of realistic perinatal research in the delivery room, we described the Neurologic and Adaptive Capacity Scoring System (NACS).[11] This evaluation is simple and benign with good inter-observer reliability, fast enough to be repeatable several times in the first days of life if necessary, with each test being formally defined and the response being grossly quantified. When we designed our NACS we believed that none of the tests in use, for example the Brazelton Neonatal Behavioral Assessment Scale (BNBAS), or the Scanlon Early Neonatal Neurobehavioral Scale (ENNS)[12] fully met these needs.

As a screening test, the NACS may be used routinely in the delivery room, in the first half-hour, just after the routine neonatal care. It can easily be performed with the mother in attendance as the examination was designed to avoid aversive stimulation such as repeated pinpricks or Moro maneuvers. Moreover, the positive effect on mother–infant interaction of demonstrating the newborn's powers has been demonstrated;[13] it is a good opportunity for young mothers to learn about the abilities of their amazing newborn.

DESCRIPTION OF THE NACS

Using 20 criteria, the NACS evaluates five general areas: adaptive capacity, passive tone, active tone, primary reflexes and general neurologic status (Table 8.4). Each criterion is given a score of 0, 1 or 2, based on whether the response to testing that criterion is absent or grossly abnormal (0), mediocre or slightly abnormal (1) or normal (2). Therefore the maximum possible score is 40.

Although the 20 items in the NACS can be tested in any order, we have listed them in the sequence that we believe to be the easiest and most logical to follow (Table 8.4). The examiner determines the neonate's best performance; if the neonate scores 1 or 0 on an item, then that item should be retested later in the examination to confirm the low score.

The complete description of each of the 20 criteria is to be found in the original publication.[11] Only some of the most important points will be described here and illustrated.

Assessment of adaptive capacity (items 1–5)

The ability of the infant to respond to the environment (adaptive capacity) is tested using five criteria that measure reactions to sensory stimuli (light and sound) and observations of consolability when the baby is agitated. This section of the NACS requires a bell and a flashlight.

The infant should be tested in a quiet environment, preferably before being unwrapped or undressed, to minimize distracting stimuli. If the infant is too sleepy or restless, the maximum response may not be elicited easily. In such instances, the neurologic portion of the examination should be completed first and the adaptive responses retested afterward. This allows the infant the opportunity to achieve an optimum score.

Evaluation of passive tone (items 6–9)

Extensibility of muscles is observed segment by segment using a number of maneuvers that evaluate the amplitude of a slow movement executed by the observer with the infant remaining passive. Two maneuvers have been selected: the scarf sign, to define passive tone in upper limbs (Fig. 8.2), and the popliteal angle, to define passive tone in lower limbs (Fig. 8.2). The recoil describes how fast a segment returns to the initial posture of flexion after being extended. The examiner can evaluate passive tone

Table 8.4

NEUROLOGICAL AND ADAPTIVE CAPACITY SCORE IN FULL-TERM NEWBORNS

NAME ______________________

Date of Birth ______________ Chart Number ________

	(not able to test : N.A.)	N.A.		0	1	2
1	RESPONSE TO SOUND			absent ;	mild ;	vigorous ;
2	HABITUATION TO SOUND			absent ;	7-12 stimuli	≤ 6 stimuli ;
3	RESPONSE TO LIGHT			absent ;	mild ;	brisk blink or startle ;
4	HABITUATION TO LIGHT			absent ;	7-12 stimuli ;	≤ 6 stimuli ;
5	CONSOLABILITY			absent ;	difficult ;	easy ;

TOTAL [ ] ADAPTIVE CAPACITY

			0	1	2
6	SCARF SIGN		encircles the neck ;	elbow slightly passes midline;	elbow does not reach midline;
7	RECOIL OF ELBOWS		absent	slow; weak;	brisk; reproducible;
8	POPLITEAL ANGLE		> 110 °	100 ° - 110 °	≤ 90 °
9	RECOIL OF LOWER LIMBS		absent	slow; weak;	brisk; reproducible ;
10	ACTIVE CONTRACTION OF NECK FLEXORS (from lying position)		absent or abnormal ;	difficult ;	good; head is maintained in the axis of the body;
11	ACTIVE CONTRACTION OF NECK EXTENSORS (from leaning forward position)		absent or abnormal ;	difficult ;	good; head is maintained in the axis of the body;
12	PALMAR GRASP *		absent ;	weak ;	excellent ; reproducible;
13	RESPONSE TO TRACTION (following palmar grasp)		absent ;	lift part of the body weight;	lift all the body weight;
14	SUPPORTING REACTION (upright position)		absent ;	incomplete ; transitory ;	strong ; support all body weight ;
15	AUTOMATIC WALKING *		absent ;	difficult to obtain;	perfect ; reproducible ;
16	SUCKING *		absent ;	weak ;	perfect ; synchronous with swallowing ;
17	MORO REFLEX *		absent ;	weak ; incomplete;	perfect ; complete ;
18	ALERTNESS		coma ;	lethargy or hyperexcitability;	normal ;
19	CRYING		absent ;	abnormal, (poor or excessive)	normal ;
20	MOTOR ACTIVITY		absent ;	diminished or excessive ;	normal ;

TOTAL [ ] NEUROLOGICAL

TOTAL SCORE [ ] AT ________ MINUTES OF LIFE

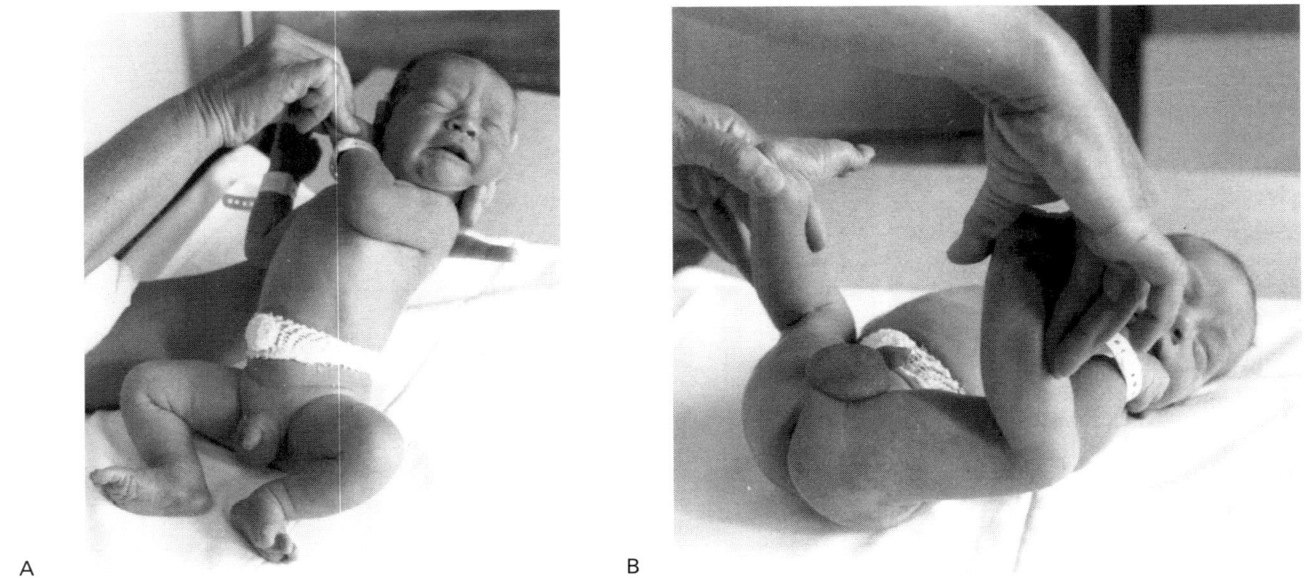

Fig. 8.2 Passive tone in upper and lower limbs. In a normal full-term newborn, the elbow does not reach the midline (scarf sign, criterion 6) and the popliteal angle is 90 or less (criterion 8).

by observing and manipulating the infant while quiet but not asleep. The maneuvers must be performed slowly and gently and to the point of meeting resistance. In case of an asymmetric response, the examiner scores the best side, since the hypotonic side may be abnormal as a result of peripheral nerve injury.

In the case of breech delivery, passive tone in the lower limbs will be modified temporarily by the intrauterine posture. The resulting apparent hypotonia of the lower limbs will therefore result in an abnormal popliteal angle and abnormal recoil of the lower extremities, effects that are unrelated to central nervous system dysfunction. Therefore, with breech presentation, these two criteria should not be tested. To complete the scoring of passive tone, the same scores as those obtained for scarf sign and recoil of elbows should be used. We believe that this is appropriate, since mild central nervous system dysfunction causes hypotonicity predominantly in the upper limbs. Thus, in the breech infant, if passive tone is normal in the upper limbs, one can assume it would also have been normal in the lower limbs had the baby been born in the vertex position.

Evaluation of active tone and primary reflexes
(items 10–17)

Active tone describes the motor performance of the infant in response to a given situation created by the examiner. As primary reflexes are often used to create this particular situation (for instance: grasp and response to traction), both groups of criteria are tested at the same time (asterisks on the grid signify primary reflexes). The comparison of contraction of the neck flexors (criterion 10) with neck extensors (criterion 11) is extremely important in a full-term newborn, as it means that the maturation of both sets of muscles is allowing a symmetrical balance at this stage (see Fig. 8.3). Various abnormalities can be observed, as described in the original paper;[11] more detailed descriptions

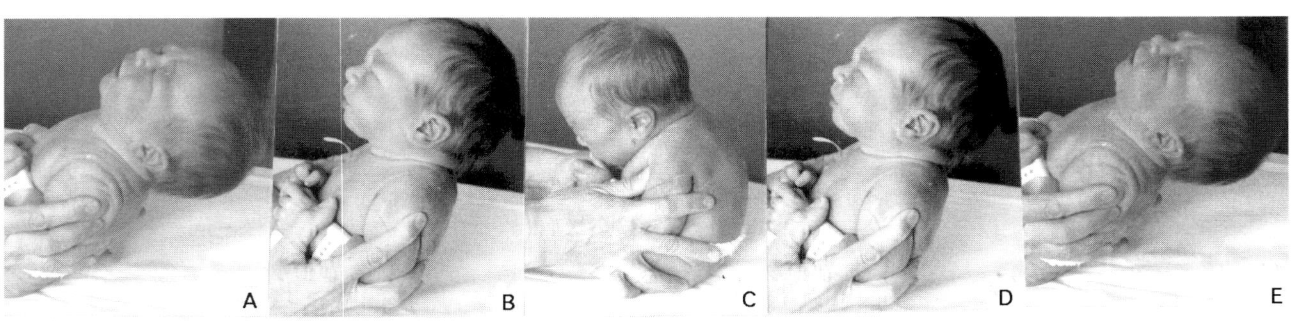

Fig. 8.3 The raise-to-sit and reverse maneuver. (A, –B, –C) Active tone in neck flexor muscles. (C, D, E) Active tone in neck extensor muscles. This perfect balance between the agonists and antagonists is reached at the full-term period (criteria 10 and 11).

of using these criteria to differentiate mild birth asphyxia and traumatic delivery from obstetric medication can be found elsewhere[3,14] and will be briefly described below.

Palmar grasp and response to traction (Fig. 8.4) are performed in sequence, the reflex activity of the fingers allowing the examiner to test the activity in the whole of the shoulder girdle. Normally infants lift their body weight completely and the head usually moves forward.

The infant must be well enough to allow manipulation of the head and trunk. If the child is crying, it is necessary to postpone testing of the neck extensors until consoled. A normal crying infant has mild hypertonicity of the neck extensors, probably due to transitory elevation of intracranial pressure.[2,14] Because the primary reflexes may also be transitorily modified by excessive crying, testing of reflexes may also need to be postponed for a few minutes.

General neurologic assessment (items 18–20)

To measure these last three criteria, experience is necessary; however, a certain degree of subjectivity must be accepted. The judgment of alertness takes into account the predominant state of consciousness during the entire examination. The quality of the cry is again estimated as a whole (screaming high-pitched versus normal). The motor activity is scored according to quantity and harmonious quality of spontaneous activity as observed during the entire testing period.

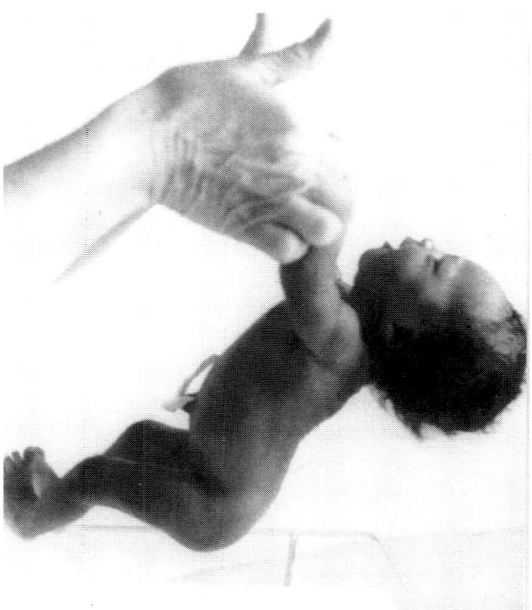

Fig. 8.4 Palmar grasp and response to traction. Strong flexion of the infant's fingers onto the examiner's index fingers is first obtained (palmar grasp, criterion 12). When the index fingers are lifted, the contraction spreads to flexor muscles of the upper limbs so that the infant can lift himself/herself completely (response to traction, criterion 13).

USE OF THE NACS

Duration of examination and inter-observer reliability

Sixty-one infants were examined 15 min after vaginal delivery with the NACS, and at 2 and 24 h after birth.[11] Mothers had received a variety of obstetric medications including opioids, pudendal block, local infiltration and inhalation analgesia. The average length of time required to perform the NACS was 4.36 + 0.1 min (SE). Each examination was scored simultaneously and independently by two observers who were unaware of the analgesic management. These observers were either anesthesiologists or staff research associates. The inter-observer reliability was 92.8%.

Total score

The NACS exam gives a total score that evolves from the sum of the scores on each individual test. As a preliminary work (unpublished data) we scored at birth 40 low-risk infants born to healthy multiparous women with no antepartum or intrapartum complications and who received no systemic medications or anesthetics within 3 h of vertex delivery and in whom no fetal distress occurred during labor. All neonates scored 35–40. Therefore, according to this preliminary evaluation, we have arbitrarily chosen the scores 35–40 to indicate neurologically vigorous neonates. Later, we compared NACS and ENNS (scores) in 61 infants and confirmed that a total score of 35 correctly defined the normal range.[11] A score of 34 or below is low enough to detect babies with possible problems, and in these cases the test must be repeated.

Recovery curve and subtests

When the first score is not optimal, both the recovery curve and the group of criteria responsible for the low score are equally important in order to determine the cause. It is not the purpose of this screening test to describe and score any CNS condition encountered in the neonatal period: a sick child will be more fully explored clinically and other investigations performed. However, the clustering of signs and symptoms may give an indication of the likely reason for the low score.

Generalized mediocre tone and poor habituation often indicate a global depression and are frequently associated with drugs and anesthetics.[12,15–18] In these cases the initial score is 34 or below but the subsequent scores steadily increase to reach the normal range within 48 h.

Hyperexcitability and *predominant tone in extensor muscles of the axis*, first increasing within the first 2 or 3 days, followed by a recovery by day 4 or 5 probably indicate mild brain edema.[14,19] These signs linked with moderate intracranial hypertension are a common consequence of birth asphyxia and/or birth trauma.

When after a few days, discrete signs persist, such as an excessive scarf sign and poor active tone in neck flexors, the hypotonicity in the upper part of the body indicates the need for a close follow-up.[3]

SOME OF THE DATA BASED ON THE NACS

In this chapter we have no intention of providing a *complete* general review on the neurobehavioral effects observed after various types of obstetric analgesia and anesthesia. This is to be found elsewhere.[20–22] We will briefly discuss the findings of the first 10 years of the use of the NACS. Several routes and types of analgesic drugs have been tested and compared, using Apgar scores, acid–base balance, the ENNS and the NACS.

Epidural anesthesia

A number of studies have indicated that continuous epidural anesthesia with small *intermittent bolus injections* of all commonly used local anesthetics for labor and delivery, including lidocaine, bupivacaine and chloroprocaine, has no adverse effects on the NACS. These studies with the NACS corroborated previous studies[23,24] in which the Scanlon ENNS was used to study neurobehavior and *did not* agree with Scanlon's original report that lidocaine did indeed compromise neurobehavioral function in the neonate.[12]

One would expect that, if local anesthetics adversely affect neonatal neurobehavior, the larger doses used for cesarean delivery would cause effects that could be determined by either the NACS or ENNS. In fact, epidural bupivacaine, chloroprocaine or lidocaine for cesarean delivery has no detrimental effects on neonatal neurobehavior.[25]

Corroborating these findings, Kileff et al,[26] using the ENNS, compared infants born by cesarean deliveries under epidural anesthesia with 2% lidocaine or 0.5% bupivacaine. Neonates in the lidocaine group scored as well as those in the bupivacaine group on all items of the ENNS. Similarly, Kuhnert et al,[27] using the BNBAS, compared neonates of mothers given chloroprocaine or lidocaine for vaginal or cesarean delivery. Only very subtle changes were attributable to lidocaine. No babies had significant hypotonia. Although the differences in effects between the two drug groups were statistically significant, they were so small as to be clinically insignificant.

An increasingly popular technique for labor epidural anesthesia is *continuous infusion* of local anesthetics with theoretical accumulation of local anesthetics in the fetus. Using the NACS, no adverse effects of this technique were found with bupivacaine, chloroprocaine or lidocaine.[28]

Epinephrine is commonly added to local anesthetics for epidural anesthesia in concentrations of 1 : 200 000 to 1 : 400 000 to decrease systemic absorption and peak blood levels of the local anesthetic, to provide a longer duration of action and to intensify motor blockade.[29–32] The use of epinephrine in obstetrics is controversial because of possible detrimental effects on uterine blood flow[33–35] and activity.[36–40] Epinephrine that is slowly absorbed from the epidural space probably would not have clinically significant effects on uterine blood flow[41–44] and fetal well-being.

These assumptions have been corroborated by the findings of no differences in the NACS whether or not epinephrine is added to 1.5% lidocaine,[45] 0.5% bupivacaine,[46] 2% chloroprocaine[47] or a mixture of bupivacaine 0.25%, butorphanol 1 mg and epinephrine.[48] Thus, for cesarean delivery in which larger doses of local anesthetic are used and more profound motor blockade is desired, the addition of epinephrine 1 : 200 000 to the local anesthetic solution may be advantageous and has no detrimental effects on the NACS.

In the USA, Nesacaine (chloroprocaine) has recently undergone a change in formulation. The sodium bisulfite has been removed as the antioxidant and replaced by EDTA. Studies of the new epidural bisulfite-free chloroprocaine with and without 1 : 200 000 epinephrine have demonstrated no detrimental effects on the NACS.[49] These findings are similar to those using the old chloroprocaine formulation.[47]

Systemic opioids

Opioids administered systemically to the mother for labor analgesia rapidly cross the placenta and potentially depress the neurobehavioral status of the newborn. A number of investigators have used both the NACS and ENNS to demonstrate a dose-dependent relationship between high doses of opioids and low neurobehavioral scores and the reversal of these findings with naloxone.[50–54]

Fentanyl, a very popular opioid in labor, has not been studied extensively. Two studies[55,56] indicate that intravenous fentanyl administration (mean dose 140 $\pm$ 32μg) has minimal effect on the NACS. However, using patient-controlled intravenous analgesia for labor, it was found that nalbuphine in doses up to 42mg produced lower NACS scores than did meperidine in doses up to 210mg.[57]

Spinal and epidural opioids

The general concern of depressant effects of maternally administered opioids on the newborn are always present. Concern for the newborn, in part, stimulated the initial interest in the use of *intraspinal opioids*: low-dose effective analgesia would pose less risk to the neonate. We found[58] that newborns delivered to mothers given 2.0, 5.0 and 7.5 mg of epidural morphine had high Apgar and NACS scores, along with normal values for umbilical arterial and venous blood gas tensions.

We documented the safe use of subarachnoid morphine with similar clinical data.[59] With such low doses of 0.5–1.0 mg, this finding is not surprising. Subarachnoid meperidine does not depress the NACS.[60] Dailey et al[61] found that a continuous maternal intravenous infusion of naloxone to decrease side-effects such as severe itching did not adversely affect the infant's NACS. We have also found that epidural fentanyl, 1 μg/kg administered to a parturient undergoing cesarean delivery, has no adverse effects on the NACS,[62] nor is the NACS adversely affected by the addition of fentanyl 50–100 μg either administered in saline or mixed with bupivacaine for labor.[63,64] Use of epidural butorphanol with either bupivacaine[65] or lidocaine[66] for labor does not adversely affect the NACS. Nor does epidural sufentanil, for labor analgesia in doses at least up to 30 μg, depress the NACS.[67]

Inhalation agents

Inhalation anesthetic agents have been studied either for analgesia for labor (the parturient receiving pain relief while awake) or for cesarean deliveries (for which deeper levels of anesthesia were required). No adverse effects on the NACS have been demonstrated with labor analgesia using nitrous oxide, enflurane or isoflurane.[68,69] However when these agents are used for elective cesarean delivery and the infants are compared with those born with spinal or epidural anesthesia, some transient depression of the NACS has been noted.[70]

Anesthesia adjuncts for Cesarean delivery

When one compares the induction of general anesthesia for cesarean delivery with midazolam (a potent benzodiazepine) in doses of 0.3 mg/kg i.v. with the standard drug, thiopental 4 mg/kg, the NACS is found to be higher following thiopental induction.[71]

We have also examined the neonatal effect of two widely used nondepolarizing muscle relaxants used as an adjunct to general anesthesia for cesarean delivery and have found very little placental transfer of the drug and no adverse effect on the NACS.[72]

Finally, prior to cesarean delivery, metoclopramide has been administered in a dose of 10 mg to attempt to decrease gastric volume and pH. No depression of the NACS has been reported.[73]

We find it very interesting that a study of 15 neonates born at risk of neurologic sequelae and 15 healthy controls using the NACS and auditory brainstem response (ABR)[74] demonstrated that the NACS is sensitive to mild but diffuse disturbances, whereas the ABR appears to reflect insults to the brainstem structures that are susceptible to damage from anoxia. This study also confirmed the validity of an arbitrary choice of a score of 35 or more to define normal range ($X^2 = 26.67, P < 0.01$).

In summary, with the introduction of the NACS, we believe that we have supplied data that allow the physician to select drugs and techniques which have the least adverse effects on the neonate, which supports the recommendations of the USA FDA and the American Academy of Pediatrics.[75]

CRITICAL VIEWS AND CONCLUSIONS

Any developmental psychologist is tortured by the idea that somewhere, somehow, someone could propose a simple neurobehavioral test for the newborn infant. It is therefore not surprising that the publication of the NACS in 1982 was preceded and followed by vigorous criticisms. The state of mind of reviewers, commentators and the chief editor of *Anesthesiology* can be summarized by a list of adjectives, in many ways paraphrasing the 'nose monologue' in *Cyrano de Bergerac*.[76]

— *Virulent*: 'Extravagant claims are made for this exam' (an anonymous reviewer for *Anesthesiology*).
— *Moral*: 'The idea of a single score or label for a baby is the most frightening thing I can think of as a clinician' (an anonymous reviewer for *Anesthesiology*).
— *Satirical*: 'The reader is forced to hit his own head in disbelief' (an anonymous reviewer for *Anesthesiology*).
— *Contemptuous*[77]: 'This examination fails to adequately conceptualize the capabilities of the neonates and the process of early development'.
— *Desperate*[77]: 'What is a neonate?... I realize that we are no closer to having an useful clinical instrument, ...'
— *Sarcastic*: 'When Virginia Apgar proposed her score, 5 items seemed too much to handle for pediatricians... Now, what will happen with the 20 items of the NACS! (L. Gluck, personal communication)
— *Cautious*[78]: 'Publication of work in a journal such as *Anesthesiology* is commonly (and properly) viewed as a form of endorsement. When it is not such, the reader must be so informed'.

But:

— *Generous*[78]: 'The considerable experience and recognized expertise of Dr. Amiel-Tison and her co-authors should be made available to our readers'.

Finally, a very important question was asked of the medical community:[79] 'Since, as Tronick points out, there is no single test available that can fully assess a neonate, should the anesthesiologist, obstetrician and pediatrician then simply measure acid–base balance and blood levels of anesthetic drugs without ever looking at the baby itself?' We believe that so much nonsense has been published in the medical and lay public literature about the deleterious effects of anesthetic medications given to the mother that an imperfect answer seemed to us better than none. According to the 'blasé' state of mind described by La Fontaine in his fable 'The Miller, His Son and the Donkey', we answered by this statement:[79]

As in many other aspects of medicine, this score is the result of a compromise, and will appear far too simple or too complicated according to the individual's personal tendencies and needs'.

REFERENCES

1. Pajot C 1882 Travaux d'obstétrique et de gynécologie. Lauwereyns, Paris, 675p
2. Amiel-Tison C 1979 Birth injury as cause of brain dysfunction in full-term newborns. In: Korobkin R, Guilleminault C (eds) Advances in perinatal neurology. Spectrum Publications, New York, pp 57–83
3. Amiel-Tison C & Grenier A 1986 Neurological assessment during the first year of life. Oxford University Press, New York, 197p
4. Amiel-Tison C & Ellison P 1986 Birth asphyxia in the full-term newborn: early assessment and outcome. Developmental Medicine and Child Neurology 28: 671–682
5. Amiel-Tison C, Sureau C, Shnider S M 1988 Cerebral handicap in full-term neonates related to the mechanical forces of labour. In: Patel N (ed) Baillère's clinical obstetrics and gynaecology, Baillère Tindall, London, Vol 2, No 1, pp 145–165
6. Amiel-Tison C, Dube R, Levy A et al 1988 Early prediction for a normal outcome based on a normal neurobehavioral assessment in the full-term newborn. XIth European Congress of Perinatal Medicine. Abstract book. CIC Editions Internazionali, Rome, p 70
7. Brazelton T B 1984 Neonatal bahavioral assessment scale, 2nd edn, Clinics in developmental medicine No 88. Blackwell Scientific Publications, London, 125p
8. Mehler J, Fox R (eds) (1985) The neonate cognition: beyond the blooming buzzing confusion. Laurence Erlbaum, London, 469p
9. Sarnat H B 1984 Anatomic and physiologic correlates of neurologic development in prematurity. In: Sarnat H B (ed) Topics in neonatal neurology. Grune & Stratton, Orlando, p 1–25
10. Sarnat H B 1989 Do the corticospinal and corticobulbar tracts mediate functions in the human newborn? Can J Neurol Sci 16: 157–160
11. Amiel-Tison C, Barrier G, Shnider S M et al 1982 A new neurologic and adaptive capacity scoring system for evaluating obstetric medications in full-term newborns. Anesthesiology 56: 340–359
12. Scanlon J W, Brown W U, Weiss J B et al 1974 Neurobehavioral responses of newborn infants after maternal epidural anesthesia. Anesthesiology 40: 121–128
13. Widmayer S M, Field T M 1981 Effects of Brazelton demonstrations for mothers on the development of preterm infants. Pediatrics 67: 711–714
14. Amiel-Tison C 1994 Does neurological assessment still have a place in the NICU? The use of axial tone as an example. In: Amiel-Tison, Stewart A (eds) The newborn infant: one brain for life. Edition INSERM, Paris
15. Corke B C 1977 Neurobehavioral responses of the newborn. The effect of different forms of maternal analgesia. Anaesthesia 32: 539–543
16. Hodgkinson R, Marx G F, Kim S S et al 1977 Neonatal neurobehavioral tests following vaginal delivery under ketamine, thiopental and extradural anesthesia. Anesth Analg 56: 548–553
17. Brackbill Y, Kane J, Manniello R L et al 1974 Obstetric meperidine usage and assessment of neonatal status. Anesthesiology 40: 116–120
18. Brit I, Lindbach E, Ingebjorg S 1979 Neurobehavioral response of infants after paracervical block during labor. Acta Obstet Gynecol Scand 58: 41–44
19. Amiel-Tison C, Korobkin R, Esque-Vaucouloux M T 1977 Neck extensor hypertonia: a clinical sign of insult to the central nervous system of the newborn. Early Hum Dev 1: 181–190
20. Cohen S E 1987 Evaluation of the neonate. In: Shnider S M, Levinson G (eds) Anesthesia for obstetrics, 3rd edn. William & Wilkins, Baltimore, pp 671–692
21. Kuhnert B R, Linn P L, Kuhnert P M 1985 Obstetric medication and neonatal behavior, current controversies. Clinics in Perinatology, W B Saunders, Philadelphia, Vol 12, No 2. pp 423–439
22. Dailey P A, Baysinger C L, Levinson G 1982 Neurobehavioral testing of the newborn infant, effects of obstetric anesthesia. Clin Perinatol 9: 191–214
23. Abboud T K, Khoo S S, Miller F et all 1982 Maternal, fetal, and neonatal responses after epidural anesthesia with bupivacaine, 2-chloroprocaine, or lidocaine. Anesth Analg 61: 638–644
24. Abboud T K, Sarkis F, Blikian A et al 1982 Lack of adverse neurobehavioral effects of lidocaine. Anesthesiology 57: A404
25. Abboud T K, Kyung C K, Noueihed R et al 1983 Epidural bupivacaine, chloroprocaine, or lidocaine for cesarean section – maternal and neonatal side effects. Anesth Analg 62: 914–919
26. Kileff M E, James F M, Dewan D M et al 1984 Neonatal neurobehavioral responses after epidural anesthesia for cesarean section using lidocaine and bupivacaine. Anesth Analg 63: 413
27. Kuhnert B R, Harrison M J, Linn P L et al 1984 Effect of maternal epidural anesthesia on neonatal behavior. Anesth Analg 63: 301–308
28. Abboud T K, Afrasiabi A, Sarkis F et al 1984 Continuous infusion epidural analgesia in parturients receiving bupivacaine, chloroprocaine, or lidocaine – maternal, fetal, and neonatal effects Anesth Analg 63: 421–428
29. Bromage P R, Robson J G 1961 Concentrations of lignocaine in the blood after intravenous, intramuscular, epidural and endotracheal administration. Anaesthesia 16: 461
30. Mather L E, Tucker G T, Murphy T M et al 1976 The effects of adding adrenaline to etidocaine and lignocaine in extradural anaesthesia. II. Pharmacokinetics. Br J Anaesth 44: 989
31. Scott D B, Jebson P J R, Braid D P et al 1972 Factors affecting plasma levels of lignocaine and prilocaine. Br J Anaesth 44: 1040
32. Bromage P R 1978 Epidural analgesia. Saunders, Philadelphia, pp 358–360
33. Rosenfeld C R, Barton M D, Meschia G 1976 Effects of epinephrine on distribution of blood flow in the pregnant ewe. Am J Obstet Gynecol 124: 156
34. Wallis K L, Shnider S M, Hicks J S et al 1976 Epidural anesthesia in the normotensive pregnant ewe: effects on uterine blood flow and fetal acid–base status. Anesthesiology 44: 481–487
35. Hood D D, Dewan D M, Rose J C et al 1983 Maternal and fetal effects of intravenous epinephrine containing solutions in gravid ewes. Anesthesiology 59: A393
36. Rucker M P 1925 The action of adrenalin on the pregnant uterus. South Med J 18: 412
37. Gunther R E, Bauman J 1969 Obstetrical caudal anesthesia. I. A randomized study comparing 1% mepivacaine with 1% lidocaine plus epinephrine. Anesthesiology 31: 5
38. Gunther R E, Bellville J W 1972 Obstetrical anesthesia. II. A randomized study comparing 1 per cent mepivacaine with 1 per cent mepivacaine plus epinephrine. Anesthesiology 37: 288–298
39. Matadial L, Cibils L A 1976 The effect of epidural anesthesia on uterine activity and blood pressure. Am J Obstet Gynecol 125: 846
40. Zador G, Nilsson B A 1974 Low dose intermittent epidural anaesthesia with lidocaine for vaginal delivery. II. Influence on labour and foetal acid–base status. Acta Obstet Gynecol (suppl) 34: 17
41. Levinson G, Shnider S M, Krames E et al 1975 Epidural anesthesia for cesarean section: effects of epinephrine in the local anesthetic solution. Abstracts of Scientific Papers, Annual Meeting, American Society of Anesthesiologists, Chicago, p 285

42. deRosayro A M, Hahrwold M L, Hill A B 1981 Cardiovascular effects of epidural epinephrine in the pregnant sheep. Reg Anesth 6: 4–7
43. Albright G A, Jouppila R, Hollmén A I et al 1981 Epinephrine does not alter human intervillous blood flow during epidural anesthesia. Anesthesiology 54: 131–135
44. Craft J B, Epstein B S, Coakley C S 1972 Effect of lidocaine with epinephrine versus lidocaine (plain) on induced labor. Anesth Analg 51: 243
45. Abboud T K, David S, Nagappala S et al 1984 Maternal, fetal, and neonatal effects of lidocaine with and without epinephrine for epidural anesthesia in obstetrics. Anesth Analg 63: 973–979
46. Abboud T K, Sheik-ol-Eslam A, Yanagi T et al 1985 Safety and efficacy of epinephrine added to bupivacaine for lumbar epidural analgesia in obstetrics. Anesth Analg 64: 585–591
47. Abboud T K, DerSarkissian L, Terrasi J et al 1987 Comparative maternal, fetal, and neonatal effects of chloroprocaine with and without epinephrine for epidural anesthesia in obstetrics. Anesth Analg 66: 71–75
48. Abboud T K, Afrasiabi A, Zhu J et al 1989 Bupivacaine/butorphanol/epinephrine for epidural anesthesia in obstetrics: maternal and neonatal effects. Reg Anesth 14: 219–224
49. Abboud T K, Mosaad P, Maker A et al 1988 Comparative maternal and neonatal effects of the new and the old formulations of 2-chloroprocaine. Reg Anesth 13: 101–106
50. Hodgkinson R, Bhatt M, Wang C N 1978 Double blind comparison of the neurobehavior of neonates following administration of different doses of meperidine to the mother. Can Anaesth Soc J 25: 405–411
51. Hodgkinson R, Bhatt M, Grewal G et al 1978 Neonatal neurobehavior in the first 48 hours of life: effect of the administration of meperidine with and without naloxone in the mother. Pediatrics 62: 294–298
52. Hodgkinson R, Hugg R W, Hayashi R H et al 1979 Double blind comparison of maternal analgesia and neonatal neurobehavior following intravenous butorphanol and meperidine. J Int Med Res 7: 224–230
53. Bonta B W, Gagliardi J O, Williams V et al 1970 Naloxone reversal of mild neurobehavioral depression in normal newborn infants after routine obstetric analgesia. J Pediatr 94: 102–105
54. Weiner P C, Hogg M I, Rosen M 1979 Neonatal respiration, feeding and neurobehavioral state. Effects of intrapartum bupivacaine, pethidine and pethidine reversal by naloxone. Anaesthesia 34: 996–1004
55. Rayburn W, Rathke, A, Leuschen M P et al 1989 Fentanyl citrate during labor. Am J Obstet Gynecol 161: 202–206
56. Rayburn W F, Smith C V, Parriott J E, Woods R E 1989 Randomized comparison of meperidine and fentanyl during labor Obstet Gynecol 74: 604–606
57. Frank M, McAteer E J, Cattermole R et al 1987 Nalbuphine for obstetric analgesia. Anaesthesia 42: 697–703
58. Hughes S C, Rosen M A, Shnider S M et al 1984 Maternal and neonatal effects of epidural morphine for labor and delivery. Anesth Analg 63: 319–324
59. Abboud T K, Shnider S M, Dailey P A et al 1984 Intrathecal administration of hyperbaric morphine for the relief of pain in labour. Br J Anaesth 56: 1351–1359
60. Talafre M L, Jacquinot P, Legagneux F et al 1987 Intrathecal administration of meperidine versus tetracaine for elective cesarean section. Anesthesiology 67: A620
61. Dailey PA, Brookshire G L, Shnider S M et al 1984 Naloxone decreases side effects after intrathecal morphine for labor. Anesth Analg 64: 658–666
62. Preston P, Rosen M, Hughes S et al 1988 Epidural anesthesia with fentanyl and lidocaine for cesarean section: maternal effects and neonatal outcome. Anesthesiology 68: 938–943
63. Murakawa K, Abboud T K, Yanagi T et al 1987 Clinical experience of epidural fentanyl for labor pain. J Anesth 1: 93–95
64. Cohen S E, Tan S, Albright G A et al 1987 Epidural fentanyl/bupivacaine mixtures for obstetric analgesia. Anesthesiology 67: 403–497
65. Abboud T K, Afrasiabi A, Zhu J et al 1989 Epidural morphine or butorphanol augments bupivacaine analgesia during labor. Reg Anesth 14: 115–120
66. Zhu J, Abboud, T K, Afrasiabi A et al 1990 Epidural butorphanol augments lidocaine analgesia during labor. Anesthesiology 73: A979
67. Little M S, McNitt J D, Choi H J, et al 1987 A pilot study of low dose epidural sufentanil and bupivacaine for labor anesthesia. Anesthesiology 67: A444
68. Stephani S J, Hughes S C, Shnider S M et al 1982 Neonatal neurobehavioral effects of inhalation analgesia for vaginal delivery. Anesthesiology 56: 351–355
69. Abboud T K, Gangolly J, Mosaad P et al 1989 Isoflurane in obstetrics. Anesth Analg 68: 388–391
70. Abboud T K, Nagappala S, Murakawa K et al 1985 Comparison of the effects of general and regional anesthesia for cesarean section on neonatal neurologic and adaptive capacity scores. Anesth Analg 64: 996–1000
71. Ravlo O, Carl P, Crawford M E et al 1989 A randomized comparison between midazolam and thiopental for elective cesarean section anesthesia. II. Neonates. Anesth Analg 68: 234–237
72. Dailey P A, Fisher D M, Shnider S M et al 1984 Pharmacokinetics, placental transfer, and neonatal effects of vecuronium and pancuronium administered during cesarean section. Anesthesiology 60: 569–574
73. Cohen S E, Jasson J, Talafre M L et al 1984 Does metoclopramide decrease the volume of gastric contents in patients undergoing cesarean section? Anesthesiology 61: 604–607
74. Eldredge L, Salamy A 1988 Neurobehavioral and neurophysical assessment of healthy and at-risk full-term infants. Child Development 59: 186–192
75. American Academy of Pediatrics 1978 Effect of medication during labor and delivery on infant outcome. Pediatrics 62: 402–403
76. Rostand E 1897 Cyrano De Bergerac, Act I, Scene IV
77. Tronick E 1982 A critique of the Neonatal Neurologic Adaptive Capacity Score (NACS) Anesthesiology 56: 338–339
78. Michenfelder J D 1982 Accept, revise, reject or punt: an example of the latter. Anesthesiology 56, 337
79. Amiel-Tison C, Barrier G, Shnider S M, Levinson G, Hughes S C, Stephani S 1982 The Neonatal Neurologic and Adaptive Capacity Score (NACS). Anesthesiology 56, 492–493

9. Uteroplacental perfusion

PART A
UTEROPLACENTAL PERFUSION: BASIC CONCEPTS

P. Youngstrom M. Hoyt

PLACENTAL STRUCTURE AND RESPIRATORY FUNCTION

The human placenta sustains two anatomically distinct circulations that function as a unit. Its purpose is to provide oxygen and nutrients from the maternal circulation and remove by-products from the fetal circulation for elimination. Comparisons have been made between the placenta as an organ of respiration and the lung,[1,2] based in large part on animal studies.[3] But different species have structurally different placentas that are likely to have functional distinctions from the human placenta.[3] Therefore, analogies must be drawn with caution. A consideration of the human condition necessarily draws heavily on animal research, a potentially important distinction that is identified throughout this discussion.

Maternal aspects

The maternal blood supply to the placenta derives principally from the uterine arteries on either side of the uterus (Fig. 9.1). From these, arcuate arteries branch and run parallel to the uterine wall, sending off perpendicular divisions toward the endometrial cavity. These divisions, called radial arteries, dilate at their terminal portions to become spiral arteries. Each spiral artery channels through the basal plate into the intervillous space and spurts blood toward the chorial plate of the placenta, from which project villi containing the fetal circulation. Blood then flows laterally, becoming quite sluggish and well deoxygenated, before returning to the basal plate and draining through gaps connected to the venous system. This design of maternal blood directly bathing fetal villi which enclose the fetal circulation describes a hemochorial placenta, which is found in primates.[2–6] Alternative arrangements in other species lead to significant differences in diffusion distance between the two circulations.[3] Although maternal and fetal cells have been known to cross this barrier, there is no direct communication between the two.[4]

The uteroplacental circulation is a low-resistance system,[7] primarily because of the inability of the spiral arteries to constrict following loss of smooth muscle to trophoblast invasion.[8] This creates near-maximal dilatation,[9,10] displacing the burden of resistance upon larger arteries, which must constrict to a greater degree than smaller vessels to achieve the same amount of resistance.[11] This low-resistance circulatory system has been likened to another anatomic variant, the arteriovenous fistula.[4] As a fistula opens, cardiac output increases in proportion to the amount of flow through it. During pregnancy, cardiac output begins to increase during the first trimester and peaks early in the third, being maintained or slightly diminished as term is reached. This hemodynamic change coincides with the onset of maternal-placental circulation at the fifth to sixth gestational week, as the spiral arteries begin to erode through the basal plate.[3] The placenta is covered with spiral arteries by the twentieth week.[4] Total uterine blood flow peaks near term at a rate of 500–700 ml/min,[12,13] of which 85% perfuses the placenta.[6,10,14] Late in pregnancy uterine blood flow may not keep pace with growth, an observation that has been theorized to be related to atrophy of spiral arteries.[4]

A maternal arterial pressure of at least 100 mmHg is recommended to maintain an adequate pressure gradient to the intervillous space, where the pressure is 10–30 mmHg.[15] Uterine contractions can increase intervillous pressure to 40 mmHg and decrease both uterine

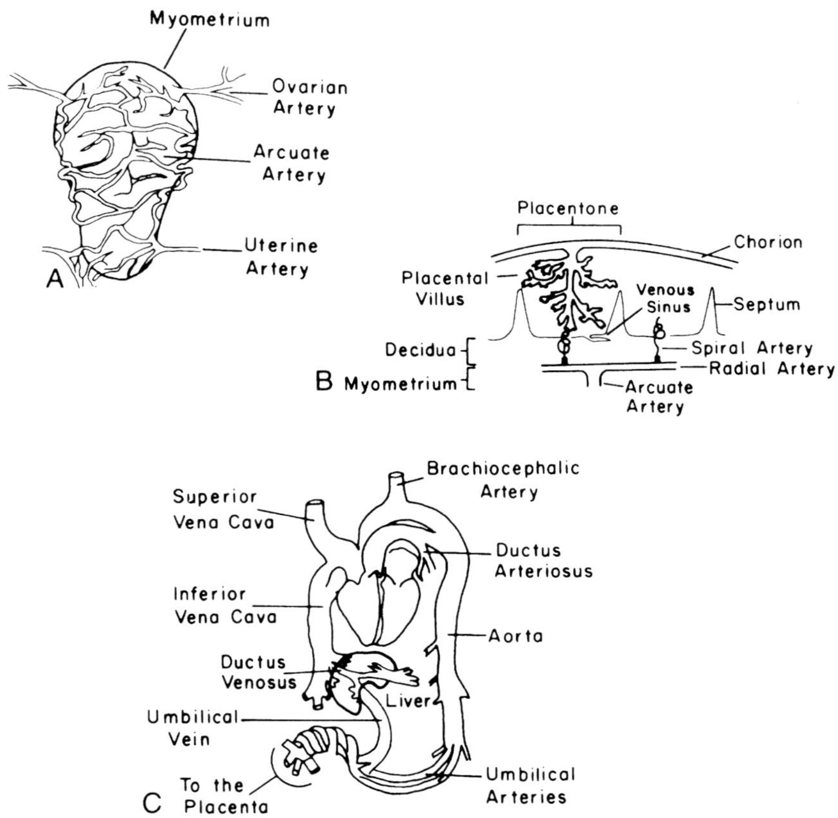

Fig. 9.1 The maternal–placental-fetal unit. (A) The maternal component. (B) The placental component. (C) The fetal component. (Reproduced with permission from Parer J T 1987 Uteroplacental circulation and respiratory gas exchange. In: Shnider S M, Levinson (eds) Anesthesia for obstetrics, 2nd edn. Williams & Wilkins, Baltimore.)

and intervillous blood flow.[6,10] Effects on oxygenation are moderated by intervillous blood, which can be likened to the functional residual capacity of the lung in that intervillous blood contributes to homeostasis during contractions or short periods of low flow just as the lung's functional residual capacity supports oxygenation during short periods of apnea.

Sheep studies suggest that the widely dilated near-term uterine vasculature has little capacity to autoregulate flow.[10,11,14] (The question of local vascular regulatory mechanisms is considered later.) This has important implications for hypotension from any cause. Importantly, a reduction in perfusion pressure, as from supine recumbency and aortocaval compression, can compromise intervillous blood flow.[16] In general, the uterine arteries vasoconstrict from neurohumoral stimuli (sympathetic nerves, vasopressors) like other peripheral vessels.[10,14] Depending upon simultaneous pressure changes, such vasoconstriction could compromise flow. However, unlike the peripheral vessels, uterine vessels are slow to relax after the stimulus is removed.[10] Lingering elevation in resistance would compromise intervillous blood flow after other vascular beds had returned to their prestimulus condition.

Fetal aspects

Fetal blood enters the placenta from two umbilical arteries at a pressure of 60–70 mmHg (Fig. 9.1).[17] These arteries divide, sending branches to perfuse the cotyledons. Smaller vessels traverse the chorial plate and protrude into the intervillous space. Each vessel branches extensively, creating a network of capillaries. As the vessel crosses the chorial plate, it is encased in three fetal tissue layers (capillary endothelium, chorial stroma, and trophoblastic synctium) and is termed a villus.

The developed villus resembles a leafless tree, in which each of the many tips contains a capillary for nutrient and waste exchange. This formation promotes exchange by increasing villous surface area,[2] estimated to be about 11–14 m^2 at term.[3] Enriched blood drains back by a similar path and ultimately enters a single umbilical vein through which it traverses the full length of the cord at low pressure (10–20 mmHg). It has been proposed that umbilical vein flow is facilitated by a pulsometer pumping system intrinsic to the cord.[17] Umbilical blood flow at term is approximately 120 ml/kg/min,[18] and sheep studies have shown a shunt of 20%.[3] Fetal circulation and villus formation begins to develop about the sixteenth day after conception and is completed by the twelfth week.[3]

Fetoplacental vessels are not innervated,[1] thereby lacking a neural means to shunt blood away from poorly oxygenated areas. However, in vitro studies suggest that this may be accomplished by a local regulatory mechanism similar to hypoxic pulmonary vasoconstriction in the lung. In isolated cotyledons exposed to a hypoxemic challenge, the fetal vasculature was shown to vasoconstrict. This condition rapidly reversed when normoxia resumed, suggesting that the fetus may be able to shunt blood away from hypoperfused or hypoxic areas to better perfused, normoxic ones.[1] In vitro studies have also shown that low oxygen tensions stimulate trophoblastic growth.[2] Local regulation of fetoplacental perfusion and potential maternal-fetal interactions are considered later.

Gas exchange

Gas exchange across the placenta is subject to many influences, such as differences between fetal and maternal hemoglobin, uterine and umbilical hemodynamics,[1,2,10,19–21] regulation of perfusion in areas of gas exchange,[1,22] and placental factors such as vascular geometry,[2,23] diffusing capacity,[3] and oxygen consumption.[3,24] Several fundamentals warrant review, with the caveat that measured oxygen and carbon dioxide gradients between the maternal and fetal circulations have not been fully explained.

The distinctive features of fetal hemoglobin play a key role in oxygen transport. Compared with adult hemoglobin, fetal hemoglobin has a higher oxygen affinity as reflected in a lower P_{50} (oxygen tension required to produce 50% hemoglobin saturation) of 19 *vs.* 27. This represents a left shift in the fetal oxyhemoglobin dissociation curve, and is associated with a reduction in fetal 2,3-diphosphoglycerate (2,3-DPG), while pregnancy affects a 30% rise in maternal 2,3-DPG. This separation between fetal and maternal oxyhemoglobin dissociation curves (or oxygen affinity) represents a driving force behind oxygen transfer.[3]

Conditions affecting the separation between the two curves can affect oxygen transfer.[3] A rise or fall in carbon dioxide tension (with a corresponding fall or rise in pH) leads to a right or left shift, respectively, in the dissociation curve (Bohr effect). At the gas-exchange interface, maternal arterial blood encounters increasing carbon dioxide tension producing a right-shift and increased oxygen unloading. Conversely, fetal venous blood encounters reduced carbon dioxide tension, leading to a left shift and increased oxygen uptake. This inverse relationship between carbon dioxide tension and oxygen affinity probably reflects carbon dioxide effect on pH.[25,26] Respiratory alkalosis (as from hyperventilation during labor) will tend to shift the maternal curve to the left, oppose the favorable carbon dioxide effect on maternal oxygen unloading at the gas-exchange interface, and impair fetal oxygenation.[21,25–28] Similarly, fetal acidosis may result in a right shift of the fetal curve, which opposes fetal oxygen uptake and depresses oxygen transfer.[3,27]

The fetus is thought to normally extract 5 ml of oxygen per 100 ml of maternal–placental blood flow,[3] and to require at least 5 ml of oxygen per kg per min.[24] Oxygen uptake and carrying capacity are enhanced by an elevated fetal hemoglobin concentration (15 g/100 ml), and in sheep studies have been shown to increase by 25% in response to chronic hypoxia.[29] The fetus is able to respond to an acute reduction in the supply of maternal oxygen to the intervillous space by redistributing flow (to brain, heart, and placenta) and decreasing oxygen consumption. However, assuming maternal and fetal placental flows are well matched, there is little capacity for increased oxygen extraction by the fetus unless maternal oxygen delivery to the intervillous space can be enhanced either by increasing intervillous flow or by elevating oxygen content of maternal blood. This is illustrated by primate studies[30,31] as well as by observations made during simultaneous maternal and fetal transcutaneous oxygen tension monitoring in humans. In one instance, within 2 mins of changing the mother's position from lateral to supine (thereby reducing intervillous perfusion and the supply of maternal oxygen to the intervillous space), maternal $P\text{O}_2$ fell from 100 to 89 mmHg and fetal $P\text{O}_2$ fell from 22 to 12 mmHg. Initial treatment was with a vasopressor (cafedrine hydrochloride) rather than lateral uterine displacement. The maternal $P\text{O}_2$ increased to 100 mmHg and the fetal to 20 mmHg. In a later observation, maternal $P\text{O}_2$ increased from 89 to 179 mmHg and fetal from 10 to 19 mmHg after administration of supplemental oxygen to the mother.[28]

Oxygen equilibration across the placenta is not normally complete as indicated by observation of a persistent oxygen gradient of 15–30 mmHg between the umbilical and uterine veins.[3,32] Shunts (anatomic and physiologic) and placental oxygen consumption contribute, but understanding of this discrepancy is not complete.

At term, for every milliliter of maternal oxygen transferred, the fetal-placental unit produces 0.8–0.9 ml of carbon dioxide for elimination.[3] Dissolved carbon dioxide diffuses readily across the placenta, but the bulk of carbon dioxide transport is accounted for by hemoglobin effects.[3] The fetal carbon dioxide–hemoglobin dissociation curve is displaced to the right of the maternal curve, meaning that fetal hemoglobin gives up carbon dioxide more readily. A rise or fall in oxygen tension leads to a right or left shift, respectively, in the dissociation curve (Haldane effect). At the gas-exchange interface, fetal venous blood takes up oxygen, leading to a right shift and enhanced carbon dioxide unloading. Conversely, maternal arterial blood deoxygenates producing a left shift and increased carbon dioxide affinity. The Haldane effect accounts for about

50% of carbon dioxide transfer.[33] Despite the apparent efficiency of this system and the ready diffusion of carbon dioxide, a persistent gradient of 3–5 mmHg exists between the umbilical and uterine veins, and remains unexplained.[32]

REGULATION OF MATERNAL–PLACENTAL PERFUSION

The search for mechanisms that control local maternal–placental perfusion has encompassed a large variety of potential regulators, some of which are discussed here. Investigations of maternal–placental perfusion have commonly used any of three measurement techniques: an electromagnetic flowmeter sited on a uterine artery, radioactive microspheres, and detection of injected radioisotope over anteriorly situated placentas.

Uterine artery flow studies in sheep have described uteroplacental flow as maximal in normal pregnancy but capable of significant reduction from sympathetic or adrenergic vasoconstriction, uterine contractions and maternal hypotension.[9] Vasodilatory beta-adrenergic responses could not be identified,[34] though Wallenberg and Hutchinson[35] demonstrated constriction and dilatation in the uteroplacental vessels of the monkey with norepinephrine and metaproterenol respectively. Further, uterine artery blood flow has been shown to be directly proportional to uterine artery pressure in pregnant sheep,[13] though Venuto et al,[36] using radioactive microspheres, found that uteroplacental flow was maintained over a wide range of perfusion pressures in the rabbit. This proportionality is dependent on a fully dilated vasculature with unchanging resistance, circumstances that frequently do not pertain clinically (Skjöldebrand et al,[37] using radioisotope detection, found no correlation between human placental blood flow and maternal blood pressure over a clinically relevant range.) Uterine artery flow measurement has been applied extensively in animal research, along with an underlying presumption that changes in uterine blood flow (UBF) have easily predictable implications for placental perfusion and fetal well-being (in normal pregnancy at term, 85% of total uterine blood flow perfuses the placenta). While such correlation is accepted following gross reductions in uterine blood flow, the relationship between variations in UBF and adequacy of placental perfusion is subject to controversy. Confounding factors include autoregulation in myometrial vessels,[15] differential responses to adrenergic stimulation between myometrial and placental vessels[34] and perhaps between species,[38,39] and potential consequences of different degrees of underlying sympathetic tone, among others (see below). Depending upon the magnitude of the stimulus under consideration and the existing hemodynamic milieu, it may not be reasonable to equate placental perfusion and uterine blood flow, and UBF results must not be overinterpreted when drawing clinical conclusions.[40,41]

Regulation of maternal-placental (rather than total uterine) perfusion has been investigated using radioactive microspheres. Reports on the effects of angiotensin II have been contradictory, depending on species and experimental conditions (both increases and decreases in flow have been reported in sheep).[42] Interestingly, Hariharan et al[43] observed a significant dose-related increase in endogenous epinephrine (but not norepinephrine) with angiotensin infusion, an increase in mean arterial pressure and systemic vascular resistance, no change in uteroplacental vascular resistance, and a significant increase in uteroplacental blood flow (almost entirely due to the increase in placental flow) in guinea pigs. Epinephrine alone in sheep was shown to vasoconstrict placental vasculature less than nonplacental, but catecholamine levels were not measured, making evaluation of dose-related epinephrine effects in this species and comparison with other species difficult.[44]

Prostaglandins have been of interest as both potential regulators and intermediaries in the control of maternal–placental perfusion. Indomethacin (an inhibitor of prostaglandin production) has been associated with placental vasoconstriction, suggesting a vasodilatory role for prostaglandins in the uteroplacental vasculature.[45] Prostacyclin was shown to significantly increase uterine artery flow in sheep,[46] but it was subsequently demonstrated with microspheres that the reduction in resistance occurred in the uterine and not placental vessels.[47] The direct vascular effects of prostaglandin E_2 are difficult to ascertain because of its ability to produce a uterine contraction. During infusion of angiotensin II (which is associated with secondary release of E-series prostaglandins) the observed reduction in uterine artery blood flow was accentuated by indomethacin.[48] However, microsphere investigation revealed that indomethacin affected resistance in uterine but not placental vessels, and provided no evidence for prostaglandin modulation of placental vasoconstriction in response to angiotensin II.[49] The placental vascular response to norepinephrine, however, was attenuated by prostaglandin E_2 and potentiated by indomethacin.[50] Further, indirect evidence has suggested that stimulation of uteroplacental kinin production, associated with secondary release of prostaglandin E_2, results in increased uterine and placental blood flow without change in systemic blood pressure or total peripheral resistance in nephrectomized rabbits treated with an angiotensin antagonist.[51] Adenosine was ineffective in modulating placental vasoconstriction induced by angiotensin II in sheep,[52] and prostacyclin heightened resistance and further decreased flow (though systemic hypotension and blood flow redistribution complicate interpretation in this situation).[53] Radioisotope detection studies in humans have demonstrated no relation between intervillous blood flow and either blood levels of vasoactive prostaglandins or infusion of prostacyclin in preeclampsia.[54,55] While vasodilatory effects for prostaglandin E_2 and kinins are suggested, the mediators and mechanisms of local control of maternal–placental perfusion are not yet understood.

Atrial natriuretic factor (ANF) has been shown to be a potent vasodilator in the placental circulation. Chemtob et al[56] demonstrated blood pressure reduction, normalization of total peripheral resistance, and increased placental blood flow after ANF in normal and hypertensive (nephrectomy and renal artery ligation) rats. Reid et al[57] observed placental vasodilation in both normal and angiotensin II-constricted sheep, while uterine (nonplacental) resistance decreased only in the latter group. It seems clear that placental vascular responses are mediated by significantly different mechanisms from those affecting nonplacental uterine vessels.

Only radioisotope detection techniques have found extensive human application, principally in the form of the ^{133}Xe clearance method of Rekonen et al[58] and Kuikka et al.[23] Briefly, a double exponential clearance curve is observed over the placenta after intravenous ^{133}Xe injection. The fast component is used to calculate blood flow per unit volume of intervillous space (but not total placental blood flow, a noteworthy distinction when evaluating adequacy of placental perfusion in abnormal pregnancy associated with decreased placental volume), while the slow component is related to myometrial flow. By this technique mean intervillous blood flow in normal pregnancy was found to be 125 ml/min/100 ml, with flow in the central placenta 55% greater than that in the marginal parts. Myometrial flow was about 17 ml/min/100 g irrespective of placental proximity. However, studies of ^{113m}In accumulation in humans,[59] clearance of ^{133}Xe from the isolated guinea pig placenta,[60] and theoretical models[61] have contested the validity of this compartmental interpretation. Nevertheless, this technique has been extensively employed for serial evaluations of intervillous blood flow in selected patients.

Severe preeclampsia and diabetes are associated with abnormalities of the uteroplacental vasculature and significant reductions in intervillous blood flow.[62] Aortocaval compression by the third-trimester uterus in the supine position has been documented angiographically[63] and may produce depressed arterial pressure, high venous pressure and reduced blood flow in the uterus. Correspondingly, intervillous blood flow was found to be lower in supine recumbency than in a left-tilted position.[15] Smoking a standard cigarette was found to elevate maternal blood pressure and heart rate while depressing intervillous blood flow for 15 mins.[64] Six minutes of exercise in the third trimester was associated with significant increases in maternal blood pressure, heart rate and cardiac output but no significant effect on intervillous blood flow.[65]

It appears that significant sympathetic and/or alpha-adrenergic activation, leading to uteroplacental vasoconstriction (more marked in the uterine than in the placental bed) and diversion of blood flow, offers a defense of threatened maternal homeostasis. Also, placental flow may vary independently from uterine (nonplacental) flow. However, despite a number of observed vascular effects, mechanisms for local regulation of maternal–placental perfusion have not yet been defined.

REGULATION OF FETAL–PLACENTAL PERFUSION

Regulation of fetal–placental blood flow may be viewed at several different levels (excluding neural control, as the umbilical arteries are devoid of autonomic innervation). It has been suggested that fetal–placental flow may be self-regulating: briefly, a reduction in flow is associated with a fall in fetal capillary fluid pressure, followed by a maternal-to-fetal fluid flux leading to an increase in fetal blood volume, central venous pressure, cardiac output, and arterial pressure, culminating in a restoration of fetal–placental flow.[66] This proposal provides an interesting backdrop to another aspect of fetoplacental blood flow regulation: subsequent observations of angiotensin II and norepinephrine effects in the umbilical vascular circulation. Neither of these agents was found to play an important role in regulation of resting umbilical vascular resistance in unstressed fetal sheep.[67] This resistance was found to have the following distribution: 37% across the umbilical arteries, 8% across umbilical veins, and 55% across the cotyledons.[68] Exogenous angiotensin II increased umbilical vascular resistance by increasing umbilical arterial resistance, and reduced placental perfusion despite an increase in fetal systemic arterial blood pressure. Reduced cotyledon arterial pressure would favor maternal-to-fetal fluid transport.

Exogenous norepinephrine increased umbilical vascular resistance principally by increasing venous resistance; rising resistance eventually balanced the systemic pressor effect so that placental perfusion was increased at first, then gradually returned to normal. Vasopressin also participates in the fetal stress response; administered exogenously, its predominant effect is to elevate fetal arterial pressure.[69,70] The elevated cotyledon arterial pressure would favor fetal-to-maternal fluid transport. While it is unclear how this potential fluid flux effect would contribute to adjustment to fetal stress, there is another notable consequence of these pressure changes. A net effect of these changes and of fetal blood flow redistribution is an increase in the volume of fetal blood in the placenta.[71] That no effect was observed on the resistance of vessels intrinsic to the cotyledon[68] may reflect the distensible nature (high compliance) of these vessels[72] and/or recruitment of vessels whose critical closing pressure has been exceeded by the increased cotyledon arterial pressure.[73] This is reminiscent of the behavior of pulmonary vascular resistance. Indeed, arterial oxygen tension and umbilical oxygen delivery in fetuses given vasopressin increased, while carbon dioxide tension and pH changes were small and dose related (tending toward acidosis at high doses).[69,70]

The relative inaccessibility of the fetal–placental vasculature presents a challenge to the investigation and understanding of its regulatory mechanisms. Much work has been done in vitro using umbilical vessels and placenta lobules. By such techniques, angiotensin II has been shown to powerfully constrict arterial resistance vessels.[74] Evidence for conversion of angiotensin I to angiotensin II in the fetal–placental vasculature indicates that angiotensin II may act locally to regulate fetal–placental perfusion.[75–77]

In vitro observations of perfusion pressure changes in human placental cotyledons have indicated pressure reduction by prostacyclin[78–81] and elevation by U46619 (a thromboxane-mimetic), PGE_2, and bradykinin.[74,78–83] The pressor effect of angiotensin II has been significantly reduced by prostacyclin and potentiated by PGE_2, thromboxane-mimetic, and indomethacin.[82] Angiotensin II has been associated with a secondary rise in both vasodilating and vasoconstricting prostaglandins,[78,84] though apparently the former normally predominate, thereby modulating angiotensin II effects in the placental vasculature.[82] Bradykinin has been observed to increase thromboxane production (an effect not mediated by angiotensin II),[83] while its pressor effect has been variably affected by indomethacin.[79,83] Leukotrienes cause vasoconstriction but are less potent than thromboxane.[85] Adenosine has a vasodilating effect that is attenuated by indomethacin.[86] Such evidence of powerful vascular effects suggests an important role for prostaglandins in mediating changes in fetal–placental blood flow.

In vivo investigation of the sheep fetus have demonstrated increased umbilical resistance after prostaglandin E_2 with a time course suggestive of secondary release of a potent vasoconstrictor.[87] This PGE_2 effect has been shown not to be mediated by alpha-adrenergic or angiotensin II receptors.[88] Indomethacin led to increased cotyledonary resistance, again with a time course suggestive of activity by a secondarily released agent.[89] The response to indomethacin could suggest release of an unknown vasoconstrictor or inhibition of a potent prostaglandin vasodilator. With respect to the latter, however, in vivo studies have failed to demonstrate placental vasodilation after prostacyclin alone or in the presence of angiotensin II or thromboxane-induced vasoconstriction.[90–92] This observation could reflect a passive change in placental resistance secondary to hypotension and decreased placental perfusion from systemic prostacyclin. This interpretation is consistent with vasodilatory changes in umbilical artery Doppler ultrasound indices after prostacyclin administration at the level of the umbilical arteries, though here too a significant decrease in fetal arterial pressure and umbilical placental blood flow was observed.[93] However, the ability of umbilical artery Doppler indices to distinguish placental vascular from umbilical venous resistance has recently been challenged,[94] as has interpretation of Doppler indices during instable circulatory changes associated with vasopressin administration.[95] While vasodilatory effects for prostacyclin and constrictor effects for other prostaglandins may be suggested, their role in local mechanisms regulating fetal–placental perfusion is undefined.

Developments in Doppler ultrasound technology have provided a noninvasive means of assessing blood flow in both fetal and maternal (arcuate) vessels with human applications. Two-dimensional, range-gated, pulsed Doppler ultrasonography describes a flow velocity curve, the area under which (the flow velocity integral), multiplied by the area of the vessel, permits calculation of flow.[96] The validity of this estimation depends on accurate measurement of vessel cross-sectional area, minimal angle between the direction of blood flow and the Doppler beam, and measurement during fetal apnea. The status of downstream resistance can be indicated by derived Doppler indices, including the ratio of peak systolic to end-diastolic flow velocity (S/D ratio), and systolic less diastolic velocity divided by mean velocity (pulsatility index). Excellent correlations have been demonstrated between results from flow velocity waveforms and measurements made with electromagnetic flow probes in fetal sheep.[97,98] Embolic occlusion of fetal sheep placental arteries and arterioles produces changes in umbilical artery flow velocity waveforms indicative of increased resistance.[99,100] These same changes have been associated with decreased numbers of small arterial vessels in human placentas following growth-retarded pregnancy.[101,102] While Doppler ultrasound studies appear to hold great promise in the clinical management of complicated pregnancies,[103,104] the breadth of their proposed application is still unresolved.[105,106] However, in light of the difficulties with Doppler interpretations alluded to above, a role for such studies in the investigation of local regulatory mechanisms in placental perfusion is unclear.

It appears that fetal-placental perfusion is capable of alteration in response to stress in the direction of maximizing umbilical oxygen delivery. Here again observations of potent vascular effects are suggestive of significant local regulation of placental perfusion, but the mechanisms involved remain unexplained.

INTERACTIONS BETWEEN FETAL AND MATERNAL–PLACENTAL PERFUSION

The prospect of potent regulation of local perfusion in

each of two distinct but intrinsically intertwined vasculatures suggests the possibility of interaction between them.[107,108] In zone 2 of the lung blood flow is thought to depend on the difference between pulmonary arterial pressure and surrounding alveolar pressure (rather than pulmonary venous pressure),[109] a mechanical effect that has also been proposed to apply to placental perfusion. In studies of the perfused sheep cotyledon and placenta, elevation of uterine outflow pressure (by compression of the inferior vena cava) increased cotyledonary inflow pressure, presumably through compression of fetal vessels by elevated maternal placental vascular (surrounding) pressure.[110,111] Consistent with this, human umbilical artery S/D ratios were found to be higher with the mother supine than in the lateral position, indicating elevated umbilical vascular resistance from presumably increased uterine venous pressure.[112] Conversely, elevation of fetal outflow pressure increased fetal inflow pressure only after a threshold of 15 mmHg (presumably the cotyledonary surrounding pressure) was exceeded. Subsequent investigation in intact sheep demonstrated effects on fetal–placental blood flow and arterial pressure from small increases in umbilical vein pressure, providing no evidence of meaningful surrounding pressure and undermining the physiologic relevance of reported mechanical effects on placental perfusion.[113] However, another study in intact sheep demonstrated a significant reduction in uteroplacental blood flow during umbilical cord occlusion, and attributed this to compression of maternal placental vessels by elevated fetoplacental vascular pressure.[114] Contradictory evidence has not yet resolved the role of mechanical effects in regulation of placental blood flows perhaps because, as in the lung, the requisite pressure relationships are not uniformly present. Additionally, observed effects might equally well be attributed to locally produced vasoactive agents involved in the maintenance of placental perfusion ratios.

Ventilation–perfusion ratios in the lung characterize the interaction of the alveolar and pulmonary vascular compartments. There are local mechanisms that normally maintain these ratios in the relatively narrow range required for effective gas exchange. Analogous perfusion–perfusion ratios and requirements may exist in the placenta. Radioactive microsphere investigation in sheep has measured maternal–fetal perfusion ratios between 0.5 and 1.5 in 70% of tissue samples, with 9% below and 21% above this range.[115] This degree of mismatching may help to explain the observed uterine-umbilical venous oxygen gradient. Experimental perturbation of the umbilical circulation by microembolization or norepinephrine in sheep demonstrated that perfusion changes in one compartment were matched by perfusion changes in the other so that perfusion–perfusion ratios were stabilized.[116] In fact, there is some evidence in a similar sheep model to suggest that during stress (maternal hypoxia or ligation of a branch of the umbilical artery) maternal and fetal perfusion become more evenly matched than at rest, thereby contributing to fetal oxygenation.[117]

It is apparent that local regulation of perfusion occurs and is important to placental gas exchange. Delineation of the regulators from among a variety of vasoactive substances will require further research. Interesting candidates include prostaglandin E_2, prostacyclin, kinins and atrial natriuretic factor, among others. For example, sheep studies have demonstrated vasoconstriction in the umbilical circulation and vasodilation in the uterine circulation after fetal administration of prostaglandin E_2.[87,118,119] Evidence for prostaglandin transfer across the human placenta, however, is conflicting.[80,108] Such mechanisms may influence both local perfusion–perfusion ratios and total placental vascular resistance, and if gone awry (e.g. preeclampsia) could have critical effects on placental gas exchange. Specific therapeutic intervention will be difficult and potentially hazardous until these regulatory mechanisms are better understood.[120,121]

REFERENCES

1. Howard R B, Hosokawa T, Maguire M H 1987 Hypoxia-induced fetoplacental vasoconstriction in perfused human placental cotyledon. Am J Obstet Gynecol 157: 1261–1266
2. Teasdale F 1978 Functional significance of the zonal morphologic differences in the normal human placenta – a morphometric study. Am J Obstet Gynecol 130: 773–781
3. Metcalfe J, Bartels H, Moll W 1967 Gas exchange in the pregnant uterus. Physiol Rev 47: 782–838
4. Burchell R C 1967 Arterial blood flow into the human intervillous space. Am J Obstet Gynecol 98: 303–311
5. Freese U E 1986 The uteroplacental vascular relationship in the human. Am J Obstet Gynecol 101: 8–16
6. Less M H, Hill J D, Ochsner III A J, Thomas C L, Novy M J 1971 Maternal placental and myometrial blood flow of the rhesus monkey during uterine contractions. Am J Obstet Gynecol 110: 68–81
7. Assali N S 1989 Dynamics of the uteroplacental circulation in health and disease. Am J Perinatol 6: 105–108
8. Pijnenborg R, Robertson W B, Brosens I Dixon G 1981 Trophoblast invasion and the establishment of hemochorial placentation in man and laboratory animals. Placenta 2: 71–91
9. Greiss F C 1967 A clinical concept of uterine blood flow during pregnancy. Obstet Gynecol 30: 595–604
10. Greiss F C 1973 Concepts of uterine blood flow. In: Wynn R (ed) Obstetrical and gynecological annual, Vol 2. Appleton Century Crofts, Norwalk pp 55–83
11. Greiss F C, Anderson S G, Still J G 1976 Uterine pressure–flow relationships during early gestation. Am J Obstet Gynecol 126: 799–808
12. Assali N S, Douglass R A, Baird W W, Nicholson D B, Suyemoto R 1953 Measurement of uterine blood flow and uterine metabolism. IV. Results in normal pregnancy. Am J Obstet Gynecol 66: 248–253
13. Metcalfe J, Romney S L, Ramsey L H, Reid D E, Burwell C S 1955 Estimation of uterine blood flow in nomal pregnancy at term. J. Clin Invest 34: 1632–1638
14. Greiss F C Pressure–flow relationship in the gravid uterine vascular bed. Am J Obstet Gynecol 96: 41–47
15. Alverez H, Caldeyro-Barcia R 1954 Normal and abnormal contractile waves of the uterus during labor. Gynaecologia 138: 190–212
16. Kauppila A, Koskinen M, Puolakka J, Tuimala R, Kuikka J 1980

Decreased intervillous and unchanged myometrial blood flow in supine recumbency. Obstet Gynecol 55: 203–205
17. Reynolds S R M 1978 Mechanisms of placentofetal blood flow. Obstet Gynecol 51: 245–249
18. Gill R W, Trudinger B J, Garrett W J, Kossoff G, Warren P S 1981 Fetal umbilical venous flow measured in utero by pulsed doppler and B-mode ultrasound. I. Normal pregnancies. Am J Obstet Gynecol 139: 720–725
19. Morishima H O, Daniel S S, Adamsons Jr K, James L S 1965 Effects of positive pressure ventilation of the mother upon the acid–base state of the fetus. Am J Obstet Gynecol 93: 269–273
20. Brownfield G L, Gilbert R D, Power G G 1987 Maternal placental vascular compliance in rabbits. Am J Physiol 234: H289–292
21. Miller F C, Petrie R H, Arce J J, Paul R H, Hon E H 1974 Hyperventilation during labor. Am J Obstet Gynecol 120: 489–495
22. Myers R E, Stange L, Joelsson I, Huzeel B, Wussow C 1977 Effects upon the fetus of oxygen administration to the mother. A study in monkeys. Acta Obstet Gynecol Scand 56: 195–203
23. Kuikka J, Käär K, Jouppila P, Pyörälä T, Rekonen A 1978 An intravenous ^{133}Xe method for measuring regional distribution of placental blood flow. Acta Obstet Gynecol Scand 57: 249–251
24. Romney S L, Reid D E, Metcalfe J, Burwell C S 1955 Oxygen utilization by the human fetus in utero. Am J Obstet Gynecol 70: 791–799
25. Motoyama E K, Rivard G, Acheson F, Cook C D 1967 The effect of changes in maternal pH and pCO_2 on the pO_2 of fetal lambs. Anesthesiology 28: 891–903
26. Levinson G, Shnider S M, deLorimier A A, Steffenson J L 1974 Effects of maternal hyperventilation on uterine blood flow and fetal oxygenation and acid–base status. Anesthesiology 40: 340–347
27. Moya F, Morishima H O, Shnider S M, James L S 1965 Influence of maternal hyperventilation on the newborn infant. Am J Obstet Gynecol 91: 76–84
28. Huch A, Huch R 1976 Transcutaneous, noninvasive monitoring of pO_2. Hospital Practice (June) pp 43–52
29. Paulone M E, Edelstone D I, Shedd A 1987 Effects of maternal anemia on uteroplacental and fetal oxidative metabolism in sheep. Am J Obstet Gynecol 156: 230–236
30. Myers R E, Mueller-Heubach E, Adamsons K 1973 Predictability of the state of fetal oxygenation from a quantitative analysis of the components of late deceleration. Am J Obstet Gynecol 115: 1083–1094
31. Khazin A F, Hon E H, Hehre F W 1975 Effects of maternal hyperoxia on the fetus. 1. Oxygen tension. Am J Obstet Gynecol 109: 628–637
32. Comline R S, Silver M 1970 Daily changes in fetal and maternal blood of conscious pregnant ewes with catheters in umbilical and uterine vessels. J Physiol 209: 567–586
33. Hill E P, Power G G, Longo L D 1973 A mathematical model of carbon dioxide transfer in the placenta and its interaction with oxygen. Am J Physiol 224: 283–299
34. Greiss F C 1972 Differential reactivity of the myoendometrial and placental vasculatures: adrenergic responses. Am J Obstet Gynecol 112: 20–30
35. Wallenberg H C S, Hutchinson D L 1979 A radioangiographic study of the effects of catecholamines on uteroplacental blood flow in the rhesus monkey. J Med Primatol 8: 57–65
36. Venuto R C, Cox J W, Stein J H, Ferris T F 1976 The effect of changes in perfusion pressure on uteroplacental blood flow in the pregnant rabbit. J Clin Invest 57: 938–944
37 Skjöldebrand A, Eklund J, Johansson H, Lunell N O, Nylund L, Sarby B, Thornström S 1990 Uteroplacental blood flow measured by placental scintigraphy during epidural anaesthesia for caesarean section. Acta Anesthesiol Scand 34: 79–84
38. Wallenberg H C S, Mazer J, Hutchinson D L 1973 Effects of a beta-adrenergic agent (metaproterenol) on uteroplacental circulation. Am J Obstet Gynecol 117: 1067–1075
39. Lippert T H, De Grandi P B, Fridrich R 1976 Actions of the uterine relaxant, fenoterol, on uteroplacental hemodynamics in human subjects. Am J Obstet Gynecol 125: 1093–1098
40. Youngstrom P, Hoyt M, Veille J C, Cohen I, Amini S, Herman M 1990 Effects of intravenous test dose epinephrine on fetal sheep during acute fetal stress and acidosis. Reg Anesth 15: 237–241
41. Ramanathan S, Grant G J 1988 Vasopressor therapy for hypotension due to epidural anesthesia for cesarean section. Acta Anaesthesiol Scand 32: 559–565
42. Naden R P, Rosenfeld C R 1981 Effect of angiotensin II on uterine and systemic vasculature in pregnant sheep. J Clin Invest 68: 468–474
43. Hariharan S, Tseng H, Myers S 1987 A comparison of the hemodynamic responses of systemic and uteroplacental vasculature to angiotensin in conscious guinea pigs. Am J Perinatol 4: 235–239
44. Rosenfeld C R, Barton M D, Meschia G 1976 Effects of epinephrine on distribution of blood flow in the pregnant ewe. Am J Obstet Gynecol 124: 156–163
45. Rankin J H G, Berssenbrugge A, Anderson D, Phernetton T M 1976 Ovine placental vascular responses to indomethacin. Am J Physiol 236: H61–H64
46. Clark K E, Austin J E, Seeds A E 1982 Effect of bisenoic prostaglandins and arachidonic acid on the uterine vasculature of pregnant sheep. Am J Obstet Gynaecol 142: 261–268
47. Landauer M, Phernetton T M, Parisi V M, Clark K E, Rankin J H G 1985 Ovine placental vascular response to the local application of prostacyclin. Am J Obstet Gynecol 151: 460–464
48. McLaughlin M K, Brennan S C, Chez R A 1978 Effects of indomethacin on sheep uteroplacental circulations and sensitivity to angiotensin II. Am J Obstet Gynecol 132: 430–435
49. Anderson D, Berssenbrugge A, Phernetton T, Rankin J H G 1978 Effects of angiotensin II on ovine placental blood flow. Proc Soc Exp Biol Med 158: 54–58
50. Berssenbrugge A, Anderson D, Phernetton T, Rankin J H G 1978 The effect of prostaglandin E_2 and indomethacin on the placental vascular response to norepinephrine. Proc Soc Exp Biol Med 159: 281–285
51. Seino M, Carretero O A, Albertini R, Scicli A G 1982 Kinins in regulation of uteroplacental blood flow in the pregnant rabbit. Am J Physiol 242: H142–H147
52. Landauer M, Phernetton T M, Rankin J H G 1986 Maternal ovine placental vascular responses to adenosine. Am J Obstet Gynecol 154: 1152–1155
53. Parisi V M, Rankin J H G 1985 The effect of prostacyclin on angiotensin II-induced placental vasoconstriction. Am J Obstet Gynecol 151: 444–449
54. Ylikorkala O, Jouppila P, Kirkinen P, Viinikka L 1983 Maternal prostacyclin, thromboxane, and placental blood flow. Am J Obstet Gynecol 145: 730–732
55. Jouppila P, Kirkinen P, Koivula A, Ylikorkala O 1985 Failure of exogenous prostacyclin to change placental and fetal blood flow in preeclampsia. Am J Obstet Gynecol 151: 661–665
56. Chemtob S, Potvin W, Varma D R 1989 Selective increase in placental blood flow by atrial natriuretic peptide in hypertensive rats. Am J Obstet Gynecol 160: 477–479
57. Reid D L, Goodfriend T L, Hollister M C, Phernetton T M, Rankin J H G 1989 Effects of atrial natriuretic factor on maternal ovine vascular resistance. J Dev Physiol 11: 25–28
58. Rekonen A, Luotola H, Pitkänen M, Kuikka J, Pyörälä T 1976 Measurement of intervillous and myometrial blood flow by an intravenous ^{133}Xe method. Br Obstet Gynaecol 83: 723–728
59. Olkkonen H, Suonio S, Lahtinen T, Penttilä I M 1977 Comparison of ^{113m}In and ^{113}Xe i.v. injection methods for evaluation of placental blood flow. Int J Nucl Med Biol 4: 179–183
60. Schröder H, Voss G, Leichtweiss H P 1984 Washout of xenon-133 from isolated guinea-pig placenta. Gynaecol Obstet Invest 17: 25–35
61. Schmitt R M, Kurz C S, Giese W W 1984 Evaluation of the Xe-133 clearance method for indirect placental blood flow determination. Placenta 5: 495–512
62. Käär K, Jouppila P, Kuikka J, Luotola H, Toivanen J, Rekonen A 1980 Intervillous blood flow in normal and complicated late pregnancy measured by means of an intravenous ^{133}Xe method. Acta Obstet Gynaecol Scand 59: 7–10
63. Bieniarz J, Crottogini J J, Curuchet E, Romero-Salinas G,

Yoshida T, Poseiro J J, Caldeyro-Baracia R 1968 Aortocaval compression by the uterus in late human pregnancy. Am J Obstet Gynecol 100: 203–217
64. Lehtovirta P, Fross M 1978 The acute effect of smoking on intervillous blood flow of the placenta. Br J Obstet Gynaecol 85: 729–731
65. Rauramo I, Forss M 1988 Effect of exercise on maternal hemodynamics and placental blood flow in healthy women. Acta Obstet Gynecol Scand 67: 21–25
66. Conrad E E, Faber J J 1977 Water and electrolyte acquisition across the placenta of the sheep. Am J Physiol 233: H475–H487
67. Rankin J H G, Phernetton T M 1978 Alpha and angiotensin receptor tone in the near-term sheep fetus. Proc Soc Exp Biol Med 158: 166–169
68. Adamson S L, Morrow R J, Bull S B, Langille B L 1989 Vasomotor responses of the umbilical circulation in fetal sheep. Am J Physiol 256: R1056–R1062
69. Rurak D W, Gruber N C 1984 The effect of vasopressin on fetal oxygenation in sheep. Can J Physiol Pharmacol 62: 27–30
70. Tomita H, Brace R A, Cheung C Y, Longo L D 1985 Vasopressin dose–response effects on fetal vascular pressures, heart rate, and blood volume. Am J Physiol 249: H974–H980
71. Linderkamp O 1982 Placental transfusion: determinants and effects. Clin Perinatol 9: 559–592
72. Erskine L 1987 Placental compliance – inferences from Doppler studies of umbilical blood flow during cardiac arrhythymia. Acta Obstet Gynaecol Scand 66: 301–304
73. Panizza V H G, Benedetti W L, Alvarez H 1976 Critical closing pressure in the fetal vessels of the human placenta in vitro. Reproduction 3: 97–105
74. Tulenko T N 1979 Regional sensitivity to vasoactive polypeptides in the human umbilicoplacental vasculature. Am J Obstet Gynecol 135: 629–636
75. Glance D G, Elder M G, Bloxam D L, Myatt L 1984 The effects of the components of the renin–angiotensin system on the isolated perfused human placental cotyledon. Am J Obstet Gynecol 149: 450–454
76. Hosokawa T, Howard R B, Maguire M H 1985 Conversion of angiotensin I to angiotensin II in the human foetoplacental vascular bed. Br J Pharmacol 84: 237–241
77. Wilkes B M, Krim E, Mento P F 1985 Evidence for a functional renin–angiotensin system in full-term fetoplacental unit. Am J Physiology 249: E366–E373
78. Tulenko T N 1981 The actions of prostaglandins and cyclo-oxygenase inhibition on the resistance vessels supplying the human fetal placenta. Prostaglandins 21: 1033–1043
79. Mak K K, Gude N M, Walters W A W, Boura A L A 1984 Effects of vasoactive autacoids on the human umbilical–fetal placental vasculature. Br J Obstet Gynaecol 91: 99–106
80. Howard R B, Hosokawa T, Maguire M H 1986 Pressor and depressor actions of prostanoids in the intact human fetoplacental bed. Prostaglandins Leukotrienes Med 21: 323–330
81. De Moura R S 1987 Effect of prostacyclin on the perfusion pressure and on the vasoconstrictor response of angiotensin II in the human isolated foetal placental circulation. Br J Clin Pharmacol 23: 765–768
82. Glance D G, Elder M G, Myatt L 1986 The actions of prostaglandins and their interactions with angiotensin II in the isolated perfused human placental cotyledon. Br J Obstet Gynaecol 93: 488–494
83. Wilkes B M, Mento P F 1988 Bradykinin-induced vasoconstriction and thromboxane release in perfused human placenta. Am J Physiol 254: E681–E686
84. Glance D G, Elder M G, Myatt L 1985 Prostaglandin production and stimulation by angiotensin II in the isolated perfused human placental cotyledon. Am J Obstet Gynecol 151: 387–391
85. Thorp J A, Walsh S W, Brath P C 1988 Comparison of the vasoactive effects of leukotrienes with thromboxane mimic in the perfused human placenta. Am J Obstet Gynecol 159: 1376–1380
86. Krygicz J, Urban J, Malofiejew M 1978 Influence of adenosine on contractility of isolated vessels of human placenta. Am J Obstet Gynecol 131: 587–589
87. Rankin J H G, Phernetton T 1976 Circulatory responses of the near-term sheep fetus to prostaglandin E_2. Am J Physiol 231: 760–765
88. Rankin J H G, Phernetton T 1978 Alpha and angiotensin receptor tone in the near-term sheep fetus. Proc Soc Exp Biol Med 158: 166–169
89. Rankin J H G, Berssenbrugge A, Anderson D, Phernetton T 1979 Ovine placental vascular responses to indomethacin. Am J Physiol 236: H61–H64
90. Parisi V M, Walsh S W 1989 Fetal vascular responses to prostacyclin. Am J Obstet Gynecol 160: 871–878
91. Parisi V M, Walsh S W 1989 Fetal placental vascular responses to prostacyclin after angiotensin II-induced vasoconstriction. Am J Physiol 257: E102–E107
92. Parisi V M, Walsh S W 1989 Fetoplacental vascular responses to prostacyclin after thromboxane-induced vasoconstriction. Am J Obstet Gynecol 160: 502–507
93. Trudinger B J, Connelly A J, Giles W B, Hales J R, Wilcox G R 1989 The effects of prostacyclin and thromboxane analogue (U46619) on the fetal circulation and umbilical flow velocity waveforms. J Dev Physiol 11: 179–184
94. van Vugt J M G, Hasaart T H M, Ruissen C J, Hoogland H J, Hoeks A P G, de Haan J 1988 Pulsatility index and its relationship to placental vascular resistance during partial umbilical venous occlusion: a study in fetal lambs. Gynecol Obstet Invest 26: 1–7
95. Maulik D, Yarlagadda P, Nathanielsz P W, Figueroa J P 1989 Hemodynamic validation of Doppler assessment of fetoplacental circulation in a sheep model system. J Ultrasound Med 8: 177–181
96. Kurjak A, Rajhvajn B 1982 Ultrasonic measurements of umbilical blood flow in normal and complicated pregnancies. J Perinat Med 10: 3–16
97. Veille J C, Tavill M, Sivakoff M, Cohen I, Ben-Ami M, Yang Y C, Jovkovsky V 1989 Evaluation of pulsed Doppler echocardiography for measurement of aortic blood flow in the fetal lamb. Am J Obstet Gynecol 161: 1610–1614
98. Nimrod C, Clapp J, Larrow R, D'Alton M, Persaud D 1989 Simultaneous use of Doppler ultrasound and electromagnetic flow probes in fetal flow assessment. J Ultrasound Med 8: 201–205
99. Trudinger B J, Stevens D, Connelly A, Hales J R, Alexander G, Bradley L, Fawcett A, Thompson R S 1989 Umbilical artery flow velocity waveform and placental resistance: the effects of embolization of the umbilical circulation. Am J Obstet Gynecol 157: 1443–1448
100. Morrow R J, Adamson S L, Bull S B, Ritachie J W K 1989 Effects of placental embolization on the umbilical arterial velocity waveform in fetal sheep. Am J Obstet Gynecol 161: 1055–1060
101. Giles W B, Trudinger B J, Baird P J 1985 Fetal umbilical artery flow velocity waveforms and placental resistance: pathological correlation. Br J Obstet Gynaecol 92: 31–38
102. McCowan L M, Mullen B M, Ritchie K 1987 Umbilical artery flow velocity waveforms and the placental vascular bed. Am J Obstet Gynecol 157: 900–902
103. Berkowitz G S, Mehalek K E, Chitkara U, Rosenberg J, Cogswell C, Berkowitz R L 1988 Doppler umbilical velocimetry in the prediction of adverse outcome in pregnancies at risk for intrauterine growth retardation Obstet Gynaecol 71: 742–746
104. Al-Ghazali W, Chapman M G, Allan L D 1988 Doppler assessment of the cardiac and uteroplacental circulation in normal and complicated pregnancies. Br J Obstet Gynaecol 95: 575–580
105. Hanretty K P, Primrose M H, Neilson J P, Whittle M 1989 Pregnancy screening by Doppler uteroplacental and umbilical artery waveforms. Br J Obstet Gynaecol 96: 1163–1167
106. Gudmundsson S, Marsal K 1988 Umbilical and uteroplacental blood flow velocity waveforms in pregnancies with fetal growth retardation. Eur J Obstet Reprod Biol 27: 187–196
107. Rankin J H G, McLaughlin M K 1979 The regulation of the placental blood flows. J Dev Physiol 1: 3–30
108. Parisi V M, Walsh S W 1986 Arachidonic acid metabolites and the regulation of placental and other vascular tone during pregnancy. Semin Perinatol 10: 288–298
109. West J B, Dollery C T, Naimark A 1964 Distribution of bloodflow in isolated lung: relation to vascular and alveolar pressure. J Appl Physiol 19: 713–724

110. Power G G, Longo S D 1973 Sluice flow in placenta: maternal vascular pressure effects on fetal circulation. Am J Physiol 225: 1490–1496
111. Power G G, Gilbert R D 1977 Umbilical vascular compliance in sheep. Am J Physiol 233: H660–H664
112. Marx G F, Patel S, Berman J, Farmakides G, Schulman H 1986 Umbilical blood flow velocity waveforms in different maternal positions and with epidural analgesia. Obstet Gynecol 68: 61–64
113. Thornberg K L, Bissonnette J M, Faber J J 1976 Absence of fetal placental waterfall phenomenon in chronically prepared fetal lambs. Am J Physiol 230: 886–892
114. Hasaart T H M, de Haan J 1985 Depression of uterine blood flow during total umbilical cord occlusion in sheep. Europ J Obstet Gynec Reprod Biol 19: 125–131
115. Power G G, Dale P S, Nelson P S 1981 Distribution of maternal and fetal blood flow within cotyledons of the sheep placenta. Am J Physiol 241: H486–H496
116. Stock M K, Reid D L, Phernetton T M, Rankin J H G 1989 Matching of maternal and fetal flow ratios in the sheep placenta. J Dev Physiol 11: 29–35
117. Power G G, Longo L D, Wagner H N, Kuhl D E, Forster R E, 1967 Uneven distribution of maternal and fetal placental blood flow, as demonstrated using macroaggregates, and its response to hypoxia. J Clin Invest 46: 2053–2063
118. Rankin J H G, Phernetton T M 1976 Effect of prostaglandin E_2 on ovine maternal placental blood flow. Am J Physiol 231: 754–759
119. McLaughlin M K, Brennan S C, Chez R A 1978 Vasoconstricive effects of prostaglandins in sheep placental circulations. Am J Obstet Gynecol 130: 408–413
120. Fidler J, Bennet M J, deSwiet M, Ellis C, Lewis P J 1980 Treatment of pregnancy hypertention with prostacyclin. Lancet 2: 31–32
121. Lewis P J, Shepard G L, Ritter J et al 1981 Prostacylin and pre-eclampsia. Lancet 1: 559

PART B
UTEROPLACENTAL AND FETAL HEMODYNAMICS: EFFECTS OF OBSTETRIC ANALGESIA AND ANESTHESIA

R. Jouppila S. Alahuhta P. Jouppila

INTRODUCTION

An adequate uteroplacental and fetal blood flow during labor and cesarean delivery is of prime importance for fetal well-being and neonatal outcome. Uteroplacental perfusion varies directly with the perfusion pressure and indirectly with the vascular resistance. During pregnancy, labor, and delivery, there are many factors which can potentially modify these components and thus the uteroplacental and fetal hemodynamics.

Maternal stress and pain during labor causes increased sympaticoadrenal activity and catecholamine secretion, which cause vasoconstriction, decreased uteroplacental blood flow and fetal distress.[1]

In high-risk pregnancies, i.e. preeclampsia, the placental blood flow is decreased[2] as a consequence of the vasoconstriction and hypovolemia typical in these patients. In addition, the fetal blood flow has been shown to be significantly decreased in pregnancies in which there is fetal growth retardation and asphyxia.[3,4]

Obstetric analgesia and anesthesia can potentially alter placental and fetal hemodynamics. The risks associated with pain relief include maternal hypotension after epidural and spinal anesthesia, direct toxic effects of the analgesic or anesthetic agents on the fetus and vasoconstriction in the uteroplacental and fetal vessels. Thus, knowledge of the effects of obstetric anesthesia on placental and fetal blood flow, is an important guideline when assessing the safety of these methods.

METHODS FOR MEASURING UTEROPLACENTAL AND FETAL BLOOD FLOW

Isotope techniques

Many of the placental blood flow studies during obstetric analgesia and anesthesia in humans have been performed using the intravenous ^{133}Xe technique described by Rekonen et al 1976.[5] This radionuclide is diffusible; the patient holds her breath for 20 s after intravenous injection of the isotope to diminish the escape of the tracer through the lungs. The radionuclide enters the placenta as a bolus. Its removal from the placental area is then registered with a scintillation detector. Both the myometrial and intervillous blood flow (IVBF) can be calculated from a biexponential clearance curve.

Another non-invasive isotope technique, functional placental scintigraphy, was described in 1983 by Nylund et al.[6] This method measures the total placental blood flow expressed as an uteroplacental blood flow index. Intravenously injected ^{113}In and computer-linked scintillation camera are used.

Doppler and color Doppler ultrasonic methods

Doppler studies have been widely used during the last few years for the examination of the uterine, umbilical and fetal circulation. It is possible to use either continuous or pulsed Doppler methods in obstetric blood flow studies. Using a pulsed system combined with real-time imaging, it is possible to measure blood flow velocities precisely from the vessel of interest by putting the 'sample volume' of the Doppler beam on the right area. Methodologically, it is preferable to a continuous wave system, as this allows a more reliable determination of velocities and flow. In the continuous method, the clinician must recognize patterns of flow and infer the location and identity of the vessels on the recognition of flow velocity pattern alone. With both systems, the Doppler shifts of the reflected signals are in correlation with the blood flow velocity and are displayed on a real-time spectrum analyzer.

Because the measurement of blood flow volume (ml/min per kg fetal body weight) in fetal vessels is subject to many potential methodologic errors, the main interest during the last few years has been focused on the examination of blood velocity waveforms in the pulsatile fetal and uterine vessels. The blood velocity waveform in the arteries is influenced by many regulatory factors such as the contraction of the heart, the compliance of the vessel walls, the distance from the heart and, especially, the peripheral vascular resistance. A typical finding for a normal physiologic condition is a low peripheral vascular resistance in the fetal vessels, which is detectable as a continuous and relatively high end-diastolic velocity. If the resistance against the bloodstream is increased, it can be recognized by decreased or absent blood flow velocity at end-diastole (Fig. 9.2). As signs of a redistribution of fetal blood flow from peripheral tissues to central circulation or as markers of increased placental resistance, these visual findings in the fetal aorta or umbilical artery form the basis for clinical evaluation. Similar calculations are also possible in the main uterine and arcuate arteries and fetal cerebral and kidney arteries. The exact evaluation of specific indices [pulsatility (PI), resistance (RI), A/B index (A/B)] gives more detailed information on the blood velocity waveforms.

The indices used in the evaluation of vascular resistance are independent of insonation angle, and so methodologic errors in the repeated examination of a vessel, e.g. the umbilical artery, are of the order of 5–10%. The use of a color Doppler technique has markedly increased the possibilities for the exact location of short and small vessels and

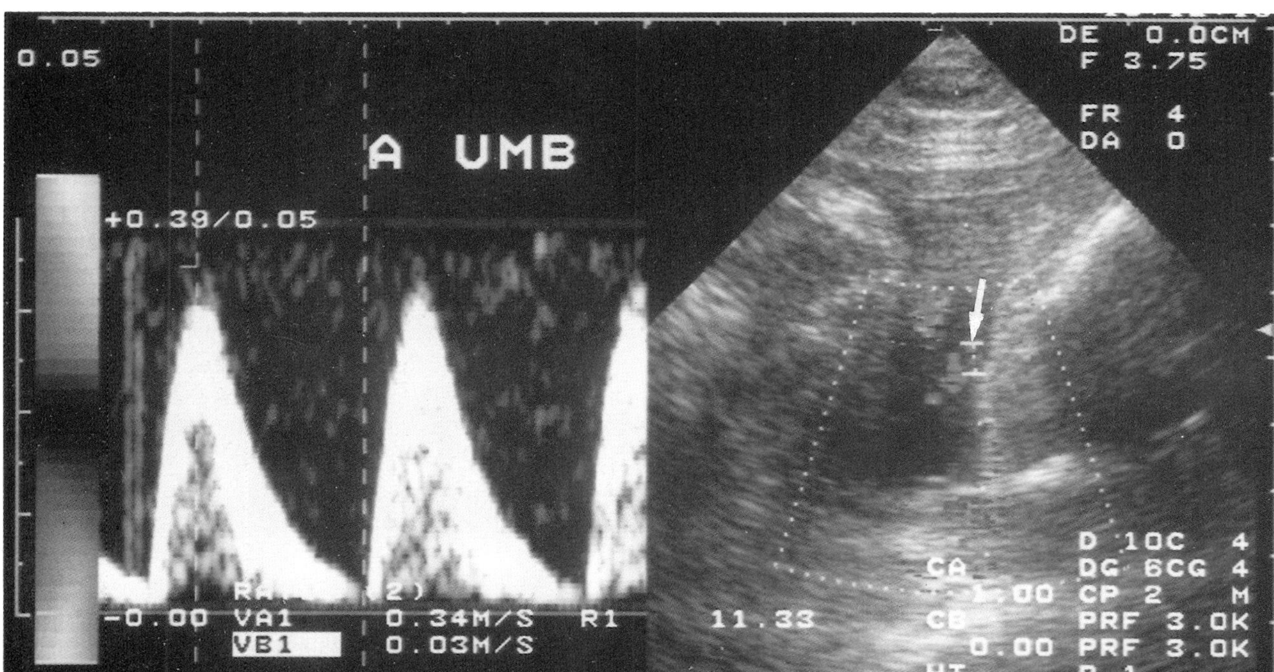

Fig. 9.2 Blood velocity waveform from the umbilical artery. The increased vascular resistance is reflected as low end-diastolic velocity. The sample volume is put on the artery (arrow) according to the information of the color display.

so has improved the accuracy of measurement. Currently, the versatile evaluation of fetal cardiac function is possible by the combination of Doppler and color Doppler methods.

Pathologically high index values in uterine and umbilical arteries have been found as a sensitive and early warning signal with a high positive predictive value for fetal distress.[7] These values have also been used in studies in which the effects of vasoactive agents given to the mother have been studied in the uterine and fetal circulation.[8] Thus, at the present time, the Doppler method is the method of choice when assessing the effects of different obstetric anesthetic methods on uteroplacental and fetal circulation.

THE EFFECT OF PAIN RELIEF DURING LABOR ON IVBF AND ON FETAL BLOOD FLOW

IVBF during epidural anesthesia in normal and preeclamptic pregnancies

The effect of epidural anesthesia on IVBF during labor has been widely studied with the ^{133}Xe method in the Oulu University Hospital, Finland. Segmental epidural anesthesia given at the T10–12 level with 4 ml of 0.5% bupivacaine plain or with bupivacaine–epinephrine did not significantly change the IVBF in normal labor.[9] The wider lumbar epidural block from T10–L3 with 10 ml of 0.25% bupivacaine or 2% chloroprocaine led to a significant improvement in IVBF in normal pregnancies.[10] In preeclamptic pregnancies, IVBF improved after segmental epidural anesthesia slightly, but insignificantly in most of the 11 parturients studied.[11] After extending the lumbar epidural anesthetic, IVBF improved significantly. The mean percentage increase was 70%.[12]

IVBF and paracervical block

The effect of a superficial and low-dosage technique of paracervical block on IVBF has been studied in 38 healthy parturients with normal pregnancy. IVBF did not significantly change after PCB with 25 mg of bupivacaine. In three cases with fetal bradycardia, the changes in IVBF were also minimal.[13]

Epidural anesthesia and umbilical and fetal blood flow measured by the Doppler ultrasonic method

The use of Doppler and color Doppler ultrasonic methods for the examination of blood flow volume and especially blood velocity waveforms in uterine, umbilical and fetal vessels have opened up many new possibilities for studies concerning the effects of obstetric analgesia and anesthesia on uteroplacental and fetal hemodynamics.

Marx et al[14] found a decrease in umbilicoplacental resistance 15 min after epidural analgesia during labor. No such effect could be verified by the work of Lindblad et al,[15] but they observed a significant increase in the volume of blood flow in the fetal descending aorta after epidural anesthesia. A similar change occurred in the group without any anesthesia. In the meperidine group, this increasing effect could not be verified and the fetal pulse frequency decreased significantly. A tendency of fetal aortic blood flow to decrease in a small group with paracervical block was observed. The authors concluded that epidural anesthesia correlated well with the fetal hemodynamic responses of normal labor.

In another study by Marx et al[16] umbilical artery blood velocity A/B ratios decreased after epidural anesthesia with 8 ml of lidocaine plain (15 cases). The injection of lidocaine with epinephrine produced identical results in fetuses with initially normal A/B ratios (10 cases). In contrast, all six fetuses with initially high A/B ratios who received the epinephrine-containing anesthetic reacted with a rise in the ratio, and two of them developed transient heart rate decelerations. The authors concluded that when there is an abnormally high umbilical artery blood flow resistance, the addition of epinephrine to epidurally administered local anesthetics increases the stress to the fetus. In the recent study of Hughes et al[17] no changes were observed in the indices of uterine and umbilical arteries when epidural anesthesia with 0.25% bupivacaine was given to healthy parturients despite the moderate fall in maternal blood pressure.

The effects of epidural opioid administration on maternal uterine and fetal umbilical artery blood flow dynamics were studied during the first stage of labor by Alahuhta et al.[18] The patients were given either 12 ml 0.25% bupivacaine or 50 μg sufentanil in a double-blind randomized fashion. The authors found no significant changes in any of the blood flow velocity waveform indices measured after the administration of either drug and concluded that epidural sufentanil can provide adequate analgesia without adverse vascular effects in the uterine and umbilicoplacental circulation.

THE EFFECT OF DIFFERENT ANESTHETIC METHODS ON UTEROPLACENTAL AND FETAL BLOOD FLOW DURING CESAREAN DELIVERY

IVBF during cesarean delivery: effect of spinal, epidural and general anesthesia

In a study by Jouppila et al[19] the effects of spinal anesthesia on IVBF using 0.5% bupivacaine after acute hydration with Ringer's lactate solution 1500–2000 ml i.v. was estimated in nine patients undergoing elective cesarean delivery. Ephedrine infusion, 50 mg in 500 ml, was instituted at the first sign of maternal hypotension in seven patients. Although significant decreases in mean maternal systolic and diastolic arterial pressure were recorded, the individual decreases in pressure were less than 30 mmHg in all except two patients. In general, IVBF did not change during spinal anesthesia, although there was a marked flow increase in one patient with toxemia of pregnancy and a decrease in one woman with diabetes mellitus.

Epidural anesthesia with 16–20 ml of 1.5% lidocaine with epinephrine 5 μg/ml after an acute infusion of 500 ml of 3.5% gelatin solution (Haemaccel) and 1 l of Ringer's solution led to a nonsignificant mean decrease (13%) in IVBF from the control value in nine healthy women undergoing elective cesarean delivery as demonstrated by Jouppila et al.[20] Huovinen et al[21] found a significant decrease in maternal blood pressure and a nonsignificant decrease in IVBF during epidural anesthesia for cesarean delivery without an acute infusion. When an acute infusion of a plasma expander (Haemaccel), 10 ml per kg body weight, was given with epidural anesthesia the maternal blood pressure and IVBF were unchanged. Hollmèn et al[22] investigating the effect of intravenous prophylactic ephedrine 15 mg during epidural anesthesia for cesarean delivery found no significant differences in IVBF before and after the initiation of the block. These patients received an acute infusion of 30 ml per kg body weight. Later Skjöldebrand[23] studied the uteroplacental blood flow during epidural anesthesia for cesarean delivery using functional placental scintigraphy by ^{113}In. He observed that by increasing the volume of acute hydration from 10 to 20 ml per kg body weight the maternal blood pressure and uteroplacental circulation was maintained during epidural anesthesia.

General anesthesia led to a significant decrease in IVBF in the study of Jouppila et al[24] in which the IVBF was measured before and after the induction of general anesthesia with thiopental in healthy mothers.

The effect of spinal and epidural anesthesia on the uterine and fetal blood flow during cesarean delivery: experiences with the Doppler method

The effect of spinal anesthesia for cesarean delivery on umbilical and fetal blood flow was first studied by Lindblad et al[25] in 15 nonlaboring parturients using pulsed Doppler ultrasonography. All patients received 2 l of lactated Ringer's solution before the subarachnoid block. An intravenous infusion of ephedrine was used to maintain maternal blood pressure within 90% of the preanesthetic level. There were no significant changes in blood flow volume after spinal anesthesia at either the fetal aorta or the umbilical vein. There was, however, a significant increase in fetal heart rate 30 mins after instituting the ephedrine infusion. The PI measured at the fetal aorta actually decreased – possibly indicating a decrease of downstream resistance in fetal peripheral arteries. A significant decrease was also observed in PI of umbilical arteries, reflecting a decrease in fetoplacental vascular resistance.

Fairlie et al[26] recorded the umbilical artery Doppler flow velocity waveforms during spinal anesthesia prior to elective cesarean delivery in 15 uncomplicated pregnancies. Although spinal anesthesia was associated with a significant fall in maternal systolic and diastolic blood pressure, there was no change in the umbilical artery PI either after actually expanding the maternal circulation with 750–1000 ml of Hartman's solution or for the first 15 mins after subarachnoid injection of 0.5% bupivacaine. The fetal heart rate fell after acute hydration, but was unchanged by the administration of bupivacaine. The investigators also found a weak negative correlation between fetal heart rate and the umbilical artery PI and concluded that in normal pregnancy spinal anesthesia has no detrimental effect on the umbilical artery PI.

Vasopressors given for the treatment of maternal hypotension due to regional anesthesia may modify the uterine and fetal circulation. Räsänen et al[27] recorded an increase in the ratios of the uterine artery blood velocity after treatment of hypotension with two vasopressors, ephedrine and etilefrine, during spinal anesthesia for cesarean delivery. Neither drug had any effect on the vascular resistance of the umbilical artery but ephedrine increased myocardial contractility in the fetal right ventricle and decreased vascular resistance in the kidney and middle cerebral arteries. Vasopressors with predominant alpha-adrenergic activity such as phenylephrine have been considered contraindicated because of a fear of uterine vasoconstriction and reduced uteroplacental perfusion. Our team[28] has measured blood flow velocity waveforms in uteroplacental and fetal vessels during the prophylactic infusion of phenylephrine and ephedrine in healthy parturients undergoing cesarean delivery under spinal anesthesia. Phenylephrine administration resulted in an increase in the Doppler ratios for the uterine and placental arcuate arteries while the indices remained unchanged in the ephedrine group. This study suggests that phenylephrine does not seem to be the ideal vasopressor due to its untoward effects on the uteroplacental circulation, and encourages the use of ephedrine as the drug of choice in treating maternal hypotension during obstetric regional anesthesia.

The effects of epidural anesthesia for cesarean delivery on the fetal hemodynamics have been studied by the Doppler method during the last few years. Lindblad et al[29] compared three anesthetic agents – 1.5% etidocaine, 0.5% bupivacaine and 0.5% bupivacaine with epinephrine in healthy mothers at elective Cesarean deliveries. No changes could be observed in the volume blood flow of the umbilical vein. In the fetal aorta, the blood flow increased in the bupivacaine with epinephrine group, but was not affected by the other anesthetic agents. Maternal blood pressure was maintained in this study by acute hydration with 500–1000 ml of a balanced electrolyte solution and ephedrine i.v. if needed. Giles et al[30] studied the effects of acute hydration with crystalloid and epidural anesthesia with 0.5% bupivacaine on the uterine arcuate and umbilical artery vascular resistance. Both acute infusion and epidural block were associated with a decrease in systolic/diastolic velocity ratios of both of these arteries. On the contrary, no changes in uterine and umbilical artery resistance were noted after epidural anesthesia or after acute volume expansion in the studies of Long and Price[31] and Petrikowski et al.[32] No alterations were also observed by Veille et al[33] and Morrow et al[34] when using bupivacaine or bupivacaine with epinephrine as anesthetic agents for cesarean deliveries. In the study of Baumann et al[35] the effects of 0.5% bupivacaine used in epidural anesthesia on the uteroplacental and umbilical blood velocities were studied. A significant decrease in maternal diastolic blood pressure was associated with the increased resistance in the uterine arteries after anesthesia. The indices in the umbilical arteries were unaffected.

Our team has recently found no changes in the maternal and fetal (umbilical, middle cerebral, kidney) hemodynamics during epidural anesthesia with either 0.5% bupivacaine plain[36] or with epinephrine[37] in healthy mothers undergoing cesarean delivery, while in hypertensive parturients the blood flow velocity waveform indices in the uterine and placental arcuate arteries increased after epidural bupivacaine with epinephrine administration[38]. The use of bupivacaine plain was not associated with any hemodynamic changes in the uteroplacental and fetal arteries and it can be recommended as a safe anesthetic technique in this respect for anesthesia in pregnancies complicated by hypertensive disorders.

CONCLUSIONS AND DISCUSSION

The studies on uteroplacental, umbilical and fetal circulation evaluate the effects of potentially vasoactive agents, such as the different forms of obstetric analgesia and anesthesia. The introduction of Doppler methods combined recently with color display has enabled investigators to pinpoint the exact location of the vessels of interest and simultaneously to provide noninvasive documentation of changes in hemodynamic events. This method has replaced the earlier isotope methods used. However, many methodologic problems exist and are also of concern with the Doppler methods. It is not possible to separate the placental and myometrial blood flow in studies on uterine circulation. The measurement of indices of blood velocity waveforms reflects the peripheral vascular resistance but the exact determination of blood flow volume in different vessels is problematic with Doppler. Physiologically, it is unclear whether or not the vasodilator and vasoconstrictor changes produced in the fetal circulation by some vasoactive agent given to the mother are beneficial to fetal homeostasis because the role of many other fetal compensatory mechanisms (changes in blood pressure, oxygen metabolism, etc.) is difficult to assess in human studies. The fetal tolerance of hemodynamic changes in the uterine circulation is individual and dependent on the primary condition of the parturient.

According to the results obtained by isotope and Doppler methods from the uterine and fetal circulation, epidural analgesia and anesthesia appear to be safe methods when used for pain relief during labor or cesarean delivery in healthy mothers. The prophylactic methods used for avoidance of maternal hypotension seem to also protect the uterine circulation from significant disturbances when spinal anesthesia is used for cesarean delivery. The preliminary results obtained by using vasopressors for the treatment of maternal hypotension have demonstrated modifying vasoactive effects on the fetal circulation. The Doppler method has opened up new areas for the study of human uterine and fetal hemodynamics and has markedly increased our knowledge of their physiologic adaptation. This method is also very suitable for testing the safety of new anesthetic methods and analgesic agents for obstetric practice.

REFERENCES

1. Redick L F 1982 Epidural analgesia. Clin Perinatol 9: 63
2. Käär K, Luotola H, Jouppila P et al 1980 Placental blood flow by an intravenous ^{133}Xe method in complicated late pregnancy. Acta Obstet Gynecol Scand 59: 7
3. Jouppila P, Kirkinen P 1984 Increased vascular resistance in the descending aorta of the human fetus in hypoxia. Br J Obstet Gynaecol 91: 853
4. Rochelson B 1989 The clinical significance of absent end-diastolic velocity in the umbilical artery waveforms. Clin Obstet Gynaecol 32: 692
5. Rekonen A, Luotola H, Pitkänen M et al 1976 Measurement of intervillous and myometrial blood flow by an intravenous ^{133}Xe method. Br J Obstet Gynaecol 83: 723
6. Nylund L, Lunell N O, Sarby B et al 1983 Functional placental scintigraphy. Acta Radiol Diagn 24: 165
7. Schulman H, Fleisher A, Stern W et al 1984 Umbilical velocity wave ratios in human pregnancy. Am J Obstet Gynecol 148: 985
8. Jouppila P, Kirkinen P, Koivula A et al 1986 Labetalol does not alter the placental and fetal blood flow or maternal prostanoids in pre-eclampsia. Br J Obstet Gynaecol 93: 543
9. Jouppila R, Jouppila P, Hollmén A et al 1978 Effect of segmental extradural analgesia on placental blood flow during normal labour. Br J Anaesth 50: 563
10. Hollmén A, Jouppila R, Jouppila P et al 1982 Effect of extradural analgesia using bupivacaine and 2-chloroprocaine on intervillous blood flow during normal labour. Br J Anaesth 54: 837
11. Jouppila R, Jouppila P, Hollmén A et al 1979 Epidural analgesia and placental blood flow during labour in pregnancies complicated by hypertension. Br J Obstet Gynaecol 86: 969
12. Jouppila P, Jouppila R, Hollmén A et al 1982 Lumbar epidural

analgesia to improve intervillous blood flow during labour in severe pre-eclampsia. Obstet Gynaecol 59: 158
13. Puolakka J, Jouppila R, Jouppila P et al 1984 Maternal and fetal effects of low-dosage bupivacaine paracervical block. J Perinat Med 12: 75
14. Marx G F, Patel S, Berman J A et al 1986 Umbilical blood flow velocity waveforms in different maternal positions and with epidural analgesia. Obstet Gynaecol 68: 61
15. Lindblad A, Bernow J, Marsal K 1987 Obstetric analgesia and fetal aortic blood flow during labour. Br J Obstet Gynaecol 94: 306
16. Marx G F, Elstein I D, Schuss M et al 1990 Effects of epidural block with lignocaine and lignocaine–adrenaline on umbilical artery velocity wave ratios. Br J Obstet Gynaecol 97: 517
17. Hughes A B, Devoe L D, Wakefield M L et al 1990 The effects of epidural anesthesia on the Doppler velocimetry of umbilical and uterine arteries in normal term labor. Obstet Gynecol 75: 809
18. Alahuhta S, Räsänen J, Jouppila P et al 1993 Epidural sufentanil and bupivacaine for labor analgesia and Doppler velocimetry of the umbilical and uterine arteries. Anesthesiology 78: 231
19. Jouppila P, Jouppila R, Barinoff T et al 1984 Placental blood flow during caesarean section performed under subarachnoid blockade. Br J Anaesth 56: 1379
20. Jouppila R, Jouppila P, Kuikka J et al 1978 Placental blood flow during caesarean section under lumbar extradural anaesthesia. Br J Anaesth 50: 275
21. Huovinen K, Lehtovirta P, Forss M et al 1979 Changes in placental intervillous blood flow measured by the 133 Xenon method during lumbar epidural block for elective caesarean section. Acta Anaesthesiol Scand 23: 529
22. Hollmén A I, Jouppila R, Albright G A et al 1984 Intervillous blood flow during caesarean section with prophylactic ephedrine and epidural anaesthesia. Acta Anaesthesiol Scand 28: 396
23. Skjöldebrand A 1989 Uteroplacental blood flow during epidural anaesthesia for caesarean section. Measurement with functional placental scintigraphy. Kungl Carolinska Medic Chirurgiska Institutet Stockholm. Dissertation p 31
24. Jouppila P, Kuikka J, Jouppila R et al 1979 Effect of induction of general anaesthesia for caesarean section on intervillous blood flow. Acta Obstet Gynecol Scand 58: 249
25. Lindblad A, Bernow J, Marsal K 1988 Fetal blood flow during intrathecal anaesthesia for elective caesarean section. Br J Anaesth 61: 376
26. Fairlie F M, Kirkwood I, Lang G D et al 1990 Umbilical artery flow velocity waveforms during spinal anaesthesia. Eur J Obstet Gynaecol Reprod Biol 38: 3
27. Räsänen J, Alahuhta S, Kangas-Saarela T et al 1991 The effects of ephedrine and etilephrine on uterine and fetal blood flow and on fetal myocardial function during spinal anaesthesia for caesarean section. Int J Obstet Anesth 1: 3
28. Alahuhta S, Räsänen J, Jouppila P et al 1992 Ephedrine and phenylephrine for avoiding maternal hypotension due to spinal anaesthesia for Caesarean section. Int J Obstet Anesth 1: 129
29. Lindblad A, Bernow J, Vernersson E et al 1987 Effects of extradural anesthesia on human fetal blood flow in utero. Br J Anaesthesiol 59: 1265
30. Giles W B, Lah F X, Trudinger B 1987 The effect of epidural anaesthesia for Caesarean section on maternal uterine and fetal umbilical artery blood flow velocity waveforms. Br J Obstet Gynaecol 94: 55
31. Long M G, Price M 1988 Uteroplacental perfusion after epidural analgesia for elective Caesarean section. Br J Obstet Gynaecol 95: 1081
32. Petrikovsky B M, Cohen M, Tancer M L 1988 Uterine and umbilical blood flow during Caesarean section under epidural anesthesia. Acta Obstet Gynaecol Scan 67: 737
33. Veille J C, Yongstrom P, Kanaan C et al 1988 Human umbilical artery flow velocity waveforms before and after regional anesthesia for Caesarean section. Obstet Gynaecol 72: 890
34. Morrow R J, Rolbin S H, Knox Ritchie J W et al 1989 Epidural anaesthesia and blood flow velocity in mother and fetus. Can J Anaesth 36: 519
35. Baumann H, Alon E, Atanassoff P et al 1990 Effect of epidural anesthesia for Caesarean delivery on maternal femoral arterial and venous, uteroplacental and umbilical blood flow velocities and waveforms. Obstet Gynaecol 75: 194
36. Alahuhta S, Räsänen J, Jouppila R et al 1991 Uteroplacental and fetal haemodynamics during extradural anaesthesia for Caesarean section. Br J Anaesth. 66: 319
37. Alahuhta S, Räsänen J, Jouppila R et al 1991 Effects of extradural bupivacaine with adrenaline for Caesarean section on uteroplacental and fetal circulation. Br J Anaesth 67: 678
38. Alahuhta S, Räsänen J, Jouppila P et al 1993 Uteroplacental and fetal circulation during extradural bupivacaine–adrenaline and bupivacaine for Caesarean section in hypertensive pregnancies with chronic fetal asphyxia. Br J Anaesth 71 (in press)

10. Placental transfer of drugs

M. Finster H. Pedersen A. C. Santos

Most drugs, including anesthetic agents, cross the placenta with ease, and the growth of information in this field has been aided by the development of highly sensitive and specific techniques for drug analysis in biological fluids and tissues.

Since 1961, with the first demonstration of lidocaine in the umbilical cord blood of newborns whose mothers had received the drug for epidural analgesia during labor,[1] clinicians began to consider the potential for untoward neonatal effects if large amounts of local anesthetic were taken up by the fetus.[2] It was soon demonstrated that following repeated lumbar epidural or caudal injections of mepivacaine, fetal drug concentrations may become sufficiently elevated to result in neonatal depression, manifested by an Apgar score of 6 or less. It is recognized today that even low concentrations of some local anesthetic drugs can cause subtle changes in neonatal adaptive, neurological, or behavioral function, without affecting the Apgar score.[3,4] Since local anesthetics are probably the most commonly used drugs in obstetric anesthesia, their pharmacokinetic properties have been most thoroughly investigated, and often serve to illustrate the principles involved in perinatal pharmacology.

PLACENTAL TRANSFER

Amongst the factors influencing the placental transfer of drugs are the physicochemical characteristics of the compound itself, maternal drug concentrations in the plasma, the properties of the placenta itself, and the hemodynamic events within the fetomaternal unit.

Anesthetic agents in the maternal circulation traverse the placenta by simple diffusion, a process mainly governed by physiocochemical factors according to the Fick principle, which states that the rate of diffusion is a function of the concentration gradient of the free (unionized, not bound to plasma proteins) substance between maternal and fetal blood, the surface available for transfer, and the thickness of the membrane. The relation is expressed by the equation:

$$Q/t = \frac{K \cdot A\, C_m - C_f}{D}$$

where Q/t is the rate of diffusion, A is the surface area available for transfer, C_m is the free drug concentration in the maternal blood, C_f is the free drug concentration in the fetal blood, D is the thickness of the membrane, and K is the diffusion constant of the drug across the membrane.

The diffusion constant (K) of the drug depends on physicochemical characteristics such as molecular size, lipid solubility, and the degree of ionization.

Compounds with a molecular weight less than 500 daltons are unimpeded in crossing the placenta, whereas those with molecular weights of 500–1000 are more restricted. Most drugs commonly used by the anesthesiologist have molecular weights that permit easy transfer, as exemplified by the commonly used local anesthetics, which range between 220 and 325.

Drugs that are highly lipid soluble cross biologic membranes more readily, and the degree of ionization is important because the unionized moiety of a drug is more lipophilic than the ionized one. Local anesthetics and opioids are weak bases, with a relatively low degree of ionization, and considerable lipid solubility. In contrast, muscle relaxants are less lipophilic and more ionized. For this reason, it was thought formerly that muscle relaxants could not cross the placenta in significant amounts. However, more recently developed analytic techniques have shown measurable, but low, concentrations of pancuronium, atracurium and vecuronium in blood specimens taken from the umbilical vessels at delivery, even after the use of clinical doses of the drug.[5–8] This raises, at least in theory, the possibility of muscle weakness occurring in the newborn following large maternal doses of relaxants used to facilitate endotracheal intubation. Similarly, studies on rhesus monkeys have shown placental transmission of succinylcholine to be more rapid and extensive than previously believed.[9] In humans, succinylcholine given to a mother with atypical serum cholinesterase can cause neonatal flaccidity and apnea in atypical homozygous babies.[10] Heterozygous infants do not seem to be seriously affected.

More recently, it has been proposed that if the blood flow to the fetal side of the placenta can be measured, as it has in some animal studies, calculating the placental clearance is the more appropriate way of expressing drug transfer to the fetus.[11] At steady state:

$$\text{Cl} = \frac{Q_u\,(C_{uv} - C_{ua})}{C_{ma}}$$

where Cl is the clearance in volume/time, Q_u is the umbilical blood flow, C_{uv} is the umbilical vein drug concentration, C_{ua} is the umbilical artery drug concentration and C_{ma} is the maternal arterial drug concentration.

The relative concentrations of drug existing in the unionized and ionized forms can be predicted from the Henderson–Hasselbalch equation:

$$\text{pH} = \text{p}K_a + \log \frac{(\text{base})}{(\text{cation})}$$

The ratio of base to cation becomes particularly important in the case of local anesthetics, since it is the unionized form that penetrates tissue barriers, while the ionized form is pharmacologically active in blocking nerve conduction.

The pK_a is the pH value at which the concentrations of free base and cation are equal. For the amide local anesthetics, the pK_a values are sufficiently close to the physiologic pH that changes in maternal or fetal biochemical status may significantly alter the proportion of ionized and unionized drug present. At equilibrium, the concentrations of unionized drug in the fetal and maternal plasma are equal. In the case of the acidotic fetus, a greater tendency for drug to exist in the ionized form, which cannot diffuse back across the placenta into the maternal plasma, results in a larger total amount of drug accumulation in the fetal plasma. This is the mechanism for the phenomenon described as 'ion trapping'.[12] It is also responsible for the enhanced accumulation of local anesthetic in the tissues of acidotic fetuses.[13] Fetal acidosis should also increase the uptake of other basic drugs such as opioids.

Maternal blood concentration of drug

The driving force for the passage of drug across the placental membranes is the concentration gradient of free drug from maternal to fetal blood. While other variables in the Fick equation are beyond the clinician's control, the maternal blood concentration can be influenced to a considerable degree. It is determined by the interaction of the dose administered, the mode and site of administration, and, in the case of local anesthetics, the use of vasoconstrictors. Maternal drug concentration will also depend on the rate of distribution, metabolism, and excretion of the drug, which may vary according to the progress of gestation.

The rapid drop in plasma drug concentrations following intravenous bolus injection (e.g. thiopental) results in a correspondingly short time of exposure of the uterine contents to high blood levels of this depressant drug.[14,15] In contrast, the more sustained maintenance of anesthetic concentrations of the various maternally administered inhalation agents is associated with continued transfer of drug to the fetus.[16]

Higher doses will usually result in higher maternal blood concentrations, as illustrated by a study in which thiamylal was administered by intravenous injection to mothers undergoing elective cesarean delivery under general anesthesia.[15]

Under the controlled circumstances of a steady-state infusion of lidocaine, maternal and fetal blood concentrations of the drug at equilibrium were found to be proportionate to the amount administered. The drug was infused at two different rates to chronically instrumented pregnant ewes. At equilibrium, animals receiving lidocaine 0.1 mg kg/min had a mean arterial blood concentration of 1.56 μg/ml, and their fetuses 0.8 μg/ml.[17] The infusion rate of 0.2 mg kg/min resulted in almost double the maternal (2.5 μg/ml) and fetal (1.5 μg/ml) blood concentrations of lidocaine.[18]

Another important factor is the route of administration. Compared with other sites of injection, an intravenous bolus will result in the highest blood concentration of drug. This was documented in a study comparing maternal and fetal plasma levels of meperidine following intravenous, intramuscular or epidural injection (2 mg/kg over 60 s) to pregnant ewes.[19] Epidural injection resulted in mean peak maternal blood concentrations similar to those following intramuscular injection. Fetuses whose mothers were given the drug intravenously had significantly higher plasma concentrations of meperidine for at least 30 min compared with those whose mothers received the drug by the intramuscular or epidural route. It has also been shown that following an intravenous injection of meperidine during labor a greater proportion of the dose administered is transferred to the fetus than following an intramuscular injection.[20]

In general, the rate of absorption from the injection site is dependent on the vascularity of the tissues. For instance, the use of lidocaine for paracervical block during labor has been shown to result in detectable maternal blood levels of the drug as soon as 1 min after the injection, the peak concentration being reached by 9–10 min.[21] Similarly, in the baboon, the highest concentration of lidocaine following paracervical block occurs within 8 min.[22] Absorption from the lumbar epidural space tends to be somewhat slower. Injection of mepivacaine resulted in detectable maternal plasma concentrations after 7 min and peak concentrations at 25–40 min.[2] Injection of local anesthetic into the caudal rather than lumbar epidural space may lead to higher blood levels,[23] but this observation is probably of little clinical consequence.

Subarachnoid administration of local anesthetics has been thought to result in negligible plasma concentrations because of the small doses used and the relatively poor vascularity of this area. However, in a study involving pregnant patients undergoing cesarean delivery under spinal anesthesia, induced with lidocaine 75 mg, maternal plasma concentrations of the drug were similar to those reported by others following epidural anesthesia.[24] Furthermore, significant levels of the drug were found in the umbilical vein at birth. In nonpregnant patients, administration of lidocaine, 75 mg, for spinal or epidural anesthesia led to similar peak blood concentrations of the drug (0.32 and 0.41 μg/ml respectively).[25]

The rise in maternal blood concentrations following repeated administration of a drug depends, in great measure, on the dose and frequency of reinjection, as well as on the kinetic characteristics of the drug. The elimination half-life of amide local anesthetic agents is relatively high, so that repeated injection may lead to accumulation in the maternal plasma.[2] It would be expected that those amides having higher clearance, such as prilocaine, would accumulate less.[26] Epinephrine reduces the peak maternal local anesthetic concentration by 30–50% with lidocaine or mepivacaine, but has little effect on peak levels of bupivacaine or etidocaine.[27] On the other hand, 2-chloroprocaine, an ester local anesthetic, undergoes rapid enzymatic hydrolysis in the presence of pseudocholinesterase. In vitro studies have shown the half-life of this drug in the maternal serum to be 21 s.[28] Following epidural injection, the half-life in the mother was 2.94 min.[29] After reinjection, 2-chloroprocaine could be detected in the maternal plasma for 5–10 min only, and no accumulation was evident.[30] The discrepancy in the half-life between in vivo and in vitro studies can be ascribed to continued absorption of 2-chloroprocaine from the epidural space.

Pregnancy itself is associated with physiologic changes that may influence maternal pharmacokinetics and the action of anesthetic drugs. Furthermore, these changes are progressive during the course of gestation. There is a marked increase in cardiac output and blood volume beginning early in the first trimester.[31,32] The extravascular water content also increases during pregnancy.[33] Simultaneously with the increase in maternal plasma volume and body water, the concentrations of plasma albumin and α_1-glycoprotein decrease.[33,34] Thus, there should be an increase in the free fraction of the agent, which would be of particular importance for highly protein-bound compounds. Indeed, pregnancy does reduce the protein binding of some drugs. For example, at high serum concentrations, binding of bupivacaine is lower in pregnant than in nonpregnant ewes,[35] whereas there is no effect on the binding of mepivacaine or ropivacaine.[36] Plasma protein binding of bupivacaine is also reduced during human pregnancy.[37]

The effects of maternal plasma protein binding of different local anesthetics on the rate and amount transferred to the fetus are not well understood. One would assume that highly bound drugs, having a lesser free fraction, would be more restricted in crossing the placenta. Indeed, animal studies have shown that the transfer rate is slower for bupivacaine than for lidocaine.[38] However, the low umbilical vein-to-maternal vein concentration ratios of bupivacaine and etidocaine are due to the difference in fetal and maternal plasma protein binding (which is higher in the mother) rather than to maternal binding alone.[39] If enough time is allowed for fetal–maternal equilibrium to be approached, substantial accumulation can occur in the fetus. Indirect evidence in humans was provided by the observation that neonates exposed in utero to bupivacaine administered for epidural anesthesia had measurable plasma concentrations and urinary excretion of the drug for at least 3 days after delivery.[40] Tucker[41] suggested that the protein binding of a local anesthetic does not significantly impede its diffusion across the placenta, because the dissociation of drug from protein is essentially instantaneous. This could not be substantiated for bupivacaine but was documented for fentanyl, an opioid bound to plasma albumin.[42]

Animal data indicate that hepatic blood flow is slightly increased during pregnancy, but there is a progressive depression in the in vitro hepatic microsomal enzyme activity.[43,44] Pretreatment with an H_2-receptor antagonist, cimetidine, to reduce the risk of acid pulmonary aspiration, may alter maternal drug metabolism since it reduces hepatic blood flow and microsomal enzyme activity.[45] Cimetidine has been shown to decrease the clearance of lidocaine but not of bupivacaine.[46] Ranitidine, another H_2-blocker, but devoid of hepatic microsomal inhibition, has no effect on the metabolism of either local anesthetic.[46]

Kinetic studies after injection of thiopental for induction of anesthesia at cesarean delivery showed a greater volume of distribution, plasma clearance, and longer elimination half-life than were obtained by the same authors in a group of nonpregnant women.[47] When methohexital was administered by intravenous injection to pregnant and nonpregnant ewes, plasma clearance was significantly higher in the former group.[48]

Alterations in ventilation and lung volumes have a significant effect on the rate of uptake and excretion of inhalation agents. Of most concern to the anesthesiologist is a 20% reduction in functional residual capacity (FRC) at term.[49] As a result, the equilibration time between the alveolar and inspired concentrations of inhalation agents is shortened. Pregnancy is also associated with a reduction in the minimal alveolar concentration of 25% for halothane, 40% for isoflurane, and 32% for methoxyflurane.[50] Maternal redistribution, metabolism, and excretion will lead to a reduction in drug concentration in the intervillous space, diminishing the transplacental diffusion gradient.

The elimination half-lives for the most frequently used local anesthetics range from $1^1/_2$ h for lidocaine to $3^1/_2$ h for bupivacaine in human volunteers.[51] Following epidural administration of bupivacaine for cesarean delivery, there was a rapid elimination phase ($t^1/_2\ \alpha = 47$ min), and a slow elimination phase ($t^1/_2\ \beta = 9$ h) from maternal blood.[52]

Placenta

As the placenta matures, the rate of drug transfer to the fetus may be altered, since the thickness of the trophoblastic epithelium decreases from 26 μm to 2 μm at term. In pregnant mice, diazepam and its metabolites are transferred more rapidly in late than in early pregnancy.[53]

In theory, uptake and biotransformation of anesthetic drugs by the placenta would decrease the amount transferred to the fetus. However, the placental drug uptake is limited, and there is no evidence to suggest that this organ significantly metabolizes any of the agents commonly used to produce anesthesia or analgesia in pregnant women.[54,55] An in vitro study has demonstrated placental biotransformation of phencyclidine (PCP), an anesthetic used in animals.[56]

Hemodynamic factors

Uterine blood flow increases during pregnancy and, at term, amounts to 500–700 ml/min or approximately 10% of resting maternal cardiac ouput; 80% perfuses the placenta and the remaining 20% supplies the myometrium and endometrium. Any factor decreasing placental blood flow such as aortocaval compression, hypotension due to sympathetic blockade, or hemorrhage can decrease drug delivery to the fetus.

Studies of drug transfer across rabbit placenta, perfused in situ, showed that a decrease in maternal blood pressure by 35% reduced the placental clearance of meperidine, but not bupivacaine.[57]

During labor, uterine contractions intermittently reduce perfusion of the placenta. Should uterine contraction coincide with the rapid decline in plasma drug concentration following an intravenous bolus injection, then by the time perfusion has returned to normal the concentration gradient across the placenta will have been greatly reduced. When women were given an intravenous injection of diazepam, one group at the onset of contraction and the other one during uterine diastole, less drug was found in infants born to mothers in the former group.[58]

On the fetal side of the placenta, the umbilical blood flow, estimated at 600 ml/min, represents at least 50% of the combined fetal cardiac output.

Studies of drug transfer across rabbit placenta, perfused in situ, indicate that a reduction in umbilical blood flow may increase the fetal–maternal concentration ratio but reduce the rate of placental transfer of drugs such as bupivacaine, lidocaine, and meperidine.[38]

The relative directions of maternal and fetal blood flows within the placenta may affect the efficiency of transfer of respiratory gases, drugs, and other substances between mother and fetus. In the human placenta, these exchanges appear to be on a 'multivillous stream' vascular pattern, in which maternal blood as it traverses the intervillous space flows successively past a large number of fetal villi. As oxygen from the maternal stream enters the fetal blood, fetal capillaries lying further downstream in the intervillous space are exposed to maternal blood of progressively decreasing oxygen tension. It is to be expected that a similar decline in concentration of drugs in the maternal bloodstream will occur.

There are several characteristics of the fetal circulation that delay the equilibration between the fetal arterial and venous blood, and thus delay the depressant effects of anesthetic agents. The liver is the first fetal organ perfused by the umbilical vein blood, which carries drug to the fetus. Substantial uptake by this organ has been demonstrated for a variety of agents such as thiopental,[59] lidocaine,[54] and halothane.[55] During its transit to the arterial side of the fetal circulation, the drug undergoes progressive dilution, as blood in the umbilical vein becomes admixed with fetal venous blood from the gastrointestinal tract, from the lower extremities, from the head and upper extremities, and finally from the lungs. Because of this unique pattern of the fetal circulation, administration of anesthetic concentrations of nitrous oxide or cyclopropane during elective cesarean deliveries was shown to result in newborn depression only if the induction to delivery interval exceeded 5–10 min.[60,61] On the other hand, administration of thiopental or thiamylal, not in excess of 4 mg/kg, resulted in fetal arterial concentrations of barbiturate below a level that would result in neonatal depression.[15] When thiopental was given during labor to two women carrying anencephalic fetuses, or to pregnant guinea pigs, drug concentrations in the newborn or fetal central nervous system were extremely low, while those in the liver were high.[59]

Changes in regional blood flow in the fetus can also affect the amount of drug taken up by individual organs. For example, it has been shown that during asphyxia and acidosis a greater proportion of the fetal cardiac output perfuses the fetal brain, heart, and placenta.[62] Infusion of lidocaine into asphyxiated baboon fetuses was associated with increased drug uptake in the heart, brain, and liver as compared with non-asphyxiated controls.[13]

Local anesthetics transferred across the placenta may

adversely affect the fetal circulatory adaptation to asphyxia, including increased placental blood flow. In the chronically instrumented pregnant ewe, lidocaine infusion resulting in clinically relevant maternal and fetal plasma levels of the drug is well tolerated by the partially asphyxiated mature fetal lamb.[63] In contrast, the preterm fetus loses its cardiovascular adaptation to asphyxia, and its condition deteriorates.[64]

FETUS AND NEWBORN

Any drug transferred across the placenta is carried to the fetal tissues, where its uptake depends on several factors, including alterations in protein binding to fetal red cells and plasma proteins, lipid solubility, degree of ionization, and the distribution of fetal circulation. The protein-binding capacity of fetal plasma for many drugs, such as local anesthetics, phenobarbital, and meperidine, has been shown to be less than that of maternal plasma, resulting in increased availability of free drug for tissue distribution at a given total blood concentration in fetal plasma.[65–67]

Uptake of lidocaine in fetal tissues was studied in pregnant guinea pigs following i.v. injection (10 mg/kg) into the mother.[54] Measurable concentrations of drug were present in the fetal blood and tissues as early as 1 min after injection, reaching their maximum at 2 min. The relatively high concentrations in fetal liver, myocardium, and brain demonstrated the rapid distribution to highly perfused fetal tissues. The liver was the only organ in which lidocaine levels in the fetus exceeded those in the mother. Substantial hepatic accumulation of other anesthetic drugs, such as thiopental[59] and halothane,[55] has also been shown. The strategic situation of the fetal liver in regard to the umbilical circulation has already been mentioned.

Any drug that reaches the fetus will undergo metabolism and excretion. In the term as well as preterm newborn, the liver contains enzymes essential for the biotransformation of amide local anesthetics.[68] A study comparing the pharmacokinetics of lidocaine among adult ewes and fetal and neonatal lambs demonstrated that the metabolic clearance in the newborn was similar to, and renal clearance greater than, that in the adult.[69] Nonetheless, the elimination half-life was higher in the newborn. This was attributed to a greater volume of distribution and tissue uptake of the drug, so that at any given time the neonate's liver and kidneys were exposed to a smaller fraction of lidocaine accumulated in the body. Similar results were reported in another study involving lidocaine administration to human infants in a neonatal intensive care unit.[68] Higher elimination half-lives in the newborn compared with the adult have been noted for other amide local anesthetics.

One drug, 2-chloroprocaine, is metabolized in the fetal blood so rapidly ($t^1/_2> = 43$ s) that substantial accumulation in the fetus is avoided even in acidosis.[28,30]

The fetus has an advantage over the newborn in that it can excrete the drug back to the mother once the concentration gradient of the free drug across the placenta has been reversed. With the use of local anesthetics, this may occur even though the total plasma drug concentration in the mother may exceed that in the fetus, because there is lower protein binding in fetal plasma.[39]

The question remains whether the fetus and newborn are more sensitive to the depressant and toxic effects of drugs than is the adult. Animal investigations have shown that the newborn is, in fact, more sensitive to the depressant effects of barbiturates and opioids. With local anesthetics, neonatal depression (Apgar 6 or less at 1 min) occurred at blood concentrations of mepivacaine or lidocaine that were significantly less than those producing toxic manifestations in the adult.[72,70] However, infants accidentally injected with mepivacaine in utero (intended for maternal caudal anesthesia) stopped convulsing when the drug concentration decreased below the threshold level for convulsions in the adult.[71] The relative central nervous and cardiorespiratory toxicity of several local anesthetics has been studied in adult ewes and fetal and newborn lambs.[18,72] The doses required to produce toxicity in the fetus and newborn were significantly higher than those required in the adult, while plasma levels were similar. In the fetus this difference was attributed to placental clearance of drug into the mother and better maintenance of blood gas tensions during convulsions. In the newborn, the larger volume of distribution is probably responsible for the higher doses needed to induce toxic effects.

Lastly, neurobehavioral studies following maternal drug administration for epidural anesthesia, have revealed subtle changes in newborn neurologic and adaptive function. In the case of most local anesthetic agents, these changes are minor and transient, lasting for only 24–48 hs.[74,73]

REFERENCES

1. Bromage P R, Robson J G 1961 Concentrations of lignocaine in the blood after intravenous, intramuscular, epidural and endotracheal administration. Anaesthesia 16: 461–478
2. Morishima H O, Daniel S S, Finster M, Poppers P J, James L S 1966 Transmission of mepivacaine hydrochloride (Carbocaine) across the human placenta. Anesthesiology 27: 147–154
3. Scanlon J W, Brown W U, Weiss J B, Alper M H 1974 Neurobehavioral responses of newborn infants after maternal epidural anesthesia. Anesthesiology 40: 121–124
4. Amiel-Tison C, Barrier G, Shnider S M et al 1982 A new neurologic and adaptive capacity scoring system for evaluating obstetric medications in full term newborns. Anesthesiology 56: 340–350
5. Abouleish E, Wingard Jr L B, De La Vega S, Uy N 1980

Pancuronium in caesarean section and its placental transfer. Br J Anaesth 52: 531–536
6. Duvaldestin P, Demetriou M, Henzel D, Desmonts J M 1978 The placenta transfer of pancuronium and its pharmacokinetics during caesarean section. Acta Anaesthesiol Scand 22: 327–333
7. Flynn P J, Frank M, Hughes R 1984 Use of atracurium in caesarean section. Br J Anaesth 56: 599–605
8. Dailey P A, Fisher D M, Shnider S M et al 1984 Pharmacokinetics, placental transfer and neonatal effects of vecuronium and pancuronium administered during cesarean section. Anesthesiology 60: 569–574
9. Drábková J, Crul J F, van der Kleijn E 1973 Placental transfer of ^{14}C labelled succinylcholine in near-term Macaca mulatta monkeys. Br J Anaesth 45: 1087–1096
10. Baraka A, Haroun S, Bassili M, Abu-Haider G 1975 Response of the newborn to succinylcholine injection in homozygotic atypical mothers. Anesthesiology 43: 115–116
11. Reynolds F, Knott C 1989 Pharmacokinetics in pregnancy and placental drug transfer. In: SR Milligan (ed) Oxford Reviews of Reproductive Biology, Vol 11. Oxford University Press, New York p 389
12. Brown W U, Bell G C, Alper M H 1976 Acidosis, local anesthetics and the newborn. Obstet Gynecol 48: 27–30
13. Morishima H O, Covino B G 1981 Toxicity and distribution of lidocaine in non-asphyxiated and asphyxiated baboon fetuses. Anesthesiology 54: 182–186
14. Finster M, Morishima H O, Moya F, Perel J M, James L S, Dayton P G 1966 Plasma thiopental concentrations in the newborn following delivery under thiopental nitrous oxide anesthesia. Am J Obstet and Gynecol 95: 621–629
15. Kosaka Y, Takahashi T, Mark L C 1969 Intravenous thiobarbiturate anesthesia for cesarean section. Anesthesiology 31: 489–506
16. Siker E S, Wolfson B, Dubnansky J, Fitting Jr G M 1968 Placental transfer of methoxyflurane. Br J Anaesth 40: 588–592
17. Morishima H O, Hiraoka H, Tsuji A et al 1983 Pharmacodynamics of lidocaine in the mature non-asphyxiated fetal lamb. Anesthesiology 59: Absract 412
18. Morishima H O, Pedersen H, Finster M et al 1981 Toxicity of lidocaine in adult, newborn and fetal sheep. Anesthesiology 55: 57–61
19. Finster M, Morishima H O, Pedersen H, Balkon J 1981 Meperidine: placental transfer after epidural, intramuscular, and intravenous injection. Anesthesiology 55: Abstract 321
20. Crawford J S, Rudofsky S 1965 The placental transmission of pethidine. Br J Anaesth 37: 929–933
21. Petrie R H, Paul W L, Miller F C et al 1974 Placental transfer of lidocaine following paracervical block. Am J Obstet Gynecol 120: 791–801
22. Morishima H O, Covino B G, Yeh M N, Stark R I, James L S 1981 Bradycardia in the fetal baboon following paracervical block anesthesia. Am J Obstet Gynecol 140: 775–780
23. Mazze R I, Dunbar R W 1966 Plasma lidocaine concentrations after caudal, lumbar epidural, axillary block and intravenous regional anesthesia. Anesthesiology 27: 574–579
24. Kuhnert B R, Philipson E H, Pimental R, Kuhnert P M, Zuspan K J, Syracuse C D 1986 Lidocaine disposition in mother, fetus and neonate after spinal anesthesia. Anesth Analg 65: 139–144
25. Giasi R M, D'Agostino E, Covino B G 1979 Absorption of lidocaine following subarachnoid and epidural administration. Anesth Analg 58: 360–363
26. Covino B G, Vassallo H G 1976 Pharmacokinetic aspects of local anesthetic agents. In: Covino B G, Vassallo H G (eds) Local anesthetics: mechanisms of action and clinical use. Grune & Stratton, New York pp 108–109
27. Covino B G, Vassallo H G 1976 Chemical aspects of local anesthetic agents. In: Covino B G, Vassallo H G (eds) Local anesthetics: mechanisms of action and clinical use. Grune & Stratton, New York p 100
28. O'Brien J E, Abbey V, Hinsvark O, Perel J M, Finster M 1979 Metabolism and measurement of 2-chloroprocaine, an ester type local anesthetic. J Pharm Sci 68: 75–78
29. Kuhnert B R, Kuhnert P M, Philipson E H, Syracuse C D, Kaine C J, Chang-hyon Y 1986 The half-life of 2-chloroprocaine. Anesth Analg 65: 273–278
30. Kuhnert B R, Kuhnert P M, Prochaska A L, Gross T L 1980 Plasma levels of 2-chloroprocaine in obstetric patients and their neonates after epidural anesthesia. Anesthesiology 53: 21–25
31. Lees M M, Taylor S H, Scott D B, Kerr M G 1967 A study of cardiac output at rest throughout pregnancy. J Obstet Gynaecol Br Cwlth 74: 319–328
32. Lund C J, Donovan J C 1967 Blood volume during pregnancy. Am J Obstet Gynecol 98: 393–403
33. Hytten F E, Thomson A M, Taggart N 1966 Total body water in normal pregnancy. J Obstet Gynaecol Br Cwlth 73: 553–561
34. Song C S, Merkatz I R, Rifkind A B, Gillette P N, Kappas A 1970 The influence of pregnancy and oral contraceptive steroids on the concentration of plasma proteins. Am J Obstet Gynecol 108: 227–231
35. Santos AC, Pedersen H, Harmon TW et al 1989 Does pregnancy alter the systemic toxicity of local anesthetics? Anesthesiology 70: 991–995
36. Santos A C, Arthur G R, Pedersen H et al 1991 Systemic toxicity of ropivacaine during ovine pregnancy. Anesthesiology 75: 137–141
37. Wulf H, Münstedt P, Maier C H 1991 Plasma protein binding of bupivacaine in pregnant women at term. Acta Anaesthesiol Scand 35: 129–133
38. Hamshaw-Thomas A, Rogerson N, Reynolds F 1984 Transfer of bupivacaine, lignocaine and pethidine across the rabbit placenta: influence of maternal protein binding and fetal flow. Placenta 5: 61–70
39. Kennedy R L, Miller R P, Bell J U et al 1986 Uptake and distribution of bupivacaine in fetal lambs. Anesthesiology 65: 247–253
40. Kuhnert P M, Kuhnert B R, Stitts B S, Gross T L 1981 The use of a selected ion monitoring technique to study the disposition of bupivacaine in mother, fetus and neonate following epidural anesthesia for cesarean section. Anesthesiology 55: 611–617
41. Tucker G T 1975 Plasma binding and disposition of local anesthetics. Int Anesthesiol Clin 13: 33–59
42. Vella M L, Knott C, Reynolds F 1986 Transfer of fentanyl across the rabbit placenta. Br J Anaesth 58: 49–54
43. Neale M G, Parke D V 1973 Effects of pregnancy on the metabolism of drugs in the rat and rabbit. Biochem Pharm 22: 1451–1462
44. Dean M E, Stock B H 1975 Hepatic microsomal metabolism of drugs during pregnancy in the rat. Drug Metab Dispos 3: 325–331
45. Feely J, Wilkinson G R, McAllister C B, Wood A J J 1982 Increased toxicity and reduced clearance of lidocaine by cimetidine. Ann Int Med 96: 592–594
46. O'Sullivan G M, Smith M, Morgan B, Brighouse D, Reynolds F 1988 H_2 antagonists and bupivacaine clearance. Anaesthesia 43: 93–95
47. Morgan D J, Blackman G L, Paul J D, Wolf L J 1981 Pharmacokinetics and plasma binding of thiopental II: studies at cesarean section. Anesthesiology 54: 474–480
48. Santos A, Morishima H O, Pedersen H et al 1985 Pharmacokinetics of methohexital in pregnant and non-pregnant ewes. Anesthesiology 63: Abstract 441
49. Prowse C M, Gaensler E A 1965 Respiratory and acid–base changes during pregnancy. Anesthesiology 26: 381–392
50. Palahniuk R J, Shnider S M, Eger E I 1974 Pregnancy decreases the requirements for inhaled anesthetic agents. Anesthesiology 41: 82–83
51. Tucker G T, Mather L T 1975 Pharmacokinetics of local anesthetic agents. Br J Anaesth 47: 213–224
52. Magno R, Berlin A, Karrlson K, Kjellmer I 1976 Anesthesia for cesarean section. IV. Placental transfer and neonatal elimination of bupivacaine following epidural analgesia for elective cesarean section. Acta Anaesthesiol Scand 20: 141–146
53. Idanpaan-Heikkila J E, Taska R J, Allen H A, Schoolar J C 1971 Placental transfer of diazepam–^{14}C in mice, hamsters and monkeys. J Pharm Exp Ther 176: 752–757
54. Finster M, Morishima H O, Boyes R N, Covino B G 1972 The placental transfer of lidocaine and its uptake by fetal tissues. Anesthesiology 36: 159–163

55. Geddes T C, Brand L, Finster M, Mark L C 1972 Distribution of halothane-^{82}Br in maternal and fetal guinea pig tissues. Br J Anaesth 44: 542–548
56. Rayburn W F, Holsztynka E F, Domino E F 1984 Phencyclidine: biotransformation by human placenta. Am J Obstet Gynecol 148: 111–112
57. Gaylard D G, Carson R J, Reynolds F 1990 Effect of umbilical perfusate pH and controlled maternal hypotension on placental drug transfer in the rabbit. Anesth Analg 71: 42–48
58. Haram K, Bakke O M, Johannessen K H, Lund T 1978 Transplacental passage of diazepam during labor: influence of uterine contractions. Clin Pharmacol Ther 24: 590–599
59. Finster M, Morishima H O, Mark L C, Perel J M, Dayton P G, James L S 1972 Tissue thiopental concentrations in the fetus and newborn. Anesthesiology 36: 155–158
60. Moya F 1962 Relationship of anesthesia to mortality in elective cesarean section. NY State J Med 62: 2169–2172
61. Finster M, Poppers P J 1968 Safety of thiopental used for induction of general anesthesia in elective cesarean section. Anesthesiology 29: 190
62. Cohn H E, Sacks E J, Heymann M A, Rudolph A M 1974 Cardiovascular responses to hypoxemia and acidemia in fetal lambs. Am J Obstet Gynecol 120: 817–824
63. Morishima H O, Santos A C, Pedersen H et al 1987 Effect of lidocaine on the asphyxial responses in the mature fetal lamb. Anesthesiology 66: 502–507
64. Morishima H O, Pedersen H, Santos A C et al 1989 Adverse effects of maternally administered lidocaine on the asphyxiated preterm fetal lamb. Anesthesiology 71: 110–115
65. Tucker G T, Boyes R N, Bridenbaugh P O, Moore D C 1970 Binding of anilide-type local anesthetics in human plasma. II. Implications in vivo, with special reference to transplacental distribution. Anesthesiology 33: 304–314
66. Ehrnebo M, Agurell S, Jalling B, Boreus L O 1971 Age differences in drug binding by plasma proteins: studies on human foetuses, neonates, and adults. Eur J Clin Pharmacol 3: 189–193
67. Szeto H H, Mann L I, Bhakthavathsalan A, Liu M, Inturrisi C E 1978 Meperidine pharmacokinetics in the maternal – fetal unit. J Pharmacol Exp Ther 206: 448–459
68. Mihaly G W, Moore R G, Thomas J, Triggs E J, Thomas D 1978 The pharmacokinetics and metabolism of the anilide local anaesthetics in neonates. Eur J Clin Pharmacol 13: 143–152
69. Morishima H O, Finster M, Pedersen H et al 1979 Pharmacokinetics of lidocaine in fetal and neonatal lambs and adult sheep. Anesthesiology 50: 431–436
70. Shnider S M, Way E L 1968 Plasma levels of lidocaine (Xylocaine[R]) in mother and newborn following obstetrical conduction anesthesia: clinical applications. Anesthesiology 29: 951–957
71. Finster M, Poppers P J, Sinclair J C, Morishima H O, Daniel S S 1965 Accidental intoxication of the fetus with local anesthetic drug during caudal anesthesia. Am J Obstet Gynecol 92: 922–924
72. Morishima H O, Pedersen H, Finster M, Feldman H S, Covino B G 1983 Etidocaine toxicity in the adult, newborn and fetal sheep. Anesthesiology 58: 342–346
73. Hodgkinson R, Marx G F, Kim S S, Miclat N M 1977 Neonatal neurobehavioral tests following vaginal delivery under ketamine, thiopental and extradural anesthesia. Anesth Analg 56: 548–553

11. Drug interactions in labor and delivery

A. Runyon-Hass

Information on drug interactions specific to pregnancy, labor and delivery is both limited and complex. While predominant obstetric advice is aimed at minimizing the drugs to which both mother and fetus are subjected during labor and delivery, it is not uncommon for a patient with a chronic disease (such as diabetes or epilepsy) to become pregnant and have an ongoing requirement for pharmacologic therapy.

A discussion of all the possible interactions between both chronically and acutely administered agents in certainly beyond the scope of this chapter. Medications other than drugs used for pain relief that are commonly administered during labor are reviewed, and the effects of these agents on anesthetic management are described.

INTERACTIONS AMONG SYSTEMICALLY ADMINISTERED AGENTS

OXYTOCICS

Oxytocics are drugs that stimulate uterine contractions. The main clinical uses for these agents are:

1. To induce or augment labor;
2. To control post-partum bleeding and uterine atony;
3. To cause uterine contraction after cesarean delivery or other uterine surgery:
4. To induce therapeutic abortion.

Oxytocin (Pitocin)

Mechanism of action

Oxytocin has a receptor-specific action on uterine smooth muscle that stimulates both the frequency and force of contractions.

Mode of delivery

Administration of oxytocin is always via continuous intravenous infusion.

1. *For augmentation of labor*: 10 IU (1.0 ml) is diluted in 1000 ml of infusate. Infusion rates vary from 1 to 10 mU/min.

2. *To minimize post-partum bleeding*: rates of 20–100 mU/min are used. Effects occur within 3 min, are maximal at about 20 min and disappear within 15–20 min after discontinuing the infusion. In practical terms, 20–40 IU is usually added to 1000 ml of fluid and administered to effect.

Hemodynamic effects

Of historical interest is that, prior to the introduction of purely synthetic oxytocin, purified extracts of human posterior pituitary gland were used as a source of oxytocin. These extracts possessed enough 'contaminant' vasopressin to cause both an independent and an additive hypertension when administered along with sympathomimetic amines.

The doses of synthetic oxytocin administered for most obstetric purposes are not sufficient to produce marked alterations of blood pressure. However, administration of large intravenous boluses of 5–10 IU results in:

1. a 50% decrease in total peripheral resistance;
2. a 30% decrease in mean arterial pressure;
3. a 30% increase in heart rate; and
4. a 30% increase in cardiac output.[1]

Drug interactions

Sympathomimetic amines. As mentioned above, the commonly administered sympathomimetic amines, ephedrine and phenylephrine, have not been associated with any incidence of malignant hypertension when used concurrently with synthetic oxytocin. When almost continuous monitoring of blood pressure (every 1–2 min) is utilized, there have been no reported cases of malignant hypertension associated with the commonly administered ephedrine doses of 5–10 mg or with the 40- to 80-μg doses of phenylephrine.

Inhaled agents. Although not specifically studied, inhaled agents will augment the hypotensive effects of large (5-to 10-IU) oxytocin boluses.

Agents that will antagonize the uterotonic actions of oxytocin. Antagonists of oxytocin include halothane, propranolol, tetracaine, quinidine and chloroprocaine.[2]

Miscellaneous effects

Both the natural and synthetic oxytocin preparations possess antidiuretic activity. In addition, induction with oxytocin has been associated with higher neonatal bilirubin concentrations.[3]

Ergot derivatives: methylergonovine (Methergine) and ergonovine maleate (Ergotrate)

Obstetric and gynecologic uses

Ergot derivatives are indicated in the management of post-partum bleeding and uterine atony and are limited only to the post-partum period. After small doses, in the nonpregnant uterus, there is an increase in force and frequency of contractions followed by a normal degree of relaxation. After large doses, or in the pregnant uterus, these agents cause contractions to become forceful and prolonged, and resting tonus is markedly increased.

Administration

A rapid and lasting response is produced with administration of 0.2–0.3 mg i.m. Onset of activity is within 10 min and increased uterine activity persists for 2–6 h.

Cardiovascular effects

Potent vasoconstriction of both arteries and veins occurs, resulting in increased peripheral resistance, decreased venous capacitance and increased mean blood pressure.[4]

Drug interactions

The only drug interactions reported have been with sympathomimetic amines.

1. Munson[4] demonstrated a 20% increase in systolic blood pressure from methergine alone and an additional 20% increase when either ephedrine or phenylephrine was given additionally to nonpregnant rabbits.
2. Numerous cases of malignant hypertension have been associated with the intramuscular administration of ergot alkaloids and the prophylactic intramuscular administration of either ephedrine or methoxamine. Severe hypertension is more likely to occur in patients who are already midly hypertensive. Unintentional intravenous administration may cause severe malignant hypertension.
3. Central nervous system sequelae to hypertension associated with methylergonovine have included retinal detachment,[5] ruptured cerebral aneurysm,[6] blurred vision, dizziness[7] and even seizures.[8]

Prostaglandins

Obstetric and gynecologic uses

Prostaglandins (PGs), primarily $PGF_{2\alpha}$, are used in the treatment of post-partum hemorrhage and for induction of mid-trimester abortion; they are currently being studied as agents for induction of labor. Treatment of uterine atony usually consists of manual uterine compression and intravenous administration of oxytocin and the intramuscular administration of methylergonovine maleate. Evaluation of the coagulation profile is also necessary because ongoing post-partum bleeding may be secondary to an underlying maternal coagulopathy.

Administration and dosage

$PGF_{2\alpha}$ or Prostin 15M, a prostaglandin analog, is given either intramuscularly or directly via intramyometrial injection. The efficacy of each is similar. However, before repeated doses are given it must be remembered that the post-partum uterus is a highly vascular structure with a potential for rapid drug absorption.

The average dose of each agent is 500 μg (two doses of 250 μg), which results in an 80–90% sustained response.

Failure, or the requirement for multiple injections, is often related to chorioamnionitis or retained placental tissue.[9]

Side-effects

Cardiovascular. Increases in heart rate, mean arterial blood pressure, pulmonary artery pressure and cardiac output without changes in peripheral vascular resistance are frequently observed.

Pulmonary. Bronchospasm, dyspnea, and pulmonary edema have been observed in patients undergoing mid-trimester abortion. Pulmonary function tests demonstrate small-airway constriction, air trapping, and reduction in maximum end-expiratory flow. Decreases in PaO_2 have also been observed and are believed to be caused by ventilation: perfusion mismatching secondary to the combined bronchoconstriction and pulmonary arteriolar constriction.[10]

MAGNESIUM SULFATE

Clinical use

Magnesium sulfate is the most frequently used agent in the management of hypertensive disorders of pregnancy.

Pharmacodynamic properties

1. Decreases presynaptic release of acetylcholine;
2. Decreases sensitivity of post-junctional membrane to liberated acetylcholine;
3. Decreases excitability of muscle cell membranes;
4. Reduces uterine blood flow and contractility;
5. Produces moderate vasodilation with a brief decrease in blood pressure;
6. Produces central nervous system depression;
7. Increases uterine blood flow and cerebral blood flow.

Administration and pharmacology

1. *Loading dose*: 20 ml of 20% magnesium sulfate (4 g) i.v. over 3 min. *Maintenance*: 1.0–1.5 g/h i.v. as a continuous infusion.

2. Clinical neurologic signs associated with the following plasma magnesium levels:

a. normal deep tendon reflexes (DTRs): 1.5–2.5 meq/L;
b. diminished DTRs: more than 4–5 meq/L;
c. absent DTRs: more than 10 meq/L;
d. respiratory paralysis: more than 12–15 meq/L.

Drug interactions

Depolarizing neuromuscular relaxants. Magnesium sulfate prolongs the duration of depolarizing neuromuscular blockade and decreases the dose of succinylcholine required to facilitate tracheal intubation by 50%.[11]

Nondepolarizing neuromuscular relaxants.

1. Magnesium sulfate alone acts as a nondepolarizing relaxant, with approximately 1/1000 the potency of d-tubocurarine.[11]

2. Magnesium potentiates activity of d-tubocurarine by a factor of 4.

3. Concurrent magnesium therapy has been shown to cause an eight fold increase in the duration of action of vecuronium.[12]

4. Calcium administration will not predictably reverse the magnesium-enhanced neuromuscular block.

Other maternal and neonatal effects

Maternal hypocalcemia resulting in complete heart block, central nervous system irritability and tetany has been observed.[13] Neonatal effects secondary to maternal administration include flaccidity, hyporeflexia, respiratory depression and weak or absent cry.[14] Marked potentiation of neuromuscular blockade by a combination of hypermagnesemia and aminoglycoside antibiotics has also been described in neonates.[15]

TOCOLYTIC AGENTS

Tocolytic agents are used to stop premature labor while other therapeutic measures such as steroid therapy are initiated to induce maturation of fetal lungs. They prevent the myometrial response to internal or external stimuli (e.g. β-sympathomimetics, prostaglandin inhibitors and calcium channel blockers) and decrease stimulus input to the uterus (e.g. ethanol).

β-Sympathomimetics

Of all the agents listed above, β-sympathomimetics have become the most widely accepted form of tocolytic therapy. However, there is increasing support for the use of magnesium sulfate.

Mechanism of action

The binding of these agents to β_2-receptors activates adenylate cyclase, eventually resulting in increased calcium uptake by the sarcoplasmic reticulum. The decreased intracellular free calcium causes a shorter duration of sarcomere contraction and less frequent contractions. The net result is a decrease in strength and frequency of contractions.

Administration and dosage

Terbutaline. Terbutaline is the most popular of the tocolytic agents and can be administered orally, intramuscularly or subcutaneously. Tocolytic therapy often involves a combination of methods of administration.

1. Our current practice is to administer three 0.25-mg doses of terbutaline s.c. over a 1-h period. This is then followed by 5 mg p.o. every 4 to 6 hours.

2. Dosages are limited by excessive heart rate increases and are withheld if the maternal heart rate is greater than 120 beats per minute (bpm) or the fetal heart rate is greater than 160 bpm.

3. Oral maintenance is then provided with 5 mg every 4–6 h until fetal lung maturity is established via amniocentesis and assessment of lecithin – sphingomyelin ratios or the 'fetal lung maturity' assay, which utilizes the surfactant – albumin ratio. Otherwise, sufficient doses of betamethasone are administered to help ensure fetal lung maturity.

Ritodrine

1. Initial dose: 0.1 mg/min i.v. for 10–20 min.
2. Dosage is adjusted by increasing by 0.05 mg/min every 10 min until contractions cease.
3. Oral maintenance: 10 mg every 2 h for 1 day, then 10–20 mg every 4–6 h.

Maternal side-effects

1. Hyperglycemia, hyperinsulinemia and lactic acidemia may occur secondary to the systemic β-sympathomimetic effects.
2. Hypokalemia occurs secondary to enhanced insulin secretion.
3. Tachycardia and hypotension: doses should be withheld if heart rate is greater than 120 bpm.
4. Tremor, palpitations, nervousness, headache, nausea, and vomiting have been observed.

Neonatal side-effects

1. Fetal tachycardia occurs commonly.
2. Neonatal insulin production is increased, resulting in neonatal hypoglycemia.
3. Hypotension and hypocalcemia are observed.

Drug interactions resulting in pulmonary edema

Glucocorticoids (e.g. betamethasone) are given frequently with tocolytics to promote fetal lung maturation. There is an increased incidence of pulmonary edema with the concurrent use of β-sympathomimetics and glucocorticoids.[16] The mechanism of this interaction is unknown, but maternal factors such as fluid overload, hypokalemia, twin gestations and sustained tachycardia greater than 140 bpm may play an active role in increasing the risk of pulmonary edema.

Calcium antagonists

Nifedipine

Although not approved for tocolytic therapy, nifedipine has been shown to be effective in abolishing uterine activity during premature labor.[17,18] The effective dose is 10 mg p.o. three times a day.

Maternal side-effects. Maternal flushing and transient increases in heart rate (10–15 bpm) are common but do not limit therapy.

Drug interactions. The hypotensive effects of inhaled anesthetics will probably be enhanced by this agent secondary to the peripheral vasodilating effects. In addition, the relatively long pharmacologic effects of nifedipine could result in post-partum uterine atony and hemorrhage that would be unresponsive to oxytocic agents.

Verapamil

Verapamil is ineffective for tocolysis at pharmacologically tolerable doses.

Ethanol

Intravenous ethanol was the most popular tocolytic agent in the USA during the late 1960s and early 1970s. Ethanol provides a tocolytic action via suppression of release of oxytocin from the posterior pituitary. Blood levels of 80–160 mg/dl produce myometrial depression but will similarly increase the incidence of nausea, vomiting and headaches. The loss of psychic control associated with the necessary ethanol doses may increase the incidence of gastric regurgitation and pulmonary aspiration.

Prostaglandin synthetase inhibitors

Indomethacin

Indomethacin has been shown in numerous clinical trials to be effective in halting premature labor. Widespread popularity has not been achieved secondary to the reported incidence of premature closure of the ductus arteriosus, resulting in pulmonary hypertension and cardiac failure in the neonate.[17]

Aspirin

Maintenance aspirin therapy has been shown to prolong the duration of pregnancy while blocking the development of hypertension in pregnancy-induced hypertension (PIH)-prone patients. Several large studies are currently being performed to evaluate the use of low-dose aspirin (60 mg/day) in the treatment of PIH.

Regional anesthesia and prostaglandin synthetase inhibitors

The question will undoubtedly arise as to whether maintenance aspirin therapy increases the associated risk of receiving regional anesthesia during labor. To date, there have been no studies that indicate an increased risk of neurologic or hematologic complications in patients receiving regional anesthesia while on aspirin or nonsteroidal anti-inflammatory drug therapy.

MISCELLANEOUS AGENTS USED SYSTEMICALLY

Trimethaphan camsylate (Arfonad)

Pharmacology and clinical uses

1. Trimethaphan is a ganglionic blocker that is used in acute treatment of hypertension associated with PIH. It does not cross the placenta and can be safely administered without central intravenous access as long as frequent blood pressure monitoring is observed.
2. It is rapidly metabolized, although its administration is associated with histamine release, tachycardia and tachyphylaxis in large doses.

3. Initial starting dose by continuous intravenous infusion in 100 μg/min. Routinely, 500 mg is mixed in 500 ml of fluid and administered to effect by intravenous infusion.

Drug interactions

Trimethaphan possesses significant interactions with both nondepolarizing and depolarizing neuromuscular relaxants.

Nondepolarizing neuromuscular relaxants. Trimethaphan has a direct effect at the neuromuscular junction, producing a 'nondepolarizing-type block' that is only a fraction of that provided by d-tubocurarine. Prolonged block will therefore be observed with concurrent use of all nondepolarizing agents.

Depolarizing neuromuscular relaxants. Trimethaphan noncompetitively inhibits plasma cholinesterase, resulting in prolonged blockade by succinycholine.[19]

Sodium nitroprusside

Sodium nitroprusside does not inhibit succinylcholine metabolism, however the possibility of fetal cyanide accumulation exists if prolonged use is required.

Dantrolene

Clinical use

Dantrolene is used in the treatment of malignant hyperthermia (MH) or for prophylaxis in MH-prone patients.

Pharmacologic properties

Dantrolene decreases the release of calcium ions from the sarcoplasmic reticulum. It causes skeletal muscle relaxation with reduction in force of contraction; this effect evens out short of total paralysis.

Administration and dosage

1. *For treatment of MH*: initial effective dose in 2.4 mg/kg IV.

a. The initial loading dose is given at 15-min intervals until relaxation of muscle rigor and control of tachycardia and arrhythmias is achieved.

b. The maximum dose is up to 10 mg per kg body weight.

c. Concomitant resuscitative measures must be carried out.

2. *Prophylaxis in MH-prone individuals*: although currently not recommended for use in either obstetric or nonobstetric patients, an oral dose of 3.4 mg/kg is roughly equivalent to an intravenous dose of 2.4 mg/kg.

Drug interactions

1. Verapamil is used for the treatment of supraventricular tachycardias and has been proposed in the treatment of MH-induced tachycardias. In animal studies, therapeutic doses of dantrolene in conjunction with verapamil have been shown to cause severe cardiovascular depression and cardiac arrest. The mechanism is unknown and this interaction has not been reported in humans.[20]

2. Concurrent use of the neuromuscular relaxants, vecuronium and dantrolene, has been shown to cause a twofold increase in the duration of neuromuscular blockade.[21]

Antibiotics

Drug interactions with anesthetic agents involve primarily potentiation of neuromuscular blockade. Virtually all of the aminoglycoside antibiotics tested show a wide range of actions. Most of these agents have combined actions on both the nerve terminals and the cholinergic receptor. When used in the presence of nondepolarizing agents, most of these effects can be reversed with either calcium or neostigmine. There have been case reports of concomitant maternal administration of vecuronium and gentamicin resulting in post-partum respiratory depression and hypotonia of the neonate.[15]

INTERACTIONS BETWEEN AGENTS ADMINISTERED IN THE EPIDURAL SPACE AND AGENTS GIVEN SYSTEMICALLY

EPIDURAL OPIOIDS

Fentanyl

Fentanyl is the most commonly administered epidural opioid at the Brigham and Women's Hospital. During labor, fentanyl is administered in combination with a local anesthetic, usually bupivacaine, via continuous infusion to provide 10–20 μg/h doses. Epidural boluses of 25–100 μg with a local anesthetic during labor or 50–100 μg in 10 ml of preservative-free normal saline or local anesthetic for post-cesarean pain relief are also administered. To date, there have been no drug interactions between epidural fentanyl and systemically administered medications noted in our practice or in the literature.

Hydromorphone (Dilaudid)

Epidural hydromorphone in a dose of 1.25 mg, in conjunction with intravenous droperidol (1.25 mg), has been shown to cause profound respiratory depression that is not responsive to naloxone but does respond to physostigmine.[22]

Acute abstinence syndrome

Acute abstinence syndrome is characterized by tachycardia, tachypnea, diaphoresis, hypotension, abdominal discomfort and agitation. In humans, acute abstinence reactions have been precipitated by the intravenous or epidural administration of opioid agonist – antagonists to patients who are physiologically dependent on narcotics. Epidural administration of butorphanol[23] and buprenorphine[24] has been observed to cause acute withdrawal.

EPIDURAL LOCAL ANESTHETICS

Cimetidine

Cimetidine, an H_2-receptor antagonist, is commonly administered intravenously, intramuscularly or orally (300 mg) to raise gastric pH as prophylaxis against aspiration pneumonitis. Cimetidine interferes with hepatic oxidative metabolism and initial distribution of amide local anesthetics. A 30% increase in the peak plasma level of amide local anesthetics administered by the intravenous or epidural route should be expected if the patient is receiving cimetidine.[25] No adverse effects of this transient increase in levels of local anesthetics have been noted in mothers or neonates.

Effects of altered plasma cholinesterase activity

1. Prolonged epidural block has been observed in a patient with abnormal plasma cholinesterase activity (dibucaine no. = 27). This individual heterozygous for plasma cholinesterase deficiency demonstrated a 90-minute block from epidural chloroprocaine.[26]
2. Grand mal seizures have been observed in a patient with absent plasma cholinesterase activity (dibucaine no. = 0) after epidural chloroprocaine.[37]
3. Although of rare concern in obstetric patients, phospholine iodide eye drops significantly affect plasma cholinesterase activity. Although the duration of local anesthesia is more dependent on the rate at which the drug is transported away from the injection site, significantly decreased cholinesterase activity can be associated with increased systemic toxicity and possibly prolonged duration of epidural block with the ester local anesthetics (e.g. chloroprocaine).[28]

INTERACTIONS BETWEEN AGENTS ADMINISTERED WITHIN THE EPIDURAL SPACE

LOCAL ANESTHETIC–OPIOID INTERACTIONS

Chloroprocaine and opioids

Chloroprocaine administered into the epidural space decreases the subsequent effectiveness of both fentanyl[29] and morphine[30] given via epidural injection. Epidural lidocaine and bupivacaine do not antagonize epidural opioids in the same manner. The mechanism for this antagonism is not known. In fact, fentanyl may potentiate the amide local anesthetics. Current research is under way to evaluate this phenomenon.

LOCAL ANESTHETIC–LOCAL ANESTHETIC INTERACTIONS

Chloroprocaine and bupivacaine

Epidural chloroprocaine will decrease the effectiveness and duration of anesthesia provided by bupivacaine. Chloroprocaine will alter bupivacaine effectiveness whether bupivacaine is given concurrently or subsequent to chloroprocaine.[31] Other local anesthetics commonly used in labor and delivery have not been shown to have this interaction.

Bupivacaine and chloroprocaine

Bupivacaine inhibits chloroprocaine hydrolysis by plasma cholinesterase. Bupivacaine administered into the epidural space will reach plasma levels sufficient to decrease chloroprocaine hydrolysis by 38%.[32]

REFERENCES

1. Weis F R Jr, Markello R, Mo B, Bechiechio P 1975 Cardiovascular effects of oxytocin. Obstet Gynecol 46: 211
2. Anderson W G, Miller J W 1975 Interaction between halothane and propranolol on oxytocin-induced uterine contractions. J Pharm Exp Ther 192: 408
3. Davies D D 1973 Neonatal jaundice and maternal oxytocin infusion. Br Med J 2: 476
4. Munson W M 1965 The pressor effect of various vasopressor-oxytocic combinations: a laboratory study and review. Anesth Analg 44: 114
5. Gombos G M, Howitt D, Shinyee C 1969 Bilateral retinal detachment occurring in the immediate postpartum period after methylergonovine and oxytocin administration. Eye Ear Nose Throat Mo 48: 45
6. Casady G N, Moore D C, Bridenbaugh D L 1960 Postpartum hypertension after use of vasoconstrictor and oxytocic drugs. J Am Med Assoc 172: 1011
7. Alper M H, Datta S 1986 Agents in obstetrics: mother, fetus, and newborn. In Smith N T, Corbascio A N (eds) Drug interactions in anesthesia, 2nd edn. Lea & Febiger, Philadelphia
8. Abouleish E 1976 Postpartum hypertension and convulsion after oxytocic drugs. Anesth Analg Curr Res 55: 813
9. O'Leary J A 1985 Prostaglandins and postpartum hemorrhage. Sem in Reprod Endocrinol 3: 247
10. Greeley W J, Leslie J B, Reves J G 1987 Prostaglandins and the cardiovascular system: a review and update. J Cardiothorac Anesth 1: 331
11. Morris R, Giesecke A H 1968 Potentiation of muscle relaxants by magnesium sulfate therapy in toxemia of pregnancy. South Med J 61: 25

12. Sinatra R S, Phillip B K, Naulty S J, Ostheimer G W 1985 Prolonged neuromuscular blockade with vecuronium in a patient treated with magnesium sulfate. Anesth Analg 64: 1220
13. Eisenbat E, Lobue C 1976 Hypocalcemia after therapeutic use of magnesium sulfate. Arch Intern Med 136: 688
14. Lipsitz P J 1991 The clinical and biochemical effects of excess magnesium in the newborn. Pediatrics 47: 501
15. L'Hommideau C S 1983 Potentiation of magnesium sulfate induced neuromuscular weakness by gentamicin, tobramycin and amikacin. J Pediatr 102: 629
16. Benedetti T J, Hargrove J C, Rosene K A 1982 Maternal pulmonary edema during preterm labor inhibition. Obstet Gynecol 59: 33s
17. Van Kets H, Thiery M, Deran R 1979 Perinatal hazards of chronic antenatal tocolysis with indomethacin. Prostaglandins 18: 893
18. Ulmsten U, Anderson K E, Wingerup L 1980 Treatment of premature labor with the calcium antagonist nifedipine. Arach Gynecol 229: 1
19. Dale R C, Schneider E T 1976 Respiratory paralysis during treatment of hypertension with trimethephan camsylate. Arch Intern Med 136: 816
20. Lynch C, Durbin C G, Fisher N A et al 1986 Effects of dantrolene and verapamil on atrioventricular conduction and cardiovascular performance in dogs. Anesth Analg 65: 252
21. Driessen J J, Wuis E W, Gielen M J 1985 Prolonged vecuronium neuromuscular blockade in a patient receiving orally administered dantrolene. Anesthesiology 62: 523
22. Cohen S E, Rothblatt A J, Albright G A 1983 Early respiratory depression with epidural narcotic and intravenous droperidol. Anasthesiology 59: 559
23. Weintraub S J, Naulty J S 1985 Acute abstinence syndrome after epidural injection of butorphanol. Anesth Analg 64: 452
24. Christensen F R, Andersen L W 1982 Adverse reaction to extradural buprenorphine. Br J Anesth 54: 476
25. Feely J, Wilkinson G R, McAllister C B, Wood A J 1982 Increased toxicity and reduced clearance of lidocaine by cimetidine. Ann Intern Med 96: 592
26. Kuhnert B R, Philipson E H, Pimental M D, Kuhnert P M 1982 A prolonged chloroprocaine epidural block in a postpartum patient with abnormal pseudocholinesterase. Anesthesiology 56: 477
27. Smith A R, Hur D, Rosano F 1987 Grand mal seizures after 2-chloroprocaine epidural anesthesia in a patient with plasma cholinesterase defiency. Anesth Analg 66: 677
28. Brodsky J B, Campos F A 1978 Chloroprocaine analgesia in a patient receiving echothiopate iodide eye drops. Anesthesiology 48: 288
29. Naulty S J, Hertwig L, Hunt C O, et al 1988 Duration of analgesia of epidural fentanyl following cesarean delivery – effects of local anesthetic drug selection. Anesthesiology 65(3): A186 1988
30. Kotelko D M, Thigpen J W, Shnider S M et al 1983 Postoperative epidural morphine analgesia after various local anesthetics. Anesthesiology 59(3): A413
31. Corke B C, Carlson C G, Dettbarn W D 1984 The influence of 2-chloroprocaine on the subsequent analgesic potency of bupivacaine. Anesthesiology 60: 25
32. Lalka D, Vicuna N, Burrow S R et al 1978 Bupivacaine and other amide local anesthetics inhibit the hydrolysis of chloroprocaine by human serum. Anesth Analg 57: 534

SECTION 2

Epidural anesthesia for obstetric pain relief

12. Anatomy of the lumbar and sacral spinal canal

*W. Luyendijk**

INTRODUCTION

Since the beginning of this century clinical interest in the epidural space has fluctuated. Interest arose as a consequence of epidurography (or canalography) during the first decades after World War II. This diagnostic procedure was intended to replace Lipiodol and Pantopaque myelography of the lumbar region in order to prevent consequent arachnoiditis.[1–8]

After the introduction of water-soluble contrast media, which were well tolerated when injected into the subarachnoid space, epidurography was replaced by caudosaccography. Despite the relative short period of application of epidurography, studies in 460 patients certainly contributed to anatomic knowledge of the epidural space.[9–11]

Clinical anatomic interest in the epidural space was again aroused by the development of epidural anesthesia during the last two decades.[12–15] This development stimulated further anatomic and physiologic studies, especially in the lumbosacral region.[16]

LUMBAR VERTEBRAE AND SACRUM

Like all other vertebrae – with the exception of the two upper cervical ones – the five lumbar vertebrae consist of a vertebral body, which is posteriorly connected to a vertebral arch (Fig. 12.1). The upper and lower surfaces of the body are kidney shaped. Its anterior, lateral and posterior sides are somewhat concave. The arch is made up of two pedicles and two laminae. The pedicles arise from the posterolateral angles of the vertebral body. From the junction between the pedicles and the laminae the transverse processes protrude laterally. At the median junction of the laminae the spinous process protrudes posteriorly, showing a slight downward angulation with respect to the plane of the upper and lower surfaces of the vertebral body.[16] The angle of the mid-lumbar spinal processes with

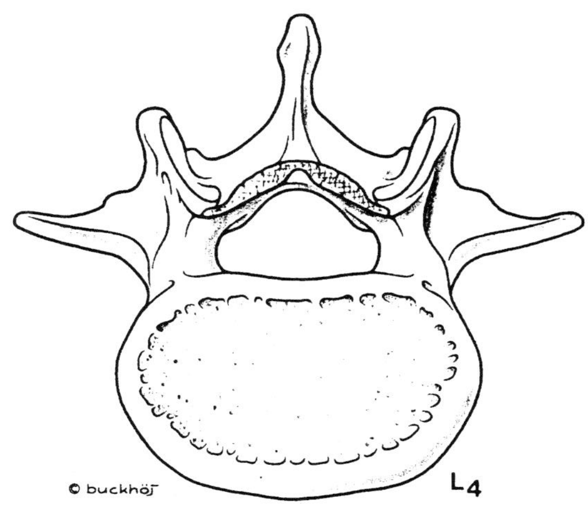

Fig. 12.1 Superior view of the fourth lumbar vertebra. The attachment of the ligamentum flavum is indicated. (Reproduced with permission from ref. 17.)

the long axis has a mean value of 70.7° and may vary from 63°–83°.[17] At the base of the laminae the superior and inferior articular processes arise more or less perpendicularly and extend over the vertebral body at both sides.

The posterior side of the vertebral body together with the arch surrounds the vertebral foramen, which in the lumbar region has the form of a flattened triangle. The anteroposterior (AP) distance of this foramen is of clinical importance. It has been proven that a small AP distance is an indication of narrowness of the lumbar canal, which may lead to neurogenic claudication.[19] Normal values as assessed by measuring the anteroposterior distance of the lumbar vertebral canal in 47 normal skeletons are as follows: L1, 14–22 mm; L2, 13–20 mm; L3, 12–27 mm; L4, 11–22 mm; and L5, 12–22 mm.[20]

The vertebrae are interconnected by (Fig. 12.2):

1. Intervertebral discs lying between the vertebral bodies. They consist of a soft, elastic nucleus pulposus surrounded by the strong fibrocartilaginous annulus fibrosus.

*This chapter contains the results of studies undertaken at the Department of Anatomy, State University of Leiden, The Netherlands.

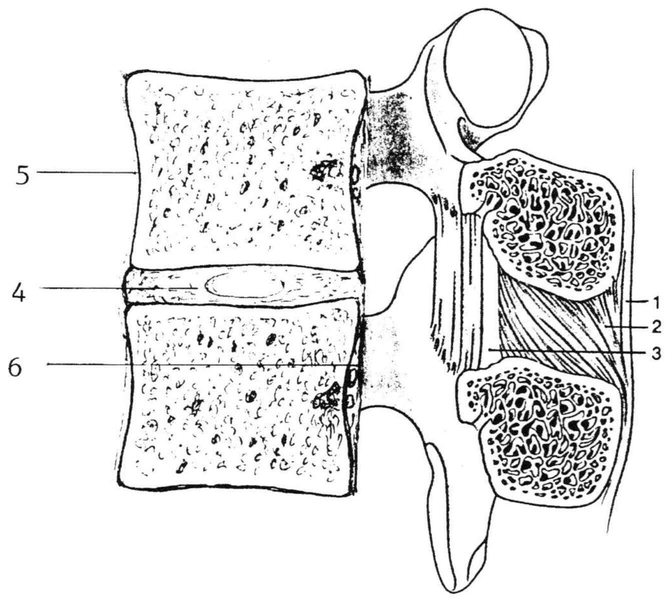

Fig. 12.2 Mid-sagittal section through the second and third lumbar vertebrae showing the connecting ligaments. Note the transverse veins between vertebral body and posterior longitudinal ligament.
1, Supraspinous ligament; 2, interspinous ligament; 3, ligamentum flavum; 4, intervertebral disc; 5, anterior longitudinal ligament; 6, posterior longitudinal ligament. (Reproduced with permission from ref. 17.)

2. Intervertebral articulations between the successive articular processes.

3. Anterior and posterior longitudinal ligaments, which partially cover the anterior and posterior sides of the vertebral bodies and the intervertebral discs (see below).

4. The ligamenta flava which connects the vertebral arches (2–5 mm thick).[17,66,69]

5. Strong inter- and supraspinous ligaments stretched between and over the spinous processes.

6. Intertransverse ligaments connecting the transverse processes.

The lumbar vertebral canal is enclosed by the vertebral foramina and completed by some of the ligamentous intervertebral connections: the intervertebral disks, the ligamenta flava and the capsules of the intervertebral articulations. Its anterior wall is partially covered by the posterior longitudinal ligament. The lateral wall of the vertebral canal has openings situated between the bases of the arches: the intervertebral foramina. They are surrounded by the pedicles, the adjacent posterolateral parts of the vertebral bodies and intervertebral discs, and the intervertebral articulations.

The construction of the lumbar column allows considerable mobility. In bending, stretching and sideward deviation of the back, the lumbar column plays an important role, and while doing so the curvature of the lumbar vertebral canal is influenced by the various postures. In the upright standing position the lumbar spinal column with its canal shows a lordosis, the degree of which varies in normal individuals of different races. In the supine position the lordosis is abolished or even changed into a slight kyphosis. In the lateral position a maximal lumbar kyphosis is attained by bending the head to the knees of flexed legs.

The bony walls of the vertebral canal are covered by periosteum. Some authors describe a thin continuous layer of connective tissue at the inner side of the periosteum and ligaments, extending throughout the whole spinal canal.[18,21,22] It is doubtful whether this stratum can easily be separated from the underlying structures in adults, but this is certainly the case in babies and infants: while performing a laminectomy in such young patients a rather firm membrane is clearly seen lying directly underneath the laminae. Inexperienced neurosurgical trainees often mistake it for the dura mater. After opening it, to their surprise, no CSF flows off, but fatty tissue comes out instead.

In the literature mention is made of two dural layers enclosing the epidural space.[23,24] In his meticulous study Hochstetter[25] made it clear that the embryonal spinal cord and its surrounding space are initially enveloped by an undifferentiated meninx primitiva extending to the perichondrium along the inside of the primordial vertebral canal. During the 10th week of development and later, the dural lamella detaches from the endorrhachis, and it is far from clear whether the dura lamella originates from the meninx primitiva only or whether the perichondrial cell layer also contributes to its formation. In any case, the existence of a double layered spinal dura mater is no longer accepted.

In the sacral region the five vertebral bodies and laminae are all fused together, except for the laminae of the fifth segment (Fig. 12.3). The absence results in an opening at the dorsal side of the sacral canal, the hiatus sacralis, which is covered by the sacrococcygeal ligaments. After closing off the hiatus these structures extend caudally to the dorsal side of the coccyx. Elaut and Verdonk[26] studied the sacrum in 120 apparently normal skeletons. In 26% the sacral hiatus reached to the third sacral segment, and in 4% even to the second one. The entrance to the sacral canal was barred by a bony bump in the region of the hiatus in 3%.

The sacral canal has a kyphotic bend; together with the lordotic lumbar canal it forms a faintly curved S when seen from the left side.

Anteriorly as well as posteriorly the sacrum shows four foramina, via which spinal nerves pass outwardly. The thickest and most important ones leave the sacral canal by the anterior foramina on their way to the sacral plexus located at the dorsal wall of the pelvis.

EPIDURAL SPACE

The epidural space is situated between the bony wall of

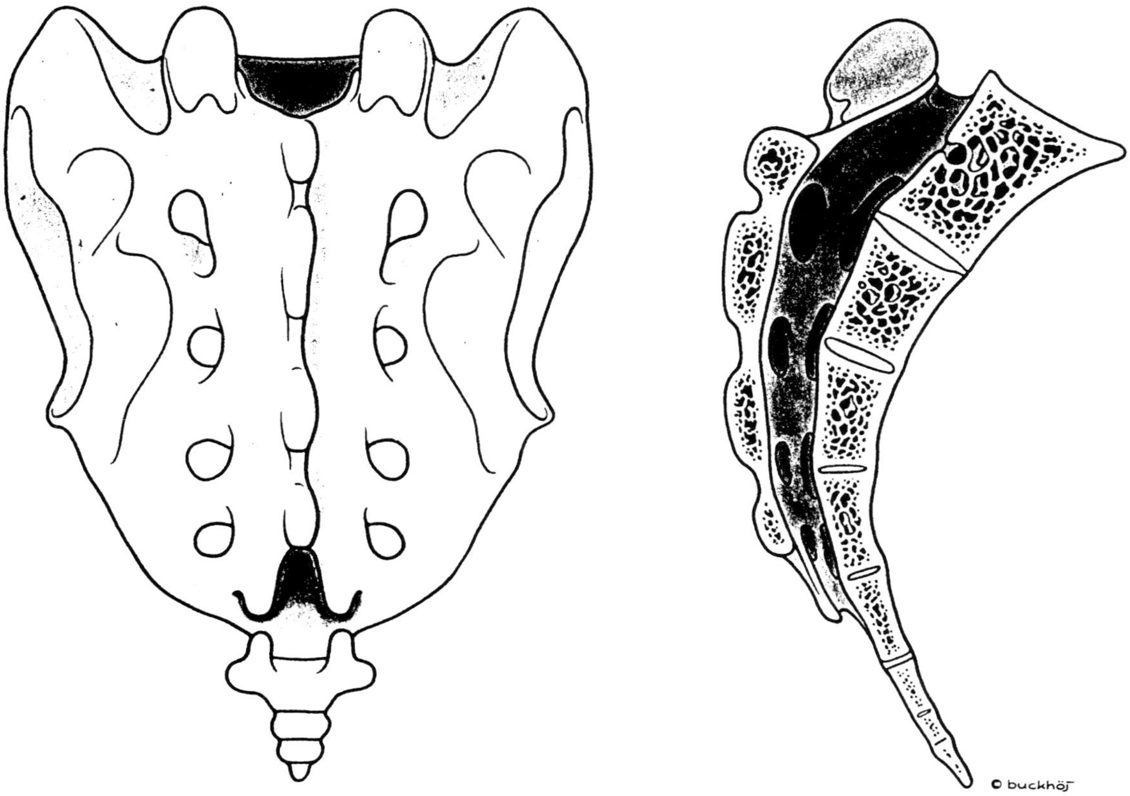

Fig. 12.3 Posterior view and sagittal section of the sacrum and coccyx. (Reproduced with permission from ref. 17.)

the vertebral canal and the spinal dura mater, i.e. the dural tube and sac. At their posterior sides the vertebral bodies and the intervertebral disks are partly covered by the relatively narrow posterior longitudinal ligament. This structure is only firmly attached to the disks and the adjacent edges of the vertebral bodies where it extends in a lateral direction. Between each discal level the posterior ligament is tapered towards the middle of the vertebral body (Fig. 12.4). There, behind the posterior and somewhat concave side of the vertebral body, it is separated from the bony surface, leaving some space for the transverse connections of the epidural veins situated immediately behind the vertebral bodies. For the other aspects of the bony wall of the vertebral canal and its coverings, see above.

At its inner side the epidural space is bounded by the dural tube and sac. The dural tube extends from the level of the foramen magnum downward. From the mid-lumbar region it gradully tapers, terminating at the caudal ending of the dural sac at the level of the second sacral segment. From there the filum durae matris extends caudally to the coccyx, where it blends with the periosteum at the dorsal side. The dural sac itself contains the spinal cord and the adjacent parts of its roots, all covered by the arachnoid and pia mater, and floating in CSF. No exact and verified data on the quantity of spinal CSF are available. Values in the literature vary from 25 to 90 ml.[24,27,28]

In adults the spinal cord is very much shorter than its total dural envelope. The cord extends from the foramen magnum to the level of the first or second lumbar vertebra only, where it ends as the terminal cone.[29] At birth, however, the well-known ascensus medullae has not yet been completed, the terminal cone being still located behind the third lumbar vertebra.[27,30] Caudal to the terminal cone the filum terminale extends onto the ending of the dural sac, where it continues within the filum durae matris.

Between the spinal dura mater and the underlying arachnoid lining a subdural space theoretically exists. This virtual space may be opened when it is erroneously punctured and injected with an anesthetic agent or a contrast medium. In myelography or epidurography this may result in misleading pictures. Such erroneous puncture is reported to occur in 1–13% of procedures.[31–33] In epidural and subarachnoid anesthesia this complication leads to an insufficient or incomplete effect.[34–36]

The blind caudal ending of the epidural space at the sacral hiatus, is firmly closed by the sacrococcygeal ligaments. Cranially the epidural space extends to the

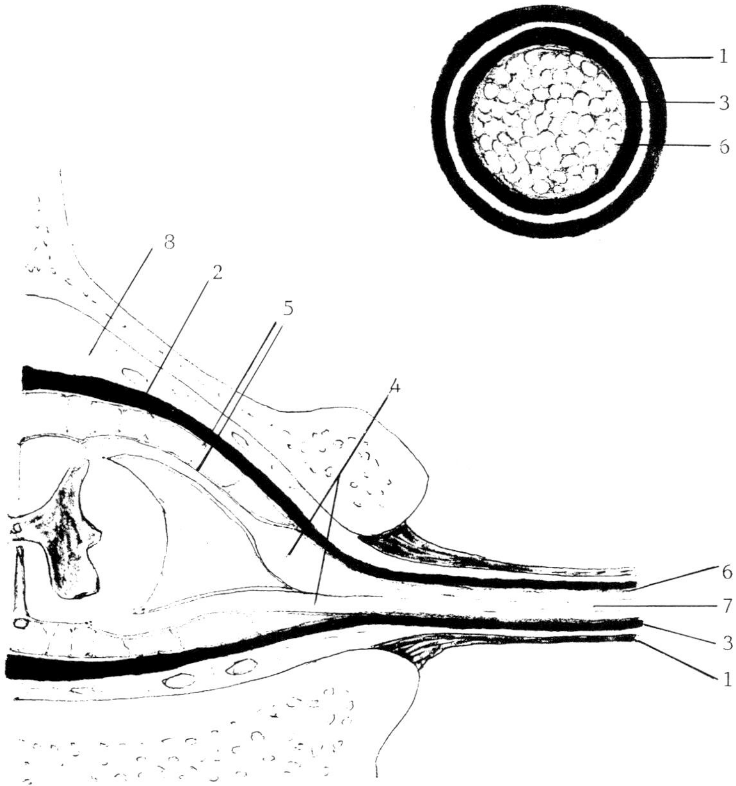

Fig. 12.4 Transverse section through the thoracic spine and intervertebral foramen, showing the spinal cord (left half), spinal roots and nerve with their envelopes. Laterally the dura mater becomes adherent to the roots and dorsal ganglion (root sleeve) and passes continuously into the epineurium of the spinal nerve; the underlying arachnoid passes into the perineurium. Beyond the intervertebral foramen the nerve with coverings is enveloped by the external tunica. The small underlying space communicates with the epidural space. In the upper right corner a cross-section of the spinal nerve is shown. 1, Tunica externa; 2, dura mater; 3, epineurium; 4, spinal roots and ganglion; 5, pia–arachnoid; 6, perineurium; 7, spinal nerve; 8, epidural space.

foramen magnum, where the dural tube unites with the periosteal lining of the vertebral canal. Opinion varies as to the exact level of the dural attachment: Charpy, for instance, described the third cervical vertebra as the place of attachment, as did several other anatomists later, with slight variations as to the exact cervical level.[37,38] However, Heile[39] obtained a quite different result. This author injected a mercury–turpentine emulsion into the epidural space in 20 human cadavers and then studied the cranial extension on radiographs. Its cranial extension appeared to have taken place largely beyond the foramen magnum, reaching as far as the cerebellar tentorium in some cases.

The width of the epidural space beneath the flaval ligament varies considerably in the different regions of the spinal column; in the lumbar region this distance is the greatest in the midline, where it amounts to 5–6 mm; as a consequence of the triangular shape of the lumbar vertebral canal it gradually narrows in the lateral direction. In the mid-thoracic region, it is 3–5 mm in the midline and very narrow laterally. In the upper thoracic region it measures 3–4 mm in anteflexion. In the lower cervical region the flava–dura mater distance is only 1.5–2 mm.[24]

Recently, Westbrook et al[17] published the results of precise measurements taken from normal MR images at the L2–3 level in 39 patients (alive, not epidurally injected). The skin–ligamentum flavum distance varied from 30–85 mm. The flavum–dura mater distances were measured at the cranial, mid-point and caudal level of the L2–3 laminar interstice. These distances had mean values of 5.97 (4–9 mm), 6.15 (4–9 mm) and 3.95 (2–7 mm) respectively,[17] and appeared to be in agreement with the results of Hogan's study on 38 cadavers using cryomicrotome techniques.[40]

The epidural space is not a closed compartment: laterally it communicates with the loosely arranged structures in the paravertebral and presacral regions via the intervertebral foramina (see below).

Capacity of the epidural space

Within the rigid walls of the vertebral canal the capacity of the epidural space is dependent on the volume and the filling of the dural tube and sac, which show a large degree of variability. It may fluctuate considerably in normal circumstances, as can be observed at neurosurgical interventions.[9,10] The greatest variations are seen in the lumbar region, where the dural sac only contains the fibers of the cauda equina, the filum terminale and CSF.

Caudad to the dural sac, the epidural space is bounded by the bony sacral canal, containing only the filum durae matris and some sacral roots.

Some topographic variations in the lumbosacral region deserve attention in regard to local epidural injections: in patients with spina bifida occulta and other forms of dysraphism, the dural sac with its contents may reach down into the sacral canal far beyond the level of the second sacral segment. In such cases the sac is considerably widened, similar to the situation in fetal stages of development.[27] Needless to say, such a configuration may easily lead to penetration of the dural membrane while unsuspectingly performing an epidural puncture in this region.

Although occult spina bifida can easily be diagnosed on radiographs, a systematic analysis is impractical and far from indicated. Some manifestations may be visible outwardly: the skin in the lumbosacral regions may show a cutaneous angiomatosis or present a superfluous hair growth. One should be alert as these small signs may indicate unknown congenital anomalies.

The total capacity of the epidural space during life is not exactly known. It was measured in fresh human cadavers by Farr,[43] who injected a sodium iodide solution epidurally. Radiographs showed that a volume of 118 ml could fill the epidural space from the sacral canal to the skull base. A volume of 89 ml was needed to fill it to the level of the fourth thoracic vertebra.[16] It is questionable however, whether these data are applicable to living people since the CSF pressure falls to zero after death. Moreover, no account was taken of contrast medium escaping to paravertebral areas via the intervertebral foramina. In addition the capacity of the epidural space will be reduced by overfilling of the epidural veins, as for example during pregnancy (see below).

Contents of the epidural space

The epidural space is everywhere filled with loosely arranged tissue and fat. The epidural fat shows a great variation in its quantity and distribution. It is doubtful whether a correlation exists with the thickness of the subcutaneous layer of fat. The epidural fat forms small pads, mainly at the dorsolateral side of the dural tube; it is particularly found between the arches of the thoracic and the lumbar vertebrae, but also ventrolateral to the dural tube just behind the vertebral bodies.[44–46] Embedded in the loosely arranged epidural tissue of the lumbosacral region various anatomic structures are present.

Spinal roots continuing their course on their way to the intervertebral foramina

In the epidural space the spinal roots are covered by a continuation of the dural membrane. This dural envelope extends to the intervertebral foramen. Beyond the foramen the dural layer passes into the epineurium of the spinal nerve. In the cervical region the roots follow a straight ventrolateral course, in the highest segments even running slightly upward. The thoracic roots have a gradually increasing downward course. In the lumbosacral area the constituent fibers of the cauda equina lie flat in the epidural space and show a steep and almost longitudinal course on their way to the low lumbar and sacral foramina.

Arteries accompanying the spinal roots

The radicular arteries enter the vertebral canal along the caudal side of each spinal root. They originate from various arterial stems in the paravertebral areas.[47–50] In the lumbar and sacral region, their sources are the lumbar, hypogastric and lateral sacral arteries. Soon after its entrance through the intervertebral foramen the radicular artery divides into three. One branch – the medial or neuromedullary branch – accompanies the spinal root in the direction of the spinal cord. The small rami along the posterior roots join the longitudinal posterior and posterolateral spinal arteries that lie on each side of the posterior root entrances. The posterior and posterolateral spinal arteries vascularize the posterior third of the spinal cord.

At the anterior side of the spinal cord the anterior spinal artery is found, running longitudinally over the anterior median fissure. Its branches enter the median fissure at more or less regular intervals before their rami penetrate into the medullary parenchyma and vascularize the anterior two-thirds of the cord. In addition, the spinal cord is covered by a pial vascular network, which also contributes to the vascularization of the cord, albeit in modest measure. Only some of the many arterial branches along the anterior spinal roots will reach the spinal cord and join the anterior spinal artery, thus participating in the medullary supply. They are distinguished as the principal arteries, which are conspicuously thicker than the rest. There are only 6–8 such arteries throughout the spinal cord.[50–52,59]

A remarkably thick principal artery enters the spinal canal in the lower thoracic or upper lumbar area, usually at the left side (in 80%). This is the great radicular artery, also called the artery of Adamkiewicz. It was drawn by Von Haller[56] but this fact was evidently not noticed in his lifetime, or completely forgotten.[51,52] Adamkiewicz[53] and Kadyi[55] gave detailed descriptions in 1885 and 1886 respectively. Mostly this artery accompanies one of the anterior roots from T8 through L2. At the anterior side of each cord segment it bends sharply caudally while joining the anterior spinal artery. Thus most of its blood is conveyed to the lumbar intumescence, which is why French anatomists call it 'l'artère du renflement lombaire'.[50–52,54,57] However, the artery of Adamkiewicz sometimes enters the spinal canal at a higher level, along one of the roots from T5–7; according to Lazorthes et al[48,50] this is the case in 15% of individuals. It is important to know that in those cases a supplementary principal artery is present and enters the spinal canal along the fifth lumbar or the first sacral root. This arterial variation eventually supplies the lower medullary segments.[48,50]

It will be clear from the foregoing survey that interruption of the principal arteries, especially of the Adamkiewicz artery or its variation, may lead to severe lesions of the spinal cord. From my own experience[58] the extent of such lesions varies widely and depends on the functional territory of the supply arteries.

Veins

The epidural space contains many venous channels. They lie ventral as well as dorsolateral to the dural tube. Together they form the internal venous plexus. This internal plexus has an abundance of connections and communications with the extensive extravertebral venous plexus (Fig. 12.5).

The complete system of richly interconnected vertebral plexuses is known as the system of Batson.[62,63] This author stressed the importance of this valveless system for the venous circulation in the body as a whole, since it can serve as a bypass of the inferior vena cava (see below).

Within the complexity of the epidural venous plexus two main longitudinal systems can be distinguished, situated on on each side of the midline:[63,64]

1. Two anterior intravertebral or internal veins, lying directly behind the vertebral bodies and the intervertebral discs. The lateral one is situated at the junction with the pedicles, while the other takes a more medial course. Both anterior internal veins are interconnected in the midline by conspicuous transversal veins lying between the somewhat concave middle of each vertebral body and the bridging posterior longitudinal ligament[60,61] (Fig. 12.6). In this way a sort of ropeladder is formed which is clearly seen on anteroposterior epidural venograms.[65–67] The anterior internal venous system is richly connected with the osseous veins of the vertebral bodies.

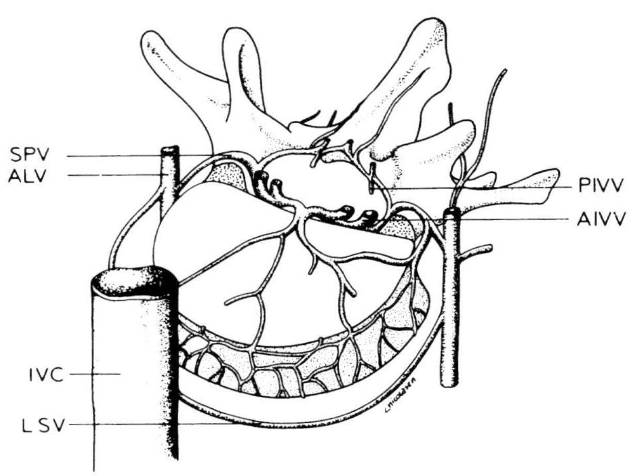

Fig. 12.5 Transverse section of the lumbar spine showing the relation between the extra- and intravertebral venous system. AIVV, anterior internal vertebral veins; ALV, ascending lumbar veins; IVC inferior vena cava; LSV, lumbar segmental vein; PIVV, posterior internal vertebral veins; SPV, suprapedicular communicating vein. (Reproduced with permission from refs 66 and 67.)

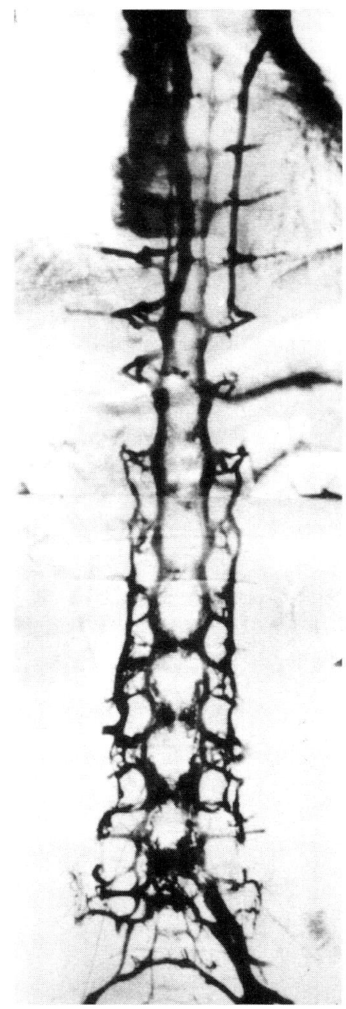

Fig. 12.6 Epidural venogram and azygogram (anteroposterior projection) showing the hexagon/ropeladder configuration of the anterior internal vertebral veins. (Reproduced with permission from refs 66 and 67.)

2. In the posterior epidural venous plexus one or two longitudinal veins are distinguished.[64] Other authors deny the existence of those longitudinal channels.[68] The posterior internal veins are situated dorsolaterally of the dural tube and sac. They show numerous communications with heterolateral posterior veins as well as with the anterior venous system.

Blood from the whole internal plexus is partly directed into the complex intraosseous system, which in turn is drained into the extravertebral subdivision of the Batson system (Fig. 12.7). A considerable part of the blood flows directly to the supra- and infrapedicular veins, which leave the epidural space via the intervertebral foramina on their way to the paravertebral venous channels. Blood from the lumbosacral area is drained to the common iliac and inferior caval veins, while blood from higher segments drains into the azygos and hemiazygos veins.

As was mentioned previously, the whole venous system of Batson has no valves; by way of its ample connections with large veins, it may serve as a bypass of the inferior vena cava in case of a partial or even complete obstruction.[70] According to Clemens and Von Quast[71] valves are only found in the radicular veins where they pass through the dura mater on their way to the epidural space and beyond. These valves are considered to serve to protect the spinal cord against venous overfilling.[71,72]

The extravertebral venous system conveys the greatest part of its blood to the superior vena cava via the azygos and hemiazygos veins. Midway the diaphragm divides this system into two parts: one part lies intra-abdominally and the other intrathoracically. It can be expected, therefore, that the alternating rise and fall of pressure during respiration will exert an influence on the drainage of blood from the Batson system. This has been clearly demonstrated experimentally by Cooper.[73]

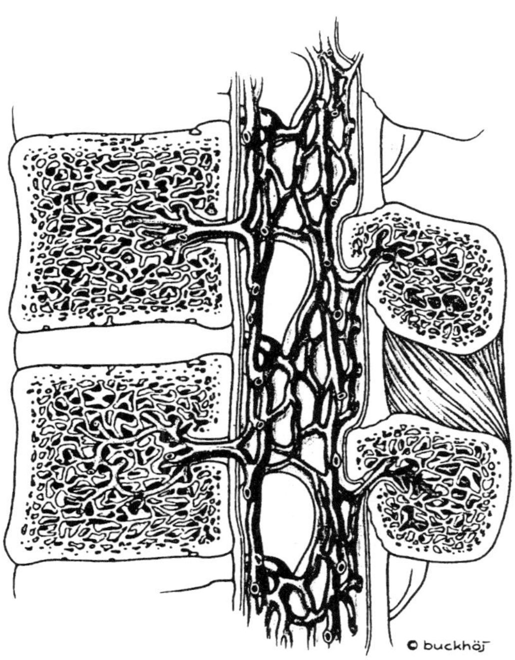

Fig. 12.7 Venous drainage of the internal venous plexus. (Reproduced with permission from ref. 17.)

Special attention should be drawn to pregnancy and delivery. During pregnancy the total blood volume gradually increases as a consequence of the increased vascularization of the uterus and the other organs in the pelvis. At the end of pregnancy the total blood volume amounts to an average of 7.7% of body weight compared with 6.3% in nonpregnant women.[74]

Backflow from the dilated uterovaginal plexus occurs via the hypogastric and sacral veins. The lumbar and sacral epidural veins participate in this overfilling and dilation, especially during the last months of pregnancy, when the regular venous return is hindered more and more by the increasing volume of the pelvic organs. In extreme situations this may even lead to compression of the inferior vena cava.[75] Distension of the epidural veins occurs along with a decrease in the effective volume of the epidural space. Consequently, the dose of epidurally injected agents can be reduced by 30% to exert the same effect as in nonpregnant women.[16] Thus it should be obvious that overfilling of the epidural veins presents a greater risk of bleeding and intravenous injection while performing an epidural anesthetic. This risk is still greater during delivery with the patient in the supine position. During labor each uterine contraction may cause a caval compression or even an obstruction. This will intensify the already existing engorgement of the pelvic and uterine veins. Each uterine contraction will squeeze out 0.3–0.5 L of blood, which has partly or completely to drain into the epidural veins, from where it is directed to the azygos and hemiazygos veins by way of the collateral Batson system.

In these circumstances any unintentional intravenous injection when performing an epidural puncture immediately before the next uterine contraction will endanger the patient as a result of bolus transport of the injected agent directly into the right atrium.[16] This complication can be avoided by placing parturients in a lateral or semilateral position, with a wedge under the right hip.[76]

Lymphatics

A network of lymphatic vessels is described as lying around the dural root sleeves. Via the intervertebral foramina, these lymph vessels run anteriorly to longitudinal channels in front of the vertebral column.[77]

Fixation of the dural tube and sac

When dissecting the lumbar epidural space very carefully, numerous fine threads can be seen connecting the dural membrane to the walls of the vertebral canal (Figs 12.8

and 12.9). These fibers are densely arranged, especially in front of the dural tube and sac; amidst the fine threads, thicker filaments and small ligaments are found, which play a mechanical role in the fixation of the dural envelope.[68] Apart from those thready connections the following elements contribute to the fixation of the dural tube and sac:

1. The spinal roots in their epidural ventrolateral course to the intervertebral foramina. Their role in fixing the dural tube is certainly important in the cervical and upper thoracic regions. It is gradually diminished in the lower parts of the vertebral column and is neglible in the lumbar and sacral areas since the long roots of the cauda equina can be compared with slack bridles.

2. Various ligamentous strands connecting the dural envelope with the walls of the vertebral canal. Such strands are regularly found in the cervical and lumbosacral regions.

3. Dorsomedian connection of the dura mater to the posterior wall of the epidural space.

Among the numerous epidural filaments, special attention should be paid to the many fine fibers that extend dorsomedially from the dural sac to the inner side of the vertebral arch and yellow ligaments, all in the medial plane. Some authors[78-80] describe this connection as a ligament or membrane. Its effect on the dural sac is not apparent in normal situations and is only observed when the subarachnoid pressure has fallen considerably or when

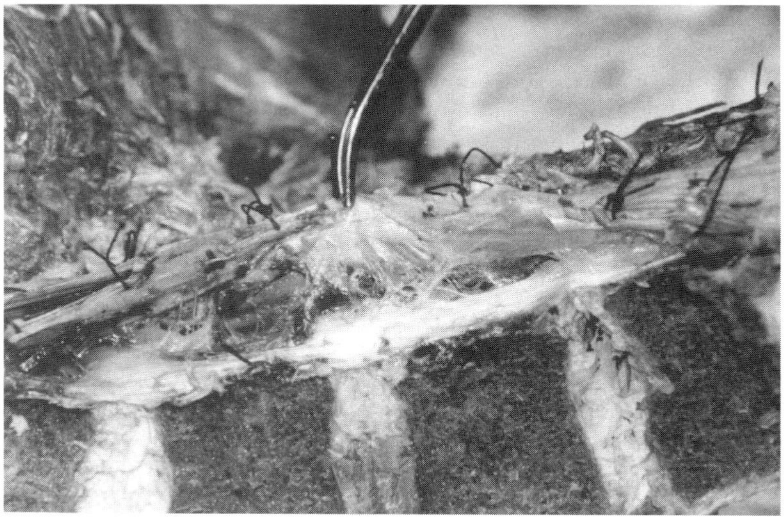

Fig. 12.8 When the dural sac is somewhat raised and pulled to the contralateral side, its cobweb-like connections to the anterior wall of the epidural space are seen.

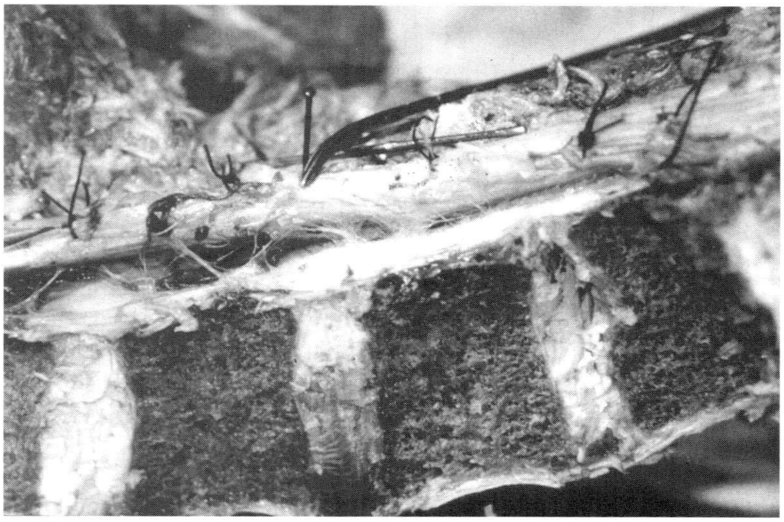

Fig. 12.9 After disruption of the many finer threads, coarser filamentous dural connections can be seen.

the pressure in the epidural space is increased artificially.[81] In such circumstances the dural sac is collapsed or compressed respectively. However, complete collapse is prevented by the dorsomedian fixation, which at the same time will instead produce a sharp dorsomedian fold in the dural membrane.

The dorsomedian fold (plica mediana dorsalis) is regularly seen during surgery to repair herniated discs by way of horizontal hemilaminectomy. Patients are placed in the 'salâam position' lying on their knees and shoulders, their low-back region being considerably raised. After removal of the yellow ligaments and the caudal brim of the lumbar arches, the dural sac comes into view. Because of the patient's position it is slack and presents the sharp dorsomedial fold resulting from its median fixation to the still intact arch of the next vertebra (Fig. 12.10). After simple interruption of this fixation the dural sac collapses completely[10,11,82] (Fig. 12.11). The dorsomedian fold can easily be demonstrated post mortem by injecting a Chinese ink and gelatin mixture into the epidural space via the sacral hiatus.[9,82]

In recent years these findings have been confirmed by epidural injections of resins.[83,84] Blomberg,[80] in his thesis on epiduroscopy, demonstrated the existence of the plica mediana dorsalis in vivo while exploring the lumbar epidural space.

Some of the foregoing anatomic data are important in relation to effective and safe epidural injection and catheterization for the following reasons. At the caudal level of the interlaminar interstice, the epidural space has a shallower extent than at the cranial level;[17] hence it may seem preferable to introduce a needle via the cranial route.

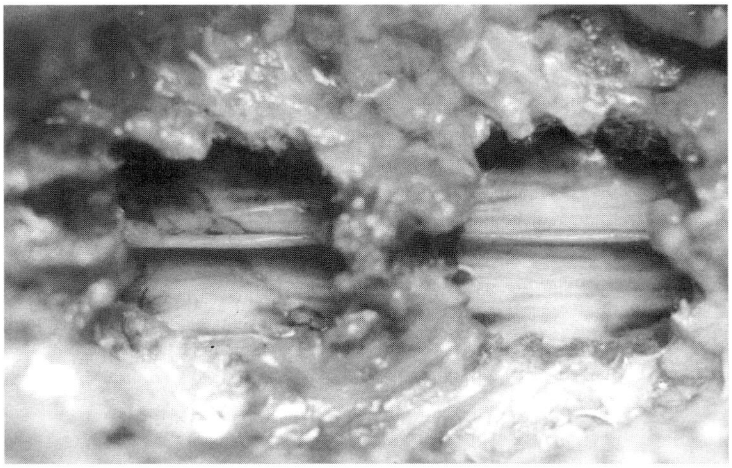

Fig. 12.10 Dorsal view of the dural sac at operation. After removal of the spinous processes and the lower brims of the lumbar arches, the plica mediana dorsalis is seen while the dural sac is otherwise slack.

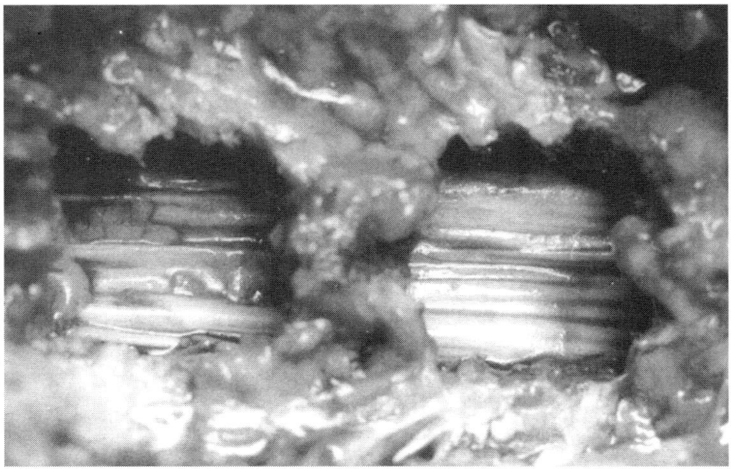

Fig. 12.11 After disruption of the dorsomedian fixations to the lumbar arches the dural sac is completely collapsed.

It has to be borne in mind, however, that many dural fixations to the inner side of the lamina may hamper a (steep) successful introduction of a needle via the cranial route, thus offering a greater risk of tenting or perforating the dura mater. For this reason it is preferable to use the caudal route, introducing the needle in a more oblique upward direction.[17]

It is also preferable to use the paramedian entrance rather than the median one. In this way the dorsomedian dura fold will be avoided while simultaneous fluid injection into the dorsolateral subcompartment of the epidural space will widen it and thus reduce any harm to the dura mater at the same time.[85–88]

Connections between the epidural and the paravertebral/presacral tissue spaces

The epidural space is far from being a closed compartment: each intervertebral foramen provides for a potential communication with the paravertebral and presacral areas of loosely arranged connective tissue.

Via the intervertebral foramina the spinal roots pass from the epidural space into the paravertebral spinal nerves. This transitional area, together with the periradicular and perineural structures, has been the subject of thorough investigations during the last three decades. The results of these studies may be summarized as follows. The spinal roots are enveloped by a lateral continuation of the dural membrane, lined on its inside by the arachnoid mater. As it nears the intervertebral foramen the dural sleeve gradually becomes thinner and more adherent to the root. Before reaching the foramen the arachnoid forms a 'cul de sac', thus enclosing the most lateral extension of the (sub) arachnoid space. The arachnoid itself continues as a thin layer underneath the periradicular dura mater. Within and beyond the intervertebral foramen the dural envelope passes into the epineurium of the spinal nerve while the underlying arachnoid continues into the perineurium which surrounds the constituent fiber bundles (funiculi) of the spinal nerve.[89]

The firm attachment of the periradicular and perineural envelopes in the transitional course, in and beyond the intervertebral foramina, prevents the introduction of a probe from the root sleeve underneath these envelopes completely. The root sleeve course has been subjected to detailed investigations since it appears to be an active region of resorption and expulsion of watery fluids as well as of large molecular and even particulate substances.[90–94] Electron microscopic studies have added many important details in this respect:

- The dural and epineural covering of the spinal root and nerve consist of a layer of longitudinal collagen fibers. This layer is freely permeable and exerts no barrier function whatsoever.

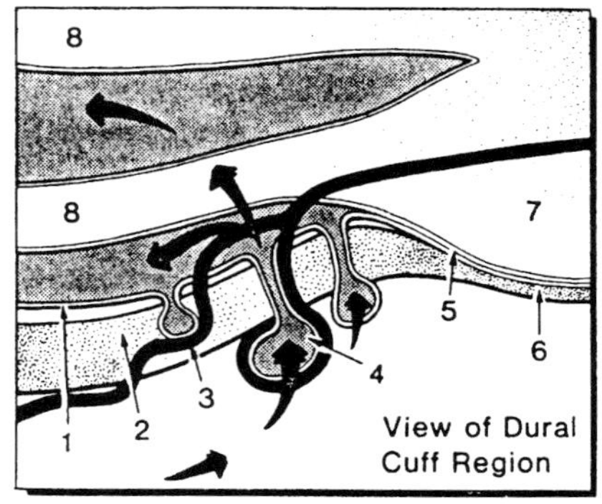

Fig. 12.12 Root sleeve with protruding arachnoid granulations. 1, Arachnoid membrane; 2, dura mater; 3, epidural vein; 4, arachnoid granulation protruding through dura and contacting epidural vein; 5, perineurium of spinal nerve in continuity with arachnoid; 6, epineurium of spinal nerve in continuity with dura; 7, dorsal root ganglion; 8, intradural spinal roots. (Reproduced with permission from ref. 24.)

- In the root sleeve (Fig. 12.12) the dural membrane is pierced by many arterial and venous channels entering or leaving the subarachnoid space. The root sleeve itself is covered all around by a rich plexus of small veins. From the inside small but sometimes large arachnoidal villi reach into or beyond the dura mater.[95,96] The larger ones invaginate the epidural space and may have close contacts with the surrounding venous plexus.[97] In man these villous formations are particularly found in the lumbosacral area.[98]
- The arachnoidea and the perineurium around the spinal root and nerve bundles are composed of several cell layers. The perineurium has 3–15 concentric layers of flattened cells with a well-defined basement membrane; they lie in a lamellar fashion around the neural funiculi.
- The cells show closed-contact (tight) intercellular junctions, which suggest the existence of an impermeable barrier to large molecular substances and particulate matters.[99–102] Nevertheless a regular penetration of those matters has been demonstrated by way of pinocytosis.[99–102] This mechanism starts with vesicular invagination of the cell membrane leading to the formation of intracellular vesicles, by which means the transcellular transport of materials takes place.
- Large molecular substances applied to the outer surface of a spinal nerve appear to penetrate the perineurium in this way within a relative short time varying from 0.5 to 6 h.[103,104]
- In the arachnoid cells large vacuoles and even pores form a cyclic dynamic system of transcellular transport.[105] This system is thought to drain CSF and macromolecular and particulate (debris) matter from the subarachnoid compartment to the subdural and epidural space.

The pia mater is a layer of connective tissue fibers running in all directions over the surface of the spinal cord and its roots. It is covered by extremely flat overlapping cells.[106] Although its fibrous layer is thin it has a tough structure, as is well-known to every neurosurgeon who performs anterolateral cordotomy. The pia mater, like the endoneurium presents no barrier to the penetration of local anesthetics and other watery solutions.

In its course through the intervertebral foramina, the root sleeve and the epineural covering of the spinal nerve are only loosely fixed to the foraminal wall and brims in a way that is similar to the fixation of the dural sac to the bony wall of the vertebral canal (see below). During the first four decades of this century it was debated whether the intraforaminal structures are able to block free communication between the epidural space and the extravertebral connective tissue areas. This question was certainly posed by Charpy, who described a condensation of periradicular fixating structures in the intervertebral foramen.[107,108] The role of this configuration, which is known as Charpy's ligament, has been considered by several authors in different ways, varying from a complete partition to a rather open passage. Forestier[107] for instance, described Charpy's ligament as a fibrous operculum closing off the intervertebral foramen almost completely:

> Mais au moment où le nerf (spinal) sort du trou (de conjugaison), avant sa division, il rencontre un plan fibreux très disséquable, qui forme en quelque sorte l'opercule fibreux de l'orifice externe du trou de conjugaison tendu sur le pourtour à la manière d'une peau de tambour sur son cadre, ou si l'on veut, comme le tympan au fond du conduit auditif.

Forestier's conclusion probably results from the fact that he studied desiccated specimens of vertebral columns and ligaments. Other authors have made an exception for the sacral foramina, where this barrier is incomplete.[39–42] On the other hand, it has been demonstrated that epidurally injected Lipiodol passes through the intervertebral foramina along the lumbar and sacral roots and nerves to the paravertebral and presacral areas.[109,110]

Careful anatomic dissection of the paralumbar and presacral areas shows that the spinal nerve with its covering epineurium is enveloped by another mantle consisting of a substantial layer of connective tissue.[21] Between this tunica externa and the spinal nerve with its epineurium some free space exists all around the nerve (Fig. 12.13). Only a small number of fine thread-like filaments connect the spinal nerve with the surrounding tunica externa. Proximally the tunica externa is firmly attached to the external brim of the intervertebral foramen and its immediate surroundings. Proceeding peripherally, the tunica gradually becomes thinner.

When the perineural configuration is compared at various levels of the vertebral column, it is obvious that the tunica externa is substantial in the lower lumbar and sacral regions, while it is thinner around the high lumbar and thoracic spinal nerves. The perineural sheath appears to have free communication with the epidural space: a probe can freely be introduced from the epidural space into the perineural sheath via the intervertebral foramen (Fig. 12.14). Such a probe meets no obstruction and can easily be inserted a considerable distance into the paralumbar and presacral areas. The same holds true for the reverse direction: after incision of the tunica externa a probe can be introduced into the perineural sheath and freely moved from there into the epidural space.

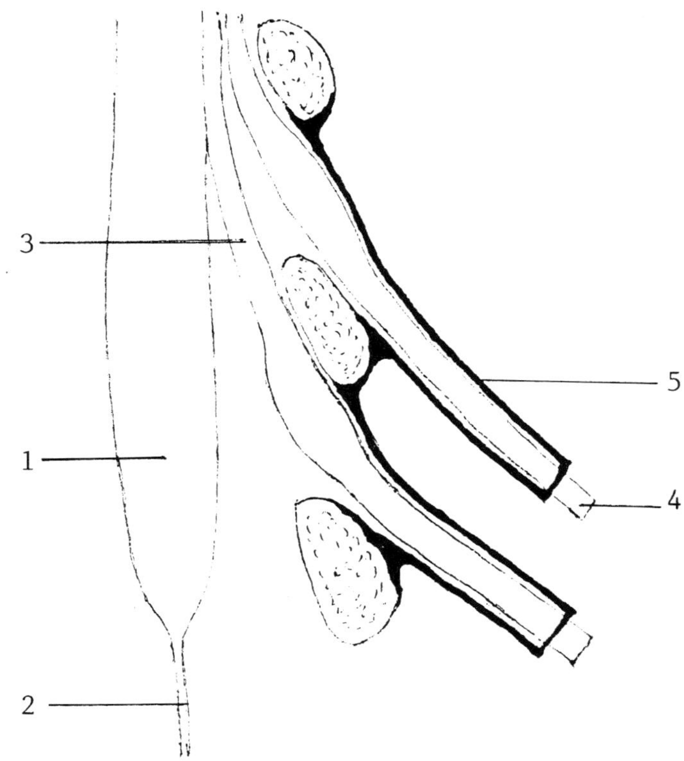

Fig. 12.13 L4 and L5 roots leaving the epidural space via the intervertebral foramina. The roots are covered by dura mater, which passes continuously into the epineurium of the spinal nerves. In its initial extravertebral course the spinal nerve with epineurium is enveloped by the tunica externa. Beyond the intervertebral foramen the epidural space is continued underneath the tunica externa. 1. Dural sac; 2. filum durae matris; 3. spinal root covered by dura mater; 4. spinal nerve covered by epineurium; 5. tunica externa.

It may be concluded from these anatomic studies that free communication between the epidural space and the extradural perineural sheath is evident. This finding is completely in accord with many experiments in the past. The spread of epidurally injected contrast media, in watery solutions as well as oily fluids, has been established by various authors; evidently those fluids could pass from the epidural space into the paravertebral tissue areas through the intervertebral foramina.[109,111]

These findings contradict the opinions of the French anatomists earlier this century, who thought that the intervertebral foramen was closed by an operculum. This operculum was reported to contain some openings for the spinal nerves and vessels, but it was described as a firm membrane similar to the eardrum.[107,110] This description has led to considerable confusion[16,18,112] and must be

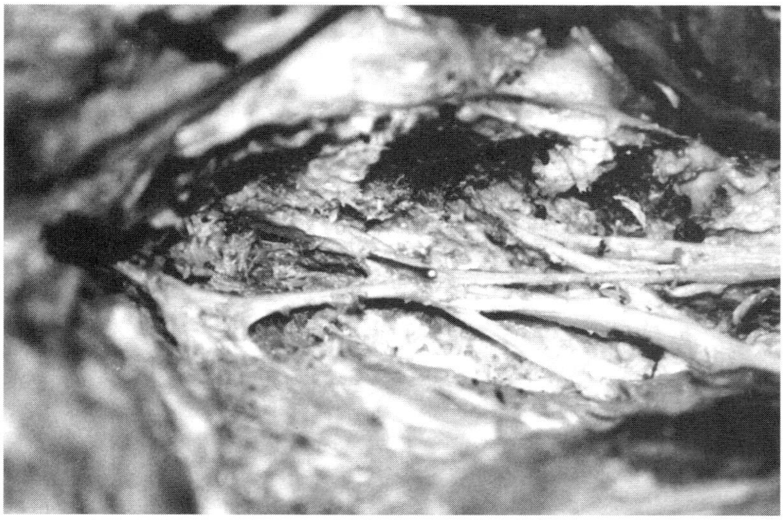

Fig. 12.14 View of the right side of the lumbar spine. A probe is easily passed from the epidural space along the L4 nerve (r.ventralis) underneath the tunica externa. The probe becomes visible after piercing the tunica externa via a small incision.

attributed to the fact that the studies were done on desiccated spinal columns.

Expansion and distribution of watery fluids injected into the epidural space

The expansion and distribution of watery fluids has been studied with epidurograms (460 cases). After epidural injections of 20 ml or more of water-soluble contrast media via the hiatus sacralis, radiographs were taken in standard projections (AP, lateral and oblique)[9,10] (Fig. 12.15). The relevant points of this study can be summarized as follows:

1. The epidural expansion in the cranial direction usually reaches a high lumbar level and sometimes even the low thoracic region. Although not included in this study pregnancy and obesity may lead to overfilling of the epidural veins, resulting in a reduction of the available space for injected fluids. In such situations smaller quantities of injected anesthetics will lead to the same results as in normal and nonpregnant individuals.[16] In case of pathology within the epidural space (e.g. disc protrusion, adhesive epiduritis etc.) the normal expansion will be locally impeded.

2. In addition to its longitudinal expansion within the epidural space, the contrast medium also spreads in the lateral direction with an extension into and beyond the intervertebral foramina. It apparently flows to the paralumbar and presacral areas along the spinal nerves. According to anteroposterior epidurograms, the intra- and paravertebral contrast deposits show an uninterrupted connection, the direction of which corresponds with the course of the spinal roots and nerves. The quantity of the extravertebral outflow shows a relation with age.

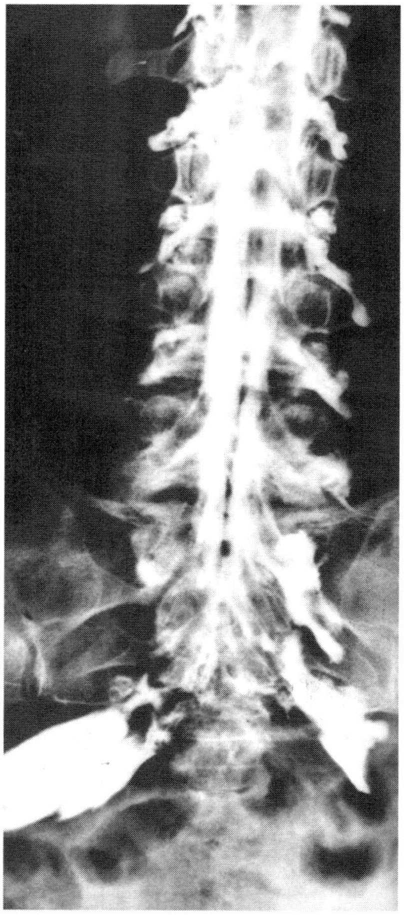

Fig. 12.15 Epidurogram in anteroposterior projection. The contrast medium, injected via the sacral hiatus, has expanded to the low thoracic region. Note the lateral outflow along the lumbar and sacral nerves. The dark midline corresponds to the dorsomedian dural fold.

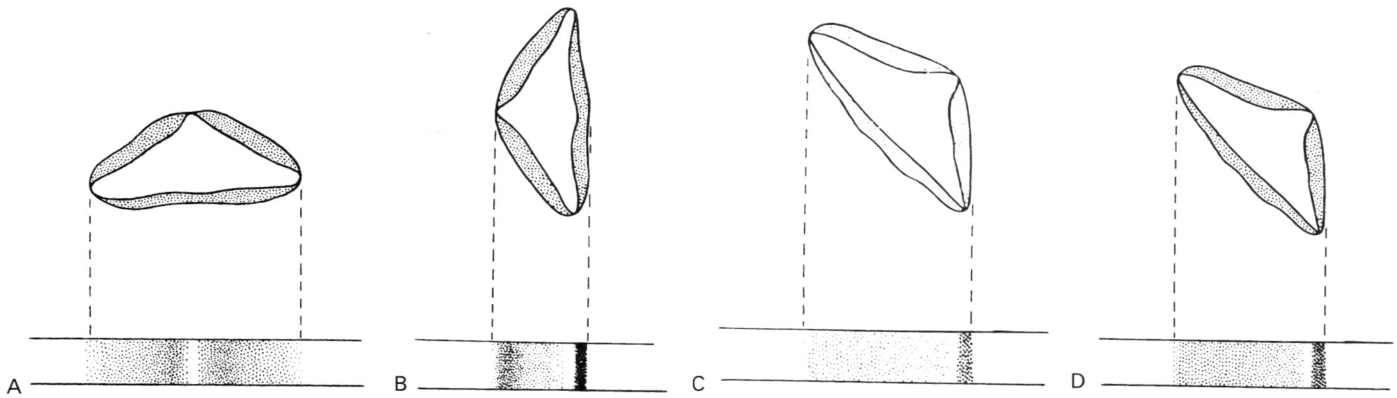

Fig. 12.16 The expansion of contrast medium in the epidural subcompartments (dotted areas) in (a) anteroposterior, (b) lateral and (c) oblique (three-quarters) projections. The white midline on AP projection corresponds to the dorsomedian dural fold. In the lateral view a lighter central area separates the broader dorsal contrast band from the narrow and intense ventral contrast shadow, while the contrast medium expanded in one of the dorsolateral subcompartments projects as a narrow strip on the oblique film.

Apparently the passability of the intervertebral foramina decreases with age (see below).[9,10]

3. Radiographs taken in various -even extreme- patient positions do not show any change in the expansion of the radiopaque substance. Evidently it is not dependent on the influence of gravitation.

4. Epidurally injected contrast solution is rather rapidly resorbed: depending on its quantity the contrast shadows fade over a period of 15–45 min. Evidently the resorption of paravertebral contrast deposits takes more time, as was demonstrated by successive epidurograms.

5. Different projections of lumbosacral epidurograms give more detailed information on the distribution of the contrast medium in the various epidural subcompartments (Fig. 12.16). In the lateral projection high-intensity filling of the anterior subcompartment is seen anterior to the dural sac. At the dorsal side the contrast shadow expands along the inner side of the vertebral arches and the interconnecting yellow ligaments without any interruption or indentation. This is also the case in the oblique (three-quarters) projection. There are only slight indications of a posterior sawtooth configuration, as is sometimes mentioned in literature.[17,23] On the epidurograms in anteroposterior projection, a white midline is seen in many cases, which apparently represents the dorsomedian dural fold. This fold separates the two dorsolateral subcompartments the filling of which is clearly demonstrated in the oblique (three-quarters) projections.[113,114] Notwithstanding some remarks in the literature, it is obvious that epidurally injected watery solutions spread easily from one subcompartment to another, thus surrounding the dural tube and sac completely. Some exceptions have been observed however:

6. In 11 of the 460 epidurograms, the sacrally injected contrast medium showed a strictly unilateral expansion in the lumbar region (2.4%). Analysis of these cases showed that the epidural space was unilaterally blocked at the level of a low-lumbar or lumbosacral disk by a large prolapse, osteochondrosis, local epiduritis, etc. (Fig. 12.17). Evidently this pathology prevented the cranial expansion of the contrast medium at that side while the contralateral contrast shadow showed a normal picture with a sharp median borderline. These pictures demonstrated that no

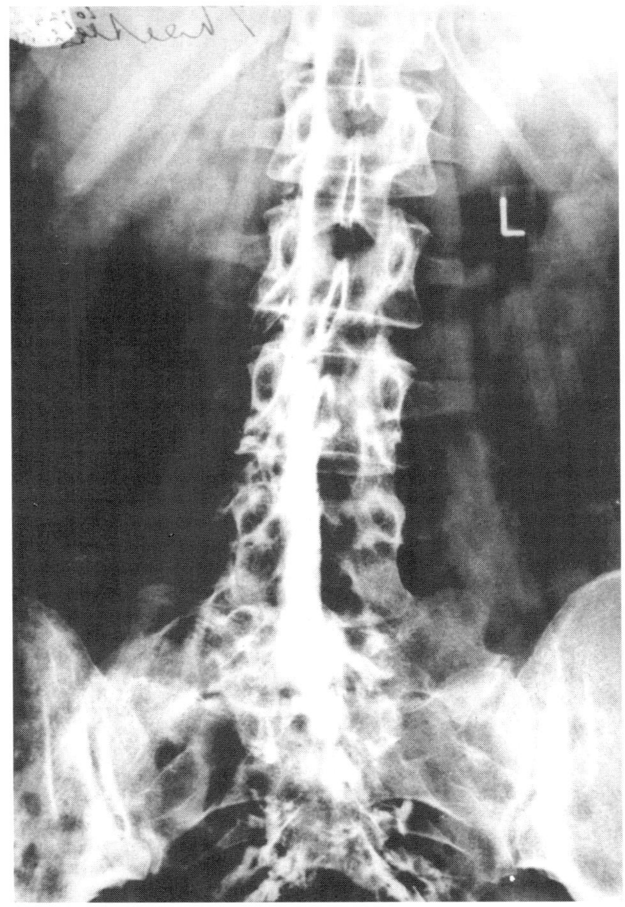

Fig. 12.17 Unilaterally expanded contrast medium from the (sacralized) L5 cranially. A large protruded disk and periduritis at L4 and L5 is evidently blocking the expansion of contrast medium at that side.

Table 12.1 Paravertebral outflow of epidural contrast medium via the lumbar intervertebral foramina: relation to age

Age (years)	Number	Positive	(%)	Doubtful/negative	(%)
20	20	19	95.0	1	5.0
21–30	58	53	91.4	5	8.6
31–40	89	72	80.9	17	19.1
41–50	89	74	83.2	15	16.8
51–60	46	38	82.6	8	17.4
61–70	12	9	75.0	3	25.0
Total	314	265		17/32	49.0
%	100	84.4		5.4/10.2	15.6

communication existed beyond a midline barrier in those cases. Further analysis made clear that this barrier had to be located between the two dorsolateral subcompartments, probably formed by the dorsomedian fold.[9,10,82] In some other cases the medial barrier appeared to exist only in the caudal part of the lumbar area, thus enabling the contrast medium to cross the midline at the level of the first or second lumbar vertebra and to expand from there downward into the dorsolateral subcompartment of the other side. In another 17 cases (3.8%) the contrast shadow showed a lower intensity on one side than on the normally filled other half of the epidural space. Although these exceptional pictures are due to extensive one-sided low-lumbar or lumbosacral pathology, they demonstrate the existence of a complete or partial median barrier between the two dorsolateral subcompartments of the epidural space in 6% of the studied cases. This finding is a probable explanation of the one-sidedness of analgesia that may unexpectedly result from a seemingly correct epidural puncture and anesthesia.[115]

7. Some workers have mentioned that the passability of the intervertebral foramina may progressively diminish with advancing age.[9,10] This was based on the assumption that the areolar tissue around the spinal root in its foraminal course should become denser with age. In order to examine this theory, 314 epidurograms were studied. The age of the patients varied from less than 10 to more than 60 (see Table 12.1). Passage of watery radiopaque solution from the epidural to the paravertebral tissue space through the intervertebral foramen was considered to occur when the contrast shadow appeared to extend beyond the lateral limits of the vertebral bodies as observed on the anteroposterior epidurograms. In patients under the age of 20 years passage did not occur or was doubtful in only 5%. This percentage gradually increased in older individuals, rising to 25% in those aged 61–70, although even in this age group the outflow could still be abundant. Although these data are not statistically significant (HR Van der Vaart, personal communication), they do seem to support the theory that there is a tendency to decreased passability of the intervertebral foramina with advancing age.

REFERENCES

1. Garland L H 1940 Effect of iodized oil on meninges of spinal cord and brain. Radiology 35: 467–476
2. Marcovich A W, Walker A E, Jessico C M 1941 Früh- und Spätfolgen der Jodölmyelographie. J Am Med Assoc 116: 2247–2254
3. Kristiansen Kr 1942 Über Jodölmyelographie und ihre Gefahren. Nord Med: 35: 43–51
4. Krayenbühl H, Lüthy F 1944 Über spinale Lipiodolschädigung. Dtsch Z Nervenheilk 156: 97–108
5. Tarlov I M 1945 Pantopaque meningitis disclosed at operation. J Am Med Assoc 129: 1014–1016
6. Lindblom K 1947 Complications of myelography by Abrodil. Acta Radiol 28: 69–73
7. Luck J C, Leith W, Burrage W S 1951 Pantopaque meningitis due to hypersensitivity. Radiology 57: 878–881
8. Hurteau E F, Baird W C, Sinclair E 1954 Arachnoiditis following the use of iodized oil. J Bone Jnt Surgery 36: 393–400
9. Luyendijk W 1962 Canalografie. Röntgenologisch onderzoek van de peridurale ruimte in het lumbosacrale deel van het wervelkanaal. Thesis, University of Leiden
10. Luyendijk W 1963 Canalografie. J Belge Radiol 46: 236–254
11. Luyendijk W, van Voorthuisen A E 1966 Contrast examination of the spinal epidural space. Acta Radiol 5: 1051–1066
12. Bromage P R 1967 Physiology and pharmacology of epidural analgesia. Anesthesiology 28: 592–622
13. Van Zundert A A J 1985 Bupivacaine 0.125% + Epinephrine 1: 800 000. The value of a low concentration of a local anesthetic drug for epidural analgesia in obstetrics. Thesis, University of Leiden
14. Van Zundert A, Vaes L, Soetens M et al 1987 Every dose given in epidural analgesia for vaginal delivery can be a test dose. Anesthesiology 67: 436–440
15. Bösenberg A T, Bland A R, Schulte-Steinberg D H, Downing J W 1988 Thoracic epidural anesthesia via caudal route in infants. Anesthesiology 69: 265–269
16. Bromage P R 1978 Epidural analgesia. W B Saunders, Philadelphia
17. Westbrook J L, Renowolen S A, Carrie L E S 1993 Study of the anatomy of the extradural regions using magnetic resonance imaging. Br J Anaesth 71: 495–498
18. Covino B G, Scott D B 1985 Handbook of epidural anaesthesia and analgesia. Schultz Medical Information, Copenhagen, pp 9–28
19. Verbiest H 1976 Neurogenic intermittent claudication. North Holland/Elsevier, New York
20. Huizinga J, van der Heiden J A, Vinken P J J G 1952 The human lumbar vertebral canal: a biometric study. Proc Kon Ned Akad Wet c55: 22–23
21. Kikuchi S 1982 Anatomical and experimental studies of nerve root infiltration. J Jpn Orthop Assoc 56: 605–614

22. Soulié A 1899 Nerfs radichiens. In: Poirier P, Charpy A (eds) Traité d'anatomie humaine. Masson, Paris
23. Leyden E 1874 Klinik der Rückenmarks-Krankheiten I. A Hirschwald, Berlin
24. Cousins M J, Bridenbaugh Ph O 1988 Neural blockade, 2nd edn. J B Lippincott, Philadelphia
25. Hochstetter F 1934 Über die Entwicklung und Differenzierung der Hüllen des Rückenmarkes beim Menschen. Gegenbauers Morphol Jahrbuch 74: 1–104
26. Elaut L, Verdonk G 1934 Anatomische Beobachtungen zur epiduralen und transsakralen Anästhesie. Zbl Chir 61: 12–19
27. Rieckenbacher J, Landolt A M, Theiler K 1982 Rücken. In: Lang J, Wachsmuth W (eds) Praktische anatomie 2.7 (T. von Lanz, W. Wachsmuth). Springer Verlag, Berlin
28. Weston P G 1916 Sugar content of the blood and spinal fluid of insane subjects. J Med Res 35: 199–207 (cited by Davson H 1970 Physiology of the cerebrospinal fluid. Churchill, London)
29. Maiuro F, Ganguni M, Gambardella A 1990 Anatomical and radiological variations of the lumbar dural sac and nerve root sheaths. Clin Neurol Neurosurg 92: 203–213
30. Theiler K 1948 Die Entwicklung der Konstruktiven Form der Rückenmarkshäute beim Menschen. Schweizer Arch Neurol Psych 61: 337–370
31. Schultz E H, Brogdon B G 1962 The problem of subdural placement in myelography. Radiology 79: 91–96
32. Jones M D, Newton T H 1963 Inadvertent extra-arachnoid injections in myelography. Radiology 80: 818–822
33. Taveras J M, Wood E H 1972 Myelography: technical errors. In: Robbins L L (Ed) Golden's diagnostic roentgenology. Williams & Wilkins, Baltimore
34. Sechzer P H 1963 Subdural space in spinal anesthesia. Anaesthesiology 24: 869–870
35. Cohen C A, Kallos T 1972 Failure of spinal anesthesia due to subdural catheter placement. Anesthesiology 37: 352–353
36. Dawkins C J M 1969 An analysis of the complications of extradural and caudal block. Anaesthesia 24: 554–563
37. Paturet G 1964 Système nerveux. In: Testut & Latarjet Traité d'anatomie humaine, 4th edn. Masson, Paris
38. Charpy A (cited in Paturet G 1964 Système nerveux. In: Testut & Latarjet Traité d'anatomie humaine, 4th edn. Masson, Paris
39. Heile B 1913 Zur Darstellung des epiduralen Raumes. Zbl Chir 40: 110–111
40. Hogan Q H 1991 Lumbar epidural anatomy. A new look by cryomicrotome section. Anesthesiology 75: 767–775
41. Cathelin F 1903 Les injections épidurales par ponction du canal sacré et leurs applications dans les maladies des voies urinaires. Baillière, Paris
42. Dogliotti A M 1939 Anesthesia local, regional, spinal. Lebour, Chicago
43. Farr R E 1926 Sacral anesthesia. Arch Surg 12: 715
44. Ramsey H J 1959 Comparative morphology of fat in the epidural space. Am J Anat 105: 219–232
45. Ramsey H J 1959 Fat in the epidural space in young and adult cats. Am J Anat 104: 345–380
46. Tretjakoff D 1926 Das epidurale Fettgewebe. Ztschr Anat 79: 110–111
47. Staemmler M 1939 Beiträge zur normalen und pathologischen Anatomie des Rückenmarkes. I. Zur Pathologie der Blutgefäsze des Rückenmarks. Ztschr Ges Neurol Psychiatr 164: 179–194
48. Lazorthes G, Poulhes J, Bastide E, Bulleau J, Chaucholte A R et al 1957 La vascularisation arterielle de la moelle. Comptes Rendues Ass Anat 58: 410–421
49. Gillilan L A 1958 The arterial blood supply of the human spinal cord. J Comp Neurol 110: 75–104
50. Lazorthes G, Gouazé A, Djindjian R 1973 Vascularisation et circulation de la moelle épinière. Masson, Paris
51. Luyendijk W 1979 The arterial supply of the spinal cord. A historical note. Surg Neurol 11: 369–372
52. Luyendijk W 1982 The arteries of the spinal cord. The history of a paradigmal shift. Acta Neurochir 61: 25–41
53. Adamkiewicz A 1885 Die Blutgefässe des menschlichen Rückenmarkes. Sitz ber d K Akademie d Wissensch Math-Naturw 85: 101–130
54. Luyendijk W, Cohn B, Rejger V, Vielvoye G J 1988 The great radicular artery of Adamkiewicz in man. Acta Neurochir 95: 143–146
55. Kadyi H 1886 Über die Blutgefässe des menschlichen Rückenmarkes. Anat Anz 1: 304–314
56. von Haller A 1754 Iconum anatomicarum, Fasc VII. Abraham van den Hoek, Göttingen
57. Tanon L 1908 Les artères de la moelle dorso-lombaire. Considérations anatomiques et cliniques. Thesis, University of Paris
58. Luyendijk W 1986 The role of arterial deficiency in spinal cord symptomatology. Progr Clinic Neurosci 2: 257–264
59. Domisse G F 1975 The arteries and veins of the human spinal cord from birth. Churchill Livingstone, Edinburgh
60. Willis T 1664 Cerebri anatome. M & J Allestry, London
61. Breschet G 1829 Recherches anatomiques physiologiques et pathologiques sur le système veineux et spécialement sur les canaux veineux des os. Thesis, University of Paris
62. Batson O V 1940 Function of vertebral veins and their role in spread of metastases. Ann Surg 112: 138–149
63. Batson O V 1957 The vertebral vein system. Am J Roentgenol 78: 195–212
64. Clemens H J 1961 Die Venensysteme der menschlichen Wirbelsäule. W. de Gruyter, Berlin
65. Helander C G, Lindblom A 1955 Sacrolumbar venography. Acta Radiologica 44: 410
66. Meijenhorst G C H 1980 Transfemoral epidural double-catheter venography in the diagnosis of lumbar disc herniation, 2nd edn. Nico de Bruyn, Deventer, The Netherlands
67. Meijenhorst G C H 1982 Computed tomograpy of the lumbar epidural veins. Radiology 145: 687–691
68. Parkin I G, Harrison G R 1985 The topographical anatomy of the lumbar epidural space. J Anat 141: 211–217
69. Zarzur E 1984 Anatomic studies on the human lumbar ligamentum flavum. Anesth Analges 63: 499–502
70. Surington C T, Jonas A F 1952 Intra-abdominal venography following inferior vena cava ligation. Arch Surg 65: 605–610
71. Clemens H J, Von Quast H 1960 Untersuchungen über die Gefäsze des menschlichen Rückenmarkes. Acta Anatom 42: 277–306
72. Oswald-Prahn K 1961 Untersuchungen über das Vorkommen von Sperrmechanismen in den Venae radiculares des Menschen. Med Inaug Diss, FU Berlin
73. Cooper E 1960 The vertebral venous plexus. Acta Anatomica 42: 333–351
74. Seitz L 1941 Die normale Schwangerschaft. In: Stoeckel W (ed) Lehrbuch der Geburtshilfe, 6th edn. Fischer, Jena, pp 100–172
75. Kerr M G, Scott D B, Samuel E 1964 Studies of the inferior vena cava in late pregnancy. Br Med J 1: 532–533
76. Van der Hoeven P C T 1935 De physiologie van de zwangerschap baring en kraambed, 4th edn. Willem Vorsselmans, Zundert, The Netherlands
77. Field E J, Brierley J B 1948 The lymphatic drainage of the spinal nerve roots in the rabbit. J Anat 82: 198–206
78. Blomberg R 1986 The dorsomedian connective tissue band in the lumbar epidural space of humans: an anatomical study using epiduroscopy in autopsy cases. Anesth Analges 65: 747–752
79. Savolaine E R, Pandya J B, Greenblatt S H, Conover S R 1988 Anatomy of the human lumbar epidural space: new insights using CT-epidurography. Anesthesiology 68: 217–220
80. Blomberg R G 1989 Endoscopy – epiduroscopy and spinaloscopy – of the lumbal epidural and subdural space. Medical Dissertation No 292, University of Linköping
81. Huson A, Luyendijk W, Tielbeek A, Van Zundert A 1988 CT-epidurography and the anatomy of the human lumbar epidural space. Anesthesiology 69: 797–798
82. Luyendijk W 1976 The plica mediana dorsalis of the dura mater and its relation to lumbar peridurography (canalography). Neuroradiology 11: 147–149
83. Husemeyer R P, White D C 1980 Topography of the lumbar epidural space. A study in cadavers using injected polyester resin. Anaesthesia 35: 7–11
84. Harrison G R, Parkin I G, Shah J L 1985 Resin injection studies of the lumbar extradural space. Br J Anaesth 57: 333–336

85. Carrie L E S 1971 The approach to the extradural space. Anaesthesia 26: 252–253
86. Baretto C, Hook R, Seah C H 1977 Use of the Tuohy needle in paramedian approach for peridural block. Anesth Analges 56: 582–584
87. Armitage E N 1976 The paramedian approach to lumbar epidural analgesia. Analgesia 31: 1287
88. Reynolds A F, Roberts P A, Pollay M, Stratemeier P H 1985 Quantitative anatomy of the thoracolumbar epidural space. Neurosurgery 17: 905–907
89. Shantaveerappa T R, Bourne G H 1962 The perineural epithelium: a metabolic active continuous protoplasmic cell barrier surrounding peripheral nerve fasciculi. J Anat 96: 527–536
90. Ivanow G, Romodanowsky K 1928 Über den anatomischen Zusammenhang der cerebralen und spinalen submeningealen Raume mit dem Lymphsystem. Z Ges Exp Med 58: 596–607
91. Mortensen O A, Sullivan W E 1933 The cerebrospinal fluid and the cervical lymph nodes. Anat Rec 56: 359–363
92. Brierley J B, Field E J 1948 The connexions of the spinal subarachnoid space with the lymphatic system. J Anat 82: 153–166
93. Brierley J B, Field E J 1949 The fate of an intraneural injection as demonstrated by the use of radio-active phosphorus. J Neurol Neurosurg Psychiat 12: 86–99
94. Brierley J B 1950 The penetration of particulate matter from the cerebro-spinal fluid into the spinal ganglia, peripheral nerves and perivascular spaces of the central nervous system. J Neurol Neurosurg Psychiat 13: 203–251
95. Attwood H D, Wooley P A 1974 Arachnoid villi in the spinal cord of Dasyurid marsupials. J Comp Neurol 155: 343–354
96. Welch K, Pollay M 1963 The spinal arachnoid villi in the monkeys *Cercopithecus aethiops sabaeus* and *Macaca Irus*. Anat Rec 145: 43–48
97. Alksne J F, Lovings E T 1972 The role of the arachnoid villus in the removal of red blood cells from the subarachnoid space. An electronmicroscope study in the dog. J Neurosurg 36: 192–200
98. Rexed B A, Wennström K G 1959 Arachnoidal proliferation and cystic formation in the spinal nerve-root pouches of man. J Neurol 16: 73–84
99. Feng T P, Liu Y M 1949 The connective tissue sheath of the nerve as effective diffusion barrier. J Cell Comp Physiol 34: 1–20
100. Haller F R, Low F N 1971 The fine structure of the peripheral nerve root sheath in the subarachnoid space in the rat and other laboratory animals. Am J Anat 131: 1–20
101. Haller F R, Haller A C, Low F N 1972 The fine structure of cellular layers and connective tissue space at spinal nerve root attachment in the rat. Am J Anat 133: 109–124
102. Crescitelli F 1951 Nerve sheath as a barrier to the action of certain substances. Am J Physiol 166: 229–240
103. Singer M 1972 Penetration of ruthenium red into peripheral nerve fibres. Anat Rec 173: 375–389
104. Krishman N, Singer M 1973 Penetration of peroxidase into peripheral nerve fibres. Am J Anat 136: 1–14
105. Tripathi B J, Tripathi R C 1974 Vascular transcellular channels as a drainage pathway for cerebrospinal fluid. J Physiol 239: 195–206
106. Morse D E, Low F N 1972 The fine structure of the pia mater of the cat. Am J Anat 133: 349–367
107. Forestier J 1922 Le trou de conjugaison vertébral et l'espace épidural. Thèse de Paris Jouve, Paris
108. Charpy A (cited in Forestier J 1922 Le trou de conjugaison vertébral et l'espace épidural. Thèse de Paris Jouve, Paris)
109. Forestier J, Sicard A, Oeconomos D 1949 Exploration radiologique des disques intervertébraux par le discolipiodol épidural introduit à la sonde. Rev Neurologique 81: 119–123
110. Sicard J A, Cestan R 1904 Etude de la traversée meningoradiculaire au niveau du trou de conjugaison. Le nerf de conjugaison (nerf radicular spinal). Quelques déductions cliniques. Bull Soc Med Hop Paris 21: 715–725
111. Haguenau J 1936 Le lipiodiagnostic sousarchnoidien est il dangereux? Monde Med 46: 825–827
112. Lazorthes G 1981 Le système nerveux périphérique, 3rd edn. Masson, Paris
113. Lewit K, Sereghy T 1975 Lumbar peridurography with special regard to the anatomy of the lumbar peridural space. Neuroradiology 8: 233–240
114. Lewit K 1976 The contributions of peridurography to the anatomy of the lumbosacral spinal cord. Folio Morphol (Praha) 24: 289–295
115. Shanks C A 1968 Four cases of unilateral epidural analgesia. Br J Anaesth 40: 999–1002

13. Pharmacology and toxicity of local anesthetics

Part A General *B. G. Covino*
Part B Ropivacaine *B. H. Minzter*

PART A
GENERAL
B. G. Covino

Local anesthetic drugs may be defined as pharmacologic agents that are capable of producing a loss of sensation in a circumscribed area of body. This localized form of anesthesia is due to an inhibition of excitation at nerve endings or to a blockade of the conduction process in peripheral nervous tissue. Regional anesthesia originated in 1884 when Koller described the topical anesthetic properties of cocaine, an alkaloid that had been isolated from the leaves of the *Erythroxylon coca* bush. Since that time numerous clinical compounds have been synthesized as local anesthetic agents. The agents which are currently employed for regional anesthesia and their primary area of clinical use are listed in Table 13.1.

PHARMACODYNAMIC CONSIDERATIONS

Mechanism of action

At rest, a negative electrical potential of approximately 60–90 mV; i.e, the resting potential, exists across the nerve membrane. When a nerve is stimulated, a relatively slow phase of depolarization occurs, during which the electrical potential within the cells becomes progressively less negative (Fig. 13.1). When the electrical potential between the interior and exterior surface of the cell membrane reaches a critical level; i.e., the threshold potential, a rapid phase of depolarization follows, resulting in a reversal of the electrical potential such that the interior of the cell becomes positively charged with respect to the exterior surface of the membrane. At the peak of the

Table 13.1 Physicochemical and pharmacologic properties and primary clinical use of local anesthetic agents

Agent	Physicochemical properties				Pharmacologic properties			
	Molecular mass (base)	pK_a (25°C)	Partition coefficient	Protein binding	Onset	Relative potency	Duration	Primary clinical use
Esters								
Procaine	236	8.9	0.02	6	Slow	1	Short	Spinal
Tetracaine	264	8.5	4.1	76	Slow	8	Long	Spinal
Chloroprocaine	271	8.7	0.14	–	Fast	1	Short	Epidural
Amides								
Prilocaine	220	7.9	0.9	55	Fast	2	Moderate	i.v. regional
Lidocaine	234	7.9	2.9	64	Fast	2	Moderate	All forms of regional anesthesia
Mepivacaine	246	7.6	0.8	78	Fast	2	Moderate	Peripheral nerve blocks
Bupivacaine	288	8.1	27.5	96	Moderate	8	Long	Epidural and spinal
Etidocaine	276	7.7	141	94	Fast	6	Long	Epidural

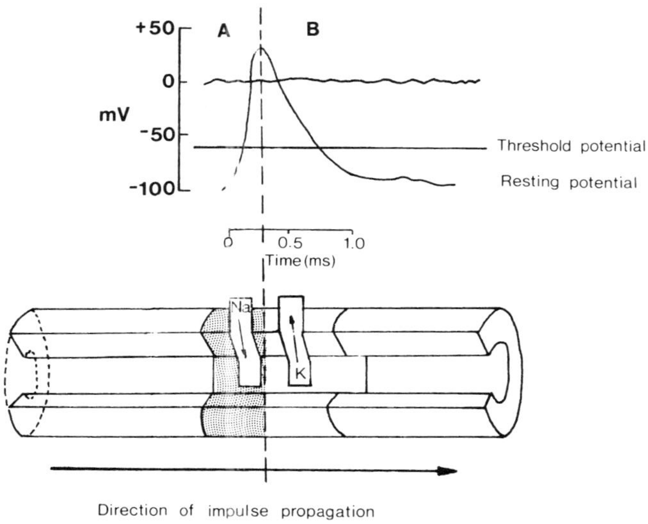

Fig. 13.1 Surface action potential recorded from an isolated nerve (upper figure). Lower portion of figures shows sodium channel activation during depolarization phase and potassium channel opening during repolarization phase.

action potential, the interior of the cell has a positive electrical potential of approximately 40 mV as compared with the exterior of the cell. The total amplitude of the action potential is approximately 100 mV. When depolarization is complete, the nerve begins to repolarize, and the interior of the cell progressively becomes more negative again until the resting potential of –60 to –90 mV is re-established. The entire process of depolarization and repolarization occurs within 1 ms. Depolarization accounts for 30% of the action potential duration, whereas the repolarization phase is slower and is responsible for the remaining 70% of the action potential duration.

These electrophysiologic events are dependent on:

1. the relative concentration of electrolytes in nerve cytoplasm and extracellular fluid; and
2. the permeability of the cell membrane to various ions, particularly sodium and potassium.

The resting potential level is intimately related to the ratio of potassium ions between the inside (K_i) and outside (K_o) of the cell membrane. At rest, a K_i/K_o ratio of approximately 30 : 1 exists. Since the cell membrane is relatively impermeable to the movement of sodium, this ion does not contribute to the resting membrane potential. Following excitation, an increase in the permeability of the cell membrane occurs and sodium ions pass from the exterior to the interior of the nerve cell through the so-called sodium channels. This inward movement of sodium ions accounts for the depolarization phase of the action potential. As the cell becomes maximally depolarized, the permeability of the cell membrane to sodium decreases (sodium inactivation) and an increased flow of potassium ions occurs from the interior to the exterior of the cell, which results in repolarization of the nerve membrane. The flux of sodium and potassium ions during excitation is a passive phenomenon since these ions are moving down their concentration gradients. At the end of the action potential, an excess of sodium ions is present within the cell and an excess of potassium ions exists outside the nerve cell. Re-establishment of the ionic gradient across the nerve membrane requires energy to extrude sodium ions against a concentration gradient. In addition, potassium ions are believed to be actively transported from the exterior to the interior surface of the nerve membrane. However, potassium ions may also move passively along an electrostatic gradient. The energy required for the active transport of sodium and potassium ions (i.e., for the 'sodium pump') is derived from the oxidative metabolism of adenosine triphosphate.

Following exposure of an isolated nerve to a local anesthetic agent, the membrane resting potential and the threshold potential remain essentially unaltered.[1] The maximum rate of rise of the nerve action potential has been shown to decrease from a control value of 190 V/s to 120 V/s following exposure to a solution of 0.005% (0.2 mM) lidocaine with no significant change in the rate of repolarization.[1]

Local anesthetic drugs have been shown to decrease the permeability of the nerve membrane to sodium. For example, at a normal sodium concentration of 116 mM, 3.2 mM cocaine produced a 50% decrease in the height of the isolated frog sciatic nerve action potential.[2] However, when the sodium concentration was lowered to 12 mM in the bathing solution, only 0.15 mM cocaine was required to cause a similar reduction in the amplitude of the action potential. Direct sodium and potassium conductance studies have demonstrated a complete loss of sodium currents[3,4] in the presence of 1 mM lidocaine. On the other hand, 3.5 mM of lidocaine caused only a 5% decrease in potassium conductance.

Most of the clinically useful local anesthetic preparations are available in the form of solutions of a salt; e.g., lidocaine is usually prepared as a 0.5–2.0% solution of lidocaine hydrochloride. In solution, the salts of these local anesthetic compounds exist both in the form of uncharged molecules (B) and as positively charged cations (BH^+). The relative proportion between the uncharged base (B) and the charged cation (BH^+) depends on the pK_a of the specific chemical compound and the pH of the solution. The relationship between these various factors can be expressed as follows: $pH = pK_a - \log (BH^+/B)$. Since pK_a is constant for any specific compound, the relative proportion of free base and charged cation will be dependent essentially on the pH of the local anesthetic solution ($BH^+ \quad B + H^+$). As the pH of the solution is decreased and H^+ concentration increased, the equilibrium will shift towards the charged cationic form. Conversely, as the pH is increased and H^+ concentration decreased, the equilibrium will be shifted towards the free base form.

Two factors are involved in the action of local anesthetics:

1. diffusion through the nerve sheath and membrane, and
2. binding at some site in the cell membrane.

In isolated nerves with an intact epineurium, an increase in the pH of the local anesthetic bathing solution–which favors the formation of the base–markedly accelerated the rate of decrease of the height of the surface action potential. However, in desheathed nerve, a less alkaline solution, in which a relatively greater amount of the charged cation is present, resulted in increased local anesthetic activity. These studies indicate that the uncharged base form is important for optimal penetration of the nerve sheath.[5,6] Following diffusion through the epineurium equilibrium recurs between B and BH^+, and at the cell membrane the charged cation is ultimately responsible for the suppression of electrophysiologic events in peripheral nerve (Fig. 13.2).

The sodium channel is the site at which local anesthetic agents exert their pharmacologic action. These agents are believed to combine with a receptor in the sodium channel, which ultimately results in sodium channel inactivation and conduction blockade.[7] Studies conducted with tertiary amide local anesthetic agents and quaternary derivatives of lidocaine have revealed that the anesthetic potency is enhanced when these compounds are applied to the internal surface of the nerve membrane.[8] Thus, it has been postulated that conventional local anesthetic agents, such as lidocaine, enter the sodium channel from the axoplasmic side.

Although the cationic form of local anesthetics is believed to be primarily responsible for conduction

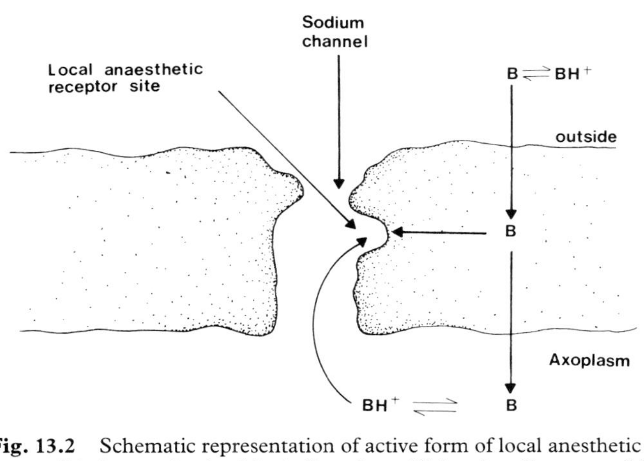

Fig. 13.2 Schematic representation of active form of local anesthetic responsible for conduction block. Base form (B) is primarily responsible for diffusion through nerve membrane into axoplasm, where it is converted to the cationic form (BH^+). The cationic form is primarily involved in combining with receptor site within the sodium channel, leading to conduction blockade.

blockade by combining with a receptor site in the sodium channel, the uncharged base may also contribute to the action of local anesthetics.[7] The uncharged base may penetrate the lipid portion of the cell membrane and cause conformational change in the lipoprotein matrix with a resultant decrease in the diameter of the sodium channels and so contribute to the inhibition of sodium conductance.

In summary, the sequence of events that results in conduction blockade in peripheral nerves by local anesthetic agents is as follows:

1. diffusion of the base form of the local anesthetic molecule across the nerve sheath and nerve membrane;
2. re-equilibrium between the base and cationic form of the local anesthetic compound on the axoplasmic surface of the nerve membrane;
3. penetration into, and attachment to, a receptor at a site within the sodium channel;
4. blockade of the sodium channel;
5. inhibition of sodium conductance;
6. decrease in the rate and degree of the depolarization phase of the action potential;
7. failure to achieve the threshold potential level;
8. lack of development of a propagated action potential; and
9. conduction blockade.

STRUCTURE–ACTIVITY RELATIONSHIP

Chemical compounds that demonstrate clinically useful local anesthetic activity possess the following chemical arrangement:

Aromatic portion – intermediate chain – amine portion

Alterations in either the aromatic portion, amine portion or intermediate chain of specific chemical compounds will modify their anesthetic activity. For example, increasing the molecular weight by lengthening the intermediate chain or by adding of carbon atoms to the aromatic or amine portion tends to increase intrinsic anesthetic potency until a maximum anesthetic potency is reached.[9] Beyond this point, a further increase in molecular weight results in a decrease in anesthetic activity. The aromatic portion of a local anesthetic molecule is usually responsible for its lipophilic properties, whereas the amine portion is associated with hydrophilicity. Changes in either the aromatic or amine portion will alter the lipid–water distribution coefficient of a specific agent. Chemical modification of either end of the molecule will also affect the protein-binding characteristics of a chemical substance which, in turn, will alter its anesthetic profile. For example, the addition of a butyl group to the aromatic end of the procaine molecule increases lipid solubility and protein binding and results in tetracaine, a compound which has a greater intrinsic anesthetic potency and longer duration of anesthetic activity (Table 13.1). The addition of a butyl group to the amine end of mepivacaine transforms this agent into the bupivacaine molecule, a more lipid soluble and more highly protein bound compound which biologically possesses a greater intrinsic potency and longer duration of action (Table 13.1). In the case of lidocaine, substitution of a propyl for an ethyl group at the amine end, and the addition of an ethyl group to the alpha-carbon in the intermediate chain yields etidocaine, which is more lipid soluble, more highly protein-bound and, biologically, a local anesthetic agent of greater potency and longer duration.

The clinically useful local anesthetics essentially fall into two chemical categories:

1. Agents with an ester link between the aromatic end of the molecule and the intermediate chain. Procaine, chloroprocaine and tetracaine are examples of amino-ester agents.
2. Compounds with an amide link between the aromatic portion and the intermediate chain. Lidocaine, mepivacaine, prilocaine, bupivacaine and etidocaine represent amino-amide drugs.

The basic difference between the ester and amide compounds resides in

a. the manner in which they are metabolized, and
b. their allergic potential.

The ester agents are hydrolyzed in plasma by pseudocholinesterase, whereas the amide compounds undergo enzymatic degradation in the liver. Para-aminobenzoic acid is one of the metabolites formed from the hydrolysis of ester-type compounds. This substance is capable of inducing allergic-type reactions in a small percentage of the general population. The amide, lidocaine-like drugs are not metabolized to para-aminobenzoic acid and reports of allergic phenomena with these agents are extremely rare.

The anesthetic profile of the amino-esters and amino-amides is dependent on their physicochemical properties;[10] i.e.,

- lipid solubility;
- protein-binding;
- pK_a.

Lipid solubility appears to be a primary determinant of instrinsic anesthetic potency. The lipid solubility of procaine, as determined by partition coefficient measurements, is less than 1, and this drug is least potent in suppressing conduction in an isolated nerve. On the other hand, the partition coefficients of bupivacaine, tetracaine and etidocaine vary from approximately 30 to 140, indicating an extremely high degree of lipid solubility. These drugs produce conduction blockade in an isolated nerve at very low concentrations such that their intrinsic anesthetic potency is approximately 20 times greater than that of procaine. The relationship of lipid solubility to intrinsic anesthetic potency is consistent with the biochemical composition of the nerve membrane. Approximately 90% of the axolemma consists of lipids. Therefore, local anesthetic agents that are highly lipid soluble penetrate the nerve membrane more easily, which is reflected biologically in increased potency.

The protein-binding characteristics of local anesthetic agents primarily influence the duration of action. Agents such as procaine are poorly bound to proteins and basically possess a relatively short duration of action. Conversely, tetracaine, bupivacaine and etidocaine are highly bound to proteins and display the longest duration of anesthesia. The relationship between protein binding of local anesthetic agents and their duration of action is again consistent with the basic structure of the nerve membrane. Proteins account for approximately 10% of the nerve membrane. Therefore, agents that penetrate the axolemma and attach more firmly to the membrane proteins will tend to possess a prolonged duration of anesthetic activity.

The pK_a of a chemical compound may be defined as the pH at which its ionized and nonionized forms are in complete equilibrium. As previously indicated, the uncharged base form of a local anesthetic agent is primarily responsible for diffusion across the nerve sheath. The onset of anesthesia is directly related to the rate of epineural diffusion which, in turn, is correlated with the amount of drug in the base form (Table 13.2). The percentage of a specific local anesthetic drug which is present in the base form when injected into tissue whose pH is 7.4 is inversely proportional to the pK_a of that agent. For example, lidocaine, which has a pK_a of 7.74, is 65% ionized and 35% nonionized at a tissue pH of 7.4. On the other hand, tetracaine, with a pK_a of 8.6, is 95% ionized and only 5% nonionized at a tissue pH of 7.4. Both in vitro and in vivo studies have confirmed that local anesthetic drugs such as lidocaine, whose pK_a is closer to tissue pH, have a more rapid onset time than agents with a high pK_a, such as tetracaine.

On the basis of differences in anesthetic potency and

Table 13.2 Relationship of pK_a to percent base form and time for 50% conduction block in isolated nerve

Agent	Chemical class	pK_a	Percent base at pH 7.5	Onset (min)
Prilocaine	Amino-amide	7.7	35	2–4
Lidocaine	Amino-amide	7.7	35	2–4
Etidocaine	Amino-amide	7.7	35	2–4
Bupivacaine	Amino-amide	8.1	20	5–8
Tetracaine	Amino-ester	8.6	5	10–15
Procaine	Amino-ester	8.9	2	14–18

duration of action, it is possible to classify the clinically useful injectable local anesthetic compounds into three categories:

Group I. Agents of low anesthetic potency and short duration of action; e.g., procaine and chloroprocaine.

Group II. Agents of intermediate anesthetic potency and duration of action; e.g., lidocaine, mepivacaine and prilocaine.

Group III. Agents of high anesthetic potency and long duration of action; e.g., tetracaine, bupivacaine and etidocaine.

PHARMACOKINETICS OF LOCAL ANESTHETICS

Local anesthetic activity and toxicity are influenced by such factors as systemic absorption from site of injection, distribution, metabolism and excretion. The development of specific and sensitive analytical methods, such as gas chromatography, for measuring the concentration of local anesthetic drugs in blood and urine has resulted in the accumulation of considerable information concerning the pharmacokinetic properties of local anesthetic agents.

Absorption

The systemic absorption of local anesthetics is a function of the site of injection, dosage, addition of a vasoconstrictor agent and the pharmacologic profile of the agent itself.[11] A comparison of the peak blood levels of lidocaine achieved following various regional anesthetic techniques reveals that the highest drug level occurs after intercostal nerve blockade, followed in order of decreasing maximum blood levels by injection into the caudal canal, paracervical area, epidural space, brachial plexus and sciatic femoral site, subcutaneous tissue and the subarachnoid space (Fig. 13.3). The high blood levels following intercostal administration may be related to the multiple injections required for intercostal nerve blocks such that a local anesthetic solution is exposed to a greater vascular area, which results in a greater rate and degree of absorption. This relationship of administration site to rate of absorption is of clinical significance, since use of a fixed dose of a local anesthetic agent may be potentially toxic in one area of administration but not in others. For example, the use of 400 mg of lidocaine without epinephrine for intercostal nerve block results in an average peak venous plasma level of approximately 7 μg/ml, which is sufficient to cause symptoms of CNS toxicity in some patients. This same dose of lidocaine employed for brachial plexus block yields a mean maximum blood level of 3.5 μg/ml, which is rarely associated with signs of toxicity.

The absorption and subsequent blood level of local anesthetic agents is related to the total dose of drug administered regardless of the site of administration. For most agents there is a linear relationship between the amount of drug administered and the resultant peak anesthetic blood level. For example, the mean venous blood level of lidocaine increased from approximately 1.5 μg/ml to 4 μg/ml as the total dose administered into the lumbar epidural space was increased from 200 to 600 mg[12]. Depending on the site of administration, a blood level of 0.5–2.0 μg/ml is achieved for each 100 mg of lidocaine or mepivacaine injected.

The peak anesthetic blood level achieved following regional anesthesia is a function of the total dose of drug administered, irrespective of the concentration or volume of the local anesthetic solution. No significant differences in lidocaine, prilocaine and etidocaine blood levels are observed following intercostal or epidural administration, provided the total dose remains constant, regardless of alterations in concentration and volume of solutions.[12]

Many commercial local anesthetic solutions contain a vasoconstrictor agent, usually epinephrine, in concentrations varying from 5 to 20 μg/ml. The addition of a vasoconstrictor to a local anesthetic solution may prolong the duration of action of certain agents. In addition, epinephrine decreases the rate of absorption of certain agents from various sites of administration and, thus, lowers their potential toxicity (Fig. 13.4). Epinephrine at a concentration of 5 μg/ml (1 : 200 000) significantly reduces the peak blood levels of lidocaine and mepivacaine,

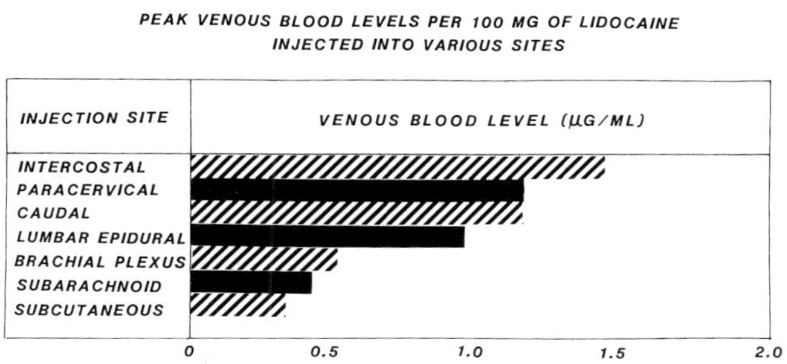

Fig. 13.3 Peak venous blood levels of lidocaine following injection of 100 mg of lidocaine into various anatomical sites.

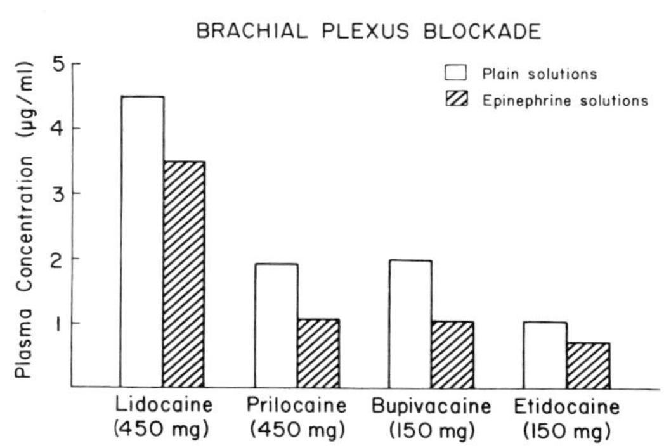

Fig. 13.4 Peak venous plasma concentrations of various local anesthetics administered with and without epinephrine for brachial plexus blockade.

irrespective of the site of administration.[12,13] On the other hand, the peak blood levels of prilocaine, bupivacaine and etidocaine are minimally influenced by the addition of a vasoconstrictor substance following epidural administration. The optimal concentration of epinephrine in the lumbar epidural space appears to be 5 µg/ml (1 : 200 000). Use of a 1 : 80 000 concentration of epinephrine failed to produce a further reduction in the peak blood level of lidocaine.[12] Other vasoconstrictor agents, such as phenylephrine and norepinephrine, have been employed in combination with local anesthetic agents. Neither phenylephrine nor norepinephrine in concentrations of 1 : 20 000 appears to be as effective in reducing the rate of absorption of lidocaine and mepivacaine as epinephrine 1 : 200 000.[14,15]

The pharmacologic characteristics of the specific local anesthetic drug also influence the rate and degree of vascular absorption. A comparison of agents of equivalent anesthetic potency reveals that lidocaine and mepivacaine are absorbed more rapidly following epidural administration than is prilocaine. Bupivacaine is absorbed more rapidly than etidocaine. These rates of absorption, particularly from the epidural space, are probably a reflection of differences in the vasodilator activity and the lipid solubility of these agents. Prilocaine produces less vasodilation than lidocaine. However, etidocaine possesses similar vasodilator activity to bupivacaine. The greater lipid solubility of etidocaine suggests a sequestration of this agent by epidural fat, which may be responsible for the decreased rate of absorption and lower peak blood level following epidural administration.

Distribution of local anesthetics

Local anesthetic agents distribute themselves throughout total body water. The rate of disappearance of local anesthetic drugs from blood (tissue redistribution), the volume of distribution and the relative uptake by various tissues are related to the physicochemical properties of the specific agents. The distribution of local anesthetic agents can be described by a two- or three-compartment model (Fig. 13.5).[16] The rapid disappearance from blood (alpha-phase) is believed related to uptake by rapidly equilibrating tissues; i.e., tissues that have a high vascular perfusion. The slower phase of disappearance from blood (beta-phase) is mainly a function of distribution to slowly equilibrating tissues and the metabolism and excretion of the compound. This secondary phase may also be subdivided into a beta-phase (distribution to slowly perfused tissue) and a gamma-phase (metabolism and excretion). A comparison of the three amide drugs of similar potency and duration of action (i.e., lidocaine, mepivacaine and prilocaine) reveals that prilocaine is redistributed at a significantly more rapid rate from blood to tissues than is lidocaine and mepivacaine. The rate of tissue redistribu-

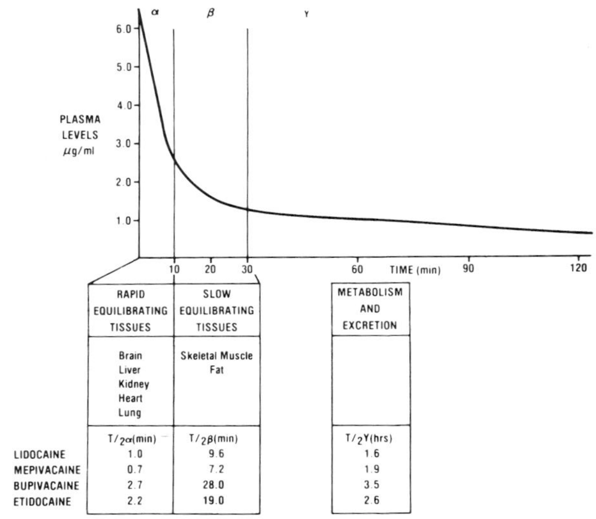

Fig. 13.5 Upper portion shows representative plasma concentration decay curve of a local anesthetic following intravenous injection. Alpha-phase represents redistribution into rapidly equilibrating tissues. Beta-phase represents redistribution into slowly equilibrating tissues and gamma-phase represents metabolism and excretion.

tion for these last two agents is similar. In addition, the beta disappearance phase from blood also occurs more rapidly with prilocaine, suggesting a more rapid rate of metabolism.[17] Differences also exist between the two more potent, longer acting amide-type local anesthetic drugs. Etidocaine possesses a shorter beta half-life than bupivacaine, which is indicative of a more rapid rate of metabolism.

Local anesthetic agents are distributed throughout all body tissues, but the relative concentration in different tissues varies.[18,19] In general, the more highly perfused organs such as lung and kidney initially show higher concentrations of local anesthetic drug than the less well-perfused organs. However, over a longer period of time the highest percentage of an injected dose of a local anesthetic agent is found in skeletal muscle. Although this tissue does not show any particular affinity for this class of drugs, the mass of skeletal muscle makes it the largest reservoir for local anesthetic agents.

Selected tissue distribution studies have been conducted in man (Table 13.3). A correlation exists between the degree of plasma protein binding and the

Table 13.3 Relationship of protein-binding capacity to plasma–RBC and fetal–maternal (U/M) distribution of various local anesthetic agents

Agent	Protein-binding capacity (%)	Plasma–RBC ratio	UV/M ratio
Prilocaine	55	0.88	1.0–1.18
Lidocaine	64	1.34–2.1	0.52–0.69
Mepivacaine	77	2.6	0.69–0.71
Etidocaine	94	7.5	0.14–0.35
Bupivacaine	95	7.8	0.31–0.44

plasma–erythrocyte (P/E) ratio of the different agents. Bupivacaine and etidocaine, which have the greatest capacity for plasma protein binding, also have the highest plasma–erythrocyte ratio. On the other hand, prilocaine shows the lowest P/E ratio and the lowest level of protein binding. Lidocaine and mepivacaine are intermediate in terms of plasma protein binding and plasma–erythrocyte distribution.[19,20] Anesthetic levels in peripheral arteries and veins are also indicative of the distributive properties of the different drugs. For example, simultaneous measurements of samples from the brachial artery and the antecubital vein show a venous–arterial blood concentration ratio of 0.73 for lidocaine and 0.47 for prilocaine.[19] Thus, the rate of diffusion into muscle is considerably faster for prilocaine than for lidocaine, which would account, in part, for the lower blood levels observed with prilocaine.

A specific distribution situation of clinical significance involves the placental transfer of local anesthetic agents. It is generally accepted that local anesthetic agents cross the placenta by passive diffusion. However, the rate and degree of diffusion vary significantly among agents and are directly correlated with the degree of maternal plasma protein binding (Table 13.3).[21] Bupivacaine and etidocaine have the lowest value for umbilical vein–maternal blood ratios (UV/M) and are the agents that are most highly protein bound. Prilocaine shows the highest UV/M ratio and is the least protein bound. Lidocaine and mepivacaine occupy intermediate positions with regard to their degree of placental transfer and their binding to plasma proteins.

Metabolism and excretion

The pattern of metabolism of local anesthetic agents varies according to their chemical classification. Those agents which belong to the ester or procaine-like class undergo hydrolysis in plasma by the enzyme pseudocholinesterase.[22] The rate of metabolism may vary markedly between agents in the same chemical class. Chloroprocaine shows the most rapid rate of hydrolysis (4.7 μmol/ml/h) as compared with a rate of 1.1 μmol/ml/h for procaine and 0.3 μmol/ml/h for tetracaine. With regard to excretion, less than 2% of unchanged procaine is found in urine.[23] Approximately 90% of para-aminobenzoic acid, which is the primary metabolite of procaine, appears in urine. On the other hand, only 33% of diethylaminoethanol, the other major metabolite of procaine, is excreted unchanged.

The local anesthetic compounds that belong to the amide or lidocaine-like series undergo enzymatic degradation primarily in the liver.[17] Prilocaine undergoes the most rapid rate of hepatic metabolism, while bupivacaine appears to be metabolized most slowly. Some degradation of the amide-type compounds may take place in tissue other than liver. The formation of certain metabolites has been observed following incubation of prilocaine with kidney slices.

The metabolism of the amide-type agents is more complex than that of the ester drugs. Although many of the metabolites have been identified, the complete metabolic pathways for all the compounds in this class have not been elucidated. Most metabolic studies have been concerned with lidocaine. The main pathway of metabolism with this agent in man appears to involve oxidative de-ethylation of lidocaine to monoethylglycinexylidide, followed by a subsequent hydrolysis of monoethylglycinexylidide to xylidine.[24]

The excretion of the amide-type local anesthetic drugs occurs by way of the kidney. Less than 5% of the unchanged drug is excreted via the kidney into the urine. The major portion of the injected agent appears in the urine in the form of various metabolites. The renal clearance of the amide local anesthetic agents appears to be inversely related to their protein-binding capacity.[25] Prilocaine, which has a lower protein-binding capacity than lidocaine, has a substantially higher clearance value than lidocaine. Renal clearance also is inversely proportional to the pH of urine, suggesting that urinary excretion of these agents occurs by nonionic diffusion.

TOXICITY OF LOCAL ANESTHETICS

Systemic toxicity

The central nervous system and cardiovascular system are particularly sensitive to the toxic effects of local anesthetic drugs (Table 13.4).

CNS effects

Local anesthetic agents readily cross the blood–brain barrier. At nontoxic blood levels, minimal CNS effects are observed. As the dose and subsequent blood level are

Table 13.4 Signs and symptoms of local anesthetic toxicity

Cardiovascular effects	CNS effects
Mild	
Minimal changes in cardiovascular parameters	Lightheadedness
	Dizziness
	Tinnitus
	Disorientation
Severe	
Prolonged PR interval	Muscle twitching
Prolonged QRS duration	Tremors of face and extremities
Sinus bradycardia	Unconsciousness
Decreased cardiac output	Generalized convulsions
Hypotension	Respiratory arrest
Asystole	

increased, electroencephalographic evidence of excitation becomes manifest. The following EEG changes have been reported in animals and man: an increased delta–theta activity, a decrease in alpha activity, particularly in the amygdaloid nuclear complex, rhythmic spindling, progressing to spike–spindle complex, spiking and, finally, ictal episodes that are correlated with overt signs of seizure activity.[26]

The initial symptoms in man consist of a generalized feeling of lightheadedness and dizziness, followed by auditory and visual disturbances, such as difficulty in focusing and tinnitus. Drowsiness, disorientation and a temporary lack of consciousness may also occur. Slurred speech, shivering, muscle twitching and tremors of the face and extremities appear to be the immediate precursors of a generalized convulsive state.

A further increase in the dose of local anesthetic agents during the excitatory period ultimately results in cessation of convulsive activity and a flattening of the brain wave pattern consistent with generalized central nervous system depression. Respiratory depression and, ultimately, respiratory arrest are the manifestations of the generalized CNS depressive state.

The signs and symptoms of CNS excitation followed by depression are related to an inhibition of cerebral cortical neurons.[27] The initial excitatory state is the result of a selective blockade of the inhibitory cortical neurons or synapses. This inhibition of inhibitory pathways allows facilitatory fibers to function unopposed, leading to excitation of the central nervous system, which is manifested as generalized convulsions. Further increases in dosage produce a depression of both inhibitory and facilitatory pathways, which ultimately causes a generalized state of central nervous system depression.

In general, the potential central nervous system toxicity of local anesthetic agents following an unintentional intravascular injection is correlated with their intrinsic anesthetic potency (Table 13.5).[28] For example, procaine is the least potent and least toxic of the clinically useful local anesthetic agents as defined by the dose which produces convulsions in 50% of animals following a rapid i.v. injection (CD_{50}). On the other hand, bupivacaine and tetracaine are the most potent compounds in terms of both intrinsic anesthetic and CNS convulsive activity.

Table 13.5 Comparison of relative in vivo anesthetic potency and convulsive dose (CD_{100}) of various local anesthetics following i.v. administration in dogs

Agent	Relative anesthetic potency	Convulsive dose (mg/kg)	Relative CNS toxicity
Procaine	1	85	1
Chloroprocaine	1	30	2.8
Prilocaine	2	30	2.8
Mepivacaine	2	30	2.8
Lidocaine	2	30	2.8
Etidocaine	4	22	4
Bupivacaine	8	11	8
Tetracaine	8	13	6.5

In clinical situations in which toxicity occurs following the extravascular administration of an excessive dose, the potential toxic effect of local anesthetic agents will be influenced by such factors as rate of absorption, tissue distribution and metabolism. For example, prilocaine and lidocaine are similar in terms of intrinsic anesthetic potency, whereas prilocaine is approximately 60% less toxic than lidocaine following subcutaneous administration. This phenomenon is due to the rapid tissue redistribution of prilocaine. Similarly, etidocaine and bupivacaine are equitoxic when administered by rapid i.v. injection, but etidocaine is only half as toxic as bupivacaine when the agents are administered subcutaneously. Among the amino-ester agents, procaine is significantly less toxic than chloroprocaine following intravenous administration. However, chloroprocaine is the least toxic of all local anesthetics following an extravascular injection due to its rapid rate of hydrolysis.

Cardiovascular effects

Local anesthetic agents can produce profound effects on the cardiovascular system (Table 13.4). The systemic administration of these agents can exert a direct action both on cardiac muscle and on peripheral vascular smooth muscle.

Cardiac effects. The primary electrophysiologic effect of local anesthetics is a decrease in the maximum rate of depolarization. This decrease in the maximum rate of depolarization is believed due to an interaction with the fast sodium channels in cardiac membrane.[29] This decrease in sodium conductance results in a decreased rate of depolarization. Action potential duration and the effective refractory period are also decreased. However, the ratio of effective refractory period to action potential duration is increased both in Purkinje fibers and in ventricular muscle.

Local anesthetic agents also exert profound effects on the mechanical activity of cardiac muscle in addition to their effect on electrical activity. Studies on isolated atria from guinea pigs have shown that all local anesthetics exert a dose-dependent negative inotropic action.[30] The ability of local anesthetic agents to depress the contractility of cardiac muscle is proportional to their ability to suppress conduction in peripheral nerves. Thus, the more potent local anesthetic agents tend to depress cardiac contractility at lower doses and concentrations than the less potent local anesthetic agents. Studies on the isolated whole rabbit heart have essentially confirmed the results observed on isolated atria.[31] Again, the more potent local anesthetics, bupivacaine, tetracaine and etidocaine, depress ventricular contractility by 25% at concentrations of approximately 1–1.5 μg/ml. On the other hand, lidocaine, mepivacaine and prilocaine require concentrations of approximately 10–15 µg/ml to cause a similar decrease of 25% in the maximum rate of tension development.

Studies in dogs in which a strain gauge arch was sutured to the right ventricle revealed that all local anesthetic agents were capable of exerting a negative inotropic action.[32] A relationship existed between the local anesthetic potency of various agents and their ability to decrease myocardial contractility in intact animals (Fig. 13.6). For example, tetracaine is approximately 8–10 times more potent than procaine in man as a local anesthetic, and similarly tetracaine was found to be approximately eight times more potent as a depressant of myocardial contractility than procaine in intact dogs.

Peripheral vascular effects. Local anesthetic agents can exert significant effects on peripheral vascular smooth muscle. These agents have a biphasic action on smooth muscle of peripheral blood vessels. Direct measurements of the diameter of arterioles in the cremaster muscle of rats prior to and following the topical application of lidocaine revealed that concentrations of lidocaine varying from 10^0 to 10^3 µg/ml produced a dose-related state of vasoconstriction varying from 88–60% of the control vascular diameter.[33] An increase in the concentration of lidocaine to 10^4 µg/ml produced approximately a 27% increase in arteriolar diameter indicative of a significant degree of vasodilation. A similar biphasic effect on vascular smooth muscle was also demonstrated with bupivacaine.[34]

In vivo studies have also confirmed the biphasic effect of local anesthetic on the peripheral vasculature.[35] For example, the intra-arterial administration of mepivacaine in human volunteers resulted in a decrease in forearm blood flow without any change in arterial pressure, which suggests that mepivacaine caused vasoconstriction, which increases peripheral vascular resistance. Similar studies with lidocaine also showed an increased tone in capacitance vessels with less consistent effect on resistance vessels. As the dose of local anesthetic agent administered and the concentration of the agent to which the vascular smooth muscle is exposed increases, the stimulatory or vasoconstrictor action of these agents changes to one of inhibition and vasodilation.

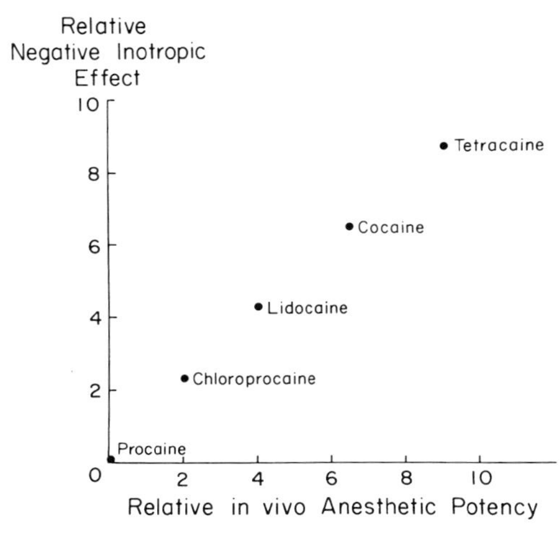

Fig. 13.6 Relationship between the relative negative inotropic effect of various local anesthetics and their relative in vitro anesthetic potency as determined on isolated nerve.

The sequence of cardiovascular events that usually occurs following the systemic administration of local anesthetic agents is as follows. At relatively nontoxic blood levels of these agents, either no change in blood pressure or a slight increase in blood pressure may be observed. The slight increase in blood pressure may be related to a slight increase in cardiac output and heart rate, which have been seen in some animal preparations and are believed due to an enhancement of sympathetic activity by these agents. In addition, the direct vasoconstrictor action of local anesthetics on certain peripheral vascular beds at low concentrations may be responsible in part for a slight increase in systemic blood pressure. Concentrations of local anesthetics which produce CNS toxicity will result in a marked increase in heart rate, blood pressure and cardiac output that is directly related to the degree and duration of convulsive activity. A further increase in dosage and blood level of local anesthetic leads to cardiovascular depression. The initial depression in blood pressure related primarily to a fall in cardiac output is transient in nature and spontaneously reversible in most patients. However, if the amount of local anesthetic administered is excessive or if additional local anesthetic agent continues to be administered, then a profound and irreversible state of cardiovascular depression occurs. The profound hypotension and cardiovascular collapse seen prior to death is related not only to the negative inotropic action of the local anesthetics, but also to the profound peripheral dilation that these agents can produce due to their direct relaxant effect on vascular smooth muscle. At high concentrations the depressant effect of these agents on the excitability of cardiac tissue will also become evident as a decrease in sinus rate and AV conduction block. Ultimately, the combined peripheral vasodilation, decreased myocardial contractility and depressant effect on rate and conductivity will lead to cardiac arrest and circulatory collapse. In addition, certain agents such as bupivacaine may precipitate fatal ventricular fibrillation.

Comparative cardiovascular effects of local anesthetics

Most of the early studies concerning the cardiodepressant effects of local anesthetics indicated that a relationship exists between the intrinsic anesthetic potency of the various agents and their relative negative inotropic activity. In recent years there has been some suggestion that the more potent local anesthetic agents such as bupivacaine may be relatively more cardiotoxic than the less potent local anesthetics, such as lidocaine.

The cardiotoxicity of the more potent agents such as bupivacaine appears to differ from that of lidocaine in the following manner.

1. The ratio of the dosage required for irreversible cardiovascular collapse (CC) and the dosage that will produce CNS toxicity (convulsions); i.e. the CC/CNS ratio is lower for bupivacaine and etidocaine than for lidocaine.
2. Ventricular arrhythmias and fatal ventricular fibrillation may occur following the rapid intravenous administration of a large dose of bupivacaine but not lidocaine.
3. The pregnant animal or patient may be more sensitive to the cardiotoxic effects of bupivacaine than the nonpregnant animal or patient.
4. Cardiac resuscitation is more difficult following bupivacaine-induced cardiovascular collapse.
5. Acidosis and hypoxia markedly potentiate the cardiotoxicity of bupivacaine.

CC/CNS ratio. The dosage and blood level of lidocaine, bupivacaine and etidocaine associated with the development of convulsive activity and cardiovascular collapse has been determined in adult sheep in which continuous intravenous infusions of these various local anesthetics were administered.[36] A CC/CNS ratio of 7.1 ± 1.1 existed for lidocaine, indicating that seven times as much drug was required to induce irreversible cardiovascular collapse as was needed for the production of convulsions (Table 13.6). In comparison, the CC/CNS ratio for bupivacaine was 3.7 ± 0.5 and for etidocaine 4.4 ± 0.9. Thus, although the central nervous system was still more sensitive to the toxic effects of the more potent local anesthetics, a smaller difference did exist between the dose to cause convulsions and that which led to irreversible cardiovascular collapse as compared with the less potent anesthetic lidocaine.

Studies in sheep in which the blood levels of various local anesthetics were determined and related to the onset of CNS and cardiovascular toxicity also reveal a narrower CC/CNS ratio for the more potent local anesthetics. For example, lidocaine was found to possess a CC/CNS blood level ratio of 3.6 ± 0.3 compared with values of 1.6 to 1.7 for bupivacaine and etidocaine (Table 13.6). Tissue levels of the various local anesthetics which were determined at the time of cardiovascular collapse indicate a greater uptake of bupivacaine and etidocaine by the myocardium compared with lidocaine. Thus, the enhanced sensitivity of the myocardium to these more potent agents appears to be due to a greater myocardial uptake.

Table 13.6 Comparative cardiovascular collapse (CC)/convulsive (CNS) ratio and cardiac tissue–blood concentration ratio of lidocaine, bupivacaine and etidocaine in adult sheep. (Data derived from Morishima et al 36.)

	Lidocaine	Bupivacaine	Etidocaine
CC/CNS Dose ratio	7.1 ± 1.1	3.7 ± 0.5	4.4 ± 1.9
CC/CNS Blood concentration ratio	3.6 ± 0.3	1.6 ± 0.1	1.7 ± 0.2
Cardiac tissue	2.6 ± 0.5	3.8 ± 0.6	3.5 ± 0.7

Ventricular arrhythmias. In recent years a number of investigators have reported the development of ventricular arrhythmias in animals exposed to toxic doses of bupivacaine.[37–39] The incidence of ventricular arrhythmias has been determined in awake dogs in which convulsant and supraconvulsant doses of lidocaine, mepivacaine, bupivacaine, etidocaine and tetracaine were administered intravenously. Ventricular arrhythmias occurred in approximately 50% of dogs following the rapid intravenous injection of a convulsant or supraconvulsant dose of bupivacaine and 20% of the animals receiving etidocaine. Ventricular arrhythmias were not observed in dogs treated with lidocaine, mepivacaine or tetracaine. The results suggest that the occurrence of ventricular fibrillation is not related to the basic piperidine ring structure of bupivacaine since mepivacaine, which contains the piperidine moiety, failed to cause these cardiac abnormalities. In addition, a precise correlation does not appear to exist between the frequency of ventricular arrhythmias and the lipid solubility and protein binding of local anesthetics. Large doses of etidocaine, which is more lipid soluble than bupivacaine and equally protein bound, may cause ventricular arrhythmias and fibrillation, but the incidence appears to be lower than that observed with bupivacaine.

The etiology of bupivacaine-associated ventricular arrhythmias is believed to be related to a prolonged inhibition of sodium conductance in the cardiac membrane. Electrophysiologic studies on isolated tissues have shown that bupivacaine can markedly depress the rapid phase of depolarization (V_{max}) of the cardiac action potential.[40,41] The recovery phase is prolonged in isolated papillary muscles exposed to bupivacaine, suggesting the possibility of unidirectional blockade of conduction pathways leading to a re-entrant type of arrhythmia. Bupivacaine has been characterized as a fast-in, slow-out type of agent whereas lidocaine is a fast-in, fast-out agent. Reiz and Nath[42] have also demonstrated that the myocardial uptake of lidocaine and bupivacaine is rapid, but lidocaine washes out of the myocardium rapidly while the washout of bupivacaine is slow.

The development of ventricular arrhythmias following the intravenous administration of bupivacaine may be due to a direct effect on the myocardium or may be indirectly related to a CNS effect, or it may result from both a direct and indirect action of bupivacaine. Ventricular arrhythmias have been produced in isolated hearts exposed to bupivacaine[43] and following the direct intracoronary injection of bupivacaine in pigs.[44] However, ventricular arrhythmias have also been observed in cats and rats following the intracranial injection of bupivacaine.[45,46] In addition, arrhythmias were not observed in anesthetized dogs in whom large intravenous doses of bupivacaine were administered.[47] Thus, bupivacaine-induced cardiac arrhythmias may be related to both a direct and indirect effect on the myocardium.

Enhanced cardiotoxicity in pregnancy. A number of the cardiotoxic reactions reported following the use of bupivacaine has occurred in pregnant patients. As a result, the 0.75% solution is no longer recommended for use in obstetric anesthesia in the USA. Studies in pregnant and nonpregnant sheep have shown that the CC/CNS dosage ratio decreased from 3.7 ± 0.5 in nonpregnant sheep to 2.7 ± 0.4 in pregnant animals.[36] However, little difference was observed in the CC/CNS blood level ratio, which varied from 1.6 ± 0.1 in nonpregnant animals to 1.4 ± 0.1 in pregnant ewes. These studies suggest that, in terms of local anesthetic dosage to produce CNS and cardiovascular toxicity, the myocardium of the pregnant animal may be somewhat more sensitive. Measurements of cardiac tissue levels have failed to demonstrate a greater myocardial uptake of bupivacaine in pregnant sheep at the time of cardiovascular collapse, which indicates that the possible enhanced vulnerability of the pregnant animal is not related to greater myocardial uptake of drug.

Cardiac resuscitation. Cardiopulmonary resuscitation is apparently extremely difficult in patients in whom cardiotoxicity has occurred following the administration of a toxic dose of bupivacaine. Studies in acidotic and hypoxic sheep have also indicated that cardiac resuscitation following bupivacaine-induced toxicity is difficult.[48] Studies in cats and dogs rendered toxic with bupivacaine indicate that resuscitation is possible if massive doses of cardiac stimulants are employed.[49,50]

Effect of acidosis and hypoxia. Changes in acid–base status will alter the potential cardiovascular toxicity of local anesthetic agents. The combination of hypoxia and acidosis markedly potentiates the cardiodepressant effects of bupivacaine in isolated atrial tissue.[51] Hypoxia and acidosis also increased the frequency of cardiac arrhythmias and the mortality rate in sheep following the intravenous administration of bupivacaine.[48] Marked hypercarbia, acidosis and hypoxia occur very rapidly in some patients following seizure activity due to the rapid unintentional intravascular injection of local anesthetic agents.[52] Thus, the cardiovascular depression observed with the more potent agents such as bupivacaine may be related in part to the severe acid–base changes that occur following the administration of toxic doses of these agents.

Local tissue toxicity

Local anesthetic agents that are employed clinically rarely produce localized nerve damage. Studies on isolated frog sciatic nerve revealed that concentrations of procaine, cocaine, tetracaine, and dibucaine required to produce irreversible conduction blockade are far in excess of the concentration of these agents used clinically.[53] A comparison of lidocaine, tetracaine or etidocaine administered subarachnoid in rabbits revealed histopathologic spinal cord changes following the use of 2% tetracaine, which is considerably greater than the maximum concentration of 1% employed for spinal anesthesia in man.[54] Chloroprocaine has been reported to cause prolonged sensory motor deficits in some patients following the epidural or subarachnoid injection of large doses of this particular drug.[55,56] Studies in animals have proven somewhat contradictory regarding the potential neurotoxicity of chloroprocaine. Paralysis has been observed in rabbits given chloroprocaine solutions subarachnoid.[57] However, the paralysis was believed to be related to the sodium bisulfite, which is employed as an antioxidant in chloroprocaine solutions. The use of pure solutions of chloroprocaine without sodium bisulfite did not cause paralysis. Isolated rabbit vagus nerve studies have revealed that commercial solutions of 3% chloroprocaine which contain the local anesthetic agent itself, 0.2% sodium bisulfite and hydrogen ions yielding a pH of approximately 3.0 resulted in irreversible conduction block.[58] The use of 3% chloroprocaine with sodium bisulfite buffered to a pH of 7.0 or a sodium bisulfite-free solution caused reversible conduction block. Application of an 0.2% sodium bisulfite solution at a pH of 3.0 resulted in irreversible conduction block, whereas the use of an 0.2% sodium bisulfite solution with a pH of 7.0 caused no conduction block. The results of these studies suggest that the combination of a low pH and the presence of sodium bisulfite may be responsible for the neurotoxic reactions observed following the use of large amounts of chloroprocaine solution. Chloroprocaine itself does not appear to be neurotoxic.

Allergic or hypersensitivity reactions

True allergic reactions to local anesthetic agents are rare. Ester derivatives of para-aminobenzoic acid, such as procaine and tetracaine, are responsible for most of the allergic phenomena associated with the use of local anesthetic agents. When the ester-type agents were the only anesthetic drugs available, dermal reactions were reported, particularly by members of the dental profession. Since the introduction of the amide-type of local anesthetic compounds, such reports have been extremely rare. In a detailed study of patients with and without a history of local anesthetic allergy, cutaneous reactions were observed in both types of patients following the intradermal injection of ester-type local anesthetic agents.[59] No cutaneous sensitivity reactions occurred following treatment with the amide-type agents even in those subjects who presented with a history of sensitivity to these specific drugs. Multiple-dose vials of some amide local anesthetic agents may contain, as a preservative, methylparaben, which is similar to para-aminobenzoic acid. This substance may cause allergic-type reactions in certain patients.[60]

SUMMARY

Local anesthetic agents may be classified chemically as either amino-ester or amino-amide compounds. In terms of their clinical anesthetic activity these agents may be divided into three groups:

1. agents of low potency and short duration; e.g., procaine and chloroprocaine;
2. agents of intermediate potency and duration; e.g., lidocaine, prilocaine and mepivacaine;
3. agents of high potency and long duration; e.g., bupivacaine, etidocaine and tetracaine.

The anesthetic profile of the various agents is primarily related to lipid solubility, protein binding and pK_a.

The blood concentration of local anesthetic agents is related to their rate of vascular absorption and their redistribution, metabolism and excretion. Absorption is a function of the site of administration, dosage, addition of vasoconstrictors and specific drug employed. The elimination of the various local anesthetic differs considerably. Among the amino-esters, chloroprocaine is hydrolyzed most rapidly, while prilocaine is the most rapidly metabolized amino-amide agent.

The toxicity of local anesthetic agents can be divided into basically three categories:

1. systemic toxic reactions due usually to unintentional intravascular injection or the administration of excessive doses of these agents;
2. miscellaneous reactions such as allergy and methemoglobinemia; and
3. local tissue toxicity.

The systemic toxicity of local anesthetic agents is primarily related to the inhibition of inhibitory fibers in the brain, resulting in signs of CNS excitation and convulsive activity. An increase in the dose and concentration of local anesthetics will result in a depressant effect on facilitatory neurons, which ultimately leads to a generalized state of CNS depression. The cardiovascular system is more resistant to the toxic actions of local anesthetics than is the central nervous system. However, if sufficient doses and blood levels of local anesthetics are achieved, signs of profound cardiovascular depression may be observed. Local anesthetics can depress the rate of depolarization of cardiac membranes and can exert a negative chronotropic and inotropic action on the heart. In addition, these agents can cause profound peripheral vasodilation. The combination of cardiac depression and peripheral vascular dilation results in profound irreversible circulatory collapse. Differences exist between local anesthetics in terms of their relative potential for cardiotoxicity. The CC/CNS ratio for bupivacaine and etidocaine is less than for lidocaine. In addition, bupivacaine may precipitate ventricular arrhythmias and ventricular fibrillation.

Miscellaneous systemic reactions include allergy and methemoglobinemia. Allergic reactions occur more frequently with the amino-ester agents due to the formation of para-aminobenzoic acid. Methemoglobinemia has been observed following the use of high doses of prilocaine.

Finally, local tissue toxicity can occur following the administration of local anesthetics. In general, neural tissue appears to be relatively resistant to the irritant effects of local anesthetic drugs. However, large dosages of chloroprocaine solutions administered subarachnoid have been associated with prolonged sensory-motor deficits in a few patients, probably due to the low pH and presence of sodium bisulfite in the chloroprocaine solutions.

REFERENCES

1. Aceves J, Machne X 1963 The action of calcium and of local anesthetics on nerve cells, and their interaction during excitation. J Pharmacol Exp Ther 140: 138–148
2. Condouris G A 1961 A study of the mechanism of action of cocaine on amphibian peripheral nerve. J Pharmacol Exp Ther 131: 243–249
3. Taylor R E 1959 Effect of procaine on electrical properties of squid axon membrane. Am J Physiol 196: 1071–1078
4. Hille B 1966 Common mode of action of three agents that decrease the transient change in sodium permeability in nerves. Nature 210: 1220–1222
5. Ritchie J M, Ritchie B, Greengard P 1965 The active structure of local anesthetics. J Pharmacol Exp Ther 150: 152–159
6. Ritchie J M, Ritchie B, Greengard P 1965 The effect of the nerve sheath on the action of local anesthetics. J Pharmacol Exp Ther 150: 160–164
7. Butterworth J F, Strichartz G R 1990 Molecular mechanisms of local anesthesia: a review. Anesthesiology 72: 711–734
8. Narahashi T, Yamada M, Frazier D T 1969 Cationic forms of local anesthetics block action potentials from inside the nerve membrane. Nature 223: 748–749
9. Takman B H, Camougis G 1970 Local anesthetics. In: Burger A (ed) Medical chemistry. John Wiley, New York.
10. Covino B G 1985 Pharmacology of local anaesthetics. Br J Anaesth 58: 701–716
11. Scott D B, Jebson P J R, Braid D P, Ortengren B, Frisch P 1972 Factors affecting plasma levels of lignocaine and prilocaine. Br J Anaesth 44: 1040–1049
12. Tucker G R, Mather L E 1975 Pharmacokinetics of local anesthetic agents. Br J Anaesth 47: (suppl): 213–224
13. Tucker G T, Moore D C, Bridenbaugh P O, Bridenbaugh L D, Thompson G E 1972 Systemic absorption of mepivacaine in commonly used regional block procedures. Anesthesiology 37: 277–287
14. Stanton-Hicks M, Berges P U, Bonica J J 1973 Circulatory effects of peridural block. IV. Comparison of the effects of epinephrine and phenylephrine. Anesthesiology 39: 308–314
15. Dhuner K G, Lewis D H 1966 Effect of local anesthetics and vasoconstrictors upon regional blood flow. Acta Anaesth Scand 23 (suppl): 347–352
16. Tucker G T 1986 Pharmacokinetics of local anaesthetics. Br J Anaesth 58: 717–731
17. Akerman B, Astrom A, Ross S, Telc A 1966 Studies on the

absorption, distribution and metabolism of labelled prilocaine and lidocaine in some animal species. Acta Pharmacol. Toxicol (Kbh) 24: 389–403
18. Katz J 1968 The distribution of ^{14}C-labelled lidocaine injected intravenously in the rat. Anesthesiology 29: 249–253
19. Eriksson E, Engelsson S, Wahlqvist S, Ortengren B 1966 Study of the intravenous toxicity in man and some in vitro studies on the distribution and absorbability. Acta CHir Scand 358 (suppl): 25–36
20. Tucker G T, Boyes R N, Bridenbaugh P O, Moore D C 1970 Binding of anilide-type local anesthetics in human plasma. I. Relationships between binding, physiochemical properties, and anesthetic activity. Anesthesiology 33: 287–303
21. Covino B G 1971 Comparative clinical pharmacology of local anesthetic agents. Anesthesiology 35: 158–167
22. Foldes F F, Davidson G M, Duncalf D, Kawabara S 1965 The intravenous toxicity of local anesthetic agents in man. Clin Pharmacol Ther 6: 328–335
23. Brodie B B, Lief P A, Poet R 1948 The fate of procaine in man following its intravenous administration and methods for the estimation of procaine and diethylaminoethanol. J Pharmacol Exp Ther 94: 359–366
24. Keenaghan J B, Boyes R N 1972 The tissue distribution, metabolism and excretion of lidocaine in rats, guinea pigs, dogs and man. J Pharmacol Exp Ther 180: 454–463
25. Eriksson E, Granberg P O 1965 Studies on the renal excretion of Citanest and Xylocaine. Acta Anaesth Scand 16 (suppl): 79–85
26. deJong R H, Robles R, Corbin R W 1969 Central actions of lidocaine – synaptic transmission. Anesthesiology 30: 19–23
27. Tanaka K, Tamasaki M 1966 Blocking of cortical inhibitory synapses by intravenous lidocaine. Nature 209: 207–208
28. Englesson S 1974 The influence of acid–base changes on central nervous system toxicity of local anesthetic agents. I. An experimental study in cats. Acta Anaesthesiol Scand 18: 79–87
29. Clarkson C W, Hohdeghem L M 1985 Mechanism for bupivacaine depression of cardiac conduction: fast block of sodium channels during the action potential with slow recovery from block during diastole. Anesthesiology 62: 396–405
30. Feldman H S, Covino B G, Sage D J 1982 Direct chronotropic and inotropic effects of local anesthetic agents in isolated guinea pig atria. Reg Anesth 7: 149–156
31. Block A, Covino B G 1982 Effect of local anesthetic agents on cardiac conduction and contractility. Reg Anesth 6: 55–61
32. Stewart D M, Rogers W P, Mahaffrey J E, Witherspoon S, Woods E F 1963 Effect of local anesthetics on the cardiovascular system in the dog. Anesthesiology 24: 620–624
33. Johns R A, DiFazio C A, Longnecker D E 1985 Lidocaine constricts or dilates rat arterioles in a dose-dependent manner. Anesthesiology 62: 141–144
34. Johns R A, Seyde W C, DiFazio C A, Longnecker D E Dose-dependent effects of bupivacaine on rat muscle arterioles. Anesthesiology 65: 186–191
35. Jorfeldt L, Lofstrom B, Pernow B, Wahren J 1970 The effect of mepivacaine and lidocaine on forearm resistance and capacitance vessels in man. Acta Anaesthesiol Scand 14: 183–201
36. Morishima H O, Pederson H, Finster M et al 1985 Bupivacaine toxicity in pregnant and nonpregnant ewes. Anesthesiology 63: 134–139
37. deJong R H, Ronfeld R A, DeRosa R A 1982 Cardiovascular effects of convulsant and supraconvulsant doses of amide local anesthetics. Anesth Analg 61: 3–9
38. Kotelko D M, Shnider S M, Kailey P A et al 1984 Bupivacaine-induced cardiac arrthymias in sheep. Anesthesiology 60: 10–18
39. Sage D J, Feldman H S, Arthur G R, Doucette A M, Norway S B, Covino B G 1985 The cardiovascular effects of convulsant doses of lidocaine and bupivacaine in the conscious dog. Reg Anesth 10: 175–183
40. Lynch C 1986 Depression of myocardial contractility in vitro by bupivacaine, etidocaine, and lidocaine. Anesth Analg 65: 551
41. Moller R A, Covino B G 1988 Cardiac electrophysiologic effects of lidocaine and bupivacaine. Anesth Analg 67: 107–114
42. Reiz S, Nath S 1986 Cardiotoxicity of local anesthetic agents. Br J Anaesth 38: 736–746
43. Tanz R D, Heskett T, Loehning R W, Fairfax C A 1984 Comparative cardiotoxicity of bupivacaine and lidocaine in the isolated prefused mammalian heart. Anesth Analg 63: 549–556
44. Nath S, Haggmark S, Johansson G, Reiz S 1986 Differential depressant and electrophysiologic cardiotoxicity of local anesthetics: An experimental study with special reference to lidocaine and bupivacaine. Anesth Analg 65: 1263–1270
45. Heavner J E 1986 Cardiac dysrhythmias induced by infusion of local anesthetics into the lateral cerebral ventricle of cats. Anesth Analg 65: 133–138
46. Thomas R D, Behbehani M M, Coyle D E, Denson D D 1986 Cardiovascular toxicity of local anesthetics: An alternative hypothesis. Anesth Analg 65: 444–450
47. Liu P L, Feldman H S, Covino B M, Giasi R, Covino B G 1982 Acute cardiovascular toxicity of intravenous amide local anesthetics in anesthetized ventilated dogs. Anesth Analg 61: 317–322
48. Rosen M A, Thigpen J W, Shnider S M, Foutz S E, Levinson G, Koike M 1983 Bupivacaine-induced cardiotoxicity in hypoxic and acidotic sheep. Anesth Analg 64: 1089–1096
49. Chadwick H S 1985 Toxicity and resuscitation in lidocaine or bupivacaine infused cats. Anesthesiology 63: 385–390
50. Kasten G W, Martin S T 1985 Bupivacaine cardiovascular toxicity: comparison of treatment with bretylium and lidocaine. Anesth Analg 64: 911–916
51. Sage D J, Feldman H S, Arthur G R, Datta S, Ferretti A M, Norway S B, Covino B G 1983 Influence of lidocaine and bupivacaine on isolated guinea pig atria in the presence of acidosis and hypoxia. Anesth Analg 63: 1–7
52. Moore D C, Crawford R D, Scurlock J E 1980 Severe hypoxia and acidosis following local anesthetic-induced convulsions. Anesthesiology 53: 259–260
53. Skou J C 1954 Local anaesthetics. II. The toxic potencies of some local anesthetics and of butyl alcohol, determined on peripheral nerve. Acta Pharmacol Toxicol 10: 292–296
54. Adams H J, Mastri A R, Eicholzer A, Kilpatrick G 1974 Morphologic effects of intrathecal etidocaine and tetracaine on the rabbit spinal cord. Anesth Analg 53: 904–908
55. Ravindran R S, Bond V K, Tasch M D, Gupta D C, Luerssen T G 1980 Prolonged neural blockade following regional analgesia with 2-chloroprocaine. Anesth Analg 58: 447–451
56. Reisner L S, Hochman B N, Plumer M H 1980 Persistent neurologic deficit and adhesive arachnoiditis following intrathecal 2-chloroprocaine injection. Anesth Analg 58: 452–454
57. Wang B C, Hillman D E, Spiedholz N I, Turndorf H 1984 Chronic neurological deficits and Nesacaine-CE – an effect of the anesthetic, 2-chloroprocaine, or the antioxidant, sodium bisulfite? Anesth Analg 63: 445–447
58. Gissen A J, Datta S, Lambert D 1984 The chloroprocaine controversy. II. Is chloroprocaine neurotoxic? Reg Anesth 9: 135–145
59. Aldrete J A, Johnson D A 1970 Evaluation of intracutaneous testing for investigation of allergy to local anesthetic agents. Anesth Analg 49: 173–183
60. Aldrete J A, Johnson D A Allergy to local anesthetics. J Am Med Assoc 207: 356–357

PART B
ROPIVACAINE
B. H. Minzter

HISTORY

The goal of obstetric anesthesia is to provide safe, effective, and enduring pain relief to the laboring parturient. The ideal local anesthetic for the management of labor pain would confer excellent analgesia with minimal to no motor block. Additionally, it should have a high therapeutic ratio, with minimal toxicity relative to its potency.

In the hundred or more years since Koller's experiments with cocaine, many local anesthetics have been synthesized and studied in animals and humans. The most recently developed amide local anesthetic, ropivacaine, is being evaluated in clinical trials for women in active labor or undergoing cesarean delivery. This section outlines the material available to date on this new amide local anesthetic, which appears to have promise for obstetric anesthesia.

In 1963, the amide local anesthetic bupivacaine was first used clinically. This agent provided excellent surgical anesthesia with relatively less motor block than lidocaine and a longer duration of action. In time, however, it was found that both bupivacaine and etidocaine, introduced in the 1970s, were relatively cardiotoxic, especially in pregnant women, and that these drugs could lead to intractable cardiovascular collapse if unintentionally injected intravascularly. There were reports, especially in pregnant women, of malignant arrhythmias occurring at plasma concentrations not much greater than those that cause seizures.[1] Fractionation of the appropriate dose of bupivacaine was advised, and, at the present time, bupivacaine is widely utilized for surgical and obstetric anesthesia, as well as for post-operative pain management.

Researchers have continued to look for a less cardiotoxic, long-acting local anesthetic. Ropivacaine was synthesized during the development of bupivacaine, but first used for clinical trials in 1988.

PHYSICOCHEMICAL CHARACTERISTICS

The amino-amide ropivacaine is a homolog of mepivacaine and bupivacaine. Bupivacaine is the butyl derivative of mepivacaine, with a methyl group, and ropivacaine is the propyl derivative (Fig. 13.7). Whereas mepivacaine and bupivacaine are prepared as racemic mixtures, ropivacaine is prepared as the *S*-isomer around its asymmetric carbon atom. In 1988, Akerman et al[2] demonstrated that isomers of local anesthetics are not as toxic as racemic compounds. Within this homologous series of compounds, ropivacaine and bupivacaine have equally high percentages of protein binding, probably contributing to their long duration of action. Their pK_a are essentially the same and, not surprisingly, they both have relatively moderate onsets of action compared with mepivacaine, with a lower pK_a. Additionally, as ropivacaine is less lipid soluble than bupivacaine, it should be expected that its potency may be somewhat less (Table 13.7).

Table 13.8 lists some of the pharmacokinetic properties of bupivacaine and ropivacaine. Essentially, these two local anesthetics share similar kinetics, so that when comparable doses are infused intravenously into dogs the mean peak plasma concentrations do not appreciably differ. However, there is a more rapid clearance of ropivacaine, resulting in a shorter half-life than bupivacaine.[3]

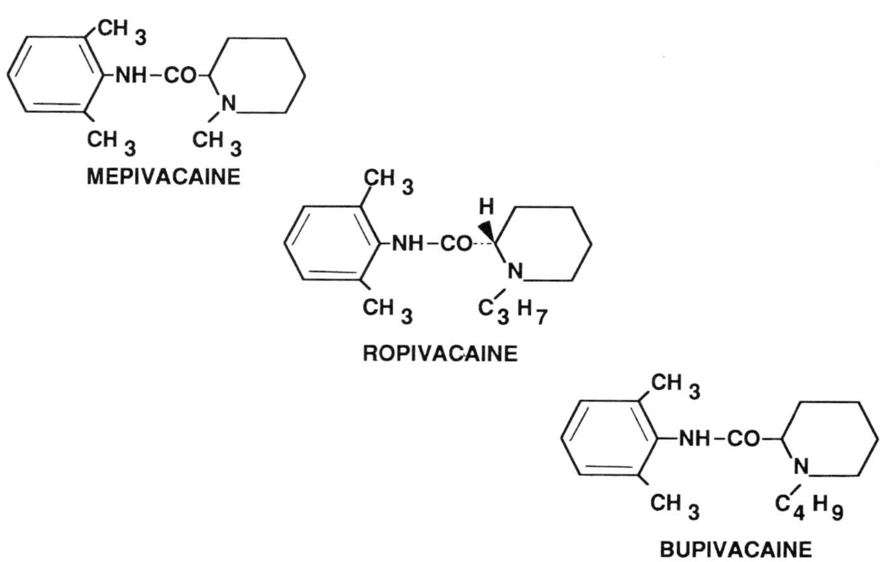

Fig. 13.7 Chemical structures of mepivacaine, ropivacaine and bupivacaine.

Table 13.7 Pharmacology

	Molecular mass	(pK_a 25°C)	Partition coefficient	Protein binding (%)	Onset	Relative potency*	Duration
Ropivacaine	274	8.0	8.5	94	Moderate	6	Long
Bupivacaine	288	8.1	27.5	96	Moderate	8	Long
Mepivacaine	246	7.6	0.8	78	Fast	2	Moderate

* As compared with procaine.

Table 13.8 Pharmacokinetic data after i.v. infusion of 3.0 mg/kg ropivacaine and 3.4 mg/kg bupivacaine (Data from Arthur et al[3])

	C_{max} (μg/ml)	Weight (kg)	$t_{1/2\beta}$ (min)	MBRT (min)	Cl (ml/min/kg^{-1})
Ropivacaine	2.41 ± 0.52	18.5 ± 1.9	25.9 ± 1.7*	27 ± 4	41.1 ± 8.2
Bupivacaine	3.35 ± 0.16	17.7 ± 1.5	39.1 ± 13.3	37 ± 13	32.3 ± 8.2

* $P < 0.05$, ropivacaine compared with bupivacaine, C_{max} was not compared. C_{max} peak concentration; $t_{1/2\beta}$ half-life of elimination; MBRT, mean body residence time; Cl, total body clearance.

This more rapid elimination of ropivacaine after an intravenous dose may contribute to a decreased toxicity.

After epidural injection of equal doses of these agents, peak concentrations of both are similar, but the half-life of ropivacaine without epinephrine appears to be slightly greater than that of bupivacaine after epidural injection (Table 13.9). There are subtle physicochemical differences between bupivacaine and ropivacaine, but overall there is no major difference pharmacologically.

ANESTHETIC PROPERTIES

It is in its anesthetic properties that ropivacaine differs from bupivacaine. Rosenberg and Heinonen[4] examined the differential effects of this new agent on various nerve fibers and found that the ability to block sensory fibers relative to motor fibers is greater for ropivacaine than for bupivacaine in vitro.

Bader et al[5] also illustrated the selectivity of ropivacaine in vitro by comparing various concentrations of bupivacaine and ropivacaine. Ropivacaine depressed the action potential amplitude of motor fibers less than did bupivacaine at the same concentration, while decreasing action potential amplitude to an equal degree in sensory fibers.

At all concentrations of the two agents, ropivacaine depressed the action potential amplitude of motor fibers less than did bupivacaine, but they caused equivalent depression of sensory fiber action potentials. Therefore, ropivacaine has a greater degree of motor–sensory dissociation than its homolog bupivacaine.

This increased degree of selectivity between motor and sensory fibers was not demonstrated in live animals, but so far it has been borne out in the initial human studies. A number of reports comparing bupivacaine and ropivacaine has shown that, at equivalent concentrations, ropivacaine is equipotent with respect to sensory anesthesia, and that it produces a less profound motor block of shorter duration after epidural administration.[6,7] In peripheral nerve blocks, 0.5% ropivacaine has been shown to produce motor and sensory block equivalent to that produced with 0.5% bupivacaine;[8] 0.25% of either is probably not adequate.[9]

Table 13.9 Pharmacokinetic data after epidural administration of ropivacaine and bupivacaine* (Data from Arthur et al[3])

	Bupivacaine		Ropivacaine	
	0.75% plain	0.75% + epinephrine	0.75% plain	0.75% + epinephrine
Dose (mg)	22.5	22.5	22.5	22.5
Weight (kg)	20.8 ± 3.1	20.8 ± 3.1	15.5 ± 3.7	15.5 ± 3.7†
$t_{1/2\beta}$ (min)	168 ± 33†	218 ± 47†	201 ± 89†	202 ± 37†
Cl (ml/min/kg)	35.3 ± 6.2	24.6 ± 4.0†	25.3 ± 7.6†	24.6 ± 5.2†
MBRT (min)	226 ± 50†	297 ± 66†	268 ± 105†	267 ± 47†
C_{max} (μg/ml)	0.36 ± 0.12	0.34 ± 0.06	0.50 ± 0.13	0.39 ± 0.11

* Values are means ± SD.
† $P < 0.05$ compared with i.v. data.

CARDIOTOXICITY

Animal data

Bupivacaine increases the tendency to develop ventricular arrhythmias in several ways. When Covino and Moller[10] evaluated the cardiac transmembrane electrophysiologic effects of ropivacaine compared with those of bupivacaine and lidocaine in an isolated rabbit Purkinje fiber–ventricular muscle preparation, they found ropivacaine to be less potent than bupivacaine but more potent than lidocaine in terms of its depressant effect on cardiac excitation and conduction. Bupivacaine altered action potential configuration and caused longer Purkinje fiber inexcitability and conduction block than ropivacaine, creating an environment ripe for ventricular arrhythmias. Furthermore, they demonstrated that not only did ropivacaine exert fewer transmembrane effects on cardiac muscle preparations that did bupivacaine, but that when such toxicity occurred recovery appeared sooner in the ropivacaine-treated fibers. These studies, however, took place in vitro. The real test was in intact animals and, ultimately, in humans.

In a series of experiments in dogs, Feldman et al[11] employed unpremedicated and unanesthetized dogs to mimic the clinical situation in which a rapid unintentional intravenous injection of a local anesthetic agent occurs in patients during an attempted regional anesthetic procedure. After inducing seizure and arrhythmias, they also attempted to resuscitate the dogs.

Their results indicated much greater lethality from bupivacaine (83% vs. 17%) when convulsant doses (CD) were infused, as well as an increased incidence of ventricular arrhythmias (83% vs. 33%), at similar peak plasma concentrations. After attempts at resuscitation, it also appeared as though bupivacaine-induced ventricular arrhythmias might be more difficult to treat than those induced by ropivacaine.[11] In a subsequent study,[12] the same authors showed that early aggressive treatment of CNS and cardiovascular toxicity is capable of reducing the incidence of mortality associated with the rapid intravenous administration of excessive doses of local anesthetics. In this study, more dogs died after 2 × CD of bupivacaine (2/6) than after 2 × CD of ropivacaine (0/6).

Human data

To determine the relative toxicity of these agents in humans, Scott et al[13] infused ropivacaine and bupivacaine intravenously in a randomized, double-blind fashion in 12 volunteers. Bupivacaine induced symptoms of mild CNS toxicity at much lower plasma concentration than did ropivacaine. Using electrocardiography and echocardiography, they measured changes in myocardial conductivity and contractility.

Ropivacaine caused fewer CNS symptoms and was at least 25% less toxic than bupivacaine in regard to the dose tolerated. Both agents increased heart rate and arterial pressure. Stroke volume and ejection fraction were reduced, and there was no change in cardiac output. Although both drugs caused evidence of depression of conductivity and contractility, these signs appeared at lower dosages and lower plasma concentrations of bupivacaine than of ropivacaine.

USE IN OBSTETRICS

While ropivacaine may offer more motor–sensory dissociation than bupivacaine, as well as affording a greater margin of safety between CV toxicity and CNS toxicity, it is important to consider the effect of this agent on uterine blood flow to ensure its safety in the parturient. Santos et al[14] recently published their conclusions that neither ropivacaine nor bupivacaine, when infused intravenously as fast as 0.2 mg/kg/min and 0.1 mg/kg/min respectively, led to any ill-effects on uterine artery blood flow or fetal well-being. This was important to determine, as it previously has been reported that ropivacaine, unlike its relative amides, had vasoconstrictive properties when administered subcutaneously in animals.[15] As pregnancy seems to enhance the cardiotoxicity of bupivacaine, the investigators had also investigated the systemic toxicity of ropivacaine during ovine pregnancy and concluded that ovine pregnancy does not enhance the systemic toxicity of ropivacaine.[16]

THE FUTURE

At the present time, clinical trials of ropivacaine in obstetric patients are under way. It appears that ropivacaine is an exciting new agent offering greater motor and sensory dissociation than bupivacaine when administered epidurally while affording an increased margin of safety when comparing its cardiac and systemic toxicities. After further studies in humans are completed, it promises to offer greater patient satisfaction and comfort, particularly when used in the management of obstetric anesthesia and post-operative pain control.

REFERENCES

1. FDA 1983 Adverse reactions with bupivacaine. FDA Drug Bulletin 13: 23
2. Akerman B, Hellberg I B, Trossvik C 1988 Primary evaluation of the local anesthetic properties of the amino amide agent ropivacaine (LEA 103). Acta Anaesthesiol Scand 32: 571–578
3. Arthur G R, Feldman H S, Covino B G 1988 Comparative pharmacokinetics of bupivacaine and ropivacaine, a new amide local anesthetic. Anesth Analg 67: 1053–1058
4. Rosenberg P H, Heinonen E 1983 Differential sensitivity of A and C nerve fibers to long-acting amide local anesthetics. Br J Anaesth 55: 163–167
5. Bader A M, Datta S, Flanagan H et al 1989 Comparison of

bupivacaine- and ropivacaine-induced conduction blockade in the isolated rabbit vagus nerve. Anesth Analg 68: 724–727
6. Brockway M S, Bannister J, McClure J H et al 1991 comparison of extradural ropivacaine and bupivacaine. Br J Anaesth 66: 31–37
7. Kerkkamp H E, Gielen M J, Edstrom H H 1990 Comparison of 0.75% ropivacaine with epinephrine and 0.75% bupivacaine with epinephrine in lumbar epidural anesthesia. Reg Anesth 15: 204–207, 1990
8. Hickey R, Hoffman J, Ramamurthy S 1991 A comparison of ropivacaine 0.5% and bupivacaine 0.5% for brachial plexus block. Anesthesiology 74: 639–642
9. Hickey R, Rowley C L, Candido K D et al 1992 A comparative study of 0.25% ropivacaine and 0.25% bupivacaine for brachial plexus block. Anesth Analg 75: 602–606
10. Moller R, Covino B G 1990 Cardiac electrophysiologic properties of bupivacaine and lidocaine compared with those of ropivacaine, a new amide local anesthetic. Anesthesiology 72: 322–329
11. Feldman H S, Arthur G R, Covino B G 1989 Comparative systemic toxicity of convulsant and supraconvulsant doses of intravenous ropivacaine, bupivacaine, and lidocaine in the conscious dog. Anesth Analg 69: 794–801
12. Feldman H S, Arthur G R, Pitkanen M et al 1991 Treatment of acute systemic toxicity after the rapid intravenous injection of ropivacaine and bupivacaine in the conscious dog. Anesth Analg 73: 373–384
13. Scott D B, Lee A, Fagan D 1989 Acute toxicity of ropivacaine compared with that of bupivacaine. Anesth Analg 69: 563–569
14. Santos A C, Arthur G R, Roberts D J et al 1992 Effect of ropivacaine and bupivacaine on uterine blood flow in pregnant ewes. Anesth Analg 74: 62–67
15. Kopacz D J, Carpenter R L, Mackey D C 1989 Effect of ropivacaine on cutaneous capillary blood flow in pigs. Anesthesiology 71: 69–74
16. Santos A C, Arthur G R, Pedersen H et al 1991 Systemic toxicity of ropivacaine during ovine pregnancy. Anesthesiology 75: 137–141

14. Pharmacology of opioids

PART A
OVERVIEW
F. Reynolds

It has long been apparent that morphine and related drugs must act on specific receptors, first, because their actions tend to be sensitive, selective and stereo-specific and, second, because highly specific competitive antagonists are available. The sensitivity of opioid drug–receptor interactions is demonstrated by the fact that a number of opioids, for example some of the fentanyl family and the veterinary drug, etorphine, act in very low doses. Selectivity implies that a characteristic pattern of drug effects is produced. This is well demonstrated with the opioids. Stereospecificity is also seen among those opioids that possess asymmetric carbon atoms, for example: l-methadone and d-propoxyphene are active isomers.

For many years both opioid receptors and the endogenous ligands for which they were intended seemed elusive. In the early 1970s, however, not only were the opioid receptors mapped, using the then new radioligand binding techniques,[1] but also endogenous opioid substances were identified,[2] resulting in a veritable explosion in our understanding of opioid behavior in the body.

SITES OF OPIOID RECEPTORS

Opioid receptors have been identified throughout brain and spinal cord[1], largely at sites that can be associated with a known action of morphine, thus:

- amygdala, limbic system } mood elevation
- thalamus, periaqueductal gray matter, median raphe nuclei, substantia gelatinosa } inhibition of pain transmission
- hypothalamus, pituitary } hormone regulation
- medullary centers
  - respiratory depression
  - cough suppression
  - area postrema: emesis[3]
- gastrointestinal tract: inhibition of peristalsis.

CLASSIFICATION OF OPIOID RECEPTORS

With the discovery of opioid receptors it was not long before it was found that the various opioid agonists differed from one another in the spectrum of effects they produced. This led to the identification of different types of opioid receptors[4,5] and inevitably to their classification into numerous subtypes. Only the simplest classification is necessary for a broad understanding of opioid behavior, thus:

μ
- analgesia to thermal *and* chemical stimuli
  - central analgesia
  - spinal analgesia
- euphoria and dependence
- respiratory depression
- pruritus

κ
- analgesia to chemical stimuli *only*
  - spinal analgesia
- sedation

δ
- gastrointestinal effects
- analgesia to thermal stimuli *only*
- ? respiratory depression

σ
- dysphoria (some doubt is cast on the existence of σ receptors).

δ and μ receptors tend to be closely associated and to subserve similar functions.[5] Intraspinal analgesia was originally thought to be principally a κ agonist effect, but it is now apparent from the effectiveness of μ agonists intraspinally that the spinal cord of the human contains many μ receptors. κ agonist drugs have been used for both systemic and intraspinal analgesia, in the hope of avoiding respiratory depression. However, they are inevitably less effective, blocking only one of the two classic types of experimental pain stimuli. More recently the desire to separate effective analgesia from respiratory depression has led, by wishful thinking, to the subclassification of μ_1 and μ_2 receptors, and while meptazinol, for example, is claimed to be selective for μ_1 receptors (see below), drugs that usefully achieve this feat of separation are rare.

PARTIAL AGONISTS

Drugs vary not only in their pattern of stimulation of different receptor types, but also in their efficacy as agonists (Table 14.1). Certain drugs such as pentazocine and buprenorphine are termed partial agonists (or agonists/antagonists), produce only a low ceiling effect and, in certain circumstances, behave as antagonists. They can reduce the effects of toxic doses of pure agonists, while buprenorphine in large doses can even antagonize itself.[6] Such drugs are said to have low *efficacy* (they cannot produce the same maximum effect as a pure agonist) but high *affinity* (they can displace an agonist from the receptor). Some such drugs appear to be partial agonists because they are principally κ agonists (for example, butorphanol and nalbuphine) and for this reason appear to have low ceiling effects.

ENDOGENOUS OPIOIDS

While the search for opioid receptors was in progress, pharmacologists in Aberdeen, UK, demonstrated that substances with opioid-like activity could selectively inhibit electrically induced activity in the guinea pig ileum and the mouse vas deferens. Using these preparations they were able to identify two pentapeptides isolated from pig brain that possess potent, naloxone-reversible opioid like activity. They have the amino acid sequences Tyr-Gly-Gly-Phe-Met and Tyr-Gly-Gly-Phe-Leu and were named met-enkephalin and leu-enkephalin.[2] They appeared to act as neurotransmitters in spinal cord and gastrointestinal tract. Later, longer peptides that also possess opioid-like activity, the endorphins, were identified. Of these the principal one appears to be β-endorphin, a pituitary hormone that possesses μ activity and contains the Tyr-Gly-Gly-Phe sequence and probably subserves a hormone-regulatory function. Since then many related endogenous peptides have been identified together with precursor substances which are made up of many more amino acid residues. These together with their favored receptors may be summarized:

pro-opiomelanocortin – β-endorphin – μ
proenkephalin – enkephalins – δ
prodynorphin – dynorphins – κ.

The enkephalins have very short half-lives, as befits neurotransmitters, but β-endorphin, which appears to possess a spectrum of activity similar to that of morphine (see below), has a longer half-life, as is more suited to its humoral role. It is found principally in the brainstem and is released into the cerebrospinal fluid.

Table 14.1 Activity of opioids at different receptors

	Receptor type		
	μ	κ	σ
Morphine	Agonist	? Agonist	
Pentazocine	Agonist/antagonist	Agonist	Agonist
Buprenorphine	Agonist/antagonist		
Butorphanol	? Agonist/antagonist	Agonist	Weak agonist
Nalbuphine	? Agonist/antagonist	Agonist	Weak agonist
Meptazinol	Agonist/antagonist	Weak agonist	

THE ACTIONS OF OPIOIDS

Both morphine and endogenous opioids appear to be able to inhibit release of substance P in substantia gelatinosa[7] and gastrointestinal tract.[8] They also inhibit acetylcholine release in brain[9] and increase dopamine turnover, while having a variable effect on release.[5] They possess a number of secondary functions that result from these actions. They promote release of vasopressin and growth hormone, as well as prolactin (a function probably secondary to inhibition of dopamine release), while release of ACTH, LH and FSH tends to be inhibited.

The important clinical effects of morphine are analgesia, sometimes somnolence, euphoria, dependence and reduced anxiety, respiratory depression, inhibition of cough, emesis – particularly in females, antidiuresis, some hyperglycemia, miosis, delayed gastric emptying and constipation. Cardiovascular effects are not prominent in the absence of severe respiratory depression, though occasional hypotension is believed to be associated with histamine release. A fall in blood pressure may also occur in association with dramatic relief of pain. Both systemic and intraspinal morphine may cause pruritus, though with systemic administration it is usually milder and confined to the nose.

In the respiratory center it appears that opioid receptors are in series with cholinergic receptors (hence opioids inhibit acetylcholine release; see above), thus physostigmine can overcome the respiratory depression associated with morphine.[10] In the chemoreceptor trigger zone it appears that dopamine receptors are in series with opioid receptors, since dopamine release is promoted rather than inhibited in the area postrema and emesis due to opioids can be blocked by the dopamine antagonists and naloxone, while that due to apomorphine (a dopamine agonist) is blocked only by the former.[3]

MECHANISMS OF ANALGESIA

Pain is transmitted from the periphery by the small A δ and C fibers, whose cell bodies lie in the dorsal root ganglia. Central projections enter the cord in the lateral division of the dorsal root, where they enter the gray matter of the dorsal horn. Except for a few A δ fibres that terminate in the marginal layer (lamina I), the remainder synapse in the substantia gelatinosa (lamina II), communicating (probably by a series of interneurons) with cells whose bodies reside in lamina V. These are mainly the wide dynamic range neurons, which respond, as their name implies, to both high-intensity stimuli provoked by pain and also to low-intensity light touch. Increased activity in these neurons results in impulse transmission in the anterolateral ascending columns (Fig. 14.1).

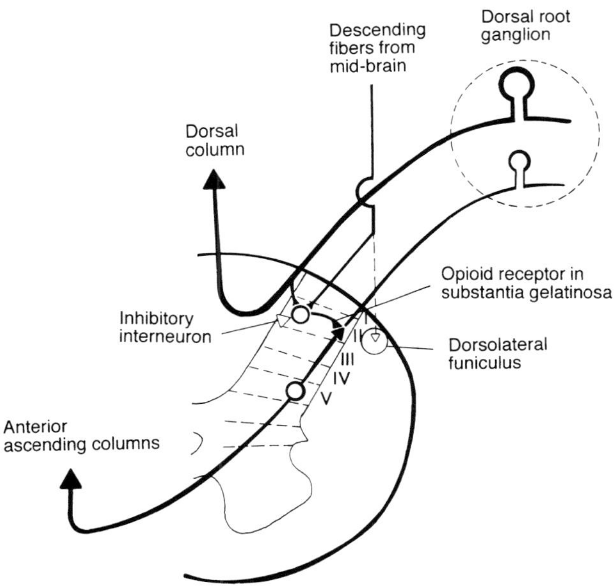

Fig. 14.1 A highly simplified representation of the pain pathways in the spinal cord. Pain is conducted by the small sensory fibers whose cell bodies are in the dorsal root ganglia and whose central projections synapse principally in lamina II. Release of transmitter at the synapse is inhibited by a relay of inhibitory interneurons and by opioid agonists. The inhibitory neurons are activated both by collaterals from the large sensory fibers which ascend in the dorsal columns and also by fibers descending in the dorsolateral funiculus from the brainstem.

Substance P, together with other peptides, appears to act as a neurotransmitter in the pain pathways. It is found in the cell bodies of the dorsal root ganglia and is released in the substantia gelatinosa in response to painful stimuli. There is a series of interneurons residing largely in lamina II, some of which are enkephalinergic and whose activity inhibits substance P release. These are activated both by collaterals from the larger sensory fibers whose central projections ascend in the dorsal column and also by descending inhibitory fibers in the dorsolateral funiculus. These arise in the midbrain in areas rich in opioid receptors and are themselves largely tryptaminergic. Stimulation of inhibitory interneurons or opioid receptors in the substantia gelatinosa would appear to act principally by reducing cyclic AMP levels in opioid-sensitive cells,[11] resulting in presynaptic inhibition of the release of substance P, and also in part by causing post-synaptic hyperpolarization of dorsal horn neurons. Thus the increase in activity in lamina V neurons and in the anterolateral ascending columns that normally results from painful stimulation is prevented. Morphine is more effective at blocking activity produced by C than by A δ stimuli.

Pain transmission can therefore be selectively inhibited by several mechanisms. Rubbing the part and transcutaneous electrical nerve stimulation activate inhibitory neurons, releasing endogenous opioids which inhibit substance P release. Stimulation of the periaqueductal gray matter and the median raphe nuclei in the midbrain produces the most intense analgesia, presumably by activating descending inhibitory pathways as well as by blocking ascending pain stimuli. Opioids can act both via the midbrain and in the substantia gelatinosa, the latter being of paramount importance with intraspinal administration. Direct application of opioids, by either subarachnoid or even epidural administration, can produce concentrations in the substantia gelatinosa many times higher than following systemic administration. It is not surprising, therefore, that intraspinal analgesia is more intense and less readily reversed by naloxone.

Uterine contraction pain is principally conducted to the cord by A δ fibers, those that also conduct pinprick sensation. Such fibers are particularly sensitive to blockade by local anesthetics. Pathologic pain, and less well-localized more aversive pain, are conducted by C pain fibers, which are less sensitive to local anesthetic block but more so to inhibition by opioids. Thus, in the presence of a uterine scar, labor analgesia should be provided by minimal doses of local anesthetic only, so as to preserve C pain fiber activity. By this means it may be possible to distinguish between uterine pain and scar pain, which is felt in an identical site. Normal pain of uterine contractions is not reliably blocked by epidural opioids alone, while a combination of local anesthetic and an opioid such as fentanyl or sufentanil is ideal.

PROPERTIES OF THE INDIVIDUAL OPIOIDS

Opioids differ from one another not only in their potency, affinity and efficacy on different receptors, but also in their ratio of agonist to antagonist activity and in physicochemical and in pharmacokinetic properties.

Physicochemical properties

The molecular weights of opioids in common use vary between 200 and 500 (see Table 14.2). All possess a basic nitrogen group which, with a very few exceptions, is in the form of a piperidine ring (a six-membered saturated, nitrogen-containing ring).

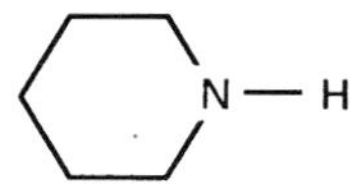

Piperidine

This ring is concealed in morphine (Fig. 14.2) and in related drugs such as buprenorphine, butorphanol, nalbuphine and naloxone, while in meperidine (Fig. 14.2) and the fentanyls it is exposed. Meptazinol contains a homopiperidine or seven-membered ring. Methadone and propoxyphene each contain a tertiary amine group. Piperidine groups and tertiary amine groups behave in a similar fashion in that each can accept one proton and so become ionized and water soluble in acid solution, while in the nonionized form they are lipid soluble and more able to penetrate lipid membranes. The extent to which the basic group is ionized at a given pH depends on the pK_a (the $\log_{10}$ of the reciprocal of the acid dissociation constant), some values of which are given in Table 14.2. All except alfentanil are more than 50% ionized at pH 7.4.

Morphine also possesses two hydroxyl groups (on the 3 and 6 positions). Nalbuphine also possesses two such groups, and most other related drugs only one. These hydroxyl groups are important in that they are weakly *acidic*. They greatly enhance the hydrophilicity of the molecule as they reduce the population of nonionized particles. Hydroxyl groups are also important in that they can be conjugated with glucuronide, most readily in the 3 position, which inactivates the molecule. Thus, the more lipid-soluble agents without a hydroxyl group, such as fentanyl, being able to penetrate lipid membranes readily, disappear rapidly from the circulation, but are much more slowly inactivated. Hence the distribution half-life of fentanyl is brief but the elimination half-life relatively prolonged, while for morphine the reverse is true and there is less difference between distribution and elimination half-lives.

Table 14.2 Physicochemical properties of opioids

	Molecular weight	pK_a of base group	Apparent oil–buffer (pH 7.4) partition coefficients		
			Octanol	Oleyl alcohol	Heptane
Morphine	285	7.9	1.4		
Meperidine	247	8.5	39	18	
Methadone	309	9.3	116	55	
Nalbuphine	357	8.7			
Buprenorphine	467	8.4			2000
Meptazinol	234	8.7			
Fentanyl	336	8.4	77	550	9
Alfentanil	416	6.5			2.9

A 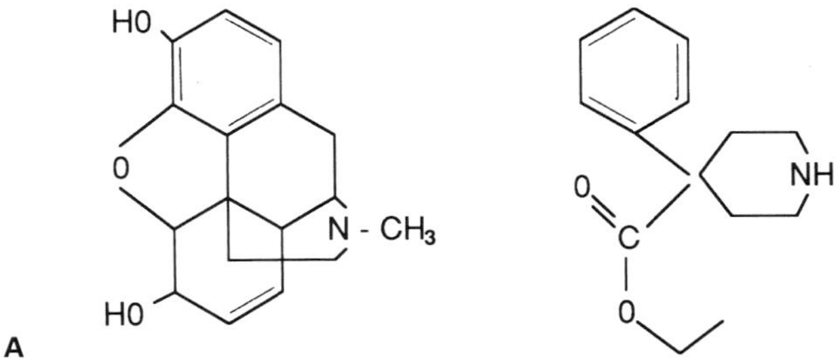 B

Fig. 14.2 Structural formulae of (a) morphine and (b) meperidine showing the piperidine ring in each.

Lipid solubility

Some values for partition coefficients between buffer and various organic solvents are given in Table 14.2. A partition coefficient, however, is not a true measure of lipid solubility (a term that, strictly speaking, denotes the maximum amount of a substance that is soluble in a lipid medium). For example, the partition coefficient of buprenorphine appears disproportionately high because it is so poorly *water* soluble. Such a figure can be said to give an indication of how a drug will partition between extracellular fluid and lipid cell membrane, and is closely associated with speed of passage across the blood–brain barrier (Fig. 14.3).

Pharmacokinetics

High lipophilicity is associated with a large volume of distribution and rapid disappearance from the circulation but with a relatively prolonged elimination half-life. Reported terminal half-lives are shown in Table 14.3.

Protein binding (Table 14.3)

Hydrophobic drugs tend to be highly protein bound. Many basic drugs are bound mainly to the acute-phase protein α_1-acid glycoprotein (AAG), and this appears true for meperidine, methadone and alfentanil. AAG possesses a single high-affinity hydrophobic binding site for which saturation and competition are not usually evident at clinical concentration.[13] The importance of AAG binding in the obstetric context is that fetal levels of this protein are always lower than maternal.[14] Thus, at equilibrium, the total concentration of a drug highly bound to AAG, such as alfentanil, is often two to four fold higher in the mother than in the fetus. There is no such consistent

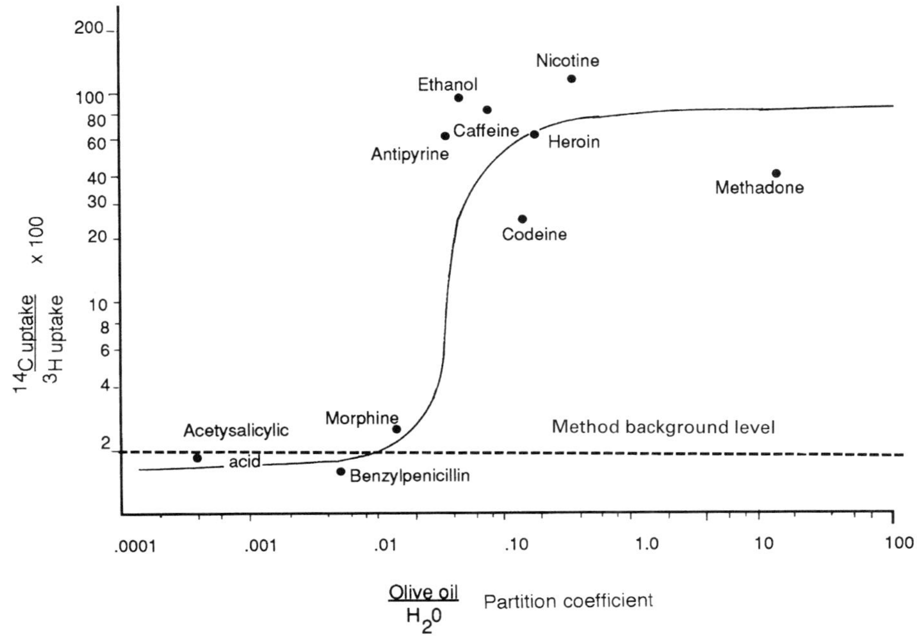

Fig. 14.3 Lipid solubility and blood brain barrier penetration. Relationship between percentage clearance of radiolabeled drug compared with that of tritiated water and oil–buffer partition coefficient. (Adapted from ref. 12 by kind permission of the author and publishers.)

discrepancy in albumin binding, fetal albumin levels at term being similar to or slightly higher than maternal.[14]

MORPHINE

Morphine is the principal alkaloid of opium, which is derived from the exudate of the seed capsule of the poppy *Papaver somniferum*. It is the most poorly lipid soluble of the opioids in common use (see above). It is commonly administered as morphine sulfate in aqueous solution, the ampule for systemic use containing preservative as it would otherwise be insufficiently stable in solution.

Morphine is the archetypal mu agonist, giving its name to the receptor. It therefore possesses the actions listed above. Given by any route its onset of action is slow since, unlike its more lipid-soluble congeners, it is unable to equilibrate across the blood–brain barrier in a single circulation[15] (Fig. 14.3). It is therefore slow to penetrate to its site of action, whether midbrain or substantia gelatinosa, and this slow onset makes it unsuitable for use in labor.

Table 14.3 Some pharmacokinetic properties of opioids

	Protein binding (%)	$T_{1/2}$ (h)
Morphine	30	1.4–4
Meperidine	30–65	3–5
Methadone	60–90	>24
Nalbuphine	34	2.4
Butorphanol	–	2.5–3.5
Buprenorphine	96	2–5
Meptazinol	30	2
Fentanyl	84	3–6
Alfentanil	90	1.6

Morphine was used systemically in the first dose of the twilight sleep regimen, which was instituted at the turn of the century. It was used in combination with hyoscine (scopolamine), the latter drug alone being repeated as necessary. In consequence, the analgesia was appalling, but the amnesia successful – an approach to pain relief that might be considered barbaric. However, morphine was considered too dangerous to repeat. Its evil reputation stemmed from the recognition that opioid addiction was detrimental to the baby.

Given intraspinally (epidurally or subarachnoid) morphine has a uniquely long action because its hydrophilicity insures its affinity for CSF, by which it is readily transported to the brain, giving rise to frequent side-effects. Given epidurally, morphine is useful in the management of chronic pain, but it is of little value in labor. The onset of action is too slow and the analgesia remarkably ineffective.[16,17] There is no potentiation of bupivacaine with morphine as there is with fentanyl.[18] Indeed, it may actually counteract the analgesia from bupivacaine.[19] Morphine is more effective subarachnoid, but onset of action may still be delayed for up to an hour,[20,21] and analgesia incomplete if less than 1 mg is used.[19] Though the duration of effect is about 8 h,[20,21] analgesia is rarely sufficient to cover the second stage. There appears to be little benefit in using a hyperbaric solution.[20] Moreover, side-effects are frequent and severe, with pruritus reported in 100% and nausea and vomiting in 75–80% of women.[21,22] A reduction in the frequency of pruritus is seen if naloxone is given.[23] Subarachnoid morphine has been used with more success after cesarean delivery, with length of hospital stay being reduced.[24] Epidural is more effective than intramuscular administration, with analgesia lasting about 20 h.[25] Both routes, however, are less popular with mothers than intravenous patient-controlled analgesia (PCA).[26,27] The addition of epinephrine has no effect on analgesia from epidural morphine.[25] The long-acting antagonist, naltrexone, has been found to reduce the frequency of all side-effects following subarachnoid hyperbaric morphine.[28] It is possible that pruritus caused by intraspinal morphine is associated with a recrudescence of herpes labialis in carriers of herpes simplex virus.[29] Delayed respiratory depression, characteristic of intraspinal morphine administration in other circumstances, is not a prominent feature in obstetrics.

Fate

Morphine is conjugated in the liver with glucuronide at the 3 and 6 positions. In general, more morphine 3-glucuronide is produced, but both conjugates are readily excreted in the urine. In renal failure, morphine occasionally has a profound and prolonged effect, and this has been found to be associated with accumulation of morphine 6-glucuronide.

MEPERIDINE

When, in the years following World War II, an analgesic agent suitable for use in labor was sought, meperidine was chosen as a supposedly safer alternative to morphine. As a comparative newcomer at the time, it was believed to be as effective as morphine but free from its side-effects. (This is a story that has been told many times.) Meperidine is probably more suitable than morphine, simply because, being more lipid soluble (Table 14.2), its onset of action is quicker regardless of the route of administration. It is also shorter acting than morphine by all routes, because of a more pronounced distribution phase rather than through any difference in elimination half-life (Table 14.2).

Meperidine, like morphine, is principally a μ agonist, but of lower potency, necessitating a dose that might be expected to be nonselective. Given as the hydrochloride salt, in a dose of 100–150 mg it has been shown to reduce the pain score in labor by about 20%.[30] At this dose it is also a powerful sedative. The increased incidence of nausea and vomiting that results can be prevented by an antiemetic such as metoclopramide, which helps prevent reflux[31] and, unlike some phenothiazines, has no antianalgesic effect.[30]

Delayed gastric emptying is a prominent feature of the use of meperidine in labor,[32] and this is only partly counteracted by metoclopramide.[33] If a woman elects to receive meperidine rather than epidural analgesia in labor, she is more likely to need general anesthesia should operative delivery be required. This argues in favor of giving a H_2-antagonist to every woman who receives meperidine in labor, to reduce the volume and acidity of the gastric contents.

Respiratory depression is not usually observed in women who receive meperidine for analgesia in labor, because contractions continue to be painful and to provoke hyperventilation. However, even during labor, hypoxic episodes have been observed more frequently with meperidine than with epidural analgesia,[34] probably associated with significant underventilation between contractions.

Fate

Unlike morphine, which is directly conjugated in the gut wall and/or liver, meperidine is first *N*-dealkylated, with a high first-pass effect, to produce nor-meperidine. The ester linkage is also hydrolyzed to yield meperidinic acid and nor-meperidinic acid, products which can be conjugated. The major metabolite, nor-meperidine, is itself active, and has convulsant properties.[34] Thus meperidine, despite its sedative properties, is unsuitable for use in fulminating preeclampsia or eclampsia, as indeed are the phenothiazines, for the same reason.

Neonatal effects

When each new opioid is introduced it is hoped it will produce minimal effects on the baby. When meperidine was first used it was thought appropriate to withhold it in late labor, to minimize neonatal effects, in keeping with the old-fashioned midwifery tradition of withholding analgesia when labor pain is reaching its peak. In fact, meperidine has a markedly depressant effect on the newborn, causing respiratory depression even in small doses,[36] reducing suckling and neurobehavioral responses.[37] Its effect is at its height when the drug is given 3–4 h before delivery, and negligible if given *only* within 1 h.[38] This is because both the parent drug and its active metabolites take time to accumulate in the fetus,[36] and it would appear that the detrimental effect is due at least as much if not more to nor-meperidine than to meperidine[40] (Fig. 14.4). Nevertheless, all the depressant effects appear to be reversible by giving naloxone to the newborn.[37] The half-life of meperidine is prolonged to about 22 h in the newborn, and naloxone should be given in a dose of

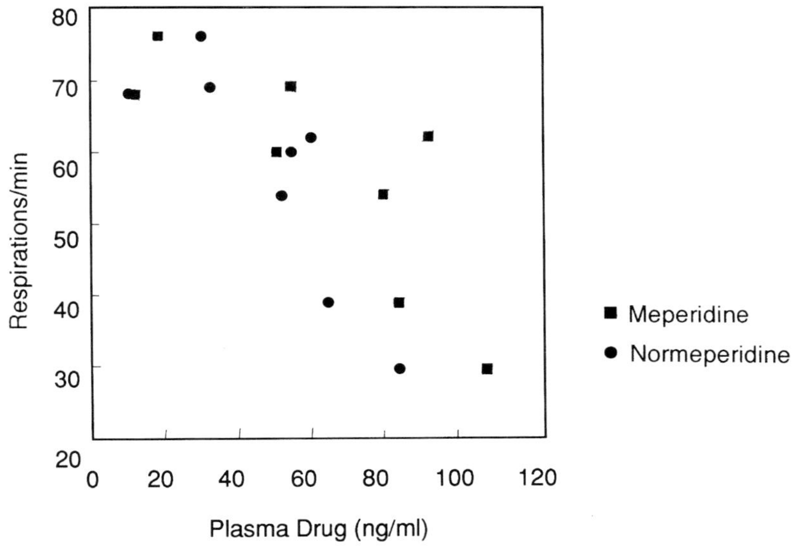

Fig. 14.4 Relationship between neonatal respiratory rate and umbilical cord meperidine (MEP) and normeperidine (NorMEP) concentrations at birth in macaque monkeys. For meperidine $r = -0.81$ and for normeperidine $r = -0.84$. (Reproduced from ref. 40 by kind permission of the authors and publishers.)

0.1 mg/kg i.v. to reverse the effects of meperidine (Recommendation of the American Heart Association and the Americans Academy of Pediatrics).

Mode of administration

Although by tradition meperidine is given by bolus intramuscular administration, even this technique results in excessive peaks and troughs in plasma and, hence, CNS concentration. PCA using 10–15 mg i.v. demand doses[41,42] or 50 mg i.m. doses[43] has been employed in an attempt to improve analgesia and iron out the fluctuations in concentration. This is generally associated with similar pain relief to that provided by nurse-administered i.m. bolus, but more patient satisfaction. Dose requirement is reported to be smaller[41] or greater.[42] Meperidine has also been used extensively epidurally, by which route its duration of action is only about 1–2 h in labor,[44,45] and though analgesia is more effective than with systemic use, dose requirement is similar. After cesarean delivery, both epidural meperidine 50 mg and i.m. meperidine 100 mg last about 4 h and produce similar side-effects,[46] although the epidural route may be preferred by mothers.[47] Epinephrine does not enhance analgesia.[48] In the large doses that are necessary (25–100 mg), local anesthetic activity contributes to the analgesic effect of epidural meperidine.[48,49]

PARTIAL AGONISTS

A succession of partial opioid agonists and selective κ agonists, supposedly producing effective analgesia but free from side-effects such as dependence, liability and respiratory depression, have been introduced over the years. Many have been tried in obstetrics in the hope that analgesia would be at least as good as that with meperidine (no big deal!) but that neonatal depression would be diminished.

Pentazocine

One of the first drugs to be developed, pentazocine is a mu agonist/antagonist but a κ and σ agonist. It has a duration of action briefer than that of meperidine. Its ceiling of analgesia and side-effects is low but dysphoria is a regrettable feature. In general, it was found to have few advantages over meperidine; however, in one trial, neonatal respiratory depression was found to be more short-lived with pentazocine.[50]

Meptazinol

Meptazinol is believed to have a high affinity for mu_1 receptors, which are thought to be responsible for analgesia but not for respiratory depression. It would appear to be a partial agonist at mu_1 receptors because it can reverse signs of morphine overdose and precipitate abstinence syndrome in morphine-dependent subjects. It has low affinity for delta and kappa receptors and would appear to be a weak kappa agonist. Also, it appears to potentiate acetylcholine in both brain and gastrointestinal tract. Its relative lack of respiratory depressant effects has been attributed variously to selective mu_1 agonist activity and to its ability to potentiate the effects of acetylcholine centrally.

In a dose of 100 mg, meptazinol produces analgesia similar to that with meperidine but lasting for only about 2 h.[51] It is more likely to produce nausea and vomiting,[52] and should not be used without an antiemetic. Neonatal effects are believed to be milder than with meperidine[53] and the half-life in the newborn may be shorter.[54]

Meptazinol has also been administered epidurally. Analgesia is more rapid in onset, more complete and longer lasting than when given intramuscularly.[55] Some sedation is reported following both routes of administration.

Nalbuphine

Nalbuphine has a spectrum of activity not unlike pentazocine, although it is a more potent kappa agonist and partial agonist at mu receptors with less effect on sigma receptors, only producing dysphoria at very high doses. Though said to be an antagonist at mu receptors, it does in fact produce a degree of respiratory depression with a ceiling at about 30 mg. It can, however, antagonize ventilatory depression following high doses of a mu agonist.[56] It would appear to be less likely to produce emesis than meptazinol and meperidine,[57] but maternal sedation is prominent, as is neonatal depression.[58]

Nalbuphine may be given in intravenous or intramuscular bolus doses of 10–20 mg about every 4 h or by PCA using 1 mg increments.[59] PCA has been associated with a smaller total dose and less need for an antiemetic, less sedation and more maternal satisfaction. Nalbuphine has not become popular for use by the epidural route.

Buprenorphine

Buprenorphine is a partial agonist acting selectively at mu receptors. It is about 20 times as potent as morphine and has a high affinity for opioid receptors and slow dissociation from them. It has a capacity for self-antagonism, which tends to produce a bell-shaped dose–response curve and in high doses a biphasic time course of action (Fig. 14.5). This may be observed for both analgesia and respiratory depression.[6,60]

It has been used both by injection and by the sublingual route, principally for post-operative analgesia, and has not become popular during labor. Sublingual buprenorphine

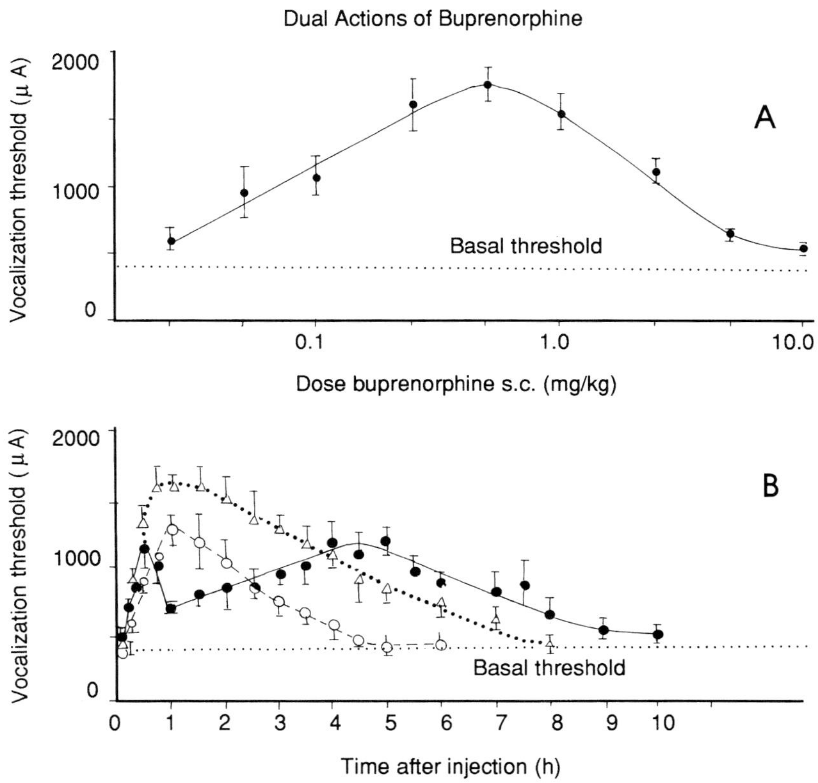

Fig. 14.5 (a) Dose–response curve for buprenorphine antinociception in rats measured 1 h after subcutaneous injection, using the vocalization threshold. (b) The time course of effect of buprenorphine 0.1 mg/kg (open circles) 0.5 mg/kg (triangles) and 5 mg/kg (filled circles). Vertical lines represents standard errors. Autoantagonism is demonstrated with the higher doses of buprenorphine at the time of maximum effect (1 h). (Reproduced from ref. 6 by kind permission of the authors and publishers.)

appears to have a long duration of action (6–12 h) and, though side-effects are rare, when nausea and respiratory depression do occur they can be exceedingly persistent and difficult to reverse. The plasma half-life of about 3 h appears to bear little relation to its long duration of action. It has been used epidurally following cesarean delivery, by which route a dose of 0.18 mg has been found to be more effective than 0.09 mg and more effective than morphine 3 mg.[61] Moreover, pruritus was less severe than with morphine though emesis occurred equally with the two drugs.

Butorphanol

Butorphanol is also a mu partial agonist and a kappa agonist. Occasional psychomimetic effects suggest that, in some individuals, it may also be a weak sigma agonist. Although only a partial agonist at mu receptors it has been shown to produce a shift in the carbon dioxide response curve parallel to that of meperidine.[62] As a kappa agonist, it produces a dose-related sedative effect.

In obstetrics it has been used most extensively by the epidural route. During labor it has been used in bolus doses of 1, 2 or 3 mg dissolved in 0.25% bupivacaine.[63–65] It can reduce the local anesthetic requirement but at the expense of producing maternal somnolence. It has also been used by continuous infusion in a concentration of 0.2 mg/ml in dilute bupivacaine.[66] By this regimen Neurologic and Adaptive Capacity Scores (NACS) are said to be normal.

It is interesting to note that when butorphanol 3 mg was added to morphine 4 mg for epidural analgesia after cesarean delivery, the side-effects of pruritus and nausea, so prominent with morphine, were actually eliminated while drowsiness was not a feature. Moreover, respiratory status as evidenced by pulse oximetry was improved by the addition of butorphanol to morphine and the duration of analgesia was about 24 h.[67]

OTHER OPIOID AGONISTS

Methadone

Methadone is an agonist with relatively low affinity for opioid receptors and a low ceiling effect but long duration of action. Thus, while it does not displace other agonists from receptors and cannot precipitate abstinence, it can maintain an opioid addict in a relatively stable state in which withdrawal symptoms are of slow onset and mild but prolonged. Its use for systemic analgesia in labor is not reported other than in heroin addicts on methadone maintenance, but being relatively lipid soluble (Table 14.2) it has been used in an attempt to provide epidural analgesia in labor[68] and after cesarean delivery[68] with only modest success.

Diamorphine

This drug, the diacetyl derivative of morphine more commonly known as heroin, is more lipid soluble hence more rapid in onset of action than is morphine. It remains legal in the UK and popular in orthodox medicine. Diamorphine itself probably acts principally as a prodrug to enable its two active metabolites, monoacetyl morphine and morphine, more readily to gain access to opioid receptors. Over the years it has been used sporadically in the UK to provide systemic analgesia during labor. Clinical impressions suggests it is more effective than meperidine. More recently it has become popular by the epidural route. When added in a dose of 5 mg to the initial bolus dose of bupivacaine it has been found to improve analgesia and reduce bupivacaine dose requirements.[70] When used alone to provide epidural analgesia following cesarean delivery, its duration of action is about twice as long as that of fentanyl.[71] Its action may be marginally prolonged by the addition of epinephrine which, however, increased the frequency of emesis.[72] Pruritus is less frequent and less severe than with epidural morphine and the duration of analgesia about 8 h.[73] Bolus epidural doses are no less effective and appear less likely to produce respiratory depression than an epidural infusion.[74]

REFERENCES

1. Snyder S H 1975 Opiate receptor in normal and drug altered brain function. Nature 257: 185–189
2. Hughes J, Smith T W, Kosterlitz H W, Fothergill L A, Morgan B A, Morris H R 1975 Identification of two related pentapeptides from the brain with potent opiate agonist activity. Nature 285: 577–589
3. Bhargava K P, Dixit K S, Gupta Y K 1981 Enkephalin receptors in the emetic chemoreceptor trigger zone of the dog. Br J Pharmacol 72: 471–475
4. Martin W R 1979 History and development of mixed opioid agonist, partial agonists and antagonists. Br J Clin Pharmacol 7: 273s–279
5. Yaksh T L 1984 Multiple opioid receptor systems in brain and spinal cord. Part 2. Eur J Anaesthesiol 1: 201–243
6. Dum J E, Herz A 1981 In vivo receptor binding of the opiate partial agonist, buprenorphine, correlated with its agonistic and antagonistic actions. Br J Pharmacol 74: 627–633
7. Jessell T M, Iversen L L (1977) Opiate analgesics inhibit substance P release from rat trigeminal nucleus. Nature 268: 549–551
8. Gintzler A R, Scalisi J A 1982 Effects of opioids on noncholinergic excitatory responses of the guinea pig isolated ileum: inhibition of release of enteric substance P. Br J Pharmacol 75: 199–205
9. Jhamandas K, Sutak M 1980 Action of enkephalin analogues and morphine on brain acetylcholine release: differential reversal by naloxone and an opiate pentapeptide. Br J Pharmacol 71: 201–210
10. Weinstock M, Davidson J T, Rosin A J, Schnieden H 1982 Effect of physostigmine on morphine induced postoperative pain and somnolence. Br J Anaesth 54: 429–434
11. Goldstein A 1979 Endorphins and pain: a critical review. In: Beers R F, Bassett E G (eds) Mechanisms of pain and analgesic compounds. Raven Press, New York, pp 249–262
12. Oldendorf W H 1974 Lipid solubility and drug penetration of the blood brain barrier. Proc Soc Exp Biol Med 147: 813–816
13. Muller W E, Ricks S, Brunner F 1986 Drug binding to human alpha-l-acid glycoprotein. Focus on a single binding site. In:

Tillement J-P, Lindeblaub E (eds) Protein binding and drug transport. F K Schattover Verlang, Stuttgart, pp 29–44
14. Krauer B, Dayer P, Anner R 1984 Changes in serum albumin and alpha-l-acid glycoprotein concentrations during pregnancy: an analysis of feto-maternal pairs. Br J Obstet Gynaecol 91: 875–881
15. Oldendorf W H, Hyman S, Braun L, Oldendrof S Z 1972 Blood–brain barrier: penetration of morphine, codeine, heroin and methadone after carotid injection. Science 178: 984–986
16. Husemeyer R P, O'Connor M C, Davenport H T 1980 Failure of epidural morphine to relieve pain in labour. Anaesthesia 35: 161–163
17. Booker P D, Wilkes R G, Bryson T H L, Beddard J 1980 Obstetric pain relief using epidural morphine. Anaesthesia 35: 377–379
18. Douglas M J, McMorland G H, Janzen J A 1988 Influence of bupivacaine as an adjuvant to epidural morphine for analgesia after cesarean section. Anesth Analg 67: 1138–1141
19. Lirzin J D, Jacquinot P, Dailland P et al 1989 Controlled trial of extradural bupivacaine with fentanyl, morphine or placebo for pain relief in labour. Br J Anaesth 62: 641–644
20. Abboud T K, Shnider S M, Dailey P A et al 1984 Intrathecal administration of hyperbaric morphine for the relief of pain in labour. Br J Anaesth 56: 1251–1360
21. Baraka A, Noueihid R, Hajj S 1981 Intrathecal injection of morphine for obstetric analgesia. Anesthesiology 54: 136–140
22. Scott P V, Bowen F E, Cartwright P et al 1980 Intrathecal morphine as sole analgesia during labour. Br Med J 281: 351–353
23. Dailey P A, Brookshire G L, Shnider S M et al 1885 The effects of naloxone associated with the intrathecal use of morphine in labor. Anesth Analg 64: 658–666
24. Stenkamp S J, Easterling T R, Chadwick H S 1989 Effect of epidural and intrathecal morphine on the length of hospital stay after cesarean section. Anesth Analg 68: 66–69
25. Youngstrom P C, Cowan R I, Sutheimer C, Eastwood D W, Yu J C M 1982 Pain relief and plasma concentrations from epidural and intramuscular morphine in post-cesarean patients. Anesthesiology 57: 404–409
26. Eisenach J C, Grice S C, Dewan D M 1988 Patient controlled analgesia following cesarean section: a comparison with epidural and intramuscular narcotics. Anesthesiology 68: 444–448
27. Harrison D M, Sinatra R, Morgese L, Chung J H 1988 Epidural narcotic and patient-controlled analgesia for post-cesarean section pain relief. Anesthesiology 68: 454–457
28. Abboud T K, Lee K, Zhu J et al 1990 Prophylactic oral naltrexone with intrathecal morphine for cesarean section: effects on adverse reactions and analgesia. Anesth Analg 71: 367–370
29. Crone L- A L, Conly J M, Storgard C et al 1990 Herpes labialis in parturients receiving epidural morphine following cesarean section. Anesthesiology 73: 208–213
30. Vella L, Francis D, Houlton P, Reynolds F 1985 Comparison of the antiemetics metoclopramide and promethazine in labour. Br Med J 290: 1173–1175
31. Hey V M F, Ostick D G, Mazumder J K, Lord W D 1981 Pethidine, metoclopramide and the gastro-oesophageal sphincter. A study in healthy volunteers. Anaesthesia 36: 173–176
32. Nimmo W S, Wilson J, Prescott L F 1975 Narcotic analgesia and delayed gastric emptying during labour. Lancet 1: 890–893
33. Murphy D F, Nally B, Gardiner J, Unwin A 1984 Effect of metoclopramide on gastric emptying before elective and emergency cesarean section. Br J Anaesth 56: 1113–1116
34. Reed P N, Colquhoun A D, Hanning C D 1989 Maternal oxygenation during normal labour. Br J Anaesth 62: 316–318
35. Kaiko R F, Foley K M, Grabinski P Y 1983 Central nervous system excitatory effects of meperidine in cancer patients. Ann Neurol 13: 180–185
36. Thalme B, Belfrage P, Raabe N 1974 Lumbar epidural analgesia in labour. I. Acid–base balance and clinical condition of mother, fetus and newborn. Acta Obstet Gynecol Scand 53: 27–35
37. Wiener P C, Hogg M I, Rosen M 1979 Neonatal respiration, feeding and neurobehavioural state. Effects of intrapartum bupivacaine, pethidine and pethidine reversed by naloxone. Anaesthesia 34: 996–1004
38. Morrison J C, Wiser W L, Rosser S I et al 1973 Metabolites of meperidine related to fetal depression. Am J Obstet Gynecol 15: 1132–1137
39. Kuhnert B R, Kuhnert P M, Tu A-S L, Lin DCK 1979 Meperidine and normeperidine levels following meperidine administration during labor. II. Fetus and neonate. Am J Obstet Gynecol 133: 909–914
40. Golub M S, Eisele J H, Kuhnert B R 1988 Disposition of intrapartum narcotic analgesics in monkeys. Anesth Analg 67: 637–643
41. Robinson J O, Rosen M, Evans J M, Revill S I, David H, Rees G 1980 Self-administered intravenous and intramuscular pethidine. A controlled trial in labour. Anaesthesia 35: 763–770
42. Rayburn W, Leuschen M P, Earl R, Woods M, Lorkovic M, Gaston-Johnsson F 1989 Intravenous meperidine during labor: a randomised comparison between nursing- and patient-controlled administration. Obstet Gynecol 74: 702–706
43. Li D F H, Rees G A D, Rosen M 1988 Feasibility of self-administered analgesia by the intramuscular route in labour. Eur J Obstet Gynecol Reprod Biol 27: 99–104
44. Perriss B W 1980 Epidural pethidine in labour. A study of dose requirements. Anaesthesia 35: 380–382
45. Perriss B W, Malins A F 1981 Pain Relief in labour using epidural pethidine with adrenaline. Anaesthesia 36: 631–633
46. Perriss B W, Latham B V, Wilson I H 1990 Analgesia following extradural and IM pethidine in post-caesarean section patients. Br J Anaesth 64: 355–357
47. Brownridge P, Frewin D B 1985 A comparative study of techniques of postoperative analgesia following cesarean section and low abdominal surgery. Anaesth Intensive Care 13: 123–130
48. Skjoldebrand A, Garle M, Gustafsson L L, Johansson H, Lunell N-O, Rane A 1982 Extradural pethidine with and without adrenaline during labour: wide variation in effect. Br J Anaesth 54: 415–420
49. Husemeyer R P, Cummings A J, Rosankiewicz J R, Davenport H T 1982 A study of pethidine kinetics and analgesia in women in labour following intravenous, intramuscular and epidural administration. Br J Clin Pharmacol 13: 171–176
50. Refstad S O, Lindbaek E 1980 Ventilatory depression of the newborn of women receiving pethidine or pentazocine. A double-blind comparative trial. Br J Anaesth 52: 265–271
51. Sheikh A, Tunstall M E 1986 Comparative study of meptazinol and pethidine for the relief of pain in labour. Br J Obstet Gynaecol 93: 264–269
52. Slattery P J, Harmer M, Rosen M, Vickers M D 1981 Comparison of meptazinol and pethidine given i.v. on demand in the management of postoperative pain. Br J Anaesth 53: 927–931
53. Nicholas A D G, Robson P J 1982 Double blind comparison of meptazinol and pethidine in labour. Br J Obstet Gynaecol 89: 318–322
54. Jackson M B A, Robson P J 1983 Preliminary clinical and pharmacokinetic experiences in the newborn when meptazinol is compared with pethidine as an obstetric analgesic. Postgrad Med J 59 (suppl 1): 47–51
55. Verborgh C, Van Der Auwera D, Camu F 1987 Meptazinol for postoperative pain relief in man. Comparison of extradural and IM administration. Br J Anaesth 59: 1134–1139
56. Moldenhauer C C, Roach G W, Finlayson D C et al 1985 Nalbuphine antagonism of ventilatory depression following high-dose fentanyl anesthesia. Anesthesiology 62: 647–650
57. Wilson C M, McClean E, Moore J, Dundee J W 1986 A double-blind comparison of intramuscular pethidine and nalbuphine in labour. Anaesthesia 41: 1207–1213
58. Wilson C M, Moore J, McClean E, Dundee J W 1986 Maternal analgesia and neonatal neurobehaviour following nalbuphine and pethidine. Br J Pharmacol 21: 613P
59. Podlas J, Breland B D 1987 Patient-controlled analgesia with nalbuphine during labor. Obstet Gynecol 70: 202–204
60. Jensen F M, Jensen N-H, Holk I K, Ravnborg M 1987 Prolonged and biphasic respiratory depression following epidural buprenorphine. Anaesthesia 42: 470–475
61. Simpson H K, Madej T H, McDowell J M, Macdonald R, Lyons G 1988 Comparison of extradural buprenorphine and extradural morphine after caesarean section. Br J Anaesth 60: 627–631

62. Kallos T, Caruso F S 1979 Respiratory effects of butorphanol and pethidine. Anaesthesia 34: 633–637
63. Naulty J S, Malinow A, Hunt C O et al 1986 Epidural butorphanol–bupivacaine for analgesia during labor and delivery. Anesthesiology 65: A 369
64. Abboud T K, Reyes A, Richardson M et al 1989 Epidural morphine or butorphanol augments bupivacaine analgesia during labor. Reg Anesth 14: 115–120
65. Hunt C O, Naulty J S, Malinow A M, Datta S, Ostheimer G W 1989 Epidural butorphanol–bupivacaine for analgesia during labor and delivery. Anesth Analg 68: 323–327
66. Rodriguez J, Abboud T K, Reyes A et al 1990 Continuous infusion epidural anesthesia during labor: a randomised double-blind comparison of 0.0625% bupivacaine/0.002% butorphanol and 0.125% bupivacaine. Reg Anesth 15: 300–303
67. Lawhorn C D, McNitt J D, Fibuch E E, Joyce J T, Leadley R J 1991 Epidural morphine with butorphanol for postoperative analgesia after cesarean delivery. Anesth Analg 72: 53–57
68. Martin C S, McGrady M, Colquhoun A, Thorburn J 1990 Extradural methadone and bupivacaine in labour. Br J Anaesth 65: 330–332
69. Beeby D, Macintosh K C, Bailey M, Welch D B 1984 Post operative analgesia for caesarean section using epidural methadone. Anaesthesia 39: 61–63
70. McGrady E M, Brownhill D K, Davis 1989 Epidural diamorphine and bupivacaine in labour. Anaesthesia 44: 400–403
71. Houlton P G, Reynolds F 1981 Epidural diamorphine and fentanyl for postoperative pain (letter). Anaesthesia 36: 1144–1145
72. Semple A J, Macrae D J, Munishankarappa S, Burrow L M, Milne M K, Grant I S 1988 Effect of the addition of adrenaline to extradural diamorphine analgesia after caesarean section. Br J Anaesth 60: 632–638
73. Patrick J A, Smith M, Cross G, Reynolds F 1991 A comparison of extradural diamorphine with intramuscular papaveretum following caesarean section. Int J Obstet Anesthesia 1: 25–28
74. Patrick J A, Meyer-Witting M, Reynolds F 1991 Lumbar epidural analgesia following thoracic surgery. Anaesthesia 46: 85–89

PART B
PLACENTAL TRANSFER
F. Reynolds

The human placenta is classified as hemomonochorial, that is a singular layer of chorionic tissue, the syncytiotrophoblast, separates maternal blood from fetal capillaries. The membrane thickness is similar to that of rodents such as the rabbit and the guinea pig but much thinner than that of the sheep. The human placenta is also described as villous, and the flow pattern is haphazard but behaves essentially as a concurrent system. By contrast, in the labyrinthine placentas of rabbit and guinea pig a more efficient countercurrent system operates. The sheep flow pattern is similar to that of the human. The placental membrane is essentially a syncytium in all these species and therefore behaves as a continuous lipid membrane for the purposes of diffusion. Hence, lipid-soluble molecules can diffuse readily across the placenta up to a molecular weight of 600–1000, while water-soluble molecules diffuse freely only up to a molecular weight of 60–100 and thereafter they are progressively impeded as the particle size increases.

Much experimental work on the distribution of drugs in the fetal–placental unit has been carried out in sheep. Because of the thickness of the sheep placenta, there is a tendency for much greater drug concentration gradients to exist and to persist, which is true particularly for poorly lipid-soluble substances. Therefore, the sheep is, in some respects, a poor model from which to extrapolate placental drug transfer to man.

Though drugs in general are constrained by the physical laws of diffusion, substances necessary for fetal growth and fetal waste products could not be expected to cross the placenta by diffusion at a rate sufficient to maintain fetal welfare. Therefore, other mechanisms are available. For example, amino acids, which are present only in low concentrations in maternal blood, are actively transported to the fetus against a concentration gradient, while dextrose is transferred from maternal blood by a process of facilitated diffusion, which takes places down a concentration gradient but at a rate more rapid than simple physical laws would normally allow.

FACTORS GOVERNING THE RATE OF TRANSPLACENTAL DIFFUSION

Placental factors

Because the rate of diffusion depends upon the transplacental gradient, blood flow on either side of the placenta, which initially helps to preserve the gradient, promotes placental transfer and speeds the approach towards equilibrium. In placentas with countercurrent flow systems, transfer rate and, therefore, approach towards equilibrium are more rapid than with less efficient flow systems. However, in all placentas there appears to be a variable element of shunting on both sides of the membrane, and this limits the ability of the drug to equilibrate across the placenta in a single circulation. The area of placental adhesion also affects the area available for exchange and hence the overall rate of approach towards the equilibrium. Placental thickness also affects the transfer rate, particularly of hydrophilic compounds.

Drug characteristics

The more lipid-soluble a drug the more readily it is able to approach equilibrium across the placental membrane in a single circuit of the placenta. Hence, the factors determining the rate of transfer of hydrophilic and lipophilic substances are different.

Flow-dependent transfer

The concentration of a substance that diffuses readily across the placental membrane approaches equilibrium across the placenta in a single circuit. Hence, as for respiratory gases across the alveolar membrane, permeability is not a limiting factor. Rather the gradient of diffusible substance determines the amount of transfer. During transit the gradient will tend to disappear; hence, the higher the blood flow on either side of the membrane, the better preserved is the gradient, and the greater the amount of drug transferred. It would appear from studies in the rabbit that, for highly protein-bound drugs of which there may be substantial stores in maternal blood, umbilical flow is a more important influence than maternal flow[1,2] (Figs 14.6 and 14.7). This is likely to be true also in the human, in whom maternal flow is about double the fetal flow, presenting a superfluity of supply.

As the particle size of drug bound to protein is too large to cross the placenta with any ease, and similarly a drug that is ionized diffuses poorly, it follows that the *diffusible*

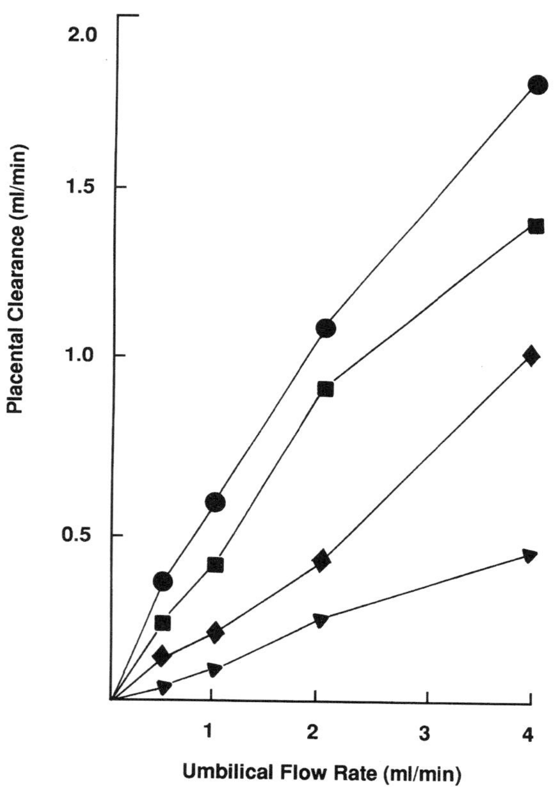

Fig. 14.6 The effect of umbilical blood flow on the placental transfer rate (as represented by placental clearance) of bupivacaine (triangles), fentanyl (diamonds), meperidine (squares), and antipyrine (circles) measured using the rabbit placenta perfused in situ with Krebs bicarbonate buffer containing dextran instead of protein to maintain the oncotic pressure. All agents show clear flow-dependent characteristics, and the difference between them is accounted for by the maternal protein binding of each. (From Vella et al,[3] by kind permission of the publishers.)

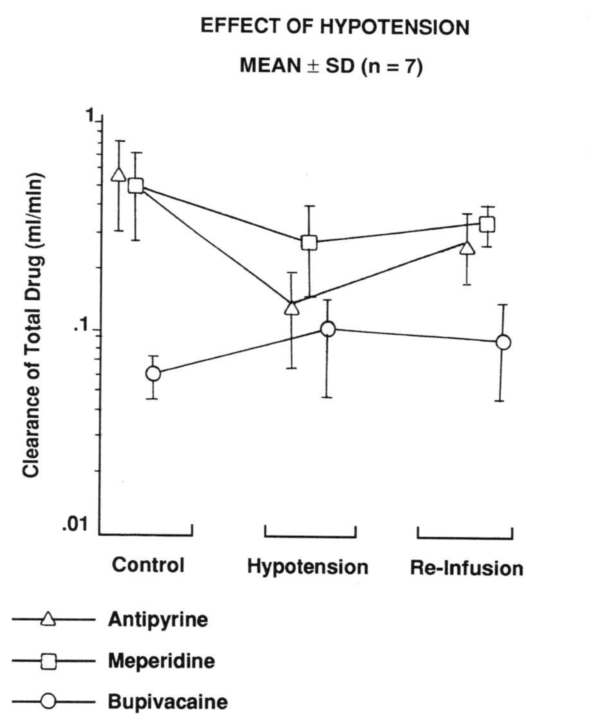

Fig. 14.7 The effect of maternal hypotension induced by hemorrhage on the placental clearance of bupivacaine (circles), meperidine (triangles), and antipyrine (squares) studied in the rabbit placenta perfused in situ with Krebs bicarbonate buffer containing dextran. Data are mean ± SD in seven rabbits. The fall in antipyrine ratio is significant and demonstrates that maternal hemorrhage results in reduced maternal blood supply to the placenta and consequent fall in antipyrine transfer. There is significant restoration of function with reinfusion of blood. Transfer of meperidine is also significantly reduced but does not rise significantly with reinfusion. There is no decline in bupivacaine transfer with maternal hypotension. Again the differences between the agents in the control period are accounted for by their maternal protein binding. (Data from Gaylard et al.[2])

gradient is that for nonionized and unbound drug, while the number of ionized and protein-bound particles on either side of the placenta determines the equilibrium distribution. However, if equilibrium is approached in a single circuit then the affinity of maternal and fetal blood for the drug may affect not only the ultimate distribution but also the rate of transfer.[2]

Ionization

There is a pH gradient across the placenta that is normally around 0.1 of a pH unit, hence, basic groups are more ionized in the more acid fetal plasma, and acidic groups more ionized in maternal plasma. Therefore, according to the Henderson–Hasselbalch equation, if the nonionized moiety equilibrates across the membrane, total free concentration of a basic substance is higher in fetus than mother, while the reverse is true for an acid. Moreover, the more extreme the pH gradient, the greater would be this ion-trapping effect. It has been demonstrated in both sheep and humans that fetal–maternal (F/M) ratios of local anesthetics are higher than normal in the presence of fetal acidosis.[4–7] These were, however, findings in intact preparations that cannot reliably indicate whether the rate of placental transfer was affected, because equilibration may only occur with recirculation. In a perfused rabbit placenta using an open nonrecirculating system it has been shown that reducing the pH of the umbilical perfusate (to mimic fetal acidosis) increases the *rate* of transfer of both meperidine and bupivacaine[2] (Fig. 14.8). Thus, fetal acidosis may enhance the fetal toxicity of basic drugs. In theory, the more acidotic the fetus, and the stronger the base, the higher the equilibrium F/M ratio (Fig. 14.9).

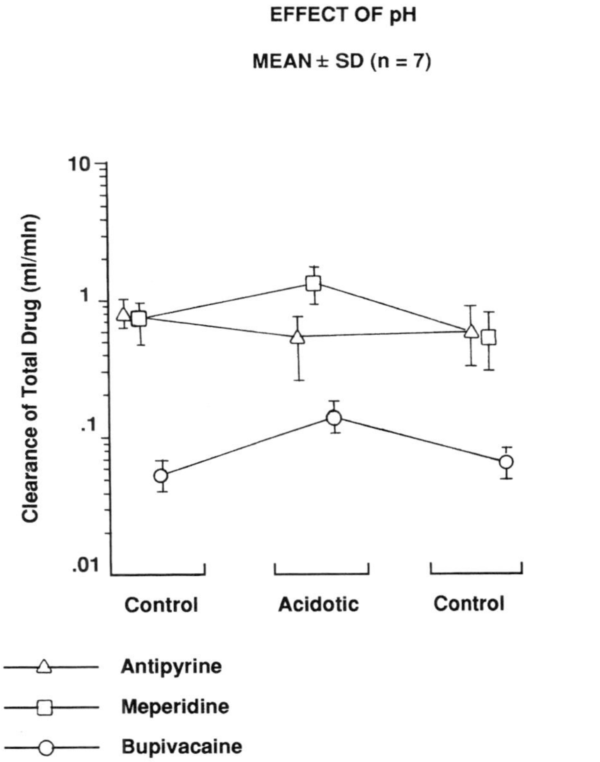

Fig. 14.8 The effect of umbilical perfusate pH on the placental clearance of bupivacaine (circles), meperidine (squares), and antipyrine (triangles) using the perfused rabbit placenta as in Figure 9.2. During the 'acidotic' period of the experiment the pH of the Krebs bicarbonate buffer was decreased to 7. Transfer of antipyrine, which is virtually nonionized, did not change significantly, demonstrating normal functioning of the placenta. The transfer of both bupivacaine and meperidine, which are weak bases, was increased significantly during acidotic perfusion, demonstrating ion trapping on the fetal side of the placenta. (Data from Gaylard et al.[2])

Protein binding

Although drugs cross the placenta principally in the unbound form, once in the fetal circulation they become bound to fetal protein. It might be expected that in a single circuit of the placenta the umbilical circulation would tend to equilibrate with maternal free drug while fetal protein content would affect only the final equilibrium. However, adding protein to the fetal side of the perfused placenta in an open system can increase transfer rate of protein-bound drugs, the more so the higher the binding[8] (Fig. 14.10).

Equilibrium distribution is strongly influenced by the relative concentrations of binding protein in mother and fetus. In a study of maternal–fetal pairs delivered at different times throughout gestation, Krauer et al[9] showed that fetal protein concentrations increased throughout gestation, but whereas albumin levels commonly rose to exceed maternal at term, those of α_1-acid glycoprotein (AAG) never attained maternal concentrations. Thus F/M ratios of albumin-bound substances such as thiopental, other acid drugs and diazepam may well exceed unity, while ratios of drugs strongly bound to AAG such as bupivacaine and alfentanil are consistently $<<1$. Indeed F/M ratios of bupivacaine correlate significantly with the transplacental AAG gradient,[10] and binding gradient affects not only the final equilibrium, if diffusion is free, it affects also the rate of transfer (see above and Fig. 14.8).

It may be said that relative protein binding is unimportant, because it is only the free drug which is active, and it is this component which tends to equilibrate across the placenta. However, high fetal binding does provide an increased store of drug in the neonatal period when albumin binding may fall and the free concentration may actually rise. Such a phenomenon has been demonstrated for diazepam.[11]

Permeability-dependent transfer

Polar drugs, such as mannitol and neuromuscular blocking agents, cross the placenta very slowly, and their rate of diffusion is limited by permeability. The perme-

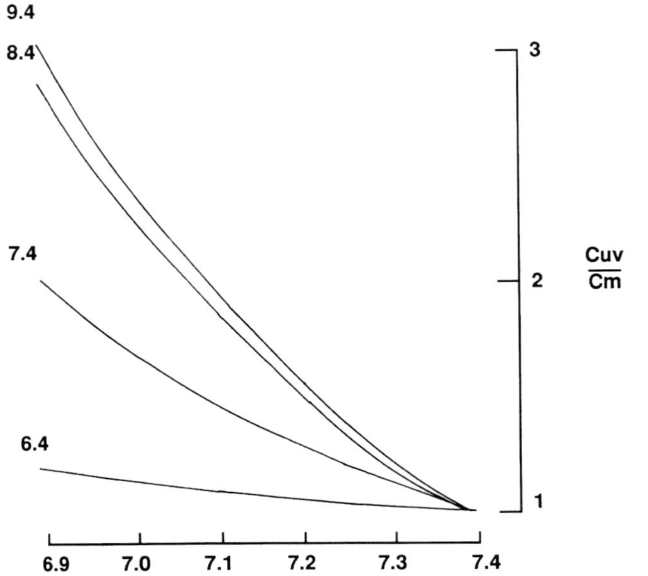

Fig. 14.9 The effect of fetal acidosis on equilibrium fetal–maternal ratios of hypothetical basic compounds, the pK_a values of which are shown on the left. The stronger the base and the more acidotic the fetus, the greater the potential for ion trapping in the fetal compartment.

ability of the placenta to a polar molecule falls as molecular weight rises.[12,13] Between the two extremes of lipophilic readily diffusible drug such as meperidine and hydrophilic compound such as mannitol are drugs such as morphine and antipyrine (Fig. 14.6) that exhibit flow-dependent transfer at low flow but whose maximum transfer rate is limited by permeability. Morphine has been shown to diffuse more readily across the primate placenta than across the much thicker membrane of the sheep.[14]

Among the factors affecting placental transfer of polar compounds, therefore, concentration gradient and flow are of less importance than with lipophilic drugs. The all-important drug characteristic is molecular size, which limits permeability, and the important placental characteristics are area and thickness of the membrane.

Fetal tissue equilibration

Even if the distribution of a drug approaches equilibrium across the placental membrane in a single circulation, equilibration throughout the entire fetal compartment is

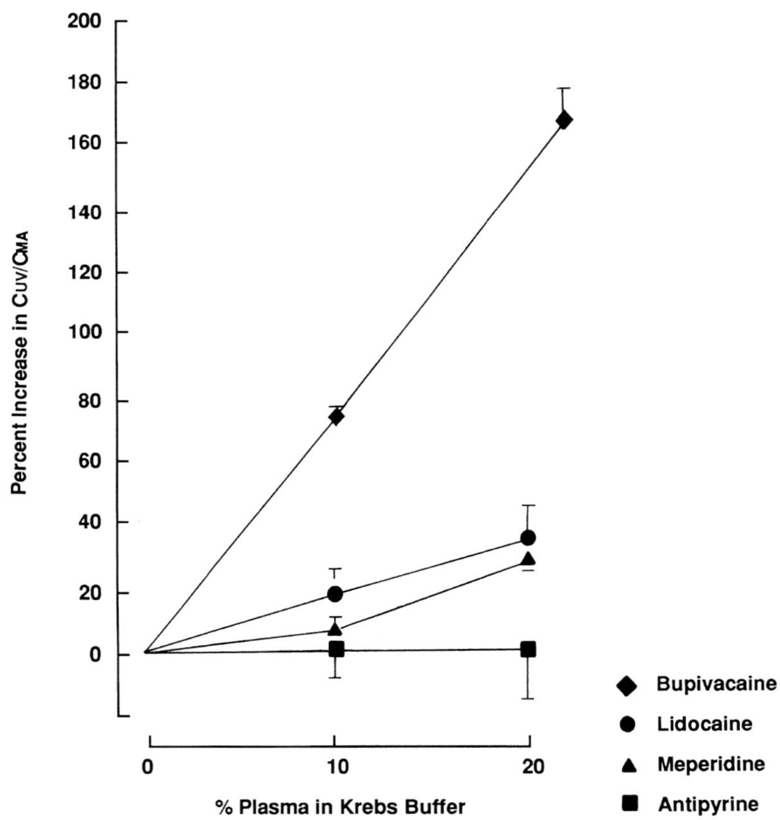

Fig. 14.10 The effect of increasing the protein content of the umbilical perfusate on the placental transfer of antipyrine (squares), meperidine (triangles), lidocaine (circles), and bupivacaine (diamonds) using the rabbit placenta perfused in situ with Krebs bicarbonate buffer to which either dextran or 10% or 20% human plasma had been added. The greater the protein binding of the ligand, the greater the increase in placental transfer with increasing protein content on the fetal side. (Data from Hamshaw-Thomas et al.[7])

always a comparatively slow process. Within the maternal environment the fetus must be classed as a very deep compartment, as maternal blood does not directly perfuse fetal organs. This may sound obvious but it is worth emphasizing, as it explains why the fetus is protected from the full force of a bolus dose of a drug given intravenously to the mother. No matter how rapidly a bolus of drug crosses the placenta, it must undergo dilution within the fetal circulation before reaching fetal organs. Approximately 50% of the umbilical venous return passes through the liver, which takes up drug before it reaches the fetal systemic circulation. This further attenuates the peak concentration of a bolus dose. If the maternal concentration of a drug is maintained then fetal concentration will rise gradually towards a theoretical equilibrium distribution. The F/M ratio of meperidine has been observed to rise with dose–delivery interval[15] (Fig. 14.11) and, while this may be associated with a falling maternal and even umbilical vein concentration, there is no doubt that total fetal dose of meperidine and active metabolites rises for some hours following a maternal dose.[16] The same relationship between dose–delivery interval and F/M ratio at delivery for bupivacaine is less apparent[17] (Fig. 14.12), as this ratio is predominantly influenced by the transplacental AAG gradient. However, umbilical artery–vein ratio is unaffected by AAG gradient, and some increase in this ratio may be observed in the first hour following bupivacaine administration. This suggests that fetal tissue equilibration takes place fairly rapidly. However, during *continued* maternal administration, bupivacaine accumulates gradually in fetus as in mother.[17]

There is little chance for polar molecules to equilibrate throughout the fetal compartment because they tend to be excreted in fetal urine much more rapidly than they cross the placenta. Though the fetus drinks amniotic fluid, charged particles and polar molecules that are swallowed are poorly absorbed through the gut wall. They thus tend to accumulate in the lumen of the gastrointestinal tract. A transplacental gradient persists but amniotic fluid concentration may come to exceed that in any other compartment, as has been demonstrated for mannitol.[18] Quarternary ammonium compounds such as neuromuscular blocking drugs and hexamethonium are fully ionized and can therefore be expected to cross the placenta only slowly. When given in normal doses for the usual brief period of time before delivery, neuromuscular blockade is not in evidence in the baby. Interestingly, hexamethonium was once used to treat hypertension in pregnancy (unsuccessfully as it is a ganglion blocker) and babies born to mothers so treated were often observed to suffer paralytic ileus resulting from a high concentration of hexamethonium in the intestinal lumen.

Fetal elimination

Though the fetus can readily eliminate drugs that are renally excreted by passing them into the amniotic fluid, drugs that are principally metabolized are less efficiently handled. It would be inappropriate for a fetus to convert drugs to more polar substances because by so doing its main route of drug elimination, back-transfer to the mother, would be prevented and the polar metabolities would become trapped in the fetal environment.

The placenta contains several types of cytochrome P450 systems, which may provide a protective barrier to endogenous substrates and related compounds such as corticosteroids, but which play a minor role compared with the fetal liver in the detoxicification of drugs. It also contains small amounts of monoamine oxidase, catechol-O-methyltransferase and cholinesterase, which limit placental transfer of maternal transmitters, but which are readily swamped by bolus doses of drugs.

The human fetal liver is able to oxidize drugs using the cytochrome P450 system from the end of the first trimester, and, at term, has the adult complement of enzymes though with only about half the activity. Thus

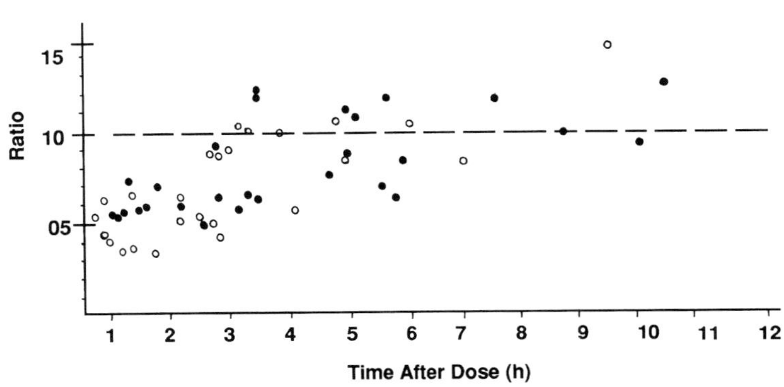

Fig. 14.11 Fetal–maternal ratios of meperidine following intramuscular injection. Umbilical vein–maternal vein, closed symbols; fetal scalp–maternal vein, open symbols. (From Tomson et al[14] by kind permission from the author and publishers.)

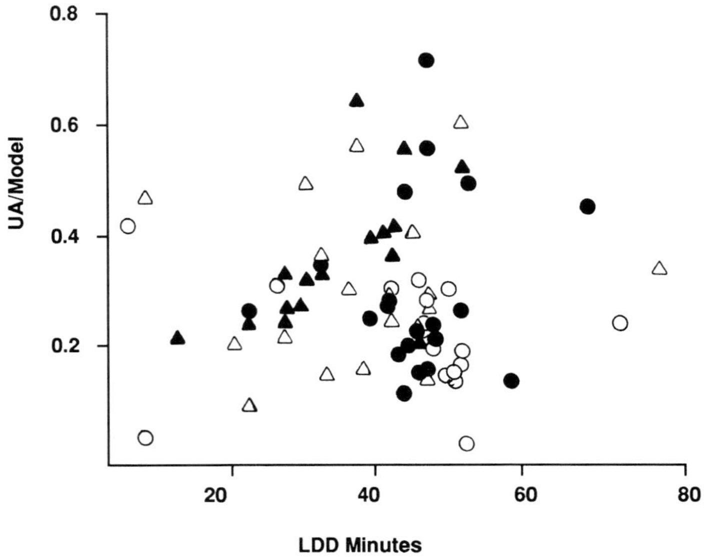

Fig. 14.12 Fetal–maternal ratios (UA/MDel) of bupivacaine related to dose–delivery interval. At time zero women received 20 ml of 0.5% bupivacaine with epinephrine (filled symbols) or alone (open symbols), either for elective Cesarean delivery (circles) or following epidural anesthesia in labor (triangles). Measuring umbilical artery concentrations should give the best indication of fetal content of bupivacaine. Time has no effect on these ratios, unlike the clear relationship seen for meperidine in Figure 9.6. (Data from Reynolds et al.[16])

first-order processes do occur but at a reduced rate, as has been shown by kinetic studies in the newborn. The half-life of meperidine may be 2–6 h in the mother but 16–20 h in the newborn.[19,20] Similarly with bupivacaine, the maternal half-life of 3–6 h compares with 24 h plus in the newborn.[21,22] The fetal liver is deficient in UDP-glucuronyltransferase activity, therefore many conjugation processes are conspicuously depressed, as witness the toxicity of chloramphenicol in the newborn. Benzodiazepines such as oxazepam and lorazepam are conjugated much more slowly in fetus than adult and all have a long and profound effect on the newborn. One exception to this rule is sulfate conjugation, which is as brisk in the fetal–placental unit as in the adult,[23] occurs principally in the placenta, and affects the handling of β-adrenoreceptor stimulant drugs.

MEASURING PLACENTAL TRANSFER

Confusion arises because placental transfer rate is sometimes erroneously taken to mean velocity of transfer from one side of the membrane to the other. Experimenters have attempted to measure the time at which a drug can first be detected in the umbilical circulation following a maternal dose. In practice, this is dependent on the maternal circulatory state and on the sensitivity of the method used to detect the drug. Therefore, it is a pointless exercise. The rate of placental transfer is more correctly taken to mean the net amount of drug crossing the placenta per unit time, which is dependent on the gradient, largely a man-made variable.

Fetal–maternal concentration (F/M) *ratios* are frequently taken to be an index of placental transfer rate but, in practice, they are influenced by a number of different factors. When considering the significance of F/M ratios, it is important to know at what point in the circulation the concentrations have been measured. In human studies umbilical vein (UV) concentration is often measured. This is directly downstream from the placenta and, therefore, a UV/M ratio measured while the umbilical artery (UA) concentration is zero, for example on first exposure to the drug or in an open system, is a function of placental transfer rate. As fetal tissue equilibration takes place, UA approaches UV concentration and transfer rate diminishes. Measuring UA and UV concentrations can indicate the direction of placental transfer and the extent of fetal tissue equilibration. Thus if UA < UV fetal tissue uptake and hence net transfer is continuing while if UA ≃ UV fetal tissue uptake is slight. In the case of bupivacaine, F/M ratios are consistently low even in the presence of UA/UV ratios near unity.[17] This indicates that the transplacental inequality is due to differences in affinity of maternal and fetal blood for the drug, and not to continuing fetal tissue uptake.

During continuous maternal drug administration, a gradient across the placenta is likely to persist. As maternal drug elimination is more rapid than fetal, once administration ceases the direction of net transfer may well be reversed. In such a case, therefore, *high* F/M ratios do not indicate rapid net transfer, still less active transfer, but simply reverse transfer. This phenomenon is well demonstrated following intravenous administration of meperidine in both sheep[24] and humans (Fig. 14.11) and of bupivacaine in sheep[25] (Fig. 14.12).

To measure the rate of transfer (T), that is the *amount* of drug crossing the placenta and arriving in the fetal environment per unit time, it is necessary to know the concentration of drug in umbilical artery (C_{ua}) and umbilical vein (C_{uv}) and the umbilical flow (Q_u). Thus:

$$T = Q_u \, (C_{uv} - C_{ua})$$

In practice, such measurements are often made when perfusing the placenta artificially, thus controlling Q_u. Moreover, if an open system is used and no drug is perfused on the fetal side $C_{ua} = 0$, therefore:

$$T = Q_u \cdot C_{uv}$$

In various reviews of placental transfer[26–28] a formula for the calculation of transfer rate quoted from Moya and Thorndike[29] and others has been given thus:

$$\text{Rate of transfer } (T) = \frac{KA\,(C_m - C_f)}{X} \qquad (1)$$

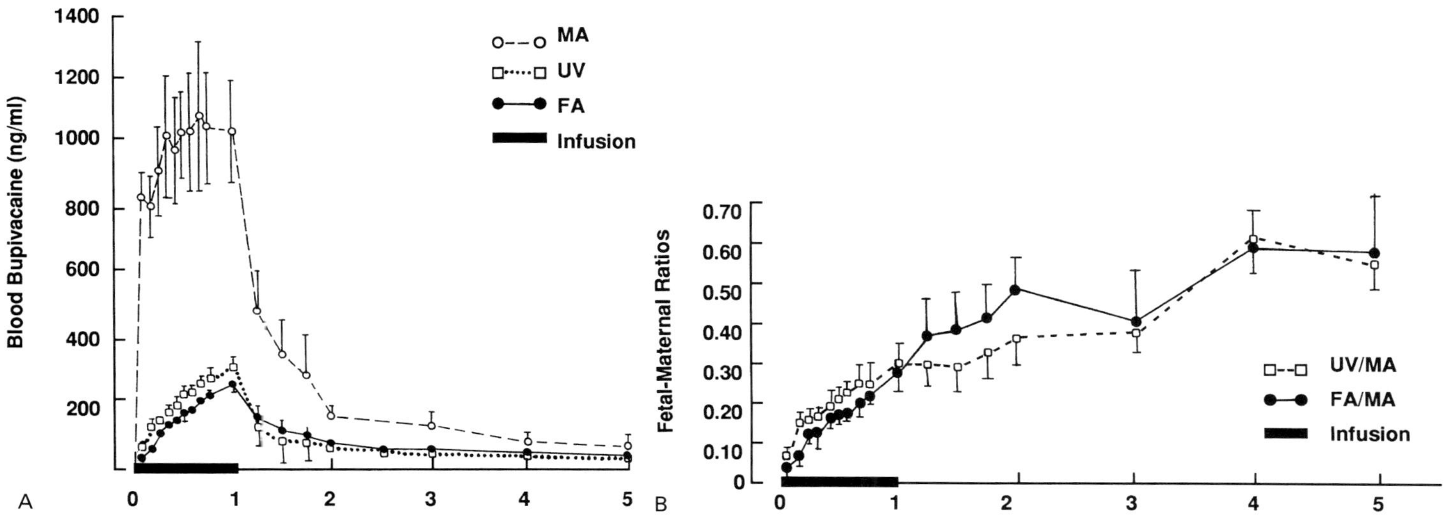

Fig. 14.13 (a) Bupivacaine concentrations (mean ± SEM) in maternal artery (open circles), umbilical vein (squares), and fetal aorta (filled circles) during and after bupivacaine infusion of 2.7 mg/kg in five ewes. (b) Fetal maternal ratios of bupivacaine (mean ± SEM) measured in the same ewes. UV/MA, open circles; FA/MA, filled circles. (Reproduced from Kennedy et al[24] by kind permission of the author and publishers.)

where A is the surface area available for transplacental exchange, now commonly referred to as S, and X is membrane thickness; C_m and C_f are said to be concentrations in mother and fetus, though whether arterial or venous and whether total concentrations or just the diffusible fraction is not stated. K is a constant said to be dependent on lipid solubility, molecular weight, and ionization. Such a formula is almost completely inapplicable. In the first place, rate of transfer is not calculated from a formula using a constant, but rather measured in order to derive the constant. As the equation is applicable *only* to permeability-dependent transfer, the constant is generally referred to as P, the permeability constant. Moreover, as surface area is generally unknown, the product of permeability and surface area (*PS*) is more usually calculated. In order to derive some uniformity from the data this may be measured per unit weight of placenta. The equation can now be rewritten:

$$PS = \frac{TX}{C_m - C_f} \qquad (2)$$

In practice, the thickness of the placenta is neglected and *PS* then becomes the rate of drug transfer (T) per unit of transplacental concentration gradient. Within very strictly defined experimental conditions P may be a constant for a *polar* compound and appears to be dependent upon molecular size.[12,13]

The gradient $C_m - C_f$ now needs to be defined. In a concurrent-flow system this is high at first point of contact but diminishes with passage through the placenta. Therefore, it would be appropriate to take the theoretical harmonic mean gradient. In practice, if a drug is poorly diffusible, the gradient may change little. In a countercurrent system such as that in rodents, the gradient changes little with transit and the readily measured gradient $C_{ma} - C_{uv}$ may be taken. Thus, from equations 1 and 2:

$$PS = \frac{Q_u(C_{uv} - C_{ua})}{C_{ma} - C_{uv}} \qquad (3)$$

PS has the dimension of volume/time, and the equation presupposes that the entire content of drug is homogenously diffusible. In calculating *PS* for a substance that is partly ionized and partly protein bound, the gradient for the unbound nonionized fraction is the principal determinant of transfer rate.

For a substance that diffuses freely across the placenta, however, and may therefore come into equilibrium in a single circuit in the absence of any shunting, $C_{ma} = C_{uv}$ and, as is appropriate, $PS = \infty$. Any attempt to measure *PS* for freely diffusible drugs simply gives a measure of the efficiency of placental exchange and of the amount of shunting that takes place rather than of permeability.

The concept of clearance (CL) may usefully be applied to the placenta. This is the volume of maternal blood cleared of drug in unit time:

$$CL = \frac{Q_m (C_{ma} - C_{mv})}{C_{ma}} \qquad (4)$$

If C_{ma} is maintained constant and if the placenta does not metabolize the drug and becomes saturated with it, then at steady state:

$$Q_m (C_{ma} - C_{mv}) = Q_u (C_{uv} - C_{ma})$$

Therefore:

$$CL = \frac{Q_u(C_{uv} - C_{ua})}{C_{ma}}$$

Like *PS*, therefore, CL also has the dimension volume/time. For a drug that equilibrates perfectly in a single circuit of a countercurrent placenta, $C_{ma} = C_{uv}$. Thus while $PS = \infty$ clearance simply increases linearly with umbilical flow. Therefore, clearance is not a pure drug characteristic but can be used to demonstrate flow dependent characteristics[1,3,8] (Fig. 14.6).

In clinical practice estimating the placental transfer rate is impractical. In the context of prolonged drug administration it is irrelevant while equilibrium F/M ratio gives an indication of fetal drug exposure. On brief exposure, however, an early F/M ratio is an index of transfer rate. If low, this may be because placental permeability is low or because the affinity of fetal blood for the drug is less than that of the mother. In either case fetal exposure will be reduced.

REFERENCES

1. Hamshaw-Thomas A H, Rogerson N, Reynolds F 1984 Transfer of bupivacaine, lignocaine and pethidine across the rabbit placenta–influence of maternal protein binding and fetal flow. Placenta 5: 61–70
2. Gaylard D G, Carson R J, Reynolds F 1990 The effect of umbilical perfusate pH and controlled maternal hypotension on placental drug transfer in the rabbit. Anesth Analg 71: 42–48
3. Vella L M, Knott C, Reynolds F 1986 Transfer of fentanyl across the rabbit placenta – effect of umbilical flow and concurrent drug administration. Br J Anaesth 58: 49–54
4. Kennedy R L, Erenberg A, Robillard J E, Merkow A, Turner T 1979 Effects of changes in maternal-fetal pH on the transplacental equilibrium of bupivacaine. Anesthesiology 51: 50–54
5. Datta S, Alper M H, Ostheimer G W, Brown W U, Weiss J B 1979 Effects of maternal position on epidural anesthesia for cesarean section, acid–base status and bupivacaine concentrations at delivery. Anesthesiology 50: 205–209
6. Datta S, Brown W U, Ostheimer G W, Weiss J B, Alper M H 1981 Epidural anesthesia for cesarean section in diabetic parturients: maternal and neonatal acid–base status and bupivacaine concentrations. Anesth Analg 60: 574–578
7. O'Brien W F, Cefalo R C, Grissom M P, Vieras S F, Golden S M, Uddin D M, Davis S E 1982 The influence of asphyxia on fetal lidocaine toxicity. Am J Obstet Gynecol 142: 205–208
8. Hamshaw-Thomas A, Reynolds F 1985 Placental transfer of bupivacaine, pethidine and lignocaine in the rabbit. Effect of umbilical flow rate and protein content. Br J Obstet Gynaecol 92: 706–713
9. Krauer B, Dayer P, Anner R 1984 Changes in serum albumin and alpha-1-acid glycoprotein concentrations during pregnancy: an analysis of feto-maternal pairs. Br J Obstet Gynaecol 91: 875–881
10. Petersen M C, Moore R G, Nation R L, McMeniman W 1981 Relationship between the transplacental gradients of bupivacaine and α-1-acid glycoprotein. Br J Clin Pharmacol 12: 859–862
11. Nau H, Luck W, Kuhnz W, Wegener S 1983 Serum protein binding of diazepam, desmethyldiazepam, furosemide, indomethacin, warfarin and phenobarbital in human fetus, mother and newborn infant. Ped Pharmacol 3: 219–227
12. Illsley N P, Hall S, Penfold P, Stacey T E 1985 Diffusional permeability of the human placenta. Contrib Gynecol Obstet 13: 92–97
13. Schneider H, Sodha R J, Progler M, Young M P A 1985 Permeability of the human placental for hydrophilic substances studied in the isolated dually in vitro perfused lobe. Contrib Gynecol Obstet 13: 98–103
14. Golub M S, Eisele J H, Anderson J H 1986 Maternal-fetal distribution of morphine and alfentanil in near-term sheep and rhesus monkeys. Dev Pharmacol Ther 9: 12–22
15. Tomson G, Garle R I M, Thalme B, Nisell H, Nylund L, Rane A 1982 Maternal kinetics and transplacental passage of pethidine during labour. Br J Clin Pharmacol 13: 653–659
16. Kuhnert B R, Kuhnert P M, Tu A-S L, Lin D C K 1979 Meperidine and normeperidine levels following meperidine administration during labor. II Fetus and neonate. Am J Obstet Gynecol 133: 909–914
17. Reynolds F, Laishley R, Morgan B, Lee A 1989 The effect of time and adrenaline on the transplacental distribution of bupivacaine. Br J Anaesth 62: 509–514
18. Basso A, Fernandez A, Althabe O, Sabini G, Piriz H, Belitzky R 1977 Passage of mannitol from mother to amniotic fluid and fetus. Obstet Gynecol 49: 628–631
19. Caldwell J, Notarianni L J, Smith R L 1978 Impaired metabolism of pethidine in the human neonate. Br J Clin Pharmacol 5: 362P–363P
20. Moreland T A, Brice J E H, Mohamdee O, Walker C H M 1983 The influence of dose-delivery time interval on neonatal plasma pethidine levels. Acta Obstet Gynecol Scand 62: 549–553
21. Caldwell J, Moffatt J R, Smith R L, Lieberman B A, Cawston M O, Beard R W 1976 Pharmacokinetics of bupivacaine administered epidurally during childbirth. Br J Clin Pharmacol 3: 956P
22. O'Sullivan G M, Smith M, Morgan B, Brighouse D, Reynolds F 1988 H_2 antagonists and bupivacaine clearance. Anaesthesia 43: 93–95
23. Rane A, Tomson G 1980 Prenatal and neonatal drug metabolism in man. Eur J Clin Pharmacol 18: 9–15
24. Shier R W, Sprague A D, Dilts P V 1973 Placental transfer of meperidine HCl. II. Am J Obstet Gynecol 115: 556–559
25. Kennedy R L, Miller R P, Bell J U, Doshi D, de Sousa H, Kennedy M J, Heald D L, David Y 1986 Uptake and distribution of bupivacaine in fetal lambs. Anesthesiology 65: 247–253
26. Vert P, Boutroy M-J, Morselli P 1984 Placental transfer of drugs. In: L Stern (ed) Drug use in pregnancy. Adis Health Science Press, Sydney, pp 45–67
27. Krauer B, Krauer F, Hytten F 1984 Drug prescribing in pregnancy. Churchill Livingstone, Edinburgh
28. Pedersen H, Morishima H O, Finster M 1985 Anesthesia during pregnancy and parturition. In: Eskes TKAB, Finster, M (eds) Drug therapy during pregnancy. Butterworths, London, pp 161–182
29. Moya F, Thorndyke V 1962 Passage of drugs across the placenta. Am J Obstet Gynecol 84: 1778–1798

PART C

EPIDURAL AND SUBARACHNOID OPIOIDS IN LABOR AND DELIVERY: USA VIEW

R. Mullins M. D. Johnson

INTRODUCTION

A wide variety of opioids have been used to provide analgesia for childbirth. However, effective pain relief requires large parenteral doses that are often associated with maternal–fetal sedation and respiratory depression.

For many years parturients have enjoyed the benefits of local anesthetic agents administered epidurally to provide pain relief for labor. While many women receive adequate pain relief by this route, there are some who have incomplete relief, severe perineal discomfort, unpleasant motor block and hypotension from sympathetic blockade. Therefore, it is understandable that anesthesiologists are enthusiastic about improved analgesia and anesthesia for childbirth through the use of epidural and subarachnoid opioids.

HISTORY

In the late 1970s Behar et al[1] reported the clinical use of epidural morphine. Wang et al[2] and Yaksh[3] reported the analgesic effects of subarachnoid opioids. Subsequently, many investigators have evaluated epidural and subarachnoid opioids for pain relief. Animal and human studies have not demonstrated neurotoxicity with any commercially available preservative-free opioid agent administered via the epidural or subarachnoid route.[4] Opioid receptors were demonstrated in the spinal cord in 1976. A number of separate opioid receptors have subsequently been identified (Table 14.4). These receptors in the spinal cord exist primarily in the substantia gelatinosa in the dorsal horn.[5] Presumably, epidurally administered opioids reach these receptors via the cerebrospinal fluid as well as passing around nerve root sleeves.[4]

Table 14.4 Opioid receptors

Receptor	Effect	Agonist	Antagonist
μ_1	Analgesia	β-endorphin Morphine μ_2 agonists	Naloxone Pentazocine
μ_2	Depressed ventilation	Morphine Fentanyl Alfentanyl Sufentanil Meperdine	Nalbuphine
δ	Modulate μ	Leu-enkephalin	Naloxone Met-enkephalin
κ	Analgesic sedation	Butophanol	
σ	Dysphoria Tachycardia Hypertonia	Pentazocine	Naloxone

Opioids given via the epidural space also diffuse into the systemic circulation with resultant measurable blood levels similar to that seen after an intramuscular injection. The rate at which these processes occur depends on the physicochemical properties of the opioid (e.g. rate is proportional to lipid solubility and inversely proportional to molecular weight).[4]

Clinically, opioids can be classified as lipid insoluble (e.g. morphine), tending to have a delayed onset of action and long duration of effect, or lipid soluble (e.g. fentanyl), tending to have a shorter onset time but shorter duration of effect. The clinical epidural–spinal ratio (i.e. the dose of opioid required to exert a clinical effect when given via the epidural route as compared with the subarachnoid route) is about 10 : 1 for morphine. Morphine is not rapidly taken up into tissue following intraspinal administration and a slow cephalad spread in the CSF can occur; this can result in delayed respiratory depression. Fentanyl, which is 600 times more lipid soluble than morphine, has a clinical epidural–spinal ratio of about 3 : 1. Since it is bound tightly within the central nervous system there is minimal CSF redistribution and thus minimal risk of respiratory depression.[4] Nevertheless, when fentanyl is administered epidurally, significant plasma levels occur that can approach those observed after parenteral administration.

Clinically effective epidural doses of morphine or fentanyl result in small but detectable blood levels of opioid. Similar doses of opioid given epidurally instead of parenterally produce more profound analgesia and are of greater duration. Thus smaller doses given less often can be used. This minimizes peak maternal plasma concentrations and resultant fetal exposure. The recent resurgence of interest in the subarachnoid route for opioids in labor may further reduce this fetal exposure.

ANALGESIA FOR LABOR AND DELIVERY

Intraspinal opioids for the management of labor pain, either alone or in combination with local anesthetics, may provide analgesia without causing motor and sympathetic block.

Subarachnoid opioids

In 1979, Yaksh et al[6] reported that subarachnoid morphine produced analgesia in pregnant rats. Early reports of subarachnoid morphine in humans for labor were enthusiastic and controversial.[7] It soon became clear that subarachnoid morphine, while useful in early labor, did not consistently provide adequate pain relief for the second stage.[8,9] Subarachnoid morphine is also associated with a high incidence of side-effects, including somnolence, severe pruritus, and nausea and vomiting. However, Brookshire et al[10] found that an intravenous infusion of naloxone could significantly reduce the side-effects without inhibiting the analgesia provided by subarachnoid morphine 1 mg.

The use of subarachnoid morphine without combination with local anesthetic has found limited application for the relief of labor pain in recent years. For example, Abboud et al[11] reported the successful use of preservative-free morphine 1 mg with 7.5% dextrose in a parturient with severe pulmonary hypertension, in whom pain relief without sympathetic blockade was essential.

The goal of providing labor analgesia with a single dose of subarachnoid opioid is laudable, and other efforts have been made. Subarachnoid opioid administration may eventually prove to be a simple method of providing at least partial analgesia for labor in hospitals in which conventional epidural coverage is unavailable or impractical. Leighton et al[12] recently reported the use of a combination of subarachnoid morphine and fentanyl. Theoretically fentanyl, because of its rapid onset, should provide rapid pain relief and morphine should provide long-term pain relief. Morphine 0.25 mg was administered with fentanyl 25 μg through a single dural puncture early in the first stage of labor. Analgesia was achieved in less than 5 min and lasted until delivery (3–3.5 h) in 60% of the patients. The remaining 40% ultimately required conventional lumbar epidural anesthesia with local anesthetics. The risk of delayed respiratory depression limits increasing the dose of subarachnoid morphine to further prolong the duration of analgesia. Perhaps a safer and more controllable approach would utilize continuous subarachnoid infusion of a highly lipid-soluble agent such as fentanyl through a subarachnoid catheter. However, until recently, only relatively large catheter (19- and 20-gauge) and needle (17- and 19-gauge) combinations were available. Dural punctures with these needles were associated with a prohibitively high rate of post-dural puncture headache. In 1989, the Food and Drug Administration (FDA) approved a 32-gauge polyimide catheter for continuous spinal anesthesia. This microcatheter (Microspinal, TEX Medical, Duluth, GA, USA) will pass through the lumen of a standard 25- or 26-gauge spinal needle and has been used successfully to provide labor analgesia with subarachnoid meperidine for a patient with a history of allergy to amide and ester local anesthetics.[13] Patient satisfaction was high in a small study utilizing continuous subarachnoid meperidine (administered through a 28-G catheter) as the sole analgesia for vaginal delivery. Of note with this method was the good to excellent expulsive efforts demonstrated by these patients, possibly a benefit of low-dose subarachnoid meperidine.[14] Meperidine is apparently unique in that it has local anesthetic as well as spinal opioid receptor activity.[15] Cesarean deliveries have been performed with subarachnoid meperidine alone.[16,17] Unfortunately, there has been recent controversy over the use of microcatheters with regard to the development of cauda equina syndrome. The rare cases of cauda equina syndrome reported were associated with local anesthetics, not opioids. This has led to a moratorium on their use in the USA pending further investigations by the FDA. After these investigations, they may prove a useful route to administer opioids. Obviously, this route would be important because of the much smaller dose of drug required.

Oyama et al[18] in 1980, reported the use of synthetic β-endorphin in obstetrics. Subarachnoid administration resulted in profound pain relief and no transplacental transmission to the fetus. Appropriate toxicity testing must be accomplished before further studies are performed.

The recent utilization of subarachnoid opioid and continuous epidural opioid plus local anesthetic takes advantage of the best of both techniques. The future of this approach for relief of labor pain appears promising.

Epidural opioids

Administration of opioids via the epidural space for labor is becoming increasingly popular. The effect of epidural opioids is complicated by the need for the drug to cross the dura and by the presence of a rich venous epidural plexus that absorbs the drug and is often distended secondary to the inferior vena caval obstruction associated with pregnancy. As a consequence of these effects, the use of epidural opioids alone has generally proved to be of limited utility as a labor analgesic.[19,20] However, they are useful in combination with local anesthetics as previously discussed.

Morphine

As the only currently approved opioid for intraspinal (epidural and subarachnoid) use, morphine is a logical choice for combination with bupivacaine for labor analgesia and anesthesia. Niv et al[21] added epidural morphine 2 mg to 0.25% bupivacaine and significantly increased the duration of pain relief before reinforcement. Pruritus was the only significant side-effect observed and no neonatal depression was seen. The slow onset of morphine (30–60 min) and relatively high incidence of side-effects (pruritus, nausea, vomiting and potential respiratory depression) will probably prevent widespread clinical acceptance of this technique.

Butorphanol

Butorphanol, a κ-agonist and weak μ-agonist–antagonist, is a commonly administered systemic opioid for labor and has been demonstrated to be safe and effective for the mother with minimal effect on the fetus/newborn. Hunt et al[23] suggested that butorphanol 2 mg added to 0.25% bupivacaine 8.5–10 ml was the optimal dose for epidural anesthesia during labor. The duration of analgesia was significantly greater and the time to onset of analgesia significantly shorter than when no butorphanol was added. The most common maternal side-effect was somnolence, which was occasionally accompanied by an altered sensorium. Care must be taken not to administer this drug to patients who are physically dependent on opioids since this agonist–antagonist drug may precipitate an acute withdrawal syndrome even when given epidurally.[23]

Nalbuphine

Nalbuphine, a κ-agonist, is now available in preservative-free solution. After appropriate testing for neurotoxicity, one can assume that nalbuphine will be administered into the epidural and subarachnoid spaces with and without local anesthetics to determine its efficacy in providing pain relief during labor, delivery and post-operatively.

Sufentanil and alfentanil

As might be expected, epidural alfentanil and sufentanil are now being studied alone or in combination with bupivacaine during labor. Heytens et al[24] used epidural alfentanil alone in 16 primiparous patients at an infusion rate of 30 µg/kg/h, with boluses of 30 µg/kg as needed. Excellent pain relief was rapidly obtained in early labor but analgesia was inadequate for the later part of stage I and stage II. The Amiel–Tison Neonatal Neurologic and Adaptive Capacity (NACS) examination revealed significant hypotonia. A preliminary report[25] suggests that combining lower-dose alfentanil with bupivacaine can provide excellent pain relief for labor with no detectable neonatal depression.

Sufentanil is attractive because of its very high lipid solubility and affinity for the µ receptor. Van Steenberge et al[26] and Philips[27] showed that sufentanil in combination with bupivacaine provided prolonged pain relief, reduced the total bupivacaine dose and gave limited motor block. However, in the epidural space, sufentanil appears to be only 2–3 times more potent than fentanyl, whereas systemically it is 5–10 times more potent. Therefore, unintentional intravascular injection of sufentanil 30 µg or more would be likely to cause respiratory depression. Van Steenberge et al did find epidural sufentanil to be associated with maternal dizziness and lowered 1 min Apgar scores, which may indicate significant systemic absorption. Sufentanil is also associated with significantly more pruritus and nausea and is more expensive then fentanyl.

Sufentanil has recently been approved for epidural use in the USA by the FDA.

Fentanyl

The most popular opioid for use in labor in undoubtedly fentanyl. Justins et al,[28] in 1982, added fentanyl 80 µg to 0.5% bupivacaine 3 ml. Since then Youngstrom et al[29] in 1984, Skerman et al[30], Vella et al[31] and Cohen et al[32] in 1987, and Cellano and Capogna[33] and Chestnut et al[34] in 1988 have touted the efficacy of the combination of bupivacaine and fentanyl. Bupivacaine concentrations as low as 0.028% combined with fentanyl 100 µg have provided adequate pain relief for labor.

Respondents to a recent survey at the annual meeting of the Society for Obstetric Anesthesia and Perinatology indicated that 56% used epidural opioids for labor, with the vast majority favoring fentanyl. The solutions most popular were fentanyl 50–100 µg in 0.25 or 0.125% bupivacaine 10 ml. About 20% of the respondents used fentanyl in an infusion, the preferred solution was fentanyl 1–2 µg/ml in 0.125% bupivacaine, which was administered at rates of 8–10 ml/h.

ANALGESIA FOR CESAREAN DELIVERY AND POST-OPERATIVE PAIN RELIEF

Even in the presence of an adequate sensory block with local anesthetic agents, significant numbers of women will experience discomfort during cesarean delivery especially during times of visceral stimulation. Opioids administered by the subarachnoid or epidural route can improve the intraoperative analgesia.[35,36]

The recommended doses of subarachnoid and epidural opioids for cesarean delivery and postoperative pain relief are listed in Table 14.5.

Subarachnoid opioids

Subarachnoid morphine has been used successfully in many types of surgery, including cesarean delivery. A high incidence of side-effects, including life-threatening respiratory depression, can be seen if doses greater than 0.5 mg are used. Chadwick and Ready[37] concluded that subarachnoid morphine sulfate in doses of 0.3–0.5 mg provides similar post-operative analgesia to epidural morphine 3 to 5 mg but with greater duration and no greater side-effects. Two especially interesting reports in 1988 by Abboud et al[38] and Abouleish et al[39] showed that morphine 0.1, 0.2 and 0.25 mg mixed with hyperbaric bupivacaine provides excellent post-operative analgesia and may cause less respiratory depression than standard subcutaneous morphine injection. Hunt et al[40] demon-

Table 14.5 Recommended doses of subarachnoid and epidural opioids for cesarean delivery and post-operative pain relief

	Dose	Onset (min)	Duration (h)
Subarachnoid			
Morphine sulfate	0.2–0.3 mg	30–45	12–15
Fentanyl	10–20 µg	5	2–4
Sufentanil	3–5 µg	3	2–4
Epidural			
Morphine sulfate	2–3 mg/up to 10 ml NS	45–60	12–18
Fentanyl	40–100 µg/10 ml NS	5	2–3
Sufentanil	25–50 µg/10 ml NS	3–5	2–4
Butophanol	1–2 mg/10 ml NS	10–15	3–5

NS, normal saline.

strated that fentanyl in doses as low as 6.25 µg is also an effective subarachnoid adjunct that provides effective post-operative analgesia for 3–4 h.

Epidural opioids

Epidural morphine, fentanyl and butorphanol have been studied for cesarean delivery. Hughes[41] reported 1700 consecutive patients who had received epidural morphine with excellent long-lasting post-operative analgesia. Four patients were noted to have respiratory depression, two required treatment with naloxone and one was seriously acidotic. The issue of monitoring patients after intraspinal morphine is controversial (see monitoring of the obstetric patient receiving intraspinal opioids, Chapter 16).

Fentanyl is the most popular opioid for epidural use in cesarean delivery. Fentanyl appears to be very safe, with 50 µg giving pain relief lasting approximately 2–3 h.[42] Fentanyl 50 µg should be diluted in 10 ml of preservative-free normal saline (or local anesthetic) for fastest onset and longest duration.[43] Epidural fentanyl augments intra-operative anesthesia with epidural bupivacaine[44] or lidocaine[45] and may reduce the incidence of peripartum shivering. Thus it is advantageous to give the epidural fentanyl once the epidural block has been established and prior to delivery. An additional dose of fentanyl 50 µg in normal saline 10 ml can be given post-operatively just prior to removal of the epidural catheter to provide several hours of analgesia after the resolution of the local anesthetic block.

While the effects of epidural lidocaine and bupivacaine[44,45] are additive with epidural fentanyl, chloroprocaine is antagonistic. Malinow et al[46] found no clinically significant period of fentanyl analgesia after 3% chloroprocaine was administered epidurally for cesarean delivery. The low pH of chloroprocaine (3.3–3.5) or some secondary metabolite may be responsible for this interaction.

Epidural sufentanil has also been studied in patients undergoing cesarean delivery. Doses of 30–50 µg diluted in preservative-free normal saline 10 ml provided analgesia with onset and duration similar to fentanyl.[47] At clinically effective doses, it is associated with a greater incidence of nausea and pruritus than fentanyl.[40] Interestingly, in epidural doses of 50 µg or greater, sufentanil can abolish shivering and effect maternal temperature control in a dose-dependent fashion.[45–49]

Epidural sufentanil appears to offer little advantage over fentanyl in the setting of cesarean delivery and it presents significantly greater risk. Should the epidural catheter end up intravascular, a dose of 30–50 µg could precipitate respiratory depression, apnea or chest wall rigidity.

Epidural butorphanol, in doses of 1–2 mg,[22] has also been studied in patients following cesarean delivery. It has an onset of 15–20 min and a duration of 3–4 h. It has not been associated with pruritus or significant respiratory depression. Naulty et al[50] reported on the uses of an epidural butorphanol–fentanyl combination to minimize side-effects of fentanyl. Epidural butorphanol can produce some maternal sedation and may affect the fetal heart rate, producing a sinusoidal-type pattern. No evidence of fetal distress has been detected by pH monitoring of scalp capillary blood. It may be most useful for post-operative analgesia after the fetus is delivered.

SIDE-EFFECTS AND COMPLICATIONS

Nausea, vomiting, pruritus, and urinary retention are side-effects that can occur with any µ agonist given by the epidural or subarachnoid route. Often these effects can be managed with small intravenous doses of naloxone, which usually can be titrated to relieve the side-effects without antagonizing analgesia. Urinary retention is not usually a problem after cesarean delivery because a urinary catheter is routinely used. Pruritus can usually be treated adequately with an antihistamine or antagonist. Butophanol, a κ-agonist, given epidurally, causes minimal nausea and pruritus and may actually be useful epidurally in combination with a µ-agonist to minimize these side-effects.[50]

Respiratory depression (usually delayed) after subarachnoid and epidural opioid administration appears to be the most serious complication. The respiratory depression can be bimodal with early respiratory depression due to blood levels and late respiratory depression due to rostral spread of the morphine. Predisposing factors for respiratory depression include use of a water-soluble opioid (morphine), high doses and concomitant use of opioids or other CNS depressants by other routes. The safety record with fentanyl is excellent and the likelihood of respiratory depression when fentanyl is administered in appropriate doses without concomitant sedative drugs is minute. Hospital staff trained to monitor and treat respiratory depression must be available when morphine is given by the subarachnoid or epidural route. A specific protocol for monitoring should be in effect. Respiratory rate appears to be the best indicator of respiratory depression. Intravenous naloxone is used to reverse respiratory depression but, since it has a short half-life, repeated doses may be necessary.[4] An unexpected side-effect appears to be the recurrence of herpes simplex labialis virus (HSV) in patients with a prior history of herpes simplex after receiving epidural morphine.[51] No studies have associated HSV recurrence with fentanyl administration. Another study[52] did not confirm a difference between the incidence of cold sores in patients receiving epidural or subarachnoid opioids compared with general anesthesia, but it is reasonable to inform patients of the possibility of reactivation after epidural morphine. Other complications include the known risks in placement of epidural and subarachnoid anesthetics including infection, hematoma formation, nerve injury and post-dural puncture headache.

FETAL TOXICITY AND INTRASPINAL OPIOIDS

The considerable advantages of intraspinal opioids must always be weighed against the possibility of fetal depression. Drugs administered to the mother are transported rapidly to the uterus and the concentrations of free drug available to cross the placenta will depend on the agent, total dose, route of administration, lipid solubility, pK_a, maternal pH, protein binding, metabolism and excretion.[4] All commercially available opioids have low molecular weights and readily cross the placenta by diffusion.[53]

Although there is an extensive literature concerning maternal effects of intraspinal morphine, evaluation of the infant has most often been confined to Apgar scores or the occurrence of apnea. Subtle effects of drugs on the neonate require subtle neurobehavioral tests. However, most investigators would agree that the risk of neonatal depression with epidural morphine appears to increase with higher doses and shorter interval between dosing and delivery time because of higher maternal blood levels of morphine.[49] The prolonged onset, the high incidence of maternal side effects, and the risk of delayed respiratory depression have limited the use of epidural morphine in laboring patients.

Fentanyl has an impressive safety record. Neonatal depression has only been reported with very high repeated epidural doses. When administered by the epidural route, fentanyl produces peak plasma levels similar to those produced by the same dose given intramuscularly. Gaffud et al[41] administered fentanyl 100 μg epidurally approximately 20 min before cesarean delivery. Theoretically this should produce near maximal fetal exposure. They found that epidural fentanyl 100 μg resulted in an average umbilical artery concentration of 0.8 μg/ml. This is below the concentration implicated in respiratory depression of the neonate. In another study, the optimal dose of epidural fentanyl in the parturient was determined to be 50 μg[40] in normal saline 10 ml, which should minimize fetal exposure and possible depression.

Phillips[26] has complied with much of the data regarding the use of epidural sufentanil. Undetectable levels in maternal venous and umbilical cord blood are consistent with very high lipid solubility of this drug. Overall, 156 parturients received sufentanil with only one study reporting a decrease in the mean Apgar scores. Unfortunately, neurobehavioral testing of the neonate has not been reported.

While the published evaluations are few, alfentanil has been associated with neonatal depression. Heytens et al[23] continuously infused epidural alfentanil alone and stopped at the onset of the second stage of labor. Although Apgar scores and umbilical blood gas values were normal, the NACS showed significant depression of active and passive tone.

Butorphanol in epidural doses of 1–2 mg is not usually associated with respiratory depression. Thus far, neonatal depression has not been seen. However, butorphanol given via epidural or other parenteral routes may be associated with low amplitude-high frequency sinusoidal-like fetal heart rate pattern.[52] This pattern usually resolves spontaneously and is usually associated wtih normal fetal scalp capillary blood pH.

CONCLUSION

Morphine is the only opioid approved for epidural or subarachnoid use by the FDA in the USA. Sufentanil has recently been approved by the FDA for epidural use. However, fentanyl appears to be the safest currently available opioid agent for intraspinal use. The risks associated with subarachnoid morphine appear higher and it would be prudent to require close attention to respiratory function for 24 h after administration.

Intraspinal opioids have specific indications when used alone for labor analgesia but when used in combination with local anesthetics can provide excellent analgesia and anesthesia. Intraspinal opioids can augment local regional anesthesia for cesarean delivery as well as provide post-operative analgesia. At the present time the epidural route is dominant in obstetric anesthesia but the future of subarachnoid administration appears promising particularly in the combined subarachnoid opioid–continuous epidural with local anesthetic with and without opioid technique.

REFERENCES

1. Behar M, Magora F, Olshwang D, Davidson J T 1979 Epidural morphine in treatment of pain. Lancet 1: 527–531
2. Wang J K, Nauss L E, Thomas J E 1979 Pain relief by intrathecally applied morphine in man. Anesthesiology 50: 149–151
3. Yaksh T 1976 Analgesia mediated by a direct spinal action of narcotics. Science 192: 1357 –1358
4. Cousins M J, Mather L E 1984 Intrathecal and epidural administration of opioids. Anesthesiology 61: 276
5. Benedetti C 1984 Intraspinal analgesia: an historical overview. Acta Anaesthesiol Scand 31 (suppl 85): 17–24
6. Yaksh T L, Wilson R P, Kaiko R F, Intrussi C E 1979 Analgesia produced by a spinal action of morphine and effects upon parturition in the rat. Anesthesiology 51: 386–392
7. Alper M H 1979 Intrathecal morphine; a new method of obstetric analgesia. Anesthesiology 51: 378–379
8. Scott P V, Bowen F E, Cartwright P et al 1980 Intrathecal morphine as sole analgesia during labour. Br Med J 281: 351–353
9. Baracca A, Noueihed R, Najj S 1981 Intrathecal injection of morphine for obstetric analgesia. Anesthesiology 54: 136–140
10. Brookshire G L, Shnider S M, Abboud T K et al 1983 Effects of naloxone on the mother and neonate after intrathecal morphine for labor analgesia. Anesthesiology 58: A417
11. Abboud T K, Raya J, Noueihed R, Daniel 1983 Intrathecal morphine for relief of labor pain in a parturient with severe pulmonary hypertension. Anesthesiology 59: 477–479
12. Leighton B L, DeSimone C A, Norris M C, Ben-David B 1989 Intrathecal narcotics revisited: the combination of fentanyl and morphine intrathecally provides rapid onset of profound, prolonged analgesia. Anesth Analg 69: 122–125
13. Johnson M D, Hurley R J, Gilbertson L I, Datta S 1990 Continuous microcatheter spinal anesthesia with subarachnoid meperdine for labor and delivery. Anesth Analg 70: 658–661
14. Swayze C R, Walker E B, Skerman J H, Sholte F G 1991 Efficacy of subarachnoid mepherdine for labor analgesia. Reg Anesth 16: 309–313
15. Famewo C E, Naguiob M 1985 Spinal anesthesia with meperidine as the sole agent. Can Anaesth Soc J 32: 533
16. Talafre M L, Jacquinot P, Legagneux F et al 1987 Intrathecal administration of meperidine versus tetracaine for elective cesarean section. Anesthesiology 67: A620
17. Camann W R, Bader A M 1992 Spinal anesthesia for cesarean delivery with meperdine as the sole agent. Int J Obst Anest 1: 156–158
18. Oyama T, Matsuki A, Taneichi T et al 1980 Beta-endorphin in obstetric analgesia. Am J Obstet Gynecol 137: 613–616
19. Husemeyer R P, O'Connor M C, Davenport H T 1980 Failure of epidural morphine to relieve pain in labour. Anesthesia 35: 161–163
20. Writer W D R, James F M, Wheeler A S 1981 Double blind comparison of morphine and bupivacaine for continuous epidural analgesia in labor. Anesthesiology 54: 215–219
21. Niv D, Rudick V, Golan A, Chayen M S 1986 Augmentation of bupivacaine analgesia by epidural morphine. Obstet Gynecol 67: 206
22. Hunt C O, Naulty J S, Malinow A M et al 1986 Epidural butorphanol bupivacaine for analgesia during labor and delivery. Anesth Analg 68: 323–327
23. Weintraub S J, Naulty J S 1985 Acute abstinence syndrome after epidural injection of butorphanol. Anesth Analg 64: 452–453
24. Heytens L, Cammu H, Cámu F 1987 Extradural analgesia using alfentanil. Br J Anaesth 59: 331–337
25. Carp H, Johnson M D, Bader A M 1988 Continuous epidural infusion of alfentanil and bupivacaine for labor and delivery. Anesthesiology 69: A687
26. Van Steenberge A, DeBroux H C, Noorduin H 1987 Extradural bupivacaine with sufentanil for vaginal delivery: a double-blind trial. Br J Anaesth 59: 1518–1522
27. Phillips G 1988 Continuous infusion of epidural analgesia in labor – the effect if adding sufentanil to 0.125% bupivacaine. Anesth Analg 67: 462–465
28. Justins D M, Francis D, Houlton P G, Reynolds F 1982 A controlled trial of extradural fentanyl in labour. Br J Anaesth 54: 409–414
29. Youngstrom P, Sedensky M, Frankmann D, Spagnuolo S 1988 Continuous epidural infusion of low-dose bupivacaine–fentanyl for labor analgesia. Anesthesiology 69: 686–692
30. Skerman J H, Thompson B A, Goldstein M R et al 1985 Combined continuous epidural fentanyl and bupivacaine in labor: a randomized study. Anesthesiology 53: A450
31. Vella L M, Willatts D G, Knott C et al 1985 Epidural fentanyl in labour Anesthesia 40: 741–747
32. Cohen S E, Tan S, Albright G A, Halpen J 1987 Epidural fentanyl/bupivacaine for obstetric analgesia. Anesthesiology 67: 403–407
33. Cellano D, Capogna G 1988 Epidural fentanyl plus bupivacaine 0.125 per cent for labour: analgesia effects. Can J Anaesth 35: 375–378
34. Chestnut D H, Owen C L, Bates J N et al 1988 Continuous infusion epidural analgesia during labor: a randomized, double-blind comparison of 0.0625% bupivacaine/0.0002% fentanyl versus 0.125% bupivacaine. Anesthesiology 68: 754–759
35. Westmore M D 1990 Epidural opioids in obstetrics – a review. Anaesth Intensive Care 1992 18: 292–300
36. Shnider S M 1992 Peridural opioids and local anesthetic for pain management in obstetrics. ASA Refresher Course, p 244
37. Chadwick H S, Ready L B 1988 Intrathecal and epidural morphine sulfate for post cesarean analgesia. Anesthesiology 68: 925–929
38. Abboud T K, Dror A, Mossad P et al 1988 Mini-dose intrathecal morphine for the relief of postcesarean section pain. Anesth Analg 67: 370
39. Abouleish E, Rawal N, Fallon K, Hernandez D 1988 Combined morphine and bupivacaine for cesarean section. Anesth Analg 67: 370–374
40. Hunt C O, Naulty J S, Bader A M et al 1987 Perioperative analgesia with subarachnoid fentanyl–bupivacaine. Anesthesiology 67: A621
41. Hughes S C 1982 Intraspinal narcotics in obstetrics.Clin Perinatol 1: 167
42. Naulty J S, Datta S, Ostheimer G W et al 1985 Epidural fentanyl for postcesarean delivery pain management. Anesthesiology 63: 694–698
43. Birnbach D J, Johnson M D, Arcario T et al 1989 Effect of diluent volume on analgesia produced by epidural fentanyl. Anesth Analg 68: 808–810
44. Gaffud M P, Bansal P, Lawton C et al 1986 Surgical analgesia for cesarean delivery with epidural bupivacaine and fentanyl. Anesthesiology 65: 331–334
45. Preston P G, Rosen M A, Hughes S C et al 1988 Epidural anesthesia with fentanyl and lidocaine for cesarean section: Maternal effects and neonatal outcome. Anesthesiology 68: 938–943
46. Malinow A et al 1988 Choice of local anesthetics effects postcesarean epidural fentanyl analgesia. Reg Anesth 13: 86–87
47. Tan S, Cohen S E, White P F 1986 Sufentanil for analgesia for cesarean section: intravenous versus epidural administration. Anesth Analg 65: 5138
48. Rosen M A, Dailey P A, Hughes S C et al 1988 Epidural sufentanil for postoperative analgesia after cesarean section. Anesthesiology 68: 448
49. Sevarino F B, Johnson M D, Lema M J et al 1989 The effect of epidural sufentanil on shivering and body temperature in the parturient. Anesth Analg 68: 530–533

50. Naulty J S, Labove P, Datta S et al 1987 Epidural butophanol/fentanyl for post-cesarean delivery analgesia. Anesthesiology 67: A463
51. Fuller J F, McMorland G H, Douglas N J, Palmer L 1990 Epidural morphine for analgesia after Cesarean Section: a report of 4,880 patients. Can J Anesth 37: 636–640
52. Weiss J H, Carney M D, Norris M C, Leighton B L, Torjmenor M 1990 Incidence of Recurrent herpes simplex virus labialis after Cesarean section. Anesthesiology 73: A951
53. Hug C C 1984 Pharmacokinetics of new synthetic narcotic analgesics. In Estafanous F G (ed) opioids in anesthesia. Butterworths, Boston p 52

PART D
EPIDURAL AND SUBARACHNOID OPIOIDS IN LABOR AND DELIVERY: EUROPEAN VIEW

A. Van Steenberge

FENTANYL

Pharmacology

Fentanyl is highly lipid soluble, has a faster onset of action than most opioids, has a short time to peak effect (5.5 min) and quickly crosses the blood–brain barrier. Rapid redistribution to non-neural tissues results in a relatively short duration of action of 2–3 h that is affected by the total dose administered as well as by the concomitant use of other anesthetic agents. Injected into the epidural space, fentanyl rapidly reaches the spinal cord receptors and nonspecific binding sites (onset time 4–6 min).

Fentanyl 100 μg injected into the epidural space crosses the placenta with an umbilical cord blood to maternal blood ratio at delivery (45 min after injection) of 0.13; when given together with epinephrine 100 μg this ratio increases to 0.32. Stoeckel et al[1] studied the effects of fentanyl in volunteers and observed secondary plasma peaks resulting in decreases in minute ventilation and reduced response to carbon dioxide. A small epidural dose (< 50 μg) and subarachnoid dose (< 10 μg) will enhance the action of local anesthetics. Overdosage with unintentional i.v. fentanyl is manifested by bradycardia, hypotension, respiratory depression and muscle rigidity. Protein binding is strongest with α_1-acid glycoprotein with 60% fentanyl bound.[2] This has very important implications for possible toxicity in the newborn, in whom the α_1-acid glycoprotein content is reduced.

Fentanyl is rapidly metabolized in the liver. Metabolites exceed the unchanged drug concentration within 30 min.[3] However, fentanyl has no active or toxic metabolites. Cirrhosis has no influence on the rate of clearance, elimination, half-life or volume of distribution of fentanyl.[4] Caution should be used when administering fentanyl to nursing mothers; however, there is no evidence that fentanyl affects neonates during breast feeding. During labor, provided no other opioid is given, one can safely administer 20–40 μg of fentanyl into the epidural space and 10–20 μg into the cerebrospinal fluid. Higher doses will not improve the analgesic benefits, while side-effects will increase. The most common side-effects are pruritus and urinary retention.

Pharmacokinetics (Table 14.6)

Fentanyl acts primarily at opioid μ receptors to produce analgesic effects.[5] This is the rationale behind its epidural and subarachnoid administration.

Table 14.6 Pharmacokinetic data for fentanyl and sufentanil

Drug	pKa	Clearance (l/h)	$t_{1/2}$ (h)	Volume of distribution (l/kg)	Protein binding (%)
Fentanyl	8.43	47	3.0	3.0	83
Sufentanil	8	44	2.6	2	93

Fentanyl has no effect on the release of histamine.[6] During surgery and under conditions of stress[7] or pain, fentanyl provides cardiovascular stability. Hemodynamic responses include a reduction in both systolic blood pressure and heart rate. Fentanyl given in anticipation of increased stress in surgery and labor tends to stabilize hemodynamic and cardiac variables.

Fentanyl can cause respiratory depression with reduced response to carbon dioxide through activity at central opioid receptors; therefore, monitoring for respiratory depression must continue until spontaneous breathing is adequate.

Secondary peak concentrations occur between 45 and 90 min after a single intravenous bolus, but are not observed after epidural (50 μg) or subarachnoid (10 μg) administration. This secondary peak, with its concomitant decreased carbon dioxide response, can last for 30–45 min. It is this potential for a second plasma or CSF peak that makes post-operative monitoring compulsory. The duration of action of fentanyl may be prolonged either by drug interactions or by hemodynamic changes resulting from surgery. However, subarachnoid and epidural administration of fentanyl in the recommended dose (< 10 μg subarachnoid and < 30 μg epidurally) should not result in respiratory depression. The neurologic effects of fentanyl after a maximum dose of 50 μg injected into the epidural space or 10 μg injected into the CSF are negligible, and the drug is therefore suitable for analgesia and light sedation during painful labor.

SUFENTANIL

Pharmacology

Sufentanil is a potent fentanyl analog which, after intravenous administration in rats, is 4521 times more potent than morphine and possesses a safety margin of 25 211. The drug is very lipid soluble and has a high affinity for μ opioid receptors. Analgesic activity after epidural sufentanil has been reported in rats, guinea pigs, cats and dogs.[8–10] In all these animals, adequate analgesia with rapid onset was reported. In rats, epidural sufentanil was demonstrated to be more than 30 times more active than morphine. Compared with meperidine, the difference was > 300. Sufentanil was at least four times more active than fentanyl and almost 100 times more active than alfentanil. In terms of duration of analgesia at equiactive doses, the relative order of the tested opioids was morphine > sufentanil > meperidine > fentanyl[11] and lofentanil > sufentanil > carfentanil > fentanyl > alfentanil.[10] The time of onset of analgesia at twice the ED_{50} for significant analgesia is 4.3 min for sufentanil and 12.0 min for morphine.[12] Peak analgesia was measured for meperidine, fentanyl, sufentanil and morphine at 14, 16, 20 and 36 min after epidural administration.[11] In terms of both potency and duration of analgesia after epidural administration, sufentanil was superior to meperidine, fentanyl and alfentanil. Compared with morphine, sufentanil is more potent and has a faster onset time[12] and a shorter latency to peak analgesia[11] but also a shorter duration of activity. Naloxone reverses the effects of sufentanil. In other animal species, including cats[8] and guinea pigs,[9] epidural sufentanil has been demonstrated to be superior to fentanyl and morphine.

In rats, epidural sufentanil has been compared with other routes of administration including subcutaneous[11,13] intravenous,[14] intraperitoneal[15] and subarachnoid administration.[12] In terms of analgesic potency, epidural sufentanil is as good as intravenous and subarachnoid sufentanil, and three times more potent than subcutaneous sufentanil. With regard to duration of analgesia, sufentanil given epidurally has a longer duration of action than after subarachnoid and intraperitoneal administration but shorter action than after subcutaneous administration. With regard to onset of analgesia, the order of latencies is subarachnoid < epidural < subcutaneous sufentanil. For the dissociation between analgesic activity and supraspinal and central effects (e.g. blockade of pinna and cornea reflexes), the epidural route is more selective than all other routes of administration. This greater selectivity is also reflected by the fact that it causes less respiratory depression than subcutaneous administration. Furthermore, epidural sufentanil results in lower levels of sufentanil in plasma and brain relative to intravenous and intraperitoneal administration, and epidural sufentanil results in lower levels of μ opioid receptor binding in the brain than does intravenous administration.

Similar effects have been reported in other animal species. In guinea pigs, epidural sufentanil has higher efficacy than subcutaneous sufentanil.[9] In cats,[8] epidural sufentanil has a longer duration of action than intravenous administration although a longer onset time was found for the epidural route. In dogs,[10] epidural sufentanil has been demonstrated to act longer than subarachnoid sufentanil and, in addition, lower plasma levels were measured after epidural administration.

At doses mostly higher than those needed to produce analgesia, all fentanyl analogs, including sufentanil, can produce secondary effects after epidural administration. These secondary changes are related to activity typical of μ opioid agonists. As compared with morphine, however, no late respiratory depression is observed with epidural sufentanil and retching or vomiting and pruritus are diminished. The relative order of specificity of various opioids after epidural administraion is: meperidine > morphine > fentanyl > lofentanil > sufentanil > carfentanil > alfentanil.

Different variables can modulate the analgesic activity of epidural sufentanil.[16,17] It has been demonstrated that increasing the diluent volume of the epidural injectate increases the duration of analgesia. Adding epinephrine or α_2 agonists to epidural sufentanil as well as testing the animals in stressful or acute and chronic pain states can increase the activity of epidural sufentanil. A pronounced potentiation of the analgesic properties of sufentanil and increased safety and specificity have been observed after adding a small quantity of the local anesthetic bupivacaine to epidurally administered sufentanil[18] and after complexation of sufentanil in hydroxypropyl-beta-cyclodextrin.[19]

Pharmacokinetics of epidural sufentanil

Unlike intravenous sufentanil in general anesthesia, the regional analgesia produced by epidural sufentanil does not depend upon the general circulation for drug transport to the sites of action. After epidural drug administration, local drug distribution kinetics within the epidural space is the most important factor, whereas the rate and the extent of absorption into the systemic circulation primarily determine the safety of an epidurally given drug. Therefore, the time profile of sufentanil concentrations in both plasma and cerebrospinal fluid after clinically relevant doses should be taken into account.

Because of its high lipophilicity, epidural sufentanil is easily distributed to the CSF. Maximal concentrations in CSF appear on average 39 min after the epidural injection. After the peak, the decay in CSF concentrations is biphasic. The initial fast decay might be related to further drug spread in the CSF, uptake in fat and local tissues and systemic absorption. The terminal half-life of sufentanil in CSF averages 165 min, indicating a high CSF clearance. Maximal concentrations in plasma are attained within 10 min of dosing and are approximately 20 times lower than those in the CSF. The elimination half-life averages 355 min. This long half-life may be partly related to a slow, sustained release of the drug from the dura, epidural fat and other local tissues around the epidural space.[20] Its limited systemic absorption in the first hours after dosing can be reduced by combination with epinephrine. A twofold decrease in the fraction systemically absorbed within the first 2–3 h has been observed.[21,22]

Clinically effective doses during labor and delivery are too low for pharmacokinetic assessments. The placental transfer of epidural sufentanil has therefore been investigated in women undergoing cesarean delivery.[23] Fetal plasma concentrations were, if measurable, on average 40% of those of the mother at the time of delivery, indicating a rapid equilibration with maternal concentrations. The negligible sufentanil concentrations in the plasma of the mother and the neonate support the clinical findings that sufentanil can be given safely in obstetrics, particularly because doses of only 10 μg sufentanil, intermittently given, are recommended for use during labor and delivery.[24]

REFERENCES

1. Stoeckel H, Schuttler J Magnussen H, Hengstmann J J Plasma fentanyl concentrations and the occurrence of respiratory depression in volunteers. Br J Anaesth 54: 1087–1095
2. Meuldermans W E G, Hurkmans R M A, Heykants J J P 1982 Plasma protein binding and distribution of fentanyl, sufentanil, alfentanil and lofentanil in blood. Archiv Pharmacodyn Ther 257: 4–19
3. Mc Clain D A, Hug Jr C C 1980 Intravenous fentanyl kinetics. Clin Pharmacol Ther 28: 106
4. Haberer J P, Schoeffler P, Couerc E, Duvaldestin P 1982 Fentanyl pharmacokinetics in anaesthetized patients with cirrhosis. Br J Anaesthesiol 54: 1267
5. Martin W R 1984 Pharmacology of opioids. Pharmacol Rev. 35: 283
6. Flacke J W et al 1987 Histamine release by four narcotics, a double blind study in humans. Anesth Analg 66: 723
7. Hall G M 1980 Fentanyl and the metabolic response to surgery. Br J Anaesth 52: 561
8. Aoki M, Senami M, Kitahata L M, Collins J G 1986 Spinal sufentanil effects on spinal pain-transmission neurons in cats. Anesthesiology 64: 225–229
9. Edwards W T, White M J, Xiao C S 1987 A comparison of epidural and systemic narcotics in modification of vocalization behavior in the guinea pig. Pain (suppl 4) S 397
10. Sabbe M, Mjanger E, Sosnowski M, Yaksh T 1988 Study on tolerance development after daily epidural injection of sufentanil in dogs. Anesthesiology 69: A392
11. Van den Hoogen R H W M, Colpaert F C 1987 Epidural and subcutaneous morphine, meridine (pethidine), fentanyl and sufentanil in the rat: analgesia and other in vivo pharmacologic effects. Anesthesiology 66: 186–194
12. Meert T F 1989 Pharmacological effect of epidural opioids. In: editor (ed) Therapeutics Today Series. Epidural use of a new opioid sufentanil. Publisher, place Niemegeers C J E, SChellekens K H L, Van Bever W F M, Janssen P A J 1976 Sufentanil, a very potent and extremely safe intravenous morphine-like compound in mice, rats and dogs. Arzneim-Forsch (Drug Res) 26: 1551–1556
13. Van den Hoogen R H W M, Bervoets K J W, Colpaert F C 1988 Enhancement by pain and stress of analgesia produced by epidural sufentanil in the rat. Anesthesiology 69: 24–28
14. Colpaert F C, Leysen J E, Michiels M, Van den Hoogen R H W M 1986 Epidural and intravenous sufentanil in the rat: analgesia, opiate receptor binding, and drug concentrations in plasma and brain. Anesthesiology 65: 41–49
15. Madej T, Immelman L, Roth S 1987 Extradural and intraperitoneal sufentanil in the rat: analgesia, antagonism and plasma drug concentrations. Br J Anaesth 59: 932P
16. Meert T F, et al 1989 Pharmacological effects of epidural opioids. In: Therapeutics today: epidural use of a new opioid: sufentanil. Proceedings of a satellite symposium of the 8th annual meeting of the European Society of Regional Anaesthesia, Lisbon, Portugal. Adis Press, USA: 1–9
17. Van den Hoogen R H W M, Bervoets K J W, Colpaert F C 1988 Respiratory effects of epidural and subcutaneous morphine, meperidine, fentanyl and sufentanil in the rat. Anesth Analg 67 1071–1078
18. Vercauteren M, Meert T, Adriaensen H 1991 Epidural sufentanil: effect of bupivacaine addition on pain relief characteristics in rats. Anesth Analg 72: S308

19. Meert T F, Mesens J, Verheyen P, Noorduin H, Vercauteren M 1991 Hydroxypropyl-B-cyclodextrin can potentiate the analgesic properties of spinal sufentanil in rats. Anesth Analg 72: S180
20. Nordberg G 1989 Pharmacokinetics of spinal opioids. In: Therapeutics Today Series. Epidural use of a new opioid sufentanil, pp 10–15
21. Verborgh C, Van der Auwera D, Noorduin H, Camu F 1988 Epidural sufentanil for post-operative pain relief: effects of adrenaline Eur J Anaesthesiol 5: 183–191
22. Hasenbos M A, Gielen M J M, Bos J, Tielbeek E, Stanton-Hicks M, van Egmond J 1988 High thoracic epidural sufentanil for post-thoracotomy pain: influence of epinephrine as an adjuvant – a double-blind study. Anesthesiology 69: 1017–1022
23. Van Steenberge A, Debroux H C 1989 Epidural sufentanil with bupivacaine 0.5% (+ adrenaline 1/200000) in cesarean section. Janssen Research Foundation, CRRR 33800/8
24. Vertommen J D, Vandermeulen E, Van Aken H et al 1991 The effects of the addition of sufentanil to 0.125% bupivacaine on the quality of analgesia during labor on the incidence of intrumental deliveries. Anesthesiology 74: 809–814

15. Maternal, fetal and neonatal effects of intraspinal opioids

Part A Maternal effects *R. J. Hurley* *M. D. Johnson*
Part B Fetal and neonatal effects *C. O. Hunt* *B. H. Minzter*

PART A
MATERNAL EFFECTS

R. J. Hurley *M. D. Johnson*

After Queen Victoria accepted chloroform during the delivery of Prince Leopold, the concept of pain relief during childbirth became more socially accepted. Opioids have been used to provide pain relief for thousands of years and a wide variety of these drugs have been employed in an attempt to provide analgesia for childbirth. However, until recently, even marginally effective pain relief for labor required relatively large parenteral doses that were often associated with maternal or fetal sedation and respiratory depression. The discovery of opioid receptors in the spinal cord presented the intriguing possibility that opioid agonists could be locally administered to specific receptors to produce analgesia, while minimizing systemic effects. Such an approach has theoretical advantages for the pregnant patient as it might significantly reduce fetal exposure to opioids.

In 1979, Behar et al[1] first used epidural morphine and Wang et al[2] reported the use of subarachnoid morphine, both in the clinical setting. Studies on the effects of epidural opioids in the pregnant patient followed in rapid succession. The epidural route has been especially attractive, as the incidence of post-dural puncture headache is increased in pregnant patients and epidural local anesthetics are being used with increasing frequency for labor and delivery.

Extensive animal and human studies have not demonstrated neurotoxicity with any commercially available, preservative-free opioid agent administered via the epidural or spinal route.[3] Epidural opioids appear to exert most of their effect on receptors in the substantia gelatinosa of the spinal cord.[4] Presumably, epidurally administered opioids reach these receptors via the cerebrospinal fluid (CSF), following direct penetration of the dura, as well as by passing around nerve root sleeves.[5] Opioids given via the epidural space also diffuse into the systemic circulation with resultant measurable blood concentrations similar to levels seen with intramuscular parenteral administration. The rate at which these processes occur depends on the physicochemical properties of the opioid (e.g. the rate is directly proportional to lipid solubility and inversely proportional to molecular weight).[3]

Clinically, opioids can be classified as lipid insoluble (e.g. morphine), which tend to have a delayed onset of action and long duration of effect, or lipid soluble (e.g. fentanyl), which tend to have a shorter onset time but shorter duration of effect. The clinical epidural–spinal ratio (i.e. the dose of opioid required to exert a clinical effect when given via the epidural route as compared with the subarachnoid route) is about 10:1 for morphine. Morphine is not rapidly taken up into tissue following intraspinal administration and a slow cephalad spread in the CSF can occur; this can result in delayed respiratory depression. Fentanyl, which is 600 times more lipid soluble than morphine, has a clinical epidural–spinal ratio of about 3:1. Since it is bound tightly within the central nervous system (CNS), there is minimal CSF redistribution and thus minimal risk of respiratory depression.[3] Nevertheless, when fentanyl is administered epidurally, significant plasma levels occur that can approach those observed after parenteral administration.

Nausea, vomiting, pruritus and urinary retention are side-effects that can occur with any μ-agonist given by the epidural or subarachnoid route. Often, these side-effects can be managed with small intravenous doses of naloxone, which usually can be titrated to relieve the side-effect without antagonizing analgesia. Butorphanol, a κ-agonist, given epidurally, causes minimal nausea and pruritus and may actually be useful epidurally in combination with μ-agonists to minimize these side-effects.[6]

Clinically effective epidural doses of morphine or fentanyl result in small but detectable blood levels of opioid. Similar doses of opioid given epidurally instead of parenterally produce more profound analgesia and are of greater duration. Thus smaller doses given less often can be used. This minimizes peak maternal plasma levels and resultant fetal exposure. The recent resurgence of interest in the subarachnoid route for opioids in labor may further reduce this fetal exposure.

ANALGESIA FOR LABOR AND DELIVERY

Spinal opioids for the management of labor pain, either alone or in combination with local anesthetics, may provide analgesia without causing motor and sympathetic block.

Subarachnoid opioids

In 1979, Yaksh et al[7] reported that subarachnoid morphine produced analgesia in pregnant rats. Early reports of subarachnoid morphine in humans for labor were enthusiastic and controversial.[8] It soon became clear that subarachnoid morphine, while useful in early labor, did not consistently provide adequate pain relief for the second stage.[9,10] Subarachnoid morphine was also associated with a high incidence of side-effects, including somnolence, severe pruritus and nausea and vomiting. However, Brookshire et al[11] found that an intravenous infusion of naloxone could significantly reduce the side-effects without inhibiting the analgesia provided by subarachnoid morphine 1 mg.

The use of subarachnoid morphine without combination with local anesthetic has found limited application for the relief of labor pain in recent years. For example, Abboud et al[12] reported the successful use of preservative-free morphine 1 mg with 7.5% dextrose in a parturient with severe pulmonary hypertension, in whom pain relief without sympathetic blockade was essential.

The goal of providing labor analgesia with a single dose of subarachnoid opioid is laudable and other efforts have been made. Subarachnoid opioid administration may eventually prove to be a simple method of providing at least partial analgesia for labor in hospitals where conventional epidural coverage is unavailable or impractical. Leighton et al[13] recently reported the use of a combination of subarachnoid morphine and fentanyl. Theoretically, the fentanyl should provide rapid onset and the morphine should provide prolonged duration of analgesia. Morphine 0.25 mg was administered with fentanyl 25 μg through a single dural puncture early in the first stage of labor. Analgesia was achieved in less than 5 min and lasted until delivery (3–3.5 h) in 60% of the patients. The remaining 40% ultimately required conventional lumbar epidural anesthesia with local anesthetics. The risk of delayed respiratory depression limits increasing the dose of subarachnoid morphine to further prolong the duration of analgesia. Perhaps a safer and more controllable approach would utilize continuous subarachnoid infusion of a highly lipid-soluble agent such as fentanyl through a subarachnoid catheter. However, until recently, only relatively large catheter (19 and 20 gauge) and needle (17 and 18 gauge) combinations were available. Dural punctures with these needles were associated with a prohibitively high rate of post-dural puncture headache. In 1989, the Food and Drug Administration approved a 32-gauge polyimide catheter for continuous spinal anesthesia. This microcatheter (Microspinal, TFX Medical, Duluth, GA, USA) will pass through the lumen of a standard 25- or 26-gauge spinal needle. We used one of these microcatheters to provide labor analgesia with subarachnoid meperidine for a patient with a history of allergy to amide and ester local anesthetics. Meperidine is apparently unique in that it has some local anesthetic as well as spinal opioid receptor activity.[14] Perineal surgery[15] and cesarean delivery[16] have been performed with subarachnoid meperidine alone.

Oyama et al,[17] in 1980, reported the use of synthetic β-endorphin administered subarachnoid to women in labor. The results were amazing. Labor pain in all 14 patients disappeared completely within 3–4 min and this analgesia lasted 12–32 h. Side effects were minimal and all infants appeared normal. The relatively large size (3300 daltons) of β-endorphin limited diffusion through the dura and necessitated subarachnoid placement of the drug. Subarachnoid administration may be advantageous, however, since it risks little or no transmission to the fetus. Unfortunately, the cost of the drug is prohibitive and appropriate toxicity testing should be accomplished before further studies are done.

Although the subarachnoid route for labor analgesia is not frequently used by the clinician today, the future of this approach for relief of labor pain with subarachnoid opioids and epidural opioid-local anesthetic combinations appears bright.

Epidural opioids

Administration of opioids via the epidural space for labor is becoming increasingly popular. The effect of epidural opioids is complicated by the need for the drug to cross the dura and by the presence of a rich venous epidural plexus that absorbs the drug and is often distended secondary to the inferior vena caval obstruction associated with pregnancy. As a consequence of these effects, epidural opioids alone have generally proved to be of limited utility as labor analgesics.[18,19] However, they are useful in combination with local anesthetics.

Morphine

As the only currently approved opioid for intraspinal use, morphine is a logical choice for combination with bupivacaine for labor anesthesia. Niv et al[20] added epidural morphine 2 mg to 0.25% bupivacaine and significantly increased the duration of pain relief before reinforcement.

Pruritus was the only significant side-effect observed and no neonatal depression was seen. The slow onset of morphine (30–60 min) and relatively high incidence of side-effects (pruritus, nausea, vomiting, and potential respiratory depression) will probably prevent widespread clinical acceptance of this technique.

Butorphanol

Butorphanol, a κ-agonist and weak μ-agonist–antagonist, is a commonly administered systemic opioid for labor and has been demonstrated to be quite safe. Hunt et al[21] suggested that butorphanol 2 mg added to 0.25% bupivacaine 8.5–10 ml was the optimal dose for epidural anesthesia during labor. The duration of analgesia was significantly greater and the time to onset of analgesia significantly shorter than when no butorphanol was added. The most common maternal side-effect was somnolence, which was occasionally accompanied by an altered sensorium. Care must be taken not to administer this drug to patients who are physically dependent on opioids since this agonist–antagonist drug may precipitate an acute withdrawal syndrome even when given epidurally.[22]

Nalbuphine

Nalbuphine, a κ-agonist, is now available in preservative-free solution. After appropriate testing for neurotoxicity, one can assume that nalbuphine will be administered into the epidural and subarachnoid spaces with and without local anesthetics to determine its efficacy in providing pain relief during labor and post-operatively.

Sufentanil and alfentanil

As might be expected, epidural alfentanil and sufentanil are now being studied alone or in combination with bupivacaine during labor. Heytens et al[23] used epidural alfentanil alone in 16 primiparous patients at an infusion rate of 30 μ/kg/h, with boluses of 30 μ/kg as needed. Excellent pain relief was rapidly obtained in early labor but analgesia was inadequate for the later part of stage I and stage II. The Amiel-Tison Neonatal Neurologic and Adaptive Capacity (NACS) examination revealed significant hypotonia. A preliminary report[24] suggests that combining lower dose alfentanil with bupivacaine can provide excellent pain relief for labor with no detectable neonatal depression.

Sufentanil should be attractive because of its very high lipid solubility and affinity for the μ-receptor. Van Steenberge et al[25] and Phillips[26] showed that sufentanil in combination with bupivacaine provided prolonged pain relief, reduced the total bupivacaine dose and gave limited motor block. However, in the epidural space, sufentanil appears to be only 2–3 times more potent than fentanyl, whereas systematically it is 5–10 times more potent. Therefore, unintentional intravascular injection of sufentanil 30 μg would be likely to cause respiratory depression and has recently been reported to have done so (GW Ostheimer, personal communication). Van Steenberge did find epidural sufentanil to be associated with maternal dizziness and lowered 1-min Apgar scores, which may indicate significant systemic absorption. Sufentanil is also associated with significantly more pruritus and nausea and is more expensive then fentanyl.

Fentanyl

The most widely used opioid for use in labor is undoubtedly fentanyl. Justins et al,[27] in 1982, added fentanyl 80 μg to 0.5% bupivacaine 3 ml. Since then, Skerman et al[28] and Vella et al[29] in 1985, Cohen et al[30] in 1987, and Youngstrom et al[31], Cellano and Capogna[32] and Chestnut et al[33] in 1988 have touted the efficacy of the combination of bupivacaine and fentanyl. Bupivacaine concentrations as low as 0.028% combined with fentanyl 100 μg have provided adequate pain relief for labor.

Respondents to a recent survey at the annual meeting of the Society for Obstetric Anesthesia and Perinatology indicated that 56% used epidural opioids for labor, with the vast majority favoring fentanyl. The solutions most popular were fentanyl 50–100 μg in 0.25 or 0.125% bupivacaine 10 ml. About 20% of the respondents used fentanyl in an infusion; the preferred solution was fentanyl 1–2 μg/ml in 0.125% bupivacaine, which was administered at rates of 8–10 ml/h.

ANALGESIA FOR CESAREAN DELIVERY AND POST-OPERATIVE PAIN RELIEF

The recommended doses of subarachnoid and epidural opioids for cesarean delivery and post-operative pain relief are listed in Table 15.1.

Subarachnoid opioids

Subarachnoid morphine has been used successfully in many types of surgery, including cesarean delivery. A high incidence of side-effects, including life-threatening respiratory depression, can be seen if doses greater than 0.5 mg are used. Chadwick and Ready[34] concluded that subarachnoid morphine sulfate in doses of 0.3–0.5 mg provided similar post-operative analgesia to epidural morphine 3–5 mg but with greater duration and no more side-effects. Two especially interesting reports in 1988 by Abboud et al[35] and Abouleish et al[36] showed that morphine 0.1, 0.2, and 0.25 mg mixed with hyperbaric bupivacaine provided excellent post-operative analgesia and may cause less respiratory depression than standard

Table 15.1 Recommended doses of subarachnoid and epidural opioids for cesarean delivery and post-operative pain relief

	Dose	Onset (min)	Duration (h)
Subarachnoid			
Morphine sulfate	0.2–0.3 mg	30–45	12–15
Fentanyl	10–20 μg	5	2–4
Epidural			
Morphine sulfate	2–3 mg/ up to 10 ml NS	45–60	12–18
Fentanyl	50–100 μg/ 10 ml NS	5	2–3
Sufentanil	25–50 μg/ 10 ml NS	3–5	2–4
Butorphanol	1–2 mg/ 10 ml NS	10–15	3–5

NS, normal saline

subcutaneous morphine injection. Hunt et al[37] showed that fentanyl in doses as low as 6.25 μg is also an effective subarachnoid adjunct that provides effective post-operative analgesia for 3–4 h.

Epidural opioids

Epidural morphine, fentanyl and butorphanol have been studied for cesarean delivery. Hughes[38] reported 1700 consecutive patients who had received epidural morphine with excellent long-lasting post-operative analgesia. Four patients were noted to have respiratory depression, two required treatment with naloxone and one was seriously acidotic. The issue of monitoring patients after intraspinal morphine is controversial.

Fentanyl is the most popular opioid for epidural use in cesarean delivery. Fentanyl appears to be very safe, with 50 μg giving pain relief lasting approximately 2–3 h.[39] Fentanyl 50 μg should be diluted in at least 10 ml of preservative-free normal saline (or local anesthetic) for fastest onset and longest duration.[40] Epidural fentanyl augments intraoperative anesthesia with epidural bupivacaine[41] or lidocaine[42] and may reduce the incidence of peripartum shivering.[43] Thus it is advantageous to give the epidural fentanyl once the epidural block has been established and prior to delivery. An additional dose of fentanyl 50 μg in normal saline 10 ml can be given post-operatively just prior to removal of the epidural catheter to provide several hours of analgesia after the resolution of the local anesthetic block.

While the effects of epidural lidocaine and bupivacaine[41,42] are additive with epidural fentanyl, chloroprocaine is antagonistic. Malinow et al[44] found no clinically significant period of fentanyl analgesia after 3% chloroprocaine was administered epidurally for cesarean delivery. The low pH of chloroprocaine (3.3–3.5) or some secondary metabolite may be responsible for this interaction.

Epidural sufentanil has also been studied in patients undergoing cesarean delivery. Doses of 30–50 μg diluted in preservative-free normal saline 10 ml provided analgesia with onset and duration similar to fentanyl.[45] At clinically effective doses, it is associated with a greater incidence of nausea and pruritus than fentanyl.[37] Interestingly, in epidural doses of 50 μg or greater, sufentanil can abolish shivering and affect maternal temperature control in a dose-dependent fashion.[42,44–47]

Epidural sufentanil appears to offer little advantage over fentanyl in the setting of cesarean delivery and it presents significantly greater risk. Should the epidural catheter become intravascular, a dose of 30–50 μg could precipitate respiratory depression or chest wall rigidity.

Epidural butorphanol, in doses of 1–2 mg,[21] has also been studied in patients following cesarean delivery. It has an onset of 15–20 min and a duration of 3–4 h. It has not been associated with pruritus or significant respiratory depression. Naulty et al[6] reported on the uses of an epidural butorphanol–fentanyl combination to minimize side-effects of fentanyl. Epidural butorphanol can produce some maternal sedation and may affect the fetal heart rate, producing a sinusoidal-type pattern. No evidence of fetal distress has been detected by scalp capillary blood pH monitoring. It may be most useful for post-operative analgesia after the fetus is delivered.

FETAL TOXICITY AND INTRASPINAL OPIOIDS

The considerable advantages of intraspinal opioids must always be weighed against the possibility of fetal depression. Drugs administered to the mother are transported rapidly to the uterus, and the concentrations of free drug available to cross the placenta will depend on the agent, total dose, route of administration, lipid solubility, pK_a, maternal pH, protein binding, metabolism and excretion.[3] All commercially available opioids have low molecular weights and readily cross the placenta by diffusion.[48]

Although there is an extensive literature concerning maternal effects of intraspinal morphine, evaluation of the infant has most often been confined to Apgar scores or the occurrence of apnea. Subtle effects of drugs on the neonate require subtle neurobehavioral tests. However, most investigators would agree that the risk of neonatal depression with epidural morphine appears to increase with higher doses and shorter interval between dosing and delivery time because of higher maternal blood levels of morphine.[49] The prolonged onset, the high incidence of maternal side-effects and the risk of delayed respiratory depression have limited the use of epidural morphine in laboring patients.

Fentanyl has an impressive safety record. Neonatal depression has only been reported with very high repeated epidural doses. When administered by the epidural route, fentanyl produces peak plasma levels similar to those produced by the same dose given intramuscularly. Gaffud et al[41] administered fentanyl 100 μg epidurally approximately 20 min before cesarean delivery. Theoretically this should produce near maximal fetal exposure. They found that epidural fentanyl 100 μg resulted in an average umbilical artery concentration of 0.8 ng/ml. This is below the concentration implicated in respiratory depression of the neonate.[50] In another study, the optimal dose of epidural fentanyl in the parturient was determined to be 50 μg[40] in normal saline 10 ml, which should minimize fetal exposure and possible depression.

Phillips[26] has compiled many of the data regarding the use of epidural sufentanil. Undetectable levels in maternal venous and umbilical cord blood are consistent with very high lipid solubility of this drug. Overall, 156 parturients received sufentanil, with only one study reporting a decrease in the mean Apgar scores. Unfortunately, neurobehavioral testing of the neonate has not been reported.

While the published evaluations are few, alfentanil has been associated with neonatal depression. Heytens et al[23] continuously infused epidural alfentanil alone and stopped at the onset of the second stage of labor. Although Apgar scores and umbilical blood gas values were normal, the NACS showed significant depression of active and passive tone. Again, subtle effects require subtle evaluations. More recent work using much lower doses of alfentanil may be promising.[51]

Butorphanol in epidural doses of 1–2 mg is not usually associated with respiratory depression. Thus far, neonatal depression has not been seen. However, butorphanol given via epidural or other parenteral routes may be associated with a low amplitude – high frequency sinusoidal-like fetal heart rate pattern.[52] This pattern usually resolves spontaneously and is usually associated with normal fetal scalp capillary blood pH.

REFERENCES

1. Behar M, Magora F, Olshwang D, Davidson J T 1979 Epidural morphine in treatment of pain. Lancet 1: 527
2. Wang J K, Nauss L E, Thomas J E 1979 Pain relief by intrathecally applied morphine in man. Anesthesiology 50: 149
3. Cousins M J, Mather L E 1984 Intrathecal and epidural administration of opioids. Anesthesiology 61: 276
4. Calvillo O, Henry J L, Neuman R S 1974 Effects of morphine and naloxone on dorsal horn neurons in the cat. Can J Physiol Pharmacol 52: 1207
5. Ketahata L M, Kosaka Y, 1974 Taub A Lamina-specific suppression of dorsal horn unit activity by morphine sulfate. Anesthesiology 41: 39
6. Naulty J S, Labove P, Datta S et al 1987 Epidural butorphanol/fentanyl for post-cesarean delivery analgesia. Anesthesiology 67: A463
7. Yaksh T L, Wilson R P, Kaiko R F, Intrussi C E 1979 Analgesia produced by a spinal action of morphine and effects upon parturition in the rat. Anesthesiology 51: 386
8. Alper M H 1979 Intrathecal morphine; a new method of obstetric analgesia? Anesthesiology 51: 378
9. Scott P V, Bowen F E, Cartwright P et al 1980 Intrathecal morphine as sole analgesic during labour. Br Med J 281: 351
10. Baraka A, Noueihed R, Najj S 1981 Intrathecal injection of morphine for obstetric analgesia. Anesthesiology 54: 136
11. Brookshire G L, Shnider S M, Abboud T K et al 1983 Effects of naloxone on the mother and neonate after intrathecal morphine for labor analgesia. Anesthesiology 59: A417
12. Abboud T K, Raya J, Noueihed R, Daniel J 1983 Intrathecal morphine for relief of labor pain in a parturient with severe pulmonary hypertension. Anesthesiology 59: 477
13. Leighton B L, DeSimone C A, Norris M C, Ben-David B 1989 Intrathecal narcotics revisited: the combination of fentanyl and morphine intrathecally provides rapid onset of profound, prolonged analgesia. Anesth Analg 69: 122
14. Famewo C E, Naguiob M 1985 Spinal anaesthesia with meperidine as the sole agent. Can Anaesth Soc J 32: 533
15. Acalouschi I, Ene V, Lorinezi E, Nicholaus F 1986 Saddle block with pethidine for perineal operations. Br J Anaesth 58: 1012
16. Talafre M L, Jacquinot P, Legagneux F et al 1987 Intrathecal administration of meperidine versus tetracaine for elective cesarean section. Anesthesiology 67: A620
17. Oyama T, Matsuki A, Taneichi T et al 1980 Beta-endorphin in obstetric analgesia. Am J Obstet Gynecol 137: 613
18. Husemeyer R P, O'Connor M C, Davenport H T 1980 Failure of epidural morphine to relieve pain in labour. Anaesthesia 35: 161
19. Writer WDR, James F M, Wheeler A S 1981 Double blind comparison of morphine and bupivacaine for continuous epidural analgesia in labor. Anesthesiology 54: 215
20. Niv D, Rudick V, Golan A, Chayen M S 1986 Augmentation of bupivacaine analgesia by epidural morphine. Obstet Gynecol 67: 206
21. Hunt C O, Naulty J S, Malinow A M et al 1989 Epidural butorphanol-bupivacaine for analgesia during labor and delivery. Anesth Analg 68: 323
22. Weintraub S J, Naulty J S 1985 Acute abstinence syndrome after epidural injection of butorphanol. Anesth Analg 64: 452–453
23. Heytens L, Cammu H, Cammu F 1987 Extradural analgesia using alfentanil. Br J Anaesth 59: 331–337
24. Carp H, Johnson M D, Bader A M 1988 Continuous epidural infusion of alfentanil and bupivacaine for labor and delivery. Anesthesiology 69: A687
25. Van Steenberge A, DeBroux H C, Noorduin H 1987 Extradural bupivacaine with sufentanil for vaginal delivery: a double-blind trial. Br J Anaesth 59: 1518–1522
26. Phillips G 1988 Continuous infusion of epidural analgesia in labor – the effect of adding sufentanil to 0.125% bupivacaine. Anesth Analg 67: 462–465
27. Justins D M, Francis D, Houlton P G, Reynolds F A 1982 controlled trial of extradural fentanyl in labour. Br J Anaesth 54: 409–414
28. Skerman J H, Thompson B A, Goldstein M T et al 1985 Combined continuous epidural fentanyl and bupivacaine in labor: a randomised study. Anesthesiology 63: A450
29. Vella L M, Willatts D G, Knott C et al 1985 Epidural fentanyl in labour. Anaesthesia 40: 741–747
30. Cohen S E, Tan S, Albright G A, Halpern J 1987 Epidural fentanyl/bupivacaine for obstetric analgesia. Anesthesiology 67: 403–407
31. Youngstrom P, Sedensky M, Frankmann D, Spagnuolo S 1988 Continuous epidural infusion of low-dose bupivacaine-fentanyl for labor analgesia. Anesthesiology 69: 686
32. Cellano D, Capogna G 1988 Epidural fentanyl plus bupivacaine 0.125 per cent for labour: analgesic effects. Can J Anaesth 35: 375–378
33. Chestnut D H, Owen C L, Bates J N et al 1988 Continuous infusion epidural analgesia during labor: a randomized, double-blind comparison of 0.0625% bupivacaine/0.0002% fentanyl versus 0.125% bupivacaine. Anesthesiology 68: 754–759
34. Chadwick H S, Ready L B 1988 Intrathecal and epidural morphine sulfate for post cesarean analgesia. Anesthesiology 68: 925–929
35. Abboud T K, Dror A, Mosaad P et al 1988 Mini-dose intrathecal morphine for the relief of postcesarean section pain. Anesth Analg 67: 137–143
36. Abouleish E, Rawal N, Fallon K, Hernandez D 1988 Combined

morphine and bupivacaine for cesarean section. Anesth Analg 67: 370–374
37. Hunt C O, Naulty J S, Bader A M et al 1987 Perioperative analgesia with subarachnoid fentanyl–bupivacaine. Anesthesiology 67: A621
38. Hughes SC 1982 Intraspinal narcotics in obstetrics. Clin Perinatol 1: 167–175
39. Naulty J S, Datta S, Ostheimer G W et al 1985 Epidural fentanyl for postcesarean delivery pain management. Anesthesiology 63: 694–698
40. Birnbach D J, Johnson M D, Arcario T et al 1989 Effect of diluent volume on analgesia produced by epidural fentanyl. Anesth Analg 68: 808–810
41. Gaffud M P, Bansal P, Lawton C et al 1986 Surgical analgesia for cesarean delivery with epidural bupivacaine and fentanyl. Anesthesiology 65: 331–334
42. Preston P G, Rosen M A, Hughes S C et al 1988 Epidural anesthesia with fentanyl and lidocaine for cesarean section: Maternal effects and neonatal outcome. Anesthesiology 68: 938–943
43. Matthews N C: 1988 Epidural fentanyl for shaking in obstetrics. Anaesthesia 43: 783–785
44. Malinow A et al 1988 Choice of local anesthetics affects postcesarean epidural fentanyl analgesia. Reg Anesth 15: 141–145
45. Tan S, Cohen S E, White P F 1986 Sufentanil for analgesia after cesarean section: intravenous versus epidural administration. Anesth Analg 65: S158
46. Rosen M A, Dailey P A, Hughes S C et al 1988 Epidural sufentanil for postoperative analgesia after cesarean section. Anesthesiology 68: 448–454
47. Sevarino F B, Johnson M D, Lema M J et al 1989 The effect of epidural sufentanil on shivering and body temperature in the parturient. Anesth Analg 68: 530–533
48. Hug C C 1984 Pharmacokinetics of new synthetic narcotic analgesics. In: Estafanous FG (ed) Opioids in anesthesia. Butterworths, Boston, p 52
49. Nybell-Lindahl G, Carisson C, Ingemarsson I et al 1981 Maternal and fetal concentrations of morphine after epidural administration during labor. Am J Obstet Gynecol 139: 20–21
50. Milon D, Bentue-Ferrer D, Noury D et al 1983 Anesthesie peridurale pour cesarienne par association bupivacaine-fentanyl. Ann Fr Anesth Reanim 2: 273–279
51. Ray N L, Datta S, Johnson M D 1989 Continuous infusion of epidural bupivacaine with fentanyl or alfentanil. SOAP Abstracts
52. Hutjis C G, Meis P J 1986 Sinusoidal fetal heart rate pattern associated with butorphanol administration. Obstet Gynecol 67: 377–380

PART B
FETAL AND NEONATAL EFFECTS

C. O. Hunt B. H. Minzter

Epidural and subarachnoid opioids have several potential advantages when used for obstetric analgesia.[1] When administered alone, there is no sympathetic block. Hypotension, a frequent problem when local anesthetics are used, is avoided. Motor block is also absent. The motor block experienced with local anesthetics may be distressing to the parturient and may decrease her expulsive efforts during the second stage of labor. However, opioids are rarely administered alone for labor and delivery as analgesia is often inadequate. To overcome this problem, administration of combinations of local anesthetics with opioids has become standard practice. These combinations administered epidurally for labor analgesia result in improved pain relief, reduced local anesthesia requirements and less motor block. For cesarean delivery, both epidural and subarachnoid administration of opioid with local anesthetic provide improved intraoperative anesthesia and post-operative analgesia.

Despite these advantages, the exposure of the fetus to opioids should be considered. The desire to avoid fetal exposure to opioids was one of the motivating forces behind the introduction of intraspinal anesthesia into obstetrics.

Placental transfer of drugs

Maternally administered drugs are rapidly transported to the uterus, which receives approximately 10% of the cardiac output. The concentration of free drug available to cross the placenta will depend on the total dose and route of administration as well as the pK_a of the drug and maternal pH, protein binding, metabolism and excretion.[2] Drugs cross the placenta by passive diffusion according to Fick's law, which states that the rate of diffusion is proportional to the concentration gradient; that is to the change in concentration per unit length in the direction of diffusion. Diffusion is enhanced by a high uterine artery concentration of a drug that has a low molecular weight and is lipid soluble, nonionized and minimally protein bound. The concentration of free drug in the umbilical artery will depend on the concentration of drug entering the fetal circulation via the umbilical vein and other factors, including fetal pH, protein binding, tissue uptake, metabolism and excretion. All opioids have low molecular weights and readily cross the placenta (Table 15.2). Differences in placental transfer can be anticipated from the differences in the physicochemical properties of the different drugs.

Table 15.2 Physicochemical factors affecting the disposition of opioid analgesics (From ref. 3 with permission)

	Molecular weight	pK_a	Percent nonionized at pH 7.40	Free fraction in human plasma at pH 7.4	Octanol–water partition coefficient (apparent at pH 7.4)
Morphine	285	7.9	23	70	1.4
Meperidine	247	8.5	7.4	30	39
Fentanyl	336	8.4	8.5	16	816
Alfentanil	417	6.5	89	7.9	89
Sufentanil	386	8.0	20	7.5	1727

Epidural opioids

Morphine

Morphine has been one of the most extensively studied opioids. In post-surgical patients, Weddel and Ritter[4] examined epidural morphine in clinically administered doses of 5 or 10 mg per 70 kg of body weight. The serum levels they reported, 28.0 ± 20.6 ng/ml after 5 mg and 49.7 ± 35.6 ng/ml after 10mg, closely correlated to those following similar doses of intramuscular morphine. Peak concentrations were found between 15 and 30 min. Wide variation from patient to patient was noted. Youngstrom et al[5] examined plasma concentrations of morphine following epidural injection (4 mg) and intramuscular morphine injection (4 mg) in post-cesarean patients. Their peak plasma levels following epidural administration were 12.5 ng/ml, approximately half that seen after intramuscular injection, 24.8 ng/ml. The difference between their levels and those of Weddel and Ritter may reflect the small number of patients studied, differences in sample times, or altered hemodynamics in the pregnant patient.

Only two studies have directly examined the placental transfer of morphine to the fetus. First, Craft et al[6] examined maternal and fetal effects of epidural morphine 5 mg in the chronically instrumented sheep. This study of 10 pregnant ewes documented stable maternal cardiovascular status. Intrauterine pressures were unaffected and uterine blood flow was maintained except for a small decrease at 120 min. Even more encouraging were the very low fetal femoral artery morphine levels. It would be tempting to conclude that placental transfer is minimal, however extrapolation of animal data to humans can be misleading. Nybell-Lindahl et al[7] examined the plasma concentration of morphine in maternal and cord blood following administration of epidural morphine 4–6 mg. The morphine concentrations were almost identical and the greatest concentrations were found with the shortest injection-to-delivery times. One of the infants experienced respiratory depression at birth and periods of apnea during the first 16 min of life.

Neonatal assessment after exposure to epidural morphine has been limited. Husemeyer et al[8] examined 10 neonates whose mothers were given epidural morphine 2 mg and commented only on the neonatal time to sustained respiration, which occurred within 1 min in all infants. Booker et al[9] reported no neonatal central nervous system or cardiovascular depression following epidural morphine 2.5 or 4 mg administered to 25 parturients. Crawford[10] studied eight patients receiving epidural morphine 2–6 mg and reported Apgar scores of 8 at 1 and 5 min in all infants. Niv et al[11] compared the combination of 0.25% bupivacaine with morphine (2 mg) with plain 0.25% bupivacaine and found improved maternal analgesia without neonatal depression as assessed by the Apgar score. However, all of these studies assessed only the vital functions of the neonate.

Subtle effects of drugs require neurologic and neurobehavioral examinations. Writer et al[12] evaluated infants whose mothers received epidural morphine 2–8 mg (mean, 3.25 mg). They found no alterations of the fetal heart rate (FHR) tracing. There was no evidence of neonatal depression as reflected by the Apgar score or umbilical cord gas data. However, at 2–6 h, six infants had ‘borderline’ Early Neonatal Neurobehavioral Scale (ENNS) examinations, which were then normal at 20–26 h. Hughes et al[13] compared patients given 0.5% bupivacaine with those given morphine 2, 5 or 7.5 mg. They found no alterations in the FHR tracing and no neonatal depression as evidenced by normal Apgar scores, cord blood gas analysis and NACS. Although the neurobehavioral assessments were encouraging, the use of the NACS has been questioned because of its abbreviated nature and reliance on the evaluation of motor tone.

In these studies, 131 patients received epidural morphine (Table 15.3). Morphine by itself provided ineffective analgesia and required the subsequent use of a local anesthetic, usually bupivacaine. One infant had evidence of respiratory depression attributed to the opioid and six infants had neurobehavioral depression when examined using the ENNS. The influence of the local anesthetic was considered to be negligible.

The risk of neonatal depression by epidural morphine appears to be greatest with high doses and when the injection-to-delivery interval (IDI) is short. The long latency of epidural morphine, the high incidence of maternal side-effects and fear of delayed maternal respiratory depression have limited its use in laboring patients.

Table 15.3 Fetal and neonatal effects of epidural morphine

Reference	Dose	No. of patients	Reported effects
7*	4–6 mg	20	One infant had respiratory depression at birth and periods of apnea for the first 16 min
8*	2 mg	10	All infants had sustained respiration within 1 min of delivery
9*	2.5 mg or 4 mg	25	No central nervous system or cardiovascular depression
10*	2–6 mg	8	All infants had Apgar scores of 8 at 1 and 5 min
11*	2 mg	30	No depression of Apgar scores
12†	2–6 mg (× 3.25)	8	No alteration of FHR tracing or depression of Apgar scores. Umbilical cord blood gas data similar to control group. Six infants with 'borderline' ENNS at 2–6 h, all normal at 20–26 h
13*	2 mg 5 mg 7.5 mg	9 10 11	No alteration of FHR tracing No depression of Apgar scores, NACS, umbilical cord blood gas data [Control group (n = 10) received 0.5% bupivacaine]

*Received supplemental bupivacaine.
†Received supplemental chloroprocaine.

Meperidine

Husemeyer et al[14] examined pregnant patients given epidural, intramuscular or intravenous meperidine. They found similar plasma levels with intravenous and epidural administration. The umbilical cord plasma meperidine concentrations were similar to the maternal venous samples that were collected at delivery (Fig. 15.1). Infants were considered depressed if the 1-min Apgar score was <7 or there were any signs of impaired respiration in the first 5 min. A total of six infants were depressed, three of whose mothers received epidural meperidine. The highest incidence of neonatal depression was seen when the drug was administered between 2 and 3 h before delivery. Neonatal depression was not correlated with umbilical cord meperidine concentration and the investigators postulated that metabolites of meperidine may have caused the depression of the infants.

As would be expected, Skjoldebrand et al[15] found much lower plasma concentrations when lower doses of meperi-

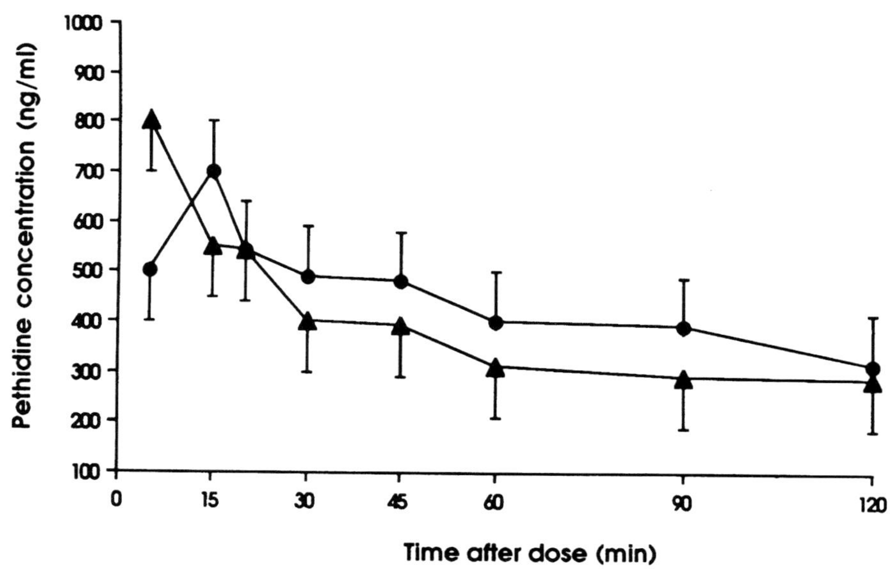

Fig. 15.1 Comparison of mean (± SD) plasma pethidine (meperidine) concentrations after intravenous (▲) and epidural (●) administration of pethidine 100 mg to patients in labor. (From ref. 14 with permission.)

dine, 25 mg, were administered epidurally. They also documented a close correlation between maternal and umbilical plasma concentrations. Two of 19 infants had 1-min Apgar scores of <7 and one of these infants had a 5-min Apgar score of <7.

Several reports including those by Perriss[16,17] and Baraka et al[18] documented the lack of changes on the FHR tracing with epidural meperidine.[19] Baraka et al[18] also evaluated Apgar scores, which were all ⩾8 at 5 min, and ENNS scores, which were normal. Hammonds et al[20] did report borderline ENNS scores, but they were not different from those whose mothers received 0.125% bupivacaine.

In these studies, a total of 89 patients received epidural meperidine, with three infants experiencing respiratory depression (Table 15.4). These mothers had been given the highest dose of meperidine 100 mg.[14] Two infants had low Apgar scores. These infants were delivered by forceps for 'threatening asphyxia'.[15] It was the opinion of most of the investigators that epidural meperidine should be administered only once and early in the course of labor to minimize the risk of neonatal depression from the cumulative effects of meperidine and its metabolites.

Fentanyl

A potential advantage of epidural fentanyl is the very low plasma concentrations produced by this form of administration. Plasma levels of fentanyl were reported by Wolfe and Davies in 1980[21] in parturients who received epidural fentanyl 100 μg following cesarean delivery. Only one of four patients had a detectable fentanyl level. However, rapid placental transfer of fentanyl has been confirmed in animal studies with rabbits and sheep.[22–24]

Carrie et al[25] reported the efficacy of epidural administration of fentanyl 150–200 μg, often as repeated doses in laboring parturients. Umbilical artery levels were much lower than maternal levels measured 30 min after administration. Unfortunately, maternal levels at delivery and I–D intervals were not reported. Neonatal evaluation was limited to the Apgar scores at 1 min, which were 7–10 in all infants except one. This infant had an Apgar score of 3 and required intubation, oxygen and naloxone. The plasma fentanyl level was 0.25 ng/ml. However, the investigators noted that other infants had similar levels and did not experience respiratory depression.

Maternal venous plasma concentrations of fentanyl following epidural or intramuscular administration of fentanyl 100 μg at the same time as the epidural test dose of bupivacaine were examined by Justins et al.[26] Although there was wide interindividual variation, the peak plasma concentrations were higher in the first 10 min with the epidural administration (Fig. 15.2). The peak plasma concentrations occurred at 5–10 min following epidural administration, whereas in the intramuscular group the plasma levels were still rising at 20 min. Unfortunately, plasma levels were measured only for the first 20 min. No neonatal respiratory depression was found with these doses.

Youngstrom et al[27] examined maternal venous and umbilical venous fentanyl concentrations in patients who received as their initial epidural injection fentanyl 150 μg either alone or with 0.125% bupivacaine. The highest maternal concentrations were found with the shortest IDI (Table 15.5). Fentanyl was not detected in any of the umbilical samples. Median Apgar scores were 9 at 1 and 5 min in both groups. Umbilical venous pHs were within normal limits.

Similarly, low concentrations of fentanyl in maternal blood were found by Skerman et al.[28] They examined fentanyl combined with bupivacaine administered as a continuous infusion. An initial level was established with 0.25% bupivacaine with fentanyl 5 μg/ml. 20 min later 0.125% bupivacaine with fentanyl 2.5 μg/ml was infused at 10 ml/h. They noted an increase in maternal plasma concentration as the duration of infusion increased,

Table 15.4 Fetal and neonatal effects of epidural meperidine

Reference	Dose (mg)	No. of patients	Reported effects
8	100	10	Three infants had respiratory depression
15*	25	19	Two infants had Apgar scores < 7 at 1 min, one infant scored < 7 at 5 min
16	50	20	No effect on the FHR tracing
17	25–100	12	No effect on the FHR tracing
18	100	13	No changes in FHR variability, one transient late deceleration All Apgar scores > 7 at 1 min, > 8 at 5 min All infants had normal ENNS (compared with 0.25% bupivacaine group)
20	25	15	No differences in ENNS, borderline scores in both groups (compared to 0.125% bupivacaine group)

* Subsequently received 25% bupivacaine.

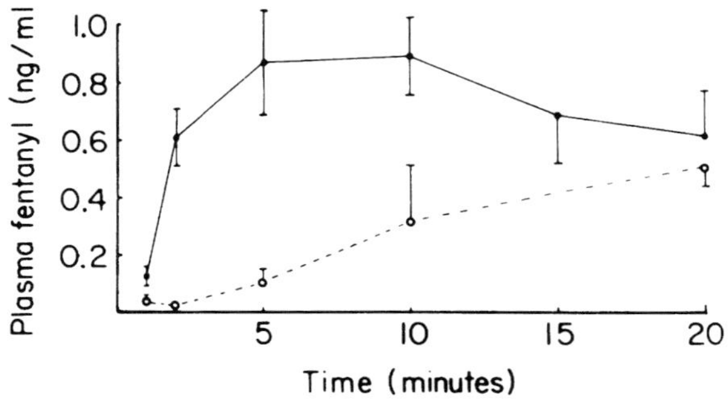

Fig. 15.2. Mean plasma concentrations of fentanyl after epidural fentanyl (-●-) and intramuscular fentanyl (-○-). Vertical bars represent standard errors. The differences between groups are significant at 1 and 10 min ($P < 0.05$) and at 2 and 5 min ($P<0.001$). (From Justins ref. 26 with permission.)

Table 15.5 Plasma concentrations after epidural fentanyl, 150 μg (Modified from ref. 27 with permission)

IDI (h)	No.of patients	Maternal concentration (ng/ml)	Cord concentration (ng/ml)
0–1	1	0.65	<0.10*
1–2	7	0.41 ± 0.18†	<0.10*
2–3	6	0.26 ± 0.06†	<0.10*
3–4	6	0.15 ± 0.03†	<0.10*
4–5	3	0.13 ± 0.04†	<0.10*
5–6	4	0.11 ± 0.05†	<0.10*
>6	7	<0.10*	

*Limit of detection 0.10 ng/ml with ± 10% precision at levels of 0.5 ng/ml.
†Mean ± standard deviation.

although exact values were not reported. Umbilical cord blood revealed undetectable fentanyl levels. There was no evidence of neonatal depression and Apgar scores were normal. Continuous epidural infusions have also been studied by Chestnut et al.[29] They found no difference in Apgar scores or umbilical cord blood gas data when 0.0625% bupivacaine with fentanyl 2 μg/ml was compared with 0.125% bupivacaine.

Several other studies of epidural fentanyl have confirmed the lack of adverse effects on the neonate. Vella et al[30] reported no neonatal depression with fentanyl administered as an epidural bolus (80 μg) or as an infusion to produce similar plasma levels. Gaffud et al[31] found no difference in Apgar scores when parturients received either 0.5% bupivacaine alone or with fentanyl 100 μg for cesarean delivery. Preston et al[32] compared two groups of patients who received 2% lidocaine epidurally for cesarean delivery with or without fentanyl (1 μg/kg). There were no differences between groups in Apgar scores or neurobehavioral examinations (NACS). Fentanyl was detected in only one umbilical venous sample (0.24 ng/ml).

Cohen et al[33] have extensively evaluated the neonate. They investigated four groups. Three groups received 0.25% bupivacaine with fentanyl 0, 50 or 100 μg. The fourth group received 0.068% bupivacaine and fentanyl 100 μg. There were several similar cases of fetal bradycardia. The only difference found was in the time to sustained respiration, which was longest in the control group. One neonate in the control group required mask ventilation. There was no difference in the incidence of low Apgar scores or low NACS. Umbilical blood gas analyses were within the normal range.

Capogna et al[34] also evaluated two groups of neonates whose mothers received bupivacaine with or without fentanyl 100 μg. There were 13 control parturients and 29 who received fentanyl. All Apgar scores were >7 at 1 and 5 min. Neonates were also evaluated with the ENNS. The fentanyl group infants were noted to have more vigorous truncal tone and placing. By 24 h, there were no differences between groups. Further, no effect was noted on the lability of state, which reflects the neonate's ability to maintain control of his reactions to environmental stimuli. The capacity to habituate, a measure of pharmacologic depression, was similar in both groups.

In these studies, fentanyl was administered to 286 parturients with only one case of neonatal depression (Table 15.6). Fentanyl appears to be the safest opioid to administer epidurally. There are very low maternal plasma levels and very little placental transfer. However, there does appear to be evidence of maternal accumulation of drug from the Skerman et al[28] infusion study. Neonatal depression has been found only with high repeated doses.

Sufentanil

Little et al[35] examined the addition of a very small dose of sufentanil, 5 μg, to an initial dose of 0.25% bupivacaine compared with 0.25% bupivacaine alone. There were no differences between groups in Apgar scores or NACS. Sufentanil levels were at or below the limits of detectability in maternal venous samples collected 2 min after the initial dose and at the time of delivery as well as in the cord blood.

Van Steenberge et al[36] examined three groups of patients who received an initial epidural injection of 10 ml of 0.125% bupivacaine with 12 μg of epinephrine combined with sufentanil 15μg, 7.5μg or 0μg. The 1-min Apgar scores were lower in the sufentanil 15 μg group with a mean of 7.9 ± 1.3 versus 8.8 ± 1.3 ($P < 0.005$) in the control group. At 5 min, there were no differences between the groups.

Phillips[37,38,39] has reported the use of sufentanil (combined with bupivacaine) as an initial bolus (1 μg/ml), intermittent boluses (1, 10, 20 or 30 μg) and continuous infusions (sufentanil 2 μg/ml). Compared with controls, he reported no differences in Apgar scores and no respiratory depression in the first 3 h. Despite administering sufentanil 40–151 μg, plasma levels were undetectable in maternal venous and umbilical cord blood. Similarly, low

Table 15.6 Fetal and neonatal effects of epidural fentanyl

Reference	Dose	No. of patients	Reported effects
25*	150–200 μg 15 repeated doses	38	One infant with 1-min Apgar score of 3 requiring resuscitation
26	100 μg	18	Mean Apgar score of 8 at 1 min, 9.3 at 5 min (no difference from i.m fentanyl groups)
26	80 μg	35	No change in FHR tracing Mean Apgar score of 7.9 ± 0.2 at 1 min, 9.4 ± 0.3 at 5 min (no difference from control group (n = 33)
27	150 mg	21 (alone) 21 (w/0.125% bupivacaine)	Median Apgar score of 9 at 1 and 5 min Umbilical vein pH 7.32 (no difference from control group (n = 23)
28	2.5 μg/ml	25	No neonatal depression No difference in Apgar score from control group (n = 25)
30	80 μg vs. i.v. infusion	20 20	Mean Apgar score of 7.6 at 1 min, 9.2 at 5 min Mean Apgar score of 7.2 at 1 min, 9.2 at 5 min
31	100 μg	10	Mean Apgar score of 7.9 at 1 min, 9 at 5 min
33	50 μg 100 μg	22 39	Similar frequency of bradycardia, low Apgar scores, low NACS
34	100 μg	29	Apgar score > 7 at 1 and 5 min At 2 h, truncal tone and placing were more vigorous in fentanyl group (control group n = 13)
29	2 μg/ml	41	No difference in Apgar scores or umblical blood gas data from control group (n = 39)
33	1 μg/kg	15	No difference in Apgar scores or NACS from control group (n = 15)

* These patients did not receive supplemental bupivacaine.

levels (less than 0.1 mg/ml) have been reported by Steinberg et al[40] when up to 50 μg of sufentanil was added to their initial dose of bupivacaine.

Unfortunately, few studies have evaluated the neonate with neurobehavioral examinations (Tables 15.7 and 15.8). Capogna et al,[41] using both the ENNS and NACS, did find a reduced NACS at 1 h in infants whose mothers received sufentanil 50 μg with the initial dose of bupivacaine. There were no differences from control at 4 h. When sufentanil 80 μg was used, mild hypotension, poor primary reflexes and reduced habituation was found at 1 and 4 h. Preliminary reports with very low doses of sufentanil have not found adverse neurobehavioral effects.[42,43]

Alfentanil

Heytens et al[44] administered epidural alfentanil as a 30μg/kg loading dose followed by a continuous infusion of 30 μg/kg/h. Top-up doses consisted of alfentanil 30 μg/kg or 0.2% bupivacaine 10 ml. The infusion was stopped at the beginning of the second stage of labor and no further drugs were given. The mean total dose of alfentanil was 198.9 μg/kg (range, 54.4–334.7 μg). Although there were

Table 15.7 Neonatal effects of epidural sufentanil

Reference	Study group	Reported effects
35	0.25% bupivacaine + 5 μg sufentanil (n = 8) vs. 0.25% bupivacaine (n = 6)	No difference in Apgar score or NACS Undetectable sufentanil group, equal at 5 min
36	15 μg sufentanil + 12.5 mg bupivacaine + 12.5 μg epi (n = 37) vs 7.5 μg sufentanil + 12.5 mg bupivacaine + 12.5 μg epi (n = 36) vs. 12.5 mg bupivacaine + 12.5 μg epi (n = 34)	Apgar scores significantly lower at 1 min in 15 μg sufentanil group, equal at 5 min

Table 15.8 Neonatal effects of epidural sufentanil (Data from refs 37, 38 and 39)

Initial dose	Subsequent doses	Neonatal effect
3 ml 1.5% lidocaine + 7 ml 0.25% bupivacaine + 1 ml saline (n = 10) or 10 μg sufentanil (n = 10) or 20 μg sufentanil (n = 10) or 30 μg sufentanil (n = 10)	Intermittent doses of 0.25% bupivacaine	No difference in Apgar scores
10 ml of 0.25% bupivacaine (n = 25) or 0.125% bupivacaine with 2 μg/ml sufentanil (n = 25)	Intermittent doses of assigned solution	No difference in mean Apgar scores: 1 min 8 (4–9) 5 min 9 (7–9) No respiratory depression in first 3 h
10–15 ml of 0.125% bupivacaine + 2 μg/ml sufentanil (n = 20)	Continuous infusion at 10 ml/h	No difference in mean Apgar score: at 1 min 8(6–9) at 5 min 9
or 10–15 ml of 0.25% bupivacaine	or 0.125% bupivacaine + 1 μg/ml suf or 0.125% bupivacaine	No respiratory depression in first 3 h Undetectable sufentanil levels

no differences in Apgar scores or umbilical cord gas analyses compared with the control group whose mothers received no analgesia, the Amiel-Tison score (a neurobehavioral evaluation similar to the NACS) showed significant depression of passive and active tone (Table 15.9). This clearly demonstrates the importance of more extensive neurologic evaluations of neonates. There was a lack of correlation between the duration of second stage and the maternal venous concentration of alfentanil in this study.

Several preliminary reports with low doses of alfentanil have not shown adverse neonatal effects.[45,46] Although these results are encouraging, more extensive double-blind studies must be done before this drug can be advocated for clinical use.

Butorphanol

Butorphanol is a strong κ- and weak μ-receptor agonist–antagonist not associated with respiratory depression and, combined with bupivacaine, has also been evaluated for labor analgesia.[47] Parturients received butorphanol 0, 1, 2 or 3 mg with their initial dose of 0.25% bupivacaine. Detectable fetal effects were found in the butorphanol 3 mg group. Four of six fetuses developed low amplitude sinusoidal-like FHR patterns which began around 10 min after drug injection and resolved spontaneously over 25 min (Fig. 15.3). Fetal scalp capillary pH samples obtained from one fetus were 7.35 and 7.31. There were no differences between groups in Apgar scores, which were ⩾7 at 1 min and ⩾9 at 5 min. Umbilical blood gas data were within the normal range for all neonates. The ENNS results were similar in all groups. The NACS results have also been evaluated following maternal administration of epidural butorphanol 1 and 2 mg.[48] No differences from the control group were noted.

Table 15.9 NACS in neonates following maternal epidural administration of alfentanil (Modified from ref. 44 with permission)

	Control group	Alfentanil group
Passive tone (max. 8)	7.31 ± 0.20	6.07 ± 0.25*
Active tone (max. 10)	7.63 ± 0.20	5.75 ± 0.52†
Primary reflexes (max. 6)	5.50 ± 0.13	5.07 ± 0.18
General assessment (max. 6)	5.63 ± 0.15	5.87 ± 0.13
Total score (max. 30)	26.06 ± 0.34	22.92 ± 0.68*

*$P < 0.005$.
†$P < 0.001$.

Subarachnoid opioids

Morphine

Scott et al[49] were among the first to investigate subarachnoid morphine for the relief of labor pain. In their pilot study, morphine 1.5 mg was administered. One infant was delivered by emergency cesarean delivery because of bradycardia and late decelerations. Three infants had Apgar scores of 6 at 1 min and all were ⩾8 at 5 min. One infant required intubation and naloxone.

Shortly thereafter, Chauvin et al[50] examined plasma concentrations of subarachnoid morphine injection in surgical patients. Even when administered in large doses, 0.2 mg/kg, lower plasma levels resulted than with epidural or intramuscular administration of the same dose. When small doses of morphine (0.02 mg/kg) were administered, the greatest plasma concentration was 13 μg/ml at 1 hour. The method used by Chauvin et al[51] measured both morphine and its metabolites.

Using a similar radioimmunoassay but separating morphine from its metabolites, Bonnardot et al[52] measured plasma concentrations of morphine obtained at delivery from maternal vein and umbilical cord blood. All mothers received subarachnoid morphine 1–1.75 mg. All plasma concentrations measured less than 6 ng/ml. As the IDI increased, maternal concentrations tended to decrease, whereas neonatal concentrations increased (Fig. 15.4). Twenty-two infants had Apgar scores of ⩾9 at 5 min.

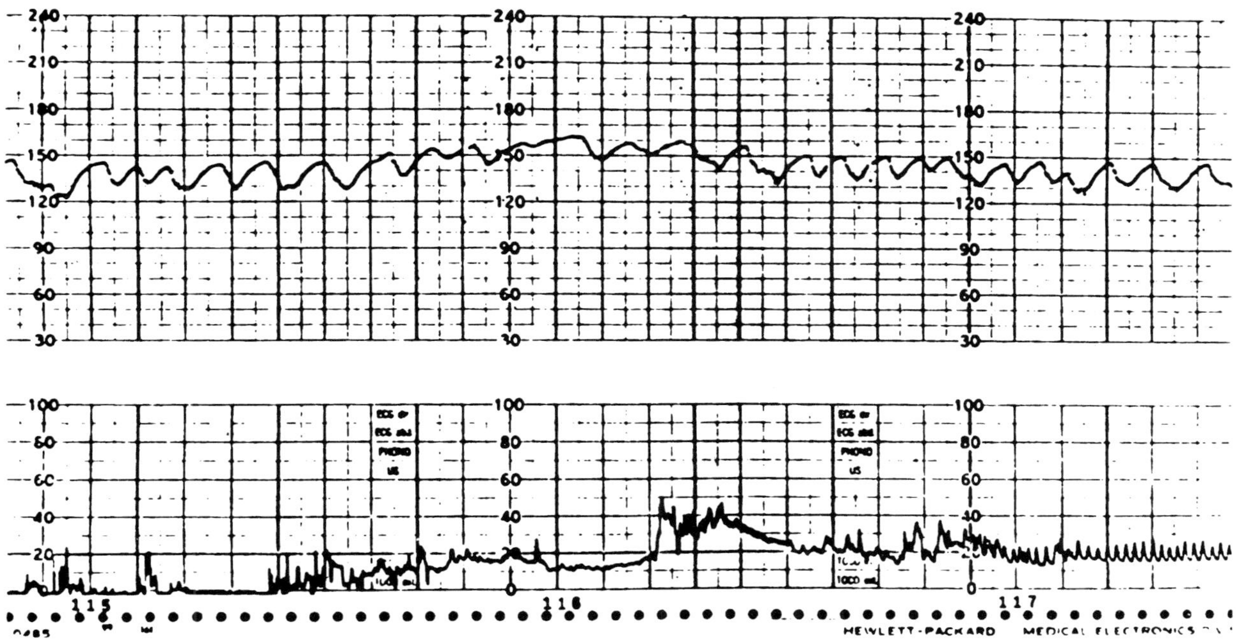

Fig. 15.3 A transient sinusoidal FHR tracing developing within 10 min of maternal epidural administration of butorphanol 3 mg.

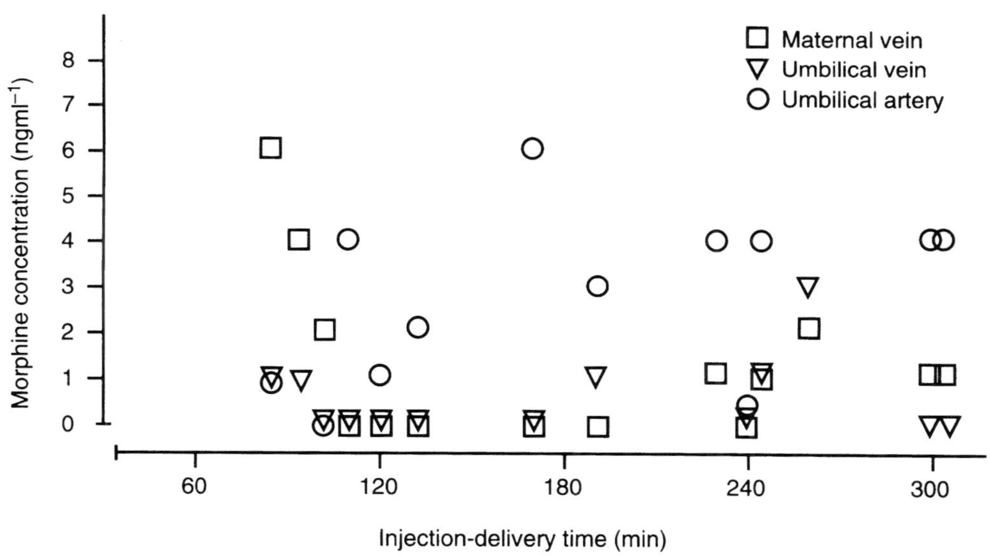

Fig. 15.4. Maternal and fetal concentrations (radioimmunoassay) after subarachnoid administration of morphine hydrochloride 0.8 mg/ml. The ratio of maternal–fetal plasma concentrations of morphine was inversely proportional to IDT, maximum rates being equal to or less than 6 ng/ml. (From ref. 52 with permission.)

Three scores of 8, 7, and 5 were attributed to umbilical cord compression.

Baraka et al[53] administered subarachnoid morphine 1 or 2 mg to 20 laboring patients. In 19 cases the FHR pattern was normal with no loss of variability. These neonates also cried immediately at birth. Apgar scores at 1 min ranged from 7 to 9 and at 5 min ranged from 8 to 10. One patient who received morphine 2 mg had a prolonged labor. The FHR tracing demonstrated bradycardia. The 1-min Apgar was 5 and the 5-min score was 7. The neonates were evaluated within 24 h using the ENNS and were all considered normal.

In 1984, Abboud et al[54] studied subarachnoid morphine 0.5 and 1 mg for labor analgesia. She observed no effect on the FHR tracing. All 30 infants had sustained respiration by 90 s. The 1-min Apgar was depressed in six infants. By 5 min all infants scored ⩾7. NACS results at 15 min were less than 35 (35–40 being normal) in eight infants, but by 24 h all were normal. The maternal doses of morphine were not specified for the depressed infants.

In an attempt to decrease the incidence of maternal side-effects of subarachnoid morphine 1 mg, Dailey et al[55] administered intravenous naloxone as a 0.4-mg bolus followed by a 0.4–0.6 mg/h infusion. Twenty-three patients received naloxone and 17 served as controls. In both groups the FHR and variability were not changed by the morphine or naloxone. One infant in the naloxone group did not have sustained respirations within 90 s. Three infants in each group had 1-min Apgar scores < 7 although all were ⩾7 at 5 min. A similar incidence of low scores on the NACS was found at 15 min. All NACS results were between 35 and 40 at 24 h. The only significant difference between the groups was in the umbilical arterial gas analyses. The naloxone group had higher pH and $P\text{O}_2$ values.

In these studies, 127 patients received subarachnoid morphine (Table 15.10). All five of these studies demonstrated fetal depression as evidenced by low 1-min Apgar and 15-min NACS scores. However, by 5 mins all Apgar scores were ⩾7. By 24 h, the neurobehavioral scores were normal. Bonnardot et al[52] attributed the low Apgar scores in their study to cord compression. The depressed infant in the Baraka et al[53] study was attributed to a prolonged labor. Abboud et al[54] suggested that forceps or cesarean delivery may have caused the early neonatal depression in their study. It should be noted that there are no data for patients not receiving analgesia, a problem shared by all investigators. Furthermore, most of these patients required additional anesthesic for the delivery; local perineal infiltration, pudendal block or epidural block was administered, and may also have influenced neonatal outcome.

A more promising use of subarachnoid morphine is the combination of very small doses with hyperbaric bupivacaine for improved intraoperative and post-operative pain relief. Abboud et al[56] administered morphine 0.1 or 0.25 mg mixed with hyperbaric bupivacaine. There were no differences between groups in Apgar scores. At 1 min, one infant in each morphine group and two in the control group had a score of >6. At 5 min, all scored ⩾7. All umbilical vein and artery pH and $P\text{O}_2$ values were within normal limits. NACS results were not different for any test items. Abouleish et al[57] also reported good Apgar scores and umbilical cord gas data when morphine 0.2 mg was added to hyperbaric bupivacaine (Table 15.11).

Table 15.10 Fetal and neonatal effects of subarachnoid morphine for labor and delivery

Reference	Dose (mg)	No. of patients	Reported effects
49	1.5	12	One fetus had bradycardia and late decelerations
52	1–1.75	25	No neonatal respiratory depression Three had low Apgar scores All plasma concentrations in mother and neonate < 6 mg/ml
53	1 or 2	20	One fetus had bradycardia Apgar scores: 7–9 (one 5), at 1 min 8–10 (one 7) at 5 min ENNS all normal
54	0.5 or 1	30	No effect on FHR tracing All had sustained respirations by 90 seconds Apgar scores: 24 ⩾ 7 at 1 min 30 ⩾ 7 at 5 min Umbilical cord blood gases within normal range NACS: 21 ⩾ 35 at 15 min All ⩾ 35 at 24 h
55	1	40	No changes of FHR tracing One infant with respiratory depression Three 1-min Apgar scores > 7, all > 7 at 5 min Three low NACS at 15 min, all normal by 24 h

Table 15.11 Neonatal effects of subarachnoid morphine–bupivacaine for cesarean delivery

Reference	Dose (mg)	No. of patients	Reported effects
56	0.25	11	No differences in incidence of low 1-min Apgar scores
	0.10	10	All 5-min Apgar scores > 7
	0	12	Umbilical blood gas data within normal range
56	0.2	17	Apgar scores:
	0	17	1 min > 7
			5 min > 8
			All umbilical blood gas data within normal range

Fentanyl

The combination of hyperbaric bupivacaine with fentanyl in doses of 0, 2.5, 5, 6.25, 12.5, 25, 37.5 and 50 μg has also been evaluated.[58] All neonates except one had Apgar scores at 1 and 5 min of ≥7. There was one depressed infant whose mother received fentanyl 12.5 μg. This mother was hypotensive prior to delivery despite administration of intravenous fluids and ephedrine. All infants had umbilical blood gas analyses within normal limits. There were no differences in ENNS results between groups on days 1 and 3.

Meperidine

In a recent case report, subarachnoid administration of meperidine provided adequate pain relief during labor and for cesarean delivery because of its local anesthetic-like properties.[59]

REFERENCES

1. Kanto J, Erkkola R 1984 Epidural and intrathecal opiates in obstetrics. Int J Clin Pharmacol Therap Toxicol 22: 316–323
2. Mirkin B L, Singh S 1978 Placental transfer of pharmacologically active molecules. In Perinatal Pharmacology and Therapeutics. Academic Press, Orlando, FL
3. Hug C C 1984 Pharmacokinetics of new synthetic narcotic analgesics. In: Estafanous F G (ed) Opioids in anesthesia. Butterworths, Boston, p 52
4. Weddel S J, Ritter R R 1981 Serum levels following epidural administration of morphine and correlation with relief of postsurgical pain. Anesthesiology 54: 210–214
5. Youngstrom P C, Cowan R I, Sutheimer C et al 1982 Pain relief and plasma concentrations from epidural and intramuscular morphine in post-cesarean patients. Anesthesiology 57: 404–409
6. Craft J B, Bolan J C, Coaldrake L A et al 1982 The maternal and fetal cardiovascular effects of epidural morphine in the sheep model. Am J Obstet Gynecol 142: 835–839
7. Nybell-Lindahl G, Carisson C, Ingemarsson I et al 1981 Maternal and fetal concentrations of morphine after epidural administration during labor. Am J Obstet Gynecol 139: 20–21
8. Husemeyer R P, O'Connor M C, Davenport H T 1980 Failure of epidural morphine to relieve pain in labour. Anaesthesia 35: 161
9. Booker P D, Wilkes R G, Bryson THL, Beddard J 1980 Obstetric pain relief using epidural morphine. Anaesthesia 35: 377–379
10. Crawford J S 1981 Experiences with epidural morphine in obstetrics. Anaesthesia 36: 207–209
11. Niv D, Rudick V, Golan A, Chayen M S 1986 Augmentation of bupivacaine analgesia by epidural morphine. Obstet Gynecol 67: 206
12. Writer W D R, James F M, Wheeler A S 1981 Double blind comparison of morphine and bupivacaine for continuous epidural analgesia in labor. Anesthesiology 54: 215
13. Hughes S C, Rosen M A, Shnider S M et al 1984 Maternal and neonataleffects of epidural morphine for labor and delivery. Anesth Analg 63: 319–324
14. Husemeyer R P, Cummings A J, Rosankiewicz J R et al 1982 A study of pethidine kinetics and analgesia in women in labour following intravenous, intramuscular and epidural administration. Br J Clin Pharmacol 13: 171–176
15. Skjoldebrand A, Garle M, Gustafsson L L et al 1982 Extradural pethidine with and without adrenaline during labour: Wide variation in effect. Br J Anaesth 54: 415–420
16. Perriss B W 1980 Epidural pethidine in labour. A study of dose requirements. Anaesthesia 35: 380–382
17. Perriss B W 1981 Pain relief in labour using epidural pethidine with adrenaline. Anaesthesia 36: 631–633
18. Baraka A, Maktabi M, Noueihid R 1982 Epidural meperidine-bupivacaine for obstetric analgesia. Anesth Analg 61: 652–656
19. Oyama T, Matsuki A, Taneichi T et al 1980 Beta-endorphin in obstetric analgesia. Am J Obstet Gynecol 137: 613
20. Hammonds W, Bramwell R S, Hag C C et al 1982 A comparison of epidural meperidine and bupivacaine for relief of labor pain. Anesth Analg 61: 187–188 (abstract)
21. Wolfe M J, Davies G K 1980 Analgesic action of extradural fentanyl. Br J Anaesth 52: 357–358
22. Vella L M, Knott C, Reynolds F 1986 Transfer of fentanyl across the rabbit placenta. Br J Anaesth 58: 49–54
23. Craft J B, Coaldrake L A, Bolan J C et al 1983 Placental passage and uterine effects of fentanyl. Anesth Analg 62: 894–898
24. Craft J B, Robinchaux A G, Kin H et al 1984 The maternal and fetal cardiovascular effects of epidural fentanyl in the sheep model. Am J Obstet Gynecol 148: 1098–1104
25. Carrie LES, O'Sullivan G M, Seegobin R 1981 Epidural fentanyl in labour. Anaesthesia 36: 965–969
26. Justins D M, Knott C, Luthman J et al 1983 Epidural versus intramuscular fentanyl. Analgesia and pharmacokinetics in labor. Anaesthesia 38: 937–942
27. Youngstrom P, Eastwood D, Patel H et al1984 Epidural fentanyl and bupivacaine in labor: double-blind study. Anesthesiology 61: A414
28. Vella L M, Willatts D G, K nott C et al 1985 Epidural fentanyl in labour. Anaesthesia 40: 741–747
29. Chestnut D H, Owen C L, Bates J N et al 1988 Continuous infusion epidural analgesia during labor: a randomized, double-blind comparison of 0.0625% bupivacaine/0.0002% fentanyl versus 0.125% bupivacaine. Anesthesiology 68: 754–759
30. Cohen S E, Tan S, Albright G A, Halpern J 1987 Epidural fentanyl/bupivacaine for obstetric analgesia. Anesthesiology 67: 403–407
31. Gaffud M P, Bansal P, Lawton C et al 1986 Surgical analgesia for cesarean delivery with epidural bupivacaine and fentanyl. Anesthesiology 65: 331–334
32. Preston P G, Rosen M A, Hughes S C et al 1988 Epidural anesthesia with fentanyl and lidocaine for cesarean section: maternal effects and neonatal outcome. Anesthesiology 68: 938–943
33. Youngstrom P, Sedensky M, Frankmann D, Spagnuolo S 1988 Continuous epidural infusion of low-dose bupivacaine-fentanyl for labor analgesia. Anesthesiology 69: 686
34. Capogna G, Celleno D, McGannon P et al 1987 Neonatal neurobehavior effects following maternal administration of epidural fentanyl during labor. Anesthesiology 67: A461
35. Little M S, McNitt J D, Choi J H et al 1987 A pilot study of low dose epidural sufentanil and bupivacaine for labor anesthesia. Anesthesiology 67: A444
36. Van Steenberge A, DeBroux H C, Noorduin H 1987 Extradural bupivacaine with sufentanil for vaginal delivery: a double-blind trial. Br J Anaesth 59: 1518–1522
37. Phillips G 1988 Continuous infusion of epidural analgesia in labor – the effect of adding sufentanil to 0.125% bupivacaine. Anesth Analg 67: 462–465
38. Phillips G H 1987 Epidural sulfentanil in labor. Anesth Analg 66: S140
39. Phillips G H 1987 Combined epidural sufentanil and bupivacaine for labor analgesia. Reg Anesth 12: 165–168
40. Steinberg R B, Powell G, Hee X, Dunn S M 1989 Epidural sufentanil for analgesia for labor and delivery. Reg Anesth 14: 225–228
41. Capogna G, Celleno P, Tomassetti M 1989 Maternal analgesia and neonatal effects of epidural sufentanil for cesarean section. Reg Anesth 14: 282–289
42. Naulty J S, Ross R, Bergen W 1989 Epidural sufentanil-bupivacaine for analgesia during labor and delivery. Anesthesiology 71: A842
43. Vandemeulen E, Vertommen J, Van Aken H et al 1989 Epidural bupivacaine with sufentanil in labor. Anesthesiology 71: A844
44. Heytens L, Cammu H, Cammu F 1987 Extradural analgesia using alfentanil. Br J Anaesth 59: 331–337

45. Carp H, Johnson M D, Bader A M 1988 Continuous epidural infusion of alfentanil and bupivacaine for labor and delivery. Anesthesiology 69: A687
46. Fernando E, Shevede K, Eddi D 1989 A comparative study of epidural alfentanil and fentanyl for labor pain relief. Anesthesiology 71: A846
47. Hunt C O, Naulty J S, Malinow A M et al 1989 Epidural butorphanol-bupivacaine for analgesia during labor and delivery. Anesth Analg 68: 323
48. Abboud T K, Reyes A, Richardson M et al 1989 Epidural morphine or butorphanol augments bupivacaine analgesia during labor. Reg Anesth 14: 115–120
49. Scott P V, Bowen F E, Cartwright P et al 1980 Intrathecal morphine as sole analgesia during labour. Br Med J 281: 351–355
50. Chauvin M, Samii K, Schermann J M et al 1981 Plasma concentrations of morphine after I. M., extradural, and intrathecal administration. Br J Anaesth 53: 911–913
51. Chauvin M, Samii K, Schermann J M et al 1981 Plasma morphine concentration after intrathecal administration of low doses of morphine. Br J Anaesth 53: 1065–1067
52. Bonnardot J P, Maillet J C, Colau J C et al 1982 Maternal and fetal concentration of morphine after intrathecal administration during labour. Br J Anaesth 54: 487–489
53. Baraka A, Noueihed R, Najj S 1981 Intrathecal injection of morphine for obstetric analgesia. Anesthesiology 54: 136
54. Abboud T K, Shnider S M, Dailey P A et al 1984 Intrathecal administration of hyperbaric morphine for the relief of pain in labour. Br J Anaesth 56: 1351–1360
55. Dailey PA, Brookshire G L, Shnider S M et al 1985 The effects of naloxone associated with the intrathecal use of morphine in labor. Anesth Analg 64: 658–666
56. Abboud T K, Dror A, Mosaad P et al 1988 Mini-dose intrathecal morphine for the relief of postcesarean section pain. Anesth Analg 67: 137–143
57. Abouleish E, Rawal N, Fallon K, Hernandez D 1988 Combined morphine for the relief of postcesarean section pain. Anesth Analg 67: 137–143
58. Hunt C O, Datta S, Hauch M et al 1989 Perioperative analgesia with subarachnoid fentanyl-bupivacaine. Anesthesiology 71: 535–540
59. Johnson M D, Hurley R J, Gilbutson L I, Datta S 1990 Continuous microcatheter spinal anesthesia with subarachnoid meperidine for labor and delivery. Anesth Analg 70: 658–661

16. Monitoring of the obstetric patient receiving intraspinal opioids

R. F. LaPorta   M. D. Johnson

ASSOCIATED RISKS

Wang et al[1] and Behar et al[2] first reported pain relief by the injection of morphine into the subarachnoid and epidural spaces, respectively, in 1979. Subsequently, intraspinal opioids have been extensively used with reasonable safety. The first application of intraspinal opioids was for patients in chronic pain who had become tolerant to substantial parenteral amounts of opioids. There were few reports of major respiratory depression in these early clinical reports. In contrast, patients acutely treated for post-operative pain who have not developed tolerance were at much greater risk.

What are the risks associated with the use of intraspinal opioids, and what options are available to reduce these risks? The only narcotic agent presently approved by the FDA for intraspinal use is preservative-free morphine (Astromorph, Duramorph). Morphine, the prototypical intraspinal opioid, is the least lipid soluble and the most hydrophilic of the opioids used at present. While it provides the longest duration of action, it has the slowest onset. When administered epidurally, only 0.3% of the total morphine dose is detectable in CSF. Much of the remainder is absorbed into the circulation and thus may cause respiratory depression. Because of low lipid and high water solubility, morphine has the greatest propensity of any opioid to sequester in CSF. Following the lumbar epidural administration of morphine it can be detected in the cervical CSF within 30–60 min[3] and detectable levels may be present for up to 24 h. Thus, in contrast to the more lipid-soluble opioids such as fentanyl and sufentanil, morphine is more likely to reach respiratory centers in the fourth ventricle by rostral flow and cause respiratory depression.

MECHANISMS OF RESPIRATORY DEPRESSION

The hydrophilic properties of morphine, though associated with increased side-effects, can be clinically useful. Diffusion of water-soluble opioids along the spinal cord may make analgesia available at areas far from the insertion site of the spinal needle or epidural catheter. However in the post-cesarean delivery patient, there is little to be gained from this effect as good pain control can be achieved with drug placed in the lumbar area. Perhaps the greatest benefit of the more water-soluble opioids is their longer duration of pain relief, especially if the anesthetic technique employs a single administration of drug. While rostral spread in the CSF may have a beneficial effect, it can also produce an insidious second peak of respiratory depression that is variable in onset, usually seen in 8–12 h although it may not occur for up to 24 h.[4]

Opioid binding at medullary and pontine respiratory centers can reduce respiratory drive by reducing the sensitivity to increased $Pa\text{CO}_2$. When the effects of intravenous and epidural morphine were compared in healthy young subjects, significantly greater depression of the slope of the ventilatory response curve to end-tidal $Pa\text{CO}_2$ and tidal volume was observed with epidural morphine. Maximum respiratory depression occurred at 30 mins after the intravenous bolus of morphine, whereas with epidural morphine this occurred after 3–22 h and lasted up to 22 h.[5] Of particular concern is the wide variability in the late onset of a second peak of respiratory depression. With an average onset time of 8–12 h, this peak may often occur at night when supervision is minimal. It is the variable nature of secondary respiratory depression that demands our vigilance. Fentanyl, despite its high lipid solubility, has been reported to cause respiratory depression when given epidurally either by bolus[6] or infusion.[7] Although the degree of respiratory depression associated with intraspinal fentanyl is extremely low at ordinary doses as compared with morphine, fentanyl has a shorter duration of action and repeated dosing may result in an additive effect.

RISK ASSESSMENT

The risk of respiratory depression has been quantified in several studies. In a retrospective survey, Gustafsson et al[8] found severe respiratory depression in 29 of some 9000 patients (0.3%) receiving intraspinal morphine. The majority of these patients were elderly and there was an association with the presence of pulmonary disease. A review by Reiz and Westberg[9] of 1200 patients receiving epidural morphine revealed four patients with a respiratory rate less than 10 breaths/min. One patient exhibited marked respiratory compromise, with the onset of hypoxemia, hypercarbia and respiratory acidosis. As these studies were conducted prior to the routine use of pulse oximetry and apnea monitoring, the incidence of respiratory depression was surely underestimated. Factors that influence late onset of respiratory depression associated with intraspinal morphine include age, chronic obstructive pulmonary disease, body position, spinal level of catheter insertion, increased intrathoracic pressure, positive-pressure ventilation, use of concurrent parenteral opioids, pre-existing tolerance to opioids, kyphoscoliosis, obstruction of the inferior vena cava and baricity of the injectate.[10]

In a recent review, Ready et al[11] treated 623 patients post-operatively with epidural morphine and 167 with intravenous patient-controlled analgesia (PCA). Patients were cared for in an ICU setting and had continuous respiratory monitoring. Four patients treated with epidural morphine developed marked respiratory depression. These were elderly, high-risk patients who had undergone prolonged operative procedures. The lowest recorded respiratory rates ranged between 8 and 12 breaths/min with $PaCO_2$ ranging from 63 to 95 mmHg. Even with an apparent adequate respiratory rate, the patients became somnolent and were not easily arousable. The lowest blood pH recorded was 7.07. Time to peak depression ranged from 2.75 to 13.5 h. Respiratory depression was reversed with naloxone. None of the patients using PCA developed signs of respiratory depression.

Cheng and Stommel[12] studied 15 subjects receiving epidural sufentanil, an opioid whose greater lipid solubility should limit the degree of respiratory depression, and had four episodes in which the oxygen saturation fell below 90% and, in three patients, end-tidal $PaCO_2$ was greater than 50 mmHg.

Cousins[13] had stated that the margin of safety of epidural morphine (i.e. the difference between an effective analgesic dose and one that will cause significant respiratory depression) is about 2 : 1. Bromage[14] reported one patient who suffered apnea and loss of consciousness 4.5 h after receiving hydromorphone 1 mg epidurally. This occurred in an ICU and the patient required intubation. Parenteral opioids and sedative tranquilizers can interact synergistically with intraspinal opioids, thus increasing the risk of respiratory depression. In addition, one needs to be concerned that drug administration errors may be increased in a non-ICU setting.

Little work has been reported concerning the respiratory effects of intraspinal opioids in the post-partum patient. Abboud et al[15] compared epidural butorphanol and morphine for post-cesarean delivery and demonstrated that the respiratory response to carbon dioxide was depressed with the use of morphine 5 mg or butorphanol 2 and 4 mg. Ventilatory depression was found to be more prolonged with morphine. Recently the use of 'mini-dose' subarachnoid morphine 0.1–0.25 mg has been described in a few patients who had prolonged pain relief with no evidence of ventilatory depression. At the Brigham and Woman's Hospital, fentanyl 10–25 µg is routinely given along with the usual dose of hyperbaric bupivacaine for subarachnoid anesthesia for cesarean delivery to blunt the discomfort felt with peritoneal tugging or exteriorization of the uterus. If epidural anesthesia has been chosen, fentanyl 50 µg is given in preservative-free normal saline 10 ml or local anesthetic post delivery. Several thousand patients have been treated in this manner with no evidence of respiratory depression.

Migration of epidural catheters into both subarachnoid[16,17] and intravascular[18,19] spaces has been reported. An analysis by Dawkins[20] suggests a prevalence of unrecognized dural puncture of 0.2% and of intravascular puncture of 2.8%. Injections of incorrect medications, including diazepam and hyperalimentation solution, into the epidural catheter have been reported, which emphasizes the importance of properly labeling the epidural catheter and syringes.

APPROPRIATE MONITORING SYSTEMS

What monitoring systems should be used to optimize patient safety when intraspinal opioids are used? Observation of respiratory rate and mental status by trained personnel is the optimal monitoring technique at present, but such labor-intensive measures are considered to be unrealistic in this time of cost containment. Even with observation of an adequate respiratory rate, tidal volume may be diminished, resulting in hypercapnia.[11] Current monitoring technology includes impedance apnea monitoring, pulse oximetry, capnography and arterial blood gas analysis. Cheng and Stommel[12] compared the efficacy of pulse oximetry and end-tidal carbon dioxide monitoring to detect respiratory depression in 15 patients given epidural sufentanil. They concluded that measurement of end-tidal carbon dioxide is a more sensitive indicator of respiratory depression than pulse oximetry but that pulse oximetry is a useful adjunct. This study and the review by Ready et al[11] suggested that capnography is the more sensitive monitoring system. While capnography may be a more sensitive monitor, nonintubated patients naturally find a tight-fitting mask to be objectionable. When the mask is not properly fitted, capnography is not reliable. Pulse oximetry is a more practical mode of monitoring because of these constraints. Although pulse oximetry is not sensitive to increasing $P\text{CO}_2$ levels, the adequacy of oxygen delivery to the peripheral tissues is assured. The pulse oximeter is less expensive, and is reliable, easy to use and readily accepted by patients. Impedance apnea monitors are simple and useful if properly adjusted to ensure a low false-positive rate; however, patient movement can often result in false alarms.

The incidence of respiratory depression (and other side effects such as pruritus, urinary retention, nausea and vomiting) can be reduced by infusions of low concentrations of naloxone (5 μg/kg/h)[21] or bolus administration of nalbuphine.[22] The antagonistic effects of these agents when used in low doses can decrease the side effects of intraspinal opioids with minimal effects on analgesia. Interesting work is being done using oral naltrexone after the use of intraspinal morphine to try to reduce the frequency of respiratory depression.

Research on alternatives to morphine for intraspinal use has branched into a number of different areas. Many opioids have been tried intraspinally. Their therapeutic ratios are now being assessed. Lipid-soluble agents such as fentanyl, while less likely to cause respiratory depression, require a more frequent dosing schedule. While lofentanil and sufentanil are more lipid soluble than fentanyl, their greater affinity for opioid receptors enables a longer duration of action. Duration of analgesia with fentanyl is about 2–3 h, whereas that of sufentanil is 4–6 h. However, there are indications that tighter receptor binding may make reversal of side-effects more difficult.

Agonist–antagonist opioids have been studied. Epidural butorphanol has provided up to 5 h of analgesia with minimal respiratory depression. Combinations of local anesthetics and opioids may reduce total dose requirements and side-effects associated with each drug.[23] Addition of epinephrine to intraspinal opioids appears to lengthen duration of analgesia but also increase the prevalence of side-effects.[24] The ideal opioid should produce no respiratory depression even with high doses. Most agents now in use are predominantly μ-agonists. The use of a κ-specific agent may decrease the incidence of respiratory depression.[25] Although the ideal agent has not been found, combinations of agents such as butorphanol and fentanyl hold promise in minimizing side-effects and maximizing analgesia.

Oyama et al[26] have shown that β-endorphins can produce profound pain relief in patients with cancer or labor pains.[27] Respiratory depression, nausea, vomiting, pruritus, reduced uterine contactility or alterations in fetal heart rate were not found. Pain relief lasted up to 33 h. Unfortunately, the cost of β-endorphins is currently prohibitive.

In summary, intraspinal administration of opioids is a powerful new and seemingly simple technique with great potential for acute and chronic pain management, but its use is associated with a small but definite risk of respiratory depression, which can occur in an unpredictable time frame. The margin of safety of epidural opioids when compared with parenteral opioids is reduced and subarachnoid catheter migration can lower this margin even more. Use of more lipid-soluble opioids such as fentanyl appears to be much safer. Small 'mini-doses' of subarachnoid morphine may provide effective and safe pain relief for long periods of time but more work must be done to quantify the possible risk.

When large doses of intraspinal opioids such as morphine are used in acute post-operative situations, monitoring is absolutely necessary and should continue for 24 h after the last dose of opioid has been given. Patients treated with continuous infusions or a repeated dosing schedule, even with the more lipid-soluble fentanyl, should also be monitored. It is possible that the use of intraspinal agonist–antagonist agents may prove to be safe and not require the use of continuous monitoring, but further studies are necessary to substantiate this concept. Whenever intraspinal opioids are administered a firm policy should be followed, allowing only the pain service or designated personnel to control the dosage and/or route of administration of any analgesic substance. Patients should be monitored in appropriate nursing situations with personnel aware of the side-effects associated with intraspinal opioids. Apnea monitors and pulse oximetry are practical, available and essential if appropriate nursing personnel are not available. Supplemental oxygen should be used when indicated. All catheters, infusions and syringes must be labeled, preferably with bright warning labels that are difficult to remove. There must be a constant alertness for possible subarachnoid, subdural or intravascular migration of epidural catheters. Naloxone must be kept at the bedside and resuscitative equipment must be immediately available. Safety may be enhanced by the use of appropriate naloxone or nalbuphine infusions. Intraspinal opioids have great potential for post-operative pain management but prudence requires conservative monitoring.

REFERENCES

1. Wang J K, Nauss L A, Thomas J E 1979 Pain relief by intrathecally applied morphine in humans. Anesthesiology 50: 149–151
2. Behar M, Olshwang D, Magora F, Davidson J T 1979 Epidural morphine in treatment of pain. Lancet 1: 527–529
3. Gourlay G K, Cherry D A, Cousins M J 1985 Cephalad migration of morphine in CSF following lumbar epidural administration in cancer patients. Pain 23: 317–326
4. Bromage P R, Camporesi E M, Durant P A C, Nielsen C H 1982 Rostral spread of epidural morphine. Anesthesiology 56: 431–436
5. Camporesi E M, Nielsen C H, Bromage P R, Durant P A C 1983 Ventilatory CO_2 sensitivity after intravenous and epidural morphine in volunteers. Anesth Analg 62: 633–640
6. Negre I et al 1987 Ventilatory response to carbon dioxide after intramuscular and epidural fentanyl. Anesth Analg 66: 707–710

7. Renauld B et al 1985 Continuous epidural fentanyl: ventilatory effects and plasma kinetics. Anesthesiology A234
8. Gustafsson L L, Schildt B, Jacobsen K 1982 Adverse effects of extradural and intrathecal opiates: report of a nationwide survey in Sweden. Br J Anaesth 54: 479–486
9. Reiz S, Westberg M 1980 Side effects of epidural morphine. Lancet 2: 203–204
10. Cousins M J, Mather L E 1984 Intrachecal and epidural administration of opioids. Anesthesiology 61: 276–310
11. Ready L B et al 1988 Development of an anesthesiology based postoperative pain management service. Anesthesiology 68: 100–106
12. Cheng E Y, Stommel K A 1988 Respiratory monitoring for post-operative patients receiving epidural opioids. Anesth Analg 67: S28
13. Cousins M J The experts opine. Surv Anesthesiol: 372
14. Bromage P R The experts opine. Surv Anesthesiol: 374
15. Abboud T K, Dror A, Mosaad P et al 1988 Mini-dose intrathecal morphine for the relief of postcesarean section pain. Anesth Analg 67: 137–143
16. Ravindran R, Albrecht W, McKay M 1979 Apparent intravascular migration of epidural catheter. Anesth Anal 58: 252–253
17. Ryan D W 1973 Accidental intravenous injection of bupivacaine: a complication of obstetrical epidural anesthesia. Br J Anesth 45: 907–908
18. Gilles I D S, Morgan M 1973 Accidental total spinal with bupivacaine. Anaesthesia 28: 441–445
19. Kim Y I, Mazza N M 1975 Massive spinal block with hermicranial palsy after a test dose of extradural analgesia. Anesthesiology 43: 370–372
20. Dawkins C J M 1969 An analysis of the complications of epidural and caudal block. Anesthesiology 24: 554–563
21. Rawal N, Wattwil M 1984 Respiratory depression following epidural morphine: an experimental and clinical study. Anesth Analg 63: 8–14
22. Henderson S K, Cohen H 1987 Nalbuphine augmentation of analgesia and reversal of side effects following epidural hydromorphone. Anesthesiology 65: 216–218
23. Skerman J H, Thompson B A, Goldstein et al Combined continuous epidural fentanyl and bupivacaine in labor: a randomized study. Anesthesiology 63: A450
24. Klepper I D et al 1987 Analgesic and respiratory effects of extradural sufentanil in volunteers and the influence of adrenaline as an adjuvant. Br J Anaesth 59: 1147–1156
25. Lander C J et al 1987 Analgesia and ventilatory characteristics of epidural Spirodoline – a specific kappa agonist. Presented at the International Symposium on Spinal Analgesia, Basic and Clinical Aspects. Munich, Germany, August 1987
26. Oyama T, Toshiro J I N, Yamaya R 1980 Profound analgesic effects of beta-endorphins in man. Lancet 2: 122–124
27. Oyama T, Matsuki A, Taheichi T et al 1980 Beta-endorphin in obstetric analgesia. Am J Obstet Gynecol 137: 613–616

17. Side effects

Part A Peripartum nausea and emesis *S. A. Lussos M. D. Johnson*
Part B Pruritus *B. H. Minzter*
Part C Urinary retention *M. A. Procopio*

PART A
PERIPARTUM NAUSEA AND EMESIS
S. A. Lussos M. D. Johnson

Vomiting, or emesis,[1] is a complex reflex characterized by the forceful expulsion of gastrointestinal contents through the mouth. Nausea is an unpleasant visceral sensation that may or may not be associated with vomiting. Retching is the labored rhythmic activity of the respiratory musculature that usually precedes or accompanies vomiting, but is not ordinarily accompanied by opening the mouth. The mouth opens immediately preceding the evacuation of the stomach whether vomiting is projectile or labored.

During elective cesarean delivery under either subarachnoid[2–5] or epidural[6] anesthesia, 40–80% of parturients may incur emetic symptoms despite aggressive and meticulous control of maternal hemodynamic variables. The parturient routinely receives little or no premedication prior to elective cesarean delivery to limit fetal exposure to drugs. Emetic symptoms in an unmedicated parturient occur frequently, tend to be an upsetting experience, place the parturient at risk for pulmonary aspiration of gastric contents and often delay or interfere with surgery. In addition, retching may transiently reduce placental perfusion and adversely affect the fetus with a marginal blood supply.

PHYSIOLOGY OF THE PARTURIENT

In 1960, Bellville et al[7] reported a threefold increase in the incidence of post-operative nausea and/or vomiting among women, with a trend toward higher levels during the third and fourth weeks in their menstrual cycle. They speculated that this resulted from elevated levels of progesterone and/or gonadotropins.[7,8] Schoeneck[9] in 1942 compared urine gonadotropin levels in parturients with and without emetic symptoms. He found them to be higher among women with emetic symptoms. The highest concentration were found during the 6th to 12th weeks of gestation, which coincides with the highest incidence of emetic symptoms during pregnancy. Cohen et al[10] found in first-trimester parturients presenting for therapeutic abortions that 63% reported a history of nausea and 45% had a history of vomiting in early stages of pregnancy. Therefore, the parturient may be more prone to emetic symptoms secondary to the physiologic changes associated with pregnancy. After the first trimester, the parturient should always be considered to have a full stomach because of pregnancy-induced hormonal changes and the mechanical effects of the gravid uterus. These changes tend to become clinically significant from 18 to 20 weeks of gestation[11] until 8–24 h post-partum. Progesterone decreases gastrointestinal motility, enhances gastrin secretion, and decreases lower esophageal sphincter (LES) tone. By the end of the first trimester, the uterus may begin to mechanically obstruct the duodenum and divide the stomach into antral and fundal pouches. The gravid uterus displaces the pylorus upward and backward, raising intragastric pressure[12] while also rendering the physiologic LES incompetent. Collectively, these mechanisms serve to delay gastric emptying, increase gastric residual volume, decrease gastric pH and predispose the parturient to gastroesophageal reflux, regurgitation and emetic symptoms.

GASTRIC EMPTYING

Pregnancy, labor and opioid administration delay gastric emptying. In the parturient gastric emptying time may be increased to twice that of the nonpregnant woman.[13] Despite this, it appears that the major cause of gastric stasis during labor is the administration of opioid analgesics.[14–16] Opioids not only delay gastric emptying, but they may stimulate the chemoreceptor trigger zone (CTZ) and sensitize the vestibular apparatus to the effects of motion. Frame et al[14] in 1984 showed that intravenous naloxone can reverse the opioid-induced delay of gastric emptying in laboring parturients given intramuscular meperidine.

THE LOWER ESOPHAGEAL SPHINCTER

The physiologic LES is considered a major barrier that protects against spontaneous gastroesophageal reflux.[17] Symptoms of heartburn and reflux of gastric acids are common during pregnancy and are often related to LES incompetence. Pregnant women have weaker LES tone than nonpregnant women. Furthermore, parturients with heartburn tend to have lower LES tone than those without heartburn.[18] The LES incompetence associated with pregnancy appears to be related to the mechanical effects of the gravid uterus and elevated progesterone levels.[19]

Drugs administered in the peripartum period may predispose the parturient to further gastric reflux and regurgitation (Table 17.1). Atropine,[20] scopolamine and glycopyrrolate[21] have been demonstrated to decrease LES tone. The antiemetic, promethazine (Phenergan), has significant anticholinergic properties and also reduces LES tone.[12,22] In contrast, prochlorperazine (Compazine) has minimal anticholinergic properties and, therefore, has a tendency to increase LES tone.[12] Even though droperidol does not change LES tone, it has been shown by pH probe detection 5 cm above the LES to increase the risk of regurgitation and reflux.[22] Opioid analgesics have also been reported to decrease LES tone.[23,24] Metoclopramide[12,17,18] domperidone,[17] prochlorperazine (Compazine) and cyclizine[12,17] are antiemetics known to increase LES tone. Metoclopramide, domperidone and prochlorperazine are dopamine antagonists that may block adrenergic inhibitory impulses to acetylcholine at the LES, thereby potentiating its effect.[12] The mechanism behind cyclizine, a piperazine phenothiazine with marked antihistamine (H_1) properties, remains unclear.[12]

Table 17.1 Factors that affect lower esophageal sphincter tone (Data from refs 12, 17, 18, 20–24)

Increase	No change	Decrease
Antiemetics	Antiemetics	Antiemetics
Metoclopramide	Droperidol	Promethazine*
Domperidone		
Prochlorperazine	H_2-antagonists	Anesthetics
Cyclizine	Cimetidine	Opioids
	Ranitidine	Thiopental
Cholinergic agonists		Halothane
Bethanechol	Muscle relaxants	Enflurane
	Atracurium	
Hormones		Anticholinergics
Gastrin		Atropine
Insulin		Scopolamine
	Glycopyrrolate	
Anticholinesterases		
Edrophonium		Foods
Neostigmine		Fat
		Chocolate
Muscle relaxants		Alcohol
Succinylcholine		Cigarettes
Pancuronium		
Vecuronium		Sedative hypnotics
		Diazepam
Miscellaneous		
α-Adrenergic stimulants		Vasodilators
Antacids (by raising gastric pH)		Sodium nitroprusside
		Nitroglycerin
		Ganglionic blockers
		Verapamil
		Vasopressors
		Dopamine
		Physiologic conditions
		Pregnancy
		Obesity
		Hiatal hernia

*Has been shown to increase gastroesophageal reflux.[19,22]

PHYSIOLOGY OF VOMITING

Vomiting center

The vomiting center is situated in the dorsal part of the lateral reticular formation of the medulla, in the midst of cell groups governing salivation and respiration.[1] Emetic episodes may result from direct stimulation of the vomiting center. Emetic prodromata such as copious salivation, swallowing and sweating and vasomotor activity such as pallor, tachycardia and weakness are related to the close proximity of autonomic nuclei to the vomiting center. Sensory information regarding emesis is processed through the nucleus tractus solitarius. The motor components of vomiting are initiated by the dorsal motor nucleus of the vagus and the nucleus ambiguus. Histamine (H_1) receptors are highly concentrated in the nucleus tractus solitarius and the dorsal motor nucleus of the vagus. Muscarinic cholinergic receptors are localized in the nucleus tractus solitarius and the nucleus ambiguus.[25] Therefore, the role of antihistamines and anticholinergic medications in preventing or treating emetic symptoms has a sound physiologic basis.

Cortical afferents

Cortical stimuli resulting from psychogenic and/or emotional disturbances or unpleasant olfactory, visual or gustatory stimuli may directly trigger the vomiting center. Evans[26] in 1928 described ‘psychic’ nausea as nausea resulting from the terrifying thoughts of an overactive mind. A well-informed patient prior to regional anesthesia and a reassuring, compassionate anesthesiologist may significantly decrease the incidence of anxiety and related emetic symptoms. If the parturient is extremely anxious, mild sedation may be considered. Diazepam 0.5–5 mg or diphenhydramine 12.5–50 mg intravenously before or after the baby is delivered usually blunts anxiety and extraneous stimuli. Blunting cortical sensory afferents may ultimately decrease signals that impinge directly on the vomiting center. This may help to minimize the incidence of emetic symptoms in the operating room during regional anesthesia.

Relative brainstem hypoxia: hypotension and arterial hypoxemia

Hypotension and the resultant hypoxemia of the brainstem vomiting center may also trigger vomiting.[2,27,28] Hypotensive episodes with systolic blood pressures less than 80 mmHg have been significantly associated with the development of nausea and/or vomiting during subarachnoid anesthesia.[27] Ratra et al,[28] in a 1972 prospective study of women undergoing gynecologic surgery under subarachnoid anesthesia, noted that the frequency of emetic symptoms increased almost twofold when the systolic blood pressure decreased below 80 mmHg (70.6% versus 37.7%). These investigators also observed that the administration of supplemental oxygen therapy significantly decreased the incidence of emetic symptoms despite the presence of hypotension. This supports the theory that hypotension and the relative cerebral hypoxia or hypoxemia of the vomiting center may trigger vomiting.[26–28] During regional anesthetic techniques for cesarean delivery, Datta et al[2] and Kang et al[3] reported a 6.6- and 7.0-fold reduction in peripartum emetic symptoms during induction of subarachnoid anesthesia by avoiding maternal hypotension (keeping systolic blood pressure above 100 mmHg or within 10–20% of baseline) with the aggressive use of intravenous ephedrine by bolus[2] or infusion.[3]

Supplemental inspired oxygen by face mask and acute hydration with 1000–1500 ml of crystalloid for the healthy parturient undergoing epidural or subarachnoid anesthesia are essential. The higher the segmental sympathetic blockade (especially greater than T4), the greater the risk of hypotension and associated emetic symptoms.[22] The rapidity with which these changes occur influences the incidence of hypotension as well as the incidence of emetic symptoms. Post-induction left uterine displacement to avoid aortocaval compression and prompt intravenous administration of ephedrine as soon as maternal blood pressure begins to fall from baseline will effectively halt further downward trends in blood pressure.[2]

Visceral autonomic afferents

During obstetric surgery, reflex triggering of emetic symptoms often results when visceral or parietal peritoneum, or viscera themselves, are overzealously handled or stretched. Sympathetic innervation to the stomach (T6–T10) may be blocked with high segmental levels of subarachnoid or epidural anesthesia. This allows relatively unopposed vagal afferent impulses to predominate in the upper gastrointestinal tract. Harsh peritoneal traction, uterine exteriorization, lower uterine segment stretching or repair by inexperienced surgeons may further increase afferent impulses over unblocked vagal segments to trigger the vomiting center.

Pederson et al[29] observed two groups of parturients given a mean dose of hyperbaric bupivacaine of either 8.41 mg or 10.89 mg for cesarean delivery. The group receiving 25% more drug per centimeter of height had reduced intraoperative intravenous opioid supplementation and 2.2 times less visceral pain, which can result when inadequate extent, duration or intensity of subarachnoid or epidural anesthesia occurs.[30] Under such circumstances, reflex visceral vagal afferents from the gastrointestinal tract or uterus can travel centrally to directly trigger the vomiting center. If emetic symptoms occur at this time, a reminder to the surgeons to handle the tissues gently may suffice. Emetic symptoms associated with visceral pain are usually brief and self-limited, often resolving as surgical stimulation diminishes. Anticholinergic medications, which have detrimental effects on the LES tone, are often impractical for therapy at this time unless given prophylactically. Furthermore, antiemetics with predominant antidopaminergic properties tend to be largely ineffective in treating emetic symptoms of visceral origin.

Visceral pain during subarachnoid anesthesia is often related to inadequate anesthesia, especially when plain local anesthetic mixtures are used.[29] During epidural anesthesia, an inadequate sacral block also predisposes the parturient to visceral pain sensations and emetic consequences. The degree of pain complaints by the patient represents the state of afferent blockade of the nociceptive fibers.[31] This can be modified by the quality and quantity of local anesthetics used during the operative procedure. The use of larger dosages of local anesthetics in the subarachnoid space provides for a more profound sensory afferent blockade. This may limit the incidence of visceral pain, as well as the incidence of viscerally mediated emetic symptoms.[27] Norris[32] demonstrated that adequate anesthesia for cesarean delivery (median level T3) could be obtained with 12 mg (1.6 ml) of hyperbaric bupivacaine regardless of patient height (4'11" to 5'8"), weight or body mass index.

Subarachnoid and epidural opioids act selectively on the nociceptive receptors in the dorsal horns at the spinal column, specifically in the substantia gelatinosa. Here, subarachnoid and epidural opioids modulate nociceptive input from small primary afferent nerves of the unmyelinated C and myelinated A-δ type.[33,34] Visceral nociceptive afferents can be blunted by subarachnoid μ- and κ-agonists, such as morphine and fentanyl. Epidurally administered fentanyl 50 μg diluted in a total volume of at least 10 ml of preservative-free normal saline has been shown to help minimize the incidence of emetic symptoms associated with uterine manipulation.[35] The μ-receptor agonist–antagonists with κ-agonist properties (nalbuphine, butorphanol and nalorphine) may similarly decrease visceral pain.[33]

Hunt et al[36] in 1989, observed that hyperbaric bupivacaine plus subarachnoid fentanyl 6.25 μg allowed for complete intraoperative pain relief during cesarean delivery, when compared with plain hyperbaric subarachnoid bupivacaine solutions. No intravenous opioid supplementation was required in the subarachnoid bupivacaine/fentanyl group versus a 67% requirement in the plain hyperbaric bupivacaine group. Therefore, subarachnoid and epidural opioids may successfully decrease the incidence of intraoperative visceral pain. Interestingly, a threefold increase in the incidence of nausea was observed in the subarachnoid bupivacaine–fentanyl group compared to the plain bupivacaine group (32.6% versus 11.0%). Obviously, there are other mechanisms responsible for triggering emetic symptoms.

Chemoreceptor trigger zone

The chemoreceptor trigger zone (CTZ) lies bilaterally on the floor of the fourth ventricle in the medulla in close proximity to the vomiting center. Impulses from the CTZ are relayed to the vomiting center and a vomiting reflex initiated (Fig. 17.1). This CTZ is richly innervated with dopaminergic (D_2) receptors.[25] This is why dopamine antagonists such as phenothiazines, droperidol,[5,36] metoclopramide,[4,6,37,38] and domperidone[38] are efficacious antiemetics (Table 17.2). Triggers of the CTZ include circulating toxins and drugs (cytotoxic drugs, opioids, digoxin and apomorphine), radiation therapy, metabolic disturbances (uremia, hypoglycemia and hyperglycemia), as well as hyperemesis gravidarum.

Impulses mediating nausea and vomiting by vestibular stimulation (motion sickness) originate principally in the utricular maculae of the labyrinth. These impulses pass by way of the eighth cranial nerve to the lateral vestibular nuclei, to the uvula and nodulus of the cerebellum, then to the CTZ, and finally to the vomiting center. The lateral vestibular nucleus is innervated by muscarinic cholinergic and histamine (H_1) receptors. Therefore, motion sickness may be managed with anticholinergics (e.g. scopolamine) and/or antihistamines (H_1) such as promethazine (Phenergan)[25] or diphenhydramine. Interestingly, intramuscular ephedrine may also have antiemetic efficacy in patients prone to motion sickness. However, its mechanism remains unclear.[39]

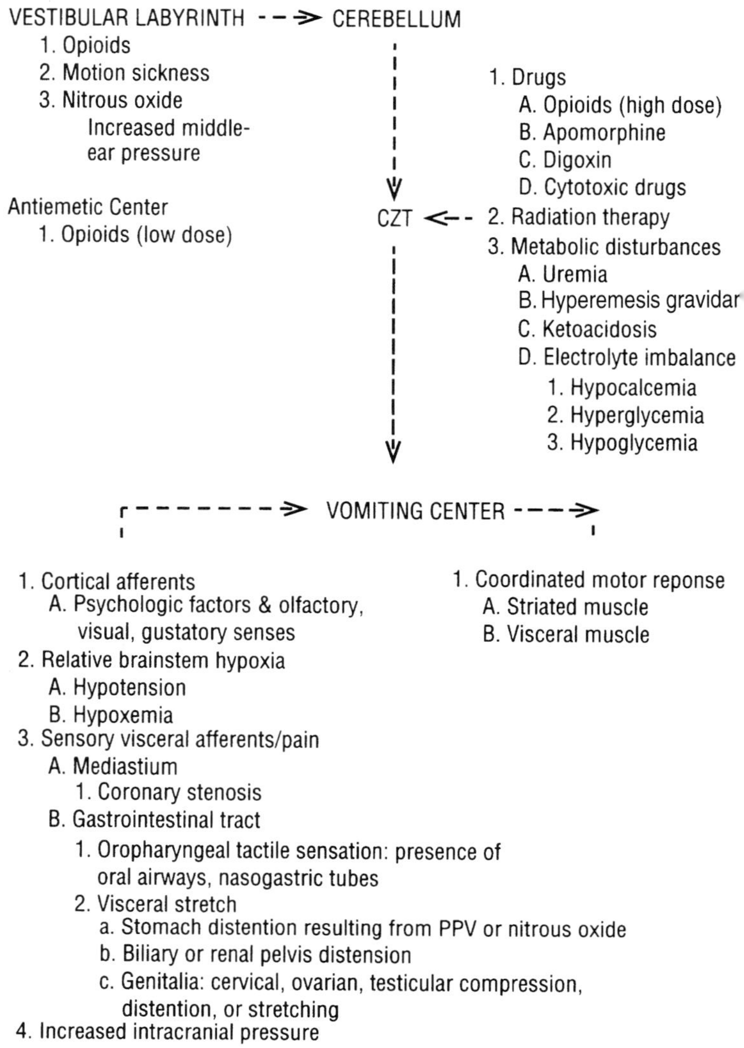

Fig. 17.1 Stimuli that cause emetic symptoms. (Data from ref. 8.)

Table 17.2 Antiemetic drug potencies at neurotransmitter receptor sites (From ref. 38 with permission)

Drug	Dopamine (D_2)	Muscarine Cholinergic	Histamine (H_1)
Anticholinergics			
Hyoscine	Negligible	+++++	Negligible
Atropine	Negligible	+++++	Negligible
Glycopyrrolate	Negligible	+++++	Negligible
H_1 Antihistamines			
Promethazine	++++	+++++	+++++
Diphenhydramine	Negligible	++++	Negligible
Cyclizine	+	+++	+++++
Phenothiazines			
Fluphenazine	+++++	++++	+++++
Prochlorperazine	+++++	+++	++++
Chlorpromazine	+++++	++++	+++++
Butyrophenones			
Droperidol	+++++	Negligible	+
Haloperidol	+++++	Negligible	+
Miscellaneous			
Metoclopramide	++++	Negligible	+
Domperidone	++++	Negligible	Negligible

PROPHYLAXIS AND TREATMENT OF EMETIC SYMPTOMS FOR THE PARTURIENT

Steps in prevention and treatment of emetic symptoms are outlined in Table 17.3.

Metoclopramide is an antiemetic[40,41] that is related to procainamide but virtually devoid of antiarrhythmic or local anesthetic activity. It accelerates gastric emptying by its direct effect on autonomic nuclei and sensitizes gastric smooth muscle to the effects of acetylcholine. In laboring primigravidas, Howard and Sharp[13] in 1973 showed an almost threefold increase in gastric emptying after 10 mg of metoclopramide was given intramuscularly following a 750-ml test fluid meal (Fig. 17.2). He also showed that metoclopramide partly reversed the delayed gastric emptying produced by meperidine in laboring patients. Murphy et al[42] similarly noted improved gastric emptying in parturients when given metoclopramide during labor and/or elective cesarean delivery. Wyner[11] demonstrated in first-trimester parturients that the preinduction administration of 10 mg of intravenous metoclopramide decreased gastric volume.

Metoclopramide's central antidopaminergic activity on the CTZ makes it a useful antiemetic whether given before[4] or after cesarean delivery.[6] Maternal and fetal safety has been well documented with metoclopramide[14,43] McGarray[37] demonstrated its antiemetic efficacy for parturients in labor when given meperidine analgesia. Lussos et al[4] reported that parturients given intravenous metoclopramide 10 mg prior to induction of bupivacaine–fentanyl subarachnoid anesthesia had a fivefold reduction in post-subarachnoid block, predelivery

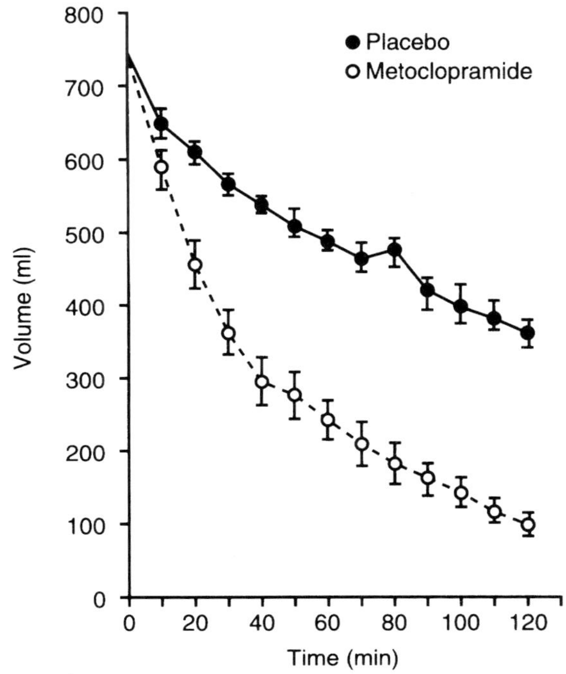

Fig. 17.2 Mean gastric volumes after a 750-ml fluid test meal remaining in laboring parturients given either metoclopramide or placebo. (From ref. 13 with permission.)

Table 17.3 Prophylaxis and treatment of emetic symptoms for the parturient during obstetric regional anesthesia

1. Full explanation of the regional anesthetic procedure and expected sensory and motor changes to be experienced following successful block.
2. 0.3 mol/L sodium citrate 30 ml PO.
3. Acute hydration with dextrose-free crystalloid solution 1.5–2.0 L.
4. Metoclopramide 10 mg IV approximately 10–15 minutes prior to induction.
5. Oxygen 6L PM by face mask.
6. Appropriate monitors applied: NIBP, SPO_2, ECG.
7. Post subarachnoid or epidural placement emetic symptoms: determine etiology.
   - A. Psychogenic/anxiety-related emetic symptoms
     - 1. Diphenhydramine 12.5–50 mg, diazepam 0.5–50 mg IV.
   - B. Relative cerebral hypoxia
     - 1. Ensure SBP > 100 or > 10–20% of baseline, check HR and level of blockade.
       - A. Bolus ephedrine in 10 mg IV increments as soon as SBP decreases from baseline.
       - B. Fluid bolus.
       - C. Ensure adequate left uterine displacement.
     - 2. Ensure adequate oxygenation: check SPO_2, oxygen source.
   - C. Visceral pain (usually occurs post-delivery)
     - 1. Inadequate anesthesia or excessive surgical visceral traction.
       - A. Ensure adequacy of regional block: extent, intensity, duration.
       - 1. Subarachnoid anesthesia
         - a. Begin block with higher dose of local anesthetic.
         - b. Add subarachnoid opioid to local anesthetic mixture.
         - c. Supplement with IV opioid after block is complete.
       - 2. Epidural anesthesia
         - a. Ensure adequate sacral block prior to incision.
         - b. Supplement block with epidural opioids.
         - c. Reassess sensory level: top-up local anesthetic, if indicated.
       - B. Glycopyrrolate 0.2 mg IV for persistent visceral pain.
   - D. Opioid induced
     - 1. Metoclopramide 10 mg IV q 4–6 h, or droperidol 0.625 mg IV q 6–8 h.
     - 2. Scopolamine patches.
     - 3. Low-dose naloxone 80 μg/h, nalbuphine 2–5 mg, butorphanol 1–2 mg IV.

emetic symptoms compared with saline controls. Chestnut et al[6] administered intravenous metoclopramide 0.15 mg/kg to parturients intraoperatively post-cesarean delivery which decreased intraoperative nausea (12% versus 36%) and resulted in no vomiting in the metoclopramide group compared with 15% in the saline placebo group. All patients received epidural morphine or hydromorphone prior to closure of the fascia. Of note was the 2.5- to 3.0-fold reduction in emetic symptoms in the metoclopramide group during the first 4 h post-operatively.

Adverse side-effects to metoclopramide are dose related and occur infrequently in the 10- to 20-mg dose ranges used clinically.[4,41] Sedation and extrapyramidal and dystonic reactions (e.g. torticollis, oculogyric crises, and trismus) are potential adverse effects of antiemetic medications. Cohen et al[10] reported that patients given droperidol 1.25 mg suffered from delayed awakening[10,39] and post-operative dizziness,[10] whereas patients given metoclopramide had less post-operative sedation and earlier discharge times. Patients with a history of dystonic reactions often benefit from pretreatment with diphenhydramine or avoidance of metoclopramide and droperidol altogether. The use of droperidol during subarachnoid anesthesia has been shown to have antiemetic efficacy in the parturient,[5] but may increase the risk of esophageal reflex and regurgitation.[22]

Timing of drug administration is important. Metoclopramide 10 mg given intravenously 5–10 min before atropine administration may counter its undesirable effects on LES tone.[44] Meperidine 1–2 mg/kg given intramuscularly can lower mean barrier pressure (barrier pressure = LES pressure – intragastric pressure) and LES tone. The subsequent administration of metoclopramide 10 mg has been shown to return mean barrier pressure toward baseline levels (Fig. 17.3).[23] Parturients with or without heartburn derive beneficial augmentation of LES tone and, therefore, increased barrier pressure when given metoclopramide.[12,18,19] This effect appears most pronounced in patients with greater intrinsic LES tone.[12]

Patients given epidural opioids (especially morphine) may develop emetic symptoms within 1 h or up to 4–10 h after administration. Early emetic symptoms may be related to the systemic absorption of opioids from the epidural space, analogous to intramuscular opioid administration. Delayed emetic symptoms reflect diffusion of epidural opioids into the cerebrospinal fluid and rostral spread to the brainstem.[45] The μ-opioid receptor agonists appear to mediate the supraspinal emetic response at the CTZ or the vestibular apparatus. Reported prevalences of emetic symptoms with subarachnoid opioids range from 20 to 50%, whereas with epidurally administered opioids prevalences range from 20 to 30%.[34]

Abouleish et al[46] observed a fivefold increase in nausea post-operatively in parturients given subarachnoid morphine 0.2 mg. Leicht et al[47] observed a 20% incidence of post-operative emetic symptoms after cesarean delivery in parturients given epidural morphine 5 mg. Abboud et al[48] demonstrated an 8.5-fold reduction in post-operative emetic symptoms (1.1% versus 9.3%) when butorphanol 2–4 mg was compared with epidural morphine 5 mg for post-cesarean delivery pain relief.

Harrison et al[49] and Eisenach et al[50] prospectively found the highest overall quality of post-cesarean analgesia with epidural morphine 5 mg when compared with patient-controlled analgesia morphine and intramuscular mor-

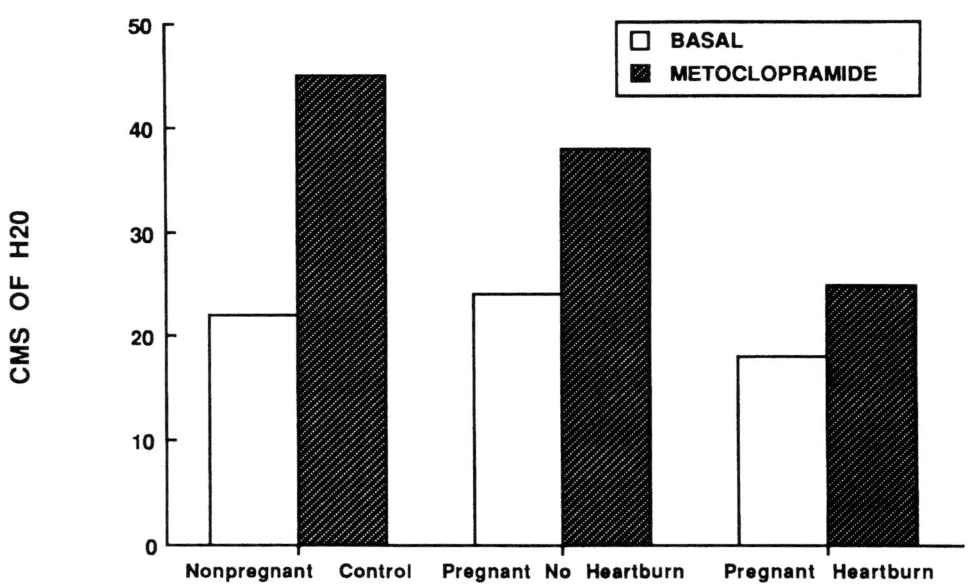

Fig. 17.3 Mean barrier pressure (LES pressure – intragastric pressure) before and after metoclopramide. (From ref. 12 with permission.)

phine. Both groups of workers failed to observe any statistically significant difference in the incidence of emetic symptoms between the three patient groups post-operatively. Interestingly, 50% of patients in Eisenach's et al[50] epidural morphine group developed nausea; 30% of these patients required antiemetic therapy. Although pruritus is usually the most common complication and late respiratory depression the most feared complication of subarachnoid or epidural opioids, perhaps emetic symptoms may leave the patient with the most lasting and unpleasant impression related to their use. Therefore, when using opioids during subarachnoid anesthesia for cesarean delivery it may be prudent to administer a preoperative antiemetic such as metoclopramide beforehand to block the CTZ.

Kotelko et al[51] demonstrated the antiemetic efficacy of transdermal scopolamine (TDS) patches in parturients receiving epidural morphine after cesarean delivery compared with placebo. Post-operative emetic symptoms remained in the 3–25% range during the first 24 h post-operatively despite TDS patches. For prolonged relief of emetic symptoms post-operatively intravenous metoclopramide 10 mg every 4–6 h, or scopolamine patches, a mixed agonist–antagonist (e.g. nalbuphine or butorphanol) or a long-acting oral opioid antagonist such as naltrexone may be used.

Finally, during transport to and from the operating room it is important to avoid abrupt movements, such as turning, and rapid head-up movements, which may trigger vestibular response and cause emetic symptoms.[8] This is especially true if the parturient has recently received opioid medications, as these can sensitize the vestibular apparatus. Adequate pain relief also has been shown to minimize the incidence of post-operative emetic symptoms.[52]

CONCLUSION

Peripartum emetic symptoms are multifactorial in nature. A management scheme to successfully reduce the incidence of emetic symptoms must anticipate those stimuli or events that may provoke or trigger this response. The parturient is unique in that hormonal changes during pregnancy, as well as the mechanical effects of the gravid uterus, predispose the patient to emetic symptoms. Labor itself, and opioid analgesics in particular, may compound this problem by causing gastric stasis.

The intensity, extent and duration of the intraspinal block cannot be overemphasized in preventing intraoperative visceral pain. Adequate local anesthetic dosages combined with subarachnoid or epidural opioids may improve the quality of sensory analgesia and modulate nociceptive sensory afferent impulses to limit visceral pain. Despite their ability to decrease the incidence of visceral pain, subarachnoid and epidural opioids may increase post-operative emetic symptoms by systemic absorption or by their rostral spread to the brainstem. They may also sensitize the vestibular apparatus to the effects of motion or trigger the CTZ directly. Efforts to obtain a high, dense segmental block must be weighed against the risk of precipitating hypotension. Forethought and aggressive prophylactic ephedrine in addition to acute hydration and left uterine displacement are essential to limit the fall of blood pressure from baseline. Supplemental oxygen and pulse oximetry are essential to protect against hypoxemia.

The ideal antiemetic for the parturient undergoing a regional anesthetic for cesarean delivery probably does not exist, especially since the etiology of pre- or post-delivery emetic symptoms may be different and may involve different pathways in triggering either the CTZ or the vomiting center. If antiemetics are utilized, proper timing and sequence of drug administration are important. Metoclopramide, which has antiemetic properties, increases LES tone and tends to reverse the gastric stasis associated with pregnancy, appears to be ideal for the parturient. Prophylactic antiemetics should be considered when the parturient describes a prior history of post-operative emetic symptoms or motion sickness, or when subarachnoid or epidural opioids are being utilized.

REFERENCES

1. Borison H L, Wang S C 1953 Physiology and pharmacology of vomiting. Pharmacol Rev 5: 193
2. Datta S, Alper M H, Ostheimer G W, Weiss J B 1982 Methods for ephedrine administration and nausea and hypotension during spinal anesthesia for cesarean section. Anesthesiology 56: 68
3. Kang Y G, Abouleish E, Caritis S 1982 Prophylactic intravenous ephedrine infusion during spinal anesthesia for cesarean section. Anesth Analg 61: 839
4. Lussos S A, Bader A M, Thornhill M, Datta S 1991 The antiemetic efficacy of prophylactic metoclopramide for cesarean delivery. Society for Obstetric Anesthesia and Perinatology; Abstracts
5. Santos A, Datta S 1984 Prophylactic use of droperidol for control of nausea and vomiting during spinal anesthesia for cesarean section. Anesth Analg 63: 85
6. Chestnut D H, Vandewalker G E, Owen C L et al 1987 Administration of metoclopramide for prevention of nausea and vomiting during epidural anesthesia for elective cesarean section. Anesthesiology 66: 563
7. Bellvile J W, Bross I D J, Howland W S 1960 Post operative nausea and vomiting. IV. Factors related to post operative nausea and vomiting. Anesthesiology 21(2): 186
8. Bellvile J W 1961 Post anesthetic nausea and vomiting. Anesthesiology 22(5): 773
9. Shoeneck F J 1942 Gonadotropic hormone concentration in emesis gravidarum. Am J Obstet Gynecol 43: 308
10. Cohen S E, Woods W A, Wyner J 1984 Antiemetic efficacy of droperidol and metoclopramide. Anesthesiology 60: 67
11. Wyner J, Cohen S E 1982 Gastric volume in early pregnancy; effect of metoclopramide. Anesthesiology 57: 209
12. Brock-Utne J G, Dow T G B, Welman S et al 1978 The effect of metoclopramide on the lower oesophageal sphincter in late pregnancy. Anaesth Intens Care 6: 26
13. Howard F A, Sharp D S 1973 Effect of metoclopramide on gastric emptying during labour. Br Med J 1: 446
14. Frame W T, Allison R H, Moir D D, Nimmo W S 1984 Effect of naloxone on gastric emptying during labour. Br J Anaesth 56: 263

15. Nimmo W S, Wilson J, Prescott L F 1975 narcotic analgesics and delayed gastric emptying during labour. Lancet 1: 890
16. Nimmo W S, Wilson J, Prescott L F 1977 Further studies of gastric emptying during labour. Anaesthesia 32: 100
17. Cotton B R, Smith G 1984 The lower oesophageal sphincter and anaesthesia. Br J Anaesth 56: 37
18. Hey V M F, Ostick D G 1978 Metoclopramide and the gastro-oesophageal sphincter: a study in pregnant women with heartburn. Anaesthesia 33: 462
19. Hey V M F, Ganguli P C, Skinner L D et al 1977 Gastro-oesophageal reflux in late pregnancy. Anaesthesia 32: 372
20. Dow T G B, Cog M R, Brock-Utne J G et al 1978 The effect of atropine on the lower eosphageal sphincter in late pregnancy. Obstet Gynecol 51(4): 426
21. Brock-Utne J G, Rubin J, Welman S et al 1978 The effect of glycopyrrolate (Robinol) on the lower oesophageal sphincter. Can Anaesth Soc J 25(2): 144
22. Brock-Utne J G, Rubin J, Welman S et al 1978 The action of commonly used anti-emetics on the lower esophageal sphincter. Br J Anaesth 50: 295
23. Hey V M F, Ostick D G, Mazumder J K, Lord W D 1981 Pethidine, metoclopramide, and the gastroesophageal sphincter. A study in healthy volunteers. Anaesthesia 36: 173
24. Hey V M F, Phillips K, Woods I 1983 Pethidine, atropine, metoclopramide and the lower esophageal sphincter. Anaesthesia 38: 650
25. Peroutka S J, Snyder S H 1982 Antiemetics: neurotransmitter receptor binding predicts therapeutic actions. Lancer 1: 658
26. Evans C H 1928 Possible complications with spinal anesthesia. Am J Surg 5(6): 581
27. Crocker J S, Vandam L D 1959 Concerning nausea and vomiting during spinal anesthesia. Anesthesiology 20: 589
28. Ratra C K, Badola R P, Bhargava K P 1972 A study of factors concerned in emesis during spinal anesthesia. Br J Anaesth 44: 1208
29. Pedersen H, Santos A C, Steinberg E S et al 1989 Incidence of visceral pain during cesarean section: the effect of varying doses of spinal bupivacaine. Anesth Analg 69: 46
30. Bonica J J, Crepps W, Monk B, Bennett B 1958 Post anesthetic nausea, retching and vomiting. Anesthesiology 19(4): 532
31. Wall P D 1989 To what would Gaston Labat be attending to today? Reg Anesth 14: 261
32. Norris MC 1988 Height, weight, and the spread of subarachnoid hyperbaric bupivacaine in the term parturient. Anesth Analg 67: 555
33. Cousins M I, Mather L E 1984 Intrathecal and epidural administration of opioids. Anesthesiology 61: 276
34. Ready L B 1990 Regional analgesia with intraspinal opioids. In Bonica J J (ed) The management of pain, 2nd edn. Lea & Febiger, Philadelphia, Ch. 95
35. Ackerman W E, Juneja M M, Colclough G W, Kaczorowski D M 1988 Epidural fentanyl significantly decreases nausea and vomiting during uterine manipulation in awake patient undergoing cesarean section. Anesthesiology 69: A679
36. Hunt C O, Naulty S, Bader A M et al 1989 Perioperative analgesia with subarachnoid fentanyl-bupivacaine for cesarean delivery. Anesthesiology 71: 535
37. McGarry J M 1971 A double-blind comparison of the anti-emetic effect during labour of metoclopramide and perphenazine. Br J Anaesth 43: 613
38. Palazzo M G A, Strunin L 1984 Anaesthesia and emesis. II. Prevention and management. Can Anesth Soc J 31: 407
39. Rothenberg D M, Parnass S M, Litwack K et al 1991 Efficacy of ephedrine in the prevention of postoperative nausea and vomiting. Anesth Analg 72: 58
40. Schulze-Delrieu K 1981 Metoclopramide. New Engl J Med 305: 28
41. Tornetta F J 1969 Clinical studies with the new antiemetic, metoclopramide. Anesth Analg 48: 198
42. Murphy D F, Nally B, Gardiner J, Unwin A 1984 Effect of metoclopramide on gastric emptying before elective and emergency caesarean section. Br J Anaesth 56: 1113
43. Bylsma-Howell M, Riggs K W, McMorland G H et al Placental transport of metoclopramide: assessment of maternal and neonatal effects. Can Anaesth Soc J 30: 487
44. Brock-Utne J G, Rubin J, Downing J W et al 1976 The administration of metoclopramide with atropine. (A drug interaction effect on the gastroesophageal sphincter in man.) Anesthesia 31: 1186
45. Bromage P R, Camporesi E M, Durant P A C, Neilsen C H 1982 Non-respiratory side effects of epidural morphine. Anesth Analg 61: 490
46. Abouleish E, Rawal N, Fallon K, Hernandez D 1988 Combined intrathecal morphine and bupivacaine for cesarean section. Anesth Analg 67: 370
47. Leicht C H, Hughes S C, Dailey P A et al 1986 Epidural morphine sulfate for analgesia after cesarean section: a prospective report of 1000 patients. Anesthesiology 65: A366
48. Abboud T K, Moore M, Zhu J et al 1987 Epidural butorphanol or morphine for the relief of post-cesarean section pain: ventilatory responses to carbon dioxide. Anesth Analg 66: 887
49. Harrison D M, Sinatra R, Morgese L, Chung J H 1988 Epidural narcotic and patient-controlled analgesia for post-cesarean section pain relief. Anesthesiology 68: 454
50. Eisenach J C, Grice S C, Dewan D M 1988 Patient-controlled analgesia following cesarean section: a comparison with epidural and intramuscular narcotics. Anesthesiology 68: 444
51. Kotelko D M, Rottman R L, Wright W C et al 1988 Transderm scop (R) decreases post-cesarean nausea and vomiting in patients receiving epidural morphine. Anesthesiology 69: A666
52. Andersen R, Krohg K 1976 Pain as a major cause of postoperative nausea. Can Anaesth Soc J 23: 366
53. Clarke R S J 1984 Nausea and vomiting. Br J Anaesth 56: 19
54. Palazzo M G A, Strunin L 1984 Anaesthesia and emesis. I. Etiology. Can Anaesth Soc J 31: 178

PART B
PRURITUS
B. H. Minzter

Epidural and subarachnoid opioids are widely utilized for anesthesia during labor and vaginal and cesarean delivery, and for post-operative pain control. While their efficacy is well documented, the associated side-effects – more specifically, pruritus – are also well documented, with a prevalence of 20–93% percent,[1] depending on the investigator and the report

The pruritus associated with opioids is seen more commonly after epidural and subarachnoid administration than after systemic administration and is more common in pregnant women than in nonpregnant patients.[2] Interestingly, the pruritus is often localized to the face,[2,3] unlike that of systemically administered opioids, in which the itching tends to be more generalized. This facial itching has recently been linked to reactivation of oral herpes simplex virus.[4,5]

The dermatomal pattern of pruritus provides valuable information regarding its mechanism, which is far from fully understood. It appears that stimulation of opioid μ-receptors may be responsible,[6] though Ballantyne et al describe several other possible mechanisms. It is essential to evaluate these mechanism(s) in an effort to better antagonize, prevent and/or treat the itching.

First, one must consider how the sensation is transmitted and then how it differs from its close companion, pain. Both share a common neuronal pathway in the ascending spinothalamic tract and both are also generated (at least partially) by polymodal nociceptor units. It remains to be defined whether itch is a primary sensation with its own system of fibers and receptors or whether the two sensations are carried by one fiber type with different patterns of nerve impulses.[2]

The term *pruritus* needs to be defined. It is a sensation that provokes the desire to scratch and can be aroused by a variety of mechanical, electrical and chemical stimuli.[2]

Pruritus, in general, may be described as either 'itchy skin', from which itch can be aroused more readily than from normal skin, or 'spontaneous itch', which occurs without any external stimulus. Keele and Armstrong compared 'itchy skin' to hyperalgesia and 'spontaneous itch' to spontaneous pain. Morphine and similar opioids are known to be chemical mediators of pruritus, presumably through the release of histamine. With epidural and subarachnoid opioids, the segmental distribution of pruritus has been encountered. This leads one to believe that the spinal cord itself and/or the spinal roots are a significant site of this opioid-induced itching.[2]

Ballantyne et al[2] have developed a hypothesis to explain intraspinal opioid-induced pruritus. It is their contention that the hyperalgesia and itch that occur after intraspinal administration are manifestations of opioid-mediated facilitation of protective reflexes.

Their claim is that both pain and itch are sensations that invoke defensive, or protective, behaviors. The immediate pain of injury produces a reflex withdrawal. The tenderness associated with such pain induces rubbing, as a means of soothing. Itch, as a sensation, induces scratching, which may itself be a protective reflex. In response to injury, then, protective reflexes are enhanced, resulting in hyperalgesia and itch. Both arise after cutaneous injury and involve the damaged tissue as well as the surrounding area. The tenderness of damaged tissue dissipates, however, if not further stimulated. It is important that an equilibrium be reached between the suppression and facilitation of noxiously induced reflexes. Ballantyne et al contend that opioids have a role in facilitating noxiously induced activity by certain mechanisms described briefly below.

Opioids have excitatory effects, facilitating hyperalgesia and itch. There are opioid receptors on primary afferent neurons in the periphery and on primary sensory ganglia. It appears that peripheral opioid receptors may mediate hyperalgesia;[8,9] when opposed, they may allow central analgesia systems to act unopposed and thus potentiate analgesia.[8]

It has also been demonstrated in animals that subarachnoid injection of high doses of morphine can result in a scratch syndrome, or *hyperalgesia* syndrome.[10] In humans, both hyperalgesia and itch can occur after subarachnoid administration of opioids, in a segmental distribution with respect to injection site.[11,12] In view of this distribution, it seems likely that the process is most localized to the spinal cord or dorsal roots.[2]

The following mechanisms of this excitation have been postulated. First, activation of peripheral opioid receptors may produce itching, as hypothesized by Van der Kooy,[9] but this mechanism remains conjectural.

Itching may occur because certain afferent fibers with a moderating influence are suppressed, leaving only unopposed excitatory activity in other fibers.[2] High concentrations of drug – in this instance, opioid – are required to block conduction of these fibers,[13] posing some problem when explaining the itch produced by small amounts of intraspinal opioid.

Ballantyne et al also proposed that the opioid, once introduced into the cerebrospinal fluid (CSF), may reach distinct sites within the cord and then facilitate noxiously induced activity. They used morphine, with its poor lipid solubility and its often-produced facial itching, as an example, and claimed that penetration to the ventral side of the spinal cord appears to predominate, at least in the cervical region.

Finally, they suggest that opioid antagonism of the inhibitory transmitter, glycine, may be responsible for the pruritus effected by opioids, and also indicate that metabolites of opioids (e.g. morphine 3-glucuronide) may induce and/or potentiate hyperalgesia and itch.[10]

TREATMENT

Treatment of the pruritus induced by intraspinal opioids, as well as by systemic administration such as patient-controlled analgesia (PCA), is variable in its efficacy.

In some reports, intravenous morphine (PCA) produces less pruritus than epidural morphine,[14,15] but if patients do experience pruritus with PCA it is often helpful to decrease the demand dose (e.g. morphine 1 mg) or modify the lockout interval (e.g. morphine every 5 min) to decrease the pruritus. Changing from one opioid to another may be prudent in some cases. Antihistamines such as hydroxyzine or diphenhydramine are also useful.[3]

Various agents have been administered for the prevention and treatment of the pruritus and other side-effects associated with subarachnoid and epidural opioids. Rosen et al[16] found that epidural sufentanil may result in a decreased incidence of pruritus compared with morphine. A continuous infusion of naloxone 0.4–0.6 mg/h can significantly decrease pruritus while maintaining analgesia following subarachnoid administration of morphine.[17] The facial pruritus experienced by some patients can be treated with naloxone, but there remains an increased risk (about 15%) of oral reactivation of herpes simplex virus after epidural morphine in obstetric patients with a positive history of herpes labialis.[4,5] Naltrexone (5 mg) has been found to diminish both the frequency and severity of pruritus, nausea and vomiting after epidural morphine 5 mg with no diminution of the quality or duration of analgesia.[18] Similarly, 6 mg has been found to be an effective oral prophylactic against the pruritus and vomiting associated with subarachnoid morphine, but it tends to decrease the duration of analgesia.[19]

Other agents with varying efficacy include nalbuphine, administered intravenously (2.5 mg) to prevent pruritus induced by epidural fentanyl.[20] Buprenorphine 0.6 mg/50 ml total was used as a replacement for morphine in an epidural infusion with 0.125% bupivacaine in a patient who complained of severe, unremitting pruritus, and the buprenorphine mixture allowed for excellent analgesia while sustaining rapid and complete relief from pruritus.[21] Most recently the mixed agonist–antagonist butorphanol (3 mg) has been combined with epidural opioids (morphine 4 mg) to effectively decrease the occurrence of pruritus and nausea without significantly increasing respiratory depression or sedation, and without adversely affecting duration of analgesia.[1]

REFERENCES

1. Lawhorn C D, McNitt J D, Fibuch E E et al 1991 Epidural morphine with butorphanol for postoperative analgesia after cesarean delivery. Anesth Analg 72: 53–57
2. Ballantyne J C, Loach A B, Carr D B 1988 Itching after epidural and spinal opiates Pain 33: 149–160
3. Bonica J J 1990 The management of pain. Lea & Febiger, Philadelphia, p 1997
4. Crone L L, Conly J M, Storgard C et al 1990 Herpes labialis in parturients receiving epidural morphine following cesarean section. Anesthesiology 73: 208–213
5. Gierarts R, Navalgund A, Vaes L et al 1987 Increased incidence of itching and herpes simplex in patients given epidural morphine after cesarean section. Anesth Analg 66: 1321–1324
6. Martin W R 1986 Clinical evidence for different narcotic receptors and relevance for the clinician. Ann Emerg Med 15: 1026
7. Keele C A, Armstrong D 1964 Substances producing pain and itch. Edward Arnold, London
8. Van der Kooy D, Nagy J I 1985 Hyperalgesia mediated by peripheral opiate receptors in the rat. Behav Brain Res 17: 203–211
9. Van der Kooy D 1986 Hyperalgesic functions of peripheral opiate receptors, In: D D Kelly (ed): Stress-induced analgesia. Ann NY Acad Sci 467: 154–168
10. Yaksh T L, Harty G J, Onofrio B M 1986 High doses of spinal morphine produce a nonopiate receptor-mediated hyperesthesia: clinical and theoretic implications. Anesthesiology 64: 590–597
11. Bromage P R, Camporesi E M, Durant P A C, Nielsen C H 1982 Rostral spread of epidural morphine. Anesthesiology 56: 431–436
12. Bromage P R, Camporesi E M, Durant P A C, Nielsen C H 1982 Non-respiratory side effects of epidural morphine. Anesth Analg 61: 490–495
13. Staiman A, Seeman P 1974 The impulse-blocking concentrations of anesthetics, alcohols, anticonvulsants, barbiturates and narcotics on phrenic and sciatic nerves. Can J Physiol Pharmacol 52: 535–550
14. Harrison D M, Sinatra R, Morgese L, Chung J H 1988 Epidural narcotic and patient-controlled analgesia for post-cesarean section pain relief. Anesthesiology 68: 454–457
15. Eisenach J C, Grice S C, Dewan D M 1988 Patient-controlled analgesia following cesarean section: a comparison with epidural and intramuscular narcotics. Anesthesiology 68: 444–448
16. Rosen M S, Dailey P A, Hughes S C et al 1988 Epidural sufentanil for postoperative analgesia after cesarean section. Anesthesia 68: 448–454
17. Dailey P A, Bookshire G L, Shnider S M et al 1985 The effects of naloxone associated with the intrathecal use of morphine in labor. Anesth Analg 64: 658–666
18. Cullen M, Altstatt A H, Kwon N J et al 1988 Naltrexone reversal of the side effects of epidural morphine. Anesthesiology 69: A336
19. Abboud T K, Lee K, Chai M et al 1989 Prophylactic oral naltrexone with intrathecal morphine for cesarean section: effects on adverse reactions and analgesia. Anesthesiology 71: A836
20. Davies G G, From R 1988 A blinded study using nalbuphine for prevention of pruritus induced by epidural fentanyl. Anesthesia 69: 763–765
21. Keaveny J P, Harper N J N 1989 Treatment of epidural morphine-induced pruritus with buprenorphine (letter). Anesthesia 44: 691

PART C
URINARY RETENTION
M. A. Procopio

The etiology of urinary retention, a common complication of delivery, can be difficult to determine. Changes in the lower urinary system that occur toward the end of gestation include increased bladder capacity and a loss of bladder tone.[1] Consequently, urinary dysfunction may occur irrespective of the method of delivery or type of anesthesia.

EFFECT OF LABOR AND DELIVERY

The most common causes of urinary dysfunction after delivery among patients who have not received a regional anesthetic were thought to be a loss of desire to micturate and pain secondary to perineal tears, sutures and bruising.[2] Early studies by Bennetts and Judd[3] using cystoscopic and cystometric measurements reported a hypotonic post-partum bladder in 86% of patients, a finding that was supported by similar results of a study by Youssef in 1965.[3,4] More recently, Kerr-Wilson et al in 1984 found normal urodynamic measurements at 48 h and again at 4 weeks after delivery. The method of delivery, infant weight and episiotomy did not affect the likelihood in a hypotonic post-partum bladder in several studies. The authors attribute these discrepancies to changes in the management of labor and the puerperium, including more frequent use of oxytocin stimulation and cesarean delivery, which shorten labor. Also, patients were catheterized 4–6 h after delivery, whereas in previous studies patients were observed for 8 h or longer prior to catheterization if no discomfort or bladder distension occurred.[5]

EFFECT OF ANALGESIA AND ANESTHESIA

More controversial is the effect of analgesia and anesthesia on the post-partum bladder. Bennetts and Judd[3] reported that antepartum analgesia did not account for their findings of bladder hypotonicity. However, 81% of their patients received scopolamine, which causes bladder relaxation through its anticholinergic effects.[3,5]

Epidural anesthesia for labor and delivery has become increasingly popular as this technique provides excellent pain relief and minimal motor block. By suppressing afferent sensory impulses from the bladder and inhibiting the reflex mechanism for micturition, epidural anesthesia may delay normal voiding.[6] Even a single episode of overdistension of the bladder may produce urethrovesicular dysfunction due to irreversible damage to the detrusor muscle.[7] Increased residual volume and urinary retention are known side-effects of epidural anesthesia. Weil et al[8] reported a significant difference in residual volume and maximum cystometric capacities from the second to the fifth days post-partum between those patients who received epidural anesthesia and those who did not. They concluded that bladder distension during or after labor with an epidural anesthetic rather than the epidural block itself may be responsible for these results since the anesthetic effect of an epidural anesthetic lasts less than 24 h.

When evaluating patients receiving epidural anesthesia for vaginal or elective cesarean delivery, both bladder compliance and maximum cystometric capacity were significantly lower in the parturients following spontaneous vaginal delivery with and without epidural anesthesia. Factors thought to be contributory include the following:

1. active labor and obstetric trauma were avoided;
2. a urinary catheter was left in place post-operatively for 12 h, thus avoiding bladder distension; and
3. an ‘irritable’ state of the detrusor muscle and bladder contributed to a reduction in voluntary capacity.[8]

EFFECT OF INTRASPINAL OPIOIDS

The addition of opioid to the local anesthetic in epidural anesthesia has become increasingly popular for pain relief during labor. Studies specific to urinary retention in this patient population receiving epidural opioids are lacking. However, a prevalence of urinary dysfunction varying from 39 to 95% following epidural morphine in general surgical patients has been reported.[9,10] It must be remembered that urinary retention is also a known side-effect of systemic opioid administration.

Rawal et al[11] reported consistent, predictable relaxation of the detrusor muscle and increased bladder capacity leading to urinary retention for 14–16 h following epidural morphine regardless of dose among groups receiving epidural morphine 2 mg, 4 mg, and 10 mg. The degree of detrusor relaxation was more marked after higher doses, whereas the duration, the increase in maximum bladder capacity and duration of urinary retention were not dose related.[11] The effects of different opioids on urinary retention have yet to be studied.

A possible mechanism of urinary retention in patients receiving epidural or subarachnoid morphine is that the morphine travels rostrally in the cerebrospinal fluid to the supraspinal structures at the level of the pons, where it causes an inhibitory effect on the primary micturition center. However, the time needed for this cephalad spread of morphine is believed to be longer than the 15–30 min it takes for epidural morphine to cause bladder relaxation. Therefore, a spinal site of action through autonomic inhibition of sacral parasympathetic outflow has been suggested. The possible presence of opioid receptors in the urinary bladder able to cause this direct effect on bladder relaxation is another possible explanation.[11]

TREATMENT

Attempts at treating urinary retention following epidural opioids have included administration of the synthetic cholinergic agonist drug, bethanechol, and the opioid antagonist, naloxone. Subcutaneous injection of bethanechol 5 mg had been recommended as initial therapy, however, intravenous naloxone 0.4 mg–0.8 mg has been more reliable in initiating micturition.[11–13]

Current recommendations for patient care during and following epidural and subarachnoid anesthesia include frequent checks to determine if bladder distension is occurring. If attempts at spontaneous voiding are unsuccessful, catheterization is necessary. In addition, all patients after cesarean delivery should have urinary bladder catheters for 12–24 h post-operatively.

REFERENCES

1. Muellner S R 1938 Physiological bladder changes during pregnancy and the puerperium. J Urol 41: 691–695
2. Grove L H 1973 Backache, headache and bladder dysfunction after delivery. Br J Anaesth 45: 1147
3. Bennetts F A, Judd G E 1941 Studies of the post-partum bladder. Am J Obstet Gynecol 42: 419–427
4. Youssef A F 1956 Cystometric studies in gynecology and obstetrics. Obstet Gynecol 8: 181–188
5. Kerr-Wilson R H J, Thompson S W et al 1984 Effect of labor on the postpartum bladder. Obstet Gynecol 64: 1, 115–117
6. Katz J, Aidinis S J 1980 Complications of spinal and epidural anesthesia. J Bone Joint Surg 62A: 1219–1222
7. Hinman F 1976 Post-operative overdistension of the bladder. Surg Gynecol Obstet 142: 901–902
8. Weil A et al 1983 Effect of lumbar epidural analgesia on lower urinary tract function in the immediate post-partum period. Br J Obstet Gynaecol 90: 428–432
9. Torda T A, Pubus D A 1981 Clinical experience with epidural morphine. Anesth Intens Care 9: 129–134
10. Lanz E, Theiss D, Riess W, Sommer V 1982 Epidural morphine for postoperative analgesia: a double-blind study. Anesth Analg 61: 236–240
11. Rawal N, Möllefors K, Alexlsson K et al 1983 An experimental study of urodynamic effects of epidural morphine and of halaxone reversal. Anesth Analg 62: 641–665
12. Cousins M J, Mather L E 1984 Intrathecal and epidural administration of opioids. Anesthesiology 61: 276–310
13. Bromage P R, Camporesi E M, Chestnut D 1980 Epidural narcotics for post-operative analgesia. Anesth Analg 59: 7, 473–480

18. Other intraspinal analgesics

H. Carp P. G. W. Cramp

The search for the ideal anesthetic technique for the parturient began centuries before the era of modern anesthesia. In 1818, Benjamin Rush described the essential characteristics of the ideal anesthetic for obstetrics.[1] He expressed the hope that 'a medicine would be discovered which should suspend sensibility altogether and leave irritability or powers of motion unimpaired'. After more than a century, the ideal anesthetic for labor analgesia has still not been found. However, recent developments in the neurophysiology and neuropharmacology of pain have led to major advances toward this goal.

PROPOSED MECHANISM OF INTRASPINAL ANALGESIA: ION CHANNELS, HYPERPOLARIZATION AND THE INHIBITION OF NERVE CELLS

The processing of pain information begins in the dorsal horn of the spinal cord and is modulated in part by the excitation of the so-called wide dynamic response neurons.[2] Although this process is not entirely understood, the primary action of most analgesics, including opioids and adrenergic agonists, is thought to involve inhibition of activation of neural pain-encoding networks by their effects on individual nerve cell ion channels. Although single nerve cells do not act independently in vivo, in vitro studies using single cells have shown that spinal analgesic agents may act to inhibit nerve cell firing by hyperpolarizing these cells as a result of increases in potassium (or chloride) ion conductance.[3]

Inhibition of nerve cells is an important modulator of nerve cell function. One example of the importance of nerve cell inhibition is the reduction in excitability of motor neurons supplying opposing muscle groups. This is brought about by the opening of chloride channels, which permits chloride to enter the cell, leading to hyperpolarization and inhibition of nerve cell excitation.[3] Interestingly, nerve cell hyperpolarization as a result of increased chloride ion conductance may be the mechanism underlying the spinal analgesic effects of benzodiazepines.

Another way to hyperpolarize nerve cells and thus inhibit firing is to open potassium channels, which will allow potassium ions to diffuse out of the cells. In fact, the bradycardic effects of acetylcholine binding to muscarinic receptors in the heart is the result of increased potassium ion conductance, which hyperpolarizes and inhibits the cardiac pacemaker and slows the heart rate.[3]

Interestingly, the bulk of experimental evidence also suggests that hyperpolarization of nerve cells, as a result of increased potassium conductance with subsequent inhibition of firing, may explain the spinal analgesic action of many drugs, including opioids and adrenergic agonists.[3] Many of the in vitro experiments that form the basis for this conclusion were carried out by Dr Alan North and his colleagues on small pieces of nerve tissue with the tip of a glass microelectrode positioned in the cell interior so that the membrane potential can be measured.[3] The results of such in vitro experiments demonstrate that opioids, norepinephrine, clonidine and somatostatin produce membrane hyperpolarization and inhibition of neuronal firing. This is shown in Figure 18.1 for an enkephalin derivative.[4]

Next, experiments to confirm the mechanism of nerve cell hyperpolarization were conducted using the voltage clamp method. The results of voltage clamp experiments

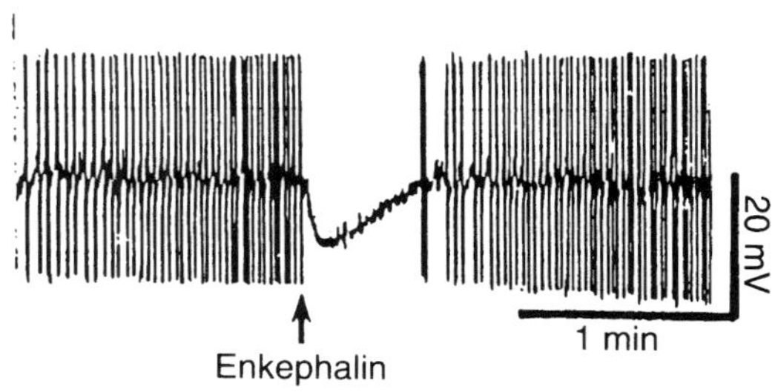

Fig. 18.1 Enkephalin inhibits nerve cell firing. An intracellular recording from a spontaneously firing locus ceruleus neuron. Enkephalin (D-Ala^2-D-leu^5-enkephalin) was applied to a pipette positioned just above the brain slice at the times indicated by the arrows. The cell hyperpolarized and the action potential discharge was transiently inhibited. (Adapted from ref. 4 with permission.)

demonstrate that the action of opioids, clonidine, norepinephrine and somatostatin[4] is to open ion channels in the membrane that are selectively permeable to potassium.[3] In the normal cellular environment this current is outward and leads to hyperpolarization and inhibition of cell firing. This may be the effector mechanism underlying the spinal analgesic action of these agents.[3]

However, increased potassium conductance following opioid or adrenergic agent receptor binding requires the subsequent activation of a signal transducer, known as a G-protein, that is linked to the ion channel.[3–5] This is summarized in Figure 18.2. Binding of an opioid or adrenergic agonist to its spinal cord receptor activates the associated G-protein. The G-protein then directly opens a potassium channel in the membrane to produce hyperpolarization of the nerve cell and inhibition of nerve cell firing in a pain-sensitive neuron with resultant analgesia.[3–5]

The interposition of a G-protein between receptor and effector allows for further diversification of the action of the particular agonist. In fact, the same G-proteins mediating increases in potassium ion conductance by spinal analgesics may also open other ion channels such as calcium or activate cellular enzymes such as adenyl cyclase, and these effects may also be important.[3–5] Interestingly, indirect evidence suggests that the action of general anesthetics may be mediated by G-proteins.[6]

In summary, based on in vitro studies, a variety of drugs capable of producing spinal analgesia interact with their specific cell surface receptors to hyperpolarize nerve cells. Hyperpolarization of nerve cells will inhibit nerve cell firing, causing a reduction in neurotransmitter release and the production of analgesia. Opioids, adrenergic agents and somatostatin may produce this effect by increasing potassium ion conductance, and benzodiazepines increase chloride conductance.

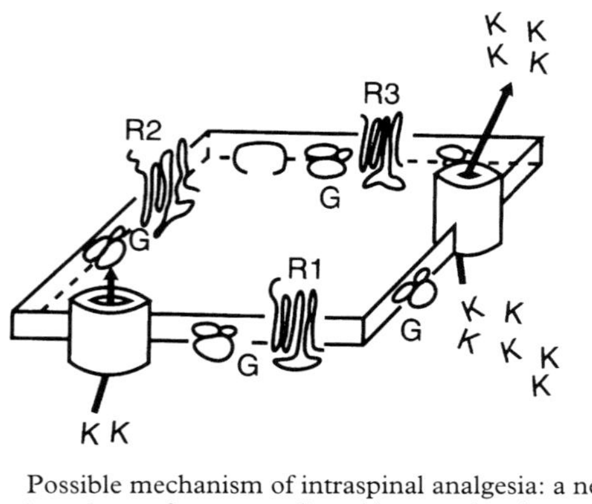

Fig. 18.2 Possible mechanism of intraspinal analgesia: a nerve cell membrane (exterior surface upward) and its associated membrane receptors and ion channels. The cellular response to intraspinal analgesic agents is initiated by binding to specific cell-surface receptors (R1, R2, R3) followed by activation of a common G-protein (G). Next, the activated G-protein directly opens potassium channels (K) to produce membrane hyperpolarization, inhibition of nerve cell firing and analgesia. R1, R2, R3, represent opioid, adrenergic agonist or somatostatin receptors.

Understanding the basic cellular mechanisms of pain and analgesia will certainly lead to the development of more effective analgesic agents and techniques capable of producing analgesia without maternal or fetal side-effects.

SPECIFIC AGENTS

Adrenergic agonists

Recent studies in experimental animals and humans demonstrate that adrenergic agonists, including epinephrine, norepinephrine and clonidine, are capable of producing profound analgesia following epidural or subarachnoid administration.[7–9]

Despite its relatively poor selectivity for the α_2-receptor, clonidine is the only α_2-agonist currently available for clinical use in this country.[7] Epidural clonidine produces analgesia by a nonopioid mechanism and may offer advantages over other agents for labor analgesia.[8] Unlike local anesthetics, clonidine does not produce motor or sensory blockade and, unlike opioids, clonidine has not been reported to produce delayed respiratory depression, nausea, pruritus or urinary retention. In fact, a recent study in pregnant ewes demonstrated that epidural clonidine in analgesic doses did not produce significant maternal or fetal side-effects.[8] Furthermore, epidural clonidine has been used to provide post-cesarean delivery analgesia in humans and was found to provide analgesia of intermediate duration with minimal maternal side-effects.[9] However, under certain conditions epidural or subarachnoid clonidine may produce hypotension, bradycardia and decreased ventilatory response to carbon dioxide.[10–12] Hemodynamic depression may limit the usefulness of clonidine in the laboring patient. However, more specific α_2-adrenergic agonists, including dexmedetomidine[7] and tizanidine,[11] may produce analgesia with fewer side-effects than clonidine. Finally, α_2-agonists may act synergistically with co-administered local anesthetic or opioid to improve the quality and duration of analgesia.[7]

α_2-Adrenergic agonists appear to be promising agents for analgesia in obstetrics.

Enkephalins

Methionine-enkephalin (met-enkephalin), a rapidly metabolized, naturally occurring opioid peptide, may be an ideal intraspinal opioid for use in obstetric anesthesia. Although met-enkephalin produces analgesia following intracerebroventricular administration,[13] preliminary studies in guinea pigs demonstrate that continuous subarachnoid infusion of met-enkephalin produces prolonged analgesia (H. Carp, unpublished observations). However, it does not produce analgesia or respiratory depression following systemic administration because of its rapid degradation by proteases contained in maternal and fetal plasma and tissues (plasma half-life, 1 min).[13] Interestingly, following acute intravenous administration of large doses of met-enkephalin to pregnant ewes, the drug was rapidly degraded in the maternal and fetal plasma and was unable to affect the fetal lambs.[14]

Subarachnoid administration of met-enkephalin to laboring patients could produce analgesia without the risk of fetal respiratory depression, because of rapid metabolism, and without the motor weakness and hypotension associated with currently used local anesthetics. This may result in improved fetal and maternal safety as well as a lesser effect on the labor process.

In contrast to the rapid degradation of met-enkephalin, metkephamid is a synthetic peptide derivative of met-enkephalin resistant to degradation and capable of producing analgesia following subarachnoid or even systemic administration in animals and man.[15] Interestingly, studies in pregnant rats and sheep have shown that metkephamid does not cross the placental barrier following maternal systemic administration of analgesic doses. Therefore, metkephamid may be an ideal analgesic agent for labor, capable of producing analgesia but unable to produce fetal depression because of an inability to cross the placental barrier.

Benzodiazepines

A number of representatives of the nonopioid, noncatecholamine drug class, including benzodiazepines, can produce intraspinal analgesia. Several studies have suggested that systemic administration of benzodiazepines may depress nociception.[16] More importantly, further studies have also shown that benzodiazepines may have profound analgesic properties following subarachnoid administration.[17–20] Lumbar subarachnoid administration of small doses of midazolam in anesthetized dogs depresses sympathetic reflexes evoked by nociceptive stimulation of the animals' hindlimbs, but not forelimbs.[17] Furthermore, subarachnoid administration of midazolam to patients with post-operative and chronic pain produced significant analgesia.[18] In that study, relatively large doses were used and significant sedation was produced. However, a more recent study clearly showed that subarachnoid administration of small doses of midazolam produced analgesia in rats.[19] In contrast, control animals receiving intraperitoneal injections of the same dose of midazolam did not demonstrate analgesia and actually developed hyperalgesia. These investigators suggested that the analgesic effect of midazolam may stem from its action at the spinal level, whereas its sedative and hyperalgesic effects are a function of its supraspinal action.

Finally, Serrao et al[20], using rats, investigated the effects of subarachnoid midazolam on the threshold for pain induced by brief passage of electric current between pairs of electrodes placed on the tail and the skin of the neck. They concluded that subarachnoid midazolam produces segmental, spinally mediated analgesia and presented indirect evidence suggesting that midazolam may produce spinally mediated analgesia by binding to nonopioid receptors in the spinal cord (i.e. benzodiazepine receptors). In support of their idea, benzodiazepine binding sites have been demonstrated in the spinal cord and endogenous benzodiazepine-like substances have been discovered in human cerebrospinal fluid.

Membrane preparations of benzodiazepine receptors have been linked with the receptors for γ-aminobutyric acid (GABA). The benzodiazepine–GABA receptor complex consists of four elongated subunits, each of which contains a central axial chloride channel outside of which is the GABA receptor and benzodiazepine receptor.[21,22] The main function of the complex is to allosterically regulate GABA receptor-mediated gating of the chloride channels. It may be that the combination of midazolam with benzodiazepine receptors in the spinal cord potentiates the effect of GABA on the chloride channel and increases chloride ion conductance so that chloride ions enter the cell, leading to hyperpolarization and inhibition of nerve cell firing and potentiation of the analgesic effect of GABA. (This effect is analogous to the hyperpolarization of nerve cells produced by opioids and clonidine as a result of increases in potassium ion conductance.)

These experimental findings with midazolam suggest that, in addition to opioids, benzodiazepines may be capable of producing intraspinal analgesia.

Progesterone

It is becoming increasingly evident that steroid hormones, including progesterone, can act on the central nervous system to produce a variety of behavioral effects, independent of their hormonal action. In fact, the anesthetic effects of steroids may be related to their ability to potentiate GABA-mediated increases in chloride ion conductance, in a manner similar to benzodiazepines.[23]

Interestingly, the subarachnoid administration of progesterone markedly potentiates the analgesic effects of neuraxial opioids in rats (H. Carp and A. Jayaram, unpublished observations). This effect of progesterone is blocked by prior administration of picrotoxin or bicuculline, agents that block GABA-mediated increase in chloride ion conductance.

These experimental results suggest that increased progesterone levels during pregnancy may potentiate the analgesic action of endogenous opioids secreted in response to labor pain and may help to explain the decreased analgesic requirements in these patients.

In addition to analgesic effects, increased progesterone levels may be related to the decrease in minimum alveolar concentration (MAC) for potent inhaled agents, as well as the increased sensitivity to local anesthetic blocks associated with pregnancy. In support of this, chronically administered progesterone decreases halothane MAC in rabbits.[24]

Calcitonin

Calcitonin is a polypeptide hormone initially detected in thyroid and recently found also in brain, pituitary and cerebrospinal fluid. In addition to its effect on calcium and phosphate metabolism, prolonged analgesia in animals and humans has been reported following calcitonin administration.[25–27] Indirect evidence suggests that calcitonin-mediated analgesia may act through the serotinergic system.

Bates et al[25] reported that subarachnoid calcitonin produced profound analgesia in a study of 56 postoperative patients with minimal side-effects. However, further experience using subarachnoid calcitonin suggests that unacceptable side-effects limit its usefulness as a spinal analgesic (M. Puig, personal communication).

Somatostatin

The nonopioid tetradecapeptide, somatostatin, was first isolated from bovine hypothalamus. The presence of somatostatin in dorsal root ganglia and small primary sensory neurons (C-afferents) suggests a possible role as a neurotransmitter or neuromodulator of pain. In fact, somatostatin has been shown to produce analgesia in experimental animals.[28] However, in some reports the analgesic action of subarachnoid somatostatin has been associated with spinal cord neurotoxicity and flaccid paralysis.[29] In humans, intracerebroventricular, subarachnoid and epidural administration of somatostatin has been reported to produce analgesia when used to treat chronic pain without evidence of neurotoxicity.[29–31]

However, there are conflicting reports of the efficacy of epidural somatostatin in the treatment of acute postoperative pain. Chrubasik et al[31] reported effective analgesia following epidural somatostatin in eight postoperative patients and further reported that epidural somatostatin produced segmental analgesia.[32] In contrast to the results obtained by Chrubasik et al, a more recent study by other investigators reported that epidural somatostatin failed to provide adequate analgesia after cholecystectomy in 24 patients.[33] This study also failed to demonstrate any cutaneous analgesia following somatostatin.

The role of somatostatin as an effective analgesic agent needs to be clarified by further study.

CONCLUSIONS

Recent developments in the neurophysiology and neuropharmacology of pain and analgesia will bring us closer to development of the ideal anesthetic for obstetrics through the discovery of drugs that are capable of altering neural transmission in such a way that analgesia results without motor, sensory or sympathetic block.

After more than a century, we are moving closer to discovering the ideal analgesic for obstetrics that in 1818 Banjamin Rush hoped would be able to 'suspend sensibility altogether and leave irritability or powers of motion unimpaired'.[1]

REFERENCES

1. Heaton C E 1946 The history of anesthesia and analgesia in obstetrics. J Hist Med Allied Sci 1: 567–572
2. Watkins D E 1986 Multiple endogenous opiate and non-opiate analgesia systems: evidence of their existence and clinical implications. Ann NY Acad Sci 467: 273–299
3. North R A 1989 Drug receptors and the inhibition of nerve cells. Br J Pharmacol 98: 13–28
4. Williams J T, Egan T M, North R A 1982 Enkephalin opens potassium channels on mammalian central neurones. Nature 299: 74–77
5. Brown A M, Birnbaumer L 1988 Direct G protein gating of ion channels. Am J Physiol 23: H401
6. Firestone S, Firestone L L 1988 Anesthetic alcohols modulate membrane-bound protein kinase C function. FASEB J 2: A1381
7. Maze M, Segal I S, Bloor B C 1988 Clonidine and other alpha-2-adrenergic agonists: strategies for rational use of these novel anesthetic agents. J Clin Anesth 1: 146–157
8. Eisenach J C, Castro M I, Dewan D M, Rose J C 1989 Epidural clonidine analgesia in obstetrics: sheep studies. Anesthesiology 70: 51
9. Viscomi C M, Eisenach J C 1989 Epidural clonidine for post cesarean section analgesia. Society for Obstetric Anesthesia and Perinatology (Abstracts) D24
10. Eisenach J C, Lysak S Z, Viscomi C M 1989 Epidural clonidine analgesia following surgery: phase 1. Anesthesiology 71: 640–646
11. Lubenow T et al 1989 Analgesic and hemodynamic evaluation of intrathecal clonidine and tizanidine. Anesthesiology 71: A648
12. Penon C, Ecoffey C, Cohen S E 1989 Ventilatory effects of epidural clonidine. Anesthesiology 71: A649
13. Buscher H H et al 1976 Evidence for analgesic activity of enkephalin in the mouse. Nature 261: 423–425
14. Lagamma E F, Itskovitz J, Abraham M R 1983 Maturation of circulatory responses to methionine-enkephalin Pediatr Res 17: 162–167
15. Frederickson R C A et al 1982 Preclinical pharmacology of metkephamid (LY 127623) a met-enkephalin analogue. In Harris L S (ed) National Institute on Drug Abuse Research Monograph p 150–156
16. Boralessa H, Senior D F, Whitwam J G 1983 Cardiovascular response to intubation. A comparative study of thiopentone and midazolam. Anaesthesia 38: 623–627
17. Niv D, Whitwam J G, Loh L 1983 Depression of nociceptive sympathetic reflexes by the intrathecal administration of midazolam. Br J Anaesth 55: 541–547
18. Rigoli M 1983 Epidural analgesia with benzodiazepines. In Tiengo M, Cousins M J (eds) Pharmacological basis of anesthesiology: clinical pharmacology of new analgesics and anesthetics. Raven Press, New York p 69–73
19. Niv D, Davidovich, S, Geller E, Urca G 1988 Analgesic and

hyperalgesic effects of midazolam: dependence on route of administration. Anesth Analg 67: 1169–1173

20. Serrao J M, Goodchild C S, Stubbs S C, Gent J P 1989 Intrathecal midazolam and fentanyl in the rat: evidence for different spinal antinociceptive effects. Anesthesiology 70: 780–786
21. Braesfrap C, Nielsen M 1982 Neurotransmitters and CNS disease: anxiety. Lancet 2: 1030–1032
22. Schoefield P R et al 1987 Sequence and functional expression of the GABA receptor shows a ligand-gated receptor superfamily. Nature 328: 221–227
23. Kavaliers M, Wiebe J P 1987 Analgesic effects of the progesterone metabolite 3 α-hydroxy-5 α-pregnan-20-one and possible modes of action in mice. Brain Res 415: 393–398
24. Datta S, Migliozzi R P, Flanagan H L, Krieger N R 1989 Chronically administered progesterone decreases halothane requirements in rabbits. Anesth Analg 68: 46–50
25. Bates R F I et al 1981 Comparison of the analgesic effects of subcutaneous and intracerebroventricular injection of calcitonin on acetic acid induced abdominal constrictions in the mouse. Br J Pharmacol 72: 575–579
26. Miralles F S et al 1987 Post-operative analgesia induced by subarachnoid lidocaine plus calcitonin. Anesth Analg 66: 615–618
27. Fraioli F et al 1982 Subarachnoid injection of salmon calcitonin induces analgesia in man. Eur J Pharmacol 78: 381–382
28. Chrabasik J et al 1984 Somatostatin: a potent analgesic substance. Lancet 2: 1208–1209
29. Gaumann D M, Yaksh T L 1988 Intrathecal somatostatin in rats: antinociception only in the presence of toxic effects. Anesthesiology 68: 733–742
30. Meynadier J, Chrubasik J, Dubar M, Wunsch E 1985 Intrathecal somatostatin in terminally ill patients. A report of two cases. Pain 23: 9–12
31. Chrubasik J, Meynadier J, Scherpereel P, Wunsch E 1985 The effect of epidural somatostatin on postoperative pain. Anesth Analg 64: 1085–1088
32. Carli P, Ecoffey C, Chrubasik J et al 1986 Spread of analgesia and ventilatory response to CO_2 following epidural somatostatin. Anesthesiology 65: suppl A216
33. Desborough J P et al 1989 Hormonal and metabolic responses to cholecystectomy: comparison of extradural somatostatin and diamorphine. Br J Anaesth 63: 508–513

19. Assessment of the effects of epidural anesthesia

Part A Maternal considerations *J. Thorburn*
Part B Fetal and neonatal considerations *A. I. Hollmén*
Part C Plasma concentrations of local anesthetics in newborns after maternal epidural administration *E. Giaufré B. Bruguerolle*

PART A
MATERNAL CONSIDERATIONS
J. Thorburn

To a healthy mother, epidural anesthesia offers relief from the pain and distress of labor, but not all mothers either wish to receive it or require it. Although it has been estimated that fewer than 1% of mothers will experience no pain in labor, 24% of mothers judge the pain of labor to be intolerable.[1] The pain of labor is perceived by the mother and her subjective experience is the result of complex and interrelated beliefs. If the parturient is a primigravid, her beliefs and aspirations are founded entirely upon education, rumor and other mothers' – including her own mother's – experiences. A first labor is a unique experience, and it has been claimed that a woman's personality may be damaged if labor is unduly prolonged.[2] The experience of labor differs from patient to patient, from obstetric unit to unit and from country to country. A mother cannot view labor objectively, but good antenatal care should ensure that she has been exposed to sensible advice regarding the management of her pain which should be comprehensive and include nonpharmacologic and pharmacologic methods of pain control as well as information about epidural anesthesia. Before the onset of labor, the mother should understand what is meant by epidural anesthesia, how it is administered, its benefits and its complications. Since pain is perceived by the mother, she must have sufficient understanding to give an informed opinion with regard to its management. In these litiginous times, the obstetrician and the anesthesiologist have a duty to explain to the mother the advantages and the limitations of all methods of pain relief, including epidural anesthesia.

Epidural anesthesia may have profound effects on the maternal physiology, the majority of which can be minimized with careful administration of the epidural anesthetic, skilled nursing care and meticulous maternal and fetal monitoring. Serious maternal risks exist but are rare and, indeed, their incidence is reassuringly low, but mothers must be informed of their existence and not led to believe that pain relief is obtained at no cost. In a series of 505 000 epidural blocks, serious but nonfatal side-effects were reported to occur in 108 mothers.[3]

To the mother, the benefits of the effective pain relief provided by epidural anesthesia will outweigh the minor effects that accompany a successful block. The type and frequency of side-effects and their influence on the mother is dependent on the type of block, whether it is continuous infusion, intermittent top-up injections, patient-controlled epidural administration, and the concentration and volume of the solutions injected. These factors are controlled by the anesthesiologist, and careful administration implies that these elements of the equation are tailored to the needs of the mother.

Effective epidural sensory anesthesia is accompanied by a feeling of warmth in the lower limbs, which occurs within a few minutes of injection. If the first dose is administered through the epidural needle, the mother will often remark on the warmth in her bottom (buttocks) if the injection was made in the sitting position. For the majority of mothers, the next stage as the block spreads is a lessening of the pain from the contractions, but, unless a large dose of local anesthetic is given, the pain is usually diminished, not eliminated. Frequently, the mother does not experience any subjective feelings other than that resulting from the pain relief. However, conducting the block demands attention to detail and frequent observation of specific physiologic variables. No mother should have an epidural anesthetic administered without an indwelling intravenous catheter and a suitable free-flowing i.v. infusion.

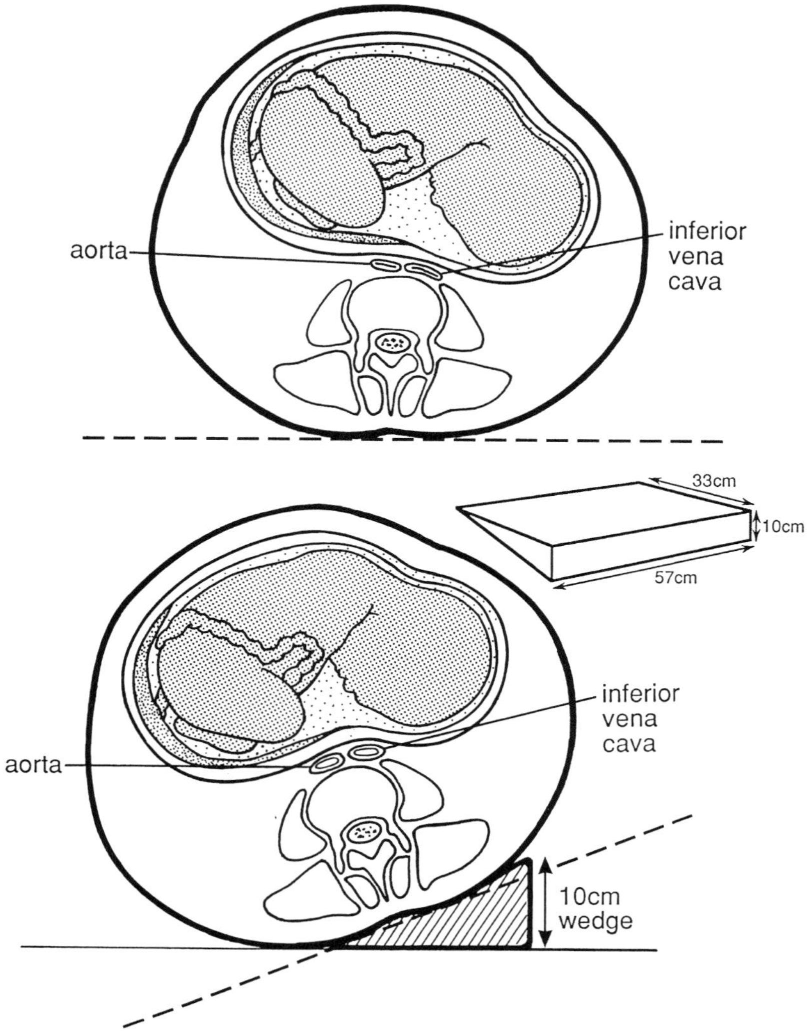

Fig. 19.1 Wedge under hip rotating pregnant uterus to the side, relieving aortocaval compression.

CARDIOVASCULAR EFFECTS

In normal pregnancy, the changes in the cardiovascular system are extensive and significant. The majority favor the neonate, to improve gas exchange at the placental level and to maintain placental blood flow, thus ensuring adequate fetal growth. The majority of these changes have occurred by 20 weeks' gestation, and are discussed in detail in Chapter 5. It is sufficient to recall here that by 30 weeks' gestation, the cardiac output has increased by more than 30% but that the rate of increase slows by term. Both the stroke volume and heart rate are increased, as is the plasma volume and red cell mass.

Vena caval occlusion

The inferior vena cava (IVC) lies slightly to the right of the midline as it passes through the abdomen. As the fetus develops, the position of gravid uterus changes. As pregnancy progresses, the uterus enlarges and, in the second and third trimester, can put pressure on the IVC that will impede the blood flow, reduce venous return and thus cardiac output if the mother lies in the supine position.[4] This may have little detectable effect in the mother, however, in a significant proportion of patients, the result is a marked reduction in maternal blood pressure resulting in the supine hypotensive syndrome. Of interest, no pregnant woman at term will choose to lie in the unmodified supine position, but will do so if asked by medical or nursing staff.

If an epidural anesthetic is functioning, the adoption of the unmodified supine position may be deleterious to both the mother and baby as the vasodilation which results from the sympathetic block will, in addition to the effect of vena caval occlusion, cause a significant decrease in venous return and, thus, cardiac output. It is impossible to overemphasize how important it is for a mother at term to avoid the use of the unmodified supine position. In the author's hospital, all beds are fitted with a Crawford wedge, a commercially manufactured product (Fig. 19.1), which is always in place, and mothers are encouraged to adopt the position that they find comfortable. This position is inevitably either sitting or lateral. With the rather more extensive block required for cesarean delivery, the dangers of the unmodified supine position are even more important. Occasionally, if profound hypotension has occurred, placing the patient in the right lateral position may decrease the hypotension, which suggests that occasionally the inferior vena cava may lie slightly to the left rather than the right.

Hypotension

In the absence of vena caval occlusion, the prevalence of hypotension, which is most frequently defined as blood pressure less than 100 mmHg or a more than 25% reduction in blood pressure, following epidural anesthesia in labor is less than 5%. If the mother is adequately hydrated and the block is sufficiently extensive to provide anesthesia in labor only, i.e., the block is not extensive and is limited to below T10, the prevalence of hypotension is low, less than 4%.

Frequently, a slight reduction in the systolic blood pressure, commonly 8–10%, accompanies the onset of a successful block. This is the result of the sympathetic blockade, which is usually more extensive than the sensory block identified by pin prick or altered temperature sensation to ice. The sympathetic block produces vasodilation below the level of the block, thus resulting in a decrease in peripheral resistance. The blood pressure reduction, if the block is not extensive, is minimized by increased sympathetic tone in the segments above the block mediated by the aortic baroreceptors. This slight alteration in blood pressure is not accompanied by any change in cardiac output, and placental perfusion pressure is well maintained.

To undertake successful cesarean delivery, the block must extend from at least T6 to S5, and the prevalence of hypotension varies from 10–45%.[5] The frequency and severity of the hypotension depends on a number of factors, but is reduced if an incremental technique is used, with the injection of 3–4 ml of local anesthetic at intervals,[6] which permits slow extension of the block. This may be effective, and it has been argued that it is safer, as it reduces the frequency of hypotension and may also reduce both the effect of an intravascular injection if the catheter is in an epidural vein and the extent of the block if the injection is unintentionally subarachnoid. The drawback, however, is that it may take a long time for the block to be effective, which may be inconvenient in a busy labor suite.

The mechanism for the development of the hypotension when the block is extensive is a combination of extensive vasodilation and the reduction in venous return, which may, in part, be attributable to vena caval occlusion. It is essential to ensure that caval occlusion does not occur by insisting that the patient is only permitted to lie in the lateral position. If the block is extensive, as for cesarean delivery, the mother should not be allowed to sit up and her movements should be limited. Transfer to theatre, if required, must be carried out gently. Minimizing the side-effects of the block required for cesarean delivery demands an almost obsessional regard for detail. If the systolic blood pressure falls below 100 mmHg then the anesthesiologist should be informed and treatment commenced. The first treatment is to increase the rate of the intravenous infusion. Ephedrine should not be withheld but aggressively given as necessary.

It should be stressed that hypotension is rare if a restricted block is present, and in these circumstances, if it follows a top-up injection, the suspicion that the catheter may be misplaced and be subarachnoid must always be considered. The prevalence of subarachnoid placement is very rare, less than 1/8000 in the Queen Mother's Hospital but, if not recognized and properly managed, the results are catastrophic. The safety record of epidural anesthetic is excellent,[3] mostly because of the overall safety of the technique, but also because of the vigilance with which such patients are monitored. However, it is not always easy to detect intravascular or subarachnoid injection: numerous anecdotal reports have testified to the failure of a negative aspiration test to identify patients at risk.[7,8] The use of an epinephrine containing test dose has been advocated,[9] but has not been universally adopted and has been the subject of criticism.[10] The ability of catheters to migrate through the dura has also been disputed, although an epidural catheter can penetrate the arachnoid,[11] and movement of an existing epidural catheter can be readily detected.[12] Subdural placement of epidural catheters has been reported,[13] but it is clear from reports of adverse reactions that the incidence of a subdural block in obstetric anesthesia is much lower. Absolute safety cannot be guaranteed, as total spinal anesthesia has occurred following injections through the epidural needle when neither CSF nor blood had been detected.[8] Thus, scrupulous vigilance and monitoring of the block are essential.

UNINTENTIONAL SUBARACHNOID INJECTION

The development of an unintentional subarachnoid block is identified by relatively rapidly ascending sensory levels of anesthesia and dyspnea, which, if associated with weakness of the hands and arms, must be aggressively managed. The only treatment is the induction of general anesthesia, with application of standard precautions including cricoid pressure and the insertion of an endotracheal tube. Intermittent positive-pressure ventilation will be required for a variable period.

In these circumstances, fetal welfare will not necessarily be compromised since hypotension does not invariably accompany a total spinal block, but it would be an unusual obstetrician who would not expedite delivery in such circumstances. By the time weakness has developed in the arms, the patient is, not surprisingly, very alarmed, and the time for response is correspondingly limited. It is essential to recognize and respond to the development of a block that appears unduly rapid and extensive. This is best achieved by ensuring that the first injection of local anesthetic through the needle and the catheter is delivered and monitored by the anesthesiologist, and ensuring that all anesthetic and nursing staff are trained to monitor all blocks carefully. This should include some crude assessment of the power in the lower limbs, which, if altered by the single injection of a small dose of local anesthetic, should raise the issue of subarachnoid injection. In this circumstance the anesthesiologist should be informed if not present (top-ups being administered by nurse anesthetist or nurse midwife).

It is now recommended by the College of Anaesthetists in the UK that an epidural top-up may be administered only if a person skilled in resuscitation is immediately available. While it is not specified that this should be an anesthesiologist, in practice, this is usually the case. In the UK, the majority of epidural blocks are administered by anesthesiologists, but, in some maternity units where supervision is strictly controlled, top-ups are administered by trained midwives.

DIRECT CARDIOVASCULAR TOXICITY

Cardiovascular toxicity from local anesthetic agents in the UK is rare. Scott and Hibbard (1990)[3] reported 21 cases of convulsions following epidural top-ups in 505 000 epidural anesthetics, due to excessive dose or intravascular injection. In the USA, recommendations for the use of 0.75% bupivacaine in obstetrics were withdrawn following the reports of a number of deaths associated with the use of that solution.[7] It was also reported that aspiration of the catheter prior to the epidural injection had not elicited blood in many instances, which suggests that aspiration of the catheter is not always reassuring if negative. During top-up injections, particularly for cesarean delivery the anesthesiologist should maintain verbal contact with the patient and ask if any numbness or tingling is experienced during the injection of the local anesthetic, as it is suggested that symptoms of toxicity will be manifest initially by altered sensation of the lips (numbness), as a result of the extremely rich blood supply.

The maternal effects of toxicity are generalized convulsions, which, in obstetrics, appear to be identical to eclamptic seizures. Increasing the total dose will ultimately cause cardiovascular toxicity, which, when caused by bupivacaine, with its high pK_a and protein binding, is prolonged.[7] Resuscitation is extremely difficult. Hypoxia and acidosis, which frequently accompany convulsions, may also have an additive effect on both the CNS and CVS toxicity of bupivacaine.[14] Emphasis must be on the safe conduct and monitoring of the epidural block, with careful assessment of all top-up injections. Cardiotoxicity is extremely rare, and in the 27 years of epidural administration at the Queen Mother's Hospital, which now numbers over 40 000 epidural blocks and almost 100 000 top-ups, cardiovascular toxicity has not been recorded, although convulsions have occurred[15] following top-up injections for cesarean delivery which exceeded the recommended maximum dose. No maternal deaths from unintentional intravascular injections of bupivacaine or from cardiovascular toxicity have occurred in the UK.

It is clear, therefore, that epidural anesthesia has an outstanding safety record if administered and monitored carefully. Mothers need have little fear that in skilled hands it is both effective and safe.

REFERENCES

1. Melzack R 1984 The myth of painless childbirth. Pain, 19: 321–323
2. O'Driscoll K, Stronge J, Minogue M 1973 Active management of labour. Br Med J 3, 135, 7–9.
3. Scott D B, Hibbard B M 1990 Serious non-fatal complications associated with extradural block in obstetric practice. Br J Anaesth 64: 537–541
4. Lees M M, Scott D B, Kerr M G 1970 A study of cardiac output at rest through pregnancy. J Obstet Gynecol Br Commonw 77: 29–34
5. Reid J A, Thorburn J 1988 Bupivacaine and lignocaine for epidural Caesarean section and the role of maternal posture. Br J Anaesth 61: 149–153
6. Crawford J S 1987 Epidural anaesthesia for elective Caesarean section. Anaesthesia 42: 555
7. Albright G A 1979 Cardiac arrest following regional anesthesia with etidocaine or bupivacaine (editorial). Anesthesiology 51: 285–287
8. Ravindran R S, Bond V K, Tasch M D, Gupta C D, Leuressen T G 1980 Prolonged neural blockade following regional analgesia with 2-chloroprocaine. Anesth Analg 59: 447–451
9. Moore D C, Batra M S 1981 Components of an effective test dose prior to epidural block. Anesthesiol 55: 693–696
10. Dain S L, Rolbin S H, Hew E M 1987 The epidural test dose in obstetrics: is it necessary? Can J Anaesth 34: 601–605
11. Hardy P A J 1986 Can epidural catheters puncture the dura mater. Anaesthesia 41: 1146–1147
12. Phillips D C, Macdonald R, Lyons G 1986 Possible subarachnoid migration of an epidural catheter. Anaesthesia 41: 653–654
13. Reynolds F, Speedy H 1990 The subdural space. The third place to go astray. Anaesthesia 45: 120–123
14. Rosen M A, Thigpen J W, Shnider S M, Foutz S E, Levinson G, Koike M 1985 Bupivacaine induced cardiotoxicity in hypoxic and acidotic sheep. Anesth Analg 64: 1089–1096
15. Thorburn J, Moir D D 1984 Bupivacaine toxicity in association with extradural analgesia for Caesarean section. Br J Anaesth 56: 551–552

PART B
FETAL AND NEONATAL CONSIDERATIONS

A. I. Hollmèn

INTRODUCTION

Maternal psychological stress caused by pain will lead to hyperdynamic cardiovascular changes and increased respiratory drive during labor as well as increased secretion of stress hormones. Epidural anesthesia (EA) relieves maternal pain effectively. It leads to decreased cardiovascular and respiratory changes and reduces the circulating level of catecholamines.[1] EA can improve uncoordinated uterine contractions caused by elevated catecholamine levels and increase intervillous blood flow.[2] The effect of EA on progress of labor is minimal and it reduces the likelihood of the infant developing metabolic acidosis during the second stage.[3]

Obstetric anesthesia may produce adverse neonatal effects. These are often complex and influenced by obstetric factors. Neonatal effects of obstetric anesthesia may be divided into direct drug effects (local anesthetics, opioids or anesthetic adjuvants such as epinephrine or ephedrine) or indirect effects caused by changes in uteroplacental blood flow, uterine tone, contractility (oxytocin infusion, etc.) and duration and mode of delivery (e.g. prolonged second stage, vacuum extraction).

EPIDURAL ANESTHESIA AND FETAL AND NEONATAL STRESS

Vaginal delivery results in mechanical stress and hypoxia in the fetus and thus triggers a strong sympathoadrenal activity that is reflected in progressively increasing fetal blood catecholamine (CA) levels and high CA levels in umbilical arterial blood. The functional role of this CA surge in utero is probably to support cardiac function during hypoxia and preserve blood supply to the vital organs. Since EA modifies maternal sympathoadrenal activity and improves intervillous blood flow, it could indirectly reduce intrauterine fetal stress and modify the fetal CA surge, which has been suggested to play an important role in neonatal adaptation to extrauterine life. High CA levels will increase absorption of lung liquid and surfactant material in the newborn. It will mobilize in the neonate extra energy (glucose and free fatty acids) and improve the ability of the left ventricle to respond to increased functional demand during the critical first hours of life.[4] It may also be important for bonding reactions and for neonatal imprinting.

Interestingly, epidural anesthesia for cesarean delivery has been shown to be associated with higher neonatal CA levels than general anesthesia.[5]

FETAL EFFECTS OF EPIDURAL ANESTHESIA

Local anesthetics

The continuous epidural infusion technique using low doses and concentrations of local anesthetic (LA) for EA results in very low fetal blood LA concentrations. It reduces the risk of maternal systemic toxic reaction and possible high fetal blood levels of LA due to unintentional intravenous injection. Properly conducted, EA has no effect on fetal heart rate and acid–base values (Figs 19.2 and 19.3). Recently the Doppler technique, used to assess fetal hemodynamic changes associated with epidural block for cesarean delivery, has shown that EA causes no change in umbilical artery blood flow–velocity waveforms[6] or a decrease in resistance.[7] Using the color Doppler technique, Alahuhta et al[8] found that in healthy parturients 0.5% bupivacaine used to achieve a level of T5 with epidural anesthesia for cesarean delivery does not change fetal

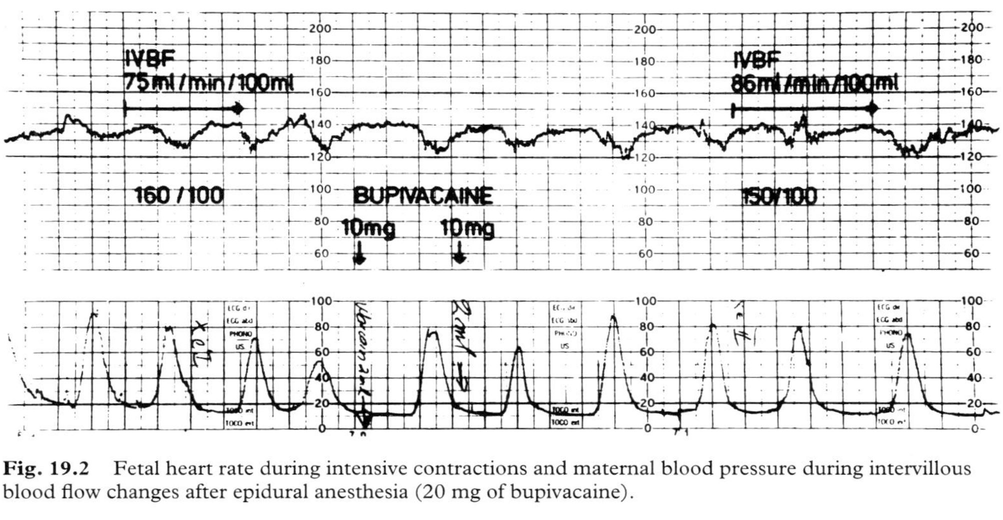

Fig. 19.2 Fetal heart rate during intensive contractions and maternal blood pressure during intervillous blood flow changes after epidural anesthesia (20 mg of bupivacaine).

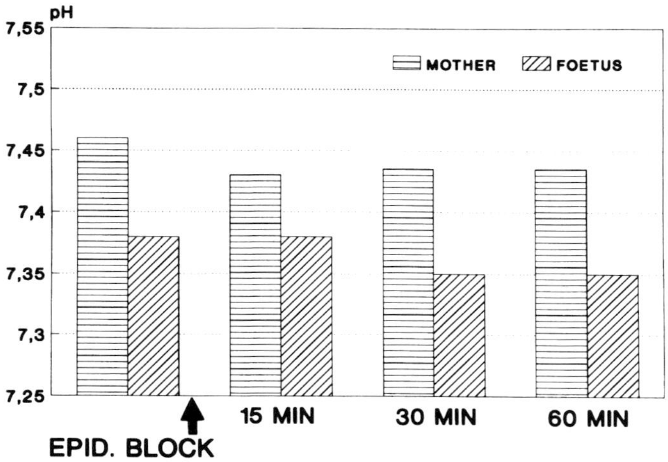

Fig. 19.3 Stable fetal pH after epidural anesthesia with bupivacaine (20 mg) (10 healthy parturients).

myocardial function or influence the velocity of blood flow in fetal umbilical, renal and middle cerebral arteries.

Epinephrine added to LA improves the quality and prolongs the duration of EA. Although animal data indicate that uterine blood flow decreases when epinephrine is used with LA, clinical studies suggest that epinephrine used during EA for labor or cesarean delivery (100μg) does not decrease intervillous blood flow.[9] Recent studies using the Doppler technique demonstrated no changes in uterine or umbilical artery blood flow waveforms after epidural bupivacaine,[10] lidocaine or chloroprocaine-epinephrine[11] used for cesarean delivery.

Ephedrine used to treat maternal hypotension during EA is a lipid-soluble substance and has been shown to cross the placenta[12] and to affect fetal heart rate and variability.[13] The Doppler technique indicates that ephedrine given as a 10-mg i.v. bolus to treat hypotension has no effect on umbilical vascular resistance.[14]

Although a healthy fetus seems to tolerate the low dose of LA presently used for EA, chronic fetal asphyxia, acute hypoxia or prematurity combined with EA could have an effect on fetal well-being. Hypoxia and acidosis will increase the blood flow and distribution of LA to the brain and heart. Animal studies indicate that in the term fetus circulatory adaptation to asphyxia is not altered by moderate plasma concentrations of lidocaine. In contrast, premature fetuses exposed to similar plasma concentrations of lidocaine lose their cardiovascular adaptation to asphyxia and their condition deteriorates.[15] Chloroprocaine is rapidly metabolized to inactive metabolites by plasma cholinesterases so that only trace amounts are transferred to the fetus, which makes this drug a good choice for EA in the situation of fetal acidosis and/or prematurity.

HOW TO EVALUATE THE RECOVERY OF THE NEONATE AFTER EA

The neonatal effects of the drugs used during obstetric pain relief can be studied through measurement of the neonatal pharmacokinetics of drugs, neurobehavioral testing and neurophysiologic methods.

Placental transfer and neonatal pharmacokinetics

Drugs are transferred across the placenta by the process of simple diffusion. Local anesthetics and opioids used for EA are very lipid soluble, have a molecular weight of approximately 300 Daltons and, at physiologic pH, a significant proportion of these drugs exists in diffusible nonionized form. Such drugs, therefore, cross the placenta easily. The rate of passage of any drug is either permeability or flow limited. Being highly permeable, the transfer of LAs and opioids is flow limited. Maternal hypotension with decreased uterine blood flow could thus limit the transfer of local anesthetics and opioids.

Factors other than drugs must be taken into account in a depressed neonate. For instance, fetal asphyxia will increase blood flow and oxygen delivery to the vital organs and increase the tissue concentration of local anesthetic (heart, brain, etc.). Circulatory adaptation to asphyxia will not be influenced by moderate concentrations of lidocaine. However, preterm asphyxiated fetuses will not tolerate similar plasma concentrations of lidocaine without losing cardiovascular adaptation resulting in deterioration in their condition.[15] Premature babies have decreased α_1-glycoprotein plasma levels, which increases the amount of free, unbound local anesthetic in plasma.

During the first hours of life any reduction in drug metabolism influences neonatal behavior. The speed of elimination of drugs in the neonate is improved if the body temperature is maintained. In the neonate, demethylation of drugs is normal, but hydroxylation, hydrolysis and conjugation are less efficient than in the adult. These functions will be even more depressed in the presence of neonatal acidosis. It is important to maintain newborn body temperature and oxygenation in order to facilitate elimination of the drugs.

Neurobehavioral evaluation

Newborns delivered with normal Apgar scores and umbilical blood acid–base values may still have slight central nervous system (CNS) depression caused by drugs used for EA. In order to study these subtler effects, neurobehavioral testing was introduced. The most popular neurobehavioral tests include the Brazelton Neonatal Behavioral Assessment Scale (BNBAS), the Scanlon Early Neonatal Neurobehavioral Scale (ENNS) and the

Amiel–Tison/Barrier/Shnider Neurological and Adaptive Capacity Scores (NACS) (see Chapter 8, part A). The comprehensiveness and the emphasis that these tests place on various aspects of neurologic function and newborn behavior differ. Generally, they evaluate muscle tone, ability to alter state of arousal, ability to suppress response to repetitive stimulation, ability to respond appropriately to external events, ability to initiate complex motor acts and the appropriateness of reflex motor responses.

The BNBAS is the most comprehensive neurobehavioral examination. Unfortunately, owing to the time required to carry out the examination and the special training necessary, the BNBAS is rarely used by anesthesiologists in their clinical studies.

The ENNS was designed to examine the early neurobehavioral changes particularly associated with the use of local anesthetics and is widely used by anesthesiologists. Since it is thought that anesthetic-related changes are primarily manifested as decreased muscle tone, this aspect is emphasized in the ENNS. The neonate's autonomic stability as well as state of orientation is not evaluated by ENNS. This is a drawback since available data suggest that these neurobehavioral tests are affected by obstetric medications.[16] Another limitation of the ENNS is that it is not designed to be repeated and to follow the recovery curve during the neonatal period.

Amiel–Tison et al[17] believe that the ENNS puts too little emphasis on neonatal muscle tone and was not designed to distinguish differences in tone between the extension and flexor muscles of the neck or differences between upper and lower parts of the body. They believe that these differentiations are important in distinguishing abnormalities that are due to birth trauma from those resulting from drug depression. Although the NACS emphasizes tone, there are few or no tests that reflect the range of state, regulation of state or autonomic stability. Thus it excludes factors known to be affected by low levels of obstetric medication (e.g. mother–infant interaction). Like the ENNS, the NACS is not designed to be repeated in the neonatal period and does not allow the recovery curve of an infant to be studied as is the case with the BNBAS. The NACS takes less than 5 mins to perform and is becoming increasingly popular with anesthesiologists.

For statistical evaluation, ENNS and NACS use nonparametric statistics, whereas BNBAS uses parametric statistics, making a false-negative result less likely.

Neurobehavioral testing has other problems, including observer subjectivity, difficulty in obtaining quantitative measurements and biases in population selection. At present a large number of publications of the effects of obstetric anesthesia on newborn behavior are available. The significance of short-term neurobehavioral alterations is unclear, but there is also a lack of prospective studies with proper control groups. Appropriate treatment of obstetric and pharmacologic confounding variables is often lacking. Therefore, comparing one study with another is difficult.

Spectral EEG

EEG reactivity to drugs has recently become a matter of considerable interest. The EEG is dependent on brain activity as well as cerebral metabolism. The electrical activity of the brain and the behavior of the organism as a whole are two different indicators of brain metabolism and biochemistry. Spectral EEG has recently been introduced as an objective and sensitive technique to detect subtle drug effects on the central nervous system (CNS). Properly analyzed, the noninvasive EEG technique gives very specific information which cannot be obtained by any other technique. The EEG can be continuously recorded and the data from a spectral EEG can be transformed into numerical values. Thus, for instance, changes in the degree of consciousness (alertness or drowsiness) show typical EEG patterns.

Hollmėn et al[18] recently reported the use of the spectral EEG to evaluate the effects of different types of anesthetic techniques on neonates after elective cesarean delivery in a controlled group of infants. As nonmedicated controls they used vaginally delivered newborns whose mothers had no pharmacologic pain relief. The three study groups of neonates were delivered from mothers who received general, epidural and spinal anesthesia. Although the conventional relative power and mean frequency parameters of the various EEG bands showed little difference, the zero band power rate (ZBPR) reflecting the dynamic rapid fluctuations in EEG showed significant differences in all frequency bands. The neonates in the epidural and control groups were similar and differed significantly from those in the general and spinal anesthesia groups.

The difference in EEG patterns between the epidural and spinal groups (plain bupivacaine was used in both groups) was suggested to be related to the use of ephedrine (a CNS stimulant) in the latter group. Later studies by Kangas-Saarela et al[19] demonstrated that ephedrine used to treat maternal hypotension has significant dose-related effects on the neonatal spectral EEG during the first hours after delivery. These changes disappear after 24 hs. Interestingly, neurobehavioral testing showed no difference between the ephedrine and nonephedrine spinal anesthesia groups. Thus, spectral EEG seems to offer a more sensitive and specific tool for study of neonatal drug effects.

Spontaneous frontal muscle EMG

The reticular formation (RAS) of the brainstem is a system responsible for correlating alertness, activity of autonomic nervous function and affective or emotional

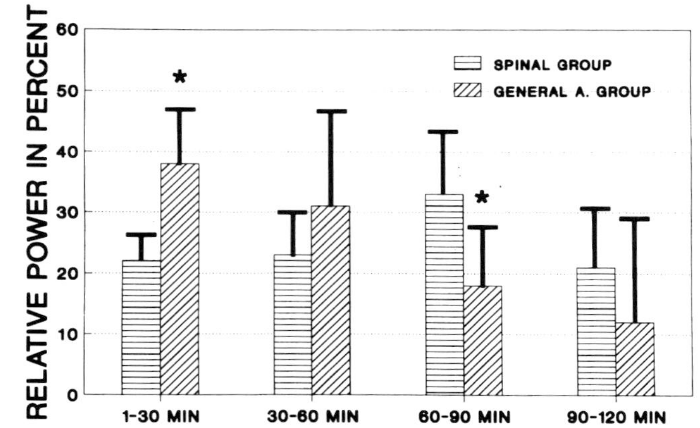

Fig. 19.4 Spontaneous frontal muscle EMG power changes during 2 h monitoring of full-term healthy neonates (10 newborns in each group) after cesarean delivery. In the spinal group 10–15 mg of ephedrine was given to mothers to treat hypotension. The EMG reflecting vigilance shows a significant increase in the spinal group, contrary to the findings in general anesthesia.

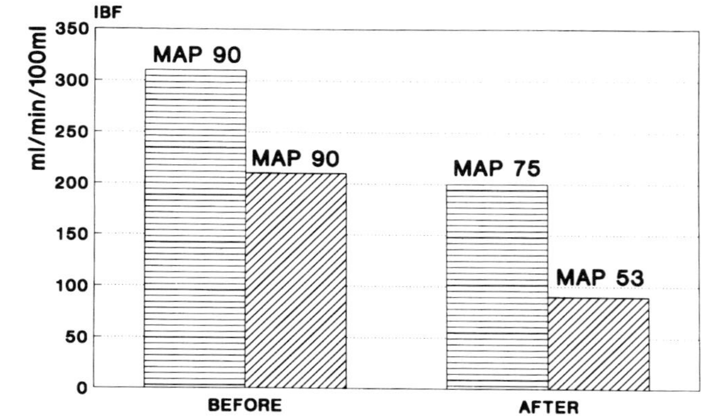

Fig. 19.5 The influence of maternal hypotension after epidural anesthesia on intervillous blood flow in two healthy parturients.

behavior with muscle tone. Stimulation of the RAS produces a nonspecific increase in cortical activity, which leads to increased cerebral consciousness and stimulation of the autonomic nervous system as well as increased muscle tone. When cerebral consciousness decreases, muscle tension also decreases. Therefore, the spontaneous frontal muscle EMG can be used to detect changes in muscle tone and has also been shown to reflect consciousness.[20]

Recording of frontal muscle tone has been used[21, 22] to compare the changes in muscle tone during a 2-h recovery period in the newborn after different types of anesthesia (epidural, spinal and general) for cesarean delivery. The epidural group compared well with the vaginally delivered control group in which no drugs were used. The difference between spinal and epidural groups was significant. The spinal group throughout the study period had higher spontaneous frontal muscle tone than the epidural group (Fig. 19.4). Also, clinical observation of the newborns indicated a difference in vigilance and alertness between spinal and other groups during the 2-h period. Since ephedrine was needed to treat maternal hypotension in the spinal but not in the epidural group, the increased muscle tone could be related to use of ephedrine.

It seems that ephedrine at doses clinically used to treat maternal hypotension can influence both neonatal EEG and spontaneous frontal muscle EMG activity, which reflects the alertness of the neonate during the first hours after delivery. The increased muscle tone could influence the interpretation of neurobehavioral scoring of muscle tone as well as the alertness of the newborn.

Editor's note: This work substantiates our clinical impression that newborns whose mothers had received large amounts of ephedrine appear to be jittery and hyperactive after birth.

EA AND NEONATAL EFFECTS

The influence of maternal hypotension on the neonate

In full-term pregnant healthy parturients, the supine position significantly decreases the intervillous blood flow (IVBF) compared with the lateral position and increases resistance in the umbilical artery.[23,24] In the supine position EA aggravates this situation and leads to fetal heart rate changes indicating fetal asphyxia.[25] Maternal dehydration or meperidine given before EA increases the likelihood of maternal hypotension. Prevention is the best treatment for hypotension: a parturient should never be placed supine.

Epidural anesthesia for vaginal delivery is much less likely to cause maternal hypotension than epidural anesthesia for cesarean delivery. Maternal hypotension leads to decreased IVBF (Fig. 19.5) and can cause fetal asphyxia. Clinical data suggest that systolic blood pressure (SBP) below 90 mmHg for several minutes leads to neonatal acidosis.[26] The most sensitive technique to detect subtle neonatal depression, namely neurobehavioral testing, indicates that mild hypotension (SBP < 90 mmHg) lasting less than 3 min will not significantly influence neurobehavioral scoring.[27] However, Corke et al[27] found that neonates of hypotensive mothers compared with those born to nonhypotensive mothers did show a trend towards weak sucking and rooting reflexes, which are sensitive indicators of neonatal depression. In case of more severe hypotension (MAP < 70 mmHg for 2–5 min) the rooting and sucking reflexes of the newborn will be significantly depressed despite normal Apgar scores and acid–base status[28] (Fig. 19.6).

While the available evidence suggests that short-lived maternal hypotension and a moderate decrease in IVBF have no deleterious effects on the fetus and neonate of a healthy mother, this is not necessarily so in cases of chronically reduced IVBF. Fetuses of parturients with toxemia

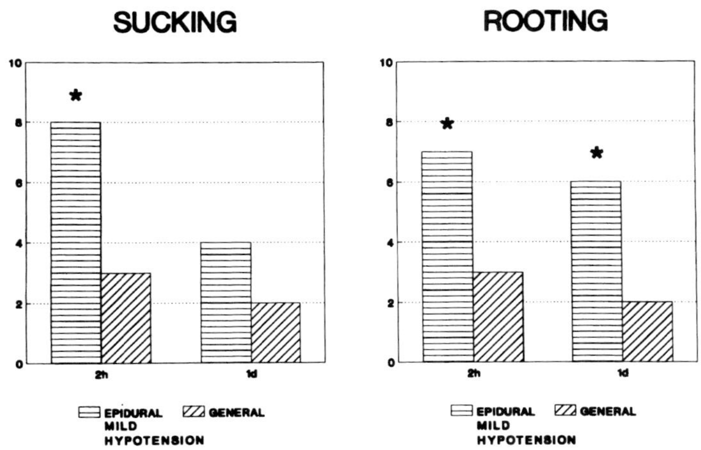

Fig. 19.6 The depressive effect of moderate short-lived maternal hypotension [MAP (intra-arterial pressure or direct arterial pressure)<70 mmHg for 2–5 min] on sucking and rooting reflexes after epidural anesthesia for cesarean delivery.

tolerate poorly any further reduction in placental blood flow. Marginal reserves in IVBF and oxygen capacity of the fetus makes these patients very vulnerable to any further reduction in IVBF. Maternal hypotension can lead to prolonged neurological recovery.[28] Fortunately, in patients with toxemia, if hypotension is avoided, EA has been shown to significantly improve IVBF.[29]

EA with local anesthetics and neurobehavioral effects

Previous studies by Scanlon et al[30,31] earlier suggested that lidocaine has transient depressive effects on neurobehavior. However, recent studies refute these findings.[16,32] It seems that local anesthetics used during properly conducted EA either in smaller amounts for pain relief during vaginal delivery or in larger quantities for cesarean delivery have minimal effects on the neurobehavioral evaluation of healthy full-term babies during the first 5 days of life. These data are based on studies using either the ENNS or NACS. Using BNBAS and observing the infants' recovery profile, subtle local anesthetic effects have been reported.[33,34] However, several confounding variables, both obstetric and pharmacologic, were not properly observed in these later studies. Recently Kangas Saarela et al[35] reported that the infants born after maternal segmental (T12–L2) EA became accustomed and responded to inanimate auditory stimuli at 1 day of age significantly better than controls, while babies born after more extensive lumbar EA demonstrated significantly better alertness at the age of 3 h, 2 days and 4–5 days than the control group.[36]

The effects of low doses of local anesthetics and opioids on the neonate

EA with local anesthetics can lead to maternal hypotension due to sympathetic blockade. The motor blockade caused by LA is frequently distressing to the parturient and may decrease expulsive efforts during the second stage of labor. To overcome this problem, combinations of local anesthetics in low concentrations and opioids have recently gained widespread popularity. The rationale of combining these drugs is that they work at different neural sites and have synergistic effects. Although opioids alone are not sufficient to achieve adequate pain relief during labor and delivery, EA using this combination results in greater pain relief of longer duration, reduced LA requirements and less motor blockade.[37]

At present, the combined use of very small doses of LA with opioids seems to provide excellent sensory anesthesia with few side-effects. Although maternal effects are well documented, in most studies the effects on fetus and neonate were not as carefully evaluated. With epidural opioids the neonate can be exposed to a significant amount of drug. High maternal arterial concentrations of opioids, which all have low molecular weights, will enhance the transfer of these drugs across the placenta to the fetus. Lipid solubility, protein binding and the degree of ionization differ from one opioid to another. The proportion of unionized opioid at pH 7.40 ranges from 49% with alfentanil to only 7.4% with meperidine. While alfentanil and sufentanil are highly protein bound, morphine is only slightly bound. Lipid solubility varies greatly between opioids, with sufentanil being the most soluble. A short time interval between the injection to the delivery leads to almost identical morphine concentrations in maternal and cord blood and has caused neonatal respiratory depression.[38]

EA using fentanyl has the advantage of very low plasma concentrations. However, the placental transfer is rapid[39] and the peak plasma concentrations occur in both mother and fetus in 5–10 min. EA using local anesthetics with 150–200 μg of fentanyl as repeated doses leads to very low maternal plasma concentrations and very little placental transfer of fentanyl (umbilical artery <0.18 ng/ml).[40] Thus fentanyl appears to be one of the safest opioids to administer epidurally. Although neurobehavioral studies comparing control groups with fentanyl and LA infusion have not shown any depressive effect,[41,42] with repeated doses there is evidence of maternal accumulation of fentanyl, and neonatal depression has been reported.[43]

A derivative of fentanyl is sufentanil, which is more lipid soluble than fentanyl, penetrates more rapidly into the spinal cord and has higher affinity for the opioid receptor. Clinical experience has shown it to be more potent, more rapid in onset and longer acting than fentanyl. The first favorable report of using 0.15% bupivacaine with epinephrine combined with a bolus of sufentanil was that by van Steenberge et al.[37] Philips[44] compared infusion of bupivacaine (0.125%) with sufentanil (1 μg/ml) with plain bupivacaine (0.125%) infusion. He reported no difference in Apgar scores and no respiratory depression in the first 3 h. Recently Capogna et al[42] studied the neonatal effects of epidural sufentanil for cesarean delivery. Patients were randomized to a saline control group and two sufentanil groups, 50 μg and 80 μg. ENNS and NACS were used for the neurobehavioral examination of infants at 1, 4 and 24 h of life. At 1 h, both 50 and 80 μg of sufentanil led to significant depression of habituation to sound and light but at 4 h of age only the 80-μg dose of sufentanil caused significant depression in muscle tone and alertness of the neonates. At 24 h of age, there were no significant changes in either ENNS or NACS evaluations. Both the Apgar scores and acid–base status were normal and no neonate exhibited respiratory depression at any time. The interesting point is that, using these two different neurobehavioral testing procedures, NACS demonstrated changes whereas ENNS showed no significant changes in either groups at any time. The 50-μg dose of sufentanil improved interoperative analgesia and provided adequate postoperative pain relief without the potential risk of neonatal depression.

Unlike the encouraging findings with fentanyl and sufentanil, use of alfentanil for EA has been associated with neonatal depression.[45] In a study of continuous bupivacaine infusion with or without alfentanil there was no difference in Apgar scores and acid–base status between the control bupivacaine group and the bupivacaine–alfentanil group.[46] However, NACS examination indicated significant depression of passive and active muscle tone. Although low doses of alfentanil have not been reported to produce neurobehavioral depression, these results clearly demonstrate the importance of neurobehavioral evaluation of neonates when opioids are used for EA.

To date, mainly μ-receptor agonists that are primarily involved with mediation of somatic pain (fentanyl, sufentanil, alfentanil, etc.) have been studied. κ-receptor agonists are involved with mediation of visceral pain, and drugs that act at these receptors should be useful in relieving labor pain. Butorphanol is a strong κ-receptor agonist and a weak μ-receptor antagonist. Hunt et al[47] using 2 mg of butorphanol with bupivacaine produced good pain relief with no adverse fetal and neonatal effects.

To date, fentanyl has been studied most extensively and has an excellent safety record. The dose should be kept as low as possible and repeated injections should be avoided if possible. The longer the time between injection of the opioids and delivery, the less will be the risk of neonatal depression. In future studies, selection of the proper testing procedure (preferably NACS and BNBAS) will be important.

Comparing anesthetic agents for obstetric pain relief as well as testing any new drug for future use should include neurobehavioral testing as a sensitive tool in evaluating the recovery of the neonate. There is presently a need for better standardization of outcome measures, scoring techniques and data analysis methods. This includes proper treatment of confounding variables including anesthetic complications such as maternal hypotension during EA, which can affect the neurobehavioral recovery. Obstetric, ante- and peri-natal stress factors will also influence the neurobehavioral recovery.

To date, neurobehavioral testing has been done for mainly healthy infants after full-term pregnancy. The results of studying these kinds of 'super babies' are not necessarily valid for all infants. One has simply to remember that complications of labor and delivery occur in about 30% of all births.

REFERENCES

1. Shnider S M, Abboud T K, Artal R, Henriksen E H, Stefani S J, Levinson G 1983 Maternal catecholamines decrease during labor after lumbar epidural anesthesia. Am J Obstet Gynecol 147: 13–15

2. Hollmèn A I, Jouppila R, Jouppila P, Koivula A, Vierola 1982 Effect of extradural analgesia using bupivacaine and 2-chloroprocaine on intervillous blood flow during normal labour. Br J Anaesth 54: 837–842
3. Zador G and Nilsson B A 1974 Low dose intermittent epidural anesthesia in labour: influence on labour and fetal acid–base status. Acta Obstet Gynecol Scand 34 (suppl): 17
4. Lagercrantz H, Bistoletti P 1973 Catecholamine release in the newborn infant at birth. Pediatr Res 11: 889–893
5. Irestedt L, Lagercrantz H, Hjemdahl P, Hägnevik K, Belfrage P 1982 Fetal and maternal plasma catecholamine levels at elective cesarean section under general or epidural anesthesia versus vaginal delivery. Am J Obstet Gynecol 142: 1004–1010
6. Baumann H, Alon E, Atanassogg P, Pasch T, Huch A, Huch R 1990 Effect of epidural anesthesia for Cesarean delivery on maternal femoral arterial and venous, uteroplacental, and umbilical blood flow velocities and waveforms. Obstet Gynecol 75: 194–198
7. Giles W B, Lah F X, Trudinger B J 1987 The effect of epidural anaesthesia for Caesarean section on maternal uterine and fetal umbilical artery blood flow velocity waveforms. Br J Obstet Gynaecol 94: 55–59
8. Räsänen J, Alahuhta S, Kangas-Saarela T, Jouppila P, Jouppila R 1991 The effects of ephedrine and etilefrine on uterine and fetal blood flow and on fetal myocardial function during spinal anaesthesia for caesarean section. Int J Obst Anesth 1: 3–8
9. Albright G A, Jouppila R, Hollmèn A I, Jouppila P, Vierola H, Koivula A 1981 Epinephrine does not alter human intervillous blood flow during epidural anesthesia. Anesthesiology 54: 131–135
10. Lindblad A, Bernow J, Vernersson E, Marsal K 1987 Effects of extradural anaesthesia on human fetal blood flow in utero. Br J Anaesth 59: 1265–1272
11. Veille J C, Youngstrom P, Kanaan C, Wilson B 1988 Human umbilical artery flow velocity waveforms before and after regional anesthesia for Cesarean section. Obstet Gynecol 72: 890–893
12. Hughes S C, Ward M M G, Levison G, Shnider S M, Wright R G, Gruenke L D, Craig J C 1985 Placental transfer of ephedrine does not affect neonatal outcome. Anesthesiology 63: 217–219
13. Wright R G, Shnider S M, Levison G, Rolbin S H, Parer J T 1981 The effect of maternal administration of ephedrine of fetal heart rate and variability. Obstet Gynecol 57: 734–738
14. Alahuhta S, Räsänen J, Jouppila R, Jouppila P, Kangas-Saarela T, Hollmèn A 1991 Uteroplacental and fetal hemodynamics during epidural anaesthesia for caesarean section. Br J Anaesth 66: 319–323
15. Morishima H O, Pedersen H, Santos A C et al 1989 Adverse effects of maternally administered lidocaine on the asphyxiated preterm fetal lamb. Anesthesiology 71: 110–115
16. Kuhnert B R, Harrison M J, Linn P L, Kuhnert P M 1984 Effects of maternal epidural anesthesia on neonatal behavior. Anesth Analg 63: 301–308
17. Amiel-Tison C, Barrier G, Shnider S M, Levinson G, Hughes S C, Stefani S J 1982 A new neurologic and adaptive capacity scoring system for evaluating obstetric medications in full-term newborns. Anesthesiology 56: 340–350
18. Hollmèn A I, Eskelinen P, Tolonen U, Arranto J, Sulg I, Jouppila R, Jouppila P 1985 Effects of anaesthesia for caesarean section on computerized EEG of the neonate. Eur J Anaesthesiol 2: 39–51
19. Kangas-Saarela T, Hollmèn A I, Tolonen U et al 1990 Does ephedrine influence newborn neurobehavioural responses and spectral EEG when used to prevent maternal hypotension during Caesarean section? Acta Anaesth Scand 34: 8–16
20. Harmel M H, Klein F F, Davis D D 1978 The EEMG: a practical index of cortical activity and muscular relaxation. Acta Anaesth Scand 70: 97–102
21. Hollmèn A I 1986 Evaluation of the condition of newborn: Neurophysiological aspects. In: Renck H (ed) Abstracts of the Fifth Congress of the European Society of Regional Anaesthesia, Malmö, Sweden. Wallin & Dalholm Boktryckeri, Lund, p 128C
22. Hollmèn A I 1988 The effects of obstetric regional anaesthesia on placental blood flow. In: Löfström J B, Sjöstrand U (eds) Local anaesthesia and regional blockade, Elsevier, Amsterdam, pp. 169–197
23. Kauppila A, Koskinen M, Puolakka J, Tuimala R, Kuikka J 1980 Decreased intervillous and unchanged myometrial blood flow in supine recumbency. Obstet Gynecol 55: 203–205
24. Marx G F, Elstein I D, Schuss M, Anyaegbunam A, Fleischer A 1990 Effects of epidural block with lignocaine and lignocaine–adrenaline on umbilical artery velocity wave ratios. Br J Obstet Gynaecol 97: 517–520
25. Huovinen K, Kivalo I, Teramo K Factors influencing the incidence of fetal bradycardia after lumbar epidural block for vaginal labour (abstract). Proceedings of the 5th European Congress of Perinatal Medicine, Uppsala, Sweden, Almqvist & Wiksell, Stockholm p 62
26. Philipson E H, Kuhnert B R, Pimentel R, Amini S B 1989 Transient maternal hypotension following epidural anesthesia. Anesth Analg 69: 604–407
27. Corke B C, Datta S, Ostheimer G W, Weiss J B and Alper M H 1982 Spinal anaesthesia for caesarean section. The influence of hypotension on neonatal outcome. Anaesthesia 37: 658–662
28 Hollmèn A I, Jouppila R, Koivisto M, Määttä L, Pihlajaniemi R, Puukka M, Rantakylä P 1978 Neurologic activity of infants following anesthesia for cesarean section. Anesthesiology 48: 350–356
29. Jouppila P, Jouppila R, Hollmèn A, Koivula A 1982 Lumbar epidural analgesia to improve intervillous blood flow during labor in severe preeclampsia. Obstet Gynecol 59: 158–161
30. Scanlon J W, Brown W U, Weiss J B, Alper M H 1974 Neurobehavioral responses of newborn infants after maternal epidural anesthesia. Anesthesiology 40: 121–128
31. Scanlon J W, Ostheimer G W, Lurie A O, Brown W U, Weiss J B, Alper M H 1976 Neurobehavioral responses and drug concentrations in newborns after maternal epidural anesthesia with bupivacaine. Anesthesiology 45: 400–405
32. Kileff M E, James F M, Dewan D M, Floyd H M 1984 Neonatal neurobehavioral responses after epidural anesthesia for cesarean section using lidocaine and bupivacaine. Anesth Analg 63: 413–417
33. Murray A D, Dolby R M, Nation R L, Thomas D B 1981 Effects of epidural anesthesia on newborns and their mothers. Child Dev 52: 71–82
34. Rosenblatt D B, Belsey E M, Lieberman B A, et al 1981 The influence of maternal analgesia on neonatal behaviour. II. Epidural bupivacaine. Br J Obstet Gynaecol 88: 407–413
35. Kangas-Saarela T, Jouppila R, Jouppila P, Hollmèn A, Puukka M, Juujärvi K 1987 The effect of segmental epidural analgesia on the neurobehavioural responses of newborn. Acta Anaesthesiol Scand 31: 347–351
36. Kangas-Saarela T, Jouppila R, Alahuhta S, Jouppila P, Hollmèn A 1989 The effect of lumbar epidural analgesia on the neurobehavioural responses of newborn infants. Acta Anaesthesiol Scand 33: 320–325
37. Van Steenberge A V, Debroux H C, Noordin H 1987 Extradural bupivacaine with sufentanil for vaginal delivery. Br J Anaesth 59: 1518–1522
38. Nybell-Lindahl G, Carlsson C, Ingemarsson I, Westgren M, Paalzow L 1981 Maternal and fetal concentrations of morphine after epidural administration during labor. Am J Obstet Gynecol 139: 20–21
39. Vella L M, Knott C, Reynolds F 1986 Transfer of fentanyl across the rabbit placenta. Br J Anaesth 58: 49–54
40. Carrie L E S, O'Sullivan G M, Scegobin R 1981 Epidural fentanyl in labour. Anaesthesia 36: 965–969
41. Cohen S E, Tan S, Albright G A, Halpern J 1987 Epidural fentanyl/bupivacaine mixtures for obstetric analgesia. Anesthesiology 67: 403–407
42. Capogna G, Celleno D, Tomassetti M 1989 Maternal analgesia and neonatal effects of epidural sufentanil for Cesarean section. Reg Anesth 14: 282–287
43. Skerman J H, Thompson B A, Goldstein M T, Jacobs M A, Gupta A, Blass N H 1985 Combined continuous epidural fentanyl and bupivacaine in labor: randomized study. Anesthesiology 63: A450
44. Phillips G H 1987 Combined epidural sufentanil and bupivacaine for labor analgesia. Reg Anesth 12: 165–168

45. Heytens L, Camu H, Camu F 1987 Extradural analgesia during labour using alfentanil. Br J Anaesth 59: 331–337
46. Carp H, Johnson M D, Bader A M, Datta S, Ostheimer G W 1988 Continuous epidural infusion of alfentanil and bupivacaine for labor and delivery. Anesthesiology 69: A687
47. Hunt C O, Naulty S, Malinow A M, Datta S, Ostheimer G W 1989 Epidural butorphanol-bupivacaine for analgesia during labor and delivery. Anesth Analg 68: 323–327

PART C
PLASMA CONCENTRATIONS OF LOCAL ANESTHETICS IN NEWBORNS AFTER MATERNAL EPIDURAL ADMINISTRATION

E. Giaufré B. Bruguerolle

Local anesthetics (LAs), like many other drugs administered to mothers, can cross the placental barrier and can thus affect the fetus or the newborn. Bromage and Robson[1] were the first to report the placental transfer of a LA, lidocaine, after epidural anesthesia. Since that time, the placental transfer of practically every LA has been reported by many authors. We would like to review these different studies from the viewpoint of a pediatric anesthesiologist involved in regional anesthesia in small infants, a viewpoint that is very different from that of the anesthesiologist specializing in obstetrics. We shall be concentrating in this chapter on the effects of one of the most commonly used regional anesthetic techniques in obstetrics: epidural block.

The chapter begins with a brief description of the pharmacologic factors involved in the placental transfer of LA and then deals with factors affecting maternal and fetal blood concentrations of LAs, and the metabolism and excretion of LAs in newborn. It concludes with a summary of the main studies on the subject, including some recent work of our own, and with a discussion of the clinical consequences for the newborn.

PHARMACOLOGIC FACTORS INVOLVED IN THE PLACENTAL TRANSFER OF LAs

The passage of LAs across the placenta depends on many pharmacologic factors[2] such as the physicochemical properties of the drugs and the characteristics of the maternal, placental, and fetal circulation. Four factors are involved in the passage of a drug (including LAs) across any biological membrane:

1. its molecular weight;
2. its lipid solubility;
3. its degree of protein binding; and
4. its degree of ionization.

Molecular weight

The molecular size of a drug is particularly important because most unionized drugs of molecular weight less than 600 daltons cross cell boundaries readily, so most LAs can traverse the placenta easily by simple (passive) diffusion, i.e. down a concentration gradient between mother and fetus.

Lipid solubility

All membranes are relatively permeable to unionized molecules, and the rate of transfer depends on the lipid solubility of the drug. Differences in lipid solubility between various LAs may explain the differences in their placental transfer.

Degree of protein binding

Only the free (unbound) fraction of LA can cross the placenta by passive diffusion: the degree of protein binding of a LA is therefore of particular importance because any variation in protein binding affects the amount of drug present in the free, unbound form. For instance, a decrease in protein binding in the mother increases the free fraction of the drug and, hence, increases passage of the drug across the placenta. Differences in protein binding (bupivacaine and etidocaine are more protein bound than mepivacaine and lidocaine) may also explain why some drugs pass more easily than others, though the high protein binding of bupivacaine and etidocaine does not seem to be a limiting factor in their placental transfer.

Degree of ionization

LAs are bases having p*K*a values ranging from 7.6 to 9.0: thus, they are largely ionized at physiologic pH. Any alteration of pH may modify the ionization of LA and, hence, may affect their placental transfer. This may have special relevance for diabetic mothers.

Factors affecting maternal and fetal blood concentration of LAs

Many factors[2–4] may affect maternal and/or fetal blood concentrations, including the site of injection, the total dose, the number of doses and the addition of epinephrine. The addition of epinephrine to a LA produces local vasoconstriction, and this may delay absorption from the site of injection. Hemodynamic factors may also play a part: reduction in uteroplacental blood flow, from whatever cause, results in decreased delivery of drug to the fetus. Fetal hypoxemia and, more importantly, a combination of hypoxemia and acidosis may affect the distribution of the fetal cardiac output, and one must bear in mind that LAs transmitted to the fetus may themselves affect its hemodynamic status.

Other factors may affect fetal tissue uptake of LA.[4,5] For example, LA uptake depends on the tissue–blood partition coefficient, and limited placental uptake of LA has been demonstrated. Rapid diffusion of LA in the fetus itself is dependent on blood flow to the highly perfused fetal organs such as the liver, brain, and myocardium. The effect of lipid solubility on fetal tissue uptake must be emphasized. As previously noted, bupivacaine and mepivacaine are more lipid soluble than lidocaine, and it seems that bupivacaine uptake in fetal liver, brain, and myocardium is greater than that of lidocaine.

Tissue acidosis in the fetus may enhance drug transfer into heart and brain, and reduction in gastric pH may lead to accumulation in the stomach.

METABOLISM AND EXCRETION IN THE NEWBORN

The fetus and the newborn may be capable of metabolizing LA,[2,4,6] but some of the enzyme systems are inefficient. The elimination half-life has been shown to be more prolonged in the newborn owing to a greater volume of distribution and tissue uptake of the drug. Mepivacaine elimination half-life is about 9 h in the neonate[7,8] compared with 2–3 h in adults; and lidocaine elimination half-life is about 3 h in the newborn as against 1.6 –1.8 h in the adult. However, data for bupivacaine are conflicting, with Brown et al[8] giving a figure of less than 2 h in the newborn compared with Tucker and Mather's[7] figure of 8 h.

REVIEW OF STUDIES CONCERNING MATERNAL AND FETAL LA PLASMA CONCENTRATIONS

Many studies have been conducted, ranging over several years, into maternal and fetal plasma LA concentrations after epidural blocks. Tables 19.1–19.7 summarize the results of some of these studies for each drug. The list is not exhaustive and it is very difficult to compare data when, for each drug, the dose, concentration, sampling method (venous or arterial), time interval between epidural injection and delivery (∂t), gestational age of the child, and the mother's clinical history (diabetes, eclampsia, etc.) are so very different. Table 19.8 summarizes our own data in this area.

For lidocaine, the ratio of umbilical to maternal venous concentrations varies between 0.51 and 0.71 with a mean around 0.55, and for mepivacaine the figures are 0.4–0.69, with a mean around 0.6. For bupivacaine the ratio is independent of the dose or technique used, and lies between 0.11 and 0.51 with a mean around 0.3, in all the studies quoted.

Thus, the ratio seems to be fairly constant for each drug, but differences are observed when the three drugs are given as a single injection. Several factors may account for this difference, including the time of delivery and the fetal tissue saturation. Normally, the time between epidural injection and delivery is too short to obtain an equilibrium between maternal and fetal tissues. Maternal and fetal pH differences, vascular shunts in the placenta, differences in maternal and fetal LA protein or red cell binding, and placental metabolism may also be involved.

Table 19.1 Characteristics of the main studies concerning epidural block with bupivacaine (single dose)

Reference	No. of subjects	Dose (mg)	Maternal level (venous, μg/ml)	Neonatal level (venous, μg/ml)	Ratio*	∂t† (min)	Comments
9	24	58	0.25	0.14	0.51	–	B 0.75% A Mixture of L + E
10	20	1.7 mg/kg	–	>0.05	–	–	B 0.5%
11	20	168	0.72 (arterial)	0.2	0.25	–	B 0.75%
12	23 7	138 138	– –	– –	0.28 0.28	– –	B 0.5% B 0.75%
13	15	12.5 26.2	– 34% higher than with B 0.125%	– 54% higher than with B 0.125%	– –	– –	B 0.125% A B 0.375% A
14	21	56 0.71 mg/kg	0.22 (arterial)	0.06 (artery) 0.08 (vein)	UV/MA 0.29	125	B 0.25% A
14	11	82 1.22 mg/kg	0.39 (arterial)	0.072 (artery) 0.098 (vein)	UV/MA 0.26	142	B 0.25%

* Neonatal/maternal levels [umbilical vein (Uv) maternal artery (MA) when indicated.]
† ∂t (i.e. span of time in minutes from injection to time of sampling). L = lidocaine; B = bupivacaine; E = etidocaine; M = mepivacaine, the number indicating the concentration of LA; A = epinephrine.

Table 19.2 Characteristics of the main studies concerning epidural block with lidocaine (single dose). Abbreviations as in Table 19.1

Reference	No. of subjects	Dose (mg)	Maternal level (venous, μg/ml)	Neonatal level (venous, μg/ml)	Ratio	∂t (min)	Comments
9	24	295	1.05	0.68	0.66	–	L + A Mixture of B + E
15	6	4 mg/kg	2.18	1.19	0.52	22	L
16	5 11	370 372	2.8 3.4	– –	0.71 0.57	– –	L L, Eclampsia
4	–	200	1.5	0.7	0.5	–	L (mixture)

Table 19.3 Characteristics of the main studies concerning epidural block with bupivacaine (multiple doses). Abbreviations as in Table 19.1

Reference	No. of subjects	Dose (mg)	Maternal level (venous, μg/ml)	Neonatal level (venous, μg/ml)	Ratio	∂t (min)	Comments
17	24	32–100	0.2–0.47	< toxic levels	–	–	B 0.25%
2	277	95	0.36	0.11	0.31	259	B
18	20	112	0.4	0.11	0.27	177	B
14	32	96.4	0.24 (arterial)	0.065 (artery) 0.082 (vein)	UV/MA 0.38	263	B + A

Table 19.4 Characteristics of the main studies concerning epidural block with lidocaine (single dose). Abbreviations as in Table 19.1

Reference	No. of subjects	Dose (mg)	Maternal level (venous, μg/ml)	Neonatal level (venous, μg/ml)	Ratio	∂t (min)	Comments
4	–	1070	4.5	4.3	–	–	L
2	439	446	2.1	1.2	0.57	151	L
19	190	409 258	1.08 0.79	0.63 0.42	0.58 0.54	206 201	L L + A
8	11 30	423 414	2.3 1.5	1.17 0.89	0.52 0.59	183 190	L L + A

Table 19.5 Characteristics of the main studies concerning epidural block with mepivacaine (multiple doses). Abbreviations as in Table 19.1

Reference	No. of subjects	Dose (mg)	Maternal level (venous, μg/ml)	Neonatal level (venous, μg/ml)	Ratio	∂t (min)	Comments
8	42	374	2.89	1.84	0.64	136	M
	11	349	2.26	1.54	0.69	261	M + A
2	221	572	3.3	2.1	0.69	164	M

Table 19.6 Characteristics of the main studies concerning epidural block with bupivacaine (continuous infusion). Abbreviations as in Table 19.1

Reference	No. of subjects	Dose (mg)	Maternal level (venous, μg/ml)	Neonatal level (venous, μg/ml)	Ratio	∂t (min)	Comments
20	16	Loading dose 16 mg/h	0.2–0.6	0.058	0.32 f/m = 0.28	–	B 0.25%
21	5	21 +23 mg/h	0.2–0.45	0.06–0.17	0.11–0.47	333.9	B 0.25%
22	10	18 mg/h	0.325	0.143	0.44	324	B 0.125%
23	13	25 mg/h	0.76	0.17	0.22	252	B 0.25%
24	12	50 12 mg/h	<0.68	–	0.44	205	B 0.25%
25	23	182	0.54	0.18	0.33	457	B 0.5%

Table 19.7 Characteristics of the main studies concerning epidural block with lidocaine (continuous infusion). Abbreviations as in Table 19.1

Reference	No. of subjects	Dose (mg)	Maternal level (venous, μg/ml)	Neonatal level (venous, μg/ml)	Ratio	∂t (min)	Comments
26	6	658	2.34	–	0.6	–	L, Eclampsia
	6	668	1.42	–	0.4	–	L
27	11	591	1.22	0.65	0.53	689	L
	11	293	0.68	0.39	0.57	636	L + A
25	19	623	2.4	1.27	0.48	457	L 1.5%

Table 19.8 Characteristics of the study of Bruguerolle et al[28] concerning epidural block with bupivacaine (single and multiple doses). Abbreviations as in Table 19.1

Technique	No. of subjects	Dose (mg)	Maternal level (venous, μg/ml)	Ratio	∂t (min)	Comments
Single dose (cesarean delivery)	25	88 1.3 mg/kg	0.20	–	40	B 0.5%
Single dose (spontaneous delivery)	20	37.1 0.56 mg/kg	0.12	–	70.5	B 0.25%
Multiple doses (2) (spontaneous delivery)	27	53.3 0.78 mg/kg	0.14	–	150	B 0.25%
Multiple doses (3) (spontaneous delivery)	9	91.5 1.25 mg/kg	0.17	–	246.2	B 0.25%
Continuous (bolus + infusion) (spontaneous delivery)	8	84 1.1 mg/kg	0.18	–	204	B 0.25%

Many factors are known to affect plasma bupivacaine concentrations, but the actual hour at which the injection is given has not been studied. Since the hour of day or night at which a drug is injected is known to modify its kinetics (chronopharmacokinetics), we investigated the influence of this on plasma bupivacaine concentrations in the newborn, and found that, in the children of mothers undergoing cesarean delivery with a single dose of bupivacaine, there was a significant correlation with the hour of injection. Maximum values were observed when bupivacaine was injected in the late afternoon.[28]

CLINICAL CONSEQUENCES FOR THE NEWBORN

The clinical consequences of LA toxicity are well known: bradycardia, apnea, hypotonia, convulsions, mydriasis, and loss of oculocephalic reflexes. Seizures due to LA toxicity begin within the first 6 h of life, in contrast to those due to hypoxia, which usually begin after 12–24 h. Apnea after LA toxicity may be due either to brainstem depression or to convulsions. Dodson[29] has reported toxic thresholds sufficient to produce bradycardia in the newborn to be 8–12 μg/ml for mepivacaine and 2.5 μg/ml for lidocaine, and 13 μg/ml for mepivacaine to cause convulsions. As far as we are aware, data for toxic thresholds in the newborn are not available for bupivacaine. The highest mean plasma bupivacaine concentration observed in our study (0.20 μg/ml) was not associated with clinical signs of toxicity.

Scanlon[18] reported that infants whose mothers received epidural block with lidocaine or mepivacaine had significantly lower scores for tests of muscular strength; when interpreting these results, one must take into account that the correlation between the plasma concentrations and the neurobehavioral scores was not studied[30] and that the scores of the infants may have been influenced by the fact that their mothers were selected to receive epidural block.

CONCLUSIONS

The results of the studies reviewed in this chapter show that low plasma concentrations of LA are produced in the newborn, but these concentrations do not reveal the real amount of LA in the tissues, and it is on the tissue concentrations that clinical signs of toxicity depend. Thus, plasma LA concentrations are an inadequate index of the situation in the tissues and one must be careful when attempting to correlate plasma concentrations with clinical signs of toxicity, such as apnea, bradycardia, or convulsions, in a neonate whose mother has received an epidural block.

REFERENCES

1. Bromage P R, Robson J G 1961 Concentrations of lignocaine in the blood after intravenous, intramuscular, epidural and endotracheal administration. Anaesthesia 16: 461–478
2. Ralston D H, Shnider S M 1978 The fetal and neonatal effects of regional anesthesia in obstetrics. Anesthesiology 48: 34–64
3. Seebacher J, Galli-Douani P, Henry M, Lefevre G, Vauthier D, Darbois Y 1990 Anesthesie péridurale et rachianesthésie en obstetrique. In: Anesthesie régionale. Arnette, Paris pp 839–892
4. Haberer J P Anesthesie péridurale en obstétrique. In: Précis d'anesthésie loco-régionale. Masson, Paris pp 205–245
5. Pedersen H, Morishima H, Finster M 1978 Uptake and effects of local anesthetics in mother and fetus. Int Anesthesiol Clin 16: 73–89
6. Haberer J P, Monteillard C 1986 Effets de l'anesthésie péridurale obstétricale sur le fetus et le nouveau-né. Ann Fr Anesth Reanim 5: 381–414
7. Tucker G T, Mather L E 1979 Clinical pharmacokinetics of local anesthetics. Clin Pharmacokinet 4: 241–278
8. Brown W U, Bell G C, Lurie A O, Weiss J B, Scanlon J W, Alper M H 1975 Newborn blood levels of lidocaine and mepivacaine in the first postnatal day following maternal epidural anesthesia. Anesthesiology 42: 698–707
9. Jullien Y, Desch G, Derodez M, Atlan S, Descomps B, Du Cailar J 1982 Maternal and fetal levels of local anaesthetics after epidural injection of a triple mixture. Ann Fr Anesth Reanim 1: 141–146
10. Jani K, McEvedy B, Harris S, Samaan A 1989 Maternal and neonatal bupivacaine concentrations after spinal and extradural anaesthesia for cesarean section. Br J Anaesth 62: 226–227
11. McGuinness G A, Merkow A J, Kennedy R L, Erenberg A 1978 Epidural anesthesia with bupivacaine for cesarean section. Anesthesiology 49: 270–273
12. Kuhnert P M, Kuhnert B R, Stitts J M, Gross T L 1981 The use of a selected ion monitoring technique to study the disposition of bupivacaine in mother, fetus and neonate following epidural anesthesia for cesarean section. Anesthesiology 55: 611–617
13. Van Zundert A, Burm A, Van Kleef J, Spierdijk J, Van der Aa P, Smolders F, Vaes L 1987 Plasma concentration of epidural bupivacaine in mother and newborn: 0.125% versus 0.375%. Anesth Analg 66: 435–441
14. Hyman M D, Shnider S M 1971 Maternal and neonatal blood concentrations of bupivacaine associated with obstetrical conduction anesthesia. Anesthesiology 34: 81–86
15. Sakuma S, Oka T, Okuno A, Yoshioka H, Shimizu T, Ogawa H 1985 Placental transfer of lidocaine and elimination from newborns following obstetrical epidural and pudendal anesthesia. Pediatr Pharmacol 5: 107–115
16. Ramanathan J, Bottorff M, Sibai B M 1985 Maternal and neonatal effects of epidural lidocaine in preeclamptic women undergoing cesarean section. Anesth Analg 64: 268
17. Schurg R, Biscopping J, Bachmann B, Jovanovic V, Hohmann M, Hempelmann G 1989 Maternal and neonatal bupivacaine plasma levels in peridural anesthesia for relief of labor pain. Geburtshilfe-Frauenheilkd 49: 952–957
18. Scanlon J W, Ostheimer G W, Lurie A O, Brown W U, Weiss J B, Alper M H 1976 Neurobehavioural responses and drug concentrations in newborns after maternal epidural anesthesia with bupivacaine. Anesthesiology 45: 400–405
19. Zador G, Englesson S, Nilsson B 1974 Low dose intermittent epidural anaesthesia with lidocaine for vaginal delivery. Acta Obstet Gynecol Scand 34: 3–16
20. Matouskova A, Hanson B 1979 Continuous miniinfusion of bupivacaine into the epidural space during labor. Acta Obstet Gynecol Scand 83: 31–41
21. Evans K R L, Carrie L E S 1979 Continuous epidural infusion of bupivacaine in labor. A simple method. Anaesthesia 34: 310–315
22. Clark M J 1982 Continuous miniinfusion of 0.125% bupivacaine into the epidural space during labor. J A M Obstet Assoc 81: 484–491
23. Rosenblatt R 1983 Continuous epidural infusion for obstetric analgesia. Reg Anesth 8: 10–15
24. Denson D D, Knapp R M, Turner P, Thompson G A 1984 Serum bupivacaine concentrations in term parturients following continuous epidural analgesia for labor and delivery. Ther Drug Monit 6: 393–398
25. Abboud T K, Afrasiabi A, Sarkis F et al 1984 Continuous infusion epidural analgesia in parturients receiving bupivacaine, chloroprocaine or lidocaine. Maternal, fetal and neonatal effects. Anesth Analg 63: 421–428
26. Ramanathan J 1987 Continuous epidural lidocaine infusion in preeclampsia: maternal and neonatal effects. Reg Anesth 12: 95–96
27. Zador G, Willdeck-lund G, Nilsson B, 1974 Continuous drip

lumbar epidural anaesthesia with lidocaine for vaginal delivery. Acta Obstet Gynecol Scand 34: 31–40
28. Bruguerolle B, Giaufre E, Rastello C, Verdot J J 1993 Concentrations de bupivacaine chez le nouveau-né aprés anesthésie péridurale maternelle. Thérapie 48: 60–61
29. Dodson W E 1976 Neonatal drug intoxication: local anesthetics. Ped Clin N Am 23: 399–411
30. Kuhnert B R, Kennard M J, Linn PL 1988 Neonatal neurobehavior after epidural anesthesia for cesarean section: a comparison of bupivacaine and chloroprocaine. Anesth Analg 67: 64–68

20. Epidural anesthesia

PART A
THE DEVELOPMENT OF EPIDURAL NEEDLES

G. W. Ostheimer C. Shea A. Van Zundert

NEEDLES FOR EPIDURAL ANESTHESIA

In Chapter 34 we describe how Corning's significant contributions of the 1880s were overlooked until early in the twentieth century, when Cathelin and Sicard administered an anesthetic via the sacral hiatus.[1]

Advances in both technique and materials continued. By the mid-1920s Fidel Pages[2] of Spain had developed the approach for lumbar epidural anesthesia. For this he used a 20-gauge, spool-hub, short-bevel spinal needle. He suffered an early death from pneumonia, a tragedy that delayed further work on the technique for nearly 10 years. Meanwhile other researchers continued to apply epidural anesthesia via the caudal route.

RENEWED INTEREST IN LUMBAR EPIDURAL ANESTHESIA

Dogliotti[3] in Turin, Italy, working during the 1930s, reawakened interest in lumbar epidural anesthesia, using a lumbar dural puncture needle of medium size, with a very short point. Another investigator, Charles Odom,[4] of Charity Hospital in New Orleans, described a technique for the lumbar approach to the epidural space, for which he used a 20-gauge short-bevel needle with a spool-hub design.

Finally, in 1941, overcoming the limitations to the duration of regional anesthesia, continuous epidural anesthesia was employed based on Lemmon's approach to the subarachnoid space by Hingson, Edwards and Southworth. Barely 3 months later came the first use of continuous caudal epidural anesthesia in obstetrics.[5,6] Subsequently, Hingson and Edwards designed a malleable stainless-steel caudal needle with a tapered hub to allow a length of rubber tubing to be attached and through which the local anesthetic was injected (Fig. 20.1). As often happens in the pursuit of science, other researchers independently developed their techniques. S. A. Manalan[7] in Indianapolis and Adams et al[8] at the Mayo Clinic simultaneously devised continuous caudal techniques involving a ureteral catheter introduced through a large-gauge needle into the sacral canal.

Hingson and Southworth[9] 1 year later extended the concept of the continuous catheter to the lumbar epidural space. As their first attempts to pass a ureteral catheter through a large-bore Barker spinal needle met with some difficulty; they then used a malleable 19-gauge spinal needle that remained in the epidural space throughout the procedure. In this technique, rubber tubing and the Lemmon mattress were used, as described for continuous spinal techniques. The first investigator to combine the Tuohy needle with a ureteral catheter for lumbar epidural anesthesia was Curbello of Havana, in 1947. Others who experimented along these lines included C.E. Flowers of Johns Hopkins, Oral Crawford at the Missouri State Sanatorium, D.B. Gershenfeld and L.E. Savel of Newark, New Jersey, and R.S. Wagner of Temple University School of Medicine in Philadelphia (Fig. 20.2).[10–13]

Peter Cheng, in Wilmington, California, became aware of the 'negative pressure' concept for the epidural space proposed by Janzen in 1926 who concluded that a blunt needle and a side orifice both appeared to result in a greater 'negative pressure'. Following intense anatomic study, Cheng fashioned a blunt, round-tipped needle having an oval directional orifice on one side and proximal to the tip. A nylon or plastic catheter could be used with this instrument for continuous anesthesia. The cannula was marked in centimeters and millimeters from the tip. A flange that was attached facilitated gripping. The flange could be slid along the cannula to aid in immobilizing the needle after epidural insertion (Fig. 20.2). Cheng used Gutierrez's 'hanging drop' for locating the epidural space with this needle.[14,15]

In more recent times Joseph Lutz (personal communication), of Livingston, New Jersey, has designed a blunt round-tipped needle having a pinhole directional orifice 1/16 inch from the tip for lumbar epidural use (Fig. 20.2). In this procedure the skin is punctured by an 18-gauge needle or needle guide, following which the 20-gauge $3\frac{1}{2}$ inch Lutz needle is inserted into the epidural space, using the loss of resistance test. It can be used for both lumbosacral anesthesia and upper abdominal surgery.

CURRENT FEDERAL SPECIFICATIONS AND REGULATIONS

Federal Specification GG-N-196[16] governs spinal needles. Cannulas are of two types: high chromium or high carbon steel. Needle points must be strong, straight and of maximum keenness, although some variation in configuration of the bevel is permitted. Hubs are to be made of brass, with either polished nickel or polished chromium plating. They must be of such shape that they will not roll. The gauge and manufacturer's mark are to be stamped on each hub. Staging is required to join hub and cannula.

The outer surface of the finished needle is to be free of pits, and the inner surface must contain no deep pits, furrows, scaling or die marks. The lumen of the cannula must be free of foreign material of any kind.

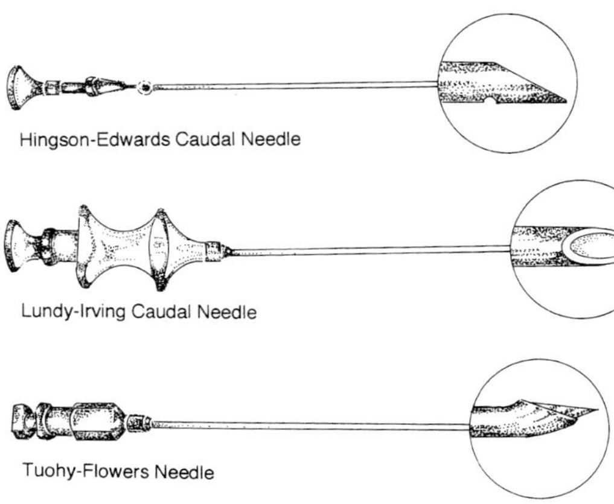

Fig. 20.1 Needles developed for use in epidural anesthesia.

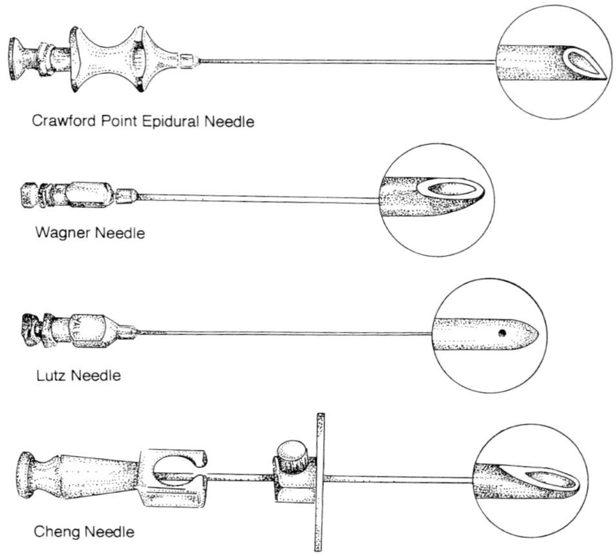

Fig. 20.2 Needles developed for use in epidural anesthesia.

Every manufactured needle must meet certain standards regarding corrosion resistance, stiffness, elasticity, swaging security, breakage resistance and tightness of fit. Packaging is also specified.

DISPOSABLE NEEDLES

Disposable spinal, epidural and caudal anesthetic needles are now available. They are made of stainless steel and, like their predecessors, must meet federal requirements. The cutting edges of the disposable needle may be dulled somewhat during the manufacturing process as an aid in both spreading rather than cutting tissues and improving the perception of dural puncture.

SPINAL NEEDLE SPECIFICATIONS AND COLOR CODING FOR IDENTIFICATION

When reviewing the specifications of spinal needles, there are several difficulties because many of the companies have developed from different regions of the world and have adopted different specifications.[17,18]

ISO (The International Organization for Standardization, Case Postale 56, CH-1211 Genève 20, Switzerland) is a worldwide federation of national organizations that provide standards. The work of preparing International Standards is normally carried out through ISO technical committees. International organizations, governmental and nongovernmental, in liaison with ISO, also take part in the work. ISO collaborates closely with the International Electrotechnical Commission (IEC) on all matters of electrotechnical standardization. Publication

Table 20.1 Color code

Nominal outside diameter of needle		
Gauge (G)	mm	Color
30 g	0.3	Yellow
29 g	0.33	Red
28 g	0.36	Blue–green
27 g	0.4	Medium gray
26 g	0.45	Brown
25 g	0.5	Orange
24 g	0.55	Medium purple
23 g	0.6	Deep blue
22 g	0.7	Black
21 g	0.8	Deep green
20 g	0.9	Yellow
19 g	1.1	Cream
18 g	1.2	Pink
17 g	1.4	Red–violet
16 g	1.6	White
15 g	1.8	Blue–gray
14 g	2.1	Pale green
13 g	2.4	Purple
12 g	2.7	Pale blue
11 g	3.0	Green–yellow
10 g	3.4	Olive-brown

as an International Standard requires approval by at least 75% of the member bodies casting a vote.

The overall objective of the standards is to specify colors to enable rapid visual identification of the outside diameter of single-use hypodermic needles, and these are documents normally used when referring to spinal needles. The colors used to 'code' needles may be applied in either opaque or transparent form, and the color code is equally applicable to normal walled, thin-walled and extra-thin-walled needles. The colors are specified by name but one must remember that this inevitably introduces a certain amount of subjectivity in the assessment of compliance. This subjectivity may be minimized by viewing the hubs under controlled lighting conditions and by the use of assessors with medically demonstrated correct color vision.

The color code for the identification of single-use hypodermic needles of nominal outside diameter in the range 0.3 mm to 3.4 mm is given in Table 20.1.[19]

The reference color samples referred to in this International Standard are available by contacting: Melab, Medizintechnik und Labor GmbH, Heimsheimer Weg 17, D-7259 Friolzheim Germany.

REREFENCES

1. Pitkin G P 1953 Conduction anesthesia, 2nd edn. Philadelphia, J. B. Lippincott Company, p 785
2. Odom C B 1936 A review of Pages' epidural anesthesia with a report of one hundred cases. New Orleans Med Surg J 88: 618–627
3. Dogliotti A M 1933 A new method of block anesthesia: segmental peridural spinal anesthesia. Am J Surg 20: 107–118
4. Odom C B 1936 Epidural anesthesia. Am J Surg 34: 547–558
5. Hingson R A, Southworth J L 1942 Continuous caudal anesthesia. Am J Surg 58: 93–96
6. Edwards W B, Hingson R A 1942 Continuous caudal anesthesia in obstetrics. Am J Surg 57: 459–464
7. Manalan S A 1942 Caudal block anesthesia in obstetrics. J Indiana Med Assn 35: 564–565
8. Adams R C, Lundy J S, Seldon T H 1943 Continuous caudal anesthesia or analgesia: a consideration of the technic, various uses, and some possible dangers. JAMA 122: 152–158
9. Hingson R A, Southworth J L 1944 Continuous peridural anesthesia. Anesth Analg 23: 215–217
10. Flowers Jr C E, Hellman L M, Hingson R A 1949 Continuous peridural anesthesia and analgesia for labor, delivery, and cesarean section. Anesth Analg 28: 181–189
11. Flowers Jr C E 1950 A technic of continuous peridural anesthesia using a blunt needle. Anesth Analg 29: 39–42
12. Crawford O B, Buckingham W W, Ottosen P, Brasher C A 1951 Peridural anesthesia in thoracic surgery: a review of 667 cases. Anesthesiology 12: 73–84
13. Crawford O B, Brasher C, Buckingham W A 1957 Peridural anesthesia for thoracic surgery. Anesthesiology 18: 241–249
14. Cheng P A 1963 Anatomical and clinical aspects of epidural anesthesia. Anesth Analg 42: 398–415
15. Cheng P A 1958 Blunt-tip needle for epidural anesthesia. Anesthesiology 19: 556–559
16. Federal Standard Stock Catalog: Federal Specifications for Needles, Hypodermic; For Luer Syringes: GG-N-196
17. ISO 7864:1988 Sterile hypodermic needles for single use. ISO, Geneva.
18. ISO 9626:1991 Stainless steel needle tubing for the manufacture of medical services. ISO, Geneva
19. ISO 6009:1992 (E) Hypodermic needles for single use – colour coding for identification. ISO, Geneva.

PART B

EPIDURAL ANESTHESIA: TECHNIQUE

G. W. Ostheimer K. A. Leavitt

ANATOMY AND LANDMARKS

The spinal cord in the adult usually does not extend below the vertebral body of L2, and more often it ends at L1 (Fig. 20.3). The dural sac, however, usually ends at the level of S1–S2. Surrounding the dural sac, delimited by the dura mater on one side and the periosteum of the vertebral bodies and the ligamenta flava on the other, is the epidural space, which extends from the foramen magnum superiorly to the sacral hiatus caudally. Therefore, in theory at least, epidural anesthesia may be given at any level between C1 and S5. The L2–L5 interspaces are usually chosen for obstetric epidural anesthesia.

The anatomic landmarks for epidural anesthesia are the same as for spinal anesthesia: an imaginary line drawn between the right and left posterior iliac crests crosses either the spinous process of the L4 vertebra or the L4–L5 vertebral interspace (Fig. 20.4). The selected vertebral interspace for the epidural block can be pinpointed by locating this interspace and then palpating the desired interspace in the cephalad direction.

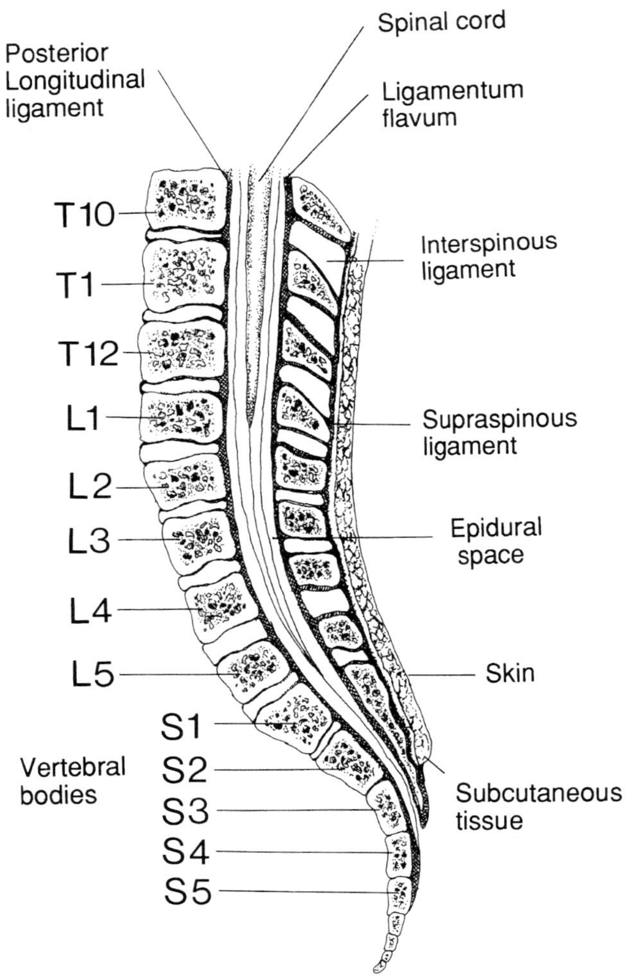

Fig. 20.3 The vertebral column.

PATIENT POSITION

The position of the patient is identical to that for spinal anesthesia: either the lateral or the sitting position, although we at the Brigham and Women's Hospital prefer the right lateral position (Fig. 20.5) in order to displace the gravid uterus from the aorta and the inferior vena cava. Additionally, upon completion of the block, the parturient can be placed in the left lateral position to avoid aortocaval compression and achieve an equivalent level of anesthesia bilaterally.

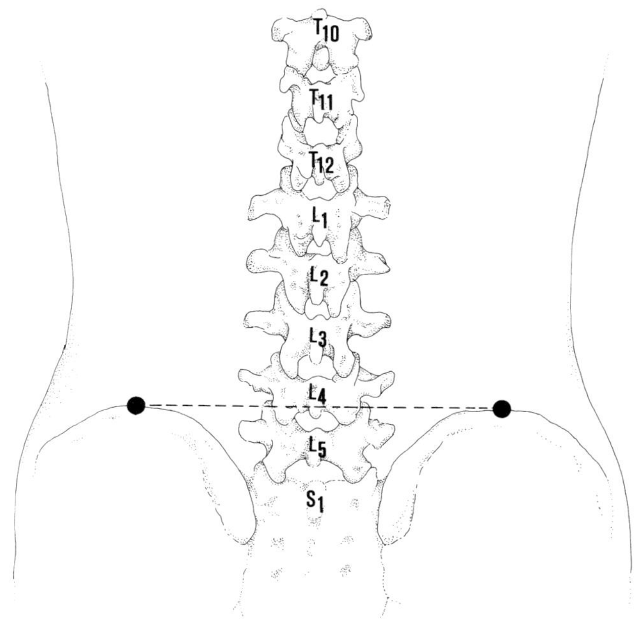

Fig. 20.4 The lumbar area. A line drawn between the right and left iliac crests crosses either the spinous process of the L4 vertebra or the L4–L5 vertebral interspace.

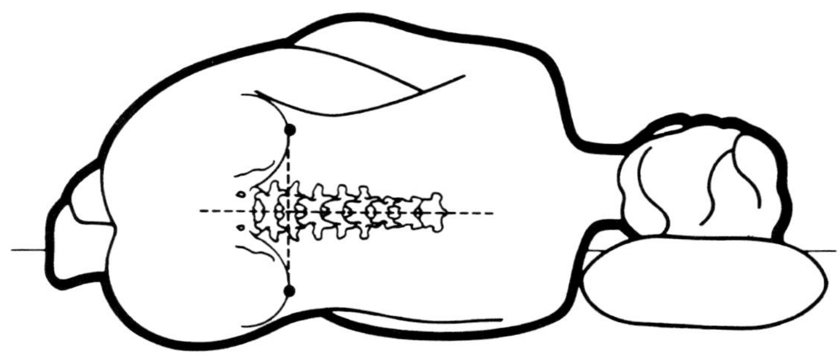

Fig. 20.5 The right lateral position for epidural and subarachnoid block.

MATERIALS

The following materials should be assembled when an epidural anesthetic is to be administered:

- One pair of sterile gloves
- Antibacterial solution for cleansing the skin
- One sterile cup for the antibacterial solution
- Forceps
- Sterile gauze pads
- Sterile towels for draping the field (if desired)
- One 25-gauge, 1.6- to 3.8-cm needle for skin infiltration
- One 21- or 22-gauge, 3.8-cm needle for deep infiltration (if desired)
- One 18-gauge needle to make an opening in the skin (if desired)
- One 17- to 19-gauge epidural needle with stylet (we prefer the 17-gauge Weiss modification of the Tuohy needle with the Huber tip)
- One 3-ml syringe
- One 5-ml glass syringe
- One 20-ml syringe
- One disposable epidural catheter.

A disposable epidural anesthetic tray usually contains all of the above items.

TECHNIQUE

Thirty milliliters of a clear antacid (0.3 mol/l sodium citrate or its equivalent) is administered before the initiation of an epidural anesthetic. No other premedication is given for vaginal delivery. For cesarean delivery, 30 ml of a clear antacid is administered (as above) and, if the patient is considered 'at risk' for any reason, metaclopramide 10 mg i.v. and cimetidine 300 mg or ranitidine 100 mg is given intramuscularly or intravenously in the 30–60 min prior to induction of the epidural block. The technique of epidural anesthesia for the parturient is similar to that for the surgical patient except that special consideration must be given to the condition of the fetus and to the maternal physiologic changes associated with pregnancy and labor.

Although arterial blood pressure must be monitored in any patient undergoing regional anesthesia, the obstetric patient must be carefully observed for changes in blood pressure. The blood pressure is determined in the supine and lateral positions before the block is initiated to check for aortocaval compression (supine hypotensive syndrome). An automatic blood pressure monitor is useful but not mandatory. The fetal heart rate (FHR) record is reviewed. Routine electrocardiographic monitoring is optional at our institution for the initiation of an epidural block for labor or cesarean delivery unless the procedure is initiated in the operating room. However, electrocardiographic monitoring is immediately available, if desired.

The parturient selected for epidural anesthesia is acutely hydrated prior to the induction of the epidural block. A large-gauge indwelling plastic catheter allows the administration of 1000 ml of warm lactated Ringer's solution or similar crystalloid solution over 10–20 min. This hydration helps to prevent the hypotension that may be caused by the sympathetic block produced by epidural anesthesia. Warm intravenous fluid diminishes pre-, intra- and postpartum shivering experienced by the parturient. The intravenous infusion is then maintained should the patient require additional hydration or intravenous medication.

The epidural tray is opened in a sterile manner and the expiration date checked. The gloved anesthesiologist prepares the skin of the lumbar area with a bactericidal preparation, wiping off the excess solution. The field may be draped with sterile towels. The desired interspace is located. Depending on the special anatomic features of the patient and the requirements of the situation, the L2–L3, L3–L4 or L4–L5 interspace may be used. We find that the L2–L3 interspace is usually the most suitable. The selected entry point into the skin is fixed by placing two fingers on either side of the interspace selected and the skin is infiltrated with a small amount of local anesthetic. The 25-gauge needle is used to create the skin wheal. Then a small amount (about 1–2 ml) of local anesthetic is injected into the subcutaneous tissue and the interspinous ligament. Some anesthesiologists will insert an 18-gauge needle through the skin wheal to create a skin opening large enough to allow the epidural needle to pass through without carrying with it a plug of skin on its way to the epidural space. We do not use this technique because the subsequent release of the skin will move the hole. If one relies on the position of the skin hole, it may be very difficult to identify the epidural space. A well-fitted stylet will prevent coring of the skin.

Various types of epidural needles are available. At our institution, the winged Weiss modification of the Tuohy needle with a Huber point (Fig. 20.6A) is preferred because it can be grasped with the index finger and the thumb of both hands while it is advanced through the tissues. Resting the middle, ring and little fingers of both hands of the anesthesiologist firmly against the patient's back gives fine control over the movement of the needle unexcelled by any other type of epidural needle. An all-purpose needle such as a 17- to 19-gauge Tuohy needle may also be used (Fig. 20.6B).

Figure 20.3 illustrates the tissue layers and ligaments that are encountered as the needle is advanced 1.2–3.7 cm to a point where the tissue resistance of the interspinous ligament is felt. For this phase of the needle replacement, the shaft of the needle is half between the thumb, index and middle fingers with the palmar aspect of the thumb resting on the head of the stylet to prevent its displacement (Fig. 20.7). We insert the needle into the interspinous ligament or ligamentum flavum with the needle bevel facing caudal or cephalad. This is done to avoid rotation

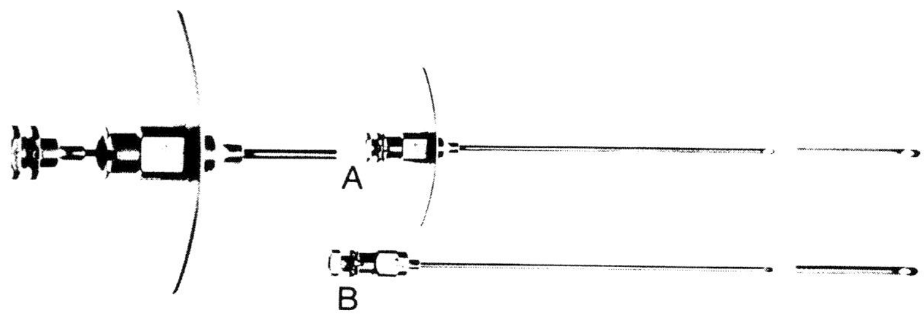

Fig. 20.6 (**A**) The winged modification of the Tuohy needle (Weiss needle). (**B**) The Tuohy needle.

of the needle once it is in the epidural space since this may result in 'coring' of the dura and the production of a dural puncture.

The needle is advanced with a smooth, continuous motion. Further movement of the needle is halted when the resistance of the ligamentum flavum changes. At this point, advancing the needle only a small distance will result in its passing through the ligamentum flavum into the epidural space, which measures only 5 mm at its widest extent (in the lumbar area). The advancing needle can easily overshoot this distance, pierce the dura and penetrate into the subarachnoid space. Therefore, it is important that the advancing movement of the epidural needle be delicately controlled.

There are two methods of identifying the epidural space. The hanging-drop method provides visual identification, whereas the loss-of-resistance method gives tactile evidence of entry.

The hanging-drop technique (Figs 20.8 and 20.9) is based on the concept of a negative pressure within the epidural space. This method was discovered by Jantzen in 1926 and rediscovered by Heldt and Moloney in 1928. In 1930, Gutierrez used negative pressure to find the epidural space by placing a drop of saline into the hub of the advancing needle. The current technique involves placing a drop of fluid into the hub of a needle that has been inserted into the interspinous ligament or ligamentum flavum.

The wings of the needle are grasped with the thumbs and index fingers and the anesthesiologist's hands are steadied by the middle, ring and little fingers resting on the patient's back, as shown in Figures 20.8 and 20.9.

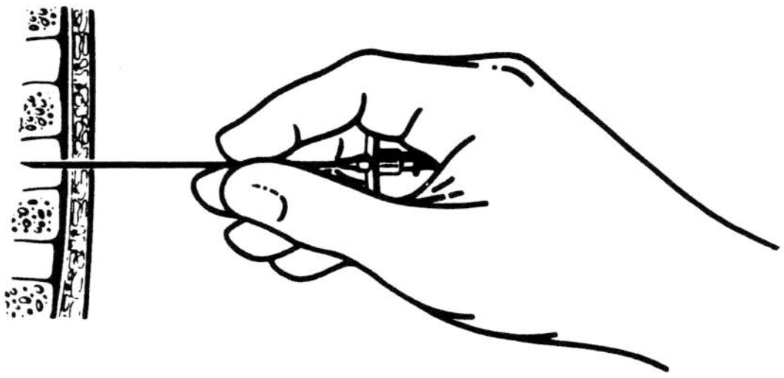

Fig 20.7 Hand position for inserting the epidural needle.

While the drop is watched constantly, the needle is slowly and continuously advanced. As soon as the ligamentum flavum is pierced and the bevel enters the epidural space, the drop is suddenly sucked into the needle as if by a negative pressure in the epidural space. Slow and continuous movement of the needle rather than a rapid intermittent or jerky motion is essential for this technique. This sign occurs about 80% of the time but the reasons for it are not clear. There are four major theories:

1. When a blunt needle impinges on the dura a cone of depression may form, creating a negative pressure. However, if this were true, the sign would occur almost 100% of the time.
2. Expansion of the thoracic cage on inspiration results in a negative pressure that may be transmitted through the paravertebral spaces and the intervertebral foraminae to the epidural space. There are no data to support this theory.

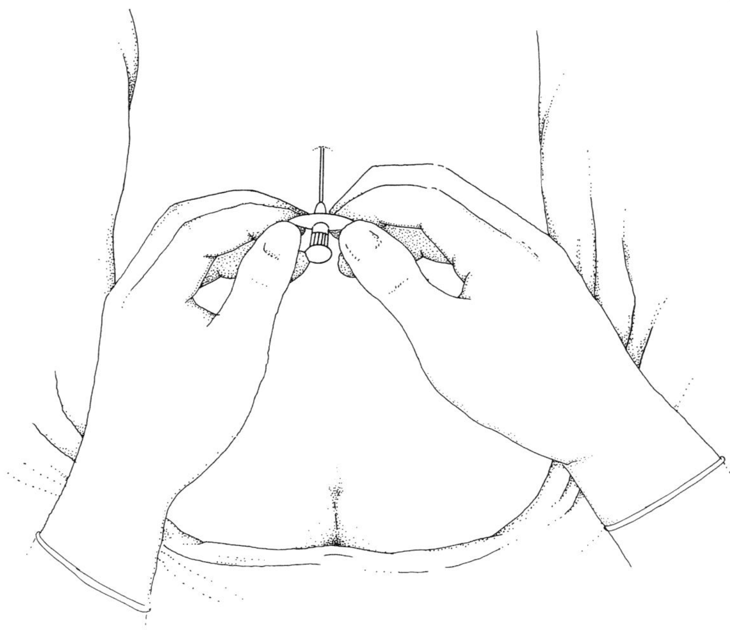

Fig 20.8 Hand position for the hanging-drop technique employed when using the winged epidural needle.

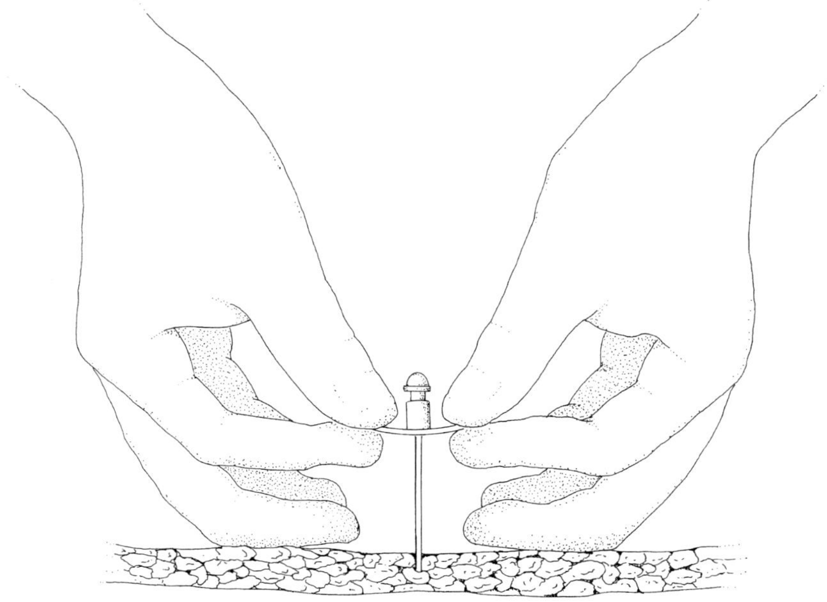

Fig 20.9 Hand position for the hanging-drop technique employed when using the winged epidural needle (cross-sectional view).

3. The epidural space may be only a potential space in the erect posture, developing only when the back is flexed and the dura mater 'separates' from the ligamentum flavum. There is some evidence for this theory.

4. The pull of the abdominal viscera on the posterior thoracic and abdominal walls can cause a negative pressure, but proof of this is lacking. The negative pressure in the epidural space is probably due to a combination of the above factors 1, 3 and 4.

Other mechanical devices can aid in the placement of the epidural needle and help reduce the failure rate of the visual technique.

At our institution, the hanging-drop technique is used with the Weiss needle, and there is additional confirmation of the position by using the loss-of-resistance technique with air and/or fluid.

The loss-of-resistance technique (Fig. 20.10), in which the anesthesiologist's thumb exerts continuous positive pressure on the end of the piston of a glass syringe containing air or preservative-free saline, depends on the sudden loss of resistance as the advancing needle point leaves the ligamentum flavum and enters the epidural space. This method was introduced by Sicard and Forestier in 1921 and was used to administer anesthesia for surgical procedures by Pages in the same year. Its success rate is greater than 90% if the dura is not entered. This technique is usually associated with Dogliotti, who popularized its use.

The needle is advanced to the level of the interspinous ligament or ligamentum flavum. The stylet is removed from the epidural needle and a small (5- or 10-ml) glass

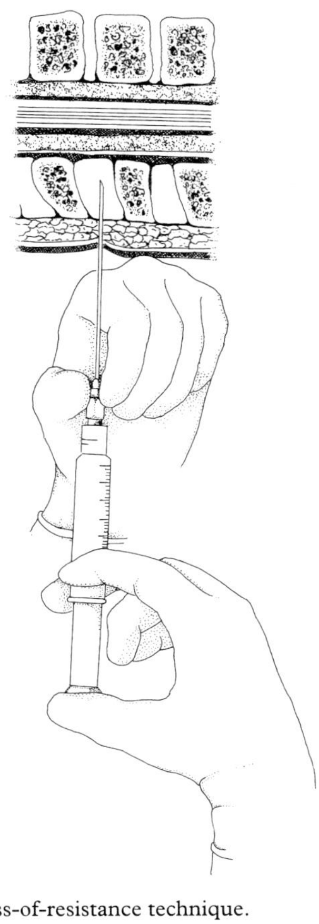

Fig 20.10 Loss-of-resistance technique.

syringe filled with air or sterile saline solution is attached. The right-handed anesthesiologist holds the epidural needle firmly between the index finger and the thumb of the left hand, as illustrated in Figure 20.10. The back of the left hand rests firmly against the patient's back. This steadies the left hand so that it has fine control over the advancement of the needle. The right hand controls the syringe; with the body of the syringe between the right index and the middle finger, the thumb applies hard, *steady* pressure to the plunger of the syringe while the left hand slowly advances the epidural needle through the tissues. None of the syringe contents will be expelled as long as the point of the needle is in the interspinous ligament or the ligamentum flavum. However, as soon as these structures are pierced and the needle enters the epidural space, this resistance suddenly disappears and the contents of the syringe are suddenly discharged. The movement of the epidural needle is halted immediately by the countertraction of the left hand.

We prefer the hanging-drop technique with the winged epidural needle over the loss-of-resistance technique because it allows better perception of the changes in tissue resistance as the needle is advanced. As their skills improve, anesthesiologists 'know' the epidural space is being entered without any movement of the hanging drop. If the loss-of-resistance technique is chosen it is recommended that fluid rather than air be used because of air's compressibility and the high incidence of false-positive results when air is used.

Regardless of which technique is used, it is advisable to perform tests to confirm that the needle is in the epidural space. The first test involves aspiration with a small (5-ml) glass syringe attached to the needle. If the aspiration test yields a bloody return, it is probable that one of the veins of the epidural plexus has been punctured. To avoid intravascular injection of the relatively large amount of local anesthetic needed for an epidural block, another interspace should be chosen and the procedure repeated. If the aspiration test results in the return of cerebrospinal fluid (CSF), another interspace should be chosen for a repeat attempt to place the needle in the epidural space. Because of this potential problem, we prefer the L2–L3 interspace. If there is a dural perforation, one can move caudad and away from the initial hole by one or two interspaces. Although it may occur, we have not seen a subarachnoid block result from an epidural block performed after the puncture of the dura at another interspace. In a surgical setting, if the dura has been punctured, it may be feasible to continue the procedure as a subarachnoid anesthetic at the same interspace.

The next confirmatory test to ensure that the needle is in the epidural space involves either the injection of 4–5 cm^3 of air or the slow injection of 3 ml of normal saline or anesthetic solution as a test dose. If air is used, a small (5-ml), empty and dry glass syringe is attached to the epidural needle and the plunger positioned at the 4- to 5-ml mark. The air is then briskly injected into the epidural space. Pressure on the plunger is released immediately after the discharge of the total air volume. Ease of injection of the air and failure of the plunger to move back more than to the 0.5- to 1.0-ml mark usually indicate that the needle point is in the epidural space. If there is resistance to the air injection or if there is significant return of air into the syringe, then the bevel of the needle may still be located in subcutaneous tissue, interspinous ligament or the ligamentum flavum. A *dry* glass syringe is utilized for this confirmatory test because a wet glass syringe without liquid contents in the barrel will become sticky and make interpretation difficult. In addition, the glass syringes in disposable epidural trays are made to be used *dry* since they are self-lubricating.

If normal saline or local anesthetic is used as a confirmatory test, we incorporate a small (0.2 cm^3) air bubble into the solution. Compression of the bubble on injection indicates that the tip of the epidural needle is still in the ligamentum flavum and not the epidural space, which is a *potential* space. Absence of bubble compression and smooth injection of the solution indicates injection into the epidural space. We also use this technique when identifying the epidural space with the loss-of-resistance technique employing normal saline.

Injecting a small amount (3 ml) of local anesthetic solution should not result in any major anesthetic effect if the needle is in the epidural space. However, if the dura mater has been pierced and the local anesthetic is injected into the subarachnoid space, extensive sensory and motor block may be noted. Three to five minutes are allowed to pass to see if any sensory anesthetic effect will appear.

It these tests indicate that the needle is in the epidural space, an aspiration test is performed before each of incremental or fractional (3- to 5-ml) doses, which are injected every 60–90 s until the total dose for a single-dose epidural block has been administered. The indicated dosages have been reduced by about 25% from those appropriate for a similar epidural block in a surgical patient (Tables 20.2 and 20.3). After the epidural needle is withdrawn, the patient is allowed to rest in a comfortable position favoring left uterine displacement – usually a semisitting position with the right hip elevated by a wedge. We prefer to initiate an epidural block with the parturient in the right lateral position. Thus, with left uterine displacement, the dependent side will receive an adequate amount of drug. Vital signs, particularly blood pressure, and the spread of anesthesia are carefully monitored.

PLACING AN EPIDURAL CATHETER

The anatomic landmarks and the initial steps for placing

Table 20.2 Local anesthetics and suggested dosages for single-dose epidural anesthesia for vaginal delivery

Local anesthetic*	Dosage† (ml)	(mg)	Clinical onset of action (min)	Duration of action (min)
Bupivacaine 0.25–0.5%	8–20	20–100	3–5	60–180
2-Chloroprocaine 2.0–3.0%	8–20	160–600	3–5	40–60
Lidocaine 1.0–2.0%‡	8–20	80–400	3–5	60–90
Mepivacaine 1.0–2.0%	8–20	80–400	3–5	60–90

* Without epinephrine.
† Dosage range depending on patient's height; total milligram dosage of the local anesthetic should not exceed manufacturer's recommendations.
‡With or without epinephrine 1:200 000.

Table 20.3 Local anesthetics and suggested dosages for single-dose epidural anesthesia for cesarean delivery

Local anesthetic*	Dosage† (ml)	(mg)	Clinical onset of action (min)	Duration of action (min)
Bupivacaine 0.5%	20–30	100–150	3–5	90–180
Chloroprocaine 3%	12–20	360–600	3–5	40–60
Etidocaine‡§ 1.0–1.5%	12–20	120–300	3–5	60–90
Lidocaine 2.0%	12–20	240–400	3–5	60–90
Mepivacaine 2.0%	12–20	240–400	3–5	60–90

* Without epinephrine.
† Dosage range depending on patient's height; total milligram dosage of the local anesthetic should not exceed manufacturer' recommendations.
‡ With or without epinephrine 1:200 000.
§ Etidocaine 1.5% is only manufactured with epinephrine 1:200 000.

an epidural catheter are the same as for the single-dose method of epidural anesthesia. An epidural needle must be selected that is large enough to admit the catheter for passage into the epidural space. The needle is positioned in the epidural space using the techniques described previously. Either the hanging-drop technique or the loss-of-resistance method may be used to identify the epidural space. We administer a test dose of 3 ml of local anesthetic through the needle before inserting the catheter into the epidural space.

The plastic catheter is examined for imperfections. The depth markings are noted and compared with the length of the epidural needle. The tubing may be inserted using a wire stylet to make the passage of the catheter through the needle easier. The wire stylet is withdrawn 2–3 cm from the tip of the catheter. The catheter is uncurled and held by the fingers of the left hand. The tip of catheter is inserted through the hub of the epidural needle by the right hand (by a right-handed anesthesiologist). As the leading point of the tubing contacts the directional bevel of the epidural needle, a sudden resistance is felt. This is usually at the first mark on the epidural catheter. This resistance is gently but aggressively overcome and the tubing is advanced through the needle so that it will project 2–3 cm beyond the bevel of the epidural needle into the epidural space. The distance can be measured by placing the plunger of the syringe against the patient's back and noting the marking on the syringe that correlates to the centimeter mark on the catheter that is at the hub of the needle. We use the back of the plunger or piston of the syringe instead of the male end to avoid contamination of the syringe with the residual antibacterial solution, and it is preferable to use a glass syringe for the initial injection through the epidural catheter. Then the needle is removed from the tissues in the following manner: the catheter is held firmly approximately 2–3 cm from the hub of the needle while the 'wings' or shaft and hub of the needle are held between the index and middle fingers and thumb of the other hand (Fig. 20.11). While the catheter is held in place with positive forward pressure the needle is carefully pulled out until the thumbs of the two hands meet. Forward pressure should be applied to the catheter at all times. The maneuver is then repeated by grasping the tubing another 2–3 cm distal to the hub of the needle and repeating the same procedure. Finally, the tip of the needle will emerge from the skin. The tubing is prevented from being dislodged by applying firm pressure with the thumb and index finger of the left hand to the tubing at the point where it emerges from the skin. The needle is then moved back over the catheter. The thumb and index finger may now move some distance up the catheter and hold the catheter firmly to prevent its dislodgement while the needle and stylet are removed from the catheter by the right hand. This should always be done close to the back to avoid dislocating the catheter. Once the needle has been

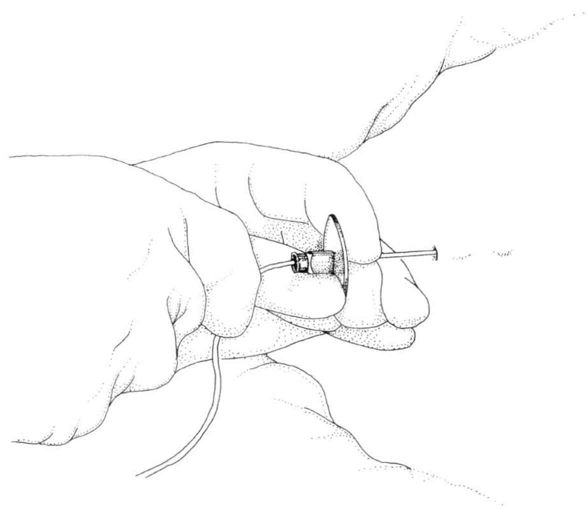

Fig 20.11 Insertion of the epidural catheter and removal of the epidural needle over the epidural catheter.

removed, a catheter is withdrawn the previously measured distance so that 2–3 cm of the catheter lies within the epidural space.

Forward repositioning of the needle is impossible once the catheter is advanced beyond the bevel. If forward repositioning is necessary, the needle and the catheter are both completely withdrawn and the procedure is repeated from the beginning. Once the catheter has advanced beyond the bevel of the epidural needle, any attempt to withdraw it can result in shearing off the catheter.

An adapter is attached to the end of the catheter, or a blunt, small-gauge needle is inserted into the tubing. Before the catheter is taped in place, an aspiration test is carefully performed to ensure that the catheter is not in the subarachnoid space or in an epidural vein. The epidural veins are thin walled; aspiration via the epidural catheter may be negative when the catheter is in an epidural vein because the aspiration has created a negative pressure that has occluded the end of the catheter with the wall of the vein. Disconnecting the syringe from a catheter adapter and holding the catheter tip *below* the level of insertion may allow blood to spontaneously appear in the lumen of the catheter as a result of venous pressure, thereby diagnosing an intravascular placement. If these tests are negative, another 3-ml test dose of local anesthetic solution is injected and the patient is observed for cardiovascular changes, sensory or motor alterations, or central nervous system toxic reaction for not less than 3 min. Sterile gauze pads are placed above and below the catheter as it emerges from the skin, and the cathether and pads are secured by pieces of tape. The entire catheter is then taped to the back of the patient and she is placed in a semisitting position with a wedge under the right hip to displace the uterus to the left.

Table 20.4 Local anesthetics and suggested dosages for continuous (intermittent) epidural anesthesia for vaginal delivery

Local anesthetic*	Dosage† First dose‡ (ml)	(mg)	Top-up dose§ (ml)	(mg)	Onset of action (min)	Duration of action (min)	Time between top-up doses (min)
Bupivacaine¶ 0.25%–0.5%	8–15	20–75	6–10	15–50	3–5	60–180	Approx. 60–120
Chloroprocaine 2.0–3.0%	8–15	160–450	6–10	120–300	3–5	40–60	Approx. 45
Lidocaine 1.0–2.0%‖	8–15	80–300	6–10	60–200	3–5	60–90	Approx. 60
Mepivacaine 1.0–2.0%	8–15	80–300	6–10	60–200	3–5	60–90	Approx. 60

* Without epinephrine.
† Total milligram dosage of the local anesthetic should not exceed manufacturer's recommendations.
‡ Dosage range depending on patient's height.
§ The top-up dose is two-thirds of the first dose if the initial dose resulted in a satisfactory level of anesthesia and if this level is to be maintained.
¶ Some have described the use of 0.125% bupivacaine for vaginal delivery but we do not use this dosage for initiation of the block, just for continuous infusion.
‖ With or without epinephrine 1:200 000.

Table 20.5 Local anesthetics and suggested dosages for continuous (intermittent) epidural anesthesia for cesarean delivery

Local anesthetic*	Dosage† First dose‡ (ml)	(mg)	Top-up dose§ (ml)	(mg)	Onset of action (min)	Duration of action (min)	Time between top-up doses (min)
Bupivacaine 0.5%	20–30	100–150	8–12	40–60	3–5	90–180	Approx. 150
2-Chloroprocaine 3.0%	12–20	360–600	8–12	240–360	3–5	40–60	Approx. 45
Etidocaine 1.0%–1.5%¶ ‖	12–20	120–300	8–12	80–180	3–5	60–90	Approx. 75
Lidocaine¶ 2.0%¶	12–20	240–400	8–12	160–240	3–5	60–90	Approx. 60
Mepivacaine 2.0%	12–20	240–400	8–12	160–240	3–5	60–90	Approx. 60

* Without epinephrine.
† Total miligram dosage of the local anesthetic should not exceed manufacturer's recommendations.
‡ Dosage range depending on patient's height.
§ The top-up dose is two-thirds of the first dose if the initial dose resulted in a satisfactory level of anesthesia and if this level is to be maintained.
¶ With or without epinephrine 1:200 000.
‖ Etidocaine 1.5% is only manufactured with epinephrine 1:200 000.

If vital signs remain satisfactory and no significant anesthesia develops after this second test dose, another aspiration test is done. Fractional doses of local anesthetic (3 to 5 ml) are administered at intervals of at least 60s until the full epidural dose is injected. We do not inject more than 5 ml of local anesthetic at a time. This translates to a maximal dose of 25mg of bupivacaine or 100 mg of lidocaine in our current practice.

To obtain continuous anesthesia from T10 to S5, the first intermittent epidural dose may be the same as for the single-dose method. When the desired level of anesthesia has been achieved with the initial dose, a subsequent 'top-up' dose of about two-thirds the initial dose will maintain this sensory level. Top-up doses are added as necessary. An aspiration test must be done prior to each reinforcement because perforation of the dura mater or one of the epidural veins by the catheter may have occurred since the last administration of the anesthetic. Fractional doses of local anesthetic (3 to 5 ml) are administered until the appropriate top-up dose has been given. Dosage schedules are listed in Tables 20.4 and 20.5. Alternatively, the patient may be placed on a continuous infusion of local anesthetic with or without opioid, as described later in this chapter.

With the patient resting comfortably, the spread of anesthesia is checked frequently by gentle repeated pinpricks or by a cotton swab moistened with alcohol. Since the loss of pain and temperature sensation progresses simultaneously, the use of alcohol to check the spread of anesthesia may be more pleasant for the patient. Repeat pinpricks may not accurately differentiate the area of complete loss of pain sensation from that of partial sensory anesthesia. However, we still prefer the 'pinprick' test. Because of the concern over blood and fluid contamination, we suggest the use of sharp plastic toothpicks to determine sensory levels. Several brands of plastic toothpicks are sharp enough to pierce olives or onions but not human skin.

PRECAUTIONS

Aspiration

Aspiration must precede the injection of local anesthetic solution in order to avoid unintentional subarachnoid injection or intravenous injection. The epidural dosage is a large multiple of that needed for subarachnoid block. Unintentional injection of such an amount of local anesthetic solution into the subarachnoid space would unavoidably result in high or total spinal block. The epidural venous plexus can be the site for an intravascular injection of a large volume of local anesthetic, which may be followed by central nervous system (CNS) excitation and convulsions. Full cardiopulmonary resuscitative equipment must be immediately available, as is customary for any regional block.

PART C
THE INTERMITTENT TECHNIQUE

L. Vaes A. Van Zundert

HISTORY

1931 could have been a great year for obstetric anesthesia: the Italian surgeon Dogliotti published in German his 'loss-or-resistance technique',[1] which is available to the English reader in a paper that cannot be praised too highly,[2] and Aburel from Rumania described a technique of continuous epidural (caudal) analgesia for the relief of pain in childbirth.[3] Unfortunately, Aburel's paper did not receive the attention it deserved. It was to be 11 years until Hingson and Edwards[4] more successfully attracted the attention of the anesthesiologist to the continuous caudal technique in labor. Their malleable caudal needle was far from practical and soon replaced by ureteral catheters. The lumbar epidural catheter technique on which current practice is based was spread throughout the world by Flowers et al in 1949.[5] Still there was the technical problem of finding a suitable catheter, and I (L.V.) remember the time when we had to cut our catheters from a roll and find a blunt needle to fit into the catheter. This practice continued into the 1970s in many units (including the Boston Hospital for Women! (G.W.O)). Then came all types of special epidural catheters, ranging from catheters with a stylet that allowed pushing, to soft, marked nylon catheters designed to slip into the epidural space. Some anesthesiologists stayed with the single-shot technique,[6] whereas others taught the Cleland[7] double-catheter technique as late as 1977.[8]

With long-acting local anesthetics such as bupivacaine 0.5% we found an easy way to keep our post-operative patients pain free with a few top-ups a day. However, this approach had a price, i.e. prolonged motor block, so we resorted to infusion pumps in order to achieve analgesia lasting several days.

For the record, the first paper on continuous epidural infusion for labor was published in 1970.[9]

For labor and vaginal delivery, all local anesthetics have been used in the intermittent techniques but, for the last decade, lidocaine, chloroprocaine and especially bupivacaine in a variety of concentrations, with or without epinephrine or opioids, have been used.

THE LOW-DOSE–LOW-CONCENTRATION TECHNIQUE

Bleyaert[10] and Soetens[11] first reported the successful use of bupivacaine 0.125% plus epinephrine 1 : 400 000 in obstetric analgesia. Stainthorp et al,[12] using no epinephrine, were far less successful in achieving satisfactory epidural analgesia for childbirth. Even lower concentrations of bupivacaine[13,14] in combination with opioids, whether or not given via a continuous-infusion technique, (next below) have been tried.

Bleyaert et al[15] and Van Zundert[16] obtained a 92% success rate with epidural bupivacaine 0.125% + epinephrine 1 : 800 000. By using a low concentration of bupivacaine in a rather large volume (10 ml), we overcame most of the potential objections to the use of epidural analgesia in childbirth. Epidural analgesia using bupivacaine 0.125% plus epinephrine 1 : 800 000 is effective and safe[17] for the control of pain during vaginal delivery. It even allows post-partum examination of the uterus and perineal repair, if necessary, without the need for any other anesthetic intervention. This dosage causes minimal or no motor block,[18] it does not lead to a prolonged expulsion time,[19] not even in breech deliveries,[20] and the maternal and neonatal plasma concentrations are well below the toxic level.[21] In 877 parturients undergoing epidural analgesia using bupivacaine 0.125% plus epinephrine 1 : 800 000, the instrumental delivery rate was 40.3% *vs.* 21.4% in a nonepidural control group.[19] Van Steenberge et al[22] were the first to demonstrate in 1987 that the addition of sufentanil to the above solution has beneficial effects. By adding sufentanil 10 μg to the aforementioned (10 ml) solution, Vertommen et al,[23] in a multicenter study, found that the duration of analgesia was longer and the quality of analgesia could be improved from 91.6% to 98.9%. The main total dose of bupivacaine was significantly less (34.3 *vs.* 42.2 mg), and the instrumental delivery rate was also significantly lower (24% *vs.* 36%). These authors have proved that variations in the epidural solution can reduce the incidence of instrumental deliveries, by using minute doses of local anesthetics (thereby avoiding or minimizing motor block) combined with small amounts of opioids. This brings us close to the ideal analgesic method, on the one hand providing effective maternal analgesia during labor and delivery using a tailored epidural analgesia technique and, on the other hand, avoiding the negative effects on the mother and the fetus of interfering with the progress of labor.

INCREMENTAL DOSES ADMINISTERED THROUGH A LUMBAR EPIDURAL CATHETER

Epidural analgesia for labor and delivery differs considerably from operative epidural anesthesia and post-operative epidural analgesia. In obstetrics the aim is selective analgesia, with minimal influence on muscle power and duration of labor, and with the lowest toxicity for the mother and the fetus. Fortunately, the pain of normal uterine contractions seems to be more readily relieved than pathologic pain. This is an important factor because it allows the use of low concentrations of local anesthetic and minimal doses of opioids.

A second important factor is the fact that the intensity and the site of analgesia vary considerably not only between parturients, but also during the course of labor in the same individual. In our opinion the goals of obstetric analgesia for vaginal delivery are best achieved with an intermittent technique, whereby for each top-up the appropriate time, dose and position can be chosen, thus flattening 'peaks and valleys' to produce a true continuous analgesia. Our choice of anesthetic is bupivacaine 0.125% plus epinephrine 1 : 800 000, combined with or preceded by sufentanil when and where it is indicated. 20 ml of this solution is obtained by mixing 5 ml of the commercially available bupivacaine 0.5% plus epinephrine 1 : 200 000 with 15 ml of sterile physiologic saline without preservative. To this 20 ml is added 0.4 ml of sufentanil 50 μg/ml to give a 1 μg/ml solution of sufentanil.

In our department, about 65% of patients undergoing vaginal deliveries receive epidural analgesia. Our experience with the low-dose–low-concentration bupivacaine technique now exceeds 18 000 cases.

We induce analgesia when the obstetrician judges that labor is established, and the woman asks for pain relief, regardless of the degree of dilation. The duration of analgesia for labor and delivery is less than 1 h in 3.5%, from 1 h to less than 2 h in 11.5%, from 2 h to less than 3 h in 11.4% and from 3 h to less than 4 h in 23.5% of parturients. In 50.5% of women, it exceeds 4 h. The duration of analgesia is longer than 7 h in less than 1% of women. A few times a year the need for analgesia exceeds 30 h.

THE INDUCTION DOSE: MAKING THE PARTURIENT PAIN FREE

What and how much will be given as a loading dose depends on the severity of pain also largely on the degree of dilation and the expected duration and progress of labor. Three groups can be defined:

1. normal, well established labor;
2. very advanced labor;
3. very early labor.

Normal, well-established labor

Although most departments will have 'treatment guidelines' and 'standard' doses, many parturients will not receive a 'standard' treatment because there exists so many variables in labor, in the experience of pain and in response to treatment. For example:

1. Moderate pain will be treated more aggressively in a more advanced stage of labor than the same degree of pain at an early stage.
2. We strongly believe that the onset of labor is more gradual when induced with oxytocin than with

prostaglandin, and pain tends to increase more sharply with prostaglandin. As a consequence, we have learned to treat pain very early in these parturients.

Our (standard) 'normal' first dose will be: 10 ml of bupivacaine 0.125% + epinephrine 1 : 800 000 + sufentanil 1 : 1 000 000 (i.e. 12.5 mg of bupivacaine + 12.5 µg of epinephrine + 10 µg of sufentanil) injected over approximately 45 s. The patient lies on her back in the Trendelenburg position (15–20°) with a pillow under her head but not under the shoulders and a cushion under the right hip to provide left uterine displacement. Blood pressure is measured every 2–3 min and the parturient is observed during the first 10 min after the injection. If she starts yawning, looks pale, feels drowsy or vomits, aortocaval compression is suspected and treated by increasing left uterine displacement. 10 min after the injection, the patient is removed from the Trendelenburg position and turned onto her (left) side.

At this point most parturients will have substantial pain relief, but it will take another 10 min before meaningful testing by cold or pinprick can be done. Full extension of skin anesthesia will take even more time.

Motor block should be tested earlier,[18] especially when pain relief is fast and complete. Indeed, this first dose can sometimes give analgesia within minutes, with skin anesthesia ranging from T8 to the sacral segments, but it will never induce a severe or complete motor block unless it was a total or partial subarachnoid administration.[24]

If the motor block on the Bromage scale is 66% or 100%, subarachnoid placement of the catheter is most likely. If this situation is confirmed by the appropriate tests, we leave the catheter in place. When a top-up is needed, we give 4 ml of our starting solution with the patient in the Trendelenburg position. If, after 15 min there is little or no pain relief, we have to consider the possibility of intravascular placement of the epidural catheter. We proceed as follows: we remove the bacterial filter and aspirate slowly with a 2-ml syringe. If negative, we connect the parturient to an ECG monitor or use the direct ECG mode of the fetal monitor[6] or the plethysmograph of an oximeter. We also apply an automatic non-invasive blood pressure monitor if not already in use. We explain to the parturient the possible signs of i.v. epinephrine and local anesthetic, such as palpitations, headache, change in taste or tinnitus. Then we inject again over 40 s 10 ml of bupivacaine 0.125% + 12.5 µg of epinephrine + 10 µg of sufentanil. If there are no signs or symptoms of i.v. placement of the catheter, we wait another 15 min for pain relief. If there is none, we replace the catheter and restart the procedure with 10 ml of our standard solution containing sufentanil.

Very advanced or rapidly progressing labor

In this case rapid treatment of the already considerable pain that exists is essential since the pain of the second stage may come before or shortly after the pain of the first stage is controlled. Hence there is a temptation 'to block everything in one shot'. We do not consider this to be safe, so our choice is the multistep procedure. When the anesthesiologist is asked for an epidural anesthetic in far advanced labor, it may be better to opt for spinal anesthesia or a sequential spinal-epidural analgesia using very fine long spinal needles through a Tuohy needle, which is placed in the epidural space. When the long spinal needle is in the subarachnoid space, the local anesthetic can be injected in order to produce a subarachnoid block with a fast onset. Then the long spinal needle is removed and an epidural catheter is introduced through the Tuohy needle into the epidural space, which allows epidural top-ups to be given when necessary.

If we use the epidural technique, our first dose will be 14 ml of bupivacaine 0.125% + epinephrine 1 : 800 000 + sufentanil 1 : 1 000 000 (i.e. 17.5 mg of bupivacaine + 17.5 µg of epinephrine + 14 µg of sufentanil). If it is necessary to provide pain relief rapidly by the epidural route or when insertion of the catheter does not go smoothly or proves to be difficult, this first dose can be given through the needle as the situation allows, and a catheter is inserted afterward. The patient lies as previously described for 10 min. During this time, she is observed closely because if this dose enters the subarachnoid space the result will be a surgical spinal anesthesia requiring a larger fluid infusion and probably a vasopressor such as ephedrine.

If after 10 min the patient is pain free, she is placed in a comfortable lateral position, and 10–15 min later skin testing can be done. If pain relief is insufficient, it is wise to make sure by questioning and vaginal examination that the beginning of the second stage is not the origin of pain. A second dose will be given regardless, but if the second stage has started it should be given in the sitting position.

If there is no pain relief, a second dose will be given in a slight Trendelenburg position, without waiting for the results of skin testing, but taking special care to detect possible i.v. administration as described previously. If this second dose does not result in a pain-free patient after 10 min, we go through the list of possible reasons for persisting pain (full bladder, full dilation, scar deshiscence after previous cesarean delivery, wrong position of the catheter, etc). If the catheter is not correctly placed, we insert a new catheter if sufficient time is left, but only repeat skin testing. We do not know yet what the safe dose of sufentanil given in a short time is so our upper limit is 30 µg.

Since 1991, we found out that 7.5 µg of sufentanil added to the 10 ml solution containing bupivacaine 0.125% plus epinephrine 1:800 000 is sufficient to obtain satisfactory analgesia, which confirms observations made by Van Steenberge.[22]

Making the parturient pain free in very early labor

Sometimes the obstetrician asks us to help a patient who, in very early labor, already complains of serious discomfort. Our experience is that at this stage 10 ml of bupivacaine 0.125% + epinephrine 1 : 800 000 with or without sufentanil may stop the contractions for some time. A reassuring talk with the parturient, placement of the epidural catheter and the promise that everything is prepared to provide for analgesia if the pain gets worse will often do a great deal of good. If this is not or no longer enough, we can make most of these women comfortable without interference with labor by the epidural administration of 10 ml of sufentanil 1 : 1 000 000.[29] Depending on the evolution of labor, this may be repeated a second time before switching to the usual local anesthetic or combination of local anesthetic plus opioid. One should keep in mind that 10 μg of sufentanil is not suitable as a test dose! The effects (pain relief) or side-effects (drowsiness, vomiting, respiratory depression, pruritus) of an unintentional i.v. injection will be weak or unobserved.[28] Subarachnoid injection will be less effective than epidural injection[29] and respiratory depression is very unlikely to occur.

THE MAINTENANCE DOSE: KEEPING THE PARTURIENT PAIN FREE

The first dose can lead to confusing results such as:

- a parturient almost without or with only unilateral anesthesia and yet perfectly pain free;
- a parturient with an ideal pattern of skin anesthesia and still having much pain;
- a parturient with a very extensive skin anesthesia, e.g. from T4 to all sacral segments, and no signs of subarachnoid injection;
- a difficult insertion of the epidural catheter and yet perfect analgesia, or the reverse: easy placement of the epidural catheter and only patchy skin anesthesia.

We still do not understand the reason for these problems! Once good analgesia has been achieved everything becomes easier: the effect of the doses becomes more predictable and the results more reliable. What we do not know in advance is *when* the maintenance doses will be needed. On average, 10 ml of bupivacaine 0.125% + epinephrine 1 : 800 000 will work for about 1 h, whereas the same dose including 10 μg of sufentanil will work for about 1.5 h, the standard deviation in both cases being approximately 45 min. These statistical data are of little help to the clinician caring for the individual parturient. So what can be done? Which indicators for the top-up dose can be used?

The top-up is the time to ask the midwife or the obstetrician about the evolution of labor. In this way the return of pain can be anticipated and analgesia adapted to the progress of labor with the standard dose of 10 ml of 0.125% bupivacaine + epinephrine 1 : 800 000. This dose will also contain 7.5 μg of sufentanil until a total dose of 30 μg of sufentanil has been administered.

There are a number of reasons for giving a top-up to a pain-free parturient. In more prolonged labors, we can learn how long a dose works in one particular individual. On a busy obstetric ward, it is preferable to give the occasional top-up dose in advance when the anesthesiologist is free than to risk having to attend three or more parturients at the same time. And with low doses, it is better to inject too early rather than too late because of the mild influence on sympathetic and motor block. Another reason is the demand for block of the sacral segments because of complaints of perineal pain or when the expulsion of the fetus is expected.

It is important to state that in our institution it is common practice to encourage the mother to push only after the cervix is fully dilated and the presenting part clearly visible.

In summary, there are three reasons for injecting the epidural dose for a parturient:

1. the induction dose;
2. the prevention of pain when it becomes apparent that the previous dose is wearing off;
3. the need for perineal analgesia if not already present.

One approach is waiting with the top-up dose until the pain returns: this is the typical 'peak and valley' method. There are strong arguments against this variant of the technique:

- A pain free labor and delivery is preferable to some pain free intervals.
- The mother will lose confidence in our ability to control her pain, a very important factor.
- It may take considerable time and effort to re-establish good analgesia once it is lost.

The other approach is the 'on-demand method' which fortunately results in good analgesia. The difference between *pain* and the return of the feeling of uterine contractions can easily be explained to the mother who indicates when she should be topped up.

We stay with the mother during the induction period so that we can explain that the first sign of effectiveness is that the painful contraction seems to shorten; the next step is feeling the next one or two contractions only at their peak of intensity. The following contraction is still perceived, but is almost or totally free of pain, and then the perception of the contractions disappears.

The mother is asked to warn the anesthesiologist when awareness of still pain-free contractions returns. That is about the time for a top-up!

REFERENCES

1. Dogliotti A M 1931 Eine neue Method der Regionären Anësthesie 'Die Peridurale segmentäre Anästhesie'. Zentrabl Chir 58: 31–41
2. Dogliotti A M 1933 Segmental peridural spinal anesthesia. Am Surg 20: 107
3. Aburel A 1931 L'anesthésie locale continue (prolongée) en obstétrique. Bull Soc Obstét Gynécol Paris 20: 35
4. Hingson R A, Edwards N B 1942 Continuous caudal anesthesia during labor and delivery. Anesth Analg Current Res 21: 301
5. Flowers C E, Hellman L M, Hingson R A 1949 Continuous peridural anesthesia and analgesia for labor, delivery and Cesarean section. Anesth Analg 28: 181
6. Hellman K 1965 epidural anesthesia in obstetrics: a second look at 26,127 cases. Can Anaesth Soc J 12: 398–404
7. Cleland I G P 1949 Continuous peridural and caudal analgesia in obstetrics. Anesth Analg 28: 61
8. Abouleish E 1977 Pain Control in Obstetrics. JB Lippincott, Philadelphia, p 285
9. Spoerel W E, Thomas A, Gerula G R 1970 Continuous epidural analgesia: Experience with mechanical injection devices. Can Anaesth Soc J 17: 37–51
10. Bleyaert A 1970 L'anesthésie péridurale en obstétrique par la bupivacaine avec adrénaline à faible dosage. Ars Medici I, Tome IX, 67–69
11. Soetens M A G 1970 Technique personelle d'analgésie péridurale en obstétrique. Ars Medici Thérapie Pratique I, 67
12. Stainthorp S F, Bradshaw E G, Chablen P D, Tobias A A 1978 0.125% bupivacaine for obstetric analgesia? Anesthesia 33: 3–9
13. Chestnut D H, Laszewski L J, Pollack K L, Bates J N, Manago N K 1990 Continuous epidural infusion of 0.0625% bupivacaine – 0.0002% fentanyl during the second stage of labor. Anesthesiology 72: 613–618
14. Rodriguez J, Abboud T K, Reyes A, Payne M, Zhu J, Steffens Z, Afrasiabi A 1990 Continuous infusion epidural anesthesia during labor: a randomized, double-blind comparison of 0,0625% bupivacaine/0.002% butarphanol and 0.125% bupivacaine. Reg Anesth 15: 300–303.
15. Bleyaert A, Soetens M, Vaes L, Van Steenberge A, Van der Donck A 1979 Bupivacaine 0.125% in obstetric epidural analgesia: experience in 3000 cases. Anesthesiology 51: 435–438
16. Van Zundert A 1985 Bupivacaine 0.125% + Epinephrine 1 : 800 000. The value of a low concentration of a local anesthetic drug for epidural analgesia in obstetrics. Thesis, Leiden, The Netherlands
17. Van Zundert A, Vaes L, Soetens M et al 1987 Every dose given in epidural analgesia for vaginal delivery can be a test dose. Anesthesiology 67: 436–440
18. Van Zundert A, Vaes L, Soetens M, De Vel M, Maesen F 1984 Measuring motor block during lumbar epidural analgesia for vaginal delivery. Obstet Anesth Digest 4: 31–34
19. Van Zundert A, Van Der Aa P, Van Der Donck A, Meeuwis H, Vaes L 1984 Motor blockade, expulsion times and instrumental deliveries with epidural analgesia for vaginal delivery. Obstet Anesth Digest 4: 152–156
20. Van Zundert A, Vaes L, Soetens M et al 1991 Are breech deliveries an indication for lumbar epidural analgesia? Anesth Analg 72: 399–403
21. Van Zundert A, Burm A, Van Kleef J et al 1987 Plasma concentrations of epidural bupivacaine in mother and newborn: 0.125% versus 0.375%. Anesth Analg 66: 435–441
22. Van Steenberge A, Debroux H C, Noorduin H 1987 Extradural bupivacaine with sufentanil for vaginal delivery. A double-blind trial. Br J Anaesth 59: 1518–1522
23. Vertommen J, Vandermeulen E, Van Aken H et al 1991 The effects of the addition of sufentanil to 0.125% bupivacaine on the quality of analgesia during labor and on the incidence of instrumental deliveries. Anesthesiology 74: 809–814
24. Van Zundert A, De Wolf A, Vaes L, Soetens M 1988 High-volume spinal anesthesia with bupivacaine 0.125% for cesarian section. Anesthesiology 69: 998–1003
25. Bromage P R 1969 An evaluation of bupivacaine in epidural analgesia for obstetrics. Can Anaesth Soc J. 16: 46–56
26. Van Zundert A, Vaes L, De Wolf A 1987 ECG monitoring of mother and fetus during epidural anesthesia. Anesthesiology 66: 584–585
27. Steinberg R B, Powel G, Hu X, Dunn S M 1989 Epidural sufentanil for analgesia for labor and delivery. Reg Anesth 14: 225–228
28. Cohen S E, Tan S, White P F 1988 Sufentanil analgesia following cesarean section: epidural versus intravenous administration. Anesthesiology 68: 129–134, 1988.
29. Donadoni R, Vermeulen H, Noorduin H, Rolly G 1987 Intrathecal sufentanil as a supplement to subarachnoid anaesthesia with lignocaine Br J Anaesth 59: 1523–1527

PART D
THE CONTINUOUS INFUSION TECHNIQUE

D. H. Chestnut

Continuous epidural infusion of local anesthetic, with and without opioid, became popular during the second half of the last decade. However, the idea of continuous epidural infusion of local anesthetic is not new.[1–6] Burn[1] and Scott and Walker[2] first described the continuous epidural infusion of lidocaine for post-operative analgesia in 1963. In 1970, Dawkins[4] reported the 'continuous drip' of local anesthetic during labor, and in 1972 Scarborough[6] first described the intrapartum use of a positive-pressure infusion pump. Early attempts to perform continuous epidural infusion of local anesthetic were constrained by the limitations of the infusion pumps available at that time. Further, some claimed that continuous epidural infusion of lidocaine (the most popular local anesthetic in obstetric practice at that time) resulted in tachyphylaxis.[5] Recently, the introduction of adjustable and reliable infusion pumps has facilitated the use of this technique. Continuous epidural infusion of local anesthetic, with and without opioid, has emerged as the intrapartum anesthetic technique of choice in many obstetric units in the USA.

ADVANTAGES

There are several purported advantages of continuous epidural infusion during labor.

A more stable level of sensory anesthesia

By providing continuous infusion of local anesthetic, one hopes to avoid fluctuation in the quality of pain relief. More important, one hopes to avoid situations when a patient loses analgesia altogether. In such cases, the patient may experience severe pain before the anesthesiologist can re-establish pain relief. Not only does continuous epidural infusion decrease the requirement for bolus injections during labor, it may also decrease the requirement for administration of local anesthetic just before delivery.[7] This is advantageous on a busy obstetric service, where the anesthesiologist may not always be able to provide additional bolus injections of local anesthetic on demand.

Greater patient safety

Decreased risk of hypotension

Some claim that the continuous epidural infusion technique reduces the risk of hypotension by avoiding fluctuation in the extent of sympathetic blockade.[8] It is unclear whether this is true in clinical practice. To my knowledge, only one study has noted a significant decrease in the incidence of hypotension with the use of continuous epidural infusion.[9] Most anesthesia care providers first establish anesthesia by performing bolus injection of a local anesthetic. Typically, the anesthesiologist does not begin the continuous epidural infusion until satisfactory sensory anesthesia has been established. Most, but not all, cases of significant hypotension occur during the first hour of epidural anesthesia. Thus, the continuous epidural infusion technique is likely to significantly reduce the incidence of hypotension.

Decreased risk of systemic toxicity

On occasion, a catheter initially positioned satisfactorily within the epidural space will migrate into an epidural vein. If this should occur during continuous infusion, there would be a slow intravenous infusion of local anesthetic, which should not cause systemic toxicity. Indeed, recession of the level of sensory anesthesia would represent evidence of intravenous administration of local anesthetic. One should suspect intravenous positioning of a catheter in situations when a patient unexpectedly complains of pain during previously satisfactory infusion of local anesthetic. Most cases of intravenous injection of local anesthetic occur during initial injection of the catheter. Use of the continuous epidural infusion technique will not prevent the intravenous injection of local anesthetic *during induction* or maintenance of epidural anesthesia.

Some claim that 'lower blood concentrations of local anesthetic . . . result from decreased absorption from the epidural space during continuous infusion'.[8] I am unaware of published data which document this advantage in obstetric patients. There have been at least six controlled comparisons of continuous epidural infusion of bupivacaine versus intermittent epidural bolus injection of bupivacaine during labor.[10–15] In each of the five studies that reported total doses of bupivacaine, the continuous-infusion group received more bupivacaine than the intermittent bolus group.[10–14] However, continuous infusion does not seem to cause dangerous accumulation of local anesthetic in the mother or fetus. Denson et al[7] measured serum bupivacaine concentrations in 12 parturients who received a bolus injection of 10 ml of 0.5% bupivacaine, followed by continuous epidural infusion of 0.0625% bupivacaine at 20 ml/h. They noted that serum bupivacaine concentrations at or just before delivery were significantly lower than the maximal concentration in all patients. They concluded that 'epidural analgesia for labor and delivery. . . . using a single 50 mg loading dose followed by a continuous infusion of 12.5 mg/h of bupivacaine will not result in maternal or fetal accumulation or toxicity'.[7]

Decreased risk of total spinal anesthesia

Proponents of continuous epidural infusion claim that, if the catheter should migrate across the dura during labor, one will see a gradual increase in the level of anesthesia rather than a sudden increase, as might occur with bolus injection of local anesthetic. However, most cases of unintentional dural puncture occur with initial placement of the catheter and the continuous epidural infusion technique will not prevent those occurences.

Decreased risk of infection

The continuous-infusion technique should result in decreased manipulation of the epidural catheter. Theoretically, this might decrease the risk of infection. This potential advantage helped motivate the early studies of continuous epidural infusion. Curiously, few authors list this as a potential advantage of continuous epidural infusion in modern obstetric anesthesia practice. Perhaps anesthesiologists now recognize that infection of the epidural space is a very rare complication of epidural anesthesia. This is both amazing and fortunate, given the unavoidable contamination that occurs with manipulation of the catheter.

Convenience for the anesthesia care provider

It is easy to understand why convenience represents a real advantage in clinical practice. With continuous epidural infusion, the anesthesiologist can often limit subsequent visits to 2–3 min, rather than spend 20 min with the patient after bolus injection of local anesthetic. But continuous epidural infusion should not be a substitute for frequent assessment of the patient. The anesthesiologist who evaluates the patient at infrequent intervals will be walking on a slippery slope and may be tempted to have the nurse adjust the rate of infusion and/or perform bolus injection of local anesthetic. Clearly, this is not safe practice. Further, continuous infusion does not obviate the availability of an anesthesiologist who can manage anesthesia-related complications.[8]

In summary, continuous epidural infusion probably results in a more stable level of sensory anesthesia when the anesthesiologist is providing care for several patients simultaneously. Undoubtedly, the continuous epidural infusion technique results in greater convenience for the anesthesiologist. It is unclear whether continuous epidural infusion results in greater patient safety.

DISADVANTAGES OF CONTINUOUS EPIDURAL INFUSION

Increased motor block

Some believe that continuous epidural infusion is associated with less motor block. Perhaps if intermittent bolus injection of 0.5% bupivacaine is compared with continuous infusion of very dilute bupivacaine, less intense motor block might be seen with continuous epidural infusion. But Bogod et al[11] observed that patients who received continuous epidural infusion of 0.125% bupivacaine had a higher incidence of leg weakness than patients who received intermittent bolus injection of 0.5% bupivacaine. Indeed, continuous epidural infusion consistently results in administration of higher total doses of local anesthetic than occurs with intermittent epidural bolus injection.[10–14] Thus, patients who receive a prolonged epidural infusion of bupivacaine are at risk for development of significant motor block.

Failure to individualize patient management

With continuous epidural infusion, anesthesiologists may be tempted to place the patient on automatic pilot. They may be less likely to individualize patient management. That is, they may try to fit the patient to the anesthetic, rather than fit the anesthetic to the patient. If anesthesiologists try to eliminate the need for 'top-up' injections, by definition, they will give some patients more local anesthetic than they need. Further, some anesthesiologists feel compelled to continue the epidural infusion of local anesthetic during the second stage in every patient, regardless of the progress of labor. Chestnut et al[16] observed that *routine* maintenance of a continuous epidural infusion of 0.125% bupivacaine until delivery prolonged the second stage of labor and increased the incidence of instrumental delivery in nulliparous patients. This study illustrates one hazard of failure to individualize patient management. With continuous epidural infusion, anesthesiologists should individualize management, just as they should do with the intermittent epidural bolus technique.

Administration of local anesthetic without the physical presence of an anesthesiologist

Some argue that one should not give local anesthetic epidurally unless an anesthesiologist is physically present with the patient. Some anesthesiologists favor the intermittent epidural bolus injection technique for this reason. They argue that when they leave a patient 20 min after bolus injection of local anesthetic there will be no further increase in the level of sensory anesthesia, no increase in the intensity of motor block, and no new onset of hypotension during their absence, unless, of course, the patient should assume the supine position and experience aortocaval compression.

EQUIPMENT AND MATERIALS

Infusion pump

First, the infusion pump should deliver the solution by

positive pressure; it should not allow gravity infusion in the event of a power failure. Second, the infusion pump should be accurate and reliable. Third, it should allow for adjustments in the rate of flow. The pump should be simple to operate, but it should not allow such adjustments to be made by accident. Fourth, some anesthesiologists recommend that the pump include a back-up power source, to be used in the event of a power failure. In my judgment, this is unnecessary. Fifth, the infusion pump should be different from the infusion pump used by the nurses to give intravenous drugs such as oxytocin and magnesium sulfate. Otherwise, a nurse may unintentionally give oxytocin or magnesium sulfate epidurally. Some anesthesiologists argue that their hospital will not purchase separate pumps for epidural infusion because of the extra cost associated with purchase of a small number of pumps. This is a small price to pay to prevent potential neurologic injury and the associated costs of litigation. Finally, one should establish strict rules regarding use of the epidural infusion pumps. In our hospital, only the anesthesiologist makes adjustments in the rate of infusion. Neither obstetricians nor labor nurses are allowed to adjust the rate of infusion, except to discontinue the infusion during patient transport or in case of maternal or fetal distress.

Tubing

The tubing which connects the infusion pump to the epidural catheter should be sufficiently long to allow for movement of the patient in bed. Further, it should not allow unintentional injection of other substances. If standard intravenous connecting tubing is used, all injection ports should be covered. Otherwise, a nurse or even the anesthesiologist may unintentionally give another drug (e.g. oxytocin, magnesium sulfate) epidurally.

Diluent

In most cases the anesthesiologist will want to dilute the solution of local anesthetic and/or opioid with saline. The diluent should be preservative-free. I prefer to use the single dose 10-ml vials of preservative-free saline.

TECHNIQUE

I first establish a T10 level with a concentration of local anesthetic approximately twice that which I plan to give by continuous infusion (e.g. establish a T10 level with 0.25% bupivacaine, followed by a continuous infusion of 0.125% bupivacaine).

Infusion rate

Some studies suggest that a large volume of a low concentration of local anesthetic is more effective than a small volume of a high concentration of local anesthetic.[17–20] The former may also result in lower plasma concentrations of local anesthetic.[21] I check the sensory level at least every hour, and adjust the rate of infusion to maintain a T10 sensory level. If the level falls below T10, I give a bolus of local anesthetic at the time that I increase the rate of infusion. Typically, one must give a bolus of at least 5 ml to increase the sensory level (i.e. a 2-ml bolus of dilute solution rarely affects the sensory level). Some turn the patient from side to side at half-hourly or hourly intervals, to increase the likelihood of symmetric sensory anesthesia. But posture does not consistently influence the spread of local anesthetic within the epidural space. I encourage patients to move at frequent intervals, not to influence the spread of local anesthetic, but to avoid having the patient remain in one position for a prolonged period.

Choice of local anesthetic

2-Chloroprocaine

From a pharmacologic point if view, 2-chloroprocaine might seem the local anesthetic of choice for continuous epidural infusion. But in my experience, it is difficult to manage a continuous epidural infusion with 2-chloroprocaine. Others have reported satisfactory results with 27–48 ml/h of 0.75% 2-chloroprocaine,[9,22] or 44ml/h of 0.5% 2-chloroprocaine.[17]

Lidocaine

Epidural infusion of 12–14 ml/h of 0.75% lidocaine provides satisfactory, though not spectacular, sensory anesthesia during the first stage of labor. It does not reliably provide pain relief during the second stage.[23] Some clain that epidural infusion of lidocaine results in tachyphylaxis.[5]

Bupivacaine

From a pharmacologic point of view, bupivacaine seems a poor choice of local anesthetic for continuous infusion. Fortunately, continuous epidural infusion does not seem to result in a progressive increase in maternal or fetal blood concentrations of bupivacaine.[7] But with the long half-life of bupivacaine, continuous infusion may result in a progressive increase in the concentration of drug within the neuraxis. Nonetheless, bupivacaine has emerged as the most popular local anesthetic for continuous infusion during labor. When 0.125% bupivacaine is given at a rate of 12 ml/h, approximately 50–70% of parturients will have surgical perineal anesthesia at delivery, without a 'perineal dose'.[16] With prolonged infusions one must beware of increased motor block.

Local anesthetic–opioid (e.g. bupivacaine–fentanyl)

The addition of opioid to local anesthetic seems most appropriate if one adds the opioid to allow administration of a decreased concentration of local anesthetic. Specifically, one might add opioid to a concentration of local anesthetic that alone would not be effective. Chestnut et al[24] observed that the addition of 0.0002% fentanyl to a solution of 0.0625% bupivacaine provided pain relief similar to that provided by a higher concentration (e.g. 0.125%) of bupivacaine-alone, with less motor block. To prepare 50 ml of this solution, mix 12.5 ml of 0.25% bupivacaine, 2 ml of fentanyl (0.05 mg/ml), and 35.5 ml of preservative-free saline. A more detailed discussion of epidural opioids is presented elsewhere within this text (see Ch. 14).

REFERENCES

1. Burn J M B 1963 A method of continuous epidural analgesia. Anesthesia 18: 78–81
2. Scott D B, Walker L R 1963 Administration of continuous epidural analgesia. Anesthesia 18: 82–83
3. Green R, Dawkins M 1966 Post-operative analgesia: the use of continuous drip epidural block. Anesthesia 21: 372–378
4. Dawkins M 1970 The relief of pain in labour by means of continuous-drip epidural block. Acta Anaesth Scand (suppl) 37: 248–250
5. Spoerel W E, Thomas A, Gerula G R 1970 Continuous epidural analgesia: experience with mechanical injection devices. Can Anaesth Soc J 17: 37–51
6. Scarborough C D 1972 Continuous lumbar epidural anesthesia in the obstetrical patient: administration by the mechanical constant infusion pump. South Med J 65: 1134–1135
7. Denson D D, Knapp R M, Turner P, Thompson G A 1984 Serum bupivacaine concentrations in term parturients following continuous epidural analgesia for labor and delivery. Therapeut Drug Monitor 6: 393–398
8. Morison D H, Smedstad K G 1985 Continuous infusion epidurals for obstetric analgesia. Can Anaesth Soc J 32: 101–104
9. Faure E A M, Bart A J, Koht A 1980 A comparison of continuous infusion epidural analgesia vs. intermittent injection technique for obstetrical pain relief (abstract). Anesthesiology 53: S294
10. Nadeau S, Elliott R D 1985 Continuous bupivacaine infusion during labor: Effects on analgesia and delivery (abstract). Can Anaesth Soc J 32: S70–S71
11. Bogod D G, Rosen M, Rees G AD 1987 Extradural infusion of 0.125% bupivacaine at 10 ml h^{-1} to women during labour. Br J Anaesth 59: 325–330
12. Gaylard D G, Wilson I H, Balmer H G R 1987 An epidural infusion technique for labor. Anesthesia 42: 1098–1101
13. Hicks J A, Jenkins J G, Newton M C, Findley I L 1988 Continuous epidural infusion of 0.075% bupivacaine for pain relief in labour. A comparison with intermittent top-ups of 0.5% bupivacaine. Anesthesia 43: 289–292
14. Smedstad K G, Morison D H 1988 A comparison study of continuous and intermittent epidural analgesia for labour and delivery. Can J Anaesth 35: 234–241
15. Lamont R F, Pinney D, Rodgers P, Bryant T N 1989 Continuous versus intermittent epidural analgesia: a randomized trial to observe obstetric outcome. Anesthesia 44: 893–896
16. Chestnut D H, Vandewalker G E, Owen C L, Bates J N, Choi W W 1987 The influence of continuous epidural bupivacaine analgesia on the second stage of labor and method of delivery in nulliparous women. Anesthesiology 66: 774–780
17. Kenepp N B, Gutsche B B 1980 Continuous infusion epidural block for analgesia in labor (abstract). Anesthesiology 53: S295
18. Kenepp N B, Cheek T G, Gutsche B B 1983 Bupivacaine: Continuous infusion epidural analgesia for labor (abstract). Anesthesiology 59: A407
19. Cheek T G, Kenepp N B, Schantz B, Dowling B L, Gutsche B B 1985 Lidocaine: Continuous infusion epidural analgesia for labor (abstract). Anesthesiology 63: A451
20. Ewen A, McLeod D D, MacLeod D M, Campbell A, Tunstall M E 1986 Continuous infusion epidural analgesia in obstetrics. Anesthsia 41: 143–147
21. Flynn R J, McMurray T J, Dwyer R, Moore J 1988 Comparison of plasma bupivacaine concentrations during continuous extradual infusion for labor. Br J Anaesth 61: 382–384
22. Abboud T K, Afrasiabi A, Sarkis F et al 1984 Continuous infusion epidural analgesia in parturients receiving bupivacaine, chloroprocaine, or lidocaine: Maternal, fetal, and neonatal effects. Anesth Analg 63: 421–428
23. Chestnut D H, Bates J N, Choi W W 1987 Continuous infusion epidural analgesia with lidocaine: efficacy and influence during the second stage of labor. Obstet Gynecol 69: 323–327
24. Chestnut D H, Owen C L, Ostman L G, Choi W W, Geiger M W 1988 Continuous infusion epidural analgesia during labor: a randomized, double-blind comparisons of 0.0625% bupivacaine/0.0002% fentanyl versus 0.125% bupivacaine. Anesthesiology 68: 754–759

PART E
PATIENT-CONTROLLED EPIDURAL ANALGESIA

F. M. Ferrante

Patient-controlled analgesia (PCA) is commonly assumed to signify the intermittent administration of intravenous opioids without physician or nursing supervision. However, 'patient-control' is really a conceptual framework for analgesic administration and not strictly related to opioids, the intravenous route or intermittent mode of administration. Recent studies suggest that analgesia under patient control may be effective when given via the sublingual,[1] transbuccal,[2] subcutaneous[3] and epidural routes.[4–7] Furthermore, the mode of administration of PCA is not restricted to intermittent boluses (*demand dosing*), but includes *constant-rate infusion plus demand dosing* (a background infusion rate is determined by a physician and may be supplemented by patient demand), and even *infusion-based PCA* (demands are granted as infusions whose rates are adjusted over time by microprocessor control).[8]

Studies of patient-controlled epidural analgesia (PCEA) as an analgesic technique have used either opioids[6,7] or bupivacaine,[4,5] alone[4,6,7] or in combination[5] by demand dosing[4,6,7] or continuous infusion plus demand dosing.[5] As compared with intravenous PCA or continuous epidural infusion (CEI) with opioids alone,[6] PCEA appears to be 'dose sparing' in nonobstetric post-operative populations. Patients using demand-dose PCEA used significantly less opioid for post-operative pain relief.[6,7]

Naturally, for a laboring population, the desired total exposure to local anesthetic and/or opioid should be as low as possible. In a randomized, single-blind placebo-controlled study using 0.125% bupivacaine via demand-dose PCEA and fixed-rate CEI, Gambling et al[4] were able to demonstrate a significant reduction in bupivacaine use with PCEA (11.2 mg/h versus 15.2 mg/h). Analgesia was similar in both groups. Unfortunately, because of the study design, these investigators made no distinction between analgesia and analgesic consumption during the first and second stages of labor.

Using the constant-rate infusion plus the demand-dose mode, Lysak et al[5] compared physician-adjusted CEI with bupivacaine (closely titrated to maintain a T10 sensory level) with three solutions administered by PCEA. The solutions contained mixtures of 0.125% bupivacaine alone; bupivacaine 0.125% with fentanyl 1 μg/ml; and 0.125% bupivacaine, fentanyl 1 μg/ml and epinephrine 1 : 400 000. Unlike the previous study, PCEA with bupivacaine alone did not decrease total local analgesic utilization or hourly infusion requirements for labor. Addition of fentanyl or fentanyl plus epinephrine did decrease hourly local analgesic use (though not total dosage necessary for vaginal delivery). Use of epinephrine-containing solutions was associated with dense motor blockade. These investigators concluded that while safe and effective for labor anesthesia, PCEA did not improve anesthesia or significantly reduce anesthetic requirements as compared with CEI.

These investigators are to be applauded for their pioneering efforts. However, a number of questions regarding the technique of PCEA still need investigation.

Patient control works via a negative-feedback loop.[9] As the patient experiences pain, local anesthetic is self-administered, thereby decreasing the immediate need for further local anesthetics. Thus, the optimal local anesthetic and/or opioid for PCEA should be of fast onset, thus avoiding transient inappropriately increased patient demands. Similarly, the optimal agent should be of intermediate duration. Agents of short analgesic duration could promote a high rate of patient demand and subsequent 'exhaustion' of the patient with the analgesic process. Agents of long duration could accumulate and eventually promote toxicity or untoward side-effects. The optimal local anesthetic or opioid (or combination) for use with PCEA has yet to be elucidated.

With respect to local anesthetics, the volume – concentration relations of the demand (bolus) dose need to be investigated, as well as the influence of the duration of the lockout intervals on local anesthetic and/or opioid analgesic efficacy and toxicity.

When using the constant-infusion plus demand-dose mode, how much local anesthetic should be supplied by infusion? As the amount of local anesthetic supplied by infusion increases, the technique becomes less under 'patient control' than under 'physician control'. Indeed, in the study by Lysak et al[5] the constant-rate infusion of the PCEA study groups delivered 50% of the hourly dose received by the CEI group. This may explain the inability to distinguish between PCEA and CEI study groups with respect to local anesthetic requirements for labor.

PCEA represents an avenue for provision of excellent pain relief for labor with the potential for utilization of lower amounts of local anesthetic agents. However, no further comment can be made on its applicability until several of the aforementioned problems with methodology have been addressed.

REFERENCES

1. Shah M V, Jones D I, Rosen M 1986 'Patient-demand' post-operative analgesia with buprenorphine. Comparison between sublingual and I. M. administration. Br J Anaesth 58: 508–511
2. Bell M D, Murray G R, Mishra P et al 1985 Buccal morphine – a new role for analgesia? Lancet 1: 71–73
3. Urguhart M L, Klapp K, White P F 1988 Patient-controlled analgesia: a comparison of intravenous versus subcutaneous hydromophine. Anesthesiology 69: 428–432

4. Gambling D R, Yu P, McMorland G H, Palmer L 1988 A comparative study of patient epidural analgesia (PCEA) and continuous infusion epidural analgesia (CIEA) during labor. Can J Anaesth 35: 249–254
5. Lysak S Z, Eisenach J C, Dobson II C E 1990 Patient-controlled epidural analgesia during labor: a comparison of three solutions with a continuous infusion control. Anesthesiology 72: 44–49
6. Marlowe S, Engstrom R, White P F 1989 Epidural patient-controlled analgesia (PCA): an alternative to continuous epidural infusions. Pain 37: 97–101
7. Sjöström S, Hartvig D, Tamsen A 1988 Patient-controlled analgesia with extradural morphine or pethidine. Br J Anaesth 60: 358–366
8. Hill H F, Mackie A M, Jacobson R C 1990 Infusion-based patient-controlled analgesia systems. In: Patient-controlled analgesia Ferrante F M, Ostheimer G W, Covino B G (eds) Blackwell Scientific Publications, Boston, p 214–222
9. White P F 1990 Patient-controlled analgesia: delivery systems. p 70–81 In: Patient-controlled analgesia. Ferrante F M, Ostheimer G W, Covino B G (eds) Blackwell Scientific Publications, Boston

21. Epidural anesthesia: complications in the obstetric patient

PART A
OVERVIEW
D. B. Scott

Epidural anesthesia has an excellent safety record when used in obstetrics. In England and Wales, detailed records of all maternal deaths have been kept for many years.[1] There were only nine deaths associated with epidural anesthesia during the 15-year period from 1970 to 1984 inclusive. During those 15 years, 127 maternal deaths associated with general anesthesia occurred. With regard to nonfatal morbidity a recent retrospective survey of over 500 000 epidural anesthetics demonstrated that an adverse effect occurred in, on average, 1 in 4500 patients.[2] Permanent damage was very rare indeed, there being a single case of multiple spinal nerve neuropathy.

However, epidural anesthesia has the potential to cause serious complications. The anesthesiologist must be aware of how complications arise, how to diagnose and treat them and, most important, how to avoid them.

COMPLICATIONS DURING THE PERFORMANCE OF EPIDURAL ANESTHESIA

Dural puncture

Dural puncture occurs when the epidural needle is advanced too far or too quickly through the ligamentum flavum. Epiduroscopy has shown that the dura mater is easily pushed away from the ligamentum flavum by the needle, and this can occur without piercing the dura. A needle striking the dura on either side of the midline can move the dura a considerable distance before perforating it. However, the perforation that might eventually be caused could be a tear rather than a puncture hole.

While experience and gentle controlled advancement of the needle will considerably reduce the possibility of dural puncture, most large institutions that have training programs declare a prevalence of 1–2%.[3]

Prevention

To locate the epidural space, a Tuohy needle or its modification in 16–18 gauge is usually employed. It must be pushed through the ligamentum flavum while using one of several means to detect the space, e.g. loss of resistance, hanging drop, etc. The slower the advancement, the less is the risk of sudden unexpected advancement as the resistance of the ligamentum flavum is overcome.

Tuohy needles vary considerably in their sharpness. A sharp needle requires less force to push it through the ligamentum flavum, but it can pierce the dura more easily than a blunt needle. A blunt needle requires more force and, as the epidural space is entered, there is likely to be a sudden forward movement as the resistance disappears. However, being blunt, it is more difficult to penetrate the dura. The anesthesiologist must be aware of the sharpness of the needle used and adjust the technique accordingly.

Diagnosis

In the great majority of cases this presents no problem, as cerebrospinal fluid (CSF) gushes unmistakeably from the needle hub. If fluid has been used to locate the space, this may drip back slowly through the needle without the dura having been penetrated. If fluid is dripping from the hub, it is customary to allow it to drop onto the skin of the anesthesiologist's forearm. If it is cold, it is the injected fluid and if it is warm it is CSF.

However, dural puncture can occur without CSF appearing at the needle hub, either because the needle point has not completely penetrated the dura or because it has invaginated the dura in such a way as to prevent CSF escaping. Though uncommon, it is still well recognized that a postdural puncture headache (PDPH) can occur following an apparently uncomplicated epidural anesthetic.

If not recognized after inserting the needle, the puncture may become manifest after the catheter has been inserted through the needle. Fluid running back through the catheter will provide the diagnosis, although the catheter end must be lowered below the point of insertion to allow the CSF to escape by gravity.

A further diagnostic aid is the use of a test dose. If the catheter tip is within the subarachnoid space, a small dose of local anesthetic will rapidly produce evidence of a developing spinal anesthesia. Because a test dose containing epinephrine is also used to diagnose intravascular placement of the catheter, a sufficient dose has to be injected, e.g. 3–5 ml of 2% lidocaine or 0.5% bupivacaine with 1 : 200 000 epinephrine. Sufficient time should be allowed (4–5 min) for a spinal block to develop. Evalution should be for numbness (sensory anesthesia) and *not* motor paralysis.

Complications of dural puncture

These are twofold, the development of a PDPH and the production of high or total spinal anesthesia (see below).

Management

Once dural puncture has been diagnosed, the anesthesiologist must decide on the course of action to be taken. The possibilities are:

1. Abandoning the epidural anesthetic.
2. Reinsertion of the needle at another intervertebral space. While this seems a logical move, there can be difficulties. There is the chance that the dura may again be punctured. CSF leaking from the first puncture may reach the needle tip – now properly placed – in the epidural space and cause considerable confusion. Local anesthetic may enter the subarachnoid space after being injected epidurally causing an unexpectedly high block.
3. Insertion of a catheter into the subarachnoid space. Once a dural puncture has occurred, the epidural has lost its major advantage over subarachnoid block, i.e. the lower prevalence of PDPH. A small dose of bupivacaine (1.0–1.5 ml of 0.5% bupivacaine) will give excellent pain relief and similar doses can be used for top-ups based on the results of the initial injection. At least, there is no question regarding the position of the catheter. Lastly, the anesthesiologist can inform the patient of the probability of a PDPH and how he/she intends to treat it. It is prudent to ensure that subarachnoid top-ups are *only* done by anesthesiologists.

High or total spinal anesthesia

This will occur if a substantial dose of local anesthetic is injected into the subarachnoid space unintentionally. Epidural anesthesia requires 8–10 times the dose used for spinal anesthesia. If dural puncture has not been diagnosed, then large amounts of drug may be deposited into the subarachnoid space, and a very high block will be produced. Such an event has been reported at top-up injections after an apparently normal epidural block with the first injection. While this is often attributed to penetration of the dura by the catheter, such an event is impossible to produce in vitro. That erosion of the dura can occur by constant movement of the catheter tip is questionable. Much more likely is that the tip of the catheter is lying in the subarachnoid space, leaving the side-holes, which are about 1 cm from the tip, in the epidural space (when a three-hole catheter is used). Advancement into the subarachnoid space could then occur with movement. Even more likely is that a catheter with three distal holes has been placed, such that the distal hole is in the subarachnoid space and the proximal holes are in the epidural space. In vitro tests show that with a slow injection, the injectate leaves through the proximal holes, i.e. into the epidural space. A fast injection on the other hand leaves through the distal hole, i.e. into the subarachnoid space (Fig. 21.1).[4]

Clinical features

A widespread block will occur very quickly, and hypotension with bradycardia is to be expected, though it may be absent. If the upper cervical spinal nerves are involved, diaphragmatic paralysis can occur, which together with intercostal paralysis will lead to inadequate respiration or apnea.

Should the local anesthetic reach the cranial subarachnoid space, then unconsciousness will occur.

Management

A patient who is unconscious, apneic, bradycardic and severely hypotensive presents an alarming clinical picture. However, the treatment is relatively easy to institute and highly effective if applied quickly.

Management consists of ventilation with oxygen and increasing the arterial pressure and heart rate with a vasopressor such as ephedrine or epinephrine. To avoid

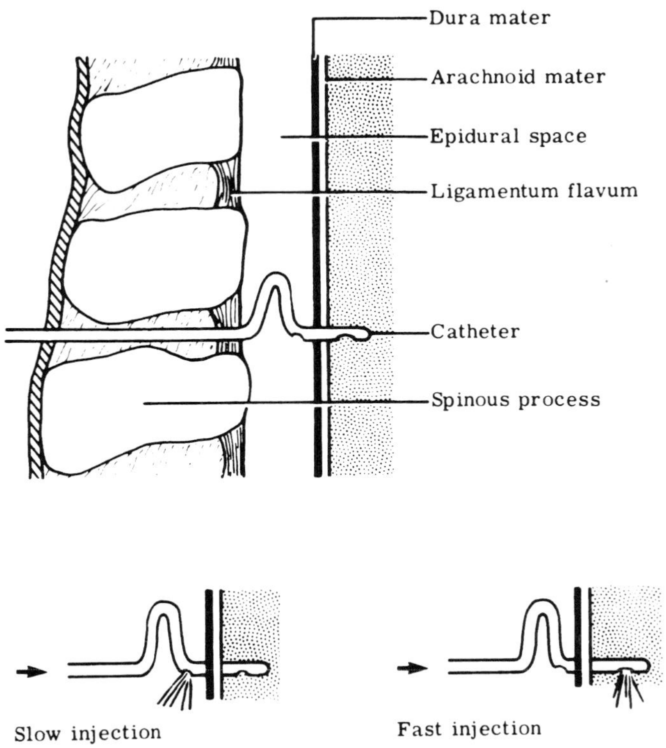

Fig. 21.1 Escape of injected fluid from multihole epidural catheters: slow injection causes escape from the proximal hole and fast injection from the distal hole.

delay do not insert a tracheal tube until the lungs have been ventilated with oxygen by positive-pressure using a bag and face mask.

Ephedrine 10–15 mg intravenously is an excellent vasopressor which works rapidly. If the effect is too little or too short-lived the dose may be repeated or epinephrine 0.1–0.5 mg may be administered i.v.

The subarachnoid block will last for the duration of the local anesthetic effect. The return of spontaneous breathing will indicate that the block is decreasing, and recovery thereafter will be quite rapid.

Subdural block

Local anesthetic injected between the dura and arachnoid mater can spread quite easily to affect a large number of spinal nerves. The development of this block tends to be slower than an unintentional spinal anesthetic, and it may be both widespread and patchy.

Treatment is similar to a high spinal anesthetic, although artificial ventilation may not be necessary.

Acute toxicity

The epidural space contains numerous veins draining blood from the spinal cord and the vertebrae. It is not uncommon for an epidural catheter, many of which have a rigid tip, to enter one of these veins. Epidural needles may also puncture veins. If blood is not seen in the catheter and the misplacement is not diagnosed, then a substantial quantity of local anesthetic may be injected intravenously, causing an acute toxic reaction.

Clincial features

Local anesthetic drugs cause toxicity by their effect on the central nervous system initially.[5] If large doses are injected, then cardiovascular effects may also appear.[6] The toxicity is due to the action of the drugs on excitable membranes in the brain and heart.

The first symptoms (Fig. 21.2) are numbness of the tongue (a local effect on the nerve endings in the tongue), lightheadedness and tinnitus. Visual disturbances can occur and the patient may start to behave and talk strangely. This can be mistaken for hysteria. Muscular twitching may be seen and presages the onset of convulsions. Unconsciousness usually precedes the convulsions, which are typical grand mal seizures. When the seizures stop, the patient may be comatose and apneic.

Cardiovascular depression involving the heart is due to the effect of the local anesthetic on myocardial conduction and contraction. Peripherally, there is vasodilation, either by a central effect or by a direct effect on the resistance vessels (or both). Together with the reduced cardiac output, this leads to profound hypotension. Cardiac arrest can occur. With the shorter acting agents, e.g. lidocaine or mepivacaine, cardiac arrhythmias are seldom seen, but the longer acting agents, e.g. bupivacaine or etidocaine, may cause ventricular fibrillation. While it is important to be aware of the cardiovascular effects, it should be remem-

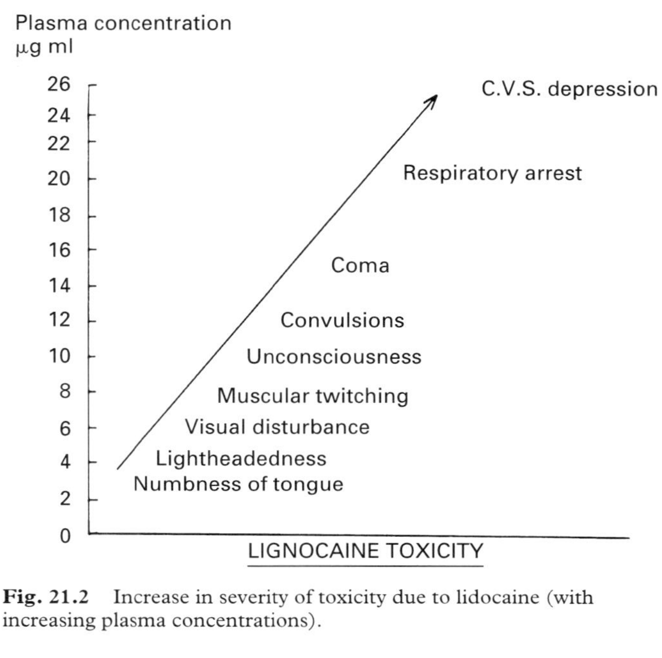

Fig. 21.2 Increase in severity of toxicity due to lidocaine (with increasing plasma concentrations).

bered that most patients who develop convulsions will not have any cardiovascular depression, (which occurs at much higher plasma concentrations), *provided* hypoxia is avoided.

Although the signs and symptoms of toxicity follow a pattern, this can be altered by the rate of injection, in that a very fast injection may produce convulsions with little in the way of premonitory signs. Rarely toxicity may occur due to overdosage rather than intravenous injection, e.g. following a bolus injection given for a cesarean delivery at the end of a long labor involving several top-ups.[7]

It has been shown when local anesthetic is injected through an epidural catheter which has entered an epidural vein that some drug may go into a vein and some may be extravasated into the epidural space.[8] This can lead to a confusing picture of mild but definite toxicity, together with a patchy and inadequate epidural block. If all the drug enters the veins, then there will be no demonstrable anesthesia.

Other conditions may confuse the diagnosis, e.g. shivering may be mistaken for muscle twitching and convulsions may be due to maternal disease such as epilepsy or eclampsia. Patients who have vasovagal syncope and become unconscious for some seconds often have a minor convulsion during the recovery of consciousness. If possible, a blood sample should be taken as soon as toxicity is suspected, to determine the plasma concentration of the local anesthetic.

Prevention

The appearance of frank blood, either at the needle hub or in the epidural catheter, makes withdrawal and reinsertion mandatory. As with CSF, the best way to test for i.v. placement is to lower the end of the catheter and allow the blood to flow by gravity.

The injection of a test dose can be unreliable unless a 'marker' such as epinephrine is added, and the heart rate and blood pressure monitored. The effect of i.v. epinephrine can be very evanescent and the heart rate must be displayed continuously preferably, using an electrocardiogram and cardiotachometer. Even then, false positives can occur in very nervous individuals.

Probably the best preventative measure is the *slow* injection of the main dose of local anesthetic. A rate of 10 ml/min should not be exceeded, and verbal contact with the patient should be maintained to elicit any of the early signs of toxicity, in which event the injection can be stopped before too large a dose has been given. The technique of injecting small volumes every few minutes will also avoid serious toxicity. *A negative test dose must not be used as an excuse to inject large doses rapidly!*

Treatment

No treatment other than oxygen inhalation is required up to the point of convulsions. The early signs will usually disappear quite rapidly if the injection is stopped. Should convulsions occur, then the patient will rapidly become hypoxic and acidotic due to apnea and the increased oxygen consumption produced by the muscular activity.[9,10]

Therefore, oxygen is the first requirement and should be given with a face mask and artificial ventilation if the patient is not breathing. Do not waste time trying to insert a tracheal tube. If the convulsions last longer than 15–20 s then an anticonvulsant should be given. Thiopental 100–200 mg will have the most rapid effect and will wear off quickly. The cardiovascular effects of such a dose are minimal. Diazepam 5–10 mg has its advocates, but it is slow both to take effect and to wear off. Succinylcholine has been recommended as an alternative to an anticonvulsant, but this commits the anesthesiologist to tracheal intubation and a general anesthetic.

Cardiovascular collapse should be treated with inotropes and vasopressors. Ephedrine 5–20 mg i.v. is a good initial agent; epinephrine 0.5–1.0 mg i.v. has support as the 'gold standard'. If cardiac arrest occurs, external cardiac compression must be applied, and often for a considerable time.

A decision on how to proceed with the patient's anesthetic and operation has to be made. All options are open if a rapid recovery of consciousness has been achieved. These options include:

1. Withdrawing the catheter and reinserting it. The subsequent injection of local anesthetic must be made with care, of course.
2. Converting to a spinal anesthetic.
3. Converting to a general anesthetic.

Awareness of the possibility of toxicity and a predetermined plan of action are invaluable in effective treatment.

COMPLICATIONS DURING EPIDURAL ANESTHESIA

Hypotension

This is the commonest complication that follows the injection of local anesthetic into the epidural space. While several factors may contribute to a decrease in arterial pressure, such as inferior vena caval (IVC) occlusion, hemorrhage or vasovagal fainting, the initial trigger to hypotension is the sympathetic blockade cause by the epidural anesthetic.

The sympathetic efferent fibers that are responsible for cardiovascular stability arise from the 14 spinal segments T1–L2. They are easily affected by epidural local anesthetic drug, either in the mixed spinal nerves or in the white rami communicantes on their way to the sympathetic chain. Thus a block to T8 will remove half the sympathetic outflow. Very high blocks involving T1–5 will also affect the cardiac sympathetics, leading to bradycardia and a reduction of myocardial inotropy.

Young nonpregnant patients seldom develop marked hypotension from sympathetic blockade alone, and IVC occlusion undoubtedly contributes to the frequency of the problem in obstetric anesthesia. Vasovagal overactivity is also common, particularly just before or during cesarean delivery.

IVC occlusion is present in most women in late pregnancy when they lie supine.[11] However, this is not apparent clinically. The venous return is often unaffected by the occlusion, blood being returned to the heart via a collateral circulation. If venous return, and thus cardiac output, is decreased, the arterial pressure is maintained by increased sympathetic tone. Thus, sympathetic blockade will 'reveal' IVC occlusion, by eliminating this compensatory mechanism.

Vagal overactivity usually occurs quite suddenly, leading to bradycardia and hypotension, accompanied by nausea, vomiting and sweating. In severe cases there is a transient cardiac arrest with loss of consciousness.

Prevention

The use of acute intravascular volume expansion of the circulation with i.v. fluids is essential.

The prophylactic use of vasopressors is not popular, as it is difficult to judge the dose and to avoid hypertension once the baby is delivered and IVC occlusion is relieved.

The avoidance of the supine position is important, and during the onset and development of the anesthetic it is best to keep the mother in the lateral position. (There is no evidence that this can cause unilateral anesthesia.) During cesarean delivery, the patient should be kept in the left lateral position, using a pelvic wedge, until the baby is delivered.

For relief of pain in labor, the dose of local anesthetic is smaller and hypotension is seldom a problem if the mother remains in the lateral position. She can, of course, move from side to side.

Frequent monitoring of the arterial pressure is necessary.

Treatment

Because vasodilation is the primary cause of the hypotension, a vasopressor is the most logical, and certainly the quickest, form of treatment. While some experts are concerned about the possibility of vasopressors reducing the uterine blood flow[12] this is not a problem with drugs such as ephedrine.[13,14] A more important problem is the development of hypertension, once the IVC occlusion is relieved at delivery, if too much vasopressor is given. Small (3–5 mg), and if necessary repeated, doses of ephedrine or a continuous infusion of phenylephrine (a short-acting alpha-adrenergic drug which may be discontinued at delivery) are preferred to a large bolus dose.

Opinions vary about the degree of hypotension that requires treatment, but a decrease in arterial pressure of over 20 mmHg provides a useful guide. Some obstetric anesthesiologists give a vasopressor as soon as a decrease in arterial pressure occurs. If bradycardia is a feature of the hypotension, ephedrine is still the best drug. Atropine is commonly used but is less effective.

Intravenous fluids are often used as the first line treatment of hypotension, but are seldom effective by themselves. Indeed, adequate treatment of hypotension is often delayed unnecessarily by giving fluids and atropine before a sympathomimetic agent.

High epidural block

It is not unusual to see an epidural block ascend to the upper thoracic or lower cervical segments. Provided the breathing and blood pressure are carefully monitored, little harm usually results. If respiratory paralysis occurs, artificial ventilation may be necessary as with a high spinal block.

Inadequate epidural block

Even experts may fail to produce 100% anesthesia for cesarean delivery in all patients. Patients should be warned to expect some discomfort, and even pain, up to the delivery.

The failure of the blockade may be total, but is more commonly partial. In the former case, there is little difficulty in diagnosing the problem *before* surgery is begun. The alternatives available to the anesthesiologist are:

1. remove the catheter and repeat the epidural anesthetic;
2. do a lumbar dural puncture and establish a spinal anesthetic;
3. convert to general anesthesia.

If the patient complains of pain after surgery has started, the cause may be:

a. Not enough time has been allowed for the block to become fully effective.
b. The epidural block is not high enough.
c. The nerve block is not profound enough to ablate all the sensory input. This is probably the commonest cause. The anesthesiologist must retain the confidence of the patient if the situation is not to deteriorate badly.

The options to be taken are:

1. Try to encourage the patient to tolerate the discomfort until the delivery. After this the pain will be less and it is possible to give i.v. opioids without risk to the baby.

2. Reinforce the block by injecting a further dose of local anesthetic, or an opioid, or both.

3. Give an i.v. opioid, while realizing that the baby must be observed carefully for respiratory depression. A very short-acting agent is advisable.

4. As a last resort, convert to a general anesthetic. Patients should always be prepared for a general anesthetic even when regional anesthesia is planned.

The use of tranquilizers, particularly the benzodiazepines, is to be deprecated because they have no analgesic properties; their amnesic properties will make it unlikely that the mother will remember the birth (often the very reason she chose an epidural); and they often convert a *cooperative* patient in pain to a very *uncooperative* patient in pain.

The experienced anesthesiologist will have a prearranged strategy worked out, and will have established a good rapport with the mother. A comment such as 'You may experience some discomfort before delivery of the baby, but it will be far less than a normal vaginal delivery' is not only truthful but puts the problem into perspective. The heightened emotional tension at a cesarean delivery especially in an unpremedicated patient, should not be underestimated. How mothers are managed in this respect is one of the greatest challenges to the 'art' of anesthesia.

LATE COMPLICATIONS OF EPIDURAL ANESTHESIA

The complications that may arise in the hours and days following epidural anesthesia are backache, post-dural puncture headache and neurologic sequelae.

Backache

While several studies have shown that backache, a common complaint after parturition, is no commoner following an epidural anesthetic,[15] there is no doubt that the insertion of a large needle into the spine (especially repeated unsuccessful insertions!) establishes a strong psychological link in the mother's mind. A recent prospective study[16] has shown that significantly more mothers who had had epidurals in labor required treatment for chronic backache than those who had not had an epidural block.

This whole problem is confounded by the fact that backache is a symptom and not a disease. It has multiple etiologies, many ill understood, and there has been no convincing mechanism advanced to explain how an epidural block could be deleterious. It is worth pointing out that epidural injections are widely used in treating chronic backache.

Post-dural puncture headache (PDPH)

PDPH usually occurs after a known dural puncture, though this is not always the case. However, it may be assumed that a typical PDPH is due to dural puncture even though this was not obvious at the time the epidural was initiated.

Pathology

The headache is related to a low CSF pressure, especially when the patient sits up or stands. The likeliest explanation is that the brain becomes less well supported within the cranium and traction is exerted on the structures supporting it. In severe cases traction may also be exerted on the cranial nerves, particularly those supplying the eye muscles, and this can lead to temporary abducens paralysis.

The condition is related to the amount of CSF leakage from the spinal subarachnoid space to the epidural space, from where it is easily absorbed. The size and shape of the hole caused by the needle puncture is of significant importance. Because epidural needles have a large outside diameter (16–18 gauge), the leakage is usually substantial and the prevalence of PDPH after epidural needle puncture of the dura is likely to be greater than 50%. This compares with 6–10% using a 22-gauge spinal needle in a similar age group. It should not be assumed that the hole is always that to be expected from a simple puncture. The dura can be 'tented' by the needle and move several centimeters before perforation occurs. This can cause tearing of the dura with the production of a very large defect. This was reported in a mother who died, during labor, of a total spinal anesthetic at the fourth top-up.[17] She had complained of severe headache soon after the 'epidural' was started and each injection of local anesthetic caused an abnormally high block with paralysis. At post-mortem the 'hole' was, in fact, a right angled tear, the sides of which were 1 cm long.

A late complication of the low CSF pressure is intracranial subdural hematoma.[18,19] Although rare, it often requires surgical intervention.

Symptoms and signs

The most important diagnostic feature is a headache that is clearly related to posture, being greatest when upright and quickly relieved by lying down. Sometimes it is accompanied by neck pain and stiffness, which may mislead by suggesting meningitis, but the headache of meningitis is not related to posture. Strabismus may be seen in severe cases, but usually has a late onset.

PDPH can be very severe and incapacitating. It is frequently accompanied by depression, the mother being unable to enjoy her new baby, receive visitors, etc.

Treatment

It is common to find anesthesiologists prevaricating quite

unnecessarily before instituting effective therapy. Simple analgesics and fluid may be effective, but it is more the exception than the rule. Such measures should not be persisted with for more than a few hours if the headache is incapacitating.

While several therapies have been tried with varying success, there is little doubt that an epidural 'blood patch' is by far the most rapid and effective treatment. This involves the injection of 10–20 ml of autologous blood into the epidural space. After identifying the space (being careful not to puncture the dura again!) venous blood is drawn with full aseptic precautions from the patient and injected through the epidural needle. Usually the PDPH is immediately relieved and the patient may start ambulating in an hour or so.

Although the term 'patch' is used to convey the idea of sealing the dural hole, it is more likely that the blood, which will clot and remain within the epidural space for several days, acts as a space 'occupier', immediately raising the CSF pressure and preventing it from decreasing to the point of causing further headache.

The success rate is high (over 90%), though the procedure may need to be repeated if the headache recurs. Complications are very rare.

Neurologic complications

Epidural anesthesia can be followed by neurologic deficit, though the incidence of this is extremely low. There are several causes of neurologic sequelae which may be temporary or permanent (Table 21.1).

Trauma

Trauma is probably the commonest cause and usually involves a single spinal nerve.[2] The needle or catheter can enter a nerve and, if an injection is made directly into that nerve, then some disruption of the fibers can occur. This may lead to a degree of neuritis, which can last for some weeks or months. In such cases the patient will usually complain of pain during insertion of the needle or catheter and at the start of the injection. When the block has worn off, the patient may complain of paresthesia in the distribution of the nerve concerned, with a partial loss of sensation and, occasionally, some motor weakness. These symptoms and signs usually disappear within a few days or weeks but occasionally last much longer.

Adhesive arachnoiditis

Adhesive arachnoiditis is a serious condition and may result in permanent loss of spinal cord function. It usually follows the injection of an irritant solution, and several compounds have been implicated, such as detergent used for cleaning syringes. The local anesthetic chloroprocaine was involved in several cases in which large quantities were injected by mistake into the subarachnoid space.[20] These reports were followed by animal studies claiming to show spinal cord damage following chloroprocaine injected into the subarachnoid space. Other animal data failed to confirm this, and many authorities are still advocating the use of the drug. The unintentional injection of a substance other than a local anesthetic or opioid should, of course, never occur, but unfortunately it does. Substances so injected have included potassium chloride, calcium chloride (in mistake for sodium chloride), thiopental and even agents for intravenous feeding.

Anterior spinal artery syndrome

Anterior spinal artery syndrome is a condition caused by failure of the blood supply in the distribution of the artery. It causes an infarct of the spinal cord with resultant permanent paraplegia. The blood supply of the cord is somewhat tenous. The anterior spinal artery, though it receives anterior radicular arteries at each vertebra, derives its main supply from the artery of Adamkiewicz. Failure of this supply may occur during aortic clamping or excessive retraction of the aorta during surgery. Atherosclerosis can

Table 21.1 Summary of various types of neurologic damage following epidural blockade

Pathology	Cause	Onset	Clinical Features	Outcome
Spinal nerve neuropathy	Trauma (needle, catheter, injection)	0–2 days	Pain during insertion of needle or catheter. Pain on injection Parasthesia, pain and numbness over distribution of spinal nerve	Recovery 1–2 weeks
Anterior spinal artery sydrome	Arteriosclerosis hypotension	Immediate	Post-operative painless paraplegia	Painless paraplegia
Adhesive arachnoiditis	Irritant injectate	0–7 days	Pain on injection Variable degree of neurological deficit. Often progressive with pain and paraplegia	May progress to severe disability with pain and paralysis
Space-occupying lesion (hematoma or abscess)	Hypocoagulation Bacteremia	0–2 days	Severe backache post-operatively with progressive paraplegia	Requires immediate surgery otherwise paraplegia

also cause a diminished blood flow which may become inadequate should hypotension occur. Induced hypotension has been blamed for the condition,[21] but hypotension by itself is an excessively rare cause of spinal cord infarction. The use of solutions containing epinephrine has also been suggested as a possible cause, and high concentrations of epinephrine have caused cord damage in experimental animals.[22] However, in the doses used clinically this would seem to be an unlikely cause of infarction.

The epidural space being a closed compartment, it is possible that infarction could follow the development of excessive pressure within the space. If this pressure were to exceed arterial pressure for more than a few minutes, a permanent lesion could result.

Space-occupying lesion

Space-occupying lesions such as hematomas, abscesses and tumors can press upon the spinal cord and cause serious cord damage. It is quite common to traumatize a vein during the course of an epidural block. This, however, will not lead to a large and dangerous hematoma in the absence of a clotting defect, which in itself is a contraindication to an epidural block. Patients given large doses of heparin to prevent coagulation during surgery could be at theoretical risk, though this should be most unlikely if the needle or catheter were inserted more than 20–30 min before the heparin was injected. The use of 'mini-dose' heparin to prevent post-operative deep venous thrombosis is held by some to contraindicate an epidural block. Others, however, have reported large series of cases without incident.[23] If there is any doubt in an individual patient, a clotting screen can be done to ensure that the heparin has not made the blood excessively hypocoagulable.

Epidural abscesses have been reported following epidural block and are thought to be due to bacteremia with colonization of an epidural hematoma.[24] In most cases the patient was suffering from a pyrexial disease. The injection of contaminated material into the epidural space appears to be amazingly rare. That epidural blocks are performed with full sterile precautions and that local anesthetics themselves are bacteriostatic or bacteriocidal may account for this rarity. Spinal tumors can, of course, cause paraplegia by direct pressure, and their presence may not be suspected until full neurologic recovery fails to occur after epidural block.

If persistent painful backache appears or the nerve block does not fully disappear in the expected time, the possibility of a space-occupying lesion should be entertained as laminectomy must be performed urgently if permanent damage is to be prevented. These cases require a full neurologic examination including scanning, and should be treated as an acute surgical emergency.

REFERENCES

1. Reports on Confidential Enquiries into Maternal Deaths in England and Wales, 1970–72, 1973–75, 1976–78, 1979–81, 1982–84. HMSO, London
2. Scott D B, Hibbard B M 1990 Serious non-fatal complications associated with extradural block in obstetric practice. Br J Anaesth 64: 537–541
3. Crawford J S 1984 Principles and practice of obstetric anaesthesia. Blackwell Scientific Publications, Oxford, p 214
4. Scott D B 1980 Test doses and catheter problems. In Doughty A (ed) Epidural analgesia in obstetrics. A second symposium. Lloyd-Luke, London. p 146–148
5. Scott D B 1986 Toxic effects of local anaesthetic agents on the central nervous system. Br J Anaesth 58: 732–735
6. Reiz S, Nath S 1986 Cardiotoxicity of local anaesthetic agents. Br J Anaesth 58: 736–746
7. Thorburn K, Moir D D 1984 Bupivacaine toxicity in association with extradural analgesia for Cesarean section. Br J Anaesth 56: 551–553
8. McKeown D W, Scott D B 1984 Bupivacaine-induced convulsions during general anesthesia. Reg Anesth 9: 207–209
9. Moore D C, Crawford R D, Scurlock J E 1980 Severe hypoxia and acidosis following local anesthetic-induced convulsions. Anesthesiology 53: 259–261
10. James M R, Marshall H, Carew-McColl M 1991 Pulse oximetry during apparent tonic–clonic seizures. Lancet 337: 394–395
11. Kerr M G, Scott D B, Samuel E 1964 Studies of the inferior vena cava in late pregnancy. Br Med J 1, 532–533
12. Greiss F C, Crandell D L 1965 Therapy for hypotension induced by spinal anesthesia during pregnancy: observations on gravid ewes. J Am Med Assoc 191: 793–796
13. Hollmen A J, Jouppila R, Albright G A, Jouppila P, Vierola H, Koivula A 1984 Intervillous blood flow during Cesarean section with prophylactic ephedrine and epidural anesthesia. Acta Anaesthesiol Scand 28, 396–400
14. Shnider A M, de Lorimer A A, Hall J W, Chapler F K, Morishima H O. Vasopressors in obstetrics 1968 I. Correction of fetal acidosis with ephedrine during spinal hypotension. An J Obstet Gynecol 102: 911–919
15. Moir D D & Davidson S 1972 Postpartum complications of forceps delivery performed under epidural and pudendal nerve block. Br J Anaesth 44: 1197–1199
16. MacArthur C, Lewis M, Know E G, Crawford J S 1990 Epidural anaesthesia and long term backache after childbirth. Br Med J 301: 9–12
17. Report on Confidential Enquiries into Maternal Deaths in England and Wales, 1973–75. HMSO, London, p 83
18. Jack T M 1979 Postpartum intracranial subdural haematoma. Anaesthesia 34: 176–180
19. Newrick P, Read D 1983 Subdural haematomata as a complication of spinal anaesthetic. Br Med J 285: 341–342
20. Covino B G, Marx G F, Finster M, Zsigmond E K 1980 Prolonged sensory and motor deficits following inadvertent spinal anesthesia. Anesth Analg 59: 399–401
21. Forrester A C 1959 Mishaps in anaesthesia. Anaesthesia 14: 388–392
22. Catherberg J, Insausti T 1964 Paraplejias consecutivas a anestesia (estudio clinico y experimental). Rev Assoc Med Argentina 78: 1–5
23. Odoom J A, Sih I L 1983 Epidural analgesia and anticoagulant therapy: experiences with one thousand cases of continuous epidurals. Anaesthesia 38: 254–259
24. Bromage P R 1978 Epidural analgesia. W B Saunders, Philadelphia p 682

PART B
SYSTEMIC TOXICITY FROM LOCAL ANESTHETICS INJECTED FOR EPIDURAL ANESTHESIA

D. C. Moore

INTRODUCTION

This chapter is based on the following experiences:

1. the author performing anesthesia for obstetric deliveries since 1942;
2. 24-h coverage of the obstetric department of the Virginia Mason Hospital with physicians (staff anesthesiologists and anesthesia residents) from 1952;[1–16]
3. fathers being present in the labor, delivery and cesarean delivery rooms from that date;[4,7,8,11] and
4. the immediate recognition and treatment of systemic toxic reactions from the esters (chloroprocaine, piperocaine, procaine, tetracaine) and the amides (bupivacaine, lidocaine, mepivacaine) or a combination of these.[17–44]

To date, in over 125 000 regional blocks (30 000 or more obstetric procedures) only one permanent sequela (mild encephalopathy) has occurred from a systemic toxic reaction. This occurred in a parturient in whom:

1. the author was supervising a resident;
2. mepivacaine was being used;
3. an intermittent caudal block was being administered; and
4. sustained convulsions resulted.[13]

The case precipitated the investigations in humans that showed amide derivatives accumulate in an intermittent-dose technique.[13]

Unfortunately, when a systemic toxic reaction from a local anesthetic results in complications, particularly permanent complications (e.g. encephalopathy or death), attention is all too often focused on one or more of the following:

a. the dosage (volume × concentration) of the local anesthetic;
b. only its concentration; or
c. the inadequacies of the package insert which describes its usage.

Systemic toxicity, followed by its known complications, is likely to occur regardless of the local anesthetic injected, if:

a. the wrong regional block is selected for a procedure;
b. the regional block chosen is appropriate but it is conducted improperly (no preparation for a complication, improper or no monitoring, no test-dose, etc);
c. a delay in treatment of the systemic toxic reaction occurs; or
d. it is treated improperly.

A prudent, vigilant anesthesiologist can avoid these iatrogenic (anesthesiologist induced) errors.

Readers should not get the impression from the references that the author does not recognize the importance of bench (laboratory) research. Nonetheless, animal and in vitro data cannot be extrapolated to humans. They are only a rough guideline to the situation in humans.[44–48] Furthermore, as stated some years previously, 'Believing in medicine is not enough, one must know'.[44,48] 'Extrapolating' and/or 'believing' are extremely dangerous, as they only lead anesthesiologists to eventually state that animal data are facts pertinent to humans, when no clinical proof exists. Perhaps most important is that doing this has, in the past, and will likely in the future, result in the twisting of facts in a medicolegal case to serve a purpose for which they may not be intended.[44,48] Therefore, the majority of the references are the results of clinical studies conducted by the Anesthesia Department of The Mason Clinic and they adhere to the following statement: 'I would have everie man write what he knows and no more' (Montaigne).*

ETIOLOGY

Systemic toxic reactions during pregnancy occur primarily from an unintentional *intravascular* injection into an epidural vein of part or all of the therapeutic dose of the local anesthetic when attempting epidural block. The reason for this is that the vertebral vein system (veins of Batson) has no valves and is a direct avenue of drainage to the heart and brain.[49] Therefore, even what are considered relatively small doses of a local anesthetic for an epidural block, e.g. bupivacaine 50–75 mg, injected intravenously result in the drug's immediate and maximum pharmacologic effect on these two organs.

PRECAUTIONS

Know the indications, contraindications and dose of the local anesthetic to be used prior to administering it

Read at least the package insert that is contained in each package (box, etc.) of a drug or *The Physician's Desk Reference* (published by Medical Economics Company, Oradell, NJ 07649, USA). These contain the minimum data required by the Food and Drug Administration for the USA for the use of a local anesthetic. They do not contain the specifics of this chapter, of which a physician (anesthesiologist, obstetrician), as well as a certified regis-

* *British Journal of Anaesthesia*, preface to editorials.

tered nurse anesthetist who administers regional anesthesia for obstetrics, should be aware.

Select the optimal block technique for the obstetric procedure

For example, intermittent-injection lumbar epidural, not caudal, block is the technique of choice for relief of pain in the first and second stages of labor for routine vaginal delivery because a significantly lower dose of the local anesthetic, which is unlikely to result in a high blood level systemic toxic reaction, can be used. On the other hand, for the same reason, single-injection spinal rather than either a single- or intermittent-injection epidural block is recommended for routine cesarean delivery, provided that an intermittent- or continuous-injection epidural block was not used to relieve the pains of labor.

Prepare resuscitation equipment and drugs

Literally within arm's reach of the anesthesiologist not down the hall, in drawers, or elsewhere, must be:

a. bag and mask suitable for ventilating the patient and connected to a source of oxygen;
b. drugs to treat complications in syringes with needles attached;
c. oral airways, tongue blades, a cuffed endotracheal tube (not in the packaged container);
d. a functioning laryngoscope; and
e. suction equipment.

Regardless of the relative toxicity or dose of the local anesthetic being injected, or where it is being administered (labor or delivery room), excuses for not being prepared for a life-threatening complication are invalid. Such a complication requires immediate and rapid treatment. Time is not available for locating and setting up equipment and drugs.

Attach appropriate monitors

Prior to, during and following the injection of a local anesthetic, the mother's vital signs should be monitored with automatic vital signs monitors, including heart rate and blood pressure; cardiac rhythm with an electrocardioscope (ECG) and/or her oxygen saturation with a pulse oximeter. In addition, the fetal heart rate and uterine contractions should be monitored with a cardiotocograph.

Start intravenous fluids

When administering a lumbar epidural block to relieve pain in the first and second stages of labor, the patient should be *acutely* hydrated with 750–1000 ml of crystalloid. For a cesarean delivery 1500–2000 ml administered prior to initiation of the block should be used. The anesthesiologist should be aware that rapid hydration can increase stroke volume by as much as 55% and place stress on the heart.[50] Therefore, if the patient has a cardiovascular disease of any magnitude, even a temporary one (pregnancy-induced hypertension) or any other disease that may contraindicate *rapid* increase of circulatory volume, acute hydration could be disastrous. In such a situation the rate of acute hydration should be based on other monitoring such as central venous, radial artery and pulmonary artery pressures.

Add epinephrine to the local anesthetic, except in high-risk pregnancies (but this opinion is not shared by all obstetric anesthesiologists)

The optimal final concentration of epinephrine is 1 : 200 000; i.e. 0.05 ml (50 μg) of 1 : 1000 epinephrine in 10 ml of a local anesthetic. This dose of epinephrine does not significantly alter uterine contractions or uterine blood flow.[51–54] Therefore, except in a markedly high-risk pregnancy, a solution containing it is routinely used for lumbar epidural block to relieve the pains of the first and second stages of labor.

Epinephrine has the following advantages when used in solutions for lumbar epidural block:

1. it slows absorption, thereby prolonging the duration of the local anesthetic (i.e. fewer doses are required), lowering the peak plasma levels of the local anesthetic, and intensifying the anesthesia;
2. its positive inotropic effect on the heart may counter the cardiac depressant effects of the local anesthetic if an unintentional intravenous injection occurs;[39] and
3. it is a necessary component of a test dose.[55]

Aspirate and observe the needle's hub or the plastic tubing for blood

Administer an effective test dose

For a test dose to give unequivocal evidence of the placement of the bevel of the needle or the opening of the plastic tubing in a blood vessel, it must contain 15 μg of epinephrine and it must be monitored by an electrocardioscope.[55] Palpating the radial pulse and/or using a pulse monitor are no substitute for the electrocardioscope. Adhering meticulously to the criteria as stated for the test dose, the author has not had a systemic toxic reaction from an epidural block since 1980, when the components of an effective test dose for this technique and its monitoring were investigated.[55–60]

Originally, the 15-μg epinephrine test dose was described for surgical patients. Its use in the patient in labor requires the following alterations.[60] When a contraction and the maternal heart rate peak and start to decrease, as monitored by the cardiotocograph and electrocardiograph respectively, the test dose is injected. At the same time, the parturient, the nurses and the family (when present) are instructed not to converse. Under these conditions, if 30 s elapse prior to the next contraction, 15 μg of epinephrine intravascularly results in the following:

1. the pulse rate shows a marked sustained increase;
2. without exception, and particularly if asked, the parturient states that her heart is pounding or that her 'heart feels like it is about to jump out of her chest', which she does not notice during a contraction; and
3. her blood pressure is elevated.

The use of 15 μg of epinephrine in pregnancy has become controversial.[56–60] Furthermore, the results of test doses have been stated to lack specificity.[61] However, test doses were not given to the parturient as stated above. Furthermore, at least the protocol of one study repeatedly cited[62] in regard to the lack of specificity is highly questionable.[59]

To date no indisputable clinical evidence in humans exists that death or brain damage to the newborn exists from: (1) 15 μg of epinephrine injected into the epidural space or a vessel in it; (2) the local anesthetic; or (3) a combination of them.

Lastly, using the test dose as previously described for obstetric epidural block and monitoring it as stated, intravascular injections of sizeable quantities of local anesthetics that could have resulted in convulsions have been avoided.

If no test dose or an ineffective one is administered, use interval dosing

Interval dosing is the administering of 3–5 ml of the local anesthetic, allowing 1–5 min to elapse before administering another 3–5 ml, and continuing such dosing until evidence of an intravascular injection or spinal block occur or the desired pain relief results.[63]

Interval dosing does not guarantee that a systemic toxic reaction will not occur or that it will not be severe – as previously stated amide local anesthetics do accumulate.

When injecting large volumes of the local anesthetic solutions, employ a syringe no larger than 10 ml

Using a 10-ml syringe, injecting at the rate of 1 ml/s through a needle or 0.2–0.3 ml/s through plastic tubing, aspirating after injecting each 5 ml, and having to refill the syringe if more than 10 ml of the local anesthetic is to be injected prevents rapid injection of large volumes of the local anesthetic and allows one circulation time to elapse, which permits the signs and symptoms of an intravascular injection to become apparent.[42]

Converse with the patient

Constant conversation with a conscious patient during and after a regional block and until time has elapsed for the peak plasma level of the local anesthetic to have been reached and recede is a simple method of ascertaining the early signs and symptoms of a systemic toxic reaction. However, it is no substitute for using the appropriate monitors.

SIGNS AND SYMPTOMS

The clinical signs and symptoms of a systemic toxic reaction are the normal, expected pharmacologic reactions to a high blood level of a local anesthetic.

Systemic toxic reactions have two types of onset, i.e. immediate and delayed. An immediate onset is the type most frequently seen by the anesthesiologist. It occurs within 30–60 s, evidently from an unintentional injection of the therapeutic dose of the local anesthetic into a blood vessel. On the other hand, an absorption reaction starts 5 min or more after completion of the injection. Its maximum severity can be expected when the blood level of the drug peaks, that is with epidural block in 15–20 min.[64,65] With an intermittent-injection technique, a delayed reaction can result after the initial injection, but it is more likely to occur from accumulation from additional doses.[13,17,18,27]

Central nervous system (CNS)

The clinical signs and symptoms are usually those of stimulation followed by depression.

The early CNS signs and symptoms of stimulation are drowsiness, restlessness, nervousness, apprehension, lightheadedness, pugnaciousness, irrationality, loquacity (talkativeness), incoherent speech (confusion), sudden headache, metallic taste in the mouth, numbness or tingling of the tongue and/or lips, roaring in the ears (tinnitus) and twitchings of small muscles, particularly those of the face. If the blood levels of the local anesthetic increase, convulsions result. Following convulsions, the CNS is depressed.

Respiratory system

At the onset of a reaction, the patient may show an increase in the rate as well as depth of respiration. But with convulsions, effective respirations cease, and hypoxia, hypercapnia and lactic acidosis develop within 30 s.[34–39]

Cardiovascular system

At the onset of a reaction, tachycardia will be observed on the electrocardioscope and the blood pressure will increase.[38,39] If the reaction progresses to convulsions, or if convulsions are the first indication of a reaction, the cardiovascular response is the same, particularly if the solution contains epinephrine. If convulsions are not treated properly and promptly within 15 s, and 1–3 min or more elapse before correct treatment, the blood pressure begins to fall and arrhythmias (asystole or fibrillation) ensue.

TREATMENT

When the therapeutic dose of the local anesthetic is administered, the anesthesiologist must be prepared to immediately treat the systemic toxic reaction where the block is performed. Having to move the patient from the induction or labor room to a delivery or operating room and then from the cart or labor room bed to the operating or delivery room table results in ineffective or no therapy of the reaction while the patient is being moved. The 2–3 min or more that elapse with ineffective or no treatment usually result in cardiac arrest, encephalopathy or death.

The 'key' to avoiding a catastrophe from systemic toxicity or any other life-threatening complication is the anesthesiologist's ability to recognize it immediately and to institute at least steps 1–7 of the following therapy within 15 s.

1. Summon additional help

If only the anesthesiologist or one other person is available to treat a severe systemic reaction, the cardiopulmonary resuscitation team should be summoned immediately regardless of whether or not it is eventually needed.

If convulsions occur, at least one knowledgeable person other than the anesthesiologist is required to treat them effectively, even with previous proper preparation and monitoring.

2. Turn the patient supine

The supine position is optimal for treatment of a systemic toxic reaction which progresses to convulsions. Trendelenburg position of 10° or more may enhance the return of blood to the heart and perfusion of the brain.

3. Avoid aortocaval pressure

In the supine position the pregnant uterus must be manually displaced, preferably to the left side. A 12.5–15 cm (5–6 inch) wedge, sandbag, roll or inflated plastic bag to elevate the right hip at a 30° angle to the bed or delivery or operating room table while the patient is convulsing is seldom effective because the patient's position on any one of these cannot be maintained. After terminating the convulsions and continuing treatment of the patient, any of these means of avoiding aortocaval compression may be effective.

Regardless of whether a complication occurs, *the uterus must never compress the vena cava or the aorta*. If a systemic toxic reaction to a local anesthetic occurs, this cardinal point is frequently overlooked.

4. Administer succinylcholine 100–120 mg intravenously within 15 s after the start of convulsions – not diazepam or barbiturates

Hypoxia, hypercarbia and lactic acidosis occur concomitantly and with convulsions. Therefore, the convulsions, which result in spasm of the vocal cords with closure of the glottis,[66] must be stopped immediately and the patient hyperventilated.

Diazepam and barbiturates administered intravenously do not consistently terminate convulsions.

5. Clear the airway

Either vomitus or saliva, or both, can prevent adequate ventilation with oxygen. If either one or both occurred and if the amount is minimal, no time is wasted in attempting to remove it. It is unlikely that it would result in preventing ventilation or result in a serious pneumonitis.

On the other hand, if the quantity is large, the secretions or vomitus would be removed rapidly with the Yankauer instrument (instrument usually employed during tonsillectomy) as soon as convulsions cease.

6. Insert an oral airway

When convulsions cease for 5–10 s or are completely stopped by succinylcholine and the vocal cords relax, ventilation may still be impossible because the tongue occludes the airway. Regardless of this, an oral airway that not only secures a patient's airway but acts as a bite block, should another convulsion occur, should be inserted at the first opportunity. When inserting the oral airway a wooden tongue blade should be used. Otherwise, during its insertion the fingers may be bitten, should the patient again convulse. Ventilation through an oral airway should not be so forceful as to pump oxygen into the stomach. The upper abdomen can be observed by the anesthesiologist and auscultated by another person during ventilation to be sure the oxygen is not entering the stomach.

Do not waste time trying to intubate. Under such circumstances, any wasted ventilation time, an endobronchial or esophageal intubation and/or the stimulation of the pharynx of a hypoxic, hypercarbic, acidotic patient can precipitate a cardiac arrest or ventricular fibrillation.

7. Hyperventilate manually with 100% oxygen

Between convulsions or when the succinylcholine terminates the muscular movements, the patient should be hyperventilated with 100% oxygen. This is the most effective way of reversing hypoxia, hypercarbia and acidosis.

Shallow respirations, which often occur prior to, between or after convulsions, or on recovery from succinylcholine, do not provide adequate ventilation. Such respirations move only the contents of the dead space of the respiratory tract (nose, mouth, pharynx, larynx, trachea, and bronchi, i.e. 150 ml). Therefore, other means of administering oxygen which deliver less than 100% oxygen and do *not* permit the anesthesiologist to hyperventilate the patient (plastic bag and mask, nasal prongs, and so forth) are *not* acceptable. Hyperventilation with 100% oxygen can be discontinued only after the patient has regained consciousness and blood gas analysis shows that his/her unassisted respirations provide adequate oxygenation.

8. Intubation

If hyperventilation cannot be accomplished without dilating the stomach, or if cardiac arrest or fibrillation occurs, then intubation is mandatory. Intubation should not be attempted until:

a. the patient is hyperventilated with oxygen;
b. the convulsions are terminated by succinylcholine; and/or
c. the patient is flaccid from cardiac failure (arrest or fibrillation).

9. Elevate the legs to avoid hypotension

Elevation of the legs will prevent pooling of blood in the lower extremities and helps prevent a decrease in cardiac output.

10. Correct hypotension

Hypotension from a systemic toxic reaction has not been observed by the author. If hypotension without bradycardia occurs, perhaps ephedrine sulfate 10–25 mg intravenously may correct it.

11. Reverse bradycardia

Ephedrine sulfate and atropine, along with rapid intravenous fluid administration, is correct treatment to reverse hypotension and bradycardia from block of the sympathetic nervous system by spinal or epidural anesthesia. However, this does not reverse bradycardia when it occurs from direct myocardial depression from a local anesthetic associated with hypoxia, hypercarbia and acidosis.

Marked bradycardia (heart rate below 40 beats per minute) during or following cessation of convulsions signals impending cardiac failure (arrest or fibrillation). Immediate treatment with epinephrine 0.1–0.2 mg intravenously and perhaps with other positive inotropic drugs (calcium chloride 500 mg) is indicated.[39] Otherwise, cardiac arrest or ventricular fibrillation is likely to result.

12. Institute cardiopulmonary resuscitation (CPR) in an attempt to reverse cardiac arrest or fibrillation

The author has yet to witness either cardiac arrest or ventricular fibrillation during a systemic toxic reaction from a local anesthetic. The following have been ascertained from review of medicolegal cases.

If the rate and rhythm of the heart which was present prior to the injection of the local anesthetic is not re-established within 30–60 s by proper treatment, encephalopathy and/or death are likely. When cardiac failure has persisted for over 1 min, further treatment, i.e. one or more of the following, has not aovided sequelae:

a. manual systole with hyperventilation;
b. defibrillation with 300–500 w s;
c. intracardiac or intravenous epinephrine 1 mg two or more times at intervals of 3–5 min;
d. calcium chloride 500–1000 mg;
e. bretylium 5–10 mg/kg;
f. lidocaine 75–100 mg rapidly; and
g. transcutaneous pacing of the heart, even if sinus rhythm is rapidly captured.

Perhaps in such a situation, a larger initial dose of a positive inotropic myocardial drug (particularly, epinephrine 2–3 mg) along with hyperventilation with 100% oxygen and effective manual systole might result in successful resuscitation.

Using a ventilator when manual systole is being performed is unacceptable. Seldom can the ventilator be synchronized with the chest compression, and, therefore, hypo- rather than hyperventilation usually results. Furthermore, manual systole performed on a patient on a soft mattress (labor room bed) is ineffective, because the mattress, not the thoracic cage, is compressed. A back board under the patient is an absolute necessity.

13. Delivery of the fetus

With one exception in the author's 48 years of performing regional block,[39] instantaneous proper treatment of local anesthetic-induced systemic toxic reactions has avoided or terminated convulsions prior to maternal cardiovascular collapse or fetal distress, thereby negating emergency delivery.[23,27,30,32–39] In this one case, 20 ml of 0.5% bupivacaine (150 mg) without epinephrine had been administered for a cesarean delivery and rapid correct treatment followed by an immediate cesarean delivery avoided maternal or fetal sequelae.[39] Whether the treatment or the rapid delivery was responsible for the outcome is unknown. However, a rapid cesarean delivery in an almost hopeless situation (not associated with a systemic toxic reaction) has resulted in survival of both the mother and the baby without sequelae.[67,68] On the other hand, from review of medicolegal cases, if treatment of the systemic toxic reaction is slow, improper, or both, and delivery is delayed, the mother, fetus or both seldom escape encephalopathy or death. Therefore, at the onset of convulsions, immediate delivery of the fetus either vaginally or abdominally must be considered, because whether maternal cardiovascular collapse or fetal depression will follow is not known.

This emphasizes the importance of a physician (obstetrician, gynecologist or surgeon) competent to perform a rapid cesarean delivery being immediately available when a lumbar epidural block is administered for a cesarean delivery or when a large therapeutic milligram dose of a local anesthetic is injected into the epidural space to relieve the pains of the first or second stages of labor, as can occur when caudal block alone, which is no longer recommended for this purpose, is employed.

14. Arterial blood gases (ABG)

When convulsions occur, an ABG determination should be obtained at the earliest possible moment. Even though the patient may be receiving 100% oxygen and the anesthesiologist 'believes' ventilation is more than adequate, an ABG usually shows hypoxia, hypercarbia and acidosis.[34,36,38] In such circumstances, more vigorous ventilation is indicated. On the other hand, particularly if respirations do not return and the patient does not regain consciousness, overventilation with resulting alkalosis could be the etiology.[69]

15. Administer sodium bicarbonate?

The acidosis that occurs concomitantly with convulsions is both metabolic and respiratory.[34,35] Knowing this has led to the administration of sodium bicarbonate empirically during or as soon as convulsions cease or when stopped by succinylcholine as well as when cardiac arrest occurs.

Bicarbonate therapy in the presence of hypoxic lactic acidosis could be detrimental. In such a situation it can increase lactic acidosis, decrease cardiac output and blood pressure and increase plasma carbon dioxide. Therefore, if used at all, it is administered '... only after proved interventions such as defibrillation, cardiac compression, support of ventilation including intubation, and pharmacologic therapies such as epinephrine and antiarrhythmics have been employed...'[70]

One ampule of sodium bicarbonate (50 mmol) will not reverse an acidosis following local anesthetic-induced convulsions – at least 2–3 ampules given as a single dose, rather than at intervals, are required.

CONCLUSIONS

To conclude:

a. systemic toxic reactions from local anesthetics can be avoided by using proper precautions and technique;

b. when they occur, rapid proper therapy avoids sequelae; and

c. when cardiac arrest, encephalopathy and/or death results, the physician (anesthesiologist, obstetrician) or certified nurse anesthetist administering the regional block is seldom faultless.

When attempting to establish innocence, he/she should remember:

'Oh what a tangled web we weave,
When first we practice to deceive!'

(Sir Walter Scott, *The Lay of the Last Minstrel*, stanza 17).

REFERENCES

1. Moore D C, Bridenbaugh L D, Owen C K, MacDougall M P, Carruthers H C 1953 Lumbar Epidural Block: the anesthetic of choice for cesarean section? A report of one hundred cases. West J Surg Obstet Gynec 61: 459–464
2. Moore D C, Bridenbaugh L D 1955 Is it practical for medical anesthetists to supply a twenty-four hour obstetrical service? West J Surg Obstet Gynec 63: 382–385
3. Moore D C 1955 Teaching residents regional nerve block on private patients for surgical operations. Anesth Analg 34: 193–201
4. Rutherford R N, Moore D C, Dare J, Rose P A 1956 Coordinated obstetric care. Obstet Gynec 8: 581–590
5. Lindstrom C, Moore D C 1957 Trends in obstetrical anesthesia following the acceptance of a twenty-four hour physician anesthesia service. West J Surg Obstet Gynec 65: 63–68
6. Nellermoe C W, Moore D C, Bridenbaugh L D, Casady G N, Braly B 1960 A clinical appraisal of 2-chloroprocaine in continuous caudal obstetrical anesthesia. Anesthesiology 21: 269–272
7. Moore D C, Bridenbaugh L D 1964 Physician anesthesia, regional block and father participation, the ultimate in care of vaginal delivery. West J Surg Obstet Gynec 72: 37–44
8. Hayden G E, Moore D C, Bridenbaugh L D 1964 Maternity care should be family centered. Mod Hosp 102: 104–105
9. Moore D C 1964 Anesthetic techniques for obstetrical anesthesia and analgesia. Charles C Thomas, Springfield, IL
10. Moore D C 1965 Anesthesia for vaginal delivery and cesarean section. In: Greenhill J P (ed) Obstetrics, W B Saunders, Philadelphia, pp 386–427
11. Moore D C 1965 Strictly personal... father participation and the physician anesthesiologist. Anesth Analg 44: 417–418
12. Moore D C 1966 Twenty-four hour coverage of obstetrical delivery by physician anesthetists. Proceedings III, Second European Congress of Anaesthesiologists. Acta Anaesth Scand (suppl) 25: 350–362
13. Moore D C, Bridenbaugh L D, Bagdi P A, Bridenbaugh P O 1968 Accumulation of mepivacaine hydrochloride during caudal block. Anesthesiology 29: 585–588
14. Moore D C, Bridenbaugh L D, Bagdi P A, Bridenbaugh P O, Stander H 1968 The present status of spinal (subarachnoid) and epidural (peridural block): a comparison of the two technics. Anesth Analg 47: 40–49

15. Bridenbaugh L D, Moore D C, Bagdi P, Bridenbaugh P O 1968 The position of plastic tubing in continuous-block techniques: an x-ray study of 552 patients. Anesthesiology 29: 1047–1049
16. Moore D C, Bridenbaugh L D, Bridenbaugh P O 1969 Twenty-four hour coverage of obstetric deliveries by anesthesiologists. Anesth Analg 48: 401–407
17. Moore D C, Bridenbaugh L D, Bridenbaugh P O, Thompson G E 1971 Bupivacaine hydrochloride: a summary of investigational use in 3274 cases. Anesth Analg 50: 856–872
18. Moore D C, Bridenbaugh L D, Bridenbaugh P O, Tucker G T 1971 Caudal and epidural blocks with bupivacaine for childbirth: Report of 657 parturients. Obstet Gynec 37: 657–676
19. Moore D C, Bridenbaugh L D, Thompson G E, Balfour R I, Horton W G 1978 Bupivacaine: a review of 11,080 cases. Anesth Analg 57: 42–53
20. Moore D C 1951 Pontocaine solutions for regional analgesia other than spinal and epidural block, an analysis of 2,500 cases. J Am Med Assoc 146: 803–808
21. Moore D C 1951 The use of hyaluronidase in local and nerve block analgesia other than spinal block: 1520 cases. Anesthesiology 12: 611–626
22. Moore D C, Green J 1956 Systemic toxic reactions to local anesthetics. Calif Med 85: 70–74
23. Moore D C, Bridenbaugh L D 1960 Oxygen: the antidote for systemic toxic reactions from local anesthetic drugs. J Am Med Assoc 174: 842–847
24. Moore D C 1966 Are systemic toxic reactions to all local anesthetic agents the same? Proceedings III, Second European Congress of Anesthesiologists. Acta Anaesth Scand (suppl) 25: 48–53
25. Moore D C, Bridenbaugh L D, Bagdi P A, Bridenbaugh P O, Stander H 1968 The present status of spinal (subarachnoid) and epidural (peridural block): a comparison of the two technics. Anesth Analg 47: 40–49, 1968
26. Moore D C 1969 Complications of regional anesthesia. In: Bonica JJ (ed) Clinical Anesthesia Series, Vol 2, Regional Anesthesia, F A Davis, Philadelphia, pp 218–251
27. Moore D C, Bridenbaugh L D, Bridenbaugh P O, Tucker G T 1970 Bupivacaine: a review of 2,077 cases. J Am Med Assoc 214: 713–718
28. Tucker G T, Boyes R N, Bridenbaugh P O, Moore D C 1970 Binding of anilide-type local anesthetics in human plasma. I. Relationships between binding, physicochemical properties and anesthetic activity. Anesthesiology 33: 287–303
29. Tucker G T, Boyes R N, Bridenbaugh P O, Moore D C 1970 Binding of anilide-type local anesthetics in human plasma II: Implications in vivo with special reference to transplacental passage. Anesthesiology 33: 304–413
30. Moore D C, Mather L E, Bridenbaugh L D, Thompson G E, Balfour R I, Lysons D F, Horton W G 1977 Bupivacaine (Marcaine®): an evaluation of its tissue and systemic toxicity in human. Acta Anaesth Scand 21: 109–121
31. Moore D C, Bridenbaugh L D, Thompson G E, Balfour R I, Horton W G 1977 Factors determining dosages of amide-type local anesthetic drugs. Anesthesiology 47: 263–268
32. Moore D C, Balfour R I, Fitzgibbons D 1979 Convulsive arterial plasma levels on bupivacaine and the response to diazepam therapy. Anesthesiology 50: 454–456
33. Moore D C 1980 Administer oxygen first in the treatment of local anesthetic induced convulsions. Anesthesiology 53: 346–347
34. Moore D C, Crawford R D, Scurlock J E 1980 Severe hypoxia and acidosis following local anesthetic drug-induced convulsions. Anesthesiology 53: 259–260
35. Moore D C 1980 Major complications from regional anesthesia in obstetrics. Excerpta Medica. International Congress Series 538: 940–943
36. Moore D C, Thompson G E, Crawford R D 1982 Long-acting local anesthetic drugs and convulsions with hypoxia and acidosis. Anesthesiology 56: 70–72
37. Moore D C 1981 Local anesthetic drugs: tissue and systemic toxicity. Acta Anaesth Belgium 32: 283–300
38. Moore D C 1983 Systemic toxicity of local anesthetic drugs. In: Katz R L (ed) Sem Anesth, Reg Anesth, 2: 62–74
39. Moore D C, Scurlock J E 1983 The possible role of epinephrine in prevention and correction of local anesthetic induced myocardial depression. Anesth Analg 62: 450–453
40. Batra M S, Bridenbaugh L D, Caldwell D B et al 1984 Bupivacaine cardiotoxicity in a pregnant patient with valve prolapse: an example of improperly administered epidural block (correspondence). Anesthesiology 60: 170–171
41. Moore D G, Bridenbaugh L D 1985 Does hyperkalemia contraindicate the use of bupivacaine or the use of succinylcholine to treat bupivacaine-induced convulsions? Anesthesiology 62: 195–197
42. Moore D C, Bonica J J 1985 Convulsions ventricular tachycardia from bupivacaine with epinephrine: Successful resuscitation – CONGRATULATIONS! (correspondence). Anesth Analg 64: 844–846
43. Moore D C 1986 Toxicity of local anaesthetics in obstetrics. IV. Management. In: Ostheimer G W (ed) Clin Anaesthesiology 4: 113–124
44. Moore D C 1991 If ventricular conduction and rhythm disorders are caused by bupivacaine, it is doubtful that intraoperative hyponatremia and hyperkalemia enhance them. (correspondence) Anesthesiology 74: 383–385
45. Yaksh T L, Collins J G 1989 Studies in animals should precede human use of spinally administered drugs. Anesthesiology 70: 4–5
46. Lasagna L 1974 A plea for the 'naturalistic' study of medicines. Eur J Clin Pharmacol 7: 153–154
47. Scott D B, Lee A, Fagan D, Bowler G M R, Bloomfield P, Lund R 1989 Acute toxicity of ropivacaine compared with that of bupivacaine. Anesth Analg 69: 563–569
48. Moore D C 1980 Administer oxygen first in the treatment of local anesthetic-induced convulsions (correspondence). Anesthesiology 53: 259–260
49. Batson O V 1957 The vertebral vein system. Am Roentgenol 78: 195–211
50. Elstein I D, Marx G F 1990 Electrocardiograph changes during cesarean section under regional anesthesia. Anesth Analg 71: 103
51. Bonica J J 1967 Principles and practice of obstetrical analgesia and anesthesia. F A Davis, Philadelphia, p 304
52. Albright G A, Jouppila R, Hollmen A L et al 1981 Epinephrine does not alter human intervillous blood flow during epidural anesthesia. Anesthesiology 54: 131–135
53. Jouppila R, Jouppila P, Hollmen A, Kuikka J 1978 Effects of segmental extradural analgesia on placental blood flow during normal labor. Br J Anaesth 50: 563–566
54. Jouppila R, Jouppila P, Juikka J, Hollmen A 1978 Placental blood flow during cesarean section under lumbar extradural analgesia. Br J Anaesth 50: 275–278
55. Moore D C, Batra M S 1981 The components of an effective test dose prior to epidural block. Anesthesiology 55: 693–696
56. Moore D C, Batra M S, Morison D H 1982 Further considerations regarding the components of an effective test dose prior to epidural block (correspondence). Anesthesiology 57: 140–141
57. Moore D C, Batra M S, Abouleish E, Bourke D 1984 Concerning the use and abuse of test doses for epidural anesthesia (correspondence). Anesthesiology 61: 345–346
58. Moore D C 1986 Epidural test-doses in obstetrics – let us face facts. Anaesthesia 41: 1152–1165
59. Moore D C, Batra M S, Bridenbaugh L D, Brown D L, Carpenter R L, Hecker B R, Ramsey D 1987 Maternal heart rate changes with a plain epidural test dose – validity of results open to question. Anesthesiology 66: 854
60. Moore D C, Leighton B L, Norris M C, Gross J B 1990 Markers other than epinephrine to avoid intravascular injection of local anesthetics in the obstetrical patient require more study. Anesthesiology 73: 576–578
61. Leighton B L, Norris M C, Sosis M, Epstein R, Chayen B, Larijani G E 1988 Limitations of epinephrine as a marker of intravascular injection in laboring women. Anesthesiology 69: 626–628
62. Cartwright P D, McCarroll S M, Antzaka C 1986 Maternal heart rate changes with a plain epidural test dose. Anesthesiology 65: 226–228
63. Covino B G, Marx G F, Finster M, Zsigmond E K 1980 Prolonged sensory/motor deficits following inadvertent spinal anesthesia. Anesth Analg 59: 399–400

64. Tucker G T, Moore D C, Bridenbaugh P O, Bridenbaugh L D, Thompson G E 1972 Systemic absorption of mepivacaine in commonly used regional block procedures. Anesthesiology 37: 277–287
65. Moore D C, Mather L E, Bridenbaugh P O et al 1976 Arterial and venous plasma levels of bupivacaine following epidural and intercostal nerve blocks. Anesthesiology 45: 39–45
66. Moore D C, Bridenbaugh L D 1956 Laryngospasm: its treatment with succinylcholine. Anesthesiology 17: 212
67. DePace N L, Betesh J S, Kotler M N 1982 'Postmortem' cesarean section with recovery of both mother and offspring. J Am Med Assoc 248: 971–973
68. Marx G 1982 Cardiopulmonary resuscitation of late-pregnant women. Anesthesiology 56: 156
69. Prentiss J E 1979 Cardiac arrest following caudal anesthesia. Anesthesiology 50: 51–53
70. Standards and guidelines for cardiopulmonary resuscitation (CPR) and emergency cardiac care (ECG). J Am Med Assoc 255: 2942

PART C
EPIDURAL ANESTHESIA: TEST DOSE

A. Van Zundert

INTRODUCTION

Anesthesiologists live daily with fail-safe principles, e.g. pin index system; color coding system for medical gases; the fluted oxygen knob and rotameters; agent-specific filling devices for volatile anesthetics; and multiple alarms on the anesthetic machine. No such thing is available in obstetric epidural practice.

Although epidural anesthesia is a very safe technique, complications are always possible. The most important complications during epidural analgesia and anesthesia are unrecognized puncture of an epidural vessel or the dura by the epidural needle or catheter.

1. An unintentional *subdural or subarachnoid injection* of local anesthetics is at best an embarrassment and at worst a life-threatening complication (possibly a high or total spinal block), which, if not recognized immediately, requires prolonged resuscitation. Large volumes of local anesthetic injected in the subarachnoid space will cause not only a total spinal block but even neurologic deficits. The prevalence of unintentional dural puncture varies between 1 and 3%.[1–13]

2. An unintentional *intravascular injection* of local anesthetic (with toxic reaction) is possible in the gravid parturient near term, in which the epidural veins are markedly dilated making entry even more likely. Unintentional perforation of an epidural vein by the needle or the catheter has a prevalence exceeding 2% and even up to 11%.[1,14–29] Accidental rapid i.v. injection of a large amount of local anesthetic will result in a grand mal convulsion[25,28] and possibly cardiovascular collapse.[15,23,24] Maternal deaths have been reported following unintentional i.v. injection during epidural anesthesia.[30–32]

3. To complicate matters further, epidural catheters that have been functioning normally at a previous injection *may migrate* into epidural veins or into the subarachnoid space.[33–40] There can be a considerable movement of the skin and soft tissues over the lumbar spine with change of position in a patient, especially in obese patients.[39] In a recent study, Bishton et al[33] found that inward or outward migration occurred in 36% of patients, even after carefully securing the epidural catheter to the back. Hazards of migration include unintentional intravenous[36,40] or subarachnoid injection[35,37] and unilateral or failed block. Therefore, as one of the safeguards against unintentional subarachnoid or intravenous injection, a test dose in recommended when initiating an epidural anesthetic. However, few topics in anesthesia have created as much controversy as have test doses for epidural anesthesia.

Numerous reports have suggested the composition and volume of test doses and numerous authors question the validity of the studies.

An epidural test dose was first recommended by Dogliotti in 1933.[41] To avoid the complication of a high spinal block, he suggested injecting a smal volume of local anesthetic through the needle in the epidural space to insure that a subarachnoid placement had not occurred prior to injecting the full epidural dose.

WHAT ARE THE COMPONENTS OF A GOOD TEST DOSE?

A good test dose in epidural analgesia and anesthesia should produce clinical evidence within a few minutes that the needle or the catheter is located either in a blood vessel or in the subarachnoid space. A test dose should be safe for mother and fetus; be easy to use; rapidly produce signs of an unintentional i.v. or subarachnoid injection and be highly specific and sensitive. False-positive and false-negative results should not occur as false-negative tests are dangerous and false positives are a considerable nuisance, as the procedure has to be repeated when, in fact, there is no incorrect placement. All test doses have limitations. Despite this, a test dose is mandatory. What kind of chemical markers have been used as a test dose? Suggestions have been made in the past to inject a *dye* that can be detected by a pulse oximeter.[42] However pulse oximetry measurements of SaO_2 may be altered by fluorescein, indocyanine green and methylene blue.[43] The last can be neurotoxic.

The intravenous injection of small volumes of *air* (1–2 ml) via a peripheral vein or via an intravenously located epidural catheter produces unmistakeable changes in Doppler heart tones.[44–46] The risk of paradoxic air embolization in patients with probe-patient foramina ovale is usually not significant in adults. Subarachnoid injection of small volumes of air is known to be safe (e.g. pneumoencephalography uses 20–30 ml of air). The Doppler test has a 2% false-positive (specificity of 98%) and no false negatives.[46] This test, however, only evaluates intravenous position, requires extra equipment and one can easily misjudge the exact location to place the Doppler probe.

An alternative that was widely practiced until 1980 is the use of a subconvulsant dose of plain local anesthetic. 100 mg of 2% or 3% chloroprocaine,[47,48] 100 mg of lidocaine,[49,50] and 25 mg of bupivacaine[43,51,52] are claimed to be good test doses for the location of epidural catheters. They should produce clinically mild systemic toxic effects if injected intravenously and an unequivocal spinal sensory block if injected in the subarachnoid space.

However, the drawbacks are many. These tests rely upon subjective symptoms, e.g. auditory changes (tinnitus, increased intensity of sound), fullness in the head, lightheadedness, warmth, numbness of the tongue or the nasopharynx, fullness in the throat, metallic taste in the mouth, thickness of the tongue, slurring of the speech, heart pounding and a variety of other sensations, which may not always be evident in a patient. The amount of the local anesthetic, however, is too much for a test dose, i.e. it may well be that the dose necessary to detect in i.v. injection may be more than the dose necessary to detect a subarachnoid injection. 3 ml of 2% chloroprocaine is not sufficient to detect i.v. placement[48] and 3 ml of 3% chloroprocaine may produce a total spinal block. If less drug is used, it may well give a false sense of safety, while, in fact, it is not a correct test dose.[48,49] It is clear that great care must be taken to avoid diagnostic error. Additionally, *chloroprocaine* may interfere with the subsequent analgesic efficacy of epidurally administered opioids.[53–56]

Nor is plain *bupivacaine* the ideal choice as a test dose. Its latent period is long,[57] it is hypobaric at body temperature and high or total spinal blocks and cardiac arrests have followed modest test doses.[30,58] Bupivacaine is more cardiotoxic than lidocaine, and this toxicity is aggravated by pregnancy.[59–61] Furthermore, up to 10 ml of 0.75% bupivacaine (75 mg) has been injected intravenously in a pregnant patient without apparent ill-effect, yet on other occasions smaller doses have had potentially fatal neurologic or cardiovascular results.[48] Subconvulsant doses of bupivacaine may produce severe ventricular arrhythmias and circulatory collapse, even in the absence of hypoxia, acidemia or hyperkalemia.[30,59,62] Resuscitation can be difficult with the need for cardiac massage for 45 min or longer.[30] Cardiac deaths have resulted from single-dose injection of 60–75 mg of 0.25%, 0.5% and 0.75% bupivacaine, indicating that dose is more important than the concentration used.[32]

Cartwright et al[63] studied in 100 healthy parturients the effect of 3 ml of 0.5% plain bupivacaine given via an epidural catheter. The maximum heart rate increased by more than 30 bpm in 12 women, which would mean that 12% of the catheters would have been removed unnecessarily (false-positive test). None of the catheters were, in fact, intravascular.

Lidocaine (100 mg) given intravenously produced symptoms with 100% sensitivity and 95% specificity in 20 healthy male volunteers.[50] In contrast to chloroprocaine it does not interfere with the efficacy of subsequent epidurally administered drugs. However, this study was not repeated in pregnant patients. 2 ml of 5% lidocaine may produce a high incidence of unacceptably high motor blocks causing respiratory difficulty in the obstetric patient.[64]

However, one should not rely on a test dose containing plain local anesthetic because the diagnosis of unintentional i.v. injection is based predominantly on the patient's subjective complaints due to CNS symptoms produced by a subconvulsant dose. Most of the time, plasma concentrations of 2 µg/ml lidocaine do not produce signs or symptoms of CNS intoxication. With the short-acting local anesthetic, lidocaine, a large difference exists between the dose needed to obtain cardiovascular depression and the dose needed to produce CNS depression. With the longer acting local anesthetic, bupivacaine, the ratio of the dose resulting in cardiovascular collapse to the convulsive dose (CC/CNS ratio) is much lower than with lidocaine. The margin of safety with regard to cardiac toxicity is less for the longer acting local anesthetics such as bupivacaine owing to a greater myocardial uptake and is further reduced in pregnancy owing to greater myocardial sensitivity.[61]

It is clear that subjective signs are unreliable. In a search for more objective signs and symptoms, *chronotropic drugs* have been used as a test dose: isoproterenol, dopamine, terbutaline, ephedrine, atropine and epinephrine.

Isoproterenol

Isoproterenol as well as dopamine and terbutaline can be used as an i.v. test dose. Baker et al[65] demonstrated that only isoproterenol 5 µg offers distinct advantages as one component of a safe and reliable test dose in obstetrics. It increases the maternal heart rate by 30%, while the uterine blood flow remains the same. However, careful monitoring is necessary.[66] A significant increase in maternal heart rate is produced, but the complicated 'peak-to-peak' analysis of heart rate is required to detect the change reliably. All chronotropic test doses suffer from two fundamental problems: poor signal-to-noise ratio and wide variation in the chronotropic responsiveness of pregnant women to beta-adrenergic agonists. Pregnant patients have a decreased sensitivity to the chronotropic effects of beta-adrenergic agonists.[67] In actively laboring women, maternal heart rate variability exceeds 20 bpm in 24–90% of patients and exceeds 30 bpm in 12–45% of patients.[66,68] Determination of a dose of a chronotropic drug that is sufficient but not excessive in all parturients may be problematic. Preeclamptic parturients are five times as sensitive to the chronotropic effect of isoproterenol as healthy pregnant women.[69] Because we lack a variety of premixed solutions, we have to make serial dilutions, with the possibility of errors. The safe use of these drugs in the subarachnoid space has yet to be defined.[70] We do not know if the efficacy of isoproterenol as an intravascular marker changes when it is combined with local anesthetic. The effect of isoproterenol on the quality and duration of concurrently and subsequently administered local anesthetic is unknown.

Larger doses of a beta-adrenergic agonist might produce a more easily detected tachycardia, but 5 µg of isoproterenol can cause a very pronounced tachycardia in some parturients.

Ephedrine

Some have suggested using the vasopressor of choice in parturients, ephedrine sulfate 15 mg,[71,72] which gives a clear indication of an intravascular injection, but again requires the complicated 'peak-to-peak' methodology for analysis of systolic blood pressure changes. Ephedrine may spare uterine perfusion during pregnancy due to a more selective constriction of systemic vessels.[73] However, because too many incorrect predictions were seen and in some patients a transient fetal tachycardia >160 bpm developed, this technique is considered unreliable.[71,72]

Epinephrine

The only vasoconstrictor commonly added to local anesthetics for obstetrics is epinephrine. In 1981 Moore and Batra[74] described the objective cardiovascular effects of 15 µg of epinephrine when injected intravascularly in normal surgical patients after its i.v. administration. The pulse rate rises unmistakeably, with the initial rise occurring at 20 s and the heart rate returning towards normal by 60 s. Monitoring of the heart rate is necessary for this technique. Subjective signs are considered as unreliable.

All kinds of combinations of local anesthetics and epinephrine have proved to be useful in the detection of a transient increase in maternal heart rate within the first minute following the administration of the test dose in both pregnant and non-pregnant patients provided adequate monitoring is applied.[52,74,76–80]

Van Zundert et al[81] found that a test dose consisting of 12.5 mg of bupivacaine plus 12.5 µg of epinephrine in 10 ml of physiologic saline, injected in a peripheral arm vein over 30 s in parturients gives a predictable and easily detectable increase in heart rate and arterial blood pressure, provided that the patient is adequately monitored.[80] This test dose even proved to be effective in detecting unintentional i.v. location of an epidural catheter in the clinical setting of a pregnant patient undergoing epidural anesthesia.[38]

This test dose is prepared by diluting 2.5 ml of bupivacaine 0.5% plus epinephrine 1 : 200 000 with 7.5 ml of sterile physiologic saline, thus producing 10 ml of bupivacaine 0.125% plus epinephrine 1 : 800 000. This test dose contains 12.5 mg of bupivacaine and 12.5 µg of epinephrine. If 10 ml of this test dose is injected intravenously in nonobstetric patients a clear but short-lived increase in heart rate and blood pressure is observed shortly after the start of the i.v. injection (40 ± 17 s) together with symptoms such as palpitations, facial pallor, headache and changes in taste and tinnitus, although these symptoms are not uniformly seen in all patients. Omitting the epinephrine and giving the plain local anesthetic (12.5 mg of bupivacaine) does not cause any signs or symptoms. When the test dose is injected into the subarachnoid space no increase in heart rate and blood pressure is seen, but the resultant subarachnoid block is sufficient to provide surgical anesthesia.[82]

When the test dose is given intravenously in obstetric patients, an increase in maternal heart rate and blood pressure is observed.[81] Graphically recording while injecting the test dose intravenously shows a short-lived but unmistakeable peak in the maternal heart rate.[80,81] As the components of subsequent doses for epidural anesthesia in vaginal delivery are the same as this test dose, every dose given to produce epidural anesthesia for vaginal delivery can be a test dose at the same time. This makes the test dose reliable, safe, and effective for obstetric practice.

The above-mentioned studies demonstrated that the components of an effective test dose (10–15 μg of bupivacaine and 10–15 μg of epinephrine) as described by Moore and Batra[74] in surgical patients are also effective in parturients.

Monitoring

However, when using a test dose containing epinephrine, monitoring is essential in order to detect unintentional intravascular injection during epidural anesthesia. Following the maternal heart rate by radial artery palpation is the easiest, but also the least reliable, method. The use of a (portable) electrocardioscope or a (cheaper) pulse meter attached on the patient's earlobe is also possible, but requires extra equipment. A fetal monitor, such as a cardiotocograph, is readily available in an obstetric suite. Abouleish and Johnson[83] described the use of the Doppler component of a fetal monitor (model 8040A, HP). Monitoring maternal heart rate (MHR) using the direct ECG mode of a model 8040A fetal monitor was suggested by Chestnut and Weiner[85] and was modified by Van Zundert et al.[89] It is this recording of the beat-to-beat MHR that allows us to identify the rapidly developing peak in MHR following the i.v. test dose. If a clear peak is observed within 1 min after injection of the test dose, and if this is accompanied by an increase in arterial blood pressure and a temporary decrease in uterine contraction intensity or contraction frequency, the anesthesiologist should be alerted. This peak is almost always easily identified, even in the presence of a highly variable MHR. If a peak in MHR is suspected but not really clearly visible, the test dose should be repeated. Rigid criteria, such as an increase in MHR of 30 bpm should *not* be applied, since this would make the use of a test dose based on changes in MHR impossible in patients having a variable heart rate, which is frequently seen in parturients.[79]

Although the literature is quite extensive about its use, epinephrine is not uniformly used as the test dose in obstetrics.[85]

There are many drawbacks to the use of epinephrine as an intravenous marker in obstetric patients:

1. epinephrine may decrease uterine blood flow (especially dangerous in case of fetal compromise);
2. epinephrine may inhibit uterine contractions;
3. no increase in MHR in response to epinephrine in patients taking beta-blocking agents;
4. lack of sensitivity/specificity.

Uterine blood flow. There are concerns about the safety of using epinephrine as a marker of i.v. injection because it decreases uterine blood flow by 3–45% for 1–5 min in pregnant sheep (10–20 μg of epinephrine) and guinea pigs (0.2 μg/kg).[86–89] However, total uterine blood flow was measured, therefore no distinction was made between myometrial and placental blood flow. Furthermore, species difference might be present, since all animals had bradycardia after i.v. epinephrine, in contrast to the tachycardia seen in humans. The authors themselves stated that the degree of uterine blood flow decrease resembles the decrease that occurs during a normal uterine contraction.[87] They also found no evidence of fetal compromise.

Wallis et al[88] reported a 14% decrease in uterine blood flow in normotensive pregnant sheep with 2-chloroprocaine and 60–80 μg of epinephrine. 45–55 μg of epinephrine added to bupivacaine given epidurally for cesarean delivery reduced the total uteroplacental blood flow, although no effect was seen on the fetus.[89] However, doses of epinephrine up to 100 μg demonstrated no significant decrease in human intervillous blood flow.[90–92] Recently Alahuhta et al[93] assessing the effects of an epidural anesthesia using bupivacaine with epinephrine 90–100 μg for cesarean delivery and measuring blood flow velocity waveforms in uteroplacental and fetal vessels demonstrated no adverse effects on vascular resistance in the uteroplacental and fetal circulation or on fetal myocardial function. Their data confirm the finding of most previous investigators that epinephrine added to the local anesthetic used in obstetric epidural anesthesia is not associated with deleterious effects on human maternal, placental and fetal circulatory parameters.[94–97] Also Abboud et al[98,99] concluded that the addition of epinephrine has no adverse effects on mother, fetus, neonate, uterine activity and the progress of labor. Leighton et al[67] demonstrated signs of transient tachycardia followed by hypertension and bradycardia and transient fetal distress in 2 out of 10 women injected with 15 μg of epinephrine intravenously. Both babies were normal at birth. Despite these concerns there has been no published report of adverse neonatal or adult outcome after intravascular injection of an epinephrine-containing test dose in humans.

Preeclampsia. However, these transient changes that have been observed might be significant in patients with compromised placental function. It has been suggested that local anesthetic solutions containing epinephrine should be avoided when performing epidural anesthesia for preeclamptic patients because hypertensive patients may be more sensitive to epinephrine administration than normal parturients and there is the possibility of adverse effects on uterine activity and blood flow.

Heller et al[100] described four cases in which epinephrine-containing solutions were used without any deterioration in the condition of the parturient or the fetus. In no case was hypertension observed. If there is a reduction in umbilical flow, it seems not to matter, implying a significant margin of safety in uterine and intervillous blood flow, and there is no reason to believe that preeclamptic parturients will not respond with vasodilation as well.[101] Dror et al[102] also was in agreement with Heller that epinephrine has no adverse effects on the mother or the neonate. Intravenously administered epinephrine can cause a dose related reduction in uterine blood flow without adversely affecting the normal fetus. Hypertension did not occur.[103]

Fetal stress and acidosis. In a study in near-term ewes, Youngstrom et al[104,105] found that intentional maternal i.v. injection of 16.5 μg of epinephrine significantly though briefly, reduced the uterine blood flow without affecting the FHR, mean arterial pressure (MAP) or arterial blood gases of nonacidotic fetal sheep. Under conditions of acute fetal compromise and acidosis (e.g. umbilical cord occlusion and partial placental infarction) inclusion of epinephrine in the epidural test dose did not significantly affect FHR, MAP or blood gases if intentionally injected intravenously. Their results did not support a relationship between small elevations in maternal epinephrine concentrations and deterioration in either the unstressed fetus or the fetus subjected to induced stress. Adding a small dose of epinephrine (5–20 μg) to the test dose to detect an unintentional i.v. injection is justified to prevent a possible catastrophe, especially in the presence of complicated labors, until another reliable and, possibly, safer marker of i.v. injection is developed.

Epinephrine in pediatrics

Unlike adults, children are frequently anesthetized (including atropine premedication) before an epidural anesthetic is initiated. In a randomized, double-blind study 65 children were given 1% halothane with nitrous oxide–oxygen(50 : 50). They received 0.1 mg/kg 1% lidocaine with or without 0.5 μg/kg epinephrine via the epidural route. Half of the children were given prior treatment with atropine 10 μg/kg i.v. The heart rate increased by less than 10 bpm in 28% of the children who received epinephrine without prior atropine and only in 5% if atropine was given.[106,107] An unintentional intravascular injection of an epidural test dose of local anesthetic containing 0.5 μg/kg epinephrine will not reliably produce tachycardia unless preceded by atropine (10 μg/kg).[107] Atropine injected i.v. prior to the test dose does not conceal the effects of the test dose and may actually improve its sensitivity.[108]

Beta-blockers

A pulse rate increase cannot be expected in response to an epinephrine-containing test dose in the presence of a moderate beta-blockade in healthy young patients. In fact, hypertension with an associated decrease in heart rate may be expected. In the normal unblocked healthy subject, tachycardia is transient (60 – 80 s) and hypertension sustained (2 min). With moderate beta-blockade, the test dose produces transient 30% hypertension (1.5 min) and a sustained bradycardia (2 min). This response is likely to be due to unopposed alpha-adrenergic stimulation and baroreceptor response to the resultant rise in blood pressure.[109] This was found in healthy volunteers,[109,110] in patients[111] as in parturients.[112] In the presence of beta-blockade the only reliable indicator of intravascular injection may be the systolic blood pressure.

Sensitivity/specificity of a test dose

Drugs such as the beta-agonists used to treat tocolysis or hydralazine used for blood pressure control and to treat fever and anxiety may result in maternal tachycardia in excess of 120 bpm, which can mask the transient tachycardia produced by a 15-μg i.v. dose of epinephrine. MHR increase during active labor and during the placement of an epidural in an apprehensive patient frequently and transiently exceeds 30 bpm.[63]

A false-negative i.v. test dose is potentially dangerous as it may give the anesthesiologist the impression that the epidural catheter is not placed in a vein. False-negative tests for i.v. placement may result from a test dose that is too low. False-negative tests for subarachnoid placement may occur as a result of an inadequate dose being used, an insufficient time being allowed for a spinal anesthetic to develop or inadequate testing for a spinal anesthetic. For example, injecting 2 ml of 0.25% bupivacaine or 1% lidocaine, waiting for 3 min and then asking the patient to move the feet or toes will give a negative result more often than a positive one if the drug has indeed been injected into the subarachnoid space.[76,113]

False-positive i.v. tests are a considerable nuisance, as the catheter is removed unnecessarily and the procedure repeated when, in fact, there is no incorrect placement.[63] Cartwright found 12% false-positive test doses, but he injected at a very fast speed (1 ml/s), whereby the jet stream exiting the catheter may cause nerve root irritation, resulting in discomfort and an elevated heart rate. Chestnut[88] reported that half of his patients in labor had spontaneous increases of heart rate of more than 25 bpm during a 15-min observation period before and after injection of a test dose.

Guinard et al[110] reported that the responsiveness to an epinephrine test dose appeared to decline with increasing age. In an earlier study, Guinard et al[42] determined the sensitivity of an epinephrine-containing epidural test dose, as well as its lowest effective dose, in healthy nonpregnant volunteers. They concluded that 10 μg of epinephrine is the lowest effective dose and that the agent is 100% sensitive in detecting intravascular injection. Colonna-Romano et al[114] confirmed the same results in laboring women: epinephrine 10–15 μg is 100% sensitive as a marker of intravenous injection, although 27–45% of epidural catheters may be unnecessarily removed in the presence of a positive test.

Gieraerts et al[115] performed a double-blind study in order to determine the specificity and sensitivity in obstetric patients undergoing lumbar epidural anesthesia (LEA). 40 obstetric patients were randomly divided into four groups and either given 10 ml of saline or 10 ml of TD (test dose) i.v. before inserting the epidural catheter or given 10 ml of saline or 10 ml of TD i.v. after the insertion of the epidural catheter. The investigator was blinded to the solution he injected. After the test dose was given, the investigator assessed whether or not he had administered normal saline or the test solution containing 12.5 μg of epinephrine. The judgments of eight other anesthesiologists resulted in an excellent specificity (99.1%) and a good sensitivity (91.9%). When only the recording of maternal heart rate was given to the anesthesiologists, the pattern of tachycardia (with a rapid rising peak, followed by a more gradual decrease to the baseline) did not always allow them to identify the solution that was administered. Information related to whether or not LEA was present did not improve the sensitivity. Knowledge about the time of injection and symptoms increased the specificity from 94.4% to more than 99%, and increased the sensitivity to 91.9% as judged by nine anesthesiologists. These results are more favorable than the results of Tom.[116]

The safety of *subarachnoid* injections of local anesthetics containing vasoconstrictors is a subject of immense clinical importance. Doses up to 200 μg used by Kozody et al[117] suggest that although dural vasoconstriction occurs there is no reduction in blood flow to the spinal cord.

A test dose, even when it contains epinephrine, has its limitations, but still may be very useful, if one considers all factors: pattern of tachycardia, increase in blood pressure, signs and symptoms of the patient and slowing of uterine contractions.

The above-proposed test dose (10 ml of bupivacaine 0.125% plus epinephrine 1 : 800 000) produces an increase in MHR that can be clearly demonstrated, provided that the patient is adequately monitored, without any untoward effect. The effects of the subarachnoid administration of the test dose were also examined in nonobstetric patients undergoing urologic surgery, in whom it caused a clearly detectable spinal anesthetic without causing significant hypotension or an excessively high dermatomal level (T7).[118] However, testing for subarachnoid migration may be difficult if one is reinjecting in a patient who already has established a high dense epidural block of the kind required for cesarean delivery.

In the obstetric population this test dose might lead to a higher level of anesthesia. In 20 patients undergoing cesarean delivery, the effectiveness and safety of the subarachnoid block using the same test dose was also evaluated.[82] A clearly detectable spinal anesthetic level and motor block were present within a few minutes, without causing an unacceptable high level of anesthesia or hemodynamic decompensation. Anesthesia was excellent in all women while hypotension was never a serious problem. Therefore, this test dose, containing 12.5 mg of bupivacaine plus 12.5 μg of epinephrine is a safe and reliable test dose to detect unintentional i.v. and subarachnoid injections, even in the obstetric population. Additionally, this test dose can be used as therapeutic dose in epidural analgesia for pain relief during vaginal delivery, and in spinal anesthesia for cesarean delivery.

CONCLUSIONS

Use a test dose containing epinephrine. The above-proposed test dose containing 12.5 mg of bupivacaine plus 12.5 μg of epinephrine can be considered as an effective and safe test dose, which can be used as the first dose and the top-up dose. In this way, every dose given in epidural analgesia for vaginal delivery can be a test dose at the same time. To this solution 10 μg of sufentanil can be added in order to improve the quality of the block.

In clinical obstetric practice using epidural analgesia/anesthesia it is advisable not to adhere to a rigid criterion and evaluate only the maternal heart rate. Both maternal heart rate and maternal blood pressure should be monitored. In the event of an equivocal response, the test dose should be repeated (e.g. when a uterine contraction begins soon after the injection of the test dose so that the increase in heart rate cannot be properly evaluated).

Test doses should be given for epidural anesthesia on the understanding that they are neither 100% sensitive nor 100% specific in preventing complications. Do not expect them to be foolproof. To date, there is no single measure that detects absolutely the two main complications of epidural anesthesia. It is even more complicated when continuous-infusion pumps are used. The test dose is not conclusive when combined spinal–epidural anesthesia techniques are used and when the subarachnoid block is administered first.

The test dose may partly reassure us that we are proceeding cautiously and trying to eliminate even rare complications. The test dose may help the trained observer to detect subarachnoid or i.v. injection but should never be considered to replace careful observation during the conduct of epidural anesthesia. It is only one more step that may help us to administer safe epidural anesthesia in obstetrics.

We have to take several precautions. Only one of them is the use of the test dose. Here are some suggestions and recommended safety procedures:

1. Always have resuscitation equipment and drugs at hand and an i.v. infusion in place before initiating the anesthetic.
2. Monitor the patient adequately: fetal heart rate, maternal heart rate and blood pressure, and uterine contractions.
3. Insert the needle (in the midline) and aspirate for blood or CSF, before and after placing the catheter.
4. Lower the epidural catheter below the operating table. Gravity may help blood to enter the epidural catheter when a vein is penetrated.
5. Perform a physical test by gentle aspiration of the catheter for blood or CSF. Before aspiration, remove the bacterial filter, if one is used. Aspiration before injecting is recommended, but this test is not very reliable as false-negative results may occur due to the viscosity of blood, blockage by air or tissue or tenting of the meninges against the catheter opening.
6. Check the epidural drug yourself. It is also a good idea to color code any connection sites and identify the tubing in order to prevent unintentional addition of medication into the epidural line.
7. Use a pharmacologic test dose containing 12.5 mg of bupivacaine and 12.5 μg of epinephrine; wait for several minutes while carefully observing the patient. Talk to the patient to detect subjective signs and symptoms.
8. Fractionate the larger dose of local anesthetic in 3–5 ml aliquots and inject slowly.
9. Allow sufficient time to elapse between the incremental doses.
10. Each subsequent dose should be preceded by a test dose because i.v. or subarachnoid migration is always possible.

There is no substitute for close observation of the patient by someone who is trained to detect adverse effects. The anesthesiologist should always be highly suspicious that, in spite of a negative result, misplacement can still be present. The test dose may help the trained observer to detect subarachnoid or intravascular injections but should never be considered to replace careful observation during the conduct of epidural analgesia/anesthesia. If one is still uncertain about the position of the epidural needle or catheter after close observation of MHR and arterial blood pressure, the test dose should be repeated.

Safety should come first in obstetric epidural anesthesia! The price of safety is eternal vigilance, and all these precautions are just step-by-step factors that are all important in performing epidural anesthesia to the benefit of both mother and fetus.

REFERENCES

1. Blomberg R G, Löfström J B 1991 The test dose in regional anesthesia. Acta Anaesthesiol Scand 35: 465–568
2. Brownridge p 1982 A three-year survey of an obstetric epidural service with top-up doses administered by midwives. Anaesth Intensive Care 10: 298–308
3. Colonna-Romano P, Shapiro B E 1989 Unintentional dural puncture and prophylactic epidural blood patch in obstetrics. Anesth Analg 69: 522–523
4. Keh-Wong E, Lubenow T, Froehlich J A, Kristof K, Ivankovich O, Ivankovich A D 1987 Subdural block following epidural injection of low-dose bupivacaine. Anesth Analg 66: S95
5. Leach A, Smith G B 1988 Subarachnoid spread of epidural local anaesthetic following dural puncture. Anaesthesia 43: 671–674
6. Lubenow T, Keh-Wong E, Kristof K, Ivankovich O, Ivankovich A D 1988 Inadvertent subdural injection: a complication of an epidural block. Anesth Analg 67: 175–179
7. McLean B, Rottman R L, Kotelko D M 1992 Failure of multiple test doses and techniques to deter intravascular migration of an epidural catheter. Anesth Analg 74: 454–456
8. Morgan B 1990 Unexpectedly extensive conduction blocks in obstetric epidural analgesia. Anaesthesia 45: 148–152
9. Norris M C, Leighton B L 1990 Continuous spinal anesthesia after unintentional dural puncture in parturients. Reg Anesth 15: 285–187
10. Okell R W, Sprigge J S 1987 Unintentional dural puncture. A survey of recognition and management. Anaesthesia 42: 1110–1113
11. Reynolds F, Speedly H M 1990 The subdural space: the third place to go astray. Anesthesia 45: 120–123
12. Russell I F 1985 Inadvertent total spinal anesthesia for cesarean section. Anaesthesia 40: 199–200
13. Stevens R A, D'Arcy Stanton-Hicks M 1985 Subdural injection of local anesthetic: A complication of epidural anesthesia. Anesthesiology 63: 323–326
14. Ahn N N, Ung D A, DeFay S, Cannelli G, Rudy T E, McKenzie R 1989 Blood vessel puncture with epidural catheters. Anesthesiology 71: A916
15. Beck H, Brassow F, Doehn M, Dziadzka A, Schulte am Esch J 1986 Epidural catheters of the multi-orifice type: dangers and complications. Acta Anesthesiol Scand 30: 549–555
16. Coventry D M 1989 Plasma bupivacaine concentrations after inadvertent intravenous injection. Anesthesia 44: 162–163
17. Crawford J S 1985 Some maternal complications of epidural analgesia. Anaesthesia 40: 1219–1225
18. Halpern S, Onayemi A, Swartz J, Rosaeg O 1987 Does an epidural test dose prevent complications of epidural catheter insertion? Anesth Analg 66: S77
19. Kasten G W, Martin S T 1984 Successful resuscitation after massive intravenous bupivacaine overdose in the hypoxic dog. Anesthesiology 61: A206
20. Lavies N G 1987 Speed of epidural injection. Anaesthesia 42: 783–784
21. McNeil M J, Thornburn J 1988 Cannulation of the epidural space. A comparison of 18- and 16-gauge needles. Anaesthesia 43: 154–155
22. Phillips D C, McDonnald R 1987 Epidural catheter migration during labour. Anaesthesia 42: 661–663
23. Prince G, McGregor D G 1986 Epidural test dose in obstetrics. Anaesthesia 41: 654–655
24. Prince G, McGregor 1986 Obstetric epidural test doses. A reappraisal. Anaesthesia 41: 1240–1250
25. Ryan D W 1973 Accidental intravenous injection of bupivacaine: a complication of obstetrical epidural anesthesia. Br J Anaesth 45: 907–908

26. Seeling W, Heinrich H 1984 Versehentlich intravasale Lage eines Periduralkatheters. Regional-Anesthesie 71: 137–139
27. Seidman S F, Marx G F 1988 Epinephrine test dose is not warranted for confirmation of intravascular migration of epidural catheter in a parturient. Can J Anaesth 35: 104–106
28. Tahir A H, Adriani J, Naraghi M 1975 Acute systemic toxicity from bupivacaine during epidural anesthesia in obstetric patients. Southern Med J 68: 1377–1380
29. Verniquet A J W 1980 Vessel puncture with epidural catheters. Anaesthesia 35: 660–662
30. Albright G A 1979 Cardiac arrest following regional anesthesia with etidocaine or bupivacaine. Anesthesiology 51: 285–287
31. Rosen M A 1986 Bupivacaine toxicity. Western J Med 144: 598–599
32. Marx G F 1986 Bupivacaine cardiotoxicity – concentration or dose. Anesthesiology 65: 116
33. Bishton I M, Martin P H, Vernon J M, Liu W H D 1992 Factors influencing epidural catheter migration. Anaesthesia 47: 610–612
34. Kenepp N B, Gutsche B B 1981 Inadvertent intravascular injections during lumbar epidural anesthesia. Anesthesiology 54: 172–173
35. Phillip J H, Brown W V 1976 Total spinal anesthesia late in the course of obstetric bupivacaine epidural block. Anesthesiology 44: 340–341
36. Ravindran R, Albrecht W, McKay M 1979 Apparent intravascular migration of epidural catheter. Anesth Analg 58: 252–253
37. Robson J A, Brodsky J B 1977 Latent dural puncture after lumbar epidural block. Anesth Analg 56: 725–726
38. Van Zundert A, Vaes L, Soetens M, De Wolf A 1988 Indentification of inadvertent placement of an epidural catheter in obstetric anesthesia. Anesthesiology 68: 142–145
39. Webster S G 1986 Migration of epidural catheters. Anaesthesia 41: 654
40. Zebrowski M E, Gutsche B B 1979 More on intravascular migration of an epidural catheter. Anesth Analg 58: 531
41. Dogliotti A M 1933 Segmental peridural spinal anesthesia. Am Surg 20: 107–118
42. Guinard J-P, Mulroy M F, Carpenter R L, Knopes K D 1990 Test doses: optimal epinephrine content with and without acute beta-adrenergic blockade. Anesthesiology 73: 386–392
43. Sidi A, Rush W R, Paulus D A, Gravenstein N, Davis R F 1986 Effect of fluorescein, indocyanine green, and methylene blue on the measurement by pulse oximetry. Anesthesiology 65: A1321
44. Leighton B L, Gross J B 1989 Air. An effective indicator of intravenously located epidural catheters. Anesthesiology 71: 848–851
45. Leighton B L, Norris M C, DeSimone C A, Rosko T, Gross J B 1990 The air test as a clinically useful indicator of intravenously placed epidural catheters. Anesthesiology 73: 610–613
46. Sleigh J W, Saddler J M 1986 Air embolus and epidural anesthesia. Anaesthesia 41: 878
47. Grice S C, Eisenach J C, Dewan D M, Mandell G 1987 Evaluation of 2-chloroprocaine as an effective intravenous test dose for epidural analgesia. Anesthesiology 67: A627
48. Harrington B E, Neal J M, Mackey D C, Mulroy M F 1988 2-Chloroprocaine and bupivacaine as indicators of intravascular injection. Anesthesiology 69: A357
49. Casey W F 1985 Epidural test doses in obstetrics. Anaesthesia 40: 226–228
50. Roetman K J, Eisenach J C 1988 Evaluation of lidocaine as an intravenous test dose for epidural anesthesia. Anesthesiology 69: A669
51. Fargas-Babjak A, McChesney J, Morison D H 1980 The efficacy of bupivacaine 0.75% as an epidural test dose. Can Anaesth Soc J 27: 500–501
52. Abouleish E, Bourke D 1984 Concerning the use and abuse of test doses for epidural anesthesia. Anesthesiology 61: 344–345
53. Malinow A M, Mokriski B L K, Wahlfield M L 1988 Anesthetic choice affects postcesarean epidural fentanyl analgesia. Anesth Analg 67: S138
54. Kotelko D M, Thigpen J W, Shnider S M, Foutz S E, Rosen M A, Hughes S C 1983 Postoperative epidural morphine analgesia after various local anesthetics. Anesthesiology 59: A413
55. Naulty J S, Hertwig L, Hunt C O, Hartwell B, Datta S, Ostheimer G W, Covino B G 1986 Duration of analgesia of epidural fentanyl following cesarean delivery – effects of local anesthetic drug selection. Anesthesiology 65: A180
56. Schlairet T J, Eisenach J C, Dobson C E 1989 Effect of catheter testing with 2-chloroprocaine on the duration of epidural morphine analgesia following cesarean section. Anesthesiology 71: A917
57. Prince G D, Shetty G R, Miles M 1989 Safety and efficacy of a low volume extradural test dose of bupivacaine in labour. Br J Anaesth 62: 503–508
58. Fine P G, Wong K C 1984 Cranial nerve block after test dose through an epidural catheter in a pre-eclamptic parturient. Can Anaesth Soc J 31: 565–567
59. Marx G F 1984 Cardiotoxicity of local anesthetics – the plot thickens. Anesthesiology 60: 3–5
60. Tanz R D, Heskett T, Loehning R W, Fairfax C A 1984 Comparative cardiotoxicity of bupivacaine and lidocaine in the isolated perfused mammalian heart. Anesth Analg 63: 549–556
61. Morishima H O, Pedersen H, Finster M et al 1985 Bupivacaine toxicity in pregnant and nonpregnant ewes. Anesthesiology 63: 134–139
62. Baker W, Eisler E A, Shnider S M, Halpern S H, Levinson G, Dailey P A, Hughes S C 1985 The lethal dose of intravenous bupivacaine in pregnant and nonpregnant rabbits. Anesthesiology 63: A447
63. Cartwright P D, McCarroll S M, Antzaka C 1986 Maternal heart rate changes with a plain epidural test dose. Anesthesiology 65: 226–228
64. Denisson B 1986 Test dose for epidurals. Anaesthesia 41: 964–965
65. Baker B W, Longmire S, Jones M, Gallen J, Palacios Q, Joyce T H, Morrow D 1987 The epidural test dose in obstetrics reconsidered. Anesthesiology 67: A625
66. Leighton B L, Norris M C, Sosis M, Epstein R, Chayen B, Larijani G E 1987 Limitations of epinephrine as a marker of intravascular injection in laboring women. Anesthesiology 66: 688–691
67. DeSimone C A, Leighton B L, Norris M V, Chayen B, Menduke H 1988 The chronotropic effect of isoproterenol is reduced in term pregnant women. Anesthesiology 69: 626–628
68. Chestnut D H, Owen C L, Brown C K, Vandewalker G E, Weiner C P 1988 Does labor affect the variability of maternal heart rate during induction of epidural anesthesia? Anesthesiology 68: 622–625
69. Leighton B L, Norris M C, DeSimone C A, Darby M J, Menduke H 1990 Pre-eclamptic and healthy term pregnant patients have different chronotropic responses to isoproterenol. Anesthesiology 72: 392–393
70. Leighton B L, DeSimone C A, Norris M C, Chayen B 1989 Isoproterenol is an effective marker of intravenous injection in laboring women. Anesthesiology 71: 206–209
71. Fong J, Gadalla F, Fiamengo S A, Druzin M, Artusio J F 1988 Ephedrine as the intravenous component of the epidural analgesia test dose in laboring parturients. Anesthesiology 69: A706
72. Cherala S R, Mehta D, Greene R 1990 Ephedrine as a marker of intravascular injection in laboring parturients. Reg Anesth 15: 15–18
73. Tong C, Eisenach J C 1992 The vascular mechanism of ephedrine's beneficial effect on uterine perfusion during pregnancy. Anesthesiology 76: 792–798
74. Moore D C, Batra M S 1981 The components of an effective test dose prior to epidural block. Anesthesiology 55: 693–696
75. Stonham J, Moss P 1983 The optimal test dose for epidural anesthesia. Anesthesiology 58: 389–390
76. Nicholas A D G 1984 The optimal test dose for epidural anesthesia. Anesthesiology 60: 79
77. Albright G A 1984 Epinephrine should be used with the therapeutic dose of bupivacaine in obstetrics. Anesthesiology 61: 217–218
78. Conklin K A, Ziadlourad F 1984 Bupivacaine: cardiotoxicity or anesthetic technique? Anesthesiology 61: 625–627
79. Chadwick H S, Benedetti C, Ready L B, Williams V 1987

Epinephrine-containing test doses – don't throw the baby out with the bath water. Anesthesiology 66: 571
80. Van Zundert A, Vaes L, De Wolf A 1987 E C G monitoring of mother and fetus during epidural anesthesia. Anesthesiology 66: 584–585
81. Van Zundert A, Vaes L, Soetens M et al 1987 Every dose given in epidural analgesia for vaginal delivery can be a test dose. Anesthesiology 67: 436–440
82. Van Zundert A, De Wolf A, Vaes L, Soetens M 1988 High-volume spinal anesthesia with bupivacaine. Anesthesiology 69: 998–1003
83. Abouleish E, Johnson K 1986 Simultaneous recording of maternal and fetal heart rate. Anesthesiology 65: 558–559
84. Chestnut D H, Weiner C P 1986 Monitoring maternal heart rate during epidural injection of a test dose containing epinephrine. Anesthesiology 64: 839–840
85. Holdcroft A 1992 Use of adrenaline in obstetric analgesia. Anaesthesia 47: 987–990
86. Hood D O, Dewan D M, Rose J C, James II F M 1983 Maternal and fetal effects of intravenous epinephrine containing solutions in gravid ewes. Anesthesiology 59: A393
87. Hood D D, Dewan D M, James F M 1986 Maternal and fetal effects of epinephrine in gravid ewes. Anesthesiology 64: 610–613
88. Wallis K L, Shnider S M, Hicks J S, Spivey H T 1976 Epidural anesthesia in the normotensive pregnant ewe. Anesthesiology 44: 481–487
89. Chestnut D H, Weiner C P, Herrig J E, Want J 1985 Effect of intravenous epinephrine upon uterine blood flow velocity in the guinea pig. Anesthesiology 63: A453
90. Chestnut D H, Weiner C P, Martin J G, Herrig J E, Wang J P 1986 Effect of intravenous epinephrine on uterine artery blood flow velocity in the pregnant guinea pig. Anesthesiology 65: 633–636
91. Jouppila R, Jouppila P, Kuikka J, Hollmen A 1978 Placental blood flow during cesarean section under lumbar extradural analgesia. Br J Anaesth 50: 275–279
92. Jouppila R, Jouppila P, Hollmen A, Kuikka J 1978 Effect of segmental extradural analgesia on placental blood flow during normal labor. Br J Anaesth 50: 563–567
93. Albright G A, Jouppila R, Hollmen A I, Jouppila P, Vierola H, Koivula A 1981 Epinephrine does not alter human intervillous blood flow during epidural anesthesia. Anesthesiology 54: 131–135
94. Alahuta S, Rasanen J, Jouppila R, Jouppila P, Hollmen A I 1991 Effects of extradural bupivacaine with adrenaline for cesarean section on uteroplacental and fetal circulation. Br J Anaesth 67: 678–682
95. Lindblad A, Bernow J, Vernersson E, Marsal K 1987 Effects of extradural anesthesia on human fetal blood flow in utero. Br J Anaesth 59: 1265–1272
96. Veille J C, Youngstrom P, Kanaan C, Wilson B 1988 Human umbilical artery flow velocity waveforms before and after regional anesthesia for cesarean section. Obstet Gynecol 72: 890–893
97. Morrow R J, Rolbin R N, Ritchie J W K, Haley S 1989 Epidural anesthesia and blood flow velocity in mother and fetus. Can J Anaesth 36: 519–522
98. Grant G J, Ramanathan S, Thurndorf H 1990 The maternal hemodynamic effects of bupivacaine-epinephrine mixture used for obstetric anesthesia. Acta Anaesthesiol Scand 34: 543–547
99. Abboud T K, Sheikh-Ol-Eslam A, Yanagi T et al 1985 Safety and efficacy of epinephrine added to bupivacaine for lumbar epidural analgesia in obstetrics. Anesth Analg 64: 585–591
100. Abboud T K, Mosaad P, Makar A et al 1988 Comparative maternal and neonatal effects of the new and old formulations of 2-chloroprocaine. Reg Anesth 13: 101–106
101. Heller P J, Goodman C 1986 Use of local anesthetics with epinephrine for epidural anesthesia in preeclampsia. Anesthesiology 65: 224–226
102. Heller P J, Goodman C 1987 Epinephrine is unsafe in the preeclamptic patient by Costin and Millikin – Reply. Anesthesiology 66: 99–100
103. Dror A, Abboud T K, Moore et al 1987 Maternal hemodynamic responses to epinephrine-containing local anesthetics in pre-eclampsia. Anesthesiology 67: A632
104. Dror A, Abboud T K, Moore J et al 1988 Makar A, Zaki N Maternal hemodynamic responses to epinephrine-containing local anesthetics in mild pre-eclampsia. Reg Anesth 13: 107–111
105. Youngstrom P, Hoyt M, Veille J C, Cohen I, Amini S, Herman M 1989 Effects of 'Test dose' epinephrine given intravenously in sheep with acute fetal stress and acidosis. Anesthesiology 71: A852
106. Youngstrom P, Hoyt M, Veille J C, Cohen I, Amini S, Herman M 1990 Effects of intravenous test dose epinephrine on fetal sheep during acute fetal stress and acidosis. Reg Anesth 15: 237–241
107. Desparmet J, Mateo J, Ecoffey C, Mazoit J X 1988 Efficacy of an epidural test dose in children anesthetized with halothane. Anesthesiology 69: A774
108. Desparmet J, Mateo J, Ecoffey C, Mazoit J X 1990 Efficacy of an epidural test dose in children anesthetized with halothane. Anesthesiology 72: 249–251
109. Narchi P, Mazoit J X, Samii K 1988 Does atropine conceal the heart rate response to an epidural test dose? Anesthesiology 69: A396
110. Hom M, Johnson P 1987 Mulroy M. Blood pressure response to an epinephrine test dose in beta-blocked subjects. Anesthesiology 67: A268
111. Guinard J P, Mulroy M F, Carpenter R L, Nadir B 1990 Epidural epinephrine test doses: influence of aging. Anesthesiology 73: A773
112. Garaud O, Samii K 1987 Dose-test pour anesthésie péridurale chez les patients traités par beta-bloquants. Ann Fr Anesth Réanim 6: 125–126
113. Popitz-Bergez F, Datta S, Ostheimer G W 1988 Intravascular epinephrine may not increase heart rate in patients receiving metoprolol. Anesthesiology 68: 815–816
114. Severn A M 1988 False positive test dose and epidural fentanyl. Anaesthesia 43: 167
115. Colonna-Romano P, Lingaraju N, Godfrey S D, Braitman L E 1992 Epidural test dose and intravascular injection in obstetrics: sensitivity, specificity, and lowest effective dose. Anesth Analg 75: 372–376
116. Gieraerts R, Van Zundert A, De Wolf A, Vaes L 1992 Ten ml bupivacaine 0.125% with 12.5 μg epinephrine is a reliable epidural test dose to detect inadvertent intravascular injection in obstetric patients. A double-blind study. Acta Anaesthesiol Scand 36: 656–659
117. Tom W C 1988 The epidural test dose and the identification of rare events. Can J Anaesth 35: 327–328
118. Kozody R, Palahniuk R J, Wade J G, Cumming M O 1984 The effect of subarachnoid epinephrine and phenylephrine on spinal cord blood flow. Can Anaesth Soc J 31: 503–508
119. Van Zundert A, De Wolf A 1988 Extent of anesthesia and hemodynamic effects after subarachnoid administration of bupivacaine with epinephrine. Anesth Analg 67: 784–787

PART D
MASSIVE SUBARACHNOID ANESTHESIA

N. Hughes

The sudden onset of hypotension with or without loss of consciousness in a parturient receiving epidural anesthesia may be due to a variety of causes.

Obstetric-related causes include:

1. hemorrhage (e.g. abruption, previa, uterine rupture, vaginal laceration, uterine atony); and
2. embolism (thromboembolism, amniotic fluid).

Epidural-related causes include:

1. massive epidural block;
2. subdural block;
3. total spinal (massive subarachnoid block); and
4. unintentional intravascular injection.

True massive epidural block involves overdosage of local anesthetic via a correctly placed needle or catheter, while subdural and total spinal block are produced by injecting appropriate amounts of local anesthetic for epidural block through an incorrectly located needle or catheter. The remainder of this section will discuss the etiology, pathophysiology, treatment and prevention of massive subarachnoid block (total spinal) during epidural anesthesia in parturients.

Unintentional high spinal or total spinal block results from the injection of appropriate amounts of local anesthetic through the epidural needle or epidural catheter into the subdural or subarachnoid space, without allowing adequate time for detection of a possible subarachnoid injection. Some anesthesiologists, particularly when administering epidural anesthesia for cesarean delivery, give much of the total dose through the epidural needle without fractionation. In the opinion of the author and editors, this procedure is unwise and certainly should not be used in inexperienced hands. Case reports describing late migration of epidural catheters into the subarachnoid space[1] serve to emphasize the necessity of aspiration through the catheter before injection of local anesthetic. In laboring patients with a continuous epidural infusion, catheter migration results in a more insidious onset of high-spinal anesthesia.

The clinical signs and symptoms of a subarachnoid block are the expected physiologic reactions of a total sympathectomy and respiratory muscle paralysis. Complete sympathectomy (T1–L1) is manifested by profound hypotension and bradycardia. Paralysis of preganglionic sympathetic fibers causes decreased systemic vascular resistance and peripheral venous pooling, which causes decreased cardiac output by a diminution of venous return to the heart.[2] Paralysis of cardioaccelerator fibres (T1–T4) causes bradycardia, which further diminishes cardiac output. Hypotension will be exaggerated if aortocaval compression is present.

Paralysis of intercostal muscles and the diaphragm (C3,4,5) results in respiratory arrest. Hypoxemia develops more rapidly in apneic parturients, partly because of a reduced functional residual capacity and an atelectatic functional residual capacity – closing capacity relationship.[3]

Loss of consciousness with high spinal or total spinal anesthesia occurs as a result of decreased cerebral blood flow (secondary to hypotension) and, in some cases, from deafferentation due to depression of the reticular networking system.[3]

The key to avoiding a catastrophe from a total spinal anesthetic is the ability of the anesthesiologist to recognize its occurrence and to immediately institute basic resuscitative measures. A total spinal block presents the anesthesiologist with an unconscious, hypoxic, hypotensive patient usually accompanied by fetal distress. Treatment involves securing and protecting the airway with a cuffed endotracheal tube, hyperventilation with 100% oxygen to reverse hypoxia, hypercapnia and lactic acidosis and circulatory support by intravenous administration of crystalloid and vasopressors. These measures may need to be continued for several hours until the total spinal block has regressed. Securing the airway with an endotracheal tube prevents aspiration and allows for prolonged mechanical ventilation. Resuscitation should also include left lateral displacement of the gravid uterus, using a 12.5–15.0 cm wedge under the right hip, to avoid aortocaval compression. Ephedrine and atropine, along with rapid fluid administration, will often reverse hypotension and bradycardia. More refractory hypotension usually responds to boluses or an infusion of phenylephrine. Epinephrine is occasionally necessary and must be available. During the resuscitation, continuous fetal monitoring is mandatory. Cesarean delivery is usually not necessary as long as prompt treatment quickly restores a normal cardiac output and maintains adequate oxygenation of the patient. Close monitoring of arterial blood pressure and blood gases is necessary until the patient can be weaned from mechanical ventilation and the sympathectomy has regressed.

Anesthesiologists performing epidural anesthesia must be constantly alert to the possibility of the occurrence of a total spinal anesthetic. This complication may be rapidly fatal for mother and fetus if is not detected and treated promptly. It should be emphasized that this condition is largely preventable by taking certain precautions and using proper technique. Use of an effective test dose[4] on initiation of the epidural block will produce prompt motor block if the catheter is in the subarachnoid space. All further local anesthetic is given by fractional dosing, i.e. administering 3–5 ml of local anesthetic, allowing 2–3 min to elapse before giving another 3–5 ml, and continuing such dosing until desired anesthesia results.[5] Before injecting, the catheter is aspirated and observed for the possibility of free flow of CSF into the syringe. It is imperative to remember that a negative aspiration test can occur with a subdural catheter[6] which, following injection, will produce excessive amounts of motor, sensory and sympathetic blockade. The last may cause a high spinal or total spinal block with standard epidural doses of local anesthetic. Where a continuous epidural infusion is in progress, the level of sensory anesthesia and blood pressure should be assessed at regular intervals. Should a total spinal block occur, proper resuscitation equipment must be immediately available. Vital equipment includes an oxygen source, suction device, a selection of cuffed endotracheal tubes, laryngoscope, Ambu (or ventilating) bag and appropriate drugs.

In summary, massive subarachnoid block is a largely preventable complication of epidural anesthesia. By adhering to proper technique and taking certain precautions, its incidence is exceedingly low. A high index of suspicion should be maintained when injecting local anesthetic epidurally, since this will allow for prompt immediate treatment if massive subarachnoid injection occurs.

REFERENCES

1. Crawford J S 1985 Some maternal complications of epidural analgesia for labor. Anaesthesia 40: 1219–1225
2. Greene N M 1992 Physiology of spinal anesthesia, 3rd edn. Williams & Wilkins, Baltimore
3. Cohen, S E 1986 Physiological alterations of pregnancy. Clin Anaesthesiol 4(1): 33–46
4. Moore D C, Batra M S 1981 The components of an effective test dose prior to epidural block. Anesthesiology 55: 693–696
5. Covino B G, Marx G F, Finster M, Zsigmond E K 1980 Prolonged sensory/motor deficits following inadvertent spinal anesthesia. Anesth Analg 59: 399–400
6. Lubenow T, Keh-Wong E, Kristof K, Ivankovich O S A 1988 Inadvertent subdural injection. Anesth Analg 67: 175–179
7. Abouleish E, Goldstein M 1986 Migration of an extradural catheter into the subdural space. A case report. Br J Anaesth 58: 1194–1197

PART E
ALLERGIC REACTIONS TO LOCAL ANESTHETICS

J. E. Arnold

Local anesthetics are an invaluable tool in the practice of obstetric anesthesia. Unfortunately, it is not uncommon for a patient to report that she is allergic to Novocain, lidocaine or even worse, all 'caines'. Frequently, this diagnosis has come from a prior exposure to one of the local anesthetics during a dental procedure or a regional nerve block. If taken at face value, this patient may be denied regional anesthesia for labor or cesarean delivery and would require general anesthesia for any surgical intervention.

Before proceeding, it is necessary to obtain a complete history from the patient about her reaction to the local anesthetic. Ideally, the patient should be referred to the anesthesiologist by her obstetrician in a timely manner before any anesthetic intervention is required. An attempt should be made to obtain any records detailing the incident in question.

Adverse reactions to local anesthetics may fall into one of four categories:[1] vasovagal reactions, epinephrine reactions, toxic reactions and allergic reactions.

Vasovagal reactions may occur in particularly anxious patients. These patients, commonly with 'needle phobias', may complain of lightheadedness or nausea at the time an anesthetic is administered. Signs include bradycardia, hypotension, pallor, diaphoresis, tachypnea and syncope. Placement of the patient in a supine position with left uterine displacement and legs elevated may be all that is needed to reverse this episode. Pharmacologic treatment is rarely needed.

Epinephrine reactions occur when a significant portion of an epinephrine-containing local anesthetic solution is absorbed systemically. Toxic effects of the local anesthetic itself may not be noticed, and the patient may complain of symptoms related to the epinephrine. These include nervousness and palpitations. Elevated blood pressure, tachycardia and extrasystoles may be present. Because of the short serum half-life of epinephrine, the episode usually subsides without intervention. Appropriate treatment is needed if conditions become life-threatening.

Toxic reactions to local anesthetics are due to an excess plasma concentration of the drug. The toxicity of these drugs involves primarily the central nervous system and the cardiovascular system. Early central nervous system effects include restlessness, tinnitus, vertigo, difficulty focusing, lightheadedness and a bitter taste in the mouth. As concentrations of the drug increase, slurred speech and skeletal muscle twitching occur. Higher blood levels result in seizures followed by central nervous system depression.

Cardiovascular effects of local anesthetics include hypotension, arrhythmias and atrioventricular heart block. Management of both central nervous system and cardiovascular system toxicity is well reviewed elsewhere.[2]

The last category of reactions to local anesthetics, true allergic reactions, are extremely rare,[3] estimated at less than 1% of all adverse reactions.[4] An allergic reaction is defined as an immune response that is exaggerated and leads to gross tissue damage.[5] The terms 'allergy', 'hypersensitivity' and 'sensitivity' are often used interchangeably in the anesthesia literature.[6]

Hypersensitivity reactions are classified according to the immune system's response. Gell and Coombs[7] defined four different types of reactions as follows: type 1, anaphylactic sensitivity; type 2, antibody-dependent, cytotoxic hypersensitivity; type 3, complex-mediated hypersensitivity; and type 4, cell-mediated or delayed-type hypersensitivity. For purposes of this review, type 2 and type 3 reactions will not be discussed in further detail since there are virtually no known occurrences of local anesthetic-induced type 2 or type 3 responses.[8]

Anaphylactic reactions (type 1) are mediated by antibodies from the immunoglobulin E (IgE) class. This is the most serious reaction and requires previous exposure to the drug or a chemically similar substance. On initial exposure to the antigenic substance, the individual's B lymphocytes are stimulated to produce IgE. The IgE antibodies then attach to receptor sites on the cell membranes of mast cells present in tissues and basophils circulating in plasma.[9] When stimulated, these 'sensitized' mast cells and basophils are capable of participating in an anaphylactic reaction. On re-exposure to the antigen, two cell-bound IgE antibodies may become cross-linked, leading to conformational changes in the cell membrane and release of granules (degranulation) from the mast cells and basophils. Degranulation of these cells leads to release of several chemical mediators, the most prominent of which is histamine. Histamine dilates terminal arterioles and increases capillary permeability leading to extravasation of intravascular fluid. Histamine also causes bronchospasm due to its role in constriction of bronchial smooth muscle. Additional chemical mediators that are released include heparin, slow-reacting substance of anaphylaxis, prostaglandins, platelet-activating factor and others.

The anaphylactic syndrome may include pruritus, erythema, flushing, urticaria, angioedema, nausea with diarrhea and vomiting, laryngeal edema, bronchospasm, hypotension, cardiovascular collapse and death, all occurring within minutes. Anaphylaxis has been reported after the raising of an intradermal wheal, injection of 1 ml of solution for a minor surgical procedure, the topical application of a small quantity of drug or the instillation of a drop or two in the conjunctival sac of the eye.[10]

Nonimmunologic stimulation of mast cells and basophils leading to the release of histamine has been termed anaphylactoid.[11] The magnitude of histamine released in this reaction is usually related to the dose of the drug and its rate of administration. In the extreme, a shock-like state may result that is indistinguishable from that of a true anaphylactic reaction.

Type 4, cell-mediated or delayed-type hypersensitivity, accounts for 90% of allergic reactions to local anesthetics.[12] This reaction involves interaction of an antigen with a primed T-lymphocyte causing tissue damage characterized by inflammation, pruritus, burning, erythematous macules and papules. There are no circulating antibodies involved and the damage is due to localized release of chemical mediators. The term delayed-type hypersensitivity is used because the symptoms may not occur for hours. Antihistamines and other such antagonistic substances are not helpful in treatment of this reaction since histamine and other circulating vasoactive substances are not involved. This type of sensitization can be detected by skin patch testing and occurs most often in individuals repeatedly exposed to a drug, for example physicians, nurses and dentists. Contact dermatitis is the most common example.

Commonly used local anesthetics fall into two distinct chemical groups, the amino-esters and the amino-amides. Amino-esters include procaine, chloroprocaine and tetracaine. Amino-amides include lidocaine, prilocaine, bupivacaine, mepivacaine and etidocaine.

Amino-ester local anesthetics are capable of producing metabolites related to para-aminobenzoic acid (PABA), which is a highly allergic substance. Most of the cell-mediated hypersensitivity reactions that were experienced by members of the dental profession were due to amino-esters.[3] These drugs may cross-sensitize and cross-react immunologically but do not cross-react with amino-amides.

Allergic reactions to amino-amide local anesthetics have been reported (refs 13 and 14 and J Arens, personal communication) but there has been only one case[15] which has had serial immunological confirmation of its nature. Other reports that have taken into account the role of preservatives[16–19] seem to present a relatively convincing picture of true allergic reactions.

Interestingly, most investigators suggest that amino-amide local anesthetics may not be substantially cross-reactive with each other.[20] A recent report about a contact sensitivity cross-reaction challenged that assertion.[21]

Allergic reactions may also be due to other chemicals or contaminants present in the local anesthetic solution. Methylparaben, a preservative for multiple-dose vials or ampules, is structurally similar to PABA. Other allergenic preservatives include methylhydroxybenzoate and bisulfites. Bisulfites are used to stabilize vasoconstrictors which are in solution. The Food and Drug Administration estimates that 5% of the nine million people with asthma in the USA may be hypersensitive to sulfites.[22] Patients with chronic atopy (allergies to foods or inhalants; bronchial asthma) are at higher risk of developing sensitization to drugs. Examples of allergic reactions due to preservatives continue to appear in the literature.[23–25]

A thorough history is essential in approaching the patient with a presumed allergy to a local anesthetic. Other types of adverse reactions, as previously discussed, should be ruled out. If the patient's history points toward a true allergic reaction, the simplest alternative may be to use a local anesthetic that is chemically unrelated to the one that is implicated. There is no simple, satisfactory and reliable method for testing for allergies to local anesthetics that a clinician may use for identifying susceptible individuals,[12] but allergy testing may be helpful.

A more complete evaluation of a patient is sometimes warranted, and this involves referral to an allergist or others who are familiar with allergy testing. The most commonly available in vivo tests for local anesthetic allergy are skin testing, incremental challenge and patch testing. Two unique in vitro tests, the leukocyte histamine release test and the platelet-activating factor (PAF) acether release test, will also be discussed.

Skin testing involves various dilutions of the preservative-free local anesthetic, applied initially to a scratch or prick in the skin and later injected in intradermal wheals. Protocols for this are well described elsewhere.[8,20,26] There are literature reports of at least 257 subjects in whom a negative skin test to a local anesthetic was followed by challenge to that drug without reaction.[27] False-negative tests have been reported in only five subjects undergoing local anesthetic testing.

Incremental challenge is used to confirm a negative skin test and should be used before a clinical trial of the drug is recommended.[27,28] This test involves subcutaneous injection of increasing dilutions and volumes of the local anesthetic. One study concluded that local anesthetics can be safely used despite the history of previous reactions if skin tests are negative and incremental challenge is used.[28]

Patch testing is the accepted method for identifying the cell-mediated hypersensitivity reaction. The drug is applied directly to the skin to detect local hypersensitivity.[29] The appearance of erythema, swelling, papules and vesicles within 24–48 h implies a positive reaction. Patch testing does not detect the types of reactions due to circulating IgE antibodies.

The leukocyte histamine release test (LHRT) is an in vitro correlate of IgE-mediated allergy.[30] The test involves incubation of washed leukocytes from the patient with and without the implicated local anesthetic. Histamine released is measured and is expressed as the percentage of total leukocyte histamine (in basophils) released into the resultant supernatant. In one study,[31] the LHRT was felt to be useful in confirming skin testing, especially negative or inconclusive skin tests. The authors felt that if both skin testing and the LHRT are negative, the likelihood of an anaphylactic reaction is small. They went on to state, though, that direct challenge in vivo, starting with low dosage and with proper monitoring and preparation for resuscitation, is the final resort in unresolved cases.

The PAF acether release test[32] is another recently described in vitro method to investigate allergic local anesthetic reactions. PAF acether is a powerful mediator of inflammation which can be released upon activation of different immune cells.[33] The PAF acether release test (PART) measures PAF acether activity in the supernatant of white blood cells which have been challenged by a specific antigen. Though this test is not the definitive in vitro test for determining a drug allergy, it may be a useful piece of information in investigating a local anesthetic allergy.

Although anaphylactic reactions to local anesthetics, especially the amino-amides, are relatively rare, prompt and aggressive treatment is necessary when this condition occurs. Many standard internal medicine or emergency medicine textbooks discuss detailed treatment protocols.[34,35] Some highlights of therapy will be discussed.

All parturients should have a large-bore intravenous line established before a regional anesthetic is administered. Clinical manifestations of an anaphylactic reaction may vary from mild to severe and the chosen therapy should vary accordingly. Early recognition is critical since irreversible anoxic organ damage or death can occur rapidly. Initial pharmacologic therapy for mild reaction is the subcutaneous injection of epinephrine, 0.2–0.5 mg, repeated every 20–30 min as necessary. If generalized urticaria or hypotension occurs, subcutaneous absorption may be upredictable and the epinephrine should be given by the intramuscular route. In the more severe reaction, the immediate goals of therapy include correction of hypoxemia, inhibition of further chemical mediator release and restoration of intravascular volume and blood pressure. Supplemental oxygen should be given and intravenous epinephrine (5 mg/kg) should be administered immediately, but cautiously[36] preferably with ECG monitoring. Avoid aortocaval compression with an appropriate wedge in the pregnant woman. In extreme circumstances, endotracheal intubation and controlled ventilation may be necessary. A crystalloid or colloid infusion should accompany the other therapeutic measures in order to replace intravascular volume. Diphenhydramine (0.5–1.0 mg/kg) is useful in reducing the likelihood that circulating histamine will bind to unoccupied receptors. Aminophylline, a 6 mg/kg loading dose over 20–30 min followed by an infusion of 0.5–1.0 mg/kg/h, may be used to relieve bronchospasm. Bronchodilation may also be achieved with an inhaler such as albuterol (Ventolin, Proventil).

In the parturient, ephedrine is still the vasopressor of choice, but other emergency drugs, including dopamine, norepinephrine, metaraminol, phenylephrine, or epinephrine may be required to maintain adequate arterial pressure. Steroids may be useful in preventing late sequelae.[37]

A full-blown anaphylactic reaction can have devastating effects. Because of this, appropriate resuscitative equipment, including the necessary medications, should be available whenever a regional anesthetic is administered.

In summary, the parturient with a history of local anesthetic allergy deserves special attention. True allergic reactions are rare and the amino-ester local anesthetics have been responsible for most reports of allergies to local anesthetics. The additives in local anesthetic solutions may also be culpable. If other adverse reactions to the anesthetics, such as vasovagal, epinephrine induced or toxic, can be ruled out, a simple approach is to substitute a chemically unrelated local anesthetic, e.g. amino-amide for amino-ester. If time permits and it is deemed necessary, the patient should be referred to an allergist or similar person for further evaluation. The results of this evaluation may not be conclusive, but may help guide the clinician in his or her decision to use a particular local anesthetic. Of greatest concern to the anesthesiologist is that patient who may have an anaphylactic reaction upon re-exposure to a particular drug. In view of this, the practitioner should have appropriate resuscitation equipment available during an anesthetic to treat that rare, though unpredictable and life-threatening, anaphylactic reaction.

REFERENCES

1. Baker J D, Blackman B B 1985 Local anesthesia. Clin Plastic Surg 12: 25–31
2. Moore D C 1986 Toxicity of local anesthetics in obstetrics. Clin Anaesthesiol 4: 113–123
3. Covino B G, Vassallo H G 1976 Local anesthetics: mechanisms of action and clinical use. Grune & Stratton, New York, pp 123–148
4. Giovannetti J A, and Bennett C R 1979 Assessment of allergy to local anesthetics. J Am Med Assoc 98: 701–706
5. VanArsdel P P 1982 Diagnosing drug allergy. J Am Med Assoc 247: 2576–2581
6. Adriani J and Naraghi M 1978 Etiology and management of adverse reactions to local anesthetics. J Am Med Wom Assoc 33: 365–372
7. Gell P G, Coombs R R 1975 Classification of allergic reactions responsible for clinical hypersensitivity and disease. In Gell P G, Coombs R R, Lachman P J Clinical aspects of immunology, 3rd edn. Blackwell Scientific Publications, Oxford, pp 761–779
8. Canfield D W, Gage T W 1987 A guideline to local anesthetic allergy testing. Anesth Progress 34: 157–163
9. Altman L C 1981 Basic immune mechanisms in immediate hypersensitivity. Med Clin North Am 65: 941–957
10. Adriani J, Zepernick R 1981 Allergic reactions to local anesthetics. South Med J 74: 669–703
11. Stoelting R 1983 Allergic reactions during anesthesia. Anesth Analg 62: 341–356
12. Adriani J 1985 Labatt's regional anesthesia: techniques and clinical applications. Warren H Green, St Louis, pp 78–88
13. Lynas R F A 1969 A suspected allergic reaction to lidocaine. Anesthesiology 31: 380
14. Morrisset L M 1957 Fatal anaphylactic reaction to lidocaine. Armed Forces Med J 8: 740
15. Brown D T, Beamish D, Wildsmith J A W 1981 Allergic reaction to an amide local anesthetic. Br J Anaesth 53: 435–437
16. Falace D A, Hill J S 1985 Allergy to lidocaine and mepivacaine: report of a case. Compendium of Continuing Education in Dentistry 6: 280–284
17. Kennedy K S, Cave R H 1986 Anaphylactic reaction to lidocaine. Arch Otolaryngeal Head Neck Surg 112: 671–673
18. MacColl S, Young E R 1989 An allergic reaction following injection of local anesthetic: a case report. Can Dent Assoc J 55: 981–984
19. Klein C E, Gall H 1991 Type IV allergy to amide-type local anesthetics. Contact Dermatitis 25: 45–48
20. Schatz M 1984 Skin testing and incremental challenge in the evaluation of adverse reactions to local anesthetics. J Allergy Clin Immunol 74: 606–616
21. Black R J, Dawson T A J, Strang W C 1990 Contact sensitivity to lignocaine and prilocaine. Contact Dermatitis 23: 117–118
22. Seng G F, Gay B J 1986 Dangers of sulfites in dental local anesthetic solutions: warning and recommendations. J Am Dent Assoc 113: 769–770
23. Fine P G, Dingman D L 1988 Hypersensitivity dermatitis following suction-assisted lipectomy: a complicaton of local anesthetic. Ann Plastic Surg 20: 573–575
24. Carr T W 1990 Severe allergic reaction to an intraurethral lignocaine preparation containing parabens preservatives. Br J Urol 66: 98
25. Dooms-Goossens A, Gidi de Alam A, Degreef H, Kochuyt A 1989 Local anesthetic intolerance due to metabisulfite. Contact Dermatitis 20: 124–126
26. Sindel L J, deShazo R D 1991 Accidents resulting from local anesthetics. True or false allergy? Clin Rev Allergy 9: 379–395
27. Schatz M, Fung D L 1986 Anaphylactic and anaphylactoid reactions due to anesthetic agents. Clin Rev Allergy 4: 215–227
28. Chandler M J, Grammer L C Patterson R 1987 Provocative challenge with local anesthetics in patients with a prior history of reaction. J Allergy Clin Immunol 79: 883–886
29. Shelley W B 1967 The patch test. J Am Med Assoc 200: 874–876
30. Assem E S K, Vickers M R 1975 Investigation of the response to some haptenic determinants in penicillin allergy by skin and in vitro allergy tests. Clin Allergy 5: 43–57
31. Assem E S K, Punnia-Moorthy A 1988 Allergy to local anaesthetics: an approach to definitive diagnosis. Br Dent J 164: 44–47
32. Dunoyer-Geindre S, Ludi F, Terki N, Gumowski P I, Girard J P 1992 PAF acether release on antigenic challenge. A method for the investigation of drug allergic reactions. Allergy 47: 50–54
33. Mencia-Huerta J M, Hosford D, Braquet P 1989 Acute and long term pulmonary effects of platelet activating factor. Clin Exp Allergy 19: 125–142
34. Lichtenstein L 1988 Anaphylaxis. In Wyngaarden J B, Smith L H (eds) Cecil textbook of medicine, Vol 2, 18th edn W B Saunders, Philadelphia, pp 1956–1958
35. Lindzon R D, Silvers W S 1988 Anaphylaxis. In Rosen P (ed) Emergency medicine: concepts and clinical practice, Vol 1, 2nd edn. C V Mosby, St Louis, pp 203–231
36. Kelley J F, Patterson R 1974 Anaphylaxis: course, mechanisms, and treatment J Am Med Assoc 227: 1431–1436
37. Wasserman S I 1983 Anaphylaxis. In Middleton E (ed) Allergy, 2nd edn. C V Mosby, St Louis pp 689–699

22. The conduct of labor under epidural anesthesia: the obstetrician's point of view

P. Defoort M. Thiery

INTRODUCTION

Lumbar epidural anesthesia (LEA), either single administration or continuous (CLEA), may influence the labor process in different ways. Throughout the first and second stages, interference with uterine motility is possible. In the second stage, there may be interference with the bearing-down effort through lack of the urge or motor ability to bear down and a modification of the tone of the muscular passageway resulting in a higher incidence of malrotation (persistent occipitoposterior position, OPP). These factors, in turn, may lead to an increased number of instrumental deliveries.

These possibilities should be kept in mind when managing labor under CLEA, so that adequate corrective steps may be taken at any time. This is of particular importance in breech delivery, multiple birth, prematurity and a scarred uterus.

EPIDURAL ANESTHESIA DURING FIRST-STAGE LABOR

There is no simple answer as to what is the influence of CLEA on uterine activity. Findings regarding the uterine response vary widely depending on a series of variables, e.g. type of anesthetic drug administered, addition of epinephrine to the solution and the timing and level of the injection.

First we wish to point out that it is a major misconception, although frequently stated in the ward by residents or midwives, that a main side-effect of CLEA is diminution of uterine activity. In vitro studies on muscle strips from gravid and nongravid human uteri demonstrate the opposite: depending on dose and agent, local anesthetics cause variable alterations of contractility, the most striking effect being *hypertonicity* accompanied by incoordinate uterine activity. The addition of epinephrine to the anesthetic solution can cause tetanic uterine contractions.[1,2] The hypertonic response of the uterus to high blood levels of local anesthetics was confirmed in animals by Greiss et al[3] and in the human by Evans et al.[4] Blood levels currently possible with the use of regional anesthesia are not generally believed to affect uterine motility,[5] although increased uterine activity has been observed, particularly with bupivacaine without epinephrine.[6–8] This increased uterine activity, especially when added to the effects of low amniotomy (Brotanek's reflex) and (hyper) stimulation through oxytocics, may have disastrous effects on the fetus. Consequently, care should be taken to dissociate in time the possible uterine effects of a topping-up injection from these or other interventions, and, therefore, it is safe to apply the top-up injection under cardiotocographic monitor control.

As a general rule, uterine *contractility* may be diminished by LEA but the effect is discrete and limited to 10–20 min at the utmost. During active labor, currently used concentrations of local anesthetics are devoid of any observable effect on uterine contractility.[9] Only during the early onset of labor (latent phase) may CLEA result in total arrest of uterine contractions, so that it is recommended to delay the start of regional anesthesia until labor is well established.[10] In other cases, adequate augmentation to maintain a satisfactory level of uterine work (active management of labor) should be considered. There is a tendency for first-stage labor to be more protracted with analgesia/anesthesia than without its use. Holm[11] studied women who, without any anesthesia/analgesia, had a significantly shorter dilation stage than those receiving either meperidine or CLEA. This was true for both multiparous (4.7 h without analgesia, 6.6 h with meperidine, 5.9 h with CLEA) and nulliparous women (6.8 h without analgesia, 8.4 h with meperidine, 8.6 h with CLEA). However, after analyzing all pertinent factors, it appears that this reflects not the type of the analgesia used, but the fact that pain relief was needed. This relates to the duration of labor, which is the result of the obstetric circumstances. The same concept is borne out by the study from Jacquemin et al.[12]

Gottschalk,[13] while identifying the difficulty of separating the complications due to the anesthesia from those due to underlying obstetric problems, points out that blaming the anesthetic for 'slowing' labor leads to a possibly deleterious delay in the diagnosis of 'other and more probable causes for arrest of labor'. A number of studies identify the occurrence of hypotension during CLEA, and the use of epinephrine as the factors most commonly associated with decreased intensity of contractions and increased duration of labor.[5]

According to De Vore,[9] provided fetal malposition and malpresentation are ruled out and, above all, hypotension is avoided, a T10 sensory level block by CLEA administered during the first stage of labor should not result in any significant effect on uterine activity or progress of labor.

In summary:

1. CLEA should not be started in very early labor unless for a medical indication. However, it may be appropriate to insert the epidural catheter at this moment.[10] The use of CLEA during the latent phase of labor will prolong the labor and require the 'active management of labor'.
2. The obstetrician should identify and correct obstetric causes for delay ('active management of labor') and monitor the fetus electronically.
3. Maternal hypotension must be avoided through acute hydration (rapid i.v. administration of fluid) and positioning (left lateral tilt). The obstetric team has its share of responsibility to maintain the correct position of the parturient.

EPIDURAL ANESTHESIA DURING SECOND-STAGE LABOR

Epidural block, depending on the concentration of the local anesthetic used, may interfere with the second stage of labor through the suppression of the bearing-down 'reflex' because of sensory and/or motor loss, and through relaxation of the pelvic muscles to an extent that interferes with the mechanics of birth (head flexion and internal rotation). These effects in turn may lead to an increase in instrumental delivery. Holm[11] reported a significant increase in the duration of the second stage in women under epidural block, using bupivacaine 0.5%, compared with women receiving meperidine and nonmedicated women, both nulliparous (50 min on average in CLEA patients compared with 43.3 and 37.6 min in patients receiving meperidine and nonmedicated patients respectively) and multiparous (26.1 min with CLEA compared with 14 and 13.2 min in the meperidine and control groups). From a randomized double-blind study, Chestnut[14] reported the time interval from 8 cm dilatation to delivery to be on average 124 min in CLEA (0.125% bupivacaine) patients compared with 94 mins in controls, and the difference is significant. Jacquemin et al[12] found the rate of instrumental delivery in women with CLEA to be almost three times higher than in controls. The difference was most pronounced in the multiparous women (three fold increase compared with a 1.3-fold increase in primiparous women). For first-stage labor, the authors acknowledge a built-in bias ascribable to the fact that CLEA tends to be administered to women more likely to have a difficult labor. Furthermore, the authors found a significant inter-obstetrician difference in readiness to resort to vacuum extraction, the incidence ranging from 17.6% to 57.1%.

Another Belgian study[15] reported a 14% prevalence of application of forceps under CLEA, compared with 4% in subjects not receiving CLEA. The author refuses to draw the simplistic conclusion that this increase in forceps extraction is 'due to' CLEA. He points out that CLEA merely simplifies the application of forceps, and that this application is, like CLEA itself, the effect of a 'programming' attitude as opposed to a 'procrastinating' attitude. It is important to note that Thoumsin[15] was able to demonstrate a decrease in the cesarean delivery rate (for difficult labor) in patients given CLEA, from 11.7% to 7.4%. Thus, as in the first stage, it is imperative that the effects of the anesthesia are dissociated from those of the underlying obstetric context. Chestnut et al[14] validated the role of the latter in a double-blind study in which women received either CLEA (bupivacaine 0.0825%) or saline. The prevalence of instrumental delivery was 31% in the CLEA group and 37% in the saline group. It would thus appear that epidural anesthesia allows the woman to cope with a number of obstetric situations that might otherwise have led to cesarean delivery, be it in part with the help of forceps or vacuum extraction.

Shnider and Cosmi[16] point out that the woman's expulsive effort depends on the motivation and ability to bear down as much as on the reflex urge to expel the fetus. In a motivated and well-assisted parturient, and while the anesthetic is balanced in such a way that, though removing the urge to push, it leaves the contractile force of the abdominal muscles intact, spontaneous delivery remains the rule. To achieve this goal, it is recommended that the perineal dose of anesthetic be withheld until descent and rotation of the fetal head have occurred, and to adjust the dose level to achieve sensory block while preserving muscular tone.[17,18] It is especially important to maintain the tone of the levator ani muscle, which plays an important role in the mechanism of internal rotation.[19] Albright[20] found that in 20% of parturients voluntarily controlled bearing-down efforts under CLEA were more efficient than involuntary bearing-down efforts without anesthesia, because intense pain may interfere with the effort.

In summary:

1. During the second stage of labor the timing and dose level of CLEA should be adjusted so as not to interfere with the mechanics of internal rotation and muscular

tone. Correct evaluation of progress of labor by the obstetrician should guide the anesthesiologist to achieve this goal.
2. If the urge to bear down is lost, the woman should be actively and competently coached to optimize her expulsive efforts. In this respect, sympathetic encouragement by the nurse (her coach) is essential.
3. Epidural anesthesia may enable the obstetrician to cope with a number of difficult labors that might have led to cesarean delivery. The underlying obstetric situation may be managed by assisted delivery.

EPIDURAL ANESTHESIA IN OBSTETRIC RISK SITUATIONS

Obstetric risk situations, e.g. breech delivery, multiple pregnancy, preterm labor, scarred uterus and toxemia of pregnancy, were originally regarded as contraindications to CLEA. We will leave the discussion of CLEA in the toxemic patient to a broader discussion from the pharmacologic and physiologic viewpoint Here we will briefly consider the more specific obstetric situations.

The anticipated diminution of the bearing-down effort, resulting in an increased incidence of extraction with subsequent morbidity and mortality, made breech extraction a relative contraindication for CLEA. However, this is not the case, because an increase in the intervention rate – be it of extraction or of cesarean delivery – is not implicit in breech delivery under CLEA. While the duration of the second stage may increase, this is not at the cost of deleterious results on either the fetal acid–base status (umbilical artery pH) or the Apgar scores. In fact, the negative influence of pelvic floor relaxation on rotation that is considered when the vertex is presenting plays no role here since the untoward effects of untimely bearing-down efforts – which frequently occur in breech delivery – are prevented.

Little and Friedman[2] found CLEA to be contraindicated for twin delivery, a viewpoint eloquently shared by Crawford.[22] In 1975, however, Crawford[23] no longer maintained his objection, having demonstrated by a controlled trial that CLEA had no deleterious effect on the second twin, while actually shortening the interval between births. The obstetric complications due to increased uterine volume and overstretching of the myometrium, caval compression and hypotonic uterus resulting in post-partum hemorrhage are likely to occur in twin pregnancies with or without CLEA, which makes prevention (acute hydration, positioning and careful post-partum observation) and treatment of the hypotonic uterus even more imperative.

Premature babies are particularly sensitive to the untoward effects of local anesthetics.[24] The blood levels of anesthetic drug with CLEA have been shown to have no deleterious effect and CLEA may be helpful in rendering the birth process less traumatic by avoiding untimely bearing down and providing relaxation of the pelvic floor, so that in premature delivery epidural anesthesia has its place.

When a uterine scar is present, there are misgivings about the safety of CLEA: it is feared that CLEA will mask the pain symptomatic of scar rupture and thus may lead to catastrophic situations. Pain, however, is not the only sign of scar dehiscence or rupture (uterine hypotonus and fetal bradycardia ensue) nor will the pain be entirely masked by CLEA since the signs of peritoneal irritation are not blocked.[11] Thus, whenever the circumstances – location of the scar, pre-existent or underlying obstetric factors (pelvic adequacy) – permit a trial of labor, CLEA may be administered provided this is done under close and constant supervision by competent staff, uterine activity and fetal heart rate are continuously monitored electronically and an available delivery room allows immediate intervention.

CONCLUSION

While CLEA during labor has possible drawbacks, these can all be prevented by correct technique and consultation between obstetrician, anesthesiologist and nursing staff. Selection of the anesthetic drug, the addition of epinephrine to the anesthetic solution, timing and amount of the injection(s) have to be considered carefully and weighed against the obstetric data. Caval compression and maternal hypotension are to be prevented by acute intravascular volume expansion and positioning of the parturient. It has to be considered whether the patient is in active labor and, in the second stage, whether descent is progressive and rotation has occurred. In particular, the motivated parturient should be coached during the bearing-down period. Active management of all stages of labor is mandatory. Breech presentation, multiple pregnancy, preterm delivery and the presence of a uterine scar call for special attention but when the above conditions are met, CLEA is a safe and rewarding technique, allowing vaginal delivery in a number of situations where this goal might otherwise not have been attained.

REFERENCES

1. McGaughey Jr H S, Corey E L, Eastwood D, Thornton Jr W N 1962 Effect of synthetic anesthetics on the spontaneous motility of human uterine muscle in vitro. Obstet Gynecol 19: 233–240
2. Munson E S, Embro W J 1978 Lidocaine, monoethylglycinexylidide, and isolated human muscle. Anesthesiology 48: 183
3. Greiss F C, Still J G, Anderson S G 1976 Effects of local anesthetic

agents on the uterine vasculature and myometrium. Am J Obstet Gynecol 124: 889–899
4. Evans J A, Chastain G M, Phillips J M 1969 The use of local anesthetic agents in obstetrics. South Med J 62: 519
5. Cosmi E V 1981 Effect of anesthesia on labor and delivery. In: Cosmi E V (ed) Obstetric anesthesia and perinatology. Appleton Century Crofts, New York, pp 365–388
6. Jouppila P, Jouppila R, Kaar K, Merila M 1977 Fetal heart rate patterns and uterine activity after segmental epidural analgesia. Br J Obstet Gynaecol 84: 481–497
7. Neumark J 1980 Die Kontinuierliche lumbale Epiduralanaesthesie. Springer, Berlin
8. Schellenberg J C 1977 Uterine activity during lumbar epidural analgesia with bupivacaine. Am J Obstet Gynecol 127: 26
9. De Vore J S 1979 Effects of anaesthesia on uterine activity and labor. In: Shnider S M, Levinson G (eds) Anesthesia for obstetrics. Williams & Wilkins, Baltimore, pp 42–52
10. Crawford J S 1978 Principles and practice of obstetric anaesthesia, 4th edn. Blackwell Scientific Publications, Oxford
11. Holm J P 1982 Epidurale analgesie bij risicobevallingen (in Dutch). Thesis, Groningen
12. Jacquemin Y, Vercauteren M, Jankie S, Adriaensen H, Buytaert P H 1989 Epidurale anesthesie en kunstverlossing (in Dutch). In: Anesthésie et analgésie en gynécologie-obstétrique (Symposium. Société Royale Belge de Gynécologie et d'Obstétrique, Brussels 1989, Proceedings). Schering, Diegem, p 69
13. Gottschalk W. Obstetric anesthesia and analgesia. In: Iffy L, Kaminetzky H A (eds) Principles and practice of obstetrics and perinatology, Vol 2: John Wiley, New York, pp 991–1016
14. Chestnut D H, Vandewalker G E, Owen C L, Bates J N, Choi W W 1987 The influence of continuous epidural bupivacaine analgesia on the second stage of labor and method of delivery in nulliparous women. Anesthesiology 66: 774
15. Thoumsin H 1989 Répercussions de l'anesthésie péridurale sur l'homéostasie foetale, le travail et l'accouchement (in French) In: Anesthésie et analgésie en gynécologie-obstétrique (Symposium. Sociéte Royale Belge de Gynécologie et d'Obstétrique, Brussels 1989, Proceedings). Schering, Diegem, pp 161
16. Shnider S M, Cosmi E V 1981 Regional anesthesia in obstetrics. In: Cosmi E V (ed) Obstetric anesthesia and perinatology. Appleton Century Crofts, New York, pp 483–505
17. Johnson W L, Winter W W, Eng M, Bonica J J, Hunter C A 1972 Effect of pudendal, spinal and peridural block anesthesia on the second stage of labor. Am J Obstet Gynecol 113: 166–175
18. Vanderick G, Geerinckx K, Van Steenberge A L, De Muylder E 1974 Bupivacaine 0.125% in epidural block analgesia during childbirth: clinical evaluation. Br J Anaesth 46: 838
19. Levinson G, Shnider S M Anesthesia for abnormal positions, presentations and multiple births. In: Shnider S M, Levinson G (eds). Anesthesia for obstetrics. Williams & Wilkins, Baltimore, pp 170–179
20. Albright G A 1978 Anesthesia in obstetrics. Maternal, fetal and neonatal aspects. Addison-Wesley Medical, Menlo Park, CA
21. Little W A, Friedman E A 1958 Anesthesia for the twin delivery. Anesthesiology 19: 515
22. Crawford J S 1971 Anaesthesia for obstetric emergencies. Br J Anaesth 43: 864
23. Crawford J S 1975 An appraisal of lumbar epidural blockade in labour in patients with multiple pregnancy. Br J Obstet Gynaecol 82: 929–935
24. David H, Rosen M 1976 Perinatal mortality after epidural analgesia. Anaesthesia 31: 1054

23. The use of obstetric epidural anesthesia from the standpoint of the infant

J. M. Hawdon M. P. Ward-Platt A. Aynsley-Green

INTRODUCTION

Epidural anesthesia has become increasingly popular as a method of pain relief during labor. It is now appropriate, and in many cases beneficial, to use epidural anesthesia in a wide range of clinical situations, for both complicated and uncomplicated deliveries. In terms of benefit and safety for mother and fetus, epidural anesthesia is the method of choice in the presence of maternal epilepsy, heart disease (apart from hypertrophic obstructive cardiomyopathy, HOCM), liver disease, pre-eclampsia and renal disease.[1] However, as with all widely used obstetric techniques, an evaluation must be made of the implications for mother, fetus and neonate. This evaluation must include a comparison with other available methods of analgesia.

PHARMACOLOGY

When considering the effects of local anesthetic agents on the fetus and neonate, pharmacokinetic data from adult studies are not always applicable. Kanto and Erkkola[2] point out the various differences between adults and neonates, which include decreased plasma protein binding of drugs, variations in fetal and neonatal acid–base balance, reduced enzyme activities, and neonatal body composition. However, animal studies[3] suggest that the gestational age of a fetus (close to term) does not affect the rate of metabolism of local anesthetic agents.

The choice of local anesthetic agent may be important, as agents appear to differ in the degree to which they cross the placenta and are metabolized by the fetus. Procaine and chloroprocaine are broken down by placental enzymes, while all other local anesthetic agents cross the placenta. Once they have crossed the placenta, amide local anesthetics are slowly metabolized by the fetus, while ester agents are rapidly metabolized. Bupivacaine, an amide, and the most commonly used agent, is rapidly transferred across the placenta, with detectable levels in the fetus at 10 mins.[4] Most authors quote an umbilical vein–maternal vein ratio (UV/MV) of 0.10–0.86 for bupivacaine, with peak fetal levels of 0.25 μg/ml.[5,6] Kanto and Erkkola[2] compared the neonatal pharmacokinetics of lidocaine, mepivacaine, bupivacaine and etidocaine. Bupivacaine had the lowest UV/MV ratio but had the longest neonatal elimination half-life, with measurable amounts of the agent and its metabolites present for 48–72 hs. Notarianni[4] quotes the fetal half-life of bupivacaine as 14 hs. In comparison, the neonatal half-life and elimination of meperidine, after maternal administration in labor, is considerably longer.[2,7]

The presence of active metabolites must be included in the consideration of fetal metabolism of local anesthetic agents because they may prolong effects seen in the fetus or neonate. Kuhnert et al,[8] using gas chromatography/mass spectrometry to measure levels of bupivacaine and its active metabolite, 2,6-pipecolylxylidine (PPX), in maternal and neonatal blood, found that levels of PPX rose and fell more slowly than bupivacaine levels, and that bupivacaine and PPX persisted in neonatal body fluids for at least 3 days. They concluded that the low UV/MV ratio of bupivacaine is due to uptake by fetal tissues. Finster and Pedersen[9] suggest that such uptake into fetal tissues is related to the lipid solubility of the drug. However, post-mortem studies found higher concentrations of bupivacaine in the lungs and the heart than in the brain.[10] Fetal acidosis increases the intracellular accumulation of bupivacaine.[10,11] Some authors have related blood gas, fetal heart rate and neonatal behavioral changes to maternal and fetal local anesthetic concentrations, but do not refer to the effect of tissue uptake of the agents.[6,12,13]

The dosage regimen, the route of administration and the addition of epinephrine to local anesthetic preparations may also affect the fetal rate of appearance and excretion of local anesthetic agents, but there appear to be no effects on neonatal outcome.[14,15] The combination of epinephrine with certain local anesthetics may prolong analgesia without increasing the concentration of local anesthetic.[16,17] However, the addition of epinephrine has been thought to result in reduced uterine activity and prolonged time to vaginal delivery.[18,19]

Lastly, it is important to recognize the role of adequate acute hydration in preventing maternal hypotension. It is crucial to administer an intravenous fluid bolus prior to both epidural and spinal anesthesia, be it with crystalloid or colloid. Spinal anesthesia, which results in lower maternal and umbilical venous bupivacaine levels than epidural anesthesia,[21] is associated with maternal hypotension more often than epidural anesthesia, and thereby generally requires a greater loading volume.[22]

ADVANTAGES OF MATERNAL EPIDURAL ANESTHESIA FOR THE FETUS AND NEONATE

Obstetric epidural anesthesia has a number of favorable effects on the fetus. First, when anesthesia or analgesia is essential, as for cesarean delivery, epidural anesthesia avoids the use of parenteral drugs with maternal and neonatal depressive effects, such as intravenous opioids or inhalation agents. Ong et al[23] compared the effects of epidural and general anesthesia on 3940 infants born by cesarean delivery. They found that, regardless of the indication for cesarean delivery, administration of epidural anesthesia to the mother was associated with a lower incidence of adverse neonatal outcome.

Second, there are indirect advantages to the fetus, as a result of administering epidural anesthesia for normal vaginal delivery. If instrumental delivery becomes necessary, it will be less traumatic for the mother if epidural anesthesia rather than local infiltration is used. Similarly, the presence of effective epidural blockade will expedite emergency delivery. Thus, epidural anesthesia minimizes the duration and stress of complicated labor, and thereby has advantages for the already compromised fetus.

Finally, epidural anesthesia may prevent changes in the mother that could have adverse effects on the fetus. For example, during normal vaginal delivery, maternal pain is associated with elevated catecholamine levels in the maternal circulation. High catecholamine levels are also found in preeclamptic mothers[24] and in the neonate after complicated deliveries.[25] It is possible that the stress represented by the elevated maternal catecholamine levels, or the catecholamines themselves, are harmful to the mother and fetus. The effects on the fetus may be secondary to changes in placental circulation (see below). The use of epidural anesthesia has been shown to reduce maternal and fetal catecholamine levels compared with a non-epidural group,[24] and to prevent the maternal rise of epinephrine seen in the second stage when no epidural anesthesia is given.[26] Epidural anesthesia also prevents the rise in maternal catecholamine levels normally seen during contractions. There is a decline in mean maternal plasma catecholamine levels after epidural block.[27]

Reports differ as to the effects of epidural anesthesia on maternal or neonatal catecholamine levels during cesarean delivery. Falconer and Lake[25] reported no differences in neonatal catecholamine levels after cesarean delivery under epidural or general anesthesia. Irestedt et al[28] reported that general anesthesia was associated with a lower maternal level of catecholamines than epidural anesthesia, while Loughran et al[29] found that the increase in maternal levels of catecholamines, cortisol, glucose and insulin seen during general anesthesia was not found during epidural anesthesia. The differences between these studies may be related to the incidence of maternal hypotension (see below). However, it must be noted that both studies reported no differences in neonatal outcome between the general and epidural anesthesia groups.

Given that pregnancy-induced hypertension has well-known risks for mother and fetus, judicious epidural anesthesia may bring about favorable circulatory changes, reducing maternal mean arterial pressure without affecting cardiac output.[30] Indeed, intervillous blood flow, as measured by Jouppila et al[31] with the ^{133}Xe technique, improved in hypertensive mothers after lumbar epidural blockade. Maternal hypertension has little effect on the metabolism of local anesthetic agents.[32]

Studies of uterine and intervillous blood flow have shown beneficial effects of epidural anesthesia for normotensive mothers. Giles et al[33] demonstrated a fall in vascular resistance (as measured by Doppler waveform) of uteroplacental circulation and umbilical artery after epidural anesthesia with adequate acute hydration. Hollmen et al,[34] measuring intervillous blood flow with ^{133}Xe technique, found increased intervillous blood flow after epidural anesthesia after adequate volume loading. There were no differences between the use of bupivacaine or 2-chloroprocaine as anesthetic agents, but a 10-ml dose of bupivacaine gave a greater increase in blood flow than a 4-ml dose. The group studied after acute hydration only had no change in intervillous blood flow. Huovinen et al[35] demonstrated the importance of acute volume expansion, in that maternal blood pressure and intervillous blood flow fell during epidural anesthesia when no acute volume expansion was performed, but rose in the group when an intravenous bolus of fluid was first given.

Epidural anesthesia appears to have no adverse effects on fetal circulation. Normal labor is associated with increases in fetal aortic diameter and blood flow. Lindblad et al[36,37] found that these increases persisted during epidural anesthesia, while no increase in fetal aortic diameter or blood flow was seen during labor when systemic prepisidine was administered to the mother. Fetal hemodynamics were stable after epidural analgesia with etidocaine plus epinephrine, bupivacaine plus epinephrine, and bupivacaine alone.

Epidural anesthesia offers particular benefits for twin deliveries. Crawford[38] studied 200 such deliveries and found that, although the second stage for the first twin was longer than without an epidural anesthetic, the mean time interval between delivery of the first and second twin was similar with and without an epidural, and epidural blockade resulted in a favorable condition of the second twin regardless of the type of delivery, compared with deliveries without epidural anesthesia. In this series, in 4.4% cases (with or without an epidural) the second twin required cesarean delivery after vaginal delivery of the first twin. In these circumstances, the presence of epidural block was helpful in expediting delivery. Weekes et al[39] found no adverse effects of epidural anesthesia on the course of labor, type of delivery or neonatal outcome in twin pregnancies. They found that when the second twin was delivered by breech extraction, the epidural group had fewer depressed neonates with low Apgar scores than the nonepidural group. In singleton breech presentations also, infants were in better clinical condition when epidural anesthesia was administered.

In terms of neonatal outcome, epidural anesthesia appears to offer advantages. A study of 6442 deliveries between 1973 and 1974[40] demonstrated a reduced perinatal mortality rate after maternal epidural anesthesia, with significantly fewer first-week deaths in infants less than 2500 g. There were no differences in intrapartum mortality. Ong et al[23] found no differences in neonatal death rate in 3940 infants born by cesarean delivery with epidural or general anesthesia.

Reports differ as to the effects of epidural anesthesia on fetal and neonatal acid–base status and metabolism, neonatal respiratory depression and the need for resuscitation. Jouppila et al[6] reported normal fetal pH after the first epidural dose of bupivacaine in normal labor. Fetal blood gas samples taken during elective cesarean delivery were similar regardless of the type of anesthesia used, but epidural anesthesia was associated with an early neonatal normalization of acidosis.[41] Pearson and Davies,[42,43] in a study of oxytocin-induced normal deliveries, found that at full dilation, fetuses in the epidural group were less acidotic than those in the control group, with the greatest rate of acidosis occurring in the control group during the second stage of labor. Similarly, Thalme et al[44,45] found that at delivery and for the next 60 mins infants in an epidural group were less acidotic and had lower blood lactate levels than those in the control group (whose mothers received alternative analgesia). Other studies comparing epidural anesthesia with no anesthesia for vaginal delivery,[46,47] and epidural anesthesia with general anesthesia for cesarean delivery[48] have found no differences in umbilical blood gases. Swanstrom and Bratteby[49] found no differences in neonatal blood fatty acids, glycerol or ketone body levels in control and epidural groups.

Similarly, no differences were found in neonatal Apgar scores after epidural or general anesthesia for cesarean delivery,[50] while other studies have shown better Apgar scores after epidural anesthesia than after general anesthesia,[51] or after no analgesia,[52] with more rapid onset of sustained respiration for infants after epidural anesthesia than after general anesthesia.[53,54]

The incidence of perinatal retinal hemorrhages has been found to be reduced after obstetric epidural anesthesia. Maltau and Egge[55] reported that there were more retinal hemorrhages, particularly of severe grades, in control infants than in infants whose mothers had epidural anesthesia. Van Zundert et al[56] reported similar findings with more severe retinal hemorrhages in control infants, although the total number of hemorrhages of all grades was similar for infants in control and epidural groups.

Finally, note must be made of the advantages of epidural anesthesia in terms of mother–infant relationship. Mothers who have experienced a traumatic and painful delivery may project negative reactions to the birth onto the infant. Mothers experience less post-natal discomfort after epidural anesthesia and will feel more able to enjoy their babies. When epidural anesthesia is used as an alternative to sedation or general anesthesia, mothers feel more involved in the birth and are more quickly able to hold and feed their babies, which is of particular importance in the establishment of breast feeding.

DISADVANTAGES OF EPIDURAL ANESTHESIA FOR THE FETUS AND NEONATE

Consideration of any adverse effects of epidural anesthesia must include, and where necessary control for, other obstetric factors that influence outcome.[57,58] Few studies have achieved this as it is difficult to identify or control for these other obstetric factors. Multiple regression analysis may identify the contribution of anesthesia to neonatal outcome.

Many of the reported adverse effects of obstetric epidural anesthesia are secondary to maternal hypotension, and thus placental hypoperfusion. These effects are manifest as pathologic fetal heart rate changes or as disordered acid–base status. Jouppila et al[18] reported fetal heart rate changes in 9% of patients 30 mins after epidural injection of bupivacaine with epinephrine, but did not comment on the presence of maternal hypotension and had no control group. Jouppila et al,[6] Lieberman et al[59] and Zilianti et al[60] noted that when fetal heart rate changes occurred in association with epidural anesthesia there was coexisting maternal hypotension or uterine hyperstimulation. In the last study,[60] fetal heart rate changes were associated with fetal acidosis. Normalization of maternal blood pressure led to resolution of the fetal heart rate changes.

McDonald et al[61] found pathologic fetal heart rate changes in the absence of maternal hypotension or fetal pH changes but had no nonepidural group for comparison. This group is alone in suggesting a direct cardio-depressive effect of local anesthetic agents. Evidence against this is provided by Belfrage et al[12] who found no relation between fetal heart rate patterns and fetal bupivacaine concentrations. Many authors report no increased incidence of abnormal heart rate patterns during epidural anesthesia when compared with controls.[19,44]

Maternal hypotension has also been associated with low neonatal Apgar scores and acidosis.[60] The potential adverse effects of maternal hypotension during epidural anesthesia are demonstrated by Antoine and Young.[62] Mothers who required treatment with ephedrine for hypotension, when compared with mothers who did not require ephedrine, had infants with lower umbilical artery pH; when high doses of ephedrine were required, umbilical vein and artery pH were low with raised neonatal lactate levels. However, there were no differences in neonatal Apgar scores between the groups.

As described above, in the absence of maternal hypotension, the effects of epidural anesthesia in the neonatal period are negligible. Swanstrom and Bratteby[48] describe a higher incidence of hypoglycemia and hyperglycemia in infants whose mothers have had epidural anesthesia, compared with controls. However, some of the mothers received glucose infusions in labor and this is known to affect neonatal blood glucose levels.[63] Thalme et al[45] found no neonatal differences between an epidural and a control group in terms of blood glucose, potassium, sodium chloride and total protein. In our own study of 24 infants born by elective cesarean delivery under general anesthesia or epidural anesthesia, with no maternal glucose infusion, there were no significant differences between the groups for umbilical pH values or concentrations of glucose and other intermediary metabolites.

The documented prolonged second stage of labor, the increased use of oxytocin and the increased incidence of instrumental deliveries associated with epidural anesthesia[40,59,62,64,65] may be disadvantages for the mother, but have not been shown to be harmful to the infant. Moreover, it cannot always be inferred that the use of epidural anesthesia has caused these complications; they may be epiphenomena, as epidural anesthesia is most likely to be used when a difficult delivery is anticipated. It has been suggested that if a longer second stage were allowed for epidural patients, with delayed onset of pushing, a lower instrumental delivery rate would be achieved without detriment to the infant.[65] Some studies have found no effect of epidural anesthesia on duration of labor.[26,54] Overall, there are no data to suggest that any effect of epidural anesthesia on duration or resolution of labor is disadvantageous for the fetus or neonate.

There is extensive literature regarding the immediate and delayed effects of epidural anesthesia on neonatal neurology and behavior. Most studies are based on neonatal behavioral assessment scales, which require training to administer.[66] The difficulties in assessing newborn infants in this way must be considered when interpreting the results of these studies. It should also be noted that many other factors affect neonatal behavior or the observer's impression of this behavior.[21,67]

Kanto and Erkkola[2] described decreased responsiveness of infants for 2–8 hs after birth when lidocaine and mepivacaine were used as local anesthetic agents, but that infants whose mothers received bupivacaine scored better than controls. Tronick et al[68] compared infants whose mothers had epidural anesthesia with infants whose mothers had systemic analgesia or minimal medication, and found poor motor organization in the epidural group in the first 12 hs, but 'behavioral recovery' on days 1–10. They found no correlations between plasma local anesthetic concentrations and behavior scores. Scanlon et al[69] found that in the first 8 hs infants of an epidural group had lower scores on tests of muscle strength, tone and rooting, but no decrease in response to pinprick, when compared with nonepidural group. They described the epidural group as 'floppy but alert'. Mepivacaine and lidocaine were used in this study, and there was no difference in their effects.

In contrast, other studies comparing infants whose mothers received epidural anesthesia with those whose mothers received no medication reported no differences at all in neonatal neurobehavior.[13,70–72] Finally, infants whose mothers have had epidural anesthesia are reported to perform better than those whose mothers had general anesthesia[73] or meperidine.[74]

ALTERNATIVE AGENTS FOR EPIDURAL ANESTHESIA

The above discussion involves only the use of local anesthetic agents. Other agents are now being introduced for epidural and spinal analgesia. Fentanyl and other opioids have been used alone and in combination with local anesthetics. Potential advantages are the lack of sympathetic blockade and reduced risk of maternal hypotension. However, there are reports[75,76] of poor pain control in labor and neonatal depressive effects. In such situations, naloxone may be required to reverse effects. The addition of fentanyl to bupivacaine has been found to increase the speed of onset and duration of analgesia, when compared with bupivacaine alone, without adverse fetal and neonatal effects.[77–80]

CONCLUSIONS

It appears that, if one avoids maternal hypotension, obstetric epidural anesthesia has few adverse effects on the fetus or neonate. In fact, it offers the advantages of rapid, controlled delivery when necessary, and is associated with a better fetal outcome than the administration of systemic medication or general anesthesia.

The importance of adequate analgesia in obstetrics is fortunately well recognized at this point in time. Epidural anesthesia has been established as the method of choice for pain control in the laboring patient. As techniques are developed with lower concentrators of drug and fewer maternal side-effects, analgesia may be optimized for maximal maternal pain relief and minimal fetal and neonatal side-effects.

REFERENCES

1. Writer W D R 1985 Anesthesia during pregnancy: Interactions with maternal disease. In: Scanlon J W (ed) Perinatal Anesthesia. Blackwell Scientific Publications, Oxford
2. Kanto J, Erkkola R 1984 Obstetric analgesia: pharmacokinetics and its relation to neonatal behaviour and adaptive functions. Biol Res Preg 5: 23–35
3. Pedersen H, Santos H C, Morishima H Q, Finster M, Plosker H, Arthur G R, Covino B G 1988 Does gestational age affect the pharmacokinetics and pharmacodynamics of lidocaine in mother and fetus? Anesthesiology 68: 367–372
4. Notarianni L J 1981 Placental transfer of pethidine and bupivacaine. Neuropharmacology 20: 1253–1258
5. Thomas J, Climie C R, Mather L E 1969 Maternal plasma levels and placental transfer of bupivacaine following epidural anaesthesia. Br J Anaesth 41: 1035–1040
6. Jouppila R, Jouppila P, Kotiniemi L, Puolokka J, Puukka M, Puukka R 1978 Maternal and fetal plasma bupivacaine concentrations in labour with segmental epidural analgesia. Ann Chir Gynaecol 67: 190–194
7. Cooper L V, Stephen G W, Aggett P J A 1977 Elimination of pethidine and bupivacaine in the newborn. Arch Dis Childh 52: 638–641
8. Kuhnert P M, Kuhnert B R, Stilts J M, Cross T I 1981 The use of selected ion monitoring technique to study the disposition of bupivacaine in mother, fetus, and neonate following epidural anesthesia for cesarean section. Anesthesiology 55: 611–617
9. Finster M, Pedersen H 1979 Placental transfer and fetal uptake of drugs. Br J Anaesth 51: 255–285
10. Muller-Holve W, von-Meyer L, Nagler P 1986 The concentration of bupivacaine in fetal organs during obstetrical epidural analgesia. J Perinat Med 14: 219–225
11. Datta S, Brown W U, Ostheimer G W, Wiss J B, Alper M H 1981 Epidural anesthesia for cesarean section in diabetic parturients: maternal and neonatal acid–base status and bupivacaine concentration. Anesth Analg 60: 574–578
12. Belfrage P, Raabe N, Thalme B, Berlin A 1975 Lumbar epidural analgesia with bupivacaine in labor. Determination of drug concentration and pH in fetal scalp blood and continuous fetal heart rate monitoring. Am J Obstet Gynecol 121: 360–365
13. McGuiness G A, Mershow A J, Kennedy R L, Erenberg A 1978 Epidural anesthesia with bupivacaine for cesarean section: neonatal blood levels and neurobehavioural response. Anesthesiology 49: 270–273
14. Bogod D G, Rosen M, Rees G A 1987 Extradural infusion of 0.125% bupivacaine at 10ml/hour to women during labour. Br J Anaesth 59: 325–330
15. Purdy G, Currie J, Owen H 1981 Continuous epidural analgesia in labour, comparison between 'on-demand' and regular 'top-up' injections. Br J Anaesth 59: 319–324
16. Reynolds F, Hargrave R L, Wyman J B 1973 Maternal and foetal plasma concentrations of bupivacaine after epidural blockade. Br J Anaesth 45: 1049–1053
17. Abboud T K, DerSarkissian L, Terrasi J, Murakawa K, Zhu J, Longhitano M 1987 Comparative maternal, fetal, and neonatal effects of chloroprocaine with and without epinephrine for epidural analgesia in obstetrics. Anesth Analg 66: 71–75
18. Jouppila P, Jouppila R, Kaar K, Mesila M 1977 Fetal heart rate patterns and uterine activity after segmental epidural analgesia. Br J Obstet Gynaecol 84: 481–486
19. Zaor G, Nilsson B A 1974 Low dose intermittent epidural anaesthesia with lidocaine for vaginal delivery. II. Influence on labour and foetal acid–base status. Acta Obstet Gynaecol Scand 34 (suppl); 17–30
20. Ramanathan S, Masih A-K, Rock I, Chalon J, Turndorf H 1983 Maternal and fetal effects of prophylactic hydration with crystalloids or colloids before epidural analgesia. Anesth Analg 62: 673–678
21. Kuhnert B R, Harrison M J, Linn P L, Kuhnert P M 1984 Effects of maternal epidural anesthesia on neonatal behavior. Anesth Analg 63: 301–308
22. Caritis S N, Abouleish E, Edelestone D 1980 Fetal acid–base state following spinal or epidural anaesthesia for cesarean section. Obstet Gynecol 56: 610–615
23. Ong B Y, Cohen M M, Palakniuk R J 1989 Anesthesia for Cesarean Section – effects on neonates. Anesth Analg 68: 270–275
24. Abboud T, Artal R, Sarkis F, Henriksen E H, Kammula R K 1982 Sympathoadrenal activity, maternal, fetal and neonatal responses after epidural anaesthesia in the preeclamptic patient. Am J Obstet Gynecol 144: 915–918
25. Falconer A O, Lake D M 1982 Circumstances affecting umbilical cord catecholamines at delivery. Br J Obstet Gynaecol 89: 44–49
26. Falconer A Q, Powles A B 1982 Plasma noradrenaline levels during labour. Influence of elective epidural lumbar blockade. Anaesthesia 37: 416–420
27. Shnider S M, Abboud T, Artal R, Henriksen M D, Stefani S J, Levinson G 1983 Maternal endogenous catecholamine release during labour after epidural anesthesia. Am J Obstet Gynecol 147: 13–15
28. Irestedt L, Lagercrantz H, Hjemdahl P, Hagnevik K, Belfrage P 1982 Fetal and maternal plasma catecholamine levels at elective cesarean section under general or epidural anesthesia versus vaginal delivery. Am J Obstet Gynecol 142: 1004–1010
29. Loughran P G, Moore J, Dundee J W 1986 Maternal stress response associated with cesarean delivery under general and epidural anaesthesia. Br J Obstet Gynaecol 93: 943–949
30. Newsome L R, Bramwell R S, Gurling P E 1986 Severe preeclampsia: haemodynamic effects of lumbar epidural anaesthesia. Anesth Analg 65: 31–36
31. Jouppila P, Jouppila R, Hollmen A, Koivula A 1982 Lumbar epidural analgesia to improve intervillous blood flow during labour in severe eclampsia. Obstet Gynecol 59: 158–161
32. Ramanathan J, Bottorf M, Jeter J N, Khalil M, Sibai B M 1986 The pharmacokinetics and maternal and neonatal effects of epidural lidocaine in preeclampsia. Anesth Analg 65: 120–126
33. Giles W B, Lah F X, Trudinger B J 1987 The effect of epidural anaesthesia for cesarean section on maternal uterine and fetal umbilical artery blood flow velocity waveforms. Br J Obstet Gynaecol 94: 55–59
34. Hollmen A I, Jouppila R, Jouppila P, Koivula A, Vierola H 1982 Effect of extradural analgesia using bupivacaine and 2-chloroprocaine on intervillous blood flow during normal labour. Br J Anaesth 54: 837–841
35. Huovinen K, Lehtovista P, Forss M, Kivalo I, Teramo K 1979 Changes in placental intervillous blood flow measured by the ^{133}Xenon method during lumbar epidural block for elective Cesarean Section. Acta Anaesth Scand 23: 529–533
36. Lindblad A, Bernow J, Marsal K 1987 Obstetric analgesia and fetal aortic blood flow during labour. Br J Obstet Gynaecol 94: 306–311
37. Lindblad A, Bernow J, Vernersson E, Marsal K 1987 The effects of epidural anaesthesia on human fetal blood flow in utero. Comparison of three local anaesthetic solutions. Br J Anaesth 59: 1265–1272

38. Crawford J S 1987 A prospective study of 200 consecutive twin deliveries. Anaesthesia 42: 33–43
39. Weekes A R L, Cheridjan V E, Mwanje D K 1977 Lumbar epidural analgesia in labour in twin pregnancy. Br Med J 2: 730–732
40. David H, Rosen M 1976 Perinatal mortality after epidural analgesia. Anesthesia 31: 1054–1059
41. Magno R, Kjellmer I, Karlsson K 1976 Anesthesia for cesarean section. III. Effects of epidural analgesia on the respiratory adaptation of the newborn in elective cesarean section. Acta Anaesth Scand 20: 73–82
42. Pearson J E, Davies P 1974 The effect of continuous lumbar epidural analgesia upon fetal acid–base status during the first stage of labour. J Obstet Gynaecol Br Cwlth 81: 971–974
43. Pearson J F, Davies P 1974 The effect of continuous epidural analgesia upon fetal acid–base status during the second stage of labour. J Obstet Gynaecol Cwlth 81: 975–979
44. Thalme B, Belfrage P, Raabe N 1974 Lumbar epidural analgesia in labour. I. Acid–base balance and clinical condition of mother, fetus and newborn child. Acta Obstet Gynaecol Scand 53: 27–35
45. Thalme B, Belfrage P, Raabe N 1974 Lumbar epidural analgesia in labour. Acta Obstet Gynecol Scand 53: 113–119
46. Jouppila R, Hollmen A 1976 The effect of segmental epidural analgesia on maternal and fetal acid–base balance, lactate, serum potassium and creatine phosphokinase during labour. Acta Anaesth Scand 20: 259–268
47. Swanstrom S, Bratteby L E 1981 Metabolic effects of obstetric analgesia and of asphyxia in the newborn infant during the first two hours after birth. III. Adjustment of arterial blood gases and acid base balance. Acta Paediatr Scand 70: 811–818
48. Marx G F, Luykx W M, Cohen S 1984 Foetal–maternal status following cesarean section for foetal distress. Br J Anaesth 56: 1009–1013
49. Swanstrom S, Bratteby L E 1981 Metabolic effects of obstetric regional analgesia and of asphyxia in the newborn infant during the first two hours after birth. II. Arterial plasma concentrations of glycerol, free fatty acids and beta-hydroxybutyrate. Acta Paediatr Scand 70: 801–809
50. Zagorzycki M T, Brinkman C R 1982 The effect of general and epidural anaesthesia upon neonatal Apgar scores in repeat Cesarean section. Surg Gynecol Obstet 155: 641–645
51. Crawford J S, Davies P 1982 Status of neonates delivered by elective Cesarean section. Br J Anaesth 54: 1015–1022
52. Wingate M, Wingate L, Iffy L, Freundlich J, Gottsegen D 1974 The effect of epidural analgesia upon fetal and neonatal status. Am J Obstet Gynecol 119: 1101–1106
53. Downing J W, Houlton P C, Barclay A 1979 Extradural analgesia for Cesarean Section: A comparison with general anaesthesia. Br J Anaesth 51: 367–373
54. Weiner P C, Hogg M I, Rosen M 1979 Neonatal respiration, feeding and neurobehavioural state. Effects of intrapartum bupivacaine, pethidine and pethidine reversed by naloxone. Anaesthesia 34: 996–1004
55. Maltau J M, Egge K 1980 Epidural analgesia and perinatal retinal haemorrhages. Acta Anaesth Scand 24: 99–101
56. Van Zundert A, Jansen J, Vaes L, Soetens M, de Vel M, Vand der Ax P 1986 Extradural analgesia and retinal haemorrhage in the newborn. Br J Anaesth 58: 1017–1021
57. Andersen H F, Auster G H, Marx G F, Merkatz I R 1987 Neonatal status in relation to incision intervals, obstetric factors and anaesthesia at cesarean delivery. Am J Perinatol 4: 279–283
58. Yudkin P L, Jonson P, Redman C W 1987 Obstetric factors associated with cord blood gas values at birth. Eur J Obstet Gynecol Reprod Biol 24: 167–176
59. Lieberman B A, Rosenblatt D B, Belsey E M et al 1979 The effects of maternally administered pethidine or epidural bupivacaine on the fetus and newborn. Br J Obstet Gynaecol 86: 598–606
60. Zilianti M, Salazar J R, Aller J, Aquero O 1970 Fetal heart rate and pH of fetal capillary blood during epidural analgesia in labour. Obstet Gynecol 36: 881–886
61. McDonald J S, Bjorkman L L, Reed E C 1974 Epidural analgesia for obstetrics; a maternal, fetal and neonatal study. Am J Obstet Gynecol 120: 1055–1065
62. Antoine C, Young B K 1982 Fetal lactic acidosis with epidural anaesthesia. Am J Obstet Gynecol 142: 55–59
63. Thomas P, Buckley P, Fox M 1984 Maternal and neonatal blood glucose after crystalloid loading for epidural Caesarean section. Anesthesiology 39: 1240–1242
64. Jaschevatzky O E, Shalit A, Levy Y, Greenstein S 1977 Epidural analgesia during labour in twin pregnancy. Br J Obstet Gynaecol 84: 327–331
65. Studd J W W, Crawford J S, Duigman N M, Rowbotham C F J, Hughes A O 1980 The effect of lumbar epidural analgesia on the rate of cervical dilatation and the outcome of labour of spontaneous onset. Br J Obstet Gynaecol 87: 1015–1021
66. Sepkoski L M 1985 Maternal obstetric medication and newborn behaviour. In: Scanlon J W (ed) Perinatal anesthesia. Blackwell Scientific Publications, Oxford
67. Harrison R F, Cullen R 1986 A comparative study of the behaviour of the neonate following various forms of maternal intrapartum analgesia and anaesthesia. Ir J Med Sci 155: 12–18
68. Tronick E, Wise S, Als H, Adamson L, Scanlon J, Brazelton T B 1976 Regional anaesthesia and newborn behaviour: effect over the first ten days of life. Pediatrics 58: 94–100
69. Scanlon J W, Brown W U, Weiss J B, Alper M H 1974 Neurobehavioural responses of newborn infants after maternal epidural anesthesia. Anesthesiology 40: 121–128
70. Abboud T K, Sarkis F, Blikian A, Varakian L, Earl S, Henriksen E 1983 Lack of adverse neonatal neurobehavioural effects of lidocaine. Anesth Analg 62: 473–475
71. Scanlon J W, Ostheimer G W, Lurie A O, Brown W U Jr, Weiss J B, Alper M H 1976 Neurobehavioural responses and drug concentrations in newborns after maternal epidural anesthesia with bupivacaine. Anesthesia 45: 400–405
72. Kangas-Saanla T, Jouppila R, Jouppila P, Hollmen A, Pukka M, Juujarvi K 1987 The effect of segmental epidural analgesia on the neurobehavioural responses of newborn infants. Acta Anaesth Scand 31: 347–351
73. Abboud T K, Najuppala S, Murakawa K, Daird S, Hasoutunian S, Zarakian M 1985 Comparison of the effects of general and regional analgesia for cesarean section on neonatal neurologic and adaptive capacity stores. Anesth Analg 64: 996–1000
74. Corke B C 1977 Neurobehavioural responses of the newborn. The effect of different forms of maternal analgesia. Anaesthesia 32: 539–543
75. Carrie I E S, O'Sullivan G M, Lugolin R 1981 Epidural fentanyl in labour. Anesthesia 36: 965–969
76. Heytens L, Cammu H, Camu F 1987 Extradural analgesia during labour using alfentanil. Br J Anaesth 59: 331–337
77. Celleno D, Capogna G 1988 Epidural fentanyl plus bupivacaine 0.125 per cent for labour: analgesic effects. Can J Anaesth 35: 375–378
78. Cohen S E, Tan S, Albright G A, Halpern J 1986 Epidural fentanyl/bupivacaine combinations for labour analgesia: effect of varying dosage. Anaesthesiology 65: A368
79. Justins D M, Francis D, Houlton P G, Reynolds F 1982 A controlled trial of extradural fentanyl in labour. Br J Anaesth 54: 409–414
80. Youngstrom P, Eastwood D, Patel H, Bhatia R, Cowan R, Sutheimer C 1984 Epidural fentanyl and bupivacaine in labor: double blind study. Anesthesiology 61: A414

24. Evaluation of the parturient for epidural analgesia and anesthesia

J. Seebacher M. Henry Y. Darbois

Epidural anesthesia for delivery is requested by the parturient to alleviate the pain of labor. The methods of epidural anesthesia described have been developed to provide safe, easily managed analgesia and anesthesia.[1–3] The benefits as well as the risks of epidural anesthesia will be outlined, as one must always be aware of the complications that may arise.

INFORMATION AND EVALUATION PRIOR TO EPIDURAL ANALGESIA

Information – examination

The parturient is informed about the administration of analgesia using an epidural catheter while the anesthesiologist takes a history and conducts a physical examination prior to administering any anesthetic.

Information

The patient should be informed of the advantages and disadvantages of epidural analgesia. This can take place in a group situation, which has the benefit of making explanations less dramatic, or individually with particularly anxious parturients. However, consent should be obtained privately.

Consultations

Anesthetic consultations have developed in France. Of course, not all parturients can be seen in the large centers, but it may be prudent to see those presenting with, for example:

1. disease likely to affect the technical intervention, such as scoliosis;
2. cardiac or hypertensive disease, which may require medical intervention, invasive cardiac monitoring or other special consideration.

If necessary, these patients may be admitted for a thorough work-up. To facilitate the selection of those patients requiring a consultation with an anesthesiologist, parturients are asked to reply to a questionnaire when they attend their first antenatal class.

The parturient should be re-examined in the labor room.

Anesthetic evaluation

The first evaluation of the parturient, after appropriate history is obtained, is clinical, with attention to potential technical difficulties and anesthetic complications. Laboratory tests, radiographs, or other information suggested by the history and physical examination should be obtained. A statement must be made about the status of the airway.

Examination

A thorough examination should include inspection of the back, looking for evidence of scoliosis or vertebral malformation. Wide variations in the different axes of the spine will be present in parturients with neurologic disease such as poliomyelitis and various myopathies. One should look for evidence of infection and coagulopathy, both contraindications to epidural analgesia.

Localized and systemic infection must be evaluated at the time of epidural placement. Similarly, one must determine the potential risk of infection in the presence of chorioamnionitis and premature rupture of membranes. At the Pitié Hospital, we agree to carry out epidural analgesia in parturients with a temperature below 38°C in the absence of maternal or fetal infection. If the patient develops fever during labor under epidural analgesia, then penicillin is administered intravenously and appropriate antibiotic therapy is continued after delivery. An infection contraindicates the placement of an epidural, while premature rupture of membranes and fever >38°C should be discussed by the anesthesia team on call. To determine the presence of an undiagnosed coagulopathy, the parturient may be questioned about incidents following cuts, menstruation or minor surgery. Some coagulation disorders existing prior to pregnancy (hereditary) may be corrected by the hypercoagulation of pregnancy. They can reappear as early as 48 hs postpartum, therefore laboratory coagulation tests are required during pregnancy and delivery in order to monitor the status of the coagulation system; when results are within normal limits, epidural placement is permissible.

If the parturient is receiving prophylactic anticoagulant treatment it can be stopped so that the epidural catheter may be placed as soon as hemostasis is normal. If the patient is receiving anticoagulant medication in curative doses this should not be stopped and an epidural block will not be administered.

Preeclampsia can accompany coagulation disorders; epidural analgesia can be administered if:

- the platelet count is greater than 100 000 and the prothrombin time and partial thromboplastin time are normal;
- if the platelet count is less than 100 000, epidural analgesia should be considered with a normal hemostatic test not more than 3 h old.

Currently, some patients receive small preventive doses of aspirin as antiaggregation therapy. Epidural analgesia can be administered if the platelet count is normal and if there are no general or obstetric hemorrhagic symptoms. An elevation of the bleeding time does not necessarily indicate poor-quality platelet aggregation.

If the history and physical examination show no signs or symptoms of coagulopathy, the patient can be considered to have normal hemostatic mechanisms. If labor progresses normally, epidural analgesia may be administered without the laboratory tests. Coagulation studies will be done when hemorrhage, regardless of the cause, is present, when there is a history of preeclampsia, aspirin therapy or anticoagulant treatment or when any doubt exists after examination.

Preparation

It is essential that the severity of a patient's disease, for example cardiac disease, be evaluated to anticipate the required monitoring and ensure the patient's safety during labor.

Contraindications/indications

Contraindications to epidural analgesia should be discussed with the obstetric team and explained to the parturient calmly, answering questions clearly. An example of a relative contraindication is multiple sclerosis.[4] At the Pitié-Salpétrière Hospital we provide epidural analgesia for these patients if all parties involved agree (e.g. the neurologist, the obstetrician, the anesthesiologist and the patient). It is necessary to give the patient adequate information about the risks associated with epidural placement; in the end, it is the patient who decides whether or not to accept this type of analgesia.

Obstetric evaluation

Epidural analgesia is administered at different stages of labor but, traditionally, analgesia is suggested when cervical dilation is 4 cm, labor is well established and the head is engaged in the pelvis.

Analgesia

At the Pitié Hospital,[5] analgesia is administered at any stage of labor. When analgesics are administered in the first stage (dilation <2 cm, spontaneous or induced contractions, non-engaged fetal head), care should be taken to avoid dystocia induced by anesthesia. At a later stage – 9 cm dilation or more – every precaution should be taken to ensure that safety is maintained throughout technical interventions.

Analgesia – induction of labor

Obstetricians often ask for epidural analgesia early for pain associated with contractions induced by oxytocin. Induction of labor is suggested:

- for medical reasons; delivery is accomplished vaginally or via cesarean delivery;
- if desired by the parturient, provided that conditions are satisfactory for induction (e.g. adequate cervical maturity).

Treatment of dystocia

Epidural analgesia is extremely useful in cases of dystocia and cervical dystocia when the cervix is rigid and dilation is painful.

To avoid bearing-down efforts

Epidural analgesia is helpful with forceps extraction and to reduce stress during delivery in patients with cardiac disease, for example.

In straightforward cases, the anesthesiologist and the obstetrician should evaluate the parturient's condition in the labor room.

MANAGEMENT ON ARRIVAL IN THE LABOR ROOM

After epidural analgesia is requested by the parturient and

obstetrician and deemed appropriate by the anesthesiologist, the parturient is acutely hydrated and the epidural catheter carefully placed.

Organization of the labor room

Epidural analgesia requires the availability of oxygen, a face mask, a blood pressure cuff and fetal monitoring. The appropriate emergency equipment must be readily available. It helps to have a spacious labor room with a bed capable of position changes.

Equipment for epidural analgesia

We use a mobile trolley to store epidural trays, local anesthetics, needles, syringes and catheters.

Equipment for supervision

Both parturient and fetus need to be monitored throughout the epidural anesthetic, primarily because of the cardiovascular changes often encountered. The blood pressure and heart rate of the mother must be monitored, as must the fetal heart rate. This may involve the use of an external or internal fetal scalp electrode.

Equipment for emergency

Each labor room should have an oxygen supply and functioning suction at all times. Resuscitation equipment should be immediately available, and must include a functioning laryngoscope, endotracheal tubes, Ambu bag and mask, as well as medications such as ephedrine, epinephrine, atropine, thiopental, benzodiazepines and muscle relaxants.

Management of the parturient

Vital signs should be recorded on an anesthetic record, with appropriate documentation of epidural placement and medication administration. An intravenous infusion of crystalloid is begun when the parturient is admitted to the labor room, and should be maintained until the patient is stable post partum.

In the parturient with major medical problems, a bolus of 500–1000 ml of crystalloid prior to epidural placement tends to eliminate hemodynamic changes. In addition, administration of 30 ml of nonparticulate antacid reduces the risk of aspiration pneumonitis in the event of a complication.

PREVENTION OF COMPLICATIONS/INCIDENTS

Arterial hypotension is rare in the first stage of labor and, when it occurs, is related to **venocaval** obstruction: the patient must be maintained in the lateral position. As doses increase and sympathetic block spreads, the effects of vasodilation should be prevented with maternal hydration and treated when necessary (arterial hypotension with variations in fetal heart rate) by repeated doses of ephedrine.

The treatment of the most serious complications or intravascular injection or extensive spinal anesthesia is outlined in several other chapters. Emergency equipment required must be immediately available.

MANAGEMENT DURING LABOR

Anesthetic and obstetric supervision

Anesthetic control is correlated with obstetric management throughout labor (Fig. 24.1). Supervision of the epidural analgesia and the obstetric situation during labor

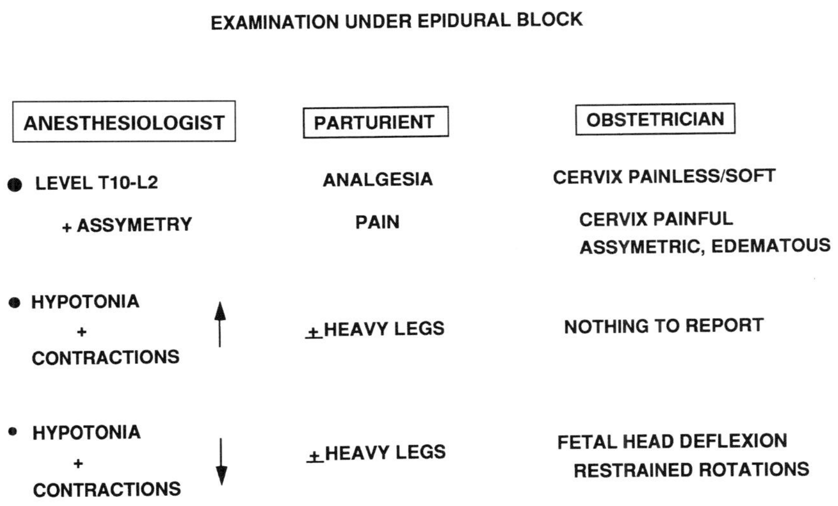

Fig. 24.1 Injection and reinjection.

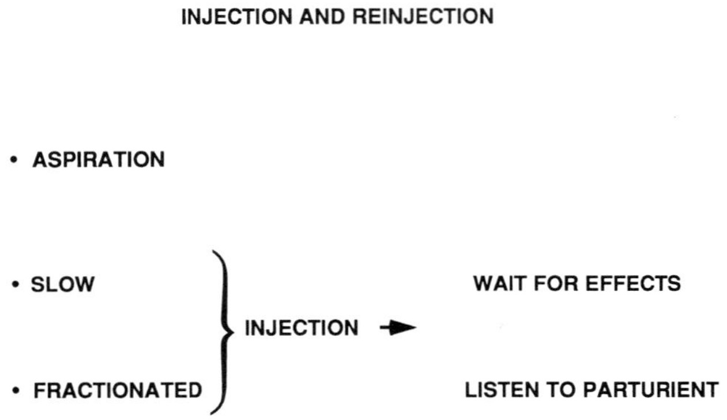

Fig. 24.2 Examination under epidural block.

is made by the midwives trained in epidural analgesia in our institution.[6] The supervision is the responsibility of the anesthesiologist and the obstetrician.

After the first anesthetic assessment, monitoring is regular and frequent. When top-ups are given, the same precautions are taken with each reinjection as with the first (Fig. 24.2). When analgesia is administered, the quality of the analgesia and degree of motor impairment should be monitored every hour, with attention to disappearance of analgesia (suspect intravascular injection) and motor impairment (suspect subarachnoid injection). If an unexpected event occurs, an anesthesiologist should be called. Hourly obstetric examination is appropriate. When dystocia is suspected, the obstetric assessment will indicate whether this is true dystocia or analgesia-induced dystocia (Fig. 24.1). Induced dystocia can, in some cases, be diminished by reducing doses of epidural analgesia or by adding opioids. The anesthesiologist should be available for readjustment and evaluation of insufficient analgesia.

EVOLUTION OF EPIDURAL ANALGESIA

At present, epidural analgesia is the most effective form of pain relief we can offer our patients. Improved knowledge of the effects of this analgesia and its interaction with obstetric management has led all teams to modify their methods.

The concentrations of local anesthetic used for epidural analgesia are decreasing, while maintaining the same beneficial effects during the course of labor. Analgesia is maintained by adding opioids at doses which have no respiratory depressant effect on either the mother or the fetus, but may sometimes induce dysphoria.

The safety of parturients is ensured by rigorous assessment, perfect technical interventions and by simple and efficient organization by a well-trained team. The obstetrician should know what to expect of the analgesia and the anesthesiologist should in turn be able to respond to the obstetric demand. In these circumstances, epidural analgesia is an effective and safe technique for the mother and the newborn.

REFERENCES

1. Bonica J J 1972 Principles and practice of obstetric analgesia and anesthesia. F A Davis, Philadelphia.
2. Bromage P R 1978 Epidural analgesia. Saunders, Philadelphia
3. Shnider S M, Levinson G, Ralston D H 1987 Regional anesthesia for labor and delivery. In: Shnider S M, Levinson G (eds) Anesthesia for obstetrics. Williams & Wilkins, Baltimore pp 135–156
4. Abouleish E 1988 Neurologic disease. In: James III F M, Wheeler A S, Dewan D M (eds) obstetric anesthesia: the complicated patient. F A Davis, Philadelphia
5. Seebacher J, Galli-Douani P, Henry M et al 1990 Anesthésie péridurale et rachianesthésie en obstétrique. In: Lecron L (ed) anesthésie loco-régionale. Arnette, Paris pp 839–886
6. Crawford J S 1984 Principles and practice of obstetric anesthesia. Blackwell Scientific Publications, Oxford

SECTION 3

Alternatives to epidural anesthesia for obstetric pain relief during labor and vaginal delivery

25. 'Prepared' childbirth – the new direction in natural childbirth: maternal considerations and psychologic approaches

D. E. Stewart

INTRODUCTION

Most women approaching labor and delivery have common fears related to their ability to bear the pain, the possibility of medical complications and the baby's health.[1,2] These fears are not limited to women in industrialized societies for virtually every culture has invented chants, incantations, rituals and pseudomedical procedures in an attempt to counteract labor pain.[3] The image of the primitive woman having a painless birth and returning to the fields is a myth. The 'natural' childbirth movement, now fortunately maturing into the 'prepared' childbirth movement in industrialized societies, is an attempt to reduce fear, anxiety, and tension by helping the pregnant woman and her partner gain some control over the pain of labor by implementing previously learned coping techniques. This sense of 'control' is central to this issue as the laboring woman fears loss of control over her body, her emotions and her birth attendants.[4] It is known from other studies on acute and chronic pain management that the implementation of previously learned coping techniques such as relaxation, attention focusing, deep breathing, cognitive coping skills, biofeedback and stress inoculation training may result in reduced perception of pain severity or less associated psychologic distress.[5] It is not surprising that many of these techniques are being applied to labor pain, which has been shown by Melzack and colleagues[3,6,7] to be among the most intense pains recorded in systematic studies with the McGill Pain Questionnaire.

HISTORIC PERSPECTIVE ON THE DEVELOPMENT OF NATURAL CHILDBIRTH PROGRAMS

To fully understand the zealous attitudes of some natural childbirth advocates it is helpful to examine the historic context in which they developed. Paralleling the transition of birth from home to hospital in North America in the middle of the nineteenth century came the arrival of the obstetrician replacing the lay midwife, and the development of obstetric analgesia/anesthesia. By 1848 the American Medical Association Committee on Obstetrics was able to proudly report the successful use of ether and chloroform in about 2000 deliveries with 'few, if any, untoward effects'.[8] By 1902 morphine and scopolamine were used to produce 'twilight sleep', and, by 1924, barbiturates were advocated to produce sedation in labor. The next 30 years saw a plethora of drugs advocated in labor often resulting in polypharmacy cocktails, administered by physicians with no special training in pain management who were often unaware of the effects of these drugs on the woman and her newborn.[9] The increased use of heavy sedation during labor and delivery was accompanied by increased and sometimes harmful and unwarranted obstetric interventions, a situation that an increasing number of women found unacceptable.[10]

The natural childbirth movement developed in the 1940s as an organized demonstration of the dissatisfaction that many women felt with their childbirth experiences. The challenge of the natural childbirth movement was that the psychologic and physical aspects of birth should both be valued, and the woman and her physician should share control of her labor and delivery.[11] It was in this social environment that Grantly Dick-Read wrote *Childbirth Without Fear*,[12] in which he described two kinds of childbirth pain: primary pain related to the mechanism of birth and secondary pain caused by fear and tension. Despite Dick-Read's enthusiasm for childbirth education, hygiene, nutrition, relaxation, and controlled breathing, he also believed there was a definite place for anesthesia–analgesia in childbirth as he felt that 'no woman in labour should be allowed to suffer pain'.[12] His followers, however, chose to disregard his support for medications, believing that adherence to their protocol would abolish the need for analgesia.

The late 1950s saw the publication by a French obstetrician, Ferdinand Lamaze, of a book called *Painless Childbirth* (psychoprophylaxis) based on a Pavlovian model of development of new conditioned reflexes.[13]

This method consisted in childbirth education plus seven cognitive or behavioral components: structured breathing, relaxation, attention focal points, self-massage (effleurage), assistance of a coach, rehearsal under stress, and systematic practice.[5] Lamaze felt that fear was the primary cause of labor pain and that with his method 'harmful drugs and anesthetics can be eliminated'.[13] A variety of other methods and modifications for natural birth were described over the next 20 years.[14–17] The Lamaze method and later modifications flourished in a social climate characterized by increased education and awareness of women about their bodies and a climate of medical and obstetric consumerism. The effects of feminism on women's assertiveness and empowerment were also vitally important in their widespread acceptance.

PRINCIPLES AND PRACTICE OF PREPARED CHILDBIRTH PROGRAMS

The 40 years between 1940 and 1980 were the zenith of the 'natural' childbirth programs. Gradually during the 1980s increasing numbers of childbirth educators and women wondered aloud whether total reliance on psychologic relaxation techniques was optimal or even adequate for all childbirths, and whether all pain could be abolished by the prescribed protocols of the current childbirth guru. There was evidence that Lamaze techniques could reduce pain by approximately 10%,[3,6,7] and that psychologic preparation was valuable, but the comfort, effectiveness, and relative safety of epidural anesthesia was also appealing for many women.[7] However, there was also a fear that to embrace wholeheartedly the medical model of childbirth would mean a return to the unacceptable state that existed prior to the advent of natural childbirth programs of the 1940s. Most modern women do not want to be unconscious and 'delivered' but rather awake, pain-free, in control and 'giving birth'. In this climate, the emphasis has gradually been changing away from 'natural' *vs.* 'medical' delivery, to how best obstetricians, anesthesiologists, prepared childbirth trainers, obstetric nurses and the woman and her partner can work together to achieve a safe, comfortable and psychologically rewarding labor and delivery.

Many childbirth educators who eschewed the doctrines of a particular method and tried to accurately present the pros and cons of obstetric interventions, obstetric anesthesia/analgesia and psychologic techniques began to refer to their practices as 'prepared childbirth programs'. Triolo[11] has pointed out that the variety of prepared childbirth methods that have evolved all share four common principles: (1) to prepare the pregnant woman for labor, delivery, and childcare; (2) to relieve anxiety and augment relaxation during labor and delivery; (3) to reduce or abolish pain or pain perception, thus reducing the need for analgesia and anesthesia; and (4) to allow the expectant mother to experience an alert state during birth, thus allowing immediate contact with the infant to facilitate bonding.

However, there continues to exist a wide variety of programs based on different assumptions, strategies, and techniques and even wide variations between different instructors in the same programs, all of which may be collected under the designation of 'prepared' childbirth.

RESEARCH ON OUTCOME OF PREPARED CHILDBIRTH EDUCATION

Beck and Hall,[18] in a 1978 review and analysis of 'natural childbirth', commented: 'With respect to psychoprophylaxis in childbirth, opinion has undergone a steady polarization almost since its introduction; it has been acclaimed as one of the most significant advances of modern medicine and as a primitive and medically unacceptable practice. Even more disturbing than the polarization itself is the fact that the process has occurred in the absence of a single adequately controlled study of the therapeutic outcome.' Little has changed in the intervening years, since most of the numerous studies that have appeared continue to suffer from serious methodologic shortcomings. Most fail to use a random assignment of patients to treatment and control groups, thus not taking into account the fact that most attenders at childbirth education classes are highly motivated, middle-class couples with positive expectations of childbirth. There is virtually never a control group who receive an attention-placebo treatment and the obstetricians are usually not blind to the preparation their patients have received. The specific details of the childbirth education programs are not given and appropriate psychologic tests used to measure pain and anxiety reduction are often not utilized. Last, but not least, many of these studies lack statistical power or fail to use appropriate statistical analyses.[18]

Beck and Hall[18] have listed a variety of claims that have been both made and refuted, including: decreased perception of pain, increased cooperation of the mother in labor, decreased incidence of post-partum depression, a more positive attitude to future pregnancies, reduced use of analgesics, reduced blood loss, reduced obstetric interventions, shorter length of labor, decreased need for neonatal resuscitation, and decreased neonatal mortality and sickness. Suffice it to say that the enormous volume of research that continues to be produced on the efficacy of prepared childbirth techniques must be analyzed carefully before drawing conclusions. One fairly robust finding by Melzack and colleagues[3,7] shows that both primiparas and multiparas who have received prepared childbirth training have lower pain scores than those who have received no training, but the average scores of trained women are still very high. Moreover, the effect varies greatly with the instructor and the particular woman.

Several variables have now been shown to correlate with reduced labor pain.[19] These include multiparity, childbirth training, older age of the mother, higher socioeconomic status, psychological factors and previous absence of painful menstrual periods. Physical factors such as obstetric presentation, pelvic architecture, size of baby and weight of the mother also play an important role. Women who give birth at night have less pain[20] as do women with previous experience of pain unrelated to labor.[21,22] Finally, a study by Melzack et al[23] shows that about 35% of women feel less front pain and 50% feel less back pain when they are in a vertical position than a horizontal position during early labor (2–5 cm). During the later stages of labor however, women find lying down more comfortable.[24] In general, labor pain is affected by many physical and psychologic factors which should be considered in effective pain relief.

COMPLICATIONS WITH NATURAL CHILDBIRTH PROGRAMS

A number of authors have commented on the unrealistic expectations of labor and delivery that are encouraged by some programs.[25] Labors are extremely variable, and the 'average' labor or amount of pain means little to the individual woman. Although two systematic studies have shown that 60–70% of primiparous women suffer 'severe' to 'intolerable' pain in labor, and only 10% suffer 'mild' pain;[3] nevertheless, some programs refuse to allow the word 'pain' to be used, insisting that 'contractions', (properly managed of course), are not painful. If labor becomes painful, it seems clear from this perspective that the woman is at fault for not having adequately learned the technique. The woman then faces not only pain but a sense of failure and guilt.[3,25] Several authors suggest that accurate realistic portrayals of what will likely happen during labor are most helpful to the pregnant woman. Lumley and Astbury[2] found that some women who attended prepared childbirth education classes actually acquired unrealistic expectations regarding pain and as a consequence developed negative attitudes towards themselves, towards childbirth, as well as towards doctors and nurses. These women then judged themselves as failures because they experienced pain. Similarly I have previously reported on several women and their partners who felt disappointed by what they perceived as 'failures' during labor and delivery (epidural anesthesia, other forms of analgesia, cesarean delivery) and, as a consequence, developed depression, anxiety, or marital/sexual problems requiring psychotherapy.[25,26] In talking with these patients it was clear that unrealistic expectations of labor and delivery had been given during prenatal training classes.[25] Occasionally one sees or hears of a woman or her partner who insists on a labor or delivery being conducted exactly as planned during childbirth preparation classes, despite intervening complications. Concern sometimes arises for the safety of the mother and/or the infant leading to difficult questions of ethics and responsibility to both mother and infant.[27] I recently treated a young nurse and her husband who insisted on a vaginal delivery of a large breech baby who had previously been classified as 'high risk'. In spite of obstetric urgings, they refused a cesarean delivery until obvious (to them) signs of fetal distress developed. An emergency cesarean delivery produced a brain-dead baby who lived 36 h, leaving behind a distraught young couple who had thought 'nature is always best'. Such tragedies are fortunately rare, but many obstetricians have tales of 'near misses'.

FUTURE DIRECTIONS FOR EFFECTIVE CHILDBIRTH PREPARATION

It is always easier to criticize what exists than to offer constructive suggestions for change. It seems clear that accurate information about labor and delivery and realistic expectations of pain are vitally important aspects of childbirth preparation.[11] The major aim of prepared childbirth programs should be to do exactly as the name suggests – 'to prepare' the couple to cope with the different possibilities they may meet in labor and delivery.[25] Similarly, the great variability of labor needs to be stressed as does the need to make mid-course corrections when labor does not proceed as planned.[27] Couples should be informed the 'average' labor is a statistical concept and that many women will deviate from this pattern. Women should be prepared for deviations that sometimes occur in labor and the possibility that they may *need* an analgesic, epidural anesthetic, or obstetric intervention.[3,11] Discussion should focus on the goal of providing the most comfortable, psychologically fulfilling, and safest labor for mother and infant.[25]

Prepared childbirth training and obstetric anesthesia are compatible and complementary procedures aimed at assisting women in childbirth to suffer less fear, anxiety, and pain.[3] A balanced view of the benefits and problems associated with the various forms of epidural anesthesia in labor should take into account the fact that labor is often extremely painful, causing reflex increases in blood pressure and oxygen consumption and liberation of catecholamines – all of which may decrease uterine blood flow.[1,26] Some of these effects of severe pain can be dangerous to the woman with cardiovascular problems, and to the fetus whose oxygen supply may be at risk during a protracted and complicated labor and delivery. Bonica[28,29] has shown that epidural anesthesia increases uterine blood flow, particularly in patients with pregnancy-induced hypertension, toxemia and other disorders that decrease placental function. Alternatively, epidural anesthesia diminishes the reflex urge to bear down and is associated with a higher rate of forceps or operative delivery. Unintentional puncture of the dura may also occur, causing postdural puncture headache, or, more seriously, the anesthetic may be injected into the subarachnoid space, resulting in an ascending level of anesthesia that may be temporarily dangerous. As approximately 10% of epidural blocks are ineffective depending on the skill and experience of the anesthesiologist, thus the unfortunate woman with a failed epidural block is often angry, disappointed, and fearful.[3] Information about analgesic/anesthetic options should preferably be presented by an anesthesiologist or, failing that, by someone who is knowledgeable and unbiased about their use in labor, as negative attitudes about the pharmacologic management of pain in labor are counterproductive.[11]

Although relaxation, structured breathing, attention focal points, coaching, and rehearsal have all been shown to be effective in increasing pain tolerance in labor,[30] a variety of newer cognitive-behavioral, biofeedback approaches are also promising but as yet unvalidated in labor.[5] These need to be further evaluated using methodologically sound designs. Melzack[3] has stated that the prepared childbirth movement's emphasis on pain has been 'misleading and unfortunate', and he sees the future of the movement resting on 'the advances of psychology in the field of individual differences, in responses to anxiety and stress, in the development and use of coping strategies and in the tendency to attribute control over events to one self or others'.

It is important that individualized programs in childbirth education are developed taking into account the woman's unique fears and preferences, pain threshold, ability to cope with stress, and education level. It is critical that accurate appraisal and evaluation of programs occur, assessing content and instructional methods, as well as basic qualifications of instructors, who at present range from untrained volunteer mothers to highly qualified nurse/educators.[11]

Finally, open honest communication is vitally important between the pregnant and laboring woman and all her health care providers. A trusting, mutually respectful setting is the most conducive environment for the woman and her partner to allow themselves the flexibility to change labor and delivery plans should the need arise. It is also the best possible setting for them to enjoy the miracle of birth.

REFERENCES

1. Bonica J J 1980 Obstetrics analgesia and anesthesia. World Federation of Societies of Anesthesiologists, Amsterdam
2. Lumley J, Astbury J 1980 Birth rites, birth rights. Sphere Books, Melbourne
3. Melzack R 1984 The myth of painless childbirth. Pain 19: 321–337
4. Lederman R 1984 Psychosocial adaptation in pregnancy. Prentice-hall, Englewood Cliffs, New Jersey pp 144–170
5. Tan S Y 1982 Cognitive and cognitive-behavioral methods for pain control: a selective review. Pain 12: 201–228
6. Melzack R, Kinch R A, Dobkin P, Lebrum M, Taenzer P 1984 Severity of labour pain: influence of physical as well as psychological variables. Can Med Assoc J 130: 579–584
7. Melzack R, Taenzer P, Feldman P, Kinch R P 1981 Labour is still painful after prepared childbirth training. Can Med Assoc J 125: 357–363
8. Speert H 1980 Obstetrics and gynecology in America: a history. Waverly Press, Baltimore pp 1380
9. Myers R E, Myers S E 1979 Use of sedative, analgesia and anesthetic drugs during labor and delivery: bane or boon? Am J Obstet 133: 83–104
10. Shorter E 1982 A history of women's bodies. Penguin, Middlesex pp 139–176
11. Triolo P K 1987 Prepared childbirth. Clin Obstet Gynecol 30: 487–494
12. Dick-Read G 1944 Childbirth without fear. Harper, New York
13. Lamaze F 1958 Painless childbirth (C B Celestin, translator). Burke, London
14. Chertok L 1967 Psychosomatic methods of preparation for childbirth. Am J Obstet Gynecol 98: 698–706
15. Leboyer F 1975 Birth without violence. Rigby Ltd, Adelaide, Australia
16. Bradley C, Brewin C R, Duncan S L 1983 Perceptions of labour. Br J Obst Gynaecol 90: 1176–1179
17. Odent M 1983 Birth under water. Lancet 1: 1476–1477
18. Beck N C, Hall D 1978 Natural childbirth. A review and analysis. Obstet Gynecol 52: 371–379
19. Melzack R 1993 Labour pain as a model of acute pain. Pain 53: 117–120
20. Harkness J, Gijsbers K 1989 Pain and stress during childbirth and time of day. Ethol Sociobiol 10: 255–261
21. Niven C, Gijsbers K 1984 A study of labour pain using the McGill Pain Questionnaire. Soc Sci Med 19: 1347–1351
22. Niven C, Gijsbers K 1989 Do low levels of labour pain reflect low sensitivity to noxious stimulation? Soc Sci Med 29: 585–588
23. Melzack R, Belanger E, Lacroix R 1991 Labor pain: effect of maternal position on front and back pain. Pain Sympt Manag 6: 476–480
24. Roberts J, Melasanos L, Mendez-Bauer C 1981 Maternal positions in labor: analysis in relation to comfort and efficacy. Birth Defects 17: 97–128
25. Stewart D E 1985 Possible relationship of post-partum psychiatric symptoms to childbirth education programmes. J Psychosom Obstet Gynecol 4: 295–301
26. Stewart D E 1982 Psychiatric symptoms following attempted natural childbirth. Can Med Assoc J 127: 713–716
27. Black J S 1983 Ethics and responsibility – experience with natural childbirth. Med J Aust 2: 116–117
28. Bonica J J 1967 Principles and practice of obstetric analgesia and anesthesia, Vols 1 and 2. F A Davis, Philadelphia
29. Bonica J J 1984 Labour pain. In: P D Wall and R Melzack (eds) Textbook of pain. Churchill Livingstone, Edinburgh
30. Worthington Jr E L, Martin G A 1980 A laboratory analysis of response to pain after training in three Lamaze techniques. J Psychosom Res 24: 109–116

26. Hypnosis

F. M. Ferrante R. C. Chantigian D. H. Wallace

Hypnosis (*hypnos*, sleep) can produce analgesia and amnesia during labor and delivery for some selected patients.[1–5]

The technique of hypnosis has been used for many centuries. Its origin is lost in antiquity. The term was coined in 1843 by James Braid, who recognized that suggestion was the basis of hypnosis.[1,2,4,6]

The subject who is hypnotized appears to be asleep. Her eyes are closed, and she appears very relaxed. In actuality, she is not asleep, but very much awake and deeply concentrating. Her eyes are closed to assist in concentration and relaxation. This state of deep concentration is called a *trance*. Once the trance state is achieved, the subject becomes highly responsive to suggestions. Suggestions are the key to hypnosis, because through them the subject can select the sensory input she wishes to obtain.[1,2,4–8]

In obstetrics, the woman who is hypnotized enters a relaxed, deeply concentrating state in which pleasurable sensations are suggested and reinforced and unpleasant sensations are transformed to more tolerable or pleasurable thoughts. For example, contractions are not pain, they are tenseness of the abdomen; bearing down is felt as pressure.[4]

The ability to reach the degree of concentration needed for labor and delivery requires a lot of time, a minimum of several training sessions, and a skilled hypnotist.[1,2,4,6] The sessions are held either in private or in groups, depending on the situation.

Those involved in the care of a patient who is hypnotized should bear in mind that she is deeply concetrating.[2] Thus, care must be taken to keep noise to a minimum and to administer sedatives and tranquilizers judiciously, as they may reduce the ability to concentrate.[8]

REFERENCES

1. Abouleish E 1977 Pain control in obstetrics. J B Lippincott, Philadelphia, p 365–382
2. Bonica J J 1967 Principles and practice of obstetric analgesia and anesthesia. F A Davis, Philadelphia
3. Bonica J J 1980 Obstetric analgesia and anesthesia. World Federation of Societies of Anesthesiologists, Amsterdam
4. Kroger W S 1979 Clinical and experimental hypnosis, 2nd edn. J B Lippincott, Philadelphia
5. Martin J 1983 Hypnosis gains legitimacy, respect, in diverse clinical specialties. J Am Med Assoc 249: 319–321
6. Collins V J 1976 Principles of anesthesiology, 2nd edn. Lea & Febiger, Philadelphia
7. Cousins M J, Bridenbaugh P O 1980 Neural blockade in clinical anesthesia and management of pain. J B Lippincott, Philadelphia
8. Gutsche B 1978 Maternal analgesia and anesthesia for vaginal delivery. Refresher Course in Anesthesiology 6: 67–80

27. Acupuncture

J. Neumark

At present, acupuncture* is practiced in few places for pain relief during labor. Acupuncture for this purpose was only introduced in the last 20 years. Traditionally, Chinese people do not use acupuncture for pain relief in labor. Several reasons for this may be speculated. It is possible that acupuncture produces a greater degree of pain relief in the extremities and cranium than in the lower abdomen and a woman in labor may often dislocate the placed needles during labor, and as a result cause frustration to the acupuncturist. Others, especially those who recommend the use of acupuncture for this purpose, believe that its lack of use by the Chinese may result from the patriarchal system of the Chinese culture, causing male acupuncturists to ignore pain due to childbirth. Thus, it has been left to Western acupuncturists of the last two decades to discover the effects of acupuncture on pregnant women. Research in animals appears to prove that acupuncture increases the circulating levels of endorphins, as demonstrated by using naloxone to antagonize the effects of acupuncture in cats.[1] However, those who believe in acupuncture view it also as a philosophy, and there seems to be no doubt that some psychologic or even placebo effect may enhance its value. It is now known that even placebos may cause endorphin release. Only a few studies have attempted to investigate whether acupuncture has a real somatic analgesic effect during labor, but these studies failed to demonstrate analgesia produced by acupuncture.[2,3]

ACUPUNCTURE IN PREPARATION FOR CHILDBIRTH

There are some acupuncturists who offer acupuncture during preparation for childbirth before the beginning of labor. They believe that acupuncture causes a regulation of the vegetative system followed by a positive influence on the initiation of labor, on the duration of the first stage of labor, and on the experience of pain.[4,5] Since preparation for childbirth has its effects mainly via psychologic preparation which is similar to natural childbirth or hypnosis, this strengthens the opinion of those who believe that acupuncture relies at least in part on psychologic and suggestive effects.

Wiesenthal[5] recommends beginning acupuncture in preparation for childbirth at about 4 weeks before the expected time of delivery. The women have needles placed once a week using the following points: S-36, K-8, B-64 and B-67*. Kubista and Kucera[4] recommend points S-36, G-34, K-8 and B-62*, while Schuler[6] uses the points GV-20, P-6, H-7 and 'Ex-6'*.

The idea of offering acupuncture in the preparation for childbirth is so new that the recommendations of different authors concerning the needling of points differ remarkably. Time will tell whether the use of acupuncture for this purpose is only a new idea of enthusiastic acupuncturists or whether it will be able to find a place in childbirth.

ACUPUNCTURE FOR PAIN RELIEF IN LABOR

Acupuncture for pain relief in labor was introduced in the last few decades. Acupuncturists who decided to try it used their own combinations of acupuncture points that they believed would achieve the best results. In published reports the location of recommended points differs.

Abouleish and Depp[2] used needle points that are used in the treatment of dysmenorrhea, including some points which are used for cesarean delivery. They used more points than the others: S-25, S-28, CV-4, CV-6, LI-4, S-36, Sp-9, Sp-6 for the first stage of labor and GV-1, CV-1 and accessory points for the second stage. The location of these points is shown in Figure 27.1. They found that the success rate was rather poor.

Wallis et al[3] asked a Chinese acupuncturist, who was a professor and supervisor for many years at the Chinese College of Acupuncture in Hong Kong, to perform this art

* When acupuncture points are mentioned in the text, the International (English) nomenclature recommended by WHO in 1984 is used rather than the different nomenclatures used by the cited authors. If any author used a point that is unknown in the international nomenclature the original nomenclature is used but enclosed in quotation marks.

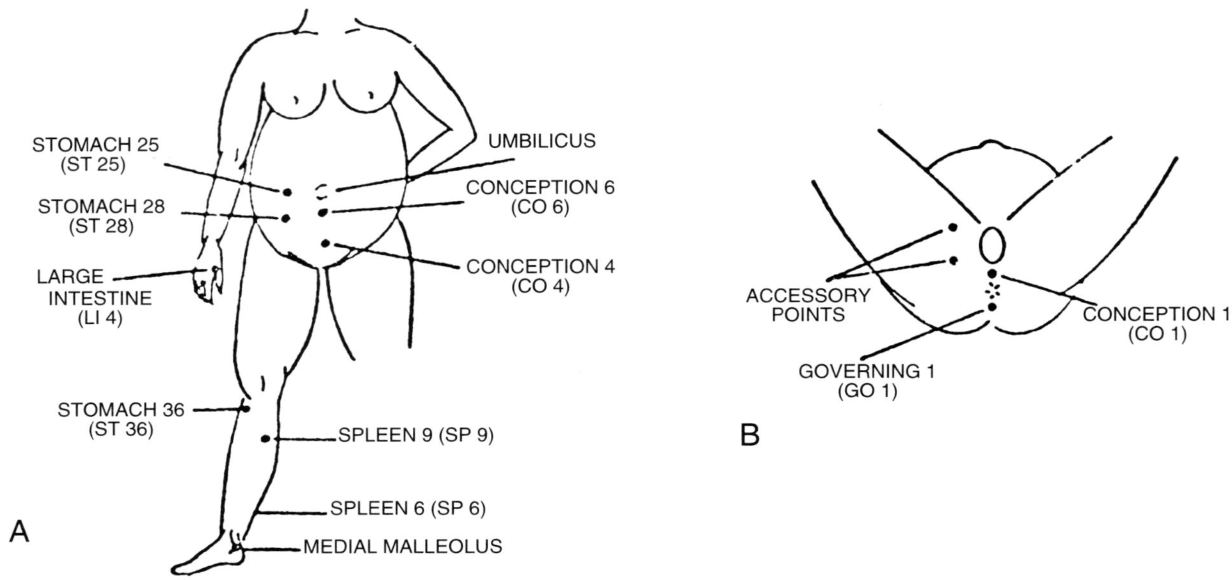

Fig. 27.1 Acupuncture points used by Abouleish and Depp[7] for pain relief in labor; reproduced with permission. (**A**) Points for uterine pain; (**B**) points for perineal pain.

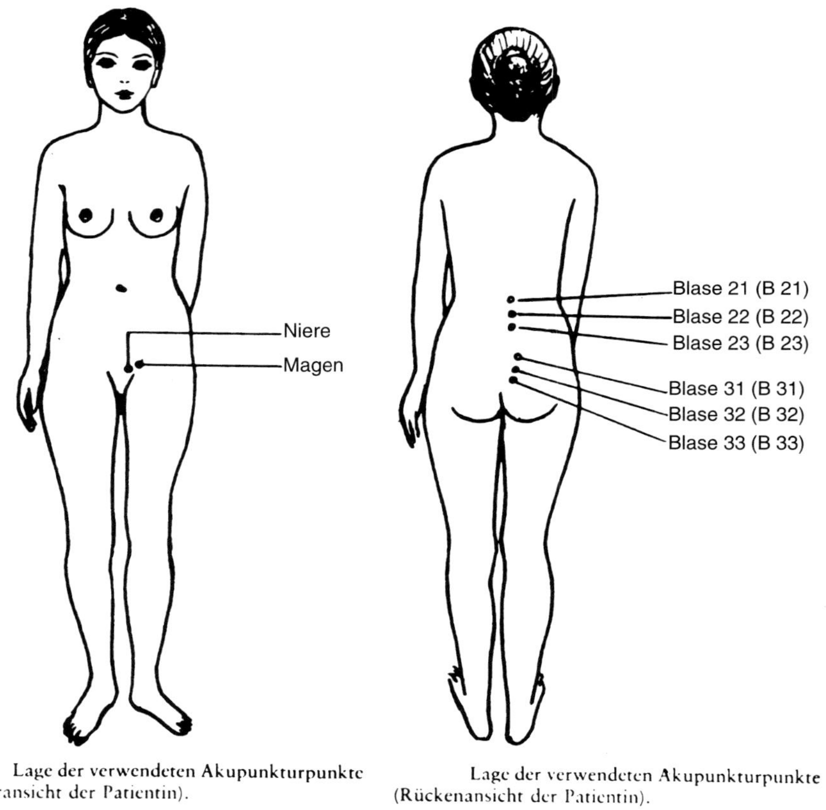

Fig. 27.2 Acupuncture points used by Kubista et al[7] for pain relief in labor; reproduced with permission.

on women in labor. They found that there was no pain relief in 19 out of 21 parturients.

On the other hand, Schuler[6] from Germany and Kubista[7] from Vienna reported a rather high success rate. Schuler does not consider acupuncture only as a somatic tool. He supports the philosophic view of acupuncture and calls his approach a 'holistic view of acupuncture'. The acupuncture points which he uses are GV-20, LI-4, 'U-Ex', Sp-6, S-36 and, in addition, G-21, G-34, Liv-3, B-37 in prolonged labor.*

Kubista[7] used points B-21, B-22, B-23, B-31, B-32, B-33, B-34, and sometimes adds S-29, CV-2, CV-3 and K-11*. The location of these points is demonstrated in Figure 27.2.

It is the author's (and the editors') conclusion that acupuncture is rather an exotic tool to provide pain relief during labor. It cannot be recommended for routine use or without any other alternative method on hand in the event it may fail to work. It may be of help in rare cases in which the patient herself believes in acupuncture and where the obstetrician is experienced in this technique and has a mental support with the philosophy of acupuncture.

ACKNOWLEDGMENTS

I would like to thank Professor Dr J Bischko, Head of the Boltzmann-Institut of Acupuncture in Vienna, for the translation of the different nomenclatures used by citated authors into the international English nomenclature recommended by WHO in 1984 and for his professional support.

REFERENCES

1. Pauser G 1980 Neurophysiologische und neuropharmakologische Untersuchungen über (mögliche) Mechanismen der peripheren Stimulationsanalgesie. Wien Klin Wschr 92 (suppl 113).
2. Abouleish E, Depp R 1975 Acupuncture in obstetrics. Anesth Analg 54: 83–88
3. Wallis L, Shnider S M, Palahniuk R J, Spivey H T 1974 An evaluation of acupuncture analgesia in obstetrics. Anesthesiology 41: 596–601
4. Kubista E, Kucera H 1973 Acupuncture preparation of primigravidae as a means of shortening labor. Am J Acupuncture 1: 181–183
5. Wiesenthal B 1987 Akupunktur zur Geburtsvorbereitung. Der Akupunkturarzt/Aurikulotherapeut 10–13
6. Schuler W 1989 Akupunktur in Geburtshilfe und Frauenheilkunde. Hippokrates, Stuttgart
7. Kubista E, Kucera H 1976 Elektroakupunktur zur Analgesie während der Geburt. Geburtsh Frauenheilkd 36: 610–613

28. Transcutaneous electrical nerve stimulation (TENS)

J. Neumark

Using nerve stimulation as a tool for pain relief is a result of the gate control theory published by Melzack in 1965.[1] This concept assumes that there is a gate-like mechanism in the dorsal column of the spinal cord. Stimulation of the thin A-δ and C fibers 'opens' the gate and enhances central transmission at the synapses, while stimulation of the thick A-β fibers 'closes' the gate and inhibits transmission at the synapses. It is believed that peripheral nerve stimulation activates the thick nerve fibers and thus inhibits the transmission of pain.

In the early 1970s electrodes were implanted directly next to the spinal cord in chronic pain patients.[2] While using transcutaneous stimulation as a test before implantation, its effect without surgical intervention became evident[3] and TENS has become a standard tool for pain relief in many pain clinics for the last two decades.[4] Currently, there is only one contraindication – the patient with a pacemaker. TENS was used for the first time for pain relief during labor in Sweden,[5,6] and subsequently investigated by others.[7–9] One author even found an improvement in placental blood flow after TENS.[10]

For pain relief during labor, the electrodes are taped to the back above the pain-transmitting afferent nerves which enter the posterior column of the spinal cord: one pair above both sides of the spinal processes from T10 to L1 (thoracic) for the first stage of labor and one pair above the spinal processes S2–S4 (sacral) for the second stage of labor (Fig. 26.1)

The stimulators deliver bipolar biphasic square-wave pulses of 4–150 Hz, depending on the product, with an intensity between 0 and 55 mA. For pain relief in labor a frequency of 40–80 Hz is recommended,[6,7] while the intensity is regulated by the patient herself during the contraction. This depends on the amount of pain she experiences and on her tolerance to the intensity of the tingling sensation from the stimulator. In my experience, this value is 25–40 mA during contractions and 5–10 mA between contractions. A disadvantage of this technique is that the electrical stimulation, especially of the sacral electrodes, interfered with electronic monitoring of the fetal heart rate.

According to the literature, pain relief after TENS during labor is achieved in 40–80% of patients, the degree of relief varying from very good to insufficient. A reduction in the need for other medication (meperidine) was also reported.[6] The best relief was obtained in back pain due to contractions, while pain relief for suprapubic and perineal pain was rather poor. Pain relief was also more successful in the first stage than in the second stage of labor. On one hand, the influence of a suggestive (placebo) effect could not be excluded, while on the other hand, there is one report which demonstrated that correct placement of the electrodes is more effective than incorrect placement.[6] Since by placing the electrodes incorrectly a placebo effect might be excluded, we performed a single-blind study in 1977.[11] Ten patients received correctly placed TENS (Fig. 28.1) while a control group received TENS with much smaller electrodes, which were placed at L4 (Fig. 28.2)

The patients in both groups received the same instructions. They were able to regulate the amount of tingling they tolerated on their back. Over a period of 70 min the patients estimated the increase or decrease of the intensity of pain of each contraction, comparing it with the previous one by marking a scale with a range of six grades. To evaluate if this type of pain monitoring is useful, five patients who refused any pain relief and five patients who received meperidine on demand, while marking their scale, were chosen to record their pain after each contraction. Since there is proven evidence of a linear correlation between progress of labor (cervical dilatation) and intensity of pain[12] during the first stage, results were calculated by a formula that included the marked grade and also the degree of the cervical dilatation. If a contraction after an increase in cervical dilatation was scored equal or lower than before this dilatation, then it was termed 'pain relief'; if a contraction was scored higher than the previous one it was termed 'no relief'. A Wilcoxon signed-rank test (a nonparametric test) revealed a statistically significant increase in the pain threshold (i.e. improved tolerance of pain) in patients with correctly placed TENS and in those patients who received meperidine. There was no statisti-

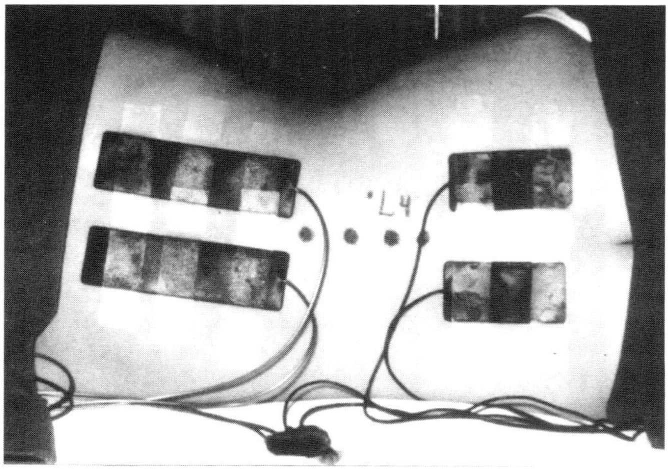

Fig. 28.1 Correct size and placement of electrodes in TENS for pain relief in labor. (Reproduced with permission from ref. 11.)

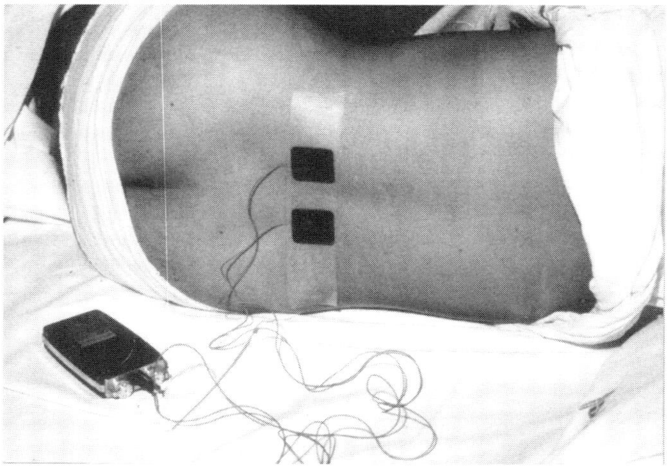

Fig. 28.2 Size and placement of electrodes in TENS in the control group. (Reproduced with permission from ref. 11.)

cally confirmed pain relief in patients receiving wrongly placed TENS and in patients who did not ask for pain relief. We believe that these results confirm the fact that TENS has a somatic effect in reducing pain. However, by asking all the patients to fill in a short questionnaire the day after delivery, it was revealed that the number of patients who believed retrospectively that they had some pain relief with the correctly placed TENS was not different from the number of patients who believed that they had pain relief with the wrongly placed TENS.

The conclusions of this study were:

1. TENS is able to increase the pain threshold and, therefore, offers some somatic pain relief which is difficult to quantitate.
2. TENS has a strong suggestive or placebo effect, because, retrospectively, there was no difference in satisfaction with the pain relief of correctly and incorrectly placed TENS.
3. The amount of the somatic effect of TENS for pain relief in labor seems to be rather poor, otherwise the retrospective satisfaction would have differed from the placebo effect. For example, a successful epidural block for pain relief in labor is retrospectively experienced quite differently than a failed epidural block, although in both cases the patient experiences the same technique.

SUMMARY

TENS is a simple tool to reduce labor pain primarily by a psychologic effect, enhanced by some true somatic effect, and as such may reduce the need for systemic medication. It is more effective in the first stage than in the second stage of labor (a pudendal block is often required for the second stage). It has no side-effects and its only disadvantage lies in the fact that it may interfere with electronic fetal heart rate monitoring. It is contraindicated in patients with pacemakers (a rare occurrence in women of child-bearing age), and additional analgesics or regional block may be necessary if pain relief is not sufficient.

REFERENCES

1. Melzack R, Wall P D 1965 Pain mechanisms: a new theory. Science 150: 971–979
2. Shealy C N, Mortimer J T, Hagfors N R 1970 Dorsal column electroanalgesia. J Neurosurg 32: 560–564
3. Shealy C N 1972 Transcutaneous electroanalgesia. Surg Forum 23: 419–424
4. Procacci P, Maresca M, Cersosimo R M 1990 Twenty years' experience with Transcutaneous Electric Stimulation. Schmerz/Pain/Doleur 11: 22–24
5. Augustinsson L E, Bohlin P H, Bundsen P, Carlsson C A, Forssman L, Sjöberg P, Tyreman N O 1977 Pain relief during delivery by transcutaneous electrical nerve stimulation. Pain 4: 59–61
6. Bundsen P, Carlsson C A, Forssman L, Tyreman N O 1978 Schmerzerleichterug während der Geburt mit transkutaner elektrischer Neurostimulation. Prakt Anästh 13: 20–28
7. Kubista E, Kucera H, Riss P 1978 Die Wirkung der transkutanen Nervstimulation auf den Wehenschmerz. Geburtsh Frauenheilk 38: 1079
8. Robson J E 1979 Transcutaneous nerve stimulation for pain relief in labour. Anaesthesia 34: 357–360
9. Stewart P 1979 Transcutaneous nerve stimulation as a method of analgesia in labour. Anaesthesia 34: 361–364
10. Kubista E 1981 Beeinflussung der Plazentafunktion durch Elektrostimulation. Probleme der perinatalen Medizin, Vol 10. Wilhelm Maudrich, Vienna
11. Neumark J, Pauser G, Scherzer W 1978 Der Wehenschmerz während der Geburt. Zur Analyse der analgetischen Wirkung der transkutanen Nervstimulation (TNS) im Vergleich mit Pethidin und Plazabos. Prakt Anaesth 13: 13–20
12. Wylie W D 1953 The practical management of pain in labour. Lloyd-Luke, London

29. Parenteral opioids

M. Harmer   M. Rosen

INTRODUCTION

The introduction into obstetric anesthetic practice of sophisticated techniques such as epidural anesthesia has largely overshadowed many of the more traditional methods of providing pain relief. Whilst accepting that epidural anesthesia provides pain relief of superior quality, it is important to bear in mind that other methods may still be widely used. In addition to efficacy, safety is an important element of any form of pain relief. Pregnancy is not a disease but a physiologic process, and thus it is unacceptable for the provision of analgesia in labor to be anything but absolutely safe. The long-standing method of intermittent intramuscular injections of an opioid analgesic, while not totally effective, has been demonstrated in millions of pregnancies to be a safe method of providing pain relief. Newer techniques such as epidural anesthesia have not had such a safety record and concern must be expressed when there is an association with even one maternal death.[1,2]

HISTORY

The use of opioid analgesic agents dates back to early Chinese civilization, where writings describe the giving of opium to relieve the pain of labor. One presumes that opium-containing 'cocktails' have continued to be used through the centuries in many societies and cultures, though there is little mention in the literature. In 1806, Sertürner isolated morphine from crude opium and, while it may have been appreciated at that time as a potent analgesic, it was not until the invention by Alexander Wood in 1853 of the hypodermic needle and syringe that it was possible to administer morphine parenterally. However, even then, morphine was injected close to a nerve from a painful site, which probably masked its general analgesic properties. It was only later that it was appreciated that the effects of morphine were achieved through systematic absorption rather than local anesthesia.

Morphine was not widely used in labor until 1902, when a combination of morphine and scopolamine was introduced by von Steinbüchel. This combination led to a state of stupor, which was further refined by Gauss in 1906 to produce the state of 'twilight sleep'. This consisted of giving a single injection of morphine and scopolamine followed by repeated injections of scopolamine alone. Although it was very popular for several decades, it could hardly be considered to be without its problems, the most common being poor analgesia and maternal confusion. Labor was long and the neonate often suffered severe respiratory depression. Its continued popularity was perhaps only due to the amnesic effect of scopolamine resulting in an inability of the mother to recall the unpleasant events!

The popularity of morphine came to an end when meperidine was synthesized in 1939 and gave indications of being less soporific than morphine. Meperidine was first used in labor in 1940 and since then has become the standard opioid analgesic in the UK for obstetric use. Since 1950 midwives have been authorized to prescribe and administer meperidine in domicillary practice.

Alternatives to meperidine have appeared and, to a large degree, disappeared over the years. The introduction of partial agonist analgesic drugs led to a belief that they might have limited side-effects, particularly respiratory depressant activity, while at the same time retaining effective analgesic properties. The two agents that have had most support are pentazocine and meptazinol, but neither has shown convincing benefits over meperidine.

While accepting that the 'ideal' drug may never be available, a great deal of work has concentrated on the mode of drug delivery. This has led to changes in dose size, the use of infusions and the development of sophisticated techniques such as patient-controlled analgesia. Such consideration of pharmacokinetic and pharmacodynamic factors has improved the effectiveness of the available opioid analgesic drugs, while at the same time maintaining their safety.

EFFECTS OF PARENTERAL OPIOIDS ON MOTHER AND FETUS/NEONATE

General considerations

The use of parenteral opioid analgesics to alleviate labor pain necessitates a compromise between using sufficient drug to provide effective analgesia and causing an increased risk of side-effects in the mother and fetus. It is the effect on the fetus that has always been the major constraint on the use of an adequate dose of analgesic as all these drugs freely cross the placental barrier and thus may have respiratory depressant effects upon the fetus.

Maternal effects of parenteral opioids

Analgesia

It has already been stated that the analgesia obtained with parenteral opioids will never challenge that produced by epidural anesthesia, but many women are able to receive a reasonable quality of pain relief. However, in general, analgesia produced by opioid analgesics is disappointing. In one study[3] 75% of mothers felt that meperidine had little or no effect on their pain although a second study of primigravidae showed that 60% were satisfied with pain relief after a combination of inhalation analgesia and parenteral opioids.[4] Further evidence of the inadequacy of analgesia was reported by Pearson and Davies,[5] who compared mothers receiving meperidine and epidural anesthesia. The $P\text{aCO}_2$ of women receiving meperidine was lower than the women who received epidural anesthesia, the cause being attributed to the increased ventilation associated with inadequate analgesia.

Respiratory system

Although in normal analgesic practice opioid analgesics cause a dose-related respiratory depression and hypoventilation, the inadequacy of analgesia associated with parenteral opioids is more likely to lead to hyperventilation. This will lead to a reduced $P\text{aCO}_2$ and, during a long labor, produce a compensatory maternal acidosis.[5] The hyperventilatory period tends to be confined to painful contractions, and hypoventilation with associated hypoxia may occur between contractions.[6] Whether this is due to the analgesic or is compensatory after a period of hyperventilation is unclear. In a study comparing oxygen saturation in mothers receiving analgesia by different methods, Zelcer et al[7] found that when opioid analgesics were given alone there was no significant fall in saturation as compared with the control group. However, if nitrous oxide was also administered, there was a significant fall. Reed et al[8] found that 49% of mothers receiving nitrous oxide and meperidine analgesia had decreases in oxygen saturation below 90% for at least 10 s.

Cardiovascular system

Unless very large doses, or standard doses given rapidly intravenously, are employed, parenteral opioids have limited clinical effect on the cardiovascular system. If a relative overdose is given it may lead to hypotension, which is further aggravated by posture and venocaval occlusion. The use of parenteral opioids to control the blood pressure swings in preeclampsia is not usually helpful, except that if an effective dose is used it may reduce the blood pressure fluctuations associated with painful contractions.

Gastrointestinal system

Gastric emptying is delayed in pregnancy and further exaggerated during labor. It is likely that much of this latter delay is due to the use of parenteral opioids like meperidine given during labor, increasing gastric emptying time to at least 5 h in 70% of women.[9] A study by O'Sullivan et al[10] using a noninvasive impedance technique to measure gastric emptying during labor showed a significant difference between groups receiving epidural anesthesia and meperidine.

Whether such delay in gastric emptying can be overcome is debatable. Metoclopramide has been shown to be ineffective in late labor in improving gastric emptying,[11] while others suggest that the time between the administration of meperidine and metoclopramide is critical in determining the possible success of metoclopramide.[12] Gastric stasis can be reduced by the combination of an opioid antagonist and the analgesic[13] but such improvement is associated with a reduction in the quality of pain relief.[14] The effect of meperidine on gastric mobility can be reversed by giving naloxone,[15] but as this will also reverse analgesia it should only be used if analgesia is being provided by another method. In addition to causing delayed gastric emptying, the parenteral opioids may also reduce the tone of the gastroesophageal sphincter, leading to a higher likelihood of gastric content regurgitation.[16,17]

In common with their use for post-operative pain relief, the parenteral opioids given during labor cause nausea and vomiting. This is central in origin and occurs in approximately 50% of patients. Some form of centrally-acting antiemetic, such as a phenothiazine, should be given with each dose of analgesic.

Uterine contractility

Parenteral opioid analgesics have no major direct effects on uterine contractility.[18–20] However, if given during a prolonged, painful labor associated with uterine incoordination, they will often lead to a more normal type of uterine action.[21] This is probably central in origin and not a direct uterine effect.

Placental transfer of parenteral opioids

All opioid analgesics cross the placenta, a fact that is predictable as they also freely cross the blood–brain barrier to produce their effects. However, there may be a difference in the ability of various opioid analgesics to cross the placenta, but the significance of this is not completely clear.

Meperidine, the most widely studied analgesic, freely crosses the placenta, with the umbilical venous blood concentration approaching that of maternal blood within 2 min of an intravenous injection. Such speed of transfer is modified by the factors that will affect the uptake of meperidine when given by the usual intramuscular route and, in this case, it may take between 2 and 5 hs to achieve unity of the fetal–maternal ratio.[22,23] Hence, after an intramuscular injection, the highest fetal concentrations are likely 2–3 hs later.[24,25]

Morphine and other opioid analgesics behave in a similar manner, but it has been claimed that some drugs do not cross the placenta to the same degree as meperidine (see below). In general, these agents are weaker analgesics and, therefore, some consideration is needed in judging the balance between their ability to provide analgesia and their potential for placental transfer.

Fetal/neonatal effects of parenteral opioids

In general, one may assume that all opioid analgesics cross the placenta and that the greater the fetal blood concentration of the drug the greater will be the effects on the fetus.

Respiratory system

The most serious effect of opioid analgesics on the neonate is respiratory depression. This is most likely to occur when the fetal blood concentration is at a peak and is likely to be most severe if delivery takes place between 2.5 and 3.5 hs after an intramuscular injection of meperidine.[26] Conversely, analgesic-induced respiratory depression is unusual if delivery takes place within 1 h of, or more than 6 hs after, an intramuscular injection. The depressant effects of a given blood concentration seem much greater in the neonate than in the mother. This may reflect the fact that the immature respiratory centre is more sensitive to the opioid analgesic, but may also be because the analgesic is less protein bound in the fetus and, therefore, more free drug is available.[27] Such protein binding and drug solubility will be further affected by variations in blood acidity since the free concentration of an analgesic in the fetus is affected by the pH of the blood.[28]

The degree to which meperidine depresses neonatal respiration has been widely studied. After a single intramuscular injection of meperidine 100 mg, the $Pa\text{CO}_2$ of the neonate may be elevated for up to 5 h,[29] and neonatal respiratory rate is generally slowed if two or more injections of meperidine are given.[30] The duration of such depression may be a result of the delayed elimination of meperidine by the neonate. Meperidine is converted initially to normeperidine, a potent respiratory depressant, and then undergoes a series of hydrolysis, demethylation and oxidation processes, all of which may be prolonged in the neonate.[31] The overall effect is that the half-life of meperidine in the neonate averages 18 hs, compared with 3–4 hs in adults. Therefore, it may take the neonate up to 3 days to excrete all the meperidine, and its metabolites, received from its mother during labor.[22]

Cardiovascular system

The normal beat-to-beat variation in the fetal heart rate may be diminished about 40 mins after the intramuscular injection of an opioid analgesic.[32, 33] The significance of this is uncertain, but it is probably innocent. Linblad et al[34] studied fetal aortic blood flow during labor using a combined ultrasonic and pulsed Doppler technique. They found that in all patients the fetal aortic flow increased during labor but the flow was decreased after the administration of meperidine.

Opioid analgesics do not tend to have any primary effect on the cardiovascular system of the neonate but may cause bradycardia secondary to opioid-induced respiratory depression.

Neurologic system

Sensitive neurobehavioral assessments show that meperidine given to the mother in labor consistently leads to abnormal behavioral patterns and depression of the reflexes in the neonate for at least 48 hs.[35,36] The time span of such alteration is very similar to the time taken by the fetus to eliminate meperidine from its body and would seem to be a residual opioid effect. Among the many abnormal behavioral patterns seen, the inability of infants to suck and breastfeed has been shown to be reversible by the opioid antagonist, naloxone.[37]

SPECIFIC OPIOID ANALGESICS (Table 29.1)

Meperidine

Meperidine was first synthesized in 1939 and rapidly became popular in obstetric practice, advanced by claims that it was less soporific than morphine or heroin. To this day it is the mainstay of parenteral opioid therapy in obstetric practice in the UK.

Traditionally, a dose of meperidine 100 mg is given intramuscularly to be repeated at approximately 3-hourly intervals as required. If more than two doses are required, as in a prolonged labor, it may be advisable to consider an

Table 29.1 Opioids used for labor analgesia and common doses. Data from Paddock et al,[38] Physicians' Desk Reference[39] and Wood & Wood[40]

Analgesia	Comparative dose	Intravenous dose	Intramuscular dose
Meperidine or pethidine (Demerol)	100 mg	25–50 mg	50–100 mg
Morphine	10 mg	2.5–5 mg	5–10 mg
Pentazocine (Talwin)	30 mg	10–20 mg	20–30 mg
Meptazinol	150 mg	30–50 mg	100–150 mg
Nalbuphine (Nubain)	10 mg	5–10 mg	10–20 mg
Butorphanol (Stadol)	2 mg	1–2 mg	1–2 mg

alternative technique in order to reduce the degree of neonatal depression. Analgesia with meperidine is often disappointing, with only 40% of women finding a dose of 100 mg helpful,[41] this figure increasing slightly to 50–60% by the use of 150 mg.[42] The use of such large doses with limited efficacy should suggest the use of an alternative analgesic drug or delivery regimen. Meperidine is known to have variable uptake characteristics when given repeatedly intramuscularly, a situation that endorses its possible unsuitability for administration by this route.[43]

As previously mentioned, there is extensive placental transfer of meperidine with consequent effects upon the neonate.

Morphine

Although having similar analgesic qualities to meperidine, morphine has the ability to allay anxiety and may retain a place in the anxious primigravid mother in early labor. Morphine is less lipid soluble than meperidine and theoretically should cross the placental barrier more slowly. This appears to be so in practice in that the fetal–maternal ratio for morphine is lower than for meperidine. However, morphine seems to have a greater ability to penetrate the infant's brain and cause depressant side-effects.[44] In view of this, morphine should only be used early in labor when delivery is not anticipated within 5–6 h.

Heroin (diamorphine)

Heroin has little place in obstetric practice except to allay anxiety in terrified patients. However, in this situation a combination of another opioid with a specific anxiolytic may be more appropriate.

Pentazocine

Pentazocine was introduced as one of the earliest partial agonist agents reputed to cause limited respiratory depression and liability to addiction. Sadly, many of its early claims have not been fulfilled. It is less lipid soluble than meperidine, crosses the placenta more slowly[45] and neonatal depression is of a briefer duration.[30] However, it is a weaker analgesic than meperidine and it is likely that similar effects in the neonate will be found if equianalgesic doses are employed. The condition of the neonate may thus be the same for meperidine and pentazocine.[46] When given by a patient-controlled analgesic technique (see later) it has been found to produce a similar level of analgesia and neonatal status as meperidine but with fewer maternal side-effects.[47]

If pentazocine has an advantage over meperidine it is in causing a much lower incidence of nausea and vomiting[41] and being free from strict prescribing restrictions.

Meptazinol

Meptazinol was claimed initially to be equipotent to meperidine while possessing less respiratory depressant activity.[48] Later work has shown that it has approximately half the analgesic potency of meperidine[49] and when used in equipotent doses to meperidine has similar respiratory depressant activity.[50] In obstetric studies[51–53] it has been found to produce a similar level of analgesia to meperidine but with marked nausea and vomiting. However, one study[54] showed improved Apgar scores in babies born to women receiving meptazinol as compared with meperidine. The explanation put forward for this observation was that the mean neonatal elimination half-life of meptazinol is 3.4 h as compared with 18 h for meperidine.[55]

A high degree of nausea and vomiting may limit the potential usefulness of this drug.

Nalbuphine

Nalbuphine has similarly been proposed as a useful analgesic with limited respiratory depression. When compared in obstetrics to meperidine it produces similar analgesia but less nausea and vomiting.[56] However, any such advantage is countered by a tendency to cause maternal dizziness. This same study demonstrated that nalbuphine crosses the placenta more rapidly than meperidine and produces a greater degree of early neonatal neurobehavioral changes. When given by a patient-controlled analgesia system (see below) nalbuphine led to better pain scores than meperidine but in other respects was similar.[57]

OPIOID ANTAGONISTS

Although it is preferable to limit the side-effects of opioid analgesics in the mother and fetus/neonate by judicious use, the opioid antagonists are capable of reversing all these effects if required. The only drug readily available is naloxone, which is able to reverse the actions of all the opioid analgesics mentioned above. If an opioid antagonist is used it must be remembered that analgesia will also be reversed, and hence it is best administered to the neonate rather than the mother. The relative short duration of action of naloxone may mean that repeated dosage is required to overcome the longer lasting effects of the analgesics.

MODE OF DRUG DELIVERY

The traditional method of delivery is by intermittent intramuscular injection. A large dose of the drug is injected into the muscle in the hope that drug absorption will result in a steady blood level that is analgesic without being so high as to cause side-effects. This is very much a 'hit or miss' philosophy which could use improvement.

Intramuscular route

As has already been discussed, the efficacy of intramuscular opioid analgesics for relief of labor pain is poor, and increasing the size of dose does not seem to improve the efficacy.[42] If one considers (Fig. 29.1a) the intramuscular

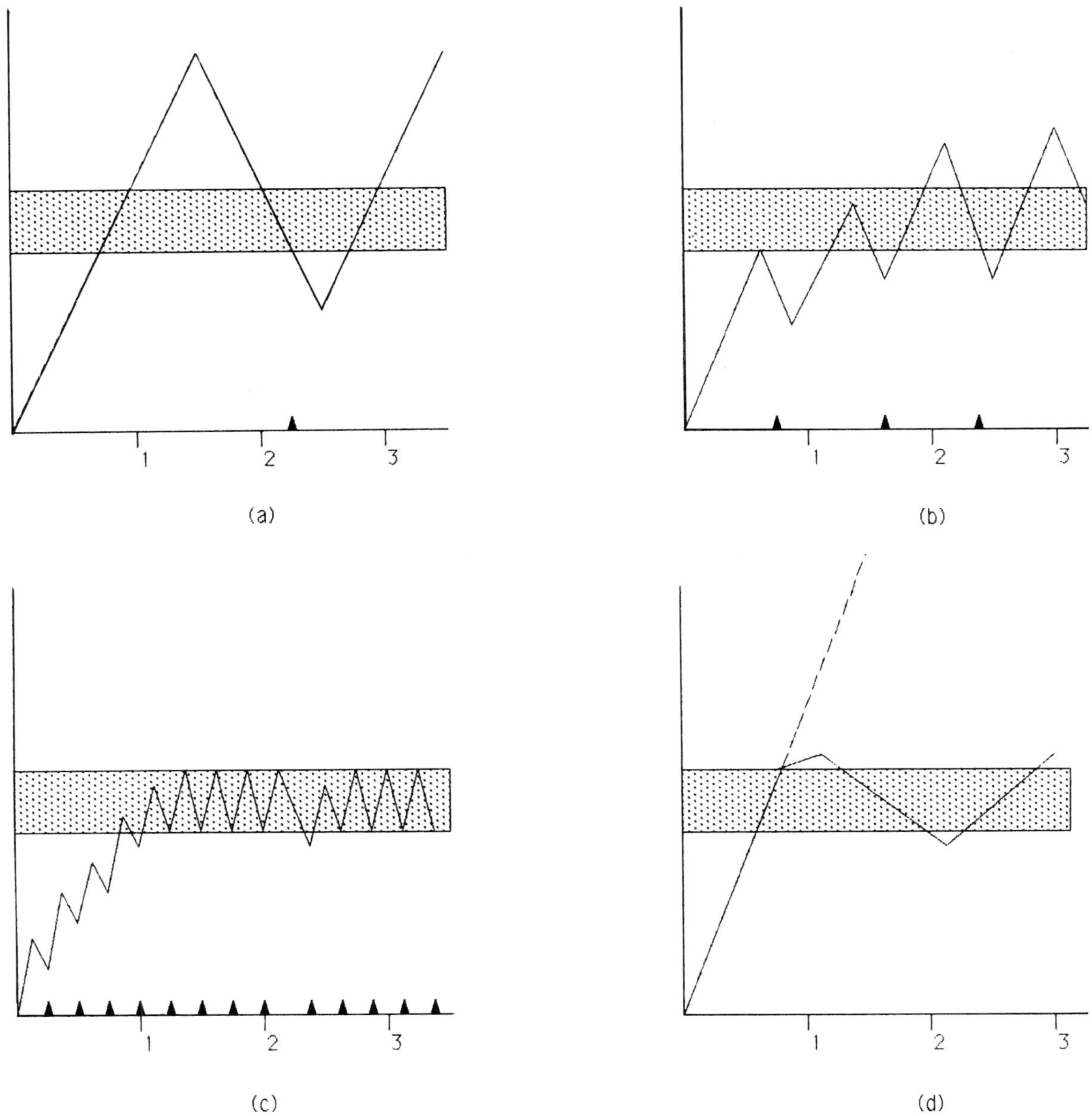

Fig. 29.1 Diagrammatic representation of four modes of analgesic administration. Graphs represent plots of blood analgesic concentration against time in hours. (a) Intermittent large-dose intramuscular injection. (b) Intermittent small-dose intramuscular injection. (c) Patient-controlled analgesia. (d) Intravenous infusion. [stippled box], effective blood analgesic concentration; ▲, administration of a dose; ----, the possible concentration if infusion continued at the original rate.

injection of a large dose of an analgesic (e.g. meperidine 150 mg), there will be a period of uptake from the muscle during which the blood concentration has not reached analgesic levels and the woman is still in pain. This will vary from patient to patient and even from injection to injection,[43] but may be as long as 40 min. On attaining a level of analgesia, the blood concentration will not plateau but will continue to rise. The period during which the blood concentration exceeds the analgesic level is 'wasted analgesia', contributing only to maternal side-effects and neonatal complications. Gradually, with time, the concentration falls until it is below the analgesic concentration, when the woman will request another dose. Once again there will be a delay in the giving and onset of analgesia. The overall effect is a delivery system producing widely separated peaks and troughs of blood concentration.

If a smaller intramuscular dose is given more frequently a different pattern will be seen (Fig. 29.1b). It may take longer and, indeed, may need a second dose to attain a satisfactory blood level, but once analgesia is attained it can be more easily maintained by regular, perhaps hourly, injections of opioid. The 'wasted' component of analgesia is reduced and there should be fewer maternal and neonatal side-effects.

If the intramuscular route is to be used, then rather than using larger doses of opioid to improve efficacy it is more logical to use smaller doses given more frequently. However, the time taken initially to attain analgesic levels can only be overcome by using a larger intramuscular loading dose or by delivering the first dose by another route, such as intravenously.

Intravenous route

By using the intravenous route, the initial delay in achieving an analgesic blood concentration can be reduced to almost zero to give an immediate effect (Fig. 29.1c). If small doses of analgesic are given as required, it is possible to accurately titrate the dose given to that required by the mother to maintain adequate analgesic without a significant degree of overshoot into 'wasted' analgesia. This could be achieved by the attendant administering small regular intravenous boluses as requested but is too labor intensive to be feasible. The concept of the patient controlling the rate at which an analgesic is given was raised by Scott[58] and was further refined by the development of a patient-activated syringe pump by Evans et al.[59] Advances in microprocessor technology have led to the development of a number of such machines, all incorporating features to allow adjustment of bolus dose, time between doses and overall drug dose limits. By allowing the mother to control analgesia it is possible to accommodate virtually all degrees of demand. This is the technique of patient-controlled analgesia (PCA), and has been shown to be superior to traditional intramuscular regimens in obstetrics.[59,60] It is usual to use PCA by the intravenous route, but it has been shown to be feasible using the intramuscular route.[61] Whilst it is still not able to match the analgesia produced by epidural anesthesia, PCA may be of particular value in units where epidural anesthesia is not readily available.[62]

The alternative to the use of PCA devices is a continuous intravenous infusion of analgesics. Various infusion regimens have been advocated from as early as 1952,[63] and, while some have been successful, many have led to maternal oversedation and lack of control. The problem that may be encountered with infusions is illustrated in Figure 29.1d. An initial high infusion rate is required to achieve analgesia, but if that rate is continued it may lead to very high blood levels with consequent deleterious effects on mother and fetus. Thus, it is vital to reduce the rate to maintain an adequate blood level. It may be very time-consuming to constantly alter the infusion rate unless the task is designated to the patient – this then effectively becomes PCA. Infusions, although theoretically better than intramuscular injections, can in practice be very difficult to control and potentially dangerous.

Other routes

There is an increasing availability of opioid preparations that can be given orally, sublingually, rectally or transdermally. Little is known of their efficacy in obstetrics, and they perhaps merit more exploratory work.

CONCLUSION

Modern obstetric analgesic practice seems to have little place for the use of parenteral opioids, but it must be remembered that not everyone has epidural anesthesia freely and readily available. To ignore the place that meperidine has played, and possibly will still play, would be to deny many mothers the chance of analgesia when other techniques are not available or are contraindicated. However, for parenteral opioids to continue to have a major place in contemporary practice, the side-effects in the mother and fetus must be reduced. The most logical method at present of providing the best results, with fewest adverse effects, is by using a delivery system such as PCA.

REFERENCES

1. Department of Health 1982 Report on Health and Social Subjects. Report on confidential enquiries into maternal deaths in England and Wales 1976–78. HMSO, London
2. Department of Health 1989 Report on Health and Social Subjects. Report on confidential enquiries into maternal deaths in England and Wales 1982–84. HMSO, London
3. Holdcroft A, Morgan M 1974 An assessment of the analgesic effect in labour of pethidine and 50 per cent nitrous oxide in oxygen (Entonox). J Obstet Gynaecol Br Cwlth 81: 603–607
4. Beazley J M, Leaver E P, Morewood J H, Bircumshaw J 1967 Relief of pain in labour. Lancet 1: 1033–1035
5. Pearson J F, Davies P 1973 The effect of continuous lumbar epidural analgesia on the acid–base status of maternal arterial blood during the first stage of labour. J Obstet Gynaecol Br Cwlth 80: 218–224
6. Huch A, Huch R, Lindmark G, Rooth G 1974 Maternal hypoxaemia after pethidine. J Obstet Gynaecol Br Cwlth 81: 608–614
7. Zelcer J, Owers H, Paull J D 1989 A controlled oximetric evaluation of inhalational, opioid and epidural analgesia in labour. Anaesth Intensive Care 17: 418–421
8. Reed P N, Colquhoun A D, Hanning C D 1989 Maternal oxygenation during normal labour. Br J Anaesth 62: 316–318
9. La Salvia L A, Steffen E A 1950 Delayed gastric emptying time in labor. Am J Obstet Gynecol 59: 1075–1081
10. O'Sullivan G M, Sutton A J, Thompson S A, Carrie L E, Bullingham R E 1987 Noninvasive measurement of gastric emptying in obstetric patients. Anesth Analg 66: 505–511
11. Nimmo W S, Wilson J, Prescott L F 1975 Narcotic analgesics and delayed gastric emptying during labour. Lancet 1: 890–893
12. Murphy D F, Nally B, Gardiner J, Unwin A 1984 Effect of metoclopramide on gastric emptying before elective and emergency Caesarean section. Br J Anaesth 56: 1113–1116
13. Wilson J 1978 Gastric emptying in labour: some recent findings and their clinical significance. J Int Med Res 6 (suppl): 54–62
14. Girvan C B, Moore J, Dundee J W 1976 Pethidine compared with pethidine–naloxone administered during labour. Br J Anaesth 48: 563–569
15. Frame W T, Allison R H, Moir D D, Nimmo W S 1984 Effect of naloxone on gastric emptying during labour. Br J Anaesth 56: 263–266
16. Brock-Utne J G, Rubin J, Downing J W, Dimopoulos G E, Moshal M G, Naicker M 1976 The administration of metoclopramide with atropine. Anaesthesia 31: 1186–1190
17. Hey V M, Phillips K, Woods I 1983 Pethidine, atropine, metoclopramide and the lower oesophageal sphincter. Anaesthesia 38: 650–653
18. Caldeyro-Barcia R, Alvarez H, Poseiro J J 1955 Action of morphine on the contractility of the human uterus. Arch Int Pharmacodynamie Therapie 101: 171–188
19. Petrie R H, Wu R, Miller F C et al 1976 The effect of drugs on uterine activity. Obstet Gynecol 48: 431–435
20. Filler W W, Filler N W 1966 Effect of a potent non-narcotic analgesic agent (pentazocine) on uterine contractility and fetal heart rate. Obstet Gynecol 28: 224–232
21. DeVoe S J, DeVoe K Jr, Rigsby W C, McDaniels B A 1969 Effect of meperidine on uterine contractility. Am J Obstet Gynecol 105: 1004–1007
22. Hogg M I J, Wiener P C, Rosen M, Mapleson W W 1977 Urinary excretion and metabolism of pethidine and norpethidine in the newborn. Br J Anaesth 49: 891–899
23. Tomson G, Garl R I M, Thalme B, Nisell H, Nylund L, Rane A 1982 Maternal kinetics and transplacental passage of pethidine during labour. Br J Clin Pharmacol 13: 653–659
24. Shnider S M, Moya F 1964 Effect of meperidine on the newborn infant. Am J Obstet Gynecol 89: 1009–1015
25. Belfrage P, Boreus L O, Hartwig P, Irestadt L, Raabe N 1981 Neonatal depression after obstetrical analgesia with pethidine. Acta Obstet Gynaecol Scand 60: 43–49
26. Roberts H, Please N W 1958 Respiratory minute volume in the newborn infant. J Obstet Gynaecol Br Emp 65: 33–40
27. Nation R L 1981 Meperidine binding in maternal and fetal plasma. Clin Pharmacol Ther 29: 472–479
28. Benson D W, Kaufman J J, Koski W S 1976 Theoretic significance of pH dependance of narcotics and narcotic antagonists in clinical anesthesia. Anesth Analg: Curr Res 55: 253–256
29. Koch G, Wendel H 1968 The effect of pethidine in the postnatal adjustment of respiration and acid–base balance. Acta Obstet Gynecol Scand 47: 27–37
30. Refstad S O, Lindbaek E 1980 Ventilatory depression of the newborn of women receiving pethidine or pentazocine. Br J Anaesth 52: 265–271
31. Caldwell J, Notarianni L J 1978 Disposition of pethidine in childbirth. Br J Anaesth 50: 307–308
32. Kariniemi V, Ammala P 1981 Effects of intramuscular pethidine on fetal heart rate variability during labour. Br J Obstet Gynaecol 88: 718–720
33. Petrie R H, Yeh S, Murata Y et al 1978 The effect of drugs on fetal heart rate variability. Am J Obstet Gynecol 130: 294–299
34. Lindbad A, Bernow J, Marsal K 1987 Obstetric analgesia and fetal aortic blood flow during labour. Br J Obstet Gynecol 94: 306–311
35. Brackbill U, Kane J, Manniello R L, Abramson D 1974 Obstetric meperidine usage and assessment of neonatal status. Anaesthesiology 40: 116–120
36. Brazelton T B 1970 Effect of prenatal drugs on behavior of the neonate. Am J Psychiatr 126: 1261–1266
37. Wiener P C, Hogg M I J, Rosen M 1977 Effects of naloxone on pethidine-induced neonatal depression. Br Med J 2: 228–229
38. Paddock R, Beer E G, Bellville J W et al 1969 Analgesic and side effects of pentazocine and morphine in a large population of postoperative patients. Clin Pharmacol Ther 10: 355
39. Physicians' desk reference, 44th edn 1990 Medical Economics Company Inc, Oradell, NJ
40. Wood M, Wood A J J 1982 Drugs and anesthesia – pharmacology for anesthesiologists. Williams & Wilkins, Baltimore
41. Moore J, Carson R M, Hunter R J 1970 A comparison of the effects of pentazocine and pethidine administered during labour. J Obstet Gynecol Br Cwlth 77: 830–836
42. Grant A M, Holt E M, Noble A D 1970 A comparison between pethidine and phenazocine (Narphen) for relief of pain in labour. J Obstet Gynecol Br Cwlth 77: 824–829
43. Austin K L, Stapleson J V, Mather L E 1980 Multiple intramuscular injections: a major source of variability in analgesic response to meperidine. Pain 8: 47–62
44. Way W L, Costley E C, Way E L 1965 Respiratory sensitivity of the newborn infant to meperidine and morphine. Clin Pharmacol Ther 6: 454–461
45. Beckett A H, Taylor J F 1967 Blood concentrations of pethidine and pentazocine in mother and infant at the time of birth. J Pharm Pharmacol 19 (suppl): 50–52
46. Duncan S L, Ginsburg J, Morris N F 1969 Comparison of pentazocine and pethidine in normal labor. Am J Obstet Gynecol 105: 197–202
47. Erskine W A, Dick A, Murell D F, Vital M, Van den Heever J 1985 Self-administered intravenous analgesia during labour. A comparison between pentazocine and pethidine. S Afr Med J 67: 764–767
48. Paymaster N J 1977 Analgesia after operation – a controlled comparison of meptazinol, pentazocine and pethidine. Br J Anaesth 49: 1139–1146
49. Slattery P J, Harmer M, Rosen M, Vickers M D 1981 Comparison of meptazinol and pethidine given i.v. on demand in the management of post operative pain. Br J Anaesth 53: 927–931
50. Slattery P J, Harmer M, Rosen M, Vickers M D 1983 Comparison of the respiratory depressant effects of i.v. meptazinol and pethidine. Br J Anaesth 55: 245P
51. Sheikh A, Tunstall M E 1986 Comparative study of meptazinol and pethidine for the relief of pain in labour. Br J Obstet Gynaecol 93: 264–269
52. Morrison C E, Dutton D, Howie H, Gilmour H 1987 Pethidine

compared with meptazinol during labour. A prospective randomised double-blind study in 1100 patients. Anaesthesia 42: 7–14
53. Osler M 1987 A double-blind study comparing meptazinol and pethidine for pain relief in labour. Eur J Obstet Gynecol Reprod Biol 26: 15–18
54. Nicholas A D G, Robson P J 1982 Double-blind comparison of meptazinol and pethidine in labour. Br J Obstet Gynecol 89: 318–322
55. Jackson M B A, Robson P J 1983 Preliminary clinical and pharmacokinetic experiences in the newborn when meptazinol is compared with pethidine as an obstetric analgesia. Postgrad Med J 59 (suppl 1): 47–51
56. Wilson C M, McClean E, Moore J, Dundee J W 1986 A double-blind comparison of intramuscular pethidine and nalbuphine in labour. Anaesthesia 41: 1207–1213
57. Frank M, McAteer E J, Cattermole R, Loughnan B, Stafford L B, Hitchcock A M 1987 Nalbuphine for obstetric analgesia. A comparison of nalbuphine with pethidine for pain relief in labour when administered by patient-controlled analgesia. Anaesthesia 42: 697–703
58. Scott J S 1970 Obstetric analgesia. A consideration of labor pain and a patient-controlled technique for its relief with meperidine. Am J Obstet Gynecol 106: 959–978
59. Evans J M, Rosen M, MacCarthy J, Hogg M I J 1976 Apparatus for patient-controlled administration of intravenous narcotics during labour. Lancet 1: 17–18
60. Robinson J O, Rosen M, Evans J M, Revill S I, David H, Rees G A D 1980 Self administered intravenous and intramuscular pethidine. A controlled trial in labour. Anaesthesia 35: 763–770
61. Li D F, Rees G A D, Rosen M 1988 Feasibility of self-administration analgesia by the intramuscular route in labour. Eur J Obstet Gynecol Reprod Biol 27: 99–104
62. Harper N J N, Thomson J, Brayshaw S A 1983 Experience with self-administered pethidine with special reference to the general practitioner obstetric unit. Anaesthesia 38: 52–55
63. Jeffcoate T N A, Baker K, Martin R H 1952 Inefficient uterine action. Surg Gynecol Obstet 95: 257–273

30. Patient-controlled analgesia

W. R. Camann

Patient-controlled analgesia (PCA) is a modality that may have some useful applications during labor. Various techniques (inhalation, intravenous and epidural) have been used, and the concept of PCA during labor is still evolving.

The technique of inhalation analgesia for labor bears some special consideration.[1] Although now largely of historical interest, inhalation analgesia was actually the first example of a self-administered (i.e. patient-controlled) modality. Virtually all inhaled agents (ether, trichloroethylene, cyclopropane, chloroform, nitrous oxide, halothane, enflurane, isoflurane and methoxyflurane) have been advocated, although only nitrous oxide is used with any regularity today. A predetermined mixture of nitrous oxide and oxygen (Entonox) is rarely used in the USA but enjoys greater popularity in the UK. The concept underlying the inhalation technique is similar regardless of which agent is used. Some sort of device (mouthpiece, inhaler, face mask or demand valve) is given to the patient, who is instructed to take several rapid breaths at the onset of a contraction. Self-administration of the agent ends when analgesia is obtained (which is often simply because the contraction has ended) or when maternal drowsiness causes inability to use the device. Inhalation analgesia is not a panacea. Excessive maternal drowsiness is clearly a problem. Some parturients are amnestic for the birth of the baby. In addition, the propensity of parturients to regurgitate and aspirate gastric contents if general anesthesia ensues without a secured airway has largely contributed to the decline in popularity of this modality. At the Brigham and Women's Hospital, inhalation analgesia during labor has not been used in over two decades.

Patient-controlled analgesia (PCA) with intravenous opioids during labor is a new and exciting development. Although first described for labor pain by Scott in 1964,[2] the technique has not gained widespread acceptance in labor units despite the fact that opioid analgesia is by far the commonest type of pain relief offered to laboring women. However, the recent blossoming of PCA as a post-surgical analgesic modality has resurrected the interest in PCA for labor pain.

Why has PCA been slow to appear in labor units? The reason is multifactorial. One of the advantages of post-surgical PCA is that the already harried surgical ward nurse will not be bothered by numerous demands for intramuscular analgesics from as many as 20 (or more!) patients. In contrast, labor nurses rarely care for more than one or two patients at a time. Hence, the inconvenience of opioid injections is minimized. One may postulate that the process of assembling the pump and infusion apparatus is a deterrent, but this has certainly not deterred the use of PCA in the surgical ward, where staff are even scarcer than in labor and delivery units. A further objection may be the concern of obstetricians that excessive opioid administration, particularly during the second stage of labor, may cause neonatal respiratory depression. This is a valid concern that bears further consideration, although preliminary studies have so far failed to document neonatal compromise.[3–5]

One must remember that although PCA is an improved method for administering systemic opioids, the ultimate result is still opioid-induced analgesia. Complete abolition of sensation (i.e. anesthesia) will not be obtained. Thus, this modality will not, and is not, designed to replace epidural anesthesia. Those patients who desire complete pain relief or who do not cope well with even moderate pain would not be suitable candidates for opioid analgesia by either bolus or PCA. However, for the subset of patients who do not desire epidural analgesia or in institutions where regional anesthesia for childbirth is unavailable, PCA offers several advantages over intermittent dosing with opioids.

First, the ability to control one's analgesic administration provides a psychological benefit. The anxiety and stress associated with childbirth are considerable, and the physical as well as emotional 'trespasses' imposed upon patients during labor can be overwhelming. Returning some degree of control to the patient is often a much-appreciated gesture.

Second, single or intermittent doses of intravenous or intramuscular opioids are usually administered during the early stages of labor. During the later stages of labor, obstetricians are often reluctant to readminister intravenous or intramuscular opioids as high peak maternal plasma levels are readily reflected in the neonate.[6] So, as labor progresses and pain intensity increases, the plasma level of opioid fades. It is in the later stages of labor that patients most need a therapeutic plasma level of opioid, and such a level is only rarely obtained with a single- or intermittent-dose technique. The ability of PCA to maintain a therapeutic plasma level of opioid while avoiding high peak levels means that the analgesic regimen will still be effective during the more painful later stages of labor. In fact, the theory behind such a dosing regimen is alluded to in a major obstetric text-book: 'In general, a small dose given more frequently is preferable to a larger one administered less often. Then, if delivery occurs during the next hour or so after injection, the infant is less likely to be depressed by the medication'.[6]

Several investigators have recently evaluated PCA for labor analgesia.[3–5] The technique originally described by Scott[2] utilized meperidine, which to this day remains the most commonly used opioid analgesic in obstetrics. However, two recent studies have evaluated nalbuphine via PCA for labor analgesia.[3,4] Nalbuphine[7] is a mixed agonist–antagonist opioid that is appealing for use in laboring women. As a k-receptors agonist, it has minimal psychomimetic effects. The incidence of gastrointestinal side-effects is lower than with pure opioid agonists. In addition, a ceiling effect for respiratory depression will theoretically enhance the safety margin of this drug when maternal safety or placental transfer to the neonate is a concern.[8]

PCA may be of use in patients in whom epidural analgesia is contraindicated. Two reports describe the use of fentanyl PCA during labor in parturients with a coagulation defect.[9,10] Satisfactory analgesia was obtained using a demand dose of 20–25 μg and a lockout interval of 3–10 minutes. Fentanyl is a useful drug during labor because of short duration of action and lack of active metabolites. It has been used safely during labor,[11] and also appears to be safe in breast-feeding women.[12] Precise dosing and lockout schedules have not been determined, and one may need to individualize these parameters for each patient's needs. Fentanyl, as well as all other opioids, will cross the placenta. Thus, appropriate monitoring is necessary to detect opioid-induced side-effects such as fetal depression, loss of beat-to-beat variability or neonatal respiratory depression.

REFERENCES

1. Bonica J J 1972 Principles and practice of obstetric analgesia and anesthesia. F A Davis, Philadelphia
2. Scott J S 1970 Obstetric analgesia: a consideration of labor pain on a patient-controlled technique for its relief with meperidine. Am J Obstet Gynecol 106: 959–978
3. Podlas J, Breland B D 1987 Patient-controlled analgesia with nalbuphine during labor. Obstet Gynecol 70: 202–204
4. Frank M, McAteer E J, Cattermole R et al 1987 Nalbuphine for obstetric analgesia. A comparison of nalbuphine with pethidine for pain relief in labour when administered by patient-controlled analgesia. Anaesthesia 42: 697–703
5. Robinson J O, Rosen M, Evans J M et al 1980 Self-administered intravenous and intramuscular pethidine. A controlled trial in labor. Anaesthesia 35: 763–768
6. Pritchard J A, Macdonald P C, Grant N F (eds) 1982 William's Obstetrics, 17th edn. Appleton-Century-Crofts, East Norwalk, CT
7. Erick J K, Heel R C 1983 Nalbuphine. A preliminary review of its pharmacological properties and therapeutic efficacy. Drugs 26: 191–201
8. Wilson S J, Erick J K, Balkon J 1986 Pharmacokinetics of nalbuphine during parturition. Am J Obstet Gynecol 155: 340–344
9. Kleiman S J, Wiesel S, Tessler M J 1991 Patient-controlled analgesia using fentanyl in a parturient with a platelet function abnormality. Can J Anaesth 38: 489–91
10. Rosaeg Op, Kitts J B, Karen G, Byford L J 1992 Maternal and fetal effects of intravenous patient-controlled fentanyl analgesia during labor in a thrombocytopenic parturient. Can J Anaesth 39: 277–81
11. Rayburn W, Rathke A, Leuschen P et al 1989 Fentanyl citrate analgesia during labor. Am J Obstet Gynecol 161: 202–6
12. Steer P L, Biddle C J, Marley W S et al 1992 Concentration of fentanyl in colostrum after an analgesia dose. Can J Anaesth 39: 231–235

31. Paracervical block anesthesia in obstetrics

P. Defoort M. Thiery

INTRODUCTION

Paracervical block anesthesia (PCB) consists of a nerve block of the Lee–Frankenhauser plexus, which conveys the nervous impulses from the uterine body and cervix to the spinal cord via the sensory nerves associated with the sympathetic chain, which enters the spinal cord with the 10th, 11th and 12th thoracic nerves. To achieve this block, the local anesthetic drug, an amide- or ester-type anesthetic, is injected through the vaginal fornices into the vicinity of the cervix. Currently, the drugs most likely to be used are the amide-type compounds bupivacaine, mepivacaine, lidocaine or prilocaine, with or without the addition of epinephrine. By 'uterosacral block' (USB) is meant a technique whereby the drug is injected not only laterally to the cervix but also more dorsally, to increase effectiveness. Radiologic studies of the diffusion of the anesthetic solution have proven that the spread is equal with PCB and USB so that the distinction between PCB and USB is artificial.

PCB was first applied as a method of pain control in labor by Gellert about 1922 and the technique was first published in 1926.[2] It was more widely introduced by Rosenfeld[3] and became popular in the mid-1950s. In 1972, Thiery and Vroman[1] were able to discuss the published evidence concerning 70 000 cases. By the 1980s, interest in the technique had decreased. Concern about fetal effects of PCB and the more ready availability of continuous lumbar epidural anesthesia (CLEA) are the determining factors in this trend. However, PCB remains a safe and effective technique in gynecologic surgery, and may still have applicability in uncomplicated obstetrics when logistics preclude the application of CLEA.

TECHNIQUE

The technique consists of injecting a dose of local anesthetic solution – usually 10–20 ml in a concentration of 0.25–1% depending upon the agent – below the mucosa of the lateral/dorsal vaginal fornices, where it will block the nerve plexus. The paracervical plexus is situated in the vicinity of the uterine artery, the venous plexus and the ureter. These structures, as well as the myometrium, placental margin and the fetus, must be avoided during injection.

To place the drug correctly, the following procedure is used. The parturient is placed in the lithotomy position; the vulva and perineum are disinfected and the woman draped. Vaginal disinfection, though much insisted upon by earlier authors, does not appear to be really effective.[1] To inject the left fornix (4 o'clock), the index and middle fingers of the gloved left hand are introduced 'diagonally' into the vagina, i.e. resting against the *right* labium majus, with the tips of the fingers introduced into the left fornix. In that way, the cervix and fetal head will be screened from the needle, while the needle tip will penetrate the tissues pointing tangentially away from the fetus and uterus. In the groove between the fingers, a guarded needle guide (needleguard, Kobak needle, Iowa trumpet) is placed to make contact with the mucosa. (An unguarded needle tends to become enmeshed in the operator's glove or to scratch the vaginal wall.) Furthermore, a guarded needle has but a limited depth of penetration. The optimal penetration depth should not be exceeded, so there should be no pressure exerted with the needle guard or fingertips. A slight resistance is felt when the needle leaves the guide and penetrates the vaginal wall. It is advisable to warn the woman of this happening as it may cause a brief feeling of pain and she should avoid startled movements.

Prior to the injection of the drug solution, it should be verified that no blood can be aspirated. If this is the case, the needle must be withdrawn and slightly redirected before reinsertion. However, even with this precaution, there is no absolute safeguard against intravascular injection.[4] The solution is then slowly (45 s to 1 min) injected into the lateral fornix. It should be confirmed intermittently that no blood can be aspirated into the syringe during the injection. After one side has been treated, the needle and guide are withdrawn. Though some authors do not insist upon it,[5,6] most find it advisable to wait a while before injection on the other side. The recommended interval varies from one or two contractions to 10–15 min in order to avoid a high concentration of drug. The contralateral fornix is then injected, using the same technique and precautions.

It is most logical to introduce the needle point not exactly laterally (3 and 9 o'clock), as the uterine arteries are most likely to be encountered at this site, but slightly laterosacral (4 and 8 or 5 and 7 o'clock). Four- and six-point injections have also been recommended, as has the 'multiple depot' technique consisting of the injection of 3-ml doses at several sites. The latter technique has been claimed to have the benefits of effectiveness (spread of drug) and safety (fractioning of the doses), but studies of the spread of radio-opaque solutions have shown that the target area is not critical to obtain satisfactory spread, and thus injecting slowly should be an effective safety measure.

The depth of the injection obtained with guarded needles may be as much as 1.5 cm or 2.0 cm. While this is not unduly deep, one must remember that the uterine artery, venous plexus and ureter are displaced cranially from the plexus during pregnancy, which still permits unintentional intrafetal injection when the cervix is nearly effaced. Radiologic studies by Jagerhorn[7] demonstrate that at 4 mm injection depth rapid intravascular spread is observed, while 2-mm-deep injection (i.e. exactly the mucosal thickness) causes a gradual lateral and cranial diffusion and minimal vascular spreading. In addition, the drug is retained for a longer period of time around the plexus. This further explains why Bloom et al[8] were able to claim 92% success, without side-effects, in patients in whom the injection was so superficial that mucosal swelling was produced.

TIMING OF THE INJECTION

Timing of a PCB is a compromise between the expected duration of drug activity and labor, and is subject to the judgement of the obstetrician. However, as Thiery and Vroman[1] state, a logical point in time to start analgesia is when the parturient asks for it. Although PCB has been advocated even in the latent phase of labor, its use is generally restricted to the acceleration phase of the first stage. As a rule, PCB is started at 4–5 cm dilation in multiparous women and at 5–6 cm dilation in nulliparous women.[5] It is not recommended to initiate the PCB too near the end of labor. There is no effective pain control from PCB during the second stage. An injection close to delivery may cause relatively high drug levels in the neonate, a potentially hazardous situation as the neonate eliminates the local anesthetic more slowly than the unborn child.

In our experience, a block covering the dilation phase up to the period of active bearing down – when most women 'push away the pain' – is usually felt to be satisfactory. While Thiery and Vroman[1] have performed up to nine blocks under internal cardiotocographic monitoring, it is mostly accepted that the number of blocks should be restricted to three or even two.[5] To provide analgesia during the second stage as well, a pudendal block may be performed ('combined block'). For sustained activity, continuous PCB may be considered.

CONTINUOUS BLOCK

'Continuous block' is the continuous infusion of the local anesthetic solution into each of the lateral fornices through a self-retaining catheter. The advantage of the method lies in dosage control and the duration of activity.[9] Several self-retaining catheter systems (barbed or coiled) have been developed, usually in combination with pudendal catheters to provide combined blocks.[10]

DRUGS USED AND DURATION OF ACTIVITY

Amide-type local anesthetics (bupivacaine, mepivacaine, lidocaine, prilocaine) are most commonly chosen for PCB, though ester-type local anesthetics (procaine, chloroprocaine, tetracaine) have also been used. The effective duration of anesthesia varies from 30 min with lidocaine to 120 min with bupivacaine with or without epinephrine. The addition of epinephrine is meant to extend the duration of action of some compounds. Pitkin and Goddard[11] doubled the duration of activity with 200 mg of lidocaine from 50 min to 100 min by adding 1:200 000 epinephrine. As bupivacaine is a long-acting drug, the advantage of adding epinephrine to the solution is not convincing. The longer duration of bupivacaine obviates the need for continuous block in many cases.

EFFICACY

Notwithstanding the amount of published material available from the 1960s and 1970s, many questions remain unanswered owing to lack of controlled studies and the use of standardized protocols. This is not only so on the matter of side-effects: the efficacy of PCB has rarely been analyzed in double-blind studies.[6] Pain relief is difficult to measure objectively. The (relatively) short duration of effectiveness and the fact that progress of labor changes the intensity and location of the pain further complicate the analysis of pain relief achieved by PCB. Moreover, in many cases, premedication or additional medication may have been administered as well.

Flu[6] found in a double-blind study that pain was significantly less with PCB than with placebo injections, as measured either by asking for the patient's feeling of relief or judging from a patient behavior scoring system. Effectiveness (with prilocaine) lasted on average for 40 min in this study.

SIDE-EFFECTS AND HAZARDS

Maternal

According to Abouleish,[5] minor effects such as vertigo, tinnitus and 'aura' have been observed in the mother in 1 in 600 cases. In 1 in 3000 cases, more serious phenomena of intoxication such as convulsions with potentially lethal outcome were reported.[4,12] The lethal cases were the result of first-trimester abortion. In view of these potential life-threatening complications, it is mandatory to keep resuscitative equipment immediately available while performing a PCB.

Paresthesiae, numbness and anesthesia of the leg can occur due to spread of the anesthetic solution to the sacral plexus. These side-effects are mostly transient. Flu[6] in his double-blind study noted no significant difference in the incidence of these effects between treated women and controls. Serious neuritis has been reported with etidocaine, and this drug has been withdrawn for PCB.[1] Hematoma of the injection site, vaginal tear and infection have been described in a few instances but should not be of major concern.

In view of the possibility of an allergic or anaphylactic reaction to the drug, some authors adhere to an intracutaneous test dose, prior to injection, while at the same time conceding the doubtful value of this test. We subscribe to the practice of asking the patient for a history of drug allergy, especially for local anesthetics, and have had no problems with this precaution. It should be noted that the so-called 'perfect block', consisting of total anesthesia with sedation of the patient may, in fact, be due to partial intravascular injection.[1] Flu[6] was unable to distinguish between treatment and control groups in the incidence of maternal hypotension and methemoglobinemia. There were no clinically significant changes in maternal pH, $P\text{CO}_2$ and base excess.

Fetal and neonatal

The fetal and neonatal effects have remained the major concern with PCB. Transient fetal bradycardia is associated with the technique in a significant number of cases. The prevalence of bradycardia varies from 2 to 70%,[13] 24% on average.[14] Differences between studies may be ascribed to the method used for detection (auscultation vs. continuous monitoring) and by the definition applied for fetal bradycardia.[1] Bradycardia is a singular phenomenon, apparently unrelated to other alterations of the fetal heart rate. Flu[6] could not demonstrate any changes in the baseline heart rate of the fetus due to PCB, nor were the number of decelerations or changes in beat-to-beat variation significantly different between treatment and control groups. In the treatment group, transient bradycardia occurred four times (10%). The start of bradycardia is observed from 1 to 12 min (6 min on average) after PCB has been given, and will last for 2–32 min (on average 8 min).[5]

The etiology of the fetal bradycardia induced by PCB is complex. It may be due to direct effects of the local anesthetic on the fetus, or decreased fetoplacental blood flow due to vascular constriction or uterine hyperactivity. Maternal hypotension through caval compression and reflex bradycardia from manipulation of the fetal head have also been incriminated.

While the amide local anesthetics have a known effect on isolated myometrial strips, their influence on actual labor is more complex to assess since labor itself is subject to a great deal of physiologic variability. Many authors from Gellert[3] onward have insisted upon oxytocic augmentation of labor to achieve as great a progress as possible while the anesthetic effect lasts. Several regimens of augmentation – with or without amniotomy – have been applied. Some hold the view that, even if uterine activity is not augmented by the block, at least the cervix is softened and may be more yielding to contractions. Flu[6] found no difference in uterine work between treatment and control groups. Thus, it cannot be maintained that transient bradycardia is mostly due to uterine hyperactivity. However, as with CLEA, coincidence of both phenomena may jeopardize the fetus.

Cibils[15] found in vitro that small concentrations of lidocaine and mepivacaine cause vasoconstriction of term uterine arteries, while the effect is much less marked in uterine arteries in pre-term pregnant women. He suggests that vasoconstriction leads to diminished uteroplacental blood flow and hypoxic bradycardia.

As evidence of a direct effect of the local anesthetic used for PCB on the fetus, authors such as Teramo and Wiedholm,[16] found a dose-related response in that the frequency of bradycardia increased from 20 to 70% as mepivacaine doses were doubled from 200 to 400 mg. The fetus can hydrolyze ester-type anesthetics, but because of hepatic immaturity is unable to readily metabolize amide-type anesthetics. In addition, metabolites of the local anesthetic can influence the fetus. Abouleish[5] points out that, in cases of bradycardia, fetal dose levels were usually higher than maternal levels. This, however, is not always the case[1] and does not conflict with the observation that bradycardia is not a constant phenomenon even in cases of intrafetal injection.

Other pharmacologic effects of local anesthetics on the fetal heart are lengthening of the atrioventricular and intraventricular conduction times.[17] On the ECG, the PR interval of the fetus is shortened and a ventricular rhythm develops. However, the QRS complex is not significantly changed, while changes in ST interval and T-peak are variable. These effects may, to some extent, be secondary to hypotensive changes. When the effect is excessive, as might be the case with direct injection and use in premature or acidotic fetuses, the QRS complex is widened and the PR interval increases, followed by complete cessation of the electric activity of the heart. Thiery and Vroman,[1] after reviewing the evidence, concluded that, within certain dose limits, it is not the absolute dose but rather the development of rapid peak levels by the drug when the block is initiated that is the underlying factor.

There are two important implications for management. First, fetal acidosis or pre-existent pathology enhances the tonic cardiac effect and may lead to a lethal vicious circle. Second, the fetus is more able to cope with the situation, by clearing the drug through the placenta, than is the neonate. As a rule, it is better not to precipitate the delivery and to wait for intrauterine fetal recovery. The measures proposed to aid recovery appear effective, as recovery is usually spontaneous.

CONCLUSIONS

1. The efficacy of PCB in providing maternal anesthesia during the acceleration phase of the first stage of labor has been documented by double-blind studies. As such, PCB is a useful tool for the obstetrician to provide effective anesthesia when an anesthesiologist is not available to initiate CLEA. PCB is not the analgesic technique of choice for a parturient wishing for complete pain control throughout the birth process.
2. While maternal side-effects occur only occasionally, are mostly benign and do not differ from those of other applications of local anesthetics, the most dangerous side-effect is the occurrence of bradycardia in the fetus. In an already compromised (acidotic, premature) fetus this may build up to a potentially lethal effect. PCB should thus be restricted in its use to term birth, in clinically normal patients, with continuous internal cardiotocographic monitoring of the fetus.

REFERENCES

1. Thiery M, Vroman S 1972 Paracervical block analgesia during labor. Am J Obstet Gynecol 113: 988–1036
2. Gellert P 1926 Aufhebung der Wehenschmerzen und Wehenuberdruck. Monatschr Geburtsh Gynaek 73: 143
3. Rosenfeld S S 1945 Paracervical anesthesia for relief of labor pains. Am J Obstet Gynecol 50: 527–532
4. Chastain G M 1969 Acute blood levels of lidocaine following paracervical block. J Med Assoc Ga 58: 426
5. Abouleish E 1977 Paracervical block. In: Abouleish E (ed) Pain control in obstetrics. J B Lippincott, Philadelphia, p 342
6. Flu P K 1977 The paracervical block during labor. Thesis (Dutch), Rotterdam
7. Jagerhorn M 1975 Paracervical block in obstetrics. An improved injection method: a clinical and radiological study. Acta Obstet Gynecol Scand 54: 9–27
8. Bloom S L, Horswill C W, Curet L B 1972 Effects of paracervical blocks on the fetus during labor: a prospective study with the use of direct fetal monitoring. Am J Obstet Gynecol 114: 218–222
9. Thiery M 1971 Continuous epidural block anesthesia during birth. (Dutch) T Geneesk 16–17: 834–841
10. Tafeen C H, Freedman H L, Harris H 1968 Combined continuous paracervical and continuous pudendal nerve block anesthesia in labor. Am J Obstet Gynecol 100: 55–62
11. Pitkin R M, Goddard W B 1963 Paracervical block in obstetrics – a controlled, double-blind study. Obstet Gynecol 21: 737–744
12. Grimes D A, Cates Jr W 1976 Deaths from paracervical anesthesia used for first-trimester abortion. New Engl J Med 295: 1397
13. Baskett J F 1974 Carson R M: Paracervical block with bupivacaine. Can Med Assoc J 110: 1363
14. Paul R H, Freeman R K 1972 Fetal cardiac response to paracervical block anesthesia: Part II. Am J Obstet Gynecol 113: 592–597
15. Cibils L A 1976 Response of human uterine arteries to local anesthetics. Am J Obstet Gynecol 126: 202–270
16. Teremo K, Wiedholm O 1967 Studies on the effects of anaesthetics on foetus. The effect of paracervical block with mepivacaine upon foetal acid-base values. Acta Obstet Gynecol Scand 46 (suppl): 1–39
17. Anderssen K E, Gennser G, Nilsen E 1970 Influence of mepivacaine on isolated human fetal hearts at normal and low pH. Acta Physiol Scand 80 (suppl 353): 34

32. Pudendal block

J. Ecker B. B. Feinberg

INTRODUCTION

First described by W. B. Muller in 1908, the pudendal nerve block has been called 'the foundation of all conduction blocks in obstetrics'.[1] In its simplicity, safety and preservation of fetal homeostasis, the pudendal block meets the essential requirements for pain control during labor and delivery. Little more than careful attention to anatomy and some basic equipment is needed for successful administration of pudendal anesthesia. Accordingly, the block has become a tool used more commonly by the obstetrician than the anesthesiologist.

INDICATIONS

With a single set of injections, the pudendal block provides satisfactory control of pain associated with delivery and permits performance of simple operative procedures. It is ideally suited for the patient who has managed the first stage of labor but requires help negotiating the discomfort of the second stage; it allows the patient to be both awake and mobile throughout the delivery. Outlet forceps deliveries and episiotomy repairs may also be performed under pudendal block without the added time, equipment and potential complications of other modalities such as spinal, epidural or general anesthesia. A pudendal block may be easily applied at times when the delivery is so imminent or the patient's discomfort is such that she cannot cooperate sufficiently for successful placement of spinal or epidural block. In its simplicity, it is also ideally suited for those situations and environments in which more experienced anesthetic help is not available.

One advantage of the pudendal block is that it is unlikely to induce the maternal hypotension that is sometimes seen after spinal or epidural anesthesia is initiated. Moreover, pudendal blocks share with other regional anesthetics a more limited risk of maternal aspiration and/or fetal depression secondary to transplacental passage of analgesic or anesthetic agents.

A pudendal block merely provides perineal anesthesia; it will not entirely eliminate the discomfort associated with contractions and, therefore, may not provide sufficient analgesia for many patients. It is inappropriate for use in operative procedures requiring deeper and more extensive manipulation such as mid-forceps deliveries or rotations. Furthermore, a pudendal block provides only a limited period of anesthesia and should be used only when the obstetrician anticipates completion of delivery and any necessary repair in less than 1–2 h, unless he wishes to reapply the block. In those situations when the obstetrician anticipates the possibility of an abdominal delivery (perhaps emergently) spinal or epidural anesthesia is a better choice.

Outside of those cases when the use of another form of anesthesia is preferable, there are few absolute contraindications to pudendal anesthesia, short of anesthetic allergies, which are exceedingly rare.

ANATOMY

Sensory innervation of the perineum is provided by three branches of the pudendal nerve, which itself arises from the fusion of branches of S2–S4 nerve roots (see Fig. 32.1). These three branches are (1) the perineal nerve with superficial and deep muscular branches providing the major nerve supply to the vulva and perineum, (2) the dorsal nerve of the clitoris providing sensation anteriorly and (3) the inferior hemorrhoidal nerve, which innervates the skin anterior and lateral to the anus as well as the lower rectum and external anal sphincter. Marginal areas of the perineum are innervated by the ilioinguinal (origin from L1), genitofemoral (origin from L1–2) and inferior pudendal nerves (a branch of the posterior femoral cutaneous nerve). It is clear that any block that targets the pudendal nerve will provide broad perineal anesthesia.

The ischial spine is the central landmark in the pudendal technique, in part because it is large and easily recognized. The techniques described below all block the pudendal nerve as it crosses the spine. The spine projects into the pelvis from the pelvic side wall to separate the

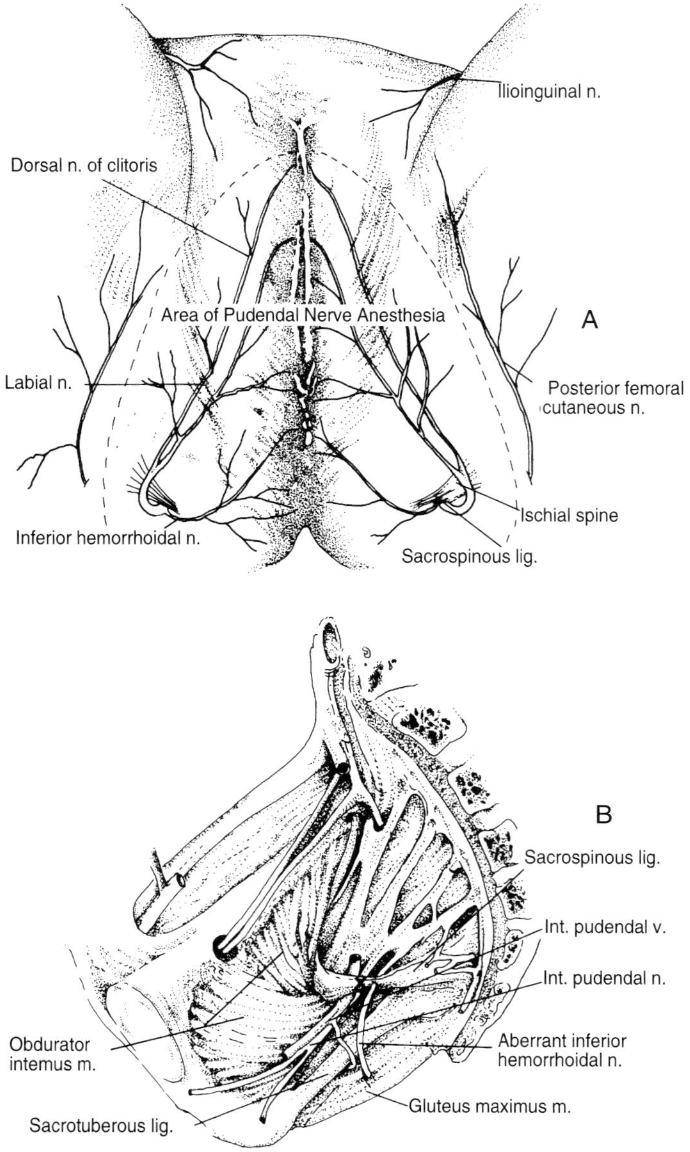

Fig. 32.1 Anatomy of pudendal nerves. (a) Internal pudendal nerve innervates entire female perineum. Its branches are dorsal nerve of clitoris, labial nerve and inferior hemorrhoidal nerve. Other nerves supplying adjacent areas but not the perineum itself are the ilioinguinal nerve and posterior femoral cutaneous nerve. (b) The main trunk of the pudendal nerve lies on the posterior surface of sacrospinous ligament just medial to ischial spine. The aberrant inferior hemorrhoidal nerve arises separately, medial to pudendal nerve, pierces the sacrospinous ligament and supplies perineum directly without entering Alcock's canal. (From ref. 1.)

greater and lesser sciatic foramina. This bony projection has a well-defined superior and inferior tip as well as anterior, posterior, superior and inferior surfaces – in essence, a wedge of bone – which are important structures and planes in the techniques described below. It is the inferior tip that projects farthest into the pelvis and is, therefore, the most easily palpable.

The pudendal nerve itself rises from S2–S4 and exits the pelvis through the greater sciatic foramen, curves around the ischial spine to cross the sacrospinous ligament, reenters the pelvis through the lesser sciatic foramen, and subsequently splits into the three branches described above (see Fig. 32.2). Of note, 50% of the time, the inferior hemorrhoidal nerve arises separately from S4 and perforates the sacrospinous ligament just medial to the spine.

Other important structures identified in relation to the spine include the pudendal canal, which contains the pudendal artery and vein lateral to the nerve, and the posterior femoral cutaneous nerve, just cephalad to the spine (lateral and posterior to the pudendal nerve). This nerve is also easily blocked by a needle directed toward the spine.

ANESTHETIC AGENTS

All varieties and types of local anesthetics have been used in placing pudendal blocks. Some of the most common agents used are listed in Table 32.1. Often these anesthetics are combined with dilute vasopressor agents such as epinephrine, which serve to retard their absorption and extend the duration of the block. In the past hyaluronidase was added to increase tissue penetration of the anesthetic;[2] however, precise placement renders such additives unnecessary.

There is little to guide one in selecting one agent over another, and undoubtedly a particular obstetrician's choice will be influenced by the usual pattern of practice at his institution.

TECHNIQUES

There are two distinct approaches to the pudendal block: transperineal and transvaginal. Both require similar basic

Table 32.1 (From Ostheimer G W 1991 Manual of obstetric anesthesia, 2nd edn. Churchill Livingstone New York)

Agent	Onset (min)	Duration (min)
Bupivacaine 0.25–0.5%	5–10	60–180
2-Chloroprocaine 1–2%	3–5	45–90
Lidocaine 0.5–1%	5–10	60–120
Mepivacaine 0.5–1%	5–10	60–120

Fig. 32.2 (a) The ischial spine: a shelf of bone with a superior and an inferior tip and anterior, posterior, superior and inferior surfaces. (b) The sacrospinous ligament, sacrotuberous ligament and obturator internus muscle forming the triangular-shaped localizing landmark shown above. (c) The pudendal nerve as it enters the lesser sciatic foramen and the pudendal canal. (d) The three main branches of the pudendal nerve trunk: (1) the inferior hemorrhoidal, (2) the perineal and (3) the dorsal clitoral nerves. (From ref. 3.)

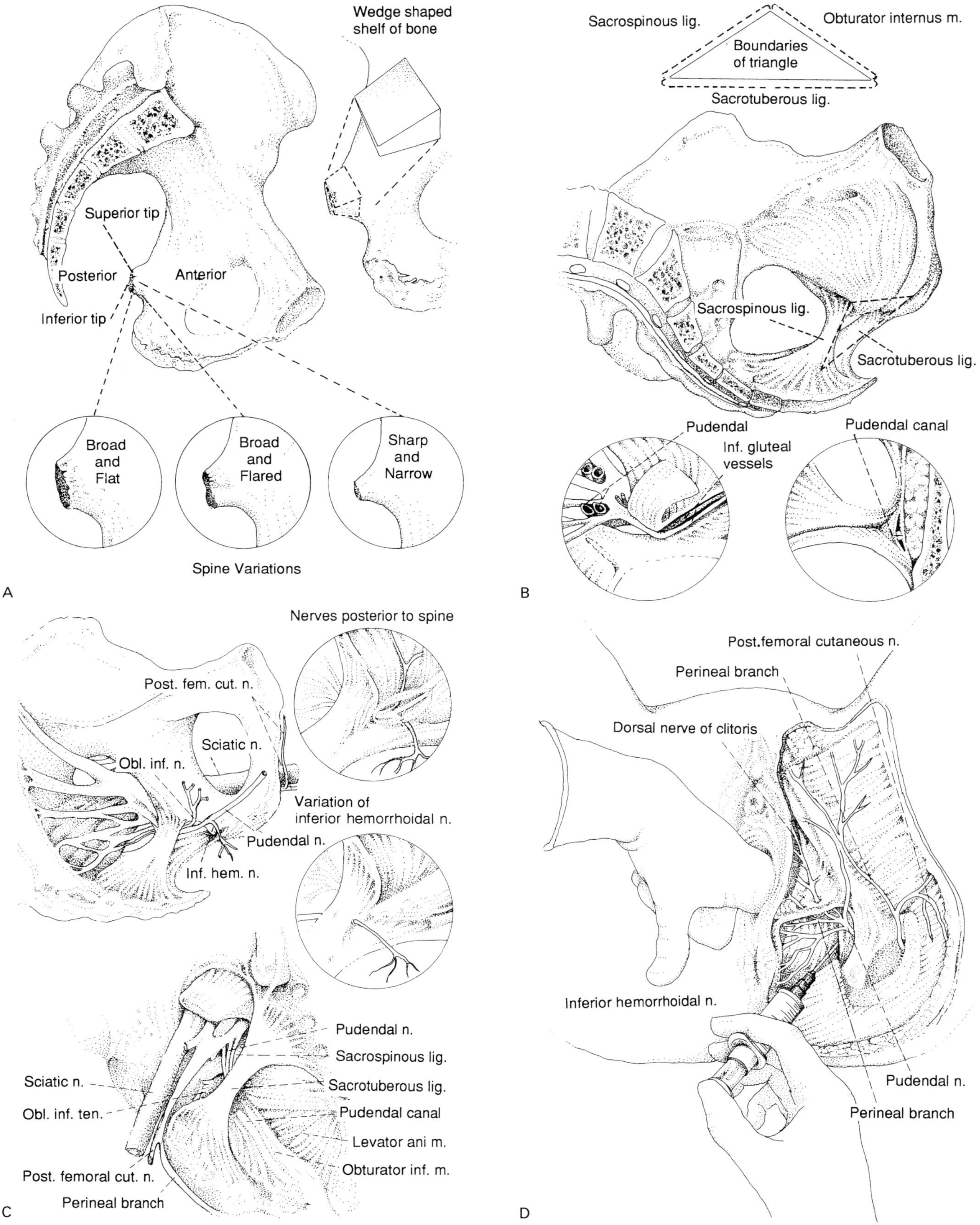
Wedge shaped
shelf of bone
Superior tip
Posterior
Anterior
Inferior tip
Broad
and
Flat
Broad
and
Flared
Sharp
and
Narrow
Spine Variations
A
Sacrospinous lig.
Obturator internus m.
Boundaries
of triangle
Sacrotuberous lig.
Sacrospinous lig.
Sacrotuberous lig.
Pudendal
Inf. gluteal
vessels
Pudendal canal
B
Nerves posterior to spine
Post. fem. cut. n.
Sciatic n.
Obl. inf. n.
Variation of
inferior hemorrhoidal n.
Pudendal n.
Inf. hem. n.
Pudendal n.
Sacrospinous lig.
Sciatic n.
Sacrotuberous lig.
Obl. inf. ten.
Pudendal canal
Levator ani m.
Obturator inf. m.
Post. femoral cut. n.
Perineal branch
C
Post.femoral cutaneous n.
Perineal branch
Dorsal nerve of clitoris
Inferior hemorrhoidal n.
Pudendal n.
Perineal branch
D

equipment: a refillable 10-ml syringe, a long narrow-gauge needle (20 gauge, 12–15 cm), betadine or other appropriate antiseptic solution and the local anesthetic itself. The transvaginal approach, in addition, requires a needle guide, such as an Iowa trumpet or Kobak guide, to protect and support the needle next to the delivering head in the mother's vagina.

Advocates of the transvaginal approach argue that this simple technique allows for a more accurate placement of the block since the needle enters the tissue directly above the central landmark – the ischial spine. Thereby, risk of both fetal puncture and damage to the rectum should be reduced.

Those who favor the transperineal approach, on the other hand, point out that this approach avoids passing the needle through the contaminated tissue of the vagina and may be used even when the fetal head is low, a position that may make the transvaginal placement difficult. The transperineal technique also allows easy block of the posterior femoral cutaneous nerve.

Whichever approach is selected, following the classic instructions laid out by Klink[3] (perineal method) and Kobak[4] (transvaginal method) the obstetrician should be able to simply effect a reproducible pudendal block.

TRANSPERINEAL APPROACH (Fig. 32.3)

To start a pudendal block via the transperineal approach, the perineum is cleaned and prepared with the patient in the lithotomy position. The needle is placed through the skin at a point halfway along a line drawn between the anus and the ischial tuberosity (which should be easily palpable). One may elect to anesthetize the skin with a small wheal before entering with the longer needle. Once through the skin, the needle is slowly advanced through the ischiorectal fossa. A finger from the other hand is place in either the vagina or rectum to guide the needle towards the ischial spine, which is usually found at a depth of 2–5 cm. When the spine is reached, 5 ml of anesthetic should be placed along the anterolateral surface to block the posterior femoral cutaneous nerve. The finger in the rectum or vagina can then be used to guide or push the needle around the spine to its posteromedial aspect. There 5 ml of anesthetic is deposited at both the inferior and superior tip of the spine. It is important to aspirate first, before injecting, as this is the location of the pudendal artery and vein as well as the nerve. Finally, the needle is advanced just beyond the spine (0.5 cm), crossing the sacrospinous ligament with a 'pop', before depositing

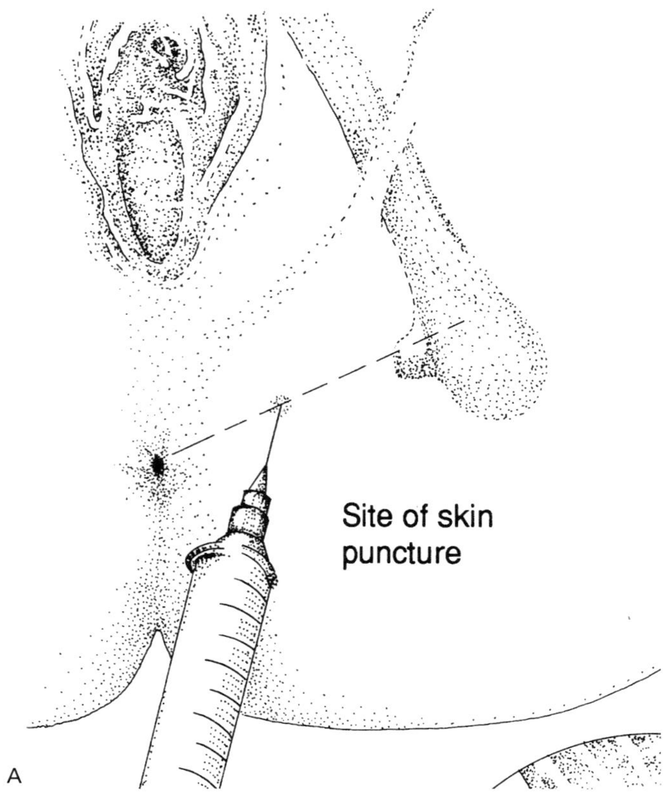

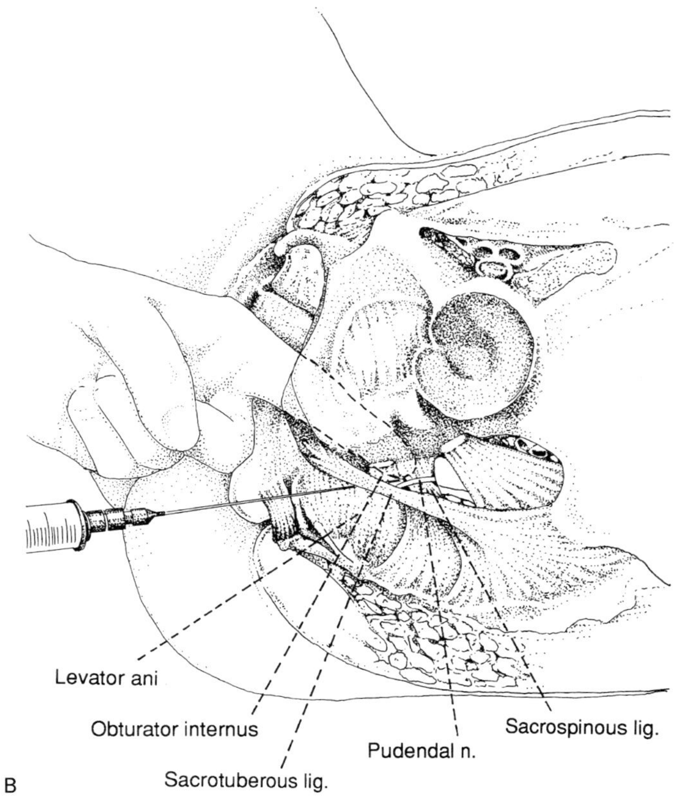

Fig. 32.3 Diagrammatic sketch of transperineal approach to pudendal nerve block. (**A**) Site of skin puncture. Injection of anesthetic solution around the main trunk of the pudendal nerve. (**B**) Insertion of the needle in the pudendal nerve block. With the finger in the vagina, both the tip of the needle and the spine are palpated. (From ref. 3.)

another 5 ml of agent; this last infiltration blocks the nerve before it branches and will also block the inferior hemorrhoidal nerve in those cases where it arises separately from the main nerve. Klink cautions that at all times the needle should move freely and easily; if the needle's motion is limited, or if one palpates a growing wheal as the anesthetic is injected, the needle may be positioned within the body of a muscle or ligament, limiting effective blockade.

Following these four injections, the needle is withdrawn and the procedure repeated on the opposite side.

TRANSVAGINAL APPROACH (Fig. 32.4)

The transvaginal approach also begins with the patient in lithotomy position. The vagina is prepared and a finger palpates the ischial spine while the other hand is used to move the guide into the vagina. The guide should be placed just medial to the spine above the point where the sacrospinous ligament attaches, which may be palpated by the vaginal finger. The needle is next pushed from within the guide through the vaginal mucosa and 3–5 ml local anesthetic is placed at the tip of the spine and just medial to the spine. The needle should then be advanced through the sacrospinous ligament (which will be crossed with a 'pop') and 5 ml injected. In all cases it is again important to aspirate before injection in order to avoid intravascular injection. The procedure is repeated on the opposite side.

With either approach, it should take between 3 and 5 mins for the block to develop. Appropriate placement can be checked by gently brushing the skin over the perineum and watching for reflex anal contracture or 'wink'. Pricking the skin with a pin or needle should be avoided until the area is adequately anesthetized to light touch. A plastic sword or towel clip may also be used.

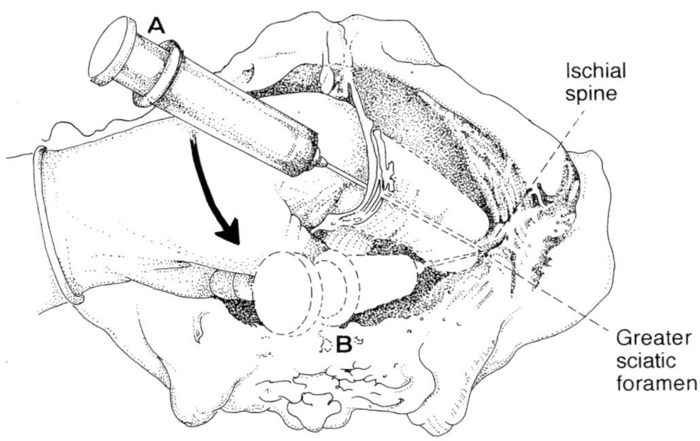

Fig. 32.4 Diagrammatic sketch of transvaginal approach to pudendal nerve block. (A) The position of the needle directed downward and laterally to pilerce the vagina just below the previous injection at the ischial spine. (B) The redirection of the needle to make it parallel with the table and the longitudinal axis of the mother as indicated by the arrows. (From ref. 4.)

COMPLICATIONS

Complications related to pudendal anesthesia may be grouped either as reactions to the anesthetic agents used or as complications resulting from the process of placing the block.

Reactions to the anesthetic agents used may result in either cardiovascular or CNS toxicities. Unintentional overdosage or intravascular injection can induce dysrhythmias and cardiovascular collapse. Accordingly, appropriate resuscitation equipment must be available whenever and wherever a pudendal block is placed. Since toxic effects depend on the cumulative dose of anesthetic delivered or on intravenous administration, one needs to include the amount of agent used elsewhere – perhaps for local infiltration or as part of a failed epidural block – in calculating the total dose delivered in order to insure that maximal safe dosages are not exceeded.

The needle used to place the pudendal block is another source of potential complication as it may unintentionally pierce and damage either the rectum, vagina or fetus. Hematomas in the ischiorectal and paravaginal spaces have been described following pudendal block. The needle may serve as a vector, introducing bacteria into previously sterile spaces; abscess and periosteal infections have been reported in association with pudendal blocks.[5,6] Sciatic neuritis has been observed following deliveries in which pudendal block was used, but it is difficult to know in such cases whether the pudendal block or the delivery and associated instrumentation was responsible for the symptoms.

Whenever drugs are used in pregnancy or during labor and delivery, one needs to consider fetal effects before labeling the agent as safe. No adverse fetal outcomes have been reported using recommended doses and placement of pudendal anesthesia.

Finally, there is nothing to suggest that the use of pudendal block impedes the progress of labor.[7] Such findings are not surprising since the block does not target innervation – either sensory or motor – of the uterus, whose muscular contractions are driving the labor towards its conclusion. Indeed, in as much as a pudendal block allows for an indicated application of forceps, it may help speed a patient's labor to a more successful outcome.

SUMMARY

Pudendal anesthesia is a valuable tool for obstetricians managing the second stage of labor. With careful attention to technique, successful placement should be common and complications few. Perhaps most important in deciding whether or not to place a pudendal block is recognizing those situations in which another anesthetic technique is more appropriate. Although the individual obstetrician will choose the technique and anesthetic agents with which he is most comfortable, the transvaginal approach is generally used as it offers the advantage of simplicity.

REFERENCES

1. Flowers C E 1967 Conduction anesthesia in obstetrics. In: Flowers C E (ed) Obstetric analgesia and anesthesia. Harper & Row, New York, p 104
2. Baum F E 1956 The use of hyaluronidase in pudendal block. Am J Obstet Gynecol 60: 1356
3. Klink E W 1953 Perineal nerve block. Am J Obstet Gynecol 1: 134
4. Kobak A J, Evans E F, Johnson G R 1956 Transvaginal pudendal block. Am J Obstet Gynecol 71: 981
5. Svancarek W, Chirino O, Schaefer G J, Blythe J G 1977 Retropsoas and subgluteal abscesses following paracervical and pudendal anesthesia. J Am Med Assoc 237: 892
6. Qvigstad E, Jerne F 1980 Severe infection following pudendal anesthesia. Int J Gynecol Obstet 18: 385
7. Johnson W L, Winter W W, Eng M, Bonica J J, Hunter C A 1972 Effect of pudendal, spinal and peridural block anesthesia on the second stage of labor. Am J Obstet Gynecol 113: 166

33. Inhalation analgesia

P. A. Clyburn

INTRODUCTION AND HISTORY

Inhalation anesthetic agents can be used in subanesthetic concentrations to provide analgesia. Such inhalation analgesia produces a degree of sedation which may progress to unconsciousness, putting the pregnant patient at risk of aspiration of regurgitated stomach contents. In addition, any sedation interferes with maternal cooperation with childbirth. However, inhalation analgesia used during the first and second stages of labor is effective, has a long and impressive safety record and is simple to administer. Despite the increasing use of regional techniques in obstetrics, inhalation analgesia still has an important role in providing pain relief for labor. Nitrous oxide analgesia, in particular, has a rapid onset and is useful to supplement regional anesthesia, either before the block is fully established or when the block is inadequate. In the UK, Entonox, a premixed supply of 50% nitrous oxide and 50% oxygen, is extensively administered by midwives both in the hospital and in the community, whilst in the USA inhalation analgesia was used in over 250 000 vaginal deliveries (estimated) in 1986.[1]

James Young Simpson, Professor of Midwifery in Edinburgh, was the first to use inhalation agents to aid childbirth. In January 1847, 3 months after the first successful general anesthetic, he administered ether to a woman in labor and noted that it was capable of removing suffering without interfering with the process of parturition.

Simpson immediately began searching for an alternative to ether. In November 1847, after first experimenting on himself and friends, he successfully used chloroform to aid childbirth. Inhalation analgesia was greatly popularized when in 1853 John Snow administered chloroform to Queen Victoria for the birth of Prince Leopold. It must have been successful because a second royal administration of chloroform was performed in 1857 for the birth of Princess Beatrice.

The first use of nitrous oxide in obstetric practice is credited to Klickowitsch of St Petersburg in 1880.[2] He found that, in addition to providing pain relief, and unlike chloroform, it did not depress uterine activity. In 1934 Minnit described his apparatus for obstetric use which delivered 35% nitrous oxide in air.[3] No doubt analgesia was aided by the hypoxia that such a mixture induces!

BASIC PRINCIPLES AND TECHNIQUE

Inhalation analgesia may be administered either continuously or intermittently. During the first stage of labor, the pain of uterine contractions is periodic, lasting around 90 s and recurring every 5–10 min. Contractions during the second stage are more frequent but remain regular and are accompanied by an urge to bear down. Such spasmodic pain is ideally treated with intermittent analgesia. However, relief is not immediate on starting inhalation; rather there is a delay or latency period.

Insoluble anesthetic agents with low blood–gas partition coefficients dissolve poorly in blood and body tissues so that equilibrium between brain and inspired concentration occurs quickly (Table 33.1). Thus, there is swift onset of analgesia and, because of low solubility in tissues, saturation is rapid with little accumulation, even after prolonged administration. When used intermittently, there is prompt excretion by the lungs so that at the start of each contraction there is little residual agent and the rate of onset of analgesia remains constant (Fig. 33.1).

In contrast, soluble anesthetic agents with high blood–gas partition coefficients, readily dissolve in body tissues (Table 33.1). Equilibration between brain and inspired concentration is delayed, leading to slow onset of analgesia. Accumulation occurs, with an increasing effect from a constant inspired concentration until the body is saturated. Even during intermittent administration, excretion by the lungs between contractions is incomplete and accumulation still occurs (Fig. 33.1). Analgesia, once established, is continued between contractions but at the expense of increased sedation.

Pregnancy causes a reduction in the functional residual capacity of the lungs and an increase in minute volume,

Table 33.1 Comparative characteristics of inhalation anesthetics

	Methoxyflurane	Halothane	Enflurane	Isoflurane	Nitrous Oxide	Desflurane	Sevoflurane
Blood: gas partition coefficient[a]	12	2.4	1.9	1.4	0.47	0.42	0.65
Brain: blood partition coefficient[a]	2	2.6	2.6	3.7	1.1	1.3	1.7
Oil: gas partition coefficient[a]	970	224	98	98	1.4	19	553.9
MAC (volumes per cent, 30–55 years old)	0.16	0.75	1.68	1.15	105–110	6–7	1.71–2.05
Vapor pressure (mmHg)							
18° Celsius	20	224	156	219	—	633	—
20° Celsius	23	224	172	240	—	669	157
22° Celsius	26	267	189	262	—	731	—
Molecular weight	165	197.4	184.5	184.5	44	168	—
Commerical preparation contains preservative	Yes	Yes	No	No	No	No	No
Stable in soda lime	No	No	Yes	Yes	Yes	Yes	No
Reacts with metal	Yes	Yes	No	No	No	No	No

[a] 37° Celsius

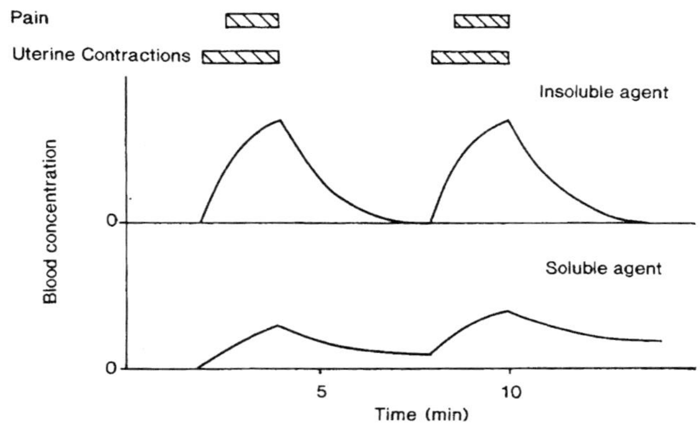

Fig. 33.1 Changes in blood concentrations of insoluble and soluble inhalation agents during intermittent inhalation.

ensuring that equilibration between inspired and alveolar concentrations occurs quickly and reducing the latency of onset of action. In addition, the minimum alveolar concentration (MAC) of inhalation anesthetic agents is reduced during pregnancy.[4] This increased sensitivity requires great care in administering inhalation agents if excessive sedation is to be avoided. Similarly, the apparatus used for delivery must be accurate and consistent in its delivered concentration.

About 50% of mothers get satisfactory pain relief from inhalation analgesia.[5–7] Success depends upon the mother being properly instructed before parturition and upon the skill of the attendant midwife or anesthesiologist in encouraging correct technique. During the antenatal period, the mother should become familiar with the apparatus and practice inhaling from a close-fitting face mask, avoiding any entrainment of air, which dilutes the analgesic effect.

In the first stage of labor, the initial 30 s of each contraction is painless, although the mother is aware of a tightening sensation. During this phase, the mother should be encouraged to inhale deeply and fairly rapidly in order that brain concentrations are adequate before the onset of pain. She should then continue deep, though slightly slower, inhalations to maintain analgesia until the end of the contraction.

In the second stage, pain is felt from the onset of the contraction as a result of distending pressure from the presenting part on the birth canal. Fortunately, contractions are at regular intervals, every 3–5 min, so that mother and midwife can anticipate each contraction and begin inhalation 30–60 s beforehand. Each bearing-down effort should last about 10 s during which the mother holds her breath. Between expulsive efforts, she should take quick, deep breaths of the agent to maintain analgesia.

APPARATUS

Inhalation analgesia is usually self-administered by the patient breathing from a hand-held face mask. This increases safety because, on becoming drowsy, the mask falls away from the mother's face, discontinuing the administration. However, the patient may position herself with the mask propped against a pillow in such a way that the mask remains fitted to the face. The mask needs to be close fitting to avoid entrainment of fresh air diluting the inhaled concentration. Approximately 30% of mothers dislike or fear the face mask. An alternative is a plastic mouthpiece which is held in place by the teeth and is preferred by many mothers.[8]

A variety of equipment is used to administer inhalation analgesia. It can be delivered from an anesthetic machine providing continuous flow, with accurate control of vapor or gas concentration adjusted to the patient's requirements by an anesthesiologist. This method is obviously unsuitable for self-administration, or for use by untrained personnel.

A number of simple drawover-type vaporizers have been designed to deliver fixed concentrations of vapor by drawing in air via an unidirectional valve. Most of these were intended for use with trichloroethylene and methoxyflurane, which are rarely used today and are mainly of historical interest. The Emotril and Tecota Mark 6 were used by British midwives to administer trichloroethylene, whilst the Cardiff inhaler was used to deliver methoxyflurane. They were sturdy, compact and reliable, incorporating temperature-compensating devices, which ensured constant concentration despite the fall in temperature caused by vaporization. Oxygen enrichment of the inspired concentration mixture was possible by means of a hood that is fitted over the Tecota or Cardiff inhalers. The Penthrane Analgizer was a simple, disposable, nontemperature-compensated vaporizer that contained a safe maximum amount of methoxyflurane (15 ml). It delivered approximately 0.3–0.9%, with the higher concentration delivered by the patient occluding a side-hole.

In 1961 Tunstall[9] suggested the use of premixed 50% nitrous oxide in oxygen (Entonox), stored in pressurized cylinders, which are color coded blue with blue and white quartered shoulders. The Entonox apparatus used for delivery consists of a pressure-reducing valve, a cylinder contents gauge and a demand flow valve developed from those used by underwater divers. The whole system is compact and eminently suitable for domiciliary use when small 500 L cylinders are used. Under usual circumstances the gases within the cylinder are thoroughly mixed and the apparatus delivers equal proportions of the two gases. However, at temperatures below −7°C, the gases separate with nitrous oxide gravitating to the bottom. Oxygen is then preferentially delivered from the top of the cylinder, leaving a potentially hypoxic concentration of nitrous oxide as the cylinder empties.[10] Because of this serious hazard, care is required in the storage and handling of Entonox cylinders. They should be maintained at temperatures above 10°C and pipeline supplies should incorporate a flow restriction to ensure that a high rate of usage does not cause excessive cooling. A flow not exceeding 300 L/min should prevent this happening.[11]

Scavenging of the expired gases is difficult and contamination of the delivery room is inevitable unless an anesthetic machine with scavenging apparatus is used for administration. For this reason, the labor room should be well ventilated with specific gas-flow patterns. For comfort, the internal resistance of any apparatus used for inhalation should be low.[12] The Entonox apparatus falls below the upper limits of acceptable resistance,[13] ensuring that breathing feels unrestricted even at high flow rates.

EFFECT ON THE FETUS

Any method of analgesia used in obstetrics should be safe to the fetus. All inhalation anesthetic agents are lipid soluble, of low molecular weight and, therefore, readily cross the placenta to reach the fetal circulation and nervous system. Agents such as methoxyflurane and trichloroethylene would be expected to accumulate in the mother and, therefore, in the fetus after prolonged administration during labor. Nevertheless, methoxyflurane does not appear to cause any neonatal depression.[14] Similarly, neurobehavioral studies during the first 24 h after delivery have failed to show any detectable effect on the neonate after analgesia with both nitrous oxide in oxygen and enflurane in oxygen had been used for vaginal delivery.[15]

Inhalation analgesic mixtures with an increased inspired oxygen concentration, such as Entonox, might be expected to improve fetal oxygenation. However, this is unlikely to be beneficial unless there is fetal distress; then an increased inspired oxygen concentration should be administered continuously and not intermittently, as is usually the case with Entonox.[16,17] It has recently been shown that Entonox, used in conjunction with intramuscular meperidine, causes a high incidence of maternal arterial oxygen desaturation,[18] and this combination is best avoided in situations of potential fetal distress.

Excessive maternal hyperventilation during labor is not uncommon, and the accompanying hypocarbia interferes with fetal oxygenation[19] by causing placental vasoconstriction[20] and a left shift in the hemoglobin–oxygen dissociation curve. It has been suggested that in such cases the mother should inhale a 50% mixture of nitrous oxide in oxygen with a low flow of carbon dioxide added to prevent hypocarbia.[21]

An advantage of inhalation analgesics is that the neonate readily excretes them via the lungs after delivery. Other systemic analgesics and sedatives, such as opioids and benzodiazepines, rely upon hepatic and renal routes of excretion, which are less reliable in the neonate.[22] Nitrous oxide, having a low blood solubility, is rapidly excreted in the lungs to the extent that the alveolar oxygen concentration may be reduced, causing diffusion hypoxia. This phenomenon is seen at the end of nitrous oxide anesthesia. Despite this theoretical risk, the nitrous oxide end-tidal concentration in the neonate is too low to cause a problem in vigorous neonates.[23] However, some infants may be adversely affected, and it is prudent to administer oxygen to infants of mothers receiving nitrous oxide immediately prior to delivery.

NITROUS OXIDE

This colorless, odorless, non-irritant gas is a relatively potent analgesic with weak anesthetic properties. For effective analgesia, concentrations approaching 50%

nitrous oxide need to be used, which if delivered in air result in a dangerously low inspired oxygen concentration. Although this combination was in common use in the past, nitrous oxide is currently delivered with oxygen. It is the commonest inhalation agent in obstetric use, principally because of the convenience of premixed Entonox.

Nitrous oxide has a low solubility (1.4) and a low blood–gas partition coefficient (0.47), so that there is rapid equilibration between inspired and brain concentrations. In practice, only 10 breaths or about 45 s are required to achieve near-maximum effect from an inspired concentration of nitrous oxide.[24] During intermittent administration, there is rapid excretion by the lungs between contractions, with little residual effect at the onset of the next contraction and, thus, minimal accumulation. The lack of significant accumulation, and the ease of maternal and neonatal excretion, suggests little need for any restriction upon the duration of inhalation.

The use of 50% nitrous oxide is a compromise between efficacy and safety. Rosen et al[25] reported that 70% of mothers derived some benefit from the use of Entonox during labor. However, other trials suggest a figure closer to 50%.[5–7] The use of 70% nitrous oxide increased the number of mothers helped to nearly 60%; however, there was a greater incidence of maternal drowsiness with decreased cooperation.[6] Jones et al[26] considered 74% nitrous oxide the optimum concentration for pain relief, but observed that this led to semiconsciousness in some patients.

The risk of aspiration during inhalation analgesia is related to the degree of sedation. Inhalation of 50% nitrous oxide did not influence the laryngeal closure reflex.[27] However, when the period of inhalation was extended to 30 min, 2 out of 10 volunteers allowed entry of radio-opaque dye into their tracheas.[28]

Despite the rapid onset of intermittent nitrous oxide analgesia, concentrations may be insufficient at the onset of the painful stage of each contraction. Arterial nitrous oxide levels at the start of Entonox inhalation were found to be very low and at the end of the contraction to be equivalent to equilibrium with only 26.4% nitrous oxide.[29] The low initial concentration can be improved by the continuous delivery of 5 L/min Entonox by means of nasal catheters,[30–32] which provides a background concentration of inhaled nitrous oxide. Thus at the start of each contraction, the mother already has an elevated end-tidal nitrous oxide level. Greater comfort can be achieved by a foam collar around the end of the catheter, and approximately 70% of mothers retain the catheter until the end of labor.[33]

Of some concern is the recent appreciation that nitrous oxide can interfere with vitamin B12 and cause bone marrow depression after prolonged administration. This has been observed mainly in sick patients requiring intensive care[34] and is of uncertain relevance to laboring mothers receiving nitrous oxide analgesia. Indeed, there is no evidence of any effect on neonates born to mothers receiving nitrous oxide for cesarean delivery.[35] Of relevance to the obstetric staff is the fact that dentists administering frequent inhalation sedation with nitrous oxide have developed mild megaloblastic bone marrow changes.[36] However, the levels of nitrous oxide to which these dentists were chronically exposed were likely to be much higher than those encountered on the labor ward. Nonetheless, as suggested earlier, it is prudent to have good ventilation in delivery rooms where nitrous oxide is administered.

METHOXYFLURANE AND TRICHLOROETHYLENE

These agents were popular for obstetric analgesia during the 1960s and 1970s but are now probably little used worldwide and are no longer available in the UK. They are more potent than nitrous oxide and can be administered in air at a concentration of between 0.2% and 0.5%. They are very soluble with high blood–gas partition coefficients (see Table 33.1) and analgesia is not achieved until 3–4 min after commencing inhalation. Accumulation occurs, even during intermittent administration, with progressively increasing effect from a constant inspired concentration. Despite this, there is evidence that mothers exhibit a degree of autoregulation,[37] subconsciously self-administering less methoxyflurane or reducing their minute volume to control end-tidal concentrations to provide sufficient analgesia without excessive sedation.

The main drawback to methoxyflurane is the fear of renal damage to mother and fetus. Methoxyflurane is metabolized to produce free fluoride ions. Urine and serum fluoride concentrations were raised for at least 48 h in neonates delivered to mothers receiving methoxyflurane analgesia during labor, but the levels were well below those considered to be nephrotoxic[38,39] and there was no evidence of renal damage in these neonates.[40] Nevertheless, it was recommended that no more than 15 ml of methoxyflurane is used for each mother during labor.[38] Trichloroethylene administration was also restricted because of fears about accumulation leading to excessive sedation in the neonate.

Both these agents have an unpleasant smell, which one-third of mothers and midwives disliked.[25]

ENFLURANE AND ISOFLURANE

The decrease in popularity and availability of trichloroethylene and methoxyflurane have encouraged a closer examination of other volatile anesthetic agents as potential inhalation analgesics.

Both enflurane (1.9) and isoflurane (1.4) have high blood–gas coefficients and speeds of onset and degrees of accumulation intermediate between those of nitrous oxide and methoxyflurane and trichloroethylene. They are fluorinated hydrocarbons and when metabolized release inorganic fluoride, which is potentially harmful to the kidneys. However, in contrast to methoxyflurane, the degree of biodegradation of enflurane[41] and isoflurane[42] is small, which minimizes the risk of renal damage.

Enflurane is capable of providing effective analgesia for childbirth[43] and proved superior to Entonox, but only at the expense of increasing drowsiness.[44] Like halothane, enflurane causes a dose-related decrease in uterine tone, though this is minimal at low concentrations.[45]

Isoflurane 0.75% in oxygen has also been shown to provide better analgesia than Entonox,[46] but, as with enflurane, there is increased maternal sedation.

FUTURE DEVELOPMENTS

The search for the ideal inhalation anesthetic agent has resulted in the development of several new volatile agents. What would be the desirable properties of any new inhalation analgesic?

1. Potent analgesia with minimal sedation.
2. Nontoxic to mother and baby.
3. Low tissue solubility and low blood–gas partition coefficient so that onset and offset of analgesia are rapid.
4. Easily vaporized with a stable molecule and long shelf-life.
5. Pleasant and nonirritant to inhale.
6. Nonflammable alone or when mixed with oxygen.
7. No effect on uterine tone.
8. No effect on cardiovascular stability.

Nitrous oxide meets many of these ideals but needs to be stored in pressurized cylinders, which makes it particularly unsuitable in developing countries, where an inexpensive, stable, volatile agent would be more desirable.

Two new volatile anesthetic agents, sevoflurane and desflurane, have low blood–gas partition coefficients similar to nitrous oxide (see Table 33.1), but both have drawbacks. Sevoflurane has a low boiling point of 23.5°C, making conventional vaporizers unsuitable. Sevoflurane is not a stable molecule and probably cannot be used with sodalime. Desflurane is now clinically available but the suitability of both agents as analgesics during labor and delivery remains to be explored. These drugs, and the development of further low-solubility volatile agents, hold promise for the future.

Table 33.1 lists the comparative characteristics of the inhalation anesthetics.

REFERENCES

1. Gibbs C P, Krischer J, Pecham B M, Sharp H, Kirschbaum T H 1986 Obstetric anesthesia: a national survey. Anesthesiology 65: 298–306
2. Klickowitsch S 1881 Arch Gynaekol 2: 81–108
3. Minnit R J 1934 Self administered anaesthesia in child birth. Br Med J 1: 501–502
4. Palahnuik R J, Shinder S M, Egar II E I 1974 Pregnancy decreases the requirement for inhaled anesthetic agents. Anesthesiology 41: 82–83
5. Holdcroft A, Morgan M 1974 An assessment of the analgesic effect in labour of pethidine and 50 per cent nitrous oxide in oxygen (Entonox). J Obstet Gynaecol Br Cwlth 81: 603–607
6. Cole P V, Crawford J S, Doughty A G et al 1970 Specifications and recommendations for nitrous oxide/oxygen apparatus to be used in obstetric analgesia. Anaesthesia 25: 317–327
7. Beazley J M, Leaver E P, Morewood J H M, Bircumshaw J 1967 Relief of pain in labour. Lancet 1: 1033–1035
8. Dolan P F, Rosen M 1975 Inhalational analgesia in labour: facemask or mouthpiece. Lancet 2: 1030–1031
9. Tunstall M E 1961 Use of a fixed nitrous oxide and oxygen mixture from one cylinder. Lancet 2: 964
10. Gale C W, Tunstall M E, Wilton Davies C C 1964 Pre mixed gas and oxygen for midwives. Br Med J 1: 732–736
11. McGregor W G, Bracken A, Flair J A 1972 Piped pre mixed 50% nitrous oxide and 50% oxygen mixture (Entonox). Anaesthesia 27: 14–24
12. Davies J M, Hogg M I J, Rosen M 1974 The resistance of Entonox valves. Br J Anaesth 46: 145–148
13. Hogg M I J, Davies J M, Mapleson W W, Rosen M 1974 Proposed upper limit of respiratory resistance for inhalational apparatus used in labour. Br J Anaesth 46: 149–152
14. Shnider S M, Steffenson J L, Margolis A J 1969 Methoxyflurane analgesia in obstetrics. Obstet Gynecol 33: 594–595
15. Stefani S J, Hughes S C, Shnider S M et al 1982 Neonatal neurobehavioral effects of inhalation analgesia for vaginal delivery. Anesthesiology 56: 351–355
16. Rosen M 1971 Recent advances in pain relief in childbirth. 1. Inhalation and systemic analgesia. Br J Anaesth 43: 837–848
17. Davies J M, Hogg M, Rosen M 1975 Maternal arterial oxygen tension during intermittent inhalational analgesia. Br J Anaesth 47: 370–378
18. Zelcer J, Owens H, Paull J D 1989 A controlled oximetric evaluation of inhalational, opioid and epidural analgesia in labour. Anaesth Intensive Care 17: 418–421
19. Fadl E, Utting J E 1969 A study of acid base state during labour. Br J Anaesth 41: 327–337
20. Morishima H O, Daniel S S, Adamsons K, James L S 1965 Effects of positive pressure ventilation of the mother upon the acid base status of the fetus. Am J Obstet Gynecol 93: 269–273
21. Argent VP 1982 Treatment of severe tetany due to hyperventilation during labour with a mixture of nitrous oxide, oxygen and carbon dioxide. Br Med J 2: 117–118
22. Kanto J, Erkkola R 1984 Obstetric analgesia: pharmacokinetics and its relationships to neonatal behavioural and adaptive functions. Biol Res Pregnancy Perinatol 5: 23–25
23. Mankowitz E, Brock-Utne J G, Downing J W 1981 Nitrous oxide elimination by the newborn. Anaesthesia 36: 1014–1016
24. Waud B E, Waud D R 1970 Calculated kinetics of distribution of nitrous oxide and methoxyflurane during intermittent administration in obstetrics. Anesthesiology 32: 306–316
25. Rosen M, Mushin W W, Jones P L, Jones E V 1969 Field trial of methoxyflurane, nitrous oxide and trichloroethylene in obstetric analgesia. Br Med J 3: 263–267
26. Jones P L, Rosen M, Mushin W W, Jones E V 1969 Methoxyflurane and nitrous oxide as obstetric analgesics. I. A comparison by continuous administration. Br Med J 3: 255–259

27. Cleaton Jones P 1976 The laryngeal closure reflex and nitrous oxide–oxygen analgesia. Anesthesiology 45: 569–570
28. Rubin J, Brock-Utne J G, Greenberg M, Bortz J, Downing J W 1977 Laryngeal incompetence during experimental 'relative analgesia' using 50 per cent nitrous oxide in oxygen. Br J Anaesth 49: 1005–1008
29. Latto I P, Molloy M J, Rosen M 1973 Arterial concentrations of nitrous oxide during intermittent patient controlled inhalation of 50% nitrous oxide in oxygen (Entonox) during the first stage of labour. Br J Anaesth 45: 1029–1034
30. Willis B A, Rosen M 1977 Entonox analgesia – a method of reducing the delay between demand and supply. Anaesthesia 32: 573–576
31. Davies J M, Willis B A, Rosen M 1978 Entonox analgesia in labour. A pilot study to reduce the delay between demand and supply. Anaesthesia 33: 545–547
32. Arthurs G J, Rosen M 1979 Self administered intermittent nitrous oxide analgesia for labour: enhancement of effect with continuous nasal inhalation of 50 per cent nitrous oxide (Entonox). Anaesthesia 34: 301–309
33. Arthurs G J, Rosen M 1981 Acceptability of continuous nasal nitrous oxide during labour. Field trial in six maternity hospitals. Anaesthesia 36: 384–388
34. Nunn J F 1988 Clinical relevance of the B12/N_2O interaction, a report of a seminar. Anaesthesia 43: 587–589
35. London M J, Toothill V J 1986 Effect of N_2O on placental methionine synthetase activity. Br J Anaesth 58: 524–527
36. Sweeney B, Bingham R M, Amos R J, Petty A C, Cole P V 1985 Toxicity of bone marrow in dentists exposed to nitrous oxide. Br Med J 2: 567–569
37. Latto I P, Rosen M, Molloy M J 1972 Absence of accumulation of methoxyflurane during intermittent self-administration for pain relief in labour. Br J Anaesth 44: 391–400
38. Creasser C W, Stoelting R K, Krishna G, Peterson C 1974 Methoxyflurane metabolism and renal function after methoxyflurane analgesia during labor and delivery. Anesthesiology 41: 62–66
39. Young S R, Stoelting R K, Bond V K, Peterson C 1976 Methoxyflurane biotransformation and renal function following methoxyflurane administration for vaginal delivery or Caesarean section. Anesth Analg 55: 415–419
40. Clark R B, Beard A G, Thompson D S 1979 Renal function in newborn and mothers exposed to methoxyflurane analgesia for labor and delivery. Anesthesiology 51: 461–467
41. Chase R E, Holaday D A, Fiserova-Bergerova V, Saidman L J, Mack F F 1971 The biotransformation of ethrane in man. Anesthesiology 35: 262–267
42. Holaday D A, Fiserova-Bergerova V, Latto I P, Zumbiel M A 1975 Resistance of isoflurane to biotransformation in man. Anesthesiology 43: 325–332
43. Abboud T K, Shnider S M, Wright R G et al 1981 Enflurane analgesia in obstetrics. Anesth Analg 60: 133–137
44. McGuinness C, Rosen M 1984 Enflurane as an analgesic in labour. Anaesthesia 39: 24–26
45. Neumark J, Faller T 1978 Halothane, Enflurane und ihr Einfluss auf die Uterusakivitat am Geburtstermin. Praktische Anaesthesie, Wiederbelebung und Intensivtherapie 13: 7–12
46. McLeod D D, Ramayya G P and Tunstall M E 1985 Self-administered isoflurane in labour: a comparative study with Entonox. Anaesthesia 40: 424–426

34. Caudal block

H. Nolte

HISTORY

In 1901 the urologist Cathelin[1] and the surgeon Sicard[2] independently described the caudal approach to the epidural space. In 1909 Stöckel[3] introduced caudal epidural anesthesia under the name 'sacral anesthesia' into gynecology and obstetrics. His first report included 141 instances of obstetric anesthetic procedures. Subsequently, uncertain effects after application of caudal anesthesia reduced its importance. However, the introduction of the continuous technique by Hingson and Edwards[4] in 1942 not only led to a revival of caudal anesthesia but may also be regarded as a milestone in the history of obstetric regional anesthesia. In the past 30 years caudal anesthesia was pushed into the background as a result of the enormous development of continuous lumbar epidural anesthesia, particularly in obstetrics.

DEFINITION

Caudal anesthesia is an epidural anesthetic procedure in which the local anesthetic is injected from 'below' via the caudal foramen of the spine into the epidural space. In order to achieve a spread similar to lumbar epidural anesthesia, higher volumes of the local anesthetic are required.

TECHNIQUE[5–8]

In obstetrics, caudal anesthesia should be performed with the patient in the lateral or knee–elbow position. The detection of the caudal foramen is relatively simple in most patients, since the cornuae caudales in general are easily palpable at the upper end of the intergluteal fold. Between both cornuae, the caudal foramen is situated in a depression. Following the common aseptic measures and local infiltrative anesthesia of the skin area, a 6- to 8-cm-long 22-gauge needle is inserted into the caudal canal. Prior to injection, careful aspiration in two quadrants has to be performed in order to avoid puncture of one of the numerous veins in the caudal canal. Some recommend the injection of 8–10 ml of air prior to the local anesthetic. If the needle is not situated properly in the caudal canal, the subcutaneous crepitations caused by the air emphysema can be felt with the flat hand lying on the os sacrum. For continuous caudal anesthesia, the introduction of a catheter through a 18-gauge or 20-gauge Crawford needle is recommended. Even more suitable are the recently developed disposable trays for continuous spinal or epidural anesthesia.

20–25 ml of a local anesthetic is sufficient for a sensory blockade to the level of T10. A reduction in volume leads to less cephalad spread of the sensory block. Appropriate local anesthetics are the medium-acting lidocaine, mepivacaine, and prilocaine in 1% solution. In the last few years, however, bupivacaine 0.25% or 0.375% has been increasingly applied owing to its long duration of action, outstanding sensory anesthetic properties and the favorable relation between maternal and fetal plasma concentrations.

SIDE-EFFECTS

Given a correct procedure and avoiding overdosages or intravascular injections, there are no significant side-effects either to the mother or to the fetus. Particularly marked hypotension will not occur if the mother is positioned adequately. An unintentional puncture of the dural sac as a result of advancing the needle too far should be avoided. Otherwise the puncture of the dura could lead to a total spinal block. Breaking of a needle or rupture of a catheter can also be avoided by appropriate care. In 1965 Sinclair et al[9] and Finster et al[10] described some cases of unintentional injection of local anesthetic into the fetal skull cap leading to severe intoxication of the fetus. These cases were reported more than 25 years ago, and by using a careful procedure this complication should no longer occur.

PHARMACODYNAMICS AND PHARMACOKINETICS

In contrast to lumbar epidural anesthesia, in which the local anesthetic spreads cephalad and caudally following injection, there is only cephalad spread of the local anesthetic with the caudal approach. Therefore, a spread of the anesthetic to the lower thoracic region can be achieved if appropriate volumes are injected at the end of the first stage. A typical feature of caudal anesthesia is its slow regression of the sensory block over a longer period of time (about 1.5–2 hours with bupivacaine). This means that with one injection only the end of the first stage and the complete second stage can be covered by caudal anesthesia (Fig. 34.1). Furthermore, post-partal measures such as episiotomies may also be performed under single-dose caudal anesthesia.

In lumbar epidural anesthesia there are differences in the number of the blocked segments between pregnant and nonpregnant women, and this is also true of the caudal approach. In unpublished investigations (we found out that between 60 and 150 mins following induction of caudal anesthesia there were significant differences between pregnant and nonpregnant patients (Fig. 34.2).

Concentrations of the local anesthetic (bupivacaine) in peripheral venous plasma demonstrated marked differences between pregnant and non pregnant women, too. As shown in Fig. 32.3, pregnant women show a 60–80% higher increase in concentrations of free bupivacaine in plasma despite low dosage per kg body weight. Following birth, plasma levels in the child are significantly lower than in the mother as expected (W Wahedi, H Nolte, F Wahedi, D Stratman, unpublished data) (Fig. 34.3).

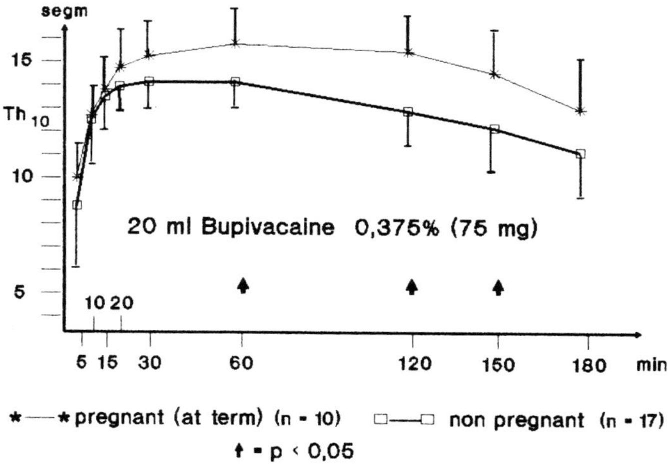

Fig. 34.2 Caudal epidural block – spread of analgesia.

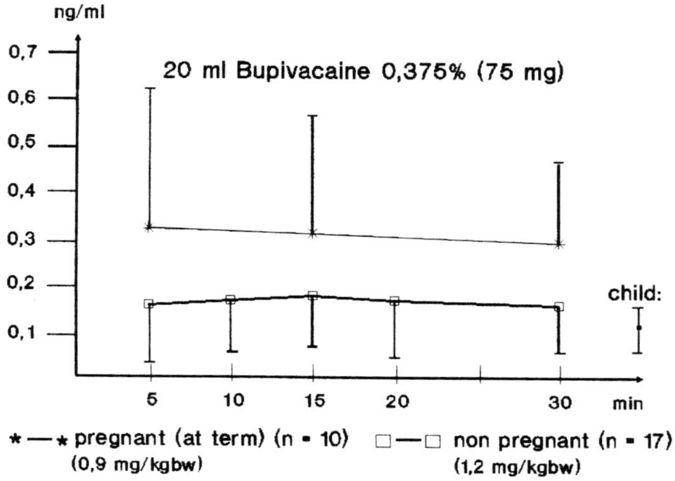

Fig. 34.3 Caudal epidural block – peripheral venous plasma levels.

INDICATIONS

Despite the fact that lumbar epidural anesthesia today is justifiably described as 'anesthesia de-luxe' for obstetrics there are some indications for caudal anesthesia as well. In cases of cervical dystocia, caudal block has proved to provide more rapid dilatation. The possibility of a single-dose caudal anesthesia has already been mentioned under the heading of Pharmacodynamics. In addition, caudal epidural anesthesia represents an alternative if, for anatomic or other reasons, a puncture of the epidural space in the lumbar region is not possible. Finally, caudal anesthesia as a single-dose method may be applied for episiotomy in the post-operative period, if the effect of the originally performed regional anesthetic procedure (e.g. pudendal block) is no longer sufficient. Table 34.1 surveys the indications for caudal anesthesia in comparison with lumbar epidural anesthesia, showing the clear advantage of lumbar epidural anesthesia in obstetrics.

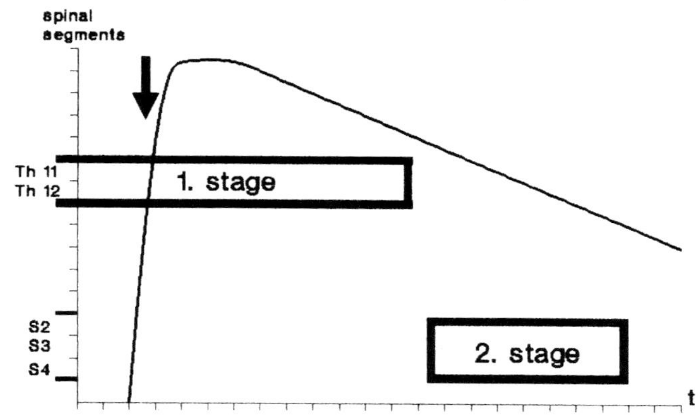

Fig. 34.1 Profile of caudal epidural block during labor.

CONTRAINDICATIONS

There are no special contraindications for caudal anesthesia, only the general contraindications valid for all regional anesthetic procedures. It goes without saying that

Table 34.1 Indications for lumbar or caudal epidural block during labor

Caudal epidural	Lumbar epidural
Cervical dystocia	All stages (I–III) of labor
Late first and second stage of labor	Cesarean delivery
Lumbar epidural puncture impossible	Early labor pain
Episiotomy	Sterilization (post-partum)

Table 34.2 Caudal epidural block for labor

Advantages	Disadvantages
Prolonged block (S1–S5)	High dose (first stage)
Subarachnoid injection very rare	Cesarean delivery excluded
Cervix dilatation	Catheter dislocation (movement of mother)

special anatomic conditions may exclude the application of caudal anesthesia, e.g. consequences of trauma or congenital defects.

CONCLUSION

Although caudal epidural anesthesia in comparison with lumbar epidural anesthesia is only regarded as an alternative method, it has some advantages over the lumbar technique (Table 34.2). In contrast to lumbar epidural anesthesia, the block is significantly prolonged in the area of the sacral segments S1–S5 (stage II). Moreover, the unwelcome and perhaps also feared unintentional dural and arachnoid perforation is very rare. Another advantage, which has already been described under the heading of Indications is effective cervical dilatation, particularly in cases of cervical dystocia. Some disadvantages should also be mentioned. A significant point is the necessary markedly higher doses of local anesthetic in comparison with lumbar epidural injection. This is particularly true for the first stage of labor. Although the continuous technique even permits a cesarean delivery under caudal anesthesia, the necessary higher concentration and volume have to be considered. The use of caudal anesthesia for cesarean delivery is therefore not recommended. Furthermore, there is at least the theoretical possibility of a catheter dislocation by maternal movement. This is because fixation is much easier with an epidural catheter than a caudal catheter.

In general, lumbar epidural anesthesia should be given priority in obstetrics over the caudal approach. It is appropriate to require that the obstetric anesthesiologist be able to perform caudal epidural anesthesia as well, since it is a true alternative if lumbar epidural anesthesia is not possible for any reason.

REFERENCES

1. Cathelin M F 1901 A new route of spinal injection: a method for epidural injections by way of the sacral canal; application to man. Compt Rend Soc Biol 53: 452
2. Sicard M A 1901 Les injections medicamenteuses extradurales par voie sacrococcygienne. Compt Rend Soc Biol 53: 396
3. Stöckel W 1909 Über sakrale Anästhesie. Zbl Gynaek 33: 1
4. Hingson R A, Edwards W B 1943 Continuous caudal analgesia. An analysis of the first ten thousand confinements thus managed with the report of the authors' first thousand cases. J Am Med Assoc 123: 538
5. Bonica J J 1967 Principles and practice of obstetric analgesia and anesthesia. F A Davis, Philadelphia
6. Moore D C 1965 Regional block, 4th edn. Charles C Thomas, Springfield I L
7. Astra Chemicals GmbH 1985 Regionalanästhesie. 2. Auflage. Gustav Fischer, Stuttgart
8. Raj P, Nolte H, Stanton-Hicks M 1988 Illustrated manual of regional anesthesia. Springer, Berlin
9. Sinclair J C, Fox H A, Lentz J F, Fuld G L, Murphy J 1965 Intoxication of the fetus by a local anesthetic. A newly recognized complication of maternal caudal anesthesia. New Engl J Med 273: 1173
10. Finster M, Poppers P J, Sinclair J C, Morishima H O, Daniel SS 1965 Accidental intoxication of the fetus with local anesthetic drug during caudal anesthesia. Am J Obstet Gynecol 92: 922

35. Spinal anesthesia

PART A
THE DEVELOPMENT OF SPINAL NEEDLES

G. W. Ostheimer C. Shea M. R. Schorr A. Van Zundert

Medicine's lengthy history includes many pages on the need for and the use of anesthesia. Nevertheless, few of those pages have been devoted to the story of the needles for regional anesthesia. Thus, they remain relatively obscure – perhaps because the needles are now so widely used as to be taken for granted. This chapter, then, presents the chronology of needles for spinal anesthesia, as a source of information for anesthesiologists whether neophyte or veteran.

EARLY ATTEMPTS IN REGIONAL ANESTHESIA

Regional anesthesia had its beginnings some 150 years ago, with the announcement by Francis Rynd, of Dublin, of his cannula and gravity-flow device for the subcutaneous administration of fluids to relieve 'painful afflictions of the nerves.'[1]

A few years later, in 1851, Charles Pravaz, of Lyon, France, fashioned a syringe and trocar with a cannula for injecting iron perchloride into an aneurysm to induce clotting. This device was notable chiefly for the composition of its components: trocar and cannula were made of gold or platinum, and the syringe was made of silver. The syringe was screwed onto the cannula after the trocar was removed, and a screw-action piston descended when the piston rod was rotated.[2,3]

Two years later, Daniel Ferguson, a British manufacturer of surgical instruments developed an interest in surgical needles. In 1853 he described his syringe and hollow trocar. The glass syringe terminated in a slender platinum tube, which in turn was encased in another somewhat longer tube, ending in a trocar-like point. Near its end was an oblique opening on one side. As the outer tube was rotated on the inner tube, their apertures could be made to correspond at the operator's will. Once the syringe was charged, the operator could rotate the outer tube so as to conceal the orifice of the inner tube completely, and thus prevent blood from entering.[4]

During the same year Alexander Wood of Edinburgh attempted to remove a nevus by injecting iron perchloride, using one of Ferguson's 'elegant little syringes'. It occurred to Wood that the instrument might be used for hypodermic injections. He first tried this procedure in November 1853, with good results. Following this, Wood injected opioids into painful areas in what he believed – erroneously – was a form of local analgesia for neurologic pains. At some later time Wood replaced the Ferguson trocar with a small hollow needle whose aperture, near the point, was 'like the sting of a wasp'. A syringe believed to be Wood's original is housed in the Museum of the Royal College of Surgeons in Edinburgh, though its authenticity is uncertain.[4]

Luer's 'modern' arrangement

Toward the end of the 1850s, Luer of Paris discarded the screw-action attachment of needle to syringe and replaced it with a conical nozzle on the syringe. This arrangement continues to be used today. Luer made two further improvements in the piston, eliminating the screw action and adding graduations.[4] Luer's syringe is regarded as the proximal forerunner of the modern hypodermic syringe;

however, the features of the attached needle and push–pull action had already become integral through the introduction of the Ferguson syringe.[2]

Cocaine in regional anesthesia

It is said that the birthdate of regional anesthesia was September 15, 1884, on which day Carl Koller of the Allgemeines Krankenhaus in Vienna conclusively demonstrated the anesthetic properties of cocaine applied to the conjunctiva. When his discovery was announced at the Heidelberg Congress later that year, he found ready acceptance by the medical world. A letter by Dr H.D. Noyes describing Koller's discovery was published in the *New York Medical Record* in October of 1884, initiating a wave of experimentation with topical cocaine.[3,5]

The news spread rapidly to the USA, where the use of cocaine in ophthalmology became widely popular. Regional anesthesia with cocaine was believed to be preferable to inhalation anesthesia because, while the pain relief was similar, less time was needed to establish the anesthesia, the ocular vessels did not become engorged – as occurred with the use of ether – and the patient was less likely to vomit.

Meanwhile W. S. Halsted in New York reported his active experimentation with cocaine. He removed a supraorbital lipoma, following cocainization of the supraorbital nerve at the supraorbital notch. His procedure conclusively demonstrated that anesthesia of the peripheral distribution of nerve trunks could be obtained following their anesthetization. In the following months Halsted proved that regional anesthesia of the extremities was practical by means of injections into the brachial plexus and posterior tibial nerve.[6]

Neurologic approach

Nearly simultaneously with Halsted, J. L. Corning of New York approached the problem of anesthesia from the neurologist's standpoint.[6] In 1885 he announced his discovery of 'spinal' (probably epidural – ed.) anesthesia.[7] However, it remained dormant but gave impetus to numerous other investigators, including Quincke and Bier of Germany, Tuffier of France and Babcock, Matas and others in USA, whose efforts brought spinal anesthesia to clinical usefulness. Then, in 1892, Francois Franck introduced the term 'nerve blocking'.[6] A few years later Cathlein and Sicard of Paris independently conceived the notion of caudal anesthesia.[1]

Regional anesthesia as we know it today was thus born – the fruit of much labor by a small army of researchers.

NEEDLES FOR SPINAL ANESTHESIA

By 1900 Corning was ready to report on the instrument he had designed for spinal anesthesia.[8] The needle was $3\frac{1}{2}$–4 inches in length and was made of gold or 'platina', both of which rendered it bendable but hardly likely to break. The introducer was $\frac{1}{2}$ inch in length, to puncture the skin. (This device was soon discarded, but was reintroduced about 20 years later.) A sliding nut with a set screw, through which the cannula passed, was fixed against the skin when the cerebrospinal fluid exited the needle hub. This maneuver prevented further advance of the needle into the spinal canal (Fig. 35.1).

The bevel of the point was short so that the needle would not penetrate the membranes too far. In this way, the solution would be deposited into the membranes.

Corning[8] had this to say:

> Uncouth needles, with a long bevel at the point, are of all things to be avoided. Only imperfect results are to be anticipated from such clumsy instruments, as, on the one hand, an overplus of penetration is requisite to insure the entry of the fluid below the membrane; and, on the other, an immoderate outflow of cerebrospinal fluid – and hence of the anesthetic – is inevitable after withdrawal of the needle.

Corning's early spinal needles were made with a tapered hub with a short length of rubber tubing attached, to join the needle to a syringe containing cocaine solution. Various alterations to the needle were incorporated, although the design remained essentially as Corning had conceived it.[9]

Rationale for use of large-bore needles

August Bier was among the early investigators who turned to larger bore needles that did not require an introducer.[10] This avoided the necessity of using introducer and dilator before inserting the needle. Bier's needle for spinal anesthesia was a 15-gauge or 17-gauge instrument (Fig. 35.1). It was widely criticized on the grounds that the large diameter was responsible for unnecessary pain and trauma to the patient; the point could leave a sizeable tear in the dura; and the distal orifice might not be entirely situated within the dura when the injection was made – all of which gave rise to unsatisfactory results.[11,12]

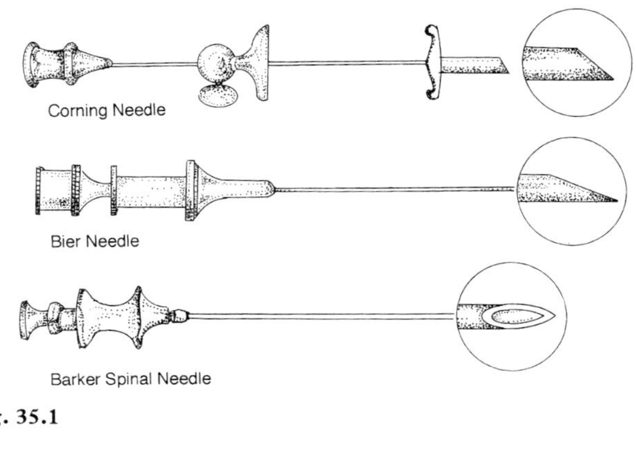

Fig. 35.1

Barker's technique

By 1907 Arthur Barker of England, considered to be the founder of hyperbaric spinal anesthesia, was ready to describe his technique for spinal anesthesia. He employed a modified Bier needle having a hollowed out point, 'so as to secure sharpness without lengthening the terminal opening too much.'[13] Barker's needle corrected the error of the Bier needle such that when the puncture was made, the entire open end of the needle would lie within the dura, without the point being pushed so far as to wound structures within the sac (Fig. 35.1).[13]

Initially Barker's needles and cannulas were made of steel with a nickel coating. They soon became blackened from constant boiling, and lost their polish. If stored when even only slightly damp, they corroded.[14] Barker therefore suggested that they be made of hard nickel, which not only proved to be the equal of the steel instruments but were also more convenient, since they could be boiled repeatedly without being changed.[14]

THE PROBLEM OF POST-SPINAL HEADACHE

Nearly 100 years ago Sicard postulated that the cause of post-dural puncture headache was leakage of cerebrospinal fluid through the dural rent.[10] Some 12 years later Greene stated that the use of finer lumbar dural puncture needles would cause only minimal side effects.[15] Then, in 1904, W. Wayne Babcock of Philadelphia recognized the advantages of the Corning needle in the following words:[16,17]

> It should be of iridized platinum or gold to avoid breakage, and have a length of 7 centimeters and a diameter of 1/10 centimeter (20 gauge). A well-fitted stylette should be provided so that the needle cannot become clogged in the introduction.

Large gauge *vs.* small gauge

Randall Hoyt of New York in 1922 proposed that a two-needle device be used for lumbar dural puncture, noting that large-gauge needles were necessary because rigidity was required so that the needle might penetrate the dense tissue. The large-gauge needle, however, caused a sizeable dural opening and led to the infamous headache. He recommended that a finer gauge inner needle be used to penetrate the dura and arachnoid. There followed a marked decrease in the frequency of post-spinal headache.[18] This may have been the reason for the use of introducers, once again, in the late 1920s.

Contemporaneously the English developed Firth–Brearly heat-tempered stainless steel, which was rust resistant but not rustproof. As if in response to that development, the Krupp steelworks in Germany manufactured V_2A, which was rustproof. Moreover, it possessed unusual resistance against breakage and it maintained its point.[19] Over time, the low-carbon steels began to be replaced by the higher-carbon rust-resistant needles; and these by the rustproof, corrosion resistant needles. By the mid-1940s most needle manufacturers in the USA were using improved V_2A steel.[19]

The Mayo Clinic's W. R. Meeker[20] in 1926 described a lightweight spinal needle made of a nickel alloy that would bend but not break. Such a needle would be superior to heavy spinal trocars of the Bier type, which were more difficult to use because their heavier 'heads' threw the needle out of balance. Needles made of platinum-iridium or gold were said to be too costly, to be readily bendable and difficult to keep sharpened.[20] Gaston Labat of Paris and later of the USA used a nickel needle, in which the shorter bevel acted as a wedge, pushing aside tissues, and a stylet that increased the rigidity of the needle (Fig. 35.2).[21]

At the University of Oregon H. M. Greene in 1923 began to experiment on cadavers, using various spinal needles.[22] This work led him to two important conclusions: post-dural puncture headache is due to trauma to the spinal dura severe enough to produce excessive leakage of cerebrospinal fluid and leave the brain without its water cushion; and a small needle having a smooth round point, similar to that of an ordinary cambric needle, would separate rather than sever the fibers of the dura.[22,23] There would be a much smaller dural opening and a much slower loss of cerebrospinal fluid. His needle was rust free and soft tempered. Its caliber was small and it would bend but not break. Routine cleaning and sharpening after each use prevented the needle from developing burrs, which could tear the dura. The first of these needles were ordinary spinal needles that were sharpened to a rounded tip by removal of the cutting edge of the bevel (Fig. 35.2).[24,25]

One year later, George Pitkin of Teaneck, New Jersey, introduced his short-bevel needle made of rustless steel.[26,27] It was less likely to break, it retained its sharp point longer and it withstood considerable manipulation

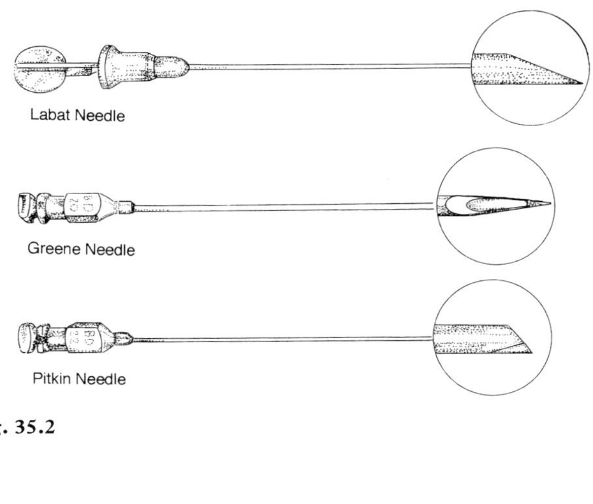

Fig. 35.2

without bending (Fig. 35.2). Pitkin made the point that the plating of certain nickel-plated needles tended to 'peel' and would not hold a point as well as those made of rustless steel.[11,12,27,28]

CONTINUOUS SPINAL ANESTHESIA

The next few years saw the emphasis placed on the perfection of the lumbar dural puncture technique and the development, introduction and use of new agents for regional anesthesia including dibucaine, piperocaine and tetracaine.

Not until the 1940s did W. T. Lemmon of Jefferson Medical College, Philadelphia, make the next contribution to spinal anesthesia: continuous spinal anesthesia.[29] Much earlier in the century the technique had been reported by Dean in the *British Medical Journal* (October 5, 1907), but if failed to gain popularity.[30] With Lemmon's description, continuous spinal anesthesia received broad acceptance and it took its rightful place in anesthesiology.

In as much as the single-dose technique of regional anesthesia imposed a time limit on the surgeon, Lemmon's continuous approach was now welcomed. He suggested the use of a malleable needle to be left in position during the procedure.[31] Lemmon used a 17-gauge or 18-gauge nickel–silver alloy needle and a length of rubber tubing to join the needle to the source of the anesthetic agent (Fig. 35.3).

Modifications and improvements to the Lemmon technique

Lemmon initially had used his technique in April of 1939. A Sise introducer was used for the initial skin and ligament puncture. The needle with its introducer was then inserted through the ligaments and into the lumbar subarachnoid space.

Robert Hingson and Charles Ferguson, working in the US Public Health Service Hospital in Staten Island in 1943, modified the Lemmon technique as follows:[32] Their needle was of stainless steel, 19 gauge, having a reinforced steel collar in place of the usual hub. This was the same type of needle they had developed for continuous caudal anesthesia. There was an extra orifice near the short-bevel point (Fig. 20.1). The proximal and distal inches of the cannula were made of rigid steel, and the middle section was annealed for malleability. The smaller caliber made for lessened trauma; the light collar aided the tubing attachment; and because the center was malleable the patient enjoyed greater mobility once the needle had been placed with its point in the subarachnoid space.

Drawing on Lemon's experience, Major E. B. Tuohy of the US Army Medical Corps (now the US Army Medical Service), made some improvements. He passed a

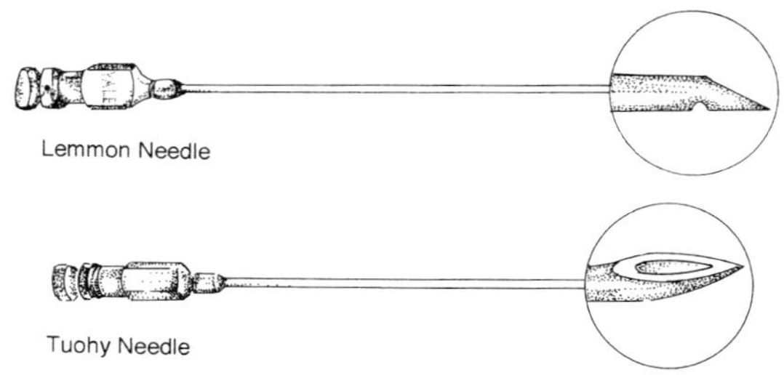

Fig. 35.3

5-French ureteral catheter through a 15-gauge lumbar puncture needle a distance of 4–5 cm into the subarachnoid space. The following year he reported on the use of a Huber point needle, which offered several advantages, among them a sharp smooth point that could pierce tissues easily. Also, with the stylet in place, tissues could not obstruct the needle, tissues were pushed aside by the closed bevel and the design of the point made it possible for the catheter to be directed either cephalad or caudad as needed (Fig. 35.3).[33–35]

NEWER SPINAL NEEDLES

The issue of post-dural puncture headache – alleviated but not entirely eliminated – continued to capture the interest of investigators.

Barnett Greene in 1950[15] described the routine use of a fine 26-gauge lumbar puncture needle that was introduced through a 21-gauge needle. This needle greatly lessened the frequency of post-dural puncture headache (the concept Hoyt had espoused in 1922).

Shortly thereafter, Hart and Whitacre[24] of the Huron Road Hospital in Cleveland in 1951 described a different needle for spinal anesthesia. At their request a manufacturer produced a 26-gauge solid-end needle that was drawn to a sharp pencil-like point, in which the orifice was on the side of the needle just proximal to the tip. There was no 'snap' when the dura was penetrated (Fig. 35.4). This suggested that the needle separated rather than

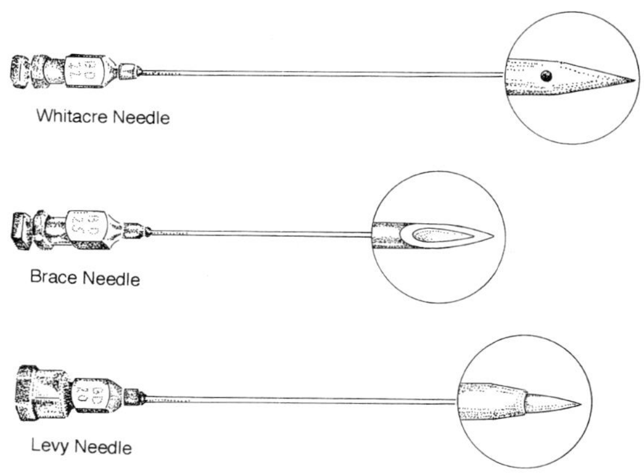

Fig. 35.4

severed the dural fibers. Several years later, in 1960, Cappe described the use of a 22-gauge Whitacre needle and claimed an extremely low incidence of post-dural puncture headache.[36] Wetchler and Brace were first to describe a short beveled 25 g needle that could be inserted without an introducer to facilitate lumbar dural puncture with a small guage needle to decrease the incidence of post dural puncture headache (Fig. 35.4).[10] Levy advocated a pencil point needle with an end orifice. In his particular design, the stylet protruded 2 or 3 mm from the cannula at its distal end (Fig. 35.4).

REFERENCES

1. Bonica J J 1953 The management of pain. Lea & Febiger, Philadelphia, pp 166–167
2. Howard-Jones N 1947 A critical study of the origins and early development of hypodermic medication. J Hist Med 2: 201–249
3. Matas R 1934 Local anesthesia: a retrospect and prospect. Am J Surg 25: 189–196
4. Blake J F 1960 Mr. Ferguson's hypodermic syringe. J Hist Med 15: 337–341
5. Koller C 1928 Historical notes on the beginning of local anesthesia. J Am Med Assoc 90: 1742–1743
6. Matas R 1934 Local anesthesia: a retrospect and prospect. Am J Surg 25: 362–379
7. Corning J L 1885 Spinal anesthesia and local medication of the cord. NY J Med 42: 483–485
8. Corning J L 1900 Some conservative jottings apropos of spinal anesthesia. Med Record 58: 601–604
9. Corning J L 1888 A further contribution on local medication of the cord. Med Record, March 17, 601
10. Wetchler B, Brace D E 1955 A technique to minimize the occurrence of headache after lumbar puncture by use of small bore spinal needles. Anesthesiology 16: 270–282
11. Pitkin G P 1928 controllable spinal anesthesia. Am J Surg 5: 537–553
12. Pitkin G P, McCormack F C 1928 Controllable spinal anesthesia in obstetrics. Surg Gynecol Obstet 47: 713–726
13. Barker A E 1907 A report on clinical experience with spinal analgesia in 100 cases, and some reflections on the procedure. Br Med J, March 23, 665
14. Barker A E 1908 A second report on clinical experiences with spinal analgesia: with a second series of one hundred cases. Br Med J, Feb 1, 244
15. Greene B A 1950 A 26-gauge lumbar puncture needle: its value in the prophylaxis of headache following spinal analgesia for vaginal delivery. Anesthesiology 11: 464–469
16. Babcock W W 1914 The technic of spinal anesthesia. Am J Surg (Quart Suppl Anesth Analg) 28: 2–7
17. Babcock W W 1914 The technic of spinal anesthesia. NY Med J 100: 699–702
18. Hoyt R 1922 Apparatus for withdrawing spinal fluid without postpuncture reaction. J Am Med Assoc 78: 428–429
19. Schwidetzky O 1944 History of needles and syringes. Anesth Analg 23: 34–38
20. Meeker W R 1924 Instrumentarium for local anesthesia. Ann Surg 79: 124–129
21. Labat G 1922 Regional anesthesia: its technic and clinical application. W B Saunders, Philadelphia, pp 15–21
22. Greene H M 1926 Lumbar puncture and the prevention of postpuncture headache. J Am Med Assoc 86: 391–392
23. Greene H M 1943 A technic to reduce the incidence of headache following lumbar puncture in ambulatory patients with a plea for more frequent examinations of the cerebrospinal fluid. Northwest Med 22: 240–245.
24. Hart J R, Whitacr R J 1951 Pencil-point needle in prevention of postspinal headache. J Am Med Assoc 147: 657–658
25. Cappe B E, Deutsch E V 1953 A needle for fractional spinal anesthesia. Anesthesiology 14: 398–404
26. Pitkin G P 1927 Controllable spinal anesthesia. J Med Soc NJ 24: 425–428
27. Pitkin G P 1953 Conduction anesthesia. J B Lippincott, Philadelphia, p 797
28. Bumpus H C 1931 History of regional anesthesia in urology. J Am Med Assoc 96: 83–88.
29. Lemmon W T 1940 A method for continuous spinal anesthesia: a preliminary report. Ann Surg 111:141–144
30. Sykes W S 1960 Essays on the first hundred years of anesthesia, Vol 1. E&S Livingstone, Edinburgh, plate XI
31. Dripps R D 1950 A comparison of the malleable needle and catheter technics for continuous spinal anesthesia. NY J Med 50: 1595–1599
32. Hingson R A, Ferguson C H, Palmer L A 1943 Advances in spinal anesthesia. Ann Surg 118: 971–981
33. Tuohy E B 1944 Continuous spinal anesthesia: its usefulness and technic involved. Anesthesiology 5: 142–148
34. Tuohy E B 1945 Use of continuous spinal anesthesia utilizing the ureteral catheter technic. J Am Med Assoc 128: 262–263
35. Tuohy E B 1945 Continuous spinal anesthesia: a new method utilizing a ureteral catheter. Surg Clin N Am 25: 834–840
36. Cappe B M 1960 Prevention of postspinal headache with a 22-gauge pencil-point needle and adequate hydration. Anesth Analg 39: 463–465

PART B
SPINAL ANESTHESIA: TECHNIQUE

G. W. Ostheimer K. A. Leavitt

ANATOMY AND LANDMARKS

The subarachnoid space may be safely entered through one of the interspaces between L2 and L5 (see Fig. 20.3). The dural sac extends to the level of S2 and the enclosed spinal cord usually extends down to L1, rarely to L2. Therefore, a puncture below this level should not encounter the spinal cord. The puncture point for insertion of the spinal needle is established in the following manner. After the most prominent point of the left and right posterior iliac crests is located, an imaginary line is drawn between these points. It usually crosses the L4 spinous process or the L4–L5 interspace (see Fig. 20.4). This interspace and the two above it are usually chosen as points of entry for subarachnoid block. The Taylor approach utilizing the interspace of L5–S1 is rarely used in obstetric anesthesia. In the midline, the entering spinal needle (see Fig. 20.3) traverses the skin, subcutaneous tissue, supraspinous ligament and interspinous ligament, and then enters the ligamentum flavum, which connects the laminae of vertebral arches. The needle then crosses the epidural space filled with loose areolar tissue containing the epidural venous plexus. Finally, the needle pierces the dura and the adherent arachnoid, thus entering the subarachnoid space.

PATIENT POSITION

The left or right lateral position (see Fig. 20.4) is generally the most comfortable for the parturient for vaginal delivery. Care must be taken that the line of the spinous processes of vertebrae is parallel to the table. To open up the vertebral interspaces, the patient is asked to flex her back by drawing her knees toward her chest. Her head is supported by a small pillow, and her neck should be flexed so that the chin touches the chest.

The obstetric patient usually requires a low block (T10–S5) for an uncomplicated vaginal delivery. At the Brigham and Women's Hospital, the lateral position is used for initiation of block using a hyperbaric solution.

The sitting position may also be used. The obese patient may be easier to approach in the sitting position because the line of the spinous processes is usually not obscured by the subcutaneous fat fold drooping over it. For the sitting position to be most effective for performing the subarachnoid block, the patient sits on the edge of the table with her feet resting on a stool. The neck is flexed so that the chin touches the chest. The arms should be folded across the upper abdomen, but they may rest loosely supported in the lap. A nurse or an assistant should steady the patient from the front to prevent the patient from falling if neurogenic syncope should occur.

It is best to inject the spinal anesthetic for cesarean delivery with the patient in the right lateral position. This prevents concentrating the hyperbaric local anesthetic solution on the left side of the dural sac. Such left-sided pooling of the anesthetic solution occurs when left uterine displacement by elevation of the right hip is used after initiating the spinal block with the parturient in the left lateral position. This 'puddling' effect may result in an inadequate block on the right side of the patient.

MATERIALS

The following materials should be ready for use when the patient is to be given a spinal anesthesia:

- One pair of sterile gloves
- Antibacterial solution for cleansing the skin
- One sterile cup for the antibacterial solution
- Forceps
- Sterile gauze pads
- Sterile towels for draping the field (if desired)
- One 25-gauge, 1.6- to 3.8-cm needle for skin infiltration
- One 21- or 22-gauge, 3.8-cm needle for preparing drugs and for deep infiltration (if desired)
- One 18-gauge needle for use as an introducer
- One 25-gauge Whitacre or 26–27 gauge Quincke, 8.9-cm spinal needle with stylet
- One 3-ml syringe
- One 5-ml glass syringe.

One disposable spinal anesthetic tray usually contains all of the above items. Several small-gauge spinal needles of varying designs are available. Small-gauge needles with or without conical points have been demonstrated to reduce the incidence of post-dural puncture headache in the parturient.

TECHNIQUE

30 ml of a clear antacid (0.3 mol/l sodium citrate or its equivalent) is administered before the initiation of the block. No other premedication is given for vaginal delivery. For cesarean delivery, the patient will receive 30 ml of a clear antacid (as above) and, if considered 'at risk' for any reason, will also receive intravenous metoclopramide 10 mg and intravenous or intramuscular cimetidine 300 mg or ranitidine 100 mg in the 30–60 min prior to induction of the subarachnoid block. The technique of anesthesia for the parturient is similar to that for the surgical patient except that special consideration must be given to the condition of the fetus and to the physiologic changes associated with pregnancy and labor.

Arterial blood pressure changes are noted in any patient undergoing regional anesthesia, but the obstetric patient must be carefully observed for these changes. The blood pressure is determined in the supine and lateral positions before the block is initiated to check for aortocaval compression (supine hypotensive syndrome). An automatic blood pressure monitor is useful but not mandatory. The fetal heart rate (FHR) record is also reviewed. Routine electrocardiography is optional in our institution for vaginal delivery in the uncomplicated pregnancy; however, it is immediately available if needed since these deliveries are accomplished in a delivery/operating room. Electrocardiographic monitoring is mandatory for cesarean delivery.

The obstetric patient receiving subarachnoid anesthesia is acutely hydrated prior to the induction of the subarachnoid block. A large indwelling plastic catheter allows the administration of warm lactated Ringer's solution or similar crystalloid solution over 10–20 min before induction of subarachnoid block (1000 ml for vaginal delivery and at least 1500 ml for cesarean delivery). This hydration helps to prevent the hypotension that may be caused by the sympathetic block produced by spinal anesthesia. Warm intravenous fluid diminishes pre-, intra- and postpartum shivering experienced by the parturient. The intravenous infusion is then maintained should the patient require additional hydration or intravenous medication. In practice, approximately 1500–2000 ml of crystalloid solution is usually administered to combat the hypotension that occurs before birth during cesarean delivery. The key to the use of major regional block in obstetrics is to maintain adequate uteroplacental perfusion, which can be indirectly monitored via maternal arterial pressure. Decreased perfusion of the intervillous space can place the fetus in jeopardy.

The spinal tray is opened in a sterile manner and the expiration date checked. The gloved anesthesiologist prepares the skin of the lumbar area with a bactericidal preparation, wiping off the excess solution. The field may be draped with sterile towels. The desired interspace is located and the correct position of the patient is checked. In the lateral position, the line of the spinous processes must be parallel to the table and the surface of the back must be vertical. This will align the spinous processes in the horizontal plane. Depending on the special anatomic features of the patient, the second, third or fourth lumbar interspace may be found most suitable for needle insertion.

The entry point into the skin is fixed by two fingers on either side of the interspace selected and the skin is infiltrated with a small amount of local anesthetic (Fig. 35.5). The 25-gauge needle is used to create the skin wheal. Then a small amount (1–2 ml) of local anesthetic is injected into the subcutaneous tissue and the interspinous ligament. When satisfactory analgesia of the entry point has been created, an 18-gauge needle is used as an introducer and is inserted through the skin wheal. The index and the middle fingers of the free hand straddle the interspace to fix the tissues of the underlying structures (Fig. 35.5). The introducer is used to create a passage for the fine spinal needle and, theoretically, prevent carrying a plug of skin or fat into the subarachnoid space. However, some anesthesiologists, including the senior author, prefer not to use an introducer and will insert the spinal needle directly. If one chooses one of the conical-point needles, it may be necessary to make a hole in the skin with the introducer needle for easier insertion.

The introducer is inserted into the interspinous area maintaining this horizontal position. An improperly inserted introducer makes it impossible to point the needle in the correct direction. A small-gauge spinal needle (26- or 27-gauge Quincke or a conical-tipped needle such as the 25-gauge Whitacre needle) should be used for the procedure. The needle must first be examined for any imperfections or weaknesses. It should be noted that the bevel of the needle is on the same side as the key notch for the stylet in the hub of the needle. Once the physician is satisfied with the needle, he or she should insert it so that the bevel does not cut across the longitudinal fibers of the dura. In practice, this may not be possible. The bevel – as indicated by the key notch – should face laterally during its passage through the dura. The spinal needle is held between the thumb, index and middle fingers and inserted through the introducer (Fig. 35.6). The spinal needle is then slowly advanced. Its progress through the tissues is followed by noting the variations in resistance as the various structures are penetrated. First, the firm resistance of the interspinous ligament and the ligamentum flavum is felt, after which a lessening of resistance is observed as the needle crosses epidural space. This is followed by the characteristic 'pop' (an abrupt disappearance of a last

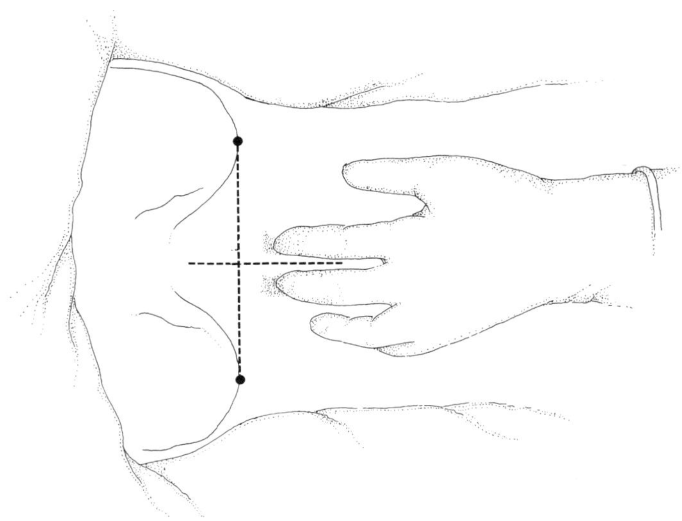

Fig. 35.5 Identification of the intervertebral space.

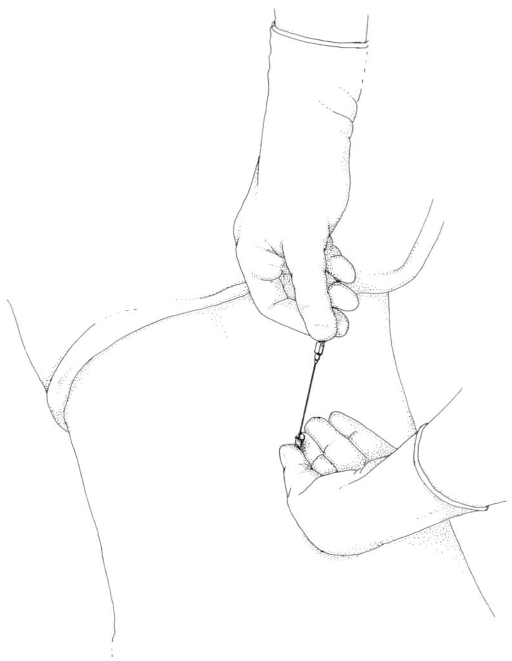

Fig. 35.6 Insertion of the spinal needle through the introducer.

resistance) as the needle pierces the dura to enter the subarachnoid space. The anesthesiologist now may check the needle's position by withdrawing the stylet to see if cerebrospinal fluid (CSF) appears (Fig. 35.7) at the hub of the needle and by aspirating with a syringe as it may not immediately appear because of the small gauge of the spinal needle.

There are several other reasons why CSF may fail to appear:

1. A nerve root or the dura may block the bevel of the needle. After withdrawing the stylet, the needle may be rotated 90 to 180° in an attempt to free the bevel of the obstruction.
2. The cerebrospinal fluid pressure may be too low to push the fluid through the needle. The anesthesiologist should always confirm the needle position by achieving free flow of CSF when aspirating with a syringe.

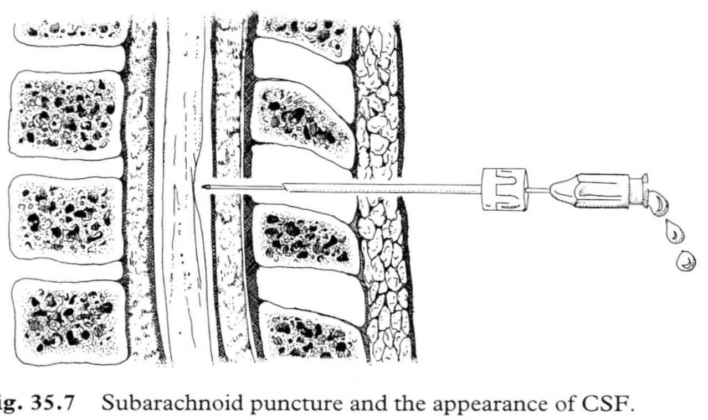

Fig. 35.7 Subarachnoid puncture and the appearance of CSF.

3. A tissue plug may be blocking the bevel. This also will be dislodged by an aspiration attempt.
4. The bevel may still be in the epidural space, at least partially. Therefore, the anesthesiologist should replace the stylet in the needle and then slowly advance the needle forward. Then the above maneuvers are repeated.

If contact with bone has been made, stop. The needle must not be forced against this resistance because the needle can be bent, the lumen of the needle can be easily blocked, and the needle point can become 'barbed'. If it appears that the needle lumen is plugged, the needle should be removed and flushed with normal saline or local anesthetic solution. Contact with bone usually means that the vertebral lamina has been encountered. This necessitates a small change of the direction of the spinal needle. To do this effectively, the needle point is withdrawn completely into the introducer and then a fresh attempt is made at a puncture in a different direction (usually cephalad). Success is indicated by the appearance of CSF in the hub of the spinal needle. When this is achieved, the hub of the spinal needle is held firmly between the index or middle finger and the thumb of the left hand of the right-handed anesthesiologist to prevent any displacement of the needle from its proper location. The back of the anesthesiologist's hand is steadied against the patient's back (Fig. 35.8). Aspiration is performed with a syringe to ascertain free flow of cerebrospinal fluid. A syringe filled with the appropriate dose of local anesthetic solution is attached to the spinal needle.

Negative pressure is applied to the syringe to withdraw a small amount of CSF to ascertain that the proper position of the needle bevel has been maintained. Mixing of the CSF and anesthetic solution will occur during aspiration and will be visible since the local anesthetic solution will have a different baricity from CSF. Then the contents of the syringe are injected into the subarachnoid space. We prefer to aspirate and reinject a small volume (about 0.2 ml) after the local anesthetic has been injected to rule out unintentional movement of the needle during the injection of the local anesthetic solution.

If aspiration is not accomplished or is difficult, we maintain the patient in position and ascertain the development of the block by testing the dependent side. If the block does not seem to be developing as expected, the spinal needle is replaced and an additional dose of anesthetic solution is administered. How much additional drug should be administered depends on the situation. The senior author administers an additional dose of 25–75% of the original volume of solution. He has not had a total spinal anesthetic using this procedure in over 25 years.

The suggested dosage of local anesthetic for the obstetric patient (Tables 35.1 and 35.2) is 30–50% lower than that given to a surgical patient. Incidentally, this

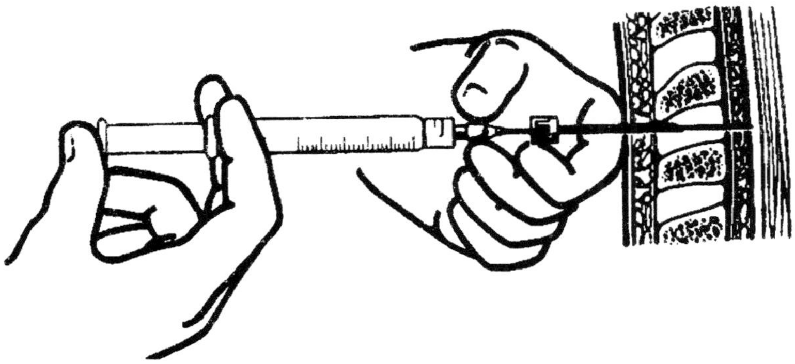

Fig. 35.8 Proper hand position during subarachnoid injection of local anesthetic.

dosage reduction is indicated for any patient with increased intra-abdominal pressure, including surgical patients with ascites or large intra-abdominal tumors.

Following the injection of the local anesthetic, the needle and the introducer are withdrawn and the patient is immediately placed in the supine position. Her uterus is displaced to the left by placing a wedge or a folded blanket under her right hip. Oxygen is administered by face mask at 6–10 l/min and the blood pressure is frequently monitored.

With the patient resting comfortably, the spread of anesthesia is checked frequently by gentle repeated pinpricks or by a cotton swab moistened with alcohol. Since the loss of pain and temperature sensation progresses simultaneously, the use of alcohol to check the spread of anesthesia may be more pleasant for the patient. Repeated pinpricks may not accurately differentiate the area of complete loss of pain sensation from that of partial sensory anesthesia. However, we still prefer the 'pinprick' test. Because of the concern over blood and fluid contamination, we suggest the use of sharp toothpicks to determine sensory levels. Several brands of plastic toothpicks are sharp enough to pierce olives or onions but not human skin. The spread of the local anesthetic depends on the specific gravity relationships between the local anesthetic solution used and CSF. Normally, the specific gravity of CSF is 1.003–1.009.

A hyperbaric solution has a higher specific gravity than that of CSF, therefore it will move to low-lying parts of the subarachnoid space. If anesthesia of just the perineal area – the frequently used 'saddle block' – is desired it is achieved by placing the patient in the sitting position as previously described.

A hypobaric solution has a specific gravity lower than CSF, therefore it will spread to higher lying areas within the subarachnoid space. An isobaric solution, with a specific gravity matching that of CSF, will tend to remain at the injection point. Both hypobaric and isobaric solutions are not used in single-dose subarachnoid block in obstetric anesthesia because of the lack of predictability of their spread in the subarachnoid space of the parturient.

RECENT DEVELOPMENTS IN DETERMINING DOSAGE FOR SPINAL ANESTHESIA

Tables 35.1 and 35.2 are meant to be a guide to the appropriate dosage of hyperbaric local anesthetic for subarachnoid block for vaginal or cesarean delivery. In a recent review article, Stienstra and Greene[1] reviewed the factors affecting the subarachnoid spread of local anesthetic solutions in nonpregnant patients. The following items have no clinically significant effect on the subarachnoid distribution of local anesthetics: patient weight, patient gender, barbotage, speed of injection, composition of CSF, circulation of CSF, pressure of CSF and the presence of vasoconstrictors in the local anesthetic solution. The most important determinants of subarachnoid distribution of local anesthetic solutions are the baricity of the local anesthetic solution, the position of the patient during injection, the dosage of the local anesthetic (to some degree) and the site of injection. Less important factors (except in extreme situations) include increasing patient age, anatomic configuration of the spinal column, the direction of the spinal needle during injection and the volume of CSF. Two controversial areas are the height of the patient and the dosage of local anesthetic (concentration $\times$ volume). Norris[2] found no difference in the spread of hyperbaric bupivacaine in term parturients regardless of age, height or body mass index. Hartwell et al[3] found no correlation between height, weight or body mass index, but did find a correlation between two vertebral length measurements, C7 to the level of the iliac crest and C7 to the sacral hiatus. These investigators believed that the length of the vertebral column gave a better indication for the dose of hyperbaric local anesthetic. In practice, it has become apparent that there is a variable relationship between height of the parturient, the dose of hyperbaric local anesthetic and the ultimate level of sensory blockade.

Table 35.1 Local anesthetics and suggested dosages for spinal anesthesia for vaginal delivery

Local anesthetic*	Dosage (patient's height) 5'	5'6"	6'0"	Onset of action (min)	Duration of action (min)
Lidocaine 5% in 7.5% dextrose in water (premixed)	40 mg (0.8 ml)	40–50 mg (0.8–1.0 ml)	50–60 mg (1.0–1.2 ml)	1–3	45–75
Bupivacaine 0.75% in 8.25% d/w (premixed)	7.5 mg (1.0 ml)	9.4 mg (1.25 ml)	11.3 mg (1.5 ml)	2–4	90–120
Bupivacaine 0.5% in hyperbaric solution†	6 mg (1.2 ml)	7 mg (1.4 ml)	8 mg (1.6 ml)	2–4	90–120
Tetracaine 1% and equal vol. 10% dextrose in water‡	5 mg (0.5 ml) and 0.5 ml	6 mg (0.6 ml) and 0.6 ml	7 mg (0.7 ml) and 0.7 ml	3–5	120–180
Total volume	1.0 ml	1.2 ml	1.4 ml		
Tetracaine 1% and equal vol. 10% procaine/water‡	4 mg (0.4 ml) and 40 mg (0.4 ml)	5 mg (0.5 ml) and 50 mg (0.5 ml)	6 mg (0.6 ml) and 60 mg (0.6 ml)	2–4	120–180
Total volume	0.8 ml	1.0 ml	1.2 ml		

* All preparations listed are hyperbaric.
† Not yet approved by the Food and Drug Administration.
‡ Rarely used any more in the USA.
d/w, dextrose in water.

Table 35.2 Local anesthetics and suggested dosages for spinal anesthesia for cesarean delivery

Local anesthetic*	Dosage (patient's height) 5'	5'6"	6'0"	Onset of action (min)	Onset of action (min)
Lidocaine 5% in 7.5% d/w (premixed)	60 mg (1.2 ml)	80 mg (1.6 ml)	100 m (2.0 ml)	1–3	45–75
Bupivacaine 0.75% in 8.25% d/w	9 mg (1.2 ml)	12 mg (1.6 ml)	15 mg (2.0 ml)	2–4	75–120
Bupivacaine 0.5% in hyperbaric solution†	8 mg (1.6 ml)	10 mg (2.0 ml)	12 mg (2.4 ml)	2–4	75–120
Tetracaine 1% and equal vol. 10% d/w‡	7 mg (0.7 ml) and 0.7 ml	9 mg (9.0 ml) and 0.9 ml	11 mg (1.1 ml) and 1.1 ml	3–5	120–180
Total vol.	1.4 ml	1.8 ml	2.2 ml		
Tetracaine 1% and equal vol. 10% procaine/water‡	6 mg (0.6 ml) and 60 mg (0.6 ml)	8 mg (0.8 ml) and 8 mg (0.8 ml)	10 mg (1.0 ml) and 100 mg (1.0 ml)	2–4	120–180
Total vol.	1.2 ml	1.6 ml	2.0 ml		

* All preparations listed are hyperbaric.
† Not yet approved by the Food and Drug Administration.
‡ Rarely used any more in the USA.
d/w, dextrose in water.

The pregnant patient is more sensitive to local anesthetics for a variety of factors that have been previously discussed (see Ch. 13). Whereas we religiously related the height of the patient to the dosage of tetracaine with glucose or procaine to produce a hyperbaric solution, such is not the situation with hyperbaric bupivacaine. Therefore, the aforementioned tables give a range and a liberal dosage scale for hyperbaric bupivacaine. We have found that the higher doses produce excellent operative anesthesia and a high level of sensory block (up to T2) does not produce the distress in the patient that was previously seen with that level produced by hyperbaric tetracaine. Clinically, we have reached the same conclusion as Norris and Hartwell et al that height is only a moderate determinant of the required dose of hyperbaric bupivacaine and probably only applies with the extremes of height.

There has been much controversy about the total volume of local anesthetic injected into the subarachnoid space and the subsequent production of a higher sensory level of anesthesia due to the altered hemodynamics of CSF in the parturient. Russell[4] recently investigated a range of volumes of local anesthetic with the same mass of drug and found that 15 mg of glucose-free 0.5% bupivacaine administered in dilutions of 3, 6, 12 or 18 ml of solution infused over 30 min produced the same final sensory levels when the parturient was turned supine. Therefore, volume does not appear to be a determinant of the sensory level of subarachnoid block with bupivacaine. Our own preliminary studies with isobaric (dextrose-free) bupivacaine demonstrated it to produce a variable but high block upon injection of 2–4 ml over a period of 1–2 min in the parturient.

Certainly the literature and our personal experience lead us to believe that the dose of hyperbaric bupivacaine is not determined by patient height or volume of injectate. Therefore, the tables presented are to be used only as a guide that should be modified by the personal experience of the anesthesiologist. The addition of preservative-free fentanyl, sufentanil or morphine makes the injectate less hyperbaric but does not appear to have a significant effect on raising the final level of sensory anesthesia.

PRECAUTIONS

To ensure safety and success of subarachnoid anesthesia, several precautions should be taken.

The entry point for the needle should be below the level of L2 so as to avoid injury to the spinal cord.

The spinal needle may on occasion puncture one of the epidural vessels, resulting in a blood-tinged return of CSF at the hub of the needle. If this occurs, the anesthesiologist should wait until the return clears. If the CSF return fails to clear, an attempt should be made to repeat the block through the same or another interspace.

The vital signs must be monitored continuously, especially in the initial 20 min (during the fixation of the block), with close attention paid to any decrease in blood pressure. In the obstetric patient, uterine displacement and intravenous hydration will help to prevent hypotension due to aortocaval compression by the uterus and subsequent uteroplacental hypoperfusion. Oxygen administered by mask to the parturient is helpful to combat cerebral hypoxia, which will manifest itself by the appearance of nausea. Since a hyperbaric solution is used, a modified head-up position, with a pillow under the head, is advisable in order to prevent an excessive cephalad spread of the block and to make the parturient more comfortable.

COMPLICATIONS

The most common complication of spinal anesthesia in obstetrics is maternal hypotension secondary to the combined effect of the decreased venous return produced by blockade of the sympathetic vascular tone and the aortocaval compression by the gravid uterus.

Should vasopressor therapy be needed, pure α-receptor-stimulating agents are usually avoided because these drugs correct the systemic blood pressure by vasoconstriction. Such an effect reduces uteroplacental perfusion and thereby compromises the fetus. However, there are exceptions to this general rule.

Ephedrine in increments of 10 mg intravenously is the best choice at present because it corrects the blood pressure predominantly by myocardial stimulation without compromising uteroplacental perfusion.

Life-threatening complications are rare and, for the most part, are due to an excessive cephalad spread of the local anesthetic causing total spinal anesthesia. This occurrence is heralded by nausea secondary to cerebral hypoxia and hypotension and can progress to respiratory and cardiac arrest. This highlights the importance of meticulous monitoring of the vital signs and the spread of anesthetic effect after the block is initiated. Standard cardiopulmonary resuscitation must be begun at once should a respiratory or a cardiac arrest occur.

Neurologic complications secondary to needle trauma are very rare but may occur if a dural puncture performed above the level of L2 results in spinal cord injury. If a paresthesia is elicited, no injection should be made. The needle should be immediately repositioned. Repeated paresthesias suggest the need to use another technique, either epidural or general anesthesia.

Minor complications include the possibility of postpartum urinary retention and postdural puncture headache. The tendency to urinary retention is present with most types of anesthesia, including general anesthesia. The condition is temporary, and it is managed by bladder assessment and catheterization until normal bladder function resumes. Postdural puncture headache occurs in a small percentage of patients and it is most troublesome when the patient must resume normal activity as soon as possible. Unfortunately, the parturient is in the group with the highest incidence of postdural puncture headache. The diagnosis is made by having the patient sit up or stand up. Headache commences within a few minutes and is relieved by lying down. Its incidence is diminished when the patient is acutely hydrated before the block and when small-gauge (25- to 27-gauge) needles are used. Persistent severe postdural puncture headache not responding to hydration, bed rest and analgesics may be treated with an epidural blood patch.

Meningitis, although rare, may result from contamination of the subarachnoid space during the initiation of spinal anesthesia in the presence of septicemia, local superficial infection of the lumbar area or contaminated equipment.

INDICATIONS

This technique provides excellent anesthesia for vaginal and cesarean delivery.

CONTRAINDICATIONS

Absolute contraindications to spinal anesthesia include infection of the meninges of the spinal cord, septicemia, local cutaneous infections at the puncture site, blood coagulopathies and acute central nervous system disease. Proven allergy to a local anesthetic agent mandates the choice of a local anesthetic drug from a different chemical family.

In other situations, such as the presence of cardiac disease, the advantage of spinal anesthesia must be weighed against potential problems arising from the cardiovascular side-effects of the block.

Several deformities of the lumbosacral spine may make spinal anesthesia technically difficult and thus the potential for trauma may be unacceptably high.

REFERENCES

1. Stienstra R, Greene N M 1991 Factors affecting the subarachnoid spread of local anesthetic solutions. Reg Anesth 16: 1–6
2. Norris M C 1990 Patient variables and the subarachnoid spread of hyperbaric bupivacaine in the term parturient. Anesthesiology 72: 478–482
3. Hartwell B L, Aglio L S, Hauch M A, Datta S 1991 Vertebral column length and the spread of hyperbaric subarachnoid bupivacaine in the term parturient. Reg Anesth 16: 17–19
4. Russell I F 1991 Spinal anesthesia for cesarean delivery with dilute solutions of plain bupivacaine: the relationship between infused volume and spread. Reg Anesth 16: 130–136

PART C
CONTINUOUS SPINAL ANESTHESIA

J. H. Skerman   R. J. Hurley   D. H. Lambert

INTRODUCTION

The idea of continuous spinal anesthesia (CSA) was first introduced in the early 1900s by the British surgeon Dean,[1] who used a spinal needle placed in the subarachnoid space and left in situ for reinjection. Because of technical difficulties, including needle trauma and breakage, this technique never gained popularity. It was not until 1944, with the invention of rubber ureteral catheters and their use by Tuohy,[2] that CSA began to evolve as new technological developments were made.

Practitioners have been using plastic and Teflon epidural catheters for many years to provide CSA for surgical procedures,[3–7] particularly in the geriatric population. Bizzarri et al[8] were the first to use a vinyl catheter for CSA in parturients.

The utilization of small-gauge 28- to 32-gauge catheters has caused a resurgence of interest in this technique. Although CSA has advantages over continuous epidural[9,10] and single-injection spinal anesthesia, until recently it was not often used in labor analgesia or during cesarean delivery because of the high incidence of post-dural puncture headache (PDPH) in pregnant women. PDPH is inversely related to age and directly related to the diameter of the needle used for lumbar dural puncture.[10] The incidence of PDPH associated with CSA when large needles and catheters were used in the pregnant woman was unacceptably high for some practitioners.[11,12] Some authorities felt the presence of a catheter through the dura may potentiate further loss of cerebrospinal fluid by a 'wick' effect.

Administration of CSA for labor and delivery with a microcatheter (32-gauge) has recently been investigated by some clinicians with good results. Huckaby et al[13] reported excellent sensory anesthesia with negligible motor block using 1% lidocaine. Other benefits noted in this study included the ability to achieve rapid sensory anesthesia and to prolong its duration as required. The density and level of anesthesia could be rapidly raised if operative delivery became necessary. In addition, the danger of central nervous system or cardiac toxicity was remote since the local anesthetic is administered in small incremental doses.

Denny et al[14] reported an incidence of PDPH of 1% after CSA performed with a 20-gauge catheter inserted through an 18-gauge Hustead needle. The average age of the patients in this study was 66 years. Unfortunately, the use of similar needles and catheters in pregnant women is not associated with the same low incidence of PDPH as

Table 35.3 Incidence of headache with continuous spinal anesthesia (Adapted from ref. 17).

Reference	Year	Needle gauge	Catheter gauge	Percent headache
14	1987	18	20	1
16	1972	20, 21	24	16*
15	1989	26	32	4
11	1989	17	20	20*
12	1990	18	20	54*

* Pregnant patients.

reported by Denny et al[14] (Table 35.3).[11,12,15,16] Nevertheless, catheters that can be inserted through 22- and 26-gauge spinal needles are now available. This recent advance in catheter technology makes CSA possible for labor and vaginal or cesarean delivery without increasing the risk of PDPH. With the ongoing improvement of microcatheter technology for CSA, the incidence of PDPH following the use of smaller catheters is probably the same as that following single-injection spinal anesthesia performed with small-diameter needles.[18]

CONTINUOUS SPINAL CATHETERS

Table 35.4 lists the catheters available for CSA and the size of the needle used to insert them. A pencil-point 24-gauge (Sprotte) needle with a lateral side port that allows passage of a 28-gauge or smaller catheter is now manufactured.[19] The pencil-point tip decreases the incidence of PDPH[20] and the Sprotte needle may prove useful for CSA in parturients.

ANATOMY AND LANDMARKS

Anatomy and landmarks are the same as previously discussed under spinal anesthesia.

PATIENT POSITION

The patient position is the same as previously discussed under spinal anesthesia. However, it should be noted that, for the parturient in early labor, the sitting position may sometimes be more advantageous, particularly for an obese patient, as it allows easier threading of the spinal catheter 1–2 cm cephalad as well as easier withdrawal of the needle without dislodgment of the catheter.

MATERIALS

The following materials should be ready for use when the patient is to be given CSA:

- One pair of sterile gloves
- Antibacterial solution for cleansing the skin
- One sterile cup for the antibacterial solution
- Forceps
- Sterile gauze pads
- Sterile towels for draping the field
- One 25-gauge, 1.6- to 3.8-cm needle for skin infiltration
- One 21- or 22-gauge, 3.8-cm needle for preparing drugs and deep infiltration (if desired)
- One 18-gauge needle for use as an introducer
- One 22-, 25-, or 26-gauge, 8.9-cm spinal needle with stylet
- One 28- or 32-gauge microcatheter
- One 3-ml syringe
- One 5-ml glass syringe
- Sterile gauze to protect the catheter
- Tape to secure the catheter.

Disposable CSA trays that contain all of the above items are commercially available.

TECHNIQUE

The technique is the same as that described for spinal anesthesia with the added steps of inserting and securing the catheter. Recently both 32-gauge catheters that can be advanced through a 25- or 26-gauge spinal needle and 28-gauge catheters that can be advanced through a 22-gauge spinal needle have become available. Most catheters have a stylet to facilitate introduction into the subarachnoid space and are marked at 1-cm intervals. Once a free flow of CSF is obtained, the catheter is advanced 1–2 cm into the subarachnoid space. After the introducer and spinal needle are removed, the catheter is secured in place with tape in a manner similar to an epidural catheter.

Table 35.4 Catheters (Adapted from ref. 17)

Type	Material	Gauge	Needle	Manufacturer
Epidural	Nylon, Teflon	19, 20	17, 18	Many
Spinal	Polyethylene	24	20, 21*	Cardiovascular and Special Instruments
Pediatric epidural	Polyurethane	24	20	Preferred Medical
Spinal	Polyurethane	27	22	Preferred Medical
Spinal	Nylon	28	22	Concord Portex
Spinal	Nylon	28	22	Kendall
Spinal	Polyimide	28	22	Rusch
Spinal	Polyimide	32	26, 27	Rusch

* Special needles

CONSIDERATIONS

The most common problem encountered when using the minicatheters (27-gauge or smaller) or the microcatheter (28- and 32-gauge) is kinking of the catheter on insertion. This difficulty is due to the catheter being advanced against tissue instead of being freely passed into CSF. Hurley and Lambert[15] describe several maneuvers that may be helpful in overcoming this problem: flushing the needle with saline, rotating the needle, rotating the needle while advancing the catheter and slowly withdrawing the needle may result in successful placement without the catheter kinking. A threading-assist adapter may also be helpful to provide lateral stabilization of the catheter within the spinal needle hub where the catheter may flex and bend upon itself during advancement. Should all of these techniques fail, another attempt should be made at another interspace.

Following successful placement, the needle is slowly withdrawn over the catheter, the catheter is padded with gauze then secured to the patient's back with tape and the local anesthetic injected. Aspiration of CSF through the large 19- or 20-gauge epidural catheter easily confirms correct subarachnoid placement, but because of the increased resistance associated with the smaller catheters aspiration may not produce CSF easily.

Some facts to be remembered when providing CSA with a mini- or microcatheter for laboring patients include the following:

1. If injection through the catheter is difficult or impossible and there is no visible evidence of occlusion, having the patient either flex or extend her back may alleviate this problem. The same technique can be utilized if difficulty is encountered during removal of the catheter.
2. Small incremental doses of local anesthetic titrated to the desired sensory level should be used. The use of both isobaric and hyperbaric agents may be needed to provide an adequate anesthetic, especially in patients with anatomic abnormalities of the spine.
3. Small doses of anesthetics with higher concentrations may provide a better block than larger doses of weaker concentrations.
4. Up to seven times more total drug may be required when using combined isobaric and hypobaric agents than with hyperbaric agents alone.

PRECAUTIONS

All precautions previously stated for spinal anesthesia should be taken with CSA.

Again, care must be taken to avoid kinking or bending of the mini- or microcatheter during placement and to avoid unintentional removal following successful insertion. There is also the danger that the catheter may be inserted directly into a blood vessel; negative aspiration of blood is not a guarantee that the catheter has not been placed or migrated into a vessel. The amount of local anesthetic used for subarachnoid anesthesia is small enough so that unintentional intravascular injection is usually without consequence but will be reflected by the lack of a developing anesthetic effect. Following surgery or delivery, it is important to remember to position the patient so that her back is either flexed or extended while the mini- or microcatheter is being removed. If the catheter seems difficult to remove, excessive force or traction should not be applied, as it may break, resulting in the need for further patient manipulation.

ADMINISTRATION AND MANAGEMENT FOR LABOR AND DELIVERY

Any of the local anesthetic agents used for single injection spinal anesthesia may be used for CSA. However, an advantage of CSA is the ability to tailor the level and duration of anesthesia. Ultra-short-acting local anesthetics are extremely useful for minimizing hemodynamic changes and subarachnoid opioids may also be added to the local anesthetics as desired.

CSA can thus be used for pain relief during labor (Table 35.5)[13,21–35] and the availability of small catheters has renewed interest in the use of this technique in obstetrics. The method was first used in 1946 with tetracaine and metycaine.[21,22] Procaine became popular in the 1950s,[16,24] and now lidocaine and bupivacaine are currently in use.[13,25,28]

In addition to local anesthetics, small doses of subarachnoid opioids have been used for labor analgesia.[27,30,32,33,36–40] Subarachnoid opioids produce an analgesic effect by binding to opioid receptors in the substantia gelatinosa. Subarachnoid morphine in doses of 0.5–1 mg has been reported to provide excellent analgesia during labor.[36–38] Side-effects include pruritus, nausea and emesis.[37] A serious side-effect is delayed respiratory depression occurring 6–10 h after administration requiring intravenous naloxone for reversal.[37] Since morphine is non-lipid soluble, the onset of respiratory depression coincides with the rostral spread of the opioid to the brain. Using a lower dose of 0.5 mg, Edwards et al[38] found subarachnoid morphine to be effective during early labor without major side-effects. Others have also reported excellent analgesia for early labor using 0.5 and 1.0 mg of hyperbaric subarachnoid morphine.[39] Side-effects include an 80% prevalence of pruritus, 53% nausea or vomiting, 43% urinary retention and 43% drowsiness. No significant respiratory depression was reported,[39] but the time to onset of effective analgesia was of concern to many participants in these studies.

In an endeavor to eliminate this concern, Leighton et al[27] combined fentanyl with morphine to hasten the onset. Shorter acting lipid-soluble opioids such as fentanyl or sufentanil may be a better choice, but since CSA is not yet

Table 35.5 Obstetric uses of continuous spinal catheters

Reference	Year	Use	Drugs
21	1945	Cesarean delivery	Procaine
22	1946	Labor analgesia	Metycaine/Tetracaine
23	1950	Eclampsia/preeclampsia	Tetracaine
24	1951	Labor analgesia	Procaine
25	1970	Labor analgesia	Lidocaine
16	1972	Cesarean delivery	Procaine
26	1988	Cesarean delivery* (difficult airway)	Bupivacaine
27	1989	Labor analgesia	Fentanyl/morphine
28	1990	Labor analgesia	Bupivacaine
15	1990	Cesarean delivery	Lidocaine/Bupivacaine
29	1990	Cesarean delivery* (kyphoscoliosis)	Bupivacaine
30	1990	Labor analgesia	Sufentanil
31	1990	Cesarean delivery* (spinal bifida)	Bupivacaine
32	1990	Labor analgesia* (Allergy)	Meperidine
13	1991	Labor analgesia	Lidocaine
33	1991	Labor analgesia	Meperidine
34	1991	Cesarean delivery	Bupivacaine
35	1992	Labor analgesia	Diamorphine/bupivacaine

* Case report.

widely utilized for labor analgesia/anesthesia the role of subarachnoid opioids for labor pain control is still evolving.

It must be remembered that morphine is approximately 10 times more potent in the subarachnoid space than in the epidural space; recommended dosages range from 0.1 to 0.5 mg for achieving 12–24 h of analgesia. The respiratory rate must be continuously monitored for 24 h because of the possibility of delayed respiratory depression associated with subarachnoid morphine administration.[30] Owing to the greater lipid solubility of fentanyl and sufentanil, there is a lower incidence of delayed respiratory depression.[40]

It seems very clear that, while subarachnoid opioids may provide good pain relief during early labor, they fail to control pain as labor intensifies during the second stage. With a mini- or microcatheter in place, the addition of low doses and low concentrations of local anesthetics subsequent to the opioids has been extremely effective in the late second stage of labor and for delivery.

Meperidine is an interesting opioid because of its local anesthetic properties. In addition to producing analgesia by interacting with spinal cord opioid receptors, it also causes neuronal conduction blockade.[32,33] Sufentanil, a highly lipid-soluble and potent opioid, is the most recently used for subarachnoid labor analgesia.[30] When 3–5 μg of sufentanil is injected through a 28-gauge catheter that is inserted through a 22-gauge needle, it produces up to 5 h of analgesia and the prevalence of PDPH is approximately 2% (J S Naulty, personal communication). The efficacy of incremental subarachnoid diamorphine for labor and delivery was tested by Kestin et al.[35] Diamorphine gave excellent anesthesia in 11 out of 20 patients. Side-effects were common, and 15 mothers had pruritus and 15 had nausea.

These results with subarachnoid opioids indicate further promise for the control of pain during early labor because they produce analgesia without motor blockade.

ADMINISTRATION AND MANAGEMENT FOR CESAREAN DELIVERY

There has been little interest in using CSA for cesarean delivery. This is probably because the operation can usually be completed within the duration of a single-injection spinal anesthetic. Furthermore, the patients are generally healthy and can tolerate the hemodynamic effects of high spinal anesthesia. It is not generally necessary to insert a subarachnoid catheter, which can be difficult and time-consuming.[15] Nevertheless, there are many recent reports of cesarean delivery performed with CSA (Table 35.5).[15,16,21,26,29,31,34] Putative advantages of CSA during cesarean delivery are the possibility of titrating the local anesthetic dose in order to limit cephalad spread. By so doing, the degree of sympathectomy is believed to be less and the hemodynamic consequences minimized. In an early study,[15] it was found that, despite injecting small doses of local anesthetics through a spinal catheter, the level of anesthesia was similar to single injection of a larger dose. However, the duration of anesthesia is shorter when small doses are given with CSA. This is of little consequence because the catheter allows renewal of the anesthetic once it begins to diminish. Another theoretical advantage of CSA over the single-injection method is that more local anesthetic can be titrated through the catheter, should the level of anesthesia be inadequate.

Kestin et al[34] also compared CSA and continuous epidural anesthesia (CEA) for elective cesarean delivery. The spinal catheter was easier and quicker to place and anesthesia was established more quickly. The maximum height of subarachnoid block was significantly higher. Hemodynamic stability was similar in both groups.

DISEASES COMPLICATING PREGNANCY

CSA is very beneficial in certain disease states that occasionally complicate pregnancy:

1. spinal deformity;
   a. kyphoscoliosis;
   b. spina bifida;
2. difficult airway;
3. obesity;
4. cardiac disease.

CSA is useful in controlling labor pain in patients with severe kyphoscoliosis.[29] The manipulation of baricity and patient position allows careful distribution of the local anesthetic, which is not possible with continuous epidural anesthesia (CEA). Nuyten and Gielen[31] used CSA for cesarean delivery in a patient with spina bifida. The patient, who desired to participate in the birth of her child, had grossly deformed vertebral anatomy that the authors believed would make successful epidural anesthesia unlikely, and instead they instituted CSA. The cesarean delivery utilizing hyperbaric bupivacaine was uneventful. Malan and Johnson[26] used CSA in a morbidly obese parturient with a difficult airway. Continuous epidural anesthesia is often difficult or impossible in the obese parturient and CSA may be easier to carry out. Furthermore, the ability to titrate the dose of local anesthetic is seen as advantageous. Parturients with cardiac disease are usually given CEA for labor and/or cesarean delivery. However, if CEA fails or is not possible in parturients with cardiac disease, the clear end-point of CSF appearing in the needle hub makes CSA a desirable and useful alternative to CEA.[41]

Years ago, Lund[23] reported on a few patients who received CSA to control the pathophysiologic effects of eclampsia and preeclampsia. Although the abnormal coagulation profiles sometimes associated with eclampsia and preeclampsia can be a relative contraindication to regional anesthesia, the technique of CSA, using initial subarachnoid opioid medications during early labor followed by administration of appropriate local anesthetic solutions for delivery, has re-emerged.

COMPLICATIONS

All complications of single dose spinal anesthesia apply to CSA. Other disadvantages associated with use of the mini- or microcatheter in CSA are mostly technical and include the following:

1. inability to thread the catheter;
2. inability to inject the anesthetic;
3. catheter breakage;
4. unitentional removal of the catheter;
5. inadequate anesthesia;
6. possible inability to aspirate CSF from the subarachnoid space owing to increased resistance;
7. mini- or microcatheters have been noted to bend, kink, twist and even knot.

The larger 19- to 21-gauge epidural catheters can usually be placed into the subarachnoid space with minimal difficulty. Since these catheters are larger and more rigid than the smaller catheters, they thread easier and are not prone to catheter lumen occlusion. The microcatheter, however, is very different. Hurley and Lambert[15] reported a 20% failure rate with their early trials during the development of the microcatheter.

Catheter breakage is always a concern with any catheter in the subarachnoid space[42,43] and may readily occur if the catheter should be withdrawn through the needle. When a catheter is unable to be advanced, both the catheter and needle must be removed together. The breakage of two microcatheters during attempted catheter removal has been reported.[15] The catheter should be protected at all times by carefully securing it in a proper manner, minimizing patient movement, especially during operating and delivery room positioning, and careful removal of the catheter with minimal force. Should a catheter break, radiographs or CT scan may be helpful in analyzing the location of the remaining fragment. Full explanation of the complication to the patient is prudent. Surgical retrieval is usually not advised unless there are neurologic findings.[42]

Except for PDPH, neurologic complications following CSA are rare. The prevalence of PDPH in parturients has been noted to be as high as 16–21% when a 19-gauge spinal needle and large catheter is used.[6,11–16,44] During CSA using a 25- or 26-gauge spinal needle and 32-gauge microcatheter, a 4% prevalence of PDPH was reported.[15] Other neurologic sequelae including adhesive arachnoiditis, transverse myelitis, cauda equina syndrome and septic meningitis are rare following CSA.

Cauda equina syndrome

Cauda equina syndrome is a prolonged and possibly permanent neurologic deficit characterized by one of the following: loss of bladder and/or bowel control; loss of perineal sensation and decreased sensation or mobility of the lower extremities. Recently in the USA (29 May, 1992) the Food and Drug Administration (FDA) issued a safety alert for the use of small-bore catheters in CSA. The

FDA had received 11 reports of cauda equina syndrome in which small-bore catheters were used to deliver 5% lidocaine with 7.5% glucose to the subarachnoid space. Recent cases had also been reported in the medical literature.[45]

Review of these reports indicated the following similarities:

1. the use of 5% lidocaine (50 mg/ml) in 7.5% dextrose;
2. less than the expected anesthetic effect for a given dose;
3. an initial lidocaine dosage of 100 mg or more to establish the spinal anesthetic;
4. a total lidocaine dosage exceeding 100 mg.

Subsequent studies and reports by many authors[46–56] have described mechanisms to account for the neural damage, while others[48–50,53,57,58] have ascribed the causative problems to inadequacies and failures in technique. Lambert et al[54] have examined the direct exposure of unsheathed nerve fibers to various concentrations of lidocaine and dextrose, while Swayze et al[58] demonstrated that a disproportionate number of experienced anesthesia personnel inserted untoward lengths of subarachnoid catheter without regard to direction or position in a model of the subarachnoid space. Meticulous attention to the details of technique related to catheter insertion along with considerations for choice of a local anesthetic agent (including volume, concentration, with or without dextrose, baricity and tonicity, maldistribution and the effect of cumulative doses) all play an important role in the successful application of CSA and the elimination of untoward and preventable neurologic sequelae.

SUMMARY

Because of the availability of small catheters that can be inserted through small-diameter needles, there is renewed interest in continuous spinal anesthesia for obstetric analgesia and anesthesia. This reduces the incidence of PDPH, which is high in parturients when a large-diameter needle is used for dural puncture. The indications for continuous subarachnoid analgesia and anesthesia in obstetrics are still evolving.

Continuous spinal anesthesia can be used to provide a rapid anesthesia for vaginal delivery, forceps application, cesarean delivery (when a catheter is already in place and functioning well), placental extraction and post-delivery episiotomy and/or laceration repairs. Since smaller doses of local anesthetics are required, serious cardiovascular and central nervous system complications are rare.

The administration of highly lipid-soluble opioids through small spinal catheters for labor analgesia is exciting and promising. Continuous spinal anesthesia has advantages over CEA in certain disease states that complicate pregnancy, particularly diseases such as kyphoscoliosis, spina bifida and obesity that distort spinal anatomy.

The history and background of continuous spinal anesthesia relative to obstetrics is thus a fascinating story and it is to be hoped that the recent excitement and advances realized with its application to obstetrics will not be subjugated by the few reports of cauda equina syndrome and the safety alert issued by the FDA in the USA. All anesthetic methods and techniques have potential for morbidity and only continued research and vigilance, along with proper application of newly developed drugs and materials subsequent to such research, will suffice to truly improve the anesthetic care and management of the parturient.

REFERENCES

1. Dean H P 1907 Discussion on the relative value of inhalation and injection methods of inducing anesthesia. Br Med J 2: 869–877
2. Tuohy E B 1944 Continuous spinal anesthesia: its usefulness and technique involved. Anesthesiology 5: 142–148
3. Lemmon W T 1940 A method for continuous spinal anesthesia. Ann Surg 111: 141–144
4. Cann J E, Wyscoff C C 1948 Continuous spinal anesthesia: a modification of the ureteral technique. Anesthesiology 9: 288–293
5. Davidson H H, Hingson R A, Helman L M 1951 Use of various plastic catheters in the subarachnoid and peridural spaces. Arch Surg 62: 540–552
6. Peterson D O, Borup J L, Chestnut J S 1983 Continuous spinal anesthesia: case review and discussion. Reg Anesth 8: 109–113
7. Shroff P K, Skerman J H, Blass N H 1988 Continuous spinal blockade: an old technique revisited. South Med J 81: 178–180
8. Bizzarri D V, Guiffrida J G, Bondoc L et al 1964 Continuous spinal anesthesia using a special needle and catheter. Anesth Analg 43: 393–399
9. Sutter P A, Gamulin Z, Forster A 1989 Comparison of continuous spinal and continuous epidural anaesthesia for lower limb surgery in elderly patients: a retrospective study. Anaesthesia 44: 47–50
10. Vandam L D, Dripps R D 1956 Long term follow up of patients who received 10,098 spinal anesthetics: III. Syndrome of decreased intracranial pressure (headache and ocular and auditory difficulties). J Am Med Assoc 161: 586–591
11. Cohen S, Daitch J S, Goldiner P L 1989 An alternative method for management of accidental dural puncture for labor and delivery. Anesthesiology 70: 164–165
12. Norris M C, Leighton B L 1990 Continuous spinal anesthesia after unintentional dural puncture in parturients. Reg Anesth 15: 285–287
13. Huckaby T, Skerman J H, Hurley R J et al 1991 Sensory analgesia for vaginal deliveries: a preliminary report of continuous spinal anesthesia with a 32 gauge catheter. Reg Anesth 16: 150–153
14. Denny N, Masters R, Pearson D, et al 1987 Postdural puncture headache after continuous spinal anesthesia. Anesth Analg 66: 791–794
15. Hurley R J, Lambert D H 1990 Continuous spinal anesthesia with a microcatheter technique: preliminary experience. Anesth Analg 70: 97–102
16. Giuffrida J G, Bizzarri D V, Masi R et al 1972 Continuous procaine spinal anesthesia for cesarean section. Anesth Analg 51: 117–124
17. Lambert D H 1992 Continuous spinal anesthesia. In: Batra M (ed) Epidural and spinal analgesia and anesthesia: contemporary issues, Vol 10. W B Saunders, Philadelphia, pp 87–102
18. Hurley R J, Lambert D H 1990 Microcatheters for continuous spinal anesthesia. Anesth Analg 71: 200–203
19. Cesarini M, Torrieli R, Lahaye F et al 1990 Sprotte needle for intrathecal anaesthesia for caesarean section: incidence of postdural puncture headache. Anaesthesia 45: 656–658

20. Carrie L E 1990 Whitacre and pencil-point spinal needles: some points to consider. Anaesthesia 45: 1097–1098
21. Ullery J C 1945 Continuous spinal and continuous caudal analgesia in cesarean section. Surg Clin N Am 25: 1382–1390
22. Gillett R E 1946 Continuous spinal anesthesia in obstetrics. Northwest Med 45: 743, 1946
23. Lund P C 1951 The role of conduction anesthesia in the management of eclampsia. Anesthesiology 12: 693–707
24. Carpenter S L, Ceravolo A J, Foldes F F 1951 Continuous-drop subarachnoid block with dilute procaine solution for labor and delivery. Am J Obstet Gynecol 61: 1277–1284
25. Elam J O 1970 Catheter subarachnoid block for labor and delivery: a differential segmental technique employing hyperbaric lidocaine. Anesth Analg 49: 1007–1015
26. Malan T P, Johnson M D 1988 The difficult airway in obstetric anesthesia: techniques for airway management and the role of regional anesthesia. J Clin Anesth 1: 104–111
27. Leighton B L, DeSimone C A, Norris M C et al 1989 Intrathecal narcotics for labor revisited: the combination of fentanyl and morphine intrathecally provides rapid onset of profund, prolonged analgesia. Anesth Analg 69: 122–125
28. Benedetti C, Tiengo M 1990 Continuous subarachnoid analgesia in labor. Lancet 335: 225
29. Moran D H, Johnson M D 1990 Continuous spinal anesthesia with combined hyperbaric and isobaric bupivacaine in a patient with scoliosis. Anesth Analg 70: 445–447
30. Naulty J S, Barnes D, Becker R et al 1990 Continuous subarachnoid sufentanil for labor analgesia. Anesthesiology 73: A964
31. Nuyten F, Gielen M 1990 Spinal catheter anaesthesia for cesarean section in a patient with spina bifida. Anaesthesia 45: 846–847
32. Johnson M D, Hurley R J, Gilbertson L I et al 1990 Continuous microcatheter spinal anesthesia with subarachnoid meperidine for labor and delivery. Anesth Analg 70: 658–661
33. Swayze C R, Skerman J H, Walker E B et al 1991 Efficacy of subarachnoid meperidine for labor analgesia. Reg Anesth 16: 309–313
34. Kestin I G, Madden A P, Mulvein J T et al 1991 Comparison of incremental spinal anaesthesia using a 32 gauge catheter with extradural anaesthesia for elective caeserian section. Br J Anaesth 68: 232–236
35. Kestin I G, Madden A P, Mulvein J T et al 1992 Analgesia for labour and delivery using incremental diamorphine and bupivacaine via a 32 gauge intrathecal catheter. Br J Anaesth 68: 244–247
36. Hee P, Stampe-Srense S, Bock J E et al 1987 Intrathecal administration of morphine for the relief of pain in labour and estimation of maternal and fetal plasma concentration of morphine. Eur J Obstet Gynecol Reprod Biol 25: 195–201
37. Abouleish E 1988 Apnoea associated with the intrathecal administration of morphine in obstetrics. Br J Anaesth 60: 592–594
38. Edwards R D, Hansel N K, Pruessner H T et al 1988 Intrathecal morphine as analgesia for labor pain. J Am Board Family Practice 1: 245–250
39. Abboud T K, Shnider S M, Dailey P A et al 1984 Intrathecal administration of hyperbaric morphine for the relief of pain in labour. Br J Anaesth 56: 1351–1360
40. Hurley R J, Johnson M D 1990 Spinal opioids in the management of obstetric pain. J Pain Symptom Management 5: 146–153
41. Johnson M D, Saltzman D H 1991 Cardiac disease. In: Datta S (ed) Anesthetic and obstetric management of high risk pregnancy. Mosby Year Book, St Louis, MO, pp 210–259
42. Schmidt S I, Moorthy S M, Dierdorf S F et al 1990 Was there a retained spinal catheter? J Clin Anesth 2: 425–426
43. Schmidt S I, Moorthy S M, Dierdorf S F et al 1990 Vanishing calibration marks on a spinal catheter. Anesth Analg 70: 462–463
44. Chen L, Fitzgerald T E, Miller F L et al 1990 Post dural puncture headache and continuous spinal anesthesia. Reg Anaesth 15: 268–272
45. Rigler M L, Drasner K, Krejcie T C et al 1991 Cauda equina syndrome after continuous spinal anesthesia. Anesth Analg 72: 275–281
46. Rosen M, Baysinger C L, Shnider S M et al 1983 Evaluation of neurotoxity after subarachnoid injection of large volumes of local anesthetic solution. Anesth Analg 62: 802–808
47. Schmidt S I, Moorthy S M, Dierdorf S F et al 1990 A series of truly failed spinal anesthetics. J Clin Anesth 2: 336–338
48. Bevacqua B K, Cleary W F, Slucky A V 1991 Catheter spinal anesthesia and cauda equina syndrome: an alternative view. Anesth Analg 73: 367–370
49. Rosenberg A L, Gold M I 1991 Catheter spinal anesthesia and cauda equina syndrome: an alternative view. Anesth Analg 73: 367–370
50. Wildsmith J A 1991 Catheter spinal anesthesia and cauda equina syndrome: an alternative view. Anesth Analg 73: 367–370
51. Rigler M L, Drasner K, Krejcie T C, et al 1991 Catheter spinal anesthesia and cauda equina syndrome: an alternative view. Anesth Analg 73: 367–370, 1991
52. Hurley R J, Lambert D H 1991 Cauda equina syndrome after continuous spinal anesthesia. Anesth Analg 72: 817–819
53. Biscoping J, Hempel V, Niesel H C et al 1992 Continuous spinal anesthesia: a statement on its practical application (editorial). DER Anaesthetist 41: 631–633
54. Lambert L A, Lambert D H, Strichartz G R 1992 Potential neurotoxity of lidocaine and dextrose solutions used for spinal anesthesia. Reg Anesth 17: S164
55. Ross B K, Coda B, Heath C H 1992 Local anesthetic distribution in spinal model: a possible mechanism of neurologic injury after continuous spinal anesthesia. Reg Anesth 17: 69–77
56. Abouleish E 1992 Cauda equina syndrome, continuous spinal anesthesia and repeated spinal block: is there a relationship? Reg Anesth 17: 356–357
57. Chan V W, Smyth R J 1992 Radiographic evaluation of catheter position in restricted sacral block after continuous spinal anesthesia. Anesth Analg 75: 449–452
58. Swayze C R, Skerman J H 1992 Cauda equina syndrome with continuous spinal anesthesia revisited. Reg Anesth 17: S1

PART D
COMBINED SPINAL-EPIDURAL ANESTHESIA
N. Rawal

INTRODUCTION

Provision of safe and effective anesthesia for abdominal surgery in the awake obstetric patient is one of the most challenging of problems. It is generally recognized that an S5–T4 block is necessary for adequate anesthesia during cesarean delivery. Such an extensive block by the epidural route requires large doses of local anesthetic drugs and may be associated with a relatively high incidence of hypotension[1,2] and a potential risk of toxic complications.[3–5] Furthermore, in spite of these large doses the block may be inadequate in 10–25% of patients, mainly because of difficulty in anesthetizing the sacral roots.[3,6,7] Spinal anesthesia is more reliable than epidural anesthesia because of its more intense motor block but the upper level of the block may be unpredictable. The technique may be associated with a high risk of precipitous maternal hypotension, which may be harmful for the neonate.[8–10] Since the catheter technique is not used, there is no possibility of providing post-operative pain relief with spinal anesthesia. Thus, in spite of their popularity, both spinal and epidural anesthesia have many disadvantages (Table 35.6).

A combined spinal–epidural (CSE) technique can reduce or eliminate some of the disadvantages of spinal and epidural anesthesia while preserving their advantages. The possibility of improving analgesia with epidural supplements and extending the analgesia well into the post-operative period is making CSE blocks increasingly popular[12–15] (Table 35.7). An array of special CSE kits and sophisticated needles designed to reduce risks of complications have also resulted in renewed interest in this technique.

The earliest reference to the technique appeared in 1937 in a manuscript in *Anesthesia* and *Analgesia*. Soresi (a New York surgeon) and colleagues used 'episubdural anesthesia' in over 200 patients; they claimed that 'by combining the two methods (epidural and spinal) many of the disadvantages of both methods are eliminated and their advantages are enhanced to an almost incredible degree'. The technique consisted of injecting local anesthetic (procaine) first into the epidural space and then into the subarachnoid space through the same fine spinal needle. The catheter technique was unknown at the time. The authors claimed that the 'perfect surgical anesthesia' of spinal anesthesia could be prolonged with epidural anesthesia to provide excellent perioperative anesthesia and prolonged post-operative analgesia lasting at least 24 h.[16]

In 1979 Curelaru[17] reported the use of combined spinal–epidural technique for upper and lower abdominal, urologic and lower extremity surgery. A total of 150 patients were studied; most were high-risk patients. The technique consisted of performing a spinal anesthetic 1–2 interspaces below the level of epidural catheter insertion. In this two-segment technique, the spinal anesthetic is performed after the epidural catheter is in place.

In 1981 Brownridge[18] described a similar technique for cesarean delivery. In about 90% of the patients, the subarachnoid block alone was adequate for cesarean delivery. The epidural catheter was available to extend the block if necessary and to provide post-operative analgesia. A modification of the technique for orthopedic surgery

Table 35.6 Relative merits of subarachnoid versus epidural anesthesia for cesarean delivery (From ref. 11 with permission)

	Subarachnoid	Epidural
Speed of onset	Very rapid	Delayed
Upper limit of block	Variable, unpredictable	Usually satisfactory to T4
Lower limit of block	Usually satisfactory to S4	Variable, sacral sparing
Density of block	Profound	Variable, agent dependent
Duration of motor block	Agent dependent; may be prolonged	Agent dependent; not usually prolonged
Systemic absorption	Negligible	Substantial; toxicity possible
Hypotension	Common, rapid onset	Variable; gradual onset
Shivering	Rare	Common
Post-dural puncture headache	Variable, unpredictable	Nil
Provision for post-operative analgesia	Nil	Ideal route for continuous analgesia

Table 35.7 Advantages of combined spinal epidural technique

- Combined advantages of epidural and spinal anesthesia for abdominal and lower extremity surgery
- Possibility of extending spinal anesthesia (for prolonged surgery)
- Possibility of extending inadequate spinal anesthesia
- Provision of prolonged post-operative analgesia by local anesthetics and/or opioids
- Treatment of PDPH should it occur (by injection of saline or autologous blood through the epidural catheter)

was reported by Coates[19] and by Mumtaz et al in 1982[20] and for cesarean delivery by Carrie and O'Sullivan in 1984.[21] These investigators described a single-space 'needle-through-needle' technique in which the epidural needle served as an introducer for a long and fine spinal needle. In 1986 Rawal[22] described a single-segment sequential CSE technique for cesarean delivery. In this technique the epidural catheter is not just a reserve catheter, it is used to gradually raise the level of an intentional low spinal block. This modification reduces the severity and frequency of maternal hypotension. Since then a large number of studies have been published.[15,23,24] In the early years CSE blocks were performed with multiple-use extra long 25–30 G spinal needles which were introduced through standard Tuohy needles. In recent years special CSE needle sets have been introduced. It is difficult to know how extensively CSE is used. One medical company sold 11 000 CSE sets in Europe during 1992 (Axel Spanholtz, B. Braun, Sweden). At present there are at least 12 medical equipment companies that distribute such specialized CSE needles world-wide.

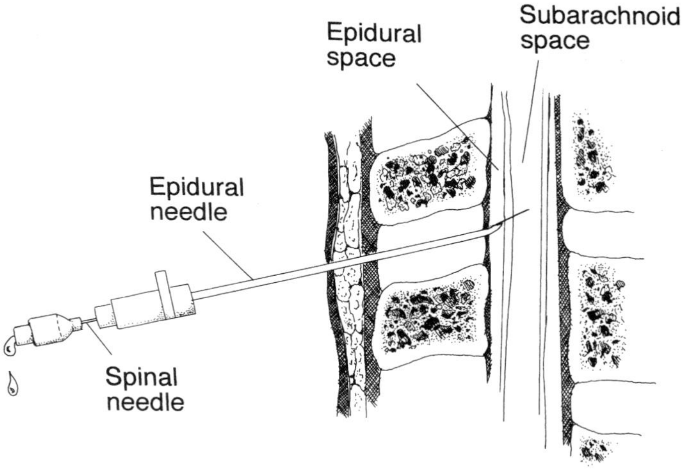

Fig. 35.9 Combined spinal–epidural anesthesia needle-through-needle technique. An extra long spinal needle is introduced through a regular Tuohy needle.

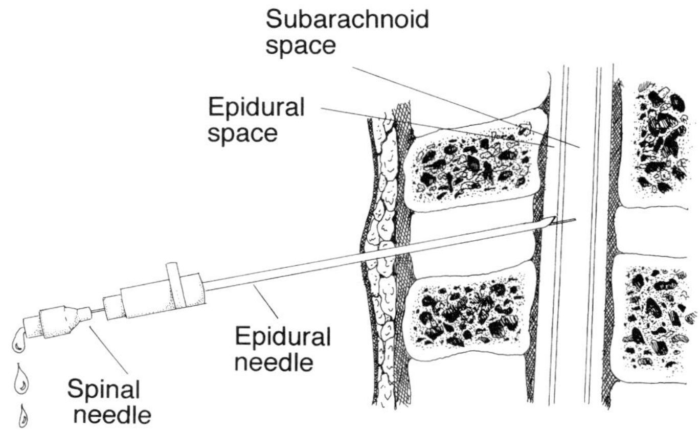

Fig. 35.10 Combined spinal–epidural anesthesia. A modified needle-through-needle technique. The spinal needle passes through a special hole near the tip of the Tuohy needle. The tip of the spinal needle does not come in contact with the inner wall of the Tuohy needle.

CSE TECHNIQUE

There are several options for performing the CSE technique (Table 35.8). The most common technique is the single-segment 'needle-through-needle' technique.

Briefly the technique is as follows. With the patient in the sitting or lateral position, the appropriate Tuohy needle is inserted at the desired intervertebral space and the epidural space identified in the usual manner. Next a long 27-gauge (or finer) spinal needle is introduced through the Tuohy needle and advanced until the tip of the spinal needle is felt to penetrate the dura (Figs 35.9 and 35.10). After correct placement of the spinal needle is confirmed by free flow of CSF, the appropriate dose of local anesthetic is injected and the spinal needle is then withdrawn. It is emphasized that at this stage the spinal needle is held in place only by the dura and therefore there is a risk of needle displacement when it is connected to the syringe or during injection of local anesthetic. This is a critical stage in the CSE technique and the most likely cause of failure of blocks. This problem can be overcome by steadying the spinal needle using the grip shown in Figure 35.11. Spinal needle displacement is not a problem in the newer special CSE kits in which the hub of the

Table 35.8 Various options for combined spinal–epidural technique

- Single needle–single interspace[16,25]
- Double needle–separate interspaces*[17,18]
- Double needle (needle-through-needle) – single interspace[19–22]
- Double needle (needle beside needle) – single interspace†
  a. spinal needle guide fixed alongside outer wall of epidural needle[26,27]
  b. spinal needle guide incorporated within epidural wall‡

* Epidural catheter insertion followed by spinal anesthesia at a lower interspace.
† Allows epidural catheter insertion before spinal anesthesia.
‡ E-SP needle. This device is FDA approved, however no clinical data are available so far.

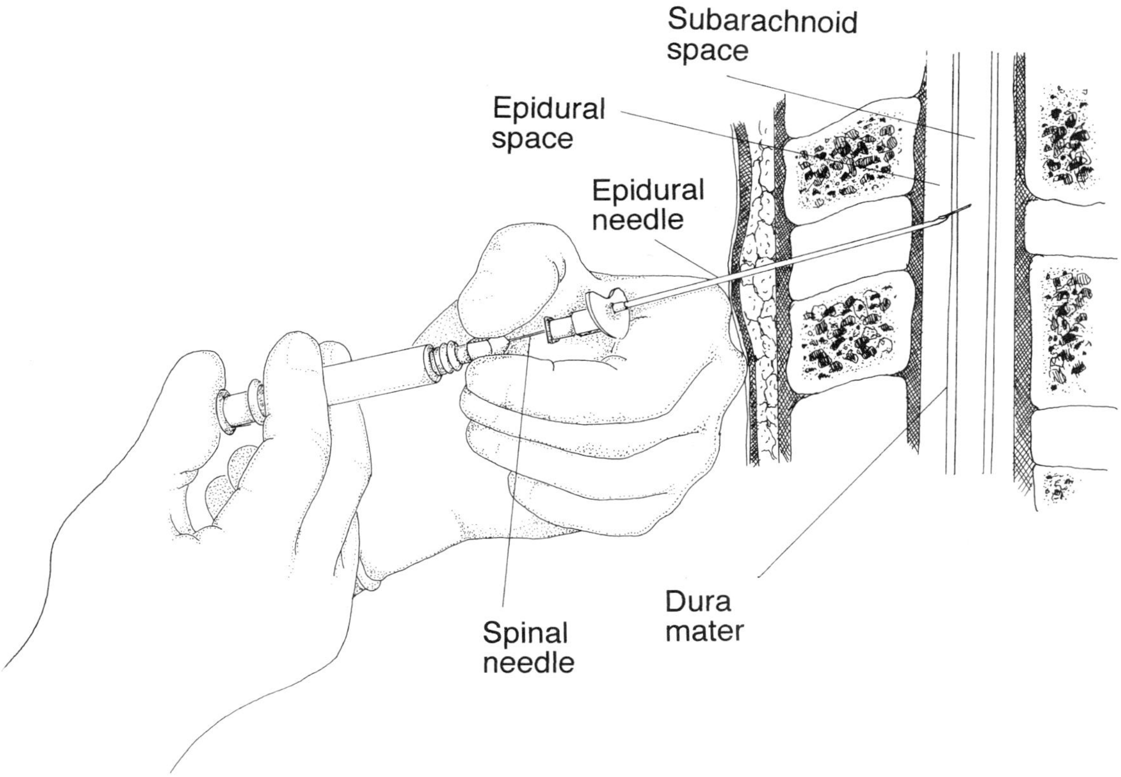

Fig. 35.11 This figure shows the importance of steadying the spinal needle in position after being introduced through the Tuohy needle. Note that one hand stays in contact with the skin on the back and the other steadies the syringe attached to the spinal needle.

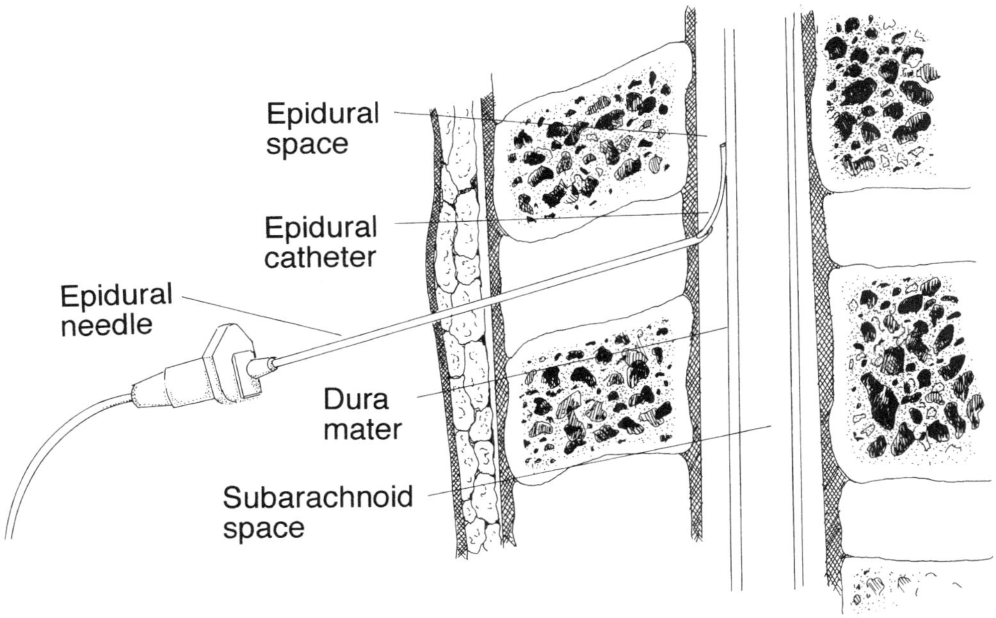

Fig. 35.12 The spinal needle is withdrawn after local anesthetic is injected through it. A catheter is now introduced into the epidural space through the Tuohy needle.

spinal needle locks into the hub of Tuohy needle. After withdrawing the spinal needle a catheter is introduced about 4 cm into the epidural space through the Tuohy needle (Fig. 35.12). Epidural catheter position is confirmed by aspiration for blood or CSF. This is followed by injection of about 1 ml of saline into the epidural catheter to test its patency. The catheter is secured firmly by tape and is now available for use during or after surgery.

SEQUENTIAL CSE TECHNIQUE FOR CESAREAN DELIVERY

Precipitous maternal hypotension remains one of the commonest problems associated with spinal anesthesia for cesarean delivery. Despite acute i.v. hydration, elastic support stockings and lateral tilt of the uterus, it may be difficult to maintain normal blood pressure. Prophylactic vasopressors are used by many. However, these drugs may have undesirable maternal and fetal effects.[8–10] Maternal hypotension may lead to maternal nausea and discomfort and may also be detrimental to the newborn. To reduce the incidence and severity of hypotension a sequential CSE technique has been described.[22,23] This technique is quite similar to that described above, the main differences are (a) the block is performed with the patient in the sitting position, (b) the dose of spinal hyperbaric bupivacaine is intentionally kept low (1.5–1.7 ml of 0.5% bupivacaine in 8% dextrose or glucose) because the aim is to achieve an S5 to T8–9 block, (c) patient is then placed supine with a left lateral tilt and (d) when the spinal anesthetic is 'fixed' (about 15 min) it is extended to T4 by injecting plain bupivacaine into the epidural catheter (1.5–2 ml for every unblocked segment) (Fig. 35.13).

Although this sequential technique will take somewhat longer than standard CSE technique it has been shown to reduce the frequency and severity of maternal hypotension when compared with the epidural technique.[23] Compared with the spinal technique the onset of maternal hypotension after CSE block is less precipitous.[28] Decreased frequency and severity of hypotension are presumably caused by less extensive sympathetic block from the low spinal anesthetic combined with the slower onset of epidural block, which allows more time for compensatory mechanisms to be effective. The sequential technique may be particularly advantageous in the high-risk parturient.

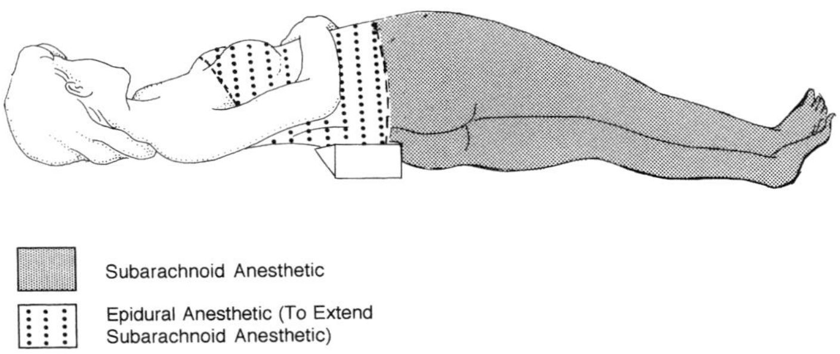

Fig. 35.13 Sequential CSE anesthesia. The figure shows the level of analgesia produced by the spinal anesthetic and extension of the block by injection of titrated doses of local anesthetic into the epidural catheter.

By positioning of the patient prior to induction of spinal anesthesia and by allowing titration with incremental epidural doses to the precise level of anesthesia desired, the CSE technique may enhance the safety of regional anesthesia for cesarean delivery.

It is emphasized that the peri-operative management of patients undergoing cesarean delivery under regional anesthesia is similar whether the block is epidural, spinal or CSE. This includes acute i.v. fluid administration, patient positioning with lateral tilt, use of elastic support stockings, frequent monitoring of blood pressure and aggressive management of maternal hypotension with vasopressor such as ephedrine.

INDICATIONS FOR CSE TECHNIQUE

CSE technique has been used for various kinds of surgery including cesarean delivery,[17,19,20,23,29] management of labor pain[30] and post-operative pain[31] (Table 35.9). It has also been used as a research tool for controlled comparison between epidural and spinal techniques. In one double-blind study epidural steroid was compared with subarachnoid midazolam for treatment of chronic low back pain.[32] The technique has been used successfully in all age groups including children above the age of 8 years (A van Steenberge, personal communication).

Although considerable literature is available and it is increasing, there is a general lack of controlled studies. The two main indications for CSE are cesarean delivery and major orthopedic surgery. In one controlled study CSE block was compared with epidural anesthesia for cesarean delivery. All patients receiving CSE block had good to excellent analgesia, whereas only 74% receiving epidural block had similar pain relief (Table 35.10). This was reflected in the requirement for additional analgesics, sedatives, or nitrous oxide–oxygen anesthesia. The muscular relaxation was also better following CSE block. The total dose of bupivacaine for a T4 block was three times higher in patients receiving only epidural anesthesia. The maternal and fetal blood bupivacaine levels were correspondingly about three times higher in the epidural group (Table 35.11). In addition, the incidence of maternal hypotension was higher in patients receiving

Table 35.9 Reported indications for the CSE technique

Orthopedic surgery (major hip and knee surgery)
Obstetrics (cesarean delivery, labor pain)
Vascular surgery*
Urologic surgery*
Gynecologic surgery*
Research tool for controlled comparison between epidural and subarachnoid techniques

* CSE block alone or in combination with light general anesthesia.

Table 35.10 Surgical analgesia following CSE and epidural block (patient, nurse anesthetist and surgeon assessment) (From ref. 23 with permission)

	CSE anesthesia Group A		Epidural anesthesia Group B	
Surgical anesthesia	Number of patients	Percentage	Number of patients	Percentage
Excellent	13	87	10	67
Good	2	13	1	7
Fair	0	–	2	13
Poor	0	–	2*	13

Table 35.11 Total dose and maternal and fetal blood levels of bupivacaine (From ref. 23 with permission)

Bupivacaine	CSE anesthesia Group A Mean ± SEM	Epidural anesthesia Group B Mean ± SEM	Statistical significance
Total dose of bupivacaine (mg)	40.2 ± 4.24*	125.0 ± 2.67	$P < 0.001$
Maternal blood concentration (ng/g)	205.3 ± 33.6	604.9 ± 51.2	$P < 0.001$
Fetal blood concentration (ng/g)	45.8 ± 8.5	186.0 ± 20.3	$P < 0.001$

* Mean total dose of 8 mg for spinal anesthesia in addition to mean total dose of 32.0 mg for epidural anesthesia.

epidural anesthesia. Apgar scores, blood gases and neurobehavioral evaluation did not show any differences between the two groups of neonates. The investigators demonstrated that CSE block was superior to epidural block for cesarean delivery and concluded that CSE block combined the reliability of spinal block and the flexibility of epidural anesthesia while minimizing their drawbacks.[23] In another controlled study epidural, spinal and CSE techniques were compared in patients undergoing major orthopedic surgery. The authors demonstrated that the analgesia and surgical conditions provided by the spinal and CSE blocks were similar and were superior to those provided by epidural anesthesia.[29] In this study the authors also demonstrated that post-operative analgesia following 0.2 and 0.4 mg of subarachnoid morphine was similar to that provided by 4 mg of epidural morphine.

RISK OF CATHETER PENETRATION THROUGH DURAL HOLE

Epidural catheter migration into the subarachnoid space is potentially very serious because failure to recognize misplacement of catheter and injection of usual epidural dose would result in total spinal anesthesia. Although CSE block has been performed in tens of thousands of patients in Europe in the last decade, there are no published reports of epidural catheter penetration through the dural hole or any other serious complications.[33] At our hospital, the CSE technique was introduced for cesarean delivery in 1984, it is now routinely used for major orthopedic (hip and knee replacement) surgery and for cesarean delivery. During 1992, CSE was used in almost 500 patients. We have not seen any epidural catheter migration or any other major complication in over 2500 patients. However, at the time of performing CSE block we have seen two cases of epidural catheter penetration into subarachnoid space; dural damage by the Tuohy needle could not be ruled out in either case. In both cases malposition of the epidural catheter was easily identified by aspiration test. Similarly, at another Swedish hospital no late catheter migration has been seen in about 4500 CSE blocks during a 10-year period (S Lindén, Uddevalla Hospital, personal communication). Thus catheter penetration into blood vessels or subarachnoid space usually occurs during the initiation of the block procedure.

Our experimental studies on isolated human dura showed that it is impossible to force an 18-gauge Portex epidural catheter through dural holes made by 26- or 27-gauge spinal needles. Also, it is quite difficult to force the catheter through holes made by spinal needles of 22- to 25-gauge diameter. 22-gauge or larger diameter spinal needles made holes large enough to permit passage of the catheter.[23] These results were confirmed by our epiduroscopic studies with video recording in fresh cadavers. In these studies epidural catheters were directed to single and multiple holes made by 25-G spinal needles and single holes made by 18-G Tuohy needles. It was impossible to force 16-or 18-G epidural catheters through dural holes made by a single dural puncture with a 25-G spinal needle. Even when five holes were made in the same area of the dura by a 25-G spinal needle epidural catheter penetration into subarachnoid space occurred in only 1 out of 20 recordings (5%). After intentional dural puncture with a Tuohy needle, epidural catheter penetration into subarachnoid space occurred in 45% of cases.[34] Nevertheless, it is emphasized that there are several reports in the literature of spontaneous catheter migration in patients who received epidural catheters.[35,36] Epidural catheters that have functioned normally at previous injection have been documented to erode into the subarachnoid space[37,38] or into epidural blood vessels.[39,40] Clearly, the risk of catheter migration can be expected to be greater if there is a hole in the dura. With routine epidural technique, Ready and Wild[41] have reported three catheter migrations in 12 000 doses of epidural opioids; all were easily detected by using an aspiration test. It is therefore important that the routine for 'top-up' doses via the epidural catheter should be clearly defined at all institutions where the CSE technique is practiced. However, the routine is not different from that for standard epidural technique and consists of confirmation of the catheter position by aspiration as well as frequent assessment of the block following injection of fractionated doses of local anesthetics. Every reinjection should be considered a test dose. Clearly, the CSE technique is not for the novice.

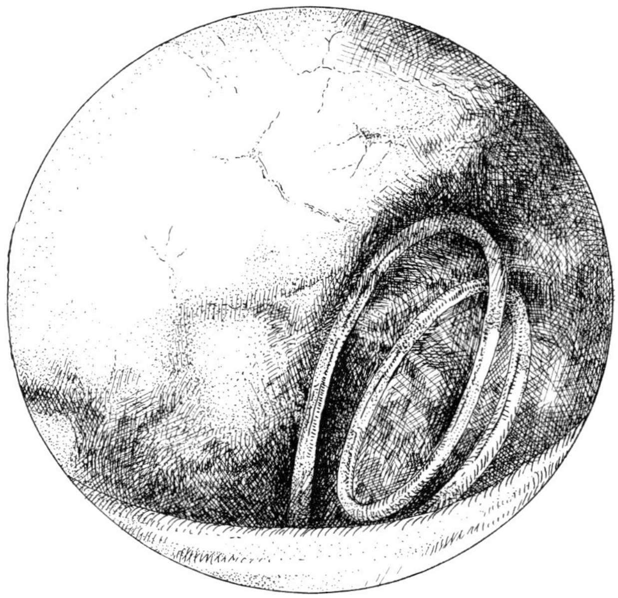

Fig. 35.14 Looping of catheter in the epidural space (epiduroscopy recording).

SEQUENCE OF DURAL PUNCTURE AND EPIDURAL CATHETER PLACEMENT (Epidural catheter before or after spinal anesthetic)

Occasionally it may be difficult to thread a catheter into the epidural space after injecting local anesthetic into the spinal needle. This could be a problem with the 'needle-through-needle' method. If some minutes are spent in replacing the epidural needle, the spinal block may become 'fixed' in the dependent area. If difficulty is experienced, catheter insertion should be abandoned or attempted after surgery. However, problems with catheter insertion through a properly positioned Tuohy needle are quite unusual. There is also the rare risk of spinal anesthetic obscuring paresthesia during epidural catheter insertion. Further, it may be difficult to verify the position of the epidural catheter. These problems can be overcome if the epidural catheter is introduced prior to the spinal anesthetic. This can be accomplished by the separate spaces technique described by Brownridge or by one of the single-segment needles described above. However, prior placement of epidural catheter has its own problems:

1. Epidural test dose makes verification of spinal block difficult.
2. A portion of epidural test dose may appear in the hub of spinal needle and create confusion.
3. The final direction of epidural catheter is unpredictable. Radiologic and video epiduroscopic studies have shown that epidural catheters may take unpredictable paths[34,37,39] (Fig. 35.14); a catheter may even tie itself in a knot.[42] Epidural catheter may divert the spinal needle or be perforated by it.
4. Since epidural catheter migration can occur over time only a recent test dose holds significance. An epidural test dose prior to subarachnoid anesthesia is of little use if the epidural catheter is to be activated after surgery.

Thus it would appear that either sequence has its advantages and disadvantages. However, the literature shows that the experienced anesthesiologist can perform both procedures safely using basic and well-accepted principles of regional anesthesia practice. As mentioned earlier, the 'needle-through-needle' technique has been used in thousands of patients without any serious complications.

EXTENSION OF SPINAL ANESTHETIC BY EPIDURAL INJECTION OF LOCAL ANESTHETIC

The difficulty in controlling the upper level of spinal anesthesia and the consequent fear of inadequate analgesia appears to have prompted the use of relatively large doses of local anesthetic for cesarean delivery. With the CSE technique the presence of an epidural catheter permits the anesthesiologist to use smaller doses for spinal anesthesia, thereby decreasing the incidence and severity of maternal hypotension. Doses of subarachnoid bupivacaine in the range of 7.5–10 mg have been shown to provide effective analgesia for most patients undergoing cesarean delivery.[15,23,43] These doses are considerably less than those reported by others.[5,44] However, in some patients additional doses of epidural local anesthetic will be necessary to extend the spinal anesthetic.[15,23]

It is unclear how relatively small doses of epidural local anesthetic can rapidly elevate the level of spinal anesthesia. The following hypotheses have been proposed:

1. leakage of epidural local anesthetic through the dural hole into the subarachnoid space;
2. continuing spread of initial subarachnoid block (unrelated to epidural injection);
3. existence of 'subclinical' analgesia at a higher level which is enhanced and becomes evident by perineural or transdural spread of epidural local anesthetic;[45]
4. compression of the subarachnoid space by the presence of the epidural catheter and by the volume of local anesthetic, resulting in a compression of the subarachnoid space and more extensive spread of local anesthetic.[23,24,46,47]

Although leakage of epidural local anesthetic into the subarachnoid space is theoretically possible, the rapidity with which extension occurs suggests some other mechanism. Furthermore, our knowledge of pressures within the epidural and subarachnoid spaces and of the role of CSF leakage in postdural puncture headache suggests that the flow of fluids is more likely to be away from the subarachnoid space rather than towards it.

The main reason for the rapid extension of subarachnoid block by epidural local anesthetics appears to be related to increased volume within the epidural space, causing a decrease in CSF volume and a cephalad shift of local anesthetic within CSF. This was demonstrated in a recent controlled study. The authors divided patients undergoing cesarean delivery into three groups: one group received 10 ml of saline epidurally, another group 10 ml of bupivacaine and the third group did not receive anything in the epidural space. A rapid progression of subarachnoid block was noted in patients receiving saline or bupivacaine, suggesting that the enhancement of subarachnoid block was due to the volume, not the nature, of injectate.[24] it should be emphasized that the extension of subarachnoid anesthesia is possible only until the block is 'fixed'; after that the influence of epidural injection on subarachnoid block is unclear. These data are consistent with the general belief that alterations in the contents of the spinal canal can influence the spread of local anesthetic. For example, in the later stages of pregnancy increased epidural vertebral venous volume leads to a reciprocal decrease in CSF volume in the distal subarachnoid space. This is believed to be one of the main reasons for the decreased requirement of local anesthetic for spinal anesthesia.[47–49] It has been demonstrated that the spread of local anesthetic in the subarachnoid space of pregnant and nonpregnant patients is more rapid following inferior vena caval compression and subsequent vertebral venous engorgement.[24,48,50] It has been shown that a bolus injection of 10 ml of local anesthetic in the epidural space transiently increased CSF pressure by 12 mmHg.[51]

CSE VERSUS CONTINUOUS SPINAL TECHNIQUE

The recent increased popularity of the continuous spinal technique is mainly a result of improved spinal needle and catheter technology and also data suggesting that the risk of PDPH is not as high as might be expected.[52] The potential risk of meningitis appears to be unfounded, especially when the technique is used during peri- and post-operative periods. However, the low risk of PDPH may be valid only for elderly patients.[53–55] It is well recognized that the incidence of PDPH decreases with age; it is also well accepted that the obstetric patient is particularly susceptible – the risk of PDPH following continuous spinal technique for cesarean delivery may be considerable.[12,55,56] The introduction of newer small-gauge catheters was expected to address this problem. However technical problems such as the inability to thread the catheter, the inability to aspirate CSF, catheter kinking and breakage have been encountered with 32-G 'microspinal' catheters.[55,57] It should be noted that inability to thread the catheter for continuous spinal anesthesia may occur in 5–15% of insertions. The reason is unclear but it is not catheter size because it occurs with all catheters.[55] The most serious setback for continuous spinal technique is related to several reported cases of the the cauda equina syndrome (perineal sensory loss and changes in sensory function).[58,59] The probable cause appears to be high local concentrations of drug in a restricted area. The risk of this complication may be higher in patients who undergo surgery in the lithotomy position. Positional stretching of the cauda equina may contribute to enhanced and selective vulnerability of nerve fibers to high concentration hyperbaric local anesthetic solutions. In a recent study, transient neurologic impairment was noted in four patients following bolus injection of hyperbaric 5% lidocaine into the subarachnoid space for surgery performed in the lithotomy position.[60] The cauda equina nerves do not have protective epineural sheaths and are, therefore, more likely to be damaged by large volumes of high-concentration local anesthetics. This is similar to the neurotoxicity that can occur if large volumes of chloroprocaine with sodium bisulfite (preservative) intended for epidural space are administered into the subarachnoid space.[61,62] The same is true if butorphanol or large doses of sufentanil intended for epidural administration are injected into the CSF.[63] The mechanism for these neural injuries is similar, i.e. too much drug injected into the wrong place.[55] These data also illustrate the efficacy of the dura mater as a remarkable barrier to the harmful effects of drugs.[63] These factors have raised doubts about the use of the continuous spinal technique. In contrast, the epidural catheter technique has been safely used for decades. Although no controlled comparisons have been made, current evidence suggests that the CSE technique is safer than the continuous spinal technique, particularly in patients undergoing cesarean delivery.

CSE AND DECREASED RISK OF POST-DURAL PUNCTURE HEADACHE (PDPH)

A high incidence of PDPH remains a major concern in the parturient; this may be as high as 10–15% even when 25- or 26-gauge spinal needles are used.[64,65] It is an important cause of post-operative morbidity. There are no data from controlled studies regarding the frequency of post-dural puncture headache associated with the CSE technique. However, several workers have commented on the very low incidence or lack of PDPH following CSE block (Table 35.12). Dennison[43] reported only two spinal headaches in 400 patients who received CSE for cesarean delivery. In another report based on experience with 300 cesarean deliveries, Kumar[15] reported two cases of mild headache; in both cases multiple dural punctures were attempted because of technical difficulties. Interestingly, in one CSE study in which the single-space 'needle-through-needle' technique was compared with the separate-spaces technique, only one PDPH was noted; this occurred in a patient in the separate-spaces group.[67] These reports suggest that the risk of PDPH in parturients, particularly if subarachnoid or epidural opioids are used as part of the technique, is very low (below 1%) or nonexistent. This is noteworthy because the risk of PDPH is considerably higher in this group of patients even when fine pencilpoint needles are used.[55] The possible reasons for this may be:

1. The Tuohy needle in the epidural space serves as an introducer and allows a meticulous puncture of the dura. Multiple attempts at identifying the subarachnoid space are thus avoided.
2. The technique allows the use of very fine-diameter spinal needles.
3. The risk of CSF leakage through the dura is decreased because of the increased pressure in the epidural space that results from the presence of an epidural catheter and from administration of epidural local anesthetics and opioids.
4. Epidural or subarachnoid opioids may have a prophylactic effect against post-dural puncture headache. This is controversial. Reports claiming[68,69] and denying[70] the prophylactic effects of spinal opioids have been published.

TECHNICAL ASPECTS OF CSE TECHNIQUE

In one study of cesarean deliveries, the technical aspects of 'needle-through-needle' versus double-space technique were compared. A high technical failure rate (13%) was noted with the former technique. This was mainly because of difficulty in establishing the subarachnoid anesthetic.[67] No other study has reported such high technical failure rates. Indeed, the spinal anesthetic is easier to perform because the Tuohy needle serves as an introducer. Since this 'introducer' needle is in the epidural space the spinal needle has only to penetrate the dura. A majority of anesthesiologists perform CSE blocks using long spinal needles (11–12 cm) of varying diameters that are introduced through 16- or 18-G regular Tuohy needles. As mentioned earlier, there is a risk of spinal needle displacement at the time of syringe connection, aspiration of CSF or injection of local anesthetic. Special devices to fix the spinal needle in place while it is in the Tuohy needle have been described.[2,7] The use of special kits and matching needles with locking mechanisms can be expected to improve the success rate. Thus, in a recent study of 150 cesarean deliveries, the failure rate with Portex CSE needles was 0.67%.[66] This is considerably lower than the failure rate for spinal anesthesia reported in recent literature.[72,73] Commenting on the technical aspects of CSE the authors concluded that the combined technique was readily learned by both senior and trainee anesthesiologists, with a high percentage of technically perfect blocks

Table 35.12 Incidence of PDPH following CSE block

Surgery	No. of patients	PDPH (%)	Spinal needle (G)	Reference
Cesarean delivery	130	0	29	5
Cesarean delivery	100	0	26	23
Cesarean delivery	200	0	26	18*
Cesarean delivery	400	0.5	–	43
Cesarean delivery	150	1.3	26	66
Cesarean delivery	100	1	26	67*
Orthopedic surgery	800	0	–	Lindén†
Cesarean delivery	300	0.7	26	15
Labor and delivery	62	4.5	26	30

* Spinal and epidural anesthetics performed at two lumbar interspaces.
† Unpublished observations.

and a low incidence of postdural puncture headache.[66] It has been commented by some that combining spinal and epidural blocks appears cumbersome. However, in experienced hands the entire procedure takes less than 4–5 min.[26,29] In one Belgian hospital about 6000 sequential CSE blocks have been performed for vaginal and cesarean deliveries; the success rate has been 99.5% (A van Steenberge, personal communication).

SPECIAL CSE SETS

In recent years several modifications of the CSE technique or needle design have been reported. Disposable CSE sets have been commercially available since 1986. At present there are at least 12 medical companies that distribute special CSE kits. One of the manufacturers (B. Braun, Melsungen AG) has modified the epidural and spinal needles to reduce the risk of catheter penetration through the dura (Fig. 35.15a) A hole at the epidural needle curve near its bevel permits the passage of the spinal needle (Fig. 35.15b). The point of dural contact by the epidural catheter is thus at some distance from the dural hole (Fig. 35.15c). A very recent innovation has been a spinal needle with a plastic sleeve (Espocan) to eliminate the risk of metal particles being shaved off the internal bore of the epidural needle (Fig. 35.15d). The tip of the spinal needle does not contact the internal wall of the epidural needle. The Portex and B-D spinal needles are pencilpoint (Figs 35.16a and b and 35.17a and b). In the technical modification described by Eldor and Olshwang a fine spinal needle is introduced alongside the outer wall of the epidural needle after a Tuohy needle is placed in the epidural space.[27] These workers have modified their needle further by brazing it with silver alloy[74] (Fig. 35.18). The needle also allows the CSE block to be performed in reverse order (i.e. the spinal block is performed after the epidural catheter is in place). An almost identical needle is the 'T-A-pair' needle, which consists of an 18-gauge epidural and a 22-gauge spinal needle welded together.

A

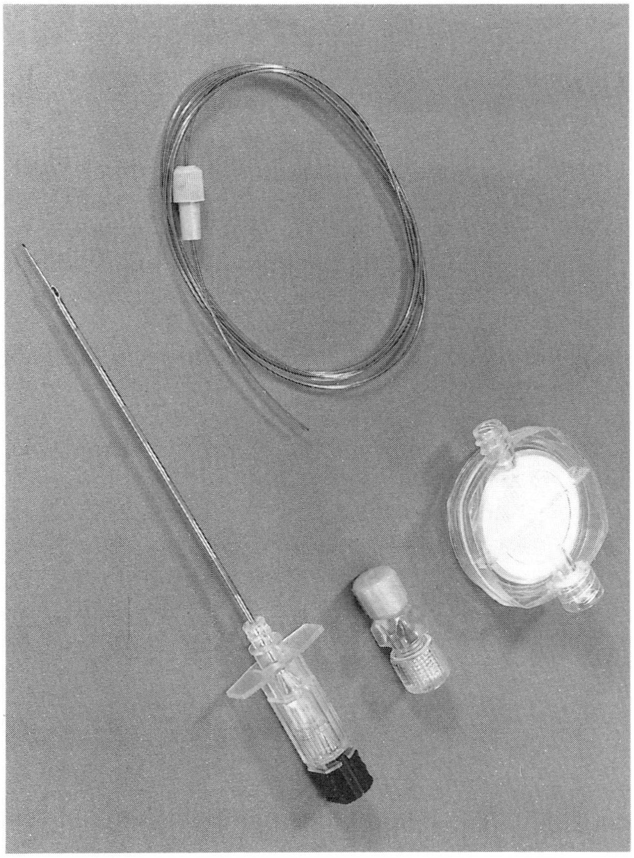

B

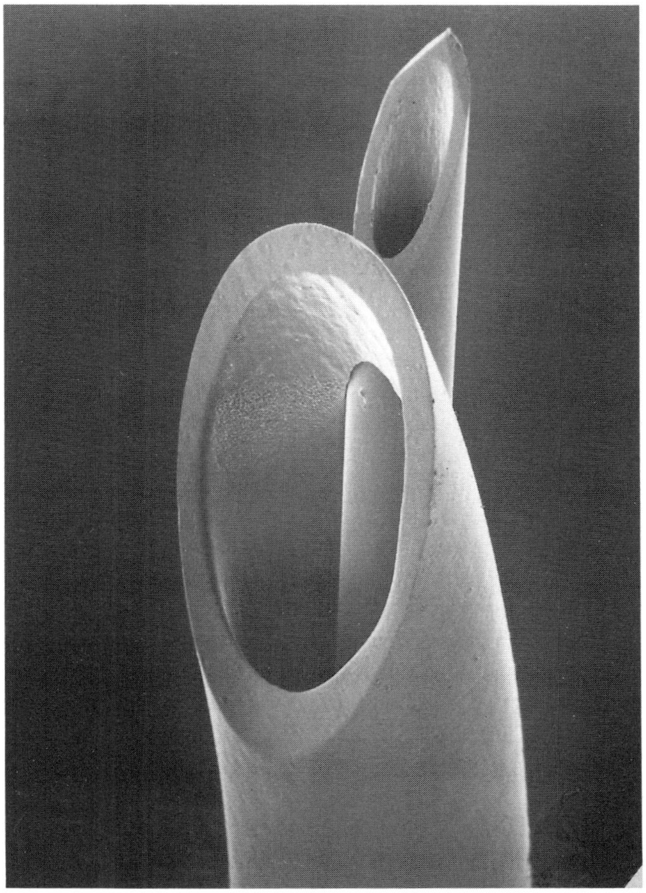

Fig. 35.15 (a) The Braun Espocan system for CSE block. (b) A hole at the epidural needle curve near its bevel permits the passage of a special spinal needle. (c) The epidural catheter passes through the regular bevel of the epidural needle. The point of dural contact by the catheter is at some distance from the dural hole. (d) Espocan spinal needle with a plastic sleeve to eliminate the risk from metal particles. The tip of the spinal needle does not come into contact with internal wall of the epidural needle.

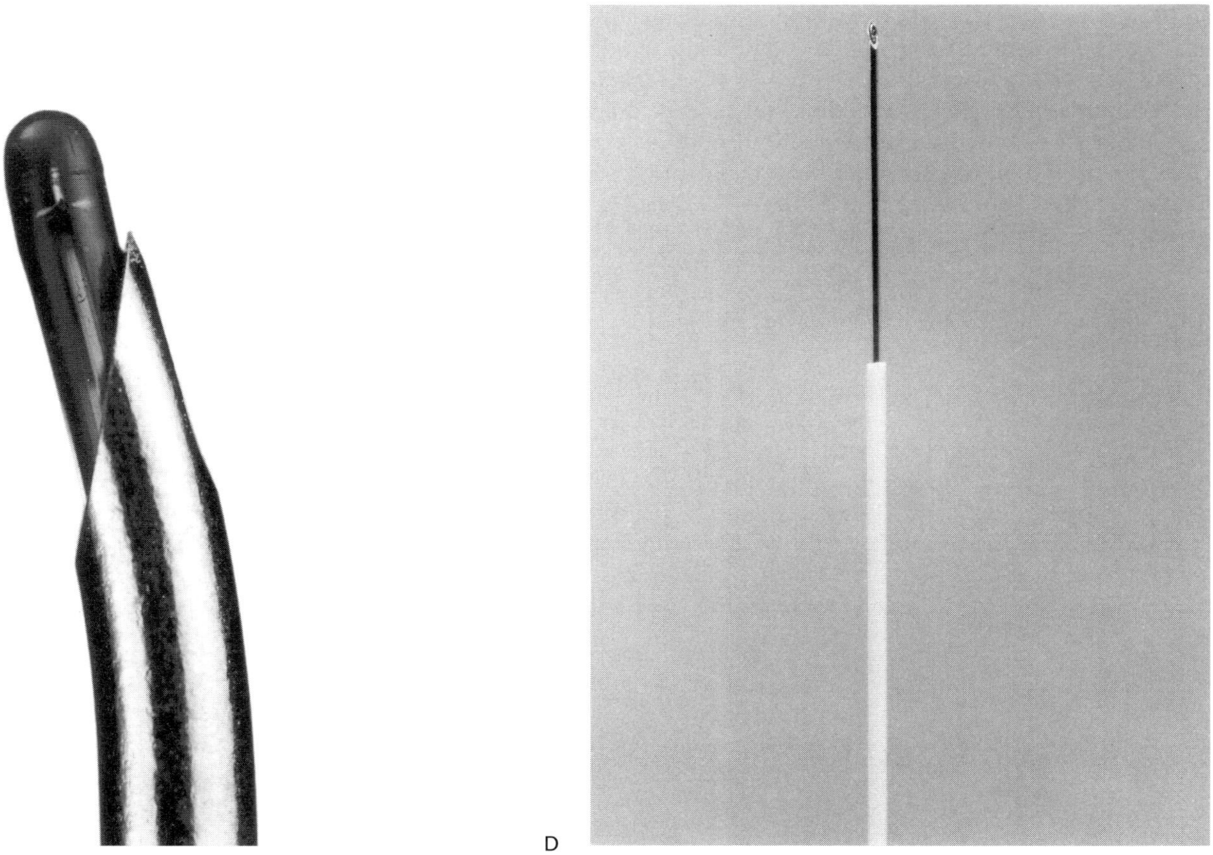

C D

Fig. 35.15 *(contd)*

The distal ends of the needles make a common tip. The epidural needle points cephalad and permits the passage of a 20-guage epidural catheter, while the bevel of the spinal needle points caudad and allows the passage of a 26-gauge or finer spinal needle.[26] The recently introduced E-SP needle (the only FDA-approved CSE device so far) (Fig. 35.19) is conceptually similar to the Eldor and T-A pair needles, the main difference being that the needle wall configuration is 'over–under' rather than parallel. With this device, it is possible to introduce the epidural catheter prior to the spinal anesthetic. The different trajectories of spinal needle and epidural catheter in some of the newer CSE kits can be expected to reduce the risk of catheter migration because the dural puncture is physically separated from the Tuohy needle tip.

Since the tip of the spinal needle may scrape against the inner wall of Tuohy needle, concern has been expressed about possible metal particles in epidural or subarachnoid space[75]. However, there is no report of any neurologic problem in any of the thousands of patients who have received CSE block by such needles. Indeed, such needles are still used for the majority of CSE blocks performed worldwide. The risk of damage to the bevel of spinal needle can be eliminated by the Braun Espocan system, which contains a spinal needle with a plastic sleeve that keeps it centrally in the epidural needle and guides it through the hole in the curve of the epidural needle tip. The spinal needle enters this hole easily and can be introduced into the dura without coming in contact with the internal wall of the epidural needle (Fig. 35.12). Some special CSE sets have locking hubs. However, with a locking mechanism the length of the spinal needle that protrudes from the tip of Tuohy needle is fixed; this may be a problem in some patients since the distance from skin to subarachnoid space is not constant. Too short a protrusion may lead to failure to puncture the dura. A protrusion of the needle tip of 8–12 mm is generally considered appropriate. None of these recently introduced special CSE needles have undergone extensive clinical testing so far.

SUMMARY

Although epidural and spinal anesthetics are well-accepted regional techniques in obstetrics they have several disadvantages. Combined spinal epidural technique reduces or eliminates these disadvantages. CSE block combines the rapidity, density and reliability of spinal anesthesia with the flexibility of continuous epidural analgesia/anesthesia to extend the duration of analgesia. It

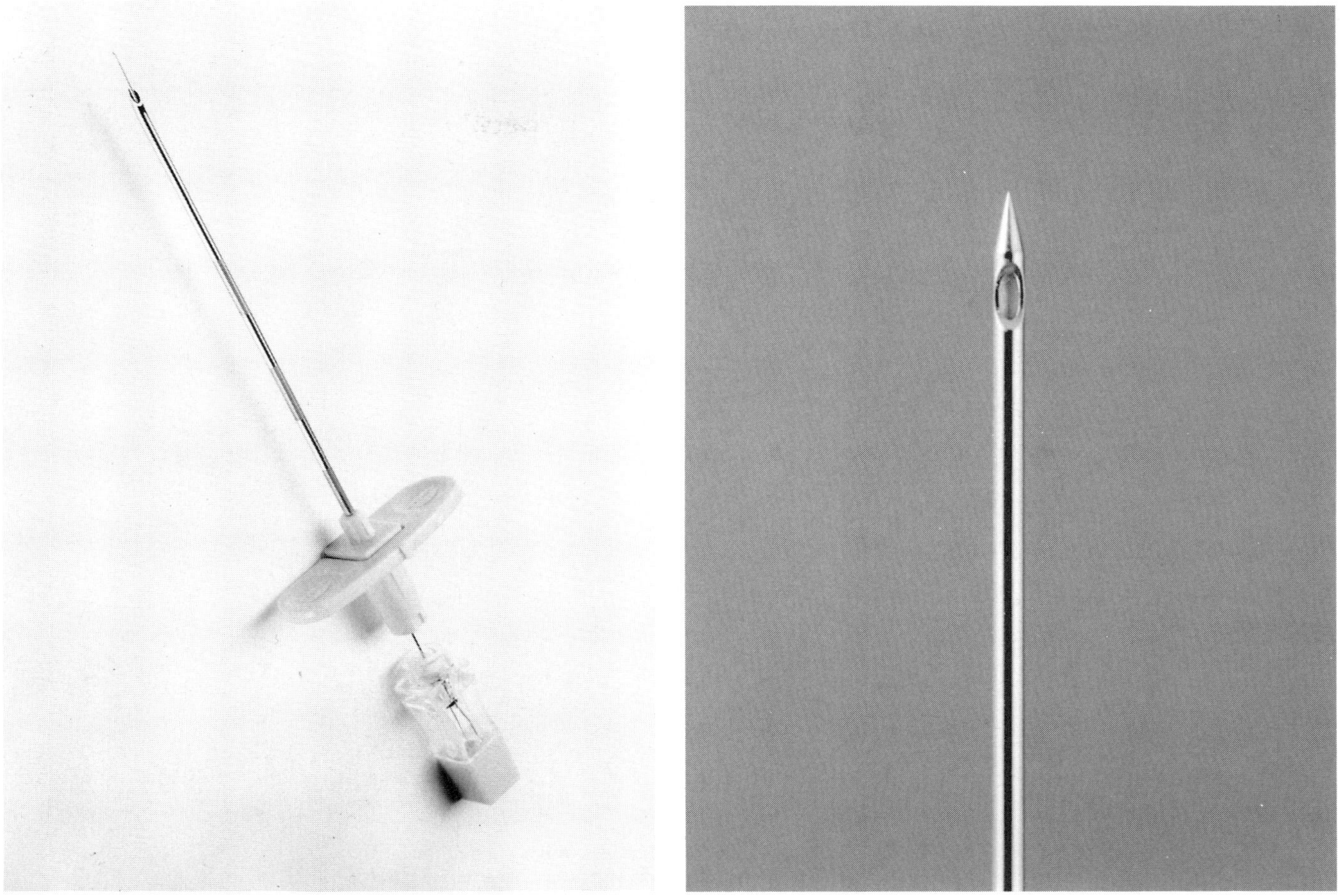

A B

Fig. 35.16 (a) The Portex CSE system. (b) The Portex spinal needle is pencilpoint.

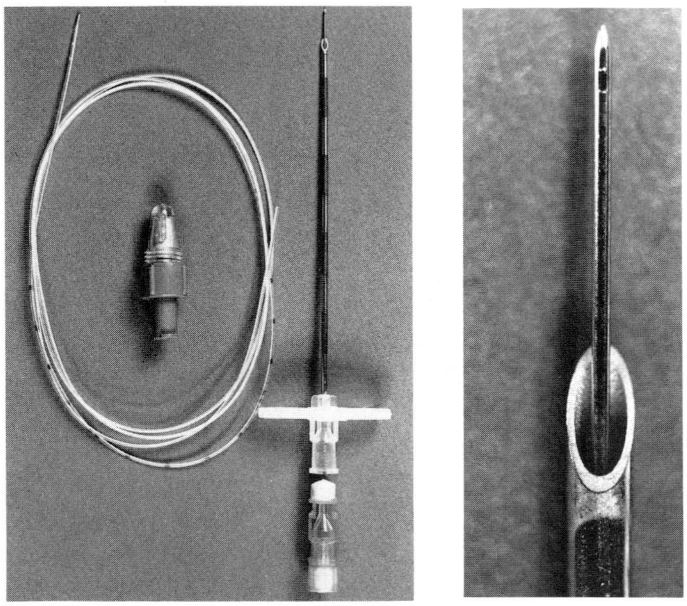

A B

Fig. 35.17 (a) The B-D CSE needle. (b) It is similar to the Portex CSE needle. The spinal needle is pencilpoint.

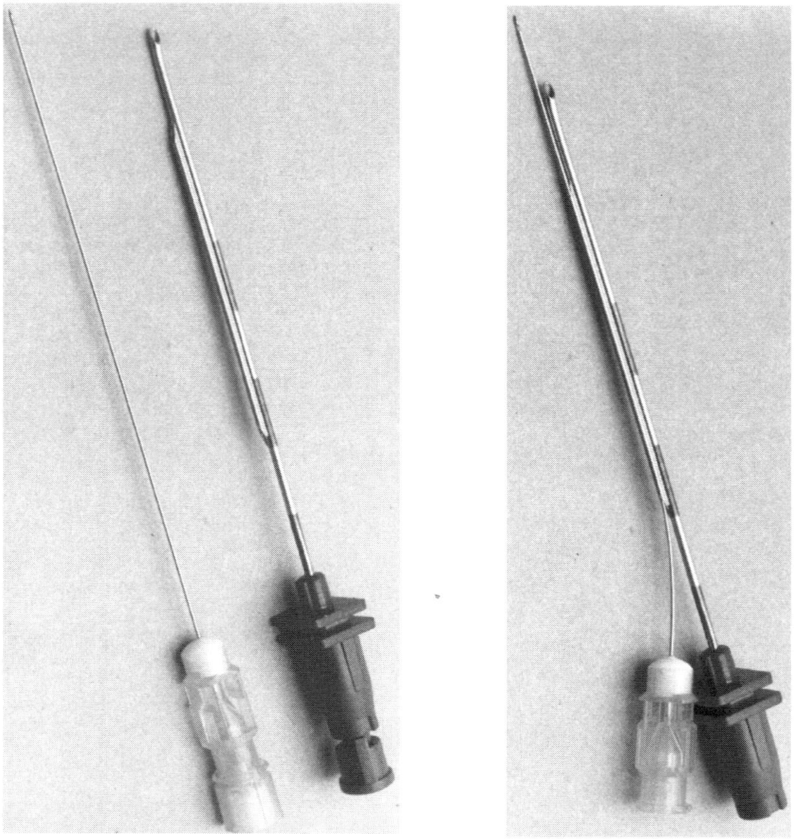

Fig. 35.18 Eldor needle. This is a double-lumen needle with separate lumens for spinal needle and epidural catheter. The epidural catheter can be introduced before initiation of spinal anesthesia.

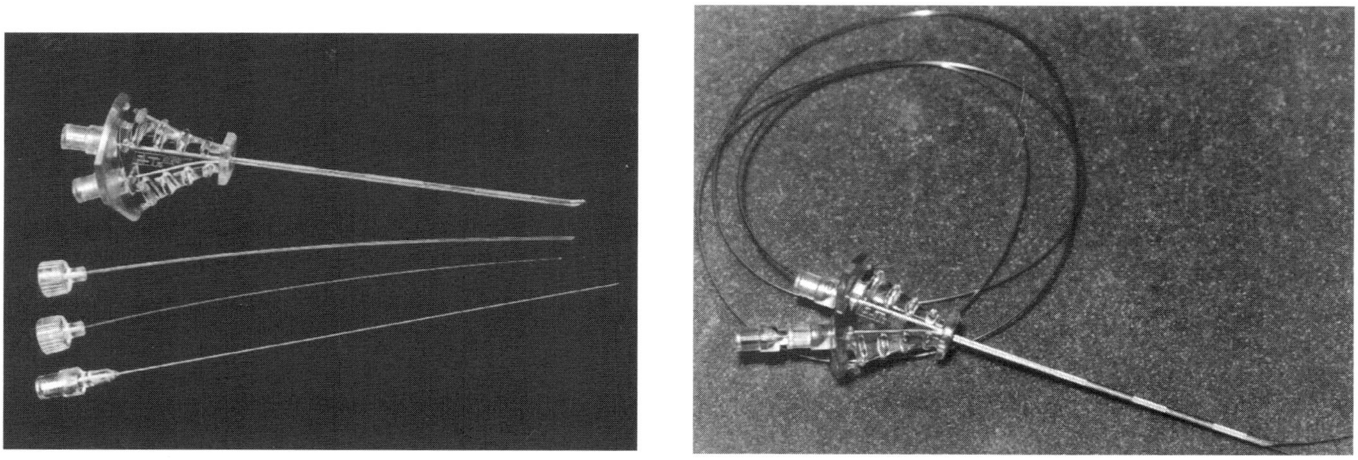

Fig. 35.19 The E-SP needle. Another dual cannula design. This needle also has separate lumens for the spinal needle and epidural catheter. It permits the introduction of the epidural catheter prior to spinal block.

has been used in thousands of patients without any reports of major problems. Catheter penetration through the dural hole though unlikely is not impossible. Before any injection via the epidural catheter, its position should always be confirmed by an aspiration test. The technique should be used only by those who are experienced in spinal and epidural blocks. CSE is an important addition to the armamentarium of the obstetric anesthesiologist.

ACKNOWLEDGEMENT

The author wishes to thank Ing-Marie Dimgren for excellent secretarial help.

REFERENCES

1. Lewis M, Thomas P, Wilkes R G 1983 Hypotension during epidural analgesia for cesarean. Anaesthesia 38: 250
2. Nikalls R W D, Dennison B 1984 A modification of the combined spinal and epidural technique. Anaesthesia 1984; 39: 935
3. Kileff M E, James F M, Dewan D M et al 1984 Neonatal neurobehavioral responses after epidural anesthesia for cesarean section using lidocaine and bupivacaine. Anesth Analg 63: 413
4. Thorburn J, Moir D D1984 Bupivacaine toxicity in association with extra-dural analgesia for cesarean section. Br J Anaesth 56: 551
5. Carrie L E S 1990 Extradural spinal or combined spinal block for obstetric surgical anaesthesia. Br J Anaesth 65: 225–233
6. Larsen J V 1982 Obstetric analgesia and anaesthesia. Clin Obstet Gynaecol 9: 685
7. Morgen B M, Aulakh J M, Barker J P et al 1983 Anesthesia for cesarean section. Br J Anaesth 55: 885
8. Clark R B, Thompson D S, Thompson C H 1976 Prevention of spinal hypotension associated with cesarean section. Anesthesiology 45: 670
9. Datta S, Alper M H 1980 Anesthesia for cesarean section. Anesthesiology 53: 142
10. Lussos S A, Datta S 1992 Anesthesia for cesarean delivery. I. General considerations and spinal anesthesia. Int J Obstet Anesth 1: 79–91
11. Cousins M J, Bridenbaugh P O (eds) 1988 Neural blockade. J B Lippincott, Philadelphia, p 629
12. Carrie L E S 1992 The combined epidural and spinal technique. The technique of the future. Third joint ESRA–ASRA Congress (abstracts) Van Zundert A (ed). Aristos Philis, Limassol, pp 324–330
13. Raj P P, Pai U, Rawal N 1991 Techniques of regional anesthesia in adults. In: Raj P (ed) Clinical practice of regional anesthesia. Churchill Livingstone, New York, pp 271–364
14. Vandermeersch E, Kick O, Möllman M, de Gouw N, van Aken H 1991 KSE–die Kombination aus Spinaler und Epiduraler Anaesthesie. Reg Anaesth 14: 108–112
15. Kumar C 1987 Combined subarachnoid and epidural block for cesarean section. Can J Anaesth 34: 329–30
16. Soresi A L 1937 Episubdural anesthesia. Anesth Analg 16: 306–310
17. Curelaru I 1979 Long duration subarachnoid anaesthesia with continuous epidural block. Prakt Anästh 14: 71–78
18. Brownridge P 1981 Epidural and subarachnoid analgesia for elective cesarean section. Anaesthesia 36: 70
19. Coates M 1982 Combined subarachnoid and epidural techniques. A single space technique for surgery of the hip and lower limb. Anaesthesia 37: 89
20. Mumtaz M H, Daz M, Kuz M 1982 Combined subarachnoid and epidural techniques. Anaesthesia 37: 90
21. Carrie L E S, O'Sullivan G 1984 Subarachnoid bupivacaine 0.5% for cesarean section. Eur J Anaesth 1: 275–283
22. Rawal N 1986 Single segment combined spinal epidural block for cesarean section. Can Anaesth Soc J 33: 254–255
23. Rawal N, Schollin J, Wesström G 1988 Epidural versus combined spinal epidural block for Caesarean section. Acta Anaesthesiol Scand 32: 61–66
24. Blumgart C H, Ryall D, Dennison B, Thompson-Hill L M 1992 Mechanism of extension of spinal anaesthesia by extradural injection of local anaesthetic. Br J Anaesth 69: 457–460
25. Sprotte G, Schedel R, Pajunk H 1987 Eine 'atraumatische' Universalkanule für einzeitge Regionalanesthesien. Reg Anaesth 10: 104–108
26. Torrieri A, Aldrete J. A 1988 The TA pair needle. Acta Anaesthesiol Belg 39: 65–66
27. Eldor J 1990 Combined spinal–epidural needle. Reg Anesth 15: 89
28. Thorén T, Holmström B, Rawal N, Schollin J, Lindberg S 1991 Spinal versus combined spinal epidural block for cesarean section. Acta Anesth Scand 35: (supply) 199
29. Holmström B, Laugaland K, Rawal N, Hallberg S 1991 Combined spinal epidural block versus spinal and epidural block for orthopedic surgery. Acta Anesthesiol Scand 35: 184
30. Abouleish E, Rawal N, Shaw J, Lorenz T, Rashad N 1991 Intrathecal morphine 0.2 mg versus epidural bupivacaine 0.125% or their combination: effect on parturients. Anesthesiology 74: 711–716
31. Dahl J B, Rosenberg J, Dirkes W E et al 1989 Prevention of postoperative pain by intraoperative spinal + epidural blockade and postoperative combined low-dose epidural bupivacaine + morphine and systemic piroxecam. In: Nuutinen L (ed) Proceedings of the European Society of Regional Anaesthesia, Oulu, Finland. Tryckeri Och Tidnug, Porvoo p 87
32. Serrao J M, Marks R L, Morley S J, Goodchild C S 1992 Intrathecal midazolam for the treatment of chronic mechanical low-back pain: a controlled comparison with epidural steroid in a pilot study. Pain 48: 5–12
33. Patel M 1992 Combined spinal and extradural anesthesia. Anesth Analg 75: 640–641
34. Holmström B, Rawal N, Axelsson K et al 1991 Epiduroscopic study of risk of catheter migration following dural puncture by spinal and epidural needles – a video presentation. Reg Anesth 15: 86
35. Crawford J S 1985 Some maternal complications of epidural analgesia for labour. Anaesthesia 40: 1219
36. Phillips D C, MacDonald R, Lyons G 1986 Possible subarachnoid migration of an epidural catheter. Anaesthesia 41: 653
37. Phillip J H, Brown W V 1976 Total spinal anesthesia late in the course of obstetric bupivacaine epidural block. Anesthesiology 44: 340–341
38. Robson J A, Brodsky J B 1977 Latent dural puncture after lumbar epidural block. Anesth Analg 56: 725–726
39. Ravindran R, Albrecht W, Mckay M 1979 Apparent intravascular migration of epidural catheter. Anesth Analg 58: 252–253
40. Zebrowski M E, Gutsche B B 1979 More on intravascular migration of epidural catheter. Anesth Analg 58: 531
41. Ready L B, Wild L M 1989 Organization of an acute pain service: training and manpower. Anesthesiol Clin N Am 7: 229–239
42. Riegler R, Pernetzky A 1983 Irremovable epidural catheter due to a sling and a knot. A rare complication of epidural anaesthesia in obstetrics (in German). Reg Anaesth 6: 19–21
43. Dennison B 1987 Combined subarachnoid and epidural block for cesarean section. Can Anaesth Soc J 34: 105–106
44. Russell I F 1987 Effect of posture during the induction of subarachnoid analgesia for cesarean section. Br J Anaesth 59: 342–346
45. Zaric D, Axelsson K, Hallgren S, Nydahl P A, Philipson L, Samuelsson L 1993 Sensory epidural blockade evaluated by qualitative and quantitative methods. In: Gielen M (ed) Proceedings of the European Society of Regional Anaesthetists, Dublin. Ponsen en Looijen – Wageningen, The Netherlands
46. Carrie L E S 1988 Epidural versus combined spinal–epidural block for cesarean section. Acta Anesthesiol Scand 32: 595–596
47. Bromage P R 1975 Mechanism of action of extradural anesthesia. Br J Anaesth 47: 199–212
48. Barclay D L, Renegar O J, Nelson E W 1968 The influence of inferior vena cava compression on the level of spinal anesthesia. Am J Obstet Gynecol 101: 792–800
49. Tunstall M E 1991 Incremental spinal anesthesia and cesarean section – relevance to the test dose for extradural analgesia. Br J Anaesth 67: 227–228
50. Russel I F 1983 Spinal anesthesia for cesarean section Br J Anaesth 55: 309–313
51. Ramsay M 1991 Epidural injection does cause an increase in CSF pressure. Anesth Analg 73: 668
52. Denny N, Masters R, Pearson D, Red J, Sihota M, Selander D 1987 Postdural puncture headache after continuous spinal anesthesia. Anesth Analg 66: 791–794
53. Makisekar U L, Winnie A P, Vasireddy A R, Masters R W 1991 Continuous spinal anesthesia and post dural puncture headache. A retrospective study. Reg Anesth 16: 107–111
54. Peterson D O, Borup J L et al 1983 Continuous spinal anesthesia. Case review and discussion. Reg Anesth 8: 109

55. Lambert D H 1992 Continuous spinal anesthesia. Third joint ESRA–ASRA Congress (abstracts) Van Zundert A (ed). Aristos Philis, Limassol, pp 339–348
56. Giufridda J G, Bizzarri D V, Masi R, Bondoc R 1972 Continuous procaine spinal anesthesia for cesarean section. Anesth Analg 51: 117–124
57. Hurley R J, Lambert D H 1990 Microcatheters for continuous spinal anesthesia (letter). Anesth Analg 71: 201
58. Rigler M L, Dranser L K 1991 Cauda equina syndrome after continuous spinal anesthesia (see comments). Anesth Analg 72: 275
59. Schell R M, Brauer F S 1991 Persistent sacral nerve root deficits after continuous spinal anesthesia. Can J Anesth 38: 908
60. Schneider M, Ettlin T, Kaufmann M, Schumacher P, Urwyler A, Hampl K, von Hochstetter A 1993 Transient neurologic toxicity after hyperbaric subarachnoid anesthesia with 5% lidocaine. Anesth Analg 76: 1154–1157
61. Ravindran R S, Bond V K et al 1980 Prolonged neural blockade following regional analgesia with 2-chloroprocaine. Anesth Analg 59: 447
62. Gissen A J, Datta S et al 1984 The chloroprocaine controversy. II Is chloroprocaine neurotoxic? Reg Anesth 9: 135
63. Rawal N, Nuutinen L, Raj P P, Lovering S, Abouleish E, Lehmkuhl L, Fallon K D 1991 Neurotoxicity of intrathecal opioids in sheep. Comparison between butorphanol, sufentanil and nalbuphine. Anesthesiology 75: 1025–1034
64. Cesarini M, Torrielli R, Lahaye F, Mene J M, Cabiro C 1990 Sprotte needle for intrathecal anaesthesia for cesarean section: incidence of postdural puncture headache. Anesthesia 45: 656–658
65. Naulty J S, Hertwig L, Hunt C O, Datta S, Ostheimer G W, Weiss J B 1990 Influence of local anesthetic solution on postdural puncture headache. Anesthesiology 72: 450–454
66. Westbrook J L, Donald F, Carrie L E S 1992 An evaluation of a combined spinal epidural needle set utilizing a 26-gauge, pencil point spinal needle for cesarean section. Anaesthesia 47: 990–992
67. Lyons G, Macdonald R, Mikl B 1992 Combined epidural spinal anesthesia for cesarean section. Through the needle or in separate spaces? Anaesthesia 47: 199–201
68. Boskovski N, Lewinski A 1982 Epidural morphine for the prevention of headache following dural puncture. Anaesthesia 37: 217–218
69. Johnson M D, Hertwig L, Vehring P H, Datta S 1989 Intrathecal fentanyl may reduce the incidence of spinal headache. Anesthesiology 71: A911
70. Abboud T, Zhu J, Reyes A et al 1992 Effect of subarachnoid morphine on the incidence of spinal headache. Reg Anesth 17: 34–36
71. Simsa J 1990 Device to maintain the position of a 29-gange spinal needle. Anesthesia 45: 593–594
72. Manchikanti L, Hadley C, Markwell S J, Colliver J A 1987 A retrospective analysis of failed spinal anesthetic attempts in a community hospital. Anesth Analg 66: 363–366
73. Tarkkila P J, Heine H, Tervo R R. Comparison of Sprotte and Quincke needles with respect to postdural puncture headache and backache. Reg Anesth 17: 283–287
74. Eldor J, Guedj P, Gozal Y 1992 Combined spinal–epidural anesthesia using the CSEN. Anesth Analg 74: 169–170
75. Eldor J, Brodsky V 1991 Danger of metallic particles in the spinal–epidural spaces using the needle-through-needle approach. Acta Anesth Scand 35: 461

36. Postdural puncture headache

Part A USA view *K. J. Mintz* *P. H. Vehring* *M. D. Johnson*
Part B European view *M. Gielen*

PART A
USA VIEW

K. J. Mintz *P. H. Vehring* *M. P. Johnson*

The first use of subarachnoid anesthesia is often attributed to Corning because of his experiments with intraspinal injections of cocaine in 1885. In 1891, Quincke reported on the diagnostic and therapeutic use of lumbar dural puncture to drain cerebrospinal fluid (CSF) from patients with hydrocephalus. The first diagnosis of postdural puncture headache (PDPH) was made by August Bier in 1898, when he observed four of six patients on whom he had performed subarachnoid anesthesia develop headaches.[1] As with many early investigators of regional anesthesia, he experimented on himself. His assistant, Dr Hildebrandt, attempted to administer a subarachnoid anesthetic to Bier using a 'fine hollow needle'. Unfortunately, the syringe did not fit properly and much CSF, along with the cocaine, was lost, resulting in an ineffective anesthetic. Bier then successfully performed a subarachnoid anesthetic on Hildebrandt.

> After these experiments on our own bodies we both went to dinner without any physical complaints. We drank wine and smoked several cigars. I went to bed at 11 o'clock and slept well throughout the night. I awoke, feeling refreshed and well the next morning, and went for a walk for an hour. Toward 3 p.m., my face turned pale; the pulse was rather faint but remained regular, and was about 70 beats per minute. Furthermore, I had the sensation of a very strong pressure in my head and felt dizzy when I arose quickly from my chair. All these symptoms disappeared as soon as I lay down horizontally but they returned when I arose in the late afternoon. Therefore, I had to go to bed, and I stayed in bed for nine days, since all the described symptoms returned whenever I tried to arise.
>
> Dr. Hildebrandt felt very well when he went to bed at 11 p.m., however, he could not fall asleep because he was affected by restlessness. At midnight, violent headaches occurred, which increased gradually to an unbearable degree. At 1 a.m. vomiting began, which recurred once during the night. Dr. Hildebrandt felt very poor the next morning, but with great physical effort he was able to do his work, which consisted mainly in operating and dressing of wounds. He had to go to bed in the afternoon, but he arose again the next morning and did his work although he still did not feel well for three or four days. He again had headaches.

Even though this experiment was performed in 1898, Bier's observations and conclusions are still valid today. He noted the headache was postural and that it was related to loss of CSF, and not to the local anesthetic itself (not in the above quote, however). Additionally, did Hildebrandt develop a chemical meningitis? The symptoms he experienced are similar.

CLINICAL FEATURES

PDPH is classically described as beginning when the patient sits or stands upright, and it is relieved upon reclining or assuming the supine position. It is aggravated by coughing and sudden movements. The headache is usually a dull aching pressure or heaviness, which characteristically begins in the occipital region and often spreads over the top of the head to the frontal region behind the eyes. Reflex spasm of the cervical muscles may occur and the pain also may radiate down the neck. It can be mild to incapacitating and the patient usually describes it as unlike any previous headache.

The onset of PDPH can occur immediately or up to several days after dural puncture. Vandam and Dripps[2] reported the average time to be within the first 48 h of the postoperative period. This may correlate with the time the patient begins to ambulate. The duration of the headache can be from hours to months (if left untreated).

However, Vandam and Dripps[2] found that most headaches resolved after 4 days.

The associated symptoms include nausea and vomiting, depression, visual changes and auditory disturbances. Vandam and Dripps[2] reported a triad that consisted of a PDPH in association with ocular and auditory dysfunction and called it 'the syndrome of decreased intracranial pressure'.[2] They noted a 0.4% prevalence of visual difficulties, including diplopia, blurred vision and photophobia. They also observed six cases of transient lateral rectus muscle paralysis. These symptoms may be secondary to cranial nerve VI (abducens) stretching associated with decreased CSF volume.[3] They also described a 0.4% percent prevalence of auditory difficulties, including decreased acuity, tinnitus and a sensation of 'ear popping'. These symptoms might also be secondary to decreased CSF pressure, as there are anatomic communications between endolymph canals and CSF.[4]

Headache in the setting of a recent dural puncture may not necessarily be a PDPH. There are other serious causes for headache that should be ruled out (Tables 36.1 and 36.2).

PATHOPHYSIOLOGY

The etiology of PDPH is complex and multifactorial. One of the major components is loss of CSF through the dural puncture site with resultant reduction in CSF pressure. Normal lumbar CSF pressure is 5–15 cmH_2O in the horizontal position. It increases to over 40 cmH_2O in the erect position, whereas the pressure in the epidural space remains close to atmospheric in either position. Therefore, in the erect position a pressure gradient of 40–50 cmH_2O exists, favoring leakage of CSF from the subarachnoid space into the epidural space.[5] Multiple studies have supported the correlation between PDPH and reduction in CSF volume (and pressure).[6–8] Kunkle et al[9] found they were consistently able to induce the symptoms of PDPH in normal human subjects in the erect position by free drainage of 20 ml of CSF. The headache could then be decreased in intensity by tipping the patient to the horizontal position, and completely relieved by artificially raising the CSF pressure to normal with a subarachnoid injection of saline solution. Other investigators have found that the headache symptoms can be relieved by raising the epidural space pressure with saline[10] or blood.[11]

The acute reduction of CSF volume reduces the CSF's cushioning effect on the brain. Theoretically, this can cause downward traction on pain-sensitive structures (intracranial sinuses, vessels, nerves and cerebral tentorium). Above the tentorium, the pain is referred via the trigeminal nerve to the frontal region of the head. Below the tentorium, the pain is referred via the vagus and glossopharyngeal nerves to the occiput. Pain in the upper neck and shoulder regions is referred via the upper three cervical nerves.[12]

Another component of PDPH may be cerebral vasodilation. The intracranial pressure is determined by the volume of three compartments within the fixed intracranial space: cerebral blood volume (5–8%), brain tissue (85%) and CSF (7–10%). A loss of CSF volume leads to a reflex vasodilation of the cerebral vessels to increase cerebral blood volume. A reduction in the volume of one of the intracranial components is balanced by an increase in the volume of another. This vasodilation may stimulate perivascular stretch receptors similar to one of the mechanisms of migraine headache.

Certain patient populations seem to be at increased risk for PDPH. These include younger patients, female patients and pregnant or post-partum patients.[2,5,13,14] The incidence of PDPH is remarkably lower in the elderly (age greater than 60 years). Although the reasons are not clearly understood, older patients do have a less dynamic CSF circulation and lower CSF pressures. A lower initial CSF pressure at the time of dural puncture may result in a reduced gradient for leakage. In addition, the cerebrospinal vessels of the elderly may be less reactive to volume changes. Finally, the constitution of connective tissue (and, possibly, the dura) changes with age, and this may aid in rapid closure of the dural leak.

The incidence of PDPH in the obstetric patient is about

Table 36.1 Differential diagnosis of headache

Meningitis
Cerebral hemorrhage (subdural, subarachnoid)
Cerebral infarction (cortical vein thrombosis)
Hypertensive crises
Migraine
Metabolic (electrolyte imbalance, hypoglycemia)
Psychogenic (post-partum)
Hormonal imbalance

Table 36.2 Evaluation of headache not caused by dural puncture

History
Characteristics
Prior history of headaches
Family history of headaches
History of depression
Associated symptoms
Physical examination
Vital signs: temperature, blood pressure, heart rate, respiratory rate
General appearance
Neck signs
Neurologic examination
Mental status
Sensory, motor and reflexes
Gait/positional alterations of headache symptoms
Laboratory work-up
Complete blood count, electrolytes, glucose, electrocardiogram
Computed tomography scan, diagnostic dural puncture, electromyelogram (neurologic consult)

twice the incidence observed in the nonobstetric population. At our institution, there has been about a 6% prevalence of PDPH after subarachnoid anesthesia in our obstetric population over a 5-year period. The higher incidence of PDPH in the obstetric patient is also multifactorial.[14] The peripartum patient is predisposed to intravascular volume depletion from diuresis, vomiting, diaphoresis, blood loss with delivery and oral fluid restriction. This may contribute to slower CSF regeneration. During labor, the CSF pressure is transiently increased with bearing down, and this may favor a leak gradient across a dural puncture site. The increase in abdominal pressure during pregnancy results in distended epidural vessels and concomitant reduction of the epidural volume. With resolution of the aortocaval compression after delivery, epidural venous engorgement subsides, resulting in a reduction of epidural space pressure. This may also favor a leakage gradient. The higher incidence of PDPH in young women persists even when obstetric patients are excluded from consideration.

PREVENTION

The use of small-gauge needles for dural puncture and needle insertion with the bevel parallel to the dural fibers are reported to reduce the incidence of PDPH. Other technical factors that may reduce the incidence of PDPH include bevel design, angle of needle approach, patient positioning, anesthetic agents used, and, possibly, the use of a catheter for continuous infusion.

Needle diameter

Many studies have correlated spinal needle diameter and the incidence of PDPH (Table 36.3). In 1968, Phillips et al[13] reviewed 10 440 subarachnoid anesthetics. This study was comparable in magnitude, data gathering and protocol to the Vandam and Dripps[2] study of 1956.

Table 36.3 Relationship of needle size to incidence of headache

Reference	Needle size (G)	Headache incidence (%)
15	20	33.3
	26	0.4
2	16	18.0
	20	14.0
	24	6.0
16	16	18.0
	19	10.0
	25	0.2
17	22	9.5
	25	5.1
13	25/26	3.5

However, Phillips et al[13] obtained a significantly lower overall incidence of PDPH (3.5% versus 11%). They attributed this difference to needle size as 82% of the spinal needles they used were 25- and 26-gauge, whereas 82% of the needles used by Vandam and Dripps were 20 and 22 gauge. Their finding was noteworthy considering the susceptibility of the patient population studied (99% were female, with a mean age of 25).[13]

Other studies have demonstrated an extremely small incidence of PDPH when 29- to 32-gauge needles are used.[18-20] These ultrafine needles require an introducer system because they are so flexible and fragile, and may have a higher failure rate.

Bevel direction

In 1926, Green[21] postulated that dural puncture with the needle bevel parallel to the dural fibers would result in a smaller defect, and that this would decrease the amount of CSF leak. Dural punctures with the bevel perpendicular to the fibers are likely to cause greater anatomic damage, thus hindering rapid closure of the leak. In 1946, Franksson and Gordh[22] confirmed this hypothesis by examining dura from patients who underwent dural puncture just prior to death. They found, using light microscopy, approximately twice the number of severed fibers when the dura was punctured at right angles.

Mihic,[23] in 1985, provided additional clinical evidence by reporting a significantly higher number of PDPH when the dura was punctured perpendicularly. In fact, he stopped piercing the dura with the bevel perpendicular after 62 patients because of the extremely high frequency of PDPH (16.1% versus 0.24%). Norris et al[24] recommend identifying the epidural space with the needle bevel oriented parallel to the dural fibers, as they found a lower incidence of PDPH if unintentional dural puncture occurred.

Bevel design

The configuration of the needle point may affect the incidence of PDPH. A needle with a cutting bevel edge may cause more damage to the dura than a conical-point needle (Whitacre). This needle may separate instead of lacerate the dural fibers, resulting in less CSF leak.[23,24] These needles have been seldom used because of the difficulty with needle positioning associated with a dull point.[25] However, our experience with disposable 25-gauge and larger Whitacre needles is extremely encouraging.

Needle angle

The angle at which the dura is pierced might influence the size and nature of the dural hole. In 1977, Hatfalvi[27]

reported a series of over 600 subarachnoid blocks using a 20-gauge needle in which he had no PDPH and attributed this finding to the paramedian approach. Using an in vitro model with samples of human dura, Ready et al[28] found that a 30° angle of approach to the dura resulted in significantly lower CSF leak rates than with a similar needle used at 60° or 90°. Since the holes made in the contiguous layers of the dura by a paramedian approach do not overlap, a seal might be formed (Fig. 36.1).

Patient position

Patients are generally placed in a flexed position to facilitate the insertion of a spinal needle through the midline. This position may place tension on the dura, resulting in an extended tear at the dural puncture site. Ash,[29] in 1955, and Rosser and Schneider,[30] in 1956, suggested that there may be an advantage to an 'unflexed back position'. Ash observed a 6% prevalence of PDPH when using the prone position to perform subarachnoid blocks. Rosser found only a 0.54% prevalence by keeping the back in a 'comfortably neutral' position (i.e. the patient was in the lateral position with the back neither flexed nor extended). These reported prevalences of PDPH are lower than expected considering both investigators used 20- to 22-gauge spinal needles and 40% of Rosser's patients were pregnant. The fact that these investigators often used the paramedian approach when the midline approach was unsuccessful (in the unflexed back position) may account for their low reported incidence of PDPH.

Agent used

In their 1956 review, Vandam and Dripps[2] concluded that the particular local anesthetic agent used for subarachnoid block had no relationship to the incidence of PDPH; this concept is still accepted. However, in a recent abstract, Naulty et al[31] suggested that certain local anesthetic agents may correlate with a higher incidence of PDPH (lidocaine > bupivacaine > tetracaine–procaine mixture). They also implicated the use of dextrose in the anesthetic solution as possibly increasing the incidence of PDPH. Other investigators have noted the addition of epinephrine[32] or fentanyl[33] may lower the incidence of PDPH.

Continuous subarachnoid anesthesia

Until recently, continuous subarachnoid anesthesia (CSA) has not been a popular technique because of the concern that dural puncture with a large-bore needle would result in an unacceptably high incidence of PDPH. However, with the exception of the Giuffrida et al[34] study in 1972, recent work has indicated that the incidence of PDPH after CSA might be surprisingly low[34–39] (Table 36.4).

It can be argued that a CSA catheter may stent open the dural puncture, resulting in greater CSF leak. Conversely, the catheter may actually occlude the dural hole while in place, thus minimizing CSF leakage into the epidural space. Finally, the catheter may precipitate an

Table 36.4 Incidence of headache following dural puncture according to needle size

Reference	Needle size (G)	Headache incidence (%)
34 (cesarean delivery patients)	21	16
35	18	0
36	18	0
37	18	<1
38 (vascular surgery patients)	21	<2
39	26	4

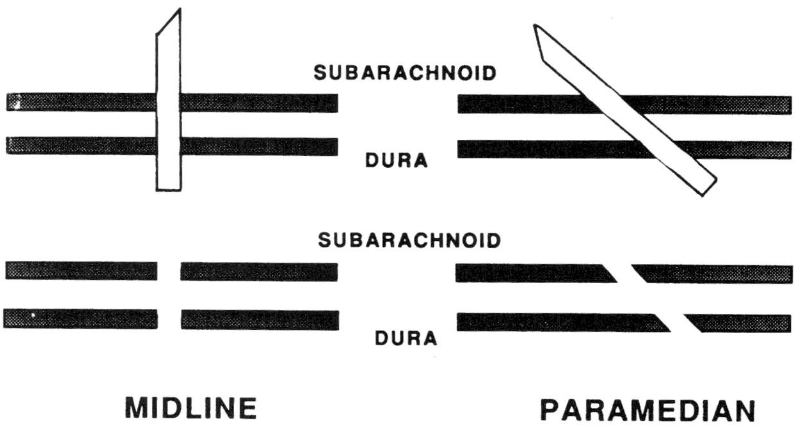

Fig. 36.1 Effect of needle angle on the size and nature of the dural hole. A 30° angle of approach results in significantly lower CSF leak rates than a similar needle used at a 60° or 90° angle.

inflammatory reaction, which may hasten the closure of the dural defect when it is removed.

The data on CSA are difficult to interpret because the patient populations vary and the group of patients selected for CSA may already have been at low risk for PDPH because of their age. Giuffrida et al[34] found a relatively high incidence of PDPH. Their patient population was pregnant women undergoing cesarean delivery.

Microcatheters (32-gauge) have being developed and tested for use with 26- and 28-gauge spinal needles, which may further diminish the incidence of PDPH,[39] although it is too early to formulate conclusions.

MANAGEMENT OF AN UNINTENTIONAL DURAL PUNCTURE ('WET TAP') AND POST-DURAL PUNCTURE HEADACHE

Unintentional dural puncture

The prevalence of unintentional dural puncture ('wet tap') associated with epidural placement is 1–2% at the Brigham and Women's Hospital, and the associated incidence of PDPH in the obstetric population is about 70%[12,40,41]. When an unintentional dural puncture occurs, the needle should be withdrawn and replaced at a more cephalad interspace with the catheter directed cephalad or at a more caudad interspace with the catheter directed caudad. Obtaining a block at a different level may reduce the incidence of PDPH. This is probably because the volume of local anesthetic in the epidural space reduces the pressure gradient between the subarachnoid space and the epidural space, minimizing CSF leak and optimizing early dural closure. In this situation, it is important to use a minimal amount of air if the loss-of-resistance technique is being used. Air injected into the epidural space may traverse across the dural puncture, resulting in an immediate, severe headache from an unintentional pneumoencephalocele. When inserting the catheter at the different interspace, it is wise to direct it away from the interspace where the unintentional dural puncture occurred. Careful observation is required as injection of local anesthetics into the epidural space may result in some local anesthetic traversing the dural hole, resulting in subarachnoid instead of epidural anesthesia.[42,43]

Postdural puncture headache

Conservative therapy

Conservative treatment is used first because PDPH is usually self-limiting and often only mild to moderate in intensity. The first rule of conservative therapy for PDPH is bed rest in the supine position. Having the patient lie flat after dural puncture will not prevent PDPH and is no longer recommended.[44–46] In fact, longer recumbency predisposes the patient to an increased incidence of nausea,[46] delayed diagnosis of PDPH and possible thromboembolism. The role for recumbency is *after* the diagnosis of PDPH is made, as most patients get excellent relief by lying supine. Other conservative therapy includes oral or intravenous hydration to allow increased CSF production and analgesics [acetominophen, ibuprofen or other nonsteroidal anti-inflammatory drugs (NSAIDs)] to relieve symptoms. The authors and the senior editor have had excellent success with NSAIDs instead of aspirin-like compounds. The senior editor does not use Fiorinal because many patients complain of a 'barbiturate hang-over'. Abdominal binders and varying the patient's position to increase venous return are not well tolerated and have not proven effective.[46,47]

Caffeine

Some investigators have reported that intravenous caffeine therapy (caffeine benzoate 500 mg) at multiple intervals reduces the duration and extent of PDPH.[48,49] Camann et al[50] used a single oral dose of caffeine (300 mg) and found improvement in PDPH, although this effect was transient in 30% of their patients. The basis of using caffeine in the treatment of PDPH comes from the observation that a loss of CSF volume leads to a reflex vasodilation in the cerebral vessels. It is postulated that the pain of PDPH is due to this reactive hyperemia and subsequent stretch of vascular receptors in the cerebral vessels, similar to the etiology of migraine headache. Therefore, caffeine may work by constricting such vessels.

Saline infusion

Studies have shown that bolus injection or continuous infusion of saline into the epidural space via epidural catheter may be effective in reducing the pain of PDPH, especially when the dural puncture is secondary to a misadventure with a 17-gauge epidural needle.[51,52] Such infusions probably work by increasing volume and, therefore, pressure in the epidural space, thereby reducing the transdural gradient and the extent of the CSF leak. Unfortunately, the rise in epidural pressure with saline is transient and the PDPH often recurs.[10] Whether given by bolus injection or continuous infusion for treatment or prophylaxis the results with epidural saline are not as good as the epidural blood patch with autologous blood.[51,53–55]

Epidural blood patch (EBP)

Use of an autologous epidural blood patch (EBP) as a treatment of PDPH was first described by Gormley in 1960 and has been widely practiced since.[14,56,57] The success rate of the EBP is excellent (above 90%). The blood should be injected in close approximation to the puncture site, if possible. There is greater cephalad spread of blood in the epidural space, therefore in the presence of more than one dural puncture the lowest puncture site should be chosen[58] (Table 36.5). Valsalva maneuvers after a recent EBP have been reported to 'blow out' the patch with resultant redevelopment of PDPH. The rate of success for repeated EBP are even better (95%), possibly because the first EBP creates a matrix to which the second can adhere. After several unsuccessful EBPs, other etiologies for headache must be pursued (e.g. cortical vein thrombosis).[59,60]

The EBP is probably effective initially because it increases pressure in the epidural space, thus reducing the pressure gradient between the subarachnoid space and epidural space. The increase in epidural pressure is transmitted across the dura to the subarachnoid space, causing an increase in the subarachnoid pressure.[11] This mechanism is probably responsible for the immediate relief of symptoms. The epidural blood occludes the dural hole via clot formation and serves as a matrix for connective tissue repair (Fig. 36.2). Epidural blood appears to be more effective than saline because its increased viscosity and hypertonicity reduces the rate of resorption into the general circulation and the clot must be resolved over time. Investigators have proposed dextran 40 to be more effective than normal saline for treatment of PDPH if one accepts the increased viscosity and hypertonicity concepts.[61]

The use of a prophylactic EBP via the epidural catheter or spinal needle has been described.[62] However, studies have shown that the incidence of PDPH does not change significantly with a prophylactic or early (sooner than 24 h) EBP.[63,64] More recent studies have challenged these earlier findings,[65,66] but no large-scale study has demon-

Table 36.5 Protocol for epidural blood patch

1. Review chart, obtain written informed consent
2. Check baseline vital signs
3. Insert i.v. line; acute hydration with warm crystalloid (about 1 l)
4. i.v. sedation/opioids prn (fentanyl, 50–100 μg, midazolam 1 mg, metoclopramide 10 mg)
5. Oxygen by mask prn (5–6 l/min)
6. Position patient slowly, preferably in lateral position to avoid worsening headache
7. Identify epidural space, preferably with loss of resistance to fluid technique. Hanging-drop technique is less preferable because the 'vacuum' in the epidural space may be lessened after a dural puncture. If using loss of resistance to air technique, use minimal amount (see text).
   a. use same space as dural puncture
   b. if more than one dural puncture, use lowest interspace
   c. preferable to use midline approach
8. Using sterile technique, withdraw 20 ml blood from arm opposite the i.v. line. It is easier to withdraw from the dependent arm
9. Maintaining sterile technique, inject blood into the epidural space about 1 ml/3–4 s. Usual dose is 10–20 ml. If pain or pressure (back, leg, buttock) is noted before 15 ml, stop and let pressure recede. Continue only if there is no exacerbation of discomfort
10. Turn patient supine; place blankets under knees to flatten lumbar lordosis
11. Let patient rest 30 min and continue i.v. fluids (remainder of first liter)
12. After 30 min, raise head of bed in stages while continually assessing patient for PDPH symptoms
13. After patient is sitting upright, post-EBP orders:
   a. avoid straining (from vomiting, stool, etc.) and heavy lifting for 5 days
   b. limited activity (encourage bed rest) first 24 h
   c. NSAIDs prn
   d. encourage oral intake
   e. tell patient to contact anesthesia department if headache symptoms recur

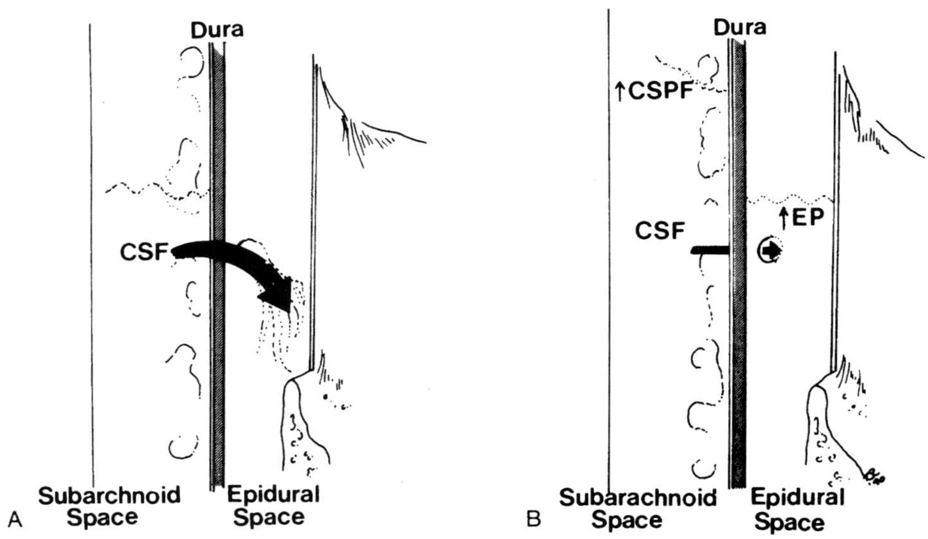

Fig. 36.2 (**A, B**) The epidural blood patch works by increasing pressure in the epidural space, thus reducing the pressure gradient between the subarachnoid space and the epidural space and causing an increase in subarachnoid pressure.

strated the efficacy of a prophylactic EBP. Since it is impossible to predict which patient will develop a PDPH, only a portion of patients with dural puncture (including unintentional epidural needle puncture) develop PDPH. Many of these patients can be treated conservatively. Therefore, the use of a prophylactic EBP is not currently performed routinely.

No permanent sequelae from a therapeutic EBP have been reported, however transient back stiffness and paresthesias are relatively common. Other rare complications include meningismus, abdominal cramps, tinnitus, vertigo, fever, epidural hematoma and subcutaneous hematoma at the injection site. Contraindications to an EBP include septicemia or local infection in the area of injection, blood dyscrasias or anticoagulation, and the presence of active central axis neurologic disease. There is no contraindication to performing epidural or subarachnoid anesthesia in patients with a previous EBP.[67,68] The success of subsequent epidural or subarachnoid anesthesia does not appear to be altered,[58] although there are a few anecdotal reports to the contrary. Since the EBP should be resorbed in a matter of days, one is hard pressed for an explanation of subsequent epidural or subarachnoid failure.

REFERENCES

1. Bier A 1989 Versuche Ober/cocaineisirung des ruckenmarkes. Deut Z Chir 51: 361
2. Vandam L D, Dripps R D 1956 Long term follow-up of patients who received 10,098 spinal anesthetics. J Am Med Assoc 161: 586
3. Wolff E 1928 A bend in the sixth cranial nerve and its possible significance. Br J Ophthalmol 12: 22
4. Hughsen W 1932 A note on the relationship of cerbrospinal and intralabrinthine pressures. Am J Physiol 101: 396
5. Tourtellotte W W, Haerer A F, Heller G L, Somers J E 1964 Post-lumbar Puncture Headaches. Charles C Thomas, Springfield, I L, p 87
6. Glesne O G 1950 Lumbar puncture headaches. Anesthesiology 11: 702
7. Jacobaeus H C, Frumerie K 1925 About the leakage of spinal fluid after lumbar puncture and its treatment. Acta Med Scand 58: 102
8. Alpers B 1925 Lumbar puncture headache. Arch Neurol 14: 806
9. Kunkle E C, Ray B A, Wolfe H G 1943 Experimental studies on headache. Arch Neurol 49: 323
10. Usubiaga J E, Brea L M, Goyena R 1967 Effect of saline injections on epidural and subarachnoid space pressure and relation to postspinal anesthesia headache. Anesth Analg 46: 293
11. Coombs D W, Hooper D 1979 Subarachnoid pressure with epidural blood 'patch'. Reg Anesth 4: 3
12. Brownridge P 1983 The management of headache following accidental dural puncture in obstetric patients. Anaesth Intens Care 11: 4
13. Phillips O C, Ebner H, Nelson A T, Black M H 1969 Neurologic complications following spinal anesthesia with lidocaine: prospective review of 10,440 cases. Anesthesiology 30: 284
14. Ostheimer G W 1979 Headache in the post-partum period. In Marx G F (ed) Clinical management of mother and newborn. Springer-Verlag, New York, p 27
15. Green B A 1950 A 26 gauge lumbar puncture needle: its value in the prophylaxis of headache following spinal anesthesia for vaginal delivery. Anesthesiology 11: 464
16. Tarrow A B 1963 Post spinal headache. Anaesthetists
17. White C W, Weiss J B, Niver E C, Heerdegen D K 1962 Anesthesia and post partum headache. Obstet Gynecol 20: 734
18. White Flaatten H, Rodt S A, Vannes J et al 1988 Postdural puncture headache using 26- or 29-gauge needles in young patients. Reg Anesth 11: 5
19. Frumin M J 1969 Spinal anesthesia using a 32 gauge needle. Anesthesiology 30: 599
20. Ditman M, Renkel F 1989 Spinal anesthesia with extremely fine needles. Anesthesiology 70: 1035
21. Green H M 1926 Lumbar puncture and the prevention of post puncture headache. J Am Med Assoc 86: 391
22. Franksson C, Gordh T 1946 Headache after spinal anesthesia and a technique for lessening its frequency. Acta Chir Scand 94: 443
23. Mihic D 1985 Postspinal headache and relationship of needle bevel to longitudinal dural fibers. Reg Anesth 10: 76
24. Norris M C, Leighton B L, De Simone C A 1989 Needle bevel direction and headache after inadvertent dural puncture. Anesthesiology 70: 729
25. Kreuscher H P, Sandmann G 1988 Prevention of postspinal headache by using Whitacre's pencil-point needle. Reg Anesth 11: 5
26. Abouleish E, Yamaoka H, Hingson R 1974 Evaluation of a tapered spinal needle. Anesth Analg 53: 258
27. Hatfalvi B I 1977 The dynamics of post-spinal headache. Headache J 17: 64
28. Ready L B, Cuplin S, Haschke R H, Nessly M 1989 Spinal needle determinants of rate of transdural fluid leak. Anesth Analg 69: 457
29. Ash W H 1955 Lateral approach for spinal anesthesia. Anesthesiology 16: 455
30. Rosser B H, Schneider M 1956 The unflexed back and a low incidence of severe spinal headache. Anesthesiology 17: 288
31. Naulty J S, Hertwig L, Datta S et al 1985 Influence of local anesthetic solution on post-dural puncture headache. Anesthesiology 63: A454
32. Gielen M J M, Meulman H, VanBeern H, Bridenbaugh P O 1986 Does the addition of epinephrine to hyperbaric bupivacaine .5% in spinal anesthesia decrease the incidence of tourniquet induced pain? Abstract F3, ESRA, Malmo, Sweden
33. Johnson M D, Hertwig L, Vehring P H, Datta S 1989 Intrathecal fentanyl may reduce the incidence of spinal headache. Anesthesiology 71: A911
34. Giuffrida J G, Bizzarri D V, Masi R, Bondoc R 1972 Continuous procaine spinal anesthesia for cesarean section. Anesth Analg 51: 117
35. Kallos T, Smith T C 1972 Continuous spinal anesthesia with hypobaric tetracaine for hip surgery in lateral decubitus. Anesth Analg 51: 766
36. Peterson D O, Borup J L, Chestnut J S 1983 Continuous spinal anesthesia case review and discussion. Reg Anesth 8: 109
37. Denny N, Masters R, Pearson D, Reed J et al 1987 Postdural puncture headache after continuous spinal anesthesia. Anesth Analg 66: 791
38. Giuffrida J G, Bizzarri D B, Dalsania J 1988 Continuous spinal anesthesia – experience with 535 patients. Abstract II, 9th World Congress of Anesthesiology, Washington, D.C.
39. Hurley R J, Lambert D H 1990 Continuous spinal anesthesia with a microcatheter technique: preliminary experience. Anesth Analg 70: 97
40. Craft C B, Epstein S, Coakley C S 1973 Prophylaxis of dural puncture headache with epidural saline. Anesth Analg 52: 228
41. Ostheimer G W 1979 Prophylactic epidural blood patch. Reg Anesth 4: 17
42. Hodgkinson R 1981 Total spinal block after epidural injection into an interspace adjacent to an inadvertent dural perforation. Anesthesiology 55: 593
43. Leach A, Smith G B 1988 Subarachnoid spread of epidural local anaesthetic following dural puncture. Anaesthesia 43: 671
44. Jones R J 1974 The role of recumbency in the prevention and treatment of post spinal headache. Anesth Analg 53: 788
45. Carbaat PAT, Crevel H V 1981 Lumbar puncture headache: controlled study on the preventative effect of 24 hours bed rest. Lancet 2: 1133
46. Vilming S T, Schrader H, Monstad F 1988 Post-lumbar-puncture headache: the significance of body posture. Cephalalgia 8: 75

47. Hander C E, Smith F R, Perkin G D, Clifford R F 1982 Posture and lumbar puncture headache: a controlled trial in 50 patients. J R Soc Med 75: 404
48. Sechzer P H, Abel L 1978 Post-spinal anesthesia headache treatment with caffeine. I. Evaluation with demand method. Curr Ther Res 24: 307
49. Jarvis A P, Greenwalt J W, Fagraeus L 1986 Intravenous caffeine for post dural puncture headache. Anesth Analg 65: 316
50. Camann W R, Murray R S, Mushlin P S, Lambert D H 1990 Effect of oral caffeine on post dural puncture headache. A double-blind placebo-controlled trial. Anesth Analg 70: 181
51. Crawford J S 1972 The prevention of headache consequent upon dural puncture. Br J Anaesth 44: 598
52. Gibson B E, Wedel D J, Faust R J, Peterson R C 1988 Continuous epidural saline infusion for the treatment of low CSF pressure headache. Anesthesiology 68: 789
53. Rice G G, Dabbs C H 1950 The use of epidural and subarachnoid injections of saline solution in the treatment of severe postspinal headache. Anesthesiology 11: 17
54. Craft J B, Epstein B S, Coakley C S 1973 Prophylaxis of dural puncture headache with epidural saline. Anesth Analg 52: 228
55. Bart A J, Wheeler A S 1978 Comparison of epidural saline placement and epidural blood placement in the treatment of post lumbar puncture headache. Anesthesiology 48: 221
56. DiGiovanni A J, Galbert M W, Wahle W M 1972 Epidural injection of autologous blood for postlumbar puncture headache. Anesth Analg 51: 226
57. Gormley J B 1960 Treatment of post-spinal headache. Anesthesiology 21: 565
58. Szeinfeld M, Ihmeidan I H, Moser M M et al 1986 Epidural blood patch: Evaluation of the volume and spread of blood injected into the epidural space. Anesthesiology 64: 820
59. Zandstra G C, Veigas O J 1989 Post partum headache following regional analgesia: a symptom of cerebral venous thrombosis. Can J Anesth 36: 705
60. Younker D, Jones M M, Adenwala J et al 1986 Maternal cortical vein thrombosis and the obstetric anesthesiologist. Anesth Analg 65: 100
61. Barrios-Alarcan J, Aldrete J A, Paragoas-Tapia D 1989 Relief of post lumbar puncture headache with epidural dextran 40: a preliminary report. Reg Anesth 14: 78
62. Ozdil T, Powell W F 1965 Post lumbar puncture headache: an effective method of prevention. Anesth Analg 44: 542
63. Loeser E A, Hill G E, Bennett G M, Sedeberg J H 1978 Time vs success rate for epidural blood patch. Anesthesiology 49: 147
64. Palahniuk R J, Cumming M 1979 Prophylactic blood patch does not prevent post-lumbar puncture headache. Can Anaesth Soc J 26: 132
65. Anderson E F 1985 Immediate blood patching after inadvertent dural puncture. Anesthesiol Rev 122: 49
66. Coldunna-Ramano P, Shapiro B E 1989 Unintentional dural puncture and prophylactic epidural blood patch in obstetrics. Anesth Analg 69: 522
67. Abouleish E, Wadhwa R K, Vega S et al 1975 Regional anesthesia following epidural blood patch. Anesth Analg 54: 634
68. Naulty J S, Herold R 1978 Successful epidural anesthesia following epidural blood patch. Anesth Analg 57: 272

PART B
EUROPEAN VIEW

M. Gielen

INTRODUCTION

Spinal anesthesia is an excellent technique for cesarean delivery and for gynecologic operations. However, post-dural puncture headache (PDPH) is a troublesome complication of spinal anesthesia and the incidence is the highest in obstetric patients, especially when unintentional dural puncture occurs during attempts to identify the epidural space to institute epidural analgesia for the pain of labor. PDPH disturbs the usually happy post-partum period and is demoralizing for the new mother. Every measure to prevent this complication should be taken. Much progress has been made in the last 5 years to reduce the incidence to an acceptable level by the use of new spinal needles.

PATHOPHYSIOLOGY

It is generally accepted that PDPH is caused by leakage of cerebrospinal fluid (CSF) through the puncture hole in the dura caused by the spinal needle.[1] The amount of CSF loss is dependent on: the pressure gradient between the subarachnoid and epidural space, which is about 40–50 cmH_2O in the sitting position; the size and shape of the dural hole and the CSF production.

The consequences of CSF loss are: a decrease in CSF pressure and a decrease in subarachnoid fluid volume. In the vertical position, the brain tends to descend as it is deprived of its fluid cushion, which leads to traction on pain-sensitive supporting structures of the brain, the venous sinuses and cerebral vessels. Moreover, as a compensatory mechanism to restore the intracranial volume relationships, dilation of intracranial vessels occurs.

SYMPTOMATOLOGY

The symptoms of PDPH are related to the neural structures stimulated by the descending brain in the upright position, and the dilation of the intracranial vessels. According to Brownridge,[2,3] pain is referred above the tentorium via the trigeminal nerve (V) to the frontal region; below the tentorium via the glossopharyngeal and vagal nerves (IX, X) to the occiput, and via the upper cervical nerves (C1, 2, 3) to the neck and shoulders. The onset of PDPH can occur any time within the first 5 days after dural puncture, but recognition is often related to the time of ambulation when the patient resumes the upright position. If PDPH occurs, it starts in 90% of patients within 3 days after dural puncture. The duration is usually 2–3 days and, in 80–85% of cases, it is over in 5 days.[4,5]

The headache is localized in the frontal region in 50% of patients, occipital in 25%, and another 25% complain of diffuse pain with neck pain or 'stiffness of the neck'. The most specific distinguishing sign in the diagnosis of PDPH is its postural character; this means that the headache is always maximal in the standing or sitting position and diminishes or disappears in the supine horizontal position. PDPH is accompanied in less than 1% of the cases by ocular symptoms such as double vision or blurred vision which are symptoms caused by traction or compression on the oculomotor or abducens nerves; and auditory symptoms such as dizziness, tinnitus and decreased hearing.[6–8] Hearing loss occurs in the few patients who have an open or partly closed cochlear aqueduct.[9]

The symptoms of spinal headache are slight in 50% of patients and do not interfere with any of the patients' normal activities. 35% have moderate complaints which are cause enough to return to bed periodically to obtain pain relief. In only 15% is the headache so severe and so painful that the patient cannot sit up long enough to eat and curative treatment is needed.[4]

DIAGNOSIS

The diagnosis of PDPH can only be made when other causes of headache are eliminated by careful interrogation and physical examination. The patient with *migraine* gives a history of headache that is unilateral, pulsatile and associated with vasomotor signs and not relieved in the supine position. *Meningitis* is extremely rare with strict aseptic spinal dural puncture technique. *Cerebral venous thrombosis* can occur in 1 : 3000–6000 pregnancies. Severe throbbing headache with increasing intensity accompanied by vegetative symptoms and even seizures will occur. The CT scan is negative, and only contrast CT scan or MRI shows abnormalities.[10–12]

Intra-, *extra-* or *subdural hematoma*, although extremely rare, can occur.

In conclusion, each time a headache after spinal anesthesia does not present the classical symptomatology, of which the postural character of the headache is essential, or does not present the classical evolution, neurologic evaluation must be undertaken without delay. A CT-scan with contrast or magnetic resonance imaging is sometimes necessary before therapeutic measures can be taken.

INCIDENCE AND PREVENTION

Of the numerous factors that influence the incidence of PDPH the most important are:

1. Age of the patient: there is a decreasing incidence of PDPH with age.[8,12,13]
2. Gender: there is a higher incidence in women and especially in parturients.[8,13,14] Several factors are responsible. First, CSF loss through the dural hole might be severe because of the increased CSF pressure caused by bearing-down efforts, although two studies have shown that this has no effect.[15,16] Second, dehydration can result from withholding fluids, blood loss during delivery and increased diuresis in the post-partum period. Third, decrease in intra-abdominal and epidural pressure after delivery with a consequent decrease in the subarachnoid fluid pressure can occur.
3. Puncture technique: the dura should be punctured at a small angle, and the needle tip of a Quincke needle should be introduced parallel to the dural fibers to reduce the incidence of PDPH.[17,18] This is confirmed in experimental studies using an in vitro model and samples of human dura.[19]
4. Needle size (see below).
5. Needle tip design (see below).

Spinal needles

Recently, most interest has been focused on needle size and on needle tip design. Apart from size there are basically six different needle tip designs: the Quincke needle, the Greene needle, the Hart and Whitacre needle, the Sprotte needle developed in 1987, the different Whitacre modifications and the Atraucan design.

1. The normal standard spinal *Quincke needle* has a sharp cutting point which cuts the dural fibers. The incidence of PDPH after the use of this needle is mostly dependent on the size of the needle. The use of a 25G Quincke needle in young patients and in obstetrics results in a prevalence of PDPH of around 15%, whereas the use of a 26G needle reduces the prevalence threefold to 5%; and using a 27G needle, the incidence is further reduced to 2.5%.[20–24] PDPH is almost non-existent when very small 29 or 30G needles are used.[25–27] Unfortunately there are disadvantages using these small-size needles: they are quite expensive, not for multiple use and cause technical problems which result in a high percentage of failures: around 8%.[28]
2. The *Greene needle* (developed in 1926) has a rounded non-cutting bevel which makes a smaller tear in the dura.[29] It was reported at that time that this needle reduces the incidence of PDPH. However, the Quincke point needle continued to be the most popular.
3. The *Hart and Whitacre needle* (developed in 1951) has a solid tip: pencilpoint with a completely rounded non-cutting bevel. The round opening is on the side, 2 mm from the tip.[30] The use of this needle reduces the incidence of headache further, but the needle has not achieved wide acceptance until recently.
4. The *Sprotte 'atraumatic' needle* was developed in 1987.[31] It is a pencilpoint-type needle with a gentle-angle

conical point with no cutting edge. The needle opening with gentle slopes is wider than the inner diameter. This needle will push aside the dural fibers, resulting in a better closure of the dural tear after removal of the needle. Most studies show that the prevalence of PDPH is very low with the use of this needle: it is around 2% using the 24G needle.[32–34]

5. *Whitacre modifications.* Different manufacturers have improved the Sprotte needle and the original Whitacre needle by changing the conical angle of the tip and the size and the place of the opening. The prevalence of PDPH with the use of these needles is also very low: using a 25G modified Whitacre needle it is around 1%. All comparative studies of these needles with the Quincke needles of the same size show a lower incidence of PDPH when Whitacre needles are used.[35–37]

6. *The Atraucan design.* The Atraucan 26-gauge spinal needle[38] has a tip designed to make a small linear cut (as opposed to a V-shaped cut) in the dura mater. The cut is smaller than the outside diameter of the needle and is dilated as the needle passes through the dura. The needle is used with a 20-gauge introducer. In vitro, it causes less leakage of cerebrospinal fluid than Quincke 26-gauge or Sprotte 24-gauge needles. A recent multicenter trial was carried out in six centers in five countries involving 362 patients undergoing spinal anesthesia. All the needles were returned to the factory and examined microscopically for damage. Spinal anesthesia was satisfactory for the planned surgery in 97%. Microscopy of the needle tips showed only a minor degree (0.01–0.19 mm) of bending in 14% and none of the tips had a 'hook'. Postdural puncture headache (PDPH) occurred in nine patients (2.5%). Thus, a new needle holds promise for producing satisfactory dural puncture with minimal PDPH.

CONTINUOUS SPINAL ANESTHESIA

It is surprising that the incidence of PDPH after continuous spinal anesthesia is very low. In three studies comprising 278 patients, most above 70 years of age, only one spinal headache occurred after the use of 18G needles to introduce the catheter. It is postulated that the prolonged presence of the catheter causes an inflammatory reaction in the dura surrounding the puncture site. When the catheter is removed, edema and fibrinous exudate resulting from the inflammatory reaction seals the hole in the dura, thus preventing leakage of CSF. However, all these studies were done in elderly subjects, in whom the incidence of PDPH is very low.

After unintentional dural puncture during an epidural procedure with a 18G Tuohy needle followed by inserting a spinal catheter, we have found a prevalence of PDPH of 37% in young patients. Continuous spinal anesthesia after unintentional dural puncture with an 18G Hustead needle did not decrease the incidence of PDPH in parturients.[40]

TREATMENT

Conservative treatment

As PDPH is mild or moderate in 85% of patients and is self-limiting, resolving within a week, the first treatment is conservative. Bed rest is advised, but bed rest should not be used as a preventive measure.[41] Optimal hydration is advisable as it is obvious that headache lasts as long as CSF loss is greater than its production. Extra fluids are not necessary.[42] Analgesics help to ameliorate the condition. Subarachnoid morphine has no effect on the incidence of PDPH.[43]

Epidural injection of saline is effective in some cases after the use of a 25G needle, but ineffective after unintentional dural puncture with a 17G Tuohy needle.[44] If an epidural catheter is in the epidural space, an infusion of 1 L of 0.9% sodium chloride can be tried for 24 h before removing the catheter, although the results of this treatment are controversial and back pain may occur.

Caffeine and theophylline have a cerebral vasoconstrictive effect and both are effective in relieving the headache caused by the painful intracranial distension. Intravenously administered caffeine (500 mg in 1 L of Ringer's lactate solution) given over 1 h and a second liter over the next 2 h results in a complete or almost complete relief of PDPH in 80% of patients.[45]

Oral caffeine 300 mg and oral theophylline 300 mg are also reported to be effective.[46,47]

Curative treatment

The most effective treatment of PDPH is the epidural blood patch (EBP). Under strict aseptic techniques, a volume of 10–20 ml of homologous blood is injected into the epidural space.[48] It is effective and successful, and free of serious complications.[49,50] There are no reasons to delay this treatment in the following conditions: when the headache is severe or does not diminish or disappear within a few days of conservative treatment or affects the time of discharge.

Prophylactic EBP should not be done immediately after dural puncture as a high failure rate will result.[51,52] It should especially not be done through an epidural catheter since blood is an excellent culture medium and epidural catheters frequently become contaminated during continuous infusion of local anesthetic with or without opioids.

Reported minor complications of EBP are backache and paresthesias during injection. A transient elevation of body temperature and backache over a few days is sometimes seen. Adhesions between the dura and the ligamentum flavum do not occur: when laminectomy is required later for other reasons no trace of clot in the epidural space was found. Also numerous epidural blocks have been performed after an EBP without problems.

Additionally, EBP can be done in HIV-positive patients.[53]

The epidural hematoma after a blood patch with 18 ml of blood has been visualized by magnetic resonance imaging (MRI).[54] It extended over four segments and out through the neural outlet foramina, which can explain transient nerve root compression after EBP. Compression of the dural sac was also seen, explaining the tamponade at the site of dural puncture. There was more spread upwards, which suggest that the ideal site for EBP may be at the level below the spinal dural puncture. Moreover, blood was seen in the subarachnoid space, which explains the mild meningitis that occurs occasionally after EBP.

Because the injection of blood into epidural space is not without complications and some patients refuse blood for religious or other reasons, the epidural injection of dextran (average dose 20 ml) is an alternative curative treatment.[54]

CONCLUSION

CSF loss has to be prevented at all times to prevent not only PDPH but all other symptoms. We are now able to do it by the use of the special spinal needles.

If, for economic reasons, a Quincke needle is used it should be of small size, preferably 27 G. When larger sizes are used, the technique is important: the needle should be introduced with the bevel parallel to the dural fibers and with a small angle to reduce the incidence of PDPH.

As the modern 25G Whitacre needle is easy to handle, results in a low failure rate with an incidence of PDPH of around 1% and is not dependent on the technique used, this needle is strongly recommended for obstetric patients.

REFERENCES

1. Gielen M J M 1989 Post dural puncture headache (PDPH): a review. Reg Anesth 14: 101–106
2. Brownridge P 1983 The management of headache following accidental dural puncture in obstetric patients. Anaesth Intensive Care 11: 4–15
3. Brownridge P 1984 Spinal anesthesia revisited: An evaluation of subarachnoid block in obstetrics. Anaesth Intensive Care 12: 334–342
4. Jones R J 1974 The role of recumbency in the prevention and treatment of postspinal headache. Anesth Analg 53: 788–796
5. Driessen A, Mauer W, Fricke M, Kossmann B, Schleinzer W 1980 Prospective studies of the postspinal headache. Reg Anesth 3: 38–41
6. De Lange J J, Stilma J S, Crezee F 1988 Visual disturbances after spinal anaesthesia. Anaesthesia 43: 570–572
7. Fog J, Wang L P, Sundberg A, Mucchiano C 1990 Hearing loss after Spinal anesthesia is related to needle size. Anesth Analg 70: 517–522
8. Vandam L D, Dripps R D 1956 Long term follow up of patients who received 10,098 spinal anesthetics. Syndrome of decreased intracranial pressure (headache and ocular and auditory difficulties) J Am Med Assoc 161: 586–591
9. Michel O, Brusis T 1992 Hearing loss as a sequel of lumbar puncture. Ann Otol Rhinol Laryngol 101: 390–394
10. Younker D, Jones M M, Adenwalla J, Citrin A, Joyce T H 1986 Maternal cortical vein thrombosis and the obstetric anesthesiologist. Anesth Analg 65: 1007–1012
11. Hubbert C H 1987 Dural puncture headache suspected, cortical vein thrombosis diagnosed. Anesth Analg 66: 285
12. Ravidran R S, Zandstra G C, Veigas O J 1989 Postpartum headache following regional analgesia; a symtom of cerebral venous thrombosis. Can J Anesth 36: 705–707
13. Rasmussen B S, Blom L, Hansen P, Mikkelsen SS 1989 Postspinal headache in young and elderly patients. Two randomised, double blind studies that compare 20- and 25-gauge needles. Anaesthesia 44: 571–573
14. Lybecker H, Moller J T, May O, Nielsen H K 1990 Incidence and prediction of postdural puncture headache. A prospective study of 1021 spinal anesthesias. Anesth Analg 70: 389–394
15. Ravindran R S, Viegas O J, Tasch M D, Cline P J, Deaton R L, Brown T R 1981 Bearing down at the time of delivery and the incidence of spinal headache in parturients. Anesth Analg 60: 524–526
16. Stride P C, Cooper G M 1993 Dural taps revisited. A 20 years survey from Birmingham Maternity Hospital. Anaesthesia 48: 247–255
17. Hatfalvi B I 1977 The dynamics of post-spinal headache. Headache 17: 64–67
18. Mihic D N 1985 Postspinal headache and relationship of needle bevel to longitudinal dural fibres. Reg Anesth 10: 76–81
19. Ready L B, Cuplin S, Haschke R H, Nessly M 1989 Spinal needle determinants of rate of transdural fluid leak. Anesth Analg 69: 457–460
20. Sarma V J, Boström U 1990 Intrathecal anesthesia for day-care surgery. A retrospective study of 160 cases 25- and 26-gauge spinal needles. Anaesthesia 45: 769–771
21. Barker P 1990 Are obstetric spinal headaches avoidable? Anesth Intensive Care 18: 553–554
22. Quanor H, Corbey M, Berg P 1990 Spinal anesthesia in day-care surgery with a 26-gauge needle. Br J Anaesth 65: 766–769
23. Hurley R J, Hertwig L M, Ostheimer G W 1990 Incidence of postdural puncture headache in the obstetric patient: 26 vs 27 gauge Quincke tip needles. Abstracts of the Society for Obstetric Anesthesia and Perinatology Annual Meeting, Boston, May 23–25
24. Crawford J S 1979 Experience with spinal analgesia in a British obstetric unit. Br J Anesth 50: 531–535
25. Dahl J B, Schultz P, Anker-Möller E, Christensen EF, Staunstrup H E, Carlson P Spinal anesthesia in young patients using a 29-gauge needle: technical considerations and a evaluation of postoperative complaints compared with general anesthesia. Br J Anaesth 64: 178–182
26. Haden R M, Scott P V, Pinnock C A 1990 Spinal obstetric anesthesia with a 29-gauge needle. Br J Anaesth 65: 294–295
27. Dittmann M, Renkl F 1989 Spinal anesthesia with extremely fine needles. Anesthesiology 70: 1035–1036
28. Flaaten H, Rodt S A, Vamnes J, Rosland J, Wisborg T, Koller M E 1989 Postdural puncture headache. A comparison between 26- and 29-G needles in young patients. Anaesthesia 44: 147–149
29. Greene H M 1926 Lumbar puncture and the prevention of postpuncture headache. J Am Med Assoc 86: 391–392
30. Hart J R, Whitacre R G 1931 Pencil-point needle and the prevention of postspinal headache. J Am Med Assoc, 147: 657–658
31. Sprotte G, Schedel R, Pajunk H 1987 Eine 'atraumatische' Universalkanule für einzeitige Regionalanesthesien. An atraumatic needle for single shot regional anesthesia. Reg Anaesth 10: 104–108
32. Cesarini M, Torrielli R, Lahaye F, Mene J M, Cabiro C 1990 Sprotte needle for intrathecal anesthesia for cesarean section: Incidence of postdural headache. Anaesthesia 45: 656–658
33. Schneider M, Schumacher PH, Kaufmann M 1992 Incidence of postdural puncture headache (PDPH) in young pregnant and non-pregnant women after spinal anesthesia with a 24 G Sprotte needle (abstract). Reg Anesth 17 (suppl): 93
34. Mayer D C, Quance D, Weeks SK 1992 Headache after spinal anesthesia for Cesarean section: a comparison of the 27-Gauge Quincke and 24-Gauge Sprotte needles. Anesth Analg 75: 377–380
35. Hurley R J, Hertwig L M, Lambert D H 1992 Incidence of post dural puncture headache in the obstetric patient: 25 gauge Whitacre vs 26 and 27 gauge Quincke tip needles (abstract). Reg Anesth 17 (suppl): 33
36. Lynch J, Arhelger S, Krings-Ernst I 1992 Post-dural puncture headache in young orthopedic in-patients: comparison of a 0.33

mm (29-gauge) Quincke-type with a 0.7 mm (22-gauge) Whitacre spinal needle in 200 patients. Acta Anaesthesiol Scand 36: 58–61
37. Shutt L E, Valentine S J, Wee M Y K, Page R J, Prosser A, Thomas T A 1992 Spinal anesthesia for cesarean section: comparison of 22-Gauge and 25-Gauge Whitacre needles with 26-Gauge Quincke needles. Br J Anaesth 69: 589–594
38. Scott D B, Morrison L M N, Dittmann M et al 1993 Atraucan[R] – a new needle for spinal anesthesia. Reg Anesth 18: 213–217
39. Denny N, Masters R, Pearson D, Read J, Sihota M, Selander D 1987 Postdural puncture headache after continuous spinal anesthesia. Anesth Analg 66: 791–794
40. Norris M C, Leighton B L 1990 Continuous spinal anesthesia after unintentional dural puncture in parturients. Reg Anesth 15: 285–287
41. Thornberry E A, Thomas T A 1988 Posture and post-spinal headache: A controlled trial in 80 obstetric patients. Br J Anaesth 60: 195–197
42. Dieterich M, Brandt T 1988 Incidence of post-lumbar puncture headache is independent of daily fluid intake. Eur Arch Psychiatr Neurol Sci 237: 194–196
43. Abbound T K, Zhu J, Reyes A et al 1992 Effect of subarachnoid morphine on the incidence of spinal headache. Reg Anesth 17: 34–36
44. Thomas D I, Suresh M S, Stride P C, Wilkey A D 1992 Prophylaxis of dural headache-epidural saline bolus versus infusion. Anesth Analg 74: S319
45. Jarvis A P, Greenwalt J W, Frageus L 1986 Intravenous caffeine for postdural puncture headache. Anesth Analg 65: 316–317
46. Camman W R, Murray R S, Lambert D H 1989 caffeine for post-dural puncture headache. Abstracts of the Society for Obstetric Anesthesia and Perinatology Annual Meeting. C–2
47. Schwalbe S S, Schiffmiller M W, Marx G F 1992 Theophylline for post-dural puncture headache (abstract). Anesthesiology 75: A 1082
48. Gromley J B 1960 Treatment of post-dural headache. Anesthesiology 21: 565–566
49. Ostheimer G W, Palahniuk R J, Shnider S M 1974 Epidural blood patch for post-lumbar puncture headache. Anesthesiology 41: 307–308
50. Abouleish E, De LA Vega S, Blendiger I, Tio To 1975 Long-term follow up of epidural blood patch. Anesth Analg 54: 459–463
51. Loeser E A, Hill G E, Bennet G M, Sederberg J H 1978 Time versus success rate for epidural blood patch. Anesthesiology 49: 147–148
52. Palahniuk R J, Cumming M 1979 Prophylactic blood patch does not prevent post lumbar puncture headache. Can Anaesth Soc J 26: 132–133
53. Tom D J, Gulevich S J, Shapiro H M, Heaton R K, Grant I 1992 Epidural blood patch in the HIV-positive patient. Review of clinical experience. Anesthesiology 76: 943–946
54. Griffiths A G, Beards S C, Jackson A, Horsman E L 1993 Visualization of extradural blood patch for post lumbar puncture headache by magnetic resonance imaging. Br J Anaesth 70: 223–225
55. Barrios-Alarcon J, Aldrete J A, Paragas-Tapia D 1989 Relief of post-lumbar puncture headache with epidural dextran 40: a preliminary report. Reg Anesth 14: 78–80

SECTION 4

Cesarean delivery

37. Epidural anesthesia

Part A USA view *R. S. F. Mackay*
Part B European view *L. M. M. Morrison*
J. H. McClure

PART A
USA VIEW
R. S. F. McKay

INTRODUCTION

With nearly one million performed annually,[1] cesarean delivery is the most frequent in-patient surgical procedure in the USA. In a recent national survey of obstetric anesthesia,[2] epidural block was reportedly used in 21% of all cesarean deliveries. In hospitals with the largest obstetric suites (>1500 births), epidural anesthesia accounted for 29% of anesthetics for cesarean delivery. An increase in the use of epidural blockade is partly a reflection of the increased availability in larger centers of anesthesiologists with training in obstetric anesthesia. Awareness of the safety, efficacy and benefits of epidural anesthesia for emergent and complicated obstetric conditions[3-7] has further increased the application of the method.

ADVANTAGES OF EPIDURAL ANESTHESIA

Versus spinal anesthesia

Epidural anesthesia offers an excellent degree of controllability with predictable levels of anesthesia when compared with single-dose spinal anesthesia. The degree of surgery, anesthesia and sympathetic block can be easily adjusted – an important feature in patients in whom rapid onset of sympathetic blockade could be detrimental. In contrast, the extent of block following a single-dose spinal anesthetic may be unpredictable. Russell and Holmqvist[8] administered 12.5 mg of isobaric 0.5% bupivacaine subarachnoid to 40 women; 17 experienced cervical levels of block at some stage and 26 developed hypotension.

The placement of an epidural catheter is a usual component of epidural block and allows the provision of anesthesia for any extension of surgery due to complications. Since the onset of the epidural is not as rapid as that of subarachnoid block, hypotension develops more slowly and is, therefore, more amenable to prevention and therapy. The reduced degree of motor block occurring with epidural sensory anesthesia, a definite advantage in the laboring gravida, may also be beneficial in women undergoing cesarean delivery. Parturients with multiple gestation may have less impairment of ventilation from the same level of epidural blockade compared to spinal blockade.[9]

Dural puncture occurs infrequently during epidural block. In patients having spinal anesthesia, Vandam and Dripps[10] reported a prevalence of headache of 10–16% during the child-bearing years. Women had twice the risk of headache. Smaller gauge needles were associated with a much lower frequency of headache; the number of *headaches* following spinal block nonetheless remained greater than the number of *dural punctures* (with or without headache) occurring during epidural anesthetics. The frequency of the latter by resident anesthesiologists was recently reported as 2.6%,[11] a figure sure to be lower in experienced hands (and in contrast to a 100% prevalence during spinal anesthesia).

Lybecker et al[12] recently performed a prospective study of 1021 patients who received spinal anesthetics and found no difference in the prevalence of headache depending on whether 22-, 25- and 26-gauge needles were used; nor did they find any gender differences (although no obstetric patients were included). Rather, the most important determinants of postdural puncture headache (PDPH) appeared to be the age of the patient and the direction of the needle bevel. Norris et al[11] demonstrated a decrease in the prevalence of headache from 50% to 19% following epidural block when the needle bevel was parallel to the axial dural fibers rather than perpendicular. However, it has been suggested that turning the epidural needle to the perpendicular position after parallel placement may increase the likelihood of dural perforation.[13] Brownridge,[14] using 25- and 26-gauge needles for dural puncture in a combined spinal-epidural technique, had a PDPH prevalence of 8.6%, although the headache was severe in only 2.3%. In 2511 parturients undergoing cesarean delivery, using a 26-gauge needle parallel to the dural fibers, Naulty et al[15] reported a PDPH prevalence of 5.85–9.54%, depending on the local anesthetic used.

Overall, the frequency of PDPH following attempted epidural block is lower than that following spinal anesthesia, despite the use of a much larger needle. The development of micro catheter continuous spinal anesthesia, while overcoming the drawbacks of controllability, duration and too rapid an onset, does involve dural puncture and is not without potential for serious complications.[16] Such complications have resulted in the mandatory withdrawal of micro catheters from the US market.[17] Epidural blockade involves the use of larger doses of local anesthetic than does spinal anesthesia, but in the vast majority of cases this is without clinical significance to either the mother or her fetus/neonate.

Finally, with the concentrations used for cesarean delivery, epidural block may result in a lesser degree of both sensory and motor blockade than spinal block. Some anesthesiologists combine spinal and epidural techniques to obtain the more rapid onset of block and the greater degree of sensory and motor blockade associated with spinal anesthesia while maintaining the ability to titrate through an epidurally placed catheter.[18] This more complicated technique needs further evaluation, with emphasis on the disposition of subsequent epidurally administered drugs and on possible complications such as subarachnoid placement of the presumed epidural catheter (no test dose is possible!). Mets et al[19] suggest spinal puncture *following* epidural anesthesia may result in dangerously high anesthetic levels. To date, however, spinal block followed by epidural anesthesia has appeared to be a safe, effective technique.

Versus general anesthesia

The advantages of regional anesthesia over general anesthesia for cesarean delivery are so numerous as to leave one to wonder why anesthesiologists in the USA still perform over one-third of cesarean deliveries using the latter method. Regional blockade avoids many problems associated with general anesthesia. It allows an awake patient who can interact with her infant and partner during the surgical procedure and who will maintain her own airway with less risk of airway complications, e.g. aspiration or difficulties with intubation. It avoids neonatal depression should the incision-to-delivery interval become prolonged (especially important in repeat cesarean deliveries and women with previous abdominal surgery). The reduction in the incidence of venous thromboses in patients receiving regional versus general anesthesia is well known. With pulmonary embolism being a frequent cause of maternal morbidity and mortality, the foregoing is of obvious importance.

The advantages of epidural block extend well into the postoperative course. By the second postoperative day, fewer epidural patients have gastrointestinal stasis or fever and more are ambulatory and breastfeeding.[20] Patients given general anesthesia tend to be wearier and have less early mother–infant contact.

General anesthesia may be administered more rapidly than regional anesthesia and, therefore, has a significant role in emergency cesarean delivery. While general anesthesia-related complications have been responsible for the majority of maternal anesthesia-related deaths, the number of deaths from epidural anesthesia is not insignificant. Indeed, a hurriedly administered epidural anesthetic without regard for proper safety may carry a higher feto-maternal risk than a general anesthetic given in the same time frame.

Neonatal status

Evans et al[21] found direct depression (low Apgar scores) of fetuses as a result of general anesthesia, especially when exposure was prolonged. No such depression was found in infants of mothers receiving epidural anesthesia for cesarean delivery. Fetal asphyxia was not a cause as no difference in acid–base status was found. Datta et al[22] found fetal acidosis in infants when the induction-to-delivery interval for general anesthesia exceeded 8 min. This study may have been flawed, however, by the effects of maternal hyperventilation, thus one is warned to avoid maternal hyperventilation during general anesthesia rather than to avoid general anesthesia itself.

CONTRAINDICATIONS TO EPIDURAL ANESTHESIA (Table 37.1)

Contraindications to epidural anesthesia include patient refusal, infection at the site of placement, severe systemic infection (septicemia), severe uncorrectable hypovolemia, increased intracranial pressure and coagulopathy. Additionally, the uncooperative patient (including the fearful or young) may place herself at too great a risk through movement during the block or through an inability or refusal to communicate necessary information to the anesthesiologist (e.g. medical history, symptoms of intravascular injection, etc.) The inability to communicate with the patient is becoming an increasing concern among US anesthesiologists as the number of non-English-speaking citizens rises. Multilanguage pamphlets may provide a partial solution, especially where translators are unavailable.[23]

Table 37.1 Contraindications to epidural anesthesia

Absolute
1. Patient refusal
2. Systemic infection
3. Infection at needle insertion site
4. Severe uncorrectable hypovolemia
5. Increased intracranial pressure
6. Most coagulopathies
Relative
1. Uncooperative patient
2. Progressive neurologic disease
3. Moderate hypovolemia
4. Mild coagulopathies
5. Certain cardiac conditions (aortic stenosis, right-to-left shunt)
6. Anatomic anomalies

Systemic infection or infection localized to the site of needle puncture is a contraindication to epidural block because:

1. little resistance to the spread of an infection along the vertical axis of the epidural space exists;
2. the potential for vessel puncture is high, which could seed blood-borne infection or nourish epidural needle-introduced infection;
3. unintentional dural puncture could compromise the blood–brain barrier and lead to CNS infection.

Herpes simplex virus infections are frequently encountered in patients presenting for cesarean delivery and, in fact, are often the reason for the operative procedure. Primary infections are accompanied by a viremia and, therefore, should probably be considered as a contraindication. Recurrent infections are localized and epidural block may be performed as long as lesions are not at the site of needle insertion. Two particular points should be made with regard to herpes viruses. First, no reports of CNS spread of a herpes virus as a result of anesthesia have been published.[24] Second, reactivation of herpes simplex virus labialis by epidural morphine has been postulated,[25,26] though the findings have been questioned.

Patients with mild coagulopathy (e.g. platelets of 100 000–150 000/mm^3) may be at a slightly increased risk for hemorrhagic complications from epidural block, but this risk may not be as significant as those imposed by other anesthetic techniques in an individual patient. Schindler et al[26] have suggested that, if bleeding time is normal, regional anesthesia is acceptable in patients with platelet counts as low as 50 000/mm^3. The usefulness of the bleeding time is suspect, however, so other techniques to evaluate platelet and coagulation function, e.g. thromboelastography and Sonoclot® analysis are now beginning to be used in the US for determination of whether to perform regional anesthesia.[28]

Some patients with progressive neurologic disease may receive a block. However, especially in the USA, they may pose a medicolegal risk should symptoms be exacerbated post delivery. Patients with multiple sclerosis, for example, have a relapse rate during the first 3 months post partum that is 2–3 times higher than during pregnancy[29] whether or not they receive epidural anesthesia. They should be informed of this relapse risk as well as the fact that studies linking epidural anesthesia to such relapses have been inconclusive. Patients with fixed neurologic lesions or pregnancy-induced neurologic symptoms (numbness and tingling in legs, etc.), in contrast, should generally not be deprived of the benefits of epidural block. However, extreme care in the performance of the block and in the subsequent management of the patient (positioning, etc.) is crucial. Anatomic abnormalities are a frequent cause of hesitation. However, women with spina bifida,[30] scoliosis (even after surgical instrumentation), and other such anomalies may generally receive successful blocks, although the possibility of failure[31,32] or complications[33] due to such pathology should be explained to the parturient.

Patients with cardiac disorders (including myocardial infarction[34–36] and transplanted hearts[37]) are generally well managed by epidural block because of the reduction in pre- and afterload and favorable effects on cardiac workload. While patients with right-to-left shunts, aortic stenosis or spinal artery disease may not tolerate the drop in afterload, Eisenmenger's syndrome (with pulmonary hypertension and right-to-left or bidirectional shunt) has been successfully managed under epidural block.[38]

OBSTETRIC CONSIDERATIONS

Epidural anesthesia is appropriate for the vast majority of elective and urgent cesarean deliveries and even some emergency cesarean deliveries (when a working epidural catheter has been previously placed).

Elective cesarean delivery

Epidural anesthesia is generally a safe, effective anesthetic method for elective cesarean delivery. Contraindications would generally be those of any regional anesthetic technique (see above).

Urgent cesarean delivery

Urgent cesarean delivery may include maternal complications that require lengthy evaluation. For example, the preeclamptic woman may need evaluation of platelet function prior to the placement of an epidural block. Nonetheless, the advantages of epidural block may outweigh the disadvantages of the time to perform such a test. Ong et al[39] recently confirmed the tenet that regional anesthesia (predominantly epidural) is generally less depressant to the neonate than general anesthesia, even in emergency cesarean delivery.

Emergency cesarean delivery

Marx et al[40] found regional anesthesia to be an acceptable alternative to general anesthesia in cases of persistent fetal distress. Yet emergent cesarean deliveries (e.g. prolapsed umbilical cord, acute fetal distress, placental abruption, amniotic fluid embolus, complicated preterm labor, etc.) most often require general anesthesia because of insufficient time to establish a regional block, maternal coagulopathy or acute maternal hypovolemia/hemorrhage. Nonetheless, emergency situations arise in women who have had prior anesthetic evaluation and have previously placed and functioning epidural catheters. If maternal homeostasis can be maintained, rapid strengthening of the block with 3% 2-chloroprocaine or 2% lidocaine may allow surgical anesthesia. Frequently, an established labor block is sufficient for commencement of surgery. Thus, enhancement of the block does not always need to precede the onset of surgery.

PHARMACOLOGIC CONSIDERATIONS

Choice of local anesthetic

Three local anesthetics are employed for epidural anesthesia for cesarean delivery in the USA: bupivacaine, lidocaine and 2-chloroprocaine. Etidocaine generally is considered to provide unreliable epidural anesthesia and is seldom used. Dutton et al[41] found that the prevalence of totally painless cesarean delivery was over 60% with bupivacaine 0.5% and 0.75% compared with only 33% with etidocaine 1.5%. Prolonged post-operative residual motor block may also be a disadvantage with the use of etidocaine. Mepivacaine is also rarely used in the USA for cesarean delivery. Recently, however, it has been shown to produce no adverse maternal or fetal effects when used for elective cesarean delivery.[42] Ropivacaine is a new amide local anesthetic structurally related to mepivacaine and bupivacaine. Of similar duration of action and potency to bupivacaine but perhaps of lesser cardiovascular toxicity, it is being evaluated for epidural use in pregnant women.[43] A preliminary study showed that epidural ropivacaine may decrease epidural blood flow in humans when compared with epidural bupivacaine.[44] Should similar vasoconstriction of uteroplacental vessels occur, ropivacaine may fail to find a place in obstetric anesthesia. A reassuring study of ropivacaine in the pregnant ewe[45] did not show adverse effects on uterine blood flow, nor on fetal wellbeing in general. There was no evidence of significant uterine artery vasoconstriction.

Bupivacaine

In a concentration of 0.5%, bupivacaine provides good surgical anesthesia for cesarean delivery when adequate time is allowed for sensory block to be established. Unfortunately, 30 mins or even more may occasionally be needed. The addition of epinephrine or an opioid (e.g. 100 μg of fentanyl) increases the quality and may decrease the onset time of surgical anesthesia. Bupivacaine 0.75% has a faster onset but is no longer used for obstetric anesthesia in the USA because of the risk of cardiotoxicity. However, Marx[46] has pointed out that the patient's peak blood level may depend not on concentration but on the actual dose injected. Onset time may be decreased by using lidocaine sequentially with bupivacaine. Some investigators have demonstrated that the alkalinization of epidural bupivacaine shortens the time of onset and lengthens the duration of sensory anesthesia with bupivacaine.[47] The addition of sodium bicarbonate and epinephrine also yields a faster onset.[48] Others, however, have not been able to find significant bicarbonate-induced changes in the onset time, duration or extent of the block.[49,50] Bupivacaine does form precipitates when sodium bicarbonate is added to raise the pH to 7.0. The combination of 2-chloroprocaine with bupivacaine, while resulting in a faster onset, may lead to reduced effectiveness of subsequent bupivacaine administration.[51] Chloroprocaine is not believed to reduce the effectiveness of epidural morphine as long as adequate analgesia is continued until the onset of morphine's analgesic action.[52]

Lidocaine

Lidocaine 2%, usually with epinephrine, is frequently used for cesarean delivery. Studies in the mid-1970s suggested that lidocaine and mepivacaine led to compromised neonatal neurobehavior, unlike bupivacaine or chloroprocaine.[53,54] Numerous studies in women undergoing cesarean delivery have now exonerated lidocaine.[55–57]

One consideration often overlooked is the effect of gestational age on the response to anesthetics. It is well established that the preterm neonate is more sensitive to depression from anesthetic agents. In several studies of lidocaine in the term and preterm fetal lamb, Morishima et al[58–60] showed that lidocaine levels following epidural block were safe for the healthy term and preterm fetus as well as the asphyxiated mature fetus. However, preterm asphyxiated fetuses exposed to lidocaine lost their circulatory adaptability to asphyxia. This alteration did not occur in mature asphyxiated fetuses exposed to lidocaine. Thus, extrapolating from the ovine model, lidocaine is likely to be an acceptable epidural anesthetic excepting preterm fetuses with distress.

2-Chloroprocaine

2-Chloroprocaine 3% provides a profound anesthetic for cesarean delivery. It has the advantage of very rapid maternal and neonatal metabolism by plasma cholinesterase should intravenous injection occur. The resultant low toxicity may make chloroprocaine the drug of choice in cases of fetal distress. The regression of sensory anesthesia is fairly sudden, and occurs after 45 min to an hour unless additional doses are given. As this is generally insufficient time for the cesarean delivery to be completed, redosing through an epidural catheter is usually required. Therefore, one will not escape a non-functioning catheter, as one might with an initial dose of bupivacaine (given through the needle). Persistent neurologic deficits following the use of earlier formulations of 2-chloroprocaine and confusion as to the cause of the problem (drug, pH, preservative) led to a decline in its use. Carefully controlled studies have determined that the deficits could be caused by either low pH, the bisulfite (0.2%) preservative or a combination thereof.[61] 2-Chloroprocaine has been reformulated into a bisulfite-free solution at a higher pH and its use is now increasing.

Chloroprocaine's safety is further enhanced in that patients reliably experience symptoms of intravascular injection. These symptoms occur less predictably with lidocaine and bupivacaine. Subarachnoid deposition of large doses (i.e. those intended for epidural administration) of chloroprocaine is still felt to be potentially hazardous. Should it occur, aspiration of CSF with replacement by preservative-free saline is prudent.

Combinations of local anesthetics

Any expectation of reduced toxicity from the use of multiple drugs has not been demonstrated. Toxicities of mixtures are additive, but are neither synergistic nor antagonistic.[62] Combinations of bupivacaine and lidocaine remain in frequent use, however, to take advantage of the more rapid onset and lower toxicity of lidocaine as well as the longer duration of bupivacaine.

Use of opioids

The addition of fentanyl 100 µg to 0.5% bupivacaine has been demonstrated to provide significantly better intraoperative pain relief.[63,64] Mild pruritus may occur, but neonatal condition appears unaffected. Sufentanil 10, 20, 30 and 50 µg was compared with fentanyl 100 µg for cesarean delivery analgesia under carbonated lidocaine epidural block by Madej and Strunin.[65] No significant advantages were found, but sufentanil 50 µg caused a significant increase in unpleasant side-effects.

Meperidine (25 mg) may be advantageous in combination with local anesthetic for cesarean delivery in that it may be more effective at reducing shivering. Given within 1 h of delivery, its neonatal effects are negligible.[66] However, a drug-to-delivery interval of 2–3 h results in maximum neonatal meperidine and high neonatal normeperidine levels.[67] Its use in epidural anesthesia for cesarean delivery may help bridge the analgesic gap between local anesthetic regression and onset of epidural morphine.

Diamorphine (heroin) is not available for medical use in the USA.

Addition of vasopressors

Epinephrine 1 : 200 000 added to bupivacaine for cesarean delivery does not reduce absorption from the epidural space in the pregnant patient but does lower the bupivacaine requirement, resulting in lower blood levels in elective cesarean deliveries but not in those following labor.[68] Epinephrine significantly prolongs the action of 2-chloroprocaine. As with bupivacaine, epinephrine has been found to have little effect on the blood levels of lidocaine during elective cesarean delivery, although it does enhance the quality of the block.[69]

Many obstetric anesthesiologists are wary of the α-adrenergic effects of epinephrine on the uterine artery. This is especially controversial when epinephrine is given in test doses to detect intravenous catheter placement. Some choose to avoid epinephrine entirely, instead relying on fractionation of doses in which every dose becomes a test dose.[70] Also, the 1 : 200 000 concentration generally used for epidural block is not necessary to obtain the effects of epinephrine on the quality of the block. Brose and Cohen[69] found a 1 : 400 000 concentration to be as effective as 1 : 200 000 with respect to quality of analgesia. Onset of anesthesia was actually more rapid with the 1 : 400 000 concentration. A recommendation of an epinephrine concentration no greater than 1 : 300 000 in obstetrics would not seem unreasonable.

Isoproterenol, having little α-adrenergic effect, has been proposed as an alternative to epinephrine for test dosing. Isoproterenol does not have the biphasic response on heart rate associated with epinephrine[71] and therefore may be more reliable. The finding that the chronotropic response in pregnant women was greatly reduced[72] led to the evaluation of a 5-µg test dose. However, the preeclamptic woman, not surprisingly, has an exaggerated response compared with her normal term pregnant counterpart, and may exhibit hypotension or exaggerated tachycardia with the same dose.[73]

PREANESTHETIC EVALUATION

The assumption that a pregnant woman is young and therefore healthy may occasionally be erroneous. A complete history and appropriate examination must be performed on each woman who presents for the procedure. The indication for cesarean delivery should not overshadow other maternal conditions, e.g. recent cocaine ingestion, which may have significant maternal and fetal/neonatal anesthetic implications. Likewise, the plan for epidural anesthesia does not allow an anesthesiologist to ignore conditions more pertinent to general anesthesia (e.g. time of last oral intake) as any epidural anesthetic may need to be converted to a general anesthetic should certain complications arise! If adequate time is not available to obtain a reasonable history, it is unlikely that adequate time is available for the performance of a regional anesthetic. Discussion of the procedure, alternatives and risks (informed consent) should precede each anesthetic.

TECHNIQUES AND DOSAGES

Preliminary comments

The choice of the particular technique for epidural anesthesia for cesarean delivery should depend on the anesthesiologist's experience and knowledge of the technique and, secondly, on the conditions placed on the anesthesiologist by the obstetric situation. The minimal dose of drug(s) to accomplish the goal of a safe and effective anesthetic should be used.

Influences on levels of analgesia

Posture plays a much smaller role in the spread of epidural anesthesia than in the spread of spinal anesthesia. Norris et al[74] and Pitkanen et al[75] found that gravity played little role in the spread of epidural anesthesia in patients placed laterally. In fact, Norris and colleagues found higher cephalad spread of sensory blockade on the nondependent side. Dosages in the sitting position usually vary little from those in the lateral position, especially if the sitting position is maintained only during the placement of the block.

INTRAOPERATIVE COMPLICATIONS

Hypotension

Uncorrected hypotension after regional anesthesia can result in fetal/neonatal acidosis. Failure to anticipate the effects of sympathetic block on vascular capacitance will generally lead to hypotension. For cesarean delivery, 30 ml/kg crystalloid will reliably prevent hypotension (H S Choi, personal communication). A smaller preload is associated with a greater incidence of hypotension. The speed of onset of block also is important. The use of bupivacaine allows a greater amount of time to compensate for the effects of sympathetic blockade. Extensive sympathetic block affecting the cardiac accelerator fibers may prevent the increase in cardiac output that normally occurs in response to hypotension.[76] Even without block of the cardiac accelerator fibers, however, relative hypovolemia (as from aortocaval compression or inadequate acute hydration) may lead to a reflex bradycardia. The slow heart rate then leads to an inadequate cardiac output and hypotension.[77] Therefore excessive levels of block, hypovolemia and aortocaval compression should be avoided. Maternal discomfort from loss of the sensation of intercostal muscle function also occurs with high levels of sensory anesthesia.

Maternal hemorrhage associated with uterine atony, surgical trauma or placenta accreta and related conditions may also readily induce hypotension. While these conditions generally follow delivery, they may threaten maternal well-being and need to be managed appropriately and promptly. Uterine atony usually responds to uterine massage and increased infusion of oxytocin. Methylergonovine is a potent uterine stimulant that should usually not be given intravenously owing to its profound α-stimulating effects, which could precipitate severe hypertension and stroke. The intramuscular administration of 0.2 mg effectively increases uterine tone while supporting the circulation. Finally, if methylergonovine is ineffective, prostaglandins may be injected directly into the uterus. 15-Methyl-$PGF_{2\alpha}$ (Prostin/15M) is currently available in the USA. An intramyometrial dose of 250 μg is used. This dose may be repeated after 15 min. Failure of these and other (surgical) measures to control blood loss can indicate the necessity for cesarean hysterectomy.

Hypotension from cardiac decompensation is a rare event during cesarean delivery but may result from fluid overload (especially after a long induction of labor with the use of oxytocics, or after excessive hydration in a preeclamptic), myocardial ischemia or any of the various embolic phenomena.

Relative hypovolemia due to patient positioning is a not an infrequent cause of hypotension, especially in the presence of an inexperienced anesthesiologist. Venocaval compression decreases venous return and will frequently cause hypotension. More importantly, aortoiliac compression also decreases uterine blood flow, without maternal signs or symptoms. It must be avoided by the use of uterine displacement. Steep head-up tilt is frequently used by inexperienced anesthesiologists to try to limit a high block. While having little effect on the level of block, it may have significant effect in regard to decreasing venous return, leading to hypotension, and, in the case of unintentional total spinal anesthesia, cardiovascular collapse.

Inadequate analgesia/sensory anesthesia

Absolute (pain at onset of surgical procedure)

When adequate anesthesia has not been established at the time of initial surgical incision, either too brief a time has been allowed for onset of the block, an inadequate dose has been given or the block has failed for technical reasons. If time allows, the anesthesiologist should determine which cause is most likely. In the case of failed block for an elective cesarean delivery, it may be wise to postpone surgery to allow blood levels of anesthetic to diminish and then to repeat the block. The addition of a spinal block allows surgery to proceed under regional anesthesia without fear of increased blood levels of anesthetic. However, there may be a significant risk of subarachnoid transfer of epidural drug resulting in excessively high sensory levels as suggested by three recent case reports.[19,78,79] Finally, if time is inadequate to establish adequate blockade, general anesthesia should be carefully induced.

Relative (pain developing intraoperatively)

Pain developing after skin incision may be from the same causes as above. However, options once surgery has started are more limited. If surgical stimuli can be stopped, more time may be allowed for the block to set up or be reinforced. If pain is limited to a certain area of the surgical field, local anesthesia may be administered to those areas. For mild to moderate pain, small doses of ketamine (10–20 mg) may allow the patient to be comfortable while surgery proceeds. If possible, intravenous opioids and amnestic agents should be reserved until after cord clamping. Many patients have discomfort, especially pressure, at the time of delivery. The vast majority need only be told of the short duration of such discomfort and will do well without medications. The arrival of their infant will then usually distract them from any mild discomfort during repair of the uterus.

Pain beginning after delivery is not uncommon, although the etiologies are sometimes uncertain. There may be increased surgical stimulation with peritoneal irritation and exteriorization of the uterus. Visceral pain during cesarean delivery is frequent during uterine exteriorization. Unfortunately, many obstetricians feel that such exteriorization is necessary to ensure adequate examination and repair of the uterus. This pain can generally be controlled by the addition of opioid to the epidural block or by small intravenous doses of opioid (25–50 μg of fentanyl). Alahuhta et al[80] compared the incidence and severity of visceral pain under spinal and epidural anesthesia and found no difference between the two techniques. Mild sedation may also be helpful. Diazepam may be superior to midazolam in that it causes less amnesia of the birth event.

As with hypotension, embolic events and cardiac ischemia may cause chest discomfort. Careful monitoring of the patient should enable the anesthesiologist to differentiate these from surgical pain. The majority of patients undergoing cesarean delivery may have Doppler changes consistent with venous air embolism.[81,82] These changes occur during uterine repair and are responsible for a significant amount of the chest discomfort and desaturation seen post delivery. Chest discomfort along with ECG changes (e.g. ST segment depression) may accompany decreases in the $Sa\text{O}_2$, suggesting ischemia as a cause of the chest discomfort. These changes nearly always resolve spontaneously and are of uncertain significance.[83–86] However, air emboli may be accompanied by hypotension or even cardiac arrest if massive (400–500 ml). Head-up tilt (5–10°) has not been shown to prevent air embolism,[82,87] but Fowler's position (head-up) should be avoided. The lower incidence in regional versus general anesthesia suggests that acute hydration is helpful.[88]

Amniotic fluid embolism

Amniotic fluid embolism (AFE) results in pulmonary vasospasm (prostaglandin $F_{2\alpha}$-related) which causes sudden pulmonary hypertension and right heart failure. The sudden decrease in pulmonary venous return decreases cardiac output. Ventilation–perfusion abnormalities cause marked hypoxia. Bronchospasm occurs only rarely. Additionally, disseminated intravascular coagulation followed by severe hemorrhage results from the release of thromboplastin-like substances from placental tissue and amniotic fluid. Uterine atony results from hypotension and decreased uterine perfusion as well as direct myometrial depression. Respiratory distress, cyanosis, cardiovascular collapse and coma generally occur, although bleeding may be the presenting sign. Management of AFE is discussed in Chapter 57.

Peripheral nerve injuries

Careful positioning of the patient should avoid these injuries in a woman undergoing cesarean delivery. Recently, injury to a radial nerve caused by an automated blood pressure machine repeated attempting to obtain a reading was reported.[89] Attention to the patient should not become lax just because she has been given a 'safe' regional anesthetic.

Extensive anesthesia

Unpredictable responses of patients may occasionally lead to a high epidural block, even when meticulous care has been taken. The cardiovascular effects of such a block are discussed above. Additionally, a patient may become short of breath as sensation to the intercostal muscles is lost. Usually, reassurance (watching chest rise, feeling air movement at mouth, breathing oxygen) is sufficient therapy. If, however, the patient develops respiratory distress, more active measures must be taken. A more stoic patient may allow mask-assisted ventilation. If this remains unsatisfactory and the reason for distress is indeed a high block and not anxiety, further sedation of the patient is not indicated as this may only result in significant respiratory depression. Rather, general anesthesia should be induced after acute oxygenation and denitrogenation. Surgical manipulations should be halted during induction to avoid gastric pressure increases.

Horner's syndrome will occasionally result from the high sympathetic block accompanying epidural anesthesia for cesarean delivery. Most often this seems limited to stuffiness of the nose and injected conjunctivae. Rarely, the complete syndrome, with ptosis, miosis, enophthalmus and vasodilation of the face, may result. Other causes of unexpectedly high block are unintentional subdural[90] or subarachnoid injections. Management is that of high or total spinal block.

POST-OPERATIVE ANALGESIA

Epidural opioids

Epidural morphine has continued to be in the forefront of post-cesarean analgesia in patients having epidural anesthesia for cesarean delivery. Significant respiratory depression from smaller doses of epidural morphine (5 mg) in the obstetric patient is very rare but appropriate monitoring of the patient is a must. Epidural morphine does have a 45–60 min latency, so must be given prior to block regression. Side-effects such as itching, nausea and vomiting can be minimized by concurrent naloxone infusion (25 µg/h); alternatively, 5 mg bolus doses of nalbuphine have been advocated.[91] This dose has little effect on the pain relief. See Chapter 41 for a more detailed discussion of epidural opioids.

Patient-controlled analgesia (PCA)

While objectively less effective than epidural morphine, patient satisfaction with PCA is very high. Problems have included the need for specialized pumps and manipulation of the boluses by people other than the patient.[92]

COMPLICATIONS

Complications which may develop during epidural anesthesia for cesarean delivery are those of epidural anesthesia in general. Toxic reactions (total spinal, seizures, cardiac arrest) may be more likely during anesthesia for cesarean delivery because greater drug concentrations and amounts are employed. Likewise, the use of epidural opioids for post-operative pain control may be associated with additional complications.

REFERENCES

1. Stafford R S 1991 The impact of nonclinical factors on repeat cesarean section. J Am Med Assoc 265: 59–63
2. Gibbs C P, Krischer J, Peckham B M, Sharp H, Kirschbaum T H 1986 Obstetric Anesthesia: a national survey. Anesthesiology 65: 298–306
3. Jouppila P, Jouppila R, Hollmén A, Koivula A 1982 Lumbar epidural analgesia to improve intervillous blood flow during labor in severe preeclampsia. Obstet Gynecol 59: 158–161
4. Duffy B L 1982 Pregnancy and triple heart valve prosthesis. Anaesth Intensive Care 10: 59–61
5. Flamm B L, Dunnett C, Fischerman E, Quilligan E J 1984 Vaginal delivery following cesarean section: use of oxytocin augmentation and epidural anesthesia with internal tocodynamic and internal fetal monitoring. Am J Obstet Gynecol 148: 759–763
6. Marx G F, Luykx W M, Cohen S 1984 Fetal–neonatal status following caesarean section for fetal distress. Br J Anaesth 56: 1009–1013
7. Marks R J, DeChazal R C S 1984 Ritodrine-induced pulmonary oedema in labour. Successful management using epidural anaesthesia. Anaesthesia 39: 1012–1014
8. Russell I F, Holmqvist E L O 1987 Subarachnoid analgesia for caesarean section: a double-blind comparison of plain and hyperbaric 0.5% bupivacaine. Br J Anaesth 59: 347–353
9. Reisner L S 1990 Anesthesia for cesarean section. Anesth Clin N Am 8: 87
10. Vandam L D, Dripps R D 1956 Long-term follow-up of patients who received 10,098 spinal anesthetics. III. Syndrome of decreased intracranial pressure (headache and ocular and auditory difficulties). J Am Med Assoc 161: 586–591
11. Norris M C, Leighton B L, Desimone C A 1989 Needle bevel direction and headache after inadvertent dural puncture. Anesthesiology 70: 729–731
12. Lybecker H, Møller J T, May O, Nielsen H K 1990 Incidence and prediction of postural puncture headache. A prospective study of 1021 spinal headaches. Anesth Analg 70: 389–394
13. Meiklejohn B H 1987 The effect of rotation of an epidural needle. An in vitro study. Anaesthesia 42: 1180–1182
14. Brownridge P 1984 Spinal anaesthesia revisited: an evaluation of subarachnoid block in obstetrics. Anaesth Intensive Care 12: 334–342
15. Naulty J S, Hertwig L, Hunt C O, Datta S, Ostheimer G W, Weiss J B 1990 Influence of local anaesthetic solution on postdural puncture headache. Anesthesiology 72: 450–454
16. Rigler M L, Drasner K, Krejcie T C, Yelich S J, Scholnick F T, DeFontes J, Bohner D 1991 Cauda equina syndrome after continuous spinal anesthesia. Anesth Analg 72: 275–281
17. United States Food and Drug Administration Safety Alert Summer 1992
18. Rawal N, Schollin J, Wesström G 1988 Epidural versus combined spinal epidural block for caesarean section. Acta Anaesthesiol Scand 32: 61–66
19. Mets B, Broccoli E, Brown A R 1993 Is spinal anesthesia after failed epidural anesthesia contraindicated for cesarean section? Anesth Analg 77: 629–631
20. Morgan B M, Barker J P, Goroszeniuk T, Aulakh J M, Reginald P W, Trojanowski A 1984 Anaesthetic morbidity following caesarean section under epidural or general anaesthesia. Lancet 2: 328–330
21. Evans C M, Murphy J F, Gray O P, Rosen M 1989 Epidural versus general anaesthesia for elective cesarean section. Effect on Apgar score and acid–base status of the newborn. Anaesthesia 44: 778–782
22. Datta S, Ostheimer G W, Weiss J B, Brown Jr W U, Alper M H 1981 Neonatal effect of prolonged anesthetic induction for cesarean section. Obstet Gynecol 58: 331–335
23. Weeks S K 1993 Overcoming the language barrier in obstetric anesthesia practice. Anesthesiology 78: 407
24. Crosby E T, Halpern S H, Rolbin S H 1989 Epidural anaesthesia for caesarean section in patients with active recurrent genital herpes simplex infections: a retrospective review. Can J Anaesth 36: 701–704
25. Crone L-A L, Conly J M, Clark K M et al 1988 Recurrent herpes simplex virus labialis and the use of epidural morphine in obstetric patients. Anesth Analg 67: 318–323
26. Gieraerts R, Navalgund A, Vaes L, Soetens M, Chang J-L, Jahr J 1987 Increased incidence of itching and herpes simplex in patients given epidural morphine after cesarean section. Anesth Analg 66: 1321–1324
27. Schindler M, Gatt S, Isert P, Morgans D, Cheung A 1990

Thrombocytopenia and platelet functional defects in pre-eclampsia: implications for regional anaesthesia. Anaesth Intensive Care 18: 169–174
28. Steer P L 1993 Anaesthetic management of a parturient with thrombocytopenia using thromboelastography and Sonoclot analysis. Canad J Anaesth 40: 84–85
29. Rolbin S H 1989 Personal communication
30. Vaaqagenes P, Fjaerestad I 1981 Epidural block during labour in a patient with spinal bifida. Anaesthesia 36: 299–301
31. Moran D H, Johnson M D 1990 Continuous spinal anaesthesia with combined hyperbaric and isobaric bupivacaine in a patient with scoliosis. Anesth Analg 70: 445–447
32. Crosby E T, Halpern S H 1989 Obstetric epidural anaesthesia in patients with Harrington instrumentation. Can J Anaesth 36: 693–696
33. McGrady E M, Davis A G 1988 Spina bifida occulta and epidural anaesthesia. Anaesthesia 43: 867–869
34. Rosenlund R C, Marx G F 1988 Anaesthetic management of a parturient with prior myocardial infarction and coronary artery bypass graft. Can J Anaesth 35: 515–517
35. Dawson P J, Ross A W 1988 Preeclampsia in a parturient with a history of myocardial infarction. Anaesthesia 43: 659–663
36. Stokes I M, Evans J, Stone M 1984 Myocardial infarction and cardiac arrest in the second trimester followed by assisted vaginal delivery under epidural analgesia at 38 weeks gestation. Case report. Br J Obstet Gynaecol 91: 197–198
37. Camann W R, Goldman G A, Johnson M D, Moore J, Greene M 1989 Cesarean delivery in a patient with a transplant heart. Anesthesiology 71: 618–620
38. Spinnato J A, Kraynack B J, Cooper M W 1981 Eisenmenger's syndrome in pregnancy: epidural anaesthesia for elective cesarean section. New Engl J Med 304: 1215–1217
39. Ong B Y, Cohen M M, Palahniuk R J 1989 Anesthesia for cesarean section – effects on neonates. Anesth Analg 68: 270–275
40. Marx G F, Luykx W M, Cohen S 1984 Fetal–neonatal status following caesarean section for fetal distress. Br J Anaesth 56: 1009–1013
41. Dutton D A, Moir D D, Howie H B, Thorburn J, Watson R 1984 Choice of local anesthetic drug for extradural caesarean section. Comparison of 0.5% and 0.75% bupivacaine and 1.5% etidocaine. Br J Anaesth 56: 1361–1367
42. Abboud T K, Moore M J, Jacobs J, Murakawa K, Soraya M, Zhu J 1987 Epidural mepivacaine for cesarean section. Maternal and neonatal effects. Reg Anesth 12: 76–79
43. Katz J A, Knarr K, Bridenbaugh P O 1990 A double-blind comparison of 0.5% bupivacaine and 0.75% ropivacaine administered epidurally in humans. Reg Anesth 15: 250–252
44. Dahl J B, Simonsen L, Mogensen T, Henriksen J H, Kehlet H 1990 The effect of 0.5% ropivacaine on epidural blood flow. Acta Anaesthesiol Scand 34: 305–310
45. Santos A C, Arthur G R, Roberts D J et al 1992 Effect of ropivacaine and bupivacaine on uterine blood flow in pregnant ewes. Anesth Analg 74: 62–67
46. Marx G F 1986 Bupivacaine cardiotoxicity – concentration or dose? Anesthesiology 65: 116
47. McMorland G H, Douglas M J, Axelson J E et al The effect of pH adjustment of bupivacaine on onset and duration of epidural anaesthesia for caesarean section. Can J Anaesth 35: 457–461
48. Tackely R M, Coe A J 1988 Alkalinised bupivacaine and adrenaline for epidural caesarean section. A comparison with 0.5% bupivacaine. Anaesthesia 43: 1019–1021
49. Benhamou D, Perrachon N, Labaille T, Bonhomme L 1989 Alkalinization of epidural 0.5% bupivacaine for cesarean section. Reg Anesth 14: 240–243
50. Stevens R A, Schubert A, Spitzer L, Chester W L, Brandon D, Grueter J A, Clayton B 1989 The effect of pH adjustment of 0.5% bupivacaine on the latency of epidural anesthesia. Reg Anesth 14: 236–239
51. Corke B C, Carlson C G, Dettbarn W D 1984 The influence of 2-chloroprocaine on the subsequent analgesic potency of bupivacaine. Anesthesiology 60: 25–27
52. Hughes S C, Wright R G, Murphy D, Preston P, Hughes W, Rosen M, Shnider S 1988 The effect of pH adjusting 3% 2-chloroprocaine on the quality of post-cesarean section analgesia with epidural morphine. Anesthesiology 69: A689
53. Scanlon J W, Brown W R, Weiss J B, Alper M H 1974 Neurobehavioral responses of newborn infants after maternal epidural anesthesia. Anesthesiology 40: 121–128
54. Scanlon J W, Ostheimer G W, Lurie A O, Brown W U, Weiss J B, Alper M H 1976 Neurobehavioral responses and drug concentrations in newborns after maternal epidural anesthesia with bupivacaine. Anesthesiology 45: 400–405
55. Abboud T K, Kyung C K, Noueihed R et al 1983 Epidural bupivacaine, chloroprocaine or lidocaine for cesarean section – maternal and neonatal effects. Anesth Analg 62: 914–919
56. Kileff M E, James F M, Dewan D M, Floyd H M 1984 Neonatal neurobehavioral responses after epidural anesthesia for cesarean section using lidocaine and bupivacaine. Anesth Analg 63: 413–417
57. Kuhnert B R, Harrison M J, Linn P L, Kuhnert P M 1984 Effect of maternal epidural anesthesia on neonatal behavior. Anesth Analg 63: 301–308
58. Morishima H O, Santos A C, Pedersen H et al 1987 Effect of lidocaine on the asphyxial responses in the mature fetal lamb. Anesthesiology 66: 502–507
59. Pedersen H, Santos A C, Morishima H O, Finster M, Piosker H, Arthur G R, Covino B 1988 Does gestational age affect the pharmacokinetics and pharmacodynamics of lidocaine in mother and fetus? Anesthesiology 68: 367–372
60. Morishima H O, Pedersen H, Santos A C, Schapiro H M, Finster M, Arthur G R, Covino B G 1989 Adverse effects of maternally administered lidocaine on the asphyxiated preterm fetal lamb. Anesthesiology 71: 110–115
61. Ford D J, Raj P P 1987 Peripheral neurotoxicity of 2-chloroprocaine and bisulfite in the cat. Anesth Analg 66: 719–722
62. Spiegel D A, Dexter F, Warner D S et al 1992 Central nervous system toxicity of local anesthetic mixtures in the rat. Anesth Analg 75: 922–928
63. Paech M J, Westmore M D, Spiers H M 1990 A double-blind comparison of epidural bupivacaine and bupivacaine–fentanyl for cesarean section. Anaesth Intensive Care 18: 22–30
64. King M J, Bowden M I, Cooper G M 1990 Epidural fentanyl and 0.5% bupivacaine for elective cesarean section. Anaesthesia 49: 285–288
65. Madej T H, Strunin L 1987 Comparison of epidural fentanyl with sufentanil. Analgesia and side effects after a single bolus dose during elective caesarean section. Anaesthesia 42: 1156–1161
66. Shnider S M, Moya F 1964 Effects of meperidine on the newborn infant. Am J Obstet Gynecol 89: 1009–1015
67. Kuhnert B R, Kuhnert P M, Tu A L, Lin D C K 1979 Meperidine and normeperidine levels following meperidine administration during labor. II. Fetus and neonate. Am J Obstet Gynecol 133: 909–914
68. Laishley R S, Morgan B M, Reynolds F 1987 Effect of adrenaline on extradural anaesthesia and plasma bupivacaine concentrations during caesarean section. Br J Anaesth 60: 180–186
69. Brose W G, Cohen S E 1988 Epidural lidocaine for cesarean section. Effect of varying epinephrine concentration. Anesthesiology 69: 936–940
70. Gutsche B B, Cheek T G Personal communication
71. Leighton B L, DeSimone C A, Norris M C, Chayen B 1989 Isoproterenol is an effective marker of intravenous injection in laboring women. Anesthesiology 71: 206–209
72. DeSimone C A, Leighton B L, Norris M C, Chayen B, Menduka H 1988 The chronotropic effect of isoproterenol is reduced in term pregnant women. Anesthesiology 69: 626–628
73. Leighton B L, Norris M C, DeSimone C A, Darby M J, Menduka H 1990 Pre-eclamptic and healthy term pregnant patients have different chronotropic responses to isoproterenol. Anesthesiology 72: 392–393
74. Norris M C, Leighton B L, DeSimone C A, Larijani G E 1988 Lateral position and epidural anesthesia for cesarean section. Anesth Analg 67: 788–790
75. Pitkanen M T, Paatero H, Rosenberg P H 1988 The effect of maternal lateral position or position change on epidural anesthesia and plasma bupivacaine concentrations. Reg Anesth 13: 157–161

76. Otton P E, Wilson E J 1966 The cardiopulmonary effect of upper thoracic epidural analgesia. Can Anaesth Soc J 13: 541
77. Jacobsen J, Søfelt S, Brocks V et al 1992 Reduced left ventricular diameters at onset of bradycardia during epidural anaesthesia. Acta Anaesthesiol Scand 36: 831–836
78. Stone P A, Thorburn J, Lamb K S R 1989 Complications of spinal anaesthesia following extradural block for caesarean section. Br J Anaesth 62: 335–337
79. Beck G N, Griffiths A G 1992 Failed extradural anaesthesia for caesarean section. Complications of subsequent spinal block. Anaesthesia 47: 690–692
80. Alahuhta S, Kangas-Saarela T, Hollmén A I, Edström H H 1990 Visceral pain during caesarean section under spinal and epidural anaesthesia with bupivacaine. Acta Anaesthesiol Scand 34: 95–98
81. Vartikar J V, Johnson M D, Datta S 1989 Precordial Doppler monitoring and pulse oximetry during cesarean delivery: Detection of venous air embolism. Reg Anesth 14: 145–148
82. Lew T W K, Tay D H B, Thomas E 1993 Venous air embolism during cesarean section: More common than previously thought. Anesth Analg 77: 448–452
83. Palmer C M, Norris M C, Guidici M C et al 1990 Incidence of electrocardiographic changes during cesarean delivery under regional anesthesia. Anesth Analg 70: 36–43
84. Trotter T N, Langton J A, Barker P, Rowbotham D J 1992 Perioperative continuous monitoring of ST-segment changes in patients undergoing elective caesarean section. Br J Anaesth 69: 352–355
85. Mathew J P, Fleisher L A, Rinehouse J A et al 1992 ST segment depression during labor and delivery. Anesthesiology 77: 635–641
86. Zakowski M I, Ramanathan S, Baratta J B et al 1993 Electrocardiographic changes during cesarean section: a cause for concern. Anesth Analg 76: 162–167
87. Karuparthy V R, Downing J W, Hussein F J, Knape K G, Blanchard J, Solomon D, Albin M S 1989 Incidence of venous air embolism during cesarean section is unchanged by the use of a 5 to 10° head-up tilt. Anesth Analg 69: 620–623
88. Fong J, Gadalla F, Pierri M K, Koff H, Artusio Jr J F 1988 Incidence of venous air embolism during cesarean section. Anesthesiology 69: A655
89. Bickler P E, Schapera A, Bainton C R 1990 Acute radial nerve injury from use of an automatic blood pressure monitor. Anesthesiology 73: 186–188
90. Collier C B 1992 Accidental subdural block: Four more cases and a radiographic review. Anaesth Intens Care 20: 215–232
91. Cohen S E, Ratner E F, Kreitzman R T et al 1992 Nalbuphine is better than naloxone for treatment of side effects after epidural morphine. Anesth Analg 75: 747–752
92. Wakerlin G, Larson Jr C P 1990 Spouse-controlled analgesia. Anesth Analg 70: 119

PART B
EUROPEAN VIEW

L. M. M. Morrison J. H. McClure

INTRODUCTION

Medical audit in the form of morbidity and mortality meetings and clinicopathologic conferences has been a feature of hospital practice in the UK for some time, but it has only recently become formalized nationally in the publications of the CEPOD (Committee of Enquiry into Perioperative Deaths).[1] However, the triennial Reports on Confidential Enquiries into Maternal Deaths in England and Wales have been published since 1952. These reports have provided information about the causes and contributing factors in maternal deaths over the past 30 years with comments about their significance and advice about methods of improvement in obstetric practice, including anesthesia.

The most recent report covers the years 1985–87 and is the first report to combine information from the four countries of the UK.[2] There has been an overall decrease in direct maternal deaths since the 1970–72 report despite an increase in the cesarean delivery rate from 5% in 1970–72 to 10% in 1982–84. Anesthesia was the commonest immediate cause of death associated with cesarean delivery, but has now moved into sixth place. Mortality is still higher among those women undergoing emergency cesarean delivery than those having this procedure electively. The condition for which the emergency cesarean delivery is performed is the most important risk factor, but the procedure is inherently more dangerous because of lack of preparation, the stressed condition of the mother and the sense of urgency engendered in the staff.

The report also draws attention to the degree of experience necessary in the obstetric anesthesiologist. In the UK most emergency cesarean deliveries are performed by junior obstetric and anesthetic staff, and it is suggested that the risks of emergency cesarean delivery could be reduced by full consultation with, and back-up from, designated consultants with expertise in obstetric anesthesia. In addition, early involvement of the anesthesiologist in any patient potentially requiring operative delivery is encouraged because this allows the anesthesiologist to discuss and plan the management of the patient in advance. The latest report also points out that the increasing use of appropriately supervised regional anesthesia has contributed to the decline in maternal mortality.

Traditionally, of the two main techniques of regional anesthesia for cesarean delivery used in the UK, epidural has been favored over spinal anesthesia. The reason for this is partly historical. Following the report from Kennedy et al (1950)[3] concerning two patients who developed spastic paraparesis after spinal anesthesia in 1947, this technique declined in popularity. Epidural anesthesia in general surgical practice using a catheter technique was popularized in the UK by Massey Dawkins in the 1960s. The technique was increasingly used in the UK to provide pain relief labor in the late 1960s and 1970s.[4]

The Obstetric Anaesthetists Association played an important role in the UK in promoting recognition of epidural anesthesia as an integral part of modern obstetric management. Although obstetric and public opinion is still somewhat ambivalent towards epidural anesthesia in normal labor, there is today no such doubt about the value of epidural anesthesia for cesarean delivery.

The ability to predict high-risk obstetric patients is clearly of value. In a prospective observational study, Morgan et al[5] found that the requirement for emergency cesarean delivery could be anticipated in 87% of 360 consecutive cesarean deliveries. In addition, the early establishment of an epidural anesthetic allowed extension to an appropriate level for surgery in 70% of the patients.

During the last 10 years most of the original contraindications to epidural block, including twin pregnancy, breech delivery and previous cesarean delivery, have been removed. The indications for the use of epidural anesthesia for cesarean delivery have for a number of years been classified into maternal, labor and, of most importance, fetal.

Epidural anesthesia is indicated in any labor in which an anticipated problem would otherwise necessitate general anesthesia with the risks of tracheal intubation or acid aspiration syndrome provided there are no contraindications per se. Therefore, prolonged labor, slow dilation of the cervix, incoordinate uterine action, failure of the presenting part to descend, twin pregnancy, breech presentation, trial of labor and previous cesarean delivery may all suggest the need for operative intervention and should therefore prompt staff to encourage these women to accept the placement of an epidural catheter.

The well-being of the fetus tends to encourage the use of epidural anesthesia in labor for premature, twin and breech deliveries regardless of whether cesarean delivery is anticipated. The place of an epidural anesthetic in cases of fetal distress is more controversial. The anesthesiologist and obstetrician involved must balance the time taken to establish the block with the urgency of delivery.

PREOPERATIVE ASSESSMENT

Assessment of patients for cesarean delivery utilizing epidural anesthesia whether elective or unplanned demands that the mother should be visited preoperatively. The media in Britain have done much to improve the awareness of women about child-bearing practices, but misconceptions do still persist. For example, Hardwick describes the fear of 'doctors attracting complications'.[6] Therefore, the visit by the anesthesiologist is intended not only to ascertain that there are no untoward physical features of the patient but also to give the anesthesiologist the opportunity to describe in detail each of the steps in the preanesthetic preparation of the mother and to reassure her. Fears about the occurrence of headache and backache after the epidural anesthetic are frequently expressed by mothers and require particular explanation and reassurance. MacArthur et al[7] claim that the relationship between backache and epidural is probably causal except when the epidural is performed for elective cesarean delivery. Postural low backache may result when the patient is placed in a position that is unusual for them for a period of time long enough to strain muscles and ligaments that are operative in low back function.

Most maternity units in Britain invite the father to be present at delivery. This, together with being able to see and touch the baby, help to prevent psychological problems developing in the post-partum period.

Premedication

Van Steenberge[8] describes the prescription of a benzodiazepine on the night before surgery, but Crawford[9] suggests that, although diazepam 5 mg can be given with premedication for excessive anxiety, it should not be a routine measure as it is 'a contradiction in terms for a mother who has asked to be awake during her operative delivery'.[9]

Antacid therapy

The legacy of maternal deaths from obstruction of the respiratory tract by semisolid material led to the introduction of low-fat, low-residue diets in early labor. In the past decade the trend has been to deny all food and drink to laboring women, partly prompted by the introduction of 'active management of labor', which has led to a reduction in the duration of labor. The elective patients will have had supper, but in the unplanned situation the mother may have been fasting throughout labor and she may have received opioid analgesia, thereby increasing the acidic residue in the stomach.

Many antacid regimens have been described in the UK and MacDonald[10] concludes that 'the existence of widely varying regimens indicates that at present there is no firm evidence that any single method is clearly superior to others in protecting the mother from acid aspiration'. Every obstetric unit should have a clear policy with regard to the use of antacids as, despite the more widespread use of epidural anesthesia, the central issue of control of gastric pH and volume remains the same.

With the introduction of H_2-receptor antagonists there is now an improved method of gastric acid control.

Cimetidine was the first to be advocated as it suppresses gastric acid secretion without adding to gastric volume. However, the shortcomings of cimetidine include low molar potency and its effect on hepatic blood flow and the cytochrome P450 enzyme systems. Cimetidine's effect on the kinetics of other drugs, especially bupivacaine, should also be considered. However, recently Kuhnert et al[11] demonstrated that cimetidine does not affect the disposition or metabolism of bupivacaine during epidural anesthesia for cesarean delivery.[11]

Ranitidine, which has less effect on liver function, is popular because it has a longer duration of action. For elective cesarean delivery either of these drugs tends to be prescribed in evening and morning doses before surgery. Flynn et al[12] have shown that neither drug affects the disposition of lidocaine used for epidural anesthesia for cesarean delivery.

For those patients in labor who are at risk of an operative delivery, an early parenteral dose of ranitidine has been recommended and may be repeated. In patients requiring emergency cesarean delivery oral antacid is still recommended. The traditional double dose of magnesium trisilicate is being questioned because of its potential for causing pulmonary damage if aspirated. Sodium citrate would appear to be a more rapidly acting agent given as a single preanesthetic dose of 30 ml less than 15 mins before surgery.

ANESTHESIA

The administration of an epidural anesthetic requires that the anesthesiologist has the attention of a skilled anesthetic assistant in the event of complication or a general anesthetic being required.

Interest has been shown recently in the site of anesthetic induction, whether for a general or epidural anesthetic, in terms of the anxiety it induces in the patient and the requirement for separate monitoring equipment localized in the anesthetic room and in the operating theater. Any patient transported to and from a theater area should be in the left lateral position. Reid and Thorburn[13] found that moving to theater a patient in whom an epidural had been established with extensive sympathetic block caused significant hypotension.[13]

Patient monitoring has been critically assessed in the UK recently, and in 1988 the Association of Anaesthetists of Great Britain and Ireland made recommendations for standards of monitoring during anesthesia. Certain items of equipment are recommended and are of particular importance to the obstetric anesthesiologist. These include efficient suction apparatus, a selection of cuffed endotracheal tubes, three laryngoscopes (normal, long and polio blades), laryngeal masks, a gum elastic bougie for difficult intubations with all the appropriate connectors and apparatus that might be required in a standard failed intubation drill. Most units keep syringes containing a 500 mg dose of thiopental and a 100 mg dose of succinylcholine drawn up in the refrigerator and changed on a regular basis (24 h). Theater tables used for cesarean delivery should be capable of rapidly producing both a Trendelenberg/reverse Trendelenberg position and a side to side tilt.

Left lateral tilt is normally used to avoid aortocaval compression, although rarely a right lateral tilt may be indicated. A 3-L inflatable plastic bag was recommended by Carrie[14] to act as a wedge under the mother's hip. It can quickly be inflated by attaching a sphygmomanometer bulb to a length of infusion tubing.

Acute hydration

The cardiovascular complications of epidural block are well recognized, and methods available to avoid them are well known. There has been some controversy over the acute intravascular volume expansion of patients before initiation of an epidural anesthetic for cesarean delivery. Wollman and Marx[15] were the first to suggest acute hydration with 1 l of crystalloid solution as prophylaxis against hypotension. In 1982 Hallworth et al[16] claimed a further reduction in incidence of hypotension by acute hydration with 0.5 l of Haemaccell and 0.5 l of Hartmann's solution. They did not promote the routine use of Haemaccell because of the recognized risk of anaphylactoid reactions, but they did suggest that acute intravascular volume expansion with 2 l of crystalloid might be just as effective. Murray et al[17] made a further comparison of colloid (1 l of hydroxyethyl starch) with crystalloid (2 l of Hartmann's solution) and found no difference in the incidence of hypotension. They concluded that acute intravascular expansion of the circulating blood volume is an unreliable method of preventing hypotension during cesarean delivery with epidural anesthesia regardless of whether colloid or crystalloid is used. Wennberg et al[18] compared 3% Dextran 70 with Ringer's acetate for acute hydration and concluded that the patients who were given crystalloid had a lower transthoracic fluid index – indicative of an increase in lung water. This suggests that increased pulmonary hydration or even edema may occur if excessive volumes of crystalloid are used for intravascular volume expansion for cesarean delivery.

Proper teaching and instruction of midwives in these concepts should form part of any training because only by applying the highest standards of anesthetic, obstetric and nursing care can the potential hazardous consequences of extensive preganglionic sympathetic block in the pregnant woman be avoided.

The value of acute intravascular volume expansion has recently been questioned. Depending on the criteria used to define hypotension, the percentage of women who still require treatment for it, despite acute hydration, is reported as between 7 and 63%. An editorial in the *Lancet* suggested that the absence of controls in many of these studies is a measure of the obligatory use of intravascular volume expansion and that to omit its use is unethical.[19] On the other hand the use of vasopressors is universally accepted, although caution should be exercised in the choice of agent. The β- and α-adrenergic stimulator, ephedrine, is the most popular agent used in the UK. It has a positive inotropic and vasoconstrictor effect and increases blood pressure by increasing cardiac output and systemic vascular resistance. It is not thought to have a significant vasoconstrictive effect on uterine arterioles. Agents such as norepinephrine, methoxamine and metaraminol are thought to have too much α-adrenergic vasoconstrictor effect and are not currently recommended.

Epidural technique

In 1973 Milne and Murray-Lawson[20] were among the first to explore epidural anesthesia for cesarean delivery. Contrary to the general impression at that time, they were impressed by the readiness with which patients accepted the technique. The technique gradually became established and two different techniques were advocated. The first is the 'incremental catheter technique' described by Thorburn and Moir[21] and quoted in many texts. With this method, after the epidural block is initiated, 10–20 ml of 0.5% bupivacaine is injected through the Tuohy needle with the patient in the sitting position. The catheter is then inserted and after 10 min the patient is placed in the supine position with a lateral tilt and the sensory level is checked. A further dose of local anesthetic is then given – 1.5 ml for every segment unblocked below T6. The disadvantage of this technique is that it is very time-consuming, requiring more than 30 min after catheter insertion before surgical anesthesia is achieved. Its advantage is that it is safer than a single bolus dose technique. Unintentional injection of small divided doses of local anesthetic agent through a misplaced catheter into the subarachnoid space or an epidural vein is less hazardous than injection of a large dose. In addition, Thompson et al[22] reported that the incremental technique was associated with lower plasma concentrations of bupivacaine. However, in review of the technique, Crawford et al[23] found that the recommended maximum dose of bupivacaine was exceeded in many cases.

When Laishley and Morgan[24] were searching for a way of reducing the total dose requirement and of shortening the induction-to-incision time they described a technique using a single 'fractionated' injection of 100 mg of bupivacaine administered through the Tuohy needle over 5 mins. Only 25% of their patients required supplementation through the catheter after assessment at 20 mins. They claimed the additional advantage of injection of the main dose through the Tuohy needle was the avoidance of unintentional dural or vascular puncture by the catheter.

Crawford[25] advised caution in attempting to hasten the procedure by injecting larger incremental doses or by injecting more anesthetic solution before the full effect of the sensory block from the previous dose has been achieved. Even worse, he claims, is that 'injecting an assumed total dose requirement as a single shot is an invitation to maternal hypotension, nausea and vomiting, with accompanying fetal acidosis'. Controversy still exists, and it is the practice of many to follow the technique described by van Steenberge[8] in 1980, which involves both the test dose and the top-ups being injected through the catheter whilst accepting an onset time of at least 30 min from first placement of the epidural catheter.

When a problem arises during established labor it is not infrequently the case that an epidural block has been inserted at an earlier stage and pain relief may have been provided by either intermittent bolus or infusion. An assessment of the height of block before a top-up is given is obligatory. Jones et al[26] suggest that, after a short period of instruction, midwives can very successfully monitor the block of women in labor by using the loss of sensation to cold stimulus as a measure. Reynolds[27] reminds us that caution must be exercised when topping up women for a cesarean delivery who have already been receiving regular local anesthetic through an epidural catheter during labor. In one study, in which topping up was used in an attempt to provide effective analgesia for cesarean delivery, 77% of women were found to have venous bupivacaine concentrations in excess of 1.6 μg/ml. Some workers believe that this value represents the threshold for systemic toxicity, although in this study none of the women exhibited any symptoms or signs. However, it is probable that it is not the absolute plasma level that is important in causing toxicity, but the rate of rise, as postulated by Scott. Crawford commented that the maximum quoted dose may be too restrictive.

In the 1980s opinion changed about the height of block that should be achieved for cesarean delivery. The highest visceral afferent fibers pass in the greater splanchnic nerves through the fifth thoracic ganglion of the sympathetic chain. Therefore a block to T5 or T4 is thought to be better than the traditional height of T6. The speed with which a woman with an epidural catheter in situ for pain relief in labor can be prepared for cesarean delivery is dependent on the intensity and level of the existing block. Reynolds[29] argues that it is not necessary to wait until an epidural block extends to T4 before proceeding to surgery. With experience, epidural top-up should not delay surgery. The analgesia for labor already provided by epidural anesthetic is usually adequate for a Pfannenstiel incision. If the epidural is topped up when the decision to operate is taken then the block should extend sufficiently while shaving and insertion of a urinary catheter takes place to allow pain-free surgery.

Regardless of the technique used to establish epidural

blockade, shivering is commonly seen. Various maneuvers including warming the infusing fluid and the local anesthetic have achieved some success. Matthews and Corser[30] used 25 µg of fentanyl added to the epidural solution and shaking ceased within 15 min in 15 out of 18 cases.

The choice of local anesthetic tends to vary from country to country. In the UK the Committee of Safety in Medicines restricts the choice to two agents: lidocaine or bupivacaine. However, bupivacaine 0.75% has been withdrawn from obstetric use following reports of cardiac toxicity. In a comparison of 0.5% and 0.75% bupivacaine given by the incremental technique, Dutton et al[31] were unable to show any advantage with the stronger concentration. Half of the patients given the stronger concentration received more than the manufacturer's recommended maximum dose without the advantage of a faster onset time. Chloroprocaine and etidocaine are not licensed for use in the UK. Ropivacaine, a new long-acting amide-type local anesthetic, is currently undergoing trials in the UK as animal studies suggest that it may be less cardiotoxic than bupivacaine.

To compensate for the lack of choice in local anesthetic, various techniques have been used to modify the speed of onset and efficacy of epidural block for cesarean delivery. Firstly, alkalinization has been used to try to increase the fraction of lipid-soluble free base and so speed the onset of block. This method is still controversial. Tackley and Coe[32] compared 0.5% bupivacaine at a pH of 5.1 and bupivacaine 0.5% in 1 : 200 000 epinephrine added freshly and corrected to a pH of 6.3 in 24 patients and found that those who received the latter were significantly more likely to be ready at 45 mins after injection than those who received the former. They found that there was also less requirement for analgesic supplementation during surgery. However, in a study of 52 patients divided into four groups comparing 0.5% bupivacaine at pH 5.3 and adjusted to pH 6.7 and 0.5% bupivacaine with 1 : 200 000 epinephrine at pH 4.8 and adjusted to pH 6.8, French workers[33] found no differences in the onset of sensory block. Similar doubts about the value of pH-adjusted solutions were raised by Stevens et al.[34] Data regarding the shortening of the latency of lidocaine with alkalinization are more convincing. However, initial optimistic results with carbonation of lidocaine to improve the latency of onset have not been confirmed.

Recently, there has been interest in the effect of warming the local anesthetic solution, mainly in an attempt to reduce the incidence of shivering. Not only does warming the local anesthetic reduce the incidence of shivering, but Howie and Dutton[35] demonstrated that warming bupivacaine to 38°C produced a reduction in onset time of about 20%.

The addition of epinephrine to the local anesthetic solution has been used to reduce onset of block, prolong its effect, improve its efficacy and to reduce the plasma levels of local anesthetic and so reduce its systemic toxicity. However, the effect of adding epinephrine to 0.5% bupivacaine for cesarean delivery is unclear. Laishley et al[36] reported a reduction in plasma levels of bupivacaine, which they ascribed to lower dosage requirements rather than reduced absorption, although they did report a greater efficacy of block with a significant reduction in the number of women requiring supplementation after an initial 100-mg dose. Thorburn[37] has demonstrated that the addition of 1 in 200 000 epinephrine to lidocaine 2% produces a quicker onset and significantly lower plasma levels because both dosage requirements and absorption are reduced. Initial fears prompted by the results of animal studies that epinephrine might affect uterine blood flow have not been borne out in human analysis using Doppler techniques and radioactive xenon.

Most UK anesthesiologists use 0.5% bupivacaine for elective cesarean delivery using an incremental technique. However, when a rapid onset for emergency delivery is required, lidocaine 2% with 1 : 200 000 epinephrine added freshly is preferred. Recently, Howell et al[38] have studied an epidural mixture of lidocaine with epinephrine and bupivacaine for elective surgery. This preliminary work suggests that this mixture produces a block as effective as bupivacaine alone and better than lidocaine with epinephrine in terms of efficacy. It is claimed that the advantage of this mixture is a reduction in bupivacaine requirements, reducing fears about cardiotoxicity.

Recent developments in Doppler ultrasound technology have enabled fetal welfare to be assessed more closely than with cardiotocography or acid–base analysis. Both the uteroplacental flow–velocity waveforms and fetal aortic blood flow have been assessed for changes following epidural block for cesarean delivery. The results at present are conflicting, although Lindblad et al[39] found that fetal aortic flow increased following epidural bupivacaine. Attention has also focused on the subtler effects of epidural block with research into the neurobehavioral responses in the newborn. These tests assess motor behavior, habituation to stimuli and attentiveness, and so far results have been equivocal. The only reliable data from studies of this type are found when epidural block is compared with general anesthesia for cesarean delivery. These data suggest that the newborn status is improved with epidural anesthesia with bupivacaine. Reynolds[40] concludes that 'provided there is no serious maternal hypotension, epidural block does not appear to have any detrimental effect on uteroplacental or fetal blood flow and is, if anything, beneficial'.

Aortocaval compression

It is becoming clear that all pregnant women in the supine position near term have complete or near complete occlusion of the inferior vena cava, and sometimes also the aorta, owing to compression between the uterus and vertebral column. Even in the left lateral tilt position the flow may not be restored completely, and the ability to compensate depends on the adequacy of the collateral circulation and peripheral vasoconstriction. The latter means of compensation is impaired to a greater extent when large doses of local anesthetic are given in preparation for cesarean delivery. Continuous monitoring of pulse and blood pressure are useful guides to this effect, and close communication with the mother is important as she will usually convey symptoms of nausea and lightheadedness if it occurs. To prevent aortocaval occlusion, a left lateral tilt is used during cesarean delivery, although this measure will not prevent it in all women, especially if the tilt is less than 45°. Kinsella et al[41] have recently described an effective noninvasive method of detecting cord compression using a Finapress digital arterial pressure monitor. They detected aortic compression in women with up to a 30° pelvic tilt and also in some women in the semirecumbent position. This was not observed when women were in the full lateral position. It is recommended that the right and left full lateral positions are used as the epidural anesthetic takes effect.

Vasoconstrictors

Lindblad et al used ultrasonography and pulsed Doppler techniques to monitor fetal aortic and umbilical blood flow during administration of ephedrine and found no reduction in either measurement.[42] They concluded that ephedrine has no harmful effects on fetal blood flow. A 5–10 mg bolus dose of ephedrine is recommended at any one time. Intramuscular ephedrine used prophylactically has been suggested, but an unpredictably high and unacceptable incidence of hypertension was associated with the injection of 50 mg of ephedrine 30 mins before inserting an epidural anesthetic.[43]

Another approach for promoting venous return, reducing pooling and the theoretical risk of venous thrombosis would be the use of elastic support stockings on the mothers' legs and slight Trendelenburg tilt. However, Lee et al[44] did not find them to be effective in preventing hypotension during epidural anesthesia for cesarean delivery.[44]

Oxytocics

Blood loss at cesarean delivery is very variable. Although cross-matching of blood is routine practice for cesarean delivery in the UK, most anesthesiologists do not transfuse blood until the loss approaches $1\frac{1}{2}$ l. Uterine blood loss following delivery appears to be equally well controlled by ergometrine and synthetic oxytocin. Syntocinon is the oxytocic of choice in the UK. Transient vasodilation and a drop in blood pressure may occur with a rapid intravenous injection of a bolus of 10 i.u. of syntocinon after delivery of the child. Syntocinon is short-acting and a bolus dose may be followed by a slow intravenous infusion of 10–20 units in 500-ml.

Inadequate anesthetic

An inadequate epidural anesthetic despite appropriate topping up procedures is distressing for the woman, anesthesiologist and obstetrician. 38 pairs of spinal nerves have to be blocked before sensory anesthesia is adequate. Anatomic studies by Luyendjik[45] help explain why some blocks may be patchy with missed segments or unilateral. He describes dorsal median folds which may compartmentalize the injected solution. The catheter tip may not be situated in the midline and local anesthetic may tend to track laterally in the epidural space in the absence of anatomic barriers. Epidural catheters may be of two types – closed-ended (three lateral holes) and open-ended (single end hole). A comparison of the two catheters in labor by Michael et al[46] recorded that the open-ended catheters caused sensory blockade to be more frequently unilateral or to have a higher incidence of missed segments. They concluded that, in spite of the theoretical advantages of detection of intravenous and subarachnoid placement, they caused an unacceptably high incidence of unsatisfactory sensory blockade.

If after repeated top-ups the block height is still inadequate there are three further possible options. A low thoracic epidural anesthetic using a small volume of local anesthetic is promoted by some workers as it frequently deposits the local anesthetic at the appropriate segment and allays the need for the other two options, namely a spinal or general anaesthetic.

Even a dense block from T4 to S5 will not modify impulses generated through the vagus nerve. Rough handling of viscera will induce nausea and dull abdominal discomfort. Swabbing the peritoneal cavity with 0.5% lidocaine has been suggested by Crawford[9] as a possible remedy. Another source of discomfort is diaphragmatic irritation caused by blood or liquor tracking under gravity and stimulating the unblocked C3–5 spinal nerves. Of interest is the recent suggestion that this symptom might be caused by venous air emboli.

It may become obvious soon after the first incision that the epidural block is not providing complete pain relief. A good rapport with the mother is essential. She must always be warned that sensation is not completely abolished and she may be aware of some discomfort. The oxygen mask that has been used to provide oxygen supplementation may be used to administer Entonox should additional analgesia be required. Intravenous opioids may be administered to treat vague discomfort following delivery. Acute distress, however, requires induction of general anesthesia.

Supplementation

Epidural opioids have been used in many fields of anesthesia since first described by Behar in 1979.[47] In obstetrics they have been used in labor, intraoperatively and for post-operative analgesia. Preoperatively they have been used to reduce the incidence of 'visceral pain', which according to Alahuhta et al[48] occurs in up to 50% of patients. Fentanyl has a rapid onset of action and is lipid soluble, which theoretically reduces its rostral spread in cerebrospinal fluid and is considered suitable for use in cesarean delivery. Milon et al[49] found that patient comfort improved by adding fentanyl to epidural bupivacaine and there was a significant reduction in onset time of the block. There have been no adverse effects reported in the neonate if doses less than 100 μg are used. Capogna et al[50] studied sufentanil in this situation as it has greater potency and longer duration of action. They compared 50 μg and 80 μg of sufentanil with lidocaine for cesarean delivery. Superior analgesia was obtained with sufentanil, but the higher dose was associated with maternal side-effects and neuromechanical depression in the newborn. In addition Madej et al[51] found, when they compared 100 μg of fentanyl with variable doses of sufentanil, that 50 μg of sufentanil caused an unacceptable frequency of side-effects and had no real advantage over fentanyl.

A recent case report by Brockway et al[52] reminds us that caution should be exercised in the use of epidural opioids. In this patient 100 μg of fentanyl was given to supplement a bupivacaine epidural anesthetic and about $1\frac{1}{2}$ h later profound respiratory depression developed in the mother, which was fortunately observed and reversed with naloxone.

After cesarean delivery of the baby with epidural anesthesia the mother can became restless with a tendency to become concerned about relatively minor irritations such as leg immobility, shoulder stiffness or even the length of time that it is taking to complete the surgery. The common practice of inviting the father into theater may help to allay this problem, as does soft music playing in the background. However, the practice of sedating these patients must only be employed when essential and, if used, caution is necessary to avoid the added risk of inhalation injury. Benzodiazepines may impair bonding and the accompanying amnesia may erase the whole birth experience from the mother's memory. The use of an intravenous opioid or self-administered 50% nitrous oxide and oxygen may be a satisfactory alternative. The risks of respiratory depression should always be considered, particularly if epidural and parenteral opioids are combined.

POST-OPERATIVE ANALGESIA

A variety of options are open to the anesthesiologist to ensure that the first 24 h after delivery are as pain-free as possible. To some extent these options are limited by the degree of monitoring that is available in the post-natal period. If epidural opioids are used most would agree that, as Morgan[53] asserts, 'some form of respiratory monitoring is mandatory'. Nausea, vomiting, somnolence, urinary dysfunction, pruritis and delayed respiratory depression have been described with all of the epidural opioids, although as a general rule side-effects are greater with higher doses and with morphine.

Morphine is the most extensively studied epidural opioid. Dosage requirements seem to be inconsistent, but certainly good analgesia has been described with much smaller doses than those given parenterally, and doses as low as 3 mg have been used effectively. In addition, the higher the dose, the greater the risk of side-effects. Because diamorphine is more lipid soluble and is more rapidly broken down to active metabolites it has been advocated for post-cesarean delivery analgesia instead of morphine. Macrae et al[54] compared 5 mg of epidural diamorphine and 2 mg of epidural phenoperidine with 5 mg of intramuscular diamorphine. They concluded that both drugs given epidurally provided more intense and long-lasting analgesia than intramuscular diamorphine. Itching was noted in 50% of the epidural patients. Similarly epidural meperidine 50 mg has been shown by Perris[55] to produce better and quicker analgesia than 100 mg of the same drug given intramuscularly, although the duration of action is equal. Of interest was the report of no itching in that study, and it was postulated that this may be related to its weak local anesthetic action. Pruritis has been described by other workers. Simpson et al[56] found no real advantage of buprenorphine over morphine, but in a comparison of morphine and methadone, Evron et al[57] found that, although both provided good analgesia, methadone produced a significantly lower incidence of urinary hesitancy requiring catheterization.

A useful increase in the duration of analgesia has been reported with the addition of epinephrine to epidural diamorphine, although this caused a high incidence of side-effects. There has also been interest in the use of combinations of epidural opioids and local anesthetics to improve the analgesia and reduce the side-effects associated with both drugs. However, results so far have been equivocal.

Infusion regimens of bupivacaine have been used in the post-operative period, but loss of bladder sensation, leg weakness and pressure sores on the heels are side-effects that must be kept in mind. Many women resent the numbness that even dilute solutions of local anesthetic can produce. This is probably because the accompanying immobility impairs the mother's ability to care for her baby. In spite of enthusiasm for the epidural route for relieving pain post-operatively one must balance its advantages and disadvantages over the same agents given parenterally. Webster et al[58] compared epidural morphine with intramuscular papaveretum and found that both groups had equivalent pain relief but the epidural morphine group required less opioid in the first 12 hs and tended to sleep better. The reported incidence of urinary retention with epidural opioids varies widely, but in a comparison between intramuscular papaveretum and epidural diamorphine Patrick et al[59] found that, although the epidural group had a higher incidence of hesitancy, the incidence of recatheterization was not increased as a result.

SPECIAL CONSIDERATIONS

There are certain situations that create problems not only for the obstetrician but also for the anesthesiologist who is faced with the problem of providing safe anesthesia for the delivery of the child and avoid causing a deterioration in the condition of the mother.

Preeclampsia

The first of these problems is the presentation for cesarean delivery of the mother who has developed preeclampsia during pregnancy. The 1985–87 Confidential Enquiry pointed out that hypertensive diseases of pregnancy are responsible for 19% of maternal deaths. These 'at-risk' patients should be identified and discussed with the obstetrician at an early stage. The blood pressure may be very labile and sensitive to the pressor effects of circulatory catecholamines. The blood pressure may already be controlled with antihypertensive therapy but it may still go up during labor, especially in response to uterine contractions. An epidural block will relieve the pain and produce a degree of sympathetic blockade dependent on the extent of thoracic spread of epidural local anesthetic. It has been established that epidural anesthesia can improve placental blood flow in the absence of hypotension. However, there may be contraindications to the use of epidural anesthesia. There may be a coagulation defect present, although this is rare unless there is severe preeclampsia. In fulminating preeclampsia, urgent cesarean delivery is indicated. If there is not enough time to establish epidural anesthesia, then the blood pressure must be controlled by using parenteral antihypertensive agents and general anesthesia.

There is an increasing tendency to deliver mothers when the preeclampsia is mild or moderate in severity to preempt any further deterioration. As a result cesarean delivery using epidural anesthesia is being offered with increasing frequency to these women. Provided special attention is paid to the increased hazards of reduced circulatory blood volume and potential synergism with antihypertensive agents such as hydralazine, these mothers should derive the same benefit from this technique as others.

Respiratory disease

Asthma is probably the commonest respiratory disorder that is dealt with in obstetric anesthetic practice. Women who suffer from this condition probably benefit from the pain relief in labor provided by an epidural anesthetic because it reduces the respiratory demand of a painful labor. In patients with severe respiratory disease the choice of anesthetic for cesarean delivery may be influenced by the degree of productive cough that is present. Opinion is divided about whether general anesthesia is better because it ensures adequate oxygenation and allows better access for tracheobronchial toilet before extubation or whether regional is better because it avoids the risk of atelectasis associated with general anesthesia. Many favor epidural anesthesia in chronic chest conditions such as cystic fibrosis with bronchiectasis or emphysematous bullae because of the fear that positive-pressure ventilation with a general anesthetic may exacerbate the condition. If pulmonary hypertension complicates a chest condition the advantages and disadvantages of an epidural anesthetic must be carefully weighed in each individual patient. This is one of the few conditions for monitoring with a pulmonary artery catheter in labor because of the acute changes seen in right and left heart pressures.

The influence of epidural anesthesia on the ability of the mother to cough has been the subject of some recent investigation. Gamil[60] found that most women maintained their peak expiratory flow rates (PEFRs) during epidural anesthesia at values consistent with effective coughing. Harrop-Griffiths et al[61] measured forced vital capacity, forced expiratory volume in one second and maximum expiratory pressure as well as PEFR in patients undergoing cesarean delivery with epidural anesthesia and concluded that, although there was a significant decrease in all the respiratory variables measured, this was unlikely to impair the normal patient's ability to cough effectively.[61] Caution should be exercised in patients who have pre-existing pulmonary disease and when the block is unintentionally high.

Cardiac

It is impossible to generalize about heart disease because of the wide variety of congenital conditions which may or may not have been corrected surgically, and all cases should be discussed with the obstetrician and a cardiologist. It is also apparent in the UK that the incidence of acquired ischemic heart disease is increasing in women of child-bearing age, and this condition may also require careful management.

There is a trend towards elective cesarean delivery patients with hemodynamically significant heart disease to avoid the strain of prolonged labor. Newman[62] measured cardiac output with transcutaneous aortovelography and found that it increased by 20% at induction of general anesthesia compared with a change of only 5% using epidural anesthesia. Robson[63] used Doppler ultrasound and cross-sectional echocardiography at the aortic valve to measure cardiac output and found that in 75% of their patients who had epidural block for cesarean delivery there was no significant change in cardiac output. However, in three of their patients, there was marked reduction in cardiac output associated with a decrease in blood pressure which was unrelated to the height of the block. The rapid and, in some cases, marked hemodynamic effect of ephedrine given to treat this complication was well tolerated, but it was suggested that this may not have been the case in subjects with cardiac disease. Acute hydration and sympathomimetics will have to be judged especially carefully in those patients who depend on maintaining their venous return and systemic vascular resistance. Difficulty can arise in deciding how to react when faced with sudden changes in their cardiovascular dynamics, which can occur perioperatively. Many anesthesiologists still consider light general anesthesia to be the safest option, especially when reports of collapse following epidural anesthesia in patients with heart disease continue to appear.[64] Whichever anesthetic technique is employed there must be close monitoring of the cardiovascular system and direct arterial pressure and pulmonary artery measurements may be indicated.

In normal delivery, synthetic oxytocin is preferred rather than ergometrine because it can aid uterine contraction without the side-effects such as hypertension, associated with ergometrine. In patients with heart disease, the use of ergometrine is even more contraindicated because of its vasoconstrictive action.

Diabetes mellitus

Another common medical problem encountered in obstetric practice is diabetes mellitus. The placental circulation is frequently compromised in mothers with this condition even if they have maintained good control of their blood glucose throughout pregnancy. Ultrasound is routinely used antenatally to identify fetal size and growth and allow the most appropriate time for delivery to be chosen. Epidural anesthesia is encouraged both for labor and if cesarean delivery becomes necessary not only because fetal acidosis is minimized but also because they avoid the use of depressant drugs. Brudenell[65] recommended that elective cesarean delivery is the safest management of these patients, although others believe that cesarean delivery should only be undertaken if there is an obstetric indication. Whatever the mode of delivery, an epidural anesthetic is advisable because it has the least effect on gastrointestinal function and blood sugar control.

Obesity

Another relatively common problem anesthesiologists encounter is the morbidly obese patient. The Confidential Enquiry into Maternal Deaths recommended the use of an epidural anesthetic in any patient in whom intubation could be expected to be difficult. In an emergency, maintenance of an airway can be very difficult and anticipation and advance preparation is advised to reduce the need for hurried intervention. If cesarean delivery seems likely, it is better performed electively when time is available to prepare these patients properly. Venous access is more difficult and the distance from skin to epidural space can be much greater than normal, making the insertion of the epidural needle and catheter a task for the most experienced. The availability of long Tuohy needles is advantageous in some cases. Hodgkinson and Husain[66] showed that the spread of a given volume of local anesthetic within the epidural space is more extensive in the obese patient, and it is recommended that smaller volumes are used.[66]

Thromboembolic disease

Thromboembolism remains an important cause of maternal death. In the most recent triennial report (1985–87) it was responsible for 21% of maternal deaths.[2] The risk is greatest in women over 35, the obese, those with preeclampsia and those who undergo cesarean delivery. Prophylactic measures used include low-dose heparin, although there is some controversy over its value. Intermittent calf compression is routinely practiced in the UK during the course of cesarean delivery. It has been suggested that epidural anesthesia itself has contributed to the decline in maternal mortality from pulmonary embolism, and various effects on blood flow and viscosity have been postulated to explain this. A prophylactic effect of the local anesthetic agent itself has been shown by Cooke et al.[67] Concern over extradural hematoma formation following vessel puncture in patients receiving heparin prophylaxis is felt by some to be a contraindication to an epidural anesthetic for cesarean delivery, but others feel that the omission of the morning dose is an adequate precaution. Another problem has arisen recently in the management of preeclamptic patients. In a survey of the obstetric units in the UK, Barker and Callandar[68] found a lack of standard practice over the use of coagulation screening in these patients. In addition, there has been a trend towards using low-dose aspirin in their management. This again presents the anesthesiologists with a dilemma as to whether it is safe to initiate an epidural block. MacDonald[69] suggests that one answer is to discontinue aspirin therapy for 7–10 days prior to surgery and the epidural anesthetic can then be safety initiated when a bleeding time of less than 10 min is obtained.

Although the mortality figures for the last 30 years reveal that there has been much progress in the anesthetic care of the pregnant woman, Scott and Hibbard[70] remind us that we need to be aware of the morbidity associated with the technique we employ. Only then can we give adequate information to quantify the risks for the inquiring mother. Their retrospective study of serious nonfatal complications indicated that the most acute and serious complications of unexpected widespread block and acute toxicity with convulsions tend to be associated with epidural anesthesia for cesarean delivery because of the larger doses involved. If the diagnosis is made quickly, no serious harm should befall the mother or child. The future of epidural anesthesia lies in reducing this morbidity even further. All anesthesiologists should be aware of the difficulties in resuscitating the mother in the supine posture and how these difficulties can be overcome. Currently many comparisons are made between flying an aircraft and giving an anesthetic. The psychologists tell us that when serious problems arise we do not resort to first principles but act on reflex. The problems arise so infrequently that our responses may not be fast or appropriate enough for the situation. One way around this is to have crisis management algorithms which are practiced regularly, possibly using computer simulation. This applies particularly in obstetrics when the slow application of what we have all learned in training may have far-reaching consequences.

REFERENCES

1. Buck N, Devlin H B, Lunn J N 1987 The report of a confidental enquiry into peri-operative deaths: The Nuffield Provincial Hospital Trust and the King's Fund, London
2. DHSS 1987 Report on confidential enquiries into maternal deaths in United Kingdom. HMSO, London
3. Kennedy F, Effron A S, Perry G 1950 The grave spinal cord paralysis caused by spinal anaesthesia. Surg Gynaecol Obstet 91: 385–398
4. Davis D M 1971 An extradural analgesia service in obstetrics. Anaesthesia 26: 494–495
5. Morgan B M, Magni V and Goroszenuik T 1990 Anaesthesia for emergency caesarean section. Br J Obstet Gynaecol 97: 420–424
6. Hardwick M 1983 Caesarean section under epidural: a personal account. Br Med J 287: 35–36
7. MacArthur C, Lewis M, Knox E G, Crawford J S 1990 Epidural anaesthesia and long term backache after childbirth. Br Med Journal 301: 9–12
8. Van Steenberge A 1980 In: Doughty A (ed) Epidural anaesthesia in obstetrics: a second symposium. Lloyd-Luke, London p 160
9. Crawford J S 1984 Obstetric analgesia and anaesthesia. Current reviews in obstetrics and gynaecology, Vol 1, 2nd edn. Churchill Livingstone, London p 97
10. Atkinson R S, Adams A P 1985. In: Atkinson R S, Adams A P (eds) Recent advances in anaesthesia and analgesia, Vol 15. Churchill Livingstone, London pp 108–133
11. Kuhnert B R, Zuspan K J, Kuhnert P M, Syracuse C D, Brashear W T, Brown D E 1987 Lack of influence of cimetidine on bupivacaine levels during parturition. Anaesth Analg 66: 986–990
12. Flynn R J, Moore J, Collier P S, Howard P J 1989 Single dose oral H_2 antagonists do not affect plasma lignocaine levels in the parturient. Acta Anaesthesiol Scand 33: 593–596
13. Reid J, Thorburn J 1988 Bupivacaine and lignocaine for epidural Cesarean section and the role of maternal posture. Br J Anaesth 61: 149–153
14. Carrie L E S 1982 An inflatable obstetric wedge. Anaesthesia 37: 745
15. Wolman S B, Marx G F 1968 Acute hydration for prevention of hypotension of spinal anaesthesia in parturients. Anesthesiology 29: 375–380
16. Halworth D, Jellicoe J A, Wilkes R G 1982 Hypotension during epidural anaesthesia for caesarean section. Anaesthesia 37: 53–56
17. Murray A M, Morgan M, Whitman J G 1989 Crystalloid versus colloid for circulatory preload for epidural caesarean section. Anaesthesia 44: 463–466
18. Wennberg E, Frid I, Haljame H et al 1990 Comparison of Ringer's acetate with 3% dextran 70 for volume loading before extradural caesarean section. Br J Anaesth 65: 654–660
19. Anon 1989 Epidural block for Caesarean section and circulatory changes (editorial). Lancet 2: 1076–1078
20. Milne M K, Murray-Lawson J I 1973 Epidural analgesia for Caesarean section. Br J Anaesth 45: 1206–1210
21. Thorburn J, Moir D D 1980 Epidural analgesia for elective Caesarean section. Anaesthesia 35: 3–7
22. Thompson E M, Wilson C M, Moore J 1985 Plasma bupivacaine levels associated with extradural anaesthesia for Caesarean section. Anaesthesia 40: 427–432
23. Crawford J S, Davies P, Lewis M 1986 Some aspects of epidural block provided for Caesarean section. Anaesthesia 41: 1039–1046
24. Laishley R S, Morgan B M 1988 A single dose epidural technique for caesarean section. Anaesthesia 43: 100–103
25. Crawford J S 1984 Obstetric analgesia and anaesthesia. Current reviews in obstetrics and gynaecology, Vol 1, 2nd edn. Churchill Livingstone, London p 105
26. Jones M J T, Bogod D G, Rees G A D, Rosen M 1988 Midwives assessment of upper sensory level; after epidural blockade. Anaesthesia 43: 557–559
27. Reynolds F, Laishley R, Morgan B, Lee A 1989 The effect of time and adrenaline on the transplacental distribution of bupivacaine. Br J Anaesth 62: 509–514
28. Scott D B 1989 Maximum recommended doses of local anasethetic drugs. Br J Anaesth 63: 373–374
29. Reynolds F 1989 Epidural anaesthesia in obstetrics. Br Med J 299: 1029
30. Matthews N C, Corser G 1988 Epidural fentanyl for shaking in obstetrics. Anaesthesia 43: 783–785
31. Dutton D A, Moir D D, Howie H B 1984 Choice of local anaesthetic drug for extradural Caesarean section. Br J Anaesth 56: 1361–1371
32. Tackley R M, Coe A J 1988 Alkalinised bupivacaine and adrenaline for epidural caesarean section. Anaesthesia 43: 1019–1021
33. Benhamou D, Perrachon N, Labaille T 1989 Alkalinisation of epidural 0.5% bupivacaine for caesarean section. Reg Anaesth 14: 240–243
34. Stevens R A, Schubert A, Spitzer L et al 1989 The effect of pH adjustment of 0.5% bupivacaine on the latency of epidural anaesthesia. Reg Anaesth 14: 236–239
35. Howie J E, Dutton D A 1990 The effect of warming bupivacaine in patients undergoing elective Caesarean section under epidural anaesthesia. In: Reynolds F (ed) Epidural and spinal block in obstetrics. Balliere Tindall, London pp 162–163
36. Laishley R S, Morgan B M, Reynolds F 1988 Effect of adrenaline on extradural anaesthesia and plasma bupivacaine concentrations during Caeserean section. Br J Anaesth 60: 180–186
37. Thorburn J 1990 In: Reynolds F (ed) Epidural and spinal block in obstetrics. Balliere Tindall, London pp 153–154
38. Howell P, Wrigley M, Tan P, Davies W, Morgan B 1990 A preliminary assessment of an epidural mixture of lignocaine and bupivacaine for elective Caesarean section. In: Reynolds F (ed) Epidural and spinal block in obstetrics. Balliere Tindall, London pp 160–161
39. Lindblad A, Bernow J, Marsal K 1987 Obstetric analgesia and fetal

aortic blood flow during labour. Br J Obstet Gynaecol 94: 306–311

40. Reynolds F (ed) Epidural and spinal block in obstetrics. Balliere Tindall, London p 207
41. Kinsella S M, Spencer J A D, Morgan B M, Whitwam J G 1990 Non-supine uterine aortic compression. Br J Anaesth 64: 395P
42. Lindblad A, Bernow J, Vernersson E, Marsal K 1987 Effect of extradural anaesthesia on human foetal blood flow in utero. Br J Anaesth 59: 1265–1272
43. Rolbin S H, Cole A F D, Hew E M, Pollard A, Virgin T S 1982 Prophylactic i.m. ephedrine before epidural anaesthesia for Caesarean section. Can Soc J 29: 148–152
44. Lee A, McKeown D, Wilson J 1987 Evaluation of the efficacy of elastic compression stockings in prevention of hypotension during epidural anaesthesia for elective Caesarean section. Acta Anaesthesiol Scand 31: 193–195
45. Luyendijk W 1976 The plica mediana dorsalis of the dura mater and its relation to lumbar peridurography. Neuroradiology 11: 147–149
46. Michael S, Richmond M N, Birks R J S 1989 A comparison between open-end and closed-end epidural catheters. Complications and quality of sensory blockade. Anaesthesia 44: 574–577
47. Behar M, Olshwang D, Magora F, Davidson J T 1979. Epidural morphine in the treatment of pain. Lancet 1: 527
48. Alahuhta S, Kangas-Saarela T, Hollman A I, Edstrom H H 1990 Visceral pain during Caesarean section under spinal and epidural anaesthesia with bupivacaine. Acta Anaesthesiol Scand 34: 95–98
49. Milon D, Bentue-Ferrer D, Noury D et al 1983 Epidural bupivacaine–fentanyl anaesthesia for Caesarean section. Annales Francaise D'anaesthesia et de Reanimation 2: 273–279
50. Capogna G, Celleno D, Tomassetti M 1989 Maternal analgesia and neonatal effects of epidural sufentanil for cesarean section. Reg Anaesth 14: 282–287
51. Madej T H, Strunin L 1987 Comparison of epidural fentanyl with sufentanil analgesia and side effects after a single dose during elective Caesarean section. Anaesthesia 42: 1156–1161
52. Brockway M S, Noble D W, Sharwood-Smith G H, McClure J H 1990 Profound respiratory depression after extradural fentanyl. Br J Anaesth 64: 243–245
53. Morgan M 1989 The rational use of intrathecal and extradural opioids. Br J Anaesth 63: 165–188
54. Macrae D J, Munishankrappa S, Burrow L M, Milne M K, Grant I S 1987 Br J Anaesth 59: 354–359
55. Perriss B W, Latham B V, Wilson I H 1990 Analgesia following extradural and i.m. pethidine in post-Caesarean section patients. Br J Anaesth 64: 355–357
56. Simpson K H, Madej T H, McDowell J M, MacDonald R, Lyons G 1988 Comparison of extradural buprenorphine and extradural morphine after Caesarean section. Br J Anaesth 60: 627–631
57. Evron S, Samueloff A, Simon A, Drenger B, Magora F 1985 Urinary function during epidural analgesia with methadone and morphine in post-Caesarean section patients. Pain 23: 135–144
58. Webster N R, Lyons G, MacDonald R 1986 Sleep and comfort after Caesarean section. Anaesthesia 41: 1143–1145
59. Patrick J A, Yoon J S L, Reynolds F 1990 Bladder function during i.m. papaveretum and epidural diamorphine analgesia following Caesarean section. In: Reynolds F (ed) Epidural and spinal block in obstetrics. Balliere Tindall, London pp 198–200
60. Gamil M 1989 Serial peak expiratory flow rates in mothers during Caesarean section under extradural anaesthesia. Br J Anaesth 62: 415–418
61. Harrop-Griffiths A W, Ravalia A, Browne D A, Robinson P N 1991 Regional anaesthesia and cough effectiveness. Anaesthesia 46: 11–13
62. Newman B 1982 Cardiac output changes during Caesarean section. Anaesthesia 37: 270–273
63. Robson S, Hunter S, Boys R, Dunlop W, Bryson M 1989 Changes in cardiac output during epidural anaesthesia for caesarean section. Anaesthesia 44: 475–479
64. Alderson J D 1987 Cardiovascular collapse following epidural anaesthesia for Caesarean section in a patient with aortic incompetence. Anaesthesia 42: 643–645
65. Brudenell J M 1978 Delivering the baby of a diabetic mother. In: Diabetes in pregnancy: a symposium. J Royal Soc Med 71: 207
66. Hodgkinson R, Husain F J 1980 Caesarean section associated with gross obesity. Br J Anaesth 52: 919–923
67. Cooke E D, Lloyd M J, Bawcock S A, Pilcher M F 1977 Intravenous lignocaine in prevention of deep vein thrombosis after elective hip surgery. Lancet 2: 797–799
68. Barker P, Callander C G 1991 Coagulation screening before epidural analgesia in pre-eclampsia. Anaesthesia 46: 64–67
69. MacDonald R 1991 Aspirin and extradural blocks. Br J Anaesth 66: 1–3
70. Scott D B, Hibbard B M 1990 Serious non-fatal complications associated with extradural block in obstetric practice. Br J Anaesth 64: 537–541

38. Subarachnoid anesthesia

Part A USA view
 I Single dose block *G. F. Marx*
 II Continuous block *J. H. Skerman, R. J. Hurley, D. H. Lambert*
Part B European view *L. E. S. Carrie*

PART A
USA VIEW
I Single dose block
G. F. Marx

Subarachnoid, i.e. spinal, anesthesia was introduced into childbirth at the turn of the century by Kreis,[1] an obstetrician at the Women's Clinic in Basle, Switzerland, to provide pain relief for labor and vaginal delivery. Two years later, Hopkins,[2] an obstetrician from Springfield, Illinois, described the 'superiority of spinal anesthesia over ether or chloroform in cases of cesarean section, because of the relaxed condition of the uterine muscles likely to obtain with the patient anesthetized by either of the two latter methods'. He reported that Doleris of Paris had also employed spinal anesthesia for 'cesarean delivery' and had spoken 'in glowing terms of the usefulness' of this technique 'because of the prompt and vigorous uterine contraction'.

During the 1930s, American anesthesiologists recognized empirically that, during the last months of gestation, a smaller dose of local anesthetic, approximately two-thirds of normal, was required to obtain the desired level of anesthesia. This knowledge increased the safety of spinal anesthesia for abdominal delivery and thus enhanced the frequency of its use, albeit more often as a substitute for local infiltration than for general anesthesia. O'Connor,[3] in 1934, reported on the 'types of anesthetics and frequency of their employment' in over 400 cesarean deliveries: ether was used in 381 cases, spinal in 31, novocaine (procaine) infiltration in 20 and 'there were no deaths directly attributable to the anesthetic'. The reduced drug requirement for spinal anesthesia in late pregnancy was subsequently confirmed by two separate studies. Assali and Prystowsky[4] used a continuous spinal technique with 0.2% procaine in 10 women, at term as well as post partum; 2 days after delivery, 3–4 times the amount of anesthetic solution was necessary to produce the same level of sensory blockade as in the prepartum period. Marx and Orkin[5] compared the effects of equal doses of spinal anesthetic (tetracaine 5 mg and dextrose 50 mg) administered under identical conditions to obstetric and young gynecologic patients; in the parturients, onset of block was significantly faster, levels higher and duration longer ($P < 0.001$).

The safety of spinal anesthesia for cesarean delivery improved further with the recognition of the benefit of acute intravenous hydration in attenuating the incidence and severity of post-block hypotension. Yet, with the increasing use of lumbar epidural block in the 1960s and 1970s, spinal anesthesia fell into disfavor – despite its advantages of reliability of technique, rapid onset of action, requirement for a low dose of anesthetic and, consequently, low maternal and fetal blood drug levels. In a comparison of bupivacaine disposition in mother and fetus during cesarean delivery, mean maternal venous drug levels after subarachnoid block (8 ± 0.5 mg) were 5% of those during epidural anesthesia (164 ± 15 mg) and mean venous cord blood levels after spinal anesthesia were 7% of those after epidural anesthesia.[6] However, the onset of epidural anesthesia is slow, and this led to the edict of the 1970s that cesarean delivery for fetal distress demands the administration of general anesthesia.

Then, in the 1980s, the pendulum started to swing the other way. First, both in the USA and in Europe, there was recognition of increased maternal mortality during general anesthesia due to difficulty with intubation or pulmonary inhalation of gastric contents. A review of anesthesia-related mortality in Michigan,[7] from 1972 to 1984 found that 'the inability to accomplish endotracheal intubation emerged as the principal cause of death in recent years', and that the emergent nature of the operation was a risk factor in most patients. Second, two scientific reports published in 1984 clearly demonstrated advantages of spinal anesthesia for both mother and infant. Brownridge[8] examined 442 cases of subarachnoid block performed in obstetric patients at Queen Victoria Hospital in Adelaide, Australia, which included 275 cesarean deliveries. He concluded that subarachnoid block 'proved to be particularly valuable when anesthesia was required urgently in the delivery suite and may even be regarded as the anesthesic of choice in these circumstances'. The second report[9] came from the Albert Einstein College of Medicine in New York City and described 126 consecutive cases of cesarean delivery undertaken for fetal distress in which fetal biochemical and neonatal clinical data were available. All operations started within 20 mins of the last scalp capillary blood pH sampling and, in all cases, umbilical vein and artery bloods were obtained prior to the infant's first breath. The choice of anesthetic was determined by the wishes of the mother. General anesthesia (induction with thiopental or ketamine–thiopental, maintenance with endotracheal 40% nitrous oxide – 60% oxygen was administered to 71 parturients, spinal anesthesia (tetracaine–dextrose) to 33 women and cephalad extension of an existing epidural block (3% 2-chloroprocaine) to 22 patients. The etiologies of fetal distress and the skin incision–delivery and uterine incision–delivery intervals were similar between the general and regional anesthesia groups. However, umbilical artery blood pH values were higher than the last scalp capillary blood pH values in 80% of the regional anesthesia cases vs. 63% in the general anesthesia cases. Furthermore, the 1-min Apgar scores were significantly better following regional as compared with general anesthesia (Table 38.1). The faster recovery of the fetal biochemical data and the better neonatal clinical conditions following the two regional techniques are explainable by the findings of lower maternal catecholamines and cortisol and higher fetal catecholamine concentrations during cesarean deliveries under regional as compared with general anesthesia, indicating decreased adrenocortical responses to stress and surgery by blockade of the afferent neurogenic pathways.[10–12] Since elevated circulating norepinephrine concentrations induce uteroplacental vasoconstriction with reduction in blood flow, the sparing effect on stress reaction is beneficial for the fetus. The markedly higher fetal catecholamine levels denote advanced sympathoadrenal activation, which promotes extrauterine adaptation.[12] Of the two regional methods, spinal anesthesia offers special advantages to the acidotic fetus because the small amount of local anesthetic utilized minimizes its 'trapping' in the low-pH blood.[13]

Table 38.1 Fetal biochemical and neonatal clinical data in 126 cases of cesarean delivery undertaken for fetal distress[9]

Anesthetic method	No.	UApH > SCpH	1-minute Apgar 8–10
Spinal	33	84%	77%
Epidural	22	75%	80%*
General	71	60%	51%*

*P < 0.01.
UApH > SCpH = umbilical artery blood pH values higher than last scalp capillary blood pH values.

Based on these recent reports, subarachnoid block is enjoying a rebirth as an anesthetic for cesarean delivery. Provided regional anesthesia is not contraindicated for medical or obstetric reasons, spinal anesthesia is considered the method of choice for emergency delivery in the following situations: anticipated airway/intubation problems, history of asthma, diagnosis of upper respiratory infection, recent solid food intake and the mother's wish to remain awake. In addition, spinal anesthesia is preferred for obese gravidas, those with an anatomically difficult back and those at risk of hematoma formation.[14] Studies in the 1980s have reaffirmed the safety of the technique for both mother and infant, with special impetus on the prevention of post-block hypotension and headache. Three local anesthetic agents are currently employed: lidocaine, 60–100 mg, duration 45–60 mins; bupivacaine, 10–15 mg, duration 60–90 mins; and tetracaine, 6–10 mg, duration 90–120 mins. The addition of a small dose of an opioid to the local anesthetic is becoming increasingly popular, as is the use of a continuous spinal anesthetic via catheter for post-operative analgesia. The incidence of post-dural puncture headache has declined greatly with the introduction of thinner needles and those of new design (e.g. the Sprotte needle).[15]

In conclusion, anesthesiologists and obstetricians have recognized the advantages of spinal anesthesia for cesarean delivery and the technique is being employed with increasing frequency and mounting satisfaction.

REFERENCES

1. Kreis O 1990 Ueber Medullarnarkose bei Gebärenden. Ctrbl Gynäkol 28: 724–729
2. Hopkins S R 1902 Case of cesarean section under spinal anesthesia. J Am Med Assoc 38: 1355
3. O'Connor C T 1934 Cesarean section. A review of four hundred and thirty-six cases. New Engl J Med 210: 948–954
4. Assali N S, Prystowsky H 1950 Studies on autonomic blockade. I. J Clin Invest 29: 1354–1366
5. Marx G F 1972 Regional analgesia in obstetrics. Anaesthesist 21: 84–91
6. Kuhnert B R, Zuspan K J, Kuhnert P M, Syracuse C D, Brown D E 1987 Bupivacaine disposition in mother, fetus and neonate after spinal anesthesia for cesarean section. Anesth Analg 66: 407–412
7. Endler G C, Mariona F G, Sokol R J, Stevenson L B 1988 Anesthesia-related maternal mortality in Michigan, 1972 to 1984. Am J Obstet Gynecol 159: 187–193
8. Brownridge P 1984 Spinal anaesthesia revisited: an evaluation of subarachnoid block in obstetrics. Anaesth Intensive Care 12: 334–342

9. Marx G F, Luykx W M, Cohen S 1984 Fetal–neonatal status following caesarean section for fetal distress. Br J Anaesth 56: 1009–1013
10. Irestedt L, Largercrantz H, Hjemdahl P, Hägnevik K, Belfrage P 1982 Fetal and maternal plasma catecholamine levels at elective cesarean section under general or epidural anesthesia versus vaginal delivery. Am J Obstet Gynecol 142: 1004–1010
11. Abboud T K, Artal R, Henriksen E H, Earl S, Kammulaa R K 1982 Effects of spinal anesthesia on maternal circulating catecholamines. Am J Obstet Gynecol 142: 252–254
12. Namba Y, Smith J B, Fox G S, Challis J R G 1980 Plasma cortisol concentrations during caesarean section. Br J Anaesth 52: 1027–1031
13. Biehl D, Shnider S M, Levinson G, Callender K 1978 Placental transfer of lidocaine. Effects of fetal acidosis. Anesthesiology 48: 409–412
14. Kotelko D M 1989 Anaesthesia for caesarean delivery in a patient with May-Hegglin anomaly. Can J Anaesth 36: 328–330
15. Sears D H, Leeman M I, O'Donnell R H, Kelleher J F, Santos G C 1990 Incidence of postdural puncture headache in cesarean section patients using the 24G Sprotte needle. Anesthesiology 73: A1003

PART A
USA VIEW
II Continuous block

J. H. Skerman R. J. Hurley D. H. Lambert

INTRODUCTION

Although continuous spinal anesthesia (CSA) has advantages over continuous epidural[1] and single injection spinal anesthesia, it is not often used in labor analgesia or during cesarean delivery. The reason for this is the high incidence of postdural puncture headache (PDPH) in pregnant women. The incidence of PDPH is inversely related to age and directly related to the diameter of the needle used for lumbar dural puncture.[2] Because it has been necessary to use a large-diameter needle to insert a catheter for CSA, the resulting high rate of PDPH has limited the use of CSA in pregnant women.

SPINAL HEADACHE

Recently, Denny et al[3] reported a prevalence of PDPH of 1% after CSA performed with a 20-gauge catheter inserted through an 18-gauge Hustead needle. The average age of the patients in this study was 66 years. Unfortunately, the use of similar needles and catheters in pregnant women is not associated with the same low prevalence of PDPH reported by Denny et al[3] (Table 38.2). Nevertheless, catheters that can be inserted through 22- and 26-gauge spinal needles are now available. This recent advance in catheter technology makes CSA possible for labor and vaginal or cesarean delivery without increasing the risk of PDPH. The incidence of PDPH following the use of smaller catheters is probably the same as that following single-injection spinal anesthesia performed with smaller-diameter needles.[9]

CONTINUOUS SPINAL CATHETERS

Table 38.3 lists the catheters available for CSA and the size of the needle used to insert them. A pencil-point 24-gauge (Sprotte) needle with lateral side port that allows

Table 38.2 Incidence of headache with continuous spinal anesthesia (Adapted from ref. 4 with permission)

Reference	Year	Needle gauge	Catheter gauge	Percent headache
3	1987	18	20	1
5	1972	20, 21	24	16*
6	1989	26	32	4
7	1989	17	20	20*
8	1990	18	20	54*

*Pregnant patients.

Table 38.3 Catheters (From ref. 4 with permission)

Type	Material	Gauge	Needle	Manufacturer
Epidural	Nylon, Teflon	19, 20	17, 18	Many
Spinal	Polyethylene	24	20, 21*	CSI
Pediatric Epidural	Polyurethane	24	20	Preferred Med.
Spinal	Polyurethane	27	22	Preferred Med.
Spinal	Nylon	28	22	Concord Portex
Spinal	Nylon	28	22	Kendall
Spinal	Polyimide	28	22	Rusch
Spinal	Polyimide	32	26, 27	Rusch

*Special needles.

passage of a 28-gauge or smaller catheter is also manufactured.[10] The pencil-point tip decreases the incidence of PDPH[11] and the Sprotte needle may prove useful for CSA in parturients.

LABOR ANALGESIA/ANESTHESIA

Continuous spinal anesthesia can be used for pain relief during labor (Table 38.4) and the availability of small catheters has renewed interest in this technique.[19] The method was first used in 1946 with tetracaine and metycaine.[13] Procaine became popular in the 1950s[15] and now lidocaine and bupivacaine are in use.[16,19] Many opioids have been used for labor analgesia.[18,23] Meperidine is an interesting opioid because of its local anesthetic properties. Beside producing analgesia by interacting with spinal cord opioid receptors, it also causes neuronal conduction blockade.[24] Sufentanil, a highly lipid-soluble and potent opioid, has recently been used for subarachnoid labor analgesia.[21] When 3–5 mg of sufentanil is injected through a 28-gauge catheter that is inserted through a 22-gauge needle, it produces up to 5 h of analgesia and the prevalence of PDPH is approximately 2% (J S Naulty, personal communication). These results with subarachnoid opioids indicate promise for the control of pain during labor because they produce analgesia without motor blockade.

Table 38.4 Obstetric uses of continuous spinal catheters

Reference	Year	Use	Drugs
12	1945	Cesarean section	Procaine
13	1946	Labor analgesia	Metycaine Tetracaine
14	1950	Eclampsia Preeclampsia	Tetracaine
15	1951	Labor analgesia	Procaine
16	1970	Labor analgesia	Lidocaine
4	1972	Cesarean section	Procaine
17	1988	Cesarean section* Difficult airway	Bupivacaine
18	1989	Labor analgesia	Fentanyl Morphine
19	1990	Labor analgesia	Bupivacaine
5	1990	Cesarean section	Lidocaine Bupivacaine
20	1990	Cesarean section* Kyphoscoliosis	Bupivacaine
21	1990	Labor analgesia	Sufentanil
22	1990	Cesarean section* Spina bifida	Bupivacaine

*Case report.

CESAREAN DELIVERY

There has been little interest in using CSA for cesarean delivery. This is probably because the operation can usually be completed within the duration of a single-injection spinal anesthetic. Furthermore, the patients are generally healthy and can tolerate the hemodynamic effects of high spinal anesthesia. It is not generally necessary to insert a subarachnoid catheter, which can be difficult and time-consuming.[6] Nevertheless, there are reports of cesarean delivery performed with CSA (Table 38.4).

Putative advantages of CSA during Cesarean delivery are the possibility of titrating the local anesthetic dose in order to limit cephalad spread. By so doing, the degree of sympathectomy is believed to be less and the hemodynamic consequences minimized. In our study,[6] we found that, despite injecting small doses of local anesthetics through a spinal catheter, the level of anesthesia was similar to single injection of a larger dose. However, the duration of anesthesia is shorter when small doses are given with CSA. This is of little consequence because the catheter allows renewal of the anesthetic once it begins to diminish. Another theoretical advantage of CSA over the single-injection method is that more local anesthetic can be given through the catheter, if the level of anesthesia is inadequate.

DISEASES COMPLICATING PREGNANCY

Continuous spinal anesthesia is beneficial in certain disease states that occasionally complicate pregnancy:

1. spinal deformity
   a. kyphoscoliosis
   b. spina bifida;
2. difficult airway;
3. obesity;
4. cardiac disease.

Continuous spinal anesthesia is useful in controlling labor pain in patients with severe kyphoscoliosis.[20] The manipulation of baricity and patient position allows careful distribution of the local anesthetic, which is not possible with continuous epidural anesthesia (CEA). Nuyten and Gielen[22] used CSA for cesarean delivery in a patient with spina bifida. The patient, who wanted to participate in the birth of her child, had grossly deformed vertebral anatomy that the authors believed would make successful epidural anesthesia unlikely and instead they instituted CSA. The cesarean delivery utilizing hyperbaric bupivacaine was uneventful. Moran and Johnson[12] used CSA in a morbidly obese parturient with a difficult airway. Continuous epidural anesthesia is often difficult or impossible in the obese parturient and CSA may be easier to carry out. Furthermore, the ability to titrate the dose of local anesthetic is considered advantageous. Parturients with cardiac disease are usually given CEA for labor and/or cesarean delivery. However, if CEA fails or is not possible in parturients with cardiac disease, the clear end point of cerebrospinal fluid appearing in the needle hub makes CSA a desirable and useful alternative to CEA.[25]

Years ago, Lund[14] reported on a few patients who received CSA to control the pathophysiologic effects of eclampsia and preeclampsia. Although this is an interesting idea, the method is no longer used. The abnormal coagulation sometimes associated with eclampsia and preeclampsia can be a relative contraindication to regional anesthesia.

SUMMARY

Because of the availability of small catheters that can be inserted through small-diameter needles, there is renewed interest in CSA for obstetric anesthesia and analgesia. This decreases the incidence of PDPH, which is high in parturients when a large-diameter needle is used for lumbar dural puncture. The indications for continuous spinal anesthesia and analgesia in obstetrics are still evolving. The administration of highly lipid-soluble opioids through small spinal catheters for labor analgesia is exciting and promising. Continuous spinal anesthesia has advantages over CEA in certain disease states that complicate pregnancy, particularly diseases, such as kyphoscoliosis, spina bifida and obesity, which distort spinal anatomy.

REFERENCES

1. Sutter P A, Gamulin Z, Forster A 1989 Comparison of continuous spinal and continuous epidural anaesthesia for lower limb surgery in elderly patients: a retrospective study. Anaesthesia 44: 47
2. Vandam L D, Dripps R D 1956 Long term follow up of patients who received 10,098 spinal anesthetics. III. Syndrome of decreased intracranial pressure (headache and ocular and auditory difficulties). J Am Med Assoc 161: 586
3. Denny N, Masters R, Pearson D, Read J, Sihota M, Selander D 1987 Postdural puncture headache after continuous spinal anesthesia. Anesth Analg 66: 791
4. Lambert D H 199x Continuous spinal anesthesia. Anesth Clin N Am in press
5. Giuffrida J G, Bizzari D V, Masi R, Bondoc R 1972 Continuous procaine spinal anesthesia for cesarean section. Anesth Analg 51: 117
6. Hurley R J, Lambert D H 1990 Continuous spinal anesthesia with a microcatheter technique: preliminary experience. Anesth Analg 70: 97
7. Cohen S, Daitch J S, Goldiner P L 1989 An alternative method for management of accidental dural puncture for labor and delivery (letter). Anesthesiology 70: 164
8. Norris M C, Leighton B L 1990 Continuous spinal anesthesia after unintentional dural puncture in parturients. Reg Anesth 15: 285
9. Hurley R J, Lambert D H 1990 Microcatheters for continuous spinal anesthesia (letter). Anesth Analg 71: 201
10. Cesarini M, Torrieli R, Lahaye F, Mene J M, Cabiro C 1990 Sprotte needle for intrathecal anaesthesia for caesarean section: incidence of postdural puncture headache (letter). Anaesthesia 45: 656
11. Carrie L E S 1990 Whitacre and pencil-point spinal needles: some points to consider (letter). Anaesthesia 45: 1097
12. Ullery J C 1945 Continuous spinal and continuous caudal analgesia in cesarean section. Surg Clin N Am 25: 1382
13. Gillett R E 1946 Continuous spinal anesthesia in obstetrics. Northwest Med 45: 743
14. Lund P C 1951 The role of conduction anesthesia in the management of eclampsia. Anesthesiology 12: 693
15. Carpenter S L, Caravolo A J, Foldes F F 1951 Continuous-drop subarachnoidal block with dilute procaine solution for labor and delivery. Am J Obstet Gynecol 61: 1277
16. Elam J O 1970 Catheter subarachnoid block for labor and delivery: a differential segmental technique employing hyperbaric lidocaine. Anesth Analg 49: 1007
17. Malan T P, Johnson M D 1988 The difficult airway in obstetric anesthesia: techniques for airway management and the role of regional anesthesia. J Clin Anesth 1: 104
18. Leighton B L, DeSimone C A, Norris M C, Ben-David B 1989 Intrathecal narcotics revisited: the combination of fentanyl and morphine intrathecally provides rapid onset of profound, prolonged analgesia. Anesth Analg 69: 122
19. Benedetti C, Tiengo M 1990 Continuous subarachnoid analgesia in labour (letter). Lancet 335: 225
20. Moran D H, Johnson M D 1990 Continuous spinal anesthesia with combined hyperbaric and isobaric bupivacaine in a patient with scoliosis. Anesth Analg 70: 445
21. Naulty J S, Barnes D, Becker R, Pate A 1990 Continuous subarachnoid sufentanil for labor analgesia (abstract). Anesthesiology 73: A964
22. Nuyten F, Gielen M 1990 Spinal catheter anesthesia for cesarean section in a patient with spina bifida. Anaesthesia 45: 846
23. Hurley R J, Johnson M D 1990 Spinal opioids in the management of obstetric pain. J Pain Symptom Manage 5: 146
24. Johnson M D, Hurley R J, Gilbertson L I, Datta S 1990 Continuous microcatheter spinal anesthesia with subarachnoid meperidine for labor and delivery. Anesth Analg 70: 658
25. Johnson M D, Saltzman D H 1990 Cardiac disease. In: Datta S (ed) Anesthetic and obstetric management of high risk pregnancy. Mosby Year Book, St Louis p 210

PART B
EUROPEAN VIEW

L. E. S. Carrie

INTRODUCTION

Some reduction in the popularity of spinal anesthesia was inevitable following the introduction of muscle relaxant drugs in the 1950s. Nevertheless, it has continued to be widely used even in more prosperous countries with a high standard of general anesthesia where its advantages of simplicity and minimal cost were less important. A notable exception was the UK where anxiety about the safety of spinal anesthesia was brought to the fore by the Woolley and Roe cases, when two men on one operating list suffered painful and permanent paraplegias after spinal block.[1] The repercussions of this occurrence resulted in the virtual disappearance of the technique, the use of which was stated in an editorial in the *British Journal of Anaesthesia* in 1975 to be confined to a few enthusiasts.[2] There was little training in spinal anesthesia for two decades and, as a result, as consultants with knowledge of the technique retired they were replaced by others with little experience of the method.

By the mid 1970s there were signs of renewed interest in the technique – a fact confirmed by two surveys carried out in Scotland in 1976 and 1981,[3,4] the second showing a considerable increase in use over the 5-year period. An unpublished survey by this author of obstetric anesthesiologists in the UK in 1978 demonstrated that, while 40% of those replying used spinal anesthesia in obstetrics, the commonest reason given for not using it was 'lack of experience in the technique'. Interest in its use has continued to increase steadily in the past 5–10 years.

Besides expertise, one of the main factors affecting usage of spinal anesthesia is the available choice of local anesthetic drugs. For many years after its introduction in 1929, hyperbaric cinchocaine (Nupercaine) was the mainstay of spinal anesthetic drugs in the UK. After the introduction of bupivacaine in the late 1960s, that drug was used to some extent in its normal (almost isobaric) formulation for spinal anesthesia.[5] When hyperbaric 0.5% bupivacaine solution was introduced in 1985, cinchocaine was withdrawn from the market. As hyperbaric solutions of prilocaine and mepivacaine, which had been available for a few years in the UK, had also been withdrawn, this left bupivacaine as the only hyperbaric solution both available and approved by the Committee on Safety of Medicines (CSM). However, 5% hyperbaric lidocaine may soon be added to the list. These two hyperbaric solutions are now in widespread use throughout Europe and Scandinavia, with some others, e.g. mepivacaine and tetracaine, having a more limited, regional popularity.

CESAREAN DELIVERY

After 20 years of increasing popularity of regional anesthesia for cesarean delivery, there are signs that the virtual monopoly of epidural anesthesia for this purpose is being steadily eroded by subarachnoid block. The explanation for this lies in both the advantages offered by the spinal technique and the limitations of epidural block. The rate of onset of spinal is quicker than epidural anesthesia (this is especially apparent in countries where 2-chloroprocaine is not available for epidural block); anesthesia is more reliable, not only because the local anesthetic agent is injected in closer proximity to the nerve roots but also because spread of the solution is easier than in the epidural space; and, unlike epidural anesthesia, drug toxicity in the mother and fetus is not a hazard.

Plain bupivacaine

Before hyperbaric bupivacaine became available, attempts were made to provide reliable anesthesia for cesarean delivery using the 0.5% plain solution.[5–7] A major theoretical advantage of this technique was that the patient could be maintained in the full lateral position, with minimal aortocaval occlusion, while the spinal anesthetic was becoming established. While this did occur in some cases, in others the solution behaved more obviously as a slightly hypobaric one, with anesthesia restricted mainly to the lumbar and sacral segments on the upper side. However, moving the patient from one full lateral position to either the opposite wedged position[6] or the other lateral position[7] almost always resulted in much more cephalad extension of the block than was necessary and, in some instances, developed into a 'total spinal' block. Russell[6] believed this to be due to some degree of vena-caval occlusion in the wedged position causing engorgement of the veins of the epidural space and consequent 'squeezing' of the dural sac. An alternative explanation, when using the technique described by Carrie and O'Sullivan,[7] was a degree of 'internal barbotage' caused by movement of the nerve roots in the subarachnoid space on turning the patient. Vena-caval occlusion was unlikely to have been an important contributory factor in their patients, as not only were they maintained in one or other lateral position, but extension of the block still occurred if the patient was turned from one side to the other through the prone position.

Whatever the reason for the increased spread of the almost isobaric bupivacaine, its unpredictable and sometimes very high spread led to its abandonment by Russell and its inclusion in a combined spinal–epidural technique by Carrie and O'Sullivan.[7]

A technique using a large volume (10 ml) of 0.125% bupivacaine with epinephrine 1:800 000 has been recommended.[8] While excellent anesthesia was reported, some of the blocks extended to the mid-cervical nerve roots and the author is not aware of this technique being practiced widely throughout Europe.

Hyperbaric bupivacaine

Hyperbaric 0.5% bupivacaine in 8% dextrose (Marcain Heavy, Astra Pharmaceuticals) remains (at present) the only hyperbaric spinal solution both available in the UK and approved by the Medicines Control Agency (MCA, formerly the CSM). When this solution was released in the UK in 1985, only two studies had been published in the world literature of its use in obstetrics. In the first of these, 12 patients were given 2.2–3.0 ml (11–15 mg) of hyperbaric 0.5% bupivacaine subarachnoid in the sitting position before being placed supine during development of the block for elective cesarean delivery.[9] Anesthesia was reported to be satisfactory in all cases. However, in the other study[10] only 1.5–2.0 ml (7.5–10.0 mg) of the same solution was injected in 22 women, also initially in the sitting position. While mean spread of analgesia was to T3, all but one patient required intravenous analgesic or sedative supplementation. Later work by Pederson et al[11] confirmed that with bupivacaine it is essential to give a large enough dose of the drug to obtain satisfactory anesthesia for cesarean delivery. Using two dose ranges (7.5–10.0 mg and 10.0–12.5 mg) of 0.5% hyperbaric bupivacaine according to patient height, they found that the prevalence of moderate to severe pain associated with peritoneal traction was reduced from 70.5% to 31.6% by increasing the dose of local anesthetic. These studies indicated that with this agent effective anesthesia of sufficient duration for cesarean delivery was only obtained with adequate 'painting' of the nerve roots by the local anesthetic.

In 1982 Chambers et al[12] demonstrated that with 0.5% hyperbaric bupivacaine solution increasing the volume (and hence the mass) of drug given from 2.0 to 4.0 ml prolonged the duration of the anesthetic block but did not increase its spread, as might be expected when the spinal curvatures are used to limit the spread of the drug. Although the only approved hyperbaric solution in the UK, few controlled studies have been carried out using the 0.5% solution in obstetrics. Two further reports confirm the better standard of pain relief obtained with larger quantities of the drug. Michie et al[13] compared the agent with 0.5% hyperbaric cinchocaine for cesarean delivery. The hyperbaric solutions were injected with all patients in the left lateral and horizontal position before being rolled supine on to a wedge under the right hip. All 20 patients given 2.5 ml (12.5 mg) of bupivacaine were pain-free during the operation and had no need for perioperative supplementation. Carrie,[14] in a study of 50 patients in whom a fixed dose of 2.8 ml (14.0 mg) of 0.5% hyperbaric bupivacaine was given to patients regardless of height as part of a combined spinal–epidural technique for cesarean delivery (see below) found excellent anesthesia from the spinal anesthetic alone in 82% of cases. In the other cases, epidural local anesthetic was given preoperatively to raise the sensory level of anesthesia to T4. These studies confirm the efficacy of 0.5% hyperbaric bupivacaine for cesarean delivery, but only if sufficient drug is given.

SUBARACHNOID OPIOIDS

There is at present a greater reluctance among European than American obstetric anesthesiologists to use intraspinal opioids by either the subarachnoid or epidural routes. Subarachnoid morphine for pain relief in labor was reported by Scott et al in 1980,[15] Baraka et al in 1981[16] and Bonnardot et al in 1982,[17] but has not been extensively used because of the high incidence of side-effects. The use of other subarachnoid opioids in labor has not been reported from Europe.

There are also, as yet, no European reports of the use of subarachnoid opioids to improve the efficacy of spinal anesthesia for cesarean delivery, but Tunstall has gained considerable experience in the addition of fentanyl to hyperbaric 0.5% bupivacaine for this purpose (M E Tunstall, personal communication). He recommends a dose of approximately 12.5 μg added to 2.25–2.75 ml of local anesthetic solution and reports a very high success rate of excellent post-operative analgesia with this technique.

COMBINED SPINAL–EPIDURAL TECHNIQUES

As experience has been gained and information collected about epidural block for cesarean delivery, it has become apparent that consistently excellent pain relief is unattainable with any of the currently available local anesthetic drugs. Better understanding of the anatomy of the epidural space derived from anatomic and surgical dissections,[18] by polyester resin cast studies,[19] by computerized tomography[20] and by epiduroscopy[21,22] has shown that, besides the normal barriers to spread of epidural solutions, e.g. fat and dura mater, there are variable bands and septa that produce varying degrees of compartmentalization of the epidural space. In extreme cases this may result in a purely unilateral block. In the USA, this has led to various modifications in epidural anesthesia to try to increase its rate of onset or improve its efficacy, the commonest of these being addition of an opioid to the local anesthetic or its pH adjustment, and one or both of these techniques is used during epidural anesthesia for the majority of cesarean deliveries. In the UK, where there has been greater reluctance to use spinal opioids and less familiarity with pH adjustment, there has been a greater tendency to turn to subarachnoid block as an alternative, and more recently to combined spinal and epidural block.

Combined spinal–epidural anesthesia was first described in 1979 by Curelaru[23] using separate lumbar interspaces for the spinal and epidural needle insertions. A similar technique was reported by Brownridge for cesarean delivery in 1981.[24] The first description of a spinal needle-through epidural needle technique using a single interspace, which is the method now usually understood by the term 'combined spinal–epidural (CSE) anesthesia', was made by Coates in 1982[25] for orthopedic use and by Carrie and O'Sullivan for cesarean delivery in 1984.[7] The basic advantages of the technique are the combination of the speed of onset, reliability and low toxicity of the spinal anesthetic with the availability of the epidural catheter to modify the subarachnoid block if it is not adequate. Additionally, CSE anesthesia allows the greatest possible flexibility in central neural axis regional anesthesia. Opioids can be given subarachnoid, alone or in combination with local anesthetic drugs, either to improve perioperative analgesia or prolong it into the post-operative period. The epidural catheter can be used for the same purposes and its presence greatly extends the possible duration of post-operative pain relief. Variations are also possible in the basic technique. Some workers[26,27] attempt to provide adequate anesthesia for cesarean delivery from the spinal block alone, using the epidural route only if required. As for any spinal anesthetic for cesarean delivery, the injection can be given in the sitting or lateral recumbent positions. Carrie[27] gives the injection in the left lateral position, but then turns the patient into the right lateral position, thus avoiding aortocaval occlusion until the patient is rolled back onto the wedge for surgery to commence. Excessive cephalad spread of the hyperbaric solution is prevented by an inflatable support under the shoulder, maintaining the uphill gradient from the thoracic to the cervical regions of the spine. Rawal,[28] on the other hand, performs the spinal injection in the sitting position, in a deliberate attempt to block only the lower spinal segments, and extends the upper level of anesthesia by use of the epidural catheter after the patient has been placed supine. The claimed advantage of this technique is a lower incidence of hypotension with the slower upward extension of the block – always a greater potential problem when the wedged rather than the full lateral position is maintained.

There are also possible indications for the CSE technique for pain relief in labor, e.g. a subarachnoid opioid can be given, followed if and when necessary by epidural anesthesia (B B Gutsche, personal communication).

The increasing popularity of the CSE technique is apparent from the ingenuity of anesthesiologists in designing and the readiness of needle manufacturers to produce equipment specifically for the technique. As the epidural needle acts as a guide for the spinal needle almost to the subarachnoid space, very fine spinal needles may be used and both 29-gauge cutting-tipped[29,30] and 26-gauge pencil-point needles[31] have proved very satisfactory for the technique. At least one special device has been manufactured which makes it possible to introduce the epidural catheter before injecting the spinal solution,[32] thus avoiding any delay which might occur in positioning the patient after injecting the drug subarachnoid if any difficulty should arise in passing the epidural catheter.

CONTINUOUS SPINAL ANESTHESIA

Fear of meningitis and an expected high incidence of post-dural puncture headache (PDPH) resulting from the large caliber of needle required to introduce a subarachnoid catheter has in Europe, as elsewhere, until recently stifled enthusiasm for continuous spinal anesthesia. Two factors may change this attitude. Firstly, a recent report by Denny et al[33] confirmed an earlier study by Kallos and Smith[34] indicating a surprisingly low prevalence (0% and 0.85% in the two studies) of PDPH following the introduction of 20-gauge catheters through 18-gauge needles. However, a warning that these figures are unlikely to be strictly extrapolable to obstetric patients with their high susceptibility to PDPH comes from a study by Giuffrida et al,[35] who reported a 16% frequency of PDPH when 24-gauge catheters were introduced through 21-gauge needles for cesarean delivery. Secondly, extremely fine 32-gauge catheters, which can be passed through 25- or even some 26-gauge needles, have recently been introduced. Experience with these catheters in Europe so far is limited to two studies, one reporting few technical difficulties,[36] but the other being less enthusiastic.[37]

Catheters of a 'compromise' size, 28 gauge, which will pass through a 22-gauge spinal needle, are now becoming available. It remains to be seen whether catheters of this caliber will have an acceptably low incidence of PDPH in obstetric patients.

Continuous spinal anesthesia using local anesthetics, opioids or mixtures of the two has many potential indications not only in the routine provision of pain relief for labor, cesarean delivery and post-operatively, but for a variety of special problem situations. While this is an area of considerable interest at present, experience with this technique and the development of special equipment is in its relative infancy.

OTHER INDICATIONS IN OBSTETRICS FOR SPINAL ANESTHESIA

Subarachnoid block provides excellent anesthesia for a variety of vaginal procedures including insertion of a cervical circumsuture and a group of semiemergency situations when an epidural catheter is not already in situ, e.g. rotational forceps delivery and manual removal of a retained placenta. Spinal anesthesia is used increasingly for these procedures in Europe, and this tendency is to be encouraged, partly to avoid the dangers of general anesthesia and partly because most women prefer to remain awake during, or become so shortly after, the delivery of their baby.

SPINAL ANESTHESIA IN OBSTETRICS AND POST-DURAL PUNCTURE HEADACHE (PDPH)

The increase in popularity of spinal anesthesia has rekindled interest in the prevention and treatment of PDPH. Because of its postural nature this complication is particularly distressing in the obstetric patient who wishes to be fully mobile to care for her new baby. Unfortunately, women of child-bearing age are highly susceptible to PDPH.

Despite many clinical and laboratory studies, there is still some doubt concerning the precise role of the various factors involved in the etiology of PDPH. Reasons for this include failure in some of these studies to control factors known to be important, e.g. needle caliber, age and sex of patients. Nevertheless, it is accepted that the headache is associated with the rate and duration of cerebrospinal fluid leak through the hole made by the spinal needle in the dura mater and that factors resulting in the early closure of that hole will be associated with a lower incidence of PDPH. Until recently, the main effort at reducing PDPH has been directed towards using finer needles, and sizes as small as 26-gauge or even smaller are now commonly used. These needles have cutting tips that most clinical studies indicate should be inserted through the dura mater with the bevel parallel to the long axis of the vertebral canal to produce the least CSF leak. Most investigators have found a prevalence of PDPH in the 3–10% range even with needles as fine as 26-gauge in obstetric patients, and some of these headaches can be severe. Even finer needles present manufacturing problems, especially with the bonding of transparent plastic hubs (so useful in the early detection of cerebrospinal fluid) to such fine shafts. There are also difficulties during use owing to bending and lack of feel.

In the last few years great interest has been rearoused in the use of needles with atraumatic, or 'pencil' points to reduce the incidence of PDPH. This concept is not new, Greene proposing the use of such needles in 1926[38] and Hart and Whitacre[39] and Haraldson in 1951.[40] The idea remained relatively dormant until a report on a new design of atraumatic needle by Sprotte et al in 1987.[41] This extraordinary study reported the use of atraumatic needles on 34 950 occasions for a wide range of indications, the majority of which were plexus blocks. However, 7175 were a mixture of spinal anesthetics and dural punctures for a variety of diagnostic and therapeutic purposes; no details of age or sex of the patients were given. Despite this, the claimed prevalence of PDPH of 0.02% using a mixture of 22- and 24-gauge needles was so impressive that other manufacturers were encouraged to produce similarly tipped needles. Now the results in more carefully selected groups of patients are beginning to appear, and neither Cesarini et al[42] using 24-gauge Sprotte needles for spinal anesthesia for cesarean delivery in 55 patients, Thomas and Noble[43] using 22-gauge Whitacre needles in a preliminary report in 19 obstetric patients nor Carrie and Donald[31] using 26-gauge atraumatic needles in 53 patients for Cesarean delivery have reported any cases of PDPH. One investigator[44] did not find any difference in the incidence of PDPH between cutting and pencil-point needles of the same caliber and, although the above reports appear optimistic, the evidence is not yet conclusive in favor of the atraumatic needles. If the substitution of atraumatic for cutting tips allows the use of larger needles without a high incidence of PDPH, this will obviate both the manufacturing and clinical difficulties.

REFERENCES

1. Cope R W 1954 The Woolley and Roe case. Anaesthesia 9: 249–270
2. Editorial 1975 Spinal anaesthesia. Br J Anaesth 47: 421–422
3. Robertson D H, Lewerentz H, Holmes F 1978 Subarachnoid spinal analgesia. A comparative survey in current practice in Scotland and Sweden. Anaesthesia 33: 913–923
4. Robertson D H 1983 Subarachnoid spinal analgesia. Changing patterns of practice. Br J Anaesth 55: 1141–1147
5. Nolte H, Schikor K, Gergs P, Meyer J, Stark P 1977 Zur frage der spinalanaesthesie mit isobarem bupivacain 0.5%. Anaesthesist 26: 33–37
6. Russell I 1983 Spinal anaesthesia for Caesarean section. The use of 0.5% bupivacaine. Br J Anaesth 55: 309–314
7. Carrie L E S, O'Sullivan G M 1984 Subarachnoid bupivacaine 0.5% for Caesarean section. Eur J Anaesthesiol 1: 275–283
8. Van Zundert A, De Wolf A M, Vaes L, Soetens M 1988 High volume spinal anesthesia with bupivacaine 0.125% for Cesarean section. Anesthesiology 69: 998–1003
9. Willdeck-Lund G, Lyrenas S, Edstrom H 1983 Spinal anaesthesia for Caesarean section. Acta Anaesthesiol Scand 27 (suppl 78): 98
10. Santos A, Pederson H, Finster M, Edstrom H 1984 Hyperbaric bupivacaine for spinal anesthesia in Cesarean section. Anesth Analg 63: 1009–1013
11. Pederson H, Santos A C, Steinberg E S, Schapiro H M, Harmon T W, Finster M 1989 Incidence of visceral pain during Cesarean section: the effect of varying doses of spinal bupivacaine. Anesth Analg 69: 46–49
12. Chambers W A, Littlewood D G, Edström H H, Scott D B 1982 Spinal anaesthesia with hyperbaric bupivacaine: effects of concentration and volume administered. Br J Anaesth 54: 75–80
13. Michie A R, Freeman R M, Dutton D A, Howie H B 1988 Subarachnoid anaesthesia for elective Caesarean section. A comparison of two hyperbaric solutions. Anaesthesia 43: 96–99
14. Carrie L E S 1989 Awake without tears: combined spinal–epidural anesthesia for Cesarean section using 29 G spinal needles. Proceedings of the Society for Obstetric Anesthesia and Perinatology. Seattle
15. Scott P V, Bowen F E, Cartwright P et al 1980 Intrathecal morphine as sole analgesic during labour. Br Med J 281: 351–355
16. Baraka A, Nouehid R, Hajj S 1981 Intrathecal injection of morphine for obstetric analgesia. Anesthesiology 54: 136–140
17. Bonnardot J P, Maillet M, Colau J C, Millot F, Deligne P 1982 Maternal and fetal concentration of morphine after intrathecal administration during labour. Br J Anaesth 54: 487–489

18. Luyendijk W 1976 The plica mediana dorsalis of the dura mater and its relation to lumbar peridurography (canalography). Neuroradiology 11: 147–149
19. Husemeyer R P, White D C 1980 Topography of the lumbar epidural space. Anaesthesia 35: 7–11
20. Savolaine E R, Pandya J B, Greenblatt S H, Conover S R 1988 Anatomy of the human lumbar epidural space: new insights using CT-epidurography. Anesthesiology 68: 217–220
21. Blomberg R 1986 The dorsomedian connective tissue band in the lumbar epidural space of humans. Anesth Analg 65: 747–752
22. Blomberg R G, Olsson S S 1989 The lumbar epidural space in patients examined with epiduroscopy. Anesth Analg 68: 157–160
23. Curelaru I 1979 Long-term subarachnoid anaesthesia with continuous epidural block. Praktische Anasthesie Wiederbelebung und Intensivtherapie 14: 71–78
24. Brownridge P 1981 Epidural and subarachnoid analgesia for elective Caesarean section. Anaesthesia 36: 70
25. Coates M B 1982 Combined subarachnoid and epidural techniques. Anaesthesia 37: 89–90
26. Nickalls R W D, Dennison B 1984 A modification of the combined spinal and epidural technique. Anaesthesia 39: 935–936
27. Carrie L E S 1989 Spinal and/or epidural blockade for Caesarean section. In: Reynolds F (ed) Epidural and spinal blockade in obstetrics. Bailliere Tindall, London p 139
28. Rawal N, Schollin J, Wesstrom G 1988 Epidural versus combined spinal epidural block for Caesarean section. Acta Anaesthesiol Scand 32: 61–66
29. Haden R M, Scott P V, Pinnock C A 1990 Spinal obstetric anaesthesia with a 29-gauge needle. Br J Anaesth 65: 294–295
30. Carrie L E S, Collins P D 1991 29-gauge spinal needles. Br J Anaesth 66: 145–147
31. Carrie L E S, Donald F A 1991 A 26-gauge Pencil Point needle for combined-epidural anaesthesia for Caesarean section. Anaesthesia 46: 230–231
32. Eldor J, Chaimsky G 1988 Combined spinal-epidural needle (CSEN). Can J Anaesth 35: 537–539
33. Denny N, Masters R, Pearson D, Read J, Sihota M, Selander D 1987 Postdural puncture headache after continuous spinal anaesthesia. Anesth Analg 66: 791–794
34. Kallos T, Smith T C 1972 Continuous spinal anesthesia with hypobaric tetracaine for hip surgery in lateral decubitus. Anesth Analg 51: 766–771
35. Giuffrida J G, Bizzarri D V, Masi R, Bondoc R 1972 Continuous procaine spinal anesthesia for Cesarean section. Anesth Analg 51: 117–124
36. Kestin I G, Madden A P, Mulvein J T, Goodman N W 1991 Comparison of incremental spinal anaesthesia using a 32-gauge catheter with extradural anaesthesia for elective Caesarean section. Br J Anaesth 66: 232–236
37. Nagle C J, McQuay H J, Glynn C J 1990 32-gauge spinal catheters through 26-gauge needles. Anaesthesia 45: 1052–1054
38. Greene H M 1926 Lumbar puncture and the prevention of postpuncture headache. J Am Med Assoc 86: 391–392
39. Hart J R, Whitacre R J 1951 Pencil-point needle in prevention of postspinal headache. J Am Med Assoc 147: 657–658
40. Haraldson S 1951 Headache after spinal anesthesia: experiments with a new spinal needle. Anesthesiology 12: 321–327
41. Sprotte G, Schedel R, Pajunk R, Pajunk H 1987 Eine “atraumatische” Universalkanule fur einzeitige Regionalanaesthesien. Reg Anaesth 10: 104–108
42. Cesarini M, Torrieli R, Lahaye F, Mene J M, Cabiro C 1990 Sprotte needle for intrathecal anaesthesia for Caesarean section: incidence of postdural puncture headache. Anaesthesia 45: 656–658
43. Thomas T A, Noble H A 1990 A re-evaluation of the Whitacre needle in obstetric practice. Anaesthesia 45: 489
44. Eckstein K L, Rogacev Z, Vicente-Eckstein A, Grahovac Z 1982 Prospectiv vergleichende Studie postspinaler ‘Kopfschmerzen bei jungen Patienten (< 51 Jahre). Reg Anaesth 5: 57–61

39. General anesthesia

Part A USA view *G. M. Bassell*
Part B UK view *G. O'Sullivan*

PART A
USA VIEW
G. M. Bassell

INTRODUCTION

Until the early 1960s, general anesthesia was preferred for cesarean delivery in the USA. Although spinal anesthesia was used frequently in some academic centers, and in some community hospitals with relatively large obstetric units, it did not account for a large proportion of the total number of anesthetics administered for the procedure nationwide. Toward the end of the decade, however, the use of spinal anesthesia began to overtake that of general anesthesia. In fact, in a survey published by the American College of Obstetricians and Gynecologists (ACOG) in 1971, spinal anesthesia accounted for 53% of the anesthetics administered for cesarean delivery, general anesthesia for 32% and epidural block for 3%.[1] In other surveys reported over the subsequent 15 years, the extent of use of general anesthesia remained fairly constant at between 35 and 43%, but the use of epidural anesthesia encroached upon territory previously held by spinal anesthesia[2,3] (Fig. 39.1).

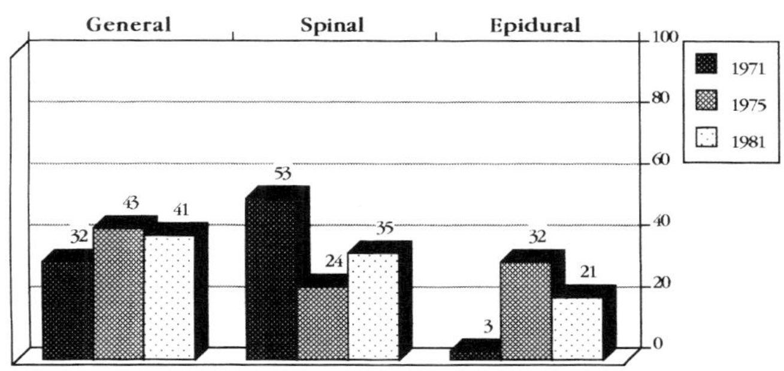

Fig. 39.1 Bar graph showing the percentage use of various anesthetic techniques for cesarean delivery as reported in surveys for the years shown.[1–3]

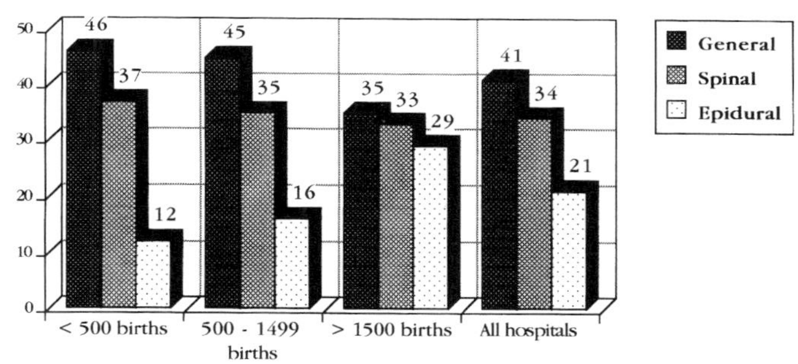

Fig. 39.2 Bar graph showing the percentage use of various anesthetic techniques for cesarean delivery in relation to number of births per hospital. (From the data of Gibbs et al.[3])

Currently, general anesthesia is still employed for a substantial number of cesarean deliveries in the USA in all sizes of obstetric suites[3] (Fig. 39.2). Despite publication of data demonstrating the safety of spinal anesthesia for urgent cesarean delivery even in the face of fetal distress,[4,5] it is probable that the vast majority of abdominal deliveries for this indication are still performed under general anesthesia. There are a number of reasons for this approach. Small labor and delivery suites that do not have 24-h, in-house, obstetric anesthesia coverage abound in the USA. Surgical deliveries in these facilities are frequently performed in the general operating suite and the anesthetic is administered by personnel who usually provide only anesthesia for cesarean delivery. Consequently, epidural and spinal anesthesia are rarely performed, and the experience necessary to maintain the level of skill required for safe, rapid administration of regional block under urgent circumstances is not attained. In many hospitals, anesthetic coverage is provided by personnel who have not had adequate training in obstetric regional anesthesia. For these and other reasons, much emphasis has recently been placed on requiring that training programs in the USA provide instruction for anesthesiology residents and student nurse anesthetists in the knowledge and skills required for the provision of safe general anesthesia for urgent cesarean delivery.

PHYSIOLOGIC CONSIDERATIONS

Some aspects of the physiology of pregnancy that form the basis for the choice of general anesthetic technique used for cesarean delivery in the USA are delineated briefly below. (An exhaustive review of maternal physiology can be found in Ch. 5.)

Aortocaval compression

It is unfortunate that the term 'supine hypotensive syndrome' is more frequently recognized than the term 'aortocaval compression'. The former is merely one manifestation of the latter, yet there is a widespread and erroneous belief that maternal position is unimportant unless there is associated hypotension. Such lack of understanding of the relationship between maternal position and uterine compression of the great abdominal vessels places both the gravida and her fetus at risk, particularly during cesarean delivery.

Uterine compression of the *inferior vena cava* when the gravida lies supine begins to be evident at around the 28th week of gestation. At term, more than 90% of parturients are affected and the interruption of vena-caval flow can be almost complete.[6] Blood returning from the pelvic organs and the lower limbs is forced to bypass the obstruction by rerouting through the dilated vertebral venous plexus to the azygous vein and, then, to the heart. However, the capacity of this alternative route is much less than that of the unobstructed vena-cava, and if venous return is forced in this direction, severe impairment of cardiac output occurs secondary to decreased cardiac filling. In the usual course of events, about 12% of the unanesthetized women affected in this manner will become hypotensive.[7] This number increases to between 60 and 80% in the presence of either regional or general anesthesia. In the remaining gravidas, substantial decreases in arterial pressure are usually avoided by reflex increments in systemic vascular resistance.[8] Unfortunately, the price of maintaining maternal homeostasis in this manner can be an associated reduction in uteroplacental blood flow. The very high incidence of supine hypotension encountered during cesarean delivery conducted under general anesthesia occurs for two main reasons. First, volatile and other anesthetics increase vascular capacitance, further reducing venous return over that resulting from compression of the inferior vena cava and, second, anesthetics interfere with the gravida's ability to employ the compensatory mechanism outlined above.

The *aortoiliac* system is also affected. Significant compression occurs in practically all gravidas who lie on their back during the third trimester.[9] In contrast to the situation that occurs with vena-caval obstruction, the degree of compression, and resultant decrease in uteroplacental blood flow, worsens as the fetal presenting part descends through the maternal pelvis. Since the obstruction to flow occurs in the abdomen and pelvis, no brachial hypotension or maternal symptoms are produced. On the contrary, aortoiliac compression by the gravid uterus when women in late pregnancy lie supine poses little risk of maternal complications apart from some reduction in renal function – the overt and immediate danger is to placental perfusion and fetal well-being.[10] General anesthesia increases the hazard by rendering the large abdominopelvic arteries more compressible.

Respiratory changes

Maternal oxygenation

The gravida's respiratory function changes progressively throughout pregnancy. Of importance to the conduct of safe general anesthesia are the increase in minute alveolar ventilation – up 70% by term – and the reduction in functional residual capacity (FRC) – down 20% by term.[11] An important effect of the reduction in FRC is the limitation it imposes on the mother's ability to maintain an oxygen reserve. This is accentuated by the increased oxygen consumption of pregnancy. Therefore, even brief periods of hypoventilation or apnea can result in significant maternal and fetal hypoxemia.[12] These incidents can occur during the relaxant-induced apneic period immediately before successful endotracheal intubation, during eclamptic convulsions, during local anesthetic-induced seizures and following excessive administration of opioid analgesics or tranquilizers. Prevention should be aimed at augmenting maternal blood oxygen tension before any predictably hazardous periods such as induction of general anesthesia. To that end, administration of 100% oxygen by face mask for 5 mins (or four deep breaths) before injection of the induction agent, and maintenance of anesthesia with no less than an inspired oxygen fraction (FIO_2) of 0.5 will enhance maternal and, thereby, fetal oxygenation.[13] In view of the heightened metabolic rate of pregnancy and associated increased oxygen consumption, enriching the maternal FIO_2 has beneficial effects on fetal oxygenation during cesarean delivery performed under regional anesthesia as well.

Maternal hypocarbia

Although respiratory rate increases by only 1–2 breaths/min over the course of pregnancy, the rise in minute alveolar ventilation is much larger (see above).[11] As a result, the partial pressure of carbon dioxide in maternal arterial blood is approximately 32 mmHg at term.[14] Any further increases in the parturient's minute ventilation, whether involuntary or deliberate, can precipitate additional falls in carbon dioxide tension and result in alkalemia. The impact on fetal oxygenation can be severe. A number of deleterious effects have been demonstrated: first, both uteroplacental and umbilical blood flow can be retarded;[15] second, the maternal oxygen cost of the hyperventilation itself reduces the amount of oxygen available for placental transmission; third, alkalosis shifts the maternal hemoglobin–oxygen dissociation curve to the left, thereby binding oxygen more tightly to maternal hemoglobin and reducing its release at the placental interface;[16] and, finally, the delicate relationship between intervillous space and fetal blood pH is disrupted. The hydrogen ion gradient across the placenta is responsible in large part for efficient transfer of oxygen from mother to fetus,[17] and when this balance is upset normal transmission deteriorates. Thus, it is incumbent upon the anesthesiologist to ensure that maternal arterial carbon dioxide tension is maintained at normal term-pregnant levels (32–34 mmHg) during cesarean deliveries conducted under general anesthesia.

Gastrointestinal changes

Regurgitation and aspiration of stomach contents are more likely to happen to women during pregnancy because of physiologic changes occurring in the gastrointestinal system over the course of gestation. These include decreased bowel motility, delayed stomach emptying, reduction of the barrier pressure usually provided by the gastroesophageal junction, increased intra-abdominal pressure and augmented gastric acid and pepsin secretion.[18]

The pain of labor, and the parenteral opioid analgesics frequently used for its treatment, slow stomach emptying further. Thus, a parturient presenting for an urgent cesarean delivery after a prolonged, painful labor can be expected to have a 'full stomach'. Often overlooked, however, is the woman scheduled for an elective cesarean delivery who has fasted for many hours. In spite of the absence of stomach intake, she, too, must be considered to be at risk for regurgitation and aspiration of gastric contents and should be prepared and treated accordingly.

Altered drug response

The reduction in FRC mentioned above affects the uptake of gaseous and volatile anesthetics. Alveolar partial pressures of inhalation anesthetics increase more rapidly so that faster induction of anesthesia with gaseous or volatile agents occurs and deep anesthetic planes are achieved with greater ease and speed than in nonpregnant women. In addition, gravidas at term are more likely to be rendered unconscious by inspired concentrations of anesthetic gases and vapors that would not produce loss of consciousness in their nonpregnant counterparts.

Over the course of pregnancy, the dose requirement for anesthetics and other drugs is lowered. Minimum alveolar concentration (MAC) of volatile anesthetics, a measure of the amount required to bring about a particular degree of insensibility to pain, is reduced by up to 40%.[19] The implication is that doses must be reduced from those used in a similarly sized nonpregnant woman. Failure to do this can be expected to increase the likelihood of the complications related to deep general anesthesia.

CLINICAL CONSIDERATIONS

Preservation of fetal oxygenation

Maintenance of uteroplacental perfusion

Maternal positioning. As previously stated, the prevalence of supine hypotension increases to 60–80% in anesthetized gravidas. Even when no blood pressure fall is observed, uteroplacental blood flow is prejudiced.[20] Consequently, it is the standard of care in the USA for the uterus to be displaced from the great vessels immediately after the parturient is placed supine on the operating table until the infant has been delivered. Such displacement of the uterus is achieved by a variety of means, most commonly by placing a wedge of folded towels or blankets under the woman's hip. Recommendations vary concerning the number of degrees (15–30°) of displacement from the vertical that must be accomplished. In the vast majority of obstetric suites in the USA, the end point tends to be when the uterus appears visually to be displaced sufficiently.

Management of maternal blood pressure. Prevention of blood pressure decreases during general anesthesia for cesarean delivery requires knowledge of the effects of anesthetics and adjuvant drugs on the maternal cardiovascular system as well as familiarity with all events in the hours preceding delivery. Thus, women whose abdominal delivery follows a lengthy period without food or fluid intake are more likely to experience episodes of hypotension than are women who have been well hydrated during an antecedent, prolonged labor.[21] Pregnant women generally depend on heightened sympathetic tone to counteract the effect of pregnancy hormones on the peripheral vasculature, so when that activity is diminished during general anesthesia, hypotension is more apt to occur. Acute intravenous volume augmentation is, therefore, indicated prior to general anesthesia as it is before regional blockade. The amount of such 'preload' or acute hydration is not usually more than 500–750 ml. This is in contrast to the 1500 ml or more commonly infused immediately prior to induction of an epidural or subarachnoid block for cesarean delivery.

A large-bore intravenous catheter (16 G) is a routine part of most obstetric anesthetics in the USA.

The guidelines for treatment of blood pressure decreases have changed in recent years. Traditionally, any drop in systolic pressure below 100 mmHg or fall from control value of 10%, 20% or 30% (depending on the publication!) or greater was deemed to require further treatment if fetal well-being was to be preserved. Although there is sufficient evidence that hypotension reduces uteroplacental blood flow and threatens fetal oxygenation, the degree of such reductions that can be tolerated by a healthy fetus was, and still is, unknown. Datta et al[22] studied 60 term parturients undergoing elective primary or repeat cesarean delivery under subarachnoid block. The indication for intravenous ephedrine was the occurrence of any drop from baseline blood pressure. Umbilical vein and artery acid–base status and 1-min Apgar scores were almost identical irrespective of whether a fall in blood pressure had been treated with intravenous ephedrine or no actual decrease had occurred. In contrast, the infants of mothers who had experienced systolic blood pressure decreases to below 100 mmHg or falls of more than 30 mmHg from baseline had significantly lower pH levels in both umbilical vein and artery blood.

Irrespective of the definition of maternal hypotension employed, treatment during cesarean delivery in the USA is relatively standard. Increasing the intravenous infusion rate, displacing the uterus further, lightening the anesthetic plane if appropriate, augmenting the inspired oxygen fraction and administering repeated, small intravenous doses (5–10 mg) of ephedrine are the mainstays of therapy. Ephedrine is the drug of choice in this situation before delivery of the infant since it is the least likely of the available pressor amines to produce alpha-agonism and a resultant decrease in uteroplacental perfusion.[23]

In recent years, investigations in the USA have suggested that small doses of phenylephrine can be used safely.[24,25] At this time, however, ephedrine remains the drug of choice for the treatment of hypotension occurring during obstetric anesthesia.

Avoidance of maternal hypocarbia. The advent of reliable, affordable capnography has rendered avoidance of excessive maternal ventilation by the anesthesiologist relatively straightforward. In the USA, measurement of end-tidal carbon dioxide is performed routinely during every general anesthetic in obstetrics, so the deleterious effects of respiratory alkalosis on placental circulation and oxygen transmission are completely preventable. The critical period is, of course, that between induction of general anesthesia and delivery of the infant. Here, manual ventilation is preferred over mechanical ventilation owing to the ability of the anesthesiologist to respond rapidly to the capnogram. Ideally, the gravida is maintained normocarbic for term pregnancy ($Pa\text{CO}_2$ = 32–34 mmHg).

The 'delivery window'. As a corollary to the dose of induction drug employed, it has long been accepted that the duration of fetal anesthetic exposure during cesarean delivery has the potential to influence neonatal outcome adversely.[26,27] Over the years, therefore, significant attention has been directed toward limiting the induction–delivery interval (IDI) by completing skin preparation and sterile draping before induction of general anesthesia. These measures have become ingrained in American obstetric practice despite the accrual of evidence showing that producing relatively high maternal oxygenation ($F\text{IO}_2$= 0.65–0.7), preventing aortocaval compression and preserving normotension can maintain normal acid–base status in the newborn for up to 30 min of anesthetic exposure.[28] However, in a study of 105 neonates whose mothers had received either general or spinal anesthesia for elective, repeat cesarean delivery, the importance of other time relationships became apparent.[29] In those infants delivered during either type of anesthesia, an IDI of more than 8 min combined with a uterine incision–delivery interval (UDI) of more than 180 s was associated with an extremely high incidence of moderate to severe depression at 1 min of extrauterine life. There was correspondingly severe umbilical artery acidosis. However, when spinal anesthesia was used, the IDI played a secondary role. As long as the UDI was less than 180 s, prolonged IDIs (mean = 22 min) had little deleterious effect, but when UDIs were greater than 180 s the most severe newborn biochemical depression occurred. In contrast, infants exposed to maternal general anesthesia experienced greater degrees of newborn depression when the IDI exceeded 8 min and the UDI surpassed 180 s. Thus, the concept of a 'delivery window' has been introduced: during general anesthesia, the ideal time for delivery is within 8 min of anesthetic induction following a UDI of less than 180 s.

Maintenance of placental oxygen transmission

Maternal hyperoxia. Avoidance of maternal hypoxemia with resultant fetal hypoxia and acidosis requires acute oxygenation before induction of general anesthesia for cesarean delivery. Additionally, augmentation of maternal arterial oxygen tension in the period before delivery enhances placental transmission of oxygen. Owing to the design of the placental and fetal circulations, maximal enhancement of fetal oxygenation occurs at maternal arterial tensions of approximately 300 mmHg. This level is achieved with an $F\text{IO}_2$ greater than 0.5 via an endotracheal tube (Table 39.1).[13]

Maternal acid–base management. The importance of the relationship between maternal and fetal hydrogen ion concentration and the efficient placental transmission of oxygen and carbon dioxide cannot be overemphasized. Deep planes of anesthesia and resultant hypotension have

Table 39.1 The relationship between maternal inspired oxygen delivered by endotracheal tube (%), maternal arterial oxygen tension (MA), umbilical artery oxygen tension (UA), and umbilical vein oxygen tension (UV). All oxygen tensions are expressed as the mean in mmHg. (From the data of Marx and Mateo.[13])

	33%	65%	97%
MA	125.0	282.6	392.8
UA	18.0	23.0	25.2
UV	28.3	35.0	42.1

the potential for producing maternal acidemia. Excessive maternal ventilation and the ensuing respiratory alkalemia can move the maternal hemoglobin–oxygen dissociation curve to the left, thereby reducing release of oxygen at the placenta. Neither situation benefits the fetus. Ideally, then, light anesthesia with ventilation adequate to maintain normal acid–base status is preferred before delivery of the infant.

Aspects of maternal safety

Prevention of the acid aspiration syndrome

Most recent efforts have been directed at chemical means of averting regurgitation by reducing gastric volume (H_2-receptor antagonists, metoclopramide) or lessening the severity of pulmonary injury following aspiration (H_2-receptor antagonists, oral antacids). Traditional preventive measures take into account the physiologic mechanisms involved. Thus, the risk of regurgitation is reduced by avoiding large doses of opioid analgesics or sedatives during labor, by exercising caution when using suprafundal pressure, and by avoiding steep head-down positioning during induction of general anesthesia. The likelihood of aspiration is lessened by employing rapid-sequence induction with cricoid pressure and the availability of a large-bore suction apparatus.

Although the practice of preventing succinylcholine-induced fasciculations by prior treatment with a small dose of nondepolarizing muscle relaxant is widespread in the USA, the technique has fallen into disfavor for cesarean delivery. The supposed advantage of the method was avoidance of the further increases in intragastric pressure caused by fasciculations of the abdominal musculature. However, the fasciculations seen in gravidas do not seem to have the intensity of those occurring in their nonpregnant counterparts.[30] Further, the propensity of small doses of the nondepolarizing muscle relaxants to reduce the effectiveness of sequentially administered depolarizing drugs increases the dose requirement for the latter, and renders attempts at endotracheal intubation much more difficult.[31]

Difficult intubation

Difficulty with endotracheal intubation, and its frequently associated accompaniment, aspiration pneumonitis, is now the leading anesthesia-related cause of obstetric death.[32] Thus, thorough airway assessment is routinely performed before every general anesthetic in obstetrics. Anticipated difficulties in airway management can be indications for regional anesthesia or awake endotracheal intubation depending on their specific type. A variety of laryngoscope blades and Guedel airways, the Datta–Briwa short-handled laryngoscope, apparatus for transtracheal ventilation, tracheostomy trays and fiber-optic laryngoscopes or bronchoscopes have all been endorsed as necessary items to be kept in labor and delivery suites. As in other parts of the world, the importance of the presence of an experienced anesthesiologist for obstetric anesthesia in avoiding intubation problems has been recognized in the USA.

Figure 39.3 describes an algorithm for the management of the difficult or failed intubation.[33]

Prevention of maternal awareness

Induction and anesthetic drugs

Thiopental remains the mainstay of general anesthetic induction drugs in the USA; etomidate and propofol may also be used. Because of the reported incidence of maternal awareness when the traditional technique of thiopental induction followed by nitrous oxide–oxygen (50 : 50) until delivery is employed, many centers employ a sequence of ketamine–thiopental to reduce wakefulness. When ketamine alone (1 mg/kg), thiopental (4 mg/kg), and a ketamine–thiopental combination (0.5 mg/kg–2 mg/kg) were compared in 36 women undergoing elective cesarean delivery, ketamine was associated with the lowest incidence of wakefulness during the anesthetic.[34] Most of the women exhibiting recall or wakefulness had received thiopental, with intermediate results seen after the combination. From induction until delivery, the women received only nitrous oxide in oxygen (70 : 30). Ketamine (1.5 mg/kg) has been used as the sole anesthetic for cesarean delivery until delivery of the infant.[35] Maternal awareness or newborn depression did not occur. The addition of a small dose of volatile anesthetic together with nitrous oxide has been shown to reduce the incidence of maternal awareness further.[36] Cardiovascular stability following induction with ketamine 1 mg/kg for cesarean delivery was significantly better than that following thiopental 4 mg/kg, and the incidence of emergence phenomena and awareness was low.[37]

Retrograde amnestics

The benzodiazepines have been shown to be effective in

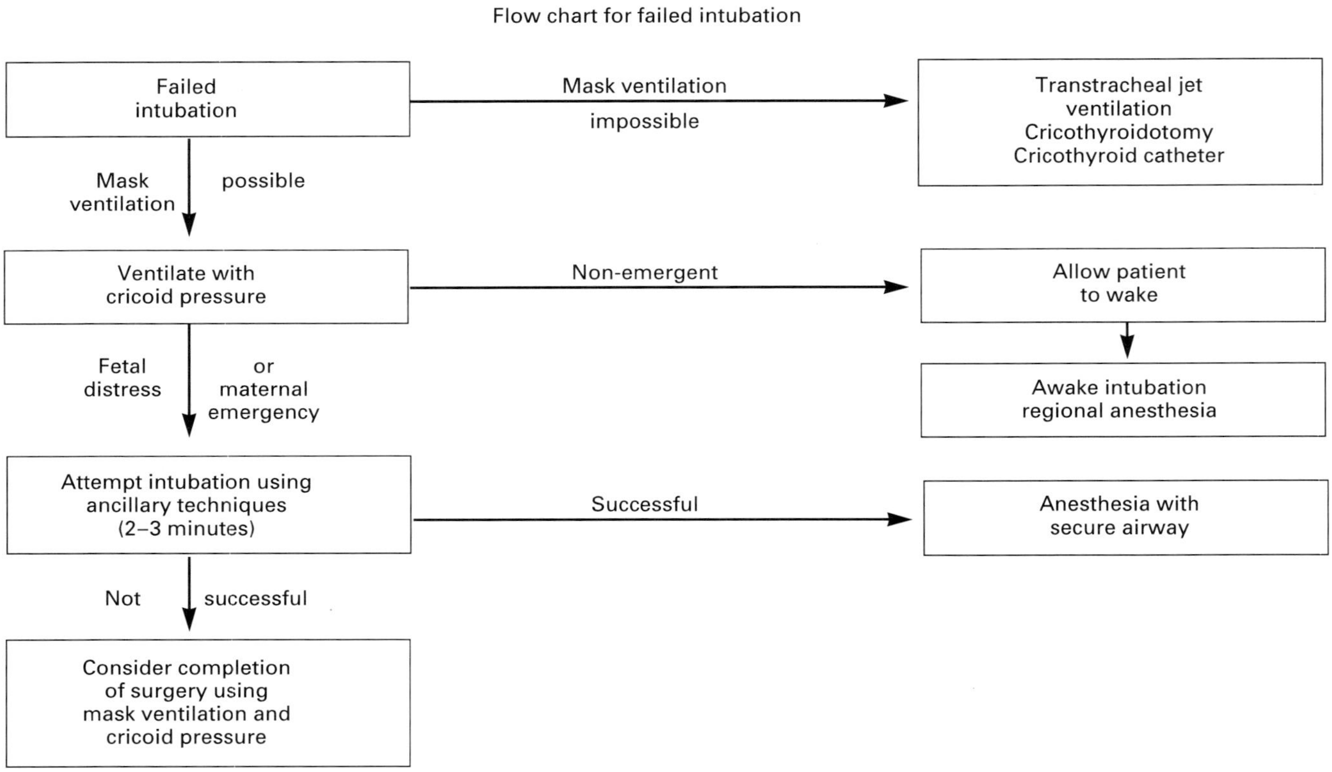

Fig. 39.3 Flow chart for failed intubation

reducing maternal awareness when administered intravenously soon after delivery of the infant.[38] Although diazepam and lorazepam have been the subject of most studies during general anesthesia in obstetrics, midazolam is employed with increasing frequency in the USA at the present time. The retrograde amnesia produced by this drug is predictable in its degree. Consequently, a combination of midazolam and opioid is commonly administered intravenously at the time of umbilical cord clamping.

Common techniques

The preanesthetic period

Sedative–hypnotic drugs or antisialogogues are no longer used as premedicants before either elective or urgent cesarean delivery. H_2-receptor antagonists such as ranitidine are often administered orally on the evening before planned cesarean delivery and again intravenously 1–2 h before anesthetic induction. At this time, intravenous metoclopramide is frequently given. Oral antacids, most commonly nonparticulate, are administered within the 30 min prior to induction. Once the parturient is positioned on the operating table with her uterus displaced, oxygen is administered by tight-fitting face mask (FIO_2 = 1.0). Monitors, including electrocardiograph, automated noninvasive blood pressure device and pulse oximeter are then applied.

Induction to delivery

Induction is usually accomplished with intravenous thiopental (4 mg/kg) alone, or a sequence of ketamine (0.5 – 0.7 mg/kg) followed by thiopental (2 mg/kg). Endotracheal intubation is accomplished with the aid of succinylcholine (1.0–1.5 mg/kg). After the injection of the induction agent, cricoid pressure is applied by an assistant and succinylcholine is administered. Cricoid pressure is not released until the endotracheal tube has been passed successfully into the trachea and the cuff has been inflated. The anesthetic is maintained until delivery with nitrous oxide in oxygen (50 : 50 or 40 : 60) and a small amount of volatile anesthetic (halothane 0.5%, enflurane 0.75%, isoflurane 0.75%). The capnograph is employed to detect carbon dioxide excretion after successful endotracheal intubation and to assist in maintaining end-tidal carbon dioxide at around 32 mmHg during manual/mechanical ventilation.

Following delivery

Once the shoulders have been delivered (or the head if a breech), synthetic oxytocin (20 IU) is added to the intravenous infusion bag. At cord clamping, mechanical ventilation may be initiated, if not already used, and the nitrous oxide concentration is increased to the desired level (usually 70%). The calculated dose of the opioid and benzodiazepine chosen is administered as an intravenous bolus, and, if desired, the volatile anesthetic can be discontinued. Continued muscle relaxation, if needed, is provided by a dilute intravenous infusion of succinylcholine (1–2 mg/ml) or by a nondepolarizing drug of moderate duration such as vecuronium or atracurium.

CONCLUSION

General anesthesia for cesarean delivery is a success when an experienced, knowledgeable anesthesiologist employing techniques appropriate to the clinical situation produces no maternal or infant morbidity related to the anesthetic. As can be seen from perinatal mortality statistics, this does not always occur. The efforts of obstetric anesthesiologists should continue to be directed toward achieving this ideal.

REFERENCES

1. American College of Obstetricians and Gynecologists 1971 National study of maternity care: survey of obstetric practice and associated services in hospitals in the United States. American College of Obstetricians and Gynecologists, Chicago
2. Hicks J S, Levinson G, Shnider S M 1976 Obstetric anesthesia training centers in the USA –1975. Anesth Analg 55: 839–845
3. Gibbs C P, Krischer J, Peckham B M, Sharp H, Kirschbaum T H 1986 Obstetric anesthesia: A national survey. Anesthesiology 65: 298–306
4. Marx G F, Luykx W M, Cohen S 1984 Fetal–neonatal status following caesarean section for fetal distress. Br J Anaesth 56: 1009–1013
5. Brownridge P 1984 Spinal anaesthesia revisited: an evaluation of subarachnoid block in obstetrics. Anaesth Intensive Care 12: 334–342
6. Kerr M G, Scott D B, Samuel E 1964 Studies of the inferior vena cava in late pregnancy. Br Med J 1: 532–533
7. Howard B K, Goodson J H, Mengert W F 1953 Supine hypotensive syndrome in late pregnancy. Obstet Gynecol 1: 371–377
8. Lees M M, Scott D B, Kerr M G, Taylor S H 1967 Circulatory effects of the supine posture in late pregnancy. Clin Sci 32: 453–465
9. Bieniarz J, Crottogini J J, Curuchet E, Romero-Salinas G, Yoshida T, Poseiro J J, Caldeyro-Barcia R 1968 Aortocaval compression by the uterus in late human pregnancy. II. An arteriographic study. Am J Obstet Gynecol 100: 203–217
10. Abitbol M M 1976 Aortic compression by pregnant uterus. N Y State J Med 76: 1470–1475
11. Bonica J J 1967 Principles and practice of obstetric analgesia and anesthesia. F A Davis, Philadelphia pp 13–39
12. Archer Jr G W, Marx G F 1974 Arterial oxygen tension during apnoea in parturient women. Br J Anaesth 46: 358–360
13. Marx G F, Mateo C V 1971 Effects of different oxygen concentrations during general anaesthesia for elective caesarean section. Can Anaesth Soc J 18: 587–593
14. Andersen G J, Walker J 1970 The effect of labour on the maternal blood–gas and acid–base status. J Obstet Gynaecol Br Cwlth 77: 289–293
15. Motoyama E K, Rivard G, Acheson F, Cook C D 1967 The effects of changes in maternal pH and PCO_2 on PO_2 of fetal lambs. Anesthesiology 28: 891–903
16. Levinson G, Shnider S M, de Lorimier A A, Steffenson J L 1974 Effects of maternal hyperventilation on uterine blood flow and fetal oxygenation and acid–base status. Anesthesiology 40: 340–347
17. Shnider S M, Moya F 1974 The hyperventilation controversy. In: Shnider S M, Moya F (eds) The Anesthesiologist, mother and newborn. Williams & Wilkins, Baltimore pp 93–99
18. Cheek T G, Gutsche B B 1987 Pulmonary aspiration of gastric contents. In: Shnider S M, Levinson G (eds) Anesthesia for obstetrics. Williams & Wilkins, Baltimore pp 300–315
19. Palahniuk R J, Shnider S M, Eger II E I 1974 Pregnancy decreases the requirements for inhaled anesthetic agents. Anesthesiology 41: 82–83
20. Kauppila A, Kokinen M, Puolakka J, Tuimala R, Kuikka J 1980 Decreased intervillous and unchanged myometrial blood flow in supine recumbency. Obstet Gynecol 55: 203–205
21. Brizgys R V, Shnider S M, Kotelko D M, Dailey P A, Levinson G 1982 The incidence and neonatal effects of maternal hypotension during epidural anesthesia for cesarean section. Anesthesiology 57: A395
22. Datta S, Alper M H, Ostheimer G W, Weiss J B 1982 Method of ephedrine administration and nausea and hypotension during spinal anesthesia for cesarean section. Anesthesiology 56: 68–70
23. Ralston D H, Shnider S M, de Lorimier A A 1974 Effects of equipotent ephedrine, metaraminol, mephentermine and methoxamine on uterine blood flow in the pregnant ewe. Anesthesiology 40: 354–370
24. Ramanathan S, Grant G J 1988 Vasopressor therapy for hypotension due to epidural anaesthesia for caesarean section. Acta Anaesthesiol Scand 32: 559–565
25. Moran D H, Perillo M, La Porta R F, Bader A M, Datta S 1991 Phenylephrine in the prevention of hypotension following spinal anesthesia for cesarean delivery. J Clin Anesth 3: 301–305
26. Hodges R J H, Bennett J R, Tunstall M E, Knight R F 1959 General anaesthesia for operative obstetrics. With special reference to the use of thiopentone and suxamethonium. Br J Anaesth 31: 152–163
27. Finster M, Poppers P J 1968 Safety of thiopental used for induction of general anesthesia in elective cesarean section. Anesthesiology 29: 190–191
28. Crawford J S, James F M, Crawley M 1976 A further study of general anaesthesia for caesarean section. Br J Anaesth 48: 661–667
29. Datta S, Ostheimer G W, Weiss J B, Brown W U, Alper M H 1981 Neonatal effect of prolonged anesthetic induction for cesarean section. Obstet Gynecol 58: 331–335
30. Datta S, Crocker J S, Alper M H 1977 Muscle pain following administration of suxamethonium to pregnant and nonpregnant patients undergoing laparoscopic tubal ligation. Br J Anaesth 49: 625–628
31. Cullen D J 1971 The effect of pretreatment with nondepolarizing muscle relaxants on the neuromuscular blocking action of succinylcholine. Anesthesiology 35: 572–578
32. Bassell G M, Marx G F 1993 Anesthesia-related maternal mortality. In: Shnider S M, Levinson G (eds) Anesthesia for obstetrics, Williams & Wilkins, Baltimore pp 455–465
33. Malan T P, Johnson M D 1988 The difficult airway in obstetric anesthesia: Techniques for airway management and the role of regional anesthesia. J Clin Anesth 1: 104–110
34. Schultetus R R, Hill C R, Dharamraj C M, Banner T E, Berman L S 1986 Wakefulness during cesarean section after anesthetic induction with ketamine, thiopental, or ketamine and thiopental combined. Anesth Analg 65: 723–728
35. Baraka A, Louis F, Dalleh R 1990 Maternal awareness and neonatal outcome after ketamine induction of anaesthesia for Caesarean section. Can J Anaesth 37: 641–644
36. Baraka A, Louis F, Noueihid R, Diab M, Dabbous A, Sibai B 1989 Awareness following different techniques of general anaesthesia for caesarean section. Br J Anaesth 62: 645–648
37. Schultetus R R, Paulus D A, Spohr G L 1985 Haemodynamic effects of ketamine and thiopentone during anaesthetic induction for Caesarean section. Can Anaesth Soc J 32: 592–596
38. Barr A M, Moxon A, Woollam C H M, Fryer M E 1977 The effect of diazepam and lorazepam on awareness during anaesthesia for caesarean section. Anaesthesia 32: 873–878

PART B
UK VIEW

G. O'Sullivan

INTRODUCTION

The Cesarean delivery rate in the UK has increased from approximately 7% in the early 1970s to 15% in 1988.[1] Obstetric, perinatal and medicolegal considerations are the main reasons for this increase. The Report on Confidential Enquiries into Maternal Deaths in England and Wales is a unique medical audit published triennally, which reviews all maternal deaths. This report indicates that anesthesia remains a common cause of maternal death, and to date over 75% of these deaths have occurred at the time of emergency general anesthesia for cesarean delivery.[2]

In most major centers in the UK the technique of general anesthesia for cesarean delivery is essentially similar: acute oxygenation/denitrogenation and a rapid-sequence induction followed by a 50:50 oxygen–nitrous oxide mixture with a volatile agent until delivery of the baby, at which time an intravenous opioid is administered and the FIO_2 is decreased to 0.3. To prevent awareness, the volatile agent is continued until the end of the procedure. At the end of the procedure the mother is extubated following the full return of laryngeal reflexes. As a result of increasing maternal demand and the belief that, even in the hands of trainee anesthesiologists, regional anesthesia is intrinsically safer than general anesthesia for cesarean delivery[3] there has been a sharp decline in the number of general anesthetics administered to the pregnant patient. For the obstetric anesthesiologist this decline in the use of general anesthesia for cesarean delivery increases the challenge in providing safe anesthesia for the mother whilst providing comprehensive teaching for the anesthesiologist in training.

GENERAL ANESTHESIA FOR ELECTIVE CESAREAN DELIVERY

General anesthesia for elective cesarean delivery should aim to provide adequate anesthesia and analgesia for the mother while avoiding the dangers of aortocaval occlusion, acid pulmonary aspiration and excessive uterine relaxation; the other paramount aim is to avoid neonatal depression.

Preoperative preparation

Medical or obstetric complications and patient refusal of regional anesthesia are the main indications for performing elective cesarean delivery under general anesthesia. The mother may be anxious about herself and her unborn baby and, therefore, will require reassurance and a full explanation of the impending events. A careful medical and obstetric history should be taken, a recent hemoglobin should be available and a sample of the patient's serum should be identified for blood group and Rh factor and saved. The ultrasonic scan should be reviewed and the site of the placenta noted. In the event of an anterior placenta previa, when blood loss can be considerable, 3–4 units of cross-matched whole blood or packed RBCs should be available before surgery begins. Sedative and opioid premedications can potentially result in neonatal depression and should be avoided. As prophylaxis against acid pulmonary aspiration (Mendelson's syndrome[4]) the mother should be medicated with an H_2-antagonist, such as ranitidine 150 mg, on the night prior to and on the morning of surgery.[5] Given electively in this manner the H_2-antagonists will significantly decrease gastric volume and increase gastric pH in most women. However, since failure of this regimen can occur, a nonparticulate antacid such as 0.3M sodium citrate should also be administered in the operating theatre immediately prior to induction of anesthesia. If the parturient is admitted to the operating suite on the day of surgery, then the H_2-antagonist may be given intravenously. A new group of compounds,[6] the substituted benzimidimazoles (e.g. omeprazole), which inhibit H^+, K^+-ATPase, the final common pathway of gastric acid secretion, are currently being evaluated as prophylaxis against acid aspiration. When taken orally, omeprazole must be enteric coated to prevent its degradation by gastric acid. The advantage of this group of drugs is their long duration of action following a single dose. Studies to date in the obstetric patient indicate that 40 mg of omeprazole taken on the night prior to and on the morning of surgery is more effective at increasing gastric pH and decreasing gastric volume[8] than either ranitidine [7] or single-dose omeprazole: in addition no maternal or fetal side-effects have been detected. Further studies of this promising compound are obviously required in the obstetric patient.

Preinduction and induction of anesthesia

In the immediate preinduction period the identity and written consent of the mother should be checked. The mother should be in the full lateral position to prevent vena-caval occlusion, which if allowed to occur can result in significant neonatal depression. Monitoring, which should include ECG, automatic blood pressure and pulse oximetry, should commence prior to induction of anesthesia. An intravenous infusion of a balanced salt solution should be established and a nonparticulate antacid such as 30 ml of 0.3 M sodium citrate should be administered. Nonparticulate antacids do not have a long duration of action and hence should only be administered immediately prior to induction of anesthesia.[9]

As the incorrect application of cricoid pressure has probably contributed to maternal mortality, the anesthesiologist must be assisted by someone trained to correctly apply cricoid pressure. An efficient high-powered suction apparatus should be available as should endotracheal tubes varying in size from 5.0 to 8.0 mm. In addition, a gum elastic bougie should be available to facilitate intubation. Laryngoscopes should ideally include one standard with both long and standard length blades, one with a short handle and one with a 'polio' blade. Further facilities to deal with a difficult intubation should also be available. Ideally the mother should remain in the full lateral position while preoperative preparations such as insertion of the intravenous catheter and the urinary catheter are being made. When the surgeon is ready to begin the mother should be placed in the supine position with left lateral tilt; this is most reliably achieved by elevating the right hip 15–30°. She should be acutely oxygenated/denitrogenated for 3–5 min prior to the induction of anesthesia, during which time skin preparation and surgical draping can be completed. In the pregnant woman at term, functional residual capacity is decreased and oxygen consumption is increased, therefore apnea results in a more rapid fall in $P\text{O}_2$ than in nonpregnant controls, a factor that will be of particular importance if intubation is difficult and prolonged.[10]

In the UK thiopental sodium is the agent most commonly used to induce anesthesia. A dose sufficient to induce anesthesia, in an unpremedicated young woman, and which should contribute to the prevention of awareness prior to delivery, should be administered (4–7 mg/kg).[11] The induction agent propofol allows rapid recovery from anesthesia and thus has not surprisingly been evaluated for cesarean delivery. Placental transfer of propofol is rapid but studies of the neonatal effects of a single induction dose of propofol are conflicting.[12,13] When a propofol infusion is used, a high infusion rate of propofol, especially if combined with a long induction-to-delivery interval, has been shown to depress neurologic and adaptive capacity scores.[14,15] Overall, however, propofol will probably prove to be a suitable induction agent for cesarean delivery. To prevent regurgitation and aspiration a rapid-sequence induction is employed, with 100 mg or 1.5 mg/kg of the short-acting depolarizing muscle relaxant, succinylcholine, being administered immediately after the induction agent. Cricoid pressure should be applied as the patient loses consciousness, as the too early application of cricoid pressure can result in uncontrolled patient movements such as coughing. As described by Sellick,[16] the cricoid cartilage should be held between the thumb and middle finger with the pressure on the cricoid being executed by the index finger. If preferred, the assistant's free hand can be placed behind the patient's neck in order to maintain it in the extended position. The assistant must remember that the patient is not lying in the supine position and adjust the cricoid pressure accordingly, otherwise the larynx will be displaced laterally, an event which frequently contributes to a difficult intubation in the pregnant patient. An adequate amount of time must be allowed for the succinylcholine to have full clinical effect. It has been shown that trainee anesthesiologists attempt laryngoscopy earlier in the obstetric patient (mean time 29.8 s) than in patients requiring general surgery (mean time 63.5 s).[17] Following insertion of the endotracheal tube the cuff should be immediately inflated. Correct placement of the endotracheal tube should be ensured before cricoid pressure is released and surgery is allowed to commence. This is best established by measuring end-tidal carbon dioxide.[18]

The increase in pulse rate and arterial blood pressure as a result of laryngoscopy and tracheal intubation can have serious implications for the patient with pregnancy-induced hypertension. Hydralazine can attenuate this response but has the disadvantage of a relatively slow onset of action. Alfentanil and magnesium sulfate have also been shown to attenuate the pressor response to tracheal intubation in the hypertensive proteinuric pregnant patient.[19] Agents with a more rapid onset of action include labetalol[20] and nitroglycerin,[21] however, a sudden rapid decrease in pressure should be avoided.

Maintenance of anesthesia

Maintenance of anesthesia must encompass the difference in anesthetic requirements in the pre- and post-delivery periods. Prior to the delivery of the infant the aim is to achieve maternal anesthesia without causing drug-induced neonatal and uterine depression or alternatively reducing placental blood flow by light planes of maternal anesthesia.[22] If general anesthesia is meticulously administered with avoidance of vena-caval occlusion, there should be no difference in the acid–base status of the neonate delivered under general anesthesia and the neonate delivered under regional anesthesia.[23,24] With general anesthesia the time to commence spontaneous respiration for the neonate has been shown to be delayed.[24] The results of studies comparing the effects of anesthetic technique for elective surgery on the Apgar score are conflicting, with some studies showing no change[25] and others showing a higher percentage of depressed Apgar scores in babies delivered under general anesthesia.[24,26] In the predelivery interval, maternal and fetal requirements are probably best fulfilled by supplementing a 50 : 50 oxygen–nitrous oxide mixture with a concentration of volatile agents sufficient to prevent awareness without causing uterine atony (halothane 0.5%, enflurane 0.6% or isoflurane 0.75%). These recommendations are based on studies which indicate that an increase in maternal FIO_2 to greater than 0.6 does not improve fetal oxygenation.[27] However, in a study in which 0.8% isoflurane was used with oxygen and nitrous oxide in either a 50:50 ratio or a 33:67 ratio, the biochemical and clinical status of the neonates studied was not significantly different.[28] Probably of equal importance to neonatal outcome is the maintenance of normocapnia. It has been demonstrated that a fresh gas flow of at least 100 ml/kg/min prevents both maternal hypocapnia and hypercapnia.[29] Hyperventilation, by decreasing placental blood flow and shifting the maternal oxygen dissociation curve, can compromise fetal oxygenation and acid–base balance. Monitoring of end-tidal carbon dioxide and oxygen saturation is mandatory during cesarean delivery. Muscle relaxation should be maintained by a relatively short-acting relaxant such as succinylcholine or the nondepolarizer, vecuronium, which is not significantly transferred across the placenta.[30] Long-acting muscle relaxants are usually inappropriate and have been implicated in maternal deaths as a result of post-operative respiratory depression.[31] Once the baby has been delivered and the umbilical cord clamped, anesthesia can be deepened. The concentration of nitrous oxide can be increased to 70% and an intravenous opioid (fentanyl 100–200 μg or Omnopon 20 mg) should be administered. This should provide intra- and early post-operative analgesia. Uterine involution is aided by intravenous oxytocin 5–10 units and maintained in the early post-operative period by an intravenous infusion of 20–30 units of oxytocin in 500 ml of balanced salt solution.

Upon completion of surgery the mother must not be extubated until laryngeal reflexes have fully returned. The quality of pain relief following general anesthesia for cesarean delivery will be inferior to that following regional anesthesia. However, reasonable analgesia can be provided with a combination of parenteral opioids and oral, rectal or parenteral nonsteroidal anti-inflammatory agents.

GENERAL ANESTHESIA FOR EMERGENCY CESAREAN DELIVERY

In the UK over 75% of maternal anesthetic deaths occur in association with emergency cesarean delivery. Difficulties with intubation and inhalation of gastric contents account for most of these deaths (Table 39.2). Whilst the anesthetic technique for emergency cesarean delivery remains unchanged from that used for the elective procedures, the urgency of the situation and the fact that in the UK the mother might be anesthetized by a trainee anesthesiologist may contribute to the greater number of problems occurring in association with emergency delivery.

Acid pulmonary aspiration

Difficulty with intubation is frequently associated with intubation of the esophagus, which can precipitate regurgitation and subsequent aspiration. Effective prophylaxis against aspiration should aim to achieve a small intragastric volume of high (basic) pH. Whilst this aim can now be achieved for elective cesarean delivery, the ideal is harder to achieve at the time of emergency surgery. In conditions such as a prolapsed cord the mother may have recently eaten, whereas those women who require surgery during labor will have a delay in gastric emptying which will be directly related to the use of opioid analgesia and the duration of labor.[32] This will result in a significant gastric residual volume and increase the risk of regurgitation and aspiration. To consistently achieve a small intragastric volume of high pH is almost impossible in the mother requiring emergency cesarean delivery. For the sudden and unexpected emergency, e.g. the prolapsed cord, a nonparticulate antacid should be administered immediately prior to induction. In the short time available it will be impossible to alter gastric volume, and thus complete reliance must then be placed upon the correct application of cricoid pressure to prevent regurgitation and aspiration. Mechanical emptying of the stomach is both traumatic for the mother and time-wasting in a serious emergency. While parenteral H_2-antagonists (ranitidine 50 mg) can and should be administered prior to induction, the time taken for them to increase gastric pH means that their protective effects will only be of value during the recovery period. Intravenous omeprazole, which has been studied in general surgery patients,[33] requires evaluation for emergency cesarean delivery. To prevent regurgitation

Table 39.2 Maternal mortality associated with anesthesia (Adapted from the ref. Z)

	1970–72	1973–75	1976–78	1979–81	1982–84	1985–87
Numbers of deaths associated with anesthesia	31	27	27	22	18	6
Percentage of direct maternal deaths due to anesthesia	10.8	11.9	12.4	12.4	13.0	4.3
Deaths due to aspiration	14	13	14	8	7	1
Deaths due to difficult intubation	5	7	16	8	10	4
Deaths due to epidural block	1	2	4	0	1	1

and aspiration in the early post-operative period the stomach should be emptied through an orogastric tube once the baby has been delivered; a further 30 ml of an antacid such as 0.3 M sodium citrate should then be instilled through the tube prior to its removal. For some women it is possible to anticipate an emergency cesarean delivery, e.g. a trial of labor following a previous cesarean delivery, malpresentation and failure of labor to progress satisfactorily. It is suggested that these women should receive 6-hourly oral or parenteral H_2-antagonists in addition to the preinduction antacid. While this regimen is not as successful as the preoperative regimen described above for the elective patient, it will significantly decrease gastric volume.[33] More importantly, these women should have an epidural catheter inserted during labor so that if surgery is required it can be performed under regional block.

Failed or difficult intubation

Failure to intubate the trachea with consequent anoxia, and the regurgitation and inhalation of gastric contents as a result of unintentional intubation of the esophagus during a difficult intubation, contribute significantly to maternal mortality (Table 39.2). In Table 39.2 patients in whom the primary event was difficult intubation but who subsequently died of Mendelson's syndrome are included in both columns. Intubation of the trachea can be more difficult and the reported incidence of failed intubation is greater in pregnant women.[35] The relatively incorrect application of cricoid pressure caused by the mother lying in a right or left lateral tilt, laryngeal edema in the preeclamptic patient, full dentition and large breasts are amongst the factors which contribute to the greater frequency of difficult intubations in the pregnant patient. Failure to intubate must be acknowledged without undue delay and a failed intubation drill should be rapidly instituted before the apneic mother becomes anoxic. Oxygen saturation must be carefully monitored during these attempts and failure must be accepted after two or three attempts involving mechanical aids such as a short-handled or polio laryngoscope, an introducer and smaller endotracheal tubes. The use of a second dose of succinylcholine should be avoided in the author's opinion but is controversial. The risk of aspiration will obviously be greatest in patients requiring emergency surgery in whom prophylactic measures against aspiration will probably not have had time to be fully effective.

Ongoing management must be discussed with the obstetrician. If surgery is not urgent the mother can be allowed to awaken and surgery carried out under regional block. In the interim cricoid pressure should be maintained, an oropharyngeal airway should be inserted and the lungs should be ventilated manually with 100% oxygen until spontaneous respiration returns. If delivery is essential then the mother should be placed in the left lateral position and should be allowed to breathe spontaneously to an adequate depth of anesthesia. The advent of the laryngeal mask may facilitate the management of the failed intubation in the obstetric patient.[36] A method whereby it can be incorporated into a conventional failed intubation drill is illustrated in Figure 39.4. Whilst the manufacturers of the laryngeal mask stress that it will not give full protection against aspiration, for some patients it should improve the safety margin in the management of a difficult or failed intubation. However, a careful prospective analysis of its use is required before it can be fully established whether or not the laryngeal mask has an effective and safe role to play in the management of a failed intubation in the obstetric patient. In some patients in whom ventilation remains impossible, airway management has been facilitated by passing an endotracheal tube into the esophagus, where it serves as an esophageal obturator.[37] In a failed intubation where ventilation becomes impossible it may be necessary to puncture the cricothyroid membrane. Facilities for transtracheal ventilation should therefore be an integral part of the 'difficult intubation' kit kept on every labor ward.

Unplanned awareness

The reported incidence of and the medicolegal costs of awareness during anesthesia for cesarean delivery have increased substantially in the UK during the past decade; in addition, media interest in the topic has been considerable. In 1969 Wilson and Turner[38] reported that approximately 8% of patients anesthetized with thiopental, oxygen, nitrous oxide and a muscle relaxant could recall intraoperative events. It was subsequently demonstrated by Moir[39] that this prevalence could be reduced to less than 1% when 200–250 mg of thiopental sodium and oxygen–nitrous oxide was supplemented with 0.5% halothane. Enflurane 0.6% and isoflurane 0.75% have similarly been shown to decrease the level of awareness during cesarean delivery.[40] When a 50 : 50 oxygen–nitrous oxide mixture is being supplemented with a low concentration of volatile agent, it is essential that the vaporizer's reliability can be guaranteed, otherwise awareness may occur. The rigid protocol has recently been criticized in a study from Leeds, UK, where between 1982 and 1985 the prevalence of recall was 1.3% when anesthesia similar to that described above was used for cesarean delivery. Abandoning this regimen, and allowing increased doses of thiopental (5–7 mg/kg) and increased concentrations of volatile agents, decreased the frequency of awareness to 0.4% in the period between 1985–89. The neonatal effects of these larger doses of anesthetic agents were not rigidly evaluated but no gross differences were detected.[11] In addition, there is now evidence that for elective cesarean delivery a reduction in FIO_2 from 0.5 to

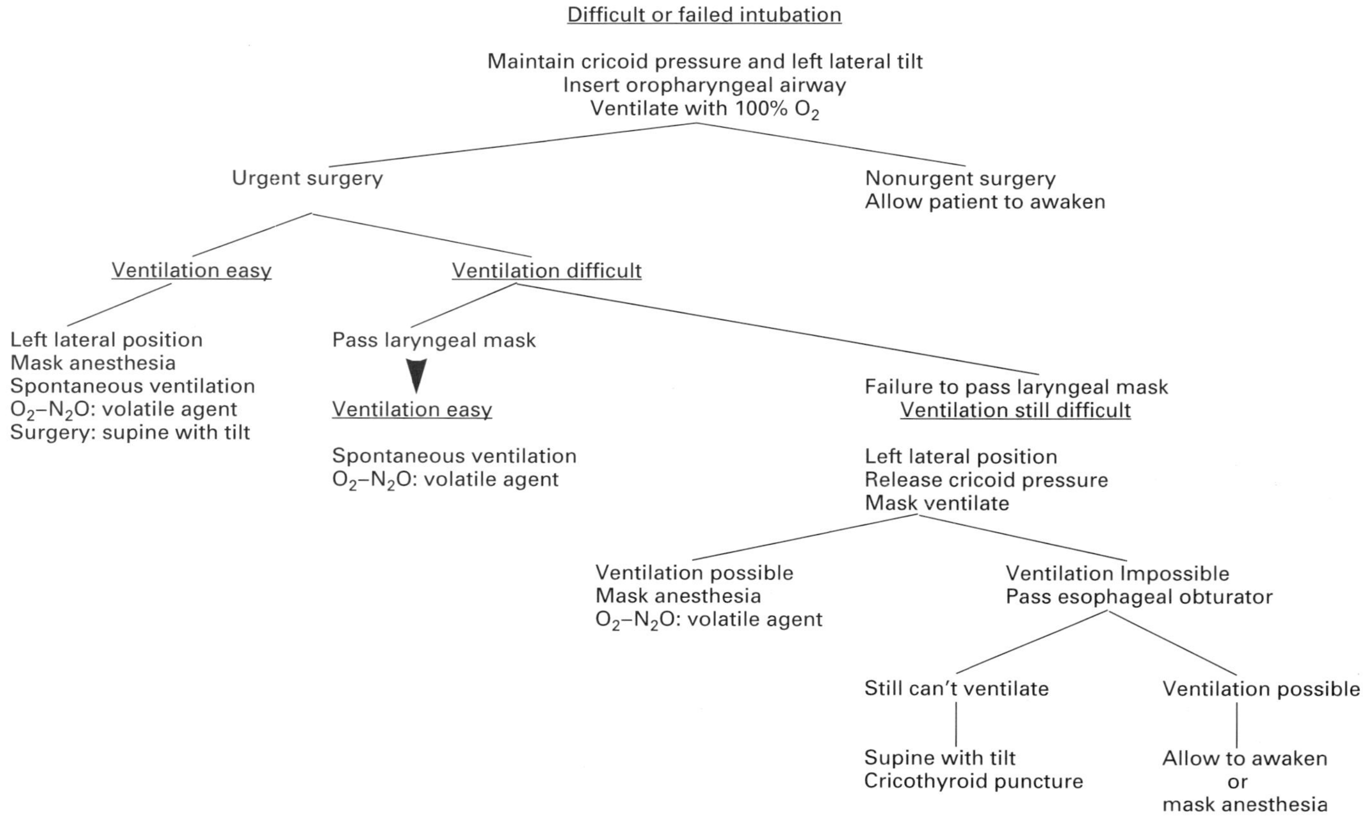

Fig. 39.4 Management of failed intubation.

0.3 has no detrimental effect on fetal outcome or acid–base status.[28] Theoretically, this higher concentration of nitrous oxide should help reduce the incidence of awareness, though obviously oxygen saturation must be continuously monitored and venocaval occlusion avoided. The use of an F_{IO_2} of 1.0 and 1.5 MAC isoflurane for mothers requiring emergency cesarean delivery has recently been evaluated.[41] The resulting increase in umbilical venous PO_2 and an improvement in Apgar scores, which was not statistically significant, probably does not justify the use of 100% oxygen because of the potential risk of awareness in the mother. What should the patient be told preoperatively about awareness? Some advocate that the possibility of awareness should be discussed with high-risk groups such as those requiring cesarean delivery[42] whilst others advocate that the risks should only be discussed if the patient is in the position to be able to choose between regional and general anesthesia.[11] However, once awareness has occurred the anesthesiologist must discuss the event with the patient.

Pulmonary embolism

A survey of maternal deaths in Massachusetts from 1954 to 1985 showed that for the years 1982–85 the commonest causes were trauma and pulmonary embolism.[43] The Report on Confidential Enquiries into Maternal Deaths in England and Wales for successive years show that pulmonary embolism and hypertensive disorders of pregnancy are the commonest causes of maternal mortality.[2,31] The risk of death from pulmonary embolism is greater in women aged over 35 years, in those with severe preeclampsia, in the obese and in those who undergo cesarean delivery. Overall, however, there has been a decline in the total number of maternal deaths from pulmonary embolism (Table 39.3). The reasons for this are probably multifactorial and include early ambulation and the avoidance of vena-caval occlusion and consequent venous stasis. Evidence from hip surgery indicates that improved peripheral blood flow resulting from the vasomotor block associated with regional anesthesia may also result in a reduction in deep vein thrombosis and subsequent pulmonary embolism.[44] This suggests, though it has never been demonstrated, that women undergoing cesarean delivery under general anesthesia could be at greater risk of pulmonary embolism. Perhaps women in the high-risk category should be strongly encouraged where possible to have their cesarean delivery performed under regional block. If general anesthesia is required low-dose heparin should perhaps be considered for high-risk patients, though this is certainly not common practice in the UK.

Table 39.3 Maternal deaths from pulmonary embolism 1970–84

Years	Deaths after vaginal delivery	Deaths after Cesarean delivery	Total
1970–72	22 (11.6)	15 (145.2)	37
1973–75	13 (7.7)	6 (59.2)	19
1976–78	20 (12.7)	9 (74.6)	29
1979–81	4 (2.3)	7 (41.9)	11
1982–84	4 (2.4)	12 (64.6)	16
1985–87	6	7	13

Table 39.4 Direct maternal deaths in England and Wales within 42 days of cesarean delivery (CD)

	1970–72	1973–75	1976–78	1979–81	1982–84
All direct deaths	343	227	217	178	138
Direct deaths from CD	81	60	61	59	44
Percentage of all direct deaths	24	26	28	33	32
Caesarean delivery rate (%)	5.16	5.63	7.14	8.90	10.09
Fatality rate 1000 CD	0.78	0.59	0.51	0.35	0.24

THE NEONATE AND GENERAL ANESTHESIA FOR CESAREAN DELIVERY

Both general and regional anesthesia, when carefully conducted, result in normal blood gases and acid–base status in babies weighing more than 2500 g.[23,24] The results of studies comparing the effects of anesthetic techniques for elective surgery on neonatal Apgar scores are conflicting, with some studies showing no change[45] and other, more recent, studies showing a higher percentage of depressed Apgar scores in babies delivered under general anesthesia.[24] In a study of emergency cesarean deliveries performed because of fetal distress, the neonatal blood gas and acid–base values were similar in both the general and regional anesthetic groups, although Apgar scores were higher in the latter.[46] A retrospective study of 3940 babies delivered by elective and emergency cesarean delivery showed that following emergency surgery Apgar scores were lower and more babies required intubation when the cesarean delivery was performed under general anesthesia.[26] Studies also indicate that the time to the onset of sustained respiration is shorter in the regional anesthetic group. Current evidence also suggests that general anesthesia reduces neurobehavioral scores in the first 24–48 hs after delivery.[23]

Thus studies to date indicate that the baby born by cesarean delivery using regional anesthesia is more alert and is quicker to establish spontaneous respiration. However the long-term effects, if any, on the baby of regional as opposed to general anesthesia remain unknown. Both are safe for the baby when optimally administered. Table 39.4 illustrates that, despite the increase in the number of operative deliveries, the mortality from cesarean delivery in England and Wales has declined. However, all obstetric anesthesiologists must be aware that the current statistics indicate that surgical delivery, particularly if a general rather than an epidural anesthetic is used, remains significantly more hazardous than vaginal delivery.

REFERENCES

1. Leading Article 1988 Holding back the tide of Caesareans. Br Med J 297: 569
2. Department of Health and Social Security 1991 Report on Confidential Enquiries into Maternal Deaths in England and Wales 1985–1987. HMSO, London
3. Morgan B M, Aulakh J M, Barker J P 1983 Anaesthesia for Caesarean section. Br J Anaesth 55: 885
4. Mendelson C L 1946. The aspiration of stomach contents into the lungs during obstetric anesthesia. Am J Obstet Gynecol 52: 191
5. O'Sullivan G M, Sear J W, Bullingham R E S, Carrie L E S 1985 The effect of magnesium trisilicate mixture, metoclopramide and ranitidine on gastric pH, volume and serum gastrin. Anaesthesia 40: 246
6. Leading Article 1990 Omeprazole – a useful new agent. Br J Anaesth 65: 607
7. Moore J, Flynn R J, Sampaio M, Wilson C M, Gillon K R W 1989 Effect of single-dose omeprazole on intragastric acidity and volume during obstetric anesthesia. Anaesthesia 44: 559
8. Gin T, Ewant M C, Yan G, Oh T E 1990 Effects of oral omeprazole on intragastric pH and volume in women undergoing elective Caesarean section. Br J Anaesth 65: 616
9. O'Sullivan G M, Bullingham R E S 1984 The assessment of gastric acidity and antacid effect in pregnant women by a non-invasive radiotelemetry technique. Br J Obstet Gynaecol 91: 973
10. Archer G, Marx G F 1974 Arterial oxygen tension during apnoea in parturient women. Br J Anaesth 46: 358
11. Lyons G, Macdonald R 1991 Awareness during Caesarean section. Anaesthesia 46: 62
12. Celleno D, Capogna G, Tomassetti M, Costantino P, Difeo G, Nisini R 1989 Neurobehavioural effects of propofol on the neonate following elective Caesarean section. Br J Anaesth 62: 649
13. Gin T, Gregory M A, Chan K, Oh T E 1990 Maternal and fetal levels of propofol at Caesarean section. Anaesth Intensive Care 18: 180
14. Yan G, Gin T, Ewant M C, Khotur C F, Leung R K W, Oh T E 1991 Propofol for induction and maintenance of anaesthesia at Caesarean section. Anaesthesia 46: 20
15. Gregory M A, Gin T, Yan G, Leung R K W, Chan K, Oh T E 1990 Propofol infusion anaesthesia for Caesarean section. Can J Anaesth 37: 514
16. Sellick B A 1961 Cricoid pressure to control regurgitation of stomach contents during induction of anaesthesia. Lancet 2: 404
17. Carmie J C, Street M K, Kumar B 1986 Emergency intubation of the tracheal facilitated by suxamethonium. Observations in obstetric and general surgical patients. Br J Anaesth 58: 498
18. Vaghadia H, Jenkins L C, Ford R W 1989 Comparison of end-tidal carbon dioxide, oxygen saturation and clinical signs for the detection of oesophageal intubation. Can J Anaesth 36: 560
19. Allen R W, James M F M, Uys P C 1991 Attenuation of the pressor response to tracheal intubation in hypertensive proteinuric pregnant patients by lignocaine, alfentanil and magnesium sulphate. Br J Anaesth 66: 216
20. Ramanathan J, Sibai B M, Mabie W C, Chanhan D, Ruiz A G 1988 The use of labetalol for attenuation of the hypertensive response to endotracheal intubation in preeclampsia. Am J Obstet Gynecology 159: 650
21. Hood D D, Dewar D M, James F M, Floyd H M, Bogard T D 1985 The use of nitroglycerin in preventing the hypertensive

response to tracheal intubation in severe preeclampsia. Anesthesiology 63: 329
22. Palahniuk R J, Cumming M 1977 Fetal deterioration following thiopentone–nitrous oxide anaesthesia in the pregnant ewe. Can J Anaesth 24: 361
23. Abboud T K, Nagappala S, Muratawa K et al 1985 Comparison of the effects of general and regional anesthesia for Caesarean section on neonatal neurologic and adaptive capacity scores. Anesth Analg 64: 996
24. Evans C M, Murphy F, Gray O P, Rosen M 1989 Epidural versus general anaesthesia for Caesarean section. Anaesthesia 44: 778
25. James F M, Crawford J S, Hopkinson R, Davies P, Naiem H 1977 A comparison of general anaesthesia and lumbar epidural analgesia for elective Caesarean section. Anesthesia and Analgesia 56: 228
26. Ong B Y, Cohen M M, Palahniuk R J 1989 Anesthesia for Caesarean section – effects on neonates. Anesth Analg 68: 270
27. Marx G F, Mateo C J 1971 Effects of different oxygen concentrations during general anaesthesia for elective Caesarean section. Can J Anaesth 18: 587
28. Lawes E G, Newman B, Campbell M J, Irwin M, Dolenska S, Thomas T A 1988 Maternal inspired oxygen concentration and neonatal status for Caesarean section under general anaesthesia. Br J Anaesth 61: 250
29. Duncan P W, Lawes E G, Bland B, Downing J W 1987 Fresh gas-flow requirements using the ADE anaesthetic system during late pregnancy. Br J Anaesth 59: 360
30. Bailey P A, Fisher D M, Shnider S M, Baysinger C L, Shinohara Y, Millar R D, Abbond T K, Kim K C 1984 Pharmacokinetics, placental transfer and neonatal effects of vecuronium and pancuronium administered during Caesarean section. Anesthesiology 60: 569
31. Department of Health and Social Security 1986 Report on Confidential Enquiries into Maternal Deaths in England and Wales 1979–1981. HMSO, London
32. Holdsworth J D 1978 Relationship between stomach contents and analgesia in labour. Br J Anaesth 50: 1145
33. Cruickshank R H, Morrison D A, Bamber P A, Nimmo W S 1989 Effect of IV omeprazole on the pH and volume of gastric contents before surgery. Br J Anaesth 63: 536
34. Colman R D, Frank M, Longhnan B A, Cohen D G, Caltermole R 1988 Use of IM ranitidine for the prophylaxis of aspiration pneumonitis in obstetrics. Br J Anaesth 61: 720
35. Samsoon G L T, Young J R B 1987 Difficult tracheal intubation, a retrospective study. Anaesthesia 42: 487
36. McClure S, Regan M, Moore J 1990 Laryngeal mask airway for Caesarean section. Anaesthesia 45: 227
37. Boys J E 1983 Failed intubation in obstetric anaesthesia. Br J Anaesth 55: 187
38. Wilson J, Turner D J 1969 Awareness during Caesarean section under general anaesthesia. Br Med J 1: 280
39. Moir D D 1970 Anaesthesia for Caesarean section. An evaluation of a method using low concentrations of halothane and 50% oxygen. Br J Anaesth 42: 136
40. Warren T M, Datta S, Ostheimer G W, Naulty J S, Weiss J B, Morrison J A 1983 Comparison of the maternal and neonatal effects of halothane, enflurane and isoflurane for Caesarean delivery. Anesth Analgesia 62: 516
41. Piggott S E, Bogod D G, Rosen M, Rees A D, Harmer M 1990 Isoflurane with either 100% oxygen or 50% nitrous oxide in oxygen for Caesarean section. Br J Anaesth 65: 325
42. Anon 1990 Awareness during anaesthesia: what should the patient be told? (leading article). Anaesthesia 45: 351
43. Sachs B P, Brown D A J, Driscoll S G, Schulman E, Acker D, Ransil B J, Jewitt J F 1987 Maternal mortality in Massachusetts. Trends and Prevention. New Engl J Med 316: 667
44. Mackenzie P J, Wishart H Y, Gray I, Smith G 1985 Effects of anesthetic technique on deep vein thrombosis: a comparison of subarachnoid and general anaesthesia. Br J Anaesth 57: 853
45. Downing J W, Houlton P C, Barclay A 1979 Extradural analgesia for Caesarean section: a comparison with general anaesthesia. Br J Anaesth 51: 367
46. Marx G F, Luykx W M, Cohen S 1984 Fetal–neonatal status following Caesarean section for fetal distress. Br J Anaesth 56: 1009

40. Local infiltration for cesarean delivery

W. H. Barth

The opinions expressed in this manuscript are those of the author and not necessarily those of the United States Air Force or the Department of Defense.

In 1975, Ranney and Stanage[1] advocated local anesthesia for cesarean delivery because 'local field block of the abdominal wall is the least complicated, most direct anesthetic technique which will provide the necessary relief from pain, yet least adversely modify the maternal-fetal physiology'. These authors cited two neonatal deaths of term infants in 1951 and 1952 as motivation for learning the technique of local anesthesia for cesarean delivery. Now, 40 years later, the availability of safe regional or general anesthetic techniques in most hospitals renders the need for local anesthesia for abdominal delivery almost obsolete. Consequently, few obstetricians or anesthesiologists in practice today have ever seen or administered local anesthesia for a cesarean delivery. Nonetheless, on rare occasions, knowledge of the procedures for local infiltration for cesarean delivery may prove life-saving for the mother and fetus.

Indications for use of local infiltration anesthesia for cesarean delivery are limited. In some hospitals, personnel trained in general or regional anesthesia may be on call from home. In such a setting, should a parturient present with severe fetal distress, the obstetrician may be required to begin delivery under local infiltration anesthesia. Also rare, but conceivable, is the parturient with an inaccessible or compromised airway combined with a failed or contraindicated regional block. While these may be very rare circumstances, the need to supplement a 'patchy' or partial intraspinal anesthetic may be the most common indication for local infiltration.

ANATOMY

Sensory innervation of the lower abdominal wall originates from the anterior division of the T7–T11 intercostal nerves. These nerves run in the neurovascular bundle beneath the inferior margin of each rib and then medially between the aponeuroses of the internal oblique and transverse abdominis muscles. As each approaches the semilunar line, or lateral margin of the rectus abdominis muscle, it turns anteriorly to penetrate the posterior aspect of the inferolateral rectus sheath (Fig. 40.1). These major fibers course medially about halfway through the rectus muscle, then again turn anteriorly to penetrate the anterior rectus sheath. These arborize to become the anterior cutaneous branches of the thoracic nerves. Additionally, each of these thoracic nerves gives off a lateral cutaneous branch that supplies the skin from the mid-axillary line to the semilunar line. The T12, iliohypogastric and ilioinguinal nerves all pass more toward the mons pubis. The iliohypogastric nerve courses between the internal and external oblique muscles to supply the skin from the anterior superior iliac crest, medially to the area just superior to the pubic bone. The ilioinguinal nerve descends within the inguinal canal, exits at the external ring and branches superficially to supply the skin over the symphysis pubis, mons and labia majora. In general, the areas near the pubic bone and mons are more densely innervated than the areas supplied by the T7–T11 nerves. Finally, regarding the relative density of nerve endings in the different layers, the skin is the most sensitive, followed by the fascia second, muscle third and subcutaneous tissue last.

METHODS FOR LOCAL AND LOCAL–REGIONAL BLOCK

Multiple techniques for local or local–regional anesthesia of the lower abdominal wall have been described. Most, however, are modifications of one of four specific techniques:

1. intercostal–paravertebral nerve block;
2. lateral intercostal–thoracoabdominal nerve block;
3. rectus abdominis block; and
4. direct local infiltration.

Intercostal–paravertebral block

As previously described, rarely the need for cesarean

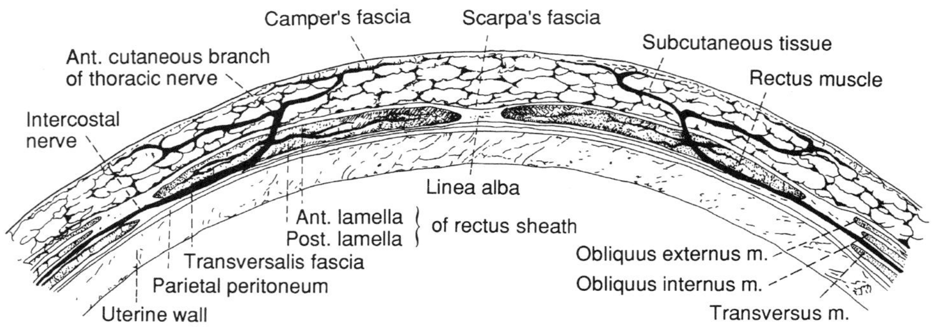

Fig. 40.1 Anatomy. Schematic diagram showing the course of the thoracic nerves as they supply the various layers of the anterior lower abdominal wall. (From ref. 2 with permission.)

delivery may arise in a patient for whom both intraspinal and general anesthesia are contraindicated. In such a circumstance, if personnel trained in regional anesthesia are available, and if the fetus is not in extremis necessitating emergent delivery, an intercostal–paravertebral block may be performed. This procedure offers the advantage of more complete anesthesia and relaxation of the abdominal wall, yet requires less total anesthetic solution than other methods. Possible complications include pneumothorax, intravascular injection and hypotension as a result of peripheral vasodilation from the paravertebral block.[2]

The procedure, as described by Bonica,[2] is performed as follows. The patient is placed on the operating table on her side such that the plane of her back makes a 45° angle with the floor, allowing access to all points required for the block (Fig. 40.2). While a number of anesthetic solutions may be used, that favored by Bonica is a mixture of 1% chloroprocaine combined with 0.1% tetracaine, which produces 2–3 h of anesthesia. Other suggested local anesthetics are given in Table 38.1. The intercostal blocks are placed at the most prominent part of the posterior aspect of each rib bilaterally at the T8, T9, T10 and T11 segments. A finger is used to protect the intercostal space and push the skin just cephalad. A short needle then is advanced to the inferior margin of the rib, the skin is released and the needle advanced another 5 mm into the neurovascular bundle, where the anesthetic is deposited. Paravertebral block is then carried out at the T11–T12 and L1 areas to block the iliohypogastric nerve, ilioinguinal nerve and fibers supplying the uterus.

To perform the paravertebral block, the patient is

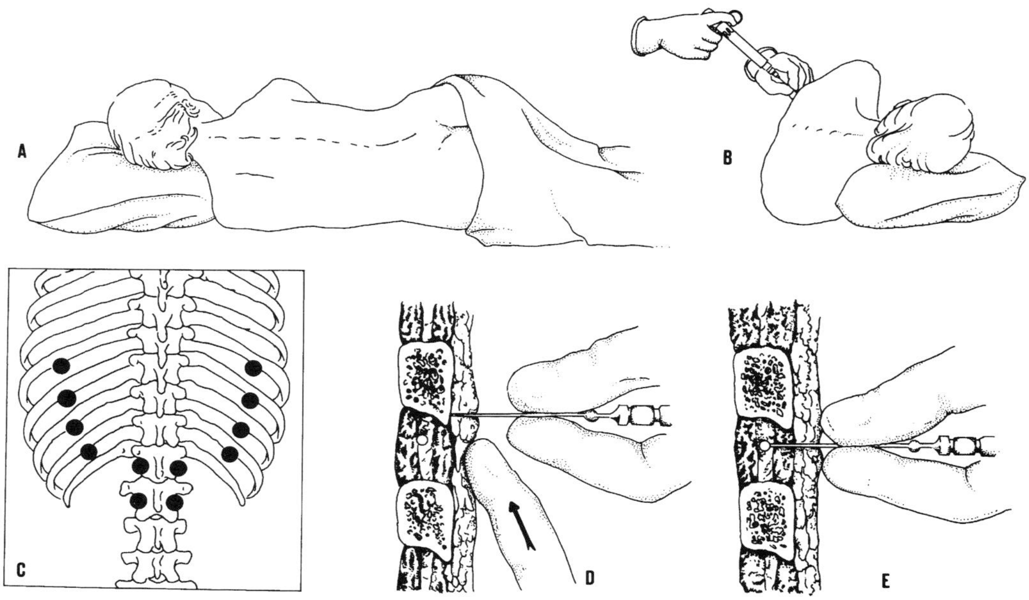

Fig. 40.2 Intercostal paravertebral block. (**A and B**) Positioning of the patient. (**C**) Points for intercostal and paravertebral injections. (**D and E**) Technique for intercostal injection. (From ref. 2, with permission.)

placed briefly in the sitting position. The spinous processes of the T11–T12 and the L1 vertebrae are located by counting cephalad from L4. This is easily palpated in a horizontal line between the iliac crests. With a marker, horizontal lines are drawn on the skin through the most cephalad point of each spinous process of the three target vertebrae. A vertical line is then drawn parallel to the spine 3.2–3.8 cm on both sides of the spine depending on the size of the patient. The resulting six intersections are the points of entry for the paravertebral block.[3] After a skin wheal is raised at each point, a 3.8-cm, 22-gauge needle is used to infiltrate directly down to the transverse process that should lie below each wheal. Next, a 7.5-cm, 22-gauge needle is advanced in the same tract until it impinges on the transverse process. At this point, a distance of 3 cm is visualized or measured from the surface of the skin and marked on the needle. With care taken to remain in the parasagittal plane, the needle is angled caudad, little by little, until it passes just beneath the transverse process, upon which the needle is advanced until the mark reaches the skin. 10-20 ml of the above local anesthetic solution should be injected in each of the six sites.

Lateral intercostal–thoracoabdominal nerve block

A second method, combining the advantages of regional and local anesthesia, is the lateral intercostal–thoracoabdominal nerve block described by Busby.[4] The advantage of this procedure over that previously described is that this method may be employed by the delivering obstetrician. The expertise needed for paravertebral block is not required.

The procedure, beginning with the arrowhead field block, is described by Busby as follows (Fig. 40.3A). A point midway between the inferior costal margin and the iliac crest is located in the mid-axillary line. A 2-inch, 22-gauge needle is used to penetrate the fascia of the internal and external oblique muscles, depositing 5–8 ml of local anesthetic to block the 11th intercostal nerve. The needle is withdrawn to just beneath the skin, angled 45° cephalad, and again advanced through the aponeuroses to access the 10th intercostal nerve. Finally, this same needle is again withdrawn to just beneath the surface of the skin, angled 45° caudad, and advanced, thus depositing the local anesthetic in the vicinity of the 12th intercostal nerve. Because the area over the mons is also innervated by the iliohypogastric and ilioinguinal nerves, these must be blocked as they exit the inguinal ring (Fig. 40.3B). To accomplish this, the skin over the pubic tubercle is pierced, angling the needle 45° down and laterally for 2–3 cm, depositing the anesthetic at the level of the external oblique fascia. The abdomen is then draped for a midline incision. A 'pigskin' wheal is raised along the line of incision with care taken to place the local anesthetic

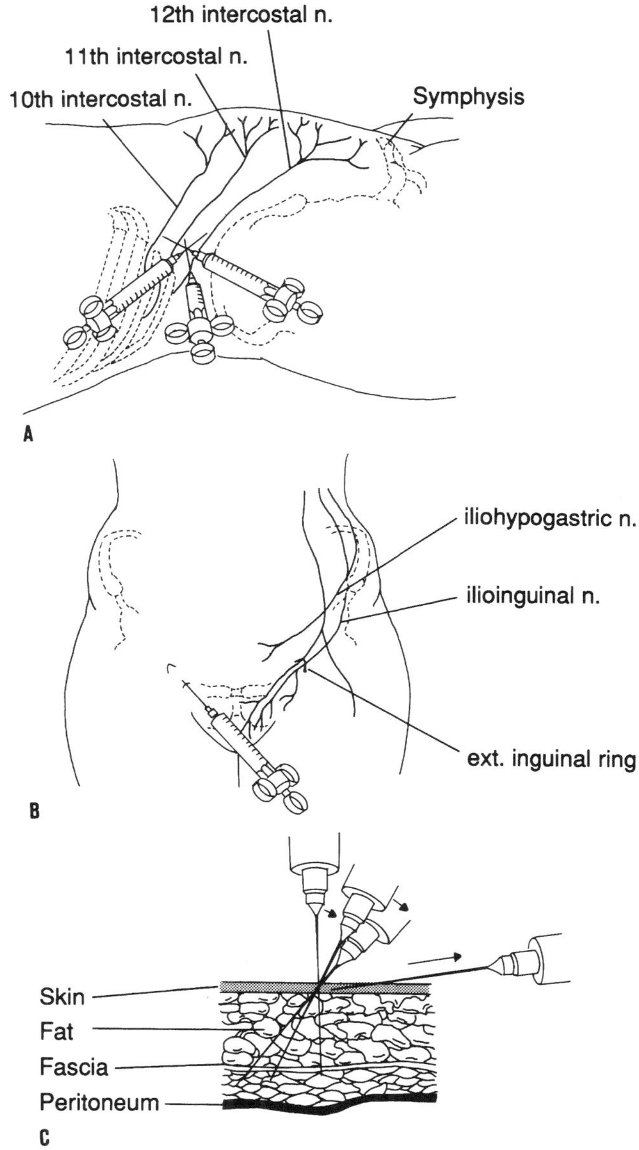

Fig. 40.3 Lateral intercostal–thoracoabdominal nerve block. (**A**) Arrowhead field block. (**B**) Injection to block the iliohypogastric and ilioinguinal nerves. (**C**) Technique for midline skin and fascial injection. (From ref. 4 with permission.)

intradermally, not in the subcutaneous fat. Next, the fascia is anesthetized by piercing the raised line and slowly injecting the local anesthetic as the needle advances through the fascia, which can be felt as a slight resistance. A small amount, roughly 1 ml, of anesthetic is deposited just below the fascia, effectively lifting the peritoneum off the undersurface of the fascia (Fig. 40.3C). The needle is withdrawn slightly, angled caudally and again advanced through the fascia, injecting slowly as the needle traverses the fascia. This is repeated until the complete line is infiltrated. After the incision has been carried through the fascia and the peritoneum has been entered, Busby advocates the placement of 10 ml of anesthetic freely into the peritoneal cavity, effectively anesthetizing the serosal surfaces in the pelvis. Although probably not necessary, a small amount of anesthetic may also be injected just beneath the proposed bladder flap to facilitate dissection of the tissue planes and provide additional visceral anesthesia.

Like the intercostal–paravertebral block, the lateral intercostal–thoracoabdominal procedure may be complicated by pneumothorax or intravascular injection. Additionally, while Busby reported reasonable results in 28 patients, others have not been able to achieve the same success with this procedure. Ranney and Stanage[1] wrote of this method, '. . . it [lateral intercostal block] seemed that more time and procaine were wasted than the process was worth'.

Rectus abdominis block

The rectus block takes advantage of the fact that the thoracoabdominal nerves course through the rectus sheath before branching to supply the lower abdominal wall. Ranney and Stanage[1] suggest that by using this technique the amount of local anesthetic required is minimal with 1% procaine 60 ml usually providing adequate cesarean anesthesia. (The author suggests the use of 1% chloroprocaine or 0.5% lidocaine.) They describe the procedure as follows (Fig. 40.4).

The anesthetic is first drawn up in 10-ml syringes fitted with 1.5-inch, 25-gauge needles. After raising a skin wheal 4 cm lateral to the umbilicus, the needle is directed just beneath the skin toward the umbilicus, infiltrating 2 ml as the needle advances. As the needle is withdrawn, the operator stops at three points to angle the tip just deep to the rectus fascia, as shown in Figure 40.4. Approximately 1 ml of anesthetic is injected at each spot. Before the needle is fully withdrawn, its point is directed toward the pelvis, advanced beneath the skin, and used to create the next skin wheal, as shown in the figure. This process is repeated down to the pubis, the same process being repeated on the contralateral side. Next, a continuous subcutaneous wheal is created in the midline without deep infiltration. Finally, after the skin and subcutaneous

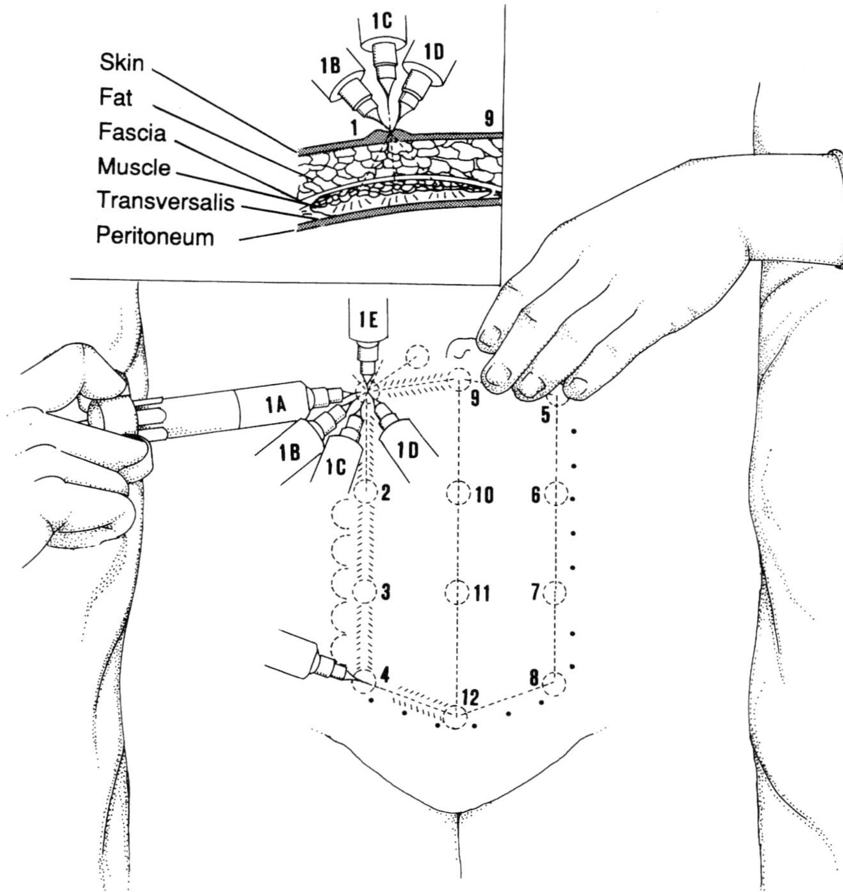

Fig. 40.4 Rectus block. Schematic diagram showing points for injection. (Inset: Detail of rectus compartment infiltration.) (From ref. 1 with permission.)

Table 40.1 Maximal recommended doses of common local anesthetics (Modified with permission from Chestnut D H, Gibbs C P 1991 Obstetric anesthesia. In Gabbe S G, Niebyl J R, Simpson J L (eds) Obstetrics: normal and problem pregnancies, 2nd ed Churchill Livingstone, New York, p 493)

Local anesthetic	Without epinephrine (mg/kg)	With epinephrine* (mg/kg)
Lidocaine	4.0	7.0
Chloroprocaine	11.0	14.0
Bupivacaine	2.5	3.0
Mepivacaine	5.0	–
Tetracaine	1.5	–

* Assumes all epinephrine concentrations are 1:200 000.

tissues are opened, the fascia is directly infiltrated and incised. The visceral peritoneum may be handled as in the previous procedures.

In experienced hands, patient acceptance of this technique is remarkable. Ranney and Stanage[1] reported that, of 141 women who had had a cesarean delivery under rectus block anesthesia, 77 underwent a repeat cesarean delivery and only three asked for a general anesthetic.[1] Despite this apparent patient approval, there are disadvantages to the rectus block. First, the procedure is associated with several complications, including toxic reactions from excessive doses or intravascular injection, unintentional injection directly into the uterus and hematomas from laceration of abdominal wall vessels.[2] Second, while the theory behind injection into the rectus sheath may sound attractive, this anatomic compartment may be very hard to identify in the pregnant woman with a distended abdomen, diastasis recti or marked obesity. In recognition of this, some authors recommend that rectus block anesthesia be performed only by persons with extensive experience with this technique in the nonpregnant patient, effectively excluding most obstetricians.[2]

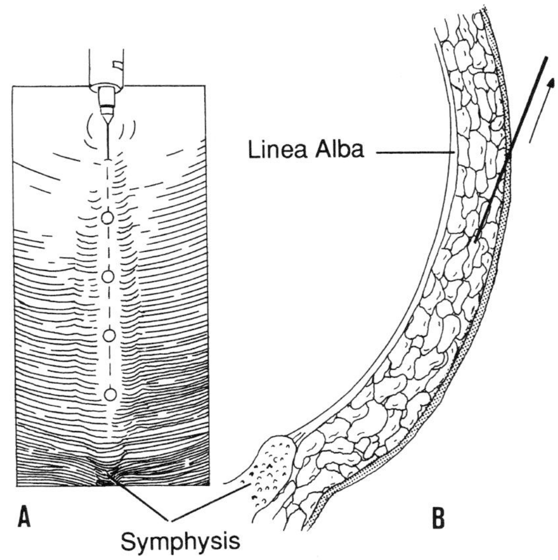

Fig. 40.5 Local infiltration of (**A**) the skin and (**B**) the subcutaneous tissue. (Modified from ref. 2 with permission.)

Direct local infiltration

When a laboring patient must be delivered emergently and no one trained in anesthesia is available, the most reliable technique for anesthetizing the lower abdominal wall is simple local infiltration. This method requires no special knowledge of regional anesthesia and is not dependent on operator experience. Because local infiltration does not require repositioning of the patient or redraping of the sterile field, the procedure may be carried out rapidly by the delivering obstetrician.

The most important consideration in local infiltration for abdominal delivery is an awareness of the maximum recommended dose of the specific agent used. The maximum recommended doses of the local anesthetic agents commonly available in labor and delivery suites are

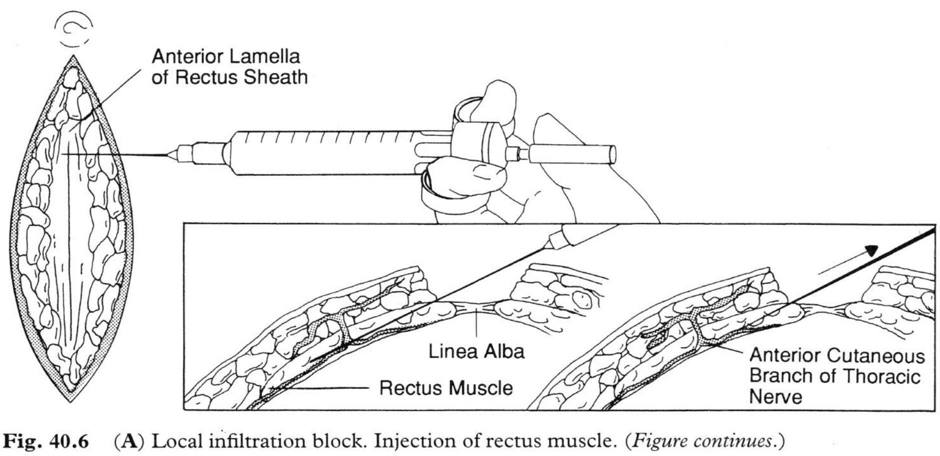

Fig. 40.6 (**A**) Local infiltration block. Injection of rectus muscle. (*Figure continues.*)

reviewed in Table 40.1. Because the limits for toxicity for most agents will be rapidly achieved with the 200–300 ml needed for adequate anesthesia, Zuspans suggests that concentration of the available solutions should be halved, noting that this will not compromise the block needed for cesarean delivery.

Local infiltration for cesarean delivery, as modified from Zuspan[5] and Bonica,[2] is begun by raising a 2-cm skin wheal just inferior to the umbilicus using a 5-cm, 25-gauge needle. Directed parallel to the skin, this needle is then used to infiltrate the intracutaneous (intradermal) tissue toward the pubis in a series of four to five injections (Fig. 40.5). Using one hand for countertraction, care is taken to keep the needle just beneath the skin, not in the subcutaneous fat. Next, using a 10-cm, 22-gauge needle, the subcutaneous tissue is infiltrated with 6–8 ml of solution, again using countertraction and direct pressure on the needle point to ensure that the tract conforms to the contour of the abdomen (Fig. 40.5). After 3–4 min, the skin may be gently incised. Lateral infiltration of the skin and subcutaneous tissue is not required. By gently separating the wound edges the fascia of the anterior medial border of each rectus sheath may be exposed for the next step. Using an 8-cm, 22-gauge needle, the rectus sheath is pierced, directing the needle laterally and down approximately 10–15° (Fig. 40.6A). The needle is advanced 3–5 cm until its point is thought to be at the lateral posterior margin of the muscle. 2 ml of solution is then injected and the needle slowly withdrawn while injecting another 1–2 ml. By repeating this step at 3-cm intervals toward the symphysis, a continuous layer of anesthetic is placed in the potential space between the muscle and the posterior fascia (Fig. 40.6B). This blocks the thoracoabdominal nerves as they traverse the rectus compartment, and produces anesthesia between the lateral margins of the two rectus muscles. After 3–5 min the fascia may be incised, exposing the parietal peritoneum. If the peritoneum is still sensitive, this may be anesthetized with direct infiltration or topical application of a local anesthetic. The visceral layers are handled as described for the previous methods.

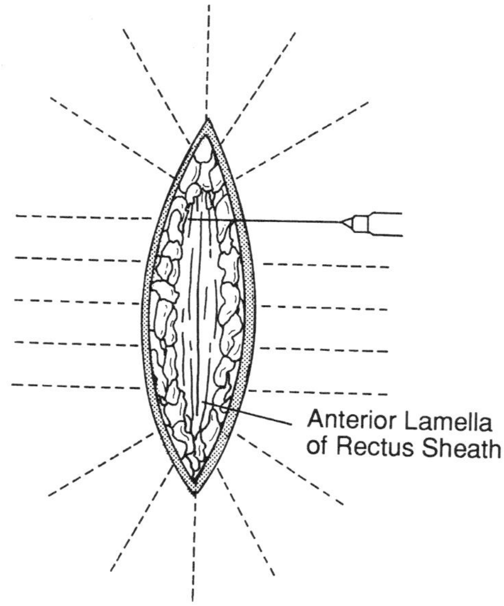

Fig. 40.6 (*Continued*). (**B**) Local infiltration block. Placement of successive rectus compartment injections. (From ref. 2 with permission.)

SURGICAL CONSIDERATIONS

Realizing that with any of these local techniques the patient will be awake, anxious and aware of her surroundings, the obstetrician has several additional responsibilities. First, he or she must ensure that all persons in the delivery room remain as quiet and calm as possible. The patient must be told to expect some minor discomfort and pressure intermittently throughout the operation. Additionally, she may experience moderate back pain with delivery of the fetus through the uterine incision. Importantly, surgical technique should be gentle. Retraction and stretching of tissues should be absolutely minimized. In modern obstetrics, there is no place for a transverse or Pfannenstiel incision when the delivery must be performed under local anesthesia. These incisions take longer, require more dissection, are associated with a greater potential for bleeding and are not suited for any of the anesthetic techniques described in this section. Finally, although the operation may have already begun, the obstetrician should ensure that someone continues to try and reach trained anesthesia personnel.

REFERENCES

1. Ranney B, Stanage W F 1975 Advantages of local anesthesia for cesarean section. Obstet Gynecol 45: 163–167
2. Bonica J J 1967 Principles and practice of obstetric analgesia and anesthesia. F A Davis, Philadelphia, p 527–538
3. Moore D C 1965 Regional block: a handbook for use in the clinical practice of medicine and surgery. 4th ed Charles C Thomas, Springfield, I L, p 206–210
4. Busby T 1963 Local anesthesia for cesarean section. Am J Obstet Gynecol 87: 399–404
5. Zuspan K J Anesthesia and analgesia. In Zuspan F P, Quilligan E J (eds): Douglas–Stromme operative obstetrics. 5th ed Appleton & Lange, East Norwalk, CT, p 123–150

41. Analgesia after operative deliveries

Part A Overview *F. B. Sevarino R. S. Sinatra*
Part B Specific therapies *M. J. Segal F. M. Ferrante*

PART A
OVERVIEW
F. B. Sevarino R. S. Sinatra

The peripartum experience is strongly influenced not only by the events of the labor and subsequent delivery, but also by the management of maternal post-operative pain. Traditional on-demand analgesia dosing involves an elaborate sequence of events that inevitably delays administration of intramuscular pain medication by 30 min to an hour. One commonly observes repetitive cycles of increased pain followed by excessive sedation and narcosis.[1]

Alternating cycles of pain and sedation may interfere with early maternal/neonatal interactions. Thus, following cesarean delivery, patients face the dilemma of electing to be either uncomfortable with pain or sedated with intramuscular doses of opioids. As in any post-surgical setting, requests for analgesics are initiated by the patient. A 'screening' of the patient's complaint then occurs in which the nurse assesses whether she requires additional pain medication. If the level of pain is deemed appropriate and requiring therapy, a further sequence of events occurs before the patient receives pain relief. Medication is signed out, prepared for injection and then finally administered to the patient. The drug must then be absorbed from the intramuscular or subcutaneous site of administration. The initial analgesic effect is followed by sedation and some degree of respiratory depression due to the erratic and prolonged absorption of the medication (Fig. 41.1).

Because of these problems, alternative techniques of opioid administration are being used with increasing frequency in many institutions. Intravenous patient-controlled analgesia (PCA) was first described by Sechzer[2]

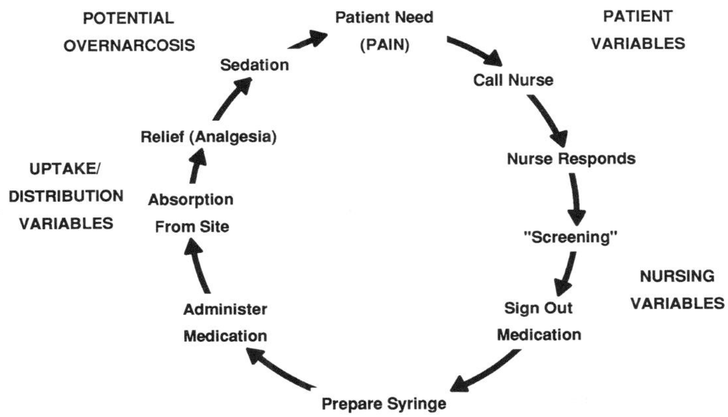

Fig. 41.1 Patient and nusring variables in pain management

in 1968. It permits the patient to effectively control post-surgical pain by intermittently self-administering opioid. The rate of administration is controlled by the patient within prescribed dose and frequency limits according to her perception of pain. In theory, PCA overcomes inter-patient variability in analgesic requirements by maintaining effective plasma concentration while avoiding periods of excessive sedation or ineffective pain control. PCA is initiated post-operatively after the patient has been given a loading dose of opioid either intraoperatively or in the post-anesthesia care unit (PACU) to provide initial analgesia for the patient. This reduces the need to have the patient 'catch up' to the degree of pain.

PCA systems work under a number of assumptions. The first assumption is that side-effects of opioids occur at higher brain concentrations than those needed to produce analgesia. While massive doses of opioid could theoretically eliminate all pain (but with unacceptable levels of respiratory depression), an adequate level of analgesia usually represents a compromise between tolerable pain and troublesome side-effects. A second assumption is that pain intensity is rarely constant. Post-operative pain is intensified by movement and coughing, and seems to have a circadian rhythm with increasing pain at night. A final assumption is that the entire spectrum of pain relief occurs within a narrow range of plasma analgesic concentration subject to individual variation.

The PCA devices available in the USA incorporate a microprocessor that allows the patient to interact with an infusion pump connected to her established intravenous infusion. The patient usually activates the pump by pressing a button connected to the apparatus. A preprogrammed amount of opioid is then administered over 10–30 s. A lockout interval is simultaneously begun after each injection, thereby preventing a second dose from being delivered within a preset time interval (usually between 5–15 min, depending upon dose and agent selected). Potential overdosage is prevented by limiting the amount of opioid delivered per bolus and limiting the number of injections over a given time interval. More sophisticated systems allow the use of a basal constant infusion rate in addition to patient activated, on-demand, boluses. This may be best utilized with rapid-acting, short-duration agents.

Neuraxial administration of opioids also provides remarkably efficacious analgesia. A major advantage of neuraxial opioids is the selectivity of the analgesic effect that occurs in the absence of motor or sympathetic blockade. In contrast to local anesthetics, the patients are able to ambulate while untoward cardiovascular effects are avoided. Morphine is the opioid most widely used in this setting, and provides up to 24 h of analgesia, while improving post-operative respiratory function and allowing early ambulation. Unfortunately, morphine is associated with a number of side-effects including pruritus, nausea and 'late-onset' respiratory depression. Epidural meperidine, methadone and hydromorphone have all been reported to give excellent post-operative analgesia;[3] however the duration of analgesia is shorter while side-effects are similar to morphine. Fentanyl and sufentanil also produce reliable post-cesarean analgesia with a lower incidence of side-effects than morphine. The duration of action, however, is shorter.[4,5]

With the availability of the alternative techniques of opioid administration discussed above, the question as to which provides the optimal pain control for the post-cesarean patient was examined. In 1988 both Eisenach et al[6] and Harrison et al[7] compared epidural morphine, patient-controlled intravenous morphine and intramuscular morphine for post-cesarean pain relief. Both teams of investigators examined not only analgesic scores but also side-effects and patient satisfaction with each of these pain control techniques[6,7,8] (Table 41.1).

Patients in both the epidural and in the PCA groups preferred their pain therapy to the traditional i.m. therapy received following their first cesarean delivery. However, patients in the PCA group were judged to be more sedated

Table 41.1 Analgesic efficacy and frequency of adverse effects with epidural, PCA and i.m. morphine

	No. of patients with good post-operative analgesia			Percentage of patients with pruritus			Percentage of patients with urinary retention	
Reference	Epidural	PCA	i.m.	Epidural	PCA	i.m.	Epidural	PCA
6	65	40	25	85	60	35	NA	NA
7	85	60	50	72	38	17	NA	NA
8	95	50	NA	73	35	NA	53	18

NA, not applicable.

in Eisenach's study, while in both studies patients receiving epidural morphine had a significantly higher incidence of pruritus. The more effective pain relief provided by the epidural morphine as compared with PCA did not result in greater patient satisfaction with this technique. As patients using PCA were 'in control', they appeared more likely to tolerate varying degrees of mild, nondistressing pain. Although epidural morphine produced more profound analgesia than PCA or i.m therapy, the analgesia was of variable duration, and inadequate amounts of parenteral opioids may be prescribed to patients receiving epidural morphine because of the concern about the risk of respiratory depression. Both authors conclude that the choice of analgesic therapy should be based in part upon patient preference and the nature of the side-effects. PCA was thus chosen by the authors as the therapy of choice because of the high degree of patient satisfaction and low incidence of side-effects.

The choice of opioid for PCA in post-cesarean patients has been addressed by Sinatra et al[9] who compared the effectiveness of morphine, meperidine and oxymorphone. They noted that all patients had similar 24-h analgesic requirements and satisfactory pain relief. Patients receiving meperidine experienced less sedation and pruritus, had lower attempt versus injection ratios, and were somewhat more satisfied with PCA therapy than those receiving morphine. Patients receiving oxymorphone experienced the most rapid onset of analgesia but had the highest (28%) incidence of nausea requiring treatment. Thus, while all three agents may be used for PCA therapy, meperidine was recommended as the opioid of choice, as it has the lowest incidence of side-effects. Hydromorphone[10] is an acceptable alternative in this setting (Table 41.2).

One final consideration with respect to the choice of PCA agent is the effect of the PCA opioid on nursing infants. Wittels et al[11] in a preliminary study suggested that PCA morphine provides equivalent maternal analgesia but significantly less infant neurobehavioral depression than did PCA meperidine in nursing mothers.

A potential disadvantage of PCA is that plasma opioid concentrations fall below analgesic levels if the infuser is

Table 41.2 Commonly used PCA medication

	Bolus dose (mg)		Lockout (min)	
Drug	Range	Usual	Range	Usual
Morphine	0.8–2	1.2	5–15	6
Meperidine	5–25	12.5	5–15	6
Oxymorphone	0.1–0.5	0.2	5–15	6
Hydromorphone	0.1–0.6	0.2	5–15	6

not activated, thereby resulting in the patient awakening at night with pain or not being prepared for an increase in pain stimulus (sudden ambulation). For this reason a basal infusion (BI) of opioid may be superimposed upon PCA. Sinatra et al[12] noted significant reduction in pain during movement and a lower total opioid usage in patients receiving either oxymorphone or morphine via PCA + BI when compared with PCA alone; however, an increased incidence of nausea and other side-effects was observed. No significant difference in patient satisfaction with respect to the agent or the mode of delivery was noted. Thus, in the post-cesarean patient the addition of a basal infusion should be reserved for the rare patient experiencing inadequate pain relief with PCA alone, such as the patient who has had a cesarean hysterectomy.

Administration of intraspinal opioids followed by PCA is the most recent trend in optimizing post-cesarean analgesia. This combination therapy offers a number of advantages in that small doses of subarachnoid or epidural opioids smooth the transition to PCA while reducing the total 24 h opioid dosage. The choice of the intraspinally administered opioid is important. Sevarino et al[4] noted that epidural fentanyl did not provide analgesia of long enough duration to impact on PCA opioid requirements. The combination of low-dose subarachnoid morphine (0.2–0.25 mg) plus PCA offers a number of advantages, including a pain-free state following cesarean delivery, which should smooth transition from the resolution of the spinal anesthesia to initiation of PCA and reduce the 24-h PCA opioid requirements.[13] Similarly, we are administering epidural meperidine (50 mg) at cord clamping and note 5 h of excellent analgesia prior to introduction of PCA.

Patient characteristics may also influence the outcome of pain therapy. Some preeclamptic patients have coagulation abnormalities and are not candidates for epidural anesthesia. Magnesium therapy may increase the sedative effect of PCA and thus a smaller PCA dose should be used. Meperidine may lower the seizure threshold, thus preeclamptic patients might better receive morphine or hydromorphone and not meperidine for PCA.

The use of PCA in substance abusers is controversial. Data collected at our institution demonstrate that, following cesarean delivery, cocaine abusers utilize PCA no differently than nonabusers. (L. Preble RN, Clinical Nurse Coordinator, Yale University/YNHH Department of Anesthesiology Acute Pain Management Service, personal communication). In narcotic abusers, we recommend oral or parenteral methadone maintenance with PCA providing only the acute pain requirements.

To summarize, superior pain control can be obtained using either i.v. PCA or epidural morphine compared with traditional i.m. therapy following cesarean delivery. Side-effects of epidural morphine result in less patient satisfaction than with PCA, and thus PCA is the preferred post-operative pain therapy in this patient population.

REFERENCES

1. Graves D, Foster A, Batenhorst R L, Bennett R L 1983 Patient controlled analgesia. Ann Int Med 99: 360–366
2. Sechzer P H 1968 Objective measurement of pain. Anesthesiology 29: 209–210
3. Naulty J S 1988 Perioperative obstetrical analgesia. Problems in Anesthesia 2: 408–421
4. Sevarino F B, McFarlane C, Sinatra R S 1991 Epidural fentanyl does not influence intravenous PCA in the post-cesarean patient. Can J Anaesth 38: 450–453
5. Naulty J S, Sevarino F B, Lema M J, Hunt C O, Datta S, Ostheimer G W 1986 Epidural sufentanil for postcesarean delivery pain management. Anesthesiology 65: 3A; A396
6. Eisenach J C, Grice S C, Dewan D M 1988 Patient-controlled analgesia following cesarean section: a comparison with epidural and intramuscular narcotics. Anesthesiology 68: 444–448
7. Harrison D M, Sinatra R, Morgese L, Chung J H 1988 Epidural narcotic and patient-controlled analgesia for post-cesarean section pain relief. Anesthesiology 68: 454–457
8. Loper K A, Ready L B 1989 Epidural morphine after anterior cruciate ligament repair: comparison with PCA. Anesth Analg 68: 350–352
9. Sinatra R S, Lodge K, Sibert K, Chung K S, Chung J H, Parker A, Harrison D M 1989 A comparison of morphine, meperidine , and oxymorphone as utilized in patient-controlled analgesia following cesarean delivery. Anesthesiology 70: 585–590
10. Urquhart M L, Klapp K, White P F 1988 Patient-controlled analgesia: a comparison of intravenous versus subcutaneous hydromorphone. Anesthesiology 69: 428–432
11. Wittels B, Scott D T, Sinatra R S 1990 Exogenous opioids in human breast milk and acute neonatal neurobehavior: a preliminary study. Anesthesiology 73: 864–864
12. Sinatra R, Chung K S, Silverman D G, Brull S J, Chung J, Harrison D M, Donielson D, Weinstock A 1989 An evaluation of morphine and oxymorphone administered via patient-controlled analgesia (PCA) or PCA plus basal infusion in postcesarean-delivery patients. Anesthesiology 71: 502–507
13. Kemper P M, Treiber H 1990 Neuraxial morphine plus intravenous patient controlled analgesia – new method in postcesarean analgesia. Anesth Analg 70: S1–S540

PART B
SPECIFIC THERAPIES

M. J. Segal F. M. Ferrante

The therapeutic choices for treatment of pain following cesarean delivery include PCA (patient-controlled analgesia) and epidural, subarachnoid and traditional intramuscular opioids. The obstetric patient's needs are different from those of the general surgical patient. After cesarean delivery, women desire to remain alert in order to bond with their neonates. Therefore, the optimal analgesic modality should provide maximum pain relief with minimal sedation in order to promote maternal– neonatal bonding.

PATIENT-CONTROLLED ANALGESIA

Intermittent i.m. dosing of opioids does not reliably produce satisfactory post-operative analgesia.[1] Variable absorption from intramuscular injection sites results in fluctuating, unpredictable plasma concentrations.[1] This uneven absorption accounts for the wide variations in peak plasma concentration (C_{max}) and the time to reach the peak plasma concentration (T_{max}) following intramuscular injections.[2] Pain relief occurs when the plasma opioid concentration reaches a minimum effective analgesic concentration (MEAC). MEAC is relatively consistent for a given patient but varies two- to fivefold among patients.[2] When opioids are given via timed, scheduled intramuscular dosing, plasma concentrations are in excess of MEAC only 35% of the time during any 4-h dosing interval.[2]

The response to PCA has been enthusiastic from both patients and obstetricians. Because PCA delivers opioids intravenously, the wide swings in plasma concentration seen with intramuscular dosing are avoided. On-demand self-administration of small amounts of opioid can accommodate highly variable analgesic requirements. PCA allows patients to 'titrate' their specific analgesic needs. The immediate accessibility of analgesia also decreases the anxiety associated with the normal delay in receiving conventional i.m. medication. Patients use PCA to maintain plasma opioid concentrations within range of their own MEAC.[3] The therapeutic window is narrow, and very small fluctuations in opioid concentration (0.05 µg/ml of meperidine) can mean the difference between discomfort and adequate analgesia.[1]

It is presently hypothesized that an individual patient's MEAC is determined by his or her preoperative endogenous opioid content in the cerebrospinal fluid (CSF).[4] Patient with low quantities of endogenous opioids in the CSF use PCA to administer liberal amounts of exogenous opioid in order to maintain higher plasma opioid concentrations. Conversely, patients with high preoperative endogenous opioid content in the CSF use PCA more sparingly to maintain lower plasma opioid concentrations. However, a recent report[5] suggest that this may not apply in obstetric patients.

At present, the most commonly used modes of administration of PCA are demand dosing (a fixed dose is self-administered) and constant-rate infusion plus demand dosing (a background infusion is supplemented by patient demand). Infusion demand modes (where demands are granted as an infusion) and variable-rate infusion plus demand dosing modes (where a microprocessor monitors demand and controls the infusion rate accordingly) are presently under study.[6]

INTRASPINAL OPIOIDS

Alternatively, intraspinal (epidural or subarachnoid) opioids may be used to provide potent analgesia after cesarean delivery. The sites of action of both epidural and subarachnoid opioids are the opioid receptors in the dorsal horn of the spinal cord.[7] Both the onset and duration of analgesia correlate with CSF opioid concentration, not plasma concentration.[8] Since epidural opioids must passively diffuse across the dura into the CSF, higher lipid solubility is associated with faster onset. Clearance from the CSF determines the duration of action. Highly lipid-soluble opioids (fentanyl, sufentanil, meperidine, methadone, butorphanol) are quickly absorbed into adjacent tissues, particularly the vasculature. Hence, a more segmental block of relatively short duration is obtained with increasing lipophilicity, as the opioid does not diffuse widely throughout the epidural and subarachnoid spaces.[9]

The low lipid solubility of morphine, by contrast, accounts for its slower onset but extremely long duration of action (12–24 h). Morphine spreads widely in the epidural and subarachnoid spaces, causing a non-segmental block. The quality of analgesia is similar with both lipophilic and hydrophilic opioids, though the onset and duration differ greatly.[9]

Concomitant with the use of morphine is the possibility for delayed respiratory depression. Late respiratory depression is due to rostral spread, which affects medullary respiratory centers. Though this feared complication is rare and usually gradual in onset, patients should be closely monitored for 24 h following injection. The lipid-soluble opioids are not associated with delayed respiratory depression because their cephalad spread is limited.[9]

COMPARISON OF TECHNIQUES FOR ANALGESIA AFTER CESAREAN DELIVERY

Epidural morphine provides analgesia superior to either PCA or intramuscular morphine following cesarean delivery.[10] (A similar trial using lipophilic opioids has not been performed.) The duration of analgesia with epidural morphine is variable, however. Approximately 40% of patients require systemic opioids within 12 h and 50% by 24 h after administration of a single bolus dose of epidural morphine.[11] Addition of parenteral opioids for breakthrough pain may increase the chance of respiratory depression when using intraspinal opioids.

Overall, patients are more satisfied with PCA-administered morphine. Although epidural morphine provides more profound analgesia, it is associated with frequent bothersome side-effects (pruritus, nausea and vomiting). The prevalence of pruritus requiring treatment may be as high as 45%, compared with 5% for patients receiving either PCA or intramuscular morphine after cesarean delivery.[10]

A significant percentage of patients may also experience pruritus with epidural administration of lipophilic opioids. This pruritus, however, is usually transient and mild and does not require treatment. The prevalence of nausea is similar among PCA, epidural and intramuscular routes.

ANALGESIC PRACTICE AT THE BRIGHAM AND WOMEN'S HOSPITAL

For alleviation of post-cesarean delivery pain at our institution, both techniques are sequentially used in combination. Because of the rare but real risk of respiratory depression, use of agents via intraspinal administration has been restricted to the lipid-soluble opioids. If cesarean delivery is performed with subarachnoid anesthesia, the opioid is given during administration of the block. If a patient chooses epidural anesthesia, a single dose of lipid-soluble opioid is administered immediately after birth. Occasionally, a second dose may be given in the post-anesthesia care unit.

The addition of opioids to local anesthetics for subarachnoid anesthesia improves both intraoperative and immediate post-operative analgesia. Subarachnoid administration of as little as 6.25 µg of fentanyl with hyperbaric bupivacaine results in 3–4 h of post-operative analgesia.[12] This is similar to the duration of analgesia obtained from epidural fentanyl but with much lower dose of opioid. For subarachnoid block, fentanyl 10–20 µg is customarily added to hyperbaric bupivacaine. In contrast, subarachnoid morphine provides approximately 24 h of post-operative analgesia.[13] This prolonged pain relief must be weighed against the risk of delayed respiratory depression.

The minimum reliably effective dose of epidural fentanyl is 50 µg, which results in 3–7 h of analgesia.[14] Dilution of fentanyl in at least 10 ml of preservative-free normal saline or local anesthetic has been shown to shorten the onset time and increase the duration of analgesia as compared with administration of lesser volumes.[15] The minimum effective dose of epidural sufentanil has not been determined, although 25–50 µg provides 3.5–5.6 h of analgesia.[16] Increasing doses of fentanyl or sufentanil will not prolong duration, but may reduce total opioid requirement for up to 24 h after cesarean delivery.[14]

After admission to the post-anesthesia care unit, a PCA infuser is connected to the patient. The patient may begin to self-administer opioids when pain is first perceived. Patients typically use PCA for 24–48 h after surgery.

REFERENCES

1. Austin K L, Stapleton J V, Mather L E 1980 Relationship between blood meperidine concentrations and analgesic response: a preliminary report. Anesthesiology 53: 460–466
2. Austin K L, Stapleton J V, Mather L E 1980 Multiple intramuscular injections: a major source of variability in analgesic response to meperidine. Pain 8: 47–62
3. Tamsen A, Hartvig P, Fagerlund C, Dahlström B 1982 Patient-controlled analgesic plasma concentrations of pethidine in postoperative pain. Clin Pharmacokinet 7: 164–175
4. Tamsen A, Sakurda T, Wahlström A et al 1982 Postoperative demand for analgesics in relation to individual levels of endorphins and substance P in cerebrospinal fluid. Pain 13: 171–183
5. Eisenach J C, Dobson C E II, Insturissi C E, Hood D D 1989 Do spinal enkephalins mediate analgesia in pregnancy? (abstract). Anesth Analg 68: S78
6. Mather L E, Owen H 1990 The pharamacology of patient-administered opioids. In Ferrante F M, Ostheimer G W, Covina B G (eds) Patient-controlled analgesia. Blackwell Scientific Publications, Boston, p 27–50
7. Game C J, Lodge D 1975 The pharmacology of the inhibition of dorsal horn neurons by impulses in myelinated cutaneous afferents in cats. Exp Brain Res 23: 75–84
8. Nordberg G, Hedner T, Mellstrand T, Dahlström B 1983 Pharmacokinetic aspects of epidural morphine analgesia. Anesthesiology 58: 545–551
9. Cousins M J, Mather L E 1984 Intrathecal and epidural administration of opioids. Anesthesiology 61: 276–310
10. Harrison D M, Sinatra R, Morgese L, Chung J H 1988 Epidural narcotics and patient-controlled analgesia for post-cesarean section pain relief. Anesthesiology 68: 454–457
11. Eisenach J C, Grice S C, Dewan D M 1988 Patient-controlled analgesia following cesarean section: a comparison with epidural and intramuscular narcotics. Anesthesiology 68: 444–448
12. Hunt C O, Naulty J S, Bader A M et al 1989 Perioperative analgesia with subrachnoid fentanyl-bupivacaine for cesarean delivery. Anesthesiology 71: 535–540
13. Rosen M A, Hughes S C, Shinder SM et al 1983 Epidural morphine for the relief of postoperative pain after cesarean delivery. Anesth Analg 62: 666–672
14. Naulty J S, Datta S, Ostheimer G W et al 1985 Epidural fentanyl for post cesarean delivery pain management. Anesthesiology 63: 694–698
15. Birnbach D J, Johnson M D, Arcario T et al 1989 Effect of diluent volume on analgesia produced by epidural fentanyl. Anesth Analg 68: 808–810
16. Rosen M A, Dailey P A, Hughes S C et al 1988 Epidural sufentanil for postoperative analgesia after cesarean section. Anesthesiology 68: 448–454

SECTION 5

The high-risk parturient and her fetus

42. Anesthetic management of obstetric emergencies

M. C. Norris B. L. Leighton

INTRODUCTION

The obstetric anesthesiologist must care for two patients at once. Little in the peripartum period can be planned in advance. Both maternal and fetal complications arise that may require urgent surgical intervention. The anesthesiologist is then faced with the task of rapidly inducing anesthesia in a potentially unstable and unknown patient.

Several steps can limit the maternal and fetal risks of emergency anesthesia. First, be prepared. Routine preoperative evaluation can predict over 80% of emergency cesarean deliveries. Continuous lumbar epidural analgesia, begun early in labor, can then be extended to provide surgical anesthesia should the need for emergent cesarean delivery arise. In one study, preoperative evaluation alone predicted the need for 87% of emergency cesarean deliveries (Table 42.1).[1] Institution of epidural analgesia early in labor allowed 70% of these patients to have operative delivery with extension of epidural blockade. We agree with the following conclusions:

1. Preoperative assessment of all patients admitted to the labor suite can identify risk factors that predispose to cesarean delivery.
2. Early epidural analgesia may avoid the need for a rushed general anesthetic if fetal distress arises.
3. Epidural block nearly eliminates the risk of maternal aspiration of gastric contents and of failed intubation; the two most common causes of maternal morbidity and mortality.[1]

Table 42.1 Factors that increase the risk of cesarean delivery

Maternal risks	Attempted vaginal birth after cesarean delivery (VBACD)
	Preeclampsia
Abnormal labor	Failure to progress
	Cephalopelvic disproportion
	Nonengaged fetal head
Abnormal presentation	Persistent occiput posterior
	Malpresentation/multiple gestation
Fetal risks	Abnormal fetal heart rate tracing
	Need for fetal scalp pH analysis
	Suspected IUGR

FETAL EMERGENCIES

More hysteria, animosity and rash decision-making occur during emergency cesarean delivery for fetal 'distress' than in any other obstetric situation. The precarious state of the distressed fetus is evident to all. However, the very real maternal hazards of rapid sequence induction of general anesthesia may be forgotten by all except the anesthesiologist.

What is 'fetal distress'?

Often used simplistically to describe a cesarean delivery done for fetal indications, the term 'fetal distress' is, unfortunately, imprecise, nonspecific and of little positive predictive value. Most babies delivered for 'fetal distress' have normal Apgar scores, are not distressed and have not suffered intrapartum asphyxia. But, the obstetric literature defines fetal distress as: 'progressive fetal asphyxia that, if not corrected or circumvented, will result in decompensation of the physiologic responses . . . and cause permanent central nervous system and other damage or death.'[2] Such a diagnosis implies significant fetal compromise and a need to proceed rapidly. Should complications develop in a neonate diagnosed as suffering from 'fetal distress', the obstetric and anesthetic management may be questioned in court.

Unfortunately, electronic fetal heart rate monitoring (EFM) is a notoriously imprecise way to diagnose fetal distress. Interpretation of fetal heart rate tracings is very subjective: experts differ widely in their interpretations of sample tracings.[3] EFM is a very sensitive yet nonspecific test. False positive diagnoses occur frequently when using EFM in populations where the incidence of fetal asphyxia is low.[4] Randomized prospective studies comparing perinatal outcome with the use of intermittent auscultation versus continuous EFM do not show any reduction in perinatal mortality with the use of continuous EFM.[5–12] Most report no difference in neonatal morbidity in terms of Apgar scores, umbilical cord blood gases, or need for resuscitation. Only severe and prolonged fetal asphyxia increases the risk of permanent neurologic dysfunction.[13,14] Most infants diagnosed with severe intrapartum asphyxia develop without any detectable neurologic deficit. Most children with neurologic disabilities displayed no evidence of perinatal asphyxia. At most, 10% of cases of cerebral palsy are associated with perinatal asphyxia.[15,16] We strongly recommend avoiding the term 'fetal distress'. It is a nonspecific, nonobjective diagnosis for which there are no uniform criteria. Few newborns delivered following such a prospective diagnosis are depressed or acidemic.

Once the obstetrician declares the need for emergency cesarean delivery, one should rapidly determine the answers to the following questions while planning the best anesthetic for both mother and fetus.

1. Can the intrauterine environment be improved enough to decrease the urgency of the cesarean delivery?

Changing the mother's body position, administering supplemental oxygen and stopping oxytocin administration can improve placental perfusion. Subcutaneous terbutaline can terminate tetanic uterine contractions and permit intrauterine resuscitation.[17] Amnioinfusion may prevent intermittent umbilical cord compression.[18] Hypotension secondary to regional anesthesia should be treated with intravenous fluids, intravenous ephedrine and altered maternal body position.[19]

Altering maternal position improves fetal blood flow by relieving aorto-caval compression or umbilical cord compression. Try right and left lateral positioning and the knee-chest position. Remember: uterine artery perfusion pressure is not accurately reflected in maternal brachial artery pressure. Maternal blood pressure measured in the arm may be entirely normal despite significant aorto-caval compression.[20]

Maternal hyperoxia improves oxygen delivery to the fetus if uterine hypoperfusion, umbilical cord compression, or uterine hypertonus have not drastically hindered fetal blood flow. Supplemental oxygen by high flow utilizing a face mask increases maternal and fetal transcutaneous PO_2 in both normal and 'high risk' parturients in labor.[21] Fetal PO_2 correlates directly with maternal PaO_2 over a wide range of values.[22] Although the rise in fetal PO_2 seems small, fetal hemoglobin lies on the steep portion of its oxyhemoglobin dissociation curve and a small increment in PO_2 greatly increases oxygen saturation and content. The increase in umbilical venous oxygen saturation from 65% to 87% can provide substantial oxygen reserve and may significantly improve the physiologic reserve of the stressed fetus. However, maternal oxygen administration will do little to improve fetal status if fetal blood supply is interrupted.

The tension developed within the myometrium during labor increases uterine vascular resistance in proportion to the intensity, frequency, and duration of contractions. Because of limited placental reserve, the stressed fetus cannot tolerate significant reductions in uterine blood flow. Thus, frequent or sustained uterine contractions often result in acute decompensation. When a nonreassuring fetal heart rate tracing or acidosis exists during labor, immediately stop exogenous oxytocin administration. In addition, β_2 sympathomimetics have been used to decrease uterine tone, abolish uterine contractions, and improve umbilical blood flow in acute intrapartum fetal distress. Either intravenous or subcutaneous terbutaline 0.25 mg significantly improves fetal acid-base status, FHR tracing, and neonatal outcome.[17,23–26] A single dose of terbutaline produces a mild maternal tachycardia, but no other side effects.[17]

Since uteroplacental blood flow varies directly with maternal arterial perfusion pressure, it is extremely important to avoid and to treat maternal hypotension rapidly. Adequate fluid infusion, left uterine displacement, use of dilute local anesthetic/opioid infusions for labor analgesia and slow, incremental titration of more concentrated local anesthetics for cesarean delivery can limit or prevent hypotension caused by sympathetic blockade from regional anesthesia.[27–30] For acute i.v. hydration, use 1–2 l of non-glucose containing isotonic crystalloid. Several studies illustrate the importance of using non-glucose containing fluids.[31–35] Philipson et al. evaluated the fetal and maternal metabolic effects of hydration with either 5% dextrose, Ringer's lactate, or isotonic saline in healthy parturients undergoing elective cesarean delivery.[31] Infusion of 1 l of 5% dextrose yields maternal and fetal hyperglycemia, and significantly decreases umbilical venous and arterial pH, and fetal oxygen saturation. Other adverse effects of fetal hyperglycemia include reactive neonatal hypoglycemia and the potential for worsened neurologic outcome after global cerebral ischemia.

2. Does the patient have an epidural anesthetic that can be extended for cesarean delivery?

If the patient had a well-functioning epidural anesthetic for labor, the block can be extended for cesarean delivery with 15–25 ml of 3% 2-chloroprocaine or 2% lidocaine with 1:400 000 epinephrine.[3] If the patient has no epidural or a poorly functioning one, we recommend inducing spinal anesthesia with 12–15 mg of hyperbaric 0.75% bupivacaine.

3. Are there contraindications to general anesthesia?

An airway examination indicating a high probability of

failure to intubate is the primary contraindication to rapid sequence induction of general anesthesia. The incidence of failed intubation is eight times higher in parturients than in general surgery patients.[36] Failed intubation is even more likely in edematous preeclamptic patients.

A contraindication to rapid sequence induction, of course, is not a contraindication to general anesthesia per se. Consider awake intubation if you anticipate a difficult intubation in a parturient.[37] Unfortunately, there is no easy, gentle, and consistently effective way to place a tracheal tube in an awake parturient as quickly as rapid sequence induction of general anesthesia. Adequate mucosal anesthesia of the mouth and pharynx is difficult to achieve in pregnant patients because of copious saliva production, mucosal edema, a hyperactive gag reflex, and the urgency of the clinical circumstances.

Nonetheless, failed rapid sequence induction of general anesthesia is the leading cause of maternal mortality and morbidity associated with anesthesia.[38] Every anesthesia practitioner caring for parturients should have a well-thought-out plan to accomplish awake intubation in a parturient and should have the equipment readily available for use in the delivery room.[37] Many practitioners prefer fiberoptic or blind nasal intubation, some like awake direct laryngoscopy or retrograde intubation. Remember, the nasal mucosa of parturients is very friable and bleeds easily in the absence of adequate vasoconstriction. Whichever plan one prefers, practice the technique in elective cases and ensure that the equipment is ready to use.

Moderate to severe asthma is a relative contraindication to general anesthesia. Regional anesthesia avoids instrumenting the airway and thus avoids mechanically-induced bronchospasm. These women tolerate high levels of epidural or spinal anesthesia. High block does not alter resting pulmonary function although the maximum forced expiratory flow rate is lower.[39] Maternal asthma can lead to several other therapeutic dilemmas. Most drugs that relax bronchial smooth muscle also relax uterine muscle. One may have to choose between not giving a drug and accepting bronchoconstriction or giving a drug and risking uterine atony and increased blood loss. Agents to avoid in the asthmatic undergoing cesarean delivery include high-dose potent inhalation agents, systemic beta agonists (both relax the uterus and may increase blood loss) and prostaglandin F_2 alpha (a potent bronchoconstrictor). Oxytocin (to contract the uterus), ketamine (to maintain anesthesia), and inhaled beta agonists (used in moderation for bronchospasm) seem to be acceptable.[40]

Attempt to avoid general anesthesia in a parturient who is malignant hyperthermia susceptible. If general anesthesia is induced, manage as if the patient is nonpregnant.

4. Are there contraindications to spinal anesthesia?

Spinal anesthesia in a parturient with uncorrected hypovolemia, especially in a patient who is continuing to hemorrhage, may produce intractable hypotension. Preeclamptic patients may become severely hypotensive during induction of spinal anesthesia. Do not pass a spinal needle through an area of active infection. The most common systemic infection in parturients is low-grade chorioamnionitis. Large case series of patients with chorioamnionitis who received epidural or spinal anesthesia suggest that the risk of meningitis or epidural abscess is not increased in these women.[41] Maternal refusal is a contraindication even if the obstetrician prefers to operate under spinal anesthesia.

Do not induce regional anesthesia in a patient with a coagulopathy; however, precise, scientifically derived guidelines, particularly for parturients, are lacking. The most common bleeding disorder in parturients is thrombocytopenia. Preeclampsia induces abnormal platelet function as well as a decrease in platelet number. Decision making based on the bleeding time used to be recommended; however, new evidence suggests that this test is such a poor measure of platelet function that the test is useless.[42]

We will usually administer spinal (or epidural) anesthesia to a patient with no clinical evidence of bleeding and a platelet count greater than 50 000. We do not administer regional anesthesia to patients with clinical evidence of coagulopathy (spontaneous bleeding, petechiae, easy bruising). In patients with no clinical evidence of coagulopathy and a platelet count less than 50 000, weigh the risks and benefits of the alternatives and discuss the matter at length with the patient (with chart documentation). If you choose regional anesthesia, use a short acting local anesthetic and follow the patient carefully for the return of full neurologic function.

5. Which anesthetic technique is best for the distressed fetus?

Anesthesiologists often use general anesthesia for emergency cesarean delivery in the absence of contraindications. However, the little data available suggest that infants born after a rapidly initiated regional anesthetic are, if anything, in better clinical condition than infants born after rapid sequence induction of general anesthesia. Marx et al allowed mothers to choose general (n=77) or regional (extension of a pre-existing epidural with 2-chloroprocaine (n=22) or spinal (n=33)) anesthesia for emergency cesarean delivery in similar fetal distress situations.[43] Five minute Apgar scores and umbilical blood gas values were similar in the two groups, while more babies in the regional group had a 1 min Apgar score greater than 7.

Why didn't the general babies do better? The regional mothers all received 800 ml of intravenous fluid and none became hypotensive. Mothers in the general anesthesia group received no fluid bolus and may have been at risk for hypotension during a thiopental induction. Uterine blood flow decreases transiently in pregnant ewes who receive intravenous thiopental followed by laryngoscopy and tracheal intubation.[44] Lastly, fetal distress is most often a slowly developing, chronic process. It is highly unlikely that an additional five minutes of intrauterine existence is the etiology of a persistent neurological deficit.

MATERNAL EMERGENCIES

Obstetric hemorrhage

Severe

The uterus receives 12% of the maternal cardiac output at term. Significant blood loss can occur quickly.[45] Obstetric hemorrhage causes 75% of maternal mortality and morbidity.[46] Two major causes of obstetric hemorrhage are increasing in incidence: placenta accreta (secondary to previous cesarean delivery) and placental abruption (secondary to cocaine use). Obstetric management requires the following:

1. Maternal resuscitation
2. Fetal delivery
3. Removal of the placenta
4. Achieving a firmly contracted uterus
5. Hysterectomy and/or repair of tissue damage, if needed.

Surgical intervention is frequently required. Hypovolemic patients and patients with brisk ongoing blood loss require general anesthesia. *Do not forget to assess the airway and act accordingly.* Regional anesthesia may be used if major blood loss is anticipated but has not yet begun. A review of 46 obstetric hysterectomies, 12 under continuous epidural anesthesia, found no difference in blood loss, crystalloid replacement, transfusion requirement or complications between patients receiving general or epidural anesthesia.[47] In this setting, however, be prepared to convert from regional to general anesthesia.[48]

Anesthetic management is dictated by the clinical circumstances but usually requires the following steps:

1. Establish adequate intravenous access (2 or more large gauge catheters)
2. Evaluate the airway; plan the anesthetic
3. Establish effective communication with the blood bank, obtain and transfuse blood products as needed
4. Continue the resuscitation and the anesthetic.

Don't forget that obstetric hemorrhage may be associated with disseminated intravascular coagulopathy, adult respiratory distress syndrome, and serious end-organ damage.

Less severe

How should one treat mild-to-moderate post-partum hemorrhage associated with low-grade uterine atony? Medical treatment should be maximized before surgical intervention is used. We use drugs in the following order:

1. Oxytocin. If rapid administration of oxytocin 20 u/l of i.v. fluid is ineffective, we infuse oxytocin 40 u/l. Remember, oxytocin is a direct-acting vasodilator and can cause hypotension and tachycardia.[49]
2. Ergonovine 0.1–0.2 mg i.m. *not* i.v. Ergonovine, especially after previous vasopressor administration, can cause severe maternal hypertension and coronary artery spasm.[50]
3. Protaglandin F_2alpha. *Beware of the side effects of this drug!* Intramuscular administration has been associated with severe bronchospasm, hypotension, bradycardia and cardiac arrest. Up to 5 doses of this drug may be administered intramuscularly into the uterus or a peripheral muscle.

Providing profound uterine relaxation

A brief period of profound uterine relaxation can facilitate delivery of a breech or second twin fetus, manual extraction of a retained placenta, or reversion of an inverted uterus. Classically, this relaxation was achieved with a potent inhalation agent administered after rapid sequence induction of general anesthesia. Three alternative agents not requiring general anesthesia have been recently described.

Nitroglycerin in intravenous bolus doses of 50–500 μg produces a sufficient degree of uterine relaxation to remove a retained placenta or revert a uterus.[51] Uterine relaxation begins 30–60 s after injection and lasts 2–3 min. Mild, clinically unimportant, hypotension has been observed, especially in hypovolemic patients. Headache or prolonged uterine relaxation have not been reported.

Terbutaline 0.25 mg SQ and intravenous *magnesium* also have been used to remove retained placentas and revert uteri.[52–53] Terbutaline is frequently associated with tachycardia and hypotension. Magnesium may be associated with chest pain, palpitations, hypotension, nausea and sedation. Magnesium has a slower onset than terbutaline or nitroglycerin. Both terbutaline and magnesium have a duration that is unnecessarily long for these situations.

Hypertensive disorders of pregnancy

In the absence of fetal distress or maternal hemorrhage, severe preeclampsia requires emergency medical, *not surgical* treatment. While it is true that evacuation of the uterus is the ultimate cure for pre-eclampsia, the disease frequently becomes more severe between 1 and 7 days following delivery. Severe maternal complications (intracranial hemorrhage, pulmonary edema, myocardial infarction) have been reported following rapid sequence induction of general anesthesia in untreated severely hypertensive parturients.[54] At a minimum, seizures must be stopped, maternal blood pressure must be under some degree of control, and the maternal hemoglobin and platelet count should be assessed while a rational anesthetic plan is being developed. The anesthesiologist must always be prepared to manage all eventualities.

REFERENCES

1. Morgan B M, Magni V, Goroszenuik T 1990 Anaesthesia for emergency caesarean section. Br J Obstet Gynaecol 97: 420
2. Parer J T, Livingston E G 1990 What is fetal distress? Am J Obstet Gynecol 162: 1421
3. Cohen A B, Klapholz H, Thompson M S 1982 Electronic fetal monitoring and clinical practice: a survey of obstetric opinion. Med Decis Making 2: 79
4. Frigoletto F D, Nadel A S 1988 Electronic fetal heart rate monitoring: why the dilemma? Clin Obstet Gynecol 31 (1): 179
5. Haverkamp A D, Orleans M, Langendoerfer S et al 1979 A controlled trial of the differential effects of intrapartum fetal monitoring. Am J Obstet Gynecol 134: 399
6. Haverkamp A D, Thompson H E, McFee J G et al 1976 The evaluation of continuous fetal heart rate monitoring in high risk pregnancy. Am J Obstet Gynecol 125: 310
7. Kelso I M, Parson R J, Lawrence G F et al 1978 An assessment of continuous fetal heart rate monitoring in labor. Am J Obstet Gynecol 131: 526
8. Renou P, Chang A, Anderson I et al 1976 Controlled trial of fetal intensive care. Am J Obstet Gynecol 126: 470
9. Wood C, Renou P, Oats J et al 1981 Controlled trial of fetal heart rate monitoring in a low risk obstetric population. Am J Obstet Gynecol 141: 527
10. Leveno K J, Cunningham F G, Nelson S et al 1986 A prospective comparison of selective and universal electronic fetal monitoring in 34,995 pregnancies. N Engl J Med 315: 615
11. MacDonald D, Grant A, Sheridan-Pereira M et al 1985 The Dublin randomized controlled trial of intrapartum fetal heart rate monitoring. Am J Obstet Gynecol 152: 523
12. Luthy D A, Shy K K, van Belle G et al 1987 A randomized trial of electronic fetal monitoring in preterm labor. Obstet Gynecol 69: 687
13. Ergander U, Eriksson M, Zetterstrom R 1983 Severe neonatal asphyxia, incidence and prediction of outcome in the Stockholm area. Acta Paediatr Scand 72: 321
14. Nelson K B, Ellenberg J H 1981 Apgar scores as predictors of chronic neurologic disability. Pediatrics 68: 36
15. Nelson K B, Ellenberg J H 1986 Antecedents of cerebral palsy. N Engl J Med 315: 81
16. Shields J R, Schifrin B S 1988 Perinatal antecedents of cerebral palsy. Obstet Gynecol 71: 899
17. Shekarloo A, Mendez-Bauer C, Cook V, Freese U 1989 Terbutaline (intravenous bolus) for the treatment of acute intrapartum fetal distress. Am J Obstet Gynecol 160: 615
18. Strong T H, Hetzler G, Sarno A P, Paul R H 1990 Prophylactic intrapartum amnioinfusion: a randomized clinical trial. Am J Obstet Gynecol 162: 1370
19. Leavitt K A 1993 Anesthesia for the stressed fetus. In: Norris M C (ed) Obstetric anesthesia. J B Lippincott, Philadelphia p 645
20. Eckstein K L, Marx G F 1974 Aortocaval compression and uterine displacement. Anesthesiology 40: 92
21. Willcourt R J, King J C, Queenan J T 1983 Maternal oxygenation administration and fetal transcutaneous PO_2. Am J Obstet Gynecol 146: 714
22. Hanowell L et al 1992 Effect of maternal inspired oxygen concentration on fetal umbilical venous oxygen tension. Reg Anesth 17: S38
23. Patriarco M S, Viechnicki B M, Hutchinson T A, Klasko S K, Yeh S Y 1987 A study on intrauterine fetal resuscitation with terbutaline. Am J Obstet Gynecol 157: 384
24. Wright J W, Patterson R M, Ridgway III L E, Berkus M D 1990 Effect of tocolytic agents on fetal umbilical velocimetry. Am J Obstet Gynecol 163: 748
25. Mendez-Bauer C, Shekarloo A, Cook V, Freese U. Treatment of acute intrapartum fetal distress by beta 2-sympathomimetics. Am J Obstet Gynecol 1987; 156: 638
26. Burke M S, Porreco R P, Day D et al 1989 Intrauterine resuscitation with tocolysis; an alternate month clinical trial. J Perinatol 9: 296
27. Hallworth D, Jellicoe J A, Wilkes R G 1982 Hypotension during epidural anesthesia for caesarean section: A comparison of intravenous loading with crystalloid and colloid solutions. Anaesthesia 37: 53
28. Lewis M, Thomas P K, Wilkes R G 1983 Hypotension during epidural analgesia for caesarean section: Arterial and central venous pressure changes after acute intravenous loading with two litres of Hartmann's solution. Anaesthesia 38: 250
29. Clark R B, Thompson D S, Thompson C H 1976 Prevention of spinal hypotension associated with cesarean section. Anesthesiology 45: 670
30. Wollman S B, Marx G F 1968 Acute hydration for prevention of hypotension of spinal anesthesia in parturients. Anesthesiology 29: 374
31. Philipson E H, Kalhan S C, Riha M M, Pimentel R 1987 Effects of maternal glucose infusion of fetal acid-base status in human pregnancy. Am J Obstet Gynecol 157: 866
32. Kenepp N B, Shelley W C, Gabbe S G et al 1982 Fetal and neonatal hazards of maternal hydration with 5% dextrose before cesarean section. Lancet 1: 1150
33. Robillard J E, Sessions C, Kennedy R L, Smith F G 1978 Metabolic effects of constant hypertonic glucose infusion in well-oxygenated fetuses. Am J Obstet Gynecol 130: 199
34. Philipps A F, Dubin J W, Matty P J, Raye J R 1982 Arterial hypoxemia and hyperinsulinemia in the chronically hyperglycemic fetal lamb. Pediatr Res 16: 653
35. Philipps A F, Porte P J, Stabinsky S, Rosenkrantz T S, Raye J R 1984 Effects of chronic fetal hyperglycemia upon oxygen consumption in the ovine uterus and conceptus. J Clin Invest 74: 279
36. Samsoon G L T, Young J R B 1987 Difficult tracheal intubation: a retrospective study. Anaesthesia 42: 487
37. Benumof J L 1991 Management of the difficult adult airway: with special emphasis on awake tracheal intubation. Anesthesiology 75: 1087
38. Department of Health 1982–84 Report on confidential enquiries into maternal deaths in England and Wales. Her Majesty's Stationery Office, London
39. Freund F G, Bonica J J, Ward R J, Akamatsu T J, Kennedy Jr W F 1967 Ventilatory reserve and level of motor block during high spinal and epidural anesthesia. Anesthesiology 28: 834
40. Schatz M, Zeiger R S, Harden K M et al 1988 The safety of inhaled β-agonist bronchodilators during pregnancy. J Allergy Clin Immunol 82: 686
41. Vaddadi A, Ramanathan J, Angel J J, Sibai B 1989 Epidural anesthesia in women with chorioamnionitis (a retrospective study). Anesthesiology 71: A863
42. Channing Rogers R P, Levin J 1990 A critical reappraisal of the bleeding time. Sem Thomb Hemostasis 16: 1
43. Marx G F, Luykx W M, Cohen S 1984 Fetal-neonatal status following caesarean section for fetal distress. Br J Anaesth 56: 1009
44. Palahniuk R J, Cumming M 1977 Foetal deterioration following thiopentone–nitrous oxide anaesthesia in the pregnant ewe. Can Anaesth Soc J 24: 367
45. Lee W, Rokey R, Cotton D B 1988 Noninvasive maternal stroke volume and cardiac output determinations by pulsed Doppler echocardiography. Am J Obstet Gynecol 158: 505
46. Chattopadhyay S K, Roy B D, Edrees Y B: Surgical control of

obstetric hemorrhage 1990 Hypogastric artery ligation or hysterectomy? Int J Gynecol Obstet 32: 345
47. Chestnut D H, Dewan D M, Redick L F, Caton D, Spielman F J 1989 Anesthetic management for obstetric hysterectomy: A multi-institution study. Anesthesiology 70: 607
48. Chestnut D H, Redick L F 1985 Continuous epidural anesthesia for elective cesarean hysterectomy. South Med J 78: 1168
49. Petty M A 1987 The cardiovascular effects of the neurohypophysial hormone oxytocin. J Auton Pharmacol 7: 97
50. Casady G N, Moore D C, Bridenbaugh L D 1960 Postpartum hypertension after use of vasoconstrictor and oxytocic drugs. JAMA 172: 1011
51. De Simone C A, Norris M C, Leighton B L 1990 Intravenous nitroglycerin aids manual extraction of a retained placenta (correspondence). Anesthesiology 73: 787
52. Kovacs B W, DeVore G R 1984 Management of acute and subacute puerperal uterine inversion with terbutaline sulfate. Am J Obstet Gynecol 150: 784
53. Grossman R A 1981 Magnesium sulfate for uterine inversion. J Reprod Med 26: 261
54. Fox E J, Sklar G S, Hill C H, Villanueva R, King B D 1977 Complications related to the pressor response to endotracheal intubation. Anesthesiology 47: 524

43. Abnormal presentations and multiple gestation

Part a USA view *B. L. Koffel*
Part B European view *Y. Darbois D. Sfoggia M. Henry D. Vauthier J. Seebacher*

PART A
USA VIEW
B. L. Koffel

Each part of this chapter includes some information relevant to the other as abnormal presentation and multiple gestation frequently coexist. Each section includes definitions of commonly used terminology, obstetric and anesthetic considerations and suggestions for anesthetic management.

Anesthesiologists and obstetricians frequently stress the need for understanding and clear communication among physicians, nurses, the parturient and the parturient's family. This is mandatory in providing optimal care for the patient with an abnormal presentation and/or a multiple gestation. Each of these conditions constitutes a complicated pregnancy and deserves special attention.

ABNORMAL PRESENTATIONS AND POSITIONS

Obstetricians determine *presentation* by the part of the fetus that can be felt through the cervix during a vaginal examination. Presentations other than the normal vertex (breech, brow, face, shoulder) are more common in multiple gestations than they are in singleton pregnancies. *Position* refers to the relationship of the presenting part to the mother's body. Terms such as occiput anterior, occiput posterior or left sacrum transverse are used to describe the position. *Lie* indicates the fetal spine alignment with the maternal spine. Both breech and vertex presentations are longitudinal lies. Oblique or transverse lies generally require abdominal delivery if external version does not produce vertex presentation. Abnormal positions, presentations and lies are all associated with increased perinatal and maternal morbidity and mortality. Anesthetic management of these problems is directly related to obstetric decisions regarding delivery (abdominal versus vaginal). The anesthetic requirements may change with only a moment's notice as the obstetric condition warrants. Thus the anesthesiologist must understand the obstetric situation and be involved with the patient as early and as frequently as possible.

Brow/face presentations

Face presentation occurs in, on average, 1 in 500 live births. 70–80% of infants with face presentation can be delivered vaginally. Vaginal manipulation, other than low forceps, is rarely successful. Although safe vaginal delivery is common, surgical intervention may be necessary if arrest of labor occurs.[1]

The infant with a brow presentation has a partially extended neck, somewhat between the usual flexed position of the normal vertex presentation and the fully extended neck of an infant with a face presentation. The frequency of brow presentation averages 1 in 1500 deliveries. Vaginal delivery has been described as unlikely but may be successful. Vaginal manipulation is contraindicated, but spontaneous neck flexion and vaginal delivery may occur. Abdominal delivery is indicated when progress is arrested.[1]

The anesthetic management of either face or brow presentations differs little from the routine anesthetic management for labor (Table 43.1). Gravidas with abnormal presentations may have more intense and earlier perineal stimulation. They may be uncomfortable if only dilute solutions of local anesthetics are used for epidural anesthesia. One must be cautious, however, when one attempts to relieve this discomfort solely with local anesthetics, as complete perineal muscle relaxation may be deemed inappropriate by our obstetric colleagues. The use of intraspinal opioids (epidural or subarachnoid) in combination with local anesthetics may provide comfort

Table 43.1 Regional anesthesia for labor

1.	Premedication: maternal administration of 30 ml of 0.3M sodium citrate or its commercial equivalent.
2.	Monitoring: maternal arterial blood pressure via Riva Rocci or continuous non-invasive.
3.	Acute intravenous hydration with 500–1000 ml of nondextrose-containing crystalloid solution.
4.	Insert epidural (or continuous spinal) catheter at L2–3 or L3–4 interspace.
5.	Semi-Fowler's position with left uterine displacement.
6.	Incremental doses of local anesthetic and/or opioid.

without extensive motor blockade. The higher incidence of operative delivery makes it mandatory to maintain vigilance and the ability to rapidly obtain surgical anesthesia.

Anesthesia for abdominal delivery of these presentations is also similar to other situations. Spinal, epidural or general anesthesia may be used safely.

Shoulder presentation

The gravida with a transverse lie requires abdominal delivery. The choice of anesthetic must be made with the usual considerations. Fetal well-being, urgency of delivery, maternal body habitus and medical problems, as well as maternal preference, must all be considered in choosing a regional or general anesthetic technique for abdominal delivery.

Breech presentation

Obstetric management of the patient with breech presentation remains controversial. Some centers favor vaginal delivery under certain conditions, while in other institutions abdominal delivery is routinely performed for all breech infants. The anesthesiologist must thus be prepared to administer anesthesia for a trial of labor and subsequent vaginal or cesarean delivery (which may be elective or emergent).

Obstetric considerations

Breech presentation occurs in approximately 4% of pregnancies. It is more than 25% in pregnancies less than 28 weeks' duration.[2] *Spontaneous breech delivery* is an entirely spontaneous vaginal delivery. In a *partial breech extraction* the infant is delivered spontaneously to the umbilicus and the remainder assisted by the obstetrician manually or with Piper forceps. In contrast, a *total breech extraction* occurs when the entire body is delivered by the obstetrician.

The causes of breech presentation are unknown. Certain conditions predispose to this presentation, notably prematurity, multiparity, uterine anomalies and multiple gestation. Other predisposing factors include hydramnios, oligohydramnios, hydrocephalus, anencephalus, placenta previa or cornual–fundal placenta. Fetal anomalies are frequently present. Many of these factors interfere with the normal process of accommodation of the fetal head, uterine cavity and maternal pelvis.[3] Three types of breech presentation are described (Fig. 43.1):

- Frank breech: lower extremities flexed at the hips and extended at the knees.
- Complete breech: lower extremities are flexed at both the hips and knees.
- Incomplete breech: one or both extremities are extended and one or both feet are present in the vagina.

About 60% of breeches are frank, 30% incomplete and 10% complete. The incidence of successful vaginal delivery is highest for a frank breech. Prolapsed umbilical cord occurs most commonly with incomplete presentation and ruptured membranes.[4]

Breech presentation is associated with an increased incidence of obstetric complications (Table 43.2). Analysis of data from studies in the 1950s and 1960s has encouraged a growing trend toward abdominal delivery for all breeches. The perinatal death rate for all breeches was increased threefold even when corrected for prematu-

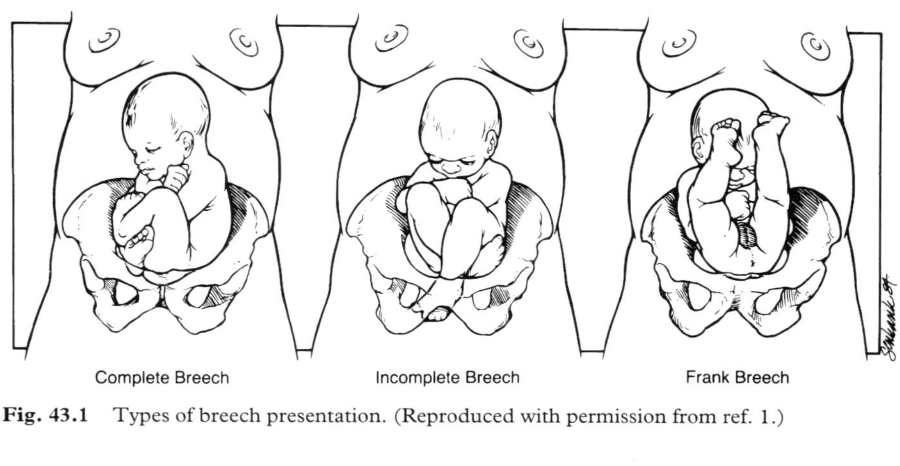

Fig. 43.1 Types of breech presentation. (Reproduced with permission from ref. 1.)

Table 43.2 Frequency of complications seen with breech presentation (Reproduced with permission from ref. 1)

Complication	Frequency
Intrapartum fetal death	Increased 16-fold
Intrapartum asphyxia	Increased 3.8-fold
Cord prolapse	Increased 5-to 20-fold
Birth trauma	Increased 13-fold
Arrest of after-coming head	8.8%
Spinal cord injuries with deflexion	21%
Major congenital anomalies	6–18%
Prematurity	16–33%
Hyperextension of head	5%

rity in a 1964 study. This same study noted an 'abrupt drop-off' in the perinatal mortality rate when infants were abdominally delivered.[5] Other frightening obstetric complications may occur with breech vaginal delivery. For breech versus vertex vaginal deliveries, cord prolapse and asphyxia are more common.[6] Head entrapment may occur in premature infants, with their relatively large head-to-body size ratio[3] or in incomplete breech presentations other than frank.[1] Compression of the after-coming head may cause intracranial hemorrhage and is a principal cause of perinatal mortality. Spinal cord injury may occur in the breech with hyperextended head. At the present time in the USA, approximately 80% of breech term infants are delivered abdominally.[7] Vaginal delivery of a breech versus vertex is associated with increased maternal morbidity due to increased incidence of cervical, uterine or perineal lacerations as well as an increased incidence of infection.[3]

However, recent studies have found that attempted vaginal delivery is successful in 72% of selected term patients without any increase in fetal or maternal morbidity and mortality.[7–9] Patients selected for trial of labor had both an adequate pelvic outlet documented by radiologic pelvimetry and an estimated fetal weight between 1500 and 3800 g. Abdominal delivery is recommended for viable fetuses weighing less than 1500 g.[10] The availability of experienced obstetricians and obstetric anesthesiologists as well as personnel skilled in neonatal resuscitation is mandatory when vaginal breech delivery is attempted. The absence of one of these essential services may require elective delivery at another time or even maternal transfer to another institution. Patients should be involved in these decisions.

While at first it may appear that trial of labor for vaginal delivery might decrease maternal morbidity and mortality, this may not be true. Sixteen – 30% of vaginal 'trials' are unsuccessful. Abdominal delivery may then become emergent rather than elective. Emergent abdominal delivery carries greater maternal morbidity and mortality than elective abdominal delivery.[11]

External cephalic version is also controversial among obstetricians. The best method, the best time to perform and the use of tocolytic agents are unresolved questions. However, when performed after 37 weeks in nonlaboring patients, success rates approximate 50–70%.[7,12,13] Gentle pressure accompanied by fetal heart rate monitoring is required. Nearly all patients with successful version have a vertex presentation at the onset of labor.[12] Vaginal delivery after successful version is about 75%.[7,12,13] The risks of external cephalic version include placental separation and cord compression, both of which can precipitate emergency abdominal delivery. Although anesthesia is not generally required for an external cephalic version, anesthesiologists should evaluate the patients scheduled for this procedure and be readily available when it is performed.

Anesthetic considerations

The anesthesiologist should evaluate the patient, review the chart and discuss with the obstetrician both the obstetric and anesthetic plan for each gravida. If this can be done on admission to the labor and delivery suite, patient care is usually optimal.

A trial of labor for breech presentation may necessitate emergency cesarean delivery. For example, umbilical cord prolapse may occur in 2% of frank breeches at term.[3] Therefore, an anesthesiologist must be immediately available. Overall, 70–84% of trials of labor result in successful vaginal delivery.[11] Reliable intravenous access should be established early in labor.

Continuous lumbar epidural analgesia/anesthesia has major advantages and few disadvantages in the patient laboring with a breech presentation. Epidural analgesia does not prolong the first stage of labor.[14,15] Although the second stage of labor may be prolonged with epidural analgesia,[15] 'expulsion time' is not prolonged with sensory anesthesia obtained with bupivacaine 0.125% with epinephrine 1:800 000.[16] Full breech extraction is not more frequent.[14] Fetal pH during the second stage and Apgar scores reveal improved condition of the fetus delivered with maternal epidural anesthesia.[14] Reduction in the bearing-down reflex may improve uteroplacental blood flow with subsequent improved fetal condition.[14] Perinatal morbidity is not increased.[15] Epidural anesthesia, by relaxation of the pelvic floor, lessens pressure on the fetal head and may decrease the likelihood of fetal trauma. In addition, surgical anesthesia can rapidly and safely be obtained in the event of fetal distress, avoiding the risks attendant to the induction of general anesthesia. For these reasons, epidural analgesia/anesthesia plays a vital role in the increasing safety of vaginal breech delivery.[17] It provides a comfortable patient who can cooperate for a controlled delivery.

Anesthetic management

Owing to the possibility of rapid change in fetal status with breech presentation, it is more important than ever to have a reliable large-bore indwelling intravenous catheter placed soon after the gravida's arrival in the labor and delivery suite. Anesthetic equipment and drugs must be checked and immediately available for the induction of general anesthesia.

External cephalic version. External version may be attempted in patients with known breech presentation prior to the onset of labor. Although anesthesia is not recommended for this procedure, immediate availability of an anesthesiologist is necessary when external version is attempted. External version has risks of fetomaternal hemorrhage, placental abruption or umbilical cord compression which may require immediate delivery.

Anesthesia for labor and vaginal delivery. Continuous lumbar epidural anesthesia may be induced after appropriate premedication and acute intravenous hydration. Epidural anesthesia is usually induced with bupivacaine 0.25% concentration or less. (see Table 43.2) The addition of a lipid-soluble opioid to a dilute solution of local anesthetic may relieve the profound 'rectal pressure' frequently noted by patients with a breech fetus. Fentanyl (50 μg), sufentanil (15μg) and butorphanol (2 mg) are commonly used. Dilute bupivacaine infusions (0.0625–0.125%) containing fentanyl (2 μg/ml), sufentanil (0.5–1 μg/ml) or butorphanol (0.1–0.2 mg/ml) may be used to provide continued analgesia if preferred over intermittent techniques. Opioids should be used with caution in the gravida with a premature infant. Premature infants are more sensitive to opioid induced respiratory depression. More concentrated solutions of bupivacaine (0.375–0.5%) may also be used to alleviate the rectal pressure but, of course, perineal muscle motor blockade will be increased. Some advocate delay in the 'block' of sacral segments to minimize motor blockade and maintain the effectiveness of maternal effort. Carbonated (or pH adjusted) lidocaine or 2-chloroprocaine may be used to rapidly produce anesthesia for breech extraction. Spinal anesthesia may be used as a continuous technique for labor or as a single-dose technique for breech extraction. Its advantages are rapid onset, good perineal relaxation and minimal fetal drug exposure. If used as a continuous technique, profound motor block may be a disadvantage.

Should uterine relaxation be required for full breech extraction, general anesthesia is indicated even if there is adequate 'anesthesia' using a regional technique. Optimally, general anesthesia should not be necessary in some situations. Aspiration prophylaxis measures including nonparticulate antacid, cricoid pressure and techniques designed to facilitate intubation such as proper positioning and the use of a short-handled laryngoscope are mandatory in this emergency situation. The gravida should breathe 100% oxygen before delivery to facilitate rapid denitrogenation if general anesthesia becomes necessary. After tracheal intubation, uterine relaxation is obtained with a volatile anesthetic agent (up to 2 MAC as needed). There is no difference in the uterine relaxation properties of halothane, enflurane and isoflurane. After delivery, volatile agents should be discontinued to allow efficient oxytocin-induced uterine contractions. Anesthesia is maintained with intravenous opioids and nitrous oxide in oxygen until extraction of the placenta and surgical repair are complete. A succinylcholine infusion (0.1%) may be used for muscle relaxation.

As an alternative to general anesthesia for uterine relaxation, amyl nitrate or nitroglycerin has been advocated.[2] An ampule of amyl nitrate may be broken into the reservoir bag of an anesthesia circle system. 100 μg of nitroglycerin can be administered as an intravenous bolus. A study involving patients with retained placentas revealed uterine relaxation within 30–40 s after nitroglycerin administration. The relaxation lasts about 1 min.[18] Published data comparing these techniques with general anesthesia for uterine relaxation in this situation are not available. Breech extraction may require a longer period of uterine relaxation than that obtained with a single dose of nitroglycerin. The maternal/fetal effects of multiple doses have not been explored.

Severe maternal hemorrhage may occur if Dührssen's incisions of the cervix are made. Bleeding into the pelvis is common. Blood exiting from the vagina is *not* the only blood loss occurring in this situation. Large-bore intravenous access is necessary. Blood for transfusion should be prepared as quickly as possible.

Anesthesia for cesarean delivery. Regional or general anesthesia may be indicated by maternal preference and/or fetal/maternal well-being. The techniques are similar to those already described. Meticulous attention to intravenous fluid administration, aspiration prophylaxis and maintenance of left uterine displacement help ensure an optimal outcome. The patient should breathe 100% oxygen before hysterotomy in case difficulty in delivering the fetus through the uterine incision is encountered. If this occurs with regional anesthesia, the anesthesiologist must be prepared to induce general anesthesia using a volatile agent to relax the uterus as described above.

Abnormal positions

During internal rotation the fetal occiput rotates from a transverse position to an *occiput anterior position*. This places the widest part of the fetal head, the occiput, toward the symphysis pubis, traversing the pelvis at its greatest dimension. When the fetal occiput rotates posteriorly toward the sacrum an *occiput posterior position* results. This occurs in about 10% of patients. Labor is likely to be prolonged with the occiput posterior position and maternal discomfort is increased. Severe back pain frequently accompanies this fetal position. Spontaneous delivery may occur but manual or forceps rotation may speed delivery and lessen perineal trauma. The persistent *occiput transverse position* may also be rotated by forceps to an occiput anterior position and subsequent delivery.

The musculature of the pelvic floor plays a role in successful internal rotation, so segmental epidural anesthesia may be useful. However, limiting local anesthetic dose in a more segmental fashion is not likely to relieve the more intense pain present with an abnormal position. The addition of opioids to a dilute local anesthetic solution may relieve pain and maintain muscle tone to facilitate rotation.

With any abnormal position, molding of the fetal head with caput formation may be deceptive. Abdominal delivery may be preferable to vaginal delivery. The obstetric anesthesiologist who prepares for that possibility early will administer the optimal anesthetic to mother and child.

Shoulder dystocia

Shoulder dystocia is an obstetric dilemma that is best prevented with consideration before vaginal delivery. Macrosomia and prolonged second stage place a pregnancy at high risk for shoulder dystocia. Shoulder dystocia, as an abnormal labor, bears some relevance to this chapter.

Shoulder dystocia is diagnosed when an infant's head is delivered and the anterior shoulder impacts against the pubic symphysis, preventing delivery. Sharp ventral rotation of both of the gravida's hips may allow delivery. Other obstetric maneuvers including suprapubic pressure, anterior rotation of posterior shoulder, delivery of posterior arm and deliberate fracture of the clavicle may be successful. Induction of general anesthesia is not generally useful in this emergency. Perineal muscle relaxation may be of some assistance as obtained with an existing epidural anesthetic. Post-partum hemorrhage is common and blood should be prepared. Large-bore intravenous access is necessary.[1,3]

MULTIPLE GESTATION

Twins occur in about 1% of all pregnancies, triplets in 0.01%. *Dizygotic twins* result when two separate ova are fertilized. Each twin develops with a separate placenta. Dizygotic twins are always diamniotic and dichorionic. *Monozygotic twins* result when a simple fertilized ovum splits after a variable number of divisions (usually before 13 days).

Placentas may be *dichorionic diamniotic*, *monochorionic diamniotic* or *monochorionic monoamniotic* (Fig. 43.2). Early monozygotic twinning (up to 2–3 days) gives a dichorionic diamniotic placenta, with later twinning (8–13 days) leading to monochorionic monoamniotic placentation. Twinning between 3 and 8 days commonly causes a monochorionic diamniotic placenta. Vascular communications occur in nearly all monochorionic placentas and are rare in dichorionic placentas.[19] The frequency of monozygotic twins is constant at about 4 per 1000 births. Dizygotic twinning varies among races and by maternal age. It is highest in Blacks, lowest in Asians and intermediate in Caucasians. The rate for women aged less than 20 is 3 per 1000 but rises to 14 per 1000 in women between 35 and 40 years. The frequency also increases with parity independent of maternal age.[20]

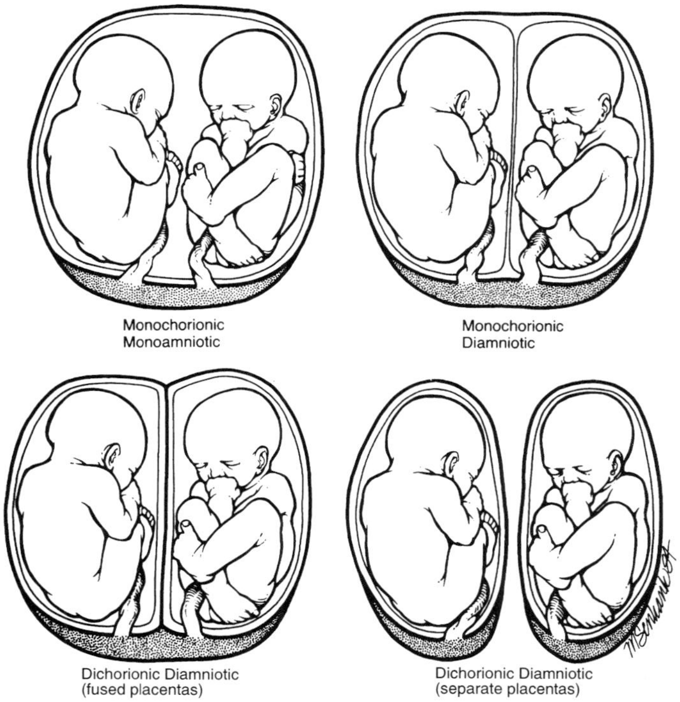

Fig. 43.2 Placentation in twin pregnancies. (Reproduced with permission from ref. 19.)

Multiple gestation (dizygotic) is becoming more common with in vitro fertilization and other assisted reproductive technology. Multiple gestation accounts for 10% of all perinatal mortality. The greatest portion of this mortality is due to prematurity.

Obstetric considerations

Multiple gestation increases maternal morbidity and mortality with an increased incidence of complications such as:

- premature rupture of membranes
- preterm labor
- prolonged labor
- preeclampsia/eclampsia

- placental abruption
- operative delivery (forceps and abdominal)
- uterine atony
- obstetric trauma
- antepartum and/or post-partum hemorrhage.

Preeclampsia/eclampsia is more severe and occurs earlier. It may occur in multiparas with no history of hypertension. Primary abdominal delivery may be as high as 50% for multiple gestations.[21]

The perinatal mortality rate in twin pregnancies is 4–6 times greater than in singleton pregnancies.[22] This is primarily because of the high incidence of preterm delivery and prematurity. Preterm labor occurs in 46% of gravidas, and about 36% deliver before 37 weeks of gestation.[23,24] Preterm delivery is more common in monozygotic than dizygotic twins.[25]

Fetal and neonatal complications occurring more frequently in multiple gestations include:

- congenital anomalies
- polyhydramnios
- cord entanglement
- umbilical cord prolapse
- intrauterine growth retardation
- twin–twin transfusion
- malpresentation.

Monozygous (as compared with dizygous) twins have increased likelihood of cord complications and twin–twin transfusion.[26] Vascular communications present in most monochorionic placentas are responsible for twin–twin transfusions.[27] The intrauterine and neonatal mortality of twin–twin transfusion is as high as 80%.[28] Suggested obstetric interventions include: decompression amniocentesis, selective feticide, administration of digoxin (for congestive heart failure in the recipient twin), selective blood letting and fetoscopic occlusion of vessels.[29] A fetoscope-directed Nd–YAG laser has been used successfully to ablate fetoplacental vascular communications in three pregnancies.[30]

Antepartum death of one twin occurs in 0.5–6.8% of twin pregnancies.[31] Morbidity in the surviving twin is common,[32] but has not been demonstrated in triplets.[33] Management of fetal death in triplets may be less of a dilemma than in twins because most triplet gestations require immediate delivery for obstetric reasons.[34] Disseminated intravascular coagulation may develop in the gravida[35,36] or the surviving fetus.[32] Carr et al [37] refute suggestions[38] that delivery early in the third trimester is indicated because of increasing perinatal morbidity and mortality. Early diagnosis with aggressive antepartum, intrapartum and post-partum management is the key to decreasing the magnitude of these problems.

Recent work contradicts the previously reported greater incidence of acidosis[39–41] or higher mortality[42] in the second twin (twin B). The acid–base status between twins[43,44] and among triplets[45] is similar. Spellacy et al[22] reported that twins A and B had identical perinatal mortality when they were similar in weight. The use and choice of anesthetic agents or the presence/absence of nuchal cord may explain the conflicting results.[43] The time interval between vaginal delivery of twin A and twin B does not influence neonatal status.[46]

Mode of delivery is an obstetric decision based primarily on gestational age and presentation. Both twins will be in the vertex position only 30–50% of the time. Some 30–40% of twin pregnancies will be in vertex/breech (twin A/twin B) position. In 10–20% of twins there will be various combinations of breech and transverse lie. Vaginal delivery is more likely if twin A is in vertex position. Indications for abdominal delivery include:

- breech presentation of twin A
- prematurity
- possibility of interlocking chins
- discordance in growth
- twin–twin transfusion
- congenital anomalies
- intrauterine death of twin A
- evidence of decreased uteroplacental reserve.

The decision-making process for breech delivery of twin A is the same as that for a breech singleton unless interlocking twins are suspected. While many obstetricians will deliver twins vaginally, few obstetricians deliver three or more infants vaginally.

Anesthetic considerations

Multiple gestation exaggerates the physiologic changes of pregnancy. The increased size of the uterus and its contents, especially near term, further decreases total lung capacity, functional residual capacity (FRC), expiratory reserve volume and residual volume. Decreased FRC allows hypoxemia to develop more rapidly, particularly in the supine parturient. Maternal weight gain is similar to singleton pregnancies until the 30th week but then increases at a greater rate.[47]

There is an increased tendency to relative or actual anemia compared with singleton pregnancies. Maternal blood volume is increased by about 500 ml more with twins.[3] Cardiovascular changes tend to occur earlier and to a slightly greater extent in multiple gestation. Cardiac output is increased. Increased myocardial contractility has been suggested by echocardiography. Cardiac reserve is limited.[48] The greater combined fetal weight and larger amount of amniotic fluid of multiple gestation predispose to aortocaval compression and supine hypotensive syndrome.

Increased gastrin production increases gastric volume and acidity. The larger uterine size may add to lower esophageal sphincter dysfunction, making aspiration pneumonitis a greater hazard. Renal, hepatic and central nervous system changes are similar to those found in a singleton pregnancy.

The larger size of the uterus may predispose to uterine atony. Increased blood loss after delivery will occur with a greater frequency. Large-bore intravenous access is essential. Cross-matched blood for transfusion should be readily available. The post-partum infusion of oxytocin may need to be increased. Methergine or prostaglandin $F_{2\alpha}$ may need to be administered.

Preterm labor is common. Therefore, many patients requesting labor pain relief or presenting for abdominal delivery will have received tocolytic agents within the previous 12 h. This drug therapy may lead to tachycardia, pulmonary edema, potentiation of neuromuscular blocking agents and/or changes in coagulation. These side-effects may strongly influence the choice of regional versus general anesthesia. Again, the premature fetus (as compared with the term fetus) is more sensitive to the depressant effects of opioids and other anesthetic drugs. Pulmonary edema associated with beta-mimetic agents is more common in multiple gestations.

Neither regional nor general anesthesia is clearly superior for abdominal delivery. Improved uterine relaxation with general anesthesia may be beneficial for intrauterine manipulation for delivery of premature fetuses and/or abnormal presentations. However, a well-conducted spinal or epidural anesthetic, with appropriate measures to prevent or immediately treat hypotension, results in good neonatal outcome at delivery.

There are clear benefits from the use of epidural anesthesia, even though labor may be prolonged in multiple gestation[43,44,49] or the frequency of forceps delivery increased.[43,49] The biochemical status of both twins delivered under epidural anesthesia is superior to that of neonates delivered without epidural anesthesia, especially if the maternal bearing-down reflex is obtunded.[43] 5-min Apgar scores, the resuscitation efforts, neonatal death, cerebral irritability, jaundice and ICU admission are also similar between twins delivered with and without epidural anesthesia.[50] Perineal relaxation and maternal cooperation decrease fetal and maternal trauma. Abdominal delivery of the second twin is necessary in 4–8% of gravidas in which the first twin was delivered vaginally.[21,43,51] If this occurs, surgical anesthesia can be rapidly obtained in a patient with epidural anesthesia for labor.

A resuscitation team for *each* fetus should be informed and immediately available. Adequate resuscitation equipment must be available for *each* fetus.

Anesthetic management

Labor

Optimal pain relief is obtained with continuous lumbar epidural anesthesia (see Table 43.1 for regional anesthesia for labor). Maternal systemic blood pressure and fetal heart rate monitoring are necessary prior to induction of anesthesia. Meticulous attention to hydration (500–1000 ml immediately prior to induction), uterine displacement and intravenous ephedrine, as necessary, will support uteroplacental perfusion. Bupivacaine 0.25–0.5% may be used to obtain anesthesia. When less concentrated local anesthetic solutions are chosen for labor, a 'top-up' with a higher concentration is advisable prior to delivery because of the frequent need for operative delivery.

Vaginal delivery

The anesthesiologist must be alert and prepared. The time between delivery of twin A and twin B is most likely to present changing obstetric and, therefore, anesthetic situations. An operative delivery may be necessary for the second twin, therefore epidural anesthesia should be maintained after the delivery of twin A.

Oxygen should be administered to the parturient to maximize fetal well-being and to prevent delay should denitrogenation and the induction of general anesthesia be required. External cephalic version of the second twin may be facilitated under epidural anesthesia due to the relaxation of the abdominal musculature.[52] Although the upper dermatomal level of epidural anesthesia may produce adequate anesthesia and facilitate internal manipulation of the second twin (i.e. version and full breech extraction), it does not produce uterine relaxation. Induction of general anesthesia is recommended for internal podalic version followed by a total breech extraction. Following rapid-sequence induction and endotracheal intubation, a potent halogenated inhalation agent is used to effect maximal uterine relaxation. As soon as delivery is completed, the agent should be discontinued. Alternative techniques for uterine relaxation as already discussed under anesthesia for vaginal breech delivery may be considered.

Abdominal delivery

Elective abdominal delivery may be performed under the anesthetic of choice considering the patient's desires and medical condition. Epidural anesthesia is perhaps preferable to spinal anesthesia because of the decreased risk of hypotension (slower onset of sympathetic blockade) in the gravida particularly susceptible to aortocaval compression. This becomes more important as the number of infants (and, thus, uterine size) increases. Simultaneous popliteal and brachial blood pressure measurement will allow detection of occult supine hypotension (decreased uterine perfusion due to aortic compression in the presence of normal maternal brachial blood pressure). Occult supine hypotension becomes more common with three or more fetuses in utero. Particular attention should be paid to administration of oxygen and aspiration prophylaxis in light of the decreased FRC and increased production of gastrin. Epidural, spinal or general anesthesia induction is otherwise similar to that for the gravida with a singleton gestation.

CONCLUSION

Care of the patient with an abnormal presentation or a multiple gestation is often a challenge to all involved. Close communication among the obstetrician, anesthesiologist, neonatologist and patient provides the optimal outcome. Lumbar epidural anesthesia is recommended for labor analgesia and delivery. However, general anesthesia may become necessary to facilitate delivery. The anesthesiologist should anticipate and be prepared for the rapidly changing obstetric and anesthetic needs of these parturients.

REFERENCES

1. Seeds J W 1986 Malpresentations. In: Gabbe S G, Niebyl J R, Simpson J L (eds) Obstetrics: normal and problem pregnancies. Churchill Livingstone, Edinburgh
2. McMorland G H, Effer S B 1991 Breech presentation, malpresentation, multiple gestation. In: Datta S (ed) Anesthetic and obstetric management of high-risk pregnancy. Mosby Yearbook, St Louis
3. Pritchard J A, MacDonald P C, Gant N F 1985 Williams Obstetrics, 17th edn. Appleton-Century-Crofts, Norwalk
4. Rovinsky J R, Miller J A, Kaplan S 1973 Management of breech presentation at term. Am J Obstet Gynecol 115: 497–513
5. Morgan H S, Kane S H 1964 An analysis of 16,327 breech births. J Am Med Assoc 187: 262–264
6. Potter Jr M G, Heaton C E, Douglas G W 1960 Intrinsic fetal risk in breech delivery. Obstet Gynecol 15: 158–162
7. Flanagan T A, Mulchahey K M, Korenbrot C C, Carol C, Green J R, Laros Jr RK, 1987 Management of term breech presentation. Am J Obstet Gynecol 156: 1492–1502
8. Collea J V, Chein C, Quilligan E J 1980 The randomized management of term frank breech presentation: A study of 208 cases. Am J Obstet Gynecol 137: 235–244
9. Gimvosky M L, Wallace R L, Schifrin B S, Paul R H 1983 Randomized management of the nonfrank breech presentation at term: a preliminary report. Am J Obstet Gynecol 146: 34–40
10. Confino E, Ismajovich B, Sherzer A, Peyser R M, David M P 1985 Vaginal versus cesarean section oriented approaches in the management of breech delivery. Int J Gynaecol Obstet 23: 1–6
11. Bingham P, Lilford R J 1987 Management of the selected term breech presentation: assessment of the risks of selected vaginal delivery versus cesarean section for all cases. Obstet Gynecol 69: 965–978
12. Van Dorsten J P, Schifrin B S, Wallace R L 1981 Randomized control trial of external cephalic version with tocolysis in late pregnancy. Am J Obstet Gynecol 141: 417–424
13. Marchick R 1988 Antepartum external cephalic version with tocolysis: A study of term singleton breech presentations. Am J Obstet Gynecol 158: 1339–1346
14. Breeson A J, Kovacs G T, Pickles B G, Hill J G 1987 Extradural analgesia–the preferred method of analgesia for vaginal breech delivery. Br J Anaesth 50: 1227–1230
15. Confino E, Ismajovich B, Rudick V, David M P 1985 Extradural analgesia in the management of singleton breech delivery. Br J Anaesth 57: 892–895
16. Van Zundert A, Vaes L, Soetens M et al 1991 Are breech deliveries an indication for lumbar epidural analgesia? Anesth Analg 72: 399–403
17. Bingham P, Hird V, Lilford R J 1987 Management of the mature selected breech presentation: an analysis based on the intended method of delivery. Br J Obstet Gynaecol 94: 746–752
18. DeSimone C A, Norris M C, Leighton B L 1990 Intravenous nitroglycerin aids manual extraction of a retained placenta. Anesthesiology 73: 787
19. Berkowitz R L 1986 Multiple gestations. In: Gabbe S G, Niebyl J R, Simpson J L(eds) Obstetrics: normal and problem pregnancies. Churchill Livingstone, Edinburgh
20. Hrubec Z, Robinette C D 1984 The study of human twins in medical research, New Engl J Med 310: 435–441
21. Redick L F 1988 Anesthesia for twin delivery. Clin Perinat 15: 107–122
22. Spellacy W N, Handler A, Ferre C D 1990 A case–control study of 1253 twin pregnancies from a 1982–1987 perinatal data base. Obstet Gynecol 75: 168–171
23. Dewan D M 1987 Anesthesia for preterm delivery, breech presentation, and multiple gestation. Clin Obstet Gynecol 30: 566–578
24. Roberts W E, Morrison J C, Hamer C, Wiser W L 1990 The incidence of preterm labor and specific risk factors. Obstet Gynecol 76: 85S–89S
25. MacGillivray I 1983 Determinants of birth weight of twins. Acta Genet Med Gemellol 32: 151–157
26. D'Alton M E, Newton E R, Cetrulo C L 1984 Intrauterine fetal demise in multiple gestation. Acta Genet Med Gemellol 33: 43–49
27. Benirschke K 1961 Twin placenta in perinatal mortality. New York State J Med 61: 1499–1508
28. Gonsoulin W, Moise Jr K J, Kirshon B, Cotton D B, Wheeler J M, Carpenter R J 1990 Outcome of twin–twin transfusion diagnosed before 28 weeks of gestation. Obstet Gynecol 75: 214–216
29. Blickstein I 1990 The twin–twin transfusion syndrome. Obstet Gynecol 76: 714–722
30. DeLia J E, Cruikshank D P, Keye Jr W R 1990 Fetoscopic neodymium: YAG laser occlusion of placental vessels in severe twin-twin transfusion syndrome. Obstet Gynecol 75: 1046–1053
31. Enbom J A 1985 Twin pregnancy with intrauterine death of one twin. Am J Obstet Gynecol 152: 424–429
32. Szymonowicz W, Preston H, Yu V Y H 1986 The surviving monozygotic twin. Arch Dis Child 61: 454–458
33. Gonen R, Heyman E, Asztalos E, Milligan J E 1990 The outcome of triplet gestations complicated by fetal death. Obstet Gynecol 5: 175–178
34. Børlum K 1991 Third-trimester fetal death in triplet pregnancies. Obstet Gynecol 77: 6–9
35. Skelly H, Marivate M, Norman R, Kenoyer G, Martin R 1982 Consumptive coagulopathy following fetal death in a triplet pregnancy. Am J Obstet Gynecol 142: 595–596
36. Romero R, Duffy T P, Berkowitz R L, Chang E, Hobbins J C 1984 Prolongation of a preterm pregnancy complicated by death of a single twin in utero and disseminated intravascular coagulation. New Engl J Med 310: 772–773
37. Carr S R, Aronson M P, Coustan D R 1990 Survival rates of monoamniotic twins do not decrease after 30 weeks' gestation. Am J Obstet Gynecol 163: 719–722
38. Rodis J F, Vintzileos A M, Campbell W A, Deaton J L, Fumia F, Nochimson D J 1987 Antenatal diagnosis and management of monoamniotic twins. Am J Obstet Gynecol 157: 1255–1257
39. Young B K, Suidan J, Antoine C, Silverman F, Lustig I, Wasserman J 1985 Differences in twins: the importance of birth order. Am J Obstet Gynecol 151: 915–921
40. James III F M, Crawford J S, Davies P, Naiem H 1977 Lumbar epidural analgesia for labor and delivery of twins. Am J Obstet Gynecol 127: 176–180
41. Laros Jr R K, Dattel B J 1988 Management of twin pregnancy: the vaginal route is still safe. Am J Obstet Gynecol 158: 1330–1338
42. Little W A, Friedman E A 1958 Anesthesia for the twin delivery. Anesthesiology 19: 515–520
43. Crawford J S 1987 A prospective study of 200 consecutive twin deliveries. Anaesthesia 42: 33–43

44. Gullestad S, Sagen N 1977 Epidural block in twin labour and delivery. Acta Anaesth Scand 21: 504–508
45. Antoine C, Kirshenbaum N W, Young B K 1986 Biochemical differences related to birth order in triplets. J Reprod Med 31: 330–332
46. Rayburn W F, Lavin J P, Miodovnik M, Varner M W 1984 Multiple gestation: time interval between delivery of the first and second twins. Obstet Gynecol 63: 502–506
47. Pederson A L, Worthington-Roberts B, Hickok D E 1989 Weight gain patterns during gestation. J Am Diet Assoc 89: 642–646
48. Veille J C, Morton M J, Burry K J 1985 Maternal cardiovascular adaptations to twin pregnancy. Am J Obstet Gynecol 153: 261–263
49. Ogbonna B, Daw E 1986 Epidural analgesia and the length of labour for vaginal twin delivery. J Obstet Gynaecol 6: 166–168
50. Jarvis G J, Whitfield M F 1981 Epidural analgesia and the delivery of twins. J Obstet Gynaecol 2: 90–92
51. Olofsson P, Rydhström H 1985 Twin delivery: how should the second twin be delivered? Am J Obstet Gynecol 153: 479–481
52. Chervenak F A, Johnson R E, Berkowitz R L, Hobbins J C 1983 Intrapartum external version of the second twin. Obstet Gynecol 62: 160–165

PART B
EUROPEAN VIEW

Y. Darbois D. Sfoggia M. Henry
D. Vauthier J. Seebacher

BREECH PRESENTATION

Breech presentation accounts for 3–5% deliveries. It is more common when the fetus is premature; spontaneous version to the vertex presentation occurs in 60% of cases during the third trimester. In 85% of cases, no cause is found. In 15% the breech presentation is associated with uterine malformation, fibromyoma, ovarian cyst, anomaly of the maternal pelvis, abnormal placental insertion, excess or insufficiency of amniotic fluid or twin pregnancy.[2,3]

There are two types of breech presentation:

1. Frank breech (75%), in which the lower limbs are extended;
2. Complete breech (25%), the fetus sitting cross-legged, with the lower limbs flexed, the feet being in the dilation zone.

Uterine dynamics in breech presentation

The contracting uterus pushes the amniotic sac downwards and dilates the cervical os. Rupture of the membranes enables engagement and descent of the presenting part in the birth canal, but the buttocks, and even more so the lower limbs, do not bear down effectively on the lower segment, leading to defective accommodation with the risk of cord prolapse. The reflex of bearing down often occurs before complete cervical dilation is achieved, especially in complete breech presentations. During the expulsion stage, uterine contractions must be coordinated with effective expulsive efforts, requiring the mother's cooperation with the birth attendant.

Obstetric mechanics in breech presentation

A breech delivery progresses as a continuum.[2,3] One essential fact is that the fetal diameters that progress through the maternal pelvis increase, whereas their deformability and accommodation decrease. The last diameter to become engaged is the vertex diameter, whereas the pelvic pole has already exited the vagina. The buttocks, shoulders, then head become engaged as one oblique diameter. The anterior buttock is delivered, followed by the posterior; the back then rotates forward, engaging the shoulders, while the arms remain pinned to the trunk. Lastly, the after-coming head, which has been flexed by the contractions, becomes fixed under the symphysis, with the occiput facing forward. It then becomes unflexed by unwinding around the symphysis and the fetal face becomes visible at the vulva.

Accidents

The complications are many but uncommon.[1,3,4] Most problems can be avoided when caution is exercised. They are summarized in Table 43.1. Complications that may cause sequelae during the expulsion stage, especially in the event of premature expulsion efforts, include:

- bilateral nuchal arms, with the upper limbs extending on either side of the head, making engagement of the head impossible;
- entrapment of the after-coming head, in which several mechanisms may be involved: insufficient diameter of the maternal pelvis, backward rotation of the back with hooking of the chin at the inlet opposite the symphysis pubis, retraction of the cervix when engagement and descent of the breech occur before complete dilation (as in very premature deliveries or in the event of expulsive efforts due to uncontrolled bearing-down reflex or arrest of fetal progression).

Management of the breech presentation

Because of its potential hazards, a breech delivery requires specific ante- and post-partum management.[2,3] The diagnosis of breech presentation must be made long before the onset of labor during the last prenatal visits. It requires cephalopelvic comparison by pelvimetry (plain x-ray pelviscan)[5] or ultrasound examination to measure the biparietal diameter. Some authors obtain a radiograph of the uterine contents to evaluate the degree of flexion of the fetal head, but this can be equally well evaluated by ultrasound.

Prophylactic cesarean delivery is proposed if the cephalopelvic proportions are unfavorable, fetal weight is above 4000 g or there is an abnormal maternal pelvis. In this case, some authors advocate external version at about 35–36 weeks after the last menstrual period,[6] or even during the prelabor stage. In contrast, the presence of a concurrent anomaly (uterine malformation, low placental insertion, prematurity, scarred uterus) is an indication for cesarean delivery .

The following criteria must be met when vaginal delivery is chosen:

- good uterine dynamics with a steady cervical dilation curve, made possible by the use of oxytocin and occasionally by the premature rupture of the membranes;
- descent and forward rotation of the back;
- controlled and appropriate expulsive efforts, coupled with appropriate uterine contractions;
- the complete team (obstetrician, anesthesiologist and neonatologist) must be present. An episiotomy is almost routine in primiparas.

Two obstetric approaches are possible for the expulsion stage:

1. *Expectant attitude*, the so-called Vermelin attitude. The fetus is delivered spontaneously under the combined pressure of uterine contraction and maternal expulsive efforts, with no obstetric assistance.
2. Other more active authors prefer *direct delivery* by gentle maneuvers. Such assistance for expulsion requires the mother's full cooperation. The Lovset maneuver assists with delivery of the shoulders, by alternate rotation of the fetal back designed to lower first one arm then the other. Bracht's maneuver accompanies delivery of the fetal head and its deflection around the symphysis, the fetus rising up against the mother's abdomen.

Forceps on an after-coming head in delayed expulsion prevent any unwanted traction on the fetal neck or mouth. The maneuvers required in the event of complications must be performed gently and without haste.

Lowering of the arms is rarely done and is difficult because it is performed after failure of Lovset's maneuver.

Head entrapment requires Mauriceau's maneuver in order to avoid inappropriate traction of the fetus. There are only a few indications for a total breech extraction, and this maneuver is usually reserved for extraction of a second twin, or in the event of fetal distress when the cervix has completely dilated. It consists of guiding every step of the breech delivery by introduction of the forearm in the uterine cavity to lower the feet. Gentle traction progressively lowers the breech by making the fetal back rotate forward. This is followed by Lovset's maneuver and by Bracht's maneuver to deliver the shoulders and the after-coming head.

Anesthesia for breech deliveries

It is essential that the anesthesiologist and obstetrician fully cooperate. The complete team (obstetrician, anesthesiologist and neonatalogist) must be present in the event of any complication. The choice of anesthetic depends on the chosen obstetric approach, the need for urgent maneuvers and the stage of labor when the woman arrives. The desired goals are always a calm and consequently more cooperative patient, preservation of expulsive efforts, the possibility of performing the necessary obstetric maneuvers without using general anesthesia in cases of extreme emergency and the nondepression of fetal vital functions.

Analgesia/Anesthesia during labor

The use of epidural anesthesia in breech pregnancies was in the past highly controversial, but is today considered by many authors as the most appropriate analgesic technique because it offers many advantages and is safe. During labor, it provides pain relief, resulting in a relaxed and thus more cooperative parturient. Although epidural anesthesia increases the duration of labor because it decreases spontaneous uterine contractions, this effect can be readily corrected by oxytocin stimulation using an electric syringe and counterbalanced by relaxation of the cervix achieved by regional anesthesia.[4,8–11] It prevents premature expulsive efforts because it suppresses the early bearing-down reflex, thus decreasing the risk of cord prolapse and entrapment of the after-coming head. During the expulsion stage, with low concentrations of local anesthetics (bupivacaine < 0.25%), expulsive efforts remain appropriate: the abdominal and diaphragmatic muscles involved in bearing down are not affected, the mother is neither tired nor in a panic and retains good motor coordination. The duration of expulsive efforts and the prevalence of obstetric maneuvers are not increased.[1] Perineal relaxation is adequate. Epidural anesthesia enables a controlled and unhurried fetal delivery and, if necessary, permits obstetric maneuvers without the need for general anesthesia. Heart rate, fetal pH and Apgar score at 0 and 5 mins are not affected by epidural anesthesia.[8,9]

In practice, the use of epidural anesthesia for breech deliveries does not pose any particular problem. However, a few specific points should be noted. During the initial stage of labor, effective analgesia is achieved with 0.25% or 0.125% bupivacaine with or without opioids. Effects on pain and on the cervix are possible with analgesia up to T 10, which may occasionally need to diffuse down to L 5 when the breech is engaged, in order to decrease the sensation of bearing down. During expulsion, to preserve appropriate motor coordination, one must avoid motor block resulting from anesthetic concentrations above 0.25% or repeated injections. It is thus often necessary to 'lighten' the anesthesia towards the end of labor by decreasing the concentration of local anesthetic used and by adding opioid to improve analgesia and decrease the stretching feeling. When deep anesthesia decreases efforts at bearing down, it is better to wait, if there are no signs of fetal distress, until perineal distension is perceived.

An alternative to an epidural anesthetic during labor is the use of meperidine with inhalation of nitrous oxide. These agents are not sufficient if maneuvers are necessary and general anesthesia requiring the full attention of the anesthesiologist is needed.

In the second stage of labor in the absence of an epidural anesthetic, the only other alternatives are spinal anesthesia or general anesthesia.

Spinal anesthesia is not toxic to the fetus. It is indicated when the patient is admitted at the last stage of labor, and when maneuvers may be necessary for expulsion. It must be limited to T 10. It has a rapid onset of action and satisfactory perineal relaxation is achieved.

General anesthesia is the last resort when obstetric maneuvers are necessary. It requires endotracheal intubation and may cause fetal depression and may aggravate fetal distress.

In the event of maneuvers, the use of halogenated compounds achieves the necessary uterine relaxation irrespective of the type of anesthetic used.

Anesthesia for cesarean delivery

The choice between general anesthesia, spinal anesthesia or epidural anesthesia depends essentially on the degree of emergency and fetal status. In the event of severe acute fetal distress, general anesthesia remains the only option. In other cases, and in particular in the event of premature extraction, regional anesthesia is preferable because it does not cause fetal depression, it allows for satisfactory abdominal and uterine relaxation and facilitates fetal extraction by hysterotomy.

Conclusions

A vaginal breech delivery, when prepared for and performed by an experienced and highly skilled team, carries little risk. Although in breech deliveries, the Apgar score at 1 min is lower than in vertex deliveries, there is no significant difference between Apgar scores at 5 min.[12–14] Furthermore, the Apgar score is not affected by the type of delivery i.e. whether vaginal or cesarean.[13] Today, it is therefore possible to reduce maternal morbidity in breech deliveries by vaginal delivery, thus avoiding unwarranted cesarean delivery, using epidural anesthesia, without increasing fetal morbidity and mortality.

TWIN PREGNANCIES

Twin pregnancies account for approximately 1% of deliveries and, because of their associated complications, contribute to perinatal morbidity and mortality. Maternal disorders are more common:[15] systemic hypertension, pyelonephritis, cholestasis, iron-deficiency anemia, premature rupture of the membranes and post-partum hemorrhage. The fetal risks are also increased: twin pregnancies are associated with a higher percentage of congenital anomalies, polyhydramnios, low placental insertion, funicular anomalies, cord prolapse, dystocia and intrauterine growth retardation and prematurity. These are the most common complications. Close monitoring throughout the entire pregnancy has led to a decrease in neonatal morbidity and mortality.

Monitoring is aimed at preventing prematurity and detecting maternal or fetal diseases by examination at monthly antenatal clinics and then twice monthly towards the end of pregnancy.[16–18] We recommend hospitalization or home monitoring, but the efficacy of this has not been demonstrated. We do not insist on ultrasound examination to screen for intrauterine growth retardation and malformations.

Twin deliveries are also associated with a certain number of difficulties. Dynamic dystocia linked to uterine distension is common, requiring the prescription of an oxytocin infusion, which has been demonstrated to be safe.[19] Expulsive efforts are poor because of the weak, distended abdominal girdle and maternal fatigue. These two factors, together with frequent fetal malpositions, often make instrumental extraction necessary.

Fetal complications include an increased risk of cord prolapse for the first twin in the event of poor accommodation.[17] The second twin is at increased risk for placental abruption and occasionally obstetric maneuvers (version, total breech extraction) are required. The Apgar score of the second twin is lower than normal at 1 min, but is not significantly different at 5 min.[20,21]

The choice of the type of delivery

At the end of pregnancy, the obstetric examination will determine the type of delivery, which depends on: maternal and fetal condition; ultrasound examination to confirm the presentations and placenta insertion; radiopelvimetry, sometimes combined with radiographic examination of the uterine contents. The accepted indications for prophylactic cesarean delivery are: fetal-pelvic disproportion, placenta previa, breech presentation of the first twin, breech presentation of the second twin with a hyperextended head, infants weighing less than 1500g and, of course, maternal disease.

Twin delivery after 37 weeks [15,19,22,23]

When vaginal delivery is acceptable, the entire team must be available at all times; this is made easier by induction of labor. Recording the contractions and the cardiac rhythm of both twins is important. The use of oxytocin during labor is common, and routine during expulsion.

Instrumental extraction of the first twin is common, as the fetal head is often poorly accommodated. After delivery of the first twin, there is a rest period without contractions during which the presentation of the second twin can be checked and oriented. Delivery of the second twin is easy when it is in the vertex presentation. If the second twin is in the breech position then, following rupture of the membranes, the fetus usually descends without any difficulty into the dilated vagina. Maintaining oxytocin infusion shortens the rest period and improves the status of the second twin. More rarely, external version (EV) may be performed followed by artificial rupture of the membranes. Total breech extraction remains controversial, with a sixfold increase in mortality. It has the advantage of shortening the interval between the deliveries of the two twins. It must be deliberately performed, after EV, before fetal distress develops, or 10 min after the birth of the first twin.

If the second twin is lying transversely, the commonly accepted procedure is to perform external version and, in the event of failure, internal version followed by total breech extraction.

A cesarean delivery of the second twin is exceptional when total breech extraction is contraindicated or when irreducible cervical retraction occurs between the delivery of the two fetuses.

The delivery of the placenta must be rapid and the mother must be closely monitored: post-partum hemorrhage is common due to uterine hypotonia secondary to overdistension and to the double placental insertion.

Manual delivery of the placenta is common but not routine. Manual exploration of the uterus is advisable before hemorrhage occurs, followed by the injection of oxytocics.

Anesthesia in twin deliveries[1–9,19–22,24–26]

Epidural anesthesia is now accepted by most. It has many advantages:

- It does not cause depression in premature infants (40% are born before 37 weeks).
- It extends the indications for induction of labor because the cervical relaxation makes it possible to modulate uterine dynamics by the use of oxytocin, thus avoiding uterine hyperkinesis and hypertonia.
- It allows instrumental extraction and painless obstetric maneuvers without requiring general anesthesia.
- It sometimes increases the duration of the first stage of labor by causing hypokinesis, but this is readily corrected by oxytocics. However, it does not increase the number of maneuvers or the time between the birth of each twins.

In practice, no specific technique is preferred, but analgesia must be achieved during the time of expulsion. These women must be very closely monitored. They are dyspneic, are only comfortable sitting and are usually hypervolemic. It is essential to prevent hypotension or venacaval compression. We will only mention general anesthesia as it is only indicated for obstetric maneuvers in the absence of epidural anesthesia.

Specific problems include unexpected premature labor. This is an emergency when the women arrives in labor before any tests have been performed. When this occurs before 31 weeks, cesarean and vaginal delivery have the same prognosis.[15]

Premature rupture of membranes

A breech presentation of the first twin in a multipara, and

growth retardation may benefit from directed labor if the cervical conditions, assessed according to the Bishop score, are favorable (score equal to or greater than 8). In the other cases, cesarean delivery is often performed for the safety of the fetuses.

Conclusions

Eutocic delivery of twin pregnancies requires increased antepartum, peripartum and post-partum maternofetal monitoring to prevent prematurity, potential handicap of the second twin and post-partum hemorrhage.

REFERENCES

1. Scott Wheeler A 1988 Breech presentation and multiple gestation. In: James F M III, Scott Wheeler A, Dewan D M (eds) Obstetric Anesthesia: the complicated patient, 2nd edn. pp 367–383
2. Barrier J 1985 La présentation du siège. In: Volkaer R (ed) Traité d'obstétrique Dories, Philadelphia Vol 2. Masson, Paris, pp 364–383
3. Puech F 1988 La présentation du siège. In: Lansac J, Brody G (eds) Pratique de l'accouchement. SIMEP, Paris, pp 95–107
4. Henry M, Vauthier D, Seebacher 1987 Anesthésie péridurale et présentation du siége Caro, Paris, pp 45–65
5. Christiane S S, Brady K, Reed J A 1990. Vaginal breech delivery: a five year prospective evaluation of a protocol using computed tumographic pelvimetry. Am J Obstet Gynecol 163: 848–855
6. Marchick R 1988 Antepartum external cephalic version with tocolysis: a study of term singleton breech presentations. Am J Obstet Gynecol 158: 1339–1346
7. Bower-Simpkins P, Ferguson J L C 1975 Lumbar epidural blocks and the breech presentation. Br J Anaesth 46: 420–424
8. Van Zundert A, Vaes L, Seotens M 1991 Are breech deliveries an indication for lumbar epidural analgesia? Anesth Analg 72: 399–403
9. Dewan D M 1987. Anesthesia for preterm delivery breech delivery and multiple gestation. Clin Obstet Gynecol 30: 566–578
10. Bingham P, Lilford R J 1988 Management of the selected term breech presentation: assessment of the risks of selected vaginal delivery versus cesarean section for all cases. Obstet Gynecol 69: 965–978
11. Gomvsky M L, Petrie R H 1989 The intrapartum management of the breech presentation. Clin Perinatol 16: 975–986
12. Bingham P, Hird V, Lilford R J 1987 Management of the mature selected breech presentation: an analysis based on the intended method of delivery. Br J Obstet Gynaecol 94: 752–756
13. Tatum R K, Orr J M, Soong S J 1985 Vaginal breech delivery of selected infants weighing more than 2000 grams. Am J Obstet Gynecol 152: 145–155
14. Rosen M G, Debanne S, Thompson K 1985 Long term neurological morbidity in breech and vertex births. Am J Obstet Gynecol, 151: 718–720
15. Puech F 1988 L'accouchement des grossesses multiples. In: Lansac J, Brody G (eds) Pratique de l'accouchement. SIMEP, Paris, pp 108–113
16. Kerbrat G, Papiernik E 1983 Surveillance des grossesses gémellaires. Mise a jour en gynécologie obstétrique. Arnette, Paris pp 249–159
17. Blanc B, Hruf C H M 1981 Accouchement de la grossesse gémellaire. Mise à jour en gynécologie obstétrique. Arnette, Paris pp 257–269
18. Poulain P, Palaric J C 1989 Grossesse gémellaire. 19e journsées nationales de médecine périnatale. Arnette, Paris, pp 247–252
19. Leroy F 1985 Les grossesses multiples. In: Volkaer R (ed) Traité d'obstétrique Vol 1. Masson, Paris, pp 616–636
20. Gocke E, Nageotte M P, Garite T 1989 Management of the non vertex second twin primary cesarean section, external version, or primary breech extraction. Am J Obstet Gynecol 161: 111–114
21. Mazor M, Leiberman J R, Dreval D 1986 Management and outcome of vertex breech and vertex–vertex presentation in twin gestation. A comparative study. Eur J Obstet Gynecol Reprod Biol 22: 69–75
22. Hays P M, Smeltzer J S 1986 Multiple gestation. Clin Obstet Gynecol 29: 264–285
23. Schoeffler P, Canis M, Monteillard C 1992 Anesthésie pour manoeuvres et situations obstétricales particulières. In: Schoeffler P (ed) Anesthésie et Analgésie en Obstetrique. Masson, Paris, pp 92–114
24. Champagne C, Pons J C, Claquin C 1987 Anesthésie péridurale et grossesse gémellaire. Expérience Résultats Caro, Paris, pp 99–115
25. Redick L F 1988 Anesthesia for twin delivery. Clin Perinatol 15: 107–122
26. Lepercq J, Slama A, Tournaire M, 1988 Effets de la péridurale sur l'accouchement. Mise en á jour en gynècologie obstétrique. Paris, pp 339–374

44. Peripartum hemorrhage: an anesthetic management plan

S. P. Gatt R. F. Smith

INTRODUCTION

Procrastination in dealing with pelvic hemorrhage only accentuates the problem. Hoping that hemorrhage will spontaneously cease is futile, and steps should be taken immediately.

Cruikshank, 1986.[1]

In the 1940s, hemorrhage was the commonest cause of maternal mortality.[2] Over the last 50 years, maternal mortality from hemorrhage has continued to decline steadily as a result of the establishment of blood banking facilities, better antenatal care, more aggressive treatment of hemorrhage and better hemodynamic monitoring.[3–6] Nevertheless, peripartum hemorrhage is still the second commonmost cause of death in pregnancy.[4] The obstetric anesthesiologist is often faced with parturients experiencing a bleeding episode. A bleeding pregnant patient presents a number of challenges peculiar to this condition – blood loss is difficult to assess, hemorrhage is often fierce and resuscitation is complicated by the supine hypotensive syndrome, altered uteroplacental blood flow and increased risk of aspiration of gastric contents.[6–9]

ANESTHETIC CONSIDERATIONS IN ANTEPARTUM HEMORRHAGE

He who sees things from the beginning will have the finest view of them.

Aristotle
384–322 BC

The commonest causes of antepartum hemorrhage are placental abruption (see Table 44.1)[6–10] and placenta previa.

Placental abruption

From the anesthesiologist's point of view, the most important aspect of resuscitation of a last-trimester patient with an abruption of the placenta is that the magnitude of

Table 44.1 Major causes of peripartum hemorrhage

	Maternal	Fetal
Antepartum	Placenta previa	
	Placental abruption	
Intrapartum	'Bloody show'	Vasa previa
	Cesarean delivery	
	Rupture of the uterus	
	'Edge bleeding'	
Post-partum	Atonic uterus	
	Retained placenta	
	Trauma to birth canal	
	Inversion of the uterus	
	Placenta accreta, increta and percreta	

vaginal bleeding may bear little resemblance to the overall degree of blood loss. A considerable proportion of shed blood (as much as 6.4 l) may be concealed behind the placenta, infiltrate the broad ligaments or uterus (Couvelaire uterus) or be sequestered in the amniotic cavity or behind the presenting part.[5,6,8,11,12] It can be assumed that, once significant abruption has been diagnosed, 1–2 l has been lost and that, if the fetus is dead, the blood loss is usually more than 2.5 l.

The bleeding is often complicated by a coagulopathy characterized by thrombocytopenia, and consumption of fibrinogen and procoagulants V, VII and VIII[8,10,13–15]. It should be realized that the coagulopathy which occurs in severe degrees of abruption is a dynamic and constantly changing process.[13] As seen in Figure 44.1, there is initially an accelerated intravascular clotting period, which is followed by an apparent normal period that precedes the onset of severe, progressive coagulopathy.[8] Disseminated intravascular coagulation (DIC) occurs in more than one-third of those with grade III abruption and a dead fetus.[12,16]

If bleeding is severe or a coagulopathy supervenes, major regional anesthesia is contraindicated. It may be possible to insert a lumbar or caudal epidural or subarachnoid block in patients with grade I placental abruption

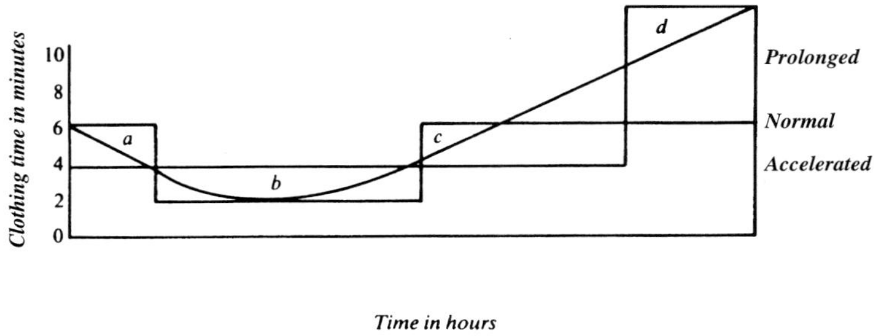

a	b	c	d
CT – N	CT – <N	CT – N	CT – ↑
Pl – N	Pl – N or <N+	Pl – <N±	Pl – ↓
CF – N	CF – N	CF – N	CF – ↓
FM – N	FM – ↑	FDP – ↑↑	FDP – ↑↑
FDP – N	FDP – ↑	F – N±	F – ↓
F – N	F – ±N	FL – N±	FL – ±N or ↑
FL – N	FL – ±N	FM – ↑	FM – ↑

CT = Clotting time
Pl = Platelets
CF = Clotting factors esp. V, VIII
FDP = Fibrin degradation products
FM = Fibrinogen monomers
F = Fibrinogen
FL = Fibrinolysins
N = Normal values for pregnancy

a = normal period

b = disseminated intravascular coagulation period (d.i.c.) (accelerated coagulation)

c = coagulation defect or coagulopathy period with the continued d.i.c. (apparent normal clotting period)

d = established coagulation defect/coagulopathy (abnormal clotting period).

Fig. 44.1 Diagrammatic representation of the progressive coagulopathy that occurs in placental abruption showing that there is a progression from accelerated intravascular coagulation to overt coagulopathy via a period of apparent quiescence during which the coagulation studies may be relatively normal. (Reproduced with permission from ref. 8)

(mild degree of separation; <250 ml blood loss; no fetal distress; no coagulopathy; no hypotension).[6,17] It should be remembered that regional and local anesthetic techniques are contraindicated if the platelet count falls below 50×10^9/l.[17,18] Above 100×10^9/l, in the absence of other coagulation defects, the Simplate II or Duke bleeding time is invariably normal and a bleeding time unnecessary.[18] In patients with platelet counts between 50 and 100×10^9/l, a bleeding time serves as a useful guide to the advisability of performing a regional block.[11,18] It should be remembered that major degrees of sympathetic blockade may be undesirable on other grounds in patients with abruption – hypovolemia with major reduction in uteroplacental blood flow, fetal distress or intrauterine death, intrauterine growth retardation, suboptimal weight gain and fetal malformations (especially in the fetal nervous system) are all relative contraindications.[6,8,15,19]

Following abruption of the placenta, fetal mortality is about 50%.[13,20] Approximately 15–25% of perinatal deaths are caused by placental abruption.[20] Perinatal mortality can be improved by delivering the infant as soon as possible after the diagnosis is established.[12,20,21] These mothers present to the anesthesiologist for urgent surgery with all its hazards – the need for rapid general anesthesia in the presence of a full stomach, fetal distress and hypovolemia. If fetal distress is diagnosed, immediate treatment should include left lateral uterine displacement (using a wedge under the right hip), oxygen enrichment, fluid volume resuscitation and blunting of uterine contractions (which may further reduce placental blood flow) with β_2-adrenergic agonists and/or magnesium sulfate, followed by immediate delivery.[6,22]

Placenta previa

When placenta previa (PP) is diagnosed at less than 36 weeks' gestation, it is usually managed in an aggressive expectant fashion with hospitalization, bed rest, repeat weekly diagnostic ultrasound examinations, periodic assessment of fetal maturity and serial monitoring of hemoglobin.[5,8,9,23,24] While conservative management is directed at reducing perinatal death, it exposes the mother to increased danger from multiple transfusion, recurrent unpredictable hemorrhage and emergency surgery occurring in less than ideal circumstances (e.g. during a period of active bleeding or after recent food intake).[20,24] About 25% of patients with significant placenta previa will have symptomatic hypovolemia accompanying their first bleed, and 10–25% develop hypovolemic shock.[5,20] It is advisable neither to examine these patients vaginally or rectally nor to pass a vaginal ultrasound probe once a diagnosis of placenta previa is made (especially in type III/IV previa.)[8,12,24,25] Only about 7% of placentae previa are type III or IV, i.e. encroach on the lower uterine segment to any significant degree.[7]

Because heavy bleeding remains a major cause of mortality in those with types III and IV previa, these patients should have a large-bore intravenous catheter in situ and should be cross-matched or grouped *and* antibody screened.[5,6,24]

Occasionally, and especially when high-quality ultrasound is not available or uncertain, the anesthesiologist is required to provide anesthesia for a 'double set-up'.[26] This procedure should not be done until the obstetrician is ready to commit the patient to delivery and requires two obstetric teams: one team performs a vaginal examination (VE); the other is scrubbed for an urgent cesarean delivery should the tentative diagnosis of PP be confirmed at VE.[12,24] The preoperative evaluation should include an assessment of degree of hemodynamic stability and fetal gestational age and 'maturity' and an estimate of blood loss (by direct measurement of shed blood, central venous pressure and urine output, from the clinical signs including magnitude of orthostatic hypotension and from ancillary investigations such as degree of inferior venacava collapse on an abdominal CT scan).[6,23,26,27] After securing adequate intravenous access and ensuring that blood is available for immediate transfusion, the anesthesiologist proceeds to rapid-sequence induction, or, if there is no hypovolemia and no active bleeding, a regional technique may be suitable (see below).[22]

It is still controversial whether an epidural anesthetic is suitable for patients with diagnosed but stable significant PP in whom the bleeding can be anticipated to be severe. The delivery may be complicated by a higher likelihood of fetal bleeding, congenital malformation, prematurity and asphyxia and maternal intrapartum (due to placenta accreta, increta and percreta) and post-partum (from lower segment 'ooze') hemorrhage.[8,28–30] Severe hypotension (which can be made more troublesome by the sympathetic block) may cause significant decreases in uteroplacental blood flow, impairment of plasma volume control, skeletal muscle vascular decompensation, coagulopathy, vertebrobasilar insufficiency and decreased maternal cerebral function (with decreased level of consciousness).[14,27,31–36] The risk is greatest in those with an anteriorly placed placenta, in whom the uterine incision must go through the placenta itself making both maternal and fetal hemorrhage much more severe.[6] On the other hand, the presence of a regional anesthetic (and its accompanying sympathetic block) allows for acute preoperative fluid loading and hemodilution, reduces the magnitude of the bleed (and the need for blood transfusion), confers some protection against the development of (prerenal) acute renal failure (the commonest severe sequela of acute bleeding in modern obstetric practice) and provides a useful monitor of cerebral perfusion.[8,37] In our practice, where a neonatologist is available to manage the baby, we are quite happy to provide epidural (but not subarachnoid) anesthesia in all grades of PP (except grade IV, anterior, in which case we prefer general anesthesia) provided that blood, vasopressors and blood products are immediately available.[5,6,17,22,38,39]

Whether regional or general anesthesia is contemplated, preoperative preparation should include adequate fasting and reduction of the risk of aspiration pneumonitis (Mendelson's syndrome) with clear antacid (e.g. 30 ml of 0.3 M sodium citrate 'on call' to the operating room) with or without an H_2 receptor blocker [e.g. 150 mg of ranitidine (Zantac) orally in two doses, 2 h preoperatively] with or without metoclopramide [e.g. 10 mg of metoclopramide (Maxolon) orally 2 h preoperatively]. Alternatively, these drugs can be administered i.v. immediately preoperatively. Special attention should be paid to denitrogenation (preoxygenation), monitoring and reduction of the impact of the supine hypotensive (inferior venacaval) syndrome with >15° left uterine displacement using a wedge under the right hip.[5,22,40]

ANESTHETIC CONSIDERATIONS IN INTRAPARTUM HEMORRHAGE

Ability of the uterus to arrest its own hemorrhage . . . is an entirely mechanical phenomenon, independent of blood coagulation.

M. H. Plumer

While 'bloody show' and 'edge bleeding' are common causes of hemorrhage during labor and delivery, in the main they are not responsible for worrisome degrees of intrapartum bleeding. Blood loss at cesarean delivery is usually about 400 ml for epidural and spinal cesarean delivery and 500–1000 ml for cesarean delivery under general anesthesia.[5]

While vasa previa can be life-threatening to the neonate, the overall blood loss is usually no more than 30–40 ml and does not require any action from an anesthesiologist not involved in neonatal resuscitation[5] (see Table 44.1).[5]

Rupture of the uterus

Uterine rupture is an uncommon (approximately 1 in 1200) but potentially lethal (5% of maternal deaths) complication of labor and delivery and is associated with a high perinatal mortality rate (>50%).[26] The spectrum of 'uterine rupture' ranges from gentle 'silent' asymptomatic dehiscence occurring over several hours and diagnosed at subsequent cesarean delivery to catastrophic rapid uterine rupture with rapid demise of the fetus and abrupt cessation of labor.

Since trial of labor following previous cesarean delivery has been proven to be an acceptable mode of delivery of low risk to mother and fetus and is becoming more widespread in obstetric practice, the incidence of cesarean delivery scar separation/dehiscence may rise in the next few years.[41–43] We may also see uterine rupture caused by the use of prostaglandins to secure middle-trimester termination of pregnancy.[42,44]

In uterine rupture, resuscitation is often complicated by vagally mediated reflexes caused by extrusion of amniotic fluid into the abdominal cavity.[5] Regional anesthesia may further confuse the issue by masking some of the clinical signs of uterine rupture, while there are some who feel that the pain associated with ruptured uterus will 'break through' a narrow segmental block and an epidural block will attenuate considerably the severe pain usually associated with a uterine rupture.[6,10,45] Indeed, there is some controversy as to whether parturients having a vaginal birth after cesarean delivery (VBACD) should be allowed epidural pain relief for labor and delivery.[42,46] In our unit, we are quite happy to institute epidural analgesia for mothers having trial of scar (labor) provided that the labor and fetal well-being are monitored continuously. Care must be taken to use the minimum concentration and volume of local anesthetic that will control labor pain. Any atypical pain (e.g. shoulder tip pain, pain occurring early after a 'top-up' or breakthrough pain associated with features of hemorrhage or shock) must be treated as being potentially due to uterine rupture.[6,47]

Once uterine rupture occurs, delivery of the asphyxiated fetus must be undertaken immediately. Immediate cesarean delivery or cesarean hysterectomy is not without hazard in a mother in shock, but rapid general anesthesia is often the only option available to the anesthesiologist.[1,5] It is worth remembering that in those parturients in whom, because of the urgency of the situation, a general anesthetic is superimposed on a pre-existing epidural anesthetic, the partial sympathetic block may make systemic arterial pressure control difficult.[5]

ANESTHETIC CONSIDERATIONS IN POST-PARTUM HEMORRHAGE

Patients who bleed Antepartum will also bleed Postpartum.

Diane Biehl, 1990

Uterine atony accounts for the majority of post-partum hemorrhage (PPH) and is also a complicating factor in a number of other causes of peripartum bleeding (e.g. placenta previa, cesarean delivery under general anesthesia, lower segment implantation). Retained placenta (or portions or cotyledons of the placenta) also accounts for a fair proportion of post-partum hemorrhage (see Table 44.1). Because diagnosis of the specific cause of post-partum bleeding is often difficult, and since the clinical picture is frequently contributed to by a number of 'pathologies' (e.g. following a difficult instrumental delivery bleeding from an atonic uterus may be complicated by bleeding from a laceration or episiotomy and made worse by an accompanying coagulopathy), the anesthetic management of all causes of PPH will be considered together.[1,18,48–50]

There are a number of factors that can contribute to PPH. Many of these are of interest to the anesthesiologist and they can be divided into four main groups:

- Coagulopathy and thrombocytopenia: preeclampsia, amniotic fluid embolism, in utero fetal death;
- Uterine atony: general anesthesia, uterine fibromyomata, grand multiparity, polyhydramnios, multiple pregnancy;
- Retained products of conception: placenta previa, intervention in third stage;
- Birth canal trauma: precipitate labor, multiple pregnancy, breech extraction.

Post-partum hemorrhage is usually described as 'more than 500 ml of blood loss following delivery of the fetus'.[51] Since average blood loss at delivery is 400–600 ml (and 800–1200 ml at elective cesarean delivery under general anesthesia), this would mean that more than 50% of parturients suffer from PPH.[5] Also, bleeding occurring in the peripartum period is notoriously difficult to measure. For the purposes of this chapter, PPH is 'bleeding sufficient to jeopardize the well-being or survival of the mother and occurring after delivery of the baby'.[52]

A number of anesthetic drugs will produce 'floppiness' (atony) of the uterus. The inhalation agents (isoflurane, enflurane, halothane and diethyl ether) can all contribute significantly to the magnitude of PPH. The same effect can be produced by the β-sympathomimetic agents (e.g. salbutamol, terbutaline, ritodrine and isoxuprine). Agents causing uterine relaxation should be withdrawn in the parturient with uterine bleeding.

The likelihood, degree, impact or severity of PPH can be reduced by a number of precautions and maneuvers undertaken during the birthing process. These are summarized below:

- Antepartum: Determine if the patient is predisposed to PPH. Correct any thrombocytopenia, anemia and coagulopathy. Investigate the source of coagulopathy and anemia. Obtain blood group.
- Intrapartum: Confirm blood group and antibody screen. Insert a 14–16 gauge intravenous catheter and ensure that hydration is maintained throughout the delivery. If analgesia or anesthesia is required for operative delivery, opt for an epidural, rather than a general anesthetic, whenever possible. Check coagulation and platelet status.

• Post-partum: Empty the uterus. If operative delivery under general anesthesia is unavoidable, minimize the use of inhalation agents after delivery. If PPH supervenes, start synthetic oxytocin and crystalloid/colloid infusion. Institute surgical means of blood loss control – suture lacerations, apply local pressure, ligate obvious bleeding points. Empty the bladder and measure urine output. Assess vital signs frequently. Obtain cross-matched blood and start transfusion. If the bleeding continues, get help, and go into 'resuscitation mode' (see below). A plan for initial resuscitation is shown in Table 44.2 and a flow diagram of subsequent management in Figure 44.3.

Control of PPH is usually achieved by a combination of surgical, mechanical, pharmacologic and angiographic techniques. These maneuvers are applied at the same time as the resuscitation is proceeding.

Surgical methods include:

• gentle and careful curretage of the endometrial cavity taking great care to avoid lateral wall or fundal perforation of the uterus.[1]

• manual exploration of the uterine cavity and removal of all or portions of the retained placenta or membranes;[5,53]

• exploration and repair of lower uterine segment, cervical, vaginal and perineal lacerations and tears;[1,54]

• bilateral ligation of the hypogastric (internal iliac) or uterine arteries;[1]

• cesarean and peripartum hysterectomy.[48,55]

It should be remembered that the main blood supply to the uterus comes from the uterine artery, a branch of the hypogastric (internal iliac) artery, while the arterial supply to the vagina is from the vaginal branch of the same artery. This means that, while hypogastric artery ligation stops hemorrhage from both uterus and vagina, uterine artery ligation does not. The mechanism whereby bleeding stops following hypogastric artery ligation is also interesting. The pulsating arterial flow is changed to a 'venous' pattern such that clots form distal to the ligations.[1]

In patients with low parity, ligation of the internal iliac arteries (hypogastric arteries) is usually preferable to hysterectomy.[49] On the other hand, if the bleeding is life-threatening, hysterectomy should not be delayed unnecessarily. Since the bulk of PPH usually comes from a poorly contracted lower segment, if an 'obstetric hysterectomy' is contemplated, a total hysterectomy more often stops the bleeding than a subtotal.[49]

Mechanical techniques aimed at temporarily arresting hemorrhage are often useful when fluid resuscitation is falling behind blood loss. They include:

- uterine fundus massage;[5,54]
- packing of the uterine cavity with a gauze pack;
- manual compression of the body of the uterus;
- application of clamps or manual compression of the aorta or iliac arteries.

The *pharmacologic* armamentarium for dealing with PPH is very extensive and includes:

• oxytocics, e.g. Syntocinon (synthetic oxytocin) given as a bolus of 5 IU followed by an infusion of 10–20 IU in 500–1000 ml of fluid (e.g. 5% dextrose or crystalloid);[2,5,30,56]

• ergot alkaloids, e.g. ergometrine (methylergobasine) 1–2 mg slowly i.v. or 4–6 mg into intrauterine muscle, or ergonovine (methylergonovine) 0.2–0.3 mg i.m. or up to 0.2 mg very slowly i.v.;[5,56]

• prostaglandins, e.g. prostaglandin $F_{2\alpha}$ 1–5 mg intramyometrially or its 15-methyl analog (Prostinfenem) 0.25 mg i.v. in 500 ml of 5% dextrose in water or 250–500 μg intramyometrially or intrauterine irrigation or vaginal (or rectal) suppositories of prostaglandin E_2;[1,54,57–59]

• epsilon aminocaproic acid (EACA), in selected patients with disseminated intravascular coagulation;[51]

• DDAVP, desmopressin acetate, in patients with thrombocytopenia or platelet function anomalies;[60]

• conjugated estrogen therapy, for mothers with delayed PPH.

Boluses of prostaglandins and oxytocics should be avoided in the hypotensive patient. Ergot alkaloids can produce hypertension from peripheral vasoconstriction (which is particularly troublesome in hemorrhaging parturients who have already received exogenous pressor agents), while synthetic oxytocin may cause vasodilation, which can further accentuate the hypotension. The use of systemic prostaglandins should be avoided because they

Table 44.2 Initial resuscitative measures in the bleeding parturient

1. Establish two venous access sites using large-bore peripheral emergency infusion devices (e.g. 6–8.5 French) or intravenous catheter (larger than 16 G).
2. Administer appropriate fluids aggressively (see later) either via an intravenous infusion set incorporating an integral, hand-compressible pressure pump or using a pressurized (40 kPa, 300 mmHg) infusor bag 'sleeve' placed around a compressible fluid bag.
3. Place the patient in the lateral position or commence left uterine displacement using a right pelvic wedge.
4. Administer oxygen by face mask (e.g. Hudson, Venturi) or nasal prongs.
5. Obtain venous blood for urgent blood group, antibody screen and full cross-match. Maintain four units of cross-matched blood in reserve at all times.
6. Initiate monitoring – oximeter, cardiotocograph, noninvasive blood pressure, ECG, indwelling urinary catheter and hourly urine measure, precordial stethoscope.
7. If surgical delivery is not indicated, evaluate the degree of blood loss, fetal gestational age and lung maturity and cause of bleeding, if surgery is contemplated,
   a. obtain a full anesthetic history;
   b. administer 10 mg of metoclopramide (Maxolon) i.v. and 50 mg of ranitidine (Zantac) i.v.;
   c. prior to induction, administer 30 ml of clear antacid (e.g. 0.3 M sodium citrate or Bicitra);
   d. upgrade monitoring (e.g. CVP, intra-arterial catheter, pulmonary artery catheter (Swan Ganz), temperature probe).

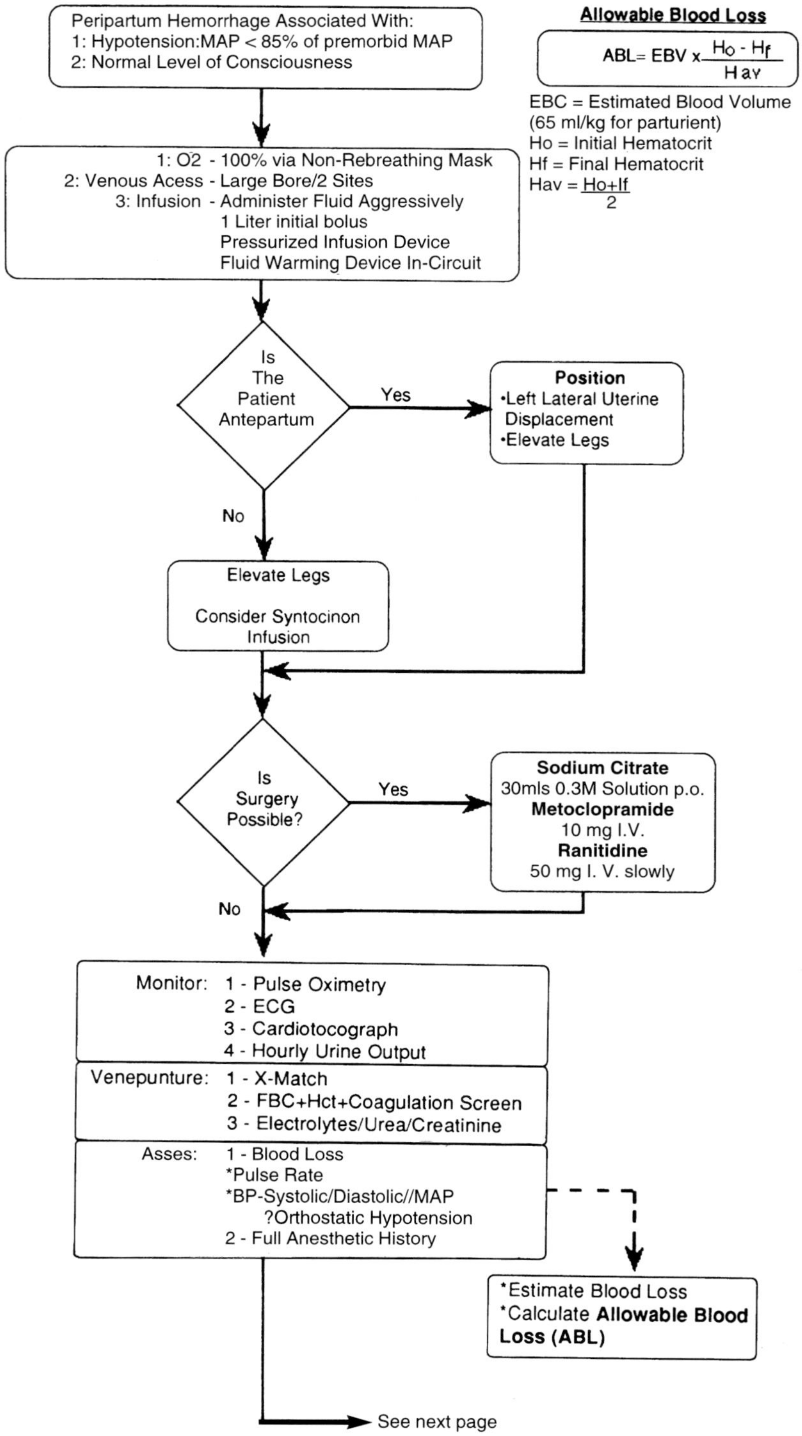

Fig. 44.2 Clinical algorithm for resuscitation in patients with peripartum hemorrhage.

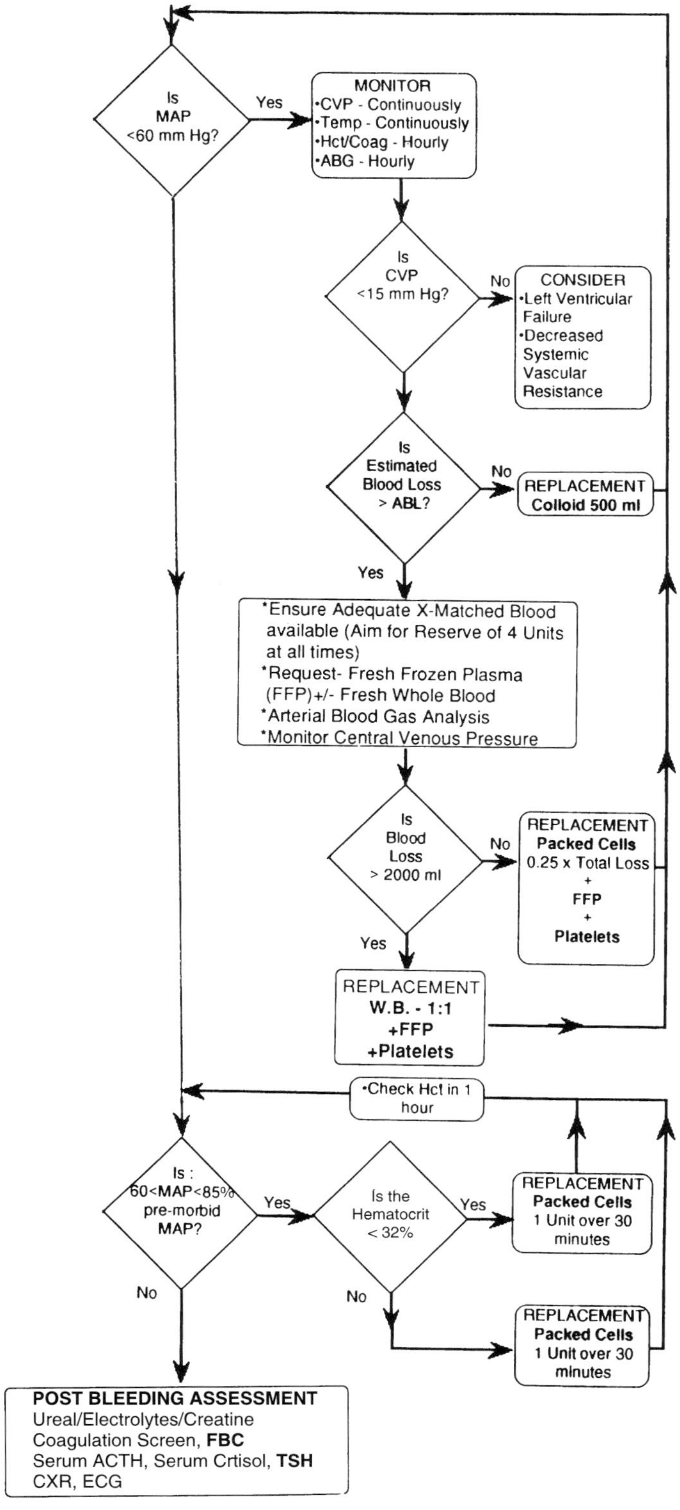

Fig. 44.2 Clinical algorithm for resuscitation in patients with peripartum hemorrhage

can cause hypo- or hypertension, bronchospasm and pulmonary edema.

Angiographic techniques are usually reserved for intractable or delayed cases in which PPH persists in spite of adequate surgical and pharmacologic measures.[52] Following pelvic angiography, vasoconstrictors or embolizing materials are infused into selected vessels.[52]

Anesthesia for PPH ranges from mild sedation in the multipara requiring removal of a placenta impacted in the cervical os to general anesthesia with intubation and artificial ventilation (intermittent positive-pressure ventilation) in the hemorrhaging, hypotensive patient with a ruptured uterus and from a caudal epidural block for repair of a perineal tear to major regional (T10–S4) blockade in a hemodynamically stable mother with a retained placenta.[5,61,62]

General anesthesia in the bleeding hypovolemic patient is not without hazard. Table 44.3 gives a standard sample anesthetic plan for management of these patients. This scheme can be modified for antepartum patients requiring emergency lower segment cesarean delivery or for patients with PPH.

MANAGEMENT OF MASSIVE BLOOD LOSS – INITIAL RESUSCITATION

As the pregnancy progresses, several changes in the hemostatic system occur, so that, by the peripartum period, several mechanisms that will protect the mother from massive hemorrhage are already in place. There is an increase in all the coagulation cascade procoagulants except XI and XIII (while the coagulation inhibitors are essentially unchanged).[50] The blood volume is increased and the procoagulants are activated to produce a 'hypercoagulable' state. The platelet count may (or may not) fall (and, in some instances, may rise).[64] This should be kept in mind when dealing with a bleeding parturient.

Blood flow to the pregnant uterus represents one-fifth of the cardiac output at term.[1,47] When torrential bleeding supervenes and massive blood transfusion is superimposed on these 'physiologic' changes, the rapidly changing dynamic process can make interpretation of the ever-expanding array of laboratory investigations difficult[50,65,66] (see Fig. 44.1). In obstetric anesthesia, the clinical picture is made even 'muddier' by resuscitative measures (e.g. pressor agents, colloids), by third-space fluid losses (and concealed or retroperitoneal and pelvic hemorrhage) and by other factors that may contribute to the shocked state (e.g. mechanical factors such as the supine hypotensive syndrome and intermittent positive-pressure artificial ventilation) and by the effect of the anesthetic which, in the main, impairs the autonomic nervous system's ability to compensate for hypovolemia.[36,39,61,67–71] At delivery, as the placental intervillous space disappears and the uterine vasculature shrinks, a volume of 300–500 ml less may be required to fill the intravascular space. This is equivalent to an effective 'autotransfusion' of 300–500 ml at delivery. The obstetric patient in the lithotomy position (e.g. during instrumental vaginal delivery) is at particular risk because

Table 44.3 An anesthetic plan for emergency general anesthesia in the hypovolemic bleeding patient (Reproduced, with modifications to include post-partum patients, from ref. 6 with permission)

Preanesthetic phase
1. Perform full preanesthetic evaluation, including assessment of the degree of blood loss, fetal gestational age, extent of maternal compensation to bleeding and etiology of bleeding.
2. Place the patient in the left lateral position.
3. Obtain venous blood for cross-match and baseline investigations.
4. Prepare and check anesthesia machine, suction apparatus, drugs, intubation and resuscitation equipment and anesthesia circuit for emergency surgery.
5. Administer 10 mg of metoclopramide (Maxolon) i.v. ± 50 mg of ranitidine (Zantac) i.v.

Immediate preoperative phase
1. In the pregnant patient, displace the uterus to the left with a right pelvic wedge or by placing the patient in the left lateral position.
2. Administer oxygen by face mask.
3. Obtain adequate intravenous access, e.g. 6–8.8 Fr emergency infusion device (EID) or 14-G venous catheter.
4. Restore blood volume aggressively with crystalloid and colloid (as described in Table 44.4).
5. Start blood transfusion when blood becomes available (along guidelines presented in Tables 44.4 and 44.5).
6. Start basic monitoring – blood pressure cuff, ECG, indwelling urinary catheter.

Preinduction phase
1. If patient is not comatose, administer 30 ml of clear antacid, e.g. 30 ml of 0.3 M sodium citrate.
2. Denitrogenate with 100% oxygen by anesthesia circle absorber system.
3. If time permits:
   - upgrade monitoring – precordial stethoscope, capnography, inhalation agent monitor, CVP catheter, automated noninvasive blood pressure cuff or Finapress 'continuous' noninvasive pressure device or intra-arterial catheter as required;
   - upgrade fluid administration apparatus – second large venous access site, integral blood pumps, pressure infusor bags or emergency pressure infusion devices, blood warmers, blood filters;
   - start infusion of colloid, blood components or blood as appropriate;
   - enlist the services of a neonatologist capable of taking care of the infant, if appropriate.
4. Identify the cricoid cartilage to the anesthetic assistant.
5. Induce the patient in the supine, left uterine displacement (not lithotomy) position.

Induction phase
1. Induce anesthesia:
   a. compensated bleeding:
      - 1.5–3 mg/kg propofol (Diprivan); or
      - 2–4 mg/kg thiopental; or
      - 0.5 mg/kg ketamine* + 2 mg/kg thiopental i.v.

   b. decompensating: 1–1.5 mg/kg ketamine* i.v.
   c. decompensated: 0.5–1.0 mg/kg ketamine* i.v.
   * If ketamine is contraindicated, e.g. severe pregnancy-induced hypertension with abruption, substitute a fentanyl (Sublimaze) – midazolam (Hypnovel) induction sequence.
   d. comatose, moribund: nothing.
2. Administer succinylcholine 1.5 mg/kg. Do not pretreat fasciculations with a nondepolarizing muscle relaxant because cesarean delivery patients do not often get muscle pain from depolarizing muscle relaxants, because fasciculations give a suitable end-point for intubation and because an increased dose of succinylcholine will be needed to guarantee intubating conditions.
3. Apply cricoid pressure (Sellick's maneuver).
4. Perform laryngoscopy and endotracheal intubation. Confirm endotracheal tube placement.

Table 44.3 *Continued*

Maintenance phase
1. Maintain anesthetic depth with an inhalation agent or an intravenous (continuous infusion or intermittent bolus) agent as appropriate.
   a. if uterine relaxation is required (e.g. manual removal of a retained placenta), introduce >2 MAC of inhalation agent as tolerated by hemodynamic parameters;
   b. if uterine relaxation is undesirable (e.g. atonic uterus), maintain depth with intravenous propofol (Diprivan) if the patient is hemodynamically stable; [62,63]
   c. for cesarean delivery in a hemodynamically unstable patient, continue 100% oxygen ± < 0.66 MAC inhalation agent;
   d. for cesarean delivery in a stable patient, start nitrous oxide – oxygen (50 : 50)± 0.75% isoflurane, 1.0% enflurane or 0.5% halothane.
2. Set alarms – circuit overpressure and disconnect, inspired oxygen tension, inhalation agent percentage.
3. Improve monitoring further – temperature probe, esophageal stethoscope, neuromuscular block twitch monitor.
4. When a train of four returns, start a nondepolarizing muscle relaxant (e.g. 15–20 mg of atracurium or 2–4 mg of pancuronium or vecuronium as dictated by arterial systemic pressure) or start a succinylcholine infusion.
5. If uterine contraction is desirable (e.g. following delivery of the infant by lower segment cesarean delivery), start 20–40 IU per 1000 ml of crystalloid by slow intravenous infusion. At cesarean delivery, following birth of the infant, administer 2 mg of midazolam (Hypnovel) ± 0.5–1.0 μg/kg fentanyl (Sublimaze), remove the hip-displacing wedge and change over to nitrous oxide–oxygen (70 : 30) if the patient is hemodynamically stable.
6. Continue aggressive resuscitation (as per Table 44.4) with cross-matched blood, packed cells, colloid and crystalloid as appropriate. Correct any coagulopathy or acid–base or temperature abnormality as it develops.

Reversal – extubation phase
1. Aspirate the stomach contents using an orogastric tube.
2. Reverse the nondepolarizer when a train of four twitch returns using neostigmine (prostigmine) + glycopyrrolate (Robinul) or atropine, or cease the succinylcholine infusion.
3. Extubate when ventilatory exchange is appropriate and the patient is cardiovascularly stable and able to guard her airway.

Post-operative phase
1. Ventilation may be required post-operatively. Transfer to the obstetric acute care unit (ACC).
2. Continue resucitation until hypovolemia and its sequelae (e.g. adult respiratory distress syndrome, coagulopathy, renal dysfunction) are corrected.

substantial blood loss can occur before tachycardia and hypotension develop.

Because quantitative estimates of blood loss in obstetrics are notoriously inaccurate, a rule of thumb is useful in determining the extent of blood loss. A parturient who has a mean arterial pressure fall and heart rate rise only on assuming the sitting position but not while lying supine has sustained a blood loss of less than 1000 ml. A post-partum patient who is hypotensive and tachycardic in the supine posture can be assumed to have an 'effective' blood loss of at least 2000 ml.

Severe hemorrhage can lead to two distinct shock syndromes:

1. Rapid blood loss leads to uncompensated or poorly compensated hypovolemia with falls in vascular volume,

vascular resistance and cardiac index and a low flow shock state.

2. Slow ongoing blood loss allows sufficient time for a compensatory plasma volume increase with anemia, hemodilution and decreased oxygen-carrying capacity.[72]

Once massive blood loss occurs, initial resuscitation may be commenced using electrolyte-containing crystalloids [e.g. normal saline, lactated Ringer's (Hartmann's) or Ringer's acetate].[73] As bleeding gets heavier, colloid may be introduced but, once the 'allowable blood loss' is reached, blood transfusion must commence. It is useful for each obstetric patient to have an end-point at which any further losses are replaced with blood. This end-point is known as the 'allowable blood loss' (ABL) (Table 44.4) The amount of blood a parturient will be allowed to lose is dependent on the predelivery hematocrit and an acceptable post-hemorrhage hemoglobin which will allow adequate oxygen-carrying capacity for an active, breast-feeding mother. A schema for fluid delivery in a bleeding parturient is given in Table 44.4 and the formula for calculation of allowable blood loss in the resuscitation algorithm (Fig. 44.2). Massive blood transfusion is defined as 'total replacement of the patient's circulating blood volume within a short period of time'.[74]

The best colloid for use in the pregnant patient remains a contentious issue. Artificial colloids can be conveniently classified into three groups:

1. modified fluid gelatins (MFGs) and urea-linked gels (e.g. polygeline, Haemaccel);
2. dextran – sucrose fermentation polysaccharides (e.g. Macrodex, Rheomacrodex);
3. hydroxyethyl starches (HESs) (e.g. Hespan).

The artificial plasma expanders are relatively contraindicated in pregnancy because all can cause anaphylactoid reactions. These reactions and associated circulatory collapse are potentially more serious and have a worse prognosis in the parturient.[75] The MFGs are probably the safest in this regard because, although anaphylactoid reactions are frequent (0.028–0.78%), they are less serious than with HESs or dextrans. Anaphylactic reactions to dextran 40, 60 and 70 can be prevented by pretransfusion with dextran 1. On the other hand, dextrans can produce a hemostatic defect so that they are contraindicated in those with a clotting disorder and the dose should not exceed 1.5 g/kg/day.[73] Dextran 40 at 10% (but not dextran 40 at 3.5% or dextran 60) can also cause renal function disturbances with anuria, histamine release, formation of IgG and IgM anti-dextran antibodies and interfere with the enzyme tests (but not blood grouping, simple cross-match or Coombs) in the cross-matching of subsequent units of blood. HESs can also produce a hemostatic defect, but less so than the dextrans.[75–77] Because most pregnant patients with massive bleeding either have, or will develop, a coagulopathy, the induction of a hemostatic defect by the plasma expander is undesirable.[49]

The colloids derived from blood fractionation include fresh-frozen plasma (FFP), cryoprotein-free plasma, plasma protein fraction (PPF) and albumin. The first two carry a significant risk of transmission of viral disease, especially non-A, non-B hepatitis. Albumin (e.g. 5% albumin) can cause pyrogenic reactions and also small falls in systemic arterial pressure from infusion of a pre–kallikrein activator (Hagemann factor fragments) and sodium acetate. The major problem with its use however is the cost. If 500 ml of 4% albumin (SPPS, sterile plasma protein solution) costs 100 'cost units', the cost of treatment that would improve the blood volume by 1500 ml is 300 cost units for albumin, 39 for dextran 60 (with preinfusion of dextran 1), 33 for dextran 40 and 30 for gelatin (MFG) or lactated Ringer's.[75,76] Nevertheless, crystalloids and SPPS remain fluids of initial choice in the bleeding

Table 44.4 Example of fluid therapy in acute blood loss

Blood loss		Intravenous replacement (ml)		
		Crystalloid (e.g. Hartmann's/ lactated Ringer's)	Colloid e.g. 5% albumin	Blood or blood products
Up to 1000 ml Crystalloid only at 4.1 × shed blood volume	at 1000 ml	4100	–	–
At 1000 ml Start colloid at 1.4 × shed blood volume Maximum volume = 500 ml	at 1350 ml	4100	500	–
At allowable blood loss (ABL) Start packed RBCs at	at 1500 ml	4100	500	375 packed cells
0.25 × total volume loss	at 2000 ml	4100	500	500 packed cells
At 2000 ml Start whole blood at 1 : 1 with total blood loss ± platelets, ± fresh plasma	at 4000 ml	4100	500	500 packed cells 2000 whole blood

parturient. Crystalloids should be infused at 4.1 × shed blood volume (SBV) and colloids at 1.4 × SBV.[78]

The place of stroma-free hemoglobin (Hb) and crystalline hemoglobin solutions (CHb) in pregnancy has never been established.[72] Stroma-free Hb carries a virus (e.g. hepatitis B) transmission risk. With CHb, the offloading of oxygen at tissue level is compromised by the high affinity for oxygen of the unmodified CHb.[72]

In situations of massive blood loss (more than one total body blood volume), as increasing blood volumes are replaced with packed cells, the platelet count and fibrinogen and factors V, VIII and IX levels progressively fall while the prothrombin (PT) and partial thromboplastin (PPT) times rise.[65,79] These patients may require additional fresh-frozen plasma and platelets.[65] If the degree of vascular loading required is more than one blood volume, FFP should be added to maintain clotting factors at more than 30%. In these patients, the use of fresh or ultrafresh blood is preferable[74] (see Table 44.5).

Table 44.5 Blood transfusion of the exsanguinated pregnant patient showing, in decreasing order of desirability, the types of unfractionated blood available (Derived, with modification, from ref. 74, with permission)

Ultrafresh blood	Within 4 h of collection; preferably unrefrigerated All components functioning normally Availability limited by the need to test for viruses (e.g. HIV)
Fresh blood	Stored <7 days RBCs will transport and deliver oxygen normally immediately after transfusion
Stored blood	Stored >7 days Needs varying periods of time (hours) for RBCs to achieve normal function
Autologous blood	
Homologous blood	
Full compatibility tested	Includes tests for incomplete antibodies
Saline-crossmatched, group-specific blood	Can be made available within 5–10 min if mother has been grouped and screened for atypical antibodies
Group O, Rh-negative, low anti-A, low anti-B hemolysin blood	Not usually immediately available in large quantity
Group O, Rh-negative packed cells reconstituted in normal saline	Circumvents the problem of high titer ABO hemolysin
Group O, Rh-negative Blood	
Group O, Rh-positive blood	Rarely necessary but do not withhold if mother likely to die
Group O uncross-matched blood	Only extremely rarely necessary

BLOOD REPLACEMENT THERAPY

Some clinical blood transfusionists advocate that all haemotherapy should be given as blood component therapy, and that there are virtually no indications for the use of whole blood. This is not my view . . .

J P Isbister, 1984

The establishment of blood banking facilities has been one of the factors that have helped reduce maternal mortality drastically in the last 50 years.[4] While banked autologous blood has several advantages – no risk of immunization, transfusion reaction or infection (especially hepatitis) and less risk of clerical error – it has its limitations in obstetric anesthesia.[80,81] Apart from the risks of the development of uterine contractions and premature labor during phlebotomy, autologous stored blood has a limited shelf-life (of 42 days at 1–6°C in Adsol). On the one hand, the need for transfusion in obstetric practice overall is quite low so that the cost–benefit ratio may not justify participation of most patients in such programs.[80] On the other hand, bleeding in obstetrics, when it does occur, is usually heavy so that storage of autologous blood does not fully protect against homologous transfusion.[80] Nevertheless, in the high-risk pregnant patient who is not anemic there is a place for banking of autologous blood (e.g. if a placenta previa is diagnosed) or, for red cell salvage immediately preoperatively, isovolemic hemodilution with 2 : 1 or 3 : 1 crystalloid–phlebotomy blood and blood retransfusion when bleeding occurs (e.g. if elective lower segment cesarean delivery is planned in a Jehovah's Witness).[80,81]

Homologous transfusion should, whenever practicable, be with 'fresh' blood. 'Fresh' blood should strictly apply to blood that has just been collected, but blood bankers have extended the term to include blood up to 1 week old.[74] When more than the patient's circulating blood volume has been replaced in less than 4 h, ultrafresh blood should be requested (see Table 44.5). It is becoming increasingly difficult to obtain truly 'ultrafresh' blood because of the need to exclude contamination of the donor sample with HIV (AIDS) virus.

The need for 'group O , negative' (or, worse still, uncross-matched) blood in modern obstetric anesthesia practice is practically nil. The administration of ABO-compatible blood remains the single most important factor in the safety of blood transfusion (Table 44.6). Since a saline cross-match can be performed in 5–10 min and virtually guarantees ABO compatibility, volume resuscitation should continue and blood should not be administered till the saline cross-match is available. If a group and antibody screen has been performed, blood can be administered remarkably safely in an urgent situation. If the antibody screen is clear, the chance of an atypical antibody being detected on cross-match is remarkably small.[74]

Table 44.6 Serological safety of blood: probability of a transfusion being compatible with the recipient (Reproduced, with permission, from ref. 74)

Randomly selected blood (untyped units, untyped recipient)	64.4%
ABO compatibility	99.4%
ABO and Rh compatibility	99.8%
ABO and Rh compatibility with negative antibody screen	99.94%
Complete pretransfusion compatibility testing	99.95%
Autologous	100%

Only in the exsanguinated patient who is likely to die should uncross-matched blood be used. The most suitable form of stored blood for use in emergency situations is shown in Table 44.5. If rhesus-positive blood is the only blood available, it should not be withheld if the patient is likely to die because, if the blood group is not known, the probability of the patient being rhesus-positive is 85%, and it is unlikely that the rhesus-negative parturient will have an anti-D antibody.[74]

CONCLUSION

This chapter is an overview of the anesthetic management of the main causes of peripartum hemorrhage. While maternal mortality continues to fall, obstetric hemorrhage is still responsible for considerable mortality and morbidity. Only careful preplanning, 'eternal vigilance' and aggressive resuscitation will allow us to further decrease morbidity from massive blood loss.

REFERENCES

1. Cruikshank S H 1986 Management of postpartum and pelvic hemorrhage. Clin Obstet Gynecol 29: 213–219
2. Prendiville W, Elbourne D, Chalmers I 1988 The effects of routine oxytocic administration in the management of the third stage of labour: an overview of the evidence from controlled trials. Br J Obstet Gynaecol 95: 3–16
3. Kaunitz A M, Hughes J M, Grimes D A, Smith J C, Rochat R W, Kafrissen M E 1985 Causes of maternal mortality in the United States. Obstet Gynecol 65: 605–612
4. Kirshon B, Hinkley C M, Cotton D B, Miller J 1990 Maternal mortality in a maternal – fetal medicine intensive care unit. J Reprod Med 35: 25–28
5. Biehl D R 1990 The anesthetic management of obstetrical hemorrhage. Int Anesthesiol Clin 28: 52–57
6. Gatt S P 1986 Anesthetic management of the obstetric patient with antepartum or intrapartum hemorrhage. Clin Anaesthesiol 4: 373–388
7. Hill D J, Beischer N A 1980 Placenta praevia without antepartum hemorrhage. Aust N Z J Obst Gynaecol 20: 21–23
8. Green Thompson R W 1982 Antepartum hemorrhage. Clin Obstet Gynecol 9: 3: 479–515
9. Silver R, Depp R, Sabbagha R E, Dooley S L, Socol M L, Tamura R K 1984 Placenta previa: aggressive expectant management. Am J Obstet Gynecol 150: 15–22
10. Paterson M E 1979 Aetiology and outcome of abruptio placentae. Acta Obstet Gynecol Scand 58: 31–35
11. Sandberg E C, McLennan C E 1974 Abruptio placentae and placenta previa. In: McLennan Ĉ E, Sandberg E C (eds) Synopsis of obstetrics, Mosby, St Louis, Vol 9: 250–266
12. Gottesfeld K R 1983 Managing the placental abruption. Contemp Obstet Gynecol 22(6): 20–22
13. Gilabert J, Estelles A, Aznar J, Galbir M 1985 Abruptio placentae and disseminated intravascular coagulation. Acta Obstet Gynecol Scand 64: 35–39
14. Maixner W, Rittenhouse E A, Barnes R W 1978 Early detection of hypovolaemia from directional arterial flow velocity. Circ Shock 5: 35–41
15. Nielsen N C 1970 Coagulation and fibrinolysis in mothers and their newborn infants following premature separation of placenta. Acta Obstet Gynecol Scand 49: 77–83
17. Datta S 1984 The High Risk Parturient. In: Ostheimer G (ed) Manual of obstetric anesthesia. Churchill Livingstone, New York, p 244
18. Schindler M, Gatt S, Isert P, Morgans D, Cheung A 1990 Thrombocytopenia and platelet functional defects in pre-eclampsia: implications for regional anesthesia. Anaesth Intensive Care 18: 169–174
19. Naeye R L 1980 Abruptio placentae and placenta praevia: frequency, perinatal mortality and cigarette smoking. Obstet Gynecol 88: 765–770
20. Abdul Karim A W, Chevli A N 1976 Antepartum hemorrhage and shock. Clin Obstet Gynecol 19: 553
21. Knab D R 1978 Abruptio placentae: an assessment of the time and method of delivery. J Obstet Gynecol 52: 625–629
22. MacDonald J S, Kryc J J 1981 Anesthetic considerations in the presence of intrapartum emergencies. Clin Perinatol 8: 145
23. McShane P M, Heyl P S 1985 Maternal and perinatal morbidity resulting from placenta previa. Obstet Gynecol 65: 176–182
24. Crenshaw C, Darnell Jones D E, Parker R T 1973 Placenta praevia: A survey of twenty years experience with improved perinatal survival by expectant therapy and Cesarean delivery. Obstet Gynecol Survey 28: 461–470
25. Neale E J, Rogers M S 1989 Vaginal ultrasound for ruling out placenta previa. Case report. Br J Obstet Gynaecol 96: 881
26. Kryc J J 1982 Anesthesia in the high risk obstetric patient. Clin Perinatol 9: 113
27. Jeffrey R B, Federle M P 1988 The collapsed inferior vena cava: CT evidence of hypovolaemia. Am Roentgenol 150: 431–432
28. Goodlin R C, Quaife M A, Dirksen J W 1981 The significance, diagnosis, and treatment of maternal hypovolaemia as associated with fetal/maternal illness. Semin Perinatol 5: 163–174
29. Nuwayhid B, Vaughn D, Brinkman C R, Assali N S 1978 Circulatory shock in pregnant sheep. IV. Fetal and neonatal circulatory responses to hypovolemia – influence of anesthesia. Am J Obstet Gynecol 132: 658–666
30. Rose J C, Morris M, Meis P J 1981 Hemorrhage in newborn lambs: effects on arterial blood pressure, ACTH, cortisol and vasopressin. Am J Physiol 240: 585–590
31. Goodlin R C 1982 Why treat 'physiologic' anemias of pregnancy? J Reprod Med 27: 639–646
32. Fortney S M, Nadel E R, Wenger C B, Bove J R 1981 Effect of acute alterations of blood volume on circulatory performance in humans. J App Physiol 50: 292–298
33. Pritz M B, Kindt G W 1981 Transient neurologic deficits associated with congestive heart failure and hypovolaemia. Surg Neurol 15: 467–470
34. Perbeck L, Hedqvist P 1982 Blood pressure responses associated with hemorrhagic shock in anesthetised rats. Acta Chirurg Scand 148: 3–8
35. Bond R F, Peissner L C, Manning E S 1977 Skeletal muscle vascular decompensation in dogs subjected to prolonged hypovolaemia. Circ Shock 4: 327–344
36. Lundvall J, Gustafsson D 1982 Impairment during marked hypotension of the plasma volume control in hemorrhage. Acta Physiol Scand 114: 371–378
37. Barkan A L 1989 Pituitary atrophy in patients with Sheehan's syndrome. Am J Med Sci 298: 38–40
38. Carp H 1990 Anesthesia for Cesarean delivery. Int Anesthesiol Clin 28: 25–29

39. Ruiz C E , Weil M H, Carlson R W 1979 Treatment of circulatory shock with dopamine. J Am Med Assoc 242: 165–168
40. Yang S C, Puri V K 1986 Role of preoperative hemodynamic monitoring in intraoperative fluid management. Am J Surg 52: 536–540
41. Eriksen N, Buttino L 1989 Vaginal birth after Cesarean section: a comparison of maternal and neonatal morbidity to elective repeat Cesarean section. Am J Perinatol 6: 375–379
42. Gellman E, Goldstein M S 1983 Vaginal delivery after Cesarean delivery. J Am Med Assoc 249: 2935–2937
43. Porreco R P, Meier P R 1984 Repeat Cesarean – mostly unnecessary. Contemporary Obstet Gynecology 24(3): 55
44. Keller F, Joyce T F 1984 Uterine rupture associated with the use of vaginal prostaglandin E_2 suppositories. Can Anaesth Soc J 31: 80–82
45. Crawford J S 1974 Epidural analgesia and uterine rupture. Lancet 1: 361
46. Eckstein K L 1973 Uterine rupture during epidural blockade. Can Anaesth Soc J 20: 566–568
47. Robson S C, Boys R J, Hunter S, Dunlop W 1989 Maternal hemodynamics after normal delivery and delivery complicated by postpartum hemorrhage. Obstet Gynecol 74: 234–239
48. Thonet R G 1986 Obstetric hysterectomy – an 11 year experience. Br J Obstet Gynaecol 93: 794–798
49. Beaudoin M, Gatt S 1986 Disseminated intravascular coagulation. In: Datta S, Ostheimer G (eds) Common problems in obstetric anesthesia, Vol 21. Year Book Medical Publications, Chicago, pp 348–361
50. Gatt S 1990 Haematological disorders responsible for bleeding in late pregnancy. Anaesth Intensive Care 18: 335–347
51. Zanini A, Norchi S, Beretta, E, Bottino S 1988 Postpartum hemorrhage – a continuing problem. Br J Obstet Gynaecol 9: 731–732
52. Feinberg B B, Resnick E, Hurt W G, Bump R C, Kubota R, Cho S R 1987 Angiographic embolisation in the management of late postpartum hemorrhage. J Reprod Med 32: 929–931
53. Plumer M H 1982 Bleeding problems. In: James F M, Wheeler A S (eds) Obstetric anesthesia: the complicated patient, Vol 9. F A Davis, Philadelphia, pp 185–208
54. Herbert N P, Cefalo R C 1984 Management of postpartum hemorrhage. Clin Obstet Gynecol 27: 139–147
55. Chestnut D H, Eden R D, Gall S A, Parker R T 1985 Peripartum hysterectomy: a review of Cesarean and postpartum hysterectomy. Obstet Gynecol 65: 365–370
56. Pedrón N, Mondragón H, Marcushamer B, Aznar R, Gallegos A J 1987 Estimates of postpartum bleeding. Contraception 35: 339–345
57. Peyser R, Kupferminc M J 1990 Management of severe postpartum hemorrhage by intrauterine irrigation with prostaglandin E_2. Am J Obstet Gynecol 162: 694–696
58. Oleen M A, Mariano J P 1990 Controlling refractory atonic postpartum hemorrhage with hemabate sterile solution. Am J Obstet Gynecol 162: 205–208
59. Granström L, Ekman G, Ulmsten U 1989 Intravenous infusion of 15 methyl-prostaglandin $F_{2\alpha}$ (Prostinfenem) in women with heavy post-partum hemorrhage. Acta Obstet Gynecol Scand 68: 365–367
60. Schindler M, Gatt S, Isert P, Morgans D, Cheung A 1990 Thrombocytopenia and platelet functional defects in pre-eclampsia: implications for regional anesthesia. Anaesth Intensive Care 18: 169–174
61. DePace N L, Betesh J S 1982 'Postmortem' Cesarean section with recovery of both mother and offspring. J Am Med Assoc 248: 971–973
62. Gin T, Gregory M A, Oh T E 1990 The hemodynamic effects of propofol and thiopentone for induction of Cesarean section. Anaesth intensive Care: 18: 175–179
63. Yau G, Gin T, Ewart M C, Kotur C F, Leung R k W, Oh T E 1991 Propofol for induction and maintenance of Anesthesia at Cesarean section. Anesthesia 46: 20–23
64. Hew-Wing P, Rolbin S H, Hew E, Amato D 1989 Epidural anesthesia and thrombocytopenia. Anaesthesia 44: 775–777
65. Murray D J, Olson J, Strauss R, Tinker J H 1988 Coagulation changes during packed red cell replacement of major blood loss. Anesthesiology 69: 839–845
66. Miller R D, Robbins T O, Tong M J, Barton S L 1971 Coagulation defects associated with massive blood transfusions. Ann Surg 175: 794–801
67. Elbert T J, Kotrly K J, Madsen K E, Bernstein J S, Kampine J P 1988 Fentanyl–diazepam anesthesia with or without N_2O does not attenuate cardiopulmonary baroreflex-mediated vasoconstrictor responses to controlled hypovolaemia in humans. Anesth Analg 67: 548–554
68. Baker D P 1982 Trauma in the pregnant patient. Surg Clin N Am 62: 275–289
69. Idvall J 1981 Influence of ketamine anestheisa on cardiac output and tissue perfusion in rats subjected to hemorrhage. Anesthesiology 55: 297–304
70. Figueras J, Weil M H 1979 Hypovolemia and hypotension complicating management of acute cardiogenic pulmonary edema. Am J Cardiol 44: 1349–1355
71. Weiss H R, Levy P J, Kleinert H D, Murthy V S 1978 Alterations in brain and muscle oxygenation during hypovolaemia and replacement with plasma substitutes in rats. Circ Shock 5: 115–124
72. Hauser C J, Shoemaker W C 1982 Hemoglobin solution in the treatment of hemorrhagic shock. Crit Care Med 10: 283 – 287
73. Modig J 1986 Effectiveness of dextran 70 versus Ringer's acetate in traumatic shock and adult respiratory distress syndrome. Crit care Med 14: 454–457
74. Isbister J P 1984 Haemotherapy for acute hemorrhage. Anaesth Intensive Care 12: 217–228
75. Fourth French Consensus Conference on Intensive care and Emergency Medicine 1990 Selection of a fluid for vascular expansion in the treatment of hypovolaemia in adult patients. Vox Sang 58: 150–151
76. Munsch C M, MacIntyre E, Machin S J, Mackie I J, Treasure T 1988 Hydroxyethyl starch: an alternative to plasma for postoperative volume expansion after cardiac surgery. Br J Surg 75: 675–678
77. Puri V K, Paidipaty B, White L 1981 Hydroxyethyl starch for resuscitation of patients with hypovolemia and shock. Crit Care Med 9: 833–837
78. Shoemaker W C 1982 Evaluation of colloids, crystalloids, whole blood, and red cell therapy in the critically ill patient. Clin Lab Med 2: 35–63
79. Goodwin T M 1989 Congenital hypofibrinogenaemia in pregnancy. Obstet Gynecol Survey 44: 157–161
80. Herbert W N P, Owen H G, Collins M L 1988 Autologous blood storage in obstetrics. Obstet Gynecol 72: 166–170
81. Davis R 1979 Banked autologous blood for Cesarean section. Anaesth Intensive Care 7: 358–361
82. Romero R 1983 The management of acquired hemostatic defect during pregnancy. In: Berkowitz R L (ed) 1983 Critical care of the obstetric patient, vol 9. Churchill Livingstone, New York, pp 219–284

45. Pregnancy-induced hypertension

Part A USA view. *J. L. Hawkins*
Part B UK view. *J. Moore*
Part C Australian view. *M. D. Westmore*

PART A
USA VIEW
J. L. Hawkins

NEW IDEAS ON ETIOLOGY AND DEMOGRAPHICS

Although the etiology of pregnancy-induced hypertension (PIH) remains elusive, a great deal is known about the demographics of the disease.[1] The young nulliparous patient who has not received adequate prenatal care is classically described as being at risk. There is a familial component as well. Compared with a 5–10% risk overall, the frequency of the disease in daughters of preeclamptic women is 28%, while in siblings the risk is 42%. Concurrent medical conditions such as diabetes, chronic hypertension, renal disease, molar pregnancy, fetal hydrops or multiple gestation also place the parturient at greater risk of PIH. The prevalence in a second pregnancy is 47% for women who had PIH during their first pregnancy compared with 8% if they were normotensive.

The etiology has been much more difficult to elucidate. Although there is a relative deficiency of prostacyclin leading to vasospasm and platelet activation,[2] this deficiency does not seem to occur until the disease is clinically evident.[3] Thus a prostacyclin–thromboxane imbalance may lead to clinical signs, but is probably not a primary cause of PIH. Abnormal immunologic response to the developing placenta has also been proposed as an etiology. Barrier contraception which prevented maternal exposure to semen was associated with a 2.37-fold increase in the risk of PIH when pregnancy occurred, implicating altered or inadequate immunoprotection of the fetoplacental unit.[4] The hypothesis that endothelial cell damage incites the vasoconstriction, intravascular fluid leakage and coagulation cascade characteristic of PIH[5] is supported by a longitudinal study examining the hemodynamics of pregnancy.[6] Women were followed throughout pregnancy with Doppler cardiac outputs, and those destined to develop PIH had significantly elevated cardiac outputs even in the first trimester, antedating development of hypertension. This hyperdynamic state may mediate end-organ damage by dilating afferent arterioles and exposing capillary beds to systemic pressures that result in diffuse endothelial damage. The damaged endothelial cells then activate the coagulation cascade and also fail to act as a barrier to extravascular fluid extravasation. The beneficial effect of beta-blockade with labetalol in ameliorating proteinuria supports this hypothesis.

ALTERED PHYSIOLOGY AND PREOPERATIVE EVALUATION

Pregnancy-induced hypertension can adversely affect every organ system, therefore a complete physical and laboratory evaluation of the patient is required. The cardiovascular profile of the patient with severe PIH has been elucidated in two large studies using invasive hemodynamic monitoring.[7,8] Both found a variety of hemodynamic profiles, but the predominant picture was one of elevated cardiac index with normal or hyperdynamic left ventricular function on Starling curves, a disproportionately elevated systemic vascular resistance and normal left ventricular filling pressures. In general, PIH is a high-output state with an inappropriately elevated systemic vascular resistance resulting in hypertension.

Edema occurs secondary to capillary endothelial defects, lower plasma oncotic pressure and increased hydrostatic pressure. Colloid osmotic pressure (COP) is reduced in parturients with PIH when compared with normotensive mothers (18 mmHg versus 22 mmHg) owing to the proteinuria associated with the disease.[9] Edema can also involve the tongue and glottis, causing airway obstruction and difficulty with intubation. A variety of smaller endotracheal tubes and alternative methods to secure the airway such as fiber-optic capability must be available. If invasive hemodynamic monitoring is in place, the COP–PCWP (pulmonary capillary wedge pressure) gradient can be used to guide fluid management. Development of pulmonary edema may be more likely when the gradient is less than 4 mmHg as a result of either an elevated PCWP or an abnormally low COP.

Thrombocytopenia is the most common coagulation abnormality, occurring in about 20% of patients with PIH. Damaged endothelium increases platelet consumption. Defects in platelet function have also been reported to occur in 12–25% of patients even when the platelet count is greater than 150 000/mm.[3,10,11] Some centers have adopted a policy of obtaining a bleeding time in all patients with PIH prior to receiving regional anesthesia, but this policy requires additional staff and equipment and the bleeding time may not represent the hematologic status of the patient. Other studies have shown that asymptomatic parturients have a 6–8% prevalence of thrombocytopenia, and many have received regional anesthesia without incident.[12,13] There is no published case of epidural hematoma occurring after epidural anesthesia in a patient with PIH. A recent review of the literature on bleeding time concluded that there is no evidence that bleeding times predict the adequacy of hemostasis or risk of bleeding elsewhere in the body.[14] Adverse outcomes must be very rare, but the use of regional anesthesia in the patient with a platelet count less than 100 000/mm^3 must be weighed against the alternatives of general anesthesia or other forms of pain relief. A rapidly falling platelet count or platelet count of less than 100 000/mm^3 should be a relative contraindication to regional anesthesia. Alterations in fibrinogen, prothrombin time (PT) or partial thromboplastin time (PTT) occur rarely, and disseminated intravascular coagulation is seen only in severe disease, usually in association with a placental abruption.

A microangiopathic hemolytic anemia may be seen in 10% of patients with severe PIH associated with thrombocytopenia and elevated liver enzymes – the HELLP (Hemolysis, Elevated Liver enzymes, Low Platelets) syndrome. This subset of patients has increased maternal and perinatal morbidity and mortality. Even in milder forms of PIH there is low-grade destruction of red cells owing to endothelial cell damage and vasospasm. The increased heme catabolism produces higher levels of carboxyhemoglobin in the parturient with PIH (2.8% versus 0.7% in the healthy mother) and causes a leftward shift of the oxyhemoglobin dissociation curve. Normal P_{50} in pregnancy is about 30 mmHg, while in PIH it is below even the nonpregnant value at 24.4 mmHg.[15] The resulting shift decreases the release of oxygen to the fetus, perhaps increasing the risk of fetal distress and intrauterine growth retardation.

Hepatic involvement is characterized by right upper quadrant pain due to capsular stretching. Elevated liver function tests are seen on laboratory examination. Subcapsular hemorrhage and liver rupture can occur and be life-threatening. Large-bore intravenous access should be maintained separate from medication infusions if hepatic involvement is suspected. When associated with the HELLP syndrome, coagulopathy and hemolysis add to maternal morbidity.

A combination of intravascular volume depletion with or without renal artery vasospasm may decrease creatinine clearance and urine output, and elevate serum blood urea nitrogen (BUN) and creatinine. Since normal values for BUN and creatinine during pregnancy are about half nonpregnant values, a creatinine > 1 mg/dl indicates significant renal insufficiency. Impaired excretion of magnesium sulfate may cause toxicity if dosages are not reduced.

PIH is the third leading cause of maternal mortality with cerebral hemorrhage as the main cause of death. Headaches, visual disturbances including cortical blindness, and seizures are symptomatic of CNS involvement. Although the etiology of seizures is unknown, pathologic examination shows numerous small hemorrhages, capillary thrombi, and small infarcts. When 44 eclamptic patients were examined by computerized tomographic (CT) scan, 26 were normal, three had cerebral thrombosis or hemorrhage, six had low-density areas in the cortical lobes and subcortical white matter and nine were classified as having cerebral atrophy with enlarged cerebral ventricles.[16] Criteria for obtaining a CT scan in an eclamptic patient are controversial, but patients who present with focal neurologic signs, decreasing level of consciousness or recurring seizures despite therapeutic levels of magnesium or phenytoin should probably be further examined.

Because of the potential for rapidly changing multisystem involvement, every patient with PIH should be evaluated with a complete blood count, platelet count, fibrinogen, PT and PTT, BUN and creatinine, liver function tests, and magnesium level every 6–8 h while in labor.

MONITORING

When and how to use invasive hemodynamic monitoring in the parturient with severe PIH is a controversial subject. At a minimum, monitoring should include a fetal scalp electrode, automated blood pressure, accurate intake and output measurements (usually requiring a urinary catheter), deep tendon reflexes for clinical signs of magnesium toxicity and close nursing supervision. The patient with moderate PIH (diastolic pressure of 100–110 mmHg) may benefit from an intra-arterial catheter for continuous observation of blood pressure trends, especially during an anesthetic or when intravenous vasodilators such as sodium nitroprusside are used. Also, if the patient is obese, accurate cuff pressures may be difficult to obtain. The patient with thrombocytopenia or other coagulopathy can avoid repeated needle sticks for laboratory blood collection when an arterial line is present.

Patients with severe PIH can present with profound hemodynamic derangements and may benefit from placement of a pulmonary artery catheter to determine their hemodynamic profile. Currently accepted guidelines for placement of a pulmonary artery catheter in the patient with PIH are:

1. diastolic blood pressure >110 mmHg unresponsive to conventional antihypertensive therapy (usually hydralazine);
2. oliguria unresponsive to fluid challenge;
3. pulmonary edema; and
4. during major regional anesthesia to guide the amount of acute hydration given and appropriate treatment of hypotension.[17]

These guidelines are useful, but can be controversial. Although it becomes much easier to choose an antihypertensive agent (i.e. beta-blocking agent versus a vasodilator) when the hemodynamic profile is known, anesthesiologists are experienced in treating hypertension in the operating room, and new drugs such as labetalol have proved to be safe for mother and fetus.[18,19] Oliguria rarely leads to renal failure in parturients, but most clinicians would prefer to maintain urine output at least 0.5 ml/$kg^{-1}.h^{-1}$. Oliguria may be unrelated to volume status, and may even be associated with high filling pressures requiring preload or afterload reduction.[20] Volume expansion may decrease systemic vascular resistance, thereby improving renal and uteroplacental perfusion, but it may also increase the risk of peripartum pulmonary or cerebral edema. Since a variety of hemodynamic profiles can be associated with oliguria, a more informed choice of therapy can be made if hemodynamic monitoring is present while avoiding the risk of volume overload. Treatment of pulmonary edema is obviously facilitated by knowledge of filling pressures and cardiac function. In addition, pulmonary edema is most likely to occur post-partum when colloid osmotic pressure falls to its lowest level and edema fluid is mobilized. Knowledge of the COP–PCWP gradient allows optimization of the Starling forces influencing edema production. Finally, the use of epidural analgesia and anesthesia in parturients with PIH is considered the preferred anesthetic technique by most obstetric anesthesiologists who deal with high-risk patients,[21] but appropriate intravascular volume expansion while slowly raising the anesthetic level is necessary to avoid unwanted hypotension, especially with the high sympathectomy produced for cesarean delivery.

Why not simply a central venous pressure (CVP) catheter? First, most of the morbidity which occurs with central monitoring (other than iatrogenic errors in interpreting and using the information) occurs during placement and includes carotid artery puncture, pneumothorax or hemothorax and dysrhythmias. These risks are similar for CVP or pulmonary artery catheter placement. Most can be decreased by use of an antecubital vein if internal jugular vein landmarks are poor, or there is a coagulopathy. Second, there is a poor correlation between CVP and PCWP data when PIH is severe. The high systemic vascular resistance often associated with severe PIH may raise left heart pressures without causing right ventricular dysfunction. A comparison of 207 simultaneous measurements of CVP and PCWP in 18 patients with severe PIH found there was no relationship between right- and left-sided pressures in 39% of patients. While 56% had a linear relationship, the gradient varied so widely there was no predictive value.[22] Although it is unlikely that a CVP <6 mmHg will be associated with an elevated PCWP, values above that may not be indicative of left-sided filling pressures.

Certainly a major consideration in the decision to use invasive monitoring is the availability of critical care nursing staff familiar with the techniques of placement, interpretation of waveforms and recording of data. Most labor and delivery nurses will not be comfortable in the intensive care unit setting (and vice versa!), and without such training these techniques may cause more harm than good.

PREOPERATIVE MANAGEMENT OF SPECIAL PROBLEMS

Seizures

When seizures occur, the first consideration is maintenance of a patent airway. Attempting to insert a tongue blade or oral airway is likely to break a tooth or induce regurgitation and should not be attempted. Place the patient on her left side with oxygen by mask and closely observe for signs of airway obstruction. A small dose of thiopental (50–75 mg) can be used to stop the seizure without further obtunding the patient, thus allowing a more accurate neurologic examination. Diazepam has a prolonged duration of action in the mother and has been associated with neonatal hypotonia and hypothermia if delivery becomes necessary. If the patient is not maintaining her airway, if regurgitation occurs or if there are recurrent seizures, the airway should be secured by endotracheal intubation after succinylcholine. The fetus will show signs of distress during and immediately after the seizure owing to maternal acidosis and hypoxia, but this does not necessitate immediate cesarean delivery before the mother is stabilized. The fetus will recover rapidly in utero if the mother is reoxygenated and aortocaval compression is prevented. If the seizure occurred despite therapeutic levels of magnesium sulfate, there should be heightened concern for a structural neurologic lesion such as intracranial bleeding. Consider further neurologic work-up and addition of another anti-seizure medication such as phenytoin.

Oliguria

Management of oliguria has been discussed above.[20] The first approach should be a fluid bolus of 500 ml of crystalloid. If the patient's hemodynamics falls in the subset of low filling pressures, hyperdynamic myocardium and high systemic vascular resistance, this should produce an increase in urine output. If this simple maneuver is unsuccessful, consideration should be given to placing a pulmonary artery catheter before further fluids are given or diuretics used. The other common hemodynamic subset in oliguric patients is high filling pressures, high cardiac index and normal systemic vascular resistance, which responds to vasodilator therapy. An occasional patient may have elevated filling pressures, depressed cardiac indices and markedly elevated systemic vascular resistance, which should respond to fluid restriction and aggressive afterload reduction. In the absence of obvious pre- or post-renal causes, low-dose dopamine therapy (1–5 μg/kg/min) has also been used successfully to increase urine output and sodium excretion.[23]

Pulmonary edema

Pulmonary edema commonly becomes manifest in the post-partum period. It may be caused by volume overload or by acute increases in afterload (often at the time of intubation) leading to cardiac dysfunction. Although noncardiogenic causes of pulmonary edema are rare, hemodynamic monitoring allows this diagnosis to be excluded while facilitating rapid optimization of hemodynamic parameters. Nitroglycerin has been used in this setting to correct the hydrostatic derangements by decreasing PCWP, although oxygenation was not improved.[24]

Hypertension

A number of antihypertensive agents have been used safely and effectively in the setting of severe acute hypertension. Drugs commonly used antepartum are hydralazine and labetalol. In the operating room, anesthesiologists are more comfortable using a rapidly acting intravenous agent such as trimethaphan, nitroglycerin or nitroprusside to prevent or treat the acute hypertension associated with laryngoscopy, intubation, and emergence. In the recovery room and during the post-partum period, parenteral d-methyldopa, sublingual nifedipine, labetalol and clonidine have all been used successfully and can be extended to long-term use if needed. Three drugs should probably be avoided in the antepartum period because of potential adverse fetal effects. In animal studies, esmolol caused prolonged beta-blockade in the fetus despite rapid decline in plasma levels.[25] Human studies are lacking. Clonidine produced maternal and fetal hypoxemia in animal studies when given parenterally while also increasing uterine tone and decreasing uterine blood flow.[26] Finally, angiotensin-converting enzyme inhibitors have been associated with neonatal hypotension, neonatal renal failure and teratogenicity.[27]

ANALGESIA FOR LABOR AND VAGINAL DELIVERY

After initial evaluation and stabilization of the mother and fetus, the obstetrician must decide on the best mode of delivery. This decision must be made in consultation with the anesthesiologist for optimal management of both patients. If a trial of labor is planned, epidural analgesia is widely used because it offers many advantages. Levels of circulating catecholamines are lowered after epidural analgesia, which may improve uterine blood flow and blood pressure control.[28] If hypotension is avoided, intervillous blood flow to the fetus is also improved.[29] Continuous epidural analgesia is a very flexible technique which can be used to provide effective analgesia or anesthesia for spontaneous vaginal delivery and forceps, or cesarean delivery as needed. Also, if there is an extensive perineal repair or cesarean delivery, post-operative analgesia can be provided with epidural opioids. A sympathectomy can also be maintained post-partum using dilute solutions of local anesthetics to buffer intravascular volume changes during fluid mobilization.

There are specific considerations when inducing a regional anesthetic in a patient with PIH. Coagulation status should be evaluated prior to the procedure, preferably with serial platelet counts and fibrinogen measurements to document any downward trend. There is still tremendous variability in the use of the bleeding time,[30,31] and its clinical usefulness remains in question. Intravascular volume status must also be evaluated to avoid adverse hemodynamic effects when the sympathectomy occurs. If there is normal urine output and hematocrit, a normal amount of acute hydration should be adequate provided the level of anesthesia is titrated slowly. Criteria for placement of invasive hemodynamic monitoring have been discussed previously.

The use of epinephrine in combination with local anesthetics is also controversial in the patient with PIH. Although normal parturients develop attenuated responses to endogenous and exogenous catecholamines,[32] preeclamptic patients do not make that adaptation.[33] The consequences of an unintentional intravascular injection of an epinephrine-containing solution of local anesthetic could be catastrophic in the hypertensive parturient.

Epidural epinephrine may also impair uteroplacental blood flow, although the data are controversial.[34,35] If epinephrine is to be added to the local anesthetic solution, the lowest concentration should be used in small incremental doses with meticulous technique to avoid intravascular injection.

Subarachnoid opioids may offer another option for early labor analgesia. Although they do not provide anesthesia for the second stage of labor or for instrumentation, good analgesia is obtained earlier in labor without sympathectomy or motor blockade.[36] Since **micro catheters** for spinal anesthesia are not currently available in the USA, the epidural space can be identified with a Tuohy needle and a single injection of subarachnoid opioid administered using the Tuohy needle as an introducer. An epidural catheter is then placed for later use.

ANESTHESIA FOR CESAREAN DELIVERY

The advantages of epidural anesthesia for cesarean delivery are similar to those for labor and vaginal delivery. When compared with general anesthesia, epidural anesthesia also avoids excessive hypertension during laryngoscopy and intubation,[37] allows the patient to maintain her own airway, reduces the risk of aspiration and allows the patient's mental status to be monitored if there is concern about neurologic involvement. For cesarean delivery, it is more important to evaluate acute hydration accurately since the sympathectomy will be more extensive. More invasive hemodynamic monitoring may be indicated. During induction of epidural anesthesia, the amount of acute fluid hydration and the selection of pressor agents can be titrated against cardiac output, filling pressures and systemic vascular resistance.

The best choice of local anesthetic for cesarean delivery is not clear. The fast onset of chloroprocaine may make hypotension more likely and it may interfere with the use of epidural opioids for post-operative pain. Bupivacaine is slow in onset and provides a less dense block with the 0.5% concentration available in the USA. Lidocaine is intermediate in onset and duration, but epinephrine is usually added to allow an adequate volume to be given without approaching a toxic dose.

If general anesthesia is required because of urgency or coagulopathy, there are special considerations. Appropriate aspiration prophylaxis should be given. Magnesium is a tocolytic and may contribute to uterine atony and blood loss. Patients with HELLP syndrome may also require blood products, so large-bore intravenous access is required. Laryngeal edema may be marked, especially if there is facial edema, hoarseness, difficulty in swallowing or recent history of an upper respiratory tract infection. Awake intubation may be required, and smaller endotracheal tubes should always be available. Hypertension at the time of laryngoscopy and intubation may be managed with a rapid-acting vasodilator such as nitroglycerin, nitroprusside or trimethaphan. Intravenous lidocaine (1.5 mg/kg), alfentanil (10 – 20 μg/kg) and magnesium sulfate (40 mg/kg) have also been used to attenuate the response to intubation without apparent effects on the fetus.[38]

During maintenance of anesthesia, recall that the P_{50} in preeclamptic patients is only 24 mmHg and any further leftward shift due to hyperventilation will decrease release of oxygen to the fetus and maternal tissues.[15] Isoflurane is probably the inhalation agent of choice. Its hemodynamic effect is primarily vasodilation, and it avoids the potential problems of further hepatic dysfunction associated with halothane and of lowered seizure threshold associated with enflurane. All nondepolarizing muscle relaxants will be potentiated by magnesium sulfate and should be carefully monitored with a nerve stimulator.[39] The duration of action of succinylcholine is not prolonged when given as a single dose, although less will be required when given by infusion[40] or when magnesium sulfate has recently been administered.

POST-PARTUM CONSIDERATIONS

Monitoring of the parturient should continue for at least 24 h post-partum. Most cases of pulmonary edema occur in the post-partum period as mobilization of fluids begins and filling pressures rise.[41] If a regional anesthetic was used, central volume will increase as the sympathetic block resolves and vascular tone returns. If the patient does not begin to diurese spontaneously, diuretics and/or low-dose dopamine can be used to improve urine output. Patients with HELLP syndrome are at particular risk of post-partum eclampsia and may also not reach the nadir of their thrombocytopenia until 2–3 days post-partum.[42] Finally, most patients will need antihypertensive medication for 6 weeks post-partum and a change from parenteral to oral medications must be made. Efficacy and compliance should be documented prior to discharge.

REFERENCES

1. O'Brien W F 1990 Predicting preeclampsia. Obstet Gynecol 75: 445–452
2. Makila U M, Viinikka L, Ylikorkala O 1984 Evidence that prostacyclin deficiency is a specific feature in preeclampsia. Am J Obstet Gynecol 148: 772–774
3. Ylikorkala O, Pekonen F, Viinikka L 1986 Renal prostacyclin and thromboxane in normotensive and preeclamptic pregnant women and their infants. J Clin Endocrinol Metab 63: 1307–1311
4. Klonoff-Cohen H S, Savitz D A, Celafo R C, McCann M F 1989 An epidemiologic study of contraception and preeclampsia. J Am Med Assoc 262: 3143–3147
5. Roberts J M, Taylor R N, Musci T J, Rodgers G M, Hubel C A, McLaughlin M K 1989 Preeclampsia: an endothelial cell disorder. Am J Obstet Gynecol 61: 1200–1204
6. Easterling T R, Benedetti T J 1989 Preeclampsia: a hyperdynamic disease model. Am J Obstet Gynecol 160: 1447–1453

7. Cotton D B, Lee W, Huhta J C, Dorman K F 1988 Hemodynamic profile of severe pregnancy-induced hypertension. Am J Obstet Gynecol 158: 523–529
8. Mabie W C, Ratts T E, Sibai B M 1989 The central hemodynamics of severe preeclampsia. Am J Obstet Gynecol 161: 1443–1448
9. Moise K H, Cotton D B 1987 Colloid osmotic pressure and pregnancy. In: Clark S K, Phelan J P, Cotton D B (eds) Critical care obstetrics. Medical Economics Books, Oradell, N J 71–90
10. Kelton J G, Hunter J S, Neame P B 1985 A platelet function defect in preeclampsia. Obstet Gynecol 65: 107–109
11. Ramanathan J, Sibai B M, Vu T, Chauhan D 1989 Correlation between bleeding times and platelet counts in women with preeclampsia undergoing cesarean section. Anesthesiology 71: 188–191
12. Burrows R F, Kelton J G 1988 Incidentally detected thrombocytopenia in healthy mothers and their infants. New Engl J Med 319: 142–145
13. Rolbin S H, Abbott D, Musclow E, Papsin F, Lie L M, Freedman J 1988 Epidural anesthesia in pregnant women with low platelet counts. Obstet Gynecol 71: 918–920
14. Rodgers R P C, Levin J 1990 A critical reappraisal of the bleeding time. Semin Thromb Hemost 16: 1–20
15. Kambam J R, Entman S, Mouton S, Smith B E 1988 Effect of preeclampsia on carboxyhemoglobin levels: a mechanism for decrease in P50. Anesthesiology 68: 433–434
16. Milliez J, Dahoun A, Boudraa M 1990 Computed tomography of the brain in eclampsia. Obstet Gynecol 75: 975–980
17. Clark S L, Cotton D B 1988 Clinical indications for pulmonary artery catheterization in the patient with severe preeclampsia. Am J Obstet Gynecol 158: 453–458
18. Eisenach J C, Mandell G, Dewan D M 1991 Maternal and fetal effects of labetalol in pregnant ewes. Anesthesiology 74: 292–297
19. Mabie W C, Gonzalez A R, Sibai B M, Amon E 1987 A comparative trial of labetalol and hydralazine in the acute management of severe hypertension complicating pregnancy. Obstet Gynecol 70: 328–333
20. Clark S K, Greenspoon J S, Aldahl D, Phelan J P 1986 Severe preeclampsia with persistent oliguria: management of hemodynamic subsets. Am J Obstet Gynecol 154: 490–494
21. Gutsche B 1986 The experts opine: is epidural block for labor and delivery and for cesarean section a safe form of analgesia in severe preeclampsia or eclampsia? Surv Anesthesiol 30: 304–311
22. Cotton D B, Gonik B, Dorman K, Harrist R 1985 Cardiovascular alterations in severe pregnancy-induced hypertension: relationship of central venous pressure to pulmonary capillary wedge pressure. Am J Obstet Gynecol 151: 762–764
23. Kirshon B, Lee W, Mauer M B, Cotton D B 1988 Effects of low-dose dopamine therapy in the oliguric patient with preeclampsia. Am J Obstet Gynecol 159: 604–607
24. Cotton D B, Jones M M, Longmire S, Dorman K F, Tessem J, Joyce T H 1986 Role of intravenous nitroglycerin in the treatment of severe pregnancy-induced hypertension complicated by pulmonary edema. Am J Obstet Gynecol 154: 91–93
25. Eisenach J C, Castro M I 1989 Maternally administered esmolol produces fetal beta-adrenergic blockade and hypoxemia in sheep. Anesthesiology 71: 718–722
26. Eisenach J C, Castro M I, Dewan D M, Rose J C, Grice S C 1988 Intravenous clonidine toxicity in pregnant ewes. Am J Obstet Gynecol 160: 471–476
27. Mehta N, Modi N 1989 ACE inhibitors in pregnancy. Lancet 2: 96–97
28. Abboud T, Artal R, Sarkis F, Henriksen E H, Kammula R K 1982 Sympathoadrenal activity, maternal, fetal, and neonatal responses after epidural anesthesia in the preeclamptic patient. Am J Obstet Gynecol 144: 915–918
29. Jouppila P, Jouppila R, Hollmen A, Koivula A 1982 Lumbar epidural analgesia to improve intervillous blood flow during labor in severe preeclampsia. Obstet Gynecol 59: 158–161
30. Voulgaropoulos D S, Palmer C M 1991 Coagulation studies in the parturient: how do we practice (Abstract)? Presented at the Society for Obstetric Anesthesia and Perinatology
31. Barker P, Callander C C 1991 Coagulation screening before epidural analgesia in preeclampsia. Anaesthesia 46: 64–67
32. Weiner C P, Martinez E, Chestnut D H, Ghodsi A 1989 Effect of pregnancy on uterine and carotid artery response to norepinephrine, epinephrine, and phenylephrine in vessels with documented functional endothelium. Am J Obstet Gynecol 161: 1605–1610
33. Leighton B L, Norris M C, DeSimone C A, Darby M J, Menduke H 1990 Pre-eclamptic and healthy term pregnant patients have different chronotropic responses to isoproterenol. Anesthesiology 72: 392–393
34. Albright G A, Jouppila R, Hollmen A I, Jouppila P, Vierola H, Koivula A. Epinephrine does not alter human intervillous blood flow during epidural anesthesia. Anesthesiology 54: 131–135
35. Marx G F, Elstein I D, Schuss M, Anyaegbunam A, Fleischer A 1990 Effects of epidural block with lignocaine and lignocaine–adrenaline on umbilical artery velocity wave ratios. Br J Obstet Gynaecol 97: 517–520
36. Leighton B L, DeSimone C A, Norris M C, Ben-David B 1989 Intrathecal narcotics for labor revisited: the combination of fentanyl and morphine intrathecally provides rapid onset of profound, prolonged analgesia. Anesth Analg 69: 122–125
37. Hodgkinson R, Husain F J, Hayashi R H 1980 Systemic and pulmonary blood pressure during caesarean section in parturients with gestational hypertension. Can Anaesth Soc J 27: 389–393
38. Allen R W, James M F M, Uys P C 1991 Attenuation of the pressor response to tracheal intubation in hypertensive proteinuric pregnant patients by lignocaine, alfentanil and magnesium sulphate. Br J Anaesth 66: 216–223
39. Baraka A, Yazigi A 1987 Neuromuscular interaction of magnesium with succinylcholine vecuronium sequence in the eclamptic parturient. Anesthesiology 67: 806–808
40. Morris R, Giesecke A H 1968 Potentiation of muscle relaxants by magnesium sulfate therapy in toxemia of pregnancy. South Med J 61: 25–28
41. Sibai B M, Mabie B C, Harvey C J, Gonzalez A R 1987 Pulmonary edema in severe preeclampsia-eclampsia: analysis of thirty-seven consecutive cases. Am J Obstet Gynecol 156: 1174–1179
42. Miles F J, Martin J N, Blake P G, Perry K G, Martin R W, Meeks G R 1990 Postpartum eclampsia: a recurring perinatal dilemma. Obstet Gynecol 76: 328–331

PART B
UK VIEW
J. Moore

INTRODUCTION

The number of women who died in England and Wales from causes related to pregnancy-induced hypertension (PIH) and the rate per million maternities for successive triennial assessments in the UK for the period 1970 to 1987 are shown in Table 45.1. The death rate from preeclampsia (PET) did not change between 1970–72 and 1985–87, whereas that for eclampsia declined. An accurate overall incidence of hypertension complicating pregnancy is not available. However, Moodley (1990),[2] by extrapolation of figures from the Oxford region, calculated that in the UK 180 cases of eclampsia per year could be expected. Their wide distribution makes it almost impossible for staff in obstetric units to gain experience in treatment and evaluation of different management regimens. A referral center in each health authority area so that intensive management facilities are available for mother and fetus/newborn has been recommended. Of the 25 deaths associated with PIH during the period 1982–84, 21 were due to cerebral hemorrhage, edema or infarction, whereas in the 1985–87 triennium 12 out of 27 deaths were attributed to pulmonary complications, nine of which were recorded as due to the adult respiratory distress syndrome. It is possible that patients who might previously have died at an earlier stage from cerebral complications are now, as a result of modern techniques of resuscitation, living long enough to develop lung pathology aggravated perhaps by fluid imbalance, leading to interference with ventilation and eventual death from hypoxia.

The decision on the mode and optimum time for delivery should be made by a management team consisting of obstetrician, neonatologist and anesthesiologist. In the majority of cases either spontaneous or induced labor with vaginal delivery will occur. Intrapartum management should involve the anesthesiologist, pain relief and sedation being his main concern. Increasing severity of PIH necessitates the use of antihypertensives and anticonvulsant/sedative treatment, and these will influence the choice and effect of analgesic therapy. In view of the physiologic increase in blood pressure as normal labor progresses, epidural analgesia/anesthesia which lessens or prevents this response would seem an obvious choice. However, this is not always available, and recourse has to be made to intravenous, intramuscular and inhalation methods of pain relief. Meperidine, 100–150 mg, is most commonly prescribed, but the patient does not obtain complete relief of discomfort. Repetitive treatments or one given within 2 h of delivery can cause infant respiratory depression. Meperidine is metabolized in the liver and one of its breakdown products, normeperidine, has convulsant effects.

Table 45.1 The absolute number of deaths and the rate per million maternities for England and Wales from PET and eclampsia from successive triennial Confidential Maternal Death reports from 1970 to 1987[1]

Triennium	Preeclampsia		Eclampsia	
	No.	Rate	No.	Rate
1970–72	14	6.1	29	12.6
1973–75	15	7.8	19	9.9
1976–78	16	9.1	13	7.4
1979–81	16	8.3	20	10.4
1982–84	11	5.8	14	7.4
1985–87	13	6.5	12	6.0

Meperidine does not prevent the hypertensive response associated with the progress of labor, so it is essential to continue both antihypertensive and anticonvulsant treatment. Methyldopa, hydralazine and diazoxide are commonly used, but the last two may cause a reflex tachycardia which may require control by a cardioselective β_1-adrenergic blocker.[3] A recent report[4] indicates that labetalol, with its α_1- and β_1-adrenergic blocking effects reduces blood pressure without inducing tachycardia or decreasing uteroplacental blood flow.

Diazepam, given as Diazemuls, is the most commonly used anticonvulsant and is usually given intravenously as a 10-mg initial bolus followed by an infusion of 40 mg in 0.5 L of 5% dextrose. Dosage is dictated by clinical response, the aim being to control irritability and hyperreflexia. Diazepam enhances meperidine analgesia but has both maternal and fetal disadvantages.[5] Life-threatening cardiorespiratory depression is less likely than with the other anticonvulsants. A specific antagonist, flumazenil, is now available. Magnesium sulfate, chlormethiazole and, more recently, phenytoin sodium are alternatives, the last having a marked anticonvulsant effect with a smaller risk of oversedation.[6] All of these drugs either alone or with opioid analgesics can cause unconsciousness with loss of airway reflexes with an associated risk of respiratory obstruction or lung soiling.

Any antihypertensive/sedative treatment requires constant nursing care and intensive cardiovascular monitoring including frequent arterial blood pressure and central venous pressure measurements. A noninvasive automatic blood pressure recorder is essential equipment for all delivery rooms. Invasive radial artery monitoring of blood pressure may be required in severe cases. The reliability of central venous pressure (CVP) measurement has been questioned and pulmonary artery catheterization has been used in severe PET.[7] However, unless inserted via a peripheral vein, serious complications can occur; thus, it is usually reserved for patients with pulmonary edema, cardiac failure or severe oliguria.

EPIDURAL ANALGESIA/ANESTHESIA

The major advantages of continuous epidural analgesia/anesthesia are better pain and stress management, easier control of maternal blood pressure, and its availability for assisted delivery should maternal or fetal condition deteriorate. Blood coagulation problems occur with PIH, and a coagulation screen is required before instituting this form of analgesia. Some women may have been treated with low-dose aspirin prophylaxis, which further complicates the situation. Contraindications are a thrombin time longer than that of the control plasma, usually by 10–15 s, and a platelet count below 100 000.[8] The reduced plasma volume in PIH predisposes the patient to dramatic hypotension as the vasodilation accompanying the autonomic blockade evolves. This complication can be reduced in severity and incidence by slow incremental injection of the local anesthetic into the epidural space, together with judicious expansion of the intravascular volume. The choice of i.v. fluid is controversial: crystalloid solutions, plasma expanders and human albumin solutions each having their advocates. Crawford[9] advocated close monitoring of the serum albumin concentration and stated that correction of deficits decreased the likelihood of pulmonary and cerebral edema in the postpartum period. Excessive use of crystalloid solutions to correct hypotension is dangerous. It is essential to ensure that the supine position is not the cause (aortocaval compression) and, if vasopressor drugs are required, an infusion of ephedrine 30 mg/250 ml should be titrated against maternal blood pressure response. Others prefer incremental dosing of 5 mg/ml. Pure α_1-adrenergic agonists can impair placental blood flow despite returning maternal blood pressure to acceptable levels. Concurrent hypotensive treatment is another cause of precipitous decreases in blood pressure and can reduce the responsiveness to vasopressor drugs. Intensive cardiovascular monitoring, including CVP measurement, greatly increases the safety of establishing epidural analgesia in severe PIH.

Epidural analgesia does not reduce the likelihood of convulsions, and careful assessment for evidence of neurologic irritability must be maintained. The anticonvulsant drugs mentioned earlier are appropriate, but if opioid analgesics have been given intramuscularly or intravenously prior to the institution of epidural analgesia the resultant complete relief of pain can be accompanied by deep sedation and respiratory depression. Opioid–local anesthetic mixtures are being used more frequently for epidural block, and the risk of respiratory depression from the cephalad spread of the opioid in the CSF is increased when anticonvulsant drugs are given.

Bupivacaine is the local anesthetic of choice, and following an initial slow incremental injection of either a 0.375% or 0.25% solution to obtain complete pain relief an infusion of 0.1% can be given at a rate of 10 ml/h. The need for top-up injections is reduced and, if required, a few milliliters of the 0.25% solution will quickly restore the analgesic state. Epidural opioids alone will give a considerable degree of pain relief in the first stage of labor and the risk of autonomic blockade is removed. Fentanyl, because of its high lipid solubility, is the most suitable, but more effective analgesia can be obtained if it is combined with a weak bupivacaine solution. A suggested regimen is bupivacaine 0.125% plus 2.0 μg/ml fentanyl infused at a rate of 8–12 ml/h after the loading of bupivacaine mentioned above. The risk of toxic effects from either drug is reduced but not eliminated. If instrumental delivery is required the epidural block may need to be intensified by a further dose of local anesthetic.

The use of epidural block for cesarean delivery in patients with PIH is controversial. Fetal compromise may rule it out entirely if it is not already established, and even so there may not be time to extend the block. Contraindications already mentioned with regard to epidural analgesia may be present. The more extensive blockade, to the T6 dermatome level or above, and the larger amount of local anesthetic required increases the likelihood of hypotension. In fulminant cases of PIH, the hyperreflexia and neurologic irritability may indicate that an eclamptic fit may occur during the operation. Oversedation can predispose to regurgitation of gastric contents and pulmonary aspiration. If these situations are not expected and adequate time is available, epidural anesthesia is a more satisfactory method. It should be induced slowly via a catheter taking at least 20 min using the incremental method advocated by Thompson et al.[10] Either bupivacaine 0.5% or lidocaine 2.0% can be used, the latter having the advantage of a shorter latent period. The addition of 5 μg/ml epinephrine is unnecessary with bupivacaine but will prolong the block with lidocaine and, if a dose exceeding 350 mg is required, it will diminish the likelihood of lidocaine toxicity. Epinephrine may cause a hypertensive response in these patients.

The usual criteria of management for epidural analgesia must be strictly observed and should include adequate i.v. hydration, availability of a vasopressor, oxygen inhalation, lateral displacement of the uterus and automatic blood pressure recording. All patients with PIH should receive routine clear antacid therapy and ranitidine 150 mg orally at 6-hourly intervals with an immediate preanesthetic dose of 30 ml of 0.3 M sodium citrate. Excessive i.v. fluid therapy to combat hypotension should be avoided and the judicious use of ephedrine by infusion, together with CVP monitoring, will avoid fluid overload. The intensity of the intraoperative block can be increased and post-operative analgesia provided by the epidural administration of 50–100 μg of fentanyl.

Contraindications to spinal anesthesia are similar to those for epidural anesthesia, but its more rapid onset means that hypotension is more likely and more severe.[1] Slight respiratory depression may be intensified and these cardiorespiratory problems can lead to a critical situation.

GENERAL ANESTHETIC MANAGEMENT

Rapid deterioration in the mother's condition or fetal distress may make general anesthesia mandatory. Maternal hyperreflexia, headache, visual disturbance, disorientation or oversedation that jeopardizes the airway as a result of either obstruction or aspiration are definite indications. Coagulation disorders may rule out epidural anesthesia. While the criteria for safe general anesthesia must be fulfilled meticulously, there are special problems to be considered when PIH complicates the pregnancy. Sedation will increase the likelihood of gastrointestinal stasis and impairment of the gastroesophageal sphincter mechanism. Regurgitation of acid gastric contents is more likely so that antacid prophylaxis is essential. H_2-receptor blockers given by the intravenous route have a delayed onset, and, even if given orally as routine management, need to be supplemented by an immediate preanesthetic dose of clear antacid. At induction, two assistants for the anesthesiologist greatly increase safety, one to apply cricoid pressure and the other to assist with instrumentation. The i.v. bolus injections of the induction agent can cause marked hypotension in the patient already treated with hypotensive drugs. Laryngoscopy and tracheal intubation have the reverse effect, almost always causing a hypertensive response. It is for these reasons that continuous blood pressure monitoring is essential by either noninvasive automatic recorder or direct measurement via the radial artery. The slow injection of the induction agent in the laterally tilted, fully oxygenated patient will do much to reduce the likelihood of hypotension, but active treatment to control the hypertensive response is necessary in the patient who has already shown resistance to blood pressure control. Hydralazine 5–10 mg i.v. for 5–10 min or lidocaine 1.5 mg/kg for 2–3 min prior to intubation or the short-acting hypotensive agents such as nitroglycerin and sodium nitroprusside have been used to effect blood pressure control. However, a safer approach may be the intravenous administration of 0.5–1 mg of alfentanil or 0.1 mg of fentanyl just prior to induction. However, as these opioids increase the risk of infant respiratory depression, an expert neonatologist should be present at delivery. Propofol has been shown to reduce hypertension during the induction–delivery interval in normal parturients, but its use in PIH has not been described.

Intubation difficulties are more likely in patients with PIH because of edema of the pharyngeal and laryngeal tissues.[12] Preoperative assessment should include examination for anatomical variants which predispose to difficulty, and all equipment necessary to deal with the unexpected situation should be available. Obesity and short stature will compound the problem. Succinylcholine is the relaxant of choice and a nondepolarizing neuromuscular blocking agent must not be given until correct placement of the tracheal tube is verified by auscultation and end-tidal carbon dioxide monitoring. Heroic attempts to intubate must not be made and the general anesthetic should continue following the principles of a failed intubation drill. Tissue oxygen saturation by pulse oximetry is a good guide to the adequacy of ventilation without an endotracheal airway. If there is no need for expediency and airway management is difficult, the patient should be awakened and a regional or local infiltration technique used. Awake intubation should be used where a very difficult intubation is anticipated and regional block is contraindicated. Maintenance of general anesthesia by conventional means is acceptable, and intensive monitoring of respiratory and cardiovascular parameters should continue. Isoflurane in low concentrations, commonly 0.75%, is preferable to halothane in view of the potential liver disturbances associated with PIH. These inhalation agents depress uterine contractility in a dose-related manner and will increase blood loss, which may necessitate transfusion. In patients with a pre-existing or borderline coagulation profile, the transfusion of stored blood may precipitate a coagulation problem. Muscle relaxation is continued with a nondepolarizing relaxant, and atracurium has the advantage of a relatively short action because it undergoes spontaneous degradation. Previous treatment with magnesium sulfate and isoflurane will prolong the myoneural block, and in these circumstances evaluation of neuromuscular transmission with a nerve stimulator is advised. Ergometrine alone or as syntometrine should be avoided because of its hypertensive effects. Syntocinon, 5 units as a bolus slowly intravenously, followed by an infusion of 20 units/L, should be used to promote uterine contraction after delivery.

Intensive recovery care is essential and, if post-operative ventilation is required, the patient should be placed in a unit familiar with this type of management. Pulmonary aspiration is still a danger and the stomach contents should have been aspirated via a wide-bore stomach tube just before the end of anesthesia. Antacid therapy should be continued, especially if sedation and antihypertensive treatment are given. The danger of convulsions in the first 24 h post partum persists, and careful assessments of neurologic and cardiovascular systems must continue. Oliguria needs careful consideration, demanding accurate fluid balance charts, monitoring of urine output and central venous pressure measurement. Furosemide is the diuretic most commonly used and should only be given if urine output does not improve following a fluid challenge with a volume expander or in the presence of adequate hydration. The probability of an alternative diagnosis for convulsions such as subarachnoid hemorrhage must always be considered.

Compared with other parts of the world the incidence of severe PIH in the UK is low, yet it remains as one of the main causes of maternal death. A safe outcome for mother and infant demands expert management by an experienced obstetric team in which the anesthesiologist has a major role.

REFERENCES

1. Confidential Enquiries into Maternal Death in England, Wales, Scotland and Northern Ireland, 1985–87 1991 HMSO, London
2. Moodley J 1990 Treatment of eclampsia. Br J Obstet Gynaecol 97(1): 99–101
3. Rubin P C 1983 Treatment of hypertension in pregnancy. Clin Obstet Gynecol 13: 307–317
4. Rogers R C, Sibai B M, Whybrew D 1990 Labetalol pharmacokinetics in pregnancy-induced hypertension. Am J Obstet Gynecol 162: 362–366
5. Moore J, Dundee J W 1983 Analgesia in labour. In: Lewis P (ed) Clinical pharmacology in obstetrics. John Wright, Bristol pp 337–359
6. Slater R M, Smith W D, Patrick J et al 1987 Phenytoin infusion in severe pre-eclampsia. Lancet 1: 1417–1421
7. Newsome L R, Bramwell R S, Curling P E 1986 Severe pre-eclampsia: hemodynamic effects of lumbar epidural anesthesia. Anesth Analg 65: 31–36
8. Letsky E 1987 Haemostasis in pregnancy. In: Morgan B M (ed) Foundations of obstetric anaesthesia. Farrand, London pp 189–207
9. Crawford J S 1987 Intensive care of the severely hypertensive woman. In: Sharp F, Symonds E M (eds) Proceedings of the 16th study group of the Royal College of Obstetricians and Gynaecologists. Perinatology Press, Ithaca, NY pp 343–348
10. Thompson E M, Wilson C M, Moore J, McCleane E 1985 Plasma bupivacaine levels associated with extradural anesthesia for Caesarean Section. Anaesthesia 40: 427–432
11. Wright J P 1983 Anesthetic considerations: anaesthetic consideration in pre-eclampsia. Anesth Analg 62: 590–601
12. Dann W L, Hutchinson A, Cartwright D P 1987 Maternal and neonatal responses to alfentanil administered before induction of general anaesthesia for Caesarean Section. Br J Anaesth 59: 1391–1396

PART C
AUSTRALIAN VIEW

M. Westmore

INTRODUCTION

The syndrome of pregnancy-induced hypertension (PIH) is encountered in obstetric practice in Australia and New Zealand with a wide variety in the degree of severity and symptomatology. There is no single 'Australian approach' to this syndrome, and the immense size of this country, with a largely coastal population, imposes special problems of its own in the transport of sick obstetric patients to tertiary referral hospitals from isolated communities. Information presented is gained from the recent Australian and New Zealand literature, and from a survey conducted of tertiary referral obstetric anesthesia departments and intensive care units in the major cities.

STATISTICS

The prevalence of PIH in primigravid pregnant women in Australia is approximately 15%.[1] The percentage of multiparas affected is lower, the overall prevalence in all deliveries being about 8% in major obstetric teaching hospitals. A higher frequency (15% and 21% at two hospitals in New South Wales) probably reflects an increased referral rate to hospitals with specialized PIH units.

Complications requiring intensive care are uncommon. Eclampsia occurs in approximately 1 in 1500–2000 deliveries, and renal failure requiring dialysis has a prevalence of about 1 in 4000. Fortunately, cerebrovascular accidents appear to be very rare.

However, PIH and eclampsia feature significantly as the major cause of maternal mortality in Australia. In the latest report from the National Health and Medical Research Council for the triennium 1982–84, 42 direct maternal deaths occurred (a rate of 5.88 per 100 000 confinements), of which seven were directly caused by PIH or eclampsia.[2] In many of the cases described, the same problems were evident as in previous triennia – failure of the patient to cooperate with the doctor, failure of the doctor to manage the disease in the early stages when it was most treatable, failure to consult where appropriate and failure to appreciate the serious implications of the fulminant case.

AREAS OF RESEARCH

The complex pathophysiologic effects of this syndrome, with hypertension but one of these, have been elucidated in a recent review by Brown.[1] The clinical spectrum of signs and symptoms is related to multiple organ involvement but, because the syndrome has been for so long associated with hypertension, other sinister presentations such as headache or epigastric pain may be misdiagnosed until eclampsia occurs. The need for a placental unit has drawn attention to this organ's possible role in the etiology of the syndrome. Genetic and immunologic influences have been considered, and reduced organ perfusion due to increased sensitivity to circulating catecholamines and activation of the coagulation cascade helps to explain the diverse range of symptoms seen in this disease.[3]

Research in the area of sodium–renin–aldosterone relationships in normal and hypertensive pregnant women[4] has shown that in those who later develop PIH, salt depletion fails to stimulate plasma aldosterone in the second trimester, when the patients are still normotensive. In addition, such women do not exhibit the 'sodium-independent' component of plasma renin activity seen in continuously normotensive parturients at a similar gestation.

Doppler studies of the umbilical and uteroplacental bed arterial flow–velocity waveforms in women suffering from severe PIH with proteinuria have revealed an abnormally elevated umbilical artery systolic–diastolic ratio in 64% of patients. An elevated umbilical artery systolic–diastolic ratio (suggesting increased resistance in the vessel and decreased perfusion) was significantly associated with small for gestational age fetuses and neonatal morbidity.[5] It is possible that as investigations with Doppler and ultrasound become more common, signs of decreased organ perfusion may be detected before clinical signs develop.

Many of the obstetric units surveyed are involved in large multicenter trials investigating the effect of low-dose aspirin (60 mg daily) in the prevention of PIH in at-risk women, or as a therapeutic maneuver when hypertension or intrauterine growth retardation is detected.

DIAGNOSIS

The diagnosis is made on a diastolic blood pressure of more than 90 mmHg after 20 weeks' gestation in women in whom no prior renal or hypertensive disease existed. Early detection of PIH should be the aim, with blood pressure measured regularly during pregnancy and other presenting signs and symptoms sought. These should be important aspects of midwifery and obstetric training, especially for general practitioner obstetricians.

HIGH-RISK ANTENATAL CLINICS

Some obstetric units surveyed have developed either specialized PIH units or high-risk antenatal clinics where a team approach is encouraged.

Members of these groups include obstetricians, perinatologists, physicians, anesthesiologists, nephrologists, neonatologists and nursing staff. Patients with PIH as well as other obstetric patients are discussed with management plans being developed (M A Brown, M Rowley, V Callanan, B L Duffy, personal communications).

In the majority of obstetric hospitals, including our own, anesthesiologists rely on referral of high-risk patients by the obstetrician or physician. This approach is more haphazard and denies other team members early input from their perspective, which may alter the overall plan of management.

The team approach is to be encouraged as it highlights the involvement of other specialists and their particular concerns, e.g. the high rate of cesarean delivery in these patients, with consequent special anesthetic hazards and problems of the premature or growth-retarded infant for the neonatologist. The system of high-risk clinics has demonstrably reduced the incidence of late referrals (M Rowley, personal communication), which may significantly affect the quality of patient care.

ANTENATAL MANAGEMENT – MILD TO MODERATE PIH

After initial diagnosis, management by the obstetrician is based on personal preference or hospital protocol.

Admission to hospital is mandatory in some units for any primigravida with an initial diagnosis of PIH (B L Duffy, personal communication). Response to bed rest is observed in conjunction with assessment of urinary protein, full blood count, electrolytes, creatinine, liver function tests and serum uric acid as well as cardiotocography (CTG) and Doppler ultrasound of the fetus.

All patients whose blood pressures fail to settle after overnight bed rest, or who have abnormal hematology or biochemistry or abnormal fetal growth or Doppler ultrasound scans, are referred by the obstetric team to the physician.

Oral antihypertensives in current use include alpha-methyldopa, hydralazine, beta-blockers (including labetalol, propranolol and oxprenolol) and nifedipine, alone or in combination.

A survey was conducted in 1982 of Fellows of the Royal Australian College of Obstetricians and Gynaecologists to determine current practice in the management of hypertensive disease of pregnancy.[6]

In the second trimester, a woman with a blood pressure of 140/95 would be treated with bed rest (36%) or hospitalization (28%) and drug treatment with an antihypertensive (45%), sedative (13%) or diuretic (3%).

In the 34th week of pregnancy, a woman with a blood pressure of 150/90 would be treated with bed rest (84%) and be hospitalized (70%). Drug treatment would include a sedative (44%) and an antihypertensive (12%), and 7% would have been started on an oral diuretic. Of those favoring antihypertensive treatment, the three drugs most favored were methyldopa, clonidine and oxprenolol.

Treatment was generally uniform amongst the states,

with the exception of sedation, which was used much more frequently by specialists who gained their qualification before 1960.

From my limited survey, I believe that the use of diuretics in this circumstance has diminished markedly in response to the recognition of the reduction in plasma volume of these patients, and the attention drawn to the hazards of diuretics with the development of renal failure and/or fetal loss.[7]

Patients continue to be monitored and can be discharged if the condition settles. Alternatively, they may be kept in hospital in an attempt to prolong the pregnancy or be given further treatment or delivered if their condition deteriorates to severe PIH.

ANTENATAL MANAGEMENT – SEVERE PIH

Diagnosis

When the diastolic blood pressure is higher than 110 mmHg or higher than 90 mmHg in conjunction with signs of other organ involvement, a diagnosis of severe PIH is made. Commonly this is referred to as preeclampsia or gestosis.[8] Baker[8] rightly points out that PIH does not adequately describe the problem, and concentrates the clinician's attention on the blood pressure, perhaps to the exclusion of other symptoms and signs. For example, patients with abdominal pain have been misdiagnosed as having gastroenteritis until eclampsia occurred. Goodlin[9] has recommended the term gestosis for this complication of pregnancy, meaning a polysymptomatic disease involving more than two organ systems occurring in pregnant women which resolves after delivery.

Maternal organ dysfunction includes:

- Neurologic — Diminished level of consciousness; Hyperreflexia with or without clonus; Subarachnoid hemorrhage
- Cardiac — Cardiac failure; Pulmonary edema
- Renal — Proteinuria; Oliguria; Increased serum urate; Increased serum creatinine
- Hematologic — Thrombocytopenia; Hemolysis
- Hepatic — Epigastric pain; Abnormal liver function

The physiologic mediators of these problems include hypertension, hypovolemia, capillary leak and thrombocytopenia. The underlying etiology of the condition still awaits elucidation.

Nursing care

Parturients should be nursed in the labor ward or in a special antenatal area in the lateral recumbent position, with fetal monitoring and frequent measurement of maternal blood pressure. Automatic oscillometric devices are inaccurate at high and low blood pressures, and manual sphygmomanometric measurement is preferred. Accurate fluid balance charts must be kept, with urinary catheterization if the patient has a diminished conscious state. Pulse oximetry should be readily available for monitoring oxygen saturation and oxygen administered accordingly.

Establishing good peripheral venous access

A cannula of at least 16 gauge should be inserted, adequate for rapid volume infusion if required.

Control of blood pressure

Rapidly acting therapy is indicated when the systolic blood pressure is higher than 170 mmHg or the diastolic blood pressure is higher than 110 mmHg.

When other organ systems are involved, treatment should be initiated at lower levels of hypertension.

In the 1982 survey of obstetricians, antihypertensive drugs used frequently for fulminating preeclampsia were diazoxide (54%), hydralazine (38%), reserpine (6%) and clonidine (4%).[6]

Current practice is varied with a range of protocols including oral or sublingual nifedipine, hydralazine and diazoxide by intravenous infusion. Extremely resistant hypertension is treated in some units with sodium nitroprusside[8] (M Rowley, B L Duffy, personal communications) and, in one, intravenous nitroglycerin is also used (B L Duffy, personal communication).

Prevention of convulsions

Phenytoin has become very popular as a prophylactic treatment. It is usually administered intravenously in a dose of 15 mg/kg over 2 h. Oral treatment may be continued if delivery is not imminent.

Other agents used include magnesium sulfate in New South Wales (S P Gatt, personal communication), South Australia (B L Duffy, personal communication) and Tasmania (D E Marsden, personal communication), and phenobarbital in South Australia (B L Duffy, P Brownridge, personal communications). This last drug has been used traditionally when patients require transport to major centers for delivery. On one occasion in our large state of Western Australia a sick Aboriginal girl with PIH living on a mission in the north of the state (over 2000 km away) took nearly 24 h to reach the tertiary referral obstetric hospital and site of the neonatal intensive care. She travelled by foot and truck before being flown by the Royal Flying Doctor Service to a regional hospital for stabilization, and was then flown on to Perth. In such situations, especially with prolonged air travel, measurement of the blood pressure is difficult; administration of drugs by infusion is almost impossible. In these cases an intramuscular long-acting drug is highly desirable.

Renal function

It is imperative that urine output be accurately measured, and this will often necessitate bladder catheterization. Plasma, and in some units urine, electrolytes, urea and creatinine should be measured.

Approximately 30–60% of patients with preeclampsia show evidence of renal involvement with elevated serum uric acid and creatinine levels.[10] In one unit, a serum urate >0.4 mmol/l is an indication for urgent delivery (A Neilson, personal communication). If oliguria occurs (<20–30 ml/h), colloid solutions are used by most units to expand the contracted circulating blood volume. Stable plasma protein solution or polygeline are the fluids nominated for this purpose, with greater preference for the former solution, perhaps because of its longer intravascular action.

Before administering any colloid solution for volume expansion, it is imperative to exclude cardiac failure (listen for gallop rhythm, crepitations and look for an elevated jugular venous pressure) and in one unit (M A Brown, personal communication) it is confirmed that the hematocrit is greater than 0.40.

Low-dose infusions of dopamine are only occasionally used (F Lah, M Fisher, personal communications) in an effort to avoid renal failure. It is surprising that this excellent renal vasodilator is not in more common use, and this may reflect lack of familiarity of obstetricians with this agent.

Coagulopathy

The relationship between severe PIH and coagulopathy is one of concern to the anesthesiologist, particularly when epidural analgesia is requested in labor, or when cesarean delivery is planned.

The actual safe lower limit for platelet count prior to epidural insertion is unknown,[11] but common practice in Australia and New Zealand is to use a cut-off point of 100 000 platelets, below which other investigations of platelet function are performed. These include a bleeding time, fibrinogen level, partial thromboplastin time, fibrinogen degradation products and measurement of monoclonal D-dimer, a specific indicator of fibrinolysis.

A recent prospective study of thrombocytopenia and platelet function defects in 40 parturients with preeclampsia[10] revealed an overall prevalence of thrombocytopenia (platelet count <150 000) of 15%; 7.5% had a platelet count of less than 100 000. Duke bleeding time was normal in all patients but one, a patient with severe preeclampsia, a platelet count of <50 000, a slightly decreased availability of platelet factor 3 and an elevated monoclonal D-dimer.

This study revealed no correlation between platelet count and blood pressure (Table 45.2) or other indices of disease severity such as birth weight, serum iron, uric acid or liver function. The authors' recommendation is that a platelet count is an adequate screening test of suitability for regional blockade. If the platelet count is between 50 000 and 100 000, a bleeding time is indicated. If the platelet count is less than 50 000, regional blockade is contraindicated.

In addition to problems for the anesthesiologist, to prevent hemorrhage (M A Brown, personal communication) the patient with severe PIH may require fresh frozen plasma if her platelet count is decreased and clotting times prolonged, and platelets if the platelet count is less than 20 000.

Liver function

Hepatic function tests should be performed, as abnormalities may be associated with coagulopathy. Epigastric pain and/or tenderness should be taken seriously.

Invasive hemodynamic monitoring

Attitudes and practices with regard to placement of intra-

Table 45.2 Maximum mean systemic pressures of patients with a platelet count $<150 \times 10^9$/l showing a lack of correlation between thrombocytopenia and severity of hypertension (from Schindler et al[10] with permission)

Maximum mean systemic pressure (mmHg)	Number of patients	Number of patients with platelet count $<150 \times 10^9$/l	χ^2
110–119	6	2	1.34
120–129	20	2	0.33
130–139	8	1	0.03
140–149	5	1	0.08
150–159	0	0	—
160–169	1	0	0.15
Total	40	6	1.93 ($P > 0.1$)

arterial lines, central venous pressure lines and pulmonary artery catheters (Swan Ganz) vary widely. In some units no suitable monitoring equipment exists. Many obstetric units are 'stand alone' (i.e. geographically isolated from intensive care units), and therefore experience in interpretation of measured pulmonary and left heart pressures may be limited, as may be the training of nursing staff.

The potential complications of central catheter placement in patients with coagulopathy needs to be weighed against the information that may be provided. Central venous lines are placed in some units if urine output is low (N Roberts, personal communication). Pulmonary artery catheters are rarely inserted in Australia, but the following are indications in patients with severe PIH:

- those hypertensives who remain oliguric in spite of a fluid challenge, especially if it occurs post-partum;[12]
- those who develop pulmonary edema;[12,13]
- when hypertension fails to respond to usual drug therapy;[12]
- when cardiomyopathy or myocardial complication occurs.[8]

If after initial investigation and treatment patients stabilize, the pregnancy is prolonged or delivery planned depending on the gestation and fetal well-being. Emergency delivery is necessary if the condition does not ameliorate.

INDICATIONS FOR DELIVERY

Delivery of the fetoplacental unit (including hydatidiform mole) is necessary to terminate PIH. However, the patient's condition may worsen after delivery, and continued monitoring in an intensive care or high-dependency unit is mandatory.

Maternal indications for delivery include inability to control the blood pressure acutely with maximum antihypertensive therapy, deteriorating liver or renal function, falling platelet count or neurologic complications.

The condition of the fetus may force the decision to deliver if an abnormal cardiotograph or severe intrauterine growth retardation is revealed.

MODE OF DELIVERY

If vaginal delivery is planned, it is important that the anesthesiologist is consulted at an early stage. The anesthesiologist may be requested to assist with intravenous line placement, provide epidural analgesia/anesthesia (see above), insert invasive hemodynamic monitoring lines and monitor fluid status, and resuscitate if eclampsia occurs.

Because of the potential for urgent delivery for maternal or fetal indications, the anesthesiologist should be familiar with the patient's family, past medical and anesthetic history, as well as the current investigations and therapy. The potential for difficult intubation must be recognized, and appropriate antacid prophylaxis instituted.

Should cesarean delivery be required, the choice of regional or general anesthesia should be discussed with the patient and surgeon. Epidural anesthesia is the technique of choice provided that there is time to extend the block if in situ and coagulopathy is not a contraindication. If eclampsia has occurred or is felt to be imminent, many anesthesiologists prefer general anesthesia.

Because of the possibility of difficult intubation, aspiration and hypertensive responses to intubation and surgical manipulations, skilled help should be on hand. Numerous antihypertensive agents are recommended in these situations, including intravenous hydralazine, sodium nitroprusside and nitroglycerin. The last two agents, because of their short duration of action, offer greater minute-to-minute control.

Ergotrate derivatives should be avoided, and blood loss assessed, as hypotension may be due to concealed losses rather than antihypertensive therapy.

MANAGEMENT POST DELIVERY

Continued monitoring of the severely preeclamptic patient should follow delivery, preferably in a high-dependency nursing unit. Hypertension may require continued intravenous therapy until oral agents are tolerated. The urine output should continue to be measured on an hourly basis. Oliguria, if it occurs, may be treated expectantly, with intravenous fluid or with diuretics. This is an area in which there is considerable variation in approach in Australasia, and is the subject of much debate. Should renal failure ensure, a consultation with a renal physician is mandatory.

After cesarean delivery, analgesia should be given either epidurally or by intravenous infusion. The platelet count should be measured before removal of the epidural catheter.

SUMMARY

Although a unified approach to all aspects of the management of PIH in Australia and New Zealand may be desirable, numerous regional differences exist. This reflects the different experiences of those involved in the treatment of this disease, and emphasizes the fact that there are many ways to treat the different systems and organs affected by this syndrome. However, despite differences in drug choices, there appears to be widespread appreciation of the need for further elucidation of the etiology of this syndrome, the need for a team approach and early consultation with anesthetic staff.

ACKNOWLEDGEMENTS

I would like to thank my colleagues who responded to my survey (not all of whom have been cited) and who assisted me in this attempt to reveal common threads in the Australasian management of pregnancy induced hypertension.

REFERENCES

1. Brown M A 1989 Pregnancy-induced hypertension: current concepts. Anaesth Intensive Care 17: 185–197
2. National Health and Medical Research Council 1988 Report on maternal deaths in Australia 1982–84. CPP Communications, Canberra
3. Roberts J M, Robert N T, Friedman S A, Goldfien A 1990 New developments in pre-eclampsia. Fetal Med Rev 2: 125–141
4. Brown M A, Nicholson E, Gallery E D 1988 Sodium–renin–aldosterone relations in normal and hypertensive pregnancy. Br J Obstet Gynaecol 95: 1237–1246
5. Trudinger B J, Cook C M 1990 Doppler umbilical and uterine flow waveforms in severe pregnancy hypertension. Br J Obstet Gynaecol 97: 142–148
6. Trudinger B J, Parik P 1982 Attitudes to the management of hypertension in pregnancy: a survey of Australian Fellows. Aust NZJ Obstet Gynaecol 22: 191–197
7. Brown M A, Child R P, O'Connor M, Williams G, Mitchell R 1989 Pregnancy-induced hypertension and renal failure: clinical importance of diuretics, plasma volume and vasospasm. Aust NZJ Obstet Gynaecol 29: 230–232
8. Baker A B 1990 Management of severe pregnancy-induced hypertension, or gestosis, with sodium nitroprusside. Anaesth Intensive Care 18: 361–365
9. Goodlin R C 1986 Expanded toxemia syndrome or gestosis. Am J Obstet Gynecol 154: 1227–1232
10. Schindler M, Gatt S, Isert P, Mogans D, Cheung A 1990 Thrombocytopenia and platelet functional defects in pre-eclampsia: implications for regional anaesthesia. Anaesth Intensive Care 18: 169–174
11. Sage D J 1990 Epidurals, spinals and bleeding disorders in pregnancy: a review. Anaesth Intensive Care 18: 319–326
12. Gatt S 1989 The cardiomyopathy of pre-eclampsia – is invasive monitoring useful? In: Gatt S, Lah F (eds) Proceedings of the inaugural meeting of Australian obstetric anaesthetists. Society of Australian Obstetric Anaesthetists Sydney, pp 47–60
13. Crowhurst J A 1989 Intensive care management of the severe pre-eclamptic. Proceedings of the inaugural meeting of Australian obstetric anaesthetists. Society of Australian Obstetric Anaesthetists, Sydney, pp 61–74

46. Cardiac disease

J. C. A. Carvalho

INTRODUCTION

Pregnancy increases both cardiac work and myocardial oxygen consumption. During the course of normal pregnancy, blood volume increases 40–50% and is accompanied by increases of 15–20% in heart rate and up to 50% in cardiac output. Additional hemodynamic changes occur during labor and are especially acute during each uterine contraction. An increase of up to 45% in cardiac output is seen during the late second stage of labor.[1–3] Such cardiovascular changes appear to be largely based on sympathetic-mediated increases in heart rate as well as in stroke volume during contractions. Cardiac output may further increase 10–20% in the immediate post-partum period as a consequence of post-partum changes in intravascular volume, which are due to release of vena caval obstruction by the pregnant uterus and the decrease in vascular capacitance associated with the delivery of the fetus and placenta and subsequent uterine contraction. Systemic vascular resistance is suddenly elevated as a result of uterine contraction after placental extraction. Such dramatic preload and afterload changes are readily accommodated by increases in cardiac output in the patient with a normal heart. However, the patient with a relatively fixed cardiac output may be unable to accommodate such hemodynamic fluctuations, and hydrostatic pulmonary edema or congestive heart failure may develop.[4] The immediate post-partum period is critical for most patients with cardiac disease as both cardiac output and systemic vascular resistance are suddenly increased, leading to extra myocardial work.

The anesthetic management of the pregnant cardiac patient should aim at cardiovascular protection against these extremely important and rapid hemodynamic fluctuations in both the intra- and the immediate post-partum period.

These cardiovascular modifications associated with pregnancy will return to nonpregnant status within 6 months post-partum, but most of this regression will occur in the first 2 weeks. Therefore, unnecessary surgical and anesthetic procedures in this high-risk group of patients, including post-partum tubal ligation, should be postponed until at least 2 weeks post-partum.

DISTRIBUTION

The distribution of cardiac disease in pregnant patients varies according to geographic regions. In Brazil, for example, it differs from that usually seen in other series (75% rheumatic heart disease, 25% congenital),[5] as a consequence of the important group of cardiomyopathies represented by Chagas' disease (Table 46.1). However, similar to that observed in such series, the most common cardiac disease presenting to the anesthesiologist is mitral stenosis, either as a sole dysfunction or in combination with mitral insufficiency, aortic insufficiency or aortic stenosis.

PLANNING THE ANESTHETIC MANAGEMENT OF THE PREGNANT CARDIAC PATIENT

The considerations which should guide the anesthetic management of pregnant cardiac patients are:

Pathophysiology

Each cardiac disease adapts to pregnancy through different mechanisms, and changes in the equilibrium between pulmonary and systemic circulation induced by stress and/or different anesthetic techniques may or may not be tolerated. From simple cases to complex cardiac dysfunctions, these patients are more appropriately managed if a comprehensive study of the case is undertaken and if the anesthesiologist knows how the following variables will affect a certain patient:

Table 46.1 Distribution of pregnant cardiac patients according to cardiac disease at the University of São Paulo in 1987–89

Rheumatic	66%
Cardiomyopathy	18%
Congenital	11%
Dysrhythmia	5%

- heart rhythm and rate;
- preload;
- afterload;
- myocardial contractility.

By using this methodical approach, it is possible to establish the desirable hemodynamic profile for the most common cardiac dysfunctions (Table 46.2), which will be an important piece of information when choosing the anesthetic technique.

Severity of heart disease

Based on the New York State Heart Association,[6] patients can be allocated into functional classes I to IV:

Class I No limitation of physical activity
Class II Symptoms with ordinary physical activity
Class III Symptoms with less than ordinary physical activities
Class IV Symptoms at rest.

Severity of heart disease based on this functional classification should not be a formal indication or contraindication for a certain anesthetic technique. Patients in functional class I could have an absolute or relative contraindication for regional anesthesia (e.g. atrial septal defect, ventricular septal defect, pulmonary hypertension, aortic and pulmonic stenosis), while there are patients in functional class IV to whom regional anesthesia could represent not only the ideal anesthetic technique but also a therapeutic tool (e.g. mitral stenosis with pulmonary edema). Severity of heart disease should never be considered without a comprehensive study of the underlying pathophysiology.

Cardiovascular adaptation to pregnancy

Detailed clinical observation of cardiac patients during prenatal care will provide useful information regarding factors involved in the improvement or in the impairment of the cardiovascular status. Some patients will benefit from the decrease in systemic vascular resistance associated with pregnancy (e.g. aortic and mitral insufficiency), while others will not tolerate increases in blood volume or in cardiac rate (e.g. mitral stenosis). The response to drugs used in the control of intercurrent dysrhythmias or other cardiac dysfunctions during pregnancy will provide a useful guide to anticipate and treat intra- and post-partum complications.

Table 46.2 Expected ideal hemodynamic features for the anesthetic techniques used in the management of pregnant cardiac patients M, maintain; SD, slight decrease; SI slight increase. (Adapted and modified from: Ranamathan S 1988 In: Ranamathan S (ed) Obstetric Anesthesia. Lea & Febiger, Philadelphia, p 191)

Disease	Heart rate	Preload	After load	Contractility
Mitral stenosis	M–SD	M–SD	M–SD	M
Mitral insufficiency	M–SI	M–SD	M–SD	M–SI
Aortic stenosis	M	M–SI	M–SI	M
Aortic insufficiency	M–SI	M–SD	M–SD	M–SI
Pulmonic stenosis	M	M–SI	M–SI	M
Pulmonary hypertension	M	M–SI	M–SI	M
Dilated cardiomyopathy	M	M–SD	M–SD	SI
Hypertrophic cardiomyopathy	M–SD	M–SI	M	M–SD
Left-to-right shunt	M	M–SI	M–SI	M
Right-to-left shunt	M	M–SI	M–SI	M
Ischemic heart disease	M	M–SD	M–SD	M–SD

Adequate documentation

Adequate documentation and accurate physical examination are absolutely essential for an understanding of the contribution of preload, afterload, cardiac rhythm and myocardial contractility to the hemodynamic status of a particular patient. Subsidiary examinations are fundamental and should include chest radiographs, electrocardiograms and, ideally, two echo Doppler cardiograms performed in the first and third trimesters of gestation.

Interpretation of the electrocardiogram in the pregnant patient should consider the changes induced by normal pregnancy:

- P-wave, PR interval and QTc interval remain stable;
- ÂQRS and ÂT are deviated to the left;
- T-wave can be negative in DIII lead and sometimes in aVF;
- ST segment depression of 0.5–1 mm is acceptable.

Echo Doppler cardiography has been extensively used in the evaluation of pregnant cardiac patients, and has been shown to be a valuable tool in their clinical and anesthetic management. An echo Doppler cardiographic profile of normal pregnant patients containing the most important variables studied can be seen in Table 46.3 and should help the reader of this chapter to understand the information contained in the case reports.[7]

Table 46.3 Echo Doppler cardiographic variables in normal pregnant patients at 24–28 weeks of gestation (P1) and at 32–36 weeks of gestation (P2) (mean ± SD) (Reproduced from ref. 7)

		P1		P2	
Mitral valve area	(cm2)	3.69	(0.48)	4.31	(0.67)
Left atrium	(cm)	2.95	(0.29)	3.25	(0.22)
Left ventricle	(cm)	4.93	(0.37)	5.06	(0.44)
Cardiac output	(L/min)	4.06	(0.54)	5.39	(1.01)
Systolic volume	(ml)	72.39	(27.25)	93.83	(29.16)
Final systolic volume	(ml)	29.70	(8.13)	34.26	(10.25)
Final diastolic volume	(ml)	116.39	(25.73)	130.35	(35.27)
Ejection fraction	(%)	0.74	(0.04)	0.76	(0.04)
Aorta	(cm)	2.85	(0.19)	3.06	(0.21)

CHOOSING THE ADEQUATE ANESTHETIC TECHNIQUE

Based on the desirable hemodynamic profile for each disease (Table 46.2) and on the expected hemodynamic effects of different anesthetic drugs and techniques, a guideline for the selection of the anesthetic technique is suggested in Table 46.4. This guideline should be used as a general approach and borderline patients should be considered individually.

REGIONAL ANESTHESIA FOR THE PREGNANT CARDIAC PATIENT

There is clear evidence in the literature that regional anesthesia is the most effective way of blocking the stress response during labor and vaginal or cesarean delivery; this is certainly highly beneficial for the cardiac patient. However, the cardiovascular changes induced by regional anesthesia must be considered for each patient depending on the underlying pathophysiology. Spinal and epidural anesthesia are associated with a small effect on conductance vessels, resulting in a small decrease in systemic vascular resistance (afterload). However, they exert a very important action on capacitance vessels, resulting in a significant pooling of blood and decrease in venous return (preload). Systemic vascular resistance can be further decreased by epidural anesthesia if epinephrine is added to the local anesthetic. Heart rate is dependent upon the reduction of both systemic vascular resistance and venous return and the concomitant use of epinephrine in association with the local anesthetic solution. For most patients, therefore, regional anesthesia may represent a cushion to the important hemodynamic fluctuations occurring during labor, delivery and post-partum period. It might, in fact, be used as a valuable therapeutic tool in the post-partum period, by extending pain control and sympathetic block for a few hours. Regional analgesia and anesthesia include the spinal or epidural administration of opioids as well as local anesthetics; if this is kept in mind, theoretically all patients would benefit from regional techniques, even those in whom the use of such techniques require very special caution, such as those presenting with pulmonary hypertension or aortic stenosis. The term 'therapeutic' would better describe the role of regional techniques in the management of the pregnant cardiac patient. However, two groups of patients must be differentiated: those in whom regional anesthesia techniques are highly beneficial and the risk is low and those in whom such techniques are also beneficial but the risk is increased and special caution is required. The latter pose some limits to regional analgesia and anesthesia, which have been re-evaluated because of the introduction of spinal and epidural opioids and the use of combined techniques (e.g. spinal opioids and pudendal block).

Table 46.4 Suggested anesthetic technique for different cardiac diseases

Mitral stenosis	Regional
Mitral insufficiency	Regional
Aortic stenosis	General
Aortic insufficiency	Regional
Pulmonic stenosis	General
Pulmonary hypertension	General
Dilated cardiomyopathy	Regional?
Hypertrophic cardiomyopathy	General
Left-to-right-shunt	General
Right-to-left shunt	General
Ischemic heart disease	Regional?

The most striking example of the benefits of regional anesthesia for pregnant cardiac patients is probably the management of the patient with mitral stenosis. Clark et al[4] reported the results of invasive monitoring utilizing a pulmonary artery catheter in a series of eight patients with mitral stenosis, in the first clinical report of this nature. Patients were functional class III or IV and delivered vaginally. A mean increase in pulmonary capillary wedge pressure of 10 mmHg was observed in the immediate post-partum period. Three of these patients received epidural anesthesia during the active phase of labor, without any significant improvement in hemodynamic status. However, Hemmings et al[8] reported the invasive hemodynamic monitoring of a functional class II parturient in whom epidural anesthesia had evident beneficial effects. Three observations were especially relevant in this case:

1. Epidural anesthesia was beneficial in the first stage of labor. When contractions became painful, pulmonary artery pressure (PAP), pulmonary vascular resistance (PVR) and systemic vascular resistance (SVR) increased and cardiac output (CO) decreased. After induction of epidural anesthesia with 0.25% plain bupivacaine, PVR, SVR and PAP decreased while CO increased toward baseline values.
2. Dramatic increases in PAP and decreases in CO were observed during bearing-down efforts in the second stage. The patient's urge to bear down was decreased by the epidural block with correction of the hemodynamic profile.
3. There was no increase in pulmonary capillary wedge pressure (PCWP) in the immediate post-partum period. The authors related this to the conservative fluid management and to the sympathetic blockade to T6.

Mostafa[9] reported the management of a parturient with severe mitral stenosis and pulmonary edema undergoing emergency cesarean delivery under spinal anesthesia, performed after unsuccessful attempts at epidural anesthesia. This case report illustrates one of the most critical situations of this group of patients, in which the understanding of the pathophysiology led to a successful clinical management. It also illustrates that the functional class of the patient by itself should not lead to the election of general anesthesia as the anesthetic technique of choice. Under such circumstances, general anesthesia, despite the beneficial effects of increasing intraalveolar pressure during intermittent positive-pressure ventilation, could lead to hypertension, tachycardia, dysrhythmias and increases in pulmonary artery pressure, associated with intubation, extubation and light anesthesia. General anesthesia would also be unable to accommodate the increased venous return during contractions or after delivery.

Patients with mild to severe mitral stenosis, mitral insufficiency or aortic insufficiency and most patients with dilated cardiomyopathy are usually safely delivered with continuous epidural anesthesia, for both vaginal and cesarean delivery (Table 46.5). Although epidural anesthesia remains the regional technique of choice for the patient with cardiac disease, as it causes less intense hemodynamic changes, spinal anesthesia has some specific indications. In patients with conduction disturbances or severe myocardial compromise (e.g. Chagas' cardiomyopathy, peripartal cardiomyopathy), in whom large doses of local anesthetics are not well tolerated, spinal anesthesia is recommended.

For a more comprehensive approach to this group of patients in whom regional anesthesia is highly beneficial and associated with low risk, a brief description of the general hemodynamic adaptive mechanisms are reviewed, and some case reports are presented to illustrate their anesthetic management.

Mitral stenosis

In normal adults the mitral valve orifice is 4–6 cm^2 and the valvular diastolic gradient is 5mmHg or less. If an obstruction to the left atrial outflow is present, a higher intra-atrial pressure is required to send the blood to the left ventricle. When the orifice is reduced to 1 cm^2, a pressure gradient of 25 mmHg is required to maintain cardiac output.

Table 46.5 Epidural analgesia and anesthesia for pregnant cardiac patients with no contraindication for regional anesthesia

Vaginal delivery
Fluid restriction
Start analgesia early
Labor in left lateral position
Continuous epidural infusion with bupivacaine plus fentanyl or sufentanil
Monitoring: pulse, NIBP, ECG, Sp_{O_2}
Cesarean delivery
Fluid restriction
Epidural with 0.5% bupivacaine plus fentanyl
Oxygen by mask
Lateral uterine displacement
Vasopressor if necessary: ephedrine (except in mitral stenosis: consider metaraminol or phenylephrine)
Monitoring: pulse, NIBP, ECG, Sp_{O_2}
Oxytocin infusion (20 i.v.) after delivery; avoid ergot derivates

NIBP: non-invasive blood pressure

Elevations in left atrial pressure raise pulmonary capillary pressure. As a complication of long-lasting severe mitral stenosis, pulmonary hypertension might result;[10] however, this is not usually seen in women of child-bearing age. Left ventricular function is normal in mitral stenosis. Right ventricular function is also normal, except when accompanied by pulmonary hypertension. Pregnancy raises both venous return and heart rate; both factors raise transvalvular gradient, thus impairing cardiac function. Pulmonary congestion and hypertension in the pulmonary venous bed are usually present; however, this state should be differentiated from hyperresistance in the pulmonary arteriolar bed, as they have different anesthetic implications (see Case report 1).

Basic rules for the anesthetic management

Heart rate. Avoid tachycardia; provide labor analgesia early to reduce pain and stress; do not use epinephrine with the local anesthetic. If hypotension occurs, use metaraminol or phenylephrine. Treat all acute dysrhythmias.

Preload. Avoid increases; sympathetic blockade will provide a reduction in venous return, especially during contractions and after delivery.

Afterload. Avoid marked decreases; do not use epinephrine with the local anesthetic

Myocardial contractility. Maintain.

Case report 1

The patient was 34 years old, gravida 6, para 3, 35 weeks of gestation. She had had a previous cesarean delivery. She suffered from severe mitral stenosis with pulmonary edema (functional class IV) and was using a beta-adrenergic blocking agent and digitalis.

ECG. Left atrial enlargement.

Echo Doppler cardiogram. Left ventricle (LV), 4.4 cm (normal); final diastolic volume (FDV), 85.0 ml (normal); systolic volume (SV), 70.0 ml (normal); final systolic volume (FSV), 16.0 ml (normal); ejection fraction (EF) 0.82% (normal); left ventricle mass (LVM), 75.0 g/m^2 (normal); volume–mass ratio (V/M), 0.65 (normal); left atrium (LA), 4.1 cm (enlarged); right ventricle (RV), normal; right atrium (RA), normal; mitral valve 1.1 cm^2 (reduced); aortic valve, normal; tricuspid valve, normal; pulmonic valve, A wave absent.

Comments and anesthetic management. This case is an example of severe pure mitral stenosis. Left ventricular cavity, volumes and function are normal. Mitral valve orifice is severely reduced and, although data are not available, transvalvular gradient pressure is probably increased; right atrium is enlarged. The absence of the A-wave in the pulmonic valve suggests pulmonary congestion. The right chambers are normal, as detected by echo cardiography and electrocardiography. Pulmonary arteriolar hypertension is not likely to be present. Cesarean delivery was performed under continuous epidural anesthesia with 100 mg of 0.5% bupivacaine plus 100 µg of fentanyl. Pulmonary edema disappeared after regional block was initiated and the patient remained asymptomatic during the surgical procedure. Upon regression of the block 4 h later, the patient again developed pulmonary edema; at that time the sympathetic blockade was extended with 60 mg of 2% lidocaine, and the patient became asymptomatic. Diuretics were then introduced and the post-operative period was uneventful.

Mitral insufficiency

In the presence of mitral regurgitation, the resistance to left ventricular emptying is reduced. There is a great outflow to the left atrium. To maintain cardiac output, the left ventricle must increase myocardial contractility. With the progression of the disease, left atrial enlargement, increased pulmonary capillary pressure and right heart failure might occur. If left ventricular function deteriorates, the left ventricle will dilate and its compliance will increase. Although cardiac function can deteriorate, the usual evolution of mitral insufficiency is benign and pregnancy is well tolerated.

Aortic insufficiency

In aortic insufficiency, the regurgitant flow during diastole can be of the same magnitude as the forward stroke volume; the major hemodynamic compensation is an increase in left ventricular end-diastolic volume, which allows the left ventricle to send a larger stroke volume and maintain ejection fraction. Different from mitral insufficiency, left ventricle enlargement occurs early. If the disease progresses, left ventricular dysfunction occurs, ejection fraction is reduced, the left atrium is enlarged and pulmonary congestion might occur.

Although there are marked differences in their pathophysiology and hemodynamic adaptations, the anesthetic considerations for *mitral* and *aortic regurgitation* can be made together (see Case report 2).

Basic rules for the anesthetic management

Heart rate. Avoid bradycardia as heart rate helps to maintain cardiac output in mitral regurgitation and reduces the degree of blood regurgitated during diastole in aortic insufficiency; careful vena caval decompression will avoid marked decreases in venous return with consequent bradycardia; if mitral stenosis is not present, epinephrine can be used in association with local anesthetics.

Preload. This should be decreased, to reduce left ventricle overdistension; sympathetic blockade will provide reduction in venous return, especially during contractions and after delivery.

Afterload. Should be decreased to reduce the regurgitant flow; early labor analgesia will avoid the pain and stress associated with marked increases in peripheral resistance; epinephrine associated with the local anesthetic is useful if mitral stenosis is not present; if hypotension occurs, use ephedrine.

Myocardial contractility. Avoid decreases; inhalation agents should be used with great caution, as these patients are extremely sensitive to them (isoflurane is preferred, if necessary).

Case report 2

The patient was 27 years old, gravida 2, para 1 at 38 weeks of gestation, undergoing cesarean delivery for fetal distress. She suffered from mitral stenosis and regurgitation plus aortic regurgitation (15-year history), was functional class II and using a beta-adrenergic blocking agent, digitalis and diuretics.

EGG. Left atrial and left ventricular enlargement.

Echo Doppler cardiogram. LV, 7.2 cm (enlarged); FDV, 373 ml (enlarged); SV, 269 ml (enlarged); FSV, 104 ml (enlarged); LV mass 160 g/m^2 (increased); volume–mass ratio, 1.42 (increased); EF, 0.72% (normal); LA, 4.9 cm (enlarged); mitral valve, 1.5 cm^2 (reduced), with regurgitant flow; aortic valve incompetent; pulmonic valve, A-wave absent.; tricuspid valve normal; right ventricle and atrium normal.

Comments and anesthetic management. An enlarged and dilated left ventricle is present, still maintaining good performance as shown by the ejection fraction. Pulmonary congestion is evident, but there are no signs of right heart involvement. Pulmonary hypertension is unlikely to be present. Cesarean delivery was performed under epidural anesthesia with 100 mg of 0.5% bupivacaine plus 100 µg of fentanyl. The patient had an uneventful intra- and post-operative course.

Dilated cardiomyopathy

The cardiac chambers, especially the left, are enlarged. The primary functional disturbance is the loss of ventricular contractile power, with a reduction in the ejection fraction. As the disease progresses, end-diastolic volume increases and cardiac output decreases. Two major representatives of this group are peripartal cardiomyopathy[11] and Chagas' disease.

Basic rules for the anesthetic management

Heart rate. Avoid bradycardia as it will raise left ventricle end-diastolic volume and compromise ejection fraction. Take care with intubation, succinylcholine and halothane.

Preload. This should be reduced; increases in venous return associated with contractions and delivery will lead to pulmonary edema; sympathetic blockade will reduce venous return and improve myocardial function.

Afterload. This should be reduced; if peripheral resistance rises, left ventricular failure might occur; early labor analgesia is suggested; if general anesthesia is required, avoid light anesthesia.

Myocardial contractility. This should be maintained or increased; large doses of local anesthetic can impair myocardial function; if a conduction disturbance is present (e.g. Chagas' disease) large doses of local anesthetic should also be avoided – epidural anesthesia is possible for labor and delivery but spinal anesthesia is preferred for cesarean delivery. Avoid inhalation agents.

If myocardial function is severely compromised, with a marked reduction in the ejection fraction, the patient should benefit from a combination of epidural and general anesthesia (see Case report 3). Epidural blockade with a low dose and concentration of local anesthetics will cause venous pooling of blood and protection against sudden increases in venous return and peripheral resistance, without further compromising left ventricular function; general anesthesia, as suggested later in this chapter, will complement the anesthetic technique.

Case report 3

The patient was 19 years old, gravida 2, para I, at 37 weeks of gestation, undergoing cesarean delivery for fetal distress. She suffered from sick sinus syndrome plus severe cardiomyopathy plus pulmonary edema. She had had a previous cesarean delivery under general anesthesia (midazolam, fentanyl, nitrous oxide–oxygen, enflurane) with post-operative pulmonary edema requiring diuretics and digitalis.

ECG. Biventricular enlargement and ventricular premature beats.

Echo Doppler cardiogram. Mitral valve insufficient; LV and RV enlarged; LV ejection fraction 0.5% (reduced).

Comments and anesthetic management. A severely compromised myocardium with extremely variable heart rate may not tolerate large doses of local anesthetics or fast-acting central neural blockade anesthesia. On the other hand, a patient receiving general anesthesia may not be able to accommodate volume overload after delivery. A combined technique was planned: epidural anesthesia was instituted with 50 mg of bupivacaine and general anesthesia was induced with etomidate, fentanyl and succinylcholine. Immediately after the initiation of epidural anesthesia the patient became asymptomatic. Upon delivery, incremental doses of furosemide were used. No complications were observed in the post-operative period.

RESTRICTIONS TO REGIONAL ANESTHESIA IN THE PREGNANT CARDIAC PATIENT

When considering patients other than those presenting with mitral stenosis, mitral insufficiency, aortic insufficiency and dilated cardiomyopathy, some restrictions to regional anesthesia may apply; under such circumstances, each patient has to be extensively evaluated before the anesthetic technique is elected. The use of regional techniques in this group of patients has been revised and increased as a result of the introduction of new concepts and techniques, which have provided us with new options. The most important restrictions to regional anesthesia in the cardiac patients are:

- anticoagulation;
- pulmonic stenosis;
- aortic stenosis;
- left-to-right and right-to-left shunts with significant hemodynamic implications;
- primary and secondary pulmonary hypertension;
- hypertrophic cardiomyopathy.

Anticoagulation

Anticoagulation is an absolute contraindication to spinal or epidural anesthesia because of the increased risk of bleeding after unintentional blood vessel trauma leading to epidural hematoma. If interruption of heparin therapy is possible, it can be safely reintroduced in the immediate post-partum period, as documented by Rao et al.[12] If heparin is discontinued for 12 h and a coagulogram is within the normal range, regional anesthesia may be used. If interruption is not recommended, pain relief with a major regional technique will not be possible, either for labor or for vaginal or cesarean delivery. Should an unusual situation occur, in which the change to heparin has not been made and the patient is still receiving oral anticoagulants (e.g. premature labor), an interval of 7–10 days is required for normal coagulation to be re-established, and regional techniques during this period are also contraindicated.

Primary and secondary pulmonary hypertension

The most striking example of the restriction to major regional techniques in obstetrics is primary pulmonary hypertension. Maternal mortality among women presenting with primary pulmonary hypertension ranges between 40 and 60% during the third trimester and post-partum period.[13] Hemodynamic features include pulmonary artery pressures (PAP) in excess of 30/15 mmHg or a mean PAP > 25 mmHg, right ventricle hypertrophy and, eventually, heart failure with a low, fixed cardiac output. Two principles must be considered in the management of patients with primary pulmonary hypertension:

1. The primary goal is to minimize increases in pulmonary vascular resistance secondary to hypercarbia, hypoxia, acidosis, stress and pain.
2. Major hemodynamic changes should be avoided, especially marked decreases in systemic vascular resistance and venous return.

There are many case reports in the literature regarding the anesthetic management of patients with primary pulmonary hypertension, with different options of anesthetic technique including combination of subarachnoid morphine and pudendal block;[14] combination of segmental epidural block with pudendal block;[15] double-catheter epidural technique;[16] continuous epidural infusion of local anesthetics and opioids.[17] All these options deserve a few comments. Subarachnoid morphine has been successfully used for pain control during labor but it is not a totally reliable technique in terms of pain relief; the double-catheter technique or the use of intermittent doses of higher concentrations of bupivacaine could lead to important hemodynamic changes; continuous local anesthetic infusion techniques may provide denser than necessary blocks and should be used with caution.

Two techniques have proven to be both effective and safe for these patients in our Institution:

1. Epidural injection of 0.125% bupivacaine, 10 ml, associated with 50–100 µg of fentanyl, reinforced if necessary; perineal anesthesia is provided by pudendal block using 1% lidocaine or by saddle block with 0.5 ml of 5% hyperbaric lidocaine. In certain patients, subcutaneous infiltration with 1% lidocaine will provide the necessary pain relief for episiotomy.
2. Bolus injection of 0.125% bupivacaine, 10 ml, plus 50 µg of fentanyl, followed by continuous infusion of 0.0625% bupivacaine plus fentanyl 1 µg/ml, at a rate of 10 ml/h.

If cesarean delivery is indicated, epidural or spinal anesthesia represents a major risk to the patient. Major regional anesthesia has been used in a few cases in the literature, under invasive central monitoring and careful titration of local anesthetics.[18] However, even when these conditions are available, it is the author's opinion that general anesthesia provides a much more stable hemodynamic situation.

When secondary pulmonary hypertension is suspected, two groups of patients should be considered. When the condition is secondary to acquired valvular heart disease, mostly mitral dysfunction, pulmonary hypertension develops later and has a more benign course. In fact, there is usually no pulmonary arteriolar hypertension with underlying anatomic modifications of the vessels and consequently no right chamber impairment. These patients are usually in a state of pulmonary congestion, with venous hypertension, and greatly benefit from the use of regional anesthesia, as it reduces venous return by causing blood pooling in the capacitance vessels. In certain cases, however, the evidence for pulmonary arteriolar hyper-resistance exists, and in such circumstances general anesthesia is preferred (see Case report 4).

Case report 4

The patient was 30 years old, gravida 1, para 0 at 36 weeks of gestation, undergoing cesarean delivery for prolonged gestation. She suffered from severe mitral stenosis, functional class II–III, and was using a beta-adrenergic blocking agent and digitalis.

ECG at term. Left atrial enlargement and right ventricular hypertrophy.

Echo Doppler cardiogram at the 26th week of gestation. LV, 4.8 cm (normal); FDV, 111 ml (normal); SV, 75 ml (normal); FSV, 36 ml (normal); LV mass, 70 gm/m^2 (normal); volume–mass ratio, 0.95 (normal); EF 0.68% (normal); mitral valve, 0.76 cm^2 (greatly reduced); mitral gradient 28/17 mmHg (maximum/median) (elevated); LA, 5.1 cm (enlarged); pulmonic valve, A-wave absent; RV, 2.1 cm (normal); tricuspid valve normal; RA normal.

Echo Doppler cardiogram at the 35th week of gestation. LV, 4.6 cm (normal); FDV, 97 ml (normal); SV, 80 ml (normal); FSV, 18 ml (normal); EF, 0.82% (normal); LV mass, 90 gm/m^2 (normal); volume–mass ratio, 0.69 (normal); mitral valve, 0.9 cm^2 (greatly reduced); mitral gradient, 47/30 mmHg (elevated); LA, 4.1 cm (enlarged); pulmonic valve, A-wave absent; RV, 2.5 cm (normal); right ventricle systolic pressure, 83 mmHg (elevated); tricuspid valve, secondary insufficiency; RA enlarged.

Comments and anesthetic management. The two echo Doppler cardiograms taken at different gestational ages illustrate the cardiovascular overload induced by pregnancy. In a patient with a critical mitral valve area, an important increase in the transvalvular gradient was observed as gestation progressed. Pulmonary congestion is evident, as the A-wave is absent in the pulmonic valve. High pressures in the right ventricle, as detected in the second echocardiogram, suggest pulmonary hyper-resistance. Although an adapted right ventricle is still present, a secondary tricuspid insufficiency has developed. With these characteristics, we managed this patient as the group with primary pulmonary hypertension. A cesarean delivery was performed under general anesthesia with an uneventful intra and post-operative period.

If pulmonary hypertension is secondary to congenital heart disease (as in Eisenmenger's syndrome), arteriolar hypertension with underlying anatomic modifications is certainly present. Preload and afterload reduction associated with major regional anesthesia may be critical for these patients, and will further increase right-to-left shunt and compromise both oxygenation and myocardial function. Patients undergoing labor and delivery should be managed as those presenting with primary pulmonary hypertension, with a combined epidural/pudendal block technique or with a continuous infusion of low-concentration bupivacaine and fentanyl. Patients undergoing cesarean delivery should receive general anesthesia (see Case report 5).

Case report 5

The patient was 22 years old, gravida 1, at 36 weeks of gestation, undergoing elective cesarean delivery. She suffered from Eisenmenger's syndrome, functional class II, and was using subcutaneous heparin. Her hemoglobin level was 16.5 g%, hematocrit 51%, arterial P_{O_2} 47 mmHg and arterial hemoglobin saturation 87%.

ECG. Biventricular enlargement.

Echo-Doppler cardiogram. Ventricular septal defect (12 mm), PAP (systolic) 115 mmHg.

Comments and anesthetic management. Long-lasting (22 years) exposure of pulmonary circulation to high blood flow led to pulmonary arteriolar hypertension and right-to-left or bidirectional shunt. Note the increased red cells and impairment of oxygenation. Regional anesthesia is contraindicated, as decreases in preload and afterload would further increase the right-to-left shunt. Cesarean delivery was performed under high-dose opioid general anesthesia, with an uneventful postoperative course.

Pulmonic and aortic stenosis

These two valvular dysfunctions can be discussed together, as they pose similar problems to the anesthesiologist. Early in the course of this disease the right or left ventricle is hypertrophic, compliance is low, the systolic volume is somewhat fixed and venous return must be always adequate in order to maintain cardiac output.

Echo Doppler cardiography has proven to be a useful tool to grade these patients according to the severity of the disease. Both valvular area and transvalvular gradients are important in defining the severity of the case (Table 46.6).

Patients with minimal aortic or pulmonic stenosis have few hemodynamic implications and can receive regional anesthesia for both labor and cesarean delivery. Patients with moderate to severe aortic or pulmonic stenosis, while undergoing labor and delivery, are managed with the technique suggested for primary pulmonary hypertension. If cesarean delivery is indicated, general anesthesia is preferred.

Table 46.6 Echo Doppler cardiogram in aortic and pulmonic stenosis

Severity of disease	Aortic gradient (mmHg)	Aortic valvular area (cm^2)	Pulmonic gradient (mmHg)
Severe	> 80	<0.7	> 80
Important	50–80	0.7–0.9	–
Moderate	30–50	1.0–1.2	40–80
Light	< 30	1.3–1.5	< 40

Hypertrophic cardiomyopathy

The basic cardiac dysfunction is a dynamic obstruction to left ventricle outflow due to increased left ventricle contractility. The left ventricle is hypertrophic and its compliance is low. Decreases in preload and in afterload are not tolerated. When undergoing labor and delivery, patients should be managed in the same way as those presenting with pulmonary hypertension. If general anesthesia is required for cesarean delivery, low-concentration halothane is beneficial in association with a high - dose opioid technique to reduce myocardial contractility. Isoflurane should be avoided, as it increases cardiac rate and reduces peripheral resistance.

Left-to-right shunt

Ventricular septal defect, atrial septal defect and patent ductus arteriosus are associated with left-to-right shunt. Small communications are not associated with marked hemodynamic changes and can be managed with regional techniques. If larger defects are present, there is a marked increase in pulmonary blood flow and pulmonary hypertension may develop. In the presence of pulmonary hypertension (Eisenmenger's syndrome), a right-to-left shunt or bidirectional shunt is associated; in such situations, regional anesthesia for labor and delivery is conducted as for primary pulmonary hypertension and cesarean delivery is performed under general anesthesia.

Right-to-left shunt

Tetralogy of Fallot is a representative of this group. The tetralogy consists of infundibular pulmonary artery stenosis, right ventricular hypertrophy, overriding aorta and a ventricular septal defect. These patients do not tolerate decreases in preload or afterload, which will further increase right-to-left shunt. Anesthetic management is similar to pulmonary hypertension if patients have not been surgically treated. For those who have been surgically treated, shunt is no longer present, and regional anesthesia is usually acceptable. A detailed evaluation of right ventricular outflow is necessary; fortunately, although a pulmonic stenosis is usually present, it is of minor importance and does not limit the use of regional techniques.[19]

Myocardial infarction

Although very uncommon, it is related to a high maternal mortality of 30–40%. The prognosis is better when myocardial infarction occurs in the first or second trimester rather than in the third trimester. All obstetric and anesthetic procedures should be postponed for at least 2 weeks after the acute event. Vaginal delivery seems to be associated with a lower incidence of complications[20] compared with cesarean delivery. Regional anesthesia can be beneficial in reducing stress response and avoiding extra cardiac work.[21] Stress response to tracheal intubation if general anesthesia is required can be a serious risk. Continuous electrocardiographic tracing in lead V5 must be carefully followed for signs of ischemia, which should be immediately treated with nitrates. If myocardial function is adequate, regional anesthesia can be utilized. If myocardial function is severely compromised as a consequence of the myocardial infarction, the restrictions to regional anesthesia apply. If cesarean delivery is required, general anesthesia is preferred.

In this important group of patients considered above, in whom a relative contraindication for regional anesthesia exists, it is possible to provide safe and effective analgesia for labor and delivery either by a continuous epidural infusion or by a combined technique. (Table 46.7). If cesarean delivery is indicated, a major regional anesthetic should be avoided and general anesthesia should be the first choice.

GENERAL ANESTHESIA FOR THE PREGNANT CARDIAC PATIENT

Opioids constitute the basis for general anesthesia in the cardiac patient, providing a rather stable hemodynamic status. The most suitable induction agent is etomidate. Low-concentration inhalation agents must be used carefully as they can seriously compromise myocardial function in some patients. Isoflurane is suitable for situations in which myocardial dysfunction is present, especially if a reduction in peripheral resistance and tachycardia are acceptable (mitral insufficiency and aortic insufficiency); however, its use is contraindicated in situations in which tachycardia and/or decrease in peripheral resistance are not tolerated, such as in Eisenmenger's syndrome, mitral and aortic stenosis and hypertrophic cardiomyopathy. Nitrous oxide can be used after delivery, unless pulmonary hypertension is present, in which situation its use is controversial. Succinylcholine to facilitate tracheal intubation must be used carefully because of the bradycardia associated with its use. It must be kept in mind that general anesthesia will not provide the perioperative hemodynamic accommodation as seen with regional anesthesia, and one should be prepared to overcome this by using vasoactive drugs to control either preload (nitroglycerin) or afterload (sodium nitroprusside) as appropriate.

Once general anesthesia has been indicated for one of the cited reasons, a standard technique based on high-dose opioid is suggested (Table 46.8), although variations in this technique could be adapted to different cases. Physiologic changes associated with pregnancy such as increased drug distribution volume, higher levels of endorphins and progesterone-stimulated respiratory center are probably responsible for the successful response of this group of patients to this high-dose opioid technique. Surgical time should be kept to the minimum necessary to avoid supplementary doses of fentanyl, thus reducing the risk of excessive sedation in the post-operative period. Neonatal respiratory depression is not usual, but it is certainly possible. Induction-to-delivery time must be as short as possible, thus reducing placental transfer according to Fick's law. Portella et al[22] have used 10 µg/kg fentanyl during general anesthesia for cesarean delivery and detected neonatal plasma levels (Table 46.9) lower than the 3.0 µg/ml known to produce respiratory depres-

Table 46.7 Labor analgesia for cardiac patients with restrictions to regional anesthesia

First Stage:
Subarachnoid morphine 0.5 mg
Epidural 0.125% bupivacaine (12.5 mg) plus fentanyl 50 –100 µg
Epidural bolus of 0.125% bupivacaine plus 50 µg fentanyl + epidural infusion (10 ml/h) of 0.0625% bupi vacaine (6.25 mg) plus fentanyl 1 µg/ml
Second stage
Local infiltration
Pudendal block
Saddle block with 50 mg of 5% hyperbaric lidocaine

Table 46.8 General anesthesia for the pregnant cardiac patient

Prepare and monitor the patient
Maintain infusion of 5% dextrose 100 ml, at minimum speed to avoid overhydration
Fentanyl 15 µg/kg + etomidate 0.2 mg/kg
Succinylcholine 0.5 mg/kg
Sellick's maneuver + tracheal intubation
Begin surgery immediately
Maintain left uterine displacement
Maintenance
Etomidate 0.05 to 0.1 mg/kg as required
Succinylcholine infusion as required
50% nitrous oxide if appropriate
Supplementary fentanyl 5 µg/kg as required
Oxytocin infusion (20 i.v) after delivery; avoid ergot derivatives

Table 46.9 Fentanyl plasma concentrations (ng/ml) in mother and neonates after general anesthesia for cesarean delivery with 10 µg/kg of fentanyl (mean + SD) (Reproduced from ref. 22)

Maternal vein (*n*=16)	7.8 ± 2.4
Maternal artery (*n*=11)	5.2 ± 0.9
Umbilical vein (*n*=16)	3.6 ± 1.2
Umbilical artery (*n*=16)	1.4 ± 0.6

sion in adults.[23] Neonatal Apgar scores varied from 6 to 9 in the first minute and from 8 to 10 in the fifth minute; all neonates had an Apgar score of 10 in the tenth minute of life.

General anesthesia plays a very important role in the management of pregnant cardiac patients. Despite our absolute preference for regional anesthesia in obstetrics, even in the presence of cardiac disease, a certain number of patients will require general anesthesia. In our institution, general anesthesia for cesarean delivery is used six times more frequently in the group of cardiac patients than in the general obstetric population (Table 46.10).

In a series of 54 cardiac patients undergoing cesarean delivery at the University of São Paulo, in 1987–89, the most frequent indications for general anesthesia were those already highlighted in this text; in some patients, however, insufficient documentation of the patient was the primary reason for avoiding regional anesthesia (Table 46.11). In this series, no major complications occurred in the groups of patients receiving regional anesthesia for cesarean delivery (34 patients) as compared with six complications in the group undergoing general anesthesia (20 patients). These results are partly due to the critical clinical conditions of the patients undergoing general anesthesia, but in some of them the anesthetic management itself may have contributed to the complication. Overhydration and the use of inhalation agents seem to be two important causes of cardiac impairment in the perioperative period (Table 46.12). Hypervolemia is a frequent intra- and post-operative complication associated with pulmonary edema. All efforts should be made to avoid excessive hydration that will contribute to further increase the naturally occurring intravascular volume shifts during labor and delivery. In patients likely to develop pulmonary congestion and pulmonary edema, diuretics should be introduced intraoperatively, immediately after delivery, so as to reduce fluid overload.

Table 46.10 Anesthesia for cesarean delivery at the University of São Paulo (1987–89)

	Overall obstetric population (n = 410) %	Cardiac patients (n = 54) (%)
Epidural	57	39
Spinal	37	24
General	6	37

Table 46.11 Contraindications to regional anesthesia in 54 cardiac patients undergoing cesarean delivery at the University of São Paulo (1987–89)

Secondary pulmonary hypertension	6
Anticoagulation	4
Severe hemodynamic instability (shock)	2
Severe pulmonic or aortic stenosis	2
Severe aortic insufficiency	2
MS + MI + aortic insufficiency	2
Mitral stenosis	1
Mitral stenosis + mitral insufficiency	1

Table 46.12 Severe maternal complications following general anesthesia for cesarean delivery of cardiac patients at the University of São Paulo (1987 – 89)

Diagnosis	Complication	Remarks
MS + MI (FC III – IV)	Pulmonary edema	Overhydration
MS + MI + pulmonary hypertension	Pulmonary edema	Overhydration Halothane
MI (FC IV)	Cardiogenic shock	Ruptured chordae tendineae
MS + atrial fibrillation	Pulmonary edema	—
MS + MI + anticoagulation	Pulmonary edema	Post-operative valve replacement
MS + MI + AoI	Cardiogenic shock	Fentanyl/midazolam

MS, mitral stenosis; MI, mitral insufficiency; FC, functional class; AoI, aortic insufficiency.

PREPARING THE PATIENT FOR SURGERY

Monitoring

The severity of the disease and the underlying pathophysiology will dictate the standard of monitoring.

NYHA functional class I and II patients can be managed with continuous non-invasive measurement of blood pressure, electrocardiogram, pulse oximetry and urinary catheter.

NYHA functional class III and IV patients should be managed with an intra-arterial catheter, electrocardiogram, central venous pressure, pulse oximetry and urinary catheter. The use of a pulmonary artery catheter is helpful when left ventricular function is severely compromised. Although the risk associated with its use is not greater in the pregnant patient than in the nonpregnant group, the Swan–Ganz catheter has been associated with significant morbidity and mortality.

Antibiotics

All patients with valvular or congenital defects either surgically corrected or not, should receive prophylactic antibiotics. The recommended prophylactic regimen includes:

- ampicillin 2.0 g i.v. 1 h before surgery;
- gentamycin 1.5 g/kg i.m. 1 h before surgery;
- repeat after 6 h

If an obstetric risk of infection is present, a therapeutic use will substitute the standard prophylactic regimen:

- cephalosporin 1.0 g/ 6 h;
- chloramphenicol 0.5 g/ 6 h

Anticoagulants

Cardiac patients likely to be using anticoagulants are those with:

- mechanic prosthesis: mitral (absolute indication), aortic (relative indication):
- primary pulmonary hypertension;
- Eisenmenger's syndrome;
- dilated cardiomyopathy;
- atrial fibrillation;
- previous thromboembolic episodes.

Oral anticoagulation is changed to heparin on the 33rd week of gestation, to avoid risks of fetal and neonatal hemorrhage. Subcutaneous heparin is then administered 5000 i.u. every 8 h (or in a higher dose), to maintain activated partial thromboplastin time (aPTT) and thrombin time (TT), at 2.5 times control values. On the day of surgery, the first dose should not be administered and the drug should be reintroduced 8–12 h after delivery.

SUMMARY

The successful management of the cardiac pregnant patient depends on the cooperative work of the cardiologist, the obstetrician and the anesthesiologist. Good prenatal care will provide the best clinical conditions and solid information on the underlying pathophysiology. Whatever the syndrome, it is essential to understand the exact contribution of preload, afterload, heart rate and myocardial contractility to the equilibrium between pulmonary and systemic circulation[5]. Regional anesthesia should be used whenever possible, as its hemodynamic effects help to accommodate the dramatic hemodynamic fluctuations occurring during labor, delivery and in the immediate post-partum period. In patients in whom regional anesthesia is associated with an increased risk, it should be used with extreme caution for pain control during labor. If cesarean delivery is indicated, general anesthesia should be preferred. If general anesthesia is indicated, a high-dose opioid anesthesia should be preferred, as it provides good cardiovascular stability. Although neonatal respiratory depression is possible with this technique, it should be viewed as a precise maternal indication. General anesthesia does not provide the hemodynamic cushion seen with regional anesthesia; fluid overload and the use of myocardial depressants are the most common causes of cardiac function impairment. Invasive monitoring is not usually and easily applicable to the pregnant patient; thus, the anesthesiologist should most appropriately rely on a comprehensive study of the case and adequate planning of the anesthetic technique.

REFERENCES

1. Ueland K, Hansen J M 1969 Maternal cardiovascular dynamics. II. Posture and uterine contractions. Am J Obstet Gynecol 103: 1–7
2. Ueland K, Hansen J M 1969 Maternal cardiovascular dynamics. III. Labor and delivery under local and caudal analgesia. Am J Obstet Gynecol 103: 8–18
3. Ueland K, Novy M, Peterson E, Metcalf J 1969 Maternal cardiovascular dynamics. IV. The influence of gestational age on the maternal cardiovascular response to posture and exercise. Am J Obstet Gynecol 104: 156–164
4. Clark S L, Phelan J P, Aldahl D, Horenstein J 1985 Labor and delivery in the presence of mitral stenosis: central hemodynamic observations. AM J Obstet Gynecol 152: 984–988
5. Mangano D T 1987 Anesthesia for the pregnant cardiac patient. In: Shnider S M, Levingson G (eds) Anesthesia for obstetrics. Williams & Wilkins, Baltimore
6. The Criteria Committee of New York Heart Association 1979 Nomenclature and criteria for diagnosis of diseases of the heart and great vessels, New York, New York Heart Association
7. Faccioli R 1990 Área da valva mitral estenótica em gestantes portadoras de doenca reumática: correlação com a prognóstico perinatal 1990 Tese de Doutoramento – Faculdade de Medicina da Universidade de São Paulo
8. Hemmings G T, Whalley D G, O' Connor P J, Benjamin A, Dunn C 1987 Invasive monitoring and anesthetic management of a parturient with mitral stenosis. Can J Anaesth 34: 182–185
9. Mostafa S M 1984 Spinal anesthesia for cesarean section management of a parturient with severe cardiovascular disease. Br J Anaesth 56: 1275–1277
10. Rapaport E 1975 Natural risk of aortic and mitral valve disease. Am J Cardiol 35: 221–227
11. O'Connel J B, Costanzo-Nordin M R, Subramanian R et al 1986 Peripartum cardiomyopathy: clinical, hemodynamic, histologic and prognostic characteristics. J Am Coll Cardiol 8: 52–56
12. Rao T L K, El-Etr A A 1981 Anticoagulation following placement of epidural and subarachnoid catheters. Anesthesiology 55: 618–620
13. Nelson D M, Main E, Crafford W, Ahumada G G 1983 Peripartum heart failure due to primary pulmonary hypertension. Obstet Gynecol 62: 58S–63S
14. Abboud T, Raya J, Noueihed R, Daniel J 1983 Intrathecal morphine for relief of labor pain in a parturient with severe pulmonary hypertension. Anesthesiology 59: 477–479
15. Sorensen M B, Korshin J D, Fernandes A, Secher O 1982 The use of epidural analgesia for delivery in a patient with pulmonary hypertension. Acta Anesthesiol Scand 26: 180–182
16. Slomka F, Salmeron S, Zetlaoui P, Cohen H, Simonneau G, Kamran S 1988 Primary pulmonary hypertension and pregnancy: anesthetic management for delivery. Anesthesiology 69: 959–961
17. Robinson D E, Leicht C H 1988 Epidural analgesia with low-dose bupivacaine and fentanyl for labor and delivery in a parturient with severe pulmonary hypertension. Anesthesiology 68: 285–288
18. Spinnato J A, Kraynack B J, Cooper M W 1981 Eisenmenger's syndrome in pregnancy: epidural anesthesia for elective cesarean section. New Engl J Med 304: 1215–1217
19. Carvalho J C A, Mathias R S, Siaulys M M, Torres M L A, Capelli E L, Gomide do Amaral R V 1993 Anesthesia for cesarean section in patients with surgically treated tetralogy of Fallot. Braz J Anesthesiol 4: 32–34
20. Hankins G D V, Wendall G D, Leveno K J, Stoneham J 1985 Myocardial infarction in pregnancy: a review. Obstet Gynecol 65: 139–146
21. Hands M E, Johnson M D, Saltzman D H, Rutherford J D 1990 The cardiac, obstetric, and anesthetic management of pregnancy complicated by acute myocardial infarction. J Clin Anesth 2: 258–268
22. Portella A A V, Reis G F F, Melo G A, Cyreno N U 1990 General anesthesia for cesarean section with fentanyl: maternal and fetal plasma concentrations. Braz J Anesthesiol Int Issue 3: 35–37
23. Stoeckel H, Schuttler J, Magnussen H, Hengstmann J H 1982 Plasma fentanyl concentration and the occurrence of respiratory depression in volunteers. Br J Anaesth 54: 1087–1095

47. Respiratory disease

Part A Chronic pulmonary disease and anesthetic technique *D. Sage J. Kolbe*
Part B Asthma: USA view *R. L. Busch*
Part C Acute adult respiratory distress syndrome in pregnancy *R. L. Busch*

PART A
CHRONIC PULMONARY DISEASE AND ANESTHETIC TECHNIQUE
D. Sage J. Kolbe

INTRODUCTION

Except for asthma, chronic respiratory disease is uncommon in young women. Generally, pregnancy has little effect on stable chronic respiratory disease and functional deterioration is not often seen – this being partly explained by the normal increase in respiratory drive of pregnancy. General anesthesia should be avoided if possible because of the $\dot{V}/\dot{Q}$ mismatch and post-operative lung atelectasis it produces. Epidural analgesia in labor is preferred and has the additional advantage of reducing maternal oxygen consumption.

This chapter discusses the common obstructive, suppurative and restrictive disorders, including kyphoscoliosis, a condition that poses unique anesthetic problems in pregnancy. While brevity demands exclusion of many rare pulmonary disorders, their anesthetic management in pregnancy can largely be extrapolated from the examples given. The reader is referred to Chapter 58 for the respiratory implications of morbid obesity. Acute lung changes caused by pulmonary embolus (Chs 55 and 56), pregnancy-induced hypertension (Ch. 45), aspiration (Ch. 48), and massive transfusion (Ch. 44).

OBSTRUCTIVE LUNG DISEASE

Asthma

Asthma is the most common chronic pulmonary disease of pregnancy. The prevalence of asthma in pregnancy has been estimated at 1% (reported range of 0.4–1.3%)[1] – a likely underestimate. Hernandez et al[2] reported that 0.15% of pregnant women required hospitalization for severe asthma. In New Zealand, asthma was the cause of nearly 5% of all maternal deaths and ranked third among fatal medical conditions after intracranial hemorrhage and cardiac disease.[3]

A universally accepted precise definition of asthma is still lacking, but most agree that a cardinal feature of this condition is nonspecific airway hyperresponsiveness (AHR) – the excessive airway narrowing following exposure to a wide variety of specific and nonspecific constrictor agents. Recent research has focused on the apparently close relationship between AHR and airway inflammation, especially eosinophilic infiltration, with subsequent management being aimed at 'modifying the disease' and reducing AHR.

Prevalence studies have found a close but not identical relationship between AHR and clinical asthma,[4] while cross-sectional and longitudinal studies show only a weak correlation between AHR and clinical features of asthma.[56] Only in a minority of individuals does AHR correlate closely with other clinical parameters,[7,8] and hence the clinical usefulness of measures of AHR remains controversial.

Effect of pregnancy on asthma

Pregnancy has an unpredictable effect on asthma[9,10] but, as a general rule, it is those with more severe asthma prior to pregnancy whose asthma tends to worsen during pregnancy. There is an increase in asthma symptoms from 29 to 36 weeks' gestation, but asthma tends to be less severe during the last 4 weeks of pregnancy.[10] It is uncommon for acute asthma to be a problem during labor and delivery. During the first 3 months post-partum, asthma reverts to its previous pattern, which argues in favor of a specific effect of pregnancy on the condition.

In a prospective study of 16 asthmatic women who conceived, there was a slight but significant reduction in AHR (improvement) during the second trimester compared with preconception values, although no consistent pattern was found. Changes in AHR were greatest in those who were most responsive initially. There was no correlation between progesterone or estriol levels and AHR, suggesting that nonhormonal factors may be responsible, but AHR returned to original preconception values in the post-delivery period.[11]

In view of a concordance rate of only 60% in the course of asthma in two successive pregnancies,[10] it would be inappropriate to advise women about the possible effects of a future pregnancy on asthma, based on their previous pregnancy experience.

Effect of asthma on pregnancy

Increased rates of prematurity, perinatal morbidity and mortality and increased maternal morbidity reported in early studies were probably due to poor control of asthma during pregnancy. Using age- and parity-matched controls, Stenius-Aarniala et al[9] demonstrated that, although asthma was associated with higher rates of preeclampsia, hypoglycemia in the infant and cesarean delivery (both elective and nonelective), there was no difference in the length of gestation, birthweight, incidence of perinatal death, frequency of low Apgar scores, neonatal respiratory difficulties, hyperbilirubinemia or malformations. Similar findings were reported by Schatz et al.[10] Although severe and/or recurrent attacks may be associated with maternal and fetal morbidity and mortality, generally the increased risk to the fetus of mothers with asthma is small and should not be overemphasized when counselling individual patients. Adverse outcomes such as low-birthweight and small-for-gestational age infants tend to be associated with episodes of acute uncontrolled asthma.[11] However, chronic impairment of maternal gestational pulmonary function (mean percent predicted FEV_1) is related to lower infant birthweights in pregnant asthmatic women,[12] owing to growth retardation rather than prematurity. Careful treatment and supervision of asthma during pregnancy and close cooperation between the obstetrician and the respiratory physician with resulting good control of asthma should prevent most obstetric and neonatal complications, even in high-risk groups.[13]

The reason for a high rate of cesarean delivery is not clear. Severe asthmatics may be regarded as high-risk patients and thus have a higher elective cesarean delivery rate. Acute cesarean delivery performed because of an exacerbation of asthma is uncommon, but asthma therapy may interfere with labor, e.g. β-agonist drug inhibition of uterine contractility, and thus increase the cesarean delivery rate.

Asthma management in pregnancy

The goals of therapy remain unchanged: to prevent death, to eliminate morbidity, allow normal exercise tolerance, eliminate symptoms and interference with daily activities and improve quality of life. No asthma medications can be considered totally safe during pregnancy, and it would be difficult, if not impossible, to conduct the appropriate well-controlled studies. Therefore, the available data must be balanced against the substantial maternal and fetal risk of uncontrolled asthma during pregnancy. Current evidence suggests that drugs used in the treatment of asthma are generally safe for the mother and do not damage the fetus; thus pregnancy alters the treatment of asthma very little.

In a prospective comparison there were no significant differences found in maternal or fetal outcome[14] between pregnant asthmatics using or not using inhaled metaproterenol and pregnant nonasthmatics. Although the antimuscarinic agent ipratropium bromide and newer β-agonists such as terbutaline, fenoterol and salbutamol (albuterol) have not been systematically evaluated, there has been no direct association between the use of these agents and congenital abnormalities.

There is no evidence of adverse effects in infants of women receiving inhaled cromolyn or theophylline during pregnancy. Theophylline clearance is lower in the third trimester than in the first and second trimesters and post-partum period.[15] As theophylline freely crosses the placenta, close monitoring of theophylline levels and a reduction in dose may be necessary in the third trimester to avoid maternal and fetal toxicity.

There is no excess of congenital malformations or neonatal or maternal deaths in asthmatic women using beclomethasone dipropionate (BDP) in 'recommended' doses during pregnancy.[16] No data are available on adverse effects associated with high doses of inhaled BDP (> 1000 μg/day), or on other types of inhaled corticosteroids, e.g. budesonide.

Biochemical evidence of adrenal suppression has been documented in nonpregnant adults inhaling > 1500 μg of BDP per day.[17,18] The clinical significance of this is unknown and it is not clear as to whether additional exogenous steroids are required to cover labor, delivery or the stress of surgical intervention in such patients, but this would seem advisable.

Prednisone and prednisolone cross poorly into the fetal circulation, and judicious use is not considered harmful to the fetus.[19,20] No evidence of neonatal adrenal insufficiency (or of fetal or neonatal loss) was found in any of 71 infants born to mothers requiring an average daily dose of 8.2 mg of prednisone for variable periods of time during pregnancy.[21]

In view of the adverse outcomes associated with uncontrolled asthma and lack of adverse effects associated with asthma drugs, it is recommended that conventional drugs and dosages be used to obtain optimal asthma control during pregnancy. A schema for the management of asthma during pregnancy is shown in Figure 47.1. It reflects the current trend of reduced reliance on bronchodilators, especially inhaled β-agonists, the earlier use of 'disease-modifying' therapy, particularly inhaled corticosteroids, and the multidisciplinary approach to the condition.

Acute attacks carry the highest risk, and management is aimed at preventing significant hypoxia or changes in acid–base balance. The management of acute asthma during pregnancy does not differ from that of the nonpregnant patient.

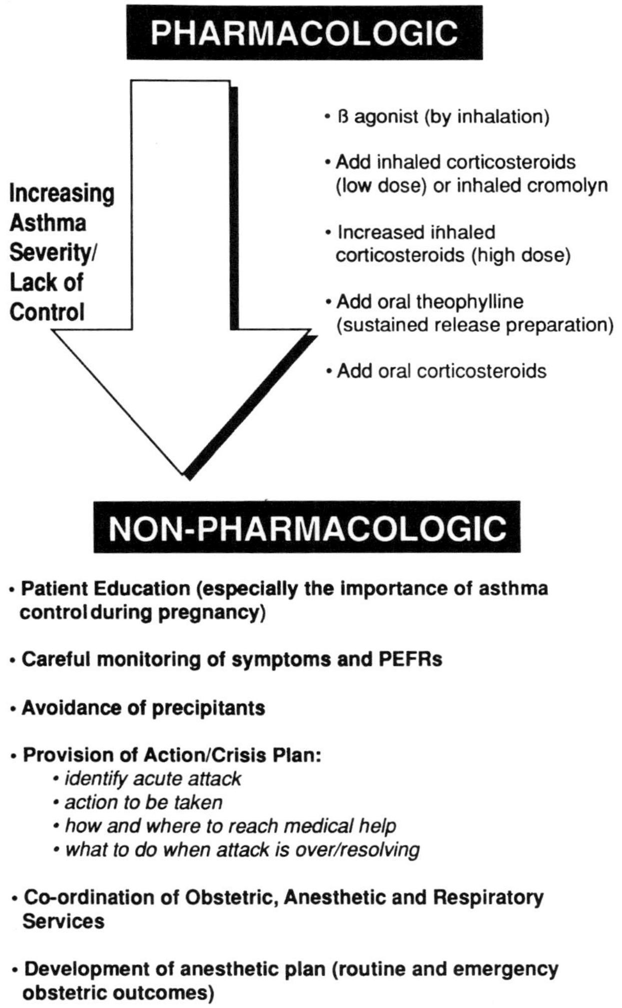

Fig. 47.1 Chronic management of asthma during pregnancy

Preanesthetic assessment of the asthmatic

Although the assessment of acute severe asthma is well documented and well validated, the same cannot be said of the preoperative assessment of the stable asthmatic who may have few signs or symptoms.

The aims of this assessment are to:

- Determine the disability/dysfunction due to asthma, i.e. asthma control. Implicit in this is an assessment of the effectiveness of therapy.
- Identify those at risk of developing acute severe asthma before, during and after anesthesia.
- Devise an anesthetic plan for different obstetric outcomes, namely analgesia in normal labor, emergency delivery, etc.

Assessment depends almost entirely upon the history. Although physical examination may demonstrate wheeze or features of chronicity such as hyperinflation or chest deformity, it is usually not helpful in achieving the above aims. Pulmonary function tests such as peak expiratory flow rate (PEFR) and FEV_1/VC are essential but are only an indication of airway caliber at that particular time. Serial PEFR measures are more useful. Chest radiographs and arterial blood gas sampling are not routinely required.

The most important predictor of outcome is the previous severity of asthma. Since no single satisfactory measure of severity exists, it is appropriate to assess the level of asthma morbidity (hospital admissions, emergency department (ED) visits, use of short courses of oral corticosteroids, etc.). In a case–control study of male and female asthma deaths, Rea et al[22] found that, compared with community controls, asthmatics who died were more likely to have had one or more ED visits or hospital admissions in the last year. This probably reflects poorly controlled asthma, for whatever reason. Also, AHR may increase following a severe attack, analogous to allergen exposure in the laboratory.[23] Following treatment of an acute attack, pulmonary function improves, although there is marked variability (diurnal and day to day) – this variability may reflect increased levels of AHR.

Rea et al[22] also found that when compared with community controls those dying of asthma were more likely to have poor medical care and exhibit noncompliance. When those admitted to hospital were used as controls, only two factors, namely psychosocial problems and a past history of 'life-threatening asthma attack', were more common in those dying of asthma.[23] (Life-threatening asthma was defined as 'an asthma attack where level of consciousness had been disturbed or appreciable hypercapnia had been recorded'.) At very high risk are those who required admission to an intensive care unit for severe asthma – the 3-year mortality is 12.5%.[24]

Also reflecting poorly controlled underlying asthma are nocturnal symptoms (a symptomatic reflection of PEFR variability), frequent use of inhaled β-agonists and frequent short courses of oral prednisone. Nonuse of 'preventive' therapy, despite continuing symptoms, reflects inadequate control and poor medical care.

These features need to be elicited in the history and are summarized in Table 47.1.

The anesthetic plan based on this assessment should be arrived at in a multidisciplinary setting that allows close consultation between respiratory physician, obstetrician, anesthesiologist and patient. The anesthetic plan for asthma management and pain relief in normal labor, as well as the anesthetic options for unexpected surgical intervention, must be documented.

Anesthetic management

In all obstetric procedures requiring general anesthesia, intubation is mandatory, but in asthmatics this carries the immediate risk of life-threatening bronchospasm. Regional anesthesia avoids this risk and is strongly preferred. Exacerbations of asthma during regional anesthesia are usually mild and easily treated, and, in labor, the medical management of asthma may be enhanced by the reduction of pain and anxiety by epidural analgesia.[25]

Table 47.1 Identification and management of the high-risk asthmatic patient

Information to be elicited from asthmatic patients during antenatal assessment

Patient factors
Social factors
Noncompliance

Disease factors
Interference with life
- Days missed from work/school
- Nocturnal symptoms

Morbidity
- Hospital admissions in last year
- Visits to ER in last year
- Visits to GP acutely in last year (particularly if recent)

Past history of life-threatening attacks
Lung function – Absolute
(PEFR) – Variability

Previous management factors
Continuity and quality of care
Knowledge and understanding
Drugs – number of classes of drugs
- Several bronchodilators in the absence of 'preventive' therapy
- Frequency of use of β-agonists
- Corticosteroids
  frequent courses
  continuous

Having identified the high-risk patient
Attempt to normalize/optimize pulmonary function (short course of oral corticosteroids);
Attempt to reduce AHR, e.g. regular inhaled corticosteroids;
Monitor peak expiratory flow rate;
Liaise with respiratory physician;
Modify the anesthetic plan.

General anesthesia is unavoidable in up to 10% of obstetric operations, and in asthmatics a number of facts related to the standard techniques should be noted:

1. Premedication with cimetidine or ranitidine should not be withheld. H_2-receptor-blocking drugs may theoretically interfere with the negative-feedback inhibition of basophil histamine release, but the clinical significance of this is unknown and is far outweighed by their proven efficacy in reducing gastric volume and acidity.

2. Awake intubation, even if time permits, almost always worsens bronchospasm, and complete loss of the cough reflex is undesirable.

3. Intravenous lidocaine (1.0–1.5 mg/kg) reduces reflex bronchoconstriction in dogs[26] and a central site of action is assumed. An intravenous bolus preceding induction and just prior to extubation appear effective in humans and has negligible morbidity. Topical lidocaine is not compatible with rapid sequence induction and may well provoke bronchospasm.[27]

4. Where rapid induction and intubation is required before deep anesthesia can be achieved, ketamine (0.5–1.0 mg/kg) is the agent of choice, maintaining anesthesia with inhalation agents and muscle relaxants. The advantages of ketamine are its bronchodilating effect, acceptably low incidence of hallucinatory side-effects and proven safety to the fetus when used for cesarean delivery.[28,29] Larger doses (2.0 mg/kg) may be associated with delivery of infants slow to breathe, but who nevertheless have excellent acid–base status.[29] Although seizure-like activity has been reported with ketamine in patients receiving aminophylline infusions, frank convulsions have not been reported.[30] In the authors' opinion aminophylline is not a contraindication to the use of ketamine. Similarly, although hypertension relatively contraindicates ketamine, short-acting vasodilators such as sodium nitroprusside, trimethaphan or trinitroglycerin by bolus or infusion can prevent an undesirable blood pressure rise at induction without apparent adverse fetal effects.

5. Neuromuscular blocking drugs all cause some histamine release, but even with the worst offender, d-tubocurarine, no uniform increase in airway resistance is found, in either normal individuals[31,32] or asthmatics.[33] Succinylcholine appears quite satisfactory in asthmatics and the current non-depolarizer of choice is vecuronium.[27] Although asthmatics do not have a higher incidence of massive histamine release following these drugs, when reactions do occur, the mortality is higher in asthmatics.[34]

6. Halothane, enflurane and isoflurane have similar bronchodilator effects in normal subjects. In the presence of increased levels of catecholamines,[35] or aminophylline,[36] isoflurane has the advantage of being less arrhythmogenic than halothane. The uterine relaxation associated with the use of low concentrations can be

overcome with a synthetic oxytocin infusion. This relative disadvantage should not deter the use of isoflurane at inhaled concentrations up to about 1 MAC both before and after delivery.

Management of intraoperative bronchospasm

Even in asthmatics, other causes for sudden 'ventilatory problems characterized by an increase in airway pressure and associated with expiratory wheeze'[37] must be excluded. These include aspiration, anaphylaxis, pneumothorax, misplaced or obstructed tracheal tube or the injection by the surgeon of prostaglandin $F_{2\alpha}$ into a flaccid bleeding uterus.

With general anesthesia, aminophylline is used only if isoflurane and salbutamol are ineffective. During cesarean delivery, both isoflurane and salbutamol relax the uterus. Delivery of the baby should be effected rapidly and oxytocin infusion commenced. Isoflurane and salbutamol can be continued judiciously, but at an early stage aminophylline bolus or infusion based on the patient's previous theophylline usage is recommended. Careful monitoring for arrhythmias and hypokalaemia is essential.

Additional measures include an appropriately high $F\text{IO}_2$, slow inspiratory flow rates, which are often only achievable with manual ventilation, and avoidance of positive end-expiratory pressure (PEEP). Intravenous hydrocortisone 100–400 mg is safe and may have a beneficial effect some hours later. Ketamine can be life-saving when oxygenation is still precarious despite all these measures.[38] In extreme cases of status asthmaticus, cesarean delivery has been undertaken for maternal or fetal reasons and anesthetic technique is merely a continuation of intensive care life support.[39]

Chronic airflow limitation

Chronic airflow limitation (CAL) [synonyms: chronic obstructive pulmonary disease (COPD), chronic obstructive airways disease (COAD)] refers to the condition of smoking-related, partially reversible chronic obstructive disease. Severe CAL is uncommon in women of child-bearing age, but may occur in predisposed individuals, e.g. those having α_1-antitrypsin deficiency. If CAL is severe, is out of proportion to the smoking history or if bullous disease is present, particularly in the lung bases, then maternal α_1-antitrypsin levels should be measured. This has implications for mother and infant, particularly as enzyme replacement therapy is now available.[40]

Cigarette smoking during pregnancy is associated with higher perinatal mortality (light smoking increases risk of fetal death by 20%, heavy smoking by 35%),[41] although low socioeconomic class, increased maternal age and parity may act as confounders. Maternal problems related to placenta and uterus are likely to be responsible for some of the increased fetal loss, which shows a dose–response relationship to cigarette consumption. Cigarette smoking is also associated with increased frequency of premature births, spontaneous abortions and low-birthweight infants, but the precise roles of carbon monoxide and nicotine are not clear. Equilibration of carboxyhemoglobin levels in the pregnant woman and fetus occurs in 5–6 h.

Smoking also induces mucus secretion. Although not necessarily a cause of physiologic abnormalities per se, mucus hypersecretion is associated with increased respiratory complications of general anesthesia and surgery. Cessation of smoking reduces perioperative morbidity[42] and, although the myocardium benefits, a substantial decline in carboxyhemoglobin levels and an increase in P_{50} are seen after 12–24 h of abstinence, 4–8 weeks are required to produce a measurable reduction in respiratory complications.[42,43]

Aims of preanesthetic assessment

1. Reduce complications
   - stop cigarettes
   - avoid other irritants
   - chest physiotherapy if productive cough
   - antibiotics to eradicate any infection
   - improve nutrition
   - optimize therapy and hence pulmonary function;
2. Assess function
   - exercise tolerance
   - lung volumes (FEV_1/VC)
   - arterial blood bases;
3. Exclude associated pulmonary pathology
   - chest radiograph.

SUPPURATIVE LUNG DISEASE

Bronchiectasis

Bronchiectasis is a permanent abnormal dilation of bronchi. Chronic cough and sputum production are the result of the combination of impairment of the cough mechanism, defective mucociliary clearance, mucus hypersecretion and chronic infection. Chronic partially reversible airflow obstruction and chronic rhinosinusitis are common accompaniments. Complications include acute infective exacerbations and pneumonia, hemoptysis, colonization by *Pseudomonas* species and empyema. In New Zealand, the incidence of bronchiectasis is much higher in Polynesians than in Europeans,[44] possibly as a result of adenovirus infection in early childhood.[45,46] The cilial ultrastructural abnormalities described in Polynesians with bronchiectasis[47] are probably secondary to infection and injury, rather than being the primary abnormality. Although the rate of decline in FEV_1 in most bronchiectatics is generally no greater than normal, there may be a subset of patients who develop progressive lung damage and eventually cor pulmonale,[48] possibly related to heavy bacterial colonization.

Generally, patients with bronchiectasis tolerate pregnancy well, without change in pulmonary function, degree of dyspnea or sputum production, and the underlying lung disease does not seem to have any adverse effect on the pregnancy.[49,50] In severe cases, intrauterine growth retardation or fetal death may occur[51] and pregnancy has reportedly precipitated maternal respiratory failure.[52]

Maternal and fetal hypoxia can be reduced by:

- stopping smoking;
- physiotherapy with postural drainage and forced expiration techniques;
- antibiotic therapy, possibly continuous;
- use of bronchodilators.

Associated inheritable conditions such as hypogammaglobulinemia, IgG subclass deficiency,[53] α_1-antitrypsin deficiency and previously undiagnosed cystic fibrosis should be excluded by appropriate tests.

Cystic fibrosis (CF)

CF is the most common lethal genetic (autosomal recessive) disorder. The gene frequency is very low in Polynesians but is as high as 1 in 25 in Europeans. In New Zealand, where routine neonatal testing is undertaken using an immunoreactive trypsin test on dried blood samples, the incidence is 1 in 3200 live non-Polynesian births.[54] Although the precise biochemical defect(s) in CF remains unknown, the discrete abnormalities in water and electrolyte fluxes across epithelial cells that occur in the nose, bronchi and sweat glands are similar. The most likely defect is decreased chloride ion conductance across apical membranes of epithelial cells.

The CF gene, which resides on the long arm of chromosome 7, has now been identified and the structure of the putative protein product (cystic fibrosis transmembrane conductance regulator) predicted. In addition, the most common (~ 70%) CF gene mutation has been identified. This leads to the loss of a single amino acid in the functional domain of the protein product. A number of less common mutations have also been identified, and these may explain the clinical heterogeneity of this condition.

Median survival rates for CF have improved dramatically in the last two decades to 20–25 years for females and 30–35 years for males. 80% of CF patients will now reach the age of 20 years.[55] Thus, many females with CF now reach reproductive age. Although fertility in these women is undoubtedly reduced for a variety of reasons, many retain the capacity to bear children.[56]

The aims of management are little different from that in the nonpregnant state, namely:

- maintain nutrition and growth by providing pancreatic enzyme replacement and, if necessary, nutritional supplements
- optimize and prevent deterioration in pulmonary function with bronchodilators, etc.;
- minimize chronic bronchopulmonary suppuration with appropriate antibiotics and chest physiotherapy;
- provide social and psychological support.

Optimal management requires close liaison between the anesthesiologist, obstetrician and the adult CF team.

Hazards of pregnancy are associated with impaired cardiopulmonary function, reduced respiratory reserve and the requirements of increased respiratory and cardiac work. The role of various factors in predicting the outcome of pregnancy in CF women is not clear, but the best predictor is likely to be the degree of pre-existing pulmonary involvement. Pregnancy in CF women with severe lung disease may be associated with significant deterioration. Although the mortality of mothers with CF after delivery was significantly increased compared with normal women, it was not different from that of nonpregnant women with CF.[57] Pregnancies in women with CF are complicated by increased frequency of prematurity and perinatal deaths but not congenital abnormalities.[57]

The complications of cystic fibrosis which are relevant to obstetric anesthesia are:

1. Respiratory
   - chronic airflow limitation, usually with a reversible component and mild AHR;
   - chronic bronchopulmonary suppuration with tenacious secretions;
   - acute 'infective' exacerbations;
   - increased risk of spontaneous pneumothoraces (may be tension and/or bilateral);
   - hemoptysis, occasionally massive;
   - *Pseudomonas* and staphylococcal colonization;
   - chronic rhinosinusitis with nasal polyps;
   - malnutrition and reduced respiratory muscle strength.
2. Gastrointestinal
   - biliary cirrhosis and portal hypertension;
   - fat-soluble vitamin deficiency, including vitamin K deficiency.
3. Other
   - diabetes mellitus;
   - altered drug metabolism.

Anesthesia (for patients with suppurative lung disease)

A regional technique is preferable, but motor block extending above T6 will seriously reduce expiratory reserve volume (ERV) and the ability to cough and clear secretions. Dehydration should be avoided. Because of impaired pulmonary function, these patients may tolerate sedative drugs poorly. Individual patients should have an obstetric emergency anesthetic plan prepared in case there is a sudden requirement for general anesthesia. Nitrous oxide can cause expansion of bullae or pneumothoraces and should be avoided, as should excessive inspired oxygen concentrations, which allow alveolar absorption collapse, and volatile agents that abolish hypoxic pulmonary vasoconstriction. Careful monitoring of oxygen saturation to determine an appropriate humidified air–oxygen mixture is ideal, with maintenance of anesthesia by intravenous agents. Although Gin and colleagues[58,59] have shown propofol to be a safe and effective induction agent for cesarean delivery, patients in their studies received nitrous oxide–enflurane maintenance prior to delivery of the infant. Predelivery maintenance of anesthesia with propofol alone has not been assessed for its effects on the fetus. Long- and short-term advantages of avoiding inhalation agents must be weighed against the possible transient depression of the newborn caused by propofol or ketamine.

RESTRICTIVE LUNG DISEASE

Sarcoidosis

Sarcoidosis is a multisystem granulomatous disorder of unknown etiology, most commonly affecting young adults and presenting most frequently with bilateral hilar lymphadenopathy, pulmonary infiltration and skin or eye lesions. Extrathoracic organ involvement is common but frequently asymptomatic.

Sarcoidosis is a common condition, and in an urban center in New Zealand the average annual incidence was 4.4/100 000 and there was no difference between Polynesians and Europeans. Community-based studies suggest that overall the outcome is good with a high rate of spontaneous resolution, a low rate of clinical involvement of vital organs and only a 2% rate of progressive pulmonary impairment leading to consequent respiratory failure.[60] Series reported from tertiary referral centers report a far higher morbidity.[61]

Apart from the rare cases of involvement of the Fallopian tubes or uterus, sarcoidosis does not usually affect fertility. Approximately 0.05% of pregnant women have sarcoidosis.[62]

Scadding and Mitchell[63] noted certain patterns of behavior of sarcoidosis during pregnancy:

- In sarcoidosis that has already undergone clinical resolution, there is no recrudescence in pregnancy or the post-partum period.
- In resolving cases, sarcoidosis continues to resolve during and after pregnancy.
- In those with stable disease, there is no change in pregnancy.
- However, in those with active sarcoidosis, reversible elements in the disease may be suppressed during pregnancy with symptomatic improvement, but in a number there is relapse towards the original state during the first few weeks after delivery, suggesting a specific beneficial effect of pregnancy.

Their conclusion was that pregnancy has no long-term effects on the prognosis of sarcoidosis.

There is no evidence that maternal sarcoidosis has an adverse effect on the fetus. Although miscarriages and congenital abnormalities have been reported in fetuses of women with sarcoidosis, the incidence of such problems is not any greater than in other women.

Although it is unusual for sarcoidosis to develop or progress during pregnancy, indications for the treatment are the same as in the non-pregnant state, namely:

- progressive and/or symptomatic pulmonary involvement;
- vital organ involvement, e.g. heart, kidneys, brain, etc.;
- hypercalcemia.

However, there is no evidence that corticosteroids influence the natural history of the disease over the long term.

Thus, sarcoidosis is most frequently a 'benign' disease; severe pulmonary impairment is rare in this group and only rarely does it become a factor in the management of pregnancy, labor or obstetric anesthesia.

The anesthesiologist should assess these patients for the presence of:

— restrictive lung disease, although an obstructive component can develop late in severe cases due to endobronchial stenoses;
— functional impairment of other vital organs, such as heart, liver and kidneys, which is rare;
— anemia, hypercalcemia;
— drugs used for its treatment – usually oral corticosteroids;
— laryngeal involvement and temporomandibular joint arthritis (rare).

CHEST WALL DISEASE

Kyphoscoliosis

This group of spinal column disorders rarely causes severe restrictive lung disease. Kyphoscoliosis is most often congenital or of early onset associated with neuromuscular disorders. The etiology of isolated scoliosis is unknown in 80% of cases, but in the remaining 20% of patients the cause is congenital or there is associated neuromuscular disease, such as poliomyelitis, cerebral palsy, neurofibromatosis or muscular dystrophies, or other causes, such as rheumatoid arthritis, trauma or infection. Spinal tuberculosis is frequently implicated in the less developed countries.

Most cases of scoliosis encountered in pregnancy will be the adolescent idiopathic form that affects females 5–8 times more often than males. Postpolio immunization surveys in the UK and North America have reported a prevalence of scoliosis in schoolchildren of 1.8–4.0 per thousand,[64,65] but if minimal degrees of scoliosis are included this figure is very much higher.[66] Only 7% of adolescents with scoliosis have any other physical abnormalities (congenital heart disease, mental retardation, upper limb anomalies[65]) although asymptomatic mitral valve prolapse is a common association.[67]

Spinal fusion using Harrington, Luque or Cofrel–Dubousset techniques are effective methods of limiting progression of idiopathic spinal curvature. In severe untreated cases there is a progressive cardiorespiratory impairment that is lethal by 30–40 years of age. An extrapulmonary restrictive pattern of pulmonary function is present in inverse proportion to the scoliosis angle. A scoliosis angle of more than 100° greatly increases the risk of respiratory failure. Abnormalities include reduced chest wall compliance, ventilation–perfusion mismatch, increased pulmonary vascular resistance and cor pulmonale and reduced ventilatory responses to hypercapnia and hypoxia.[68,69]

Although slow progression of the idiopathic scoliosis following skeletal maturity often occurs, pregnancy itself does not increase the risk of progression of the curve.[70] The skeletal abnormality does not affect the bony pelvis and the obstetric outcome is normal. Difficulty in achieving spinal anesthesia in two patients was the only obstetric problem related to the scoliosis in 175 women.[70] The cesarean delivery rate was 7.4%, for which the indications were unrelated to scoliosis. Most series report a similarly good outcome,[71–73] although increased perinatal mortality has been reported.[74,75]

With the availability of orthopedic correction and the eradication of poliomyelitis, the rare cases of severe kyphoscoliosis in pregnancy are due to early-onset causes. Successful delivery without major problems of several such patients with vital capacities of less than 1 l have been reported.[75,76] In seven women with vital capacities as low as 580 ml in whom pregnancy precipitated respiratory failure and the need for artificial ventilation, there was a universally good obstetric outcome.[77,78] Early-onset kyphoscoliosis, muscular weakness, vital capacity of less than 1.25 l, hypoxemia and pulmonary hypertension were common features in these patients.

Management of anesthesia

Severe restrictive lung disease with significant cardiorespiratory impairment, due to scoliosis, is rare in the 35–45 year age range, but these patients require detailed work-up by their physician and obstetrician. Most anesthetic experience comes from spinal fusion surgery and preoperative assessment has been reviewed.[68,79] The aim of the antenatal assessment is to determine:

- whether respiratory failure is likely as pregnancy progresses;
- whether epidural analgesia in labor is likely to be a viable option; and
- which of the three anesthesia options for cesarean delivery (regional anesthesia, general anesthesia, local anesthetic infiltration) will be possible should the need arise.

Careful examination of the spine is essential. Both spinal and epidural techniques may be difficult because of abnormal anatomy further distorted by spinal fusion operations and patient positioning difficulties. Incomplete local anesthetic spread can produce epidural failures, although the insertion of a second catheter at another vertebral level may overcome this problem.[80] Fortunately, the lower lumbar vertebrae are often spared and epidural catheterization can often be achieved with resulting adequate anesthesia, although insertion complications are more likely. Crosby and Halpern[82] noted that in four of nine obstetric patients with scoliosis and Harrington rods, one or more of the following occurred:

- — failure to identify the epidural space;
- — blood vessel trauma;
- — dural puncture;
- — failure to obtain analgesia; or
- — the need for multiple attempts at insertion.

Chronic back pain is often present in these patients, and some will justifiably resist any further interference with their back by an anesthesiologist. Continuous spinal anesthesia[83] is an option when epidural anesthesia is unsatisfactory. Similarly, local anesthetic infiltration for cesarean delivery is another safe option when both regional and general anesthetic techniques are undesirable.[84]

Kyphoscoliosis patients can react abnormally to general anesthetic drugs. Both idiopathic scoliosis and various muscular dystrophies are associated with an increased risk of malignant hyperpyrexia. If a neuromuscular disorder is present, then specific information must be obtained about its effect on muscle relaxant pharmacodynamics. For example, succinylcholine is associated with problems of sustained muscle contraction (myotonic dystrophy), hyperkalemia, myoglobinuria and cardiac arrhythmias (muscular dystrophies). Where succinylcholine is contraindicated, a nondepolarizing drug (e.g. vecuronium) can be used for intubation in the acute situation, but only in circumstances in which the possibility of inability to intubate is remote.

RESPIRATORY INSUFFICIENCY/COR PULMONALE

Pregnancy in women with severely limited respiratory

reserve or overt respiratory failure is uncommon – mainly because chronic respiratory insufficiency usually only becomes manifest later in life. It is, however, occasionally encountered in association with CF, bronchiectasis, diffuse interstitial lung disease and kyphoscoliosis.

Although guidelines are proffered, no reliable predictors regarding pulmonary function exist. Gaenster et al[85] studied seven women with moderate or severe restrictive ventilatory defects resulting from tuberculosis or its treatment. Pregnancy did not affect their already significantly reduced vital capacity and they tolerated pregnancy without difficulty. Severe restrictive defects due to kyphoscoliosis are also remarkably well tolerated in pregnancy (see above). However, it is probably unreasonable to extrapolate from these studies the outcome of patients with markedly different pathophysiology such as severe chronic airflow limitation or diffuse interstitial fibrosis.

Overall, it is those patients with the most severe preexisting pulmonary impairment who will be the most likely to deteriorate during pregnancy. Although it has been stated that a vital capacity of 1 l is necessary to maintain a normal pregnancy, there is little objective support for this particular value.

There is also little information regarding the effect of pre-existing maternal hypoxia or hypercapnia on the mother's ability to maintain a normal pregnancy. Reduced maternal $P\text{aO}_2$ has surprisingly little effect on fetal $P\text{aO}_2$, which seems more adversely affected by maternal respiratory alkalosis, perhaps related to constriction of uterine arteries. However, hypoxia has been shown to be directly associated with lower birthweight in women living at high altitudes.[86]

Maternal mortality in primary pulmonary hypertension has been reported to be higher than 50%,[87] but this figure does not necessarily apply to cor pulmonale.

Thus, few useful guidelines can be formulated for obstetric anesthetic planning. Each patient must be considered individually, based on whether the anesthetic intervention is for analgesia in labor or for a surgical procedure. Where possible the anesthesiologist should evaluate the rate of progress of the respiratory disease, measure FEV_1, VC and resting arterial blood gases, obtain noninvasive assessment of pulmonary artery pressures and right heart function and review the patient with the obstetrician. Appropriately detailed patient monitoring and access to intensive care facilities are mandatory regardless of the anesthetic technique chosen.

REFERENCES

1. Greenberger P A, Patterson R 1985 Management of asthma during pregnancy. New Engl J. Med 312: 897–902
2. Hernandez E, Angell C S, Johnson J W C 1980 Asthma in pregnancy: current concepts. Obstet Gynecol 55: 739–743
3. Holst P E 1984 The problem patient: management of asthma in pregnancy. New Ethicals 21: 71–80
4. Pattemore P K, Asher M I, Harrison A C, Mitchell E A, Rea H H, Stewart A W 1990 The inter-relationship among bronchial hyper-responsiveness, the diagnosis of asthma and asthma symptoms. Am Rev Respir Dis 142: 549–554
5. Ryan G, Latimer K M, Dolovich J, Hargreave F E 1982 Bronchial responsiveness to histamine: relationship to diurnal variation in peak flow rate, improvement after bronchodilator and airway calibre. Thorax 37: 423–429
6. Rubinfeld A R, Pain M C 1977 Relationship between bronchial reactivity, airway calibre and severity of asthma. Am Rev Respir Dis 115: 381–387
7. Josephs L K, Gregg I, Mullee M A, Holgate S T 1989 Non-specific bronchial reactivity and its relationship to the clinical expression of asthma: a Longitudinal Study. Am Rev Respir Dis 140: 350–357
8. Kolbe J, Balemi A, Richards G N, Fenwick J, Rea H H 1991 Relationship of non-specific airway responsiveness to measures of peak expiratory flow variability. Presented at the Annual Scientific Meeting of the Thoracic Society of Australia and New Zealand, Lome, Victoria, 7–11 April 1991
9. Stenius-Aarniala B, Piirila P, Teramo K 1988 Asthma and pregnancy: a Prospective study of 198 pregnancies. Thorax 43: 12–18
10. Schatz M, Harden K, Forsythe A et al 1988 The course of asthma during pregnancy, post-partum and with successive pregnancies: a prospective analysis. J Allergy Clin Immunol 81: 509–517
11. Juniper E F, Daniel E E, Roberts R S, Kline P A, Hargreave F E, Newhouse M T 1989 Improvement in airway responsiveness and asthma severity during pregnancy: a prospective study. Am Rev Respir Dis 140: 924–931
12. Schatz M, Zeiger R S, Hoffman C P et al 1990 Intra-uterine growth is related to gestational pulmonary function in pregnant asthmatic women. Chest 98: 389–392
13. Apter A J, Greenberger P A, Patterson R 1989 Outcomes of pregnancy in adolescents with severe asthma. Arch Intern Med 149: 2571–2575
14. Schatz M, Zeiger R S, Harden K M et al 1988 The safety of inhaled β agonist bronchodilators during pregnancy. J Allergy Clin Immunol 82: 686–695
15. Carter B L, Driscoll C E, Smith G D 1986 Theophylline clearance during pregnancy. Obstet Gynecol 68: 555–559
16. Greenberger P A, Patterson R 1983 Beclomethasone diproprionate for severe asthma during pregnancy. Ann Intern Med 98: 478–480
17. Smith M J, Hodson M E 1983 Effects of long term inhaled high dose beclomethasone diproprionate on adrenal functions. Thorax 38: 676–681
18. Ebden P, Jenkins A, Houston G, Davies B H 1986 Comparison of two high dose corticosteroid aerosol treatments, beclomethasone diproprionate (1500 μg/day) and budesonide (1600 μg/day) for chronic asthma. Thorax 41: 869–874
19. Fitzsimons R, Greenberger P A, Patterson R 1986 Outcome of pregnancy in women requiring corticosteroids for severe asthma. J Allergy Clin Immunol 78: 349–353
20. Arad I, Landau H 1984 Adrenocortical reserve of neonates born of long-term, steroid-treated mothers. Eur J Pediatr 142: 279
21. Schatz M, Patterson R, Zeitz S, O'Rourke J, Melam H 1975 Corticosteroid therapy for the pregnant asthmatic patient. J Am Med Assoc 233: 804–807
22. Rea H H, Scragg R, Jackson R, Beaglehole R, Fenwick J, Sutherland D C 1986 A case–control study of deaths from asthma. Thorax 41: 833–839
23. Carter A, Thompson N C, Frith P A, Roberts R, Hargreave F 1982 Allergen-induced increase in bronchial responsiveness to histamine: relationship to the late asthmatic response and change in airway calibre. J Allergy Clin Immunol 70: 170–177
24. Kolbe J, Every S, O'Hagan A, Richards G N, Garrett J E, Rea H H 1990 Outcome following a severe life-threatening attack (SLTA) of asthma: influence of asthma clinic. Aust NZ J Med 20 (suppl 1): 515
25. Younker D, Clark R, Tessem J, Joyce III T H, Kubicek M 1987 Bupivicaine–fentanyl epidural analgesia for a parturient in status asthmaticus. Can J Anaesth 34: 609–612

26. Downes H, Gerber N, Hirshman C A 1980 I.V. Lignocaine in reflex and allergic broncho-constriction. Br J Anaesth 52: 873–878
27. Morgan C, Gillbe C 1985 Anaesthetising the asthmatic. Br J Hosp Med 34: 326–328
28. White P F, Way W L, Trevor A J 1982 Ketamine – its pharamacology and therapeutic uses. Anesthesiology 56: 119–136
29. Downing J W, Mahomedy M G, Jeal D E, Allen P J 1976 Anesthesia for cesarean section with ketamine. Anesthesiology 31: 883–892
30. Hirshman C A, Krieger W, Littlejohn G, Lee R, Julien R 1982 Ketamine–aminophylline-induced decrease in seizure threshold. Anesthesiology 56: 464–467
31. Westgate H D, Gordon J R, Van Bergen F H 1962 Changes in airway resistance following intravenously administered D-tubocurarine. Anesthesiology 23: 65–73
32. Gerbershagen H U, Bergman N A 1967 The effect of D-tubocurarine on respiratory resistance in anesthetized man. Anesthesiology 78: 981–984
33. Shnider S M, Papper E M 1961 Anesthesia for the asthmatic patient. Anesthesiology 22: 886–892
34. Fisher M M, More D G 1981 The epidemiology and clinical features of anaphylactoid reactions in anaesthesia. Anesth Intensive Care 9: 226–234
35. Eger E 1981 Isoflurane: a review. Anesthesiology 55: 559
36. Stirt J A, Berger J M, Sullivan S F 1983 Lack of arrhythmogenicity of isoflurane following administration of aminophylline in dogs. Anesth Analg 62: 568–571
37. Olsson G L 1987 Bronchospasm during anesthesia. A computer-aided incidence study of 136 929 patients. Acta Anaesth Scand 31: 244–252
38. Fung D L 1985 Emergency anesthesia for asthma patients. Clin Rev Allergy 3: 127–141
39. Gelber M, Sidi Y, Gassner S et al 1984 Uncontrollable life-threatening status asthmaticus – an indicator for termination of pregnancy by cesarean section. Respiration 46: 320–322
40. Crystal R G 1990 Alpha 1 antitrypsin deficiency, emphysema and liver disease: genetic basis and strategies for therapy. J Clin Invest 85: 1343–1352
41. Meyer M B, Tonascia J A 1977 Maternal smoking, pregnancy complications and perinatal mortality. Am J Obstet Gynecol 128: 494
42. Pearce A C, Jones R M 1984 Smoking and anaesthesia: pre-operative abstinence and peri-operative morbidity. Anesthesiology 61: 576–584
43. Warner M A, Divertie M B, Tinker J H 1984 Pre-operative cessation of smoking and pulmonary complications in coronary artery bypass patients. Anesthesiology 60: 380–383
44. Hinds J R 1958 Bronchiectasis in the Maori. NZ Med J 57: 328–332
45. Long W R, Hawden C W, Laws J, Burton J F 1969 Bronchopneumonia with serious sequelae in children with evidence of adenovirus type 21 infection. Br Med J 1: 73–79
46. Becroft D M D 1971 Bronchiolitis obliterans, bronchiectasis and other sequelae of adenovirus type 21 infection in young children. J Clin Pathol 24: 72–82
47. Wakefield S, Waite D 1980 Abnormal cilia in Polynesians with bronchiectasis. Am Rev Respir Dis 121: 1003–1010
48. Cochrane G M 1985 Chronic bronchial sepsis and progressive lung damage. Br Med J 290: 1026–1027
49. Teirstein A S 1965 Bronchiectasis. In: Ravinsky J J, Guttmocher A F (eds) Medical, surgical and gynecologic complications of pregnancy. Williams & Williams, Baltimore, pp 144–149
50. Howie A D, Milne J A 1978 Pregnancy in patients with bronchiectasis. Br J Obstet Gynaecol 85: 197–200
51. Templeton A 1977 Intra-uterine growth retardation associated with hypoxia due to bronchiectasis. Br J Obstet Gynaecol 84: 389–390
52. Thaler I, Bronstein M, Aubin A E 1986 The course and outcome of pregnancy associated with bronchiectasis. Case report. Br J Obstet Gynaecol 93: 1006–1008
53. French M A H, Harrison G 1987 Serum IgG sub-classes in patients with an increased susceptibility to respiratory tract infections. Aust NZ J Med 17: 402–406
54. Wesley A W, Stewart A W 1985 Cystic fibrosis in New Zealand: incidence and mortality. NZ Med J 98: 321–323
55. Mellis C M 1985 Cystic fibrosis. Med J Aust 143: 227–228
56. Larsen Jr J W 1972 Cystic fibrosis and pregnancy. Obstet Gynecol 39: 880–883
57. Cohen L F, d'Sant Agnese P A, Friedlander J 1980 Cystic fibrosis and pregnancy – a national survey. Lancet 2: 842
58. Gin T, Gregory M A, Oh T E 1990 The haemodynamic effects of propofol and thiopentone for induction of cesarean section. Anaesth Intensive Care 18: 175–179
59. Gin T, Gregory M A, Chan K, Oh T E 1990 Maternal and fetal levels of propofol at cesarean section. Anaesth Intensive Care 18: 180–184
60. Komer F K 1982 Presentation of sarcoidosis and outcome of pulmonary changes. Don Med Bull 29: 27–32
61. Mayock R L, Bertrand P, Morrison C E, Scott J H 1963 Manifestations of sarcoidosis: analysis of 154 patients with a review of 9 series selected from the literature. Am J Med 35: 67–89
62. Grossman J H, Littner M R 1977 Severe sarcoidosis in pregnancy. Obstet Gynecol 50: 81s–84s
63. Scadding J G, Mitchell D N 1985 The genito-urinary system. In: Scadding J G, Mitchell D N (eds) Sarcoidosis, 2nd edn. Chapman & Hall Medical, London, pp 381–385
64. Shands A R, Eisberg H B 1955 The incidence of scoliosis in the State of Delaware. J Bone Joint Surg 37A: 1243–1249
65. Wynn-Davies R 1968 Familial (idiopathic) scoliosis: a family survey. J Bone Joint Surg 50B: 24–30
66. Drummond D S, Rogala E, Gurr J 1979 Spinal deformity: natural history and the role of school screening. Ortho Clin North Am 10: 761–768
67. Hirschfield S S, Rudner C, Nasch C L 1982 The incidence of mitral valve prolapse in adolescent scoliosis and thoracic hypokyphosis. Paediatrics 40: 451
68. Kafer E R 1980 Respiratory and cardiovascular functions in scoliosis and the principles of anesthetic management. Anesthesiology 52: 339–351
69. George C F, Kryger M H 1987 Sleep in restrictive lung disease. Sleep 10: 409–418
70. Betz R R, Bunnell W P, Lambrecht-Mulier E, MacEwen G D 1987 Scoliosis and pregnancy. J Bone Joint Surg 69A: 90–96
71. Manning C W, Prime F J, Zorab P A 1967 Pregnancy and scoliosis. Lancet 2: 792–795
72. Riseborough E J, Herndon J H 1975 Scoliosis and other deformities of the axial skeleton. Little, Brown, Boston: pp 76–77
73. Siegler D, Zorab P A 1981 Pregnancy in thoracic scoliosis. Br J Dis Chest 75: 367–370
74. Kopenhager T 1977 A review of 50 pregnant patients with kyphoscoliosis. J Obstet Gynecol 84: 585
75. Lao T T, Yeung S, Leung B F H 1986 Kyphoscoliosis and pregnancy. J Obstet Gynecol 7: 11–15
76. de Swiet M 1989 Diseases of the respiratory system. In: de Swiet M Medical disorders in obstetric practice, 2nd edn. Blackwell Scientific, Edinburgh, pp 1–47
77. Sawicka E H, Spencer G T, Branthwaite M A 1986 Management of respiratory failure complicating pregnancy in severe kyphoscoliosis: a new use for an old technique? Br J Dis Chest 80: 191–196
78. McKim D A, Dales R E, Lefebvre G G, Proulx M 1988 Nocturnal positive-pressure nasal ventilation for respiratory failure during pregnancy. Can Med Assoc J 139: 1069–1071
79. Gibbons P A, Lee I S 1985 Scoliosis and anesthesia. Int Anesthesiol Clin 23: 149–161
80. Schachner S M, Abram S E 1982 Use of two epidural catheters to provide analgesia of unblocked segments in a patient with lumbar disc disease. Anesthesiology 56: 150–151
81. Feldstein G, Ramanathan S 1985 Obstetric lumbar epidural anesthesia in patients with previous posterior spinal fusion for kyphoscoliosis. Anesth Analg 64: 83–85
82. Crosby E T, Halpern S H 1989 Obstetric epidural anaesthesia in patients with Harrington instrumentation. Can J Anaesth 36: 693–696
83. Moran D H, Johnson M D 1990 Continuous spinal anesthesia with combined hyperbaric and isobaric bupivacaine in a patient with scoliosis. Anesth Analg 70: 445–447

84. Cooper M G, Feeney E M, Joseph M, McGuinness J J 1989 Local anaesthetic infiltration for cesarean section. Anaesth Intensive Care 17: 198–201
85. Gaenster E A, Patton W E, Verstraetin J M et al 1953 Pulmonary function in pregnancy. III. Serial observations in patients with pulmonary insufficiency. Am Rev Tuberc 67: 797–799
86. Moore L G, Rounds S S, Jahnigen D, Graves R F, Reeves J T 1982 Infant birthweight is related to maternal arterial oxygenation at high altitude. J Appl Physiol 52: 695–699
87. Demas N W 1973 Maternal death due to primary pulmonary hypertension. Trans Pac Coast Obstet Gynecol Soc 40: 64–67

PART B
ASTHMA: USA VIEW

R. L. Busch

Asthma affects more than 1 in 20 of the population in the USA, yet it remains underdiagnosed and untreated. The number of asthma-related deaths has risen in the last decade.[1]

Asthma has classically been considered a disease characterized by bronchospasm, however asthma has an inflammatory component.[2] In many patients with asthma there is a late-phase inflammatory response that plays an integral role in the pathogenesis of severe and chronic asthma and may precipitate bronchospasm. This finding dictates the need to re-evaluate our therapeutic approach and suggests the need for more aggressive management of the late-phase response. A step care approach to the management of asthma should be employed.[3,4]

During pregnancy, both physiologic and hormonal changes occur that affect the patient with asthma. Although there is no marked change in the total lung capacity or vital capacity, there is an upward displacement of the diaphragm that contributes to a reduction in the expiratory reserve volume and residual volume. The overall effect is a reduction in functional residual volume by about 20%.

With an increase in serum concentration of progesterone, which is a respiratory stimulant, respiratory rate, tidal volume and, therefore, minute ventilation all increase. Oxygen consumption increases by approximately 20%. The combination of a reduction in pulmonary reserve with an increase in oxygen consumption makes exacerbations difficult for the asthmatic patient to tolerate.

Approximately 1% of pregnant women have asthma, and 10–15% of these women will require hospitalization for an acute attack at some time during their pregnancy. It is estimated that 50% of women with asthma will have no change in their condition during pregnancy; 25% will improve and 25% will worsen. A number of studies have shown that preterm delivery, low-birthweight infants and perinatal death occur with more frequency in pregnancies complicated by asthma.[5–7] Hemorrhage, hyperemesis, toxemia and the need to induce labor also occurred more frequently in these women.

DRUGS

The goal of therapy for asthmatic pregnant women is to prevent bronchospastic episodes causing maternal and fetal hypoxia. Although some of the drugs used have possible teratogenic effects, the fetus is at less risk than if exposed to repeated episodes of maternal bronchospasm and hypoxia.[8]

Beta-sympathomimetics

There are very few data available concerning the teratogenic effects of these drugs in humans. High-dose therapy for uterine relaxation during premature labor may cause tachycardia, hypotension and acute pulmonary edema. Albuterol, a β_2-sympathomimetic, has been associated with uterine hemorrhage during spontaneous abortion. Despite these risks, the β_2-selective sympathomimetics for bronchodilation are extremely useful when used in conjunction with a nebulizer or a hand-held inhaler in management of the pregnant patient with asthma.

Stimulation of β_2-adrenergic receptors in the lung leads to the activation of adenylate cyclase, which catalyzes the breakdown of ATP to form cAMP. cAMP then activates protein kinase, leading to the phosphorylation of certain proteins within the cell. These cause the uncoupling of actin–myosin in smooth muscle fibers, causing bronchial smooth muscle relaxation.

Corticosteroids

The safety of corticosteroid use during pregnancy is yet undetermined. Recent studies suggest that women who are steroid-dependent asthmatics are at increased risk for gestational diabetes as well as operative (cesarean) delivery.[9] Some studies have shown an association between steroid use and an increase in stillbirths, intrauterine growth retardation and cleft palate, while others have shown no increased risk. Again, the prevention of fetal hypoxia by adequately treating the mother is the primary concern and outweighs the small likelihood of teratogenic effects. The systemic effects of inhaled steroids are markedly reduced in the nonpregnant patient and inhaled steroids have now become an integral component in the step care approach to asthma. Beclomethasone by inhaler will decrease systemic absorption and limit adverse side-effects in the mother. If systemic steroids are needed, the lowest effective dose should be used, preferably given every other day.

Intravenous steroids are effective but take hours to work, so if needed in acute asthma they should be given early. The mechanism of action is believed to be direct dilation of large and small bronchi and by interference with the synthesis and action of biochemical mediators of asthma.

Theophylline

Widely used and effective in treating asthmatic patients theophylline is falling into disfavor because of its adverse systemic side-effects, concern about maintenance of therapeutic levels, and the need to monitor drug levels to prevent toxicity. Theophylline compounds appear to be free of teratogenic effects. Pregnancy doses should be continued throughout parturition. Since clearance of the drug may be unchanged or decreased during pregnancy, close monitoring of blood levels for evidence of toxicity is essential. Theophylline is a potent relaxant of uterine musculature and as such may prolong labor. However, prevention of bronchospasm certainly outweighs the risk of prolonging labor. Since theophylline easily crosses the placenta, fetal heart tracings may lose their pattern of variability. Approximately 10% of neonates will have transient tachycardia and jitteriness (even though serum concentrations are therapeutic). The elimination half-life of theophylline is prolonged in neonates, so they should be closely monitored for signs of toxicity if exposed to the drug in utero.

Magnesium sulfate

Magnesium has pharmacologic properties that are only recently being understood and may have value not only in the treatment of preeclampsia/eclampsia but also in the treatment of asthma.[10,11] The role of magnesium in preeclampsia/eclampsia is largely for its anticonvulsant properties.

Magnesium has no influence on the central ventilatory drive. However, it has been shown to be an effective bronchodilator[12] and has been useful in the treatment of severe asthma[13] where it may have an ever increasing role in the treatment of bronchospasm including the parturient.[14]

Magnesium has a role in hundreds of enzymatic processes. Its mechanism of action is thought to be as a regulator of intracellular calcium levels by activation of membrane pumps as well as a cofactor in oxidative phosphorylation. It also appears to inhibit catecholamine-induced arrhythmias, and may play a dual role in that it may increase the effectiveness of β-agonists. The ventilatory depressant effect of magnesium is probably due to the neuromuscular block that may occur at increased serum levels.

Cromolyn

The mechanism of action of cromolyn is poorly understood. It is not a bronchodilator. The role of cromolyn therapy is in the prophylaxis of asthma. It works by protecting against various indirect bronchoconstrictor stimuli. When used appropriately it may inhibit both the immediate and late inflammatory components of asthma. It is not efficacious in all patients and it is difficult to predict which patients will respond. No significant problems have been noted with cromolyn sodium used during pregnancy. If effective prior to pregnancy it should be continued through the pregnancy.

Antihistamines

Antihistamines have been used during pregnancy with apparent safety. However, in premature infants, a strong association between retrolental fibroplasia and maternal antihistamine use during the last 2 weeks of pregnancy has been established. Therefore, these drugs should be avoided during the last 2 weeks of pregnancy.

ACUTE ASTHMA

As mentioned above, slight exacerbations of asthma in the pregnant patient may lead to life-threatening hypoxemia. Patients present with chest tightness, dyspnea, cough and wheezing. In cases of severe asthma, wheezing may not be present if very little air is being expelled with ventilation. The $P\text{CO}_2$ in the pregnant patient normally ranges from 30 to 35 mmHg. A $P\text{CO}_2$ above 35 mmHg may signify a tiring patient with impending respiratory failure. Supplemental oxygen should be the first priority in treatment. A β_2-sympathomimetic such as albuterol or metaproteronol may be administered by metered dose inhaler or nebulizer. If prompt relief is not obtained subcutaneous epinephrine, 0.3 ml of a 1 : 1000 solution, or terbutaline 0.25 mg should be given. Parenteral steroid administration should be considered if the patient fails to respond by the β-sympathomimetics. Hydrocortisone may be administered intravenously, 100–200 mg every 4–6 h. Aminophylline may be added if the patient is still unresponsive to the above therapies. The loading dose is 5–6 mg/kg over 20 min, to a maximum of 400 mg. If the patient has been taking theophylline but has inadequate levels, 2.5 mg/kg over 20 min is infused. A continuous infusion is then begun at a rate of 0.5 mg/kg/h in normal patients. If the mother is a smoker, 0.7 mg/kg/h is infused; in patients with coexisting heart or liver disease the dose should be reduced to 0.3 mg/kg/h.

LABOR AND DELIVERY

Epidural analgesia is the preferred method of pain relief during labor. This has the effect of decreasing stress, anxiety and hyperventilation, which may be stimuli for bronchospasm in the asthmatic patient. Low concentrations of local anesthetics are used to prevent excessive motor block. A continuous epidural infusion of 0.125% bupivacaine with fentanyl 1–2 μg/ml is used to maintain adequate sensory analgesia. Anti-asthmatic medication can be continued throughout labor on the understanding that it will decrease uterine contractility and may retard the progress of labor.

CESAREAN DELIVERY

Regional anesthesia is the technique of choice for the parturient undergoing cesarean delivery. It is preferable to use a controlled continuous epidural or spinal anesthetic to prevent a high block from developing. Spinal anesthesia has the disadvantage of producing motor blockade at a level two or three segments higher than epidural anesthesia. This may decrease expiratory reserve volume and lessen the ability to cough. Because a less dense block is achieved with an epidural, patients may experience more discomfort with uterine and peritoneal traction. Fentanyl 50 μg diluted in 10 ml of preservative-free normal saline or local anesthetic injected epidurally will relieve this discomfort. Adequate hydration and supplemental oxygen are required with all regional anesthesia. Sedation and other respiratory depressants should be avoided or minimized.

GENERAL ANESTHESIA

If needed, general anesthesia utilizing a rapid-sequence induction and cricoid pressure must be performed to prevent the likelihood of regurgitation and gastric aspiration. 30 ml of sodium citrate 0.3 M is administered po prior to induction. Thiopental 4 mg/kg may be used for induction; however, ketamine may prevent or reverse bronchospasm and is the induction agent of choice. When used in conjunction with aminophylline, it does not increase the incidence of arrhythmias but will lower the seizure threshold. Emergence reactions can occur but are sufficiently reduced with small amounts of a benzodiazepine. A bolus of succinylcholine during induction and for maintenance of muscle relaxation is recommended. D-tubocurarine, metocurine and atracurium should be avoided because of their histamine-releasing properties. Potent inhalation agents (halothane, isoflurane, and enflurane) all have excellent bronchodilating effects and should be used for maintenance of anesthesia. The patient is extubated only after demonstrating the ability to protect her airway with intact reflexes.

CIGARETTE SMOKING

Women who continue to smoke are treated similarly to asthmatics in that they have very reactive airways. Regional anesthesia is preferred for labor and vaginal or cesarean delivery. If general anesthesia is necessary, the same precautions should be taken as with asthmatic patients with special attention to the management of secretions with an antimuscarinic agent.

REFERENCES

1. Sly R M 1984 Increases in death from asthma. Ann Allergy 53: 20–25
2. Lemanske R F, Kaliner M 1988 Late-phase IgE mediated reactions. J Clin Immunol 8: 1–13
3. Bone R C 1988 A step care strategy for asthma management. J Respir Dis 9(11): 104–117

4. Bone R C 1988 Step care for asthma. J Am Med Assoc 260: 543
5. Schaefer G, Silverman F 1961 Pregnancy complicated by asthma. Am J Obst Gynecol 82: 182–191
6. Gordon M, Niswander K R, Berendes H, Kantor A G 1970 Fetal morbidity following potentially anoxigenic obstetrical conditions. VIII. Bronchial asthma. Am J Obstet Gynecol 106: 421–429
7. Bahna S L, Erkedalt B J 1972 The course and outcome of pregnancy in women with bronchial asthma. Acta Allergy 27: 397–406
8. Sinaiko R J, German D F 1979 Perspective on asthma in pregnancy. West J Med 131: 315–316
9. Perlow J H 1992 Severity of asthma and perinatal outcome. Am J Obstet Gynecol 167: 963
10. Skobeloff E M, Spivey W H, McNamara R M, and Greenspon L 1989 Intravenous magnesium sulfate for the treatment of acute asthma in the emergency department. JAMA 262(9): 1210–3
11. Mathew R, Altura B M 1991 The role of magnesium in lung diseases: asthma, allergy and pulmonary hypertension. Magnes Trace Elem 10 (2–4): 220–8
12. Haury V G 1938 The brocho-dilator action of magnesium and its antagnostic action (dilator action) against pilocarpine, histamine, and barium chloride. J Pharmacol Exp Ther 64: 58–64
13. Okayama H, Aikawa T, Okayama M, Sasaki H, Mue S, Takishima T 1987 Bronchodilating effect of intravenous magnesium sulfate in bronchial asthma. JAMA 257: 1076–8
14. Skobeloff E M, Kim D, Spivey W H 1993 Magnesium sulfate for the treatment of bronchospasm complicating acute bronchitis in a four month's-pregnant woman. Ann Emerg Med 22(8): 1365–7

PART C
ACUTE ADULT RESPIRATORY DISTRESS SYNDROME IN PREGNANCY

R. L. Busch

Acute adult respiratory distress syndrome (ARDS) caused by acute respiratory failure (ARF) develops in patients of all age groups including parturients. An organized approach to the possible etiologies and laboratory presentation of this condition is mandatory. The majority of clinicians now agree that, in the absence of an intracardiac shunt, respiratory failure is present when the $Pa\text{O}_2$ is less than 50 mmHg and/or the $Pa\text{CO}_2$ exceeds 50 mmHg, the patient is dyspneic or the arterial pH reflects significant respiratory acidemia. Patients with acute lung disease fall into two major categories:

1. The majority, who develop atelectasis, pulmonary edema and small airway closure but have no increase in pulmonary microcirculatory permeability. This group of patients have acute respiratory failure (ARF).
2. Patients who develop diffuse capillary membrane injury and carry the diagnosis of acute respiratory distress syndrome. The adult respiratory distress syndrome (ARDS), is a syndrome of acute respiratory failure that presents as a sequence of pathophysiologic events that develop secondary to direct and indirect lung injury.

The parturient[1–3] may be especially susceptible to the sequence of events leading up to ARDS. Aspiration pneumonitis, preeclampsia/eclampsia, hemorrhage, infection,[4–5] viral or bacterial pneumonia,[7] amniotic fluid embolism,[8] intrauterine fetal death, pulmonary embolus, bacterial sepsis, major trauma, medications[9] including tocolytics[10] and shock are known causes of this injury.[11,12] While controversial, the pulmonary edema that occurs at times with the use of tocolytics is self-limited and usually has a benign course.[13]

The precise mechanism of lung injury remains obscure and, despite supportive treatment with mechanical ventilation and pharmacologic intervention, more than one-half of ARDS patients die. Clinically, ARDS is characterized by decreased lung compliance, hypoxemia and bilateral or diffuse pulmonary infiltrates. It is interesting to note that the injury is not global but consists of spared regions of relatively well-preserved normal lung.

At times, ARDS may contribute to the nosocomial complications that protract the clinical course and lead to multisystem end-organ involvement. The most common second organ to fail is the kidney. This may well be due to the septic problems that usually accompany this devastating syndrome. Survival from combined respiratory and anuric renal failure is rare. There has been little improvement in outcome over the past 10 years in patients with moderate to severe ARDS. There have been no major advances in outcome since the routine use of mechanical ventilation and the employment of positive end-expiratory pressure (PEEP). Furthermore, iatrogenic causes of lung injury which include oxygen toxicity and barotrauma amplify the difficulties of treating this syndrome.

It is essential to aggressively treat these patients underlying disease(s) in order to prevent the development of ARDS and aid recovery from the acute lung injury. Supportive therapy is unsuccessful if the etiologic agent for the acute lung injury is not corrected. Unnecessary delay may contribute to lung damage, increasing the need for larger tidal volumes, higher $F\text{IO}_2$, and higher airway pressures in order to adequately maintain gas exchange. In all patients with moderate to severe ARDS, a marked reduction in functional residual capacity (FRC) is seen. In a parturient who already has a decrease in her FRC this may be catastrophic.

PATHOPHYSIOLOGY

Early ARDS

Pulmonary venous and capillary congestion is a characteristic feature and is often accompanied by cellular swelling and necrosis of the endothelium. Within days most patients develop pulmonary artery hypertension, i.e. mean pulmonary artery pressure >20 mmHg, with pulmonary vascular resistance increasing two- or threefold. In early ARDS, the lung interstitium fills with plasma exudate and reversible vascular compression occurs. This is usually followed by distal airway closure, producing arterial hypoxemia. Employing PEEP markedly decreases the right-to-left shunt and presumably recruits and opens closed airway segments as evidenced by increasing FRC. In the short term the extent of lung damage is not altered by the use of PEEP, as demonstrated by no reduction in extravascular lung water.[14]

Hypoxic vasoconstriction may play a major role in shunting blood from segments with a low V/Q ratio to better ventilated ones. This protective mechanism could reduce the shunt and improve $P\text{aO}_2$, but may further increase the pulmonary vascular resistance and pulmonary artery pressures. However, with intensive pulmonary therapy, lung function may indeed improve, as demonstrated by improvement in lung mechanics and clearing of radiographic infiltrates.

It remains obscure as to whether microthromboembolism constitutes the common pathologic event in ARDS or is a secondary phenomenon owing to intravascular thrombosis within severely damaged lung parenchyma. Normal pregnancy is a hypercoagulable state in which enhanced clotting coupled with an increased incidence of thrombotic events occurs. All coagulation factors with the exception of factors XI and XIII are elevated in pregnancy. Coagulopathies are common in patients with severe ARDS, as in parturients with HELLP syndrome. Thrombocytopenia due to shortened platelet lifespan is common.[15]

Hyaline membranes are commonly seen within 3–4 days of the initial insult. Type I pneumocytes which are responsible for 90% of the gas-exchange surface area, are exceedingly vulnerable to injury and incapable of reproduction. This induces a vigorous hyperplasia of type II cells, which are the progenitors of the type I cells. Continued swelling and edema of the interstitial space is widespread. Surprisingly, leukocytes and macrophages are not a prominent feature in most early cases of ARDS. It is probable that the pulmonary interstitial edema accounts for the acute lung injury. Others have argued that it is the colloid osmotic pressure/microvascular gradient that produces the ongoing compromise of pulmonary function.

Late changes

Thrombi are abundant in the small and medium-sized pulmonary arteries. It is at this time that endothelial cell necrosis is seen. With the continued hyperplasia of type II pneumocytes, the alveolar lining features cuboidal epithelium and probably represents the regenerative efforts of the lung. There is continued increase in connective tissue matrix, particularly in fibrillar collagen as well as diminished elastic tissue.

It is the diffuse but focal nature of the pulmonary vascular insult and alveolar injury that produces the striking alterations in ventilation and perfusion. The accompanying pulmonary hypertension eliminates the classic zones 1 and 2 described by West.[16]

TREATMENT

Patients who develop pulmonary capillary leak due to tocolytic therapy, post-ictal pulmonary edema and pulmonary edema associated with air emboli usually do quite well with diuresis and supplemental oxygen. If mechanical ventilation is required it is usually for a short time.

However, other causes of ARDS require more aggressive management.

PHARMACOLOGIC INTERVENTION

The pathophysiology of ARDS is quite complex and the mechanism(s) of lung injury at the cellular level is incompletely understood. Many different agents have been tried empirically, but there is no magic bullet.

Heparin

Thrombocytopenia due to shortened platelet lifespan is

common. The role of heparin anticoagulation or fibrinolytic agents in ARDS remains controversial. No randomized or prospective studies have been reported to date.

Prostaglandin inhibition or administration

Many clinical studies as well as animal models have suggested a place for prostaglandin mediators in the development of acute lung injury.[17] Inhibitors of cyclooxygenase, such as the nonsteroidal antiinflammatory drugs (NSAIDs), have been proposed to be beneficial. The NSAIDs that are inhibitors of cyclooxygenase and thus thromboxane A_2 have been studied because of their ability to reduce the aggregation of platelets as well as neutrophils. There is some evidence for the use of ibuprofen[18] in patients with severe sepsis; however, further data are lacking. The use of NSAIDs at this time should be considered investigational and is not a mainstay therapy.

Prostaglandin E_1 (PGE_1) was thought to have some efficacy in ARDS because of its ability to dilate the pulmonary arterioles, inhibit neutrophil chemotaxis and inhibit platelet aggregation. While in theory this use appears sound, recent clinical trials do not support its use.[19]

Corticosteroids

Steroids have been tried in almost all disorders. They have been tried in ARDS as well with the thinking that administration would limit neutrophil mediated injury. When large doses of methylprednisolone were used, on the order of 30 mg/kg every 6 hours for a day, they did not prevent ARDS or reduce mortality when compared to placebo.[20] Steroids will probably continue to be used but there is not clear efficacy to their use in ARDS.

Surfactant

Surfactant replacement has been considered as a potential therapy for this syndrome, but to date there are no studies that reflect efficacy in the treatment of ARDS. This therapy is widely becoming popular in the treatment of neonates, but until more studies are undertaken in adults this should be considered experimental.

Phosphodiesterase inhibitors

Pentoxifylline is known to inhibit neutrophil activation, and chemotaxis has been thought to be of potential benefit in ARDS. Animal studies have suggested that pentoxifylline may protect against endotoxin-induced injury when the etiology of ARDS is sepsis.[21] Human studies have not supported its use and should be considered investigational.

New pharmacologic agents

No wonder drug exists for the treatment of ARDS. As research intensifies, perhaps combinations of agents and the development of specific anti-tumor necrosis factor antibodies when used as prophylaxis may be of benefit. This is an intensive area of both bench and clinical research.

Ventilatory support

The most important factor in treatment of a patient who has developed the constellation of signs and symptoms of ARDS is to treat the inciting event. Maximal oxygen therapy by rebreathing mask may be tried before endotracheal intubation; however, intubation not only facilitates mechanical ventilation but provides a pathway for pulmonary toilet. Elective intubation should be considered early in the course of this syndrome to permit the use of PEEP and provide rest for the patient. In patients with extreme hypoxemia, paralysis, only after sedation, will reduce the oxygen consumption by decreasing the work of breathing. Initial ventilatory settings are chosen to maximize oxygenation while minimizing the risk of oxygen toxicity and barotrauma. This may best be accomplished by using smaller tidal volumes (8 ml/kg) and higher respiratory rates (20/min). By providing smaller tidal volumes one may avoid further lung injury and continued capillary leak associated with larger tidal volumes while facilitating the use of higher levels of PEEP to reduce shunt without excessive pressures. PEEP will recruit alveoli and diminish the shunt, thereby decreasing the oxygen requirement. PEEP does not reduce lung water but rather causes a redistribution into the peribronchiovascular space. Caution must be exercised in discontinuing PEEP even for short periods as the result may be rapid alveolar flooding and prompt and dramatic deterioration of oxygenation. One should keep the disconnections to an absolute minimum and employ ventilation tubing that facilitates suctioning without disconnection. It should be noted that the patient's hemodynamics must also be taken into account as PEEP is known to reduce cardiac output by decreasing venous return to the heart. The above is only a guide; each patient must be individually assessed as to the optimal formula for mechanical ventilation.

The mode of ventilation[22,23] is unlikely to reverse the progression of the lung disease. No specific therapy has yet proven to be effective in the treatment of ARDS other than treating the underlying initiating event. Prevention is the best cure; for instance, the use of cricoid pressure to prevent aspiration during intubation and prompt aggressive therapy with antibiotics to treat any underlying infectious process. ARDS in pregnancy is associated with a maternal mortality similar to the nonpregnant patient. The primary etiology in pregnancy is infection, toxemia and hemorrhage. The beneficial effect on ventilation from delivery of the patient with adult respiratory distress syndrome cannot be overemphasized.[24,25]

As the syndrome of ARDS continues to be a therapeutic dilemma, new therapies are being developed which are aimed at blocking the acute-phase reactions of the disease, especially those that are implicated in the destruction of the underlying lung architecture.[26] Improving our understanding of the basic pathophysiology of this syndrome will direct us toward new therapies and, hopefully, increase the survival rate of patients with ARDS.

REFERENCES

1. Mabie W C, Barton J R, Sibai B M 1992 Adult respiratory distress syndrome in pregnancy. Am J Obstet Gynecol 16: 950–957
2. Anderson H F, Lynch J P, Johnson Jr T R 1980 Adult respiratory distress syndrome in obstetrics and gynecology. Obstet Gynecol 55: 291–295
3. Smith J L, Thomas F, Orme Jr J F, Clemmer T P 1990 Adult respiratory distress syndrome during pregnancy and immediately postpartum. West J Med 153: 508–510
4. Towers C V, Kaminskas C M, Garite T J, Nageotte M P, Dorchester W 1991 Pulmonary injury associated with antepartum pyelonephritis: can patients at risk be identified? Am J Obstet Gynecol 164: 974–980
5. Boucher M, Yonekura M L, Wallace R J, Phelan J P 1984 Adult respiratory distress syndrome: a rare manifestation of *Listeria monocytogenes* infection in pregnancy. Am J Obstet Gynecol 149: 686–688
6. Wilkins I, Mezrow G, Lynch L, Bottone E J, Berkowitz R L 1989 Amnionitis and life-threatening respiratory distress after percutaneous umbilical blood sampling. Am J Obstet Gynecol 160: 427–428
7. MacDonald D, Alguire P C 1990 Adult respiratory distress syndrome due to blastomycosis during pregnancy. Chest 98: 1527–1528
8. Hooper D J, Sherer D M, Abramowicz J S, Papadakos P J 1991 Extensive pulmonary embolism presenting as severe adult respiratory distress syndrome after surgical resection of a cornual pregnancy. Am J Obstet Gynecol 165: 41–42
9. Stratta P, Canarese C, Colla L, Dogliani M, Ragni R, Malcangi A, Vercellone A 1989 Adult respiratory distress syndrome following administration of nitroprusside in postpartum acute renal failure (letter). Clin Nephrol 31: 117–118
10. Bowen R E, Dedhia H V, Beatty J, Schiebel F, Koss W, Grandos J 1983 ARDS associated with the use of sympathomimetics and glucocorticoids for the treatment of premature labor. Crit Care Med 11: 671–672
11. Hollingsworth H M, Irwin R S 1992 Acute respiratory failure in pregnancy. Clin Chest Med 13: 723–740
12. Kaufman B S, Kaminsky S J, Rackow E C, Weil M H 1987 Adult respiratory distress syndrome following orogenital sex during pregnancy. Crit Care Med 15: 703–704
13. Pisani R J, Rosenow E C 1986 Pulmonary edema associated with tocolytic therapy. Ann Intern Med 146: 801
14. Hopewell P C, Murray J F 1976 Effects of continuous positive pressure ventilation in experimental pulmonary edema. J Appl Physiol 40: 568–574
15. Schneider R, Zapol W M, Carvalho A 1980 Platelet consumption and sequestration in severe acute respiratory failure. Am Rev Respir Dis 122: 445–451
16. West J 1977 Pulmonary pathophysiology: the essentials. Williams & Wilkins, Baltimore
17. Goldstein G, Luce J 1990 Pharmacologic treatment in the adult respiratory distress syndrome. Clin Chest Med 11: 773
18. Bernard G R, Reines H D, Metz C A et al 1988 Effects of a short course of ibuprofen in patients with severe sepsis (abstract). Am Rev Respir Dis 137: A138
19. Holcroft J W, Vasser M J, Webber C J 1986 Prostaglandin E_1 and survival in patients with the adult respiratory distress syndrome. Ann Surg 203: 371
20. Luce J M, Montgomery B, Marks J D et al 1988 Ineffectiveness of high-dose methylprednisolone in preventing parenchymal lung injury and improving mortality in patients with septic shock. Am Rev Respir Dis 138: 62
21. Welsh C H, Lien D, Worthon G S et al 1988 Pentoxifylline decreases endotoxin-induced pulmonary neutrophil sequestration and extravascular protein accumulation in the dog. Am Rev Respir Dis 138: 1377
22. Turner J S, Evans T W, Hunter D N et al 1990 Adult respiratory distress syndrome. Advances in diagnosis and ventilatory management (clinical conference) 301 (6760): 1087–1089
23. Gattinoni L, D'Andrea L, Pelosi P, Vitale G, Pesenti A, Fumagalli R 1993 Regional effects and mechanism of positive end-expiratory pressure in early adult respiratory distress syndrome. Journal 269: 2122–2127
24. Daily W H, Katz A R, Tonnesen A, Allen S J 1990 Beneficial effect of delivery in a patient with adult respiratory distress syndrome. Anesthesiology 72: 383–386
25. Le Guennec J C, Bard H, Teasdale F, Doray B 1980 Elective delivery and neonatal respiratory distress syndrome. Can Med Assoc J 122: 307–309
26. Fratacci M D, Frostell C G, Chen T Y, Wain Jr J C, Robinson D R, Zapol W M 1991 Inhaled nitric oxide. Anesthesiology 75: 990–999

48. Maternal aspiration

C. A. Burchman

By 1846, inhalation analgesia was utilized for parturition in the United States. An anesthetic morbidity/mortality treatise of the era *might* have read like this:

> . . . and the next patient was a stout young woman of 19, in the childbirth, in whom the vapour was inhaled for four minutes whilst she delivered. From wailing, she had a fit of coughing, and was then unconscious of pain. Her vomit went to her airway, we believe, and rightly caused her pulse to fall, her hands to get cold, and complete consciousness never to return.

A scenario 140 years later would read along these lines:

> . . . a 20 year old full-term pregnant woman is rushed to the operating room for emergency cesarean delivery because of fetal distress. After rapid-sequence induction with thiopental and succinylcholine, the patient vomited and aspirated. She was extubated in the recovery room. Six hours later, she was found dyspneic and cyanotic on the floor, and soon thereafter, died of cardiac arrest.

The practice of obstetric anesthesia has obviously changed tremendously over the past 150 years. Something has not changed, however. Aspiration is still a killer of pregnant women.

Hall[1] first associated the inhalation of gastric contents with obstetric patients in 1940. He coined the term *chemical pneumonitis*. Mendelson[2] went on to highlight the severe sequelae associated with gastric aspiration in 1946. This unfortunate phenomenon remains a major source of anesthesia-related maternal mortality.

Pregnant patients must be considered to have a full stomach because of several factors that contribute to the retention of gastric fluid and risk of regurgitation.

INCIDENCE OF MATERNAL ASPIRATION

The documentation of incidence is erratic, mainly because clinically insignificant aspirations frequently go unnoticed. If dye is placed in the stomachs of general surgical patients prior to the induction of anesthesia, the prevalence of staining of the oropharynx (regurgitation) ranges from 7–16%. Of those patients with regurgitation, 8–16% have dye in their trachea.[3] We must assume that the parturient undergoing a general anesthetic lies at least within this category of risk.

The incidence of clinically significant aspiration is also unknown, mainly because only maternal *deaths* from aspiration are reported. The most recent retrospective study was done by Olsson in 1986.[4] He reviewed over 185 000 anesthetics for all types of surgical procedures and noted a prevalence of aspiration of 1 : 2131 or 0.05%. Owing to the enormous sample size and problems associated with documenting such events, accuracy regarding incidence will continue to be problematic.

The Confidential Enquiries into Maternal Deaths in England and Wales examined virtually all maternal deaths over a 30-year period from 1952 to 1981. While absolute maternal mortality decreased by more than 90%, from 99 to 9 deaths per 100 000, no such reduction occurred in deaths from 'anesthesia', the majority of which were due to inhalation of gastric contents.[5–7] In fact, over this 30-year period, the percentage of true maternal anesthetic deaths increased threefold! Certainly what we are achieving is better management of high-risk obstetric cases. As such, our 'figures' are telling us that we are doing a better job in some avenues, while no improvements are being made in others.

MORBIDITY AND MORTALITY

What factors affect the severity of the pneumonitis following aspiration? The initial response to the introduction of gastric material into the respiratory tree is a function of the content and character of the aspirate.[8–10] Particles of food, particularly large chunks, can lodge in bronchi and cause asphyxiation in minutes.

The acidity of the aspirate is probably the single most damaging component. Nonacid liquid has been well demonstrated to produce a mild and transient hypoxia without parenchymal damage. In such a situation, the hypoxia is a result of bronchospasm and atelectasis. Increasing acidity, either alone or with food, inflicts a severe inflammatory response resulting in tracheal muscosal and lung parenchymal injury.[11] From Teabeaut's landmark 1952 study, an inference has been made that an aspirate with a pH greater than 2.5 is relatively benign.[12] Recent animal studies contradict this. Aspiration of liquids with a pH greater than 2.5 may result in a lethal outcome.[13]

Another myth of the current literature is the notion that an aspirate volume of greater than 0.4 ml/kg is uniformly fatal.[14] This 'critical volume' concept was modeled after a rhesus monkey study in which highly acidic material was instilled. More valid are the results of a study by James[15] which suggest that 'critical volume' is a function of pH. In other words, for a given volume of aspirate, even though small, a lower pH will cause a higher mortality.

Partially digested food causes the worst of all possible problems. The pulmonary shunt fraction is increased and the Pa_{O_2} falls secondary to alveolar hypoventilation.[16] Frequently, alveolar architecture is destroyed as inflammation, hemorrhage and edema ensue.

SIGNS, SYMPTOMS AND CLINICAL COURSE

Hypoxemia is the final common pathway after severe aspiration. The signs and symptoms are highly variable, depending on the volume and pH of the aspirated material.[17] One may or may not see gastric contents in the oral cavity. One may or may not hear bronchospasm or observe coughing. There may be tachypnea or pulmonary vasoconstriction, with associated pulmonary hypertension. Radiographic findings may occur early or as late as 12 h post insult. Such evidence is most often seen in the right lower lobe.

Patients sustaining a severe aspiration can be categorized into three groups by outcome.[15] One group, 10–15%, will deteriorate rapidly, with circulatory shock an early sign. Of the remaining patients, two-thirds will improve rapidly after a 1- to 4-day illness. One-third will proceed to develop a bacterial pneumonia and require antibiotic therapy. Most will eventually improve.

HOW PREGNANCY INFLUENCES RISK

The parturient is a member of the population susceptible for aspiration because of the character, quantity and 'environment' of her gastric contents. The high circulating levels of progesterone during pregnancy cause increased gastrin release and, as a result, higher basal acid secretion rates. The parturient has a delayed gastric emptying time, also a humoral effect.[18] The gravid uterus presses upward against the stomach and poses a mechanical obstruction to the duodenum. The expanding uterus actually displaces the esophageal barrier to reflux superiorly, making the segment extra-abdominal. In addition, progesterone decreases lower esophageal sphincter tone.[19]

There are other 'risk factors' introduced iatrogenically. Parenteral opioids decrease gastrointestinal motility. Increased intra-abdominal pressure encouraged during 'pushing', as well as manual pressure upon the lower abdomen during delivery, will serve to increase intragastric pressure.

Overlay all of these factors upon a patient for whom consciousness is impaired or ablated with anesthetics, in whom intubation may be difficult, and one must appreciate why the acid aspiration syndrome described over 50 years ago continues to account for conspicuous mortality in obstetric practice.

THERAPY

Following an acute aspiration, airway management is of paramount importance. Any evident liquid or particulate matter should be immediately evacuated via suction. Placing the patient into the head-down and left lateral posture immediately following the acute event has been recommended by some investigators. This may decrease the degree of pulmonary soilage, but this has not been proven and is frequently impractical. Copious saline lavage of the trachea and bronchi has been tried but studies demonstrating its efficacy are lacking. In fact, it may be detrimental. Liquid gastric aspirate is distributed rapidly to the periphery of the lungs. Such washings may help disseminate the material further. Most of the instilled liquid will not reach the already disbursed gastric material.[9] One may attempt to measure the pH of the gastric aspirate as this will give an indication as to the pH of the inhaled material. Expeditious intubation, positive pressure ventilation with supplemental oxygen and positive end-expiratory pressure are the most critical first measures. Intravenous β_2-agonists may effectively relieve bronchospasm. While acid-injured lungs are susceptible to secondary bacterial infections, no evidence supports the prophylactic administration of antibiotics, which has been shown not to decrease the incidence of infection or alter the outcome after aspiration of gastric fluid.[17]

The use of systemic glucocorticoids is also debatable. Some animal studies suggest a reduction in pulmonary damage if corticosteroids are given immediately following aspiration of acidic gastric material. Conversely, other data demonstrate an enhancement in the development of Gram-negative pneumonia, inhibition of healing and reduction in macrophage activity.[20]

Despite the absence of substantial evidence, it is not uncommon that an empiric dose of methylprednisolone (30 mg/kg) or dexamethasone (1 mg/kg) be given. If hypoproteinemia is present, as protein-rich edema fluid exudes across the alveolar epithelium, albumin may be administered. This approach is controversial, however, as it may exacerbate the pulmonary edema.

PROPHYLAXIS

The most significant treatment measure is *prevention*. A considerable amount of morbidity could be avoided if pregnant patients did not eat just prior to their arrival in the labor and delivery suite. This author has personally been told by 'prepared childbirth' class coordinators that women *should* eat prior to coming to the hospital because 'once you are there, they will not feed you'. Anesthesiologist and obstetrician alike must make an impact on this misinformation through education.

One approach toward minimizing risk is by minimizing exposure to general anesthesia. This is already accomplished throughout most of North America and western Europe, where general anesthesia for a normal spontaneous vaginal delivery is the increasingly rare exception and not the rule.

When general anesthesia is indicated, a number of steps must be applied to either decrease the chance of aspiration or decrease the risk associated with an aspiration event.

A classic full-stomach precaution remains the technique of denitrogenation with 100% oxygen to provide a buffer for the apnea that ensues with induction and laryngoscopy. End-tidal nitrogen is less than 4% within 2.5–3 min in patients without significant pulmonary disease.[21] Recently, Norris and Dewan[22] demonstrated that four maximally deep inspirations of 100% oxygen over 30 s results in a $Pa\text{O}_2$ on a par with that after 3 min of 100% oxygen inhalation.

There is an ongoing controversy as to the necessity of a pretreatment dose of a nondepolarizing muscle relaxant prior to succinylcholine administration.[23] Succinylcholine-induced muscle fasciculations produce inconsistent elevations in intragastric pressure. This rise, however, occurs concurrently with an increase in lower esophageal sphincter pressure. Furthermore, the degree of muscle fasciculations in pregnant patients is minimal. While pretreatment with nondepolarizing muscle relaxants attenuates this response, skeletal muscle relaxation takes longer, and thus apneic time is prolonged.

Application of cricoid pressure is an easy and effective maneuver in preventing aspiration via passive regurgitation during induction of general anesthesia.[24,25] The pressure should not be released until the intubation is confirmed and the endotracheal tube cuff is inflated.

In 5% of obstetric general anesthetics, intubation is difficult.[26] If difficult intubation is anticipated, an awake laryngoscopy should be performed after satisfactory topical anesthesia. If the glottis is observed, intubation may proceed as planned following induction. However, if the glottic structures are not appreciated, and regional anesthesia is not an option, an awake intubation should be performed. If intubation warranted an awake or 'rapid-sequence' protocol, an awake extubation is appropriate.[27] Extubation should only ensue once the patient regains consciousness and responds appropriately to commands. Coughing and bucking on the tube may imply that the gag reflex has returned, but it may also mean that the patient is in the excitement stage of recovery. In this stage, protective airway mechanisms may be hyperexcitable and laryngospasm is a real possibility.

The assessment of the airway, management of the failed intubation and alternative techniques have been discussed.

Antacids

There are numerous pharmacologic approaches to minimizing the severity of maternal aspiration. Antacids remain the most reliable means of neutralizing the acidic gastric fluid.[28] Originally, particulate antacids were used, and while they were effective, if they themselves were aspirated, there was the potential for development of chronic pulmonary granulomas.[29] The alternative is a water-soluble antacid. The two most well-studied soluble antacids are 0.3 mol/l sodium citrate and Bicitra (sodium citrate and citric acid). They contain the same amount of sodium citrate and have similar neutralizing capacities, although Bicitra is slightly more acidic. 30 ml of either agent, or 30 ml of water with two Alka-Seltzer Gold tablets, given prior to induction, will increase the gastric fluid pH. The patient should be rotated to her right and left following administration to allow for adequate mixing. The efficacy of the clear water-soluble antacid in raising gastric pH is immediate, but there is controversy about the duration of action. Therefore, it is essential to administer the water-soluble antacid immediately prior to or within 30 min of induction for maximal effect.

Some recent studies suggest that if there is evidence of normal gastric motility at the time of antacid administration the soluble antacids may pass beyond the stomach at a time when the production of gastric acid is ongoing.[30] A valid concern remains as to whether these agents are protective at the time of extubation.[31]

Histamine-2 antagonists

Histamine has a major role in the production of hydrochloric acid by gastric parietal cells. This effect is mediated by histamine-2 (H_2) receptors. Numerous studies have evaluated this class of agents, primarily cimetidine and ranitidine, as premedicants.[32–35]

Cimetidine is the most widely studied H_2-blocker. The safety and efficacy of cimetidine prophylaxis in obstetric anesthesia have been reported by many investigators. In fact, cimetidine has been studied more in obstetric patients than in any other group. In single- or double-dose therapy, no maternal complications attributable to cimetidine have been demonstrated nor have any adverse effects been noted in infants whose mothers received cimetidine based on Apgar scores and neurobehavioral assessments.[36]

The timing of administration of H_2-blockers is important. Following oral administration, a significant effect is seen in 60–90 min, whereas following intravenous administration efficacy is realized in 45–60 min. The delay in onset somewhat limits cimetidine's utility in an emergent situation but, if given an hour prior to induction of anesthesia, it is effective. A single 300-mg dose at bedtime results in 6–8 h of significantly decreased gastric acidity and gastric juice volume. An additional 300 mg given on the morning of surgery (either orally or intravenously) has resulted in an even greater increase in gastric pH.

Inhibition of drug metabolism by cimetidine is an important drug interaction.[37] Microsomal drug metabolism in the liver appears to be inhibited. Hepatic blood flow is also decreased. It is well documented that even after one or two doses the elimination half-life for drugs such as warfarin, barbiturates, benzodiazepines, theophylline and propranolol will be prolonged. A few reports exist relating cimetidine administration to a delay in awakening from anesthesia.[38]

Ranitidine is more potent than cimetidine and has a longer duration of action. It inhibits the hepatic mixed-function oxidase system to a lesser degree.[39] A 150-mg dose on the evening prior to surgery can provide gastric antisecretory effect well through the morning, and a morning dose should allow for similar conditions into the extubation/recovery period.

Famotidine is a new H_2-antagonist. It can inhibit gastric acid secretion for up to 10–12 h and has a faster onset of antisecretory effect (30 min). Studies are lacking on its use in the obstetric population.[39]

Metoclopramide

Metoclopramide possesses three characteristics that make it potentially very useful for aspiration prophylaxis.[40]

1. it is an antiemetic;
2. it increases lower esophageal sphincter pressure; and
3. it shortens gastric emptying time.

It does not directly affect gastric pH. It is equally efficacious orally or parenterally, although variable blood levels are attained following oral administration secondary to a wide range in first-pass metabolism. Metoclopramide is more effective in emptying the stomach after a 'light' or liquid meal than solid food. A decreased gastric volume can be demonstrated within 20 min of intravenous administration. The common adult dose is 10 mg i.v. or p.o. There are isolated reports of hypotension and arrhythmias following parenteral administration. In obstetric patients, it does not appear to affect the progress of labor. Metoclopramide freely crosses the placenta, although infants born to mothers who received it demonstrated no significant change in Apgar scores or neurobehavioral assessments.

Anticholinergics

In addition to histamine and gastrin, acetylcholine is an endogenous secretagogue. Anticholinergic agents have been found to inhibit gastric fluid production, but only in a variable fashion. Of the anticholinergic agents available, glycopyrrolate has the most pronounced effects upon gastric secretion and pH. This class of drugs, however, has some potential drawbacks. They may decrease lower-esophageal sphincter pressure and delay gastric emptying. Practically speaking, these drugs are of limited benefit.[17]

REFERENCES

1. Hall G C 1940 Aspiration pneumonitis as an obstetric hazard. J Am Med Assoc 114: 728
2. Mendelson C L 1946 Aspiration of stomach contents into lungs during obstetric anesthesia. Am J Obstet Gynecol 53: 191
3. Turndorf H, Rodis I D, Clark T S 1974 'Silent' regurgitation during general anesthesia. Anesth Analg 53: 700
4. Olsson G L, Hallen B, Hambraeys-Jonzon K 1986 Aspiration during anesthesia: a computer-aided study of 185, 358 anaesthetics. Acta Anaesth Scand 30: 84
5. Hunter A R, Moir D P 1983 Editorial — confidential enquiry into maternal deaths. Br J Anaesth 55: 267
6. Morgan M 1987 Anaesthetic contribution to maternal mortality. Br J Anaesth 59: 842
7. Rosen M 1981 Editorial — maternal aspiration. Anaesthesia 36: 145
8. LeFrock L J, Clark T S, Davies B, Klainer A S 1979 Aspiration pneumonia: a ten year review. Am Surg 45: 305
9. Vandam L D 1965 Aspiration of gastric contents in the operative period. New Engl J Med 273: 1206
10. Gibbs C P, Schwartz K J, Wynne J W et al 1979 Antacid pulmonary aspiration in the dog. Anesthesiology 51: 380
11. Bynum L J, Pierce A K 1976 Pulmonary aspiration of gastric contents. Am Rev Resp Dis 114: 1129
12. Teabeaut J R 1952 Aspiration of gastric contents. Am J Pathol 28: 51
13. Schwartz D J, Wynne J W, Gibbs C P et al 1980 The pulmonary consequences of aspiration of gastric contents at pH values greater than 2.5. Am Rev Resp Dis 121: 119
14. Hammelberg W, Bosomworth P P 1964 Aspiration pneumonitis: experimental studies and clinical observations. Anesth Analg 43: 669
15. James C F, Modell J H, Gibbs C P et al 1984 Pulmonary aspiration: effects of volume and pH in the rat. Anesth Analg 63: 665
16. Wynne J W, Hood C I 1980 Hypoxemia in the first hour after aspiration (abstract). Chest 78: 546
17. Gibbs C P 1986 Gastric aspiration: prevention and treatment. Clin Anesth 4(1): 47
18. Wyner J, Cohen S E 1982 Gastric volume in early pregnancy. Anesthesiology 57: 209
19. Ulmsten U, Sundstrom G 1978 Esophageal manometry in pregnant and nonpregnant women. Am J Obstet Gynecol 132: 260
20. Wynne J W, Reynolds J C, Hood C I et al 1979 Steroid therapy for pneumonitis induced in rabbits by aspiration of food-stuff. Anesthesiology 51: 11
21. Hamilton W K, Eastwood D W 1955 A study of denitrogenation with some inhalational anesthesia systems. Anesthesiology 16: 861

22. Norris M C, Dewan D M 1985 Preoxygenation for cesarean section: a comparison of two techniques. Anesthesiology 62: 826
23. Miller R D, Way W C 1971 Inhibition of succinylcholine-induced increased intragastric pressure by non-depolarizing muscle relaxants and lidocaine. Anesthesiology 34: 185
24. Sellick B A 1961 Cricoid pressure to control regurgitation of stomach contents during induction of anesthesia. Lancet ii: 404
25. Sellick B A 1982 Rupture of the oesophagus following cricoid pressure? Anaesthesia 37: 213
26. Malinow A M, Ostheimer G W 1987 Anesthesia for the high-risk parturient. Obstet Gynecol 69: 951
27. Thomas J L 1969 Awake intubation: indications, techniques, and a review of 25 patients. Anaesthesia 24: 28
28. Abboud T K, Curtis J, Earl S et al 1984 Efficacy of clear antacid prophylaxis in obstetrics. Acta Anaesthesiol Scand 28: 301
29. Eyler S W, Cullen B F, Murphy M E, Welch W D 1982 Antacid aspiration in rabbits. Anesth Analg 61: 288
30. O'Sullivan G M, Bullingham R E 1985 Noninvasive assessment by radiotelemetry of antacid effect during labor. Anesth Analg 64: 95
31. Roberts R B, Shirley M A 1974 Reducing the risk of acid aspiration during cesarean section. Anesth Analg 53: 859
32. Hodgkinson R, Glassenberg R, Joyce T H et al 1983 Comparison of cimetidine with antacid for safety and effectiveness in reducing gastric acidity before elective cesarean section. Anesthesiology 59: 86
33. Howe J P, McGowan W A W, Moore J et al 1981 The placental transfer of cimetidine. Anaesthesia 36: 371
34. Manchikanti L, Kraus J W, Edds S P 1982 Cimetidine and related drugs in anesthesia. Anesth Analg 61: 595
35. Stoelting R K 1978 Gastric fluid and pH in patients receiving cimetidine. Anesth Analg 57: 675
36. McGowan W A W 1979 Safety of cimetidine in obstetric patients. J R Soc Med 72: 902
37. Feely J, Wilkinson G R, Wood A J J 1981 Reduction of liver blood flow and propranolol metabolism by cimetidine. New Engl J Med 305: 28
38. Lam A M, Parkin J A 1981 Cimetidine and prolonged post operative somnolence. Can Anaesth Soc J 28: 450
39. McCammon R L 1988 What's new in drugs that affect the gastrointestinal tract? Anesth Clin North Am 6(2): 40
40. Cohen S E, Jasson J, Talafre M et al 1984 Does metochlopramide decrease the volume of gastric contents in patients undergoing cesarean section? Anesthesiology 61: 604
41. Blysma-Howell M, McMorland G H, Rurak D W et al 1983 Placental transport of metochlopramide: assessment of maternal and neonatal effects. Can Anaesth Soc J 30: 487

49. Diabetes mellitus

S. Datta

Diabetes is the most common medical problem faced by the maternal and neonatal care team. In this chapter the important pathophysiologic changes that place both the mother and the baby at high risk and the appropriate anesthetic management for labor and delivery are described.

PATHOPHYSIOLOGY

Placental insufficiency is a major problem in this disease state. Nylund et al[1] compared uteroplacental blood flow in diabetic parturients with normal pregnant patients in the last trimester of pregnancy using indium-113. There was a 35–45% decrease in placental blood flow in diabetic subjects and this problem was further aggravated by the presence of high blood glucose (uncontrolled patients). Hemoglobin A_{1c} (HbA_{1c}), a poor transporter of oxygen, is increased in diabetic parturients. Determinations of HbA_{1c} concentration have been used clinically for some time to assess the degree of glycemic control among diabetics. Maternal oxygen saturation and oxygen tension is inversely related to HbA_{1c} concentrations.[2] There will be derangement of maternal oxygen transport as well as neonatal oxygen extraction in the presence of uncontrolled diabetes associated with high HbA_{1c} concentrations. It is important to remember that hypotension following regional anesthesia will further decrease placental perfusion and fetal oxygenation, causing neonatal acidosis. Ketoacidosis has become a rare entity because of aggressive prenatal care. However, it still poses a significant threat to fetal well-being and remains the major cause of neonatal mortality. Uncontrolled diabetes-associated infection and treatment with β-mimetic drugs and dexamethasone for prematurity will increase the chance of ketoacidosis.

Besides these important pathologic changes, some important obstetric conditions are more commonly associated with the diabetic pregnancy (e.g. pregnancy-induced hypertension, premature labor, placenta abruption, macrosomia and other major fetal congenital anomalies). The anesthesiologist should always be prepared to take care of the emergency situations that might necessitate urgent cesarean delivery.

CLASSIFICATION

In 1949, Dr Priscilla White[3] proposed a classification of diabetic pregnancy based on criteria that could be identified at the time of the patient's first prenatal visit, including the age of onset and duration of diabetes and the presence or absence of micro- or macrovascular complications. Recently, White's classification has undergone some modifications and the present classification can be summarized as follows:

- Class A: Abnormal carbohydrate tolerance in the nonpregnant state, not requiring insulin either prior to or during the pregnancy
- Class B: Duration of diabetes less than 10 years
- Class C: Duration of diabetes 10–20 years
- Class D: Duration more than 20 years
- Class F: Associated diabetic nephropathy
- Class R: Associated retinitis proliferans
- Class T: Associated renal transplant
- Class H: Insulin-requiring diabetes associated with coronary artery disease.

ANESTHETIC MANAGEMENT

Labor and delivery

Early labor pain can be controlled with small doses of intravenous opioids with or without a tranquilizer. Epidural anesthesia should be used for proper control of well-established labor pain and, provided there is no associated maternal hypotension, this technique has distinct advantages. Because the pain and anxiety of labor associated with increased catecholamine levels can further decrease the placental perfusion, epidural anesthesia, by decreasing catecholamine release, will increase placental perfusion.[4] Epidural anesthesia will reduce the maternal lactic acid production and, hence, fetal acidosis.[5] Epidural anesthesia will provide excellent sensory anesthesia for forceps delivery as well as appropriate anesthesia for emergent cesarean delivery for fetal distress. Subarachnoid anesthesia can also be used for forceps or cesarean delivery. A separate intravenous line for the rapid infusion of nondextrose-containing crystalloid solution to prevent hypotension may be necessary. Maternal hypotension should be treated aggressively in these patients with ephedrine.

Cesarean delivery

Anesthetic management of the diabetic parturient requires meticulous attention to avoid anesthesia-related problems. In 1977, Datta and Brown[6] observed a higher incidence of fetal acidosis in infants of diabetic mothers (IDM) compared with normal infants when their mothers received subarachnoid anesthesia instead of general anesthesia. The effect of maternal hypotension was significantly more profound in these IDM. In a subsequent study by Datta et al[7] using epidural anesthesia, fetal acidosis was found to be related to both the severity of maternal diabetes and the presence of maternal hypotension. The genesis of fetal acidosis is complex; however, a number of factors may be related. An in vitro study has demonstrated increased lactic acid production from the human placenta in the presence of hypoxia, especially in the presence of higher glycogen content, which is normal in the placentas of diabetic parturients. Clinically, hypoxia can occur in association with hypotension following regional anesthesia. Hyperglycemia in the presence of hypoxia can produce lactic acidosis.

In our first two studies regarding diabetic parturients, we used acute intravascular volume expansion with 5% dextrose in Ringer's lactate solution, as this was the solution of choice for volume expansion at that time. Hypotension following regional anesthesia in the presence of hyperglycemia might have produced lactic acidosis and consequent fetal acidosis. An experimental study in animals has shown that infusion of insulin into the umbilical artery will increase glucose utilization, causing reduced fetal oxygenation and, ultimately, fetal acidosis.[8] This condition can exist if the diabetes of these mothers is not properly controlled, because this will increase fetal glucose concentrations and consequently fetal insulin secretion.

In 1982, Datta et al[9] repeated their previous study using subarachnoid anesthesia in diabetic parturients following a strict protocol that included (1) rigidly controlled diabetic parturients (80–120 mg/dl for fasting blood glucose), (2) nondextrose-containing solution for volume expansion (Ringer's lactate) and (3) aggressive treatment of maternal hypotension so that none of the maternal systolic blood pressures fell below 100 mmHg. In this particular study, the neonatal acid-base values in IDM were similar to those in infants of normal parturients.

Both subarachnoid and epidural anesthesia, if properly performed, can be used for these parturients and provide good neonatal outcome; however, epidural anesthesia might be preferable in patients with severe diabetes (class F, R, T, H) because of a higher incidence of abrupt hypotension associated with subarachnoid anesthesia. Separate intravenous lines may be necessary for acute intravascular volume expansion with nondextrose-containing crystalloid solution. For general anesthesia, one should be aware of a number of important issues; for example, the increased gastric stasis in diabetic patients and juvenile-onset diabetic patients may be associated with 'stiff joint syndrome' and the possibility of difficult intubation.

Neonatal resuscitation is very important for the IDM because of increased chances of macrosomia, respiratory distress syndrome, hypoglycemia and other major congenital anomalies.

Finally, one should be aware of the dramatic decrease in insulin requirement immediately after delivery of the diabetic parturient.[10] Determination of blood glucose in the recovery room is mandatory.

REFERENCES

1. Nylund L, Lunell N O, Lewander R et al 1976 Uteroplacental blood flow in diabetic pregnancy: measurements with indium-113m and a computer linked gamma camera. Am J Obstet Gynecol 144: 298
2. Madsen H, Ditzel J 1982 Changes in red blood cell oxygen transport in diabetic pregnancy. Am J Obstet Gynecol 143: 421
3. White P 1949 Pregnancy complicating diabetes. Am J Med 7: 609
4. Shnider S M, Abboud T, Artal R 1983 Maternal endogenous catecholamine decrease during labor after epidural anesthesia. Am J Obstet Gynecol 147: 13
5. Pearson J F 1968 The effect of continuous lumbar epidural block on maternal and fetal acid–base balance during labor and at delivery. In Proceedings of the Symposium on Epidural Analgesia in Obstetrics. H K Lewis, London p. 26
6. Datta S, Brown W U 1977 Acid–base status in diabetic mothers and their infants following general or spinal anesthesia for cesarean section. Anesthesiology 47: 272
7. Datta S, Brown W U, Ostheimer G W et al 1981 Epidural anesthesia for cesarean section in diabetic parturients: maternal and neonatal acid–base status and bupivacaine concentration. Anesth Analg 60: 574
8. Milley J R, Rosenberg A A, Phillips A F et al 1984. The effect of insulin on ovine fetal oxygen extraction. Am J Obstet Gynecol 149: 673
9. Datta S, Kitzmiller J L, Naulty J S et al 1982 Acid–base status of diabetic mothers and their infants following spinal anesthesia for cesarean section. Anesth Anagl 61: 662
10. Soler N G, Malins J M 1978 Diabetic pregnancy: management on the day of delivery. Diabetologica 15: 441

50. Neurologic disease

M. Thornhill A. M. Bader

Controversy surrounds the choice of anesthesia for the obstetric patient with pre-existing disease of the nervous system. If the patient's neurologic condition changes postoperatively, the cause may be unclear and the anesthetic technique or drug may be blamed. In order to develop a rational anesthetic plan, an understanding of the patient's neurologic and general medical condition is needed. Unfortunately, the anesthetic literature available on most of these conditions is limited.

CHRONIC BACK PROBLEMS

Ligamentous strain from the lumbar lordosis of pregnancy results in up to 50% of pregnant women reporting chronic back pain, often associated with symptoms of pain radiating down the legs.[1] Parturients may also present with a history of intervertebral disc disease. There is no evidence that regional anesthesia will exacerbate these problems. Post-partum back pain can be minimized by assuming proper placement in the lithotomy position with the hips supported and the lordotic curvature maintained but not aggravated.

In patients having undergone previous back surgery for disc disease or scoliosis, performing regional anesthesia may be difficult because of altered anatomy or adhesions. In many cases, epidural anesthesia can be performed successfully. However, the patient should be aware that the epidural block may be patchy and inadequate because of alterations in the epidural space from previous surgery. The possibility of unintentional dural puncture may be increased. For cesarean delivery, subarachnoid anesthesia may be easier to perform and have more predictable results.

MULTIPLE SCLEROSIS

Multiple sclerosis is a major cause of neurologic disability in young and middle-aged adults, with a frequency of about 0.5 per thousand.[2,3] The disease is characterized by random and multiple sites of demyelination in the brain and spinal cord. The disease does not affect the peripheral nervous system. The course consists of remissions and exacerbations of symptoms at unpredictable time intervals over years. The relapse rate during the first 3 months post-partum has been reported to be about three times as high as in the nonpregnant patient.

The literature regarding the effects of anesthesia is controversial. Several studies have implicated anesthesia in the exacerbation of multiple sclerosis during the post-operative period for the nonobstetric patient. However, the numbers of actual relapses reported in these studies are very small and the relationship of the relapses to the anesthetic technique is unclear, since other conditions in the postoperative period such as hyperpyrexia may also predispose to relapse. Later studies in both obstetric and nonobstetric patients have reported the use of both subarachnoid and epidural anesthesia in these patients without neurologic complications.

Therefore, although there is no evidence that women who receive epidural or subarachnoid anesthesia have a higher relapse rate overall, the patient should be informed that there is a higher incidence of relapse in the post-partum period, regardless of the use of anesthesia. The anesthesiologist should be aware that there is no absolute contraindication to the use of regional anesthesia for labor and delivery in these patients.

MYASTHENIA GRAVIS

Myasthenia gravis is an autoimmune disorder causing destruction of the acetylcholine receptor resulting in chronic neuromuscular fatigue.[4-6] Anticholinesterase medications are the treatment of choice. During the course of therapy, patients may present with global weakness and respiratory insufficiency due either to inadequate anticholinesterase effect or to relative anti-cholinesterase overdose.

Management of the pregnant myasthenic includes close surveillance of both mother and fetus. A careful history of the course of the disease, the medications taken and an assessment of the severity of the disease should be documented. Particular attention should be paid to the patient's motor strength and respiratory function. Ideally, these patients should be referred for anesthetic consultation early in the course of the pregnancy. The anesthesiologist may wish to obtain pulmonary function tests, including spirometry and peak expiratory flow rate. Evidence of significant restrictive lung disease should be further evaluated with arterial blood gases. Anticholinesterase medications should be continued throughout pregnancy and delivery. An intramuscular or intravenous preparation of the anticholinesterase medication can be given during the time that the patient is fasting.

During the course of labor, these patients need to be continually assessed for increasing muscle weakness, which may require adjustment of their anticholinesterase dosage. The anesthesiologist may wish to perform serial spirometries to help with this evaluation. An easy way to do this is to measure three consecutive vital capacities. Increasing fatiguability is indicated by progressive reductions in the second and third vital capacity measured.

Large doses and high concentrations of local anesthetics should be avoided. If there is concern about the patient's respiratory status, slowly raising the anesthetic level with a continuous technique may be preferable to a single-dose technique. When regional anesthesia is used, it is recommended that large doses of ester-type local anesthetics such as chloroprocaine be avoided because the anticholinesterases given for treatment of the disease may prevent metabolism of the ester-type anesthetics, theoretically increasing maternal and fetal toxicity.

If general anesthesia is chosen as the anesthetic technique for a cesarean delivery, careful monitoring of neuromuscular function is critical because the effect of muscle relaxants on these patients may be unpredictable. The duration of succinylcholine used for intubation is obviously prolonged because of the anticholinesterase therapy. Usually no other muscle relaxants are required for cesarean delivery. If, at the end of anesthetic, there is any question about the patient's ventilatory capacity, the patient should remain intubated until adequacy of ventilation can be confirmed by pulmonary function testing in the recovery room.

EPILEPSY

The patient with epilepsy may have complications due to side-effects of anti-seizure medication or to the seizures themselves.[7] Epileptic patients do not have an increased sensitivity to local anesthetics and regional anesthesia can be safely administered. If general anesthesia is required for cesarean delivery, agents such as enflurane and ketamine that can increase central nervous system excitability should be avoided. If anticonvulsant medication has been continued during the pregnancy, serum levels should be monitored to avoid subtherapeutic or toxic levels. Several anticonvulsants, notably phenobarbital and phenytoin, are known to interfere with vitamin K metabolism in the infant.

MIGRAINE HEADACHE

70% of migraine sufferers are women of child-bearing age. There are no studies currently reporting an increase in the incidence or severity of migraine headaches in women who have received regional anesthesia for labor and delivery. Administration of preparations containing ergot is the common treatment for these patients. Theoretically, giving ephedrine to a patient taking an ergot preparation may cause an exaggerated rise in blood pressure. The dose of vasopressor used should be carefully titrated in these patients.

VIRAL DISEASE

Herpes

There has been concern that performing regional anesthesia in a patient with a history of herpes has the risk of contaminating the patient's cerebrospinal fluid with herpesvirus particles and causing meningitis.[8] However, the patient is viremic only during the primary infection. During recurrent attacks, even when vesicles are present, patients are not viremic and subarachnoid or epidural anesthesia can be administered.

Polio

Opinions vary regarding the use of regional anesthesia in the patient with a past history of polio.[9,10] Case reports of a recrudescence of symptoms after subarachnoid anesthesia exist. However, epidural anesthesia has been used successfully for labor and delivery and epidural or subarachnoid anesthesia has been used for cesarean delivery without post-partum complications.

SPINAL CORD INJURY

Regional anesthesia can be extremely beneficial to the obstetric patient with spinal cord injury.[11,12] If the lesion is below the level of T10, patients will experience labor pain. In patients with spinal cord injuries above the level of T6, there is an increased susceptibility for the syndrome of autonomic hyperreflexia. This sympathetic response can be elicited by cutaneous or visceral stimulation below the level of spinal cord transection. Since there is no inhibition of sympathetic tone from higher centers because of the transection, patients exhibit severe hypertension, headache and flushing above and blanching below the level of the lesion. It can also be triggered by distension of the bladder or rectum, or by uterine contractions during labor. Therefore, these patients need anesthesia for labor and delivery even though they lack sensation in these areas.

Regional anesthesia is an excellent choice for preventing autonomic hyperreflexia. Performing these blocks may be technically difficult if the spine is deformed and it may be difficult to position the patient who is paraplegic. However, there should be no fear of exacerbating neurologic damage in a patient with a complete spinal cord transection. Epidural anesthesia has been reported to be extremely reliable for preventing the autonomic hyperreflexia that may be initiated by uterine contractions. Usually, only a low concentration of local anesthetic agent or opioid is required.

If epidural anesthesia alone does not completely prevent or control the hypertension, intravenous agents such as labetalol, hydralazine, trimethaphan or sodium nitroprusside may be used successfully. Cesarean delivery may be indicated if these methods do not satisfactorily control the hypertension during labor.

CEREBROVASCULAR ACCIDENTS

Cerebral hemorrhage can be seen in association with aneurysms, arteriovenous malformations and pre-eclampsia or eclampsia.[13] Hypertension should be treated aggressively and abrupt changes in blood pressure avoided. For the parturient with a history of a cerebrovascular accident, epidural anesthesia is a good choice for labor and vaginal or cesarean delivery. If general anesthesia is required, the hypertensive response to intubation may be avoided by intravenous lidocaine; other antihypertensive medications such as labetalol, hydralazine, trimethaphan, or sodium nitroprusside; and adequate dosage of induction agents.

REFERENCES

1. Moir D D, Davidson S 1972 Post-partum complications of forceps delivery performed under epidural and pudendal nerve block. Br J Anaesth 44: 1197–1199
2. Crawford J S 1983 Epidural analgesia for patients with neurologic disease. Anesth Analg 62: 621–622
3. Bader A M, Hunt C O, Datta S et al 1988 Anesthesia for the obstetric patient with multiple sclerosis. J Clin Anesth 1: 21–24
4. Plauche W C 1983 Myasthenia gravis. Clin Obstet Gynecol 26: 592–604
5. Plauche W C 1979 Myasthenia gravis in pregnancy: an update. Am J Obstet Gynecol 88: 691–679
6. Baraka A 1992 Anaesthesia and myasthenia gravis. Can J Anaesth 39: 476–86
7. Abouleish E 1988 Neurologic diseases. In James F M, Wheeler A S, Dewan D M (eds) Obstetric anaesthesia: the complicated patient. F A Davis, Philadelphia p 149–154
8. Ramanathan S, Sheth R, Turndorf H 1986 Anesthesia for cesarean section in patients with genital herpes infections: a retrospective study. Anesthesiology 64: 807–809
9. Crawford J S, James F M, Nolte H et al 1981 Regional anesthesia for patients with chronic neurologic disease and similar conditions. Anaesthesia 36: 821
10. Vandam L D, Dripps R D 1956 Exacerbation of pre-existing neurologic disease after spinal anesthesia. New Engl J Med 255: 843–849
11. Stirt J A, Marco A, Conklin K A 1979 Obstetric anesthesia for a quadriplegic patient with autonomic hyperreflexia. Anesthesiology 51: 560–562
12. Baraka A 1985 Epidural meperidine for control of autonomic hyperreflexia in a paraplegic parturient. Anesthesiology 62: 688–690
13. Minielly R, Yuzpe A A, Drake C G 1979 Subarachnoid hemorrhage secondary to ruptured cerebral aneurysm in pregnancy. Obstet Gynecol 53: 64–70

51. Renal disease and pregnancy

K. Amundson

Renal disease during pregnancy potentially poses serious risks to the parturient and fetus. Progression of renal dysfunction may occur, increasing maternal morbidity and creating a suboptimal fetal environment. Thus, it is important to diagnose and treat/control renal disorders early in their course. Mild impairment may be asymptomatic. As the disease progresses, signs and symptoms include hypertension, edema, fatigue and dyspnea. Clinical suspicion of kidney disease warrants gross and microscopic analysis of the urine, 24-h creatinine clearance and protein, blood urea nitrogen and serum uric acid. Renal function should be evaluated frequently since the kidney undergoes significant anatomic and physiologic changes as the result of pregnancy.

Renal blood flow (RBF) and the glomerular filtration rate (GFR) begin to rise at about 15 weeks and remain elevated 50% above nonpregnant values until 4–6 weeks before term, when a slight decrease occurs. RBF and GFR may decrease by as much as 20% when the patient is supine compared with the left lateral position. Etiologic factors regarding the change in RBF and GFR include a parallel increase in cardiac output, a decrease in peripheral vascular resistance and an increase in circulating volume. Blood urea nitrogen (BUN) and creatinine necessarily decrease, reflecting the change in the GFR. Normal values for BUN range between 7 and 9 mg/dl and creatinine between 0.35 and 0.55 mg/dl.

Tubular resorption increases proportionately to the filtered load to maintain an almost normal sodium and water balance; however, it is not unusual to see glucosuria, amino-aciduria and proteinuria. Serum uric acid levels decrease during a normal pregnancy (mean 300 mg/dl) and are considered a sensitive indicator of tubular function.

In addition to functional changes, the kidney undergoes anatomic changes. It increases in weight and size consistent with increases in vascular and interstitial volume. Dilation of the collecting system extends to the pelvic brim. Functionally, this represents a dead space of approximately 200 ml and must be taken into account when interpreting tests of renal function.

Some controversy exists regarding the effect of pregnancy on the natural course of kidney disease. Generally speaking, mild renal dysfunction in the absence of hypertension is usually not adversely affected by pregnancy.[1] Once serum creatinine is greater than 1.8 mg/dl are accompanied by poorly controlled hypertension, acceleration of renal insufficiency is more likely.[2]

Fetal prognosis is also related to the extent of disease and degree of hypertension. Pregnancy in the presence of mild disease (creatinine less than 1.4 mg/dl) without other complications such as hypertension or proteinuria is generally not associated with adverse effects on the fetus.[1]

Moderate renal insufficiency (creatinine greater than 1.8–2.0 mg/dl) combined with significant hypertension greatly increases fetal risk for preterm labor, intrauterine growth retardation and stillbirth. Although it has not been shown conclusively that adequate blood pressure control preserves renal function or improves fetal outcome, management of hypertension is currently a key element of therapy.

TYPES OF RENAL DISORDERS

Diseases of the glomerulus may be primary or secondary to underlying systemic disease. Often glomerular disease is accompanied by proteinuria, hypertension, or both. The prevalence of preeclampsia in this group of patients is as high as 50%.[1] Renal function may deteriorate with the development of preeclampsia.

Nephrotic syndrome (proteinuria in excess of 3.5 g/24 h) commonly results from glomerular disease; rarely it may be caused by renal vein thrombosis or amyloidosis. Preeclampsia is the most common cause of nephrotic syndrome arising de novo in pregnancy. Major physiologic alterations include hypoproteinemia, which alters drug binding and decreases effective circulating volume, marked edema formation and hyperlipidemia. Occasionally, IgG deficiency and/or hypothyroidism results from loss of immunoglobulins or thyroglobulins.

Proteinuria alone does not affect prognosis if renal function is preserved and hypertension is absent.

Patients with type I diabetes of more than 10 years' duration are likely to have some degree of renal impairment. Glomerular function is primarily affected but renal tubules may also be involved. The incidence of asymptomatic bacteruria is increased in diabetic women. Antibiotics should be prescribed to prevent progression to acute pyelonephritis. Proteinuria may increase during pregnancy, but renal function can remain stable as long as hypertension is not severe.

Up to 50% of patients with active lupus associated with nephropathy near the time of conception may experience deterioration of renal function. There is also an increased likelihood of spontaneous abortion, growth retardation, stillbirth (live birth rate is 50–85%)[3] and neonatal lupus. Patients with quiescent disease for at least 6 months prior to conception fare much better with live birth rates of 85–95%.[3]

Acute renal failure

The prevalence of acute renal failure (ARF) in pregnancy is approximately 1 per 10 000,[1] and is usually related to complications occurring late in pregnancy such as abruption or other causes of hemorrhage, amniotic fluid embolus or preeclampsia/eclampsia. However, ARF may occur as the result of the superimposition of the stress of pregnancy on patients with pre-existing renal disease. Rarely, it may be caused by post-partum hemolytic uremic syndrome. Measures to treat renal failure are largely supportive, such as correcting the precipitating factors and close monitoring of fluid and electrolyte and acid–base status. Central venous pressure and/or pulmonary arterial monitoring may be necessary to adequately assess circulating volume and guide hydration. An intra-arterial catheter is helpful if vasoactive drugs are used to control hypertension and if frequent blood sampling is required. Dialysis may be needed until kidney function returns. Drug doses must be adjusted in accordance with renal function. Systemic effects of renal failure on the heart (pericardial effusion, congestive heart failure), lung (interstitial edema), central nervous system (central nervous system depression with uremia), platelets (decreased lifespan, dysfunctional) and bone marrow (anemia) need to be considered when planning anesthetic care.

Renal transplantation

There have been more than 2000 pregnancies in transplant recipients. These pregnancies have been complicated by preterm labor (50%), growth retardation (25%) and hypertension, preeclampsia or both (30%).[4] The incidence of rejection or progressive renal dysfunction is probably not significantly different from nonpregnant counterparts.

Ideally, women are encouraged to wait 2 years following transplant in order to recover from surgery, allow graft function to stabilize and progress to only maintenance doses of immunosuppressives.

Immunosuppressive therapy can predispose the mother to infection and cause premature rupture of membranes, fetal malformation, growth retardation and neonatal lymphopenia during the first few weeks of life. Azidothymidine (AZT) reverses the effects of nondepolarizing neuromuscular blockers, potentiates succinylcholine and increases excitability of skeletal muscles because it inhibits phosphodiesterase. Cyclosporin can cause renal and hepatic toxicity, convulsions, hyperglycemia and hemolytic–uremic syndrome. It potentiates the effects of barbiturates, opioids, atracurium and vecuronium.

Patients may deliver vaginally; only rarely will dystocia occur secondary to ectopic placement of the transplanted kidney. Supplemental doses of hydrocortisone should be given at the time of delivery.

ANESTHETIC MANAGEMENT

Regional anesthesia

Anesthetic management of the parturient with renal disease presents a challenge to the anesthesiologist. Usual drug doses may require adjustment, renal blood flow should be optimized and systemic effects of altered renal function must be recognized. Regional anesthesia has the least effect on RBF and GFR provided hemodynamic stability is maintained. Continuous epidural anesthesia (CEA), in most cases, remains the method of choice for labor and delivery. Easing the pain of labor should decrease catecholamine release, thereby reducing renovascular resistance and increasing blood flow to the kidney and uterus. The advantage of CEA over subarachnoid anesthesia is that the level of sympathetic blockade can be obtained gradually, thus usually avoiding significant hypotension, which interferes with renal and uteroplacental perfusion. Ephedrine in 5–10 mg increments administered intravenously can be used to treat hypotension should it occur. Acute intravenous hydration prior to the induction of anesthesia should be approached carefully in a patient with impaired renal function. Central venous pressure monitoring in addition to clinical evaluation may be helpful in judging intravenous volume replacement. Tonicity and composition of the intravenous fluid chosen will depend on specific abnormalities in blood chemistries and the degree of renal impairment.

Caution should be exercised when using regional anesthesia in patients treated long-term with β-adrenergic blockers. Beta-adrenergic agonists such as ephedrine are less effective in correcting bradycardia and hypotension resulting from sympathetic blockade and relative hypovolemia. Clotting abnormalities may preclude the use of regional anesthesia. Because it is not uncommon for coagulopathies to be associated with renal disease, bleeding time, prothrombin time, partial thromboplastin time, fibrinogen and platelet count should be obtained to assist in the preanesthetic evaluation.

Amide local anesthetics are metabolized by the liver and as such are generally safe for use in patients with renal disease. Ester-type local anesthetics are degraded by plasma cholinesterases and therefore are also safe. In patients with pre-existing uremic neuropathy, chloroprocaine solutions with sodium bisulfite should not be used.[5]

General anesthesia

General anesthesia should be routinely avoided except in certain emergency circumstances or when regional techniques are specifically contraindicated. Inhaled anesthetics cause varying degrees of myocardial depression and vasodilation, which result in an increase in renovascular resistance and a decrease in RBF and GFR by as much as 30–50%. An increase in intrapulmonary shunt coupled with anemia (seen in both pregnancy and renal disease) may predispose the patient to severe reductions in tissue oxygen delivery. Although elimination of inhaled agents does not depend on renal excretion, similar to the once used methoxyflurane, enflurane and the relatively new agent, sevoflurane, are metabolized to some extent, yielding nephrotoxic fluoride ions. Short-term exposure (2 h or less), however, probably has little clinical significance. The metabolism of isoflurane is minimal. Halothane, in combination with electrolyte and acid–base abnormalities, can provoke myocardial irritability leading to arrhythmias.

Intravenous induction doses of barbiturates may need to be reduced to reflect hypoalbuminemia, acid–base status, which changes the ratio of ionized to nonionized drug, and impaired biotransformation in the liver in patients who are severely debilitated. Ketamine stimulates catecholamine release, which increases renovascular resistance and decreases RBF.

The muscle relaxant of choice for a rapid-sequence induction in the parturient with renal disease and serum potassium exceeding 5.5 mmol/l is vecuronium 0.28 mg/kg, as only 15% of the drug is excreted by the kidney. It may cause muscle weakness in the neonate, which requires intervention at the time of delivery. In normokalemic patients, succinylcholine can probably be used safely. Patients receiving magnesium sulfate will be much more sensitive to neuromuscular blocking agents and will require a reduction in the usual dose.

Blood pressure control during general anesthesia, especially the response to laryngoscopy and incision, can be achieved with small doses of hydralazine, realizing that excretion is prolonged when renal dysfunction is severe. Alternatively, labetalol can be used. Methyldopa is almost exclusively excreted in the urine and, therefore, the dose must be reduced. Nitroglycerin, nitroprusside and trimethaphan may be necessary for short-term antihypertensive management.

REFERENCES

1. Schrier R, Gottsschalk C, Diseases of the kidney, 5th edn. Little Brown, Boston
2. Jungers P, Houillier P, Forget D et al 1991 Specific controversies concerning the natural history of renal disease in pregnancy. Am J Kidney Dis 17(2): 166–172
3. Hayslett J 1991 Maternal and fetal complications in pregnant women with systemic lupus erythematosus. Am J Kidney Dis 17(2): 127–132
4. Davison J 1991 Dialysis, transplantation and pregnancy. Am J Kidney Dis 17: 2
5. James F, Wheeler A S 1988 Obstetric anesthesia: the complicated patient. F A Davis, Philadelphia
6. Katz J, Benumof J, Kadis L 1990 Anesthesia and uncommon diseases. 3rd edn. W B Saunders, Philadelphia
7. Burrow G, Terris T 1988 Medical complications during pregnancy. W B Saunders, Philadelphia
8. Brenner B, Floyd R 1991 The kidney, 4th edn. W B Saunders, Philadelphia
9. Gebbe S, Niebyl J, Simpson J L 1991 Obstetrics: normal and problem pregnancies. 2nd edn. Churchill Livingstone, New York

52. Liver disease

A. M. De Wolf

INTRODUCTION

Liver disease can occur in many forms in the pregnant patient, and the severity may range from mild dysfunction to fulminant hepatic failure.[1–5] Even normal hepatic function can be affected significantly by pregnancy, and it may be difficult to distinguish these changes from mild liver disease.

Pregnancy can now occur in patients with existing liver disease thanks to improvements in the management of chronic liver diseases. Most often, however, the liver disease that occurs during pregnancy is coincidental (such as viral hepatitis). But sometimes liver dysfunction is caused, at least in part, by the pregnant state (such as intrahepatic cholestasis and liver diseases associated with preeclampsia). A few life-threatening liver diseases may occur during pregnancy (such as those associated with preeclampsia or fulminant hepatitis) and require prompt diagnosis and treatment. Liver disease severe enough to cause jaundice during pregnancy is uncommon; it occurs in about 1 in 1500 pregnancies.[6]

To provide optimal anesthesia and analgesia for labor and delivery for patients with liver disease, the anesthesiologist must understand the physiologic and pathophysiologic changes. Anesthetic considerations for vaginal and operative deliveries in patients with liver disease are presented. Finally, transplantation has become a therapeutic option in patients with severe liver disease, and therefore the relation between liver transplantation and pregnancy will be described.

HEPATIC PHYSIOLOGIC CHANGES DURING PREGNANCY

Liver size and hepatic blood flow do not change with pregnancy.[7] Because blood volume and cardiac output increase during pregnancy, the fractional blood flow to the liver declines by about 35%.[8] This may lead to a reduction in clearance of certain drugs or substances from the blood [indocyanine green, bromosulfophthalein (BSP), galactose].

Fasting gallbladder volume and residual volume after contraction are increased (sluggish gallbladder of pregnancy). This decrease in smooth muscle motility of the gallbladder correlates with increases in serum progesterone values; progesterone receptors are present in the gallbladder wall. Studies of biliary lipids and bile acid kinetics during pregnancy have shown an increase in the lithogenic index of bile: there is an increase in biliary cholesterol secretion, a decrease in the synthesis of chenodeoxycholic acid relative to cholic acid and a reduced enterophepatic bile acid pool. As a result, women who have been pregnant have an increased risk of gallstones.[9]

Some changes in the results of standard laboratory tests are expected during normal pregnancy. The increase in blood volume is reflected in a decrease in hemoglobin concentration. Serum levels of all proteins synthesized by the liver are affected by pregnancy. Total protein and albumin concentrations and the albumin-to-globulin ratio decrease. Alpha- and beta-globulins may increase, but gamma-globulins decrease for reasons that are unclear. The synthesis of fibrinogen and other coagulation factors (VII, VIII, IX, and X) is increased, and fibrinolytic activity is mildly reduced. The balance of clotting changes toward a state of increased coagulability with decreased fibrinolysis. Ceruloplasmin and transferrin levels are increased, but haptoglobin concentration is unaltered. Plasma cholinesterase levels are slightly reduced during pregnancy and in the immediate post-partum period.[10,11] Serum lipids change drastically, with a 50–100% increase in serum cholesterol and a threefold increase in serum triglycerides, probably as a result of increased synthesis.[12] Therefore, hypercholesterolemia cannot be considered to be evidence of cholestasis during pregnancy. Estrogens increase the retention of BSP after a single bolus administration. The excretion capacity into bile decreases, but the hepatic storage capacity for BSP increases.[7,13,14] The change in BSP clearance is also caused at least in part by the increased binding of BSP to plasma albumin during pregnancy.[15]

Liver function tests are normal during the entire course of pregnancy with a single exception: the alkaline phosphatase level increases 2–4 times because of the presence of a heat-stable fraction of placental origin. Although serum glutamic oxaloacetic transaminase (SGOT or AST), serum glutamic pyruvic transaminase (SGPT or ALT), lactic dehydrogenase and ornithine transcarbamylase can increase slightly during normal pregnancy, they remain within the normal range.[16,17] Serum gamma-glutamyltranspeptidase (GGPT) has been reported to increase during the third trimester of pregnancy.[18] Any consistent increase in transaminase or bilirubin is an indication of possible liver disease.

Hepatic histology is not significantly altered by pregnancy.[19] However, nonspecific changes may be seen, such as alterations in the size and shape of hepatocytes, degree of lymphocyte infiltration in the portal areas and glycogen and fat content.[20]

PHYSIOLOGIC CHANGES DUE TO LIVER DISEASE

The pathophysiologic changes in patients with severe liver disease have been described previously.[21] Briefly, patients with severe liver disease have a hyperdynamic circulatory system, with increased cardiac output and decreased systemic vascular resistance, due to the presence of arteriovenous shunts and circulating vasodilators. Coagulopathy is due to a decreased synthesis of coagulation factors by the liver, thrombocytopenia and platelet dysfunction. Liver disease also results in intrapulmonary shunting, leading to hypoxemia. Pleural effusions, ascites and impaired hypoxic pulmonary vasoconstriction may contribute to hypoxemia. Portal hypertension may lead to gastrointestinal bleeding and ascites. Renal dysfunction is due, in part, to a decrease in effective plasma volume and hormonal changes. Electrolyte disorders, acid–base imbalance, hypoglycemia and hepatic encephalopathy may all be present in patients with severe liver disease.

LIVER DISEASE AND PREGNANCY

Liver disease occurring coincidentally during pregnancy

Viral hepatitis

The most common liver disease in pregnancy is viral hepatitis, which makes up approximately 40% of all liver diseases associated with pregnancy.[1,2,22] Hepatitis A is the most common form of viral hepatitis. Hepatitis may occur more frequently in pregnant women than in nonpregnant women or in men,[23] possibly because of alterations in T-cell function.[24] Viral hepatitis in general has a minimal effect on the course of pregnancy, and pregnancy has little effect on the course of viral hepatitis.[1,2,25] Exposure to viral hepatitis during pregnancy does not cause teratogenesis.[25] Although somewhat controversial, studies have indicated a slightly increased risk of premature birth.[25,26] Treatment is supportive and hospitalization is rarely necessary.[22] The incidence of severe complications (such as acute fulminant hepatic failure) is not increased in pregnant patients. The exception is herpes simplex, which has been associated with fulminant hepatic failure in pregnant women.[27]

A small percentage of patients with viral hepatitis may develop acute fulminant hepatic failure with massive hepatocellular necrosis, encephalopathy, coagulopathy and renal failure. Patients with these complications have a high mortality rate.[2,28] It is sometimes difficult to differentiate viral hepatitis from acute fatty liver of pregnancy during the third trimester,[29] although patients with acute fatty liver of pregnancy usually have only mildly elevated transaminase levels (< 500 U/I).[2,29] The role of termination of pregnancy in severe hepatitis during the last trimester is unclear. In extremely severe cases with massive necrosis, liver transplantation should be considered.

Hepatitis A is a highly contagious but benign disease without significant risk to mother or fetus. Women with hepatitis A may transmit the disease to the fetus if they are viremic at or around the time of delivery. Although clinical hepatitis in the newborn is mild and there is no carrier state, immune serum globulin may be administered to the infant.[30] However, the fetus is often protected by maternal antibodies, which readily cross the placenta. Except in fulminant hepatitis A, there are no serious sequelae or chronic forms of this disease. Treatment consists of supportive measures, and patients improve within 2–3 weeks.

Hepatitis B virus infection in women during early pregnancy does not seem to be more severe than in nonpregnant women and is without significant implications for mother and infant. The hepatitis B virus normally does not cross the placental barrier. When the infection occurs during the third trimester of the disease, however, there is a high risk (90%) of transmission to the newborn during delivery, probably by ingestion of infected material.[30–34] Some of these infants may develop severe hepatitis at 30–120 days of age.[33] Most of them (80–90%) become chronic carriers of hepatitis B surface antigen (HBsAg) developing chronic hepatitis, cirrhosis or hepatomas. The newborn should be protected by passive and active immunization, i.e. intramuscular administration of hepatitis B immune globulin (HBIG) within 24 h after birth, and hepatitis B vaccine (within 24 h and again at 1 and 6 months).[32,34–36]

5–10% of infants infected at birth have acquired the disease by the transplacental route,[32] and little can be done to prevent this kind of transmission. In addition, there may be women who are still in the incubation period of the disease at the time of delivery.

Non-A, non-B hepatitis during pregnancy may be associated with increased morbidity and mortality rates compared with rates in nonpregnant patients.[23] Because serologic identification of hepatitis non-A, non-B, cytomegalovirus and Epstein–Barr virus has become available only recently, the non-A, non-B hepatitis category in this comparison may have included other diseases, such as cholestasis of pregnancy or acute fatty liver of pregnancy. Whether non-A, non-B hepatitis is transmitted to the newborn or affects neonatal survival is unclear.[30] Some infants born to mothers with non-A, non-B hepatitis have elevated liver enzymes at birth but do not seem to develop chronic liver disease.[30]

Other liver diseases

Although pregnancy decreases gallbladder motility and increases the lithogenicity of bile; cholelithiasis and cholecystitis are not more common during pregnancy. Cholelithiasis is not a common cause of jaundice during pregnancy.[6,37] Furthermore, acute cholecystitis that is unresponsive to conservative medical treatment is uncommon in pregnancy, and, therefore, cholecystectomy during pregnancy is a rare procedure.[38,39] If necessary, however, cholecystectomy can be performed during pregnancy without an increase in morbidity for either mother or fetus. Acute pancreatitis during pregnancy is usually caused by cholelithiasis.[40,41] Drug-induced jaundice during pregnancy is responsible for <2% of cases, and has recently been reviewed extensively.[42]

Effects of pre-existing liver disease on pregnancy

Most patients with liver disease are not of child-bearing age, and most women with severe liver disease are infertile. However, pregnancy can occur in women with mild to moderate liver disease, thanks to improvements in the treatment of chronic liver diseases.[43,44]

Liver cirrhosis

Liver cirrhosis can be due to post-necrotic cirrhosis, Laennec's cirrhosis, primary biliary cirrhosis or chronic active hepatitis. Pregnancy in the presence of cirrhosis is still uncommon. The treatment of cirrhotic liver disease in pregnant patients is the same as that of nonpregnant patients, but the pregnancy can present some special problems. In pregnant patients with liver cirrhosis, worsening jaundice with progressive liver failure, ascites and hepatic coma have been reported.[45,46] It is unclear, however, whether the exacerbation of liver dysfunction is caused by the pregnancy. Most patients with cirrhosis have sustained pregnancy without any worsening hepatic function,[45,47] and, in general, there is little evidence that pregnancy worsens the underlying liver disease.[46] However, cirrhosis seems to be associated with an increased incidence of stillbirths and premature delivery, although there is no increased incidence of congenital malformations.[43,45,47,48] Maternal complications include anemia, preeclampsia and post-partum hemorrhage. The most significant complication is variceal bleeding, which may occur during the second or third trimester, or during or shortly after labor. Severe bleeding is associated with increased fetal and maternal mortality rates.[43,44,48–50] Variceal bleeding may be precipitated by worsening of pre-existing portal hypertension due to the marked increase in blood volume and azygos flow seen in normal pregnancy. Patients with a past history of variceal hemorrhage who have received a portacaval shunt have a lower incidence of hemorrhage during pregnancy.[43] There are reports of successful shunt surgery without fetal wastage during pregnancy.[48] Although the role of sclerotherapy in the prevention of esophageal varices remains unclear in this patient population, it seems to be a reasonable approach in the pregnant patient with bleeding varices. Aggressive blood replacement and intensive therapy are obviously mandatory when variceal hemorrhage occurs.

Specific liver diseases with cirrhosis

Hepatitis B can be transmitted from mother to infant at delivery. Carrier mothers transmit the virus to their infants at a rate of only 5%, which is significantly lower than the infection rate for mothers with acute hepatitis.[31] Infants develop serologic markers for hepatitis B infection 1–2 months after birth, suggesting a low incidence of transplacental transmission. Because chronic hepatitis B infection in adults can be asymptomatic, it has been recommended that all pregnant women be tested routinely for HBsAg during an early prenatal visit.[36] However, these recommendations do not optimally identify women at risk at the time of delivery. Therefore, many obstetricians screen all women for HBsAg at the time of delivery, although this is probably not necessary or cost-effective in a private obstetric population, where screening could be done based on the presence of risk factors.[51] Protection of the newborn has been discussed already.

Pregnancy in patients with *Laennec's cirrhosis* is extremely rare.[45] Chronic alcohol abuse leads to an increased incidence of miscarriages and, unlike other diseases leading to cirrhosis, is associated with an increased incidence of congenital abnormalities (fetal alcohol syndrome).[52]

Other liver diseases

Chronic persistent hepatitis does not affect the outcome of pregnancy, and no worsening in liver dysfunction is seen. In *chronic active hepatitis*, however, pregnancy is rare and, if it occurs, is frequently associated with a worsening in liver function. The effects of *Wilson's disease* on pregnancy have been studied. The use of penicillamine to treat this disease does not increase risks for the fetus or mother.[53–55] In general, patients should continue to take the medications controlling their liver disease. In some patients with Wilson's disease, symptoms have improved during pregnancy, possibly as a result of increases in ceruloplasmin levels associated with pregnancy. Because steroids have been associated with an increased risk of congenital deformities,[47] the lowest effective dose should be used. *Autoimmune hepatitis* can be controlled during pregnancy with continued use of medications (azathioprine or corticosteroids).[56] *Hepatic adenomas* or tumors of focal nodular hyperplasia associated with oral contraceptive agents have been reported to enlarge or to rupture during pregnancy and, therefore, should be resected prior to conception or during pregnancy. Mild hepatic dysfunctions such as *familial hyperbilirubinemia* and *Gilbert's syndrome* (unconjugated hyperbilirubinemia) have not been found to complicate pregnancies. Patients with conjugated hyperbilirubinemia (*Dubin–Johnson syndrome*) have a temporary worsening of their disease. *Familial intrahepatic cholestasis*, *Alagille's syndrome* (arteriohepatic dysplasia) and *Byle's syndrome* (congenital absence of bile ducts) are all worsened by pregnancy.[57]

Liver disease as a result of pregnancy

Some liver diseases are clearly related to pregnancy.

Hyperemesis gravidarum

Nausea and vomiting are common in pregnancy, particularly in the first trimester. If severe, liver dysfunction, presenting as a mild increase in bilirubin, an increase in transaminase levels and a prolongation of BSP clearance, may occur.[58] The histology is normal or shows modest cholestasis with hepatocyte necrosis. Treatment is symptomatic with correction of fluid, electrolyte and acid–base balance, and should result in complete recovery.

Intrahepatic cholestasis of pregnancy

Several cholestatic states can occur during late pregnancy:

1. normal late pregnancy, an altered physiologic state characterized by a minimal to modest degree of cholestasis;
2. generalized pruritus of pregnancy (pruritus gravidarum), a syndrome with a more pronounced level of cholestasis than in normal pregnancy, greater abnormalities in tests of liver function and symptoms of persistent itching, but with no icterus; and
3. idiopathic or recurrent jaundice of pregnancy, which is the most severe form of cholestatic disorder in pregnancy.[59]

Intrahepatic cholestasis may occur in otherwise healthy women during pregnancy. Because the syndrome has also been observed in patients taking oral contraceptives, ethinyl estradiol is suspected to be involved.[13] The precise mechanism remains undefined; abnormal estrogen metabolism in the liver may be involved. The disease occurs preferentially in certain ethnic groups (Scandinavians, Chileans), and there is evidence that it is an inherited disease.[60] Half of the patients have a family history of jaundice during pregnancy or oral contraceptive therapy. Similar symptoms, although of different severity, tend to occur in subsequent pregnancies.[60]

Intrahepatic cholestasis may occur as early as the first trimester, although it most often occurs in the last trimester. Pruritus is the dominant and most disturbing symptom, and jaundice is present only in the most severe form of the disease (recurrent jaundice of pregnancy). Any abnormality on physical examination (abdominal pain, hepatic tenderness, hepatosplenomegaly) rules out intrahepatic cholestasis; nausea, vomiting, and arthralgias are absent. The gallbladder becomes more distended, and there is a 10- to 100-fold increase in serum bile acids[61] and a 7- to 10-fold increase in alkaline phosphatase. Bilirubin levels remain normal or are slightly increased (in about 20% of patients).[62] A liver biopsy shows pure cholestasis with dilation of the bile ducts, accumulation of bile pigment, and minimal nonspecific abnormalities.

In general, this is a fairly benign condition for the mother except for fat malabsorption. Coagulopathy due to decreased vitamin K absorption may develop when malabsorption is severe and when cholestyramine is administered. An increased incidence of stillbirths, prematurity, low birth weight and perinatal complications has been reported.[63–67] There is an increased prevalence of fetal distress (22%),[67] possibly caused by a reduction in placental blood flow,[68] leading to an increased incidence of cesarean deliveries. Abnormalities in the placenta have been observed, such as alterations in terminal villi with a reduction of intervillous spaces and syncytial and cytotrophoblastic hyperplasia, which may lead to impaired fetal oxygenation.[69] These infants require close monitoring.[63,64,67] In the absence of administration of exogenous maternal vitamin K, fetal prothrombin time is abnormal. Such an infant is at great risk of intracranial hemorrhage during delivery, and, if delivered alive, is often neurologically impaired.

Therapy is directed at alleviating pruritus in the mother. Treatment includes cholestyramine and phenobarbital, as in other cholestatic syndromes.[59,64,70,71] However, these drugs have limited and variable success, and cholestyramine may worsen the fat malabsorption. All these patients should receive parenteral vitamin K. The syndrome disappears completely after delivery, usually within 1–2 weeks. It is totally reversible, leaving no sequelae.[6,59]

Liver disease associated with preeclampsia and eclampsia

Preeclampsia is a multisystem disease with a broad clinical spectrum.[72] Although it is described in detail elsewhere, it is discussed again here because liver dysfunction is frequently associated with preeclampsia and eclampsia. Hypertension, generalized edema and proteinuria are the hallmarks of preeclampsia and eclampsia, which may be caused by imbalances in prostaglandin metabolism[73] resulting in increased sensitivity to vasoconstrictive substances and endothelial cell damage. Intravascular coagulation (rarely disseminated) plays a role in their pathophysiology, and is possibly initiated by platelet adherence at sites of endothelial damage. Microangiopathic hemolysis is frequently present and may contribute to the jaundice.

Mild disturbances in liver function are found in approximately 50% of patients with preeclampsia.[6,74] Bilirubin increases in about 10% of patients with preeclampsia.[75] The liver may be involved in preeclampsia or eclampsia as a part of the generalized vascular disorder. Edema and reduction in hepatic blood flow (due to arterial vasospasm and fibrin deposits in sinusoids) may lead to hepatocyte ischemia and dysfunction. More sophisticated techniques (immunofluorescence) showed the presence of fibrin deposits in the sinusoids in all patients with preeclampsia, with periportal hemorrhage and patchy areas of necrosis in several of these patients.[76–78] Fibrin deposits are seen in other tissues, such as the kidneys, as well. Severe liver dysfunction occurs in only a few patients with preeclampsia and eclampsia. Indeed, there is a broad range of liver dysfunction associated with preeclampsia and eclampsia, including sinusoidal fibrinogen deposits, periportal hemorrhage, hepatic infarction, spontaneous rupture of the liver and the HELLP syndrome (see below).[74–79] Recently, acute fatty liver of pregnancy has been classified as a complication of preeclampsia and eclampsia, rather than as a separate entity.[1,80,81] However, not everyone agrees with this new classification.[82] Interestingly, these complications of preeclampsia and eclampsia may be associated with only mild hypertension and proteinuria,[78,83–86] and sometimes liver dysfunction may develop after delivery.[86]

If hepatic complications are minor, no special therapy is required other than the standard treatment for preeclampsia and eclampsia. Therapy for severe preeclampsia includes expeditious delivery (cesarean delivery is not absolutely necessary), magnesium sulfate for seizure prophylaxis, selective use of antihypertensives and strict fluid control. Antibiotics are reserved only for infection prophylaxis in patients who undergo cesarean delivery. These patients should be monitored and treated before and for at least 48 h after delivery, if possible in an intensive care unit. Recently, a thromboxane synthetase inhibitor (dazoxiben) has been used.[73] Patients with significant hepatic involvement due to preeclampsia and eclampsia require treatment in an intensive care facility, preferably in a tertiary care center.

Specific liver complications may occur with preeclampsia and eclampsia. *Fibrinogen deposits* in the hepatic sinusoids can be seen in women with uncomplicated preeclampsia.[76] Liver function tests remain normal. *Periportal hemorrhage* is the lesion classically associated with preeclampsia and eclampsia. Histologically, periportal fibrin deposits and hemorrhage are seen. Liver function tests are abnormal, and periportal hemorrhage may be complicated by thrombocytopenia, disseminated intravascular coagulation (DIC), hemolysis and the HELLP syndrome.[87] If severe, periportal hemorrhage may lead to the development of an intrahepatic or subcapsular hematoma. These hematomas are frequently missed, but can be diagnosed using computed tomography.[88] Every patient with preeclampsia should be monitored for evidence of hepatic hematoma or hemorrhage. Hemorrhage under the liver capsule without frank rupture may be treated conservatively,[88] but subcapsular hematomas may enlarge, sometimes resulting in spontaneous rupture. Therefore, extensive subcapsular hematomas should always be treated surgically.[89]

Spontaneous rupture of the liver, a complication of periportal hemorrhage and subcapsular hematoma, is more common in older women and in multiparous women.[90] It has also been reported in patients with acute fatty liver of pregnancy.[91] Usually the sudden development of systemic hypotension and a distended abdomen in the presence of preeclampsia make the diagnosis likely, and hepatic angiography is rarely necessary to confirm the diagnosis. Differential diagnosis includes uterine rupture, which also reveals blood on a peritoneal lavage. In either situation, immediate surgery is warranted. Obviously, vigorous resuscitation is required, combined with aggressive surgical control of the bleeding.[92] Intra-abdominal packing and drainage are usually sufficient, and lobectomy should be used only with total disruption of a segment or lobe and inability to control hemorrhage.[89] Sometimes hepatic artery ligation or embolization of the hepatic artery is required.[89,93,94] Surgical hemostasis can be difficult in the presence of multiple areas of infarction and hematoma, especially in the presence of coagulopathy. Even with aggressive treatment, mortality rates remain high.

The HELLP syndrome – (hemolysis, elevated liver enzymes, hepatic dysfunction and low platelets).

Thrombocytopenia[83] is found in about 12% of patients with preeclampsia[95] and in patients with typical acute fatty liver of pregnancy.[80] Some confusion still exists regarding the terminology, incidence, diagnosis and management of this disease.[86,87] On liver biopsy, fibrin deposits in the sinusoids and areas of hemorrhagic necrosis are frequently seen. These may develop into macroscopic hematomas. A peripheral blood smear may reveal schistocytes or spherocytes due to microangiopathic hemolysis, perhaps as a result of the passage of red blood cells, which may have membrane alterations, through small blood vessels with damaged intima and fibrin deposits.[96] Some degree of disseminated intravascular coagulation (DIC) is found.[97] The low platelet count is the result of increased platelet consumption or destruction. Intensive care and anesthetic treatment for patients with the HELLP syndrome have been presented recently.[98,99] Therapy is similar to that for acute fatty liver of pregnancy. Complications include renal insufficiency, DIC, intracerebral hemorrhage, pulmonary edema, infectious diseases, hypoglycemia and liver rupture. The perinatal mortality rate is high (10–60%), and the maternal mortality rate is between 0% and 5%.[77,83,84,87,99]

Acute fatty liver of pregnancy was first described in 1940 by Sheehan. It was described as a catastrophic illness complicating the third trimester of pregnancy, and was often fatal.[100] Initially, this syndrome had a very high maternal (85%) and fetal (50%) mortality rate, but more recently mortality rates have decreased dramatically. The increased survival rates may be due to improved intensive care of these patients, with careful attention to bleeding problems and aggressive treatment of sepsis,[80] as well as to a more widespread recognition of the disease, leading to early diagnosis and treatment of less severe cases.[101]

Acute fatty liver of pregnancy occurs more commonly in young women who are pregnant for the first time and in those with twin pregnancies. Although this disease is said not to recur in subsequent pregnancies,[101–104] one recurrence has been reported recently.[105] Symptoms appear during the later part of the third trimester. Signs of preeclampsia seem to be present in all patients. Clinical features typically include anorexia, nausea, vomiting, malaise, headache and weight loss. Diffuse abdominal pain may be present or may be limited to the right upper quadrant. Jaundice may be the initial complaint or appear several days after the other symptoms. Pruritus is rarely present. Clinically, liver function can deteriorate rapidly, leading to hepatic encephalopathy, coagulopathy, hypoglycemia, pancreatitis, renal failure and thrombocytopenia. With the appearance of diffuse bleeding or somnolence, fatal outcome is usual without rapid intervention. However, the syndrome seems to have varied symptoms, and the degree of hepatic dysfunction may range from clinically unapparent to typical acute hepatic failure.[101]

Patients frequently have laboratory test results compatible with preeclampsia. A decrease in intravascular volume may lead to increases in hemoglobin, blood urea nitrogen and uric acid. Liver function tests almost always show increased levels of transaminase, especially SGOT (AST), alkaline phosphatase, and bilirubin.[106] PT and PTT are frequently prolonged, and a marked reduction in antithrombin III is often seen.[107–109] In severe cases, there is frequently evidence of DIC with thrombocytopenia, low fibrinogen levels and increased fibrinogen degradation products.[110] Coagulopathy, therefore, is the result of increased consumption of procoagulants and impaired production of coagulation factors by the liver. Giant platelet forms (megakaryocytes), signs of increased platelet consumption or destruction, have been reported.[110] Other complications of hepatic failure frequently seen are hypoglycemia, hyperammonemia, hepatic coma and acute pancreatitis.

There is no evidence that tetracycline is the cause of this disease, but tetracycline may induce a syndrome in pregnant and nonpregnant patients that is very similar to fatty liver of pregnancy.[80] The exact pathogenic mechanism remains unknown, but it seems clear that fatty liver of pregnancy is associated with preeclampsia.[101] It has been speculated that abnormalities in mitochondria or intermediary metabolism of fatty acids may cause the fatty liver.[101]

Liver biopsy confirms the diagnosis, but may not always be possible because of coagulopathy seen in the late stage. Histologically, there is microvesicular fatty infiltration, which is most prominent in the pericentral region.[111] Usually the periportal areas are spared or have a much less prominent fatty change. The histology may vary significantly, ranging from cells that are ballooned and vacuolated but without apparent fat[80,111] to severe microvesicular fatty infiltration often associated with severe hepatic failure.[104] However, the fatty changes frequently are missed if special stains (oil red O stain) or electron microscopy are not used; the histology report then reads 'hepatitis, either viral or toxic in origin'.[77,80] Because the histologic findings are easily misinterpreted, the diagnosis may be frequently incorrect. There is usually little necrosis or inflammatory cell infiltration, except in severe cases.[111] Other organs, such as the pancreas, brain, heart, bone marrow and kidneys, may also show vacuolar changes.[111–115] The kidneys can have lesions typical of preeclampsia.[111]

Early after the delivery, recovery starts with a decrease in the number of cells demonstrating fatty changes. There is a temporary increase in cholestasis, in bile- and pigment-laden macrophages and in portal inflammatory cells, which reflects recovery after acute injury. Biopsies performed months after delivery are generally normal, without fibrosis.[101]

The diagnosis of acute fatty liver of pregnancy, or any

other hepatic manifestation of preeclampsia, should be considered when liver disease in the third trimester is associated with elevations in serum transaminase levels, leukocytosis and thrombocytopenia. Areas of decreased density in the liver parenchyma can be seen on computed tomograms.[116]

Intensive medical support before and after delivery has significantly improved survival rates in patients with severe hepatic dysfunction and multiorgan involvement. Such complications may require administration of glucose or transfusion of blood, coagulation factors and platelets. Hypertension of preeclampsia should be vigorously treated. Hepatic encephalopathy is treated with protein restriction and oral lactulose or neomycin. Hemodialysis has been used in patients with acute renal failure. Delivery is essential in the treatment of these patients, because clinical improvement does not start until the pregnancy is interrupted. The most important factor in the successful treatment of fatty liver of pregnancy is early recognition and delivery as soon as the diagnosis is established, although patients with minimal liver dysfunction could be treated more conservatively.[101] Rapid delivery of the fetus may be achieved with induced labor or cesarean delivery.[112] Reversal of the clinical symptoms and laboratory abnormalities follows delivery, and there are no signs of chronic liver disease. In extremely severe cases, however, the sequelae of hepatic failure may worsen, and post-partum treatment may be complicated.[110] These few patients should be considered candidates for hepatic transplantation.[117]

Vascular thrombosis

Both pregnancy and the use of oral contraceptive agents are associated with a hypercoagulable state.[118,119] Thrombosis of the hepatic artery has also been reported at the end of gestation, resulting in massive hepatic infarction.[120]

Budd–Chiari syndrome (hepatic vein thrombosis) has been associated with pregnancy and the use of oral contraceptives, as well as with many other diseases.[121–123] When associated with pregnancy, it usually occurs within a few weeks after delivery.[121] Although the disease may have a slow progression, most frequently an acute onset is seen, presenting as abdominal pain with hepatomegaly and ascites.[123] The disease quickly leads to portal hypertension, bleeding varices, severe ascites and hepatic failure. If portal vein thrombosis is also present, hepatocellular necrosis is massive. The diagnosis can be confirmed by hepatic scintiscan, ultrasonography or computerized tomography.[123] Palliative and temporary therapy consists of decompression of the congested liver by the creation of a portacaval shunt,[124] but when hepatocellular function deteriorates liver transplantation should be performed.[125]

Primary hepatic pregnancy

Very rarely, the inferior surface of the right lobe of the liver is the site for implantation of an ectopic pregnancy.[126] There is significant abdominal pain and bleeding into the abdominal cavity. Immediate surgery to repair the liver is required.

Diagnosis of liver disease in the pregnant patient

The diagnosis of liver disease is frequently difficult to make in the pregnant woman. Jaundice and pruritus are early signs of liver disease; however, liver disease may be present in the absence of these symptoms. Other vague symptoms (abdominal pain, fatigue) may be early manifestations of liver disease. Physical examination is rarely helpful. Palmar erythema and spider angiomas commonly develop during uncomplicated pregnancy. If liver disease is suspected, appropriate laboratory studies should be ordered. The stage of pregnancy is frequently helpful in determining the diagnosis. Although infectious hepatitis can occur at any stage, other diseases occur preferentially at a certain stage (hyperemesis gravidarum during the first trimester, cholestasis of pregnancy during the second and third trimesters, complications of preeclampsia and eclampsia during the third trimester).[2] More extensive testing may be done if time and the patient's condition allow it. Ultrasound and computed tomograms can be very helpful, but liver biopsy remains the 'gold standard' despite the sometimes difficult interpretation of the histology.

The three most important diagnoses to consider are viral hepatitis, liver disease with preeclampsia and cholestasis of pregnancy. Because liver disease in the pregnant woman implies risk to the patient and to the fetus, the evaluation should be rapid. If the disease is associated etiologically with pregnancy, the pregnancy should be terminated unless the disease is very mild.

ANESTHETIC CONSIDERATIONS FOR VAGINAL DELIVERY

Patients with only mild hepatic dysfunction and without coagulopathy can be treated as normal parturients. Even in patients with preeclampsia, epidural anesthesia is not associated with an increased incidence of systemic hypotension if acute intravascular volume expansion is optimized and if the anesthetic is administered slowly.[127] Since small doses of local anesthetics are used during epidural anesthesia for vaginal delivery, a decreased biotransformation of local anesthetics in the liver should not be a major concern. In patients with esophageal varices secondary to liver cirrhosis, Valsalva maneuvers should be avoided; this could be accomplished by a continuous epidural anesthetic technique. Forceps extraction should be used in these patients during the second stage of labor.

If coagulopathy is present, it should be corrected (fresh-frozen plasma, platelet transfusion) before performing a regional anesthetic technique. However, if coagulopathy is severe, complete correction is difficult and regional anesthesia should not be used. Small doses of intravenous analgesics or inhalation analgesia could be used as alternatives to regional anesthesia.

ANESTHETIC CONSIDERATIONS FOR OPERATIVE DELIVERY

Patients with only mild liver dysfunction and with normal coagulation status can be treated as normal pregnant patients undergoing cesarean delivery and should have regional anesthesia in most cases.

When liver dysfunction is more severe but not associated with coagulopathy, decreased metabolism and decreased protein binding of amide local anesthetics should be considered when epidural anesthesia is used.[128] Although chloroprocaine can decrease maternal blood pressure more than bupivacaine in normotensive parturients during epidural anesthesia for elective cesarean delivery[127] chloroprocaine is probably the better choice in patients with hepatocellular dysfunction because of its ester structure. Optimization of preload prior to the administration of epidural anesthetic is essential. Spinal anesthesia can result in more significant hemodynamic changes than epidural anesthesia, especially if the intravascular volume status is not optimized. However, spinal anesthesia remains a reasonable second choice after epidural anesthesia.

Sicker patients undergoing cesarean delivery can present multiple problems. Patients with significant obstetric complications (preeclampsia and eclampsia) or with severe liver disease should have invasive monitoring, including direct arterial and central venous pressure monitoring. A pulmonary artery catheter may be required when left ventricular dysfunction is suspected. Adequate blood products should be available, including fresh-frozen plasma and platelets, to correct coagulopathy aggressively. Patients with esophageal varices or coagulopathy should have adequate intravenous access to allow volume resuscitation if necessary. Because these patients frequently have coagulopathy, which is difficult to correct completely, a general anesthetic technique should be used for the cesarean delivery. General anesthesia can be induced with thiopental and succinylcholine, using a rapid sequence technique. Halothane should be avoided, because it can reduce hepatic blood flow. Low concentrations of isoflurane ($<1\%$) are probably safe in these circumstances. Although plasma cholinesterase activity is reduced during normal pregnancy and in the immediate postpartum period,[10,11] this reduction may be more significant in patients with liver disease; however, moderate doses of succinylcholine are usually metabolized easily.[130,131] The duration of action of nondepolarizing muscle relaxants is prolonged in severe liver disease, except for atracurium. A nerve stimulator should be used if muscle relaxants are administered. Finally, hyperventilation should be avoided, because it reduces both liver blood flow and placental perfusion.

PREGNANCY AND ORTHOTOPIC LIVER TRANSPLANTATION

Liver transplantation during pregnancy

Hepatic failure requiring orthotopic liver transplantation during pregnancy is a very rare event. Fulminant hepatic failure during pregnancy may occur with fulminant viral hepatitis, drug-induced hepatic toxicity or acute fatty liver of pregnancy. Currently, only three liver transplantations have been performed in pregnant patients; two of these procedures are being reported.[132,133] One patient underwent transplantation for fulminant hepatic failure due to hepatitis B and required retransplantation 3 days later for primary graft nonfunction. Another patient had fulminant hepatitis (presumably viral in origin) and underwent successful transplantation.

Anesthesia for the pregnant transplant patient is complicated: this procedure should be performed only in experienced transplantation centers. Major emphasis is on preserving maternal life, while maintaining uterine perfusion. The effects of medications on the fetus should also be considered. Potentially teratogenic drugs should be avoided. Uterine blood flow can be maintained by preserving cardiac output and arterial blood pressure and by avoiding increases in inferior vena cava pressure (especially during the anhepatic stage when the inferior vena cava is cross-clamped) by the use of a venovenous bypass system.[134] Alpha-adrenergic agents should probably be avoided.

Pregnancy after liver transplantation

Liver transplantation has resulted in long-term survival, and more patients are able to return to normal lifestyles. Women may have the desire to have children after a successful liver transplantation, despite concerns associated with the long-term use of immunosuppressive medications.

Amenorrhea, a recognized complication of end-stage chronic liver disease, is probably a result of hypothalamic–pituitary dysfunction.[135] This complication is reversible after successful liver transplantation, and regular menstruation returns within 10 months.[135]

Patients who have had liver transplantation can safely have children, although there may be an increased risk of preeclampsia, worsening hypertension, preterm delivery and fetal growth retardation.[135–137] Intrauterine growth retardation may be related to the use of immunosuppressants (prednisone, azathioprine, cyclosporine);[135–140] cyclosporine has been shown to cross the placental barrier.[141] However, there does not seem to be an increased risk of congenital abnormalities or birth defects.[135–137] There is a high incidence of cesarean deliveries; indications have included preeclampsia and premature rupture of membranes.[137] Elevated liver enzymes were seen in 35% of the patients during their pregnancy, but overall the liver function remained adequate.[137]

ACKNOWLEDGMENTS

Special thanks are extended to Drs Steven Laifer and Yoogoo Kang for reviewing this manuscript; to Lisa Cohn for editorial assistance; and to Mary Trusso for secretarial assistance.

REFERENCES

1. Riely C A 1987 The liver in pregnancy. In: Schiff L, Schiff E R (eds) Diseases of the liver, 6th edn. J B Lippincott, Philadelphia pp 1059–1073
2. Fallon H J 1988 Liver diseases. In: Burrow G N, Ferris T F (eds) Medical complications during pregnancy, 3rd edn. W B Saunders, Philadelphia pp 318–344
3. Van Thiel D H, Stone B G 1986 Hepatic changes and complications in pregnancy. In: Rustgi V K, Cooper J N (eds) Gastrointestinal and hepatic complications in pregnancy. Wiley, New York pp 162–178
4. Varma R R 1987 Course and prognosis of pregnancy in women with liver disease. Semin Liver Dis 7: 59–66
5. Rustgi V K 1989 Liver disease in pregnancy. Med Clin North Am 73: 1041–1046
6. Haemmerli U P 1966 Jaundice during pregnancy, with special emphasis on recurrent jaundice during pregnancy and its differential diagnosis. Acta Med Scand 179 (suppl 444):1–111
7. Combes B, Shibata H, Adams R, Mitchell B D, Trammell V 1963 Alterations in sulfobromophthalein sodium-removal mechanisms from blood during normal pregnancy. J Clin Invest 42: 1431–1442
8. Rovinsky J J, Jaffin H 1966 Cardiovascular hemodynamics in pregnancy. III. Cardiac rate, stroke volume, total peripheral resistance, and central blood volume in multiple pregnancy. Synthesis of results. Am J Obstet Gynecol 95: 787–794
9. Rådberg G, Friman S, Svanvik J 1990 The influence of pregnancy and contraceptive steroids on the biliary tract and its reference to cholesterol gallstone formation. Scand J Gastroenterol 25: 97–102
10. Shnider S M 1965 Serum cholinesterase activity during pregnancy, labor and the puerperium. Anesthesiology 26: 335–339
11. Kambam J R, Perry S M, Entman S, Smith B E 1988 Effect of magnesium on plasma cholinesterase activity. Am J Obstet Gynecol 159: 309–311
12. Potter J M, Nestel P J 1979 The hyperlipidemia of pregnancy in normal and complicated pregnancies. Am J Obstet Gynecol 133: 165–170
13. Kreek M J, Weser E, Sleisenger M H, Jeffries G H 1967 Idiopathic cholestasis of pregnancy: the response to challenge with the synthetic estrogen, ethinyl estradiol. New Engl J Med 277: 1391–1395
14. Reyes H, Ribalta J, González M C, Segovia N, Oberhauser E 1981 Sulfobromophthalein clearance tests before and after ethinyl estradiol administration, in women and men with familial history of intrahepatic cholestasis of pregnancy. Gastroenterology 81: 226–231
15. Crawford J S, Hooi H W Y 1968 Binding of bromsulphthalein by serum albumin from pregnant women, neonates and subjects on oral contraceptives. Br J Anaesth 40: 723–729
16. McNair R D, Jaynes R V 1960 Alterations in liver function during normal pregnancy. Am J Obstet Gynecol 80: 500–505
17. Scholtes G 1979 Liver function and liver diseases during pregnancy. J Perinat Med 7: 55–68
18. Cerutti R, Ferrari S, Grella P, Castelli G P, Rizzotti P 1976 Behavior of serum enzymes in pregnancy. Clin Exp Obstet Gynecol 3: 22–24
19. Antia F P, Bharadwaj T P, Watsa M C, Master J 1958 Liver in normal pregnancy, pre-eclampsia and eclampsia. Lancet 2: 776–778
20. Ingerslev M, Teilum G 1945 Biopsy studies on the liver in pregnancy. II. Liver biopsy in normal pregnant women. Acta Obstet Gynecol Scand 25: 352
21. Kang Y G, Gelman S 1987 Liver transplantation. In: Gelman S (ed) Anesthesia and organ transplantation. W B Saunders, Philadelphia pp 139–185
22. Rustgi V K, Hoofnagle J H 1987 Viral hepatitis during pregnancy. Sem Liver Dis 7: 40–46
23. Khuroo M S, Teli M R, Skidmore S, Sofi M A, Khuroo M I 1981 Incidence and severity of viral hepatitis in pregnancy. Am J Med 70: 252–255
24. Sridama V, Pacini F, Yang S L, Moawad A, Reilly M, DeGroot L J 1982 Decreased levels of helper T cells: a possible cause of immunodeficiency in pregnancy. New Engl J Med 307: 352–356
25. Hieber J P, Dalton D, Shorey J, Combes B 1977 Hepatitis and pregnancy. J Pediatr 91: 545–549
26. Smithwick E M, Pascual E, Go S C 1972 Hepatitis-associated antigen: a possible relationship to premature delivery. J Pediatr 81: 537–540
27. Goyert G L, Bottoms S F, Sokol R J 1985 Anicteric presentation of fatal herpetic hepatitis in pregnancy. Obstet Gynecol 65: 585–588
28. Shabot J M, Jaynes C, Little Jr H M, Alperin J B, Snyder N 1978 Viral hepatitis in pregnancy with disseminated intravascular coagulation and hypoglycemia. South Med J 71: 479–481
29. Brown M S, Reddy K R, Hensley G T, Jeffers L J, Schiff E R 1987 The initial presentation of fatty liver of pregnancy mimicking acute viral hepatitis. Am J Gastroenterol 82: 554–557
30. Tong M J, Thursby M, Rakela J, McPeak C, Edwards V M, Mosley J W 1981 Studies on the maternal–infant transmission of the viruses which cause acute hepatitis. Gastroenterology 80: 999–1004
31. Gerety R J, Schweitzer I L 1977 Viral hepatitis type B during pregnancy, the neonatal period, and infancy. J Pediatr 90: 368–374
32. Beasley R P, Hwang L Y, Lee G C Y et al 1983 Prevention of perinatally transmitted hepatitis B virus infections with hepatitis B immune globulin and hepatitis B vaccine. Lancet 2: 1099–1102
33. Delaplane D, Yogev R, Crussi F, Shulman S T 1983 Fatal hepatitis B in early infancy: the importance of identifying HBsAg-positive pregnant women and providing immunoprophylaxis to their newborns. Pediatrics 72: 176–180
34. Stevens C E, Toy P T, Tong M J et al 1985 Perinatal hepatitis B virus transmission in the United States. J Am Med Assoc 253: 1740–1745
35. Hsu H M, Chen D S, Chuang C H et al 1988 Efficacy of a mass hepatitis B vaccination program in Taiwan: studies on 3463 infants of hepatitis B surface antigen-carrier mothers. J Am Med Assoc 260: 2231–2235
36. Centers for Disease Control 1988 Recommendations of the Immunization Practices Advisory Committee: Prevention of

perinatal transmission of hepatitis B virus: prenatal screening of all pregnant women for hepatitis B surface antigen. Morbidity Mortality Weekly Reports 37: 341–351
37. Landers D, Carmona R, Crombleholme W, Lim R 1987 Acute cholecystitis in pregnancy. Obstet Gynecol 69: 131–133
38. Hill L M, Johnson C E, Lee R A 1975 Cholecystectomy in pregnancy. Obstet Gynecol 46: 291–293
39. Printen K J, Ott R A 1978 Cholecystectomy during pregnancy. Am Surg 44: 432–434
40. Jouppila P, Mokka R, Larmi T K 1974 Acute pancreatitis in pregnancy. Surg Gynecol Obstet 139: 879–882
41. McKay A J, O'Neill J, Imrie C W 1980 Pancreatitis, pregnancy and gallstones. Br J Obstet Gynaecol 87: 47–50
42. Lewis J H, Zimmerman H J 1986 Drug-induced jaundice during pregnancy. In: Rustgi V K, Cooper J N (eds) Gastrointestinal and hepatic complications in pregnancy. Wiley, New York pp 226–276
43. Schreyer P, Caspi E, El-Hindi J M, Eschar J 1982 Cirrhosis – pregnancy and delivery: a review. Obstet Gynecol Surv 37: 304–312
44. Varma R R, Michelsohn N H, Borkowf H I, Lewis J D 1977 Pregnancy in cirrhotic and noncirrhotic portal hypertension. Obstet Gynecol 50: 217–222
45. Borhanmanesh F, Haghighi P 1970 Pregnancy in patients with cirrhosis of the liver. Obstet Gynecol 36: 315–324
46. Schweitzer I L, Peters R L 1976 Pregnancy in hepatitis B antigen positive cirrhosis. Obstet Gynecol (suppl) 48: 53S–56S
47. Whelton M J, Sherlock S 1968 Pregnancy in patients with hepatic cirrhosis. Management and outcome. Lancet 2: 995–999
48. Cheng Y S 1977 Pregnancy in liver cirrhosis and/or portal hypertension. Am J Obstet Gynecol 128: 812–822
49. Soto-Albors C E, Rayburn W F, Taylor L, Musselman M 1984 Portal hypertension and hypersplenism in pregnancy secondary to chronic schistosomiasis. A case report. J Reprod Med 29:345–348
50. Britton R C 1982 Pregnancy and esophageal varices. Am J Surg 143: 421–425
51. Kuller J A, Meyer M P, Leonhard K R, Harger J H 1991 Efficacy of hepatitis B screening in a private obstetrical population. J Perinatol 11: 164–167
52. Clarren S K, Smith D W 1978 The fetal alcohol syndrome. New Engl J Med 298: 1063–1067
53. Dreifuss F E, McKinney W M 1966 Wilson's disease (hepatolenticular degeneration) and pregnancy. J Am Med Assoc 195: 960–962
54. Walshe J M 1977 Pregnancy in Wilson's disease. Q J Med 46: 73–83
55. Toaff R, Toaff M E, Peyser M R, Streifler M 1977 Hepatolenticular degeneration (Wilson's disease) and pregnancy. Obstet Gynecol Surv 32: 497
56. Steven M M, Buckley J D, Mackay I R 1979 Pregnancy in chronic active hepatitis. Q J Med 48: 519–531
57. Romero R, Reece E A, Riely C, Hobbins J C 1983 Arteriohepatic dysplasia in pregnancy. Am J Obstet Gynecol 147: 108–109
58. Larrey D, Rueff B, Feldmann G, Degott C, Danan G, Benhamou J P 1984 Recurrent jaundice caused by recurrent hyperemesis gravidarum. Gut 25: 1414–1415
59. Kreek M J 1987 Female sex steroids and cholestasis. Semin Liver Dis 7: 8–23
60. Holzbach R T, Sivak D A, Braun W E 1983 Familial recurrent intrahepatic cholestasis of pregnancy: a genetic study providing evidence for transmission of a sex-limited, dominant trait. Gastroenterology 85: 175–179
61. Heikkinen J 1983 Serum bile acids in the early diagnosis of intrahepatic cholestasis of pregnancy. Obstet Gynecol 61: 581–587
62. Heikkinen J, Mäentausta O, Ylöstalo P, Jänne O 1981 Changes in serum bile acid concentrations during normal pregnancy, in patients with intrahepatic cholestasis of pregnancy and in pregnant women with itching. Br J Obstet Gynaecol 88: 240–245
63. Ämmälä P, Kariniemi V 1981 Short-term variability of fetal heart rate in cholestasis of pregnancy. Am J Obstet Gynecol 141: 217–220
64. Shaw D, Frohlich J, Wittmann B A K, Willms M 1982 A prospective study of 18 patients with cholestasis of pregnancy. Am J Obstet Gynecol 142: 621–625
65. Reyes H 1982 The enigma of intrahepatic cholestasis of pregnancy: lessons from Chile. Hepatology 2: 87–96
66. Wilson B R I, Haverkamp A D 1979 Cholestatic jaundice of pregnancy: new perspectives. Obstet Gynecol 54: 650–652
67. Fisk N M, Storey G N B 1988 Fetal outcome in obstetric cholestasis. Br J Obstet Gynaecol 95: 1137–1143
68. Käär K, Jouppila P, Kuikka J, Luotala H, Toivanen J, Rekonen A 1980 Intervillous blood flow in normal and complicated late pregnancy measured by means of an intravenous ^{133}Xe method. Acta Obstet Gynecol Scand 59: 7–10
69. Costoya A L, Leontic E A, Rosenberg H G et al 1980 Morphological study of placental terminal villi in intrahepatic cholestasis of pregnancy: histochemistry, light and electron microscopy. Placenta 1: 361–368
70. Espinoza J, Barnafi L, Schnaidt E 1974 The effect of phenobarbital on intrahepatic cholestasis of pregnancy. Am J Obstet Gynecol 119: 234–238
71. Laatikainen K 1978 Effect of cholestyramine and phenobarbital on pruritus and serum bile acid levels in cholestasis of pregnancy. Am J Obstet Gynecol 132: 501–506
72. Goodlin R C 1976 Severe pre-eclampsia: another great imitator. Am J Obstet Gynecol 125: 747–753
73. Van Assche F A, Spitz B 1988 Thromboxane synthetase inhibition in pregnancy-induced hypertension. Am J Obstet Gynecol 159: 1015–1016
74. Steven M M 1981 Pregnancy and liver disease. Gut 22: 592–614
75. Long R G, Scheuer P J, Sherlock S 1977 Pre-eclampsia presenting with deep jaundice. J Clin Pathol 30: 212–215
76. Arias F, Mancilla-Jimenez R 1976 Hepatic fibrinogen deposits in pre-eclampsia: immunofluorescent evidence. New Engl J Med 295: 578–582
77. Rolfes D B, Ishak K G 1986 Liver disease in toxemia of pregnancy. Am J Gastroenterol 81: 1138–1144
78. Aarnoudse J G, Houthoff H F, Weits J, Vellenga E, Huisjes H J 1986 A syndrome of liver damage and intravascular coagulation in the last trimester of normotensive pregnancy. A clinical and histopathological study. Br J Obstet Gynaecol 93: 145–155
79. Krueger K J, Hoffman B J, Lee W M 1990 Hepatic infarction associated with eclampsia. Am J Gastroenterol 85: 588–592
80. Riely C A, Latham P S, Romero R, Duffy T P 1987 Acute fatty liver of pregnancy. A reassessment based on observations in nine patients. Ann Intern Med 106: 703–706
81. Minakami H, Oka N, Sato T, Tamada T, Yasuda Y, Hirota N 1988 Preeclampsia: a microvesicular fat disease of the liver? Am J Obstet Gynecol 159: 1043–1047
82. Bynum T E 1986 Miscellaneous hepatic disorders. In: Rustgi V K, Cooper J N (eds) Gastrointestinal and hepatic complications in pregnancy. Wiley, New York pp 216–225
83. Weinstein L 1982 Syndrome of hemolysis, elevated liver enzymes, and low platelet count: a severe consequence of hypertension in pregnancy. Am J Obstet Gynecol 142: 159–167
84. Weinstein L 1985 Preeclampsia/eclampsia with hemolysis, elevated liver enzymes, and thrombocytopenia. Obstet Gynecol 66: 657–660
85. Schwartz M L, Brenner W E 1983 Pregnancy-induced hypertension presenting with life-threatening thrombocytopenia. Am J Obstet Gynecol 146: 756–759
86. Sibai B M 1990 The HELLP syndrome (hemolysis, elevated liver enzymes, and low platelets): much ado about nothing? Am J Obstet Gynecol 162: 311–316
87. Sibai B M, Taslimi M M, El-Nazer A, Amon E, Mabie B C, Ryan G M 1986 Maternal-perinatal outcome associated with the syndrome of hemolysis, elevated liver enzymes, and low platelets in severe preeclampsia–eclampsia. Am J Obstet Gynecol 155: 501–509
88. Manas K J, Welsh J D, Rankin R A, Miller D D 1985 Hepatic hemorrhage without rupture in preeclampsia. New Engl J Med 312: 424–426
89. Smith Jr L G, Moise Jr K J, Dildy III G A, Carpenter Jr R J 1991 Spontaneous rupture of liver during pregnancy: current therapy. Obstet Gynecol 77: 171–175
90. Jewett J F 1977 Eclampsia and rupture of the liver. New Engl J Med 297: 1009–1011

91. Minuk G Y, Lui R C, Kelly J K 1987 Rupture of the liver associated with acute fatty liver of pregnancy. Am J Gastroenterol 82: 457–460
92. Henny C P, Lim A E, Brummelkamp W H, Buller H R, Ten Cate J W 1983 A review of the importance of acute multidisciplinary treatment following spontaneous rupture of the liver capsule during pregnancy. Surg Gynecol Obstet 156: 593–598
93. Loevinger E H, Vujic I, Lee W M, Anderson M C 1985 Hepatic rupture associated with pregnancy: treatment with transcatheter embolotherapy. Obstet Gynecol 65: 281–284
94. Terasaki K K, Quinn M F, Lundell C J, Finck E J, Pentecost M J 1990 Spontaneous hepatic hemorrhage in preeclampsia: treatment with hepatic arterial embolization. Radiology 174: 1039–1041
95. MacKenna J, Dover N L, Brame R G 1983 Preeclampsia associated with hemolysis, elevated liver enzymes, and low platelets – an obstetric emergency? Obstet Gynecol 62: 751–754
96. Cunningham F G, Lowe T, Guss S, Mason R 1985 Erythrocyte morphology in women with severe preeclampsia and eclampsia. Preliminary observations with scanning electron microscopy. Am J Obstet Gynecol 153: 358–363
97. VanDam P A, Renier M, Baekelandt M, Buytaert P, Uyttenbroeck F 1989 Disseminated intravascular coagulation and the syndrome of hemolysis, elevated liver enzymes, and low platelets in severe preeclampsia. Obstet Gynecol 73: 97–102
98. Duffy B L 1988 HELLP syndrome and the anaesthetist. Anaesthesia 43: 223–225
99. Wulf H 1990 Anaesthesia und intensivtherapie bei Schwangeren mit HELLP-syndrom. Anaesthesist 39: 117–121
100. Sheehan H L 1940 The pathology of acute yellow atrophy and delayed chloroform poisoning. J Obstet Gynaecol Br Emp 47: 49–62
101. Riely C A 1987 Acute fatty liver of pregnancy. Semin Liver Dis 7: 47–54
102. Varner M, Rinderknecht N K 1980 Acute fatty metamorphosis of pregnancy. A maternal mortality and literature review. J Reprod Med 24: 177–180
103. Davies M H, Wilkinson S P, Hanid M A, Portmann B, Brudenell J M, Newton J R, Williams R 1980 Acute liver disease with encephalopathy and renal failure in late pregnancy and the early puerperium. A study of fourteen patients. Br J Obstet Gynaecol 87: 1005–1014
104. Kaplan M M 1985 Acute fatty liver of pregnancy. New Engl J Med 313: 367–370
105. Barton J R, Sibai B M, Mabie W C, Shanklin D R 1990 Recurrent acute fatty liver of pregnancy. Am J Obstet Gynecol 163: 534–538
106. Pockros P J, Peters R L, Reynolds T B 1984 Idiopathic fatty liver of pregnancy: findings in ten cases. Medicine 63: 1–11
107. Hellgren M, Hägnevik K, Robbe H, Björk O, Blombäck M, Eklund J 1983 Severe acquired antithrombin III deficiency in relation to hepatic and renal insufficiency and intrauterine fetal death in late pregnancy. Gynecol Obstet Invest 16: 107–118
108. Liebman H A, McGehee W G, Patch M J, Feinstein D I 1983 Severe depression of antithrombin III associated with disseminated intravascular coagulation in women with fatty liver of pregnancy. Ann Intern Med 98: 330–333
109. Mosvold J, Abildgaard U, Jenssen H, Andersen R 1982 Low antithrombin III in acute hepatic failure at term. Scand J Haematol 29: 48–50
110. Burroughs A K, Seong N H, Dojcinov D M, Scheuer P J, Sherlock S V P 1982 Idiopathic acute fatty liver of pregnancy in 12 patients. Q J Med 204: 481–497
111. Rolfes D B, Ishak K G 1985 Acute fatty liver of pregnancy: a clinicopathologic study of 35 cases. Hepatology 5: 1149–1158
112. Cano R I, Delman M R, Pitchumoni C S, Lev R, Rosenthal W S 1975 Acute fatty liver of pregnancy. Complication by disseminated intravascular coagulation. J Am Med Assoc 231: 159–161
113. Hatfield A K, Stein J H, Greenberger N J, Abernethy R W, Ferris T F 1972 Idiopathic acute fatty liver of pregnancy: death from extrahepatic manifestations. Dig Dis 17: 167–178
114. Breen K J, Perkins K W, Mistilis S P, Shearman R 1970 Idiopathic acute fatty liver of pregnancy. Gut 11: 822–825
115. Slater D N, Hague W M 1984 Renal morphological changes in idiopathic acute fatty liver of pregnancy. Histopathology 8: 567–581
116. Mabie W C, Dacus J V, Sibai B M, Morretti M L, Gold R E 1988 Computed tomography in acute fatty liver of pregnancy. Am J Obstet Gynecol 158: 142–145
117. Ockner S A, Brunt E M, Cohn S M, Krul E S, Hanto D W, Peters M G 1990 Fulminant hepatic failure caused by acute fatty liver of pregnancy treated by orthotopic liver transplantation. Hepatology 11: 59–64
118. Hyde E, Joyce D, Gurewich V, Flute P T, Barrera S 1973 Intravascular coagulation during pregnancy and the puerperium. J Obstet Gynaecol Br Cwlth 80: 1059–1066
119. Lowe G D O, Drummond M M, Forbes C D, Barbenel J C 1980 Increased blood viscosity in young women using oral contraceptives. Am J Obstet Gynecol 137: 840–842
120. Dammann H G, Hagemann J, Runge M, Klöppel G 1982 *In vivo* diagnosis of massive hepatic infarction by computed tomography. Dig Dis Sci 27: 73–79
121. Khuroo M S, Datta D V 1980 Budd–Chiari syndrome following pregnancy. Report of 16 cases, with roentgenologic, hemodynamic and histologic studies of the hepatic outflow tract. Am J Med 68: 113–121
122. Tiliacos M, Tsantoulas D, Tsoulias A et al 1978 The Budd–Chiari syndrome in pregnancy. Postgrad Med J 54: 686–691
123. Maddrey W C 1987 Hepatic vein thrombosis (Budd–Chiari syndrome): possible association with the use of oral contraceptives. Semin Liver Dis 7: 32–39
124. Orloff M J, Girard B 1989 Long term results of treatment of Budd–Chiari syndrome by side to side portacaval shunt. Surg Gynecol Obstet 168: 33–41
125. Halff G, Todo S, Tzakis A G, Gordon R D, Starzl T E 1990 Liver transplantation for the Budd–Chiari syndrome. Ann Surg 211: 43–49
126. Brlum K G, Blom R 1988 Primary hepatic pregnancy. Int J Gynaecol Obstet 27: 427–429
127. Moir D D, Victor-Rodrigues L, Willocks J 1972 Epidural analgesia during labour in patients with pre-eclampsia. J Obstet Gynaecol Br Cwlth 79: 465–469
128. Ramanathan J, Bottorff M, Jeter J N, Khalil M, Sibai B M 1986 The pharmacokinetics and maternal and neonatal effects of epidural lidocaine in preeclampsia. Anesth Analg 65: 120–126
129. James F M, Dewan D M, Floyd H M et al 1980 Chloroprocaine vs. bupivacaine for lumbar epidural analgesia for elective Cesarean section. Anesthesiology 52: 488–491
130. Blitt C D, Petty W C, Alberternst E E, Wright B J 1977 Correlation of plasma cholinesterase activity and duration of action of succinylcholine during pregnancy. Anesth Analg 56: 78–83
131. Leighton B L, Cheek T G, Gross J B et al 1986 Succinylcholine pharmacodynamics in peripartum patients. Anesthesiology 64: 202–205
132. Merritt W T, Dickstein R, Beattie C, Burdick J, Kline A 1991 Liver transplantation during pregnancy: anesthesia for two procedures in the same patient with successful outcome of pregnancy. Transplant Proc 23: 1996–1997
133. Zaballos J, Perez-Cerda F, Riano D et al 1991 Anesthetic management of liver transplantation in a pregnant patient with fulminant hepatitis. Transplant Proc 23: 1994–1995
134. Shaw Jr B W, Martin D J, Marquez J M et al 1984 Venous bypass in clinical liver transplantation. Ann Surg 200: 524–534
135. Cundy T F, O'Grady J G, Williams R 1990 Recovery of menstruation and pregnancy after liver transplantation. Gut 31: 337–338
136. Laifer S A, Darby M J, Scantlebury V P, Harger J H, Caritis S N 1990 Pregnancy and liver transplantation. Obstet Gynecol 76: 1083–1088
137. Scantlebury V, Gordon R, Tzakis A et al 1990 Childbearing after liver transplantation. Transplantation 49: 317–321
138. Scott J R 1977 Fetal growth retardation associated with maternal

administration of immunosuppressive drugs. Am J Obstet Gynecol 128: 668–676
139. Pickrell M D, Sawers R, Michael J 1988 Pregnancy after renal transplantation: severe intrauterine growth retardation during treatment with cyclosporine A. Br Med J 296: 825
140. Reinisch J M, Simon N G, Karow W G, Gandelman R 1978 Prenatal exposure to prednisone in humans and animals retards intrauterine growth. Science 202: 436–438
141. Venkataramanan R, Koneru B, Wang C C P, Burckart G J, Caritis S N, Starzl T E 1988 Cyclosporine and its metabolites in mother and baby. Transplantation 46: 468–469

53. Endocrine disease

E. P. Lynch

The anesthesiologist is often confronted with a parturient with endocrine disease who requires anesthesia for vaginal or cesarean delivery or surgical removal of an endocrine gland. It is important to be aware of the normal changes in endocrine physiology that occur during pregnancy and the specific abnormalities associated with hyposecretion or hypersecretion in disease states. This section focuses on the clinical manifestations and anesthetic considerations related to particular disease states.

THYROID DISEASE

Thyroid disease is one of the more common endocrine disorders occurring during pregnancy. The normal physiologic changes that occur during pregnancy can confuse the clinical presentation of thyroid disease and make the diagnosis of pathologic states more difficult.[1]

Nontoxic goiter

A simple nontoxic goiter may increase in size during pregnancy because of a relative iodine deficiency that is caused by an increased glomerular filtration rate and renal excretion of iodide.[2]

Clinical presentation

Clinical manifestations may include dyspnea, dysphagia and changes in phonation.

Anesthetic considerations

The potential for airway obstruction exists if the gland has extended retrosternally or has enlarged significantly. Accordingly, regional anesthesia may be a preferred technique for vaginal or cesarean delivery.[2]

Hyperthyroidism

Graves' disease, also known as diffuse toxic goiter, is the most frequent cause of thyrotoxicosis during pregnancy. Other causes include toxic nodular goiter, toxic multinodular goiter, hydatidiform moles and choriocarcinoma.[1]

Clinical presentation

The euthyroid pregnant patient may have many of the hyperdynamic signs and symptoms typically associated with hyperthyroidism. Common findings include amenorrhea, tachycardia, systolic flow murmur associated with increased cardiac output, heat intolerance, increased skin temperature, diarrhea and nervousness. Weight gain as a result of pregnancy may obscure weight loss associated with hyperthyroidism. Eye changes, including exophthalmos and lid lag, are typical of Graves' disease. These changes, however, do not necessarily suggest a thyrotoxic state. Hyperemesis gravidarum may be the presenting sign of thyrotoxicosis in the parturient. The laboratory diagnosis of hyperthyroidism in pregnancy is difficult since estrogen-induced increases in thyroxine-binding globulin result in elevations of plasma thyroxine concentrations and a tri-iodothyronine resin uptake in the hypothyroid range.[1]

Anesthetic considerations

Elective surgery should be deferred until the parturient is clinically euthyroid. If emergency surgery is necessary in the thyrotoxic patient, the anesthesiologist should avoid the administration of medications that stimulate the sympathetic nervous system and should achieve an adequate depth of anesthesia prior to surgical stimulation.[3] Plasma concentrations of catecholamines are not elevated in the hyperthyroid patient. The hyperdynamic circulatory state of hyperthyroidism was thought to result from increased sensitivity to catecholamines. However, it is generally accepted that sensitivity to catecholamines is not changed by thyroid dysfunction.[4]

Adequate premedication is important in order to decrease unnecessary catecholamine release. A benzodiazepine is a reasonable choice.[5] Generally, the use of an anticholinergic drug is contraindicated since these drugs may aggravate tachycardia and inhibit heat loss.[2]

A thiobarbiturate is an accepted choice for induction because its thiourea structure has antithyroid properties. However, the clinical significance of the thiobarbiturate's antithyroid activity has not been demonstrated.[6] Ketamine is a poor choice because it can stimulate the sympathetic nervous system. With regard to muscle relaxants, pancuronium should be avoided because of its ability to increase the heart rate and stimulate the sympathetic nervous system. Drugs that minimally affect the cardiovascular system are the most rational choices.[5]

General anesthesia in the obstetric patient requires intubation of the trachea. Regional anesthesia is an attractive technique for the hyperthyroid parturient, because the potential for airway obstruction or inability to secure an airway due to an enlarged thyroid gland may be avoided. Historically, intraspinal anesthesia has been used in combination with general anesthesia in thyrotoxic patients to achieve a decreased heart rate and blood pressure during surgery. A sensory level of T4–T5 was achieved with the purpose of blocking the sympathetic innervation of the adrenal medulla and decreasing secretion of epinephrine.[6] The sympathetic blockade associated with a regional technique may be desirable. The potential disadvantage, however, is hypotension requiring pharmacologic support. Hyperthyroid patients may have an exaggerated response to sympathomimetic drugs. Although phenylephrine is a recommended direct-acting vasopressor, any vasopressor should be titrated to desired effect.

Superficial and deep cervical plexus block combined with local infiltration is an excellent choice for thyroid surgery in the pregnant patient. However, the addition of epinephrine to local anesthetics may precipitate unwanted hemodynamic responses associated with its systemic absorption and should be avoided.[5]

Hemodynamic problems in the thyrotoxic parturient in labor or undergoing surgery include tachycardia, hypertension and increased cardiac output, which may result in cardiac decompensation and arrhythmias. β-blockers are effective in attenuating manifestations of excess sympathetic activity. Other emergency drugs include lidocaine for ventricular arrhythmias, steroids and hypotensive agents such as sodium nitroprusside.[2]

An increased basal metabolic rate and oxygen consumption[7] in the parturient warrant continuous monitoring of oxygen saturation and arterial blood gases as needed. Capnography is essential during general anesthesia. A cooling blanket, cold intravenous fluids and ice should be available to treat intraoperative hyperthermia.[2]

Thyroid storm

Thyroid storm is a dangerous exacerbation of hyperthyroidism. Precipitating factors include stresses such as labor, cesarean delivery and infection.[1]

Clinical presentation

Clinical manifestations of thyroid storm include hyperpyrexia, severe dehydration, tachycardia, atrial fibrillation, extreme anxiety, altered consciousness and hemodynamic instability leading to cardiovascular collapse.[2]

Anesthetic considerations

The anesthetic considerations are the same as those described for hyperthyroidism.

Hypothyroidism

Hypothyroidism is uncommon in term pregnancy because it is associated with an increased incidence of spontaneous abortion. It is usually iatrogenic following surgery or radioactive iodine therapy.[1]

Clinical presentation

Pregnant euthyroid women have many of the signs and symptoms associated with hypothyroidism. Mild hypothyroidism may be difficult to diagnose until the increased requirements for thyroid function during pregnancy stress the parturient.[2] Usual symptoms include fatigue, cold intolerance, cool dry skin, coarse hair, periorbital edema, hoarseness, constipation and a decreased ability to concentrate. Delayed deep tendon reflexes, edema, cardiomegaly and congestive heart failure secondary to decreased myocardial contractility may be present.[7] Pleural and pericardial effusions, mild anemia and hypercholesterolemia also are consistent with the diagnosis. An electrocardiogram may demonstrate a sinus bradycardia and low-voltage complexes.[2]

Anesthetic considerations

The hypothyroid parturient may present for emergency vaginal or cesarean delivery. These patients may be more sensitive to opioids, sedatives and general anesthesia. Hypoxic ventilatory drive is decreased in both hypothyroid and myxedematous patients. A decreased hypercapnic ventilatory drive has been documented in patients with myxedema; however, it is not significantly depressed in patients with hypothyroidism. Although there is little evidence that decreased ventilatory drive alone causes respiratory failure, when combined with other factors, for example sedatives or opioids, respiratory failure may occur.[8] Metabolism of drugs, particularly opioids, may be slowed.[5] These patients demonstrate bradycardia and decreased myocardial contractility,[7] resulting in a decreased cardiac output. When cardiac output is decreased, the anesthesiologist should anticipate a delayed induction with intravenous agents as well as a more rapid induction with inhaled agents.

Hypothyroid patients typically have decreased intravascular fluid volume. Accordingly, the risks of hypotension secondary to blood loss or a sympathetic blockade from a regional anesthetic are increased. Careful preoperative hydration is recommended. Ephedrine is a useful drug to treat hypotension.[5]

When managing the hypothyroid patient, the usual doses of muscle relaxants may result in a prolonged neuromuscular block. In addition, hypoglycemia may develop secondary to thyroid hormone replacement.[5] In longstanding or severe disease, adrenal suppression may occur, requiring steroid supplementation. Moreover, these patients have an impaired clearance of free water, resulting in hyponatremia. They are also prone to develop hypothermia, which may be prevented by warming intravenous fluids, using a heating blanket, increasing the room temperature and humidifying gases during general anesthesia.[2]

ADRENAL DISORDERS

Pheochromocytoma

The occurrence of pheochromocytoma during pregnancy is rare and coincidental. However, the associated maternal and fetal morbidity and mortality are extremely high.[1]

Clinical presentation

The severity of symptoms is related to the amount of catecholamines released. Both α-adrenergic and β-adrenergic effects may be present. Classic symptoms include anxiety, headache, diaphoresis, palpitations with arrhythmias, blurred vision, heat intolerance and excessive weight loss.[1] Paroxysmal hypertension is not usually associated with proteinuria or edema. The patient may present with hypotension.[9] Prolonged α-adrenergic stimulation may result in decreased plasma volume with orthostatic hypotension and a falsely elevated hematocrit.[10] Episodic attacks may be precipitated by a mechanical effect of the uterus, uterine contractions, fetal movement or changes in posture.[2]

Anesthetic considerations

The parturient with a pheochromocytoma that is well controlled by medical therapy may deliver vaginally at term or by elective cesarean delivery followed by excision of the tumor. The safety of adrenergic-blocking drugs during pregnancy has not been established. However, it may be assumed that fetal survival is improved with adequate control of maternal hypertension with α-blockers.[11] In the nonobstetric population, commonly used α-blockers include phentolamine, phenoxybenzamine and prazosin.[9] Once α-adrenergic blockade is established, tachycardia and arrhythmias may be controlled with β-blockers. Suggested β-blockers include propranolol, labetalol and esmolol. β-blockers may decrease the fetal heart rate and increase uterine activity.[12]

It is important to avoid factors that precipitate catecholamine release, including hypoxia, hypercarbia and hypotension. Hypotension associated with epidural or subarachnoid anesthesia may precipitate catecholamine release and a hypertensive crisis. Therefore, careful intravascular volume expansion is essential prior to initiating a regional technique. Cousins and Rubin[13] reported the successful use of epidural sympathetic blockade combined with a light general anesthetic in a young patient for surgical removal of a pheochromocytoma. The claimed advantages include cardiovascular stability by deafferentation of the operative site, sympathetic blockade and systemic effects of local anesthetics. In contrast to deep general anesthesia, myocardial contractility is preserved and the myocardial and peripheral circulation are able to respond appropriately to catecholamines following tumor removal.

It is essential to maintain uterine displacement in the obstetric patient. Prudent monitoring includes the standard intraoperative monitors, direct arterial and central venous pressure monitoring and a Foley catheter for urinary output.[9]

It is reasonable to avoid those drugs that have been known to cause a pressor response or tachycardia. Drugs that have been implicated include droperidol, anticholinergic drugs, succinylcholine and drugs that release histamine, pancuronium and halothane.[9] Halothane has a greater propensity to cause arrhythmias in the presence of elevated catecholamines compared with enflurane and isoflurane. Drugs that have been used safely in the nonobstetric population include fentanyl, alfentanil, etomidate and vecuronium.

Sodium nitroprusside, nitroglycerin, prazosin and magnesium sulfate have all been advocated for the control of hypertension during surgery.[9]

Patients with a pre-existing cardiomyopathy may experience cardiac failure and hypotension following removal of the pheochromocytoma and source of catecholamines.[2]

Cushing's syndrome

Excess circulating glucocorticoids secondary to adrenal adenomas, adrenal hyperplasia or exogenous corticosteroid therapy result in Cushing's syndrome.[1] In general, ovulation and pregnancy are rare in patients with Cushing's syndrome.[2]

Clinical presentation

Clinical manifestations of Cushing's syndrome closely resemble changes in normal pregnancy. Classic signs and symptoms include weight gain, hypertension, abdominal striae, edema and increased pigmentation.[2] Other features include hypokalemia, hypernatremia, hyperglycemia, skeletal muscle weakness, central obesity, moon-shaped faces, 'buffalo hump', hirsutism, osteoporosis, easy bruise-ability and psychosis.

Anesthetic considerations

General considerations for the parturient with Cushing's syndrome include appropriate management of hypertension, normalization of volume status, regulation of serum glucose concentrations with insulin therapy and maintenance of normal electrolyte balance. Hydralazine and labetalol has been recommended as antihypertensive therapy. Hypokalemia can occur secondary to an increased excretion of potassium, resulting in muscular weakness and a decreased ability to cough post-operatively. Spironolactone, a potassium-sparing diuretic, is a rational choice for normalization of volume status.[2]

Preoperative steroid coverage is required in spite of increased cortisol levels because of an impaired pituitary-adrenal response to stress.[2]

The potential for a difficult airway exists because the patient may be obese and have a thick stature. One should consider an awake intubation using topical anesthesia. Regional anesthesia may be technically difficult secondary to obesity and vertebral osteoporosis. Care must be taken in moving and positioning the patient to avoid pathologic fractures.[2]

The incidence of spontaneous abortion, stillbirths and premature deliveries is increased in this patient population.[1]

Adrenocortical insufficiency

Adrenal insufficiency, also known as Addison's disease, is the most common disorder of the adrenal gland to occur in pregnant patients.[2] Adrenal insufficiency may occur as a result of destruction of the adrenal cortex or as a result of a deficiency of adrenocorticotrophic hormone (ACTH). It also commonly occurs in patients on long-term steroid therapy who are exposed to an acute stress or abruptly stop their medications.[5]

Clinical presentation

Addison's disease may have an indolent course or present acutely with life-threatening cardiovascular collapse. Nonspecific symptoms include malaise, weight loss, nausea and vomiting, constipation, weakness and increased skin pigmentation. These findings may be confused with changes in normal pregnancy. Other symptoms include hypotension, syncope, abdominal pain and hypoglycemia.[2] These patients have a decreased intravascular volume and cardiac output and decreased renal perfusion.[1] Addison's disease may be tolerated better than expected during pregnancy because of the placental transfer of corticosteroids from the fetus to the mother.[14] The diuresis and dehydration that occur post-partum may precipitate an addisonian crisis.[1] Metabolic abnormalities include hyponatremia, hyperkalemia, increased urinary excretion of sodium and low plasma steroid levels.[5]

Anesthetic considerations

Addisonian patients are hypovolemic.[1] Prior to inducing general anesthesia or employing a regional technique, intravascular volume expansion and steroid supplementation are essential. Dextrose-containing crystalloid solutions are a reasonable choice given patients' propensity to develop hypoglycemia.[2] These patients are also especially sensitive to drug-induced myocardial depression. Invasive monitoring of arterial and central venous pressure is reasonable to consider. An effort should be made to measure electrolyte concentrations and maintain normal electrolyte balance. Initial doses of muscle relaxants should be reduced because of these patients' baseline muscle weakness.[5]

PARATHYROID DISORDERS

Hyperparathyroidism

Parathyroid adenoma is the most common cause of hyperparathyroidism in pregnancy. Labor and delivery usually proceed uneventfully, however the incidence of spontaneous abortions, stillbirths, premature labor and neonatal tetany is increased.[2]

Clinical presentation

Clinical manifestations of hyperparathyroidism include hyperemesis, generalized weakness, anorexia, lethargy, polyuria, polydypsia, hypertension and constipation. Complications also include renal calculi, pancreatitis and psychiatric disorders. Signs of hypercalcemic crisis include mental deterioration, coma, renal failure, arrhythmias and congestive heart failure. In the normal parturient, serum calcium levels are decreased. The decrease in serum calcium levels has been attributed to hypoalbuminemia of pregnancy, the transfer of calcium to the fetus and the increase in renal blood flow and glomerular filtration of calcium. Therefore, serum calcium levels may be normal in the hyperparathyroid patient.[1]

Anesthetic considerations

Anesthetic management includes maintaining adequate hydration and urine output. Electrocardiographic monitoring may detect hypercalcemia by a decreased QT interval. Patients should be carefully positioned because of osteoporosis and susceptibility to pathologic fractures. There is no evidence that specific anesthetic drugs or techniques are better than others. Patients seem to have an unpredictable response to neuromuscular blockers, therefore, monitoring with a peripheral nerve stimulator is prudent.[5]

Hypoparathyroidism

Hypoparathyroidism is uncommon in pregnancy and is usually a consequence of unintentional parathyroidectomy during thyroid surgery. Symptoms may become obvious during pregnancy because of fetal calcium demands.[2]

Clinical presentation

Signs and symptoms include paresthesias, fatigue, muscle weakness, numbness, tetany with carpopedal spasms, convulsions and laryngeal stridor. Other clinical features include mental status changes, dry rough skin, patchy hair distribution and cataracts. The electrocardiogram may show a long QT interval and myocardial contractility is often depressed.[5]

Anesthetic considerations

Anesthetic management should be directed at preventing further decreases in plasma calcium concentration. A metabolic or respiratory alkalosis can rapidly decrease plasma ionized calcium concentrations.[5] Continuous epidural anesthesia can prevent hyperventilation associated with labor, consequently decreasing the likelihood of tetany associated with alkalosis and decreased ionized calcium.[2] One should also consider small doses of an intravenous sedative to decrease anxiety. Hypocalcemia accompanying blood transfusion is usually a transient phenomenon.[13] Rational calcium replacement during transfusion should be based on calcium measurements.[15]

PITUITARY DISORDERS

Hypopituitarism

Panhypopituitarism can result from necrosis of the pituitary gland following shock or hemorrhage associated with delivery. Post-partum pituitary necrosis, or Sheehan's syndrome, is the most common cause of anterior pituitary insufficiency.[1]

Clinical presentation

The clinical picture depends on the extent of damage and is related to the deficiency of hormones secreted by the ovaries, adrenal gland and thyroid gland.[2] The presentation may be insidious, with manifestation of disease at a time of stress. The earliest sign may be failure to lactate, with breast involution post-partum. Other signs and symptoms include abnormal menses, sparse axillary and pubic hair, pale and waxy skin, fatigue and cold intolerance.[1]

Anesthetic considerations

The major complications associated with hypopituitarism are adrenal insufficiency and hypothyroidism. Anesthetic management is discussed in the appropriate parts of this chapter.

REFERENCES

1. Burrow G N, Ferris T S 1988 Medical complications during pregnancy, 3rd edn. W B Saunders, Philadelphia
2. James F M, Wheeler A S 1981 Obstetric anesthesia: the complicated patient. F A Davis, Philadelphia
3. Stehling L C 1974 Anesthetic management of the patient with hyperthyroidism. Anesthesiology 41: 585–595
4. Murkin J M 1982 Anesthesia and hypothyroidism: a review of thyroxine physiology, pharmacology and anesthetic implications. Anesth Analg 61: 371–383
5. Stoelting R K, Dierdorf S F, McCammon R L 1988 Anesthesia and co-existing disease, 2nd edn. Churchill Livingstone, New York
6. Knight R T 1945 The use of spinal anesthesia to control sympathetic overactivity in hyperthyroidism. Anesthesiology 6: 225–230
7. Amidi M, Leon D F, deGroot W J et al 1968 Effect of the thyroid state on myocardial contractility and ventricular ejection in rate in man. Circulation 38: 229–239
8. Zwilch C W, Pierson D J, Hofeldt F D et al 1975 Ventilatory control in myxedema and hypothyroidism. New Engl J Med 292: 662–665
9. Hull C J 1986 Phaeochromocytoma diagnosis, preoperative preparation and anesthetic management. Br J Anaesth 58: 1453–1468
10. Leak D, Carroll J J, Robinson D C, Ashforth E J 1977 Management of pheochromocytoma removal. Can Med Assoc J 116: 371–375
11. Barash P G, Cullen B F, Stoelting R D 1989 Clinical Anesthesia. J B Lippincott, London
12. Langer A et al 1974 Adrenergic blockade: a new approach to hyperthyroidism during pregnancy. Obstet Gynecol 44: 181–186
13. Cousins M J, Rubin R B 1974 The intraoperative management of pheochromocytoma with total epidural sympathetic blockade. Br J Anaesth 46: 78–81
14. Milkovic K et al 1973 Maintenance of the plasma corticosterone concentration of adrenalectomized rate by the fetal adrenal glands. Endocrinology 93: 115–118
15. Denlinger J K, Nahrwold M C, Gibbs P S, Lecky J P 1976 Hypocalcemia during rapid blood transfuction in anesthetized man. Br J Anaesth 48: 995–1000

54. Autoimmune disease

M. D. Popitz

There are three basic types of autoimmune disease mechanisms that damage the host body. In the first type the combination of target antigen and a circulating autoantibody stimulates release of inflammatory mediators, triggering the complement pathway and activating cytotoxic cells (killer T cells and macrophages), both of which cause cytolysis. This antibody–antigen complex can bind to certain cell-surface receptors, thereby stimulating, inhibiting or destroying them. In the second type of mechanistic action this same antibody–antigen complex accumulates in various tissues; then, fixing complement, it can cause inflammation with resultant tissue damage. The final mechanism is one in which certain sensitized T cells damage tissue and/or release lymphokines, which then initiate a superinflammatory syndrome.

Although the maternal immune system in the healthy parturient seems to be intact, some immunosuppression at the level of the fetoplacental unit allows the pregnancy to continue to term in the majority of cases.[1] Progesterone inhibits the immune response of T lymphocytes.[2] A few serum proteins have been isolated in parturients and their levels seem to correlate with flare-up and remission of some of the autoimmune diseases.[3,4,5] They are pregnancy-associated globulin (2-PAG) and pregnancy zone protein (PZP). 2-PAG (also known as pregnancy-associated plasma protein A, PAPP-A) is an immunosuppressive glycoprotein that effects the complement system and lymphocyte transformation in normal patients and in those with autoimmune disease. 2-PAG inhibits antibody receptor function and circulating lymphocytic and monocytic human lymphocytic antigen-direct reacting (HLA-DR) antigenic expression.[1] Uromodulin is an immunosuppressive glycoprotein, isolated from normal urine, that also inhibits T-cell and macrophage activity of the parturient or the 'host' organism against the fetal 'graft'.[6] The interplay between the maternal and fetal immune systems in patients with autoimmune disease still needs to be worked out. In this chapter, some of the effects of autoimmunity on the obstetric patient are reviewed.

When informed of a pregnant patient with an autoimmune disease on the obstetric service, one should begin immediately to evaluate:

1. The clinical presentation in pregnancy.
2. Anesthetic considerations involving the airway and cardiopulmonary system (often the chest radiograph does not correlate with the degree of pulmonary impairment); if low compliance and increased restrictive disease are found, a high $F\text{IO}_2$ is needed. If placed on intermittent positive-pressure ventilation, lower total volume and higher respiratory rates are needed. Because of the decreased compliance and other pulmonary defects, regional techniques are often preferred. Rapid-sequence induction and full stomach precautions are warranted. Also of concern are renal, vascular, central nervous system, hematologic and neonatal syndromes; patient positioning; and preoperative laboratory tests (including preoperative pulmonary function tests and arterial blood gas data if time permits).

RHEUMATOID ARTHRITIS

Pathophysiology

Rheumatoid arthritis (RA) is a chronic, systemic and nonorgan-specific autoimmune disease of unknown etiology in which antibodies are formed against a myriad of gamma globulins and Epstein–Barr virus-related antigens. The end result of antigen–antibody complexing in RA is an inflammatory disorder, with its hallmark finding of ubiquitous, although not always synchronous, inflammation of synovial joints. Current dogma expresses an infectious synovitis that induces antigenic change and thus stimulates the autoimmune, body-wide havoc.

There is a female preponderance in the over five million cases in the USA. It occurs in young women three times more frequently than in young men. The disease rarely occurs during pregnancy, however, when it does, it is most serious during the puerperium. Pregnancy seems to suppress RA, perhaps by the increases in circulating adrenocorticoids, especially during the last trimester, when there is a rise in the plasma cortisol.[7] The usual scenario is for a post-partum relapse, commonly in the first 2–4 months.[8–12] Lactation appears to prolong remission.[10]

The most usual finding of RA is the synovitis, along with its accompanying pain and limitations to daily activities. However, many other findings are important factors in the delivery of an anesthetic to the parturient with this disease.

Anesthetic considerations

In the healthy parturient, several physiologic factors affect airway management, thus making it more difficult than in the nonpregnant patient, including an edematous airway (increasingly so toward term), as well as the fact that the patient is at risk for aspiration secondary to the relatively relaxed lower esophageal sphincter and increased intra-abdominal pressure. In the patient with RA, however, the additional factors that influence airway management include the possibility of:

1. mandibular hypoplasia;
2. temporomandibular joint (TMJ) arthritis or growth failure in juvenile RA patients, which leads to micrognathia and, hence, difficult intubation;
3. unstable/immobile cervical spine with possible fusions and/or subluxation (especially atlantoxial);
4. cricoarytenoid arthritis;
5. laryngeal rotation.

Therefore, these patients should be considered as presenting difficult intubation. Extreme sniffing positions should be avoided. A fiber-optic endoscope should be available for intubation at all times.

A pericardial effusion is quite common in the pregnant patient, however it is usually asymptomatic. The most common form of cardiac disease in the RA patient is pericarditis, usually associated with an exudative effusion that can progress rapidly to a tamponade. Rheumatoid nodules can be found on the epicardium, myocardium and heart valves. Less commonly found are coronary arteritis and focal interstitial myocarditis.[14]

Above and beyond the pulmonary impairments associated with normal pregnancy (decreased functional residual capacity and total volume), there are seven basic forms of lung disease found in patients with RA: airway disease (with a low maximum mid-expiratory flow rate and a low maximum expiratory flow rate at 50% forced vital capacity), pleuritis (usually subclinical), interstitial fibrosis (with a decrease in diffusing capacity of the lung of carbon monoxide, with fine, dry rales on auscultation and patchy infiltrates or a fine reticulonodular pattern on chest radiograph), nodular lung disease (Caplan's disease), pneumonitis, pulmonary arteritis (although pulmonary hypertension is rare) and intrapulmonary rheumatoid nodules (which can rupture spontaneously, yielding a pneumothorax or a pyopneumothorax).

SYSTEMIC LUPUS ERYTHEMATOSUS

Pathophysiology

Systemic lupus erythematosus (SLE) is another devastating autoimmune disease, in which the antibody targets are intranuclear: double- and single-stranded DNA, Sm1 ribonucleoprotein, lymphocytes, erythrocytes, neurons, and gamma-globulins.[13] The anti-cardiolipin antibody is one of many antiphospholipid antibodies present in a large percentage (20–65%) of patients with SLE. This disease prevalence is of the order of 4–250 per 100 000 population, with an 8–10 : 1 female–male ratio. Its peak onset is in the second to fourth decade, and it occurs in approximately 1 in 5000 pregnancies.[15] Approximately 20% of cases are diagnosed at the onset of pregnancy through routine obstetric screening.[15] Usually the course of the disease is not influenced by pregnancy; however, in contrast to patients with RA, the severity and frequency of flare-ups can approximately double in 50% of patients with SLE.[16–21] If a patient falls into a remission during her pregnancy, the chances are that she will remain so for the duration. Pregnancy is contraindicated in patients with advanced cardiac, central nervous system and/or renal disease. Those with active lupus nephritis often have a flare-up during pregnancy and tend to develop preeclampsia.[22] Usually the SLE parturient presents with constitutional symptoms, symmetric arthritis, myalgias and muscle weakness. However, a preeclampsia-like syndrome can be observed in this patient population, with hypertension, edema and proteinuria without the normal SLE symptomatology. It is usually insidious in onset, but can be abrupt and is associated with hypocomplementemia.[18,23–25]

Anesthetic considerations

As in patients with RA, the prevalence of pericardial effusions greatly increases (affecting 25% of patients) and the effusions can become quite symptomatic in SLE patients. In SLE, pericardial effusions are caused by an acute or a constrictive pericarditis, and can be manifest in many forms, from an asymptomatic friction rub to a pleuritic chest pain, from atrial arrhythmias to right heart failure from a tamponade.[26] Electrocardiographic changes can be anything from a persistent tachyarrhythmia to those consistent with a myocardial infarction. The valvulopathy most often seen is Libman–Sacks endocarditis, in which small vegetations form near the rings, resulting in valvular dysfunction.[13,26–29]

The lungs and pleura are involved in approximately

30–70% of SLE patients. The pulmonary manifestations include interstitial (chronic lupus) pneumonitis; fibrinous pleuritis, often with a bilateral pleural effusion; acute pulmonary vasculitis or advanced arteriosclerosis; focal alveolar hemorrhages; and bronchopneumonias. Rarely, a patient can present with a massive pulmonary hemorrhage. Pulmonary function tests usually show mixed obstructive/restrictive indices with decreased lung volumes, a decreased diffusing capacity of the lung to oxygen, and a decreased compliance. Arterial blood gas data usually display a low $P\text{aO}_2$ with a normal or slightly decreased $P\text{aCO}_2$.

Lupus nephritis occurs in about one-half of patients with SLE, presenting on urinalysis as hematuria and proteinuria. If the nephrotic syndrome develops, end-stage renal failure and acidosis may result. Arterial hypertension is a possible finding.[17,30]

Often one will find a slightly elevated partial thromboplastin time in the course of the preoperative hematologic evaluation. This is usually due to a circulating anticoagulant known as the lupus anticoagulant,[31–33] which, in the patient with SLE, is caused by the presence of either an anti-phospholipid antibody or a specific anti-clotting factor antibody.

If antibodies against multiple clotting factors are present, the risk of bleeding is increased. Unless the patient is transfused with the appropriate factor just prior to the administration of a regional anesthetic, this procedure should be considered to be contraindicated.[31] If the disease is associated with the formation of anti-cardiolipin antibody, there is an increased incidence of thrombocytopenia, arterial thromboses (with the possibility of cerebrovascular accident, peripheral gangrene, coronary thrombosis and myocardial necrosis, renal artery occlusion, and avascular bone necrosis), venous thromboses and intravascular clot formation (including in the placenta).[34,35] The platelets in these patients exhibit increased adhesiveness and aggregation. These patients are given anticoagulation therapy with heparin and then switched over to warfarin (Coumadin).[36,37] Raynaud's phenomenon is found in approximately 15% of patients with SLE.[38]

Preoperatively, in addition to the routine studies for patients with SLE, one should consider obtaining an echocardiogram to rule out pericardial effusions and valvulopathies (Libman–Sacks endocarditis); pulmonary function tests if the patient complains of dyspnea out of proportion to her pregnant state; and coagulation tests to screen for circulating lupus anticoagulant. If the patient is receiving chronic steroid maintenance, one should administer steroid coverage.[39,40]

The choice of anesthetic technique depends on the extent of the disease and the systems it involves. With a general anesthetic, there is the increased risk of aspiration pneumonitis and worsening underlying organ dysfunction, including increased mental confusion, depressed pulmonary and cardiac function and poor renal, hepatic and, especially, uteroplacental blood flow. Although there is an increased risk of bleeding from a regional technique, there is also a decrease in the risk of aspiration and a possible increase in the uteroplacental blood flow.

Fetal and neonatal considerations

In SLE patients, there is an increased incidence of premature labor, miscarriage and stillbirth, especially in those mothers with positive anti-phospholipid antibodies.[17,19,41–44] Patients treated with antiplatelet drugs, such as aspirin[45], or with subcutaneous heparin regimens have increased perinatal survival.[38,46] Transient abnormalities can be found in the offspring of mothers with SLE (the neonatal lupus syndrome). The neonatal lupus syndrome includes findings of cytopenias, a discoid rash and cardiac conduction defects (i.e. third-degree atrioventricular block, sometimes requiring a pacemaker).

MYASTHENIA GRAVIS

Pathophysiology

Myasthenia gravis (MG) is an organ-specific autoimmune disease in which the ACh receptor and skeletal muscle are targeted. The end-effect is skeletal muscle weakness and defective neuromuscular transmission. The MG patient has approximately one-quarter of the usual number of acetylcholine receptors because of an augmented rate of degradation and occupation of these receptors by the blocking antibody. Smooth muscle (e.g. the myometrium) is unaffected by MG. The muscle weakness is progressive and increases with exertion, especially of the muscles of the face, tongue, throat, neck, arms and respiratory system. The prevalence of this disease is approximately 3 per 100 000, with a female–male ratio of 3 : 1. The peak prevalence is in the third decade, well within the child-bearing years. It is frequently associated with thymoma or thymic hyperplasia, and occurs in patients with various connective tissue disorders.[47] Approximately 33% of patients improve during pregnancy, whereas another third worsen and the remainder do not change clinically. The patients usually tolerate labor well, as their muscles are already somewhat relaxed because of their disease state. They tend to have a prolonged second stage of labor, and forceps deliveries are common.[48] Those patients who have already undergone a thymectomy appear to fare better during their pregnancy than those who have electively retained their thymus. The anticholinesterase therapy needs to be continued during labor. Oral doses of these agents should be converted to intramuscular dosing, which is usually one-tenth of the oral dose. Approximately 30 min prior to delivery, an intramuscular dose of anticholinesterase agent should be administered to maximize the patient's pushing ability.[49–52]

Anesthetic considerations

For vaginal deliveries, regional techniques are preferred (i.e. a low subarachnoid anesthetic, preferably with a catheter for better control, or a lumbar epidural anesthetic). Because of the respiratory muscle weakness in these patients, extra care must be taken to avoid hypoventilation if a subarachnoid or epidural anesthetic is administered for a cesarean delivery. Ester local anesthetics are relatively contraindicated because chronic neostigmine or pyridostigmine therapy greatly inhibits plasma cholinesterase activity. For cesarean delivery of the patient in remission, a regional technique is preferred; however, if the disease is in a flare state, a general anesthetic should be considered.[52] Because of the initial resistance and prolonged duration of succinylcholine, 40% of the usual dose is sufficient for endotracheal intubation although patients in remission may not be resistant to succinyldicholine.[53,54] Hypokalemia, magnesium sulfate, scopolamine, and large doses of muscle relaxants are contraindicated. Short or intermediate-duration nonderrolarizing muscle relaxants can be used with careful titration by bolus or infusion dosing techniques. A nerve stimulator should always be used to monitor these patients. Muscle relaxants should be reversed with atropine or glycopyrrolate and neostigmine. Neostigmine can be beneficial in increasing muscle strength during labor. Edrophonium can lead to forceful uterine contractions.

In MG, one can find flares during the first trimester or in the first 2 weeks post-partum, the so-called myasthenic crises, in which the need for mechanical ventilation is not unusual.

Since occasional focal myocardial necrosis is found in these patients, a preoperative 12-lead electrocardiogram is imperative for post-operative comparison.

Neonatal considerations

Neonatal myasthenia can occur in 25–33% of babies born to MG mothers. The anesthesiologist or neonatologist must be aware of the increased possibility of emergent neonatal intubation, however the symptoms usually occur between 12 and 48 h post-partum.

PROGRESSIVE SYSTEMIC SCLEROSIS (SCLERODEMA)

Pathophysiology

Progressive systemic sclerosis (PSS), or scleroderma, is another systemic autoimmune disease in which antibodies are formed against gamma globulins, SCL-70 protein, the centromere and SS-A (Ro) and SS-B (La) antigens, with the end-result of abnormal proliferation and overdeposition of fibrous connective tissue. The damage can be local (e.g. coup de sabre) or ubiquitous. The CREST syndrome incorporates the findings of calcinosis, Raynaud's phenomenon, esophageal dysmotility, sclerodactyly and telangectasias.

These related disease entities occur at all ages, however the incidence peaks in middle-aged women (30–65 years of age). There are 50 000–100 000 known cases in the USA. Symptoms usually appear in the third to fifth decades. This disease spectrum is 3–4 times more common in women than in men. Usually pregnancy does not worsen the disease state, however the gastrointestinal symptoms and cardiopulmonary dysfunction of the disease can make an already difficult pregnancy much more difficult for the patient. Pregnancy normally ends in spontaneous vaginal delivery unless the scleroderma changes produce dystocia, which requires cesarean delivery.

Anesthetic considerations

The anesthetic considerations for patients with PSS involve several body systems.

Respiratory tract involvement

Respiratory tract involvement includes tight perioral skin, or 'mauskopf'; TMJ involvement; and cervical arthritis. One needs to be able to perform a blind or fiber-optic intubation. Also, there exists an increased risk of aspiration, secondary to gastrointestinal tract involvement.

Cardiac involvement

With cardiac fibrosis, one sees varying heart blocks and arrhythmias more frequently, as the fibrotic tissue replaces normal myocardium. With this cardiomyopathy, one can also see episodes of congestive heart failure, myocardial Raynaud's phenomenon (small coronary arterial vasospasm), occasional pericarditis with effusions and, rarely, cardiac tamponade. The cardiac failure is also in part a result of chronic hypertension and left ventricular hypertrophic dysfunction, and usually presents as dyspnea on exertion, orthopnea, and pedal edema. On occasion, a patient presents with angina pectoris.

Pulmonary involvement

Because of the increased prevalence of fibrosis of the pulmonary arterial intima, pulmonary hypertension can be quite common. Diffuse interstitial and alveolar fibrosis may result in fine bibasilar rales, end-stage respiratory insufficiency or cor pulmonale. The most common symptom is exertional dyspnea. Pleuritis is much less common. The diffusing capacity of the lung usually is subnormal. The chest radiograph usually shows a lineoreticular or a lineonodular density pattern. Pulmonary function testing shows a chronic restrictive disorder with decreased forced vital capacity and total lung capacity. These patients can also present with rapidly progressive respiratory failure.

Gastrointestinal involvement

As a result of hypokinesis (severely decreased or no peristalsis) and dilation of the esophagus, there may be delayed gastric emptying, gastroesophageal reflux, esophagitis, strictures and dysphagia. Aspiration pneumonia becomes much more common. Along with a dilated small and large intestine, all of these findings require the use of a rapid-sequence induction if general anesthesia is used, and continued surveillance during regional techniques. Nonparticulate antacids, histamine (H_2) blockers and metoclopramide should be administered preoperatively and a 30° head-up position maintained. Patients often present with complaints of severe bloating, abdominal cramps and diarrhea from bacterial overgrowth of the bowel. There is also an increased prevalence of primary biliary cirrhosis in these patients.

IDIOPATHIC THROMBOCYTOPENIC PURPURA

Idiopathic thrombocytopenic purpura (ITP), or autoimmune TP (ATP), is another organ-specific autoimmune disease, one of the most common in pregnancy, wherein platelets are the antibody target of choice. This results in increased platelet destruction. In the chronic form, the female–male ratio is approximately 3 : 1. It exists as an incidental finding in an otherwise healthy patient or as a symptomatic thrombocytopenia with various bleeding presentations.

Central nervous system hemorrhage is the most serious complication of the disease for both the mother and the newborn child; however, it is, fortunately, rare.

Half of ATP mothers give birth to neonates with thrombocytopenia. The antiplatelet antibody can cross the placental barrier passively, leading to varying degrees of fetal thrombocytopenia and related sequelae.[55] The fetal diagnosis is risky in itself, involving measurements of antepartum platelet counts from scalp venous or percutaneous umbilical blood specimens. Although mothers can be treated prenatally with intravenous corticosteroids or gamma globulins, their response does not correlate with that of the fetus. Approximately half of neonates born to mothers with the disease are thrombocytopenic, although usually subclinically.[56] At the other end of the spectrum of presentation is catastrophic intracranial hemorrhage. In the recent study by Samuels et al,[57] 54% of thrombocytopenic patients studied had a history of ITP (79% of whom were positive for antiplatelet antibodies), 45% had low platelet counts for the first time during their initial pregnancy, 23% had offspring born thrombocytopenic (92% of whom were born to mothers who carried a diagnosis of ITP), and 11% had children with severe thrombocytopenia (platelets less than 50 000/mm^2). These investigators concluded that mothers with a history of ITP and positive autoantibodies were likely to deliver a child with thrombocytopenia.[57]

On hematologic examination, one usually finds an increased bleeding time, thrombocytopenia and usually iron-deficiency anemia from low-grade, chronic bleeding. Patients often take corticosteroids or intravenous gammaglobulins to increase their platelet count prior to delivery. A controversy exists as to whether cesarean delivery is safer than vaginal delivery because it avoids the increased risk of intracranial neonatal hemorrhage secondary to the vaginal vault pressure on the baby's head at the time of delivery.

POLYMYOSITIS/DERMATOMYOSITIS

Polymyositis/dermatomyositis is also a nonorgan-specific disease in which the antibody targets include the nuclei; the Jo-1, Mi-2, PM-1, Ku, and PL-7 proteins; and myosin. The usual end-result is that a severe, inflammatory perivasculitis causes diffuse damage to the skeletal muscles and/or the skin of these patients. There are between 8 and 15 per million new cases per year, with a female–male ratio of 2 : 1. Patients with this disorder are most commonly found to have symmetric, proximal muscle weakness. The skin manifestations include erythematous, scaly lesions of the face, neck, shoulders, knees, elbows, ankles and metacarpophalangeal and proximal interphalangeal joints.[14] There is a high incidence of spontaneous abortion and perinatal death. Exacerbations of the disease are not uncommon during pregnancy.[58–61]

Although rare, cardiac involvement does occur in patients with polymyositis or dermatomyositis. It usually presents subclinically as electrocardiographic findings of pericarditis, arrhythmias or conduction defects. Occasionally patients present with congestive heart failure. It is rare, however, for these patients to have respiratory muscle weakness, especially in the dermatomyocytic patient group.

REFERENCES

1. Ansar S A, Penhale W J, Talal N 1985 Sex hormones, immune responses, and autoimmune diseases: mechanism of sex hormone action. Am J Pathol 121: 531–551
2. Beck I, Griffin J F 1987 Lymphocyte responses in systemic lupus erythematosus in pregnancy. Am J Med 82: 179–180
3. Silver R M, Branch D W 1992 Autoimmune disease in pregnancy. Bailleres Clin Obstet Gynaecol 6: 565–600
4. Varner M W 1991 Autoimmune disorders and pregnancy. Semin Perinatol 238–250
5. Dombrowski R A 1989 Autoimmune disease in pregnancy. Med Clin North Am 73: 605–621
6. Billingham R E, Beer A E 1984 Reproductive immunology: past, present and future. Perspect Biol Med 27: 259–275
7. Ostensen M, Husby G 1983 A prospective study of the effect of pregnancy on rheumatoid arthritis and ankylosing spondylitis. Arthritis Rheum 26: 1155–1159
8. Stein G H, Cantor B, Panush R S 1980 Adult Still's disease associated with pregnancy. Arthritis Rheum 23: 248–250
9. Persellin R H 1977 The effect of pregnancy on rheumatoid arthritis. Bull Rheumat Dis 27: 922–927
10. Ørtensen M, Aune B, Husby G 1983 Effect of pregnancy and hormonal changes on the activity of rheumatoid arthritis. Scand J Rheumatol 12: 69–72
11. Bulmash J M 1978 Rheumatoid arthritis and pregnancy. Obstet Gynecol Annu 8: 223–279
12. Kaplan D, Diamond H 1965 Rheumatoid arthritis and pregnancy. Clin Obstet Gynecol 8: 286–292
13. Rodman G P, Schumacher H R (eds) 1989 Primer on the rheumatic diseases. 9th edn. Arthritis Foundation, Atlanta
14. Askari A D 1984 Cardiac abnormalities. Clin Rheumat Dis 10: 131–149
15. Zurier R B 1975 Systemic lupus erythematosis and pregnancy. Clin Rheum Dis 1: 613
16. Kaufman R L, Kitridou R C 1982 Pregnancy in mixed connective tissue disease: comparison with systemic lupus erythematosis, J Rheumatol 9: 549–555
17. Hayslett J P, Lynn R I 1980 Effect of pregnancy in patients with lupus nephropathy. Kidney Int 18: 207–220
18. Hayslett J P 1982 Effect of pregnancy in patients with systemic lupus erythematosus. Am J Kidney Dis (July) 2 (1 Suppl 1): 223–228
19. Garsenstein M, Pollack V E, Kark R M 1962 Systemic lupus erythematosus and pregnancy. New Engl J Med 267: 165
20. Gimovsky M L, Montoro M, Paul R H 1984 Pregnancy outcome in women with systemic lupus erythematosus. Obstet Gynecol 63: 686–692
21. Morris W K 1969 Pregnancy in rheumatoid arthritis and systemic lupus erythematosis. N Z J Obstet Gynecol 9: 136
22. Varner M W 1983 Pregnancy in patients with systemic lupus erythematosis. Am J Obstet Gynecol 15: 1025–1040
23. Lockshin M D, Jarpel P C, Druzin M L, et al 1985 Lupus pregnancy. II. Usual pattern of hypocomplementemia and thrombocytopenia in the pregnant patient. Arthritis Rheum 28: 66–68
24. Buyon J P, Cronstein B N, Morris M et al 1986 Serum complement values (C3 and C4) to differentiate between systemic lupus activity and preeclampsia. Am J Med 81: 194–200
25. Estes D, Larson D L 1965 Systemic lupus erythematosis and pregnancy. Clin Obstet Gynecol 8: 307
26. Knobel B, Melamud E, Kishon Y 1984 Peripartum cardiomyopathy. Isr J Med Sci 20: 1061–1063
27. Gibbs P S, Kim K C 1988 Skin and musculoskeletal diseases. In Stoelting R K, Dierdorf S F, McCammon R L (eds) Anesthesia and co-existing disease. 2nd edn. Churchill Livingstone, New York, p 611
28. Haselby K A 1988 The immune system. In Stoelting R K, Dierdorf S F, McCammon R L (eds) Anesthesia and co-existing disease, 2nd edn. Churchill Livingstone, New York, p 695
29. Campbell C, Ravindran R S 1988 The pregnant patient. In Stoelting R K, Dierdorf S F, McCammon R L (eds) Anesthesia and co-existing disease 2nd, edn Churchill Livingstone, New York, p 749
30. Bear R 1976 Pregnancy and lupus nephritis. Obstet Gynecol 47: 715
31. Malinow A M, Rickford W J, McKriski B L, Saller D N, McGuinn W J 1987 Lupus anticoagulant: implications for obstetric anaesthetists. Anesthesia 42: 1291–1293
32. Lubbe W F, Liggins G C 1985 Lupus anticoagulant and pregnancy. Am J Obstet Gynecol 159: 322–327
33. Lockshin M D, Druzin M L, Goei S et al 1985 Antibody to cardiolipin as a predictor of fetal distress or death in patients with systemic lupus erythematosis. New Engl J Med 313: 152–156
34. Rosove M H, Brewer P M 1992 Antiphospholipid thrombosis: clinical course after the first thrombotic event in 70 patients. Ann Intern Med 117: 303–308
35. Mueh J R, Herbst K D, Rapaport S I 1980 Thrombosis in patients with the lupus anticoagulant. Ann Intern Med 92: 156–159
36. Feinstein D I 1985 Lupus anticoagulant, thrombosis and fetal loss. New Engl J Med 313: 1348
37. Harris E N, Ashecron R A, Gharavi A E, Morgan S W, Derve G, Hughes G R 1985 Thrombocytopenia in systemic lupus erythematosis and related autoimmune disorders: association with anticardiolipin antibody. Br J Haematol 59: 227–30
38. Elias M, Elder A 1984 Thromboembolism in patients with the 'lupus' type circulating anticoagulant. Arch Intern Med 144: 510–516
39. Zulman J I, Talal N, Hoffman G S et al 1980 Problems associated with the management of pregnancies in patients with systemic lupus erythematosis. J Rheumatol 7: 37
40. Zurier R B, Argyros T G, Urman J D et al 1978 Systemic lupus erythematosis: management during pregnancy. Obstet Gynecol 51: 178
41. Landy H J, Kessler C, Kelly W K, Weingold A B 1992 Obstetric performance in patients with the lupus anticoagulant and/or anticardiolipin antibodies: Am J Perinatol 9: 146–151
42. Branch D W, Scott J R, Kochenour N K et al 1985 Obstetric complications associated with the lupus anticoagulant. New Engl J Med 313: 1322
43. Lockshin M D 1985 Lupus pregnancy. Clin Rheumat Dis 11: 61
44. Tozman E C S, Urowitz M B, Gladman D D 1980 Systemic lupus erythematosis and pregnancy. J Rheumatol 7(5): 624–30
45. Barton J R, Sibai B M 1991 Low-dose aspirin to improve perinatal outcome: Clin Obstet Gynecol 34: 251–261
46. Stuart M J, Gross S J, Eliuel H, Graeber G 1982 Effects of acetylsalicyic acid ingestion on maternal and neonatal hemostasis. New Engl J Med 307: 909
47. Lisak R P 1985 Myasthenia gravis: mechanisms and management. Hosp Pract 18(3): 101–103
48. Fennel D, Ringel S 1987 Myasthenia gravis and pregnancy. Obstet Gynecol Surv 41: 414–416
49. Luz-Tobias A, Ramilo N, Yu K, Rigor B 1987 Anesthetic management of a parturient with myasthenia gravis. J Kentucky Med Assoc 85(2): 78–80
50. Plauche W C 1983 Myasthenia gravis. Clin Obstet Gynecol 26: 593–595
51. Eden R D, Gall S A 1983 Myasthenia gravis and pregnancy: a reappraisal of thymectomy. Obstet Gynecol 62: 328–332
52. Rolbin S H, Levinson G, Shnider S M, Wright R G 1978 Anesthetic considerations for myasthenia gravis and pregnancy. Anesth Analg 57: 441–447
53. Baraka A 1992 Anaesthesia and myaesthenia gravis. Can J Anaesth 39: 476–486
54. Abel M, Eisenkraft J B, Patel N 1991 Response to suxamethonium in a myasthenic patient during remission. Anaesthesia 46: 30–32
55. Scott J R, Rote N S, Cruikshank D P 1987 Antiplatelet antibodies and platelet counts in pregnancies complicated by autoimmune thrombocytopenic purpura. Am J Obstet Gynecol 145: 932–936
56. Burrows R F, Kelton J G 1988 Incidentally detected thrombocytopenia in healthy mothers and their infants. New Engl J Med 319: 142–144
57. Samuels P, Bussel J B, Braitman L E, Tomaski A, Druzin M L, Mennuti M T, Clines D B 1990 Estimation of the risk of thrombocytopenia in the offspring of pregnant women with presumed immune thrombocytopenic purpura. New Engl J Med 323: 229–244

58. Bauer K A, Seigler M, Lindheimer M A 1979 Polymyositis complicating pregnancy. Arch Intern Med 139: 449–452
59. Baines A B, Link D A 1983 Childhood dermatomyositis and pregnancy. Am J Obstet Gynecol 145: 335–341
60. Tsai A, Lindheimer M D, Lamberg S I 1973 Dermatomyositis complicating pregnancy. Obstet Gynecol 41: 570–576
61. Gutierrez G, Dagnino R, Mintz G 1984 Polymyositis/dermatomyositis and pregnancy. Arthritis Rheuma 27: 291–295

55. Thromboembolism and hemorrhagic disorders in obstetrics

Part A Thromboembolism *J. Conard M. M. Samama*
Part B Hemorrhagic disorders *M. Dreyfus G. Tertian G. Tchernia*

PART A
THROMBOEMBOLISM

J. Conard M.-M. Samama

INTRODUCTION

Thromboembolism is a rare, important and well-known complication of pregnancy, but it has become an increasing subject of interest in recent years. Indeed, new antithrombotic drugs have become available and congenital deficiencies associated with a high risk of thrombosis related to pregnancy have been documented.

INCIDENCE

Pregnancy is classically associated with an increased risk of thromboembolism, and pulmonary embolism has been considered as the leading cause of maternal death.[1] Death from obstetric pulmonary embolism has declined more than 50% in the USA from 1970 to 1985; however, some subgroups of women remain at higher risk (1.3 and 4.2 deaths per 100 000 live births in Caucasians and Blacks respectively).[2]

In many studies, the morbidity may have been overestimated because diagnosis was mainly by clinical criteria, and is probably unreliable. The risk of venous thrombosis is 5–6 times greater in pregnant than in nonpregnant women.[3] An overall prevalence of thromboembolic complications associated with pregnancy of 0.09% has been reported.[1] Studies based on objective methods to confirm clinical suspicion of deep venous thrombosis (DVT) suggest a prevalence of 0.07%.[4,5]

Thrombosis is more frequent during the post-partum period after normal delivery than during pregnancy. Prevalences of superficial thrombophlebitis of 0.016–0.15% ante partum and 0.08–1.35% post-partum, and of DVT of 0.11–0.36% antepartum and 0.15–3.0% post-partum have been reported.[6] Pulmonary embolism was found in 1 of 2000 pregnancies.[6] A prospective study using 125 I-labeled fibrinogen identified calf thrombi in 3% of cases in the post-partum period.[7]

All these data suggest that several women develop deep venous insufficiency associated with symptomatic or asymptomatic DVT during pregnancy or the post-partum period.

Some conditions related to pregnancy favor thrombosis (Table 55.1). Indeed, elements of the Virchow's triad, such as venous stasis and hypercoagulability, are present. Pressure of the gravid uterus is responsible for the decreased venous return and also for the increased peripheral venous pressure. Proximal thrombi are more common and, for anatomic reasons (compression of the left proximal iliac vein by the right iliac artery), left-sided thrombosis is more frequent than right-sided.[8]

Some additional factors are also probably important in the development of thrombosis, for example increasing age and parity, as well as prolonged bed rest and obesity.

After cesarean delivery, the prevalence of thrombosis has been reported to be as high as 2–5% and a risk about 20 times greater than following spontaneous vaginal delivery has been suggested.[8,9] In a study using plethysmography before and 1 week following cesarean delivery, thrombi were found in 1.8%.[8]

Table 55.1 Risk factors for thrombosis related to pregnancy

Age
Parity
Bed rest
Obesity
Cesarean delivery
Ovarian hyperstimulation syndrome
Previous history of thrombosis
Congenital deficiency of AT III, protein C, Protein S
Lupus anticoagulant

Another cause of thrombosis has been recently identified: the *ovarian hyperstimulation syndrome*. Severe ovarian hyperstimulation syndrome (OHSS) may be observed after induction of ovulation with clomiphene citrate, pregnant mare's serum gonadotropin, pituitary gonadotropins or human menopausal gonadotropins. Venous or arterial thrombosis is a rare complication of this syndrome. Reported cases often involved occlusions localized to the head and neck,[10] but also deep venous thrombosis of the lower limbs.[11] Thromboses were usually observed 4–6 weeks after induction of ovulation, when patients were pregnant.

The etiology of thrombotic episodes associated with ovarian hyperstimulation is still unclear. Hemoconcentration is a good indicator of the severity of the hyperstimulation syndrome, and it results in an increase in blood viscosity. In addition, coagulation is reported to be impaired with increased levels of platelets, fibrinogen and factor V.[12] Decreased levels of antithrombin III have also been observed.[13,14]

Prophylactic anticoagulant treatment may be offered to women with severe ovarian hyperstimulation and also to women with history of thrombosis having induction of ovulation.

COAGULATION AND FIBRINOLYSIS ABNORMALITIES RELATED TO NORMAL PREGNANCY

Coagulation and fibrinolysis abnormalities occur during normal pregnancy and some of them may predispose to venous thrombosis.

During pregnancy

Platelets

Although the platelet count has been reported to be unchanged in normal pregnancy, a reduction may be observed and has been mostly attributed to hemodilution.[15] In a recent study,[16] a platelet number below 150 000/mm^3 was observed in 15 of 4048 pregnant women (0.37%), but in a prospective study a mild thrombocytopenia (range 97–150 $\times$ 10^9) was found in 8.3% of healthy women admitted to an obstetric unit.[17] In the post-partum period, platelets are significantly increased.

Discrepancies have been observed concerning aggregation of platelets. Increased aggregability has been reported by different authors, but serum production of thromboxane A_2 is unchanged.[18] In contrast, another study found hypoaggregability and was considered, together with a decreased platelet count and an increase in circulating platelet aggregates, to be a sign of platelet activation.[19] This last hypothesis is supported by the fact that the levels of platelet-specific proteins, such as β-thromboglobulin and platelet factor 4, which increase in the plasma when platelets are activated, are elevated during pregnancy.[20]

Coagulation

Clotting factors. Some plasma factors are increased during pregnancy, such as fibrinogen, factors VII, VIII C, X and von Willebrand factor.[21] These factors are elevated as soon as 11–15 weeks' gestation and their levels are higher than those observed in post-partum or in nonpregnant women.[21] These increased levels are probably at least in part mediated by estrogen levels, since they are also observed after estroprogestogens intake.

Placenta may act as a source of tissue factors with a consequent formation of thrombin via the extrinsic pathway.

Physiologic anticoagulants. Concentrations of some physiologic inhibitors are decreased: antithrombin III (AT III),[21] protein S activity and free protein S antigen.[22,23] In contrast, the protein C level is not decreased, or even increased.[23] Heparin Co-factor II[24] and tissue factor pathway inhibitor (TFPI), also called LACI or EPI,[25] are also increased, but the clinical importance of these inhibitors is still unclear.

The consequence of the alterations of blood coagulation described above is activation of coagulation as judged by the increased levels of fibrinopeptide A (FPA)[20,26] and thrombin–antithrombin III complexes. The progressive decrease in factor II during pregnancy has also been considered to be the result of its utilization in thrombin generation.[27]

Fibrinolysis

It has been known for many years that fibrinolytic activity is reduced during pregnancy: euglobulin lysis times and whole-blood clot lysis times are greatly prolonged both before and after stimulation (venous occlusion for instance).[21,28]

Hypofibrinolysis is also associated with increased levels of fibrinolysis inhibitors, and especially plasminogen activator inhibitors, PAI-1 and -2.[29,30]

In the post-partum period

Coagulation factors and inhibitors normalize in 3–6 weeks,[22,30] while fibrinolytic activity returns to normal much more rapidly: 30 min after separation of the placenta, lysis times are normal.[28] PAI-1 levels decrease sharply and normalize within 3 days,[30] while the PAI-2 level remains elevated for a longer period.

It has been observed that the fibrinogen/AT III ratio is increased in the first 2 weeks post-partum, as reported in patients with post-operative thromboembolism.[31] In addition, protein S is lower in the early post-partum period than at the end of pregnancy[22] and FPA is higher.[26]

In summary, coagulation and fibrinolysis modifications occurring during pregnancy suggest hypercoagulability and hypofibrinolysis. Normalization is observed by about 6 weeks post-partum. However, the risk of thromboembolism is generally higher in the post-partum period than during pregnancy: development of some abnormalities (e.g. increase in platelet count, decrease in protein S levels) during the first week post-partum may play a role.

PRE-EXISTING RISK FACTORS OF THROMBOSIS

Congenital deficiency of coagulation inhibitors and the presence of acquired circulating anticoagulants such as lupus anticoagulants are well-known conditions predisposing to venous thrombosis.

AT III deficiency

Congenital AT III deficiency associated with thrombosis has been found in 1 in 4000–5000 normal individuals and 2–4% of patients with history of venous thrombosis. It is transmitted as an autosomal dominant trait. Heterozygous affected patients have an AT III level that is approximately 50% of normal and suffer from thromboembolic episodes. An additional triggering factor is often found, such as pregnancy, oral contraceptive intake, surgery, and bed rest.[32]

Pregnancy greatly enhances the risk of thrombosis in AT III-deficient women: approximately 45–65% develop thrombosis during pregnancy or post-partum.[33,34] Thrombosis is more frequent in the post-partum period, but it can even occur early during pregnancy (first trimester) or after abortion.

Protein C deficiency

Congenital protein C (PC) deficiency is more frequent than AT III deficiency in patients with history of thrombosis (4–8%). It has been estimated to be present in 1 in 15 000 normal individuals.[35]

Classically, the deficiency is transmitted as an autosomal dominant trait and affected heterozygotes suffer recurrent episodes of venous thrombosis. Homozygotes with undetectable levels of protein C have been detected at birth with purpura fulminans or massive thromboses.[36] Another group of homozygotes have mild deficiencies (PC level about 20%) and have a late onset of clinical symptoms with no thrombosis at birth.

In pregnant heterozygous protein C-deficient women, the risk of developing thrombosis is close to 25%. It is low during pregnancy (7%) and higher in the post-partum period (19%).[34]

Protein S deficiency

The prevalence of congenital protein S (PS) deficiency is still unknown in the normal population, while in thrombotic patients its prevalence is about the same as PC deficiency and higher than AT III deficiency.[37]

Although thrombosis has been reported during pregnancy in PS-deficient women, we have found that it is more frequently observed in the post-partum period than during pregnancy (17% vs. 0%) in a series of 17 patients (44 pregnancies).[34] We are continuing the study and three thromboses (two DVT, one superficial vein thrombosis) have been observed during pregnancy (25 women, 60 pregnancies), i.e. a frequency of 7%.

Lupus anticoagulant

Lupus anticoagulant was first found in patients with systemic lupus erythematosus (SLE) but also occurs in the absence of SLE. It can be detected by the prolongation of the activated partial thromboplastin time, not corrected by addition of normal plasma. Anticardiolipin and/or antiphospholipid antibodies may be simultaneously present.

Lupus anticoagulant has been associated with repeated miscarriages and with thromboses.[38]

DIAGNOSIS OF THROMBOSIS

Diagnosis of thrombosis is essential because it will be a guide for the type, the intensity and the duration of the treatment required during pregnancy and after delivery at the time of thrombosis, and possibly also for future pregnancies. It is of special importance since anticoagulant treatment is associated with different risks for the fetus and the mother and since a false-negative diagnosis of venous thrombosis and the absence of anticoagulant treatment exposes the mother to pulmonary embolism.

Clinical diagnosis is notoriously unreliable. More than 50% of pregnant women with unilateral leg swelling or pain have no venous thrombosis[39] and would have unnecessary anticoagulant treatment if the diagnosis were made on clinical grounds only.

Diagnostic tests that can be used during pregnancy are Doppler flow measurement, impedance plethysmography and contrast venography. The labeled fibrinogen uptake test is contraindicated during pregnancy.

Venography can be performed with relative safety if there is adequate shielding of the uterus. The interpretation of venography during pregnancy may be difficult because of extrinsic compression of the pelvic vessels by the gravid uterus. It has been noticed that, in nonpregnant patients, the clot usually starts in the calf and propagates proximally, while in pregnant women it may start in the iliac or femoral veins and then propagate distally.[40]

Noninvasive diagnostic methods are often preferred. Impedance plethysmography is very sensitive and specific for proximal vein thrombosis.[41]

Doppler sonography is also very useful in detecting popliteal, femoral and iliac thromboses. It has a disadvantage compared with impedance plethysmography, related to technician error. If one of these two tests is positive and the patient is more than 20 weeks' pregnant, confirmation by venography may be required before initiating anticoagulant therapy. If a patient has a suspected pulmonary embolism (PE), perfusion lung scanning should be performed. When its results are normal, PE is excluded; if not, ventilation–perfusion lung scan and pulmonary angiography are considered.[27]

ANTICOAGULANTS DURING PREGNANCY

Anticoagulant therapy may be needed during pregnancy either because of an established thrombosis or for prophylaxis. Its administration is often difficult owing to potential adverse effects in the mother and fetus.[42,43]

Standard heparin

Heparin does not cross the placenta and is considered as the anticoagulant of choice during pregnancy. In addition, it is not excreted in breast milk.

Heparin is a mucopolysaccharide with a mean molecular weight of 15 000 daltons. It has the ability to catalyze the inhibition of thrombin (anti-IIa activity) and activated factors X and IX by antithrombin III. It may also react with platelets. The mean biologic half-life of heparin is 60–90 min but there are individual variations. Moreover, the half-life is dose dependent, decreasing when the dose is increased.

Heparin can be administered by intravenous or subcutaneous injections. When the subcutaneous route is used, injections should be into the subcutaneous tissue of the abdominal wall or laterally above the iliac crest, but when this is not possible heparin can be injected in the lateral upper part of the thigh or the arm.[39]

Although suggested by some authors, heparin treatment does not seem to cause adverse fetal/infant outcomes, such as prematurity or fetal or neonatal deaths.[43]

The prolonged administration of heparin during pregnancy is associated with osteoporosis, the incidence being unknown.[42] It seems that there is a dose effect, and the majority of cases of heparin-associated osteoporosis have been reported in patients treated with more than 15 000 units daily for more than 6 months.[44]

Thrombocytopenia is a well-known complication of heparin treatment, and at least two cases have been reported during pregnancy.[45,46]

A complication of heparin is bleeding, and anesthesiologists usually refuse epidural anesthesia to patients receiving heparin, whatever the heparin level.[47]

Thus, although heparin is said to be the anticoagulant of choice, it is far from the ideal.

Low molecular weight heparin (LMWH)

Different types of LMWH have been prepared. Their mean molecular weight is approximately 5 000 daltons and their activity is more anti-Xa than antilla (ratio 2:5). Consequently, the laboratory monitoring of LMWH and of standard heparin is different.

Although LMWH has been said to induce less bleeding than standard heparin for an equivalent antithrombotic effect, bleeding may be observed at high doses. The relative bleeding risk of the two types of heparin is still being discussed.

Concerning osteoporosis, the effects of LMWH and standard heparin are very similar in rats,[48] and no data are presently available in humans.

LMWH has been demonstrated to have fewer effects on platelets than standard heparin and it has been administered in patients with heparin-induced thrombocytopenia. However, a low platelet count may persist despite LMWH treatment,[49] and few reports of thrombocytopenia initially induced by LMWH have been recently published.[50] Thus, this adverse effect cannot be ruled out.

During pregnancy, if LMWH were equally effective and had fewer adverse effects, it would be advantageous in anticoagulant treatment. In addition, the reduction of the number of subcutaneous injections required and the absence of the decrease in AT III during LMWH administration would be beneficial.

However, at present, the use of LMWH is not yet clearly recommended in pregnancy, although LMWH does not appear to cross the placenta.[51] It has been administered to a few women without any complication.[52, 53]

Oral anticoagulants

Oral anticoagulants cross the placenta and can have adverse effects on the fetus throughout the antenatal period. Fetopathic effects include embryopathy and central nervous system abnormalities.[42, 43]

Warfarin embryopathy consists of nasal hypoplasia and/or stippled epiphyses when the treatment is given during the first trimester of pregnancy,[54] and especially during the first 6–12 weeks. In a study of pregnant women with valvular heart disease, embryopathy was present in 10 of 35 infants born to women who received warfarin between 6 and 12 weeks of gestation, while no case of embryopathy was observed when heparin was substituted for warfarin during this period.[55]

Central venous system abnormalities (fetal optic atrophy, cerebellar atrophy) may be due to multiple small intracerebral hemorrhages and can occur following administration of warfarin during any trimester.

Oral anticoagulation may also complicate the obstetric situation if premature placental separation occurs or if cesarean delivery or instrumental delivery is urgently required.

For all these reasons, there is now a general tendency not to use oral anticoagulants during pregnancy for treatment or prophylaxis, but some cardiologists still use oral anticoagulants in the second trimester of pregnancy in women with mechanical heart valves. As a rule, if a woman is already being treated with oral anticoagulants, she should be carefully counseled and the risks explained before pregnancy occurs. In this case, two options can be considered. The first is to perform pregnancy tests as soon as menses are delayed, and to substitute heparin if the test is positive: this assumes that warfarin is safe during the first 4–6 weeks of gestation.

The second option is to replace warfarin by heparin before conception, but then, if the patient does not quickly become pregnant, there will be a prolonged exposure to heparin and an increased risk of osteoporosis and of local intolerance.

For a long time, oral anticoagulants were not recommended for nursing mothers. Recently, it has been shown that warfarin does not induce an anticoagulant effect in the infant.[56,57] The same is reported for acenocoumarin.[58]

TREATMENT OF ESTABLISHED THROMBOSIS

Deep vein thrombosis or pulmonary embolism occurring during pregnancy is usually treated with heparin. Thrombolytic agents have been administered, but these are associated with an increased risk of bleeding. Venocaval interruption using the Greenfield filter has been reported in pregnancy.[59]

Standard heparin

Heparin is preferably administered as a continuous intravenous infusion at a dose of 30 000–40 000 units per day, after a starting i.v. bolus of 5000 units. The dose is then adapted by laboratory monitoring to maintain a heparin level of 0.2–0.4 units/ml and an activated partial thromboplastin time (APTT) at about 1.5 times the control level (depending on the reagent used). This treatment is given for 7–10 days followed by subcutaneous heparin until term to maintain the APTT at 1.5 times the control 6 h after injection.[42] Laboratory monitoring should be repeated throughout pregnancy because a relative resistance to heparin usually develops. A platelet count has to be performed regularly. Heparin should be discontinued immediately before delivery and started again postpartum. After about 7 days, oral anticoagulants are frequently substituted for heparin for 4–6 weeks postpartum.

Low molecular weight heparins or heparinoids

Isolated cases of treatment with these drugs have been reported. A pregnant woman with a massive iliofemoral venous thrombosis was initially treated with standard heparin from the 11th to the 13th week of pregnancy. She then received Enoxaparin at a dose of 60–80 mg daily throughout pregnancy.[52]

A low molecular weight heparinoid (Org 10172, Organon International, Oss, The Netherlands) has also been administered for a short period to a pregnant woman. She had proximal deep vein thrombosis during the first trimester, developed heparin-induced thrombocytopenia, was given warfarin and received Org 10172 from the weeks 36 to 37.5, when delivery was induced.[46]

PROPHYLACTIC ANTICOAGULANT TREATMENT

Prophylactic therapy with anticoagulants has to be considered in pregnant women with past history of thromboembolism occurring during pregnancy or in the post-partum period because the risk of recurrent thrombosis has been found to be greater in these pregnant women than in women without thromboembolic antecedents.

The risk is even higher if a congenital thrombotic disorder such as AT III, protein C or protein S deficiency or an acquired thrombotic disorder such as lupus anticoagulant is present. Screening for these coagulation abnormalities should be performed in young women with thromboembolic antecedents, especially if these were recurrent and if the family history is positive. Interpretation of the results should take into account the possible modifications induced by pregnancy itself, and it is sometimes difficult to distinguish between acquired and congenital defects (for protein S deficiency for instance).

History of thrombosis without congenital or acquired coagulation anomaly

In this group of patients the risk of thrombotic episodes during pregnancy has been found to be enough to consider long-term administration of anticoagulants during the ante- and the post-natal periods.[59]

The risk of recurrence during pregnancy without prophylactic treatment has been estimated to be 4–12%,[60] in contrast to 0.1% in normal women. These studies were based on small study populations. However, the side-effects of long-term anticoagulants also have to be considered, and the risk of prophylactic treatment must be weighed against the risk of thromboembolism.

Recent studies[61] have not reached a definite conclusion

regarding thromboprophylaxis during pregnancy. In particular, the hazards of prophylaxis with heparin, such as bone demineralization, which could be irreversible, and the risk of heparin-induced thrombocytopenia, although rare, are well documented. As mentioned above, oral anticoagulants are associated with embryopathy when administered between the weeks 6 and 12 of gestation, and with intracerebral bleeds in the fetus, which could be responsible for central nervous system abnormalities.

Prophylactic treatment is started during the first, second or third trimester of pregnancy, the decision being made case by case according to the severity of the thrombotic disease and possible existence of an additional risk factor, such as bed rest, etc. Treatment is mandatory in the post-partum period.

The dose of heparin required for the prophylaxis of venous thromboembolism is increased in pregnancy: a dose of 7500 to 10 000 units b.i.d. has been recommended, but the dose and the level of anticoagulation required are not well defined. Anti-Xa determination has been said to be more appropriate for monitoring.[62]

In Europe, at least in France, LMW heparins have been used in some pregnant women,[53] but more work is required before establishing this treatment.

Women with congenital or acquired thrombotic tendency

Pregnancy is generally considered as a high-risk state in this category of thrombophilic patients, and the risk is probably more important in women with previous thrombosis (symptomatic) than in asymptomatic ones. The correct approach to the prevention of thromboembolic episode during pregnancy is problematic because reliable information is not available.

Women with AT III deficiency seem to have the higher prevalence of thrombosis related to pregnancy (approximately 50%).[33,34] A few reports have mentioned that recurrence of DVT in untreated women can occur very early in the first trimester, suggesting that in both symptomatic and asymptomatic patients prophylaxis is indicated. The time for starting heparin prophylaxis and the optimal dose are ill defined.

Different approaches have been recommended:[39]

1. moderate doses of unfractionated heparin: 5000 IU b.i.d. during the first two trimesters, the dose being increased in the third trimester aiming at an APTT 1.5–2 times control;
2. full dose of unfractionated heparin for the entire duration of pregnancy;
3. moderate or full dose of unfractionated heparin, starting in the third trimester.

Option 1 or 3 should be considered in asymptomatic patients, whilst option 2 should be considered in symptomatic patients. In order to improve local tolerance of long-term treatment with s.c. heparin one should consider the use of LMWH, since it is commonly observed that ecchymoses at the site of injection are less frequent with LMWH than with unfractionated heparin, especially if a single injection per day is sufficient. The dose to be used is not well defined and it can be only deduced from anecdotal reports. More work is required in order to make recommendations.

All patients should be encouraged to wear compression stockings. Frequent surveillance of the venous system of the legs with noninvasive methods such as impedance plethysmography and/or duplex ultrasound imaging has been recommended.

In women with protein C or protein S deficiency, the risk of thrombosis during pregnancy is probably lower than in AT III-deficient patients, but in the post-partum period it is suggested to be similar.[34]

In pregnant women with a lupus anticoagulant, the choice between options 1 and 2 above should be discussed with the consultant in internal medicine since in some patients with recurrent abortions a special therapeutic protocol is used that includes aspirin and prednisone.[63] In the post-partum period prophylaxis with s.c. heparin and/or oral anticoagulants for 4–6 weeks is highly recommended in these patients.

Finally, if long-term heparin treatment is given, an adjunct treatment for the prevention of osteoporosis should be considered.

Patients with an artificial heart valve

It is generally accepted that oral anticoagulants provide protection against thromboembolic accidents in patients with an artificial heart valve. However, as mentioned above, oral anticoagulants are contraindicated in the first trimester and during the last weeks of pregnancy. Their use could be accepted in the second trimester, but subcutaneous heparin is more and more often preferred because it is safer for the fetus.[43]

The first encountered problem is how to plan a pregnancy in a woman with a mechanical heart valve since she will be receiving long-term oral anticoagulant treatment and there is a consensus to aim at an International Normalized Ratio (INR) ranging between 2.5 and 3.5. Some doctors will switch to heparin therapy, while some others will stop oral anticoagulants as soon as the pregnancy test performed regularly every month becomes positive. This second approach seems more practical. Although the risk of fetopathy is said to be maximum in the weeks 6–12 of pregnancy, one cannot be certain that the risk does not exist during the first 2 weeks of pregnancy.

The second problem is the correct dose of s.c. heparin to be given. It has been demonstrated that a low dose such as 5000 units twice a day is not protective.[55] Even at higher doses, anecdotal reports of treatment failure are available, and the authors of this report[55] have been encouraged to use warfarin between weeks 12 and 36 in their patients. Once again, because anticoagulants can produce some bleeding in the fetus, laboratory monitoring should be very strict in order to prevent overdosing. Probably an INR adjusted to 3 rather than to 4.5 is desirable but this is pure speculation.

The optimum dose of heparin is not well established. It has been recommended that during heparin therapy a PTT level 1.5–2 or 2.5 times above normal would be evidence of sufficient anticoagulation with blood being collected midway betweeen two consecutive injections.

REFERENCES

1. Letsky E, de Swiet M 1984 Thromboembolism in pregnancy and its management. Br J Haematol 57: 543–552
2. Franks A L, Atrash H K, Lawson H W, Colberg K S 1990 Obstetrical pulmonary embolism mortality, United States, 1970–85. Am J Public Health 80: 720–721
3. Seigel D G 1972 Pregnancy, the puerperium and the steroid contraceptive. In: Foster D (ed) The epidemiology of venous thrombosis. Milbank Memorial Fund Q 50: 15
4. Kierkegaard A 1983 Incidence and diagnosis of deep vein thrombosis associated with pregnancy. Acta Obst Gynecol Scand 62: 239–243
5. Bergqvist A, Bergqvist D, Hallbröök T 1983 Deep vein thrombosis during pregnancy. A prospective study. Acta Obstet Gynecol Scand 62: 443–448
6. Weiner C P 1985 Diagnosis and management of thromboembolic disease during pregnancy. Clin Obstet Gynecol 28: 107–118
7. Friend J R, Kakkar V V 1970 The diagnosis of deep vein thrombosis in the peurperium. J Obstet Gynaecol Br Cwlth 77: 820–826
8. Bergqvist D 1983 Postoperative thromboembolism: frequency, etiology, prophylaxis. Springer, Berlin, p 16
9. Treffers P E, Huidekoper B L, Weenik G H, Kloosterman G S 1983 Epidemiological observations of thrombo-embolic disease during pregnancy and in the puerperium in 56,022 women. Int J Gynaecol Obstet 21: 327–331
10. Fournet N, Surrey E, Kerin J 1991 Internal jugular vein thrombosis after ovulation induction with gonadotropins. Fertil Steril 56: 354–356
11. Boulieu D, Ninet J, Pinede L, Didier-Laurent J F, Franco A 1989 Thrombose veineuse précoce de siège inhabituel, en début de grossesse après hyperstimulation ovarienne. Contraception – Fertilité – Sexualité 17: 725–727
12. Phillips L L, Gladstone W, Wiele R V 1975 Studies of the coagulation and fibrinolytic systems in hyperstimulation syndrome after administration of human gonadotropins. J Reprod Med 14: 138–143
13. Kim H C, Kemmann E, Shelden R M, Saidi P 1981 Response of blood coagulation parameters to elevated endogenous 17 β-estradiol levels induced by human menopausal gonadotropins. Am J Obstet Gynecol 140: 807–810
14. Kaaja R, Siegberg R, Tiitinen A, Koskimies A 1989 Severe ovarian hyperstimulation syndrome and deep venous thrombosis. Lancet 2: 1043 (letter)
15. Lamparelli R D V, Baynes R D, Atkinson P, Bezwoda W R, Mendelow B V 1988 Platelet parameters. Part 1. Platelet counts and mean platelet volume in normal and pregnant subjects. S Afr Med J 73: 36–39
16. How H Y, Bergmann F, Koshy M, Chediak J, Presperin C, Gall S A 1991 Quantitative and qualitative platelet abnormalities during pregnancy. Am J Obstet Gynecol 164: 92–98
17. Burrows R F, Kelton J G 1988 Incidentally detected thrombocytopenia in healthy mothers and their infants. New Engl J Med 319: 142–145
18. Louden K A, Broughton Pipkin F, Heptinstall S, Fox S C, Mitchell J R A, Symonds E M 1990 A longitudinal study of platelet behaviour and thromboxane production in whole blood in normal pregnancy and the puerperium. Br J Obstet Gynaecol 97: 1108–1114
19. O'Brien W F, Saba H I, Knuppel R A, Scerbo J C, Cohen G R 1986 Alterations in platelet concentration and aggregation in normal pregnancy and preeclampsia. Am J Obstet Gynecol 155: 486–490
20. Gerbasi F R, Bottoms S, Farag A, Mammen E 1990 Increased intravascular coagulation associated with pregnancy. Obstet Gynecol 75: 385
21. Stirling Y, Woolf L, North W R S, Seghatchian M J, Meade T W 1984 Haemostasis in normal pregnancy. Thromb Haemost 52: 176–182
22. Fernandez J A, Estelles A, Gilabert J, Espana F, Aznar J 1989 Functional and immunologic protein S in normal pregnant women and in full-term newborns. Thromb Haemost 61: 474–478
23. Warwick R, Hutton R A, Goff L, Letsky E, Heard M 1989 Changes in protein C and free protein S during pregnancy and following hysterectomy. J Royl Soc Med 82: 591–594
24. Massouh M, Jatoi A, Gordon E M, Ratnoff O D 1989 Heparin cofactor II activity in plasma during pregnancy and oral contraceptive use. J Lab Clin Med 114: 697–699
25. Sandset P M, Hellgren M, Uvebrandt M, Bergstrom H 1989 Extrinsic coagulation pathway inhibitor and heparin cofactor II during normal and hypertensive pregnancy. Thromb Res 55: 665–670
26. De Boer K, Ten Cate J W, Sturk A et al 1989 Enhanced thrombin generation in normal and hypertensive pregnancy. Am J Obstet Gynecol 160: 95–100
27. Sipes S L, Weiner C P 1990 Venous thromboembolic disease in pregnancy. Semin Perinatol 14: 103–118
28. Conard J, Ciavarella N, Samama M 1972 Fibrinolytic activity induced by venous stasis before and after childbirth. Ricerca 2: 439
29. Nilsson I M, Felding P, Lecander I, Lenner C, Astedt B 1986 Different types of plasminogen activator inhibitors in plasma and platelets in pregnant women. Br J Haematol 62: 215–220
30. Kruithof K O, Tran-Thang C, Gudinchet A, Hauert J, Nicoloso G, Genton C, Welti H, Bachman F 1987 Fibrinolysis in pregnancy: a study of plasminogen activator inhibitors. Blood 69: 460–466
31. Dahlman T, Hellgren M, Blombäck M 1985 Changes in blood coagulation and fibrinolysis in the normal puerperium. Gynecol Obstet Invest 20: 37–44
32. Thaler E, Lechner K 1981 Antithrombin III deficiency and thromboembolism. In: Prentice C R M (ed) Clinics in haematology. Saunders, London pp 369–390
33. Hellgren M, Tengborn L, Abildgaard U 1982 Pregnancy in women with congenital antithrombin III deficiency: experience of treatment with heparin and antithrombin. Gynecol Obstet Invest 14: 127–141
34. Conard J, Horellou M H, Van Dreden P, Lecompte T, Samama M 1990 Thrombosis and pregnancy in congenital deficiencies in AT III, protein C or protein S: study of 78 women. Thromb Haemost 63: 319–320
35. Broekmans A W, Conard J 1988 Hereditary protein C deficiency. In: Bertina R M (ed) Protein C and related proteins. Churchill Livingstone, Edinburgh pp 161–181
36. Marlar R A, Montgomery R R, Madden R M 1988 Homozygous protein C deficiency. In: Bertina R M (ed) Protein C and related proteins. Churchill Livingstone, Edinburgh pp 182–185
37. Briet E, Broekmans A W, Engesser L 1988 Hereditary protein S deficiency. In: Protein C and related proteins. In: Bertina R M (ed) Churchill Livingstone, Edinburgh pp 203–212
38. Lechner K 1987 Lupus anticoagulants and thrombosis. In: Verstraete M, Vermylen J, Lijnen R, Arnout J (eds) Thrombosis and Haemostasis. Leuven University Press, Leuven pp 525–547
39. Hirsh J, Ginsberg J, Turner C, Levine M N 1990 Management of thromboembolism during pregnancy: risks to the fetus. In: Bern M M, Frigoletlto F D J (eds) Hematologic disorders in maternal–fetal medicine, Wiley–Liss pp 523–543
40. Bergqvist A, Bergqvist D, Hallbrook T 1983 Deep vein thrombosis during pregnancy: a prospective study. Acta Obstet Gynecol Scand 62: 443–448
41. Hull R D, Hirsh J, Carter C et al 1985 Diagnostic efficacy of

impedance plethysmography for clinically suspected deep-vein thrombosis: a randomized trial. Ann Intern Med 102: 21
42. de Swiet M 1987 Anticoagulants. Br Med J 294: 428–430
43. Ginsberg J S, Hirsh J 1989 Use of anticoagulants during pregnancy. Chest 95 (suppl): 156S–160S
44. de Swiet M, Dorrington Ward P, Fidler J et al 1983 Prolonged heparin therapy in pregnancy causes bone demineralisation (heparin-induced osteopenia). Br J Obstet Gynaecol 90: 1129–1134
45. Meyres D, Ayalou H, Virag I, Weisbort Y, Zakut H 1986 Heparin induced thrombocytopenia and recurrent thrombosis in pregnancy. A case report. J Reprod Med 31: 993–996
46. Henny C P, Ten Cate H, Ten Cate J W, Prummel M F, Peters M, Buller H H 1986 Thrombosis prophylaxis in an AT III deficient pregnant woman: application of low molecular weight heparinoid. Thromb Haemost 68: 122–140
47. Crawford J S 1978 Principles and practice of obstetric anaesthesia, 4th edn. Blackwell Scientific Publications, Oxford pp 182–183
48. Matzsch T, Bergqvist D, Hedner U, Nilsson B, Ostergaard P 1990 Effects of low molecular weight heparin and unfragmented heparin on induction of osteoporosis in rats. Thromb Haemost 63: 505–509
49. Horellou M H, Conard J, Lecrubier C et al 1984 Persistent heparin induced thrombocytopenia despite therapy with low molecular weight heparin. Thromb Haemost 51: 134
50. Lecompte T, Luo S K, Stieltjes N, Lecrubier C, Samama M 1991 Thrombocytopenia associated with low molecular weight heparin. Lancet 2: 1217
51. Forrestier F, Daffos F, Rainaux M, Toulemonde F 1987 Low molecular weight heparin (CY 216) does not cross the placenta during the third trimester of pregnancy. Thromb Res 57: 234
52. Priollet P, Roncato M, Aiach M, Housset E, Poissonnier M H, Chavinie J 1986 Low molecular weight heparin in venous thrombosis during pregnancy. Br J Haematol 63: 605–606
53. Borg J Y, Vasse M 1991 Thrombosis prophylaxis in protein C and S deficient pregnant women: low molecular weight heparin management using prethrombotic markers as compared to normal pregnancies. Thromb Haemost 65: 1233
54. Hall J G, Pauli R M, Wilson K M 1980 Maternal and fetal sequelae of anticoagulation during pregnancy. Am J Med 68: 122–140
55. Iturbe-Alessio I, del Carmen Fonseca M, Mutchinik O, Santos M A, Zajarias A, Salazar E 1986 Risks of anticoagulant therapy in pregnant women with artificial heart valves. New Engl J Med 315: 1390–1393
56. Orme M, Lewis L E, de Swiet M J, Sibeon R, Baty J D, Breckenbridge A M 1977 May mothers given warfarin breast-feed their infants? Br Med J 1: 1564–1565
57. McKenna R, Cole E, Varsan L 1983 Warfarin sodium contra-indicated in the lactating mother? Pediatrics 103: 325–355
58. Fondevilla C G, Meschengieser S, Blanco Penalva L, Lazzari M A 1989 Effect of acenocoumarine on the breast-fed infant. Thromb Res 56: 29–36
59. Hux C H, Wapner R J, Chayen B, Rattan P, Jarrell B, Greenfield L 1986 Use of the Greenfield filter for thromboembolic disease in pregnancy. Am J Obstet Gynecol 155: 734–737
60. Lao T T, de Swiet M, Letsky E, Walters B N J 1985 Prophylaxis of thromboembolism in pregnancy: an alternative. Br J Obstet Gynaecol 92: 202–206
61. Badaracco M A, Vessey M 1974 Recurrence of venous thromboembolism disease and use of oral contraceptives. Br Med J 1: 215–217
62. Hellgren M, Hahn L, Dahlman T 1990 Thromboprophylaxis during pregnancy. Am J Obstet Gynecol 162: 1338–1339
63. Lubbe W F, Butler W S, Palmer S J et al 1983 Fetal survival after prednisone suppression of maternal lupus anticoagulant. Lancet 1: 1361–1363
64. Hirsh J, Dalen J E, Deykin D, Poller L 1992 Oral anticoagulants: mechanism of action, clinical effectiveness and optimal therapeutic range. Chest 102: 3125–3265

PART B
HEMORRHAGIC DISORDERS

M. Dreyfus G. Tertian G. Tchernia

INTRODUCTION

Dramatic changes occur in the platelet, coagulation and fibrinolytic systems during pregnancy, delivery and the post-partum period which reduce the inherent risk of hemorrhage resulting from the hemochorial system of human placentation. Knowledge of vascular and hemostatic changes developing throughout normal pregnancy and delivery provides a rational approach for diagnosis and treatment of pregnancy-associated hemorrhagic disorders.

PHYSIOLOGY OF THE HEMOSTATIC SYSTEM

Hemostasis depends upon the interaction of blood vessels, platelets and circulating blood proteins. It results from a complex interrelationship between activating and inhibitory pathways of both clot production and lysis.

The first triggering event is usually vascular injury, leading to the release of the endothelial constituents. The vascular endothelium plays a key role in hemostasis as it is an important source of serotonin, kinins, prostacyclin (PGI_2), von Willebrand factor (vWF), tissue factor, tissue plasminogen activator (tPA), and plasminogen activator inhibitors (PAIs).

Following vascular injury, vasoconstriction is achieved by contraction of precapillary sphincters or of the smooth muscles of small arteries and veins.

Hemostatic plug formation includes several steps outlined in Figure 55.1. Platelets, which do not react with intact vascular endothelium, *adhere* after vessel injury to subendothelial components. *Platelet activation* usually follows adhesion but can be triggered by circulating aggregating agents, such as thrombin generated during the coagulation process. Activated platelets undergo several changes leading to *secretion* of their components: mainly adenoisine diphosphate (ADP), which is involved in further platelet aggregation and serotonin, which induces vasoconstriction. There is a modification of the **repartition** of the membranous phospholipids leading to the external exposure of platelet factor 3, which is thereby available for the coagulation process. Platelet stimulation also triggers the activation of phospholipases present on the platelet membrane and the generation of arachidonic acid, with the subsequent initiation of the thromboxane A_2 (TXA_2) pathway (Fig. 55.2). TXA_2 is a potent aggregating and vasoconstricting agent that is secreted by stimulated platelets. To balance its activity, prostacyclin (PGI_2), a potent vasodilatator and antiaggregating agent, is simulta-

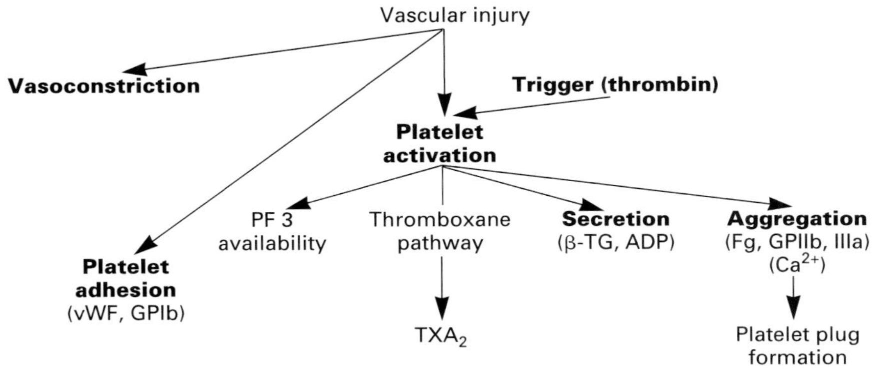

Fig. 55.1 First steps in hemostasis – platelet plug formation.

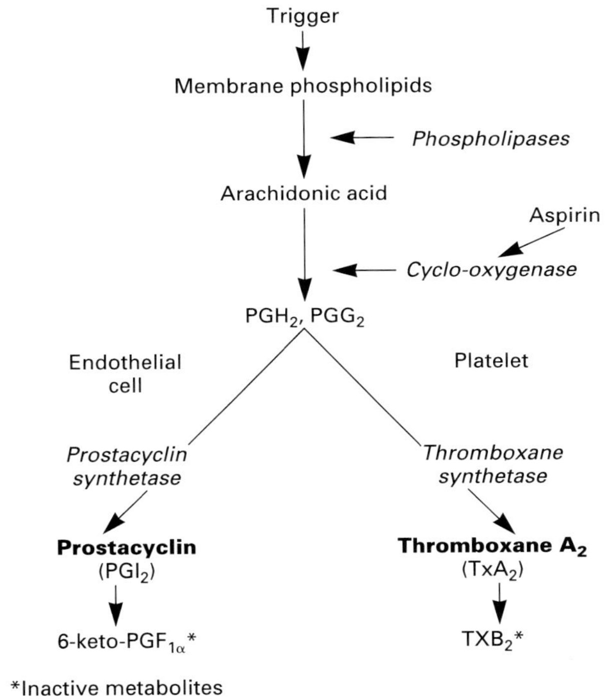

Fig. 55.2 Prostaglandin synthetic pathway in platelets and vascular endothelial cells.

neously produced by stimulated endothelial cells. *Platelet aggregation* is an active process resulting in an increase of the platelet plug at the site of injury and, therefore, in cessation of bleeding.

Blood coagulation is the result of complex enzymatic reactions involving plasma proteins called coagulation factors. They circulate as inactive zymogens that are transformed into enzymes upon activation, except factors V and VIII, which even after activation act only as co-factors in the enzymatic reactions. Owing to the very low plasma concentration of the clotting factors, most of these reactions take place on the surface of either activated platelets or endothelial cells, which allows concentration of coagulation factors.

Figure 55.3 shows the two different coagulation pathways and the successive steps leading to clot formation. The *extrinsic pathway* is triggered by tissue factor, either released from injured tissues or exposed at the surface of stimulated cells such as vascular endothelial cells. The *intrinsic pathway* is initiated by contact of blood with a foreign surface, such as basement membrane. The extrinsic and intrinsic systems lead to the activation of factor X. From this point on, they share the same pathway, leading to *thrombin formation*. Thrombin is a very potent, multifunctional enzyme: it not only induces fibrin formation but also activates factor XIII, responsible for fibrin clot stabilization. Thrombin causes platelet activation and aggregation and activates factors V and VIII, thus stimulating its own production. *Fibrin formation* is the last step of the coagulation process.

Coagulation regulation is achieved by potent inhibitors described extensively in Chapter 76. *Antithrombin III* neutralizes all the active coagulation enzymes except activated factor VII. As these reaction rates are increased in the presence of heparin, it is also called heparin co-factor. *Activated protein C* neutralizes activated factors V and VIII, the reaction being facilitated by the presence of phospholipids, Ca^{2+} and *protein S*, which is a plasmatic co-factor. Protein C activation requires thrombin, and *thrombomodulin*, a cellular co-factor present at the surface of endothelial cells.

Fibrinolysis is the dissolution of fibrin clots. It is achieved by the enzymatic digestion of fibrin by plasmin. Plasmin is a powerful proteolytic enzyme that is generated from plasminogen, an inactive plasma precursor. Plasminogen activators are of either plasma or tissue type (Fig. 55.4). Fibrin degradation products are released from fibrin clot after plasmin action.

The fibrinolysis system is also regulated by plasminogen activator inhibitors (PAIs) and plasmin inhibitors. PAI-1 in synthesized mainly by endothelial cells and megakaryocytes; PAI-2 is specifically synthesized by the placenta. The main plasmin inhibitor is α_2-antiplasmin.

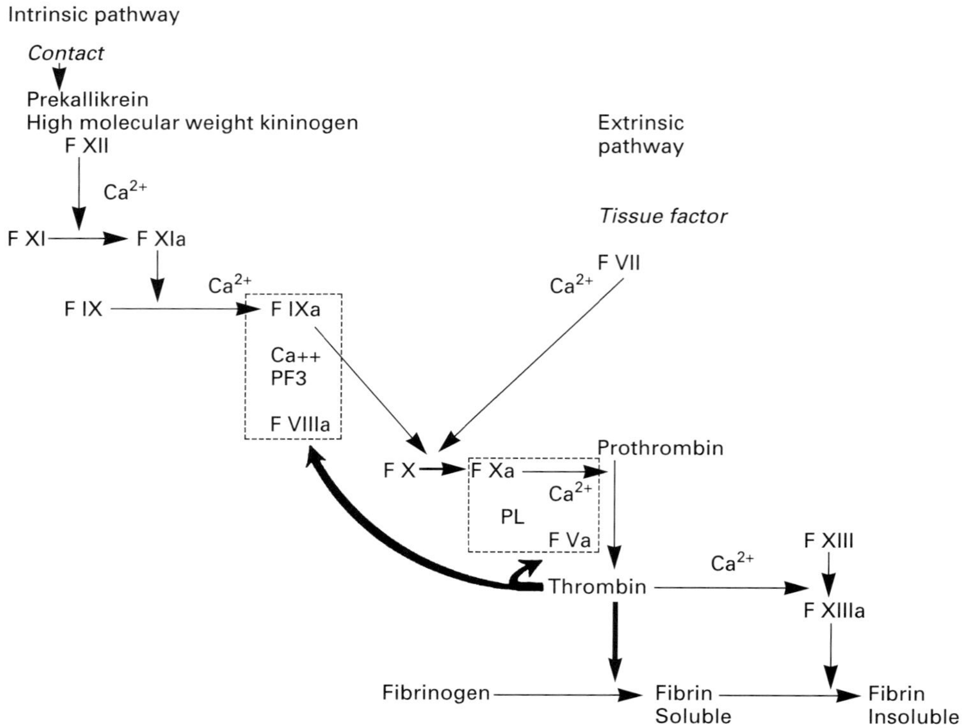

Fig. 55.3 Coagulation system.

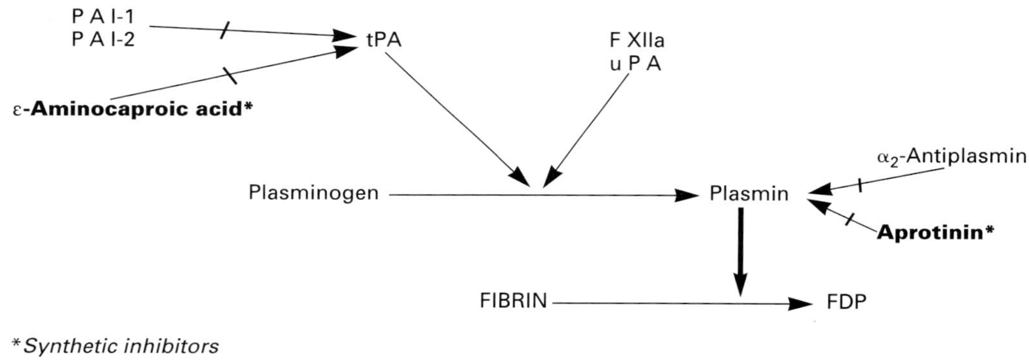

Fig. 55.4 Fibrinolysis.

HEMOSTATIC CHANGES OCCURRING DURING PREGNANCY

During pregnancy, the spiral arteries, which supply maternal blood to the placenta, undergo major changes: their elastic lamina and smooth muscle are replaced by a matrix containing mainly fibrin. These changes induce expansion of the lumen, allowing an increase in blood flow as pregnancy proceeds and facilitating the collapse of the terminal part of the spiral arteries during and after placental separation by the contraction of the myometrium.

From the end of the first trimester on, a dramatic rise in most of the clotting factors, mainly fibrinogen and factor VIII–vWF (Table 55.2),[1–3] is associated with an increase in platelet response to several aggregating agents, owing to an increased capacity of platelets to produce TXA_2.[4] There is a parallel decrease in protein S[5,6] and in fibrinolytic potential. PAI total activity increases consistently during the third trimester as a result of an increase in PAI-1 and the placental synthesis of PAI-2.[7,8] These modifications continue up to the termination of pregnancy, when they create an hypercoagulable state.[9]

During and immediately after delivery, the hemostatic system is activated, leading to a state very similar to mild compensated disseminated intravascular coagulation (DIC). Simultaneously, fibrinolytic activity returns to normal 15 min to 1 h after placental separation as a result of a dramatic decrease in PAI-1 and PAI-2.[7,10,11] These changes are thought to be needed to cope with the

Table 55.2 Major hemostatic changes during normal pregnancy

		Gestation (weeks)					
Ref.		11–15	26–30	36–40	Post-delivery	Post-natal	Non pregnant
1	Factor VII	111	158	171	134	94	
	(range)	(60–206)	(75–332)	(87–336)	(70–255)	(52–171)	
1	Factor VIII	122	188	212	206	95	
	(range)	(53–283)	(67–528)	(79–570)	(74–569)	(46–193)	
1	vWF Ag	133	203	376	421	89	
	(range)	(56–318)	(84–492)	(133–1064)	(169–1042)	(29–272)	
1	Fibrinogen	363	378	423	461	265	
	(range mg/100 1)	(264–500)	(267–535)	(290–615)	(298–714)	(171–411)	
2	Factor XI	93	77	64	56	76	94
	SD	23	18	8	14	10	15
3	Factor XIII			(35–75)			(75–125)
5	Protein S						
	(mg/1)	6.2	4.4		3.7	6.5	8.3
	SD	1.6	1.4		0.9	1.4	1.4

For factors VII, VIII, XI, XIII, and vWF Ag mean, range and SD values are expressed as a percentage of normal plasma.

modification of placental vasculature and with the hemorrhage of delivery. However, they can predispose pregnant women to develop either bleeding or thrombosis if the balance between clotting and fibrinolysis is disrupted by any abnormal condition.

HEMORRHAGIC DISORDERS

Hemorrhage has been for years the main cause of death in laboring women. Although the mortality rate has dropped dramatically in developed countries, and is low compared with the number of deaths from thromboembolism and hypertensive disease, hemorrhagic disorders remain important in terms of morbidity.[12–14]

HEMORRHAGIC DISORDERS OCCURRING DURING ABNORMAL PREGNANCIES

Disseminated intravascular coagulation (DIC)

Definition

Disseminated intravascular coagulation is the consequence of abnormal triggering of hemostatic and fibrinolytic systems. Depending on the triggering event, it can range in severity from a compensated state with no clinical manifestations but evidence of coagulation and fibrinolysis activation, to life-threatening, massive, uncontrollable hemorrhage with very low or undetectable levels of fibrinogen. In this syndrome, hemorrhage is obvious and often impressive. It may be associated with thrombosis, which although often insidious can lead to irreversible organ damage or death.

Mechanisms

Recent experimental data indicate that the pathophysiologic pathway of DIC is relatively homogenous in all disease states, and results mainly from the release or availability of tissue thromboplastin (TTP) or TTP-like substances.[15] TTP may be released from the placenta after premature separation; TTP-like substances may be infused into the maternal circulation during parturition in the case of amniotic fluid embolism or released from the fetus 3–5 weeks after intrauterine death.

During infections, the triggering event is more likely to be an insult to the vascular endothelium, resulting in the release from injured endothelial cells of factors inducing vasoconstriction, clotting and fibrinolysis activation. Such insult also exposes the subendothelial structures to the flowing blood, thereby promoting platelet adhesion and activation.

Whatever the triggering event, it leads to platelet, coagulation and fibrinolytic activation as outlined in Figure 55.5. Clinical and biological consequences of DIC are shown in Figure 55.6.

Platelet activation leads to formation of platelet plugs and thrombocytopenia. *Coagulation activation* leads to formation of fibrin monomers, which can associate either with fibrinogen or with fibrin degradation products (FDPs) to generate soluble fibrin complexes. When there is an overproduction of fibrin monomers, or if stasis occurs, the monomers accumulate and form fibrin fibers. Coagulation factors consumed in coagulation (factor V, factor II, factor VIII and fibrinogen) are decreased, whereas thrombin formation may be evident by the detection of thrombin–antithrombin complexes (TAT) and fibrinopeptide A (FPA). Inhibitors may also be consumed during the coagulation process, leading to a decrease in AT III and/or protein C.

Fibrin formation, together with platelet plug formation, results in micro- or macrovascular obstruction and thrombosis. Schizocytes detected on blood smears are indicative of red blood cell fragmentation on fibrin fibers.

The concomitant *activation of fibrinolysis* leads to throm-

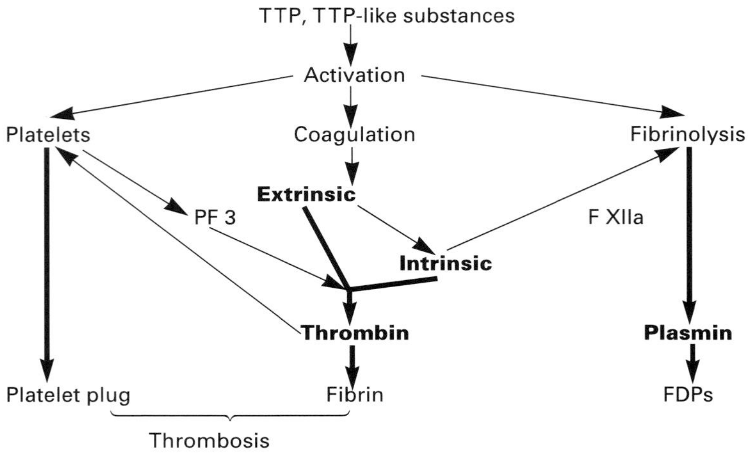

Fig. 55.5 Interrelationships between platelet, coagulation and fibrinolytic systems.

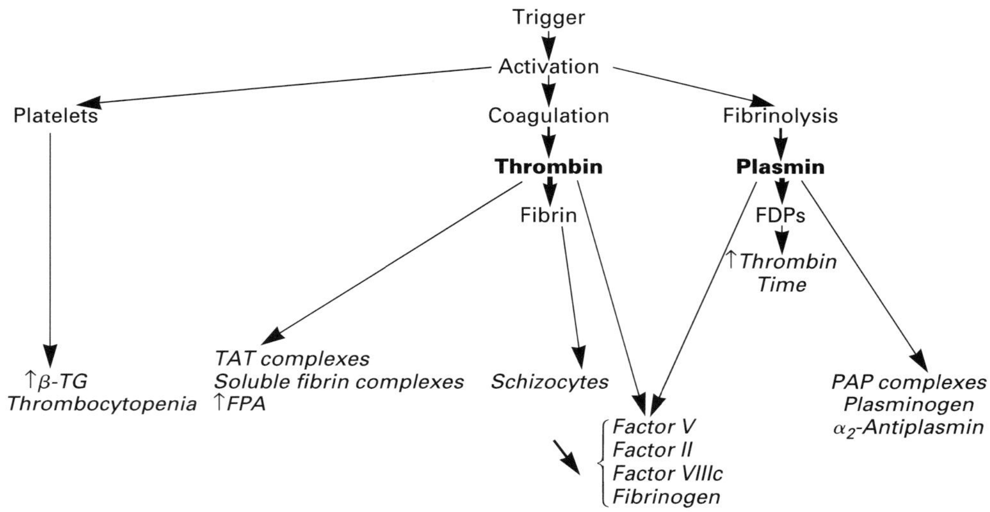

Fig. 55.6 DIC-induced biologic abnormalities.

bolysis, but also to plasmin-induced degradation of coagulation factors, thereby enhancing their depletion in plasma. Plasminogen and α_2-antiplasmin are depleted during this process and plasmin–antiplasmin complexes (PAP) may be detected. Fibrin degradation products can be assessed specifically using antibodies to cross-linked fragment D (D-dimer). FDPs induce specific inhibition of platelet aggregation and fibrin polymerization. They therefore enhance the bleeding tendency due to hemostatic failure.

Factors indicating a poor prognosis

- Defective reticuloendothelial capacity associated with pregnancy has been shown experimentally to be an aggravating factor in DIC.
- Venostasis is also present during pregnancy and allows the stagnation of activated platelets and of fibrin monomers thereby favoring the formation of platelet aggregates and fibrin polymerization.
- Decreased levels of free protein S and the defective fibrinolytic system associated with the late stages of pregnancy further contribute to lowering the mechanisms of defense.

Hence, all the factors that contribute to the severity of DIC are associated with the late stages of pregnancy.

Diagnosis

Biologic diagnosis is very often prompted in emergency situations, under circumstances that do not allow performance of long or sophisticated hemostatic studies. However, an accurate diagnosis can be achieved using simple tests that can be reliably carried out in any center. In our hands, a decrease in the fibrinogen level (< 2.7g/1) has proved to be the earliest and more constant sign of

DIC. Its association with one of the following abnormalities allows one to ascertain the diagnosis:

- Thrombocytopenia ($< 150 \times 10^9$/l) may be absent at the onset of the syndrome, especially during acute DIC associated with placental abruption. It is usually moderate and transient, disappearing within a few days after delivery and resolution of coagulation abnormalities. The occurrence of severe ($< 50 \times 10^9$/l) and prolonged thrombocytopenia is highly suggestive of infection.
- A low level of factor V (< 60%), or an elevated level of FDP (> 40 μg/ml) or D-dimer (> 1 μg/ml).
- When available, thrombin time can be of great help, as thrombin time prolongation is highly suggestive of the presence of FDPs.
- In contrast, prothrombin time (PT) and activated partial thromboplastin time (aPTT) are often normal during the early stages of DIC. Because of the high level of most clotting factors in the late stages of pregnancy, even a marked decrease may result in values that would be considered as normal in nonpregnant women.
- A decrease in antithrombin III activity has been reported to be the most sensitive indicator, with decreased levels in 89% of patients with DIC;[16] an AT III assay may thus be useful to ascertain the diagnosis when it is not obvious.

These biologic abnormalities usually progress very rapidly (within a few hours), to an acute state in which fibrinogen is no longer detectable. Early detection of DIC onset, which can be achieved by monitoring platelet and fibrinogen levels in complicated pregnancies, is mandatory.

Clinical signs

The clinical disorders induced by DIC are associated with those of the underlying disease (listed in Table 55.3) and constitute a wide spectrum of different clinical pictures that have recently been extensively reviewed.[13,16] Our aim is to focus on the main clinical features that should lead to suspicion of hemostatic failure.

Abnormal bleeding from exposed wounds, such as the site of venipuncture, cesarean delivery or the placental bed, is most likely to occur in fulminant DIC. It can be associated with bruising or hematomas, epistaxis or hemorrhage of central venous system or gastrointestinal tract. Placental abruption or premature placental separation, in which blood continues to flow to the placental site at a rate of 500–800 ml/min can provoke a state of hypovolemic shock which is fatal within a few hours after the onset of the symptoms if treatment is not prompt.

Thrombosis is rare but may be prominent in patients with septicemia or hypotension. It involves microvessels and may result in lesions resembling those of purpura fulminans, localized to the extremities and sometimes to the face. It may lead to necrosis of the tips of fingers or toes, and sometimes of nose or ears.

Ischemic damage of various organs suggested by diffuse cerebral symptoms or renal failure may occur. It is often difficult to determine whether it is due to extensive microvascular thrombosis or hypoperfusion during hypovolemic shock. Whatever the etiology, the outcome may be irreversible organ damage or death.

Table 55.3 Obstetric conditions associated with DIC

Placental abruption, premature separation of the placenta
Eclampsia–preeclampsia
Sepsis
Placenta accreta
Amniotic fluid embolism
Retention of a dead fetus
Hydatidiform mole

Treatment

Owing to the wide range of biologic and clinical abnormalities, the treatment of obstetric DIC is far from standardized. Nevertheless, there is general agreement concerning the guidelines for therapy.

1. As DIC is always secondary to an obstetric complication, the best treatment lies in the removal or treatment of the triggering process. Therefore, its identification is of primordial importance: when no obvious etiology is discovered, uterine inspection and revision must be carried out, looking for a small undiagnosed vaginal or uterine laceration likely to keep stimulating the DIC. At the same time, broad-spectrum antibiotics must be administered, even though no clinical symptoms of infection arise.

   Treatment of the cause of DIC can be achieved in most cases after emptying the uterus. This must be done as an emergency procedure, whatever the stage of pregnancy, as maternal DIC will most probably worsen with time and fetal distress will undoubtably ensue. Myometrial contraction greatly reduces bleeding from the placental site and spontaneous correction of the hemostatic defects occurs – usually shortly after delivery. However, persistence of clots filling up the uterus may contribute to the development of uterine atony, thereby enhancing the bleeding tendency. That is why delivery must be associated with procedures favoring uterine contraction such as massage of the uterus or injection of oxytocics or prostaglandins (PGF_2).[17]
2. Prevention of hypovolemic shock can be achieved using blood derivatives and/or plasma expanders.
3. Replacement therapy aimed at correcting at least

partly the hemostatic failure is still controversial, some authors fearing to 'add fuel to fire'. However, in most patients with acute DIC, with little if any detectable fibrinogen, massive blood transfusions using only packed red blood cells and plasma expanders will induce a dilution, thereby further aggravating the hemostatic failure. In these cases, replacement therapy of missing hemostatic factors is proposed, using either viro-activated fresh-frozen plasma (FFP) or plasma concentrates devoid of activated factors such as some types of fibrinogen concentrates. **The use of prothrombin complex concentrates (PCCs), which contain activated factors, is definitely contraindicated**. Transfusion of platelet concentrates should be restricted to patients with severe thrombocytopenia ($< 50 \times 10^9$ or $< 80 \times 10^9$/l in case of associated surgery).

4. Injection of aprotinin, an analog of α_2-antiplasmin, may prove useful in reducing the hemorrhagic tendency as it corrects the plasma anti-plasmin deficiency without inhibiting tissue plasmin generation.
5. The use of heparin is very controversial. It has been proved to be ineffective in preventing necrosis induced by infectious DIC.[18] Furthermore, in obstetric situations associated with life-threatening hemorrhages or with abnormal placental insertion, it should be delayed till cessation of bleeding and correction of hemostatic failure. It should therefore be restricted to low-grade DIC, especially when the onset occurs a long time prior to delivery, such as when there is retention of a dead fetus. In contrast, heparin therapy must be used for the prevention of secondary thromboembolic disease, initiated soon after DIC recovery.
6. Infusion of antithrombin III concentrates has been advocated; limited information suggests that it may be effective, but more data are needed before this can be confirmed.[19]
7. The occurrence of DIC in the mother is associated with a high incidence of severe complications in the fetus. Usually this is because of a deficient nutrient supply to the fetus as a result of an impaired placental circulation. Hence, hypovolemic shock occurring in infected or bleeding mothers or premature placental separation may result in acute fetal distress and death; DIC-induced placental microthrombi may lead to chronic fetal distress with intrauterine growth retardation and stillbirth. Therefore, assessment of the fetal status is of primary importance and includes:

   - Monitoring of the fetal heart rate. Detection of abnormalities must promptly lead to emergency cesarean delivery, which can be life-saving for the fetus.
   - At birth, blood coagulation must be assessed in an attempt to detect signs of DIC. It has been established experimentally that neither TTP, TTP-like substances, activated factors nor degradation products can be transferred from the mother to the fetus through the placenta.[20] Thus, neonatal DIC is due to an underlying neonatal disease, such as fetal distress or infection, which must be detected. In the absence of any obvious etiology, maternofetal infection is suspected and treatment with antibiotics must be initiated, before availability of the results of the bacteriologic studies.

Preeclampsia and eclampsia

Hemostatic changes reported in women with preeclampsia suggest hemostasis activation and a mild degree of DIC, thus supporting the theory of Roberts[21] that preeclampsia could be secondary to an endothelial cell injury.

Markers of platelet activation and consumption (thrombocytopenia, increased level of circulating β-thromboglobulin) are associated with signs of mild DIC such as an increased vWF Ag to VIIIC ratio and a decreased level of AT III.[22,23] The latter has recently been demonstrated to be the result of an increased consumption, leading to a reduction in the half-life of infused AT III.[24] Furthermore, preeclamptic women have been reported to have a reduced fibrinolytic potential as compared with normal pregnant women. Recent data show that this is due to an increase in the level of PAI-1, resulting in increased PAI capacity. These abnormalities correlate well with the severity of placental damage as assessed by the degree of infarction and by the placental weight, and with the intrauterine growth retardation assessed by the infant birth weight.[8]

An increased ratio of TXA_2 to prostacyclin has also been described, and some recent data suggest a major role for the imbalance of the prostaglandin system in pregnancy-induced hypertension,[25] since treatment with low-dose aspirin has a favorable preventive effect on women supposed to be at high risk.[26,27]

Most patients are readily treated by delivery and recovery is usually rapid and complete.

HELLP syndrome

The HELLP syndrome was described for the first time by Weinstein[28] as a variant of severe preeclampsia associating mechanical hemolysis (H) with an elevated liver enzyme level (EL) and a low platelet count (LP). Whether it is a variant of severe preeclampsia or an early form of the disease is still controversial. An analysis of 300 cases has recently been published, allowing a more precise description of this syndrome:[29,30]

- Its prevalence is 9% among patients with eclampsia or preeclampsia.
- It usually occurs (69%) before term (< 36 weeks). However, its onset may be delayed till the first four post-partum days.
- It typically develops in women around 25 years of age. Most of them complain at admission of malaise, epigastric or right upper-quadrant pain, sometimes associated with nausea, vomiting and headache; clinical and biologic signs of eclampsia and preeclampsia may be few or absent.
- Biologic abnormalities include a low platelet count ($< 100 \times 10^9/1$), mechanical hemolysis evidenced by the presence of fragmented red blood cells on the peripheral smear, increased bilirubin and lactate dehydrogenase levels, and increased liver enzymes (serum glutamate oxaloacetic transaminase more than 3 SDs (standard deviation) higher than the normal local mean). Associated DIC has been reported in 38% of patients.
- There is a high maternal and perinatal rate of morbidity and mortality: the mortality prevalence ranges from 0–24% in mothers and from 7.7–60% in newborns.
- Owing to the poor outcome, patients with HELLP syndrome associated with DIC should be delivered within 48 h, irrespective of gestational age. In the absence of signs of DIC and fetal lung maturity, treatment may be initiated in an attempt to postpone delivery. This will include bed rest, infusion of plasma expanders, antithrombotic agents and corticosteroid administration in order to promote fetal lung maturation. However, serial maternal and fetal assessments have to be repeated during this period in order to perform immediate delivery in case of maternal or fetal distress.

Thrombotic thrombocytopenic purpura

This is defined by a pentad of biological and clinical findings including thrombocytopenia, microangiopathic hemolytic anemia, neurologic dysfunction, fever and renal failure. Over 40 cases have been described, occurring at any stage of the pregnancy.[31] Some patients may relapse during subsequent pregnancies having been asymptomatic in the interim. This syndrome shares with eclampsia and preeclampsia the characteristics of thrombotic microangiopathy.[32] Though they are almost impossible to differentiate on the basis of clinical findings or biopsy specimens, DIC is present only in preeclampsia. An accurate diagnosis is mandatory as the treatment is completely different, and in the absence of early adequate therapy placental infarcts will develop, leading to intrauterine growth retardation and fetal death. Plasma therapy, perhaps coupled with corticosteroids or anti-platelet agents, is the treatment of choice for thrombotic thrombocytopenic purpura. Recently, pregnant women treated this way have carried to term with the delivery of healthy infants.[33]

HEMORRHAGIC DISORDERS OCCURRING DURING NORMAL PREGNANCIES

They are mainly due to congenital or acquired hemorrhagic diseases.

Constitutional hemostatic disorders

Platelet disorders

Pregnancy in patients with constitutional platelet disorders raises two problems:

1. Management of pregnancy and delivery in the mother. A few pregnancies in women with Glanzmann's thrombasthenia have been reported.[34] Bleeding problems occur mainly during and after delivery and can be overcome by the transfusion of platelet concentrates. The same therapy can be used in women with other kinds of platelet dysfunctions or constitutional thrombocytopenia; in these cases, transfusion of platelet concentrates can be prescribed depending on the degree of the hemostatic failure assessed by a standardized bleeding time.
2. Management of the newborn. When transmission of the platelet disorder is autosomal, it can be inherited by the newborn, thereby resulting in a theoretical risk of hemorrhage at childbirth. Therefore, cesarean delivery should be performed when there is a prolonged labor or a risk of traumatic delivery. Anti-platelet antibodies directed against specific platelet antigens that are lacking in Glanzmann's disease, such as HPA-1a (human platelet antigen), HPA-3a, can develop after platelet transfusions in mothers. The mother's serum must be checked for the presence of such antibodies, which can induce severe alloimmune thrombocytopenia in the offspring.

Plasma disorders

The most frequent plasma disorder is *von Willebrand disease* (vWd), characterized by qualitative or quantitative abnormalities of von Willebrand factor (vWF). vWF is involved in the first step of platelet plug formation (Fig. 55.1). It circulates in plasma as a multimeric complex, associated with factor VIIIC. vWd is heterogeneous and has been classified into several types according to the multimeric structure of vWF;[35] the largest multimers are the most active in promoting platelet adhesion. In type I, the multimeric composition of vWF is normal and there is a concomitant decrease in factor VIIIC and vWF whether it is assessed by immunologic (vWF Ag) or functional techniques (bleeding time or ristocetin co-factor activity, vWF RCO). Type II vWd is characterized by the absence of large multimers of vWF circulating in blood; factor VIIIc and vWF Ag may be normal or only slightly decreased, contrasting with a low undetectable level of vWF RCO. Type II has been further subdivided into subtypes, of which type IIB is characterized by an increased affinity of vWF for GPIb, its platelet receptor: it results in spontaneous platelet clumping and thrombocytopenia.

During pregnancy, the progressive increase in factor VIIIC/vWF leads in classic (type I) vWd to a partial or complete correction of biologic abnormalities. In contrast, in vWd variants (type II), the increase in abnormal forms of vWF results in persistence of biologic abnormalities, and a risk of hemorrhage during or after delivery. Marked thrombocytopenia has been described in type IIB variants, which can be misleading in women whose vWd was unknown before pregnancy.[36]

Correction of most of the biologic abnormalities, including thrombocytopenia in variant IIB, can be achieved before delivery or in the case of bleeding by the infusion of concentrates containing highly polymerized vWF.[37]

As transmission is autosomal dominant, the fetus may inherit the same type of disease in a more or less severe form; hence, route of delivery must be decided in order to avoid any birth trauma. Bleeding in the newborn can also be treated by infusing vWF concentrate.

Because of the physiologic increase in factor VIII or IX occurring during pregnancy, *hemophilia carriers* are at no risk of bleeding at delivery. Nevertheless, their status has to be considered, as bleeding prevention in the infant at birth may be necessary. In addition, the parents may require genetic counseling.

In contrast, the physiologic decrease in *factor XIII* and *factor XI* observed during pregnancy may cause problems in pregnant women who are deficient, even in those with mild deficiency.

Acquired bleeding defects

Autoimmune thrombocytopenic purpura (AITP)

Chronic AITP is related to inappropriate synthesis of anti-platelet antibodies resulting in an exaggerated destruction and phagocytosis of antibody-coated platelets by macrophages, mostly in the spleen.

Diagnosis may be difficult to establish during pregnancy as the half-life study of radiolabeled platelets, which is actually the most specific diagnostic tool, cannot be performed. Increased levels of platelet-associated immunoglobulins (PAIgG), detected in 90% of patients, are not specific to AITP. Serum anti-platelet antibodies can be detected in 50% of patients. A suspicion of this diagnosis arises in the absence of a previous history of AITP, when an isolated thrombocytopenia is discovered at an early stage of an uncomplicated pregnancy. Other causes of thrombocytopenia, such as systemic lupus erythematosus, viral infections (human immunodeficiency virus, Epstein – Barr virus, cytomegalovirus), or drugs, must be ruled out in order to support the diagnosis.

The association of pregnancy with AITP raises several problems.

The prevention of hemorrhagic accidents in mothers. Management of thrombocytopenic mothers has considerably improved since the 1950s. At that time the maternal mortality rate was high and the issues were whether or not these patients should be advised not to conceive and whether pregnancy should be terminated or emergency splenectomy performed. Now most of the maternal problems have been resolved and no thrombocytopenia-related maternal deaths have been reported in the last three decades.

Pregnancy may increase the severity of thrombocytopenia, particularly during the last weeks of pregnancy, with a rapid increase to basic pre-pregnancy level within a few days after delivery. In contrast, AITP does not seem to influence the course of pregnancy, though some cases of intrauterine fetal death have been reported, but with no evidence of any relationship with the hematologic disorder.[38]

Correction of platelet count must be attempted before delivery in order to prevent hemorrhagic complications. It can be achieved either by initiating steroid therapy at least 1 week prior to delivery or by infusing intravenous IgG.[39,40] Different schedules of intravenous IgG have been proposed: all provide a frequent and rapid, though transient, improvement and are usually very well tolerated.

In the case of failure of these treatments, cesarean delivery appears to be the safest method, supported by platelet infusions, although their efficiency is very poor in such cases. Furthermore, because of the short half-life of platelets, infusions have to be repeated 2–3 times a day.

The detection of fetal thrombocytopenia. Maternal anti-platelet antibodies, when they are of the IgG class, can cross the placenta and induce thrombocytopenia in the fetus. When severe, thrombocytopenia carries a risk of hemorrhagic complications. Antenatal bleeding seems to be very rare, far less frequent than in alloimmune thrombocytopenia. In contrast, the trauma linked to labor and childbirth may lead to intracerebral hemorrhage and thus to death or severe neurologic impairment. Therefore, efforts have been made to predict, to prevent, or to detect, a severe neonatal thrombocytopenia.

Is fetal thrombocytopenia predictable? The maternal platelet count does not give any indication; it has been shown that it does not correlate with fetal platelet count. Severe thrombocytopenia can be observed in the offspring of mothers with either mild thrombocytopenia or normal platelet count. This status can be the result of a compensatory increased bone marrow platelet production, masking the ongoing increased destruction mediated by anti-platelet antibodies. For this reason, a past history of platelet disorders or bleeding episodes should be sought by all anesthesiologists even though the routine biologic status appears to be normal. Women who have experienced AITP in the past (including during infancy) should be advised that subsequent pregnancies, even after years of normalization of platelet count, will require an adapted follow-up.

- The rate of thrombocytopenia in offspring is the same whether or not the mother has undergone splenectomy in the past.
- Maternal PAIgG level has no predictive value.
- Anti-platelet antibody titer in mothers' serum has been shown by some authors to correlate with the degree of fetal thrombocytopenia,[41] but this finding has not yet been confirmed.[42]

In conclusion, there is no reliable maternal parameter that will predict the occurrence and severity of fetal thrombocytopenia.

Is fetal thrombocytopenia preventable? Antenatal maternal treatment, if shown to be effective, without any adverse effect in mothers or fetuses, would be ideal. Unfortunately, the results of trials have, to date, been rather disappointing.

Low doses of steroid administered to the mother have been claimed to be effective in preventing fetal thrombocytopenia in a small group of patients.[43] Subsequently, many groups have experienced negative results using the same protocol. Moreover, it has been shown that such a treatment might not only decrease PAIgG but also increase free serum anti-platelet antibody that could cross the placenta and aggravate thrombocytopenia in the fetus.[44]

High-dose intravenous IgG infused into thrombocytopenic mothers prior to delivery, although efficient in elevating maternal platelet count, have no effect on fetal platelet count.[44] However, it has been suggested that the failure of this treatment might be attributed to the very slow transplacental transfer of IgG. Thus, a more rigorous and prolonged antenatal treatment with intravenous IgG could be more efficient.

Owing to the low prevalence of severe thrombocytopenia at birth, the efficacy of antenatal treatment can only be assessed by comparing platelet counts in fetal samples drawn before and after treatment. Such controls have been performed in small series and failed to demonstrate any effect of either steroid or intravenous IgG therapies.[42]

Is fetal thrombocytopenia detectable? The prevalence of severe thrombocytopenia (platelets $< 50 \times 10^9$/l) in the offspring of mothers with AITP has been estimated to be 10–20%. In order to protect these infants from labor or injuries during vaginal delivery, some authors have proposed performing cesarean delivery in all parturients who have had AITP. This attitude has led to many unnecessary cesarean deliveries. Therefore, during the past 5 years, techniques have been developed to diagnose severe fetal thrombocytopenia before delivery:

- Scalp blood sampling, described by Ayromlooi in 1978,[45] has been widely used since. It can be used to obtain a fetal platelet count during labor. However, this procedure has its drawbacks: it does not prevent potential fetal injury caused by the start of labor and may be irrelevant when delivery occurs while waiting for the results. Furthermore, fetal scalp blood samples are often contaminated with amniotic fluid and/or vernix caseosa, leading to in vitro platelet activation and to spuriously low platelet counts. The incidence of artifactual thrombocytopenia increased in most of the groups when fetal scalp blood sampling was done routinely, and there is now general agreement that this procedure should be abandoned.
- Percutaneous umbilical blood sampling (PUBS) was first described in 1983.[46] It can be performed during the last weeks of pregnancy prior to the onset of labor. It is reliable as the results correlate well with those of cord blood or post-natal samplings.[42] However, it is an invasive procedure with an overall estimated fetal lethal risk ranging from 0–2%; it can only be performed in reference tertiary centers and must be undertaken in a labor or delivery suite so that an emergency cesarean delivery can be performed if necessary.

Finally, there is no general agreement concerning the need to detect fetal thrombocytopenia. Several authors have argued that the low prevalence of severe thrombocytopenia and the low frequency of intracranial bleeding mean that no active procedure is necessary.[47]

The management of newborns with thrombocytopenia. Whatever the platelet count at birth, it may decrease during the first post-natal days, with a nadir on days 4–6. Thrombocytopenia is always transient and disappears spontaneously when maternal antibodies are eliminated, within 10–60 days. Platelet counts must be performed every other day until a significant increase is observed.

Post-natal bleeding is usually rare, moderate and easy to control. When moderate bleeding is associated with severe thrombocytopenia, intravenous IgG infusions may be successful in elevating the platelet count.[48]

Infants at risk of developing severe intracranial hemorrhage are those who exhibited severe antenatal thrombocytopenia and who have undergone a traumatic labor; intrauterine growth retardation and prematurity are additional risk factors. In such cases treatment with intravenous infusions (0.4 g kg^{-1} day^{-1} for 5 days or 1 g kg^{-1} day^{-1}) is mandatory. Low doses of steroids can be considered as they may have a protective effect by enhancing the vascular tone.

In the most severe cases, when there is an obvious life-threatening hemorrhage, blood exchange must be performed, using fresh blood, where platelets are still functional.

Pregnancy-associated thrombocytopenia

Some pregnant women exhibit a moderate, unexplained thrombocytopenia. It occurs mainly during the last trimester and resolves spontaneously after delivery, but may recur at any time during the course of another pregnancy. As no clinical effect has been demonstrated in mother or child, it has been called either asymptomatic thrombocytopenia (AST) or pregnancy-associated thrombocytopenia (PAT).[49,50] The reported prevalence ranges from 2–4% in normal pregnancies. Its management remains a matter of controversy, mainly because there is no reliable way of distinguishing it from AITP detected during the course of pregnancy. It has been suggested that women should be considered to be at risk of having AITP if their platelet count is lower than 70 × 10^9/1.[50] In contrast, women developing a moderate thrombocytopenia during the last trimester of their pregnancy should be considered to have AST or PAT: in these cases, the avoidance of any invasive procedure and vaginal delivery is recommended.

Drug-induced hemostatic abnormalities

Heparin and aspirin are well known to induce hemostatic abnormalities which have to be assessed repeatedly. However, we would like to point out the side-effects of other drugs, listed in Table 55.4, which may also result in the development of hemostatic abnormalities in mothers and/or newborns.

Table 55.4 Drugs inducing hemostatic abnormalities

In mother and fetus	
Rifampicin	Vitamin K deficiency
Cholestyramine	
Paraffin oil	
Latamoxef	
Aspirin	Inhibition of platelet aggregation
In mother alone	
Heparin	Anti-thrombin, anti-Xa activities
In fetus alone	
Anti-convulsants	Vitamin K deficiency
Barbiturates	

CONCLUSION

In conclusion, early detection of hemostatic disorders is the best way to prevent hemorrhagic complications. Because of the physiologic changes occurring during pregnancy, detection of inherited moderate abnormalities may be difficult before delivery. For this reason we would advise performance of a two-step hemostatic study.

The first step should take place during the first trimester and include standard preoperative tests such as platelet count, prothrombin time and activated partial thromboplastin time. More specific tests such as specific clotting factor assays or bleeding time should be performed in addition when a personal or familial bleeding tendency has been disclosed by a previous questionnaire and/or physical examination.

The second step should be devoted to the detection of hemostatic disorders acquired during pregnancy whether or not they are linked with obstetric pathology. A platelet count and fibrinogen assay should be performed in all patients, associated with other tests in when a specific pathology is suspected.

Information drawn from this two-step study should provide a good assessment of potential hazards linked to epidural anesthesia and delivery in mothers, and to birth in newborns.

CASE REPORT (to illustrate possible problems)

A 31-year-old, primigravida, nulliparous woman was admitted in the 41st week of an uneventful pregnancy. Owing to an inefficient labor associated with signs of acute fetal distress, she underwent cesarean delivery. Abnormal bleeding occurred during surgery and persisted for 4 h after delivery, necessitating massive blood transfusions. A preoperative coagulation study showed evidence of thrombocytopenia and hypofibrinogenemia (Table 55.5),

Table 55.5 Coagulation studies in the mother

	Prior to surgery	Post surgery				
		Hour 1	Hour 9	Day 3	Day 4	Day 5
Platelets (× 10^9/1)	80	270	80	65	60	150
PT (%)	75	37	34	65	66	80
Factor V (%)	ND	42	40	62	100	100
Factor II (%)	ND	40	58	66	67	85
Fibrinogen (mg/100 ml)	220	95	175	345	470	440
FDPs (μg/ml)	ND	600	80	ND	ND	ND

↑ FFP (after surgery)
Iniprol, Platelet concentrates ←→ (Hour 1 to Hour 9)

ND = not done.

Table 55.6 Coagulation studies in the newborn

	Hour 7	Normal range
Platelets ($\times 10^9$/l)	100	200–400
Factor V (%)	78	56–116
Factors VII and X (%)	34	26–70
Factor II (%)	40	24–88
Fibrinogen (mg/100 ml)	130	160–400
FDPs (μg/ml)	5	<10

whereas intra- and post-operative results exhibited all the features of typical DIC. In the absence of clinical signs of infection, eclampsia–preeclampsia or any other pregnancy-associated complication, the DIC remained unexplained. The hemorrhaging was controlled with the transfusion of 8 units of packed red blood cells (pRBC), 7 units of fresh-frozen plasma (FFP) and 10 units of platelet concentrates. In the meantime, aprotinin therapy was initiated with Iniprol injections: a starting dose of 3 million units followed by serial injections of 1 million units every half hour, then every hour.

The offspring was a girl weighing 3440 g, whose Apgar score was 5 at 1 min and 9 at 5 min. At 3 h of age, her status suddenly deteriorated, and she was transferred to the neonatal intensive care unit. Hemostasis tests performed at hour 7 were suggestive of the onset of DIC (Table 55.6). Shortly thereafter she experienced irreversible shock, leading to death.

Bacteriologic samples from mother and infant were retrospectively found to be positive for *Escherichia coli.* The maternal course was further complicated by the occurrence of secondary infected hematomas, requiring additional surgery.

In this case, the absence of any obvious etiology should have prompted the suspicion of maternofetal infection and the initiation of broad-spectrum antibiotic therapy in mother and child. This experience led us to introduce our current protocol, which includes:

- Systematic broad-spectrum antibiotics in mothers and children in cases of unexplained maternal DIC;
- Systematic coagulation studies in infants born to mothers exhibiting DIC prior to delivery.

REFERENCES

1. Stirling Y, Woolf L, North W R S, Seghatchian M J, Meade T W 1984 Hemostasis in normal pregnancy. Thromb Haemost 152: 176–182.
2. Hellgren M, Blombäck M 1981 Studies on blood coagulation and fibrinolysis in pregnancy, during delivery and in the puerperium. I. Normal condition. Gynecol Obstet Invest 12: 141–154
3. Hathaway W E, Bonnar J 1978 Perinatal coagulation. Grune & Stratton, New York
4. Andrews N P, Broughton Pipkin F, Heptinstall S 1985 Blood platelet behaviour in mothers and neonates. Thromb Haemost 53: 428–432
5. Comp P C, Thurnau G R, Welsh J, Esmon C T 1986 Functional and immunologic protein S levels are decreased during pregnancy. Blood 68: 881–885
6. Malm J, Laurell M, Dahlbäck B 1988 Changes in the plasma levels of vitamin K-dependent proteins C and S and of C4b-binding protein during pregnancy and oral conceptions. Br J Haematol 68: 437–443
7. Jorgensen M, Philips M, Thorsen S, Selmer J, Zeuthen J 1987 Plasminogen activator inhibitor-1 is the primary inhibitor of tissue-type plasminogen activator in pregnancy plasma. Thromb Haemost 58: 872–887
8. Estelles A, Gilabert J, Aznar J, Loskutof D J, Schleef R R 1989 Changes in the plasma levels of type 1 and type 2 plasminogen activator inhibitors in normal pregnancy and in patients with severe preeclampsia. Blood 74: 1332–1338
9. Gerbasi F R, Bottoms S, Farag A 1990 Increased intravascular coagulation associated with pregnancy. Obstet Gynecol 75: 385–389
10. Dahlman T, Hellgren M, Blombäck M 1985 Changes in blood coagulation and fibrinolysis in the normal puerperium. Gynecol Obstet Invest 20: 37–44
11. Gerbasi F R, Bottoms S, Farag A, Mammen E F 1990 Changes in hemostasis activity during delivery and the immediate postpartum period. Am J Obstet Gynecol 162: 1158–1163
12. Boulton F E, Letsky E 1985 Obstetric haemorrhage: causes and management. Clin Haematol 14: 683–728
13. Finley B E 1989 Acute coagulopathy in pregnancy. Med Clin Nth Am 73: 723–743
14. Hathaway W E, Bonnar J 1987 Hemostatic disorders of the pregnant woman and newborn infant. Elsevier, New York
15. Müller-Berghaus G 1989 Pathophysiologic and biochemical events in disseminated intravascular coagulation: dysregulation of procoagulant and anticoagulant pathways. Semin Thromb Hemost 15: 59–87
16. Bick R L 1988 Disseminated intravascular coagulation and related syndromes: a clinical review. Semin Thromb Hemost 14: 299–338
17. Cruikshank S H 1986 Management of post partum and pelvic hemorrhage. Clin Obstet Gynecol 29: 213–219
18. Corrigan Jr J J 1977 Heparin therapy in bacterical septicemia. J Pediatr 91: 695–700
19. Owen J 1991 Antithrombin III replacement therapy in pregnancy. Semin Hematol 28: 46–52
20. Bishop A J, Israels L G, Chernick V, Israels E D 1971 Placental transfer of intravascular coagulation between mother and fetus. Pediatr Res 5: 113–125
21. Roberts J M, Taylor R N, Musci T J et al 1989 Preeclampsia: an endothelial cell disorder. Am J Obstet Gynecol 161: 1200–1204
22. Gibson B, Hunter D, Neame P B, Kelton J G 1982 Thrombocytopenia in preeclampsia and eclampsia. Semin Thromb Hemost 8: 234–247
23. Inglis T C M, Stuart J, George A J, Davies A J 1982 Haemostatic and rheological changes in normal pregnancy and preeclampsia. Br J Haematol 50: 461–465
24. Weinar C P, Herrig J E, Pelzer G D, Heilskov J 1990 Elimination of antithrombin III concentrate in healthy pregnant and eclamptic women with an acquired antithrombin III deficiency. Throm Res 58: 395–402
25. Walsh S W 1985 Preeclampsia: an imbalance in placental prostacyclin and thromboxane production. Am J Obstet Gynecol 152: 335–340
26. Beaufils M, Uzan S, Donsimoni R, Colan J C 1985 Prevention of preeclampsia by early antiplatelet therapy. Lancet 1: 840–842
27. Schiff E, Peleg E, Goldenberg M et al 1989 The use of aspirin to prevent pregnancy-induced hypertension and lower the ratio of thromboxane A2 to prostacyclinin in relatively high risk pregnancies. New Engl J Med 321: 351–356
28. Weinstein L 1985 Preeclampsia/eclampsia with hemolysis, elevated liver enzymes, and thrombocytopenia. Obst Gynecol 66: 657–660
29. Sibai B M, Spinnato J A, Dottie L 1984 Pregnancy outcome in 303 cases with severe preeclampsia. Obstet Gynecol 64: 319–325
30. Sibai B M 1990 The HELLP syndrome (hemolysis, elevated liver enzymes, and low platelets): much ado about nothing? Am J Obstet Gynecol 165: 311–316
31. Pinette M G, Vintzileos A M, Ingardia C J 1989 Thrombotic

thrombocytopenic purpura as a cause of thrombocytopenia in pregnancy: literature review. Am J Perinatol 6: 55–57
32. Weiner C P 1987 Thrombotic microangiopathy in pregnancy and the postpartum period. Semin Hematol 24: 119–129
33. Ezra Y, Mordel N, Sadovsky, Schenker J G, Eldor A 1989 Successful pregnancies of two patients with relapsing thrombotic thrombocytopenic purpura. Int J Gynecol Obstet 29: 359–363
34. Sundquist S-B, Nilsson I M, Svanberg L, Cronberg S 1981 Pregnancy and parturition in a patient with severe Glanzmann thrombasthenia. Scand J Haematol 27: 159–164
35. Zimmerman T S, Ruggieri Z M 1982 von Willebrand's disease. In: Spaet T H (ed) Progress in hemostasis and thrombosis, Vol 6. Grune & Stratton, New York pp 202–236
36. Valster F A A, Feijen H L M, Hutten J W M 1990 Severe thrombocytopenia in a pregnant patient with platelet-associated IGM, and known von Willebrand disease: a case report. Eur J Obstet Gynecol Reprod Biol 36: 197–201
37. Ieko M, Sakurama S, Sagawa A et al Effect of a factor VIII concentrate on type IIB von Willebrand's disease associated thrombocytopenia presenting during pregnancy in identical twin mothers. Am J Hematol 35: 26–31
38. Andrew M, Kelton J G 1984 Neonatal thrombocytopenia. Clin Perinatol 11: 359–391
39. Tchernia G, Dreyfus M, Laurian Y, Derycke M, Mirica C, Kerbrat G 1984 Management of immune thrombocytopenic purpura in pregnancy. Response to infusions of immunoglobulins. Am J Obstet Gynecol 148: 225–226
40. Lavery J P, Koortz W L, Liu Y K, Howell R 1985 Immunologic thrombocytopenia in pregnancy: use of antenatal immunoglobulin therapy: case report and review. Obstet Gynecol 66: 41–43
41. Samuels P, Bussel J B, Braitman L E et al 1990 Estimation of the risk of thrombocytopenia in the offspring of pregnant women with presumed immune thrombocytopenic purpura. New Engl J Med 323: 229–235
42. Kaplan C, Daffos F, Forestier F et al 1990 Fetal platelet counts in thrombocytopenic pregnancy. Lancet 336: 979–982
43. Karpatkin M, Porges R F, Karpatkin S 1981 Platelet counts in infants of women with autoimmune thrombocytopenia: effect of steroid administration to the mother. New Engl J Med 305: 936–939
44. Cines D B, Dusak B, Tomaski A, Menruti M, Schreiber A D 1982 Immune thrombocytopenic purpura and pregnancy. New Engl J Med 306: 826–831
45. Ayromlooi J 1978 A new approach to management of thrombocytopenic purpura in pregnancy. Am J Obstet Gynecol 130: 235–236
46. Daffos F, Capella-Pavlosky M, Forestier F 1983 A new procedure for fetal blood sampling in utero: preliminary results. Am J Obstet Gynecol 146: 985–987
47. Burrows R F, Kelton J G 1989 Idiopathic thrombocytopenic purpura during pregnancy: intervention for the fetus is not required. Blood 74 (suppl 1): 187a
48. Chirico G, Duse M, Ugazio A, Rondini G 1983 High dose intravenous gamma-globulin therapy for passive immune thrombocytopenia in the neonate. J Pediatr 103: 654–656
49. Burrows R F, Kelton J G 1990 Thrombocytopenia at delivery. A prospective survey of 6715 deliveries. Am J Obstet Gynecol 162: 731–734
50. Matthews J H, Benjamin S, Gill D S, Smith N A 1990 Pregnancy associated thrombocytopenia: definition, incidence and natural history. Acta Haematol 84: 24–29

56. Venous air embolism

A. M. Malinow D. N. Schneeweiss

Venous air embolism (VAE) is a recognized complication in many surgical procedures. Classically, VAE has been associated with neurosurgical procedures performed with the patient in the sitting position.[1] However, VAE has also been reported as a complication of abdominal, orthopedic, plastic, urologic, thoracic and head and neck surgery. Many of these procedures were performed with the patient in the prone, supine or lateral position.[1,2]

Numerous case reports of VAE during cesarean delivery appeared in the medical literature as early as the nineteenth century. Deaths from VAE during cesarean delivery have been reported as recently as the 1980s.[2] Nonetheless, it was not until 1987 that the occurrence of VAE during cesarean delivery was systematically studied.[3] Subsequently, several studies have documented the occurrence of VAE during cesarean delivery[4–6] as well as during the placement of epidural catheters.[7] VAE may account for signs (e.g. arterial oxygen desaturation, arrhythmias and hypotension) and symptoms (e.g. dyspnea and chest pain) commonly found in patients during cesarean delivery.[3–6] VAE may even be as common during cesarean delivery as it is during neurosurgical procedures in the sitting position.[1,3,4,6]

PREVALENCE

Precordial Doppler monitoring can detect as little as 0.1 ml of intracardiac air.[1] There is 100% correlation between echocardiographic and Doppler evidence of VAE during cesarean delivery, thus demonstrating the specificity of precordial Doppler monitoring.[4] The prevalence of Doppler-evident VAE during cesarean delivery is 11–66%.[3–6] The majority of these patients received continuous lumbar epidural anesthesia. In patients receiving general anesthesia for cesarean delivery, the prevalence of VAE is 28–71%.[4,6] VAE may occur throughout the procedure but seems to occur most commonly during hysterotomy or repair of hysterotomy.[3,4,6]

PATHOPHYSIOLOGY

Open venous sinuses and a negative pressure gradient between the surgical wound and heart facilitates entrainment of air into the central venous circulation.[1,2] Gradients as small as -5 cmH_2O have been shown to allow significant amounts of air to enter the venous circulation.[1,8] Routine positioning of patients for cesarean delivery with 10–15° of left lateral tilt creates a -10 to -15 cmH_2O pressure gradient between the uterus and the heart.[5] Hysterotomy exposes the uterine sinuses, which may be particularly susceptible to the entrainment of air.[6] Exteriorization of the uterus and traction applied during repair of hysterotomy may distend collapsed veins and exaggerate the pressure gradient with the right heart.[3,6] Although use of a 5–10° reverse Trendelenburg position does not affect the incidence of VAE during cesarean delivery,[4] use of the Trendelenburg position may further exaggerate the negative pressure gradient.[5,6,9] A decreased central venous pressure increases the risk of venous air entrainment.[2] Factors that decrease central venous pressure include absolute hypovolemia from hemorrhage (placenta previa or placental abruption) and a contracted intravascular volume (prolonged labor with NPO status or pregnancy-induced hypertension) and relative hypovolemia from inadequate acute hydration before the initiation of regional anesthesia with resultant sympathetic block and vasodilation.[2,5–7,9]

Morbidity and mortality resulting from VAE depend on the amount of air entrained, the rate of entrainment and the site to which the air embolism travels. Small volumes of air entrained slowly are tolerated well without clinical signs or symptoms.[1] However, as little as 0.5 ml/kg/min has been shown to cause symptoms.[7] Large volumes of air (3–8 ml/kg) injected rapidly are quickly fatal.[1,6] The most likely cause of death with large VAE is an air lock causing obstruction of the pulmonary outflow tract.[1,2] Smaller amounts of air can result in ventilation–perfusion mismatching with hypoxemia, hypercapnia, right heart failure, arrhythmias and hypotension.[1,2]

Paradoxical air embolism (i.e. air entering the systemic circulation) can cause coronary or cerebral ischemia, infarction and death or permanent neurologic deficit.[1] Air may enter the systemic circulation via a patent foramen ovale (10–25% of the population) or other intracardiac shunts.[1]

CLINICAL PRESENTATION

Massive VAE can present as a devastatingly dramatic event heralded by hypotension, arterial hypoxemia and electromechanical dissociation leading to cardiac arrest.[9] The clinical picture is routinely much less profound, presumably because of the small volume of VAE.

The etiology of chest pain during cesarean delivery is unclear and is, almost certainly, multifactorial. Complaints of chest pain during cesarean delivery are often dismissed by anesthesiologists and obstetricians as being secondary to surgical traction on the peritoneum. However, it has been demonstrated that there is an association of VAE with subsequent complaints of chest pain by otherwise healthy parturients at routine, elective cesarean delivery.[3,6] 20–50% of women with Doppler-evident VAE during cesarean delivery will complain of chest pain.[3,6] Less than 2% of women will complain of chest pain during cesarean delivery without previous Doppler-evident VAE.[3,6] Patient complaints of chest pain during cesarean delivery should not be ignored. The association of chest pain with VAE should alert the clinician to look for other diagnostic signs.[3,10] The attention of the anesthesiologist should be directed toward making the diagnosis of VAE, a potentially treatable entity.

Arterial oxygen desaturation and dyspnea are associated with VAE.[1,3,4,6,9] Arterial oxygen saturations less than 92% are reported in up to 25% of parturients during cesarean delivery with Doppler-evident VAE.[6] Dyspnea is present in 20–40% of parturients during cesarean delivery with Doppler-evident VAE.[3,6] Dyspnea associated with arterial oxygen desaturation is unusual in parturients during cesarean delivery without evidence of VAE.[4,6] Other less frequent clinical presentations associated with VAE during cesarean delivery include cardiac arrhythmias (most often ventricular arrhythmias),[4,9] gasping respirations[2,9] and hypotension.[2,4,9]

RECOMMENDATIONS

It is evident that VAE is relatively common during cesarean delivery. Although significant mortality and morbidity is rare, about 1% of maternal deaths are attributed to VAE.[10]

Given the remote possibility of significant morbidity and mortality, it would seem overly cautious to *mandate* precordial Doppler monitoring in all patients undergoing cesarean delivery. Perhaps, though, certain groups of patients warrant special attention. Those patients especially prone to develop VAE or in whom otherwise insignificant volumes of VAE would probably cause significant mortality or morbidity might benefit from special preoperative preparation and intraoperative monitoring.

Hypovolemic patients are especially at risk for developing VAE.[2,5,9] A contracted blood volume and low central venous pressure, which enhance entrainment of venous air, could potentially be corrected before delivery.[2] Precordial Doppler monitoring should strongly be considered, if time allows for proper placement before delivery. Patients with a pre-existing intracardiac shunt (e.g. patent foramen ovale, atrial septal defect or ventricular septal defect) require special consideration because of their risk for developing paradoxical air embolism possibly resulting in coronary or cerebral ischemia.[1,2] In these patients, routine precordial Doppler monitoring as well as placement of a multiorificed central venous pressure (CVP) catheter in the upper right atrium to facilitate aspiration of air should be strongly considered.[2]

It is wise to avoid the Trendelenburg position during cesarean delivery because of the increased negative pressure gradient that occurs as well as the associated adverse cardiac and respiratory consequences.[2,6] Flexing the operating room table (dropping the level of the wound toward the level of the heart) before surgery begins might decrease the pressure gradient that would favor venous air entrainment.[2]

Treatment of VAE, either Doppler evident or clinically suspected, should include the following:

1. Further entrainment of air should be prevented by having the obstetricians flood the operative field. Placing the patient in the reverse Trendelenburg position will eliminate the gradient between the heart and the surgical wound. Positioning the patient with the chest tilted to the left will decrease the chance of air lock in the right ventricular outflow tract.[2]
2. Administer 100% oxygen to the patient.[2] Discontinue nitrous oxide (if it is being administered).
3. If the patient continues with symptoms of VAE or signs of clinical instability appear, a multiorificed CVP catheter should be inserted and aspiration of intracardiac air attempted. This may be life-saving whenever serious cardiovascular compromise is observed.[2,5]
4. If cardiovascular collapse occurs, immediate delivery of the baby should be accomplished as cardiopulmonary resuscitation according to advanced cardiac life support guidelines is being performed.[2]
5. Any patient who becomes comatose or fails to awaken from general anesthesia should be evaluated for intracerebral air with a computed tomographic scan. Hyperbaric pressure oxygen therapy is the only definitive means of treating intracerebral air.[2]

REFERENCES

1. Michenfelder J D 1983 Air embolism. In Orkin F K, Cooperman L H (eds) Complications in anesthesiology. JB Lippincott, Philadelphia, p 268
2. Robinson D A, Albin A S 1987 Parturition and venous air embolism. Obstet Anesth Dig 7: 38
3. Malinow A M, Naulty J S, Hunt C O et al 1987 Precordial ultrasonic monitoring during cesarean delivery. Anesthesiology 66: 816
4. Fong J, Gadalla F, Pierri M K et al 1988 Incidence of venous air embolism during cesarean section (abstract). Anesthesiology 69: A655
5. Karuparthy V K, Downing J W, Husain F J et al 1989 Incidence of venous air embolism during cesarean section is unchanged by the use of a 5 to 10 degree head-up tilt. Anesth Analg 69: 620
6. Vartikar J V, Johnson M D, Datta S 1989 Precordial Doppler monitoring and pulse oximetry during cesarean delivery: detection of venous air embolism. Reg Anesth 14: 145
7. Naulty J S, Ostheimer G W, Datta S et al 1982 Incidence of venous air embolism during epidural catheter insertion. Anesthesiology 57: 410
8. Babinski M F, Gilbert J, Smith S L 1983 Venous air embolism is not restricted to neurosurgery! (correspondence). Anesthesiology 59: 151
9. Younker D, Rodriguez V, Kavanaugh J 1986 Massive air embolism during cesarean section. Anesthesiology 65: 77
10. Kaunitz A M, Hughes J M, Grimes D A et al 1985 Causes of maternal mortality in the United States. Obstet Gynecol 65: 605

57. Amniotic fluid embolism

J. H. Skerman T. Huckaby

Amniotic fluid embolism is a rare, unpredictable and unpreventable obstetric catastrophe. It is initiated by entry of amniotic fluid into the maternal circulation and is characterized by the sudden onset of severe dyspnea, tachypnea and cyanosis during labor, delivery or the early puerperium.

Amniotic fluid embolism was first reported by Meyer[1] in 1926. It was reported again in an experiment on laboratory animals by Warden in 1927.[2]

The importance of this condition and these early studies was not established until 1941, when Steiner and Lushbaugh[3] noted the clinical and pathologic findings of eight women who died suddenly during or just after labor. They performed experimental studies on laboratory animals that produced the same severe disturbances of cardiopulmonary function following the entry of amniotic fluid into maternal circulation. Their study was documented with pathologic findings of pulmonary embolism caused by amniotic fluid particulate matter. Schneider et al[4] in 1968 showed that lethal qualities of human amniotic fluid infused intravenously into dogs were enhanced greatly by the addition of meconium. This description by Steiner and Lushbaugh of a patient with amniotic fluid embolism is classic in its detailed brevity:

> Profound shock coming on suddenly and unexpectedly in a woman who is usually in severe labor or has just finished such a labor, especially if she is an elderly multipara with an excessively large, perhaps dead, fetus and with meconium amniotic fluid, should lead to a suspicion of the possibility. If, also, the shock is introduced by a chill which is followed by dyspnea, cyanosis, vomiting, restlessness and the like and is accompanied by a pronounced fall in blood pressure and a rapid, weak pulse, the picture is more complete. If pulmonary edema now develops quickly in the known absence of previously existing heart disease the diagnosis is reasonably certain.

Their description is complete except for the development of disseminated intravascular coagulation (DIC) in patients surviving the initial pulmonary insult.

PREVALENCE

The prevalence of amniotic fluid embolism has been reported to be between 1 in 8000 and 1 in 80 000 pregnancies; a more realistic figure is probably between these two extremes.[3,5,6] The mortality rate is very high. Although it is a rare occurrence, it still remains a leading cause of maternal and fetal death. Morgan[7] in 1979 reviewed 272 cases documented in the British medical literature and reported a mortality rate of 86%. From the same study, 25% of the deaths occurred within the first hour of the onset of symptoms, indicating that, even with optimum critical care management, a high mortality rate persists. Not all sudden deaths in late pregnancy are due to amniotic fluid embolism. We must be careful not to let this diagnosis become the wastebasket for cases of unexplained death in labor, especially without confirmation by autopsy.

ETIOLOGY

Predisposing factors for amniotic fluid embolism include advanced maternal age, multiple pregnancies, fetal macrosomia, short duration of labor and intense contractions often augmented with an uterine muscle stimulant such as oxytocin.[8] Others suggest that fetal demise, meconium staining of amniotic fluid, amniotomy, pregnancy-induced hypertension (PIH), cesarean delivery, placental abruption, placenta previa, ruptured uterus, amniocentesis, insertion of an intrauterine pressure catheter and pregnancy at term with an intrauterine device present are also causative factors. Recent reviews have documented a significant association of amniotic fluid embolism with advanced maternal age.[7] Documentation of amniotic fluid embolism has also been reported following intrauterine injection of hypertonic saline to induce abortion. Recently a case was reported after use of vaginal prostaglandin E_2.[9]

Amniotic fluid embolus syndrome has been reported in association with a myriad of conditions. These conditions include first- and second-trimester abortion with saline, prostaglandins and urea, and hysterotomy. It has occurred during labor, at delivery, just after delivery, and in one case even 32 h post-partum. Most reported cases of amniotic fluid embolism occur during labor; a pattern of vigorous labor or hypertonic uterine contractions or labor further stimulated by use of oxytocin often has been implicated in the pathogenesis. Evidence for this association (use of an oxytocic) is primarily anecdotal and must be regarded with skepticism. In a review of this subject, Morgan[7] concluded: 'In view of the very wide use of accelerated labor and the rarity of amniotic fluid embolism, it must be concluded that there is no direct association between the two.' Placental abruption is present in up to 50% of cases and may contribute to the pattern of uterine hypertonus associated with amniotic fluid embolism. In 40% of cases, fetal death is reported prior to the acute clinical presentation.

In an analysis of data collected in another study,[10] the range of age was from 18 to 43 years, with 22 patients being 30 years old or older; 12 patients were over 35 years of age. The parity of patients ranged from one to eight, with the majority of patients greater than three; however, there were four cases documented in primiparous women. The duration of gestational age of the pregnancies in the patients who subsequently died ranged from 38 to 44 weeks. This excludes those patients who died from amniotic fluid embolism secondary to saline or other fluids injected intra-amniotically to induce abortion.

The characteristics of the labor pattern varied. However, it is of interest to note that four patients developed amniotic emboli without evidence of labor. The majority of patients were in various stages of either spontaneous or augmented labor (in 22% labor had been induced and in 11% labor had been augmented with an oxytocic agent). The augmentation or induction of labor was instituted for the usual reasons: ruptured membranes without consistent uterine contractions, post-maturity, PIH and elective induction. In 10%, labor was augmented because of poor progress. Of patients who labored spontaneously, 44% had tumultuous and unusually short labors averaging less than 1 h in duration. No comparably short labors or precipitous deliveries were identified in the patients who received oxytocic stimulation, nor were tetanic contractions reported.

The membranes were documented to be intact in three patients at the time the embolism or onset of symptoms occurred. In most cases studied, the membranes had ruptured either spontaneously or by amniotomy prior to the onset of symptoms. There is documentation, however, indicating that simultaneous rupture of membranes and meconium stained amniotic fluid with onset of symptoms of amniotic fluid embolus and meconium fluid was present in approximately 75% of these patients.[3]

Concerning fetal factors, no clear pattern of fetal presentation, position or engagement could be ascertained; most cases documented indicate a vertex presentation. There was generally a lack of documentation associating station of the presenting part with onset of symptoms. It could be assumed, since the onset of symptoms occurred just prior to or during delivery, that the fetal presenting part was engaged.

The size of the infant varied from 5 to 11 pounds, but unfortunately the data particular to the exact weight of all infants were not available. There is a high incidence of demise and intrapartum death of infants and, unfortunately, of those few infants born alive, a very high percentage expire during the neonatal period. In one study of 21 infants on whom information was available, there were nine diagnoses of demise with five occurring as intrapartum deaths. Ten live births were recorded in this particular study; however, only two infants were documented to have survived. There is a disproportionately large number of stillbirths, and some researchers feel that the presence of fetal demise reduces the strength of the membranes as well as greatly increases the quantity of particulate matter in the amniotic fluid.[3]

In order for amniotic fluid embolism to occur, the fluid must enter into the maternal circulation. Currently, three recognized conditions must exist for this to result: amniotomy, laceration of endocervical or uterine vessels, and a pressure gradient sufficient to force the fluid into the maternal circulation.

A tear or rent in the membranes such as occurs with amniotomy has been associated with proven embolism.[11] Various sites of entry of amniotic fluid into maternal circulation have been suggested. Laceration of endocervical veins can occur during the normal process of cervical dilation and effacement, although more severe lacerations may occur with a very rapid and tumultuous labor or vigorous cervical manipulation associated with vaginal examination. Uterine vessels can be damaged through surgical procedures such as cesarean delivery or amniocentesis. Trauma is also responsible for causing damage of the uterine vessels. According to Landing,[12] an abnormal opening of the uterine vessels, either decidual or myometrial, which occurs with uterine rupture, placenta accreta, cesarean delivery or retained placenta may provide a portal of entry for amniotic fluid. Placental abruption, whether marginal or complete, as well as any degree of placenta previa, could also provide a route of entry. If amniotic fluid finds an open maternal venous sinus, it could be pumped by a vigorous contraction through the disrupted amniotic membrane with resultant embolization.

Intra-amniotic injections of fluid (i.e. hypertonic saline, saline or urea) cause a rise in intrauterine pressure that may be greater than that associated with normal labor. Frost[13] in 1967 reported a patient with a hydatidiform mole who died from trophoblastic embolization of the lungs following injection of intra-amniotic hypertonic saline. A review of deaths following legal abortions in the USA from 1972 to 1978 revealed that 15 (12%) were due to amniotic fluid embolus; all of these followed intra-amniotic injections, and none followed uterine curettage.[14] Clinically, the symptoms exhibited in these patients were the same as in those with embolism occurring at term. This study also revealed gestational age to be a significant factor. No deaths occurred below 12 weeks of gestation, however the mortality was 7.2 per 100 000 at 21 weeks or more, representing a risk factor 24 times greater after 21 weeks gestation.[14]

Because of the rarity of the condition combined with the fact that diagnosis is often made during the postmortem examination, it is difficult to determine a definite cause and effect with this catastrophic obstetric event.

PATHOPHYSIOLOGY

The two life-threatening consequences of amniotic fluid embolism, cardiopulmonary collapse and DIC, may occur in sequence or together. The physiology of amniotic fluid embolism results in acute pulmonary hypertension with a sudden reduction of blood flow to the left heart, decreased left ventricular output and subsequent peripheral vascular collapse. The sudden development of elevated pulmonary artery pressure could precipitate acute cor pulmonale or right ventricular failure. The derangement of the ventilation-perfusion ratio of the lungs produces hypoxemia and acidemia, which in the pattern of a vicious circle further enhances pulmonary artery vasospasm. If severe pulmonary vascular obstruction and cor pulmonale are not immediately fatal, hemorrhage may soon become evident.

The etiology of DIC is controversial. Evidence suggests that the potent thromboplastin action of amniotic fluid causes disseminated deposition of fibrin clots and activation of the lysis system. These hemodynamic processes defibrinate the blood,[15] resulting in afibrinogenemia, coagulopathy and subsequent hemorrhage.[16] The powerful thromboplastin effects of trophoblast are well established; systemic release of the trophoblastic material may play an even greater role in the coagulopathy of amniotic fluid embolism than has been appreciated.

Kitzmiller and Lucas[16] have shown that amniotic fluid collected during labor (as compared with fluid collected prior to labor) has greater toxicity when infused into rabbits. The particular substance mediating this reaction is still unknown. Prostaglandins and leukotrienes produce many of the hemodynamic and hematologic effects present in patients with amniotic fluid embolism and have been implicated by some researchers.[17] These metabolites of arachidonic acid are present in increased quantities during labor.[18]

The toxicity of intravenously infused amniotic fluid appears to vary remarkably depending on the particulate matter it contains. This is especially true of meconium-stained fluid. The particulate materials found in amniotic fluid and especially in meconium-stained fluid, according to some investigators, may account for the cause of sudden death associated with this syndrome.[19]

Some researchers postulate that an acute anaphylactoid reaction may play a part in the development of the cardiovascular collapse.[20] For a true anaphylactic reaction to occur, sensitization is required, but evidence for prior sensitization of the parturient to amniotic fluid is lacking. Stefanini and Turpini,[21] in their experiment, noted that an intravenous injection of 15 ml of homologous amniotic fluid in dogs produced no effect, but 1 month later further administration of a 15 ml aliquot of the same fluid, which had been kept frozen, resulted in hypotension, hypofibrinogenemia and thrombocytopenia. Therefore, it was suggested the animal had become sensitized to amniotic fluid; this might occur in humans as well. It is possible that penetration of amniotic fluid into the systemic circulation during the antepartum period causes a state of sensitization in humans, and subsequent entry into the circulation during labor and delivery could induce an acute anaphylactic reaction. However, the absence or rarity of pruritus, urticaria, laryngospasm or wheezing in case reports does not indicate a mast cell-mediated mechanism.

In a recent review on amniotic fluid embolism, Clark[22] concluded the following: some 'normal' amniotic fluid may innocuously enter the maternal circulation of many pregnant women. However, amniotic fluid embolism may develop after maternal infusion of 'abnormal' amniotic fluid, that is fluid containing an abnormal substance, possibly one of the arachidonic acid metabolites.

The most significant pathologic findings at autopsy are limited to the lungs. Grossly, the lungs show evidence of pulmonary edema (70% in one study),[23] alveolar hemorrhage and pulmonary embolization of amniotic fluid materials. The presence of embolic particles is essential for diagnosis, but these may be missed on histologic search because of their small size.[19] Amniotic emboli are composed of amorphous debris, fetal epithelial squamous cells (squames), fetal hairs, vernix caseosa and mucin (from meconium). The emboli tend to lodge in small arteries, arterioles and capillaries of the lungs.[15] Since uterine trauma is a significant factor in the pathogenesis, signs of uterine laceration or uterine rupture may be evident.[24] Acute right ventricular dilation is usually present. Amniotic fluid elements are sometimes found in the right side of the heart as well as within uterine vessels. Careful evaluation of the other organs may also identify the magnitude of embolization when particulate matter is identified in the maternal brain, kidneys, liver, spleen and even the hypothalamus.

CLINICAL AND LABORATORY DIAGNOSIS

In a small percentage of patients the onset of symptoms occurred before labor was clinically evident. The majority of patients developed symptoms during the latter part of the first stage of labor and a lesser number became acute during birth. There have been two cases documented that were associated with delivery of the placenta, and one case occurred 32 h post delivery. In one series, 45% of cases were associated with placental abruption of varying degrees. Many investigators believe this to be one of the primary catalysts in the development of amniotic fluid embolism.

In a review of obstetric patients who developed amniotic fluid embolism,[7] the most common complications that were already present or that developed during delivery are listed in order of frequency of occurrence: severe amnionitis, moderate to severe PIH, cephalopelvic disproportion and traumatic mid-forceps delivery.

Prodromal symptoms in amniotic fluid embolism are sudden chills, shivering, sweating, anxiety and coughing, followed by signs of respiratory distress, shock, cardiovascular collapse and convulsions. All patients were conscious during the onset of symptomatology. Respiratory difficulty, manifested as cyanosis, tachypnea and bronchospasm, frequently progresses to fulminant pulmonary edema. Hypoxemia explains the cyanosis and probably accounts for the restlessness, convulsions and unconsciousness. Reflex tachypnea results from the initial decreased arterial oxygen saturation. Cardiovascular collapse, as heralded by hypotension, tachycardia and arrhythmias, may end in cardiac arrest. Convulsions may be an early manifestation of central nervous system involvement secondary to cerebral ischemia and may eventually progress to coma and death. If the patient survives this initial episode, bleeding may occur secondary to DIC and uterine atony. In all cases studied, bleeding was never documented as one of the first symptoms.

A definitive diagnosis is usually made at post-mortem examination by demonstration of amniotic fluid material in the maternal circulation and the small arteries, arterioles and capillaries of the pulmonary vessels. In the living patient, diagnosis may be made by identification of lanugo or fetal hair and fetal squames in an aspirate of blood from the right heart.[25] Fetal squames have been recovered in the maternal sputum in some cases.[26] Additional diagnostic tools for confirmation of amniotic fluid embolism suspected by the classic clinical picture include:

1. Chest radiograph, which may show enlargement of the right atrium and ventricle, a prominent proximal pulmonary artery (in massive pulmonary embolism), and pulmonary edema.
2. Lung scan, which may demonstrate some areas of reduced perfusion.
3. Central venous catheterization, which reveals an initial rise due to acute pulmonary hypertension and eventually a profound decrease due to severe hemorrhage.
4. Measurement of blood coagulation factors.

Normally, in pregnancy, blood coagulation factors are increased. However, with amniotic fluid embolism and DIC, the blood fails to clot.

In the differential diagnosis of amniotic fluid embolism, the following entities are to be considered:[27]

1. Pulmonary thromboembolism most often develops post delivery, is usually caused by a thrombus originating from the lower extremities or pelvic veins, and is usually associated with chest pain.[28]
2. Air embolism may occur following a ruptured uterus, blood transfusion under pressure, or manipulation of placenta previa during labor or cesarean delivery. It is associated with chest pain, but an important differentiating factor from amniotic fluid embolism is the auscultation of a typical 'water-wheel' murmur over the pericardium.[29]
3. Aspiration of gastric contents into the lungs causes cyanosis, tachypnea, coughing, tachycardia, hypotension and pulmonary edema. However, acid aspiration usually occurs in an unconscious patient with loss of the cough reflex,[28] or during induction or emergence from general anesthesia.
4. Eclamptic convulsions and coma in a pregnant patient may resemble amniotic fluid embolus syndrome, but the presence of hypertension, proteinuria and edema[29] in the eclamptic patient differentiates these two conditions.
5. Convulsions from a toxic reaction to local anesthetics may be confused with this syndrome, but the close temporal relationship between the onset of symptoms and administration of the drug is the differentiating factor.[29] Also, hypertension is usually present in the early clinical picture of drug toxicity.
6. Acute left heart failure is most commonly seen in pregnant patients with rheumatic heart disease, but the history of rheumatic fever with electrocardiographic changes and other clinical symptoms (i.e. cardiac murmur) helps in the diagnosis.
7. A cerebrovascular accident may be considered in the differential diagnosis, but it is distinguished from amniotic fluid embolism by the absence of cyanosis, hypotension and pulmonary edema. Also, examination of cerebrospinal fluid should aid in the diagnosis.
8. Hemorrhagic shock in an obstetric patient may be associated with placental abruption, placenta previa, or ruptured uterus. Post-delivery hemorrhage may develop from uterine atony, an unrepaired cervical laceration, retained products, or uterine inversion. A careful history and physical examination, absence of central cyanosis and low central venous pressure (if hemodynamic monitoring

is used) should guide one to the correct diagnosis and therapy.

OBSTETRIC AND ANESTHETIC MANAGEMENT

To prevent amniotic fluid embolism, trauma to the uterus must be avoided during maneuvers such as insertion of an intrauterine pressure catheter or amniotomy. Unintentional incision of the placenta during cesarean delivery should be avoided if at all possible.[7] Because one of the most frequent predisposing factors is considered to be tumultuous labor, excessively strong and frequent uterine contractions should be controlled by administration of intravenous β-adrenergic drugs[7] or magnesium sulfate with the patient laboring on her left side. Oxytocics, which might precipitate tetanic uterine contractions, should be used appropriately and judiciously.

In most cases, no therapy has been proven effective. Whenever unexplained cyanosis and shock develops during labor, a diagnosis of amniotic fluid embolism should be considered.[30] Assuming a diagnosis could be made prior to death, supportive measures should be focused at cardiopulmonary resuscitation, blood volume replacement, and treatment of coagulopathy.

Resuscitation should begin with endotracheal intubation and mechanical ventilation using inspired oxygen concentrations of 100% delivered by positive pressure and positive end-expiratory pressure (PEEP). With the use of PEEP, functional residual capacity should increase and, if oxygenation improves, as evidenced by pulse oximetry or arterial blood gas data, a lower PEEP setting may be tried. Careful observation is essential while the patient is receiving high PEEP, as a decrease in cardiac output due to increased intrathoracic pressure may develop and subsequently decrease tissue perfusion. It is hoped that improved oxygenation will reduce pulmonary capillary fragility and thereby decrease the severity of pulmonary edema. To date, there has been no documentation of the use of hyperbaric oxygen, but some feel it would be worth a try in treating the severe tissue hypoxia provided there was time. Careful hemodynamic monitoring is essential. Placement of two large intravenous lines to deliver large volumes of fluid and an intra-arterial catheter to monitor blood pressure, arterial blood gases and other pertinent chemistries, as well as a central venous or Swan–Ganz catheter to monitor cardiac status, pulmonary pressures and state of hydration, are of enormous value.

The causes of pulmonary edema have been variably ascribed to vigorous fluid resuscitation, increased pulmonary capillary permeability and cardiac decompensation due to hypoxia and tachycardia. The severity of pulmonary edema certainly plays an important role in the initial gas exchange abnormality and duration of the aberration. Hemodynamic monitoring is very helpful in preventing fluid overload and directing fluid therapy.

At present there is no clear regimen of drug therapy to reverse the symptoms and complications of amniotic fluid embolism. Drug therapy and other treatment are supportive and aimed at improving the ventilation–perfusion ratio, maintenance of adequate blood pressure and treatment of DIC.

The drug used to treat pulmonary complications such as bronchospasm and vasoconstriction of pulmonary arterioles is terbutaline, especially if the patient is undelivered with a viable fetus. Isoproterenol also relieves pulmonary vasoconstriction and improves cardiac function, although it can cause peripheral vasodilation, which will exacerbate the hypotension. Dopamine may be preferable to isoproterenol because it improves cardiac function and increases peripheral and renal perfusion unless given in too large a dose, which would result in decreased renal perfusion. Administration of aminophylline for its bronchodilation and cardiac stimulation effects is controversial, mainly because of the tachycardia it produces. Hydrocortisone in doses up to 2 g/24 h reduces pulmonary vasospasm and pulmonary edema and potentiates the cardiac response to catecholamines. In the event of heart failure, treatment with intravenous inotropes such as dobutamine is recommended, or digitalization with intravenous digoxin may be instituted.[31] Diuretics can be used if pulmonary capillary wedge pressure is elevated. Indomethacin has been effective in treating severe pulmonary hypertension in laboratory animals and should be considered for use. In a condition with such a high mortality, there would be nothing to lose.

Hypotension should be treated first by left uterine displacement if the patient is undelivered. This can be accomplished easily by insertion of a wedge under the right hip. The vasopressor of choice is ephedrine because it does not decrease uterine perfusion. However, if the fetus has expired or perhaps is already delivered, isoproterenol or dobutamine can be used. The fluid of choice should be lactated Ringer's solution, because its pH is most near that of blood; the rate of infusion will depend on the hemodynamic monitoring. If acidosis is present, as evidenced by arterial blood gas values, sodium bicarbonate should be administered.

Treatment of the bleeding diathesis requires blood replacement using fresh whole blood (when available), as the clotting factors so badly needed are intact. Otherwise, packed red cells and fresh-frozen plasma are usually more available and will retain some clotting factors, but the longer they are stored, the more the clotting factors deteriorate. Cryoprecipitate and platelet infusions are also required to help combat the coagulopathy. Heparin therapy is controversial; some patients have been documented to survive with its use, but there is documentation of survival without using heparin.

Uterine bleeding in a patient already delivered should

be controlled by massage and use of intravenous oxytocin. If uterine bleeding is unresponsive to these methods, one should consider exploration for retained placenta or membranes, or a search for cervical or uterine lacerations. Methylergonovine is also a strong uterine stimulant and can be given intramuscularly or very slowly via intravenous push if considered to be necessary in this life-threatening circumstance. The use of prostaglandins (Hemabat,® Upjohn and Co.) to control hemorrhage is controversial and may cause bronchospasm and/or pulmonary hypertension. The use of ε-aminocaproic acid and aprotinin is not well documented in the treatment of amniotic fluid embolus, but these agents might be used when rapid reversal of the lytic state is needed before delivery. Aprotinin (Trasylol) should be the drug of choice if the fetus is still viable because it does not cross the placenta as does ε-aminocaproic acid, which is teratogenic as well.

When amniotic fluid embolism occurs, the accompanying respiratory distress, cardiovascular collapse and hemorrhagic tendency are contraindications to any regional techniques, and if severe shock develops a general anesthetic must be administered with extreme caution. Because immediate delivery is indicated, emergency cesarean delivery is usually required. The choice of anesthetic agents will depend on the patient's condition, and aggressive cardiopulmonary resuscitation may be all that the anesthesiologist can provide.

REFERENCES

1. Meyer J R 1926 Embolia pulmonar amnio-caseosa. Braz Med 2: 301–303
2. Warden M R 1927 Amniotic fluid as possible factor in etiology of eclampsia. Am J Obstet Gynecol 14: 292–300
3. Steiner P E, Lushbaugh C C 1941 Maternal pulmonary embolism by fluid as a cause of obstetric shock and expected deaths in obstetrics. J Am Med Assoc 117: 1245–1254
4. Schneider C L, Henry M M, Chaplick M J 1968 Meconium embolism in vivo. Pulmonary and systemic microcirculation (as in maternal amniotic embolism). Am J Obstet Gynecol 101: 909–914
5. Liban E, Raz S 1969 A clinicopathologic study of fourteen cases of amniotic fluid embolism. Am J Clin Pathol 51: 477–486
6. Abouleish E 1974 Amniotic fluid embolism: report of a fatal case. Curr Res Anesth Analg 53: 549–553
7. Morgan M 1979 Amniotic fluid embolism. Anaesthesia 34: 20–32
8. Courtney L D 1974 Amniotic fluid embolism. Obstet Gynecol Surv 29: 169–177
9. Less A, Goldberger S B, Bernheim J et al 1990 Vaginal prostaglandin E_2 and fatal amniotic fluid embolus. J Am Med Assoc 263: 3259–3260
10. Anderson D G 1967 Amniotic fluid embolism: a re-evaluation. Am J Obstet Gynecol 98: 336–348
11. Schenken J R, Slaughter G P, DeMay G H 1950 Maternal pulmonary embolism of amniotic fluid. Am J Clin Pathol 20: 147–152
12. Landing B J 1950 The pathogenesis of amniotic fluid embolism. II. Uterine factors. New Engl J Med 243: 590–596
13. Frost A C G 1967 Death following intrauterine injection of hypertonic saline solution with hydatiform mole. Am J Obstet Gynecol 101: 342–344
14. Guidotti RJ, Grimes D A, Cates W 1981 Fatal amniotic fluid embolism during legally induced abortion in the United States: 1972–1978. Am J Obstet Gynecol 141: 257–261
15. Russell W S, Jones W N, Nicholson J 1965 Amniotic fluid embolism. A review of the syndrome with a report of 4 cases. Obstet Gynecol 26: 476–485
16. Kitzmiller J L, Lucas W E 1972 Studies on a model of amniotic fluid embolism. Obstet Gynecol 39: 626–627
17. Azegami M, Mori N 1986 Amniotic fluid embolism and leukotrienes. Am J Obstet Gynecol 115: 1119–1124
18. Karim S N, Devlin J 1979 Prostaglandin content of amniotic fluid during pregnancy and labor. J Obstet Gynaecol Br Cwlth 74: 230–234
19. Holland A J C 1968 Amniotic fluid embolism. Anaesthesia 23: 273–278
20. Dutta D, Bhargava K C, Chakravarti R N et al 1974 Therapeutic studies in experimental amniotic fluid embolism in rabbits. Am J Obstet Gynecol 106: 1201–1208
21. Stefanini M, Turpini R A 1959 Fibrinogenopenic accident of pregnancy and delivery: Syndrome with multiple etiological mechanism. Ann NY Acad Sci 75: 601–625
22. Clark S L 1990 New concepts of amniotic fluid embolism: a review. Obstet Gynecol Surv 45: 360–368
23. Peterson E P, Taylor H B 1970 Amniotic fluid embolism: An analysis of 40 cases. Obstet Gynecol 35: 787–793
24. Josey W E 1966 Hypofibrinogenemia complicating uterine rupture: relationship to amniotic fluid embolism. Am J Obstet Gynecol 94: 29–34
25. Lumley J, Owen R, Morgan M 1979 Amniotic fluid embolism. A report of 3 cases. Anaesthesia 34: 33–36
26. Schaerf R H M, deCampo T, Civetta J 1977 Hemodynamic alterations and rapid diagnosis in a case of amniotic fluid embolus. Anesthesiology 46: 155–157
27. Ziadlourad F, Conklin K A 1987 Amniotic fluid embolism. Semin Anesth 6: 171–175
28. Abouleish E 1977 Amniotic fluid embolism and disseminated intravascular coagulopathy. In Abouleish E (ed) Pain control in obstetrics. J B Lippincott, Philadelphia, p 160–185
29. Shnider S M, Moya F 1961 Amniotic fluid embolism. Anesthesiology 22: 108–119
30. Phillips O C, Weigel J E, McCarthy J J 1964 Amniotic fluid embolus. Fundamental considerations and a report of 2 cases. Obstet Gynecol 24: 431–435
31. Mulder J I 1985 Amniotic fluid embolism. An overview and case report. Am J Obstet Gynecol 152: 430–435

58. Morbid obesity

G. F. Fanciullo M. D. Johnson

Obesity is the most common nutritional disorder in the USA. It is estimated that one-fourth of the population is 30% or more over their desirable weight. The term *morbid obesity* has been coined to define a subset of obese persons who are at least twice their ideal body weight. Ideal body weight can be determined by using Broca's index, according to which ideal body weight (in kilograms) for males is equal to the height in centimeters minus 100. For females, ideal body weight (in kilograms) is equal to the height in centimeters minus 105. Another frequently used estimate of ideal body weight is the body mass index, which is equal to the weight in kilograms divided by the height in meters, squared. The normal body mass index is 25, whereas the index for the morbidly obese is considered to be greater than 30. The anesthetic management of the morbidly obese parturient requires an understanding of the physiologic changes associated with both pregnancy and obesity. Morbidly obese pregnant patients have an increased risk of perioperative respiratory failure and arrest, aspiration of gastric contents, cardiovascular failure and collapse, pulmonary embolism, infection, metabolic disturbances and hepatic and renal dysfunction. These patients have an increased incidence of oxytocic induction and repeat cesarean deliveries. They tend to be older, to have higher parity and to have increased antepartum frequency of hypertension, diabetes mellitus, twin gestations and an increased perioperative mortality.[1]

PATHOPHYSIOLOGY

Airway management is often difficult in morbidly obese patients and therefore should be a major concern.[2] Nearly 10% of morbidly obese parturients can be described as having sleep apnea and have an elevated resting $P\text{aCO}_2$. Laryngoscopy is complicated by the presence of suprasternal fat pads, large breasts, compromised cervical spine extension and redundant pharyngeal tissue. Obtaining a good mask fit often requires two hands and, on occasion, two people. These patients exhibit a restrictive pattern of pulmonary dysfunction on spirometry. They have a decreased functional residual capacity (FRC) and expiratory reserve volume (ERV) and increased closing volumes (CV). Their FRC is often less than their closing capacity, resulting in atelectasis and increased shunting.[3] These patients have an increased oxygen consumption and carbon dioxide production. They have decreased chest wall compliance and a markedly increased work of breathing. In fact, one has described breathing in the morbidly obese pregnant patient in the supine position as breathing with an 80-pound weight on one's chest. These defects are exaggerated in the supine position and amplified in the Trendelenburg position.[4] Most healthy morbidly obese patients have a residual gastric volume greater than 25 ml and a gastric pH less than 2.5.[5] Cardiac output increases proportionately with weight and total blood volume is increased in these patients. Insulin resistance and an elevation in cholesterol and triglycerides is frequently seen. Fatty infiltration of the liver associated with disturbances of liver function is common.[6] The physiologic changes of pregnancy compound the medical problems associated with obesity and further stress already minimal reserves.

Fetal monitoring may be more difficult in the morbidly obese, and aortocaval compression may occur even in the left lateral position. These patients should labor in a semisitting position, receive supplemental oxygen, wear support stockings and have an internal monitoring electrode placed on the fetus as soon as possible during labor.

PREANESTHETIC EVALUATION

Preoperatively, in addition to the usual preanesthetic evaluation, these patients should all have arterial blood gas measurements on room air. Patients with an increased $P\text{aCO}_2$ are at an increased risk for post-operative apnea. A baseline electrocardiogram should be obtained and a blood sample should be sent to the blood bank for type and screen. A complete blood count, blood urea nitrogen, creatinine, serum osmolarity and liver function tests should be obtained as well as a urinalysis with specific gravity and urine osmolarity. The status of the patient's hydration should be carefully evaluated since these patients can sequester large volumes of fluid in their interstitial spaces and can be intravascularly volume depleted while still appearing normovolemic on physical examination by skin turgor and tongue moisture. A central venous pressure (CVP) catheter should always be considered for this reason as well as the fact that intravascular access can be extremely difficult to obtain in these patients. Pulmonary function tests can be useful. If intraspinal anesthesia is a consideration or if there is a history of venous stasis or thromboembolic disease, coagulation studies should be obtained.

MATERNAL MONITORING

Maternal monitoring should consist of an electrocardiogram, pulse oximeter and an intra-arterial catheter to monitor blood pressure and to obtain blood specimens from the patient from whom blood may be impossible to obtain in a crisis and in whom the technical difficulties of obtaining cuff pressures may be insurmountable.[7] As already mentioned, a CVP catheter should always be considered in these patients. The Trendelenburg position should be avoided during line placement because of the risk of aspiration as well as a decrease in FRC. If indicated, a pulmonary artery catheter should be used without hesitation. It must be stressed that because fetal distress could necessitate an emergency cesarean delivery at any time, all preparations for such an event should be carried out well in advance. Two large peripheral intravenous catheters or one peripheral and a CVP catheter should be placed. These patients should be NPO (nil by mouth) and should receive 30 ml of a nonparticulate antacid every 4 h, cimetidine or ranitidine every 6 h and metoclopramide every 6 h.[8] An operating room should be ready for emergency delivery. The problems and management plan should be reviewed with the patient, the anesthesia care team, the nursing staff, the obstetric team, and the recovery room staff.

ANESTHESIA FOR LABOR AND VAGINAL DELIVERY

Epidural anesthesia is the obvious choice for labor and delivery. Initiation should be carried out with the patient in the sitting position to maintain maximum respiratory function and to obtain adequate spinal flexion. If the epidural is not readily accomplished, a continuous spinal anesthetic should be considered. Continuous subarachnoid anesthesia (CSA) offers several advantages over single-dose subarachnoid or continuous epidural anesthesia (CEA).[2] The technique provides the advantages of a single-dose subarachnoid block (i.e. rapid onset, consistent effectiveness and the ability to use low doses of local anesthetic) with the advantages of a CEA (i.e. controllable duration and controllable level). CSA should theoretically decrease complications such as a high motor block compromising respiratory function, total spinal anesthesia and systemic toxicity from local anesthetics. However, there will be an incidence of post-dural puncture headache with this technique. This is a manageable complication and, with the introduction and further development of microcatheters, the incidence of post-dural puncture headache should decrease. With whatever technique is chosen, the local anesthetic must be administered slowly since the level obtained with a given dose is unpredictable and may vary considerably from patient to patient. In fact, we have seen the level abruptly rise following delivery of the baby. Hypotension should be aggressively treated with both crystalloid solution and ephedrine, and, if necessary, phenylephrine. The Trendelenburg position should be avoided because, although it does increase venous return, it will decrease FRC and increase the risk of regurgitation. The anesthetic level should be kept at or below T6 since higher levels will impair the patient's ability to use her intercostal muscles for respiration. Uterine displacement should be maintained at all times, and this may be difficult to accomplish.

ANESTHESIA FOR CESAREAN DELIVERY

General anesthesia

Many authorities would argue that anesthesia for cesarean delivery necessitates the use of general anesthesia and endotracheal intubation. Cesarean delivery requires the patient to be supine with uterine displacement and involves manipulation of the abdomen. Morbidly obese pregnant patients do not tolerate intra-abdominal manipulation because of their already impaired respiratory status and their tendency to vomit and, possibly, aspirate. A high level of epidural and subarachnoid anesthesia alone will impair intercostal muscle function and further compromise respiratory status. A total spinal anesthetic can be disastrous. Thus, general endotracheal anesthesia may be necessary to support ventilation and to protect the airway. If the airway examination suggests the likelihood of a difficult intubation, an awake, sedated fiber-optic intubation in the semisitting position is warranted. Another option is to use topical anesthesia on the tongue and oropharynx in order to perform direct laryngoscopy to visualize what structures can be seen before induction of general anesthesia. If direct laryngoscopy and intubation is attempted, a rapid-sequence induction with continuous cricoid pressure is mandatory. An extra (or third) person should be available to assist in the procedure. A short-handled laryngoscope can be very helpful. A large-bore suction apparatus must be available and an assortment of small endotracheal tubes (internal diameter 5, 6 and 7 mm) with stylets in place must be ready. If, after induction, the patient is found to be unintubatable and ventilation with cricoid pressure cannot be maintained, an emergency cricothyrotomy must be performed. This involves an incision through the cricothyroid membrane with the insertion of a small (5 mm) endotracheal tube and subsequent inflation of the cuff to obtain a seal. This may be very difficult to accomplish in the morbidly obese parturient. If the mother can be ventilated but not intubated, she should be allowed to awaken. A controlled awake direct or fiber-optic intubation can then be accomplished. A blind nasal intubation is an option but should usually be avoided because of the friability of the nasal mucosa in parturients and the increased difficulty accomplishing any type of intubation when the pharynx is awash in blood. Maternal safety outweighs fetal considerations at this time and surgery should not be permitted to commence until an adequate airway has been established.

Increased cardiac output and an increase in compartment size will increase the requirement for volatile agents as well. Prior to induction, these patients should be acutely oxygenated and well denitrogenated for several minutes. A rapid-sequence induction with cricoid pressure should be accomplished with thiopental and endotracheal intubation facilitated with succinylcholine. Cricoid pressure must be maintained until endotracheal tube position is verified. Capnography is the 'gold' standard in this regard. The endotracheal tube should be well secured and an orogastric (Salem-sump) tube inserted *orally* and gastric contents emptied. Temperature should be monitored as well. The electrocardiogram should be monitored for rhythm and ST changes. Appropriate cardiac medications should be available. Isoflurane is the volatile agent of choice because it undergoes the least biodegradation. Anesthesia is maintained with at least 50% oxygen supplemented with nitrous oxide and isoflurane as needed. Pulse oximetry or arterial blood gases data will help guide the required oxygen concentration. A succinylcholine infusion can be used for neuromuscular blockade, however these patients may be predisposed to a type II block because of the large volumes of drug necessary to maintain paralysis. A better choice for neuromuscular blockade after endotracheal intubation might be an intermediate-acting nondepolarizing drug, particularly atracurium, in patients with hepatic or renal impairment. The volatile agent is usually discontinued after the fetus is born because of the degree of uterine relaxation that these drugs can cause and a nitrous–opioid–relaxant technique is used. If $Sa\text{O}_2$ is impaired by the increase in nitrous oxide, the nitrous oxide concentration must be decreased and a volatile agent reinstituted. Opioid supplementation is appropriate at this time. Some authorities would suggest that the amount of uterine relaxation from 0.2–0.4% isoflurane is minimal (or absent) and that this drug should be maintained for amnesia alone. Positive end-expiratory pressure (PEEP) can be used to reduce atelectasis, although high intrathoracic pressures can also reduce venous return.

There may be occasions when the risks of general anesthesia outweigh the risks of delivering the infant of a morbidly obese woman by regional anesthesia alone. In these situations a continuous epidural or continuous subarachnoid technique should be chosen. The sensory level should not be raised above T6. Epidural or subarachnoid opioids such as fentanyl can be administered to make the patient more comfortable intra- and post-operatively and to allow the surgery to proceed without impairing the patient's respiratory status, as may occur with high thoracic levels.

Intraspinal plus 'light general' anesthesia offers several advantages over general anesthesia alone. It allows adequate airway protection and ventilation while reducing intravenous and volatile anesthetic requirements. It also allows for the use of the epidural or subarachnoid catheter to provide post-operative pain control.

Emergency cesarean delivery

If an emergency cesarean delivery is necessary, a general anesthetic with a rapid-sequence induction with cricoid pressure can be undertaken (see earlier discussion of technique). A epidural or subarachnoid catheter can be placed post-operatively for pain management. This scenario should not emerge often, however, since an elective epidural or continuous subarachnoid catheter should have been placed already during labor.

Post-operative care

If the preoperative room air $Pa\text{CO}_2$ is elevated, if there is any question of the patient's ability to protect or ensure her airway, or if there is cardiovascular instability, the patient should remain intubated overnight. The patient can be monitored in the recovery room or intensive care unit and ventilated with PEEP on an intermittent mandatory ventilation mode as necessary. She should be kept in the sitting position on an $F\text{IO}_2$ of 50% and be continuously monitored with an electrocardiograph and pulse oximeter and observed closely by the nursing staff.

The post-partum morbidly obese patient is at high risk for respiratory failure and arrest.[8] In addition to all the reasons mentioned previously, the parturient now has an abdominal incision that may cause her to splint and take shallow breaths. There may be residual anesthetic agents present. In the pregnant state, high progesterone levels cause respiratory stimulation. Post-partum, these levels fall and respiratory stimulation decreases.

Intramuscular, subcutaneous, or more frequently 'intrafat' opioid injections should be avoided. The absorption of these drugs is unreliable under optimal conditions and these patients are often cold and peripherally vasoconstricted. The obese parturient appears to have a decreased tolerance for pain and may require large doses of opioids post-operatively, which contributes to the multiple factors already described that can cause post-operative respiratory depression. Morbidly obese parturients will require large doses of pain-relieving medications; these drugs should not be given intramuscularly as they will be sequestered in adipose tissue. In the early post-operative period, if continuous epidural or subarachnoid anesthesia has been utilized, the catheter should be maintained and post-operative pain relief provided by subarachnoid or epidural opioids and/or local anesthetics. If general anesthesia has been administered, intravenous opioids must be utilized, either on demand or by patient-controlled analgesia. Change over to oral pain medications may not be feasible for 2–3 days. Intraspinal opioids or a combination of opioids and local anesthetics is the best method of pain control. Alternatively, intravenous opioids can be titrated on an hourly basis. These patients require frequent overnight checks. All post-partum morbidly obese patients should be monitored in the recovery room or intensive care until overnight on the first post-operative night. They should be maintained in the head-up position and receive oxygen by face mask at 6–10 l/min. They should be monitored using pulse oximetry with alarms set at an $Sa\text{O}_2$ of 90%. They should have continuous electrocardiographic monitoring, frequent, if not continuous, blood pressure monitoring and frequent temperature checks. Urine output and osmolarity as well as hematocrit should be followed. Shivering should be avoided and treated with small doses of intravenous opioids as necessary. These patients should also be treated with minidose heparin. Once they are transferred to the floor, their arterial lines, CVP lines and epidural or subarachnoid catheters can be removed. They should still be maintained in the head-up position and administered 50% oxygen by face mask. Vital signs should be checked and recorded every 2 h for 8 h. An intravenous line should be kept in place until discharge. Early ambulation should be vigorously encouraged.

The risks of caring for the post-partum morbidly obese patient are often not fully appreciated by nursing or medical staff members. In addition to all of the usual obstetric post-operative complications, these patients are at increased risk of respiratory failure and arrest, venous stasis and emboli, cardiovascular failure, hypertension, hypovolemia and infection.

REFERENCES

1. Gross T, Sokol R J, King K C 1980 Obesity in pregnancy: risks and outcome. Obstet Gynecol 56: 446–450
2. Malan T P, Johnson M D 1988 The difficult airway in obstetric anesthesia: techniques for airway management and the role of regional anesthesia. J Clin Anesth 1: 104–111
3. Luce M J 1980 Respiratory complications of obesity. Chest 78: 626–631
4. Paul D R, Hoyt J L, Boutros A R 1976 Cardiovascular and respiratory changes in response to change of posture in the very obese. Anesthesiology 45: 73–78
5. Vaughan R W, Bauer S, Wise L 1986 Volume and pH of gastric juice in obese patients. Anesthesiology 65: 684–687
6. Braillon A, Capron J P, Herve M A et al 1985 Liver in obesity. Gut 26: 133–139
7. Berlines K, Fujy H, Lee D H et al 1961 Blood pressure measurements in obese persons: comparison of intraarterial and auscultatory measurements. Am J Cardiol 8: 10–13
8. Vaughan R W, Englehart R C, Wise L 1974 Postoperative hypoxemia in obese patients. Ann Surg 180: 877–882

59. The difficult airway: management of failed intubation

M. D. Johnson   T. P. Malan Jr

Failed endotracheal intubation is a principal cause of anesthesia-related maternal morbidity and mortality. In England and Wales from 1979 to 1981, 24% of maternal deaths related to anesthesia were directly related to difficulties with tracheal intubation.[1] The prevalence of failed intubation in obstetric anesthesia is not known, but has been estimated to be approximately 1 in 300.[2] This prevalence is significantly higher than that for non-pregnant patients.

The optimal approach to failed intubation is prevention. With thorough preoperative evaluation of the airway and utilization of current techniques for endotracheal intubation, the incidence of failed intubation can be minimized. However, failed endotracheal intubation after induction of general anesthesia may still occur.

Although many approaches to failed intubation in obstetrics have been proposed,[3–8] there are few objective data on which to base a protocol. However, despite these limitations, each clinician *must* formulate a plan for management of failed intubation that will help to minimize the confusion and faulty decision-making associated with an emergent, stressful situation. The plan should include an immediate assessment of the airway, alternative approaches to intubation, options for foreseeable contingencies and specific limits for how long to persist with intubation attempts. Our approach is illustrated in Figure 59.1 and summarized below.

MANAGEMENT OF FAILED INTUBATION

If intubation fails, the lungs should be ventilated while cricoid pressure remains applied. The prompt decision to

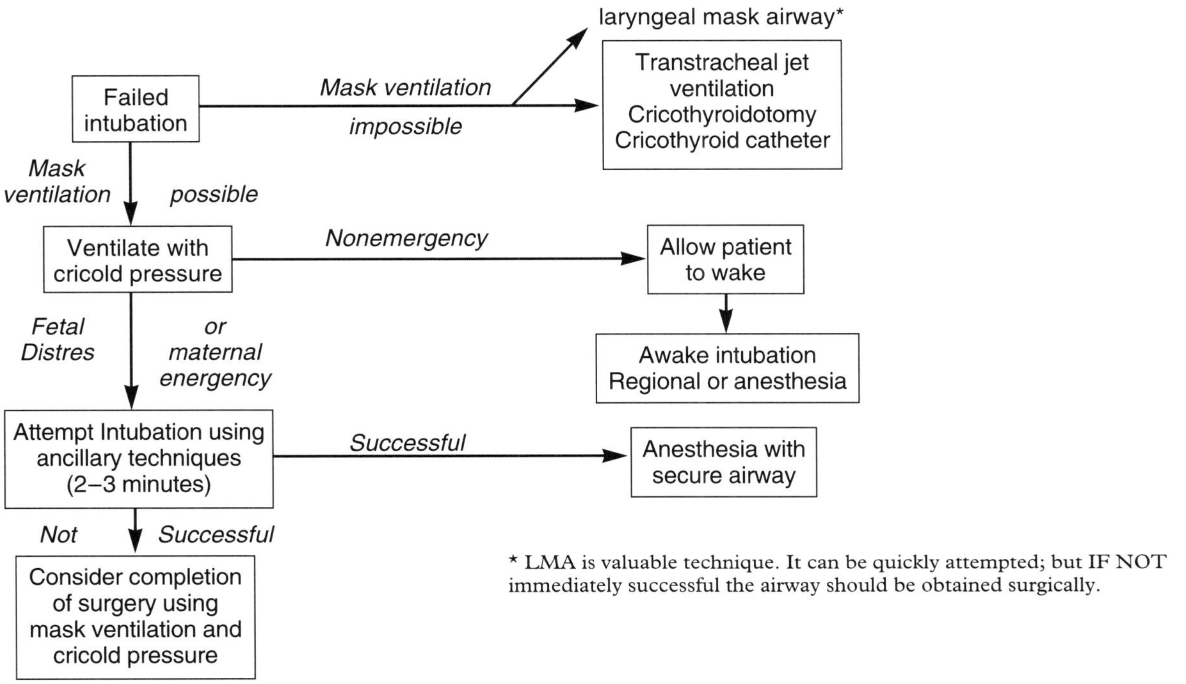

Fig. 59.1 Sample protocol for failed intubation. (Modified from ref. 9 with permission.)

abandon the first intubation attempt and ventilate the lungs by mask is critical. Scott[10] has argued that patients do not die from failure to intubate, they die from failure to stop trying to intubate. The oxygen saturation of the parturient at term will decline very rapidly when the patient is apneic. In addition, prolonged attempts at intubation may provoke retching, vomiting and subsequent aspiration of gastric contents.

Subsequent attempts at intubation should be limited and well conceived in order to minimize airway trauma. Alternative methods, such as the use of the lighted stylet or fiber-optic endoscope, should be considered. Additional anesthetic or neuromuscular blocking agents should not be administered unless (1) successful intubation is considered to be certain with an additional attempt or (2) it is elected to proceed with general anesthesia and a mask airway.

If intubation fails, one must decide whether to awaken the patient and employ an alternative anesthetic approach, such as awake intubation or regional anesthesia, or to proceed with general anesthesia and a mask airway. If the fetus does not require emergent cesarean delivery for fetal distress, the patient should be allowed to awaken. If the fetus is at risk, the decision must be based on the clinical situation and the philosophy of the individual practitioner. Most medical and legal doctrine favors overlooking the fetus before putting the mother at risk so it is prudent to allow the patient to awaken in most cases.

Some investigators propose the use of lateral or head-down positions, laryngeal masks, esophageal obturator airways or gastric suctioning in managing failed intubation. We do not routinely utilize these maneuvers because changes in patient position or manipulation of the pharynx and esophagus might interfere with ventilation, interfere with the competency of the lower esophageal sphincter or stimulate vomiting or retching.

FAILURE OF INTUBATION AND VENTILATION

If the trachea cannot be intubated and the lungs cannot be ventilated via mask, two options exist: either an airway can be established by cricothyroidotomy or the lungs can be ventilated using transtracheal jet ventilation.

The utility of transtracheal jet ventilation in the management of the difficult airway has recently been reviewed.[11] This technique has been shown to provide excellent oxygenation and ventilation in experimental animals, in elective surgical patients and in patients with complete upper airway obstruction. Using a driving pressure of 50 p.s.i, a gas flow of 500 ml/s can be delivered through a 16-gauge catheter. This gas flow is sufficient for adequate ventilation.

Benumof and Scheller[11] have described in detail three acceptable systems for transtracheal jet ventilation. These are, in descending order of preference, a jet injector powered by regulated wall or oxygen tank pressure, a jet injector powered by unregulated wall or tank oxygen pressure and an anesthesia machine flush valve using noncompliant tubing from the fresh gas outlet. The last system can be constructed from materials available in most operating rooms for a cost of approximately $6. Therefore, it is feasible to prepare this simple system for every obstetric operating room. Other methods proposed for transtracheal ventilation, such as using the anesthesia machine flush valve with the anesthesia circle system corrugated tubing or using the anesthesia machine reservoir bag with the circle system, do not reliably achieve adequate ventilation.

If transtracheal jet ventilation is utilized, it may be continued until the patient regains consciousness, the airway is secured by orotracheal or nasotracheal intubation, or cricothyroidotomy or tracheostomy is performed. Although transtracheal jet ventilation is a very useful technique, it does not provide protection of the airway from aspiration of gastric contents, a significant concern in the parturient.

Cricothyroidotomy is more complex and invasive than transtracheal jet ventilation, but has three potential advantages. First, insertion of a cuffed tube protects the airway from aspiration. Second, insertion of an appropriately sized tube allows tracheal suctioning. Third, there may be less likelihood of barotrauma and emphysema than with transtracheal jet ventilation. Therefore, this technique should be considered, particularly if prolonged ventilatory support is anticipated.

Although cricothyroidotomy is an invasive procedure, it is one that every anesthesiologist should be prepared to perform. Many approaches and techniques have been described. Although several adjunctive or percutaneous devices have been developed, none has found widespread use.

REFERENCES

1. Turnbull A C, Tindall V R, Robson G et al 1986 Report on Confidential Enquiries into Maternal Deaths in England and Wales 1979–1981. HMSO London
2. Morgan M 1987 Anaesthetic contribution to maternal mortality. Br J Anaesth 59: 842–855
3. Tunstall M E 1976 Failed intubation drill. Anaesthesia 31: 850
4. Boys J E 1983 Failed intubation in obstetric anesthesia. Br J Anaesth 55: 187–188
5. Campbell W I 1983 Failed intubation in obstetric anesthesia. Br J Anaesth 55: 1040 (letter)
6. Sivaneswaran N, McGuiness J J 1984 Modified mask for failed intubation at emergency Caesarean section. Anaesth Intensive Care 12: 279–280
7. Tunstall M E, Sheikh A 1986 Failed intubation protocol: oxygenation without aspiration. Clin Anesthesiol 4:171
8. Rosen M 1985 Difficult and failed intubation in obstetrics. p 152.

In Latto I P, Rosen M (eds) Difficulties in tracheal intubation. Balliere Tindall, London
9. Malan Jr T P, Johnson M D 1988 The difficult airway in obstetric anesthesia: techniques for airway management and the role of regional anesthesia. J Clin Anesth 1: 104–111
10. Scott D B 1986 Endotracheal intubation: friend or foe? Br Med J 292: 157–158
11. Benumof J L, Scheller M S 1989 The importance of transtracheal jet ventilation in the management of the difficult airway. Anesthesiology 71: 769–778

60. Use of the laryngeal mask in obstetric anesthesia

A. I. J. Brain

The Laryngeal Mask (LMA) is a new kind of airway for use in anesthetized, fasting patients in the form of a miniature inflatable mask attached to a tube (Fig. 60.1). It is inserted blindly into the hypopharynx where it forms a low-pressure seal around the laryngeal inlet. It requires neither laryngoscopy nor neuromuscular block for insertion. Invented in 1981, it was launched on the British market in 1988 and has now come to occupy a significant place in British anesthesia, replacing both the facemask and the endotracheal tube in a high proportion of routine uncomplicated cases. The device has also proved popular in Europe, Australia and Canada and is currently sold in 60 countries. It has recently become available in the United States, where the FDA has ruled that it should be regarded as a pharyngeal airway, not a replacement for the endotracheal tube. The inventor is entirely in agreement with this cautious approach.

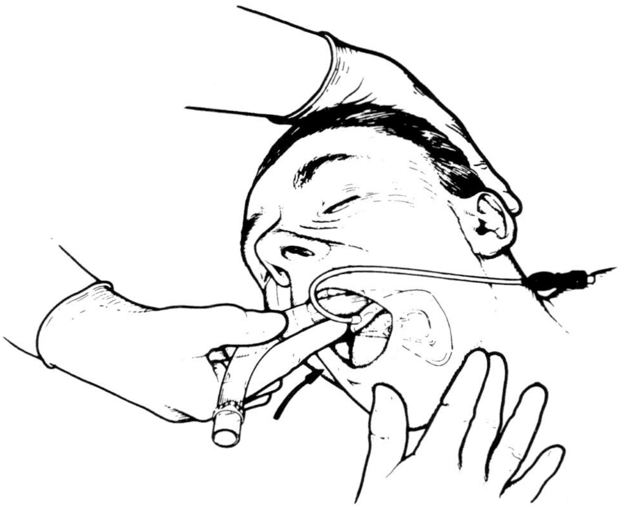

Fig. 60.1

MORTALITY AND THE AIRWAY IN OBSTETRIC ANESTHESIA

British data published by the Department of Health show a steady decline in anesthesia-related mortality during pregnancy in England and Wales, from 12.8 per million in the years 1970–1972 down to 1.9 per million in the years 1985–1987. However, the incidence of obstetric deaths associated with intubation does not show the same trend. In the triennium 1982–1984, eight out of 18 anesthetic deaths were due to intubation problems. There were only eight obstetric anesthetic deaths in the United Kingdom during the triennium 1985–1987; but of these, six were due to intubation problems. This latest report[1] expresses concern that, although only one of these eight deaths was due to inhalation of gastric contents, oral and intravenous ranitidine and oral sodium citrate had been correctly administered, cricoid pressure correctly applied and no difficulty experienced with intubation in this one particular case.

The lessons appear to be, first and most importantly, that death is more likely to be caused by hypoxia associated with failure to intubate than by pulmonary aspiration; second, that problems with intubation remain undiminished in spite of improvements in other areas, and third, that intubation, even when it is easily and correctly accomplished, does not always guarantee against aspiration occurring at some stage in the procedure. Indeed, recent evidence from a large retrospective survey of patients undergoing general anesthesia indicates that 68% of aspirations occur in association with either laryngoscopy or extubation.[2]

The British report lists the LMA[3] amongst equipment that should be available in case intubation proves to be impossible. It is noted that it does not protect the airway against regurgitated gastric contents and recommends the use of continuous cricoid pressure if it is used in obstetric patients. More recently, a multicenter study in the UK has shown that the LMA can be used by paramedics to provide effective ventilation in cardiac arrest prior to the arrival of personnel capable of intubation.[4] In a pilot study, it was used successfully in three cardiac arrest patients who could not be intubated.[5]

The LMA is currently used in some degree in all UK hospitals in which general anesthetics are carried out. For example, a recent audit from the Ambulatory Surgery Center at Addenbrooke's hospital in Cambridge, UK, shows it is used in 47% of all cases requiring general anesthesia. The indications cover most routine and a growing number of specialized operative procedures. Many cases of successful use in failed intubation have been described in the international literature. There are currently more than 400 publications on the LMA worldwide of which approximately 16% are concerned with its use in relation to difficult intubation.

ROLE OF THE LMA IN FAILED OBSTETRIC INTUBATION

The efficacy of the LMA in failed obstetric intubation has been substantiated by Chadwick[6] and McClune.[7] Chadwick notes that familiarity with the technique is important, a point which the inventor has stressed.[8] McClune commented that it was life-saving in the case he describes. Neither author refers to the associated use of cricoid pressure. Evidence to indicate cricoid pressure is effective when used in conjunction with the LMA is limited to a study on cadavers.[9] There is a theoretical risk that external pressure against the cricoid might squeeze the mask tip out of the hypopharynx which might in turn result in airway obstruction by anterior displacement of the arytenoids. The phenomenon of anterior arytenoid displacement has been noted by Payne.[10] The same author records seeing the esophagus through the mask aperture on occasion. However, this statement, which has been cited in support of the lack of protection offered by the LMA, may be a reflection of incorrect positioning of the device, as can be seen by the correct and incorrect positions demonstrated radiographically by Nandi,[11] whose paper illustrates the importance of correct insertion techniques as detailed by White[12] and Brain.[13] Füllekrug has noted the esophagus becomes visible in 10% of cases if airway pressure is allowed to exceed 25 cm H_2O.

Another potential difficulty arises from the position of the mask tip. When correctly inserted this should lie immediately posterior to the cricoid cartilage. If pressure is applied to the cricoid *during* insertion, it might prove difficult to pass the mask tip fully into position behind it, so that the tip remains opposite the laryngeal opening, where it could in theory cause total obstruction. This is a possible cause of the failure to ventilate an obstetric patient with an LMA described by Christian[14] and indicates, as suggested by Heath,[19] that cricoid pressure should be released momentarily to permit passage of the LMA to the correct depth. However, there is conflicting evidence on this subject;[15,16] it may be that the correctly deflated mask tip forms a stiff enough wedge to cleave behind the cricoid ring when pressure is applied to this structure. To investigate this supposition further, the pressures applied would need to be controlled.

REGURGITATION AND LMA USE

What is still lacking is evidence that optimal technique influences the incidence of unexpected regurgitation. Before the technique had been fully developed by the inventor, he encountered four cases of unexpected regurgitation in technically fasted non-obstetric patients during seven years of development work with prototypes – all without complications. Fluid was seen within the LMA tube and was suctioned after putting the patient in the Trendelenberg position, deepening anesthesia and increasing FiO_2. A number of other cases have been described in non-obstetric patients managed with the LMA,[17,18] but without mortality. No obstetric cases of aspiration using the LMA have been described to date.

It should be remembered that the 66 cases of acid aspiration described by Mendelson in 1946 resulted in no deaths from pneumonitis – the two deaths he described were due to obstructive hypoxia from aspiration of solid food particles,[20] a situation much less likely to arise today.

How often do non-obstetric patients in whom the LMA is used aspirate when known contraindications are avoided? A recent survey from the Royal Berkshire Hospital[21] of 2359 operations carried out using the LMA included 609 routine gynecologic cases. There was an overall incidence of regurgitation of 0.08% but no aspiration was recorded. In one district general hospital in the UK which was the first to use the commercial LMA, senior anesthetic staff were choosing it after the first year in 63% of all non-emergency general anesthetics, including 53% of all gynecologic procedures. One and a half years later, the LMA had been used in more than 7000 cases.[22] Only one case of aspiration is known to have occurred with the LMA in this hospital and this was due to unintentional use in a patient with a hiatal hernia – a known contraindication. There were no serious sequelae in this case, although life-threatening pneumonitis has been reported where the LMA has been used inappropriately.[23]

HOW SAFE IS THE LMA?

It is estimated that the LMA has been used more than 5 million times in the UK. No medico-legal claims have yet arisen in connection with its use in the UK to the inventor's knowledge. Properly used, it would appear to be a very safe device. However, *this does not mean it should ever be considered as a first choice in obstetric patients who are at risk from aspiration.* It is too early to quantify the risk of aspiration when it is used to overcome impossible intubation in this situation.

On the other hand, it is of interest that a pilot study[5] of LMA use by specially trained nurses in cardiac arrest cases occurring on general wards found no evidence of aspiration in association with use of the LMA (n=41). The explanation may lie in the speed and reliability with which control of the airway can be achieved. From the time the cardiac arrest was logged by the hospital switchboard, the investigators reported that ventilation was being achieved in 2.9 min (range 2–5) compared to 8 min (range 5–14) for endotracheal intubation. These preliminary findings have been substantiated by a larger British study involving four hospitals.[4] The low incidence of regurgitation when the LMA is used in patients who have suffered cardiac arrest raises the question as to whether, in the context of anesthesia, there may be other avoidable factors in the etiology of unexpected regurgitation. For example, high pressure differences may be generated across the esophageal sphincters associated with inspiratory efforts against an obstructed upper airway, or straining in an inadequately anesthetized patient.

USING THE LMA AS A GUIDE FOR TRACHEAL INTUBATION

Heath has shown[19] that the LMA can be used as a guide to intubation, with a success rate of over 90%, using a 6 mm cuffed tube. In Heath's hands, this maneuver was achieved within 30 s. The LMA does not need to be removed but is left in place, since it may also have a role in preventing difficulties following extubation. The option of using the LMA as a guide has been discussed by Benumof[24] and might be considered in the obstetric failed intubation. However, it requires confidence born of practice. It has been suggested that the LMA tube should be split to allow passage of a larger endotracheal tube and easier removal of the LMA.[25,26] However, as stated, problems with extubation may be more likely if intubation has been difficult, so a more rational choice might be to leave the LMA in situ until after extubation. A dedicated intubating LMA is in process of development (see below and Fig. 60.2).

HOW TO AVOID PROBLEMS WITH LMA USE

It should be remembered that seal pressures of the LMA against the laryngeal inlet are of the order of 2 kPa (20 cm H_2O) so that it is always necessary to employ a ventilatory pattern which will permit gas flow at pressures below this limit to avoid leaks at the mask to larynx interface.[27] In the author's experience, it is wise to apply only very gentle manual bag pressure after insertion, no matter how urgent the need to inflate the lungs. The inexperienced user will find it very hard to overcome the desire to inflate the lungs vigorously after successfully inserting the LMA in a patient who is already desaturated. This temptation must be resisted, because it introduces the danger of forcing gas into the stomach and may increase the risk of inhalation if regurgitation has occurred. It is important to appreciate that the correctly inserted LMA will almost always come to lie in the correct position, so that failure to achieve an airway with it is usually due to either inadequate anesthesia or inadequate neuromuscular blockade. Moreover, it has been shown that the airway tends to remain clear even with gross malposition of the device, provided anesthesia is adequate.[11]

It should be noted that insertion should not be

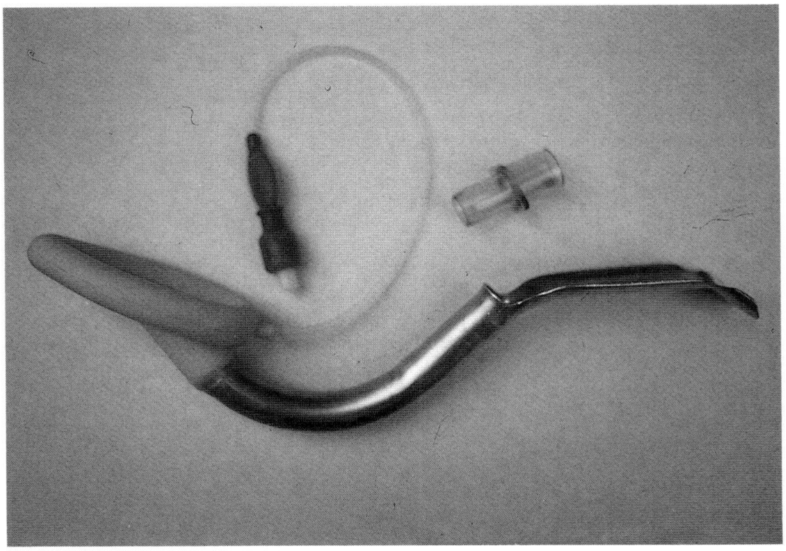

Fig. 60.2 Intubating laryngeal mask

attempted immediately after thiopental or etomidate used alone in the absence of neuromuscular block. The author does not recommend the use of etomidate with the LMA because of the tendency of patients to vomit. Propofol, however, provides good insertion conditions when given at 2.5–3.0 mg/kg. Occasionally, complete inability to ventilate through the LMA occurs when it is inserted immediately after propofol. This is due to the provocation of glottic closure as part of an uncoordinated swallowing reflex. This occurrence is easily confused by the inexperienced with malposition or laryngeal spasm but, unlike laryngeal spasm, it wears off after about 20 s, with a characteristic rapid transition from complete airway closure to complete airway patency.[27] The addition of fentanyl 2.5 μg/kg before induction reduces the likelihood of this occurrence. Fentanyl also permits insertion with normal induction doses of thiopental if propofol is not available.

USING THE LMA WITH POSITIVE PRESSURE VENTILATION

It can be argued that the low seal pressures of the LMA compared with the endotracheal tube constitute a limitation to its use for positive pressure ventilation. However, if low flow rates and moderate tidal volumes are used, leaks can usually be avoided and it is not difficult to achieve normo- or hypocapnia. The pressure limitations of the system may also constitute an important safety valve, making barotrauma unlikely. In the Royal Berkshire Hospital Survey mentioned above, 41% of all LMA cases were paralyzed and ventilated.

THE LMA IS NOT AN ENDOTRACHEAL TUBE!

The anatomical position occupied by the LMA means that, unlike the endotracheal tube, it can only fit into the space it is designed to fill – the hypopharynx. The two greatest dangers of intubation, accidental entry into the esophagus or into a main bronchus are unlikely. Moreover, the hypopharynx is adapted to accept foreign bodies in the form of food. Indeed, just as the correctly inserted mask imitates the swallowing of a bolus of food, the swallowing reflex can be seen to be provoked as anesthesia lightens. Significant pressure trauma does not apparently occur with normal use of the LMA. However, the mobility of the hypopharynx does give it one disadvantage as a space in which to form an airway seal, in that it may allow leakage of gastric contents around the mask if regurgitation occurs. Thus the suspected presence of acid gastric contents remains the most important contraindication to use of the LMA in normal circumstances. Those who become adept at the technique for routine surgery, however, are likely to acquire a level of skill and confidence which may allow a rapid solution to the problem of impossible obstetric intubation, thereby reducing the risk of disaster due to hypoxia.

WHEN AND HOW TO USE THE LMA IN FAILED INTUBATION

Once an airway is achieved by this means, which in experienced hands will be of the order of a few seconds and in inexperienced hands has been shown to be around 20 s,[28] the immediate aim of correction of hypoxia is best achieved with the provision of 100% oxygen administered with *gently* assisted manual bag inflation. However, this will be quite impossible if the patient is straining. A level of anesthesia sufficient to abolish reflex response is essential at this point, but is easily forgotten in the patient who has been subjected to repeated attempts of intubation using succinylcholine.

If this drug wears off as the surgeon applies the knife, laryngeal spasm is likely to occur. Airway resistance may be high in the inadequately anesthetized, highly stressed patient even when neuromuscular block is adequate, making effective ventilation through the LMA impossible. In the author's experience of managing non-obstetric moderately obese patients with chronic airway disease, where the LMA has been used electively, similar problems may arise following induction associated with poor uptake of volatile anesthetics. Intravenous propofol appears to be an effective way of rapidly deepening anesthesia and thus overcoming this problem; it is certainly a better drug for insertion of the LMA than thiopental.[29]

WHEN AND HOW TO USE THE LMA IN FAILED OBSTETRIC INTUBATION

At what point should the LMA be used if intubation fails at induction for cesarean delivery? In the case described by McClune,[7] saturation had dropped to 37% before the device was used. In view of the evidence[1] that hypoxia is the greatest danger when intubation fails, it might be wise for the experienced user to insert an LMA before such low levels are reached, even if only to gain time while considering other options, which will also be influenced by the degree of obstetric urgency. Benumof has placed the LMA in the difficult airway management algorithm[30] and Brimacombe has suggested an algorithm for its use in patients with a full stomach, in whom intubation fails.[31] It has been suggested the LMA be available wherever airway problems are likely to arise.[32]

USE OF THE LMA IN ROUTINE GYNECOLOGIC SURGERY

The Royal Berkshire Survey mentioned above demonstrates that routine gynecological procedures are the second most common reason for using the LMA (29% all cases). Their

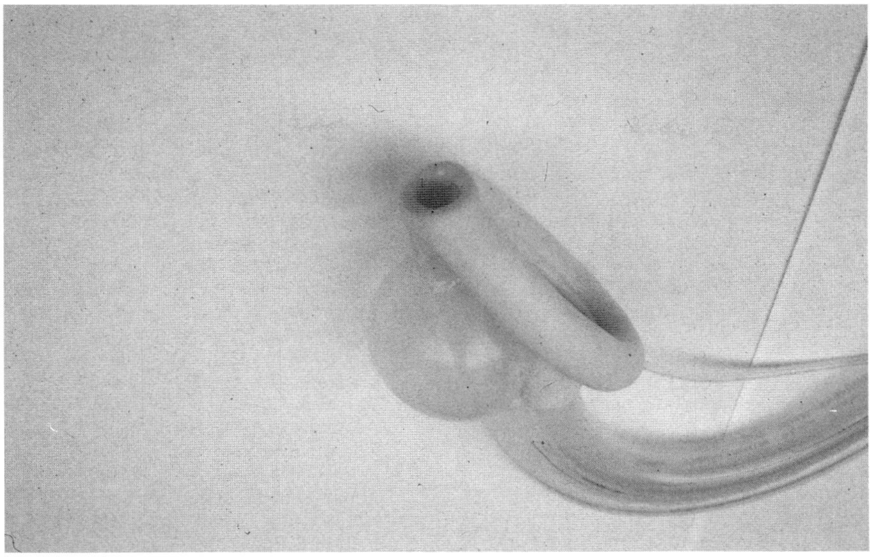

Fig. 60.3 Combined laryngeal and oesophageal mask

series included 253 laparoscopies, none of which showed evidence of regurgitation, in contrast to the findings of Duffy's 1979 study of 93 cases of which two regurgitated.[33] However, pharyngeal secretions were not tested for acidity in the Royal Berkshire Survey and Duffy's conclusion that laparoscopic patients should receive metoclopramide preoperatively would appear to be a sensible precaution. It has been suggested patients are more likely to be exposed to inadequate anesthetic depth during prolonged anesthesia and that this may increase the risk of intraoperative regurgitation.[34] The relative brevity of British surgical techniques is a feature of UK practice which should be taken into account when assessing the significance of British studies on the LMA from a transatlantic or European viewpoint. It should be remembered that the grossly obese and those with hiatus hernia symptoms should always be excluded from routine LMA use, as should any patient with a history suggestive of possible intraoperative regurgitation. However, even fasted, apparently ideal patients may have some gastric fluid[34] and the anesthesiologist has a responsibility to ensure adequate anesthesia when using the LMA.

THE FUTURE: THE ILM AND THE GLM

Two new forms of LMA are undergoing preliminary trials. The intubating laryngeal mask (Fig. 60.2) is an instrument with a short rigid wide-bore tube terminating in a standard LMA at one end and a rigid handle at the other end. This is designed to facilitate intubation using an 8 mm endotracheal tube passed through the LMA tube. The handle enables the user to alter the angle and position of the mask relative to the glottis and to stabilize the device while pushing the endotracheal tube into position through it.

The second new device is a combined laryngeal and esophageal mask (Fig. 60.3). This device is also fitted with a second posteriorly-acting cuff which provides a much higher seal pressure around the glottis. However, its principal feature is a drainage tube which forms a sealed connection with the upper esophageal sphincter. This avoids the hazards and invasiveness of intubating the esophagus but provides a passage which is sealed around its entrance, thus possibly offering a measure of protection in case of regurgitation. These and other new forms of laryngeal masks are still being developed by the inventor.

REFERENCES

1. Department of Health 1991 Report on Confidential Enquiries into Maternal Deaths in the United Kingdom 1985–1987. HMSO London, and Blackwells Scientific Publications, Oxford: pp 74–78
2. Warner M A, Warner M E, Weber J G 1993 Clinical significance of pulmonary aspiration during the perioperative period. Anesthesiol 78: 56–62
3. Brain A I J 1983 The laryngeal mask – a new concept in airway management. Br J Anaesth 55: 801–4
4. Stone B T et al 1991 Use of the laryngeal mask by nurses during cardiopulmonary resuscitation. Results of a Multicentre Trial. Anaesth (in press)
5. Alexander C A, Leach A B, Stone B 1993 The laryngeal mask in cardiopulmonary resuscitation in a district general hospital: a preliminary communication. Resuscitation 65: 245–248
6. Chadwick I S, Vohra A 1989 Anaesthesia for caesarean section using the laryngeal airway. Anaesth (corresp) 44: 261–262
7. McClune S, Moore J 1990 Laryngeal mask airway for caesarean section. Anaesth 45: 227–228

8. Brain A I J 1991 Studies on the laryngeal mask: first, learn the art. Anaesth (corresp) 46: 417–418
9. Strang T I 1992 Does the LMA compromise cricoid pressure? Anaesth 47: 829–831
10. Payne J 1989 The use of the fiberoptic laryngoscope to confirm the position of the laryngeal mask. Anaesth (corresp) 44: 865
11. Nandi P R, Nunn J F, Charlesworth C H, Taylor S J 1991 Radiological Study of the laryngeal mask. Eur J Anaesthesiol (supp) 4: 33–39
12. White D C 1991 The laryngeal mask – a non-invasive airway. Eur J Anaesthesiol (supp) 4: 1–4
13. Brain A I J 1990 Proper technique for insertion of the laryngeal mask. Anesthesiol 73: 1053
14. Christian A S 1990 Failed obstetric intubation. Anaesth (corresp) 45: 995
15. Brimacombe J 1991 Cricoid pressure and the laryngeal mask airway. Anaesth (corresp) 46: 986–987
16. Ansermino J M, Blogg C E 1992 Cricoid pressure may prevent insertion of the laryngeal mask airway. Br J Anaesth 69: 465–467
17. Griffin R M, Hatcher I S 1990 Aspiration pneumonia and the laryngeal mask airway. Anaesth 45: 1039–1040
18. Wilkinson P A, Cyna A M, MacCleod D M, Campbell J R 1990 The laryngeal mask – cautionary tales. Anaesth (corresp) 45: 137–139
19. Heath M L 1991 Endotracheal intubation through the laryngeal mask – helpful when laryngoscopy is difficult or dangerous. Eur J Anaesth (supp) 4: 41–45
20. Mendelson C L 1946 Aspiration of stomach contents into the lungs during obstetric anaesthesia. Am J Obstet Gynecol 52: 191–205
21. Verghese C, Smith T G C, Young E 1993 Prospective survey of the use of laryngeal mask airway in 2359 patients. Anaesth 48: 58–60
22. Leach A B, Alexander C A 1991 The laryngeal mask – an overview. Eur J Anaesth (supp) 4: 19–31
23. Nanji G M, Maltby J R 1992 Vomiting and aspiration pneumonitis with the laryngeal mask airway. Can J Anaesth 39: 69–70
24. Benumof J L 1992 Use of the laryngeal mask airway to facilitate fiberscope-aided tracheal intubation. Anesth Analg 74: 313–314
25. Maroof M, Khan R M, Khan H, Stewart J, Mroze C 1992 Evaluation of modified laryngeal mask airway as an aid to fiberoptic intubation. Anesthesiol 77: 3A: A1062
26. Brimacombe J, Johns K 1991 Modified intavent LMA. Anaesth & Intens Care (corresp) 19: 616
27. Brain A I J 1991 The intavent laryngeal mask instruction manual, 2nd edn. Intavent International S A, Cedar Court, 9–11 Fairmile, Henley-on-Thames, Oxon, England
28. Davies P R F, Tighe S Q M, Greenslade G L, Evans G H 1990 Laryngeal mask airway and tracheal tube insertion by unskilled personnel. Lancet 336: 977–979
29. Brown G W, Patel N, Ellis F R 1991 Comparison of propofol and thiopentone for laryngeal mask insertion. Anaesth 46: 771–772
30. American Society of Anesthesiologists 1993
31. Brimacombe J, Berry A, White A 1993 An algorithm for use of the laryngeal mask airway during failed intubation in the patient with a full stomach. Anesth Analg 77: 398–399
32. Hett D A, Bailey A R 1993 Use of the laryngeal mask airway in resuscitation. Anaesth (corresp) 48: 733
33. Duffy B L 1979 Regurgitation during pelvic laparoscopy. Br J Anaesth 51: 1089–1090
34. Maroof M, Khan R M, Siddique M S 1993 Intraoperative aspiration pneumonitis and the laryngeal mask airway. Anesth Analg 77: 409–410

61. Anesthetic and neonatal considerations in preterm delivery

Part A USA view *E. I. Abouleish B. Gonik*
Part B European view *J. Hamza*

PART A
USA VIEW
E. I. Abouleish B. Gonik

DEFINITION

Preterm labor (prematurity) is defined as delivery beyond 20 weeks' and before 37 weeks' gestation, irrespective of birthweight.[1] Abortion is interruption of pregnancy before 20 weeks' gestation. The determination of preterm labor based on weight (less than 2500 g) is not valid because decreased weight per se can be due to intrauterine growth retardation.

Importance

Prematurity is now the leading cause of perinatal death despite all efforts to prevent and stop preterm labor. In the USA, although preterm birth occurs in about 7.5% of all deliveries, it accounts for 75% of perinatal deaths.[2] Since there are about 3 500 000 deliveries per year in the USA, the number of premature babies born annually is about 250 000. It is unfortunate that many of those who survive require prolonged expensive intensive care and may suffer from permanent neurologic deficits. The main problems facing preterm babies include:

Asphyxia

The hemoglobin concentration and oxygen-carrying capacity are reduced. The lungs are immature and surfactant is decreased, and thus preterm babies are liable to develop respiratory distress syndrome (RDS). Although the development of artificial surfactants brings hope of the prevention and treatment of RDS, many of these drugs are still in their trial stages.

Vascular injury

Preterm babies and their blood vessels are fragile; thus, they may suffer from intracranial injury or ventricular hemorrhage.

Retrolental fibroplasia

This complication may follow respiratory distress syndrome when there is a need for prolonged ventilatory support with increased concentrations of oxygen.

Patent ductus arteriosus

Fetal circulation may persist after birth, with the ductus arteriosus remaining patent. This leads to increased pulmonary arterial pressure and may require surgical correction to which must be added the potential dangers of anesthesia.

Poor homeostasis

Preterm infants have difficulty in maintaining homeostasis, e.g. regulating temperature and maintaining glucose, appropriate concentrations of calcium, etc, along with proper feeding.

Apnea and periodic breathing

The lives of preterm infants are endangered by apneic episodes leading to sudden death or cerebral damage from hypoxia.

Infection

Intrapartum infection can occur secondary to chorioamnionitis. Post-partum, the development of infections such as pneumonia, sepsis and meningitis is common because of significant reduction in cellular and tissue immunity.

Necrotizing enterocolitis

This life-threatening complication increases both the mortality and morbidity of these neonates.

PREDISPOSING FACTORS

The following conditions predispose to preterm labor:

1. Overdistension of the uterus, e.g. polyhydramnios and multiple gestation.[3] The higher the number of gestations, the greater is the possibility of prematurity and the shorter is the gestation.[4]

2. Uterine and cervical factors, e.g. multiple fibroids and septate uterus. Also, certain factors can lead to incompetent internal cervix, as for example:

   a. congenital factors: antenatal exposure to diethylstilbestrol (DES);

   b. trauma: spontaneous, precipitous delivery, or iatrogenic, e.g. dilatation and curretage;[5]

   c. hormonal factors: increased secretion of relaxin.[6]

3. Infection. Subtle infection causing vaginitis, cervicitis, chorioamnionitis or urinary tract infection increases the possibility of preterm labor.[7]

4. Maternal illness. This includes preeclampsia, severe cardiac disease, severe renal disease, or thyrotoxicosis.

5. Premature rupture of the fetal membranes.

6. Trauma to the abdomen such as occurs in a motor vehicle accident.

7. Abdominal surgery, especially in the lower abdomen, where surgical manipulations may irritate the uterus and initiate uterine contractions leading to preterm labor.

8. Stress. This can theoretically lead to termination of pregnancy, whether abortion or preterm labor.

9. Smoking. This can lead to intrauterine growth retardation and/or preterm labor.

10. Extremes of maternal age. Teenage pregnancy or first conception at or above 35 years of age is said to predispose to preterm labor. Late conception has recently been refuted as a cause of premature labor.

11. Low socioeconomic status. Poor antenatal care and personal hygiene does increase the risk of prematurity.

12. Previous history of preterm labor. The chances are higher in this group of patients than in the general population.

13. Fetal anomalies.

14. Uteroplacental insufficiency, e.g. caused by preeclampsia, diabetes. This may lead not only to prematurity, but also to intrauterine growth retardation.

15. Multiple factors. More than one factor is usually associated with preterm labor. However, in many instances no apparent predisposing factor can be identified.

DIAGNOSIS

Preterm labor is defined by gestation more than 20 weeks and less than 37 weeks, uterine contractions occurring at a frequency of equal to or more than 4 per 20 min or 8 per 60 min, and/or ruptured fetal membranes. If the membranes are intact, the cervix should be ≥ 2 cm dilated and 80% or more effaced in primiparous patients.

PREVENTION

Prevention of preterm labor is better than treatment.[8] It is based on:

- identification of patients at risk;
- frequent antenatal visits;
- education, e.g. to ask for help when symptoms start, such as uterine contractions (even painless), abdominal or backaches, menstrual cramps or pelvic pressure;
- sexual and physical activity restrictions;
- the use of ambulatory uterine contraction monitor for early detection of premature uterine contractions;
- positive support system for the mother by her physician, nurse and family;
- treating any underlying cause, e.g. urinary or genital infection, anemia;
- surgical treatment of incompetent internal os by a cerclage operation at 13 –15 weeks' gestation, i.e. before onset of preterm labor.

TREATMENT

Because of the seriousness of preterm labor, our obstetric colleagues endeavor to stop preterm labor. However, there are *contraindications* to prolong pregnancy. The absolute contraindications include fetal distress, severe intrauterine growth retardation, severe maternal or fetal hemorrhage, chorioamnionitis and severe congenital anomalies incompatible with life, such as anencephaly. The relative contraindications include ruptured fetal membranes and severe maternal disease. The use of tocolytic drugs to stop labor is a double-edged sword. Although they may abort the uterine contractions, they expose the mother and fetus to various new risks depending on the type of tocolytic drug. There are many drugs that are used for tocolysis, including β-adrenergic agonist drugs, magnesium sulfate, calcium channel-blocking agents, prostaglandin synthatase inhibitors and ethanol.

β-ADRENERGIC AGONIST DRUGS (RITODRINE OR TERBUTALINE)

Mechanism of action

The mechanism of action of the β-adrenergic agonist (B-A-A) drugs is by direct stimulation of the β-receptors located in the uterine muscle cells. This leads to an increase in cyclic AMP, increased uptake of calcium by the sarcoplasmic reticulum and subsequent decrease in intracellular calcium.

Pharmacological actions

When these B-A-A drugs were first introduced, it was thought that their pharmacologic actions would be limited to β_2-adrenergic receptors, i.e. causing uterine relaxation, bronchodilation, vasodilation, increased renin–aldosterone secretion, which causes fluid and sodium retention, augmentation of glycolysis and increased insulin secondary to hyperglycemia and direct stimulation of the islets of Langerhans. However, with clinical administration, especially by the intravenous route, they exert significant β_1-adrenergic stimulation manifested by tachycardia, palpitations, increased stroke volume, increased cardiac output, arrhythmias, chest pain, tremors, increased irritability, decreased bowel movement, increased lipolysis and ketosis. The administration of B-A-A drugs is associated with significant biochemical and metabolic changes. The serum glucose level increases, while serum K^+ level decreases. This hypokalemia is due to increased insulin secretion with a shift of K^+ to the intracellular compartment; thus, the total K^+ in the body does not change and usually there is no need for K^+ infusion. However, some authorities recommend K^+ infusion if the K^+ level decreases below 3 mEq/l for fear of cardiac dysrhythmia. As a result of the lipolysis, there is increased circulation of fatty acids. The hyperglycemia and ketosis create a problem only for a diabetic patient, that is why B-A-A drugs must be administered with great caution in severe diabetics. The maternal hyperglycemia will be associated with fetal and neonatal hyperglycemia followed by reactive neonatal hypoglycemia. Therefore, the blood glucose in the neonate should be closely monitored. There is also a decrease in maternal colloid osmotic pressure caused by fluid retention and fluid administration. The oxygen requirement of the patient is increased because of the increased metabolic rate.

Complications

Acute pulmonary edema is a particular problem with administration of these drugs.[9,10] The contributing factors for this disorder are:

1. High-output cardiac failure secondary to the marked tachycardia and vasodilation. During pregnancy, the cardiac output and blood volume increase by 25–50% above prepregnancy levels. Therefore, further stimulation of the heart by B-A-A drugs may precipitate acute heart failure. Multifetal gestations have a higher risk of pulmonary edema because of the further rise in cardiac output and blood volume above those in a singleton gestation.[11]

2. Fluid overload. This is due to two factors: first, the administration of fluid concomitant with the i.v. infusion of these drugs and, secondly, the antidiuretic effect of these drugs.

3. Combination of B-A-A with corticosteroids. If time allows, corticosteroids are administered to accelerate fetal lung maturity. Some of these corticoids may cause fluid retention, and they mask infection such as chorioamnionitis. The role of corticosteroids in predisposing to pulmonary edema has recently diminished because of the use of drugs that have minimal sodium and water retention.[12]

4. Infection. Toxins increase the permeability of the pulmonary vascular bed, thus contributing to pulmonary edema.[13] Chorioamnionitis is important because it does not only lead to premature labor, but also adds to the risk of intrauterine fetal infection and to the hazard of acute pulmonary edema.

5. Decrease in colloid osmotic pressure (COP). The factors leading to decrease in COP are pregnancy, excessive fluid retention due to the i.v. fluid administration and the antidiuretic effect of these drugs, and the use of corticosteroids. COP becomes critical when decreasing from the normal of 25 mmHg to 12 mmHg.

6. Increased capillary permeability. It is postulated that B-A-A agents increase capillary permeability. But experimental studies, in the absence of infection, do not prove such a concept.[14]

Pulmonary edema with a B-A-A drug usually follows the i.v. administration and rarely the oral route. The treatment of pulmonary edema is to stop the tocolytic drug, administer a diuretic and give oxygen by face mask or by endotracheal tube with or without positive end-expiratory pressure (PEEP) depending on oxygen saturation as determined by using a pulse oximeter. In a small percentage of patients, invasive monitoring is required, e.g. pulmonary arterial catheter to regulate fluid intake and an arterial line for repeated studies of blood gases and blood chemistry.

Fetal and neonatal effects

β-adrenergic agonists cross the blood–placental barrier, causing fetal tachycardia, increased beat-to-beat variability and fetal hyperglycemia. Fetal acidosis may also occur subsequent to maternal acidosis. After delivery, the neonate may develop a reactive hypoglycemia. However, no lasting harmful effects on the neonate are attributed to those drugs provided these problems are recognized and treated accordingly.

Elimination

Following cessation of ritodrine i.v. infusion, the half-life of the α-phase of its elimination is 15–20 min, that of its β-phase is 1.5–2.5 h.[15–17]

MAGNESIUM SULFATE

Mechanism of action

Magnesium sulfate, as a tocolytic agent, acts by decreasing actin–myosin interaction in the uterine muscle.[18] Such an action is produced by decreasing the influx of calcium into the uterine muscle cell. Magnesium sulfate acts also on striated muscle fibers by decreasing acetylcholine release at the myoneural junction, increasing the threshold of depolarization of the motor end-plate to acetylcholine, and blocking the post-junctional membrane.

Pharmacologic actions

Magnesium sulfate potentiates the action of depolarizing and especially nondepolarizing muscle relaxants.[19,20] Thus, the dose of nondepolarizing muscle relaxants should be reduced by one-third, a nerve stimulator should be used to regulate the dosage and recurarization after reversal should always be considered. With succinylcholine, the full dose (1.5 mg/kg) should be administered prior to intubation to ensure complete relaxation at such a critical event. The therapeutic plasma level of magnesium sulfate is 4–8 mg/dl. Above 10 mg/dl the deep tendon reflexes are lost; above 15 mg/dl respiration is depressed, mainly due to a peripheral action; and above 20 mg/dl clinical myocardial depression is manifested by varying degrees of ECG blockade such as prolonged P–R interval and widening of QRS plus decrease in cardiac output. Magnesium sulfate is eliminated by the kidneys; thus repeated evaluation of magnesium blood levels are essential in patients with impaired renal function. The deep tendon reflexes are useful clinically in determining the degree of magnesemia: if they are normal, this indicates a safe therapeutic level, while their absence indicates an overdosage. With epidural anesthesia, the commonly used patellar reflex should be replaced by biceps and triceps reflexes, since reflexes in the lower limbs could be affected by the epidural block.

Administration

Magnesium sulfate is usually administered intravenously by injecting a loading dose of 4–6 g in 20 min, followed by a maintenance dose of 1.5–3 g/h.

Fetal and neonatal effects

Magnesium sulfate crosses the blood–placental barrier, causing loss of beat-to-beat variability. The neonatal effects of hypermagnesemia include lethargy, abdominal distension, skin vasodilation, hypotension and hypotonia. That is one of the reasons a neonatologist should be present at the delivery of a preterm baby. With adequate renal function, the neonatal effects disappear within 48 h.

Role

Magnesium sulfate therapy is indicated when the use of B-A-A drugs is not advisable, e.g. in cardiac, diabetic or thyrotoxic patients. It can also be used alone or in combination with other tocolytic drugs.[18] Following stabilization of the patient, i.v. magnesium sulfate is replaced by other oral tocolytic drugs.

Calcium channel-blocking agents

The release of calcium is important for uterine contractions. Thus calcium channel-blocking agents have been used in the treatment of preterm labor.[21] The commonly used drugs are verapamil and nifedipine. Their use with B-A-A drugs reduce the stimulating effect of the latter while adding to the tocolytic effect. Their prolonged use may cause intrauterine growth retardation of the fetus.

Prostaglandin synthetase inhibitors

Prostaglandins are important for initiating uterine contractions and maintaining them by increasing intracellular calcium. By inhibiting prostaglandin synthesis these drugs can stop preterm labor.[22] An example is indomethacin[23] which has the advantage of maternal cardiovascular stability. However, certain potential dangers are associated with its use. Indomethacin can cause premature closure of the ductus arteriosus in the fetus, leading to pulmonary hypertension and acute heart failure. Since the sensitivity of the ductus arteriosus to contract in response to indomethacin is increased with gestational age, it is recommended that it be used only in the early part of pregnancy, e.g. below 34 weeks' gestation. It can also cause bleeding in the mother and fetus by decreasing platelet aggregation and reducing factor XII activity. Before use of major regional anesthesia, a platelet count and a bleeding time should be obtained. Indomethacin should not be used in patients with a bleeding disorder, renal or hepatic disease, bronchial asthma or peptic ulcer. These agents have been associated with transient renal dysfunction and oligohydramnios.

Ethanol

Ethanol decreases uterine activity through a central action on the pituitary causing reduction of oxytocin release. It also has a peripheral action by directly depressing the uterine muscle. Ethanol, however, is no longer used with prematurity because it causes inebriation, increased gastric acidity, vomiting and potential danger of aspiration. It also causes fetal and neonatal depression.

Combinations

Some obstetricians resort to a combination of tocolytic drugs rather than using a single one in order to reduce the side-effects while enhancing the therapeutic actions,[24,25] e.g. B-A-A drug, may be used together with either magnesium sulfate or a calcium channel-blocking agent.

OBSTETRIC MANAGEMENT

An early suspicion for onset of premature labor, especially in a high-risk patient, is essential if it is to be treated on time. A mother with preterm labor should be transferred to a tertiary care hospital where adequate obstetric, anesthetic, neonatal, and nursing services are available. The initial treatment includes proper hydration, sedation and bed rest.

An external fetal monitor is applied to document fetal heart rate and uterine contractions. Ultrasonography is used to determine the well-being of the fetus, including respiration, movement and tone as well as the volume of the amniotic fluid.

The drug of choice to stop premature labor is ritodrine. Prior to its administration, one should obtain a baseline of the patient's weight, ECG, vital signs, and laboratory tests including hemoglobin concentration, complete blood count, serum electrolytes, serum glucose, colloid osmotic pressure and urine analysis. Such tests should be repeated every 6–12 h after the start of therapy to determine and correct in time any undesirable side-effects of the B-A-A drug. With i.v. ritodrine administration, glucose rather than normal saline is chosen as the carrying fluid to minimize salt and water retention. A fluid chart should be established and the total fluid intake should not exceed 2500 ml per 24 h. The colloid osmotic pressure is watched closely to ensure that it remains above 15 mmHg.

After the condition is controlled, i.v. ritodrine is stopped and is usually replaced by oral administration of the drug. Tocolysis is terminated once the gestation reaches 37 weeks, i.e. the fetus has reached maturity.

ANESTHETIC MANAGEMENT

The patient's chart is reviewed and, if time allows, the case is discussed with the obstetrician on admission to confirm the status of labor, the fetal condition and the expected obstetric management.

Anesthesia for cesarean delivery

General anesthesia

In case of an emergency, e.g. prolapsed cord, general anesthesia is indicated. As is well known, every obstetric patient in labor should be considered to have a full stomach. With B-A-A drugs, there is decreased intestinal motility, which adds to the risk of aspiration. An antacid such as 30 ml of 0.3 M sodium citrate is administered orally as soon as the need for cesarean delivery is known. The administration of an antacid does not eliminate the risk of aspiration pneumonitis, but decreases the damage if it occurs.

The application of cricoid pressure is an essential procedure because it occludes the upper end of the esophagus by compressing it between the cricoid cartilage and the sixth cervical vertebra. Cricoid pressure, being very important, should be performed by a person who is aware of the problem of aspiration, can mentally visualize the effect of cricoid pressure and thus applies the proper pressure, and knows the site of the cricoid cartilage; otherwise its position should be marked on the skin. The patient should be warned of feeling pressure at that site during induction.

Cricoid pressure should not be started until thiopental is injected. I personally do not apply cricoid pressure until the patient is about to lose consciousness, as evidenced by the initial hyperventilation following thiopental injection. This delay in applying cricoid pressure is less frightening to the patient and eliminates the sense of suffocation if the pressure is applied too early. This is particularly important in the apprehensive and agitated patient on B-A-A drugs. By doing so, the risk of aspiration is not increased because regurgitation or vomiting does not occur at this initial stage of hyperventilation. There is no need to precurarize these patients prior to succinylcholine administration: by increasing the intra-abdominal pressure, the fasciculations increase the intragastric pressure as well as the intra-esophageal pressure, and thus the gradient across the gastric sphincter remains unchanged. Moreover, fasciculations do not occur in parturients who have received magnesium sulfate. Thus precurarization in these patients is not required and may cause partial paralysis, manifested as difficulty in breathing or diplopia, a frightening experience for these patients.

A nerve stimulator, that monitors the decrease of fasciculations if they occur, heralds the onset of optimum muscular paralysis for intubation. It is only after the endotracheal tube has been inserted, the cuff inflated and no leakage around the endotracheal tube has been confirmed that cricoid pressure is released. Surgery should not commence until the proper position of the endotracheal tube has been verified by equal expansion and equal breath sounds on both sides of the chest and carbon dioxide exhalation is evident by capnography or mass spectrometry. If it is impossible to intubate the patient, wake her up and then either intubate while awake or use regional anesthesia.

In a conflicting situation, the welfare of the mother

comes first, before that of her infant.[26] It is important not to be overzealous and compromise maternal life to save a premature fetus with a doubtful outcome. Performing surgery without securing the airway or futile attempts to intubate the mother may lead to the demise of not only the mother, but also the baby. The most common cause of maternal death under anesthesia in the USA is failure to intubate the trachea; and in the UK it is maternal aspiration, which is usually associated with difficult intubation and/or esophageal intubation. Avoiding drugs that exacerbate the tachycardia, e.g. atropine, ketamine and pancuronium, is important. The uterus is displaced to the left until delivery.

For induction of anesthesia, thiopental, 4 mg/kg, is administered i.v.; doses of 6 mg/kg or less are not depressant to the neonate. CNS depressants should be used with caution, particularly in case of prematurity. The protein binding capacity of preterm babies is reduced, their respiratory centers are immature and their capacity to metabolize CNS depressants may be impaired. However, barbiturates may decrease the cerebral oxygen demand and may have a place in the delivery of a premature baby who will definitely require artificial ventilation.

Following thiopental, succinylcholine (1.5 mg/kg) is injected i.v. Anesthesia is maintained by nitrous oxide – oxygen (50:50) supplemented by half the minimum alveolar concentration (MAC) of a potent inhalation agent. Thus, adequate oxygenation of the baby is ensured by the high $F\text{IO}_2$ and by the improved intervillous space perfusion due to the tocolytic effect of the potent inhalation anesthetic. After umbilical cord clamping, the intravenous injection of an opioid, such as 10 mg of morphine and a tranquilizer, such as 5 mg of diazepam will have minimal cardiovascular effects while allowing the anesthesiologist to reduce the potent inhalation anesthetic concentration, thus permitting better uterine contraction and providing smooth recovery from anesthesia due to the residual analgesic effect of opioid post-operatively. A muscle relaxant, e.g. a succinylcholine infusion (500 mg in 500 ml), is used to maintain muscle paralysis while respiration is being controlled. The tidal volume of 10 ml/kg and a respiratory rate of 10 breaths per minute are adequate to maintain a $P\text{aCO}_2$ level that is normal for pregnant patients. In cases of a 'STAT Delivery', 100% oxygen and one MAC of the potent inhalation anesthetic can be utilized. In the presence of appreciable blood levels of B-A-A, halothane is not advisable because of the increased possibility of cardiac arrhythmias. Therefore, either enflurane or isoflurane is used. While the patient is still under the influence of B-A-A drugs, tachycardia is evident before and during anesthesia. The patient has a rather 'fixed' tachycardia, which should not be interpreted as due to dehydration or inadequate analgesia.[27] Otherwise, excessive fluid infusion will lead to pulmonary edema, and excessive opioid administration will cause post-operative respiratory depression. Post-partum hemorrhage is a potential complication of B-A-A drugs or any other tocolytic agent. Multifetal gestations or chorioamnionitis increase the possibility of post-partum hemorrhage. However, the uterus usually contracts well in response to oxytocin.

In certain conditions, even when no urgency is indicated, general anesthesia is considered the method of choice with prematurity. These conditions have a common element of reduced amniotic fluid with the uterus clamping down on the fetus, e.g. prolonged rupture of the membranes, early prematurity where the lower uterine segment is ill-defined or transverse lie of the fetus. The relaxing effect of a potent inhalation anesthetic on the uterine musculature is essential for atraumatic delivery of these fragile preterm infants. The uterine incision, regardless of its type, should be large enough to allow for atraumatic delivery of the fetus.[28] It does not make any sense to choose cesarean delivery in order to minimize the trauma associated with vaginal delivery in such a fragile preterm baby, then use excessive force and manipulations to deliver him/her through a tiny uterine incision.

Delaying surgery for about 2 h after discontinuing ritodrine, if possible, decreases appreciably the level of B-A-A and reduces the chances of adverse interactions with anesthetic drugs or their adjuvants.[28] The hypotension associated with spinal or epidural block may be more profound than that with general anesthesia if the block is induced early while the patient is under the influence of B-A-A.[29] However, in pregnant ewes, epidural anesthesia was found to be safe for the mother and fetus following the termination of ritodrine by at least 15 min since the maternal blood pressure, cardiac output and uterine blood flow as well as fetal blood pressure and acid–base status did not differ from control animals in which saline was infused.[30] The residual cardiac stimulation by ritodrine played an important role in maintaining the cardiac output and uterine blood flow.

Spinal anesthesia

If the B-A-A has been discontinued for more than 2 h before cesarean delivery, and in the absence of fetal distress or the specific conditions mentioned earlier requiring maximum uterine relaxation, spinal or epidural anesthesia is preferred over general anesthesia because the conscious patient can maintain her own airway. The presence of chorioamnionitis is not a contraindication to spinal or epidural anesthesia unless the patient has septic shock. Subarachnoid block is performed using hyperbaric bupivacaine (0.75%) 8–12 mg at the L2–3 interspace, with the patient in the lateral position. The dose is based on patient's height, 1.1 ml for 150 cm (5 feet) height with the addition of 0.1 ml for every 7.5 cm (3 inch) variation. In the sitting position an extra 0.2 ml is added to compensate for loss by gravity to the sacral region. We add 0.2 mg of epinephrine to hyperbaric bupivacaine to improve the quality of the block and increase its duration,[31] and 0.2 mg of morphine to increase the intraoperative analgesia and produce prolonged post-operative analgesia.[32] The uterus is displaced to the left until delivery occurs. The patient is closely monitored and hypotension is prevented and corrected early and adequately. To prevent hypotension, in addition to left uterine displacement, adequate acute hydration should be used. Albumin 5% rather than electrolyte solution is the preferred solution to reduce the required volume (500 ml vs. 1000 ml) and to maintain the COP. Other important points with subarachnoid block are proper monitoring of the pulse, blood pressure and ECG, and correcting any maternal hypotension early and adequately.

In experimental animals, phenylephrine decreases the uterine blood flow despite restoring the maternal blood pressure, and thus should not be used as the first choice for treating maternal hypotension. Ephedrine, in 5–10 mg increments or as continuous i.v. infusion[33] is the drug of choice. However, if the administration of ephedrine in this particular case is associated with significant tachycardia and hypotension, phenylephrine in small increments (100 μg) or as a continuous infusion (10 mg in 1000 ml of electrolyte solution) is indicated to correct both the hypotension and tachycardia. The required dose of phenylephrine is relatively small because the blood volume is already increased by fluid infusion, and the circulation is stimulated by ephedrine and any residual effect of β-adrenergic agonist. The elevation of the blood pressure due to phenylephrine usually causes reflex bradycardia, or more precisely decreases the tachycardia, thus allowing for better filling of the heart and better coronary perfusion. The danger of uterine vasoconstriction as a result of administration of phenylephrine is minimal under these circumstances because the uterine blood vessels are kept dilated due to residual tocolytic drug action, subarachnoid block and/or ephedrine. The risk of sustained maternal hypotension to the mother and fetus is greater than that of any uterine vasoconstriction produced by phenylephrine. The increase in uterine tone due to the α-sympathomimetic effect of phenylephrine is counteracted by the β-sympathomimetic effect of ephedrine and the β-adrenergic agonist. Thus the intervillous circulation is maintained.

Epidural anesthesia

Epidural anesthesia is indicated only if the patient has had continuous epidural technique during labor, the expected duration of surgery is more than 2 h, or the patient has an advanced systemic disease that may deteriorate under spinal anesthesia due to the hypotensive and muscular paralyzing effects of subarachnoid block, e.g. advanced cardiovascular, respiratory or muscular disease. For epidural anesthesia, our drug of choice is 3% chloroprocaine (15–20 ml) combined with 75 μg of fentanyl. Any hypotension with epidural anesthesia could also be prevented and corrected in the same manner as described for subarachnoid block.

Anesthesia for vaginal delivery

Vaginal delivery is indicated when tocolysis fails, the intrauterine environment is no longer safe or the patient arrives in the hospital in advanced labor. Under these circumstances, epidural analgesia is the method of choice for pain relief.

Epidural anesthesia

The advantages of epidural anesthesia are:

1. Stress is eliminated, thus decreasing further increases in cardiac output.
2. The peripheral vasodilation shifts blood from the pulmonary circulation, thus reducing the chance of pulmonary edema.[34]
3. Delivery is controlled and a wide episiotomy can be performed, thus eliminating precipitous labor and decreasing the incidence of intracranial hemorrhage caused by sudden decompression of the fetal head.
4. Epidural anesthesia can be extended to provide for abdominal delivery when required.

The combination of an epidural opioid, e.g. fentanyl and a low concentration of a local anesthetic, e.g. 0.0625% bupivacaine minimizes the incidence of hypotension and motor weakness.[35] Another modification of regional anesthesia is the use of combined subarachnoid and epidural block (CSE), which has the advantage of reducing not only the total dose of the local anesthetic drug but also the opioid required.[36] The technique involves identification of the epidural space, insertion of a long spinal needle to puncture the dura, injection of a small opioid dose subarachnoid, e.g. 0.2 mg of morphine, withdrawal of the spinal needle, insertion of an epidural catheter and continuation as a regular epidural technique. If rapid onset of analgesia is required, 10 μg sufentanil or 25 μg fentanyl can be administered subarachnoid in place of, or in addition to, 0.2 mg morphine. At the time of delivery, a relatively high concentration of local anesthetic (e.g. 2% choroprocaine, 15 ml) is injected epidurally to achieve complete perineal anesthesia and relaxation required for atraumatic delivery.

Spinal anesthesia

A subarachnoid block can be used when delivery is expected within 10–20 min. The drugs that can be used are 40 mg of 5% hyperbaric lidocaine (0.8 ml) or 6 mg of 0.75% hyperbaric bupivacaine (0.8 ml). The use of continuous spinal technique in lieu of continuous epidural anesthesia for both labor and delivery is still experimental. Nevertheless, it is a promising technique based on the advantages of spinal anesthesia mentioned earlier including rapid onset of analgesia, simple technique, and minimal drug dosage.

Pudendal nerve block

When major regional block is contraindicated or refused, pudendal nerve block with or without inhalation analgesia can be used.

Paracervical block

Paracervical block is contraindicated in cases of prematurity because of the high incidence of fetal bradycardia and death.

Cervical cerclage

Cervical cerclage has become the standard treatment of incompetent cervix despite the lack of objective scientific evidence of its efficacy.[6] It is usually performed at 13–15 weeks' gestation. It is contraindicated in the presence of ruptured membranes, active labor, cervical or uterine infection, major fetal anomalies or uterine bleeding of unknown etiology. The principle of the operation is to place a suture at or near the internal os. It has many variations, e.g. Shirodkar cerclage, McDonald cerclage, etc. It may be performed as an outpatient procedure. The diagnosis of cervical incompetence occasionally will not be made until the patient presents with advanced effacement and dilation of the cervix and with the membranes at the level of the external os or bulging into the vagina. Under these circumstances, the prognosis of preserving the gestation decreases significantly, but cerclage may still be placed in the absence of abruptio placentae, chorioamnionitis or active labor. Prophylactic tocolysis may be applied prior to the procedure.

Anesthesia

Subarachnoid block is the anesthetic method of choice because it provides ideal surgical conditions with almost no transfer of drugs to the growing fetus and smooth postoperative recovery. 50 mg of 5% hyperbaric lidocaine or 7.5 mg (1 ml) of 0.75% hyperbaric bupivacaine is injected subarachnoid at the L2–3 interspace using a conical shaped 26- or 27-gauge spinal needle or a 24G Sprotte needle to minimize the possibility of post-dural puncture headache. The aim is to provide sensory anesthesia to the T8 level. The lithotomy position helps to maintain the maternal blood pressure by increased venous return. The use of vasopressors is rarely needed to maintain a normal blood pressure.

REFERENCES

1. Creasy R K 1989 Preterm labor and delivery. In: Creasy R K, Resnik R (eds) Maternal-fetal medicine, principles and practice, 2nd edn. WB Saunders, Philadelphia pp 477–504
2. Quilligan E J, Little A B, Oh WM 1983 An elevation and assessment of the state of the science. In: Pregnancy, birth and infant. National Institute of Health, NIH Publication No. 82-02304, Bethesda, MD
3. Gonik B, Creasy R K 1986 Preterm labor: its diagnosis and management. Am J Obstet Gynecol 154: 3–8
4. McKeown T, Record R 1952 Observations on fetal growth in multiple pregnancies. J Endocrinol 8: 386–401
5. Linn S, Schoenbaum S, Manson R 1983 The relationship between induced abortion and outcome of subsequent pregnancies. Am J Obstet Gynecol 146:136–140
6. Parisi V M 1988 Cervical incompetence and preterm labor. Clin Obstet Gynecol 31: 585–598
7. Gravett M G, Nelson H P, DeRouen T 1986 Independent associations of bacterial vaginosis and chlamydia trachomatis infection with adverse pregnancy outcome. J Am Med Assoc 256: 1899–1903
8. Iams J D, Johnson F F, Creasy R K 1988 Prevention of preterm birth. Clin Obstet and Gynecol 31: 599–615
9. Wheeler A S, Patel K F, Spain J 1980 Pulmonary edema during beta-tocolytic therapy. Anesth Analg 60: 695–696
10. Benedetti T J 1983 Maternal complications of parenteral betasympathominetic therapy for premature labor. Am J Obstet Gynecol 145:1–6
11. Crosby E T, Elliott R D 1988 Anaesthesia for Caesarean section in a parturient with quintuplet gestation, pulmonary edema and thrombocytopenia. Can J Anaesth 35:417–421
12. Robertson P A, Herrin M, Katz M, Creasy R K 1981 Maternal morbidity associated with isoxuprine and terbutaline tocolysis. En J Obstet Gynecol Reprod Biol 11: 371–378
13. Gabel J C, Drake R E, 1984 Effects of endotoxin on lung fluid balance in unanesthetized sheep. J Appl Physiol 56: 489–494
14. Zavisca F G, Drake R E Abouleish E, Smith B, Laurie G E, Cotton D, Gabel J C 1984 Ritodrine does not increase lung capillary permeability in sheep. Anesthesiology 61: A399
15. Post L C 1977 Pharmacokinetics of beta-adrenergic agonist. In: Anderson P A, Beard R D, Brudenell J M, Dunn P A (eds) Pre-term labour. Proceedings of the Fifth Study Group of the Royal College of Obstetricians and Gynaecologists
16. Barden T P, Peter J B, Merkatz I R 1980 Ritodrine hydrochloride: A betaminmetic agent for use in preterm labor. Obstet Gynecol 56: 1–6
17. Caritis S N, Lin L S, Venkataramanan R, Wong L K 1988 Effect of pregnancy on ritodrine pharmacokinetics. Am J Obstet Gynecol 159: 328–332
18. Elliot J P 1983 Magnesium sulfate as a tocolytic agent. Am J Obstet Gynecol 147–277
19. Sinatra R S, Phillip B K, Naulty J S, Ostheimer G W 1985 Prolonged neuromuscular blockade with vecuronium in a patient treated with magnesium sulfate. Anesth Analg 64: 1220–1222
20. Ghoneim M M, Long J P 1970 The interaction between magnesium and other neuromuscular blocking agents. Anesthesiology 32: 23
21. Forman A, Anderson K E, Ulmsten U 1981 Inhibition of myometrial activity by calcium antagonist. Semin Perinatol 5: 288–294
22. Niebyl J R, Blake D A, White R D et al 1980 The inhibition of premature labor with indomethacin. Am J Obstet Gynecol 136: 1014–1019
23. Dudley D K L, Hardie M J 1985 Fetal and neonatal effects of indomethacin used as a tocolytic agent. Am J Obstet Gynecol 151: 181–184

24. Ferguson J E, Hensleigh P A, Kredenster D 1984 Adjunctive use of magnesium sulfate with ritodrine for preterm labor tocolysis. Am J Obstet Gynecol 148: 166–171
25. Hatjis C G, Swain M, Nelson L H, 1987 Efficacy of combined administration of magnesium sulfate and ritodrine in the treatment of preterm labor. Obstet Gynecol 69: 317
26. Abouleish E 1988 Some thoughts from the other side of the ether screen. Am J Obstet Gynecol 159: 1020–1021
27. Gerris J, Van Den Abeele G, Behiels A M, Camu F 1983 Anesthesiological problems related in the use of beta-sympathomimetic drugs for chronic and acute tocolysis. Acta Anaesthesiol Belg 34: 77-85
28. Shin Y K, Kin Y D 1988 Ventricular tachyarrhythmias during cesarean section after ritodrine therapy interaction with anesthetics. South Med J 81: 528–530
29. Muller H, Gips H, Brahler A, Kunzel W, Hempelmann G 1985 Haemodynamic effects of fenoterol for labour inhibition during spinal or epidural anaesthesia. Gynecol Obstet Invest 19: 64–72
30. Chestnut D H, Pollack L K, Thompson C S, DeBryyn C S, Weiner C P 1990 Does ritodrine worsen maternal hypotension during epidural anesthesia in gravid ewes? Anesthesiology 72: 315–321
31. Abouleish E 1987 Epinephrine improves the quality of spinal hyperbaric bupivacaine for cesarean section. Anesth Analg 66: 395–400
32. Abouleish E, Rawal N, Fallon K, Hernandez D 1988 Combined intrathecal morphine and bupivacaine for cesarean section. Anesth Analg 66: 370–374
33. Kang Y G, Abouleish E, Caritis S 1982 Prophylactic intravenous ephedrine infusion during spinal anesthesia for cesarean section. Anesth Analg 61: 839–842
34. Marks R J, DeChazal R C 1984 Ritodrine-induced pulmonary oedema in labour. Successful management using epidural anaesthesia. Anaesthesia 39: 1012–1014
35. Chestnut D H, Owen C L, Bates J N, Ostman L G, Choi W W, Geiger M W 1988 Continuous infusion epidural analgesia during labor: randomized, double-blind comparison of 0.0625% bupivacaine/0.0002% fentanyl versus 0.125% bupivacaine. Anesthesiology 68: 754–759
36. Abouleish E, Rawal R, Shaw J, Lorenz T, Rashad M N 1991 Intrathecal 0.2 mg morphine versus epidural 0.125% bupivacaine or their combination: effects on parturients. Anesthesiology 74: 711–716

PART B
EUROPEAN VIEW

J. Hamza

Preterm birth, defined as birth before 37 weeks of completed gestation, occurs in nearly 10% of deliveries.[1] Prematurity remains one of the leading causes of perinatal morbidity and mortality in developed countries, accounting for more than 75% of perinatal deaths.[2,3]

Survival rate for the premature neonate increases with increasing gestational age; it is more than 90% for the neonate delivered after 32 weeks of gestation, decreasing to less than 50% when gestational age is less than 26 weeks.[4]

The prevention of preterm birth is thus a major public health goal in many developed countries and is both cost-effective[5] and efficient in reducing the incidence of preterm birth (decrease from 7.2% to 5.6% in France between 1972 and 1981).[6] It is therefore essential that the obstetric anesthesiologist be fully aware of some important obstetric and neonatal considerations when involved in preterm labor and delivery.

OBSTETRIC CONSIDERATIONS

The currently accepted definition of preterm labor is the occurrence of uterine contractions of at least 30 s duration at a rate of at least 6/h associated with cervical effacement and dilation. When faced with a preterm labor, the obstetrician should determine and treat underlying causes, evaluate the fetus and decide if tocolysis should be used.

Determination and treatment of underlying causes

Incompetent cervix caused by previous surgical manipulation may be treated by cervical suturing during the second trimester of pregnancy.

Uterine malformations are not often surgically treatable during pregnancy, but recognizing these problems allows treatment before future pregnancies.

Vaginal or urinary tract infections are often associated with premature rupture of membranes and preterm labor,[7,8] which may lead to intra-amniotic infection. Conversely, asymptomatic intra-amniotic infection is believed to be a significant risk factor for premature labor.[9] Recent work[10] indicates that early erythromycin treatment may be useful in reducing the incidence of preterm labor.

Medical problems, such as poorly controlled diabetes or pregnancy-induced hypertension, are also risk factors for preterm birth and should be actively treated.

Nevertheless, more than 40% of preterm labors have no medical or obstetric cause. Socioeconomic factors and workload have been identified as important risk factors in some large epidemiologic studies.[11] These factors, best recognized when the pregnant patient is regularly seen during the entire pregnancy, allow, through a scoring system,[11] specific preventive measures including social measures for at-risk women to be taken.

Evaluation of the fetoplacental unit

Diagnostic ultrasound

Gestational age, fetal weight and growth are best evaluated when the actual diagnostic ultrasound may be compared with an ultrasound study performed early in the pregnancy. Placental abnormalities and fetal malformations may be detected as well as presentation of the fetus.

Amniocentesis and evaluation of fetal pulmonary maturity

The lecithin–sphingomyelin (L/S) ratio and more recently the presence of phosphatidylglycerol (PG) in the amniotic fluid are reliable indicators of fetal lung maturity. In current practice, an L/S ratio above 2 and/or the presence of PG in the amniotic fluid indicate a low risk of infant respiratory distress syndrome (IRDS). Corticosteroids, to enhance fetal lung maturity, are currently given at the start of tocolysis.

Tocolysis

Tocolytic therapy, widely used to treat preterm labor, is not always effective in reducing the incidence of preterm birth.[12] One of the reasons is the numerous contraindications to beta-sympathomimetic agents, which are summarized in Table 61.1.

Beta-sympathomimetic agents

Stimulation of the uterine beta-2 receptor induces smooth muscle relaxation. Ritodrine and salbutamol are the two drugs commonly used in France and other European countries, whereas terbutaline, commonly used in the USA, is rarely, if ever, used.

Complications of beta-sympathomimetic therapy are essentially cardiovascular and metabolic. The cardiovascular complications include tachycardia, pulmonary edema, which occurs in up to 5% of patients, particularly in the case of twin pregnancies, myocardial ischemia due to increased myocardial oxygen demand[13] and arrhythmias (premature ventricular contraction, atrial fibrillation).[14] Metabolic complications are hypokalemia and hyperglycemia, mainly due to insulin-induced movement of potassium and glucose from the extracellular to the intracellular space. Whereas insulin administration may be required to treat hyperglycemia, especially in diabetic parturients, it is not recommended to treat hypokalemia as the serum potassium level returns rapidly to normal within a few hours following cessation of beta-adrenergic therapy.[15]

Other side-effects of this therapy are tremors, headache, nausea and vomiting.

Practical considerations. Before instituting beta-adrenergic therapy, careful examination of the cardiovascular status including previous history, chest auscultation and the ECG is necessary, as well as determination of hematocrit, serum potassium and blood glucose.

Beta-2 agonist therapy is usually given by continuous intravenous infusion starting at 50 μg/min (for ritodrine) and increasing every 10 min until cessation of uterine contractions or maternal side-effects occur (palpitations, for example). When labor stops, the infusion rate is decreased during the following 24–48 h and an oral beta-2 agonist is used.

Table 56.1 Evaluation of contraindications for tocolysis

Absolute
- Severe pregnancy-induced hypertension
- Severe cardiac disease
- Severe bleeding and coagulopathy
- Chorioamnionitis
- Fetal death
- Fetal anomalies incompatible with life

Relative
- Premature rupture of membranes without chorioamnionitis
- Stable placenta previa

Prostaglandin synthetase inhibitors

Prostaglandins E_2 and $F_{2\alpha}$ activate myometrial contractions and cause cervical softening. Prostaglandin synthetase inhibitors, such as aspirin or indomethacin, may be effective in reducing the incidence of preterm delivery in more than 70% of the patients treated.[16,17]

The main side-effects are the risk of premature closure of the ductus arteriosus in utero with occasional fetal death[18] and the risk of development of neonatal pulmonary hypertension, as shown in fetal lambs in late gestation.[19] These effects in theory are less important as gestational age decreases because of a reduced sensitivity of the ductus arteriosus to prostaglandins.[20] However, this opinion was recently challenged by Moise et al,[21] who has demonstrated that constriction of the ductus did occur in fetuses of fewer than 32 weeks' gestation whose mothers receive indomethacin.

The main maternal side-effect of prostaglandin synthetase inhibitors is the effect on platelet function (inhibition of platelet aggregation). These effects last 7–10 days with aspirin but are transient and dissipate within a few days with indomethacin.[22]

The main indication for the use of the prostaglandin synthetase inhibitors is in patients who are unsuitable for treatment with beta-2 agonists. In our practice they are used only before 34 weeks of gestation, when delivery does not appear to be imminent and never for longer than 3 weeks.

Calcium channel blockers

Calcium channel blockers alter calcium uptake by the myometrial cells, leading to a decrease in the cytoplasmic free calcium and subsequently a decrease in myometrial contractility. They appear to be as effective as beta-2 agonists as tocolytics[23] but with fewer side-effects.[24]

To date, no serious maternal or fetal side-effects have been reported in humans. Nevertheless, some cases of unexplained fetal death after use of these drugs in the sheep model have been observed.

In our practice, nifedipine is used when there is a contraindication to beta-2 agonists or when preterm labor is associated with pregnancy-induced hypertension.

Magnesium sulfate

Magnesium sulfate is an effective tocolytic[25] that prevents smooth muscle contraction by decreasing calcium entry into the myometrial cells.

Magnesium sulfate is never used in France to treat preterm labor, so we have no experience of the efficacy and side-effects which are largely described in American publications.

Magnesium sulfate appears to be as effective as beta-2 agonist therapy in treating preterm labor[26] with no more side-effects. However, a recent double-blind randomized study[27] concluded that magnesium sulfate is not better than a placebo in treating preterm labor.

Reported side-effects such as pulmonary edema,[28] chest pain or nausea are similar to those seen with beta-2 agonist therapy. Furthermore, the combined association of the two treatments significantly increases the incidence of serious side-effects (46%) when compared with treatment with beta-2 agonists (ritrodine) alone (6%).[29]

Other tocolytic drugs

Ethanol was used with some effect a decade ago but is no longer used in clinical practice because of maternal side-effects.

In contrast, an oxytocin analog has been studied[30] and appears promising. In this study, it was found to be more efficacious than other usual treatments and devoid of cardiovascular effects.

Maturation of fetal lungs

The lack of alveolar surfactant observed before the 34th week of gestation explains why the preterm neonate is predisposed to the development of hyaline membrane disease.

It has been demonstrated that maternal administration of betamethasone or dexamethasone 48 h before delivery[31] increases surfactant production and significantly decreases respiratory morbidity[32] in preterm neonates delivered after 30 weeks' gestation.

Obstetric plan for delivery

Preterm fetus tolerance to labor and delivery

The preterm fetus has a lower oxygen-carrying capacity than the normal term fetus (lower hemoglobin concentration) and is therefore less well adapted to cope with asphyxia during labor and delivery.[33]

In addition, the preterm fetus has a fragile head and easily torn subependymal veins, which are responsible for the high incidence of intracranial hemorrhage. This is particularly so in the presence of asphyxia which induces a loss of the normal autoregulation of the cerebral blood flow.[34]

What is the best method of delivery?

The incidence of breech in preterm delivery is eight times higher than in full-term delivery. Therefore, prolapse of the umbilical cord and entrapment of the fetal head, particularly in a fetus weighing less than 1500 g, are the main risks associated with vaginal delivery in the preterm fetus.

ANESTHETIC CONSIDERATIONS

Interaction between tocolytic drugs and anesthesia

Beta-2 agonists

When patients receive beta-2 agonists which may be present for anesthesia, some problems may occur, particularly if general anesthesia is chosen. As halothane sensitizes the heart to sympathomimetic drug-induced ventricular arryhthmias, it is better to choose isoflurane or enflurane if a potent halogenated agent is necessary. Atropine should be avoided as severe tachycardia and systolic hypertension have been associated with its use in pregnant patients receiving ritodrine therapy.[35] As beta-2 agonists alter pulmonary hypoxic vasoconstriction, the risk of maternal hypoxia is increased at the time of induction of general anesthesia. Acute oxygenation/denitrogenation is particularly useful in this circumstance.

The ideal time interval between discontinuation of beta-2 agonist therapy and general anesthesia should be at least 30 min for intravenous administered therapy and 12 h for oral-administered therapy.

Regional anesthesia appears a better choice in these

patients as they usually present with a fluid overload which may help to reduce the risk of hypotension. However, as the need for ephedrine therapy may dramatically increase the tachycardia, it is important to carefully titrate epidural administration of local anesthetic in order to avoid dramatic changes in arterial pressure and the need for massive fluid replacement with subsequent pulmonary edema.

Prostaglandin synthetase inhibitors

With the use of prostaglandin synthetase inhibitors within 2 days of an operative procedure, some anesthesiologists believe that bleeding time should be measured prior to performing major regional anesthesia. When aspirin has been used, some avoid the use of a regional block if the time interval between discontinuation of aspirin and delivery is less than 7 days. However, most anesthesiologists consider the number (>100 000/ml) and function of the platelets to be the sine qua non to rule out bleeding tendencies.

In addition, the inhibition of myometrial contraction may be a risk factor for post-partum bleeding.

Calcium channel blockers (CCBS)

The negative cardiovascular effects of interactions between CCBS and halogenated agents have been demonstrated in experimental studies. At equianesthetic potency, enflurane combined with CCBS decreases myocardial contractility and arterial pressure more than halothane or isoflurane.[36] Diltiazem or verapamil combined with halothane decreases cardiac function more than nifedipine.[37] Furthermore, nifedipine combined with halogenated agents does not change atrioventricular conduction or intraventricular conduction.[38]

These experimental studies, extrapolated to humans, seem to suggest that:

1. Enflurane should probably be avoided.
2. Nifedipine (the CCB used to inhibit preterm labor) is safer than verapamil or diltiazem.
3. Lower than usual inspired concentrations of halothane may be sufficient as it has been shown that CCBS decrease the MAC of halothane.

With these suggestions and despite the few clinical studies reported, we agree with Merin[39] that low inspired concentrations of halogenated agents may be used in these patients.

It is important to remember that the negative inotropic effects of the combination of CCBS with halogenated agents may be reversed by calcium chloride[40] but potentiated by magnesium.[41]

CCBS combined with local anesthetics can enhance the cardiac toxicity of the local anesthetic.[42,43] It is particularly important to avoid intravascular injection when performing an epidural block (use an appropriate test dose) and to reduce the likelihood of high local anesthetic plasma levels by carefully titrating the total local anesthetic dose.

The interaction between CCBS and neuromuscular relaxants shown in experimental studies was not seen in humans as smaller doses were used.[44]

Another potential problem is the lack of effect of oxytocin and prostaglandin $F_{2\alpha}$ in restoring uterine activity in rats treated with nifedipine.[45] This may indicate the possibility of persistent uterine atony and hemorrhage in humans.

Analgesia for vaginal delivery

Continuous lumbar epidural analgesia appears to be the better form of analgesia for preterm birth for many reasons:

- fetal protection against pain-induced increased levels of maternal catecholamines which are known to decrease uterine blood flow;
- minimal interactions between the local anesthetic and the tocolytic drugs used;
- absence of fetal depression, as the human preterm fetus has the ability to metabolize all local anesthetics;
- better control of delivery as the mother is pain-free and conscious;
- ability to rapidly extend the epidural block should an emergency cesarean delivery become necessary.

There is no controlled clinical study comparing epidural analgesia for vaginal delivery with no analgesia or inhalation analgesia or opioid-induced maternal analgesia, but a large retrospective Canadian study has shown a threefold lower neonatal mortality rate when epidural anesthesia was used as compared with no anesthesia.[46]

When epidural analgesia is contraindicated, maternal analgesia may be achieved with inhalation of nitrous oxide in oxygen and/or low doses of ketamine (0.25 mg/kg).

Anesthesia for cesarean delivery

For the reasons previously discussed, epidural or spinal anesthesia is the best choice both for the mother and the preterm fetus. For the mother, major regional anesthesia minimizes the usual risks associated with general anesthesia (aspiration of gastric contents, failed intubation) and the interactions of tocolytic therapy with anesthetic drugs. For the preterm fetus, major regional anesthesia is a better choice because the preterm fetus is particularly vulnerable to the depressant effects of systemic medications for the following reasons: low protein-binding capacity, poorly developed blood–brain barrier and decreased ability to metabolize and to excrete some drugs, particularly opioid, sedative and hypnotic drugs.

The rationale for choosing the safest local or general anesthetic technique for the neonate is described in the next section.

NEONATAL CONSIDERATIONS

Effect of tocolytic drugs

Beta-2 agonists

Fetal tachycardia[47] and hyperglycemia[48] with a reactive neonatal hypoglycemia are observed during beta-2 agonist therapy. In the neonate, the incidence of respiratory distress syndrome and hypotension is significantly correlated with plasma drug concentration in the umbilical cord at delivery.[49] Neonatal renal function is also altered, insulin clearance being only two-thirds of the normal in neonates exposed to maternal ritodrine.[50]

Other drugs

Prostaglandin synthetase inhibitors may induce primary pulmonary hypertension in neonatal lambs if used in late gestation.[51] Some case reports of pulmonary hypertension have been also reported in the newborn after maternal administration of indomethacin.[52]

To date, there is no clinical report of adverse human neonatal outcome after the use of calcium channel-blocker agents to inhibit preterm labor.

Effects of anesthesia

Regional anesthesia

Major attention must be given to the prevention and treatment of sympathetic blockade with its resultant hypotension (by acute intravascular volume expansion, uterine displacement and vasopressors). If this mandate is accomplished, there is no harmful effect of regional anesthesia on the premature fetus.

Theoretically, 2-chloroprocaine (not available in many European countries) is particularly suitable for use in the preterm fetus as its rapid metabolism is reputed to be similar as in the term fetus.[53]

Bupivacaine seems theoretically better than lidocaine as the protein binding of bupivacaine is higher. However, in absence of asphyxia, the pharmacokinetics and pharmacodynamics of lidocaine in preterm fetal sheep are not affected by gestational age.[54] In the presence of asphyxia, the normal fetal sheep cardiovascular adaptation to hypoxia is altered by the usual plasma concentrations of lidocaine, resulting in a significant decrease in mean arterial pressure and blood flow to vital organs, such as brain, heart and adrenals.[55] Therefore, it seems logical to choose bupivacaine rather than lidocaine when cesarean delivery is indicated for asphyxia in preterm fetuses.

General anesthesia

There are no available publications concerning the specific clinical consequences of general anesthesia upon the preterm neonate when compared with the term neonate. However, the well-known deleterious effects of high dosages or concentrations of potent anesthetic agents and of the duration of induction to delivery interval may only be worse in a preterm neonate with less cardiovascular and metabolic reserve than a term neonate.

Owing to the frequency of asphyxia, the use of a halogenated agent in 100% oxygen is probably better in the potentially asphyxiated preterm fetus than a lower oxygen concentration with nitrous oxide, as recently shown[56] in normal-term fetuses.

The care of the preterm neonate

Immediate measures

All the neonatal facilities for rapid resuscitative measures should be checked before delivery of a preterm neonate. The main requirements for adequate neonatal care of the preterm neonate are as follows:

- Rapid and effective oxygenation through bag and mask ventilation ensuring adequate pulmonary expansion is essential.
- The indications for early endotracheal intubation are many in tiny preterm neonates as respiratory distress syndrome rapidly produces respiratory fatigue and asphyxia.
- Hypothermia develops very rapidly and is a major factor responsible for persistent fetal circulation with subsequent hypoxia due to right-to-left blood shunting through the ductus arteriosus. Drying the neonate and placing the baby under a radiant heat source are essential.
- Hypoglycemia is a frequent occurence, particularly when asphyxia is associated with preterm birth: early intravenous glucose administration is essential to prevent hypoglycemia.

An important consideration is the frequent need for rapid antibiotic therapy as silent chorioamnionitis is a frequent cause of failure of tocolytic therapy.[57] Our usual practice is to give antibiotic therapy to the neonate in the first hour of life if the direct microscopic examination of placenta and neonatal gastric juice indicates bacterial contamination. This approach may reduce the incidence of neonatal death due to fulminant sepsis frequently seen with group B beta-hemolytic streptococcal infections.

After-resuscitation measures

Monitoring of neonatal oxygenation with either a pulse oximeter or a transcutaneous oxygen monitor is essential to rapidly detect hypoxia as well as to avoid prolonged hyperoxia which may cause retrolental fibroplasia and pulmonary oxygen toxicity.

Monitoring of neonatal arterial pressure with an automated oscillometric method is also critical as wide fluctuation in arterial pressure may induce either cerebral ischemia or intraventricular hemorrhage as cerebral blood flow is frequently arterial pressure dependent in the preterm neonate.[34]

Emotional support of the parents and adequate explanation about their baby are also essential to preserve the parent–infant relationship in the future. It is our routine practice to allow parents to see and to touch the neonate before transfer to the neonatal intensive care unit, even when he or she is intubated.

CONCLUSION

Premature birth remains a major public health problem in developed countries, where it contributes to more than two-thirds of perinatal mortality. Among preventive measures, frequent outpatient consultations during the entire pregnancy and educational and social support for all pregnant patients, whatever their socioprofessional status, is essential in most countries (for example, in France the reduction of incidence of preterm labor in immigrant women from 17.4% in 1972 to 6.4% in 1981 was mainly due to free access to obstetric outpatient consultation services). Various tocolytic agents are used and all of them may have serious anesthetic interactions which are important to understand.

To date, the best anesthetic technique for either vaginal or cesarean delivery is epidural anesthesia, which allows minimal depression of the preterm neonate with greater comfort for the mother and the obstetricians. Spinal anesthesia has the same features but is most often used for cesarean delivery and only rarely for vaginal birth. General anesthesia may be safely administered if pharmacologic interactions between anesthetic drugs and tocolytics are well understood and fetal oxygenation optimized, particularly in the case of fetal asphyxia. Involvement of the anesthesiologist in the care of the preterm neonate is of great importance as proper obstetric and anesthetic care provide the basis for subsequent neonatal care.

REFERENCES

1. U S Department of Health and Human Services, Public Health Service, National Center for Health Statistics. 1984 Vital statistics of the United States, 1980, Vol 1. Hyattsville, MD
2. Brans Y W, Escobedo M B, Hayashi R H, Huff R W, Kagan-Hallet K S, Ramamurthy R S 1984 Perinatal mortality in a large perinatal center. Five-year review of 31,000 births. Am J Obstet Gynecol 148: 284–289
3. Rush R W, Keirse M J N C, Howat P et al 1976 Contribution of preterm delivery to perinatal mortality. Br Med J 2: 965–968
4. Goldenberg R L, Nelson K G, Hale C D, Wayne J, Bartolucci A A, Koski J 1984 Survival of infants with low birth weight and early gestational age, 1979 to 1981. Am J Obstet Gynecol 149: 508–511
5. Korenbrot C C, Aalto L J, Laros R K 1984 The cost effectiveness of stopping preterm labor with beta-adrenergic treatment. New Engl J Med 310: 691–696
6. Rumeau-Rouquette C, Dumazaubrun C, Rabarison Y 1984 Naître en France. Ed. INSERM, DOIN, Paris.
7. Duff P, Kopelman J N 1987 Subclinical intra-amniotic infection in asymptomatic patients with refractory preterm labor. Obstet Gynecol 69: 756–759
8. Romero R, Oyarzun E, Mazor M, Sirtori M, Hobbins J C, Bracken M 1989 Meta-analysis of the relationship between asymptomatic bacteruria and preterm delivery/low birth weight. Obstet Gynecol 73: 576–582
9. McGregor J A, French J I, Richter R, Franco-Buff A, Johnson A, Hillier S 1990 Antenatal microbiologic and maternal risk factors associated with prematurity. Am J Obstet Gynecol 163: 1465–1473
10. McGregor J A, French J I, Richter R et al 1990 Cervicovaginal microflora and pregnancy outcome. Results of a double-blind, placebo controlled trial of erythromycin treatment. Am J Obstet Gynecol 163: 1580–1591
11. Papiernik E 1984 Proposals for a programmed prevention policy for preterm birth. Clin Obstet Gynecol 27: 614–635
12. Eggleston M K 1986 Management of preterm labor and delivery. Clin Obstet Gynecol 29: 230–239
13. Michalak D, Klein V, Marquette G P 1983 Myocardial ischemia: a complication of ritodrine tocolysis. Am J Obstet Gynecol 146: 861–862
14. Benedetti T 1983 Maternal complications of parenteral beta-sympathomimetic therapy for premature labor. Am J Obstet Gynecol 154: 1–6
15. Hurlbert B J, Edelman J D, David K 1981 Serum potassium levels during and after terbutaline. Anesth Analg 60: 723–725
16. Zuckermann M, Reiss U, Rubinstein I 1974 Inhibition of human premature labor by indomethacin. Obstet Gynecol 6: 787–792
17. Zuckermann M, Shale V, Gilad G, Katzunki E 1984 Further study of the inhibition of premature labor by indomethacin. Double blind study, Parts I and II. J Perinat Med 12: 19–29
18. Niebyl J R, Witter F R 1986 Neonatal outcome after indomethacin treatment for preterm labor. Am J Obstet Gynecol 155: 747–749
19. Rudolph A M, Heymann M A 1978 Hemodynamic changes induced by blockers of prostaglandin synthesis in the fetal lamb in utero. Adv Prostaglandin Thromboxane Res 4: 231–237
20. Sharpe G L 1975 Indomethacin and closure of the ductus arteriosus. Lancet 1: 693
21. Moise K J, Huhta J C, Sharif D S, Ou C N, Kirshon B, Wasserstrum N, Cano L 1988 Indomethacin in the treatment of premature labor: effects on the fetal ductus arteriosus. New Engl J Med 319: 327–331
22. Kocsis J J, Hernandovich J, Silver M J, Smith J B, Ingerman C 1973 Duration of inhibition of platelet prostaglandin formation and aggregation by ingested aspirin or indomethacin. Prostaglandins 3: 141–144
23. Janky E, Leng J J, Cormier P H, Salamon R, Meynard J 1990 Etude randomisée de traitement de la menace d'accouchement prématurée: nifedipine versus ritodrine. J Gynecol Obstet Biol Reprod 19: 478–482
24. Ferguson J E, Dyson D C, Schutz T, Stevenson D K 1990 A comparison of tocolysis with nifedipine or ritodrine: analysis of efficacy and maternal, fetal and neonatal outcome. Am J Obstet Gynecol 163: 150–151
25. Hollander D I, Nagey D A, Pupkin M J 1987 Magnesium sulfate and ritodrine hydrochloride: a randomized comparison. Am J Obstet Gynecol 156: 631–637
26. Wilkins I A, Lynch I, Mehalek K E, Berkowitz G S, Berkowitz R L 1988 Efficacy and side effects of magnesium sulfate and ritodrine as tocolytic agents. Am J Obstet Gynecol 159: 685–689

27. Cox S M, Sherman M L, Leveno K J 1990 Randomized investigation of magnesium sulfate for prevention of preterm birth. Am J Obstet Gynecol 163: 767–772
28. Elliott J 1983 Magnesium sulfate as a tocolytic agent. Am J Obstet Gynecol 147: 277–284
29. Ferguson J E, Hensleigh P A, Kredenster D 1984 Adjunctive use of magnesium sulfate with ritodrine for preterm labor tocolysis. Am J Obstet Gynecol 148: 166–171
30. Akerlund M, Stromberg P, Hauksson A et al 1984 Inhibition of uterine contractions of premature labour with an oxytocin analogue – results from a pilot study. Br J Obstet Gynaecol 94: 1040–1044
31. Liggins G C, Howie R N 1972 A controlled study of antepartum glucocorticoid treatment of the respiratory distress syndrome in premature infants. Pediatrics 50: 515–525
32. Morales W J, Diebel D, Lazar A J, Zadrosny D 1986 The effect of antenatal dexamethasone administration on the prevention of respiratory distress syndrome in preterm gestations with premature rupture of membranes. Am J Obstet Gynecol 154: 591–595
33. Bowes Jr W A 1981 Delivery of the very low birth weight infant. Clin Perinatol 8: 183–195
34. Lou H C, Lassen N A, Friis-Hansen B 1979 Impaired autoregulation of cerebral blood flow in the distressed newborn infant. J Pediatr 94: 119–121
35. Sheybany S, Murphy J F, Evans D, Newcombe R G, Pearson J F 1982 Ritodrine in the management of fetal distress. Br J Obstet Gynaecol 89: 723–726
36. Kapur P A, Bloor B C, Flacke W E, Olewine S N 1984 Comparison of cardiovascular responses to verapamil during enflurane, isoflurane or halothane anesthesia in the dog. Anesthesiology 61: 156–160
37. Kates R A, Zaggy A P, Norfleet E A, Neath K R 1984 Comparative cardiovascular effects of verapamil, nifedipine and diltiazem during halothane anesthesia in swine. Anesthesiology 61: 10–18
38. Atlee J L, Hamann S R, Brownlee S W, Kreigh C 1988 Conscious state comparisons of the effects of the inhalation anesthetics and diltiazem, nifedipine or verapamil on specialized atrioventricular conduction times in spontaneously beating dog hearts. Anesthesiology 69: 519–528
39. Merin R G 1987 Calcium channel blocking drugs and anesthetics: is the drug interaction beneficial or detrimental? Anesthesiology 66: 111–113
40. Lehot J J, Leone B J, Foex P 1987 Calcium reverses global and regional myocardial dysfunction caused by the combination of verapamil and halothane. Acta Anaesthesiol Scand 31: 441–447
41. Gallo J A, Kobata R, Cork R C, Brown R B 1986 Verapamil–halothane–calcium–magnesium interactions on max dp/dt in guinea pig atria. Anesthesiology 65: A459
42. Kapur P A, Grogan D L, Foumier D J 1988 Cardiovascular interactions of lidocaine with verapamil or diltiazem in the dog. Anesthesiology 68: 79–85
43. Howie M B, Candler E, Mortimer W, Silver M, Frolicher D, McSweeney T 1985 Does nifedipine enhance the cardiovascular toxicity of bupivacaine? Anesthesiology 63 (suppl): A225
44. Bell P F, Mirakhur R K, Elliott P 1989 Onset and duration of clinical relaxation of atracurium and vecuronium in patients on chronic nifedipine therapy. Eur J Anaesthesiol 6: 343–346
45. Csapo A L, Puri C P, Tarro S, Henzi M R 1982 Deactivation of the uterus during normal and premature labor by the calcium antagonist nicardipine Am J Obstet Gynecol 142: 483–491
46. Ontario Perinatal Mortality Study Committee: Second Report of the Perinatal Mortality Study in Ten University Teaching Hospitals. 1967 Section 1, 1961. Supplement to 2nd Report, Tables 108–124. Department of Health, Toronto
47. Caritis S N, Lin L S, Toig G, Wong L K 1983 Pharmacodynamics of ritodrine in pregnant women during preterm labor. Am J Obstet Gynecol 147: 752–759
48. Ingemarsson I, Westgren M, Lindberg C, Ahren B, Lundquist I et al 1981 Single injection of terbutaline in term labour, placental transfer and effects on maternal and fetal carbohydrate metabolism. Am J Obstet Gynecol 139: 697–701
49. Brazy J E, Little V, Grimm J 1981 Isoxsuprine in the perinatal period. II. Relationships between neonatal symptoms, drug exposure and drug concentration at the time of birth. J Pediatr 98: 146–151
50. Hansen N B, Oh W, Larochelle F, Stonestreet B S 1983 Effects of maternal ritodrine administration on neonatal renal function. J Pediatr 103: 774–780
51. Levin D L, Mills L J, Weinberg A G 1979 Hemodynamic, pulmonary vascular, and myocardial abnormalities secondary to pharmacologic constriction of the fetal ductus arteriosus. Circulation 60: 360–364
52. Manchester D, Mayolis H S, Sheldon R E 1976 Possible association between maternal indomethacin therapy and primary pulmonary hypertension of the newborn. Am J Obstet Gynecol 126: 467–469
53. Kuhnert B, Kuhnert P, Reese A, Phipson E, Rosen M 1982 Maternal and neonatal eliminators of CABA after epidural anesthesia with 2-chloroprocaine during parturition. Anesth Analg 61: 638
54. Pedersen H, Santos A C, Morishima H O, Finster M, Plosker H, Arthur G R, Covino B G 1988 Does gestational age affect the pharmacokinetics and pharmacodynamics of lidocaine in mother and fetus? Anesthesiology 68: 367–372
55. Morishima H A, Pedersen H, Santos A C, Shapiro H M, Finster M, Arthur R, Covino B G 1989 Adverse effects of maternally administered lidocaine on the asphyxiated preterm fetal lamb. Anesthesiology 71: 110–115
56. Piggott S E, Bogod D G, Rosen M, Rees G A D, Harmer M 1990 Isoflurane with either 100% oxygen or 50% nitrous oxide in oxygen for Caesarean section. Br J Anaesth 67: 325–329
57. Hameed C, Tejani N, Verma U L, Archibald F 1984 Silent chorioamnionitis as a cause of preterm refractory to tocolytic agents. Am J Obstet Gynecol 149: 726–731

62. Post-term pregnancy and post-maturity

M. J. Paech

DEFINITIONS

Although a confusing number of terms and definitions are used, pregnancy is usually considered 'post-term' when it exceeds 294 days or 42 weeks gestation. 'Post-dates' may be synonomous or, with 'prolonged pregnancy', used to refer to gestation beyond 280 days (40 weeks) from the last menstrual period.

'Postmaturity' (rarely referred to as 'dysmaturity') is a descriptive term for a clinical fetal condition or neonatal syndrome characterized by signs of impaired placental function and late onset fetal growth retardation. There is no convincing evidence that this condition is actually more common in the post-term pregnancy.

DIAGNOSIS AND INCIDENCE

Post-term pregnancy

It is reported that about 25% of pregnancies extend 7 days beyond the expected date of delivery, becoming post-term in 10–20% of cases[1,2] and continuing beyond 43 weeks in 5–7% of cases.[1,3] The incidence varies with the population and particularly the diagnostic criteria used to estimate gestational age. Estimates based on traditional dating methods are imprecise and based on early ultrasonography, the probability that an infant born after term (based on dating of the last menstrual period) is actually post-term, is only 12%.[4]

Data based on both menstrual and early ultrasonographic dating suggest the incidence of post-term pregnancy is about 5%.[2,5,6] For further details, including etiology and diagnosis, the reader is referred to comprehensive reviews.[1,7,8]

Post-maturity

Most fetuses show continued growth at a normal rate during prolonged pregnancy,[9] so that large birthweight and macrosomic (> 4000 g) neonates are more common and comprise approximately 25% of post-term neonates.[10,11]

A physiologic reduction in some placental transport processes begins at 36 weeks and in animal studies arterial haemoglobin oxygen saturation declines from term. Reduced intervillous blood flow may accompany variable histopathologic changes in the placenta and amniotic fluid volume decreases from 37 weeks, with a 33% weekly fall after 42 weeks. There is a relationship between oligohydramnios and increased fetal heart rate decelerations. Thus, in some pregnancies, placental respiratory, nutritive and metabolic exchange functions deteriorate such that fetal growth and subsequently even survival may be jeopardized by compromised substrate availability and uptake.[1,7,8]

In 1902 Ballantyne[12] reported that the post-term infant was usually excessive in size and in 1954 Clifford[13] described the clinical characteristics of the 'post-mature' infant. These characteristics included increased body length in relation to weight giving a long, thin limbed, wasted appearance; reduced subcutaneous fat and muscle; wrinkled skin, absent vernix caseosa and, later, meconium or bile staining or desquamation. Subsequently, when it was noted that this syndrome was also seen at or prior to term, the term 'dysmaturity' was coined. The post-mature infant is said to comprise 10–20% of post-term fetuses.[1,13,14]

PERINATAL IMPLICATIONS

Perinatal mortality

Early epidemiologic data showed a relationship between increasing gestational age and rising perinatal mortality, which doubled at 43 weeks and was fourfold by 44 weeks.[15] This mortality rate was substantially greater in the presence of obstetric risk factors (e.g. pregnancy-induced hypertension or diabetes) or in the post-mature fetus.[1–3,16] Recent data indicate the magnitude of risk is less. For example, in Sweden, perinatal mortality rose from 2.3 and 2.4 per 1000 at 40 and 41 weeks to 3 at 42 weeks and 4 at 43 weeks gestation.[17] Small series using careful antenatal surveillance report no increase.[2,5,18]

Perinatal morbidity

Perinatal morbidity is significantly increased, even in the absence of additional risk factors,[1,2,14,18] although it may begin to rise before the post-term period.[19] Fetal macrosomia confers a risk of shoulder dystocia and birth trauma (e.g. nerve palsies and upper limb fractures). Post-partum hemorrhage may also be more common, presumably because of uterine hypotonus secondary to overdistension.[7] In the post-mature fetus, perinatal mortality and morbidity is mainly related to hypoxia and acidosis from antepartum and intrapartum events. The latter, particularly cord accidents associated with oligohydramnios, may produce 'fetal distress' and are thought to be major contributors to hypoxic fetal death in utero.

Neonatal problems are common and may require intensive resuscitation and neonatal special care. These include meconium aspiration, hypoglycemia, hypothermia and polycythemia.[20] Other difficulties may persist beyond the neonatal period.

The interested reader is again referred to comprehensive reviews of the perinatal implications of post-term pregnancy.[7,8]

OBSTETRIC MANAGEMENT

There is no unanimity of opinion regarding optimal obstetric management.[17,21] Clinical management is aimed at identification of the fetus at risk of an adverse outcome so that delivery can be expedited – or conversely, identification of those deemed safe to allow pregnancy to continue. There is no clear evidence that careful antenatal surveillance may improve perinatal outcome, although small studies indicate that this is possible.[18] A normal fetal biophysical profile and amniotic fluid volume are considered the best predictors of fetal well-being. The relative risks of expectant management versus intervention must be balanced, with the principal choices being routine induction of labor at 42 weeks or selective induction based on favorable cervical condition and fetal surveillance. Meta analysis of studies comparing expectant management and induction indicate that the latter does not increase the incidence of either instrumental or cesarean delivery and may reduce both fetal heart rate abnormalities and low Apgar scores.[17] However, each woman should be dealt with individually, based on accuracy of dates, suitability for induction, fetal status and other factors.

During labor about a third of fetuses will have meconium present and 5–20% develop 'fetal distress'[5,22] and thus continuous fetal heart rate monitoring will frequently be indicated. Good neonatal services by staff experienced in neonatal resuscitation and the management of meconium aspiration are essential.

ANESTHETIC CONSIDERATIONS

INDUCTION OF LABOR

Early consultation between the obstetrician, anesthesiologist, neonatologist and parents is desirable to formulate a management plan. Induction of labor or cesarean delivery on the grounds of fetal macrosomia is often proposed.

Prostaglandins

Prostaglandins are frequently used for cervical ripening, with intravaginal PGE_2 probably the simplest, safest and most effective.[23,24] This may produce gastrointestinal disturbances, particularly nausea and vomiting. The anesthesiologist should be aware of these symptoms when considering acid aspiration prophylaxis during labor.

Intramyometrial $PGF_{2\alpha}$ and PGE_2 are also effective therapeutic drugs for refractory post-partum hemorrhage, however PGF2α, a bronchoconstrictor and pulmonary vasoconstrictor, should be used with caution in those with asthma, hypertension and cardiovascular disease.[23,24] After intramyometrial injection, severe arterial oxygen desaturation, hypotension and pulmonary edema have been reported.[25–27] Intravascular absorption via various routes has caused severe multisystem effects and even maternal death. Intravaginal administration for induction of labor has rarely been associated with life-threatening maternal and neonatal complications.[28–30]

Prostaglandins should thus only be administered in the hospital, where resuscitation facilities and access to pulse oximetry and direct blood pressure monitoring are readily available. The anesthesiologist must have a sound knowledge of prostaglandin pharmacology and be prepared to provide supportive treatment with oxygen, bronchodilators, arteriolar vasodilators and anti-arrhythmic drugs.

Oxytocin

Synthetic oxytocin, an octapeptide identical to the posterior pituitary hormone, is frequently used for labor induction. It has potent myometrial stimulant activity, maximal near term, and uterine hypertonicity is a complication which not infrequently leads to 'fetal distress'. In the usual labor induction dose ranging from 10–40 mIU per minute, side effects are rare. In contrast to vasodilatation and potentially adverse changes in myocardial blood flow after bolus oxytocin, infusions have little effect on arterial blood pressure.[31] However, because of structural similarity to vasopressin, oxytocin has intrinsic antidiuretic activity and retention of free water is evident at usual dose rates, being maximal at 40 mIU per minute.[32] This may predispose to maternal overhydration and water intoxication syndrome,[33] with subsequent neonatal convulsions secondary to hyponatremia.[34,35] Free water solutions should not be used as diluent, and dose increases made by preparation of a more concentrated solution.

An association between neonatal hyperbilirubinemia and oxytocic administration in labor has been described, possibly due to neonatal hypo-osmolality and enhanced erythrocytic osmotic fragility.[36]

Fluid management

Inappropriate fluid management during labor is not uncommon and may result in maternal and perinatal morbidity. The pregnant woman undergoes many physiologic changes related to fluid and electrolyte balance, such that problems are most likely to occur following excessive administration of electrolyte-free intravenous fluid.[37] Many post-term women receive intravenous fluid for labor induction with oxytocin, in association with epidural block, and for concurrent drug infusion. Both oxytocin and systemic opioids have an antidiuretic effect.

Salt-free solutions should be infused with caution since they rapidly lower serum sodium, and maternal dilutional hyponatremia may lead to fetal hyponatremia, with possible neonatal sequelae including respiratory abnormalities, feeding difficulties, convulsions and death.[38–40] Glucose solutions increase fetal insulin secretion and may contribute to fetal lactic acidosis, fetal hyperglycemia (both of which contribute to more severe pathophysiologic effects resulting in central nervous system hypoxia) and neonatal hypoglycemia. These solutions should be avoided or restricted to rates that do not result in increased fetal insulin levels (about 10 g per hour) and total fluid input restricted to less than 3000 ml in 24 hours.[41,42]

CONDUCT OF LABOR

Pain relief

The adverse effects of severe pain during labor have been extensively reviewed.[43] These pain-induced physiologic changes are normally tolerated by the healthy fetus, due to adequate oxygen reserves and compensatory increases in umbilical circulatory and vital organ flow. In the post-mature or otherwise compromised post-term fetus, impairments of placental blood gas exchange may be critical, leading to perinatal morbidity and even mortality. Systemic and inhalation analgesia are only partially effective in counteracting these changes and, in addition to the neonatal effects of opioid analgesia, both methods may occasionally contribute to severe episodic maternal hypoxemia.[44–46] Epidural analgesia is the method which best prevents or reduces adverse maternal physiologic effects, with potential benefits for the compromised fetus.[43]

Epidural analgesia

There are no controlled studies of the effects of analgesia or anesthesia on the post-term fetus. Nevertheless, it can be argued that well-conducted epidural analgesia may be advisable in the post-mature or otherwise compromised post-term fetus, which may be physiologically less well adapted to tolerate the stress of labor and delivery.

That continuous epidural analgesia improves placental blood flow in laboring preeclamptic women[47] has been confirmed by Doppler flow velocimetry, where elevated systolic/diastolic (S/D) flow ratios are reduced.[48] However, in both compromised and normal post-term fetuses, the uteroplacental and umbilical artery S/D flow ratios are similar. This suggests that the deterioration in placental function which results in the post-mature infant occurs in the presence of normal resistance to blood flow, in contrast to early growth-retardation.[49,50] On this basis it appears unlikely epidural analgesia would similarly benefit uteroplacental flow in the post-term pregnancy.

The use of epinephrine-containing solutions in obstetrics remains controversial, especially in the compromised fetus. Solutions containing small doses of epinephrine have no significant effect on hemodynamics or fetal outcome in mild preeclampsia[51] or on uteroplacental blood flow in normal pregnancy. Animal work indicates significant falls in intervillous flow may occur with the unintentional intravenous administration of epinephrine. However, although possible deterioration in the human fetus has been reported,[52] the healthy fetus probably tolerates such reductions in flow well[53] and investigation of the effect of a small dose of intravenous epinephrine in the acidotic fetal lamb is reassuring.[54]

CONDUCT OF OPERATIVE DELIVERY

Operative risks may be increased in the post-term pregnancy because of both fetal post-maturity (and the risk of fetal hypoxia during labor), fetal macrosomia (and cephalopelvic disproportion with shoulder dystocia at vaginal delivery), or failed induction of labor. Extra vigilance with regard to the prevention of aortocaval compression is important and preparation for emergency cesarean delivery and the management of post-partum hemorrhage recommended if the fetus is macrosomic.

Since there is no specific data on the effect of anesthesia on the post-mature infant or for the post-term pregnancy, the choice of regional versus general anesthesia for cesarean delivery should be based on usual obstetric and anesthetic considerations. Unless contraindicated medically or rendered impractical because of extreme urgency, regional anesthesia can be recommended on both maternal and fetal grounds.[56] Comparative studies show advantages for the healthy, term fetus delivered under regional anesthesia. For example: better 1 minute Apgar scores (and hence less need for active resuscitation), acid-base balance and neurobehavioral scores.[57–59] In addition to avoiding the pharmacologic effects of general anesthetic agents (particularly nitrous oxide), well-managed epidural anesthesia using local anesthetic with or without epinephrine does not significantly alter normal uteroplacental (or fetal umbilical) flow,[60,61] compared to a 35% decrease with general anesthesia.[62] In the presence of 'fetal distress', regional block may also have advantages.[63,64] Epidural anesthetics can be safely and rapidly extended for emergency cesarean delivery[65] and spinal anesthesia, although possibly associated with greater neonatal acidemia despite prophylactic ephedrine infusion,[66] may also be used with excellent fetal outcome.[63,67]

CONCLUSION

The post-term pregnancy may be one of increased perinatal risk, being potentially complicated by fetal post-maturity (characterized by poor or deteriorating placental function) or, more frequently, the large birth weight or macrosomic fetus at risk of delivery trauma and complications.

Optimal obstetric management of prolonged pregnancy and its implications for perinatal outcome remain controversial. However, induction of labor, often preceded by pharmacologic cervical ripening, is a common intervention. In some cases, instrumental or cesarean delivery is more likely. The anesthesiologist must be cognizant of the pharmacologic effects of prostaglandins and oxytocics, be vigilant that peripartum fluid management is appropriate, understand the fetal effects of obstetric analgesia and anesthesia and be prepared to manage aortocaval compression and post-partum hemorrhage. Anesthetic services may be required for epidural analgesia in labor, instrumental or operative delivery, or the control of post-partum hemorrhage. Although unproven, it can be argued that in selected cases well-conducted epidural analgesia may be of benefit during labor and will also allow rapid conversion to anesthesia, thus enhancing both maternal and fetal safety. Specific research into the effects of analgesia and anesthesia on the post-mature infant, or in post-term pregnancy in general, has not been conducted and would be of interest.

REFERENCES

1. Vorrher H 1975 Placental insufficiency in relation to postterm pregnancy and fetal postmaturity. Evaluation of placental function, the management of the postterm gravida. Am J Obstet Gynecol 123: 67–103
2. Sachs B P, Friedman E A 1986 Results of an epidemiological study of postdate pregnancy. J Reprod Med 31: 162–166
3. Zwerdling M A 1967 Factors pertaining to prolonged pregnancy and its outcome. Paediatrics 40: 202–212
4. Kramer M S, McLean F H, Boyd M E, Usher R H 1988 The validity of term, preterm and postterm gestations. JAMA 260: 3306–3308
5. Usher R A, Boyd M E, McLean F H, Kramer M S 1988 Assessment of fetal risk in postdate pregnancies. Am J Obstet Gynecol 158: 259–264
6. Goldenberg R L, Davids R O, Cutter G R 1989 Prematurity, postdates and growth retardation: the influence of the use of ultrasonography on reported gestational age. Am J Obstet Gynecol 160: 462–470
7. Vorrher H, Messner R H 1983 Identification and management of the postterm pregnancy-postmaturity. In: Zuspan F P, Christian C D (eds) Reid's Controversy in Obstetrics and Gynecology, vol III. W B Saunders, Philadelphia pp 246–265
8. Phelan J P 1989 Postdatism. In: Pitkin R M, Scott J R (eds) Clin Obstet Gynecol. J B Lippincott Co, Philadelphia 32: 219–302
9. Crang-Svalenius E, Jorgensen C, Mariscal U B 1990 Intrauterine growth of the fetus at term. A prospective and longitudinal study with real-time ultrasound. J Ultrasound Med 9: 35–38
10. McLean F H, Boyd M E, Usher R H, Kramer M S 1991 Postterm infants: too big or too small? Am J Obstet Gynecol 164: 619–624
11. Chervenak J L, Divon M Y, Hirsch J, Girz B A, Langer O 1989 Macrosomia in the postdate pregnancy: is routine ultrasonographic screening indicated? Am J Obstet Gynecol 161: 753–756
12. Ballantyne J W 1902 The problem of the postmature infant. J Obstet Gynaecol Br Comm 2: 521
13. Clifford S H 1954 Postmaturity with placental dysfunction: Clinical syndrome and pathologic findings. J Pediatrics 44: 1–13
14. Schneider J M, Olson R W, Curet L B 1978 Screening for fetal and neonatal risk in the postdate pregnancy. Am J Obstet Gynecol 131: 473–478
15. McClure-Browne J C 1963 Postmaturity. Am J Obstet Gynecol 85: 573–582
16. Eden R D, Seifert L S, Winegar A, Spellacy W N 1987 Postdate pregnancies: A review of 46 perinatal deaths. Am J Perinatol 4: 284–287
17. Boylan P, McParland P 1991 Fetal assessment in postterm pregnancy. Curr Opin Obstet Gynecol 3: 41–44
18. Freeman R K, Garite T J, Modanlou H, Dorchester W, Romma I C, Devaney M 1981 Postdate pregnancy: utilization of stress testing for primary fetal surveillance. Am J Obstet Gynecol 140: 128–133
19. Guidetti D A, Divon M Y, Langer O 1989 Postdate fetal surveillance: Is 41 weeks too early? Am J Obstet Gynecol 161: 91–93
20. Mannino F 1988 Neonatal complications of postterm gestation. J Reprod Med 33: 271–276
21. Herabutya Y, Prasertsawat P O, Tongyai T, Isarangura-Na-Ayudthya N 1992 Prolonged pregnancy: the management dilemma. Int J Obstet Gynecol 37: 253–258
22. Eden R D, Gergely R Z, Schifrin B S, Wade M E 1982 Comparison of antenatal testing schemes for the management of the postdate pregnancy. Am J Obstet Gynecol 144: 683–692
23. Wilson L, Hodgkinson R 1985 The prostaglandins. Obstet Anesth Digest 5: 164–168
24. Spielman F J, Herbert W N 1988 Maternal cardiovascular effects of drugs that alter uterine activity. Obstet Gynecol Survey 43: 516–522
25. Hankins G D, Berryman G K, Scott Jr R T, Hood D 1988 Maternal arterial desaturation with 15-methyl prostaglandin F2 alpha for uterine atony. Obstet Gynecol 72: 367–369
26. Veeckman L, Muller E, Van Aken H 1989 Epidural anaesthesia and high-dose local prostaglandin administration in obstetrics. A dangerous combination. Reg Anaesth 12: 76–79
27. Douglas M J, Farquharson D F, Ross P L E, Renwick J E 1989 Cardiovascular collapse following an overdose of prostaglandin F2 alpha: a case report. Can J Anaesth 36: 466–469
28. Phelan J P, Meguiar R V, Matey D, Newman C 1978 Dramatic pyrexia and cardiovascular response to intravaginal prostaglandin E2. Am J Obstet Gynecol 132: 28–31
29. Stronge J, Monaghan J, Lenehan P 1987 A neonatal and maternal death following the administration of intravaginal prostaglandin. J Obstet Gynecol 7: 271–272

30. Maymon R, Haimovich L, Shulman A, Pomeranz M, Holtzinger M, Bahary C 1992 Third-trimester uterine rupture after prostaglandin E2 for use for labor induction. J Reprod Med 37: 449–452
31. Hendricks C H, Brenner W E 1970 Cardiovascular effects of oxytocic drugs used postpartum. Am J Obstet Gynecol 108: 751–759
32. Abdul-Karim R, Assali N S 1961 Renal function in normal pregnancy. V. Effects of oxytocin on renal haemodynamics and water and electrolyte excretion. J Lab Clin Med 57: 522–532
33. Whalley P J, Pritchard J A 1963 Oxytocin and water intoxication. JAMA 186: 601–603
34. Schwartz R H, Jones R W 1978 Transplacental hyponatraemia due to oxytocin. Br Med J 1: 152–153
35. Eggers T R, Fliegner J R 1979 Water intoxication and syntocinon infusion. Aust NZ J Obstet Gynaecol 19: 59–60
36. Singhi S, Singh M 1979 Pathogenesis of oxytocin-induced neonatal hyperbilirubinaemia. Arch Dis Child 54: 400–402
37. Lind T 1983 Fluid balance during labour: a review. J Royal Soc Med 76: 870–875
38. Tanow-Mondi W O, Shaw J C, Liu D, Gardner D A, Flynn F V 1981 Iatrogenic hyponatraemia of the newborn due to maternal fluid overload: a prospective study. Br Med J 283: 639–642
39. Alstatt L B 1965 Transplacental hyponatraemia in the newborn infant. J Paediatr 66: 985–988
40. Burnell R H, Dahlenburg G W 1979 Iatrogenic hyponatraemia in mother and infant. Med J Aust 2: 254
41. Sieber F E, Smith D S, Traystman R J, Wollman H 1987 Glucose: A reevaluation of its intraoperative use. Anesthesiology 67: 72–81
42. Morton K E 1993 Fluid management during labour: a British view. Int J Obstet Anesth 2: 147–151
43. Bonica J J 1986 Pain of parturition. Clin Anesthesiol 4: 1–31
44. Huch A, Huch R, Lindmark G, Rooth G 1974 Maternal hypoxaemia after pethidine. J Obstet Gynaecol Br Comm 81: 608–614
45. Reed P N, Colquhoun A D, Hanning C D 1989 Maternal oxygenation during normal labour. Br J Anaesth 62: 316–318
46. Zelcer J, Owers H, Paull J D 1989 A controlled oximetric evaluation of inhalational, opioid and epidural analgesia in labour. Anaesth Intens Care 17: 418–421
47. Jouppila P, Jouppila R, Hollmen A, Koivula A 1982 Lumbar epidural analgesia to improve intervillous blood flow during labour in severe pre-eclampsia. Obstet Gynecol 59: 158–161
48. Ramos-Santos E, Devoe L D, Wakefield M L, Sherline D M, Metheny W P 1991 The effects of epidural anesthesia on the Doppler velocimetry of umbilical and uterine arteries in normal and hypertensive patients during active term labor. Obstet Gynecol 77: 20–25
49. Guidetti D A, Divon M Y, Cavalieri R L, Langer O, Merkatz I R 1987 Fetal umbilical artery flow velocimetry in postdate pregnancies. Am J Obstet Gynecol 157: 1521–1523
50. Stokes H J, Roberts R V, Newnham J P 1991 Doppler flow velocity waveform analysis in postdate pregnancy. Aust NZ J Obstet Gynaecol 31: 27–30
51. Dror A, Abboud T K, Moore J et al 1988 Maternal hemodynamic responses to epinephrine-containing local anesthetics in mild pre-eclampsia. Reg Anesth 13: 107–111
52. Leighton B L, Norris M C, Sosis M, Epstein R, Chayen B, Larijani G E 1987 Limitations of epinephrine as a marker of intravascular injection in laboring women. Anesthesiology 66: 688–691
53. Colonna-Romano P, Lingaraju N, Godfrey S D, Braitman L E 1992 Epidural test dose and intravascular injection in obstetrics: sensitivity, specificity and lowest effective dose. Anesth Analg 75: 372–376
54. Youngstrom P, Hoyt M, Veille J C, Cohen I, Amini S, Herman M 1990 Effects of intravenous test dose epinephrine on fetal sheep during acute fetal stress and acidosis. Reg Anesth 15: 237–241
56. Spielman F J, Corke B C 1985 Advantages and disadvantages of regional anesthesia for cesarean section. J Reprod Med 11: 832–840
57. Evans C M, Murphy J F, Gray O P, Rosen M 1988 Epidural versus general anaesthesia for elective Caesarean section. Effect on Apgar score and acid-base status of the newborn. Anaesthesia 44: 778–782
58. Kangas-Saarela T, Koivisto M, Jouppila R, Jouppila P, Hollmen A 1989 Comparison of the effects of general and epidural anaesthesia for cesarean section on the neurobehavioural responses of newborn infants. Acta Anaesthesiol Scand 33: 313–319
59. Ong B Y, Cohen M M, Palahniuk R J 1989 Anesthesia for cesarean section-effects on neonates. Anesth Analg 68: 270–275
60. Jouppila R, Jouppila P, Kuikka J, Hollmen A 1978 Placental blood flow during cesarean section under lumbar extradural analgesia. Br J Anaesth 50: 275–278
61. Giles W B, Lah F X, Trudinger B J 1987 The effect of epidural anaesthesia for cesarean section on maternal uterine and fetal umbilical artery blood flow velocity waveforms. Br J Obstet Gynecol 94: 55–59
62. Jouppila P, Kuikka J, Jouppila R, Hollmen A 1979 Effect of induction of general anaesthesia for cesarean section on intervillous blood flow. Acta Obstet Gynaecol Scand 58: 249–253
63. Marx G J, Luykx W M, Cohen S 1984 Fetal-neonatal status following cesarean section for fetal distress. Br J Anaesth 56: 1009–1013
64. Ramanathan J, Ricca D M, Sibai B M, Angel J J 1988 Epidural vs general anesthesia in fetal distress with various abnormal fetal heart rate patterns. Anesth Analg 67: S180
65. Price M L, Reynolds F, Morgan B M 1991 Extending epidural blockade for emergency cesarean section. Int J Obstet Anesth 1: 13–18
66. Ratcliffe F M 1990 Neonatal acid-base status after general, spinal or extradural anaesthesia for cesarean section. Br J Anaesth 64: 381P
67. Jani K, McEvedy B, Harris S, Dossetor J F 1989 Neonatal outcome after spinal or epidural bupivacaine 0.5% for elective cesarean section. Anesthesiology 71: A866

63. The inner city parturient: drug addiction and acquired immunodeficiency syndrome

Part A Drug addiction in the parturient *D. J. Birnbach*
Part B Neonatal effects *F. Shahrivar*

PART A
MATERNAL EFFECTS
D. J. Birnbach

INTRODUCTION

The use of illicit drugs has become endemic in our society and, as a result, anesthesiologists are now seeing a dramatic increase in the number of patients who are using recreational drugs. Despite anti-drug programs such as drug education in schools and the well-publicized cocaine-related deaths of several famous athletes, there is an increasing incidence of drug abuse. Although substance abuse is being seen in all socioeconomic groups, it is still a problem of particular concern when treating the 'inner city' patient. For the past several years, there have been increasing numbers of reports of substance abuse during pregnancy.[1–3] Recreational drugs that have been reported as being abused in pregnancy include cocaine, crack (alkaloidal cocaine), amphetamines, narcotics (opioids), alcohol, marijuana and phencyclidine. If drugs are being used, there is often evidence of multiple drug use.[4] Substance abuse in the parturient affects both mother and fetus and impacts on the care provided by the perinatologist, neonatologist and anesthesiologist.

COCAINE/CRACK

Cocaine ($C_{17}H_{21}N_4$; benzoylmethylecgonine) is an alkaloid obtained from the plant *Erythroxylum coca*. Cocaine use in the USA is a major problem that occurs in all segments of the population. In 1985, it was estimated that over 30 million Americans (approximately 10% of the population of the USA) had used cocaine at least once and over 5 million were chronic users.[5] Because of the lower cost and increased availability of cocaine when it is alkalinized ('crack'), the number of cocaine/crack users is likely to be much greater today than the previous estimate. The number of pregnant patients who are using cocaine is also growing.[6] At St. Luke's–Roosevelt Hospital Center (New York), which has a large 'inner city' patient population, more then 70% of unregistered patients are cocaine positive on toxicology screen. Additionally, a majority of the parturients, while testing positive, deny drug use when asked by the anesthesiologist.[7]

Since cocaine is absorbed through all mucous membranes, there are multiple possible routes of administration. Routes of ingestion include smoking, snorting and intravenous or subcutaneous injection. Oral and rectal administration have also been reported.[8,9] The mixing of cocaine with other drugs is quite common. Little et al[4] estimated that two-thirds of their patients using cocaine were also using other drugs. Oro and Dixon[10] have reported that combining drugs results in higher perinatal morbidity compared with single-drug abuse.

EFFECT OF COCAINE ON THE MOTHER

Cocaine acts principally by inhibiting nerve conduction and via alterations of the neurotransmitters-norepinephrine, dopamine and serotonin.[11,12] The cocaine-induced increase in circulating norepinephrine causes many of the complications seen after cocaine administration. Cocaine can have far-reaching effects on the cardiac, pulmonary, central nervous, and gastrointestinal systems (Table 63.1). The increased norepinephrine levels resulting from cocaine abuse cause a reduction of cardiac electrical stability, thus predisposing these patients to malignant arrhythmias. In the pregnant patient, cocaine may also cause maternal–fetal vasoconstriction, hypertension and tachycardia. Cocaine use has been reported as causing maternal hypertension and other symptoms of vasoconstriction that may be confused with the onset of preeclampsia.[13,14] There is a large prevalence of substance abuse, particularly cocaine, in patients admitted in preterm labor.[15,16] Cocaine has

Table 63.1 Signs and symptoms of cocaine use

Hypertension	Hyperpyrexia
Tachycardia	Metabolic acidosis
Convulsions	Emotional lability
Hyperreflexia	Dilated pupils
Tremors	

also been reported by several investigators as causing an increase in the incidence of placental abruption.[17,18] Although it is a common misconception that the placenta protects the fetus from maternally ingested cocaine, it does not. It has been shown that maternally administered cocaine crosses the placenta and can have adverse neonatal effects due to direct and indirect actions.[19] Woods et al[20] have demonstrated that the administration of cocaine to pregnant ewes causes marked fetal hypoxia, hypertension and tachycardia. These physiologic changes are due not only to placental passage of the drug but also to decreased uterine blood flow associated with cocaine-induced hemodynamic perturbations. Moore et al[21] found a dose-related decrease in uterine blood flow of up to 40%. Transplacental passage of cocaine is not only seen in the laboratory, it has also been reported in humans.[19] Infants whose mothers used cocaine just prior to delivery excreted cocaine 12–24 h after delivery and continued to excrete the cocaine metabolite, benzoylecgonine, for 5 days. The slow metabolism of cocaine in the neonate demonstrated by the persistence of benzoylecgonine in the neonate for this lengthy period is thought to be due to low fetal plasma cholinesterase activity.[22]

Cocaine affects all major organ systems and may cause patient morbidity and mortality. Death after cocaine ingestion is most often due to cardiac abnormalities including malignant ventricular arrhythmias, myocardial infarction and cardiac asystole.[23–25] Other causes of death have also been reported, including convulsions and aspiration, bronchospasm, pulmonary edema, stroke and subarachnoid hemorrhage.[26,27] Intestinal ischemia following ingestion of cocaine has been described.[28] Pneumomediastinum, pneumopericardium and pneumothorax have also been reported after cocaine use.[29] A summary of the most common symptoms of cocaine intoxication and the relevant therapy is given in Table 63.2.

The American College of Obstetricians and Gynecologists (ACOG) has recently made suggestions relating to the management of pregnant patients who abuse cocaine.[30] These recommendations include that the obstetrician should obtain a drug history at the first prenatal visit, and the patient should be warned about the dangers of drugs in pregnancy. Additionally, they suggest that the obstetrician should consider testing of the mother or the neonate in cases of unexpected preterm labor or unexplained fetal growth retardation or placental abruption.

Table 63.2 Therapy for cocaine intoxication

Symptom	Therapy
Hypertension/tachycardia	Labetalol
Convulsions	Benzodiazepines; control airway
Tremors/CNS excitation	Benzodiazepines
Anginal syndromes	
Associated with hypertension	Labetalol
Associated with ECG changes	i.v. nitroglycerin
Ventricular fibrillation	Verapamil
Psychosis	Lithium

Although it is a difficult task, it is desirable for the anesthesiologist to clearly identify cocaine abuse before delivery. It has recently been reported that cocaine abusers have a much greater risk of developing life-threatening perturbations under anesthesia.[31] Since a majority of cocaine abusers deny their drug abuse to physicians,[7,32] toxicology testing may be necessary to make the diagnosis. Current methods of urine toxicology include gas chromatography, mass spectrometry, and radioimmunoassay. Unfortunately, most of the currently available tests all take a minimum of 24–72 h to process, and so results are of little help to the obstetric anesthesiologist who meets the patient and is asked to administer anesthesia within minutes. OnTrak Abuscreen (Roche Diagnostics, Branchburg, NJ, USA), is a newly developed assay for benzoylecgonine which allows physicians to instantly test urine for cocaine. The OnTrak assay is a latex agglutination test which provides a result in less than 4 min and therefore allows the perinatal team to make the appropriate clinical decisions regarding the care of the patient. We have evaluated the OnTrak assay at St. Luke's–Roosevelt Hospital Center and have found a 100% correlation with the laboratory results.[33] The OnTrak test had a 100% sensitivity and 100% specificity when compared with the standard toxicology testing. The major differences between the methods was that the OnTrak was not only faster (4 min vs. 48 h) but was also a fraction of the cost (<$3 vs. >$60). Although a more established method, such as gas chromatography or mass spectrometry, may be used to confirm the result, this test, because of its speed and ease of use, allows the anesthesiologist to ascertain the patient's cocaine status before administering an anesthetic, even in an emergency situation.

ANESTHETIC IMPLICATIONS OF COCAINE ABUSE

Unfortunately, obstetric anesthesiologists are often confronted by a call for an emergency cesarean delivery for an unregistered, cocaine-abusing patient in the middle of the night. The time to consider the possible ramifications of cocaine abuse and the appropriate treatment of the abusing parturient is long before the patient arrives on the labor floor in distress. Depending on the clinical setting, the anesthesiologist must decide between regional and general anesthesia. Occasionally, there will be no choice. For example, general anesthesia is needed in the hemodynamically unstable patient who has lost a massive amount of blood as a result of placental abruption. At St. Luke's–Roosevelt Hospital Center in New York, we have had success with the administration of regional anesthesia to cocaine-abusing parturients. In fact, a recent study performed at our institution[31] has shown that cocaine-abusing parturients have a statistically significant risk of developing life-threatening complications during the administration of anesthesia for cesarean delivery. We found that the risk of life-threatening events was much greater under general anesthesia than under regional anesthesia. Most of the complications associated with general anesthesia were due to hypertensive crises or arrhythmias after laryngoscopy and intubation. If general anesthesia is chosen, the anesthesiologists should be prepared to treat hypertension, malignant arrhythmias and ischemia. Hughes et al[34] have evaluated the use of labetalol for the treatment of cocaine-induced hypertension in ewes and have found that it may be preferable to hydralazine for the treatment of the acutely intoxicated parturient. Propranolol is relatively contraindicated for the treatment of cocaine-induced hypertension, since β-blockade may cause unopposed α-adrenergic receptor stimulation and worsened hypertension.[35] Drugs which sensitize the myocardium to catecholamines, such as halothane, as well as drugs which release catecholamines, such as ketamine, should also be avoided in the cocaine-abusing patient. The minimum alveolar concentration (MAC) for general anesthetic agents may be decreased in chronic cocaine addicts as a result of depletion of catecholamines. Cocaine has also been reported to alter the response to succinylcholine.[36]

Regional anesthesia, although not without risk, presented far fewer risks in our study population.[31] The major risk associated with the use of epidural or spinal anesthesia in the cocaine abuser is the potential for development of hypotension which is unresponsive to treatment with ephedrine. Therefore, the anesthesiologist should prepare a dilute solution of phenylephrine for use in treating ephedrine-resistant hypotension. Additionally, we observed a correlation between cocaine abuse and thrombocytopenia and therefore the anesthesiologist should ascertain that the known or suspected cocaine abuser has normal coagulation profile prior to initiation of the regional anesthetic.

Another potential problem facing the anesthesiologist who is using regional anesthesia for the cocaine abuser is the potential for complaints of pain despite an adequate sensory level of spinal or epidural anesthesia. In a study performed at this hospital, we observed that 87% of cocaine-positive women vs. 47% of cocaine-negative women required intraoperative opioid administration during anesthesia for cesarean delivery.[7]

Cocaine abusers often combine other drugs with cocaine. Sometimes this is intentional, as in the case of speedballs, in which a mixture of heroin and cocaine supposedly improves their experience.[37] Sometimes this is unintentional, however, such as when the cocaine is cut with a variety of pharmacologic (amphetamines, lidocaine) and nonpharmacologic adulterants (talc) which may cause toxic cardiovascular, pulmonary and neurologic complications. If single-drug abuse is suspected, the anesthesiologist should be prepared to treat the effects of multiple drugs.

AMPHETAMINES

Amphetamines are commonly abused both individually and in combination with other drugs. A recent study demonstrated that between 1986 and 1987 10% of the toxicologic screens performed in San Diego were positive for amphetamines.[38] Acute ingestion of amphetamines causes a release of catecholamines from adrenergic nerve terminals, being both an alpha- and beta-adrenergic agonist. Like cocaine, amphetamines inhibit the reuptake of catecholamines. Signs and symptoms of amphetamine use resemble those of 'crack' use and include confusion, tremors, hyper-reflexia, fever, hypertension, tachycardia, arrhythmias and pulmonary edema.[39] As with cocaine, hypertension may occur after only small doses and has been reported as causing cerebral hemorrhage and stroke. The combination of hypertension, convulsions and proteinuria resulting from ingestion of amphetamines has been mistaken for eclampsia.[40] Acute amphetamine intoxication has also been reported to increase intracranial pressure.[41] The MAC for volatile agents is increased; however, this has been shown to revert to normal during hyperventilation.[42]

Chronic use of amphetamines causes depletion of neuronal catecholamines as well as impaired response to sympathomimetics.[43] Cardiac arrest during anesthesia for cesarean delivery has been reported in patients chronically abusing amphetamines.[44] Pulmonary edema has also been reported following general anesthesia for cesarean delivery in an amphetamine abuser.[45] There may be a high incidence of psychoses associated with the use of amphetamines.[46] Such behavior may complicate the management of obstetric patients, especially those patients who are to remain awake during operative deliveries under regional anesthesia.

ALCOHOL ABUSE

The alcoholic parturient poses many problems to the anesthesiologist. During the preoperative evaluation, a history of the quantity and type of alcohol consumed, the duration of abuse, the time of the last consumption and the use of other drugs should be elicited by the anesthesiologist. The medical history and review of systems should include the neurologic, cardiac, hepatic and hematologic systems. If the patient appears intoxicated, a blood alcohol level should be obtained. A level of 100 mg/10 ml is the legal limit of intoxication. If the alcohol-abusing parturient does not present with symptoms of alcoholic peripheral neuropathy, regional anesthesia should be considered, thereby avoiding some of the potential problems associated with general anesthesia in the alcoholic patient.

Prior to initiation of regional anesthesia, the absence of peripheral neuropathies should be documented. Although regional anesthesia is not absolutely contraindicated in the alcoholic parturient with a neuropathy, it is at the very least a relative contraindication and the anesthesiologist should have a clear understanding of the neurologic involvement prior to anesthetic placement. Regional anesthesia may present other problems in the alcoholic since these patients may have a contracted blood volume and muscle wasting and, therefore, may develop hypotension and respiratory failure after initiation of the block. In the event that a general anesthetic becomes necessary, thiobarbiturates should be used with caution since they may be potentiated by ethanol. General anesthesia presents many dangers in these patients since they may react to anesthetics in unexpected ways. Additionally, the alcoholic may have a cardiomyopathy and hypoalbuminemia, both of which may cause untoward responses to general anesthetics.[47] If the patient is intoxicated, the risk of aspiration is greatly increased and decreased amounts of anesthetic will be needed to produce general anesthesia.[48] The response to neuromuscular blockade may also vary in alcoholics. Duvaldestin et al[49] have demonstrated that in alcoholic cirrhosis the initial dose required to produce relaxation is higher than normal, whereas the duration of action is prolonged in these patients. Because ethanol inhibits antidiuretic hormone, hypovolemia and fluid imbalance may be seen. The commonly seen manifestations of alcoholism and their anesthetic implications are reviewed in Table 63.3.

Table 63.3 Symptoms of alcoholism and their anesthetic implications

Symptom	Implications to anesthesiologist
Peripheral neuropathy	Regional anesthesia relatively contraindicated
Cardiomyopathy	Avoid cardiodepressant anesthetics
Increased gastric acid	Give antacid/rapid-sequence induction
Decreased albumin	Neuromuscular blockade abnormalities
Coagulation defects	Regional anesthesia contraindicated (patient may need fresh-frozen plasma, platelets, vitamin K)
Esophageal varices	Caution with nasogastric tubes, esophageal stethoscope, temperature probe
Ascites	Avoid sodium solutions
Cirrhosis	Avoid halothane
Convulsions	Avoid ketamine, enflurane
V/Q mismatch	Avoid general anesthesia if possible

NARCOTIC (OPIOID) ABUSE

Although there appears to be a decreased prevalence of opioid abuse in pregnant women in the USA, opioid abuse continues to be a frequent problem seen in inner city hospitals. Opioids being abused include morphine, heroin, meperidine and fentanyl. It has been estimated that 250 000 women in the USA abuse intravenous opioids.[50]

Perinatal opioid abuse is associated with multiple difficulties. These include acquired immunodeficiency syndrome (AIDS), hepatitis, endocarditis, pulmonary emboli, pulmonary edema, anemia, renal disease, cardiac arrhythmias and hypotension.[51] Heroin sold on the street is routinely 'cut' with a high proportion of adulterants such as talc.[52] These substances, used as fillers, may actually cause more damage than the opioid. A report has described the increasing incidence of subarachnoid/epidural abscess and disc space infection in drug-abusing patients.[53] There is an increase in the incidence of preeclampsia in the pregnant opioid abuser and therefore, the possibility of opioid abuse should be considered in the inner city parturient presenting with hypertension.[54] Electrocardiographic changes have also been noted in opioid abusers.[55]

Anesthesiologists must be able to recognize both maternal opioid overdose and withdrawal. Acute withdrawal syndrome begins at about 12 h and can present as anxiety, tremors, muscle pains, nausea, vomiting, anorexia, gastrointestinal pain, mydriasis, dehydration, tachycardia, hypertension and tachypnea. These symptoms peak at 48–72 h. Most opioid withdrawal symptoms are the result of sympathetic hyperactivity and may be modified by the administration of the α_2-agonist clonidine.[56]

The anesthetic of choice in the narcoticopioid-addicted parturient is often regional anesthesia, thus avoiding the administration of opioids. Unfortunately, regional anesthesia may be contraindicated because of coagulopathy, neuropathy or sepsis or in an uncooperative patient. Narcotic addicts often show a decreased pain tolerance, and a relative failure of regional anesthesia has been reported in these patients.[57] Pure antagonist or agonist–antagonist drugs must be avoided as they may precipitate acute withdrawal syndrome.[58] The use of epidurally administered agonist–antagonist agents is also contraindicated because of the risk of precipitating acute withdrawal.[59]

If general anesthesia becomes necessary in the opioid-abusing parturient, the anesthesiologist should take adequate precautions because of the high risk of AIDS in this patient population. Additionally, the narcotic addict may have delayed gastric emptying. Therefore, to avoid the occurrence of gastric regurgitation and the development of aspiration pneumonitis under general anesthesia, a rapid-sequence induction with cricioid pressure must be performed regardless of the time of last meal.[60,61] The anesthesiologist should also consider prophylaxis with metoclopramide and H_2-blockers such as cimetidine because of the increased risk of pulmonary acid aspiration in these patients. Severe hypotension reported to have occurred in narcotic addicts under general anesthesia has been treated with an injection of morphine.[62] Because many opioid abusers have abnormalities of liver function, drugs that are hepatotoxic or detoxified in the liver must be used cautiously in these patients. Provided that the patient's physiologic opioid requirements are met, cross-tolerance is not a problem in the maintenance of anesthesia.[63]

Post-operative analgesia may also present a problem in the opioid addict. The use of epidural anesthesia in the post-operative period can provide adequate post-operative pain relief while avoiding the use of opioids. New drugs, such as ketorolac,[64] a parenteral nonsteroidal anti-inflammatory drug, may prove to be superior for post-operative pain relief in the narcotic opioid addict.

MARIJUANA ABUSE

It is estimated that up to 37% of pregnant women use marijuana.[65] Marijuana used during pregnancy may cause arrest of labor, failure of spontaneous placental delivery, increased incidence of meconium and low birthweight.[66] Marijuana use has several implications for the anesthesiologist. Cardiac abnormalities, including tachycardia, arrhythmias and electrocardiographic abnormalities, may be seen. Agitation may be seen in the marijuana-smoking parturient and together with mental status changes may make regional anesthesia difficult to perform. Carbon monoxide levels five times greater than in tobacco smokers as well as major changes in bronchi may also be seen after marijuana smoking.[67] These pulmonary changes, including hypercarbia and increased carbon monoxide levels, may interfere with fetal oxygenation. Abnormal halothane metabolism due to marijuana-induced microsomal dechlorinase activity has been reported, therefore volatile agents other than halothane should be used in these patients[68] (Table 63.4).

Table 63.4 Management of the marijuana abuser

Symptom	Treatment
Tachycardia	Propranolol
Agitation	Benzodiazepine
Hypotension	Ephedrine
Hypotension/tachycardia	Phenylephrine
Bronchoconstriction	Avoid thiopental

VAPOR SNIFFING

Recreational inhalation of toluene-based solvents has been reported in pregnancy and may be associated with intrauterine growth retardation and perinatal death.[69] Maternal problems associated with the inhalation of solvents include renal failure, electrolyte disturbances and cardiac arrhythmias.

CIGARETTE SMOKING

Despite worldwide strides to decrease the prevalence of cigarette smoking, it is still a preventable cause of maternal and perinatal morbidity. Sloan et al[70] have demonstrated 46% use of cigarettes during pregnancy in a rural US population. The majority of women who smoke prior to pregnancy will continue to smoke during pregnancy[71] and the heavy smokers are less likely to stop.

Cigarette smoke affects the respiratory, cardiovascular and immune systems. Respiratory consequences of cigarette smoking include increases in mucus secretion, decrease in ciliary transport and small airway narrowing.[72] 4–6 weeks of abstinence from cigarette smoking is required to allow a decrease in the risk of post-operative respiratory morbidity; however, any period of abstinence will improve the patient's readiness for anesthesia.

Some authors have advocated the use of nicotine replacement therapy in women who have difficulty in stopping smoking during pregnancy.[73] Although nicotine is harmful to the fetus, transdermal nicotine therapy allows the patient to receive nicotine without exposure to all the other toxic chemicals found in cigarette smoke.

ACQUIRED IMMUNODEFICIENCY SYNDROME

History

Our knowledge of acquired immunodeficiency syndrome (AIDS) began in 1980 and 1981, when opportunistic infections in homosexual men were noted in New York, San Francisco and Los Angeles. The first report described four previously healthy homosexual men who presented with *Pneumocystis carinii* pneumonia (PCP) and were found to be immunodeficient.[74] A second paper published in 1981 suggested that drug abusers and homosexuals were at high risk for PCP.[75] It quickly became evident that this previously unrecognized disease could present with a myriad of symptoms that had devastating effects, the common denominator being an alteration in the immune system function and the subsequent development of opportunistic infections. In June 1982 the CDC named this syndrome the acquired immunodeficiency syndrome[76] and defined it as the occurrence of a disease indicative of immunodeficiency in a person without a condition known to be associated with an increased incidence of diseases related to cellular immunodeficiency.[77] Although it was assumed that AIDS did not exist prior to the 1980s, a recent review of a case and frozen serum from 1968 revealed a patient with opportunistic infections and a virus related to human immunodeficiency virus. Therefore, it is now assumed that AIDS was present in the USA as early as the 1960s.

The actual virus that causes AIDS, now termed human immunodeficiency virus (HIV), was described in 1983–84 by Barre-Sinoussi et al,[78] Gallo et al[79] and Levy et al.[80] This pathogen is a retrovirus that utilizes reverse transcriptase to copy its genome into DNA. It was initially named HTLV-III (human T-cell lymphotropic virus), then renamed as HTLV-III/LAV, and finally simplified as HIV. Two variants of this virus have thus far been identified, HIV-1 and HIV-2.[81] Although both of these viruses can cause immunodeficiency, and have been identified in the USA, HIV-1 is thought to be responsible for the vast majority of cases of AIDS in the USA and Europe.

AIDS, which can be considered as the final stage of the continuum that begins with HIV infection, affects only a small portion of the patients infected with HIV. Patients who are HIV positive may be asymptomatic for a long period of time. However, they do have a progressive disease that is, in all probability, terminal. Moss et al[82] followed 288 HIV-seropositive patients and estimated that the median duration of infection was 6 years. The projected rate of progression to AIDS is 50% at 6 years. It is thought that the majority of seropositive patients will develop AIDS within 10–15 years after infection.[83,84]

The CDC classification of HIV infection is based on clinical manifestations. HIV-infected persons are placed into one of four categories:

1. Acute infection;
2. Asymptomatic but seropositive;
3. Generalized lymphadenopathy;
4. Symptomatic HIV disease
   a. Constitutional disease
   b. Neurologic disease
   c. Secondary infectious disease.

Incidence and prevalence

As of July 1988, the World Health Organization reported over 100 000 cases of AIDS in 138 countries.[85] Although AIDS has been reported in all 50 states of the USA, it is seen mostly in several large cities, including New York, San Francisco, Los Angeles, Houston and Washington, D.C.[86] The New York City and State departments of health have reported that 1 in every 62 children born in New York City has antibodies to AIDS. New York is particularly hard hit, with the largest AIDS population in the USA. It was estimated that in 1992 there were 10 000 AIDS-related deaths in New York. It is also estimated that over 1000 HIV-infected infants will be born in New York this year, each carrying a major medical expense and what, at this point, amounts to a fatal disease.

The high-risk groups for the development of AIDS are male homosexuals, intravenous drug abusers, hemophiliacs receiving transfusion therapy, Haitians, blood recipients (especially prior to the blood screening for HIV) and any person having sexual contact with someone in a high-risk group. It was estimated that by the end of 1990 nearly 10% of all AIDS patients will be women.[87]

Detection of anti-HIV antibodies is now routinely being performed by enzyme-linked immunosorbent assay (ELISA),[88] which, although considered highly sensitive and specific, does have some deficiencies. ELISA screening for HIV-1 does not always reveal the presence of antibodies to HIV-2.[89] Additionally, false-positive results have been found to occur. Causes of false-positive ELISA include collagen vascular disease, malaria and chronic hepatitis. Other more highly specific tests such as immunofluorescence assay (IFA) or Western blot tests are utilized if ELISA is positive.[90]

Although transfused blood is now being screened for the presence of HIV, the screening test is not foolproof. The window time (during which there is virus positivity but negativity of antibody screening) can be as long as 14 months.[91] It has been estimated that the risk of a virus-positive but antibody-negative blood transfusion is 26 per 1 million units.[92]

In addition to blood, HIV has also been isolated in seminal fluid, tears, saliva, synovial fluid and CSF.[93,94] There is no evidence that saliva or tears act as a vector in the transmission of HIV. However, the anesthesiologist must still take precautions when dealing with any patient considered at risk. Since it is estimated that 1.5 million Americans harbor the virus, some now consider all patients as potential carriers. Discriminating behavior on the part of the anesthesiologist is, however, not warranted. Despite the large numbers of infected patients, the occupational risk of HIV transmission is very low and can be further reduced by careful adherence to simple 'universal precautions'.[95] Standard sterilization and disinfection of anesthesia equipment has been shown to prevent HIV transmission. The CDC has published guidelines to decrease the risk of HIV transmission. Guidelines 'universal precautions' that may be related to the practice of anesthesiology include the use of gloves for cases in which secretion contact may be occur (intubation, extubation, handling of blood or other body fluids), avoidance of needle resheathing, use of puncture-resistant 'sharps' containers and use of protective eye coverings.[96]

Clinical manifestations of HIV infection

HIV causes a variety of clinical manifestations resulting from defects in immunologic function. The clinical condition can vary from that of asymptomatic carrier to the end stages of fatal illness. Clinical manifestations of AIDS are outlined in Table 63.5.

AIDS and regional anesthesia

Anesthetic implications of HIV infection are outlined in Table 63.6.

Although it has been suggested that intraspinal anesthesia may exacerbate some of the neurologic manifestations of AIDS,[105] this has not been substantiated in the anesthesia or neurology literature. The present consensus of opinion is that regional anesthesia may be performed in the AIDS parturient if she does not have nervous system symptoms. The HIV virus has been isolated from the CSF of AIDS patients,[106] therefore transdural passage during intraspinal anesthesia should not cause new CNS symptoms.

Regional anesthesia is relatively contraindicated in the AIDS parturient who has active neurologic symptoms, such as encephalitis, vacuolar degeneration of the spinal cord, meningitis or peripheral neuropathy. Regional anesthesia is also contraindicated if the AIDS patient has a coagulopathy. Since HIV has been isolated from CSF, the anesthesiologist performing regional anesthesia must take certain precautions. An example of such a precaution would be the situation in which there may have been a dural puncture during placement of an epidural anesthetic. Allowing the unknown fluid to drop on the anesthesiologist's skin to determine its temperature should no longer be performed. Instead, the unknown fluid can be combined with sodium thiopental; the resultant precipitate will demonstrate local anesthetic rather than CSF. Since saline or diluted fentanyl can be misinterpreted, the superior method of identification would be by testing for the presence or absence of glucose.

Table 63.5 Commonly seen clinical manifestations of AIDS

Opportunistic infections, including *Pneumocystis carinii* pneumonia (PCP)
Kaposi's sarcoma, Hodgkin and non-Hodgkin lymphoma
Respiratory disease, including *Pneumocystis carinii* pneumonia and virulent mycobacterial infection
Tuberculosis
Coagulation disorders, including thrombocytopenia
Cardiac abnormalities, including myocarditis, chronic heart failure and ventricular tachycardia
Central nervous system and psychiatric disease, including cerebral toxoplasmosis infection, encephalitis, meningitis, dementia and schizophrenia
Peripheral nervous system, including polyneuropathy
Diffuse adenopathy, including tonsillar and adenoidal hypertrophy

Table 63.6 Anesthetic implications of HIV infection

Presence of pulmonary disease may cause decreased functional residual capacity and, therefore, faster desaturation[97]
Presence of tonsillar and adenoidal hypertrophy may make endotracheal intubation difficult[98]
Presence of cerebral toxoplasmosis may cause increased intracranial pressure[99]
Psychiatric disorders, including acute psychoses, may preclude regional anesthesia[100]
Presence of cardiac manifestations of AIDS may predispose the patient to arrhythmias and chronic heart failure[101]
Coagulation disorders (e.g. disseminated intravascular coagulation) may occur. Need to check coagulation status prior to placement of regional anesthesia.[102]
Presence of PCP may limit gas exchange during general anesthesia[103]
Regional anesthesia may be contraindicated because of neuropathies[104]

AIDS therapy

Since AIDS may present with a variety of symptoms there are several different drugs being used in the treatment of this disease. The immunocompromise may be treated with azidothymidine (Zidovudine or AZT), which enhances immune function. This drug has been found to decrease the mortality from and the frequency of opportunistic infections.[107] AZT is converted to a triphosphate form that inhibits HIV reverse transcriptase. This drug does cross the placenta and blood–brain barrier and can be obtained in the CSF. AZT therapy may cause multiple side-effects, which include nausea, vomiting, headache, myalgias and meningoencephalitis. Hematologic abnormalities include anemia, leukopenia and granulocytopenia.[108] AZT, while inhibiting HIV replication, has no activity against AIDS-associated opportunistic infections, therefore there is need for alternative therapy.

Acyclovir is being used to treat herpes zoster and granciclovir is being used for cytomegalovirus treatment. Tuberculosis, which may be very virulent in AIDS patients, is treated with the usual triple therapy of isoniazid, rifampin and ethambutol. Candidal infections are treated with cotrimoxazole or amphotericin B. Renal function may be altered by amphotericin B. PCP is often treated with pentamidine and cotrimoxazole, both of which are associated with severe side-effects. Phenytoin (Dilantin), which is often used to treat seizure disorders associated with central nervous system disease, can cause hepatic dysfunction.

Table 63.7 describes the anesthetic implications of AIDS therapy.

AIDS in pregnancy

Transmission of HIV from mother to child is well documented and can occur via several possible routes.[109] The mother can infect the fetus transplacentally at any time during pregnancy.[110] Since intrapartum exposure has been found to occur, cesarean delivery does not prevent fetal transmission.[111] It has also been suggested that transmission via breast milk occurs.[112,113]

Perinatal transmission of HIV cannot be prevented, although the transmission from mother to fetus is not a

Table 63.7 Anesthetic implications of AIDS therapy

Drug	Implications to anesthesiologist
AZT	Nausea/vomiting: aspiration prophylaxis needed Seizures: avoid enflurane and hyperventilation Anemia: check complete blood count preoperatively
Isoniazid	Nausea/vomiting: as above Hepatic dysfunction: avoid hepatotoxic drugs, halothane; avoid hepatically metabolized drugs Thrombocytopenia: check coagulation profile prior to use of regional anesthesia
Rifampin	Nausea/vomiting: as above Hepatitis: as above Acute renal failure: avoid drugs with renal metabolism Thrombocytopenia: as above Dyspnea: avoid respiratory depressants or secure airway
Ethambutol	Optic neuritis: ophthalmology consultation Nausea/vomiting: as above Hepatic dysfunction: as above
Amphotericin B	Nephrotoxicity: as above Hypokalemia: check potassium preoperatively; avoid hyperventilation Muscle weakness: monitor neuromuscular blockade Cardiovascular toxicity: avoid cardiodepressants
Pentamidine	Cardiotoxicity: as above ECG abnormalities: preoperative ECG Hypotension: check blood pressure frequently Hypoglycemia: monitor intraoperative glucose
Cotrimoxazole	Allergic myocarditis: avoid cardiodepressants Aplastic anemia: check complete blood count preoperatively Thrombocytopenia: check platelets before initiation of regional anesthetic
Phenytoin	Hepatic dysfunction: as above Nausea/vomiting: as above Thrombocytopenia: as above Gingival hyperplasia: care with intubation

certainty.[114] Minkoff et al[102] noted that only 36% of children born to mothers who had previously given birth to a baby with evidence of HIV infection were HIV positive.[115]

Several retrospective studies have suggested that pregnancy may accelerate the course of HIV infection because of a pregnancy-induced immune suppression.[116] Because of the risk to both mother and fetus, the CDC have recommended that HIV-positive women postpone pregnancy until more information is available regarding the transmission and treatment of perinatal infection.

AIDS and health care workers

Several reports have described health care workers who have been contaminated with HIV.[117] Hirsch et al,[118] in an overly optimistic 1985 report, followed 30 health care workers having 31 needle sticks in whom none developed AIDS. Several other reports have found occupational transmission of HIV and as of last year more than 20 cases had been reported. In 1988, the CDC found a seroprevalence rate of 0.47%, a rate of seroconversion of 1:100 to 1 : 200 following needle stick. A recent report estimates that following exposure to blood from HIV-positive patients, the seroprevalence rate was 0.42%. Because of this alarmingly high risk, the CDC suggests that all patients be considered as potential hazards to health care workers. The American Society of Anesthesiologists Committee on Occupational Health has made recommendations to decrease the risk to health care workers. Suggestions include methods for decreasing accidental needle sticks, such as punctureproof containers and policies for nonrecapping of needles. Since needle stick is the only method of transmission thus far proven to cause seroconversion in health care workers, maximal precautions must be taken to remove this hazard.

Although emphasis has been placed on the risk to health care workers who care for AIDS patients, recently there has been discussion about the transmission of HIV from doctor to patient. Since there have been numerous reports of the transmission of hepatitis B from infected surgeons to their patients, there is growing concern that HIV may also be transmitted from physician to patient. The CDC, in their 1987 guidelines, stated that decisions about infected health care workers performing invasive procedures should be made on a case-by-case basis by the infected health care worker's personal physician and hospital. These guidelines are presently being revised following the news that an HIV-infected dentist probably transmitted the virus to a patient during oral surgery. An epidemiologic study of that patient failed to reveal any AIDS risk factors or behavior that might put her at risk. Additionally, viral DNA samples from the dentist and patient showed a high degree of similarity, thereby suggesting that this actually represents a doctor to patient transmission.

REFERENCES

1. Silverman S 1989 Scope, specifics of maternal drug use, effect on fetus are beginning to emerge from studies. J Am Med Assoc 261: 1688–1689
2. Matera C, Warren W B, Moomjy M et al 1990 Prevalence of use of cocaine and other substances in an obstetric population. Am J Obstet Gynecol 163: 797–801
3. Clayton R R 1985 Cocaine use in the US: in a blizzard or just being snowed. In: Kozel N J, Adams E H (eds) Cocaine use in America: epidemiology and clinical perspectives. NIDA Research Monograph series 61. Rockville, MD, US Dept of Health and Human Services, pp 8–32
4. Little B B, Snell L M, Palmore M K et al 1988 Cocaine use in pregnant women in a large public hospital. Am J Perinatol 5: 206
5. Abelson H I, Miller J D 1985 A decade of trends in cocaine in the

household population. NIDA Research Monograph Series 61. Rockville, MD, US Dept of Health and Human Services, p 35
6. Chasnoff I J, Burns W J, Schnoll S H, Burns K A 1985 Cocaine use in pregnancy. New Engl J Med 313: 666–669
7. Birnbach D J, Grunebaum A, Weiss W 1989 Epidural anesthesia for cesarean section in cocaine abusing parturients (abstract). Society for Obstetric Anesthesia and Perinatology, F–6
8. Gawin F H, Ellinwood E H 1988 Cocaine and other stimulants. Actions, abuse, and treatment. New Engl J Med 318: 1173–1182
9. Van Dyke C, Jatlow P, Ungerer J 1978 Oral cocaine plasma concentration and central effects. Science 200: 211–213
10. Oro A S, Dixon S D 1987 Perinatal cocaine and methamphetamine exposure. Maternal and neonatal correlates. Pediatrics 111: 571–578
11. Gold M S, Washton A M, Dackis C A 1985 Cocaine abuse: neurochemistry, phenomenology, and treatment. NIDI Research Monograph Series 61. Rockville, MD, US Dept of Health and Human Services, pp 130–150
12. Pitts D K, Marwah J 1989 Autonomic actions of cocaine. Can J Physiol Pharmacol 67: 1168–1176
13. Towers C V, Pircon R A, Nageotte M P et al 1993 Cocaine intoxication presenting as preeclampsia and eclampsia. Obstet Gynecol 81: 545–547
14. Birnbach D J, Stein D J, Grunebaum A 1993 An instant approach to the differential diagnosis between preeclampsia and cocaine abuse (abstract). Am J Obstet Gynecol 168: A429
15. Ney J A, Dooley S L, Keith L G 1990 The prevalence of substance abuse in patients with suspected preterm labor. Am J Obstet Gynecol 162: 1562–1567
16. MacGregor S N, Keith L G, Chasnoff I J et al 1987 Cocaine use during pregnancy. Adverse perinatal outcome. Am J Obstet Gynecol 157: 687
17. Keith L G, MacGregor S, Friedell S et al 1989 Substance abuse in pregnant women. Obstet Gynecol 73: 715
18. Acker D, Sachs B P, Tracey K J, Wise W E 1983 Abruptio placentae associated with cocaine use. Am J Obstet Gynecol 146: 220–221
19. Bingol N, Fuchs M, Diaz V et al 1987 Teratogenicity of cocaine in humans. J. Pediatr 110: 93–96
20. Woods J R, Plessinger M A, Clark K E 1987 Effect of cocaine on uterine blood flow and fetal oxygenation. J Am Med Assoc 257: 957–961
21. Moore T R, Sorg J, Miller L et al 1986 Hemodynamic effects of intravenous cocaine on the pregnant ewe and fetus. Am J Obstet Gynecol 155: 883–888
22. Stewart D J, Inaba T, Lucassen M et al 1979 Cocaine metabolism: Cocaine and norcocaine hydrolysis by liver and serum esterases. Clin Pharm Ther 25: 464–468
23. Isner J M, Estes N A M, Thompson P D et al 1986 Acute cardiac events temporally related to cocaine abuse. New Engl J Med 315: 1438
24. Howard R E, Hueter D C, Davis G J 1985 Acute myocardial infarction following cocaine abuse in a young woman with normal coronary arteries. J Am Med Assoc 254: 95–96
25. Schachne J S, Roberts B H, Thompson P D 1984 Coronary artery spasm and myocardial infarction associated with cocaine use. New Engl J Med 310: 1665–1666
26. Wetli C V, Wright R K 1979 Death caused by recreational cocaine use. J Am Med Assoc 241: 2519–2522
27. Lichtenfield P J, Rubin D B, Feldman R S 1984 Subarachnoid hemorrhage precipitated by cocaine snorting. Arch Neurol 41: 223–224
28. Nalbandian H, Sheth N, Dietrich R et al 1985 Intestinal ischemia caused by cocaine ingestion: report of 2 cases. Surgery 97: 374–376
29. Adrouny A, Magnusson P 1985 Pneumopericardium from cocaine inhalation. New Engl J Med 313: 48–49
30. American College of Obstetrics and Gynecology. Committee on Obstetrics 1992 Maternal and fetal medicine. Cocaine in pregnancy. Committee Opinion No. 114
31. Birnbach D J, Stein D J, Thomas K et al 1993 Cocaine abuse in the parturient: what are the implications to the anesthesiologist? (abstract). Society for Obstetric Anesthesia and Perinatology, p 61
32. Knisely J S, Spear E R, Green D J et al 1991 Substance abuse patterns in pregnant women. NIDA Research Monograph 108: 280–281
33. Birnbach D J, Thomas K, Stein D J et al 1993 Instant recognition of the cocaine abusing parturient. A new method of identification. Society for Obstetric Anesthesia and Perinatology, p 62
34. Hughes S C, Vertommen J D, Rosen M A et al 1991 Cocaine induced hypertension in the ewe and response to treatment with labetalol (abstract). Anesthesiology A1075
35. Ramoska E, Sacchetti A 1985 Propranolol induced hypertension in the treatment of cocaine intoxication. Ann Int Med 14: 1112–1113
36. Jatlow P, Barash P G, Van Dyke C et al 1979 Cocaine and succinylcholine sensitivity: a new caution. Anesth Analg 58: 235–238
37. Samuels J, Schwalbe S S, Marx G F 1991 Speedballs. A new cause of intraoperative tachycardia and hypertension. Anesth Analg 72: 397–398
38. Bailey D N 1987 Amphetamine detection during toxicology screening of a university medical center population. J Clin Toxicol 25: 399–409
39. Ong B H 1962 Hazards to health: Dextroamphetamine poisoning. New Engl J Med 266: 1321–1322
40. Elliot R H, Rees G B 1990 Amphetamine ingestion presenting as eclampsia. Can J Anaesth 37: 130–133
41. Michel R, Adams A 1979 Acute amphetamine abuse. Anesthesia 34: 1016–1019
42. Johnston R R, Way W L, Miller R D 1972 Alteration of anesthetic requirement by amphetamine. Anesthesiology 36: 357–363
43. Caldwell J, Stevens P S 1974 The biochemical pharmacology of abused drugs. Clin Pharmacol Ther 16: 625–638
44. Samuels S I, Maze A, Albright A 1979 Cardiac arrest during cesarean section in a chronic amphetamine abuser. Anesth Analg 58: 528–530
45. Smith D S, Gutsche B B 1980 Amphetamine abuse and obstetrical anesthesia. Anesth Analg 59: 710–711
46. Geerlings P J 1972 Social and psychiatric factors in amphetamine users. Psychiatr Neurol Neurochir 75: 219–224
47. Rubin E 1979 Alcoholic myopathy in heart and skeletal muscle. New Engl J Med 301: 28–33
48. Bruce D L 1983 Alcoholism and anesthesia. Anesth Analg 62: 84–96
49. Duvaldestin P, Agoston S, Henzel D et al 1978 Pancuronium pharmacokinetics in patients with liver cirrhosis. Br J Anaesth 50: 1131–1136
50. Hoegerman G, Schnoll S 1991 Narcotic use in pregnancy. Clin Perinatol 18: 51–76
51. Giuffrida J G 1970 Anesthetic management of drug abusers. Anesth Analg 49: 272–278
52. Gross E M 1978 Autopsy findings in drug addicts. Pathol Annual 13: 35–67
53. Koppel B S, Tuchman A J, Mangiardi J R, Daras M et al 1988 Epidural spinal infection in intravenous drug abusers. Arch Neurol 45: 1331–1337
54. Connaughton J G 1975 Current concepts in the management of the pregnant opiate addict. Addictive Dis 2: 21–35
55. Lipski J, Stimmel B, Donoso E 1973 The effect of heroin and multiple drug abuse on the electrocardiogram. Am Heart J 86: 663–668
56. Gold M S, Pottash A L C, Extein I, Kleber H D 1980 Clonidine in acute opiate withdrawal. New Engl J Med 302: 1421–1422
57. Scheutz F 1982 Drug addicts and local anesthesia: effectivity and general side effects. Scand J Dental Res 90: 299–305
58. Tornabene V W 1974 Narcotic withdrawal syndrome caused by naltrexone. Ann Intern Med 81: 785–787
59. Weintraub S J, Naulty J S 1985 Acute abstinence syndrome after epidural injection of butorphanol. Anesth Analg 64: 452–453
60. Mendelson C L 1946 The aspiration of stomach contents into the lungs during obstetric anesthesia. Am J Obstet Gynecol 52: 191

61. Sellick B A 1961 Cricoid pressure to control regurgitation of stomach contents during induction of anesthesia. Lancet 2: 404
62. Mark L C, Marx G, Arkins R E et al 1966 Hypotension during anesthesia in narcotic addicts. NY State J Med 66: 2685–2686
63. Wood P R, Soni N 1989 Anesthesia and substance abuse. Anesthesia 44: 672–680
64. Power I, Noble D W, Douglas E, Spence A A 1990 Comparison of IM ketorolac trometamol and morphine sulphate for pain relief after cholecystectomy. Br J Anaesth 65: 448–455
65. Tennes K 1984 Effect of marijuana on pregnancy and fetal development in the human. NIDI Research Monograph Series 44. Rockville, MD, US Dept of Health and Human Services pp 115–123
66. Greenland S 1981 The effects of marijuana use during pregnancy. Am J Obstet Gynecol 143: 408–413
67. Wu T C, Tashkin D P, Djahed B et al 1988 Pulmonary hazards of smoking marijuana. New Engl J Med 318: 347–351
68. Berman M L, Bochantin J F 1972 Effect of delta 9 tetrahydrocanabinol on liver microsomal dechorinase activity. Anesth Analg 51: 929–932
69. Wilkins-Haug L, Gabow P A 1991 Toluene abuse during pregnancy: Obstetric complications and perinatal outcomes. Obstet Gynecol 77: 504–509
70. Sloan L B, Gay J W, Snyder S W, Bales W R 1992 Substance abuse during pregnancy in a rural population. Obstet Gynecol 79: 245–248
71. Prager K, Malin H, Spiegler D et al 1984 Smoking and drinking behavior before and during pregnancy of married mothers of live-born infants and stillborn infants. Public Health Rep 99: 117–127
72. Pearce A C, Jones R M 1984 Smoking and anesthesia: preoperative abstinence and perioperative morbidity. Anesthesiology 61: 576–584
73. Benowitz N L 1991 Nicotine replacement therapy during pregnancy. J Am Med Assoc 266: 3174–3177
74. Gottlieb M S, Schroff R, Shanker H M et al 1981 Pneumocystis carinnii pneumonia and mucosal candidiasis in previously healthy homosexual men. New Engl J Med 305: 1425–1431
75. Masur H, Michelis M A, Greene J B et al 1981 An outbreak of community acquired pneumocystis carinii pneumonia. New Engl J Med 305: 1431–1438
76. CDC Update on AIDS 1982 MMWR 31: 507
77. CDC Update on AIDS 1985 MMWR 34: 245
78. Barre-Sinousi F, Chermann J C, Rey F et al 1983 Isolation of a T-lymphotropic retrovirus from a patient at risk for acquired immune deficiency syndrome. Science 220: 868–871
79. Gallo R C, Salahuddin S Z, Popovic M et al 1984 Frequent detection and isolation of cytopathic retroviruses (HTLV-III) from patients with AIDS. Science 224: 500–503
80. Levy J A, Hoffman A D, Kramer S M, Landis J M 1984 Isolation of lymphocytopathic retroviruses from San Francisco patients with AIDS. Science 225: 840–842
81. Evans L A, Moreau J, Odeehouri K et al 1988 Simultaneous isolation of HIV-1 and HIV-2 from an AIDS patient. Lancet 2: 1389–1391
82. Moss A R, Bacchetti P, Osmond D, Kranpf W et al 1988 Seropositivity for HIV and the development of AIDS or AIDS related condition. Br Med J 296: 745–750
83. Carne C A, Weller I V, Loveddy C et al 1987 From persistent generalized lymphadenopathy to AIDS. Br Med J 299: 866–869
84. Eyster M E, Gail M H, Ballard J O 1987 Natural history of human immunodeficiency virus infection. Ann Intern Med 107: 1–6
85. Mann J M, Chin J 1988 AIDS a global perspective. New Engl J Med 319: 302–303
86. CDC Update on AIDS 1987 MMWR 36: 1
87. Public Health Service Report 1986 Public Health Serv Rep 101: 341
88. Update 1988 Serologic testing for antibody to human immunodeficiency virus. MMWR 36: 833–845
89. Brun-Vezinet F, Rey M A, Katlama C et al 1984 Lymphadenopathy-associated viral antibody in AIDS. New Engl J Med 311: 1269
90. Centers for Disease Control 1989 Interpretation and use of the Western blot assay for serodiagnosis of human immunodeficiency virus type 1 infection. MMWR 38 (S7): 1
91. Curran J W, Lawrence D, Jaffe H et al 1984 Acquired immunodeficiency syndrome associated with transfusions. New Engl J Med 310: 69–75
92. Ward J W, Holmberg S D, Allen J R 1988 Transmission of HIV by blood transfusion screened as negative for HIV antibody. New Engl J Med 318: 473–478
93. Friedland G H, Klein R S 1987 Transmission of the human immunodeficiency virus. New Engl J Med 317: 1125–1135
94. Seifert M H 1988 Transmission of HIV. New Engl J Med 318: 1203
95. Cantineau J P 1989 AIDS and implications for anesthesiologists. Cur Opin Anaesthesiol 2: 349–355
96. Anon 1988 Update: universal precautions for the prevention of transmission of human immunodeficiency virus, hepatitis B virus, and other bloodborne pathogens in health-care settings. MMWR 37: 377–378
97. Varteresian-Karanful L, Josephson A, Fikrig S et al 1988 Pulmonary infection and cavity formation caused by mycobacterium Tb in a child with AIDS. New Engl J Med 319: 1018–1019
98. Brazan L, Carbone A, Saracchini S et al 1989 Nasopharyngeal lymphatic tissue hypertrophy in HIV infected patient. Lancet 1: 42
99. Black P H 1985 HTLV-III, AIDS, and the brain. New Engl J Med 313: 1538–1540
100. Atkinson J H, Grant I, Kennedy C J et al 1988 Prevalence of psychiatric disorders among men infected with human immunodeficiency virus. Arch Gen Psych 45: 859–864
101. Reilly J M, Cunnion R E, Anderson D W et al 1988 Frequency of myocarditis, left ventricular dysfunction and ventricular tachycardia in the acquired immunodeficiency syndrome. Am J Cardiol 62: 789–793
102. Krilov L R, Rubin L G, Frogel M et al 1990 Disseminated adenovirus infection with hepatic necrosis in patients with human immunodeficiency virus infection and other immunodeficiency states. Rev Infect Dis 12: 303–307
103. Gotta A W 1990 AIDS and its implications to the anesthesiologist. In Stoelting RK (ed) Advances in anesthesia, Vol 7. CV Mosby, St Louis/Year Book, Chicago
104. So Y T, Holtzman D M, Abrams D I et al 1988 Peripheral neuropathy associated with AIDS. Arch Neruol 45: 945–948
105. Greene E R 1986 Spinal and epidural anesthesia in patients with the acquired immunodeficiency syndrome. Anesth Analg 65: 1090–1091
106. Ho D D, Rota T R, Schooley R T et al 1985 Isolation of HTLV-III from cerebrospinal fluid and neural tissues of patients with neurologic syndromes related to AIDS. New Engl J Med 313: 1493–1497
107. Fischl M A, Richman D D, Grieco M H et al 1987 The efficacy of AZT in the treatment of patients with AIDS and AIDS-related complex. New Engl J Med 317: 185–191
108. Richman D D, Fischl M A, Grieco M H et al 1987 The toxicity of azidothmidine (AZT) in the treatment of patients with AIDS and AIDS related complex. New Engl J Med 317: 192–197
109. The European Collaborative Study 1988 Mother to child transmission of HIV infection. Lancet 2: 1039
110. LaPointe N, Michaud J, Pekovic D et al 1985 Transplacental transmission of HTLV-III virus. New Engl J Med 312: 1325–1326
111. Jousisas E, Koch M A, Schafer et al 1982 LAV/HTLV-III in a 20 week fetus. Lancet 2: 1129
112. Friedland G H, Klein R S 1987 Transmission of the human immunodeficiency virus. New Engl J Med 317: 1125–1135
113. Thiry I, Sprecher-Goldberger S, Jonckheer T, Levy J 1985 Isolation of AIDS virus from cell free breast milk of three healthy virus carriers. Lancet 2: 891–892
114. Ziegler J B, Cooper D A, Johnson R O et al 1985 Post natal transmission of AIDS associated retrovirus from mother to infant. Lancet 1: 896–898
115. Minkoff H, Nanda D, Menez R et al 1987 Pregnancies resulting in

infants with acquired immunodeficiency syndrome. Obstet Gynecol 69: 288–291
116. Scott G B, Fischl M A, Klinas N et al 1985 Mothers of infants with acquired immunodeficiency syndrome. Evidence for both symptomatic and asymptomatic carriers. J Am Med Assoc 253: 363–366
117. Marcus R 1988 Surveillance of health care workers exposed to blood from patients infected with human immunodeficiency virus. New Engl J Med 319: 1118
118. Hirsch M S, Wormser G P, Schooley R T et al 1985 Risk of nosocomial infection with HTLV-III. New Engl J Med 312: 1–4

PART B
NEONATAL EFFECTS
F. Shahrivar

DRUG ABUSE

During the past two decades substance abuse in the USA has reached epidemic proportions and the incidence of addiction in women of child-bearing age has been increasing. The National Institute on Drug Abuse 1988 National Household Survey revealed that 8.8% of women of child-bearing age have used illicit drugs and approximately 1 in 10 infants may be exposed to illicit drugs during pregnancy,[1] and this exposure produces short-term and long-term effects on developing fetus and newborn infants. Commonly used illicit drugs are described below.

Opioids (heroin and methadone)

History and Metabolism

Perlstein in 1947[2] wrote an article entitled 'Congenital morphinism', which reported the effect of morphine on the fetus and subsequent withdrawal syndrome and convulsions. By the 1950s and 1960s, heroin and morphine were the most common opioids to cause withdrawal syndrome. Dole and Nyswander, in 1965,[3] reported on the effectiveness of oral methadone for the maintenance treatment of heroin addicts. Many pregnant women started using methadone liberally, and most often in very high dosages; therefore, methadone was used during pregnancy for a long time without much scientific investigation regarding its safety and its effects on the metabolism of the developing fetus and newborn.

Opium[4] is obtained from the poppy plant, *Papaver somniferum*. When it dries, the juice of the plant's seed turns into a powdered form of opium. In 1806, Surturner reported the isolation of a substance from opium and he named it 'morphine' after Morpheus, the Greek god of dreams. Heroin,[4,5] a diacetyl morphine, is a highly euphoriant and analgesic drug; the acetyl group causes a reduction in polarity and thus heroin can cross the blood–brain barrier and placental membrane much faster than morphine. In the body, heroin is rapidly hydrolyzed to 6-monoacetylmorphine and is excreted in urine as morphine.

Maternal effects

Heroin-dependent mothers receive little or no perinatal care and usually neglect their general health care and nutrition during pregnancy and, thus experience more complications than nondrug abusers or controlled drug users. Ostrea and Chavez[6] reported increased antenatal problems, such as anemia, bleeding, premature rupture of membranes and premature labor, and Fulroth et al[7] observed a higher prevalence of meconium-stained amniotic fluid in heroin users (36%) than in controls (10%).

Neonatal effects

Infants born to heroin- or methadone-addicted mothers are small for gestational age, or growth retarded. This is most likely due to the inhibitory effect of heroin on fetal body growth. Taeusch et al[8] found a 9% birthweight reduction after injection of heroin in pregnant does and fetal rabbits. Smaller head circumference and lower birthweight is a frequent finding in drug-exposed infants.[6,7,9] These infants also show abnormal signs and symptoms known as neonatal withdrawal or abstinence syndrome. Onset of withdrawal varies from infant to infant, and is mostly related to the time, route and dosage of drug used by the mother. Withdrawal can occur at the time of birth, with a peak 2–4 days after birth, or after as long as 2–6 weeks. Common signs and symptoms are tremors, jitteriness, high-pitched cry, feeding difficulties, lack of effective sucking reflex, gastrointestinal disturbances such as vomiting, regurgitation and diarrhea and also autonomic nervous system symptoms such as yawning, sneezing, sweating and mottling skin in the acute phase of withdrawal.

Methadone withdrawal is more severe than heroin withdrawal, with an increased incidence of sleep disorders, respiratory problems and convulsions. Glass et al[10] reported a decreased incidence of respiratory distress syndrome (RDS) in premature infants exposed to heroin in utero. Taeusch et al[8] confirmed this finding by studying lung maturation in fetal rabbits after exposure to heroin.

Neurodevelopmental outcome

There are conflicting reports regarding neurologic and psychomotor development in infants exposed to opioids. Brain sonography shows small, slit-like lateral ventricles,[11] and perinatal administration of morphine to pups has demonstrated interruption in neuronal growth in the developing brain.[12] In general, these infants have been found to be within the normal range for mental development, but their attention span is shorter and they have poor fine motor coordination.[8,13,14]

Cocaine

Cocaine abuse has increased dramatically during the past decade. In the late 1970s, cocaine gained prominence as a recreational drug and was used at high social gatherings. However, in recent years because of the wide availability and cheapness of pure cocaine from Central and South America, it has become the most popular illicit drug among all age groups in the USA – especially in the young of minority groups and women of child-bearing age.

History and metabolism[15,16]

Cocaine is classified as a stimulant drug and is also known as the first local anesthetic. It was purified by Niemann in 1860. Sigmund Freud used it as a maintenance drug for morphine withdrawal, for which it was effective but also addictive. Cocaine was used as a local anesthetic for dental and ophthalmologic surgery. Work by Einhorn and colleagues resulted in the synthesis of procaine from cocaine in 1905 and procaine became the premier local anesthetic agent.

Cocaine is derived from the leaves of *Erythroxylon coca* and it is extracted as a paste. It is an ester of benzoic acid with a molecular weight of 339.81, is highly lipid soluble, has a low degree of ionization at physiologic pH, is absorbed easily through mucous membranes and readily crosses the placenta by simple diffusion. Once in the circulation it is metabolized by hepatic and plasma cholinesterases to inactive compounds such as benzoylecgonic and ecgonic methyl esters, which are excreted in urine and used as markers for a screening test. Cholinesterase activity is diminished during pregnancy and there is especially low activity in the fetus. As a result, excretion of cocaine metabolites in urine is delayed and they remain in the body for a longer time.[17,18]

Maternal effects

Cocaine, by blocking presynaptic uptake of monoamines such as dopamine, serotonin and norepinephrine, increases circulating catecholamines, and, as a result, body temperature, heart rate and blood pressure will rise. An increase in the incidence of placental abruption and precipitous labor could be the result of maternal hypertension and tachycardia.[19,20] In addition, an increase in the incidence of premature labor and spontaneous abortion has been reported after cocaine usage.[20–22]

Fetoplacental effects

Woods[23] measured the effects of cocaine on uteroplacental blood flow by giving different doses of cocaine to pregnant ewes. The study demonstrated a dose-dependent response with increases in maternal blood pressure, decreases in uterine blood flow and a marked increase in uterine vascular resistance. Cocaine crosses the placental barrier and stimulates catecholamine response in the fetus as it does in the mother. Vasoconstriction of fetoplacental circulation results in a reduction in fetal oxygenation, leading to fetal distress, passage of meconium and low Apgar scores.[7,20,21,24]

Neonatal effects

Growth. Cocaine-exposed infants are more likely to be premature, of low birthweight, small for gestation age and have microcephaly.[7,8,24] It has been hypothesized that growth retardation is a result of fetal hypoxemia and maternal nutritional deficiency.

Neonatal withdrawal syndrome. In many cases the effects of cocaine withdrawal are mild and in some infants not even appreciable. Tremors, hyperirritability, lethargy and apnea have been reported; however cocaine may have devastating effects on different organs of exposed infants.

1. *Cardiovascular system.* Transient tachycardia and hypertension are due to circulating fetal catecholamines and down-regulation.[7,25,26] Right ventricular conducting delay and evidence of myocardial ischemia on electrocardiography have also been reported.[27]

2. *Central nervous system.* Chasnoff et al[25,28] reported cerebral infarction in a neonate at 24 h of age, and Dixon and Bejar[29] reported structural abnormality of the brain, along with hemorrhagic infarction secondary to the vasoconstrictive and hypertensive effects of cocaine.[29]

3. *Neurodevelopment.* Cocaine-exposed infants show impairment of orientation, motor tone, and homeostatic behavior on the Brazelton Neonatal Behavioral Assessment Scale.[19,22–30] Prolongation of auditory brainstem responses (ABR) and delayed brainstem transport time (BTT) are probably due to impairment of brain myelination.[31] Doberczak et al[32] reported transient neurobehavioral and electroencephalographic abnormalities in these infants, which were not apparent by 1 year of age.[32]

4. *Gastrointestinal system.* Gastrointestinal symptoms such as vomiting, loose stools, delayed gastric emptying and feeding problems are not as common as in opioid-exposed infants. In my institution a slight increase in the incidence of necrotizing enterocolitis in cocaine-exposed infants has been noticed.[33] This was also reported by Telsey et al,[34] most likely due to vasoconstrictive effects of cocaine producing ischemic colitis.

5. *Malformation.* Despite conflicting reports regarding the teratogenicity of cocaine, there is speculation that infants exposed to cocaine have a higher incidence of malformations, especially of skull, eyes, genitourinary tract, and of cardiac anomalies, especially ventricular septal effects.[20,27,35–38]

Chavez et al[39] reported an increased risk of urinary tract malformation without any effect on genital organs. Madden et al[40] found no evidence of teratogenicity in their study population.

Data from animal studies are also conflicting, Fantel et al[35] did not find any increased incidence of malformation in rats and mice but the study confirmed that the cocaine can cause growth retardation. Burkett et al[20] reported an increase in the incidence of skeletal defects in cocaine-exposed rats.

6. *Respiratory system.* In the late 1970s, Glass et al[10] reported a decreased incidence of RDS in infants of opioid-abusing mothers. In our institution, a lower incidence of RDS in cocaine-exposed infants has also been found.[33] Cocaine-exposed infants seem to have higher rate of respiratory pattern abnormalities.[41] Davidson-Ward et al[42,43] reported an increased incidence of symptomatic apnea before sudden infant death syndrome (SIDS) in 22% of cocaine-exposed infants versus 5.4% of controls.[44] There is speculation that a high level of circulating catecholamines and alteration in neurodevelopment activity may result in abnormal arousal responses and other ventilatory pattern abnormalities, which could be contributing factors in the increasing incidence of SIDS in infants exposed to cocaine in utero.[22,41–43,45] In contrast, Buckner et al[44] did not find any significant increase in SIDS in cocaine-exposed infants.

Marijuana

The name marijuana is derived from the Spanish word 'maraguany', meaning 'intoxicating substance'. It is formed from dried particles of the leaves of the hemp plant (*Cannabis sativa*).[46] It is also called grass, weed, pot or dope and it is smoked in cigarettes called joints or reefers. Stronger preparations called hashish or charas are also available.[47] The principal psychoactive compound in marijuana is Δ^9-tetrahydrocannabinol, the concentration of which varies in different products from 2 to 7%.[17,47]

Marijuana is very popular and was once called the nation's (USA) second recreational drug (second to alcohol); one-third of all adult Americans have tried the drug. The National Institute of Drug Abuse[48] reported that 10% of Americans over age 12 had used marijuana 1 month prior to interview. The effect of the recreational use of marijuana is dependent upon the concentration of tetrahydrocannabinol (THC) in the smoke and depth of inhalation. Marijuana is fat soluble and crosses the placenta easily; its half-life after smoking a cigarette containing 2% THC, is about 72 h. Smoking/inhalation of marijuana is the most common and effective form with a 50% absorption rate, versus 5 to 19% absorption if it is ingested.[49] After inhalation it enters the bloodstream and it has been shown to impair function of male and female sex hormones such as follicle-stimulating hormone, luteinizing hormone and testosterone. It also increases the heart rate and blood pressure.[17,49,50] Animal studies have demonstrated that THC in pregnant mice impairs body growth and weight regulation and, in rats, there is accumulation in tissue with very slow release. Marijuana is metabolized in the liver, but it remains in the body tissues for almost 30 days and may cause precipitous labor and premature contractions.[17,50] Infants born to marijuana users are smaller in all parameters of growth (height, weight, head circumference). Growth retardation is attributed to fetal hypoxemia secondary to increased carbon monoxide levels in the blood after smoking marijuana.[50,51] Marijuana is not known to cause a significant withdrawal syndrome, but mild irritability, restlessness, poor feeding and excessive crying have been attributed to cannabinol exposure. Poor habituation to visual stimuli and abnormal sleep patterns and arousal have been observed among the infants of marijuana users.[52] Marijuana has not been found to have teratogenic effect in humans.[49–52]

Amphetamines

Amphetamine drugs are not very popular at present, but in the early 1970s they were the third recreational drug after alcohol and marijuana. According to a report from the National Institute of Drug Abuse in 1986[48], approximately 2 million Americans over 25 years of age were using this drug. Amphetamine is called various names by drug users: speed, meth, crystal, crack and white cross.[47] Amphetamine and amphetamine-like drugs were approved by the FDA in 1930 and were used as decongestants; their abuse started in the 1970s when they were widely used as a diet pills and stimulants.[49] Amphetamine is a racemic 3-phenylisopropylamine, with similar effects to cocaine in releasing neurotransmitters such as dopamine, norepinephrine and serotonin, resulting in increased heart rate and blood pressure.[15,17,49,53,54] Studies in the USA and Sweden have shown an increase in the incidence of toxemia of pregnancy, premature labor and other perinatal complications in amphetamine users. Oro et al[55], reported an increased incidence of intrauterine growth retardation in amphetamine-exposed infants. These infants may show signs of mild withdrawal syndrome, such as hyperirritability, jitteriness, feeding problems and drowsiness.[55–57] Dixon and Bejar[58,59] reported abnormal echoencephalographic findings indicating cerebral injuries in infants exposed to amphetamines. Follow-up for 1 year did not show developmental and psychomotor delays, but signs of emotional disturbances were more common in infants who were separated from their biological parents and placed in foster homes.[56,57]

AIDS/HIV

Oleske et al[60] reported their first pediatric patient with AIDS in 1978 and suggested that there have been sporadic cases of pediatric AIDS not diagnosed since the 1970s. In 1982, only a year after identification of adult AIDS cases, the first cases of pediatric AIDS were reported.[61] The United States Public Health Service estimates that by 1991 there will be more than 3000 children with AIDS.[62] In 1988 the New York State Screening Program reported that 1.5% of all newborns in New York City were seropositive for human immunodeficiency virus.[63] In our hospital, with over 5000 deliveries per year, the rate of seropositivity is 1.9% for all infants, 10% for infants of drug abuse mothers and 17% for those born to i.v. drug users. New York City health information reports that there are 600 children with AIDS in New York City, and the Center for Disease Control has reported that 53% of children with AIDS are Black and 23% are Hispanics.[62]

Etiologic agent[61,64,66]

A retrovirus as a cause of AIDS was identified in 1983 by Barre-Sinousi et al[67] at the Pasteur Institute in Paris and in 1984 by Gallo et al[68] in the USA. This virus, which is known as human immunodeficiency virus type 1 (HIV-1), was previously called human T-cell lymphotropic virus type III (HTLV-III), lymphadenopathy-associated virus (LAV) or AIDS-associated retrovirus.[64] HIV-2, a new member of the HIV family, has been identified in African patients with AIDS.[64,66] HIV is an enveloped virus and is a member of the retrovirus family that can infect T cells bearing CD4 receptors, causing abnormalities of lymphocyte functions, which eventually lead to cellular and humoral immune deficiency.[61,64]

Transmission

Perinatal acquisition of HIV is the most common mode of transmitting AIDS to children; 80% of children with AIDS are reported to have acquired infection perinatally.[65,66,67,70] In the USA 79% of women with HIV infection are of child-bearing age[71] and contracted the infection either through sexual contacts or by sharing contaminated needles.

Mother-to-infant transmission may occur via the following routes:

Intrauterine

The time of transmission is not known but passage of the virus may take place in early gestation. AIDS virus has been identified in fetuses of 15 weeks and 20 weeks.[72,73] The virus has been found in the thymus of a 20-day-old premature infant born at 28 weeks of gestation.[65,66] The viral antigen has been detected in cord blood in 21% of infants born to seropositive mothers.[65]

During delivery

The infant is exposed to infected maternal blood and cervical secretions while passing through the birth canal.[74,75] There are conflicting reports regarding the protective effect of cesarean delivery in preventing viral transmission. Semprini et al[76] reported equal transmission rates for vaginal versus cesarean delivery.

Breast milk

There are documented cases of HIV transmission from mother to infant via breast milk and the AIDS virus has been isolated from cell-free human milk.[77]

Transmission rate

Owing to transfer of antibody from mother to fetus during gestation, infants of mother infected with AIDS virus will be seropositive at birth. This antibody may last 15 months or longer, but only infants who remain seropositive or show evidence of illness are considered infected. Therefore prediction of transmission rates in early infancy and in asymptomatic children is difficult, and the rate varies between studies in the range 25–50%.[64,66,78]

The mechanism of transmission is also unknown, but a few cases of monozygotic twin pregnancies in which only one of the twins was infected in utero have been reported.[79] Thomas et al[80] observed that large numbers of twins were born to women with AIDS in New York City; however, whether maternal HIV infection increases the rate of twinning is not known.

Clinical manifestations

The incubation period for perinatally acquired (congenital) infection is usually much shorter than transmission of the disease via blood transfusion or breast milk.[77,78] Lymphadenopathy and hepatosplenomegaly have been reported in neonates born to seropositive mothers.[66,80,81] Although prematurity and low birthweight are not associated in AIDS patients reported in the USA and Europe, infants born to seropositive mothers in Zaire were more premature, growth retarded and had higher mortality rate than controls.[66] In general, these infants remain symptom free for the first few months of life, but approximately 50% are diagnosed as having AIDS by 1 year of age[82] and they suffer from frequent bacterial infections, interstitial pneumonitis, chronic diarrhea and failure to thrive.[64,82,83]

AIDS embryopathy

There are conflicting reports regarding the validity of AIDS dysmorphism in infants born to mothers with HIV infection. Marion et al[84] reported identifying specific characteristics in a group of HIV-exposed infants in the Bronx, New York. Most of these infants appeared to be microcephalic, with prominent foreheads, hypertelorism and a prominent patulous lip.

Iosubi et al[85] also observed similar dimorphic features, but Qazi et al[86] could not confirm the presence of these characteristics in 30 children perinatally exposed to HIV. Other investigators also failed to confirm this syndrome.[78,79]

Diagnosis

1. presence of maternal risk factors and HIV antigen/antibodies;
2. P24 antigen detection from cord blood[78] and body fluid;[88]
3. proviral sequence HIV, DNA detection in leukocytes;[89]
4. serologic screening: ELISA, ELISPOT, and also elevation of anti-HIV IgM or IgA antibodies in serum;
5. abnormality in cellular and humoral immune system.

Prognosis

Perinatally acquired HIV infection has a very poor prognosis and a short survival time.

The prognosis is much worse in a child with the onset of disease under the age 1 year and after *Pneumocystis carinii* infection.[90]

VIRAL HEPATITIS

Advances in technology and the discovery of different serologic markers have resulted in better understanding of this disease and its transmission, diagnosis and prevention. Four types of hepatotrophic agents are known to cause acute or chronic hepatitis in humans.

Hepatitis A virus

This is a 27-nm RNA virus that is mainly transmitted by the fecal–oral route, therefore maternal-fetal (vertical) transmission of this virus is quite unusual.[91]

Hepatitis D virus (Delta)

This is a 35–37 nm virus which cannot survive alone and is dependent on hepatitis B virus (HBV) for replication and transmission. Its association with HBV increases the severity of the disease.[89]

Hepatitis C virus (non-A, non-B)

These viruses are transmitted via blood transfusion only.

Hepatitis B virus (HBV)

This 42-nm doubled-shelled, DNA virus is carried by approximately 300 million people throughout the world. Intact virus particles consists of several associated antigens, such as:

1. Hepatitis B surface antigen (HBsAg), the primary marker for HBV, is usually detectable 30–120 days after viral exposure and disappears when patient is in the icteric phase. If detectable for more than 6 months, the patient is considered to be in a carrier state.[91,92]

2. Hepatitis B core antigen (HBcAg) is not detectable in the serum.

3. Hepatitis e Antigen (HBeAg) when present, indicates that infection is highly infective, transmissible and the patient is in the acute stage of disease.

4. DNA polymerase is a marker for viral replication and indicates the acute stage of infection.

Epidemiology and transmission (HBV)

The HBSAg carrier rate in the USA is 0.1–0.4%. In Taiwan 30–40% of pregnant women are carriers of HBV and 3–5% of all infants are reportedly infected by HBV.[91]

Hepatitis B virus is generally transmitted via sexual contact, exchange of body fluids, transfusion of blood and blood products and also by the perinatal (vertical) route.

Perinatal (maternal–fetal or vertical) route

This route is the most common method of transmission in children. In utero transmission of HBV is very rare, possibly because of the large molecular size of the virus, making the transplacental passage difficult, but this mode of transmission has occurred and has been reported in a few cases when the fetus is exposed to the virulent virus as a result of placental leakage.[91–93] HBV transmission most likely occurs during labor and at the time of delivery, either by passage of virus via maternal–fetal transfusion or by exposure to infected blood and secretion during passage through the birth canal. Studies by Lee et al[94] demonstrated that in 95% of infants born to mothers who were positive for both HBsAg and HBeAg the gastric juice contained HBsAg. This antigen was also detectable in 33% of amniotic fluid samples, 50% of cord blood samples and 71% of breast milk samples. There is a 60% chance of transmission of virus to the infant if the mother acquired the infection in late third trimester or at time of delivery.[92] Infants who are born to mothers who are positive for both HBsAg and HBeAg have a 90% chance of becoming infected, and 80–90% of these children eventually become hepatitis carriers. If the mother is HBsAg positive, HBe antibody-positive transmission to infant is only 12% with less chance of becoming a carrier.[92,95]

Clinical presentation

Intrauterine infection is rare, and it is thought that those infants whose cord blood is positive for surface antigen may have acquired the disease during early gestation, and as a result are more likely to be premature and of low birthweight.[96]

In general, most infants do not manifest any clinical abnormalities at birth and remain asymptomatic for at least 1–3 months. They may then show mild changes in liver function tests. Others may show signs and symptoms of mild to acute hepatitis and chronic active hepatitis.

Prevention

Cesarean vs. vaginal delivery

To prevent fetal contact with infected maternal secretions at the time of delivery, cesarean delivery was suggested as a better mode of delivery to reduce exposure, but this has not been found to be effective in reducing the transmission rate.[92,94]

Perinatal screening

In the USA, an estimated 16 500 births occur to HBsAg-positive mothers annually, with 4300 also positive for 'e' antigens. Approximately 3500 of these infants will become chronic carriers; therefore, identification of antigen-positive mothers would allow treatment of these offspring with immune globulin and hepatitis vaccine as recommended by the Immunization Advisory Committee.[97,98]

Hepatitis B immune globulin (HBIg) must be given soon after birth, since delay in administration to hepatitis B-exposed infants will decrease its effectiveness in preventing infection and reducing carrier rates. Addition of hepatitis vaccine is shown to be very effective, and the combination of hepatitis immune globulin and three vaccines (birth, 1 month and 6 months of age) should prevent 85–90% of chronic hepatitis B infection.[95] Recombinant vaccine is more effective than plasma-derived vaccine, and up to 95% of infants exposed to hepatitis B virus can be protected by using this vaccine.[100]

REFERENCES

1. AAP Committee on Substance Abuse 1990 Drug exposed infants. Pediatrics 86: 639–642
2. Perlstein M A 1947 Congenital morphinism, a rare cause of convulsion in the newborn. J Am Med Assoc 135: 633–634
3. Dole V P, Nyswander M 1965 A medical treatment for diacetyl morphine (heroin) addiction, a clinical trial with methadone hydrochloride. J Am Med Assoc 193 (8): 80–84
4. Jaffe H J, Martin R W 1990 Opioid analgesics and antagonists. In: Gilman A G, Goodman L S, Gilman A (eds) Pharmacological basis of therapeutics, 8th edn. Macmillan, New York, pp 485–521
5. Clark W G, Barter D C, Johnson A R 1988 Narcotic (opioid) analgesic drugs. In: Goth S (ed) Medical pharmacology, 12th edn. C V Mosby, St Louis, Missouri, pp 328–331
6. Ostrea M E, Chavez J C 1979 Perinatal problems (excluding neonatal withdrawal) in maternal drug addiction. A study of 830 cases. J Pediatr 94: 292–295
7. Fulroth R, Phillips B, Durand J D 1989 Perinatal outcome of infants exposed to cocaine/heroin in utero. Am J Dis Child 143: 905–910
8. Taeusch H W, Carson H S, Wang S N, Avery E M 1973 Heroin induction of lung maturation and growth retardation in fetal rabbits. J Pediatr 82: 869–875
9. Chasnoff I J, Burns W J, Hatcher R 1982 Polydrug and methadone addicted newborns. A continuum of impairment. Pediatrics 70: 210–215

10. Glass L, Rajegowda B K, Evans H E 1971 Absence of RDS in premature infants of heroin addicted mothers. Lancet 2: 685–686
11. Kaltenback A K, Finnegan P L 1989 Perinatal narcotic exposure: perinatal and developmental effect. Neuro-toxicology 10: 597–604
12. Hammer P R, Ricaldo A A, Seatsig V J 1989 Effects of opiates on brain development. Neuro-toxicology 10: 475–484
13. Chasnoff I J, Burns K A, Burns W J 1986 Perinatal drug exposure effects on neonatal and infant growth and development. Neuro-toxicology Teratology 8: 357–362
14. Wilson S S, Desmond M M, Wait B R 1981 Follow up of methadone treated and untreated narcotic dependent women and their infants. Health, developmental and social implications. J Pediatr 98: 316–322
15. Ritchie M J, Green N M 1990 Local anesthetics. In Gilman A G, Goodman L S, Gilman A (eds) Pharmacological basis of therapeutics, 8th edn. Macmillan, New York, pp 311–312
16. Moferson C H, Caraccio R T 1987 Cocaine. Pediatric Annals 16: 864–874
17. Farrer C H, Kearns L G 1989 Cocaine: clinical pharmacology and toxicology. J Pediatr 115: 665–675
18. Stewart D J, Inaba T, Lucassen M, Kalow W 1979 Cocaine, metabolism, cocaine and norcocaine hydrolysis by liver and serum esterase. Clin Pharmacol Ther 25: 464–481
19. Chasnoff I J, Burns A K, Burns J W 1987 Cocaine use in pregnancy, perinatal, morbidity and mortality. Neuro-toxicology Teratology 9: 291–293
20. Burkett G, Yasin S, Palow D 1990 Perinatal implications of cocaine exposure. J Reprod Med 35: 35–42
21. MacGregor N S, Keith G L, Chasnoff J I, Rosner A M, Chisum M G, Shaw P, Manogue P J 1987 Cocaine use during pregnancy, adverse perinatal outcome. Am J Obstet Gynecol 157: 686–691
22. Chasnoff I J, Burns W J, Schull S H, Burns A K 1985 Cocaine use in pregnancy. New Engl J Med 3132: 666–669
23. Woods J R 1987 Effects of cocaine on uterine blood flow and fetal oxygenation. J Am Med Assoc 257: 957–961
24. Little B B, Snell M C, Klein R V, Gilstrap J I I 1989 Cocaine abuse during pregnancy; maternal fetal implications. Obstet Gynecol 73: 157–160
25. Chasnoff I J, Burns E M, Savitch R, Stack M C 1986 Perinatal cerebral infarction and maternal cocaine use. J Pediatr 108: 456–459
26. Ostrea E M, Kresback P, Knopp D K, Simkowski K 1987 Phosphokinase in addicted neonates. Neuro-toxicology Teratology 9: 305–309
27. Lipshultz E S, Frassica J J, Orav J E 1991 Cardiovascular abnormalities in infants perinatally exposed to cocaine. J Pediatr 118: 44–51
28. Chasnoff I J 1987 Perinatal effects of cocaine. Contemporary Obstet Gynecol 30: 163–174
29. Dixon D S, Bejar R 1990 Brain lesion in cocaine and amphetamine exposed neonates. Pediatr Res 27 (suppl): 405A
30. Chasnoff I J, Griffith D R, MacGregor S et al 1989 Temporal patterns of cocaine use during pregnancy, perinatal outcome. J Am Med Assoc 261: 1741–1744
31. Salamy A, Eldredge L, Anderson J, Bull D 1990 Brain stem transmission time in infants exposed to cocaine in utero. J Pediatr 113: 627–629
32. Doberczak T M, Shanzer S, Senie R T, Kandell R S 1988 Neonatal neurologic and electroencephalographic effects of intrauterine cocaine exposure. J Pediatr 113: 354–358
33. Klein J F, Shahrivar F 1990 Effects of intrauterine cocaine exposure on the prenatal morbidity of preterm infants. Pediatr Res 27: 211A
34. Telsey A M, Merrit J A, Dixon S D 1988 Cocaine exposure in neonate, necrotizing enterocolitis and complications. Clin Pediatr 27: 547–550
35. Fantel A G, Macphail B A 1982 Teratogenicity of cocaine. Teratology 26 (17): 17–18
36. Bingol N, Fuchs M, Diaz V, Stone R, Gromisch S D 1987 Teratogenicity of cocaine in humans. J Pediatr 110: 93–96
37. Mahalic M P, Gautieri R F, Mann Jr D E 1980 Teratogenic potential of cocaine hydrochloride in CF-I mice. J Pharm Sci 69: 703–706
38. Chasnoff I J, Chisum G M, Kaplan W E 1988 Maternal cocaine use and genito-urinary tract malformation. Teratology 37: 201–204
39. Chavez G F, Malinae J, Cordero J R 1989 Maternal cocaine use during early pregnancy a risk factor for congenital urogenital anomalies. J Am Med Assoc 262: 795–798
40. Madden J D, Payne F T, Miller S 1986 Maternal cocaine abuse and effect on the newborn. Pediatrics 77: 209–211
41. Chasnoff I J, Hunt C E, Kletter R 1989 Prenatal cocaine exposure is associated with respiratory pattern abnormalities. Am J Dis Child 143: 483–587
42. Davidson-Ward L S, Schultz S, Warchsman L et al 1991 Elevated plasma norepinephrine levels in infants of substance abuse. Am J Dis Child 145: 44–48
43. Davidson-Ward L S, Bautista D, Rpet B A et al 1990 Sudden infant death syndrome in infants of substance abusing mother. J Pediatr 117: 876–881
44. Buckner H, Zuckerman B, McClane M, Frank D, Fried L E, Kayne H 1988 Risk of SIDS among infants with in utero exposure to cocaine. J Pediatr 113: 831–834
45. Durand D J, Espinozor A M, Nikerson B H 1990 Association between prenatal cocaine exposure and SIDS. J Pediatr 117: 909–911
46. Schwartz H R 1984 Marijuana, a crude drug with spectrum of under appreciated toxicity. Pediatrics 73: 445–458
47. Clark W G, Barter D C, Johnson A R 1988 Contemporary drug abuse. In: Goth S (ed) Medical pharmacology, 12th edn. C V Mosby, St Louis, Missouri, p 348–349
48. National Institute on Drug Abuse 1988 Medical review officer's manual. US Department of Health and Human Services, Washington D C
49. Kulberg A 1986 Substance abuse clinical identification and management. Pediatr Clin N Am 33: 869–875
50. Hatch E Z, Braken B M 1986 Effects of marijuana use in pregnancy on fetal growth. Am J Epidemiol 124: 986–993
51. Zukerman B, Frank A D, Hingson R et al 1989 Effect of maternal marijuana and cocaine use on fetal growth. New Engl J Med 320: 762–768
52. Fried P 1989 Cigarettes and marijuana: are there measurable long term, neuro-behavioral, teratogenic effects? Neuro-toxicology 10: 557–584
53. Hoffman B B, Lefkowitz J R 1990 Catecholamine and sympathomimetic drugs. In Gilman A G, Goodman L S, Gilman A (eds). Pharmacological basis for therapeutics, 8th edn. Macmillan, New York, pp 210–212
54. Clark W G, Barter D C, Johnson A R 1988 Drug acting on the adrenergic neuron. In: Goth (ed) Medical pharmacology, 12th edn. C V Mosby, St Louis, Missouri, p 172–175
55. Oro A S, Dixon S D 1987 Perinatal cocaine and methamphetamine exposure maternal and neonatal correlates. J Pediatr 111: 571–578
56. Eriksson M, Larsson G, Winblodh B, Zettersstrom R 1978 The influence of amphetamine addiction on pregnant women and newborn infants. Acta Pediatr Scand 67: 95–99
57. Billings L, Eriksson M, Larsson G 1980 Acta Pediatr Scand 69: 675–680
58. Dixon S, Begar R 1989 Echoencephalographic findings in neonates associated with maternal cocaine and amphetamine use: incidence and clinical correlation. J Pediatr 115: 770–778
59. Dixon S, Bejar R 1990 Brain lesions in cocaine and amphetamine exposed neonates. Pediatr Res (suppl) 27: 405A
60. Oleske M J, Connor M E, Blond M G 1988 A perspective on pediatric AIDS. Pediatr Ann 17: 319–321
61. Rogers F M 1988 Pediatric HIV infection. Epidemiology, E-Thiropathogenesis and Transmission. Pediatr Ann 17: 324–331
62. Center for Disease Control 1988 Distribution of AIDS cases by racial, ethnic group and exposure category. MMWR 37 (55–3): 1
63. Chavkin W, Driver C R, Forman P 1989 The crisis in New York City perinatal services. NY State J Med 89: 658–663
64. Falloon J, Eddy J, Wiener L, Pizzo A P 1989 Human immune deficiency virus infection in children. J Pediatr 114: 1–30
65. Ryder R W, Wato N S A, Hassig S E et al 1989 Perinatal

transmission of the HIV type I to infants of seropositive women in Zaire. New Engl J Med 320: 1637–1642

66. Lapointe N, Michand J, Pekovic D, Chaussen S P, Dupuy J M 1985 Transplacental transmission of HTLV-III virus. Lancet 2: 1325
67. Center for Disease Control 1987 AIDS weekly surveillance report AIDS in pregnancy, August 10
68. Barre-Sinousi F, Chermann J C, Rey F et al 1983 Isolation of a T-lymphocytic retrovirus from a patient at risk for acquired immune deficiency syndrome. Science 220: 868
69. Gallo R C, Salahuddin S Z, Popovic M et al 1984 Frequent detection and isolation of lymphocytopathic retroviruses from San Francisco patients with AIDS. Science 225: 840
70. Cowan M J, Helman J D, Chadwin D 1984 Maternal transmission of acquired immune deficiency syndrome. Pediatr 73: 382–386
71. Guman M C 1987 Epidemiology of AIDS in women in US (1981–1986). J Am Med Assoc 25: 2039–2042
72. Sprecher S, Soumenkoff G, Puissant F, Deguldre M 1986 Vertical transmission of HIV in 15 week fetus. Lancet 2: 288
73. Jovaisar E, Koch A M, Schafer A, Stauber M, Lowenthal D 1985 LAV/HTLV-III in 20 week fetus. Lancet 2: 1129
74. Vogt M W, Witt D J, Craven E D et al 1987 Isolation patterns of HIV from cervical secretion during menstrual cycle of women at risk for AIDS. Ann Intern Med 106: 380–382
75. Wofsy C B, Cohen J J, Hauer L B, Padian S N, Michaelis B A, Evans L A, Levey A J 1986 Isolation of AIDS associated retrovirus from genital secretion of women with antibodies to the virus. Lancet 1: 527–529
76. Semprini A E, Vucetich A, Pardi G, Cossu M M 1987 HIV infection and AIDS in newborn babies of mothers positive for HIV antibody. Br Med J 294: 610
77. Thiry L, Sprecher-Goldberger S, Jonckbeer J, Levy J, Van de Perre P, Henrivaux P, Cogniaux-LeClerc J 1985 Isolation of AIDS virus, from cell free breast milk. Lancet 2: 891–892
78. Blanche S, Rouzioux C, Morcato M L G 1989 Prospective study of infants born to women seropositive for human immune deficiency virus Type I. New Engl J Med 1320: 1643–1648
79. Menez-Bautista R, Fikrig S W, Pahava S 1986 Monozygotic twin discordant for the acquired immunodeficiency syndrome. Am J Dis Child 140: 678–679
80. Thomas A P, Ralston J S, Bernard M, Williams R, O'Donnell R 1990 NY City Department of Health. Pediatrics 86: 774–777
81. Scott G M, Buck B E, Letterman J G 1984 AIDS in infants. New Engl J Med 310: 78–81
82. Adam H 1989 Epidemiology of pediatric HIV infection. Pediatric AIDS 20th Ross report, Ross Laboratories, Columbus, Ohio, pp 4–14
83. Pahwa S 1988 Human Immunodeficiency virus infection in childen, nature of immunodeficiency, clinical spectrum and management. Pediatr Infect Dis, J, 7: S61–S71
84. Marion W R, Wiznia A A, Hutcheon G R, Rubenstein A 1986 HTLV III embryopathy. A new syndrome associated with HTLV III infection. Am J Dis Child 140: 638–640
85. Iosubi S, Banji M, Stone K R, Gromisch S D, Wasserman E 1987 More on human immunodeficiency virus embryopathy. Pediatrics 80: 512–516
86. Qazi H Q, Sheikh M T, Fikrig S, Menikoff H 1988 Craniofacial dysmorphism in perinatal HIV infection. J Pediatr 112: 7–11
87. Embee J E, Brodelick M, Dalla P et al 1986 Lack of correlation of maternal HIV infection with neonatal malformation. Pediatr Infect Dis J 8: 700–704
88. Borkowzky W, Krasinski K, Paul D et al 1989 Human immunodeficiency virus Type I antigenemia in children. J Pediatr 114: 940–945
89. Rogers B F, Ou Y E, Rayfield M et al 1989 Use of polymerase chain reaction for early detection of proviral sequence of human immunodeficiency virus in infants born to seropositive mother. New Engl J Med 320: 1649–1654
90. Scott E B, Mutto C, Makureh R W et al 1989 Survival in children with perinatally acquired human immune deficiency virus, Type I infection. New Engl J Med 321: 1791–1796
91. Balistreri F W 1988 Viral hepatitis. Pediatr Clin N Am 35: 637–669
92. Synderman O R 1985 Hepatitis in pregnancy. New Engl J Med 313: 1398–1401
93. Lee A K Y, Wong W C W 1980 Transmission of hepatitis B antigen from symptom free carrier mothers to the fetus and infant. Br J Obstet Gynaecol 87: 958–965
94. Lee A K Y, Ip M M H, Wong W C W 1978 Mechanism of maternal fetal transmission of hepatitis B virus. J Infect Dis 138: 668–671
95. Krugman S 1988 Hepatitis virus. Ann NY Acad Sci 5: 129–134
96. Gerety J R, Schweitzer L I 1977 Viral hepatitis Type B during pregnancy. The neonatal period and pregnancy. J Pediatr 90: 368–373
97. Committee on prevention medicine 1989 Hepatitis B virus, prenatal screening of all pregnant women for HBsAg. NY State J Med 89: 351–354
98. Immunization practices advisory committee 1984 post exposure prophylaxis of hepatitis B virus. MMWR 33: 285–290
99. Nair P V, Weissman Y J, Tong M J, Thursby W M, Paul H R, Henneman E C 1984 Efficacy of hepatitis B immunoglobulin in prevention of prenatal transmission of HBV. Gastroenterology 87: 293–298
100. Steven C E, Taylor P E, Tong M J et al 1987 Yeast recombinant hepatitis B vaccine, efficacy with hepatitis B immunoglobulin in prevention of perinatal hepatitis B virus transmission. J Am Med Assoc 257: 2612–2616

64. Malignant hyperthermia

J. V. Vartikar

Malignant hyperthermia (MH) is a rare but potentially devastating clinical syndrome triggered by exposure to certain anesthetic agents. MH can be considered an inherited subclinical myopathy that becomes manifest in the presence of potential inhalation anesthetics and/or depolarizing neuromuscular blocking agents.[1] Exposure to these anesthetic agents sets in motion a sequence of events that results in a massive increase in metabolism and production of heat, carbon dioxide and lactic acid.[2]

MH presents as a variable and diverse constellation of signs and symptoms, each of which is itself nonspecific, but the combination of which is highly suggestive of the syndrome (Table 64.1).[3] The exact presentation in each case depends on the triggering agents employed, the presence of other drugs and individual variation in severity of the disease. The first sign of an MH crisis may be muscle rigidity. Rigidity may first become manifest in the jaw muscles, which may make endotracheal intubation difficult or impossible. Tachycardia, often with hypertension, is a consistent early feature of MH and is often the presenting symptom. Another consistent early sign is a marked increase in carbon dioxide production, which leads to tachypnea if the patient is not mechanically ventilated. The first sign is a rise in the mixed venous carbon dioxide tension, which is then followed by changes in the arterial blood gas. In addition, marked diaphoresis, mottled cyanosis and coagulopathy are usually evident. The combination of cyanosis and tachycardia in a well-oxygenated, previously healthy patient is highly suggestive of MH.

Table 64.1 Presenting physical and biochemical signs of an MH crisis

Rigidity*	↑ ET CO_2*
Tachycardia*	↑ Central venous CO_2*
Tachypnea*	↓ Arterial O_2
Cyanosis*	↑ Metabolic and respiratory acidosis*
Skin mottling	↑ Creatinine phosphokinase
Diaphoresis	Hyperkalemia
Arrhythmias	Myoglobinuria
Hypertension/unstable blood pressure	
Hyperthermia	

* Most frequent signs of an MH crisis.

Early diagnosis is imperative if one is to avoid the morbidity and mortality associated with delay in treatment. MH should be suspected in an anesthetized patient who develops any of the following symptoms: tachypnea, muscle rigidity, diaphoresis, mottling, cyanosis or hyperthermia. During anesthesia, the most rapid method of detecting MH is with capnography. If the $ETCO_2$ is markedly increased during constant ventilation and mechanical causes can be ruled out, the diagnosis of MH can be assumed. Confirmation of the diagnosis can be made with central venous and arterial blood gas monitoring. Under normal conditions, the difference between $P\text{vCO}_2$ and $P\text{aCO}_2$ is 5 mmHg. During an MH crisis, a difference of 15 mmHg or greater is observed. In addition, if the arterial blood gas data demonstrate either a $P\text{aCO}_2$ greater than 60 mmHg with a base deficit of at least 5 eq./c or a pH less than 7.15, the diagnosis of MH is confirmed.

The determination of patient risk for MH is essential prior to anesthetic induction so that adequate precautions may be taken. The clearest indication of susceptibility is a prior MH reaction, although even an uneventful prior anesthetic induction does not rule out MH susceptibility. In addition, patients with various musculoskeletal abnormalities may be at increased risk for MH (Table 64.2).[4] To evaluate susceptibility, muscle biopsy contracture studies must be performed. This test is considered the gold standard in diagnosis and is more than 95% reliable. Other less invasive tests have been developed but have not yet achieved validity for predicting MH susceptibility.

Triggering agents for MH include the volatile inhalation anesthetics and the depolarizing muscle relaxants. Contrary to prior reports, present evidence indicates that amide local anesthetics are safe to use in MH-susceptible patients.[5,6] Several environmental stresses have been implicated in the precipitation or potentiation of an MH crisis, including exercise, heat prostration, anoxia, apprehension and excitement. Thus all susceptible patients

Table 64.2 Associated diseases and abnormalities

Associated diseases	Associated abnormalities
Central core disease	Ptosis
King–Denborough syndrome	Strabismus
Duchenne muscular dystrophy	Joint hypermobility
Arthrogryposis	Dislocated joints
Becker's muscular dystrophy	Kyphoscoliosis
Sudden infant death syndrome*	Clubfeet
Neuroleptic malignant syndrome*	Hernia
Osteogenesis imperfecta*	Intolerance to heat and exercise
Myotonia congenita*	Muscle cramps
	Muscle swelling
	Muscle weakness
	High fevers
	Febrile convulsions
	Blackouts
	Anxiety

* Controversial association.

should be kept as comfortable as possible before, during and after surgical procedures. Although awake MH crisis is common in swine, it is not common in humans.

The only known therapeutic agent effective in MH is dantrolene. It must be administered early in the MH crisis while muscle perfusion is still adequate. The temporal profile of plasma concentrations of prophylactic dantrolene following an intravenous dose in a parturient suggests that pregnancy does not alter the pharmacokinetics of the drug. Placental transfer of dantrolene does occur and is dependent on placental factors such as area of transfer and diffusion distance as well as the difference in the maternal and fetal drug concentrations.[7] In MH-susceptible patients who received prophylactic dantrolene during labor and delivery, the uterine vein/maternal vein ratio was 0.29–0.51.[8] The infants of these mothers were vigorous and showed no adverse effects.

MANAGEMENT OF THE OBSTETRIC MH-SUSCEPTIBLE PATIENT

The MH-susceptible patient in the obstetric setting poses a unique challenge for the anesthesiologist. There have been three reported cases of MH during delivery; in each instance a cesarean delivery was performed under general anesthesia using a known triggering agent.[9–12] There have been no reported cases of MH in an obstetric patient with the use of nontriggering agents for general or regional anesthesia, nor have there been any published reports of awake triggering during delivery. The fact that so few cases of MH during delivery have been published has led some investigators to speculate that pregnancy may exert some protective influence over the MH-susceptible patient. However, there are no in vitro, animal or human studies to support this postulate. Thus, until proven otherwise, it would be prudent to consider a pregnant MH-susceptible patient to be at equal risk for the disease as any other surgical candidate.

The emotional and physical stresses of labor and delivery may act to potentiate or provoke an MH crisis, although such an event has not been documented. However, these considerations should influence the timing of anesthesia as well as the choice of monitors employed. In addition, pregnancy-induced disease such as chorioamnionitis or toxemia can add to the stresses of pregnancy and conceivably influence the onset of an MH crisis. Furthermore, the drugs used to induce, augment or depress labor may also complicate the diagnosis and treatment of MH. It must be remembered that the child born to an MH-susceptible mother may also possess the trait and may be at risk during and after the delivery. This applies to children of MH-susceptible fathers as well.

Prophylaxis

Several cases of dantrolene prophylaxis prior to uneventful labor and delivery have been reported. However, dantrolene pretreatment is no longer considered necessary. Dantrolene is not without side-effects, which may become manifest in the mother and the neonate. The neonate may experience muscle flaccidity and respiratory difficulties. In addition, uterine atony has been reported after dantrolene pretreatment.[13] Thus the routine use of dantrolene prophylaxis is not indicated, especially in the obstetric setting.[14]

Nontriggering anesthetic agents

All local anesthetics, with or without epinephrine, are now considered safe for use in MH-susceptible patients. For general anesthesia, a large armamentarium of agents is available. Nontriggering general anesthetic agents include barbiturates, nondepolarizing muscle relaxants, opioids, tranquilizers, nitrous oxide and ketamine (Table 64.3).

Preoperative preparation

All known or suspected MH-susceptible patients should have a preoperative anesthetic consultation during early pregnancy, inclusive of a complete history and physical examination. Particular emphasis should be placed on obtaining a detailed description of any previous anesthetic reactions or untoward perioperative events involving the patient or any family members. The patient should be educated about the disease and the anesthetic plan explained to her. One copy of the completed consultation form should be sent to the referring obstetrician, one copy placed in the patient's chart and one copy placed in a department register of high-risk obstetric patients. The patient should be instructed to alert the nurse upon arrival to the labor and delivery (L&D) floor, and all involved

Table 64.3 Nontriggering anesthetic agents

Barbiturates Thiopental (Pentothal) Methohexital (Brevital) Thiamylal (Surital)	Local anesthetics: amides Lidocaine (Xylocaine) Mepivacaine (Carbocaine) Bupivacaine (Marcaine) Etidocaine (Duranest) Prilocaine (Citanest)
Narcotics (opioids) Morphine Meperidine (Demerol) Hydromorphone (Dilaudid) Fentanyl (Sublimaze) Sufentanil (Sufenta) Alfentanil (Alfenta)	Local anesthetics: esters Procaine (Novocaine) Chloroprocaine (Nesacaine) Tetracaine (Pontocaine) Muscle relaxants Pancuronium (Pavulon) Atracurium (Tracrium) Vecuronium (Norcuron)
Anticholinesterases Neostigmine (Prostigmine) Pyridostigmine (Regonol) Edrophonium (Tensilon)	Tranquilizers Diazepam (Valium) Midazolam (Versed)
Other Ketamine (Ketalar) Droperidol (Inapsine) Nitrous oxide	Anticholinergics* Atropine Glycopyrrolate (Robinul)

* Controversial association

anesthesia personnel should be notified immediately so that the appropriate preparations can be made.

A cart containing the necessary drugs and equipment for treatment of MH-susceptible patients should be made available on the floor and should be checked to ensure that it is fully stocked. (Table 64.4).

A cesarean birth/delivery room should be designated for this patient and held for her until she delivers. The room should contain a dedicated MH 'clean' machine, one free of vapor contamination. If such a special unit is not available, the standard anesthesia machine should be prepared for the patient by cleaning it of all residues of vapor anesthetic agents. The breathing circuit, reservoir bag, soda lime and carbon dioxide absorber should be changed, as should the fresh gas hose from the machine. The anesthesia machine should be flushed with oxygen at 10 l/min for 10–15 min.[15] These precautions should be instituted as soon as the patient arrives on the L&D floor, as the need for emergency cesarean delivery can arise at any time.

Anesthesia for labor and delivery

All patients should have a large intravenous catheter placed on admission to the L&D floor. Regional anesthesia, unless contraindicated, should be performed on all obstetric MH-susceptible patients in order to decrease the stress of labor and delivery. Epidural anesthesia instituted early in labor via a continuous infusion is the most effective means of maintaining a constant level of sensory anesthesia through all stages of labor and delivery. Perineal anesthesia should be assured at the onset of the second stage of labor, when the patient is presumably most vulnerable to MH. Subarachnoid anesthesia given prior to delivery is an alternative to epidural anesthesia, but it is less preferable since it does not protect during the early stages of labor.

Table 64.4 Suggested minimum contents for an MH cart

Medications
Dantrolene – at least 50 20-mg ampules
Procainamide – 500 mg/ml and 100 mg/ml
Furosemide – at least 200 mg
Mannitol 25% – at least 100 ml
Dextrose 50% – 100 ml
Chlorpromazine – 250 mg
Sodium bicarbonate – at least 10 50-ml ampules
Solutions
Sterile water for injection – at least 2000 ml (for reconstituting dantrolene)
Normal saline for injection – at least 20 1000-ml bags (left cooled in refrigerator)
Normal saline for irrigation – at least five 3000-ml bags (left cooled in refrigerator)
Cooling
Availability of continuous supply of crushed ice
Cooling blanket and console
Stomach and rectal tubes
Irrigating Foley catheter with collecting bags
Monitoring
Electronic temperature probes – two
Extra electronic thermometer
Oral and rectal glass thermometers
Central venous access kits – two
Pulmonary artery catheter
Esophageal stethoscope
Blood gas kits
Blood collection tubes of all types, with appropriate labels
General
New anesthesia breathing circuit and carbon dioxide absorber cannisters
Syringes – all sizes, including 50 60-ml syringes specifically for dantrolene
Intravenous catheters – all sizes
Needles – all sizes
Alcohol sponges, gauze, tape, instruments, needle disposal bucket, log sheets, etc.

Anesthesia for cesarean delivery

Regional anesthesia is preferred to general anesthesia for cesarean delivery. In addition to the well-recognized benefits of regional anesthesia for cesarean delivery in normal patients, awake triggering of MH has never been reported in obstetric patients. Epidural anesthesia should be administered using a continuous catheter technique. The catheter allows the regional anesthetic to be continued should surgery be prolonged and also can be used for pain relief in the post-operative period. Single-dose or continuous subarachnoid anesthesia can also be utilized. For regional anesthesia, patient monitoring during cesarean delivery should include electrocardiogram (ECG), pulse oximeter, temperature, noninvasive blood pressure and urine output. For general anesthesia, capnography is necessary in addition to the monitors used in regional anesthesia. An arterial catheter may be placed, if desired, for continuous blood pressure and arterial blood gas monitoring.

If general anesthesia is necessary, it can be safely administered using the agents mentioned in Table 64.3. Although succinylcholine is the agent of choice for muscle relaxation during rapid-sequence induction, its use in MH-susceptible patients is contraindicated. The only alternatives are the nondepolarizing muscle relaxants. Unfortunately, in the recommended doses, these agents require 3–5 min for suitable endotracheal intubating conditions. This long onset time can be decreased by increasing the induction dose. Vecuronium when given in high doses provides rapid endotracheal intubating conditions with minimal effects on the autonomic nervous system. In doses of 0.25–0.4 mg/kg vecuronium has been used without significant hemodynamic changes. At these doses, vecuronium usually provides excellent intubating conditions within 1 min without greatly increasing the duration of action.[16]

Vecuronium, because of its highly ionized state, should not cross the placenta in significant amounts if the usual doses are given. However, with the high doses needed for faster onset of muscle relaxation, vecuronium may cross the placental barrier and may result in neonatal muscle weakness or paralysis.

In the recovery room, the patient should be monitored closely for any signs of an MH crisis. She should have normal laboratory tests and stable vital signs for at least 4 h prior to discharge from the recovery room. Thereafter, vital signs, including temperature, should be monitored hourly for 24 h. Explicit instructions should be given to notify the anesthesiologist for increases in temperature, heart rate or respiratory rate.

TREATMENT OF AN MH CRISIS (Table 64.5)

Effectiveness of therapy is contingent on early recognition of the MH crisis.[17] The triggering anesthetic agent should be discontinued immediately and the patient ventilated with 100% oxygen. The anesthesia machine can be replaced by one free of contamination from inhalation agents. The surgeon should be informed of the patient's condition and requested to expedite and terminate the procedure. Help from additional personnel should be requested.

The MH cart should be brought immediately to the room. Several people should be designated to prepare the dantrolene. An initial dose of 2.5 mg/kg should be administered as soon as possible at a rate of 1 mg/kg/min. The dose may be repeated every 5 min until the symptoms are reversed (the temperature, muscle tone and heart rate should decline) or until a total dose of 10 mg/kg is achieved. After the crisis, intravenous dantrolene should be continued at a dose of 1 mg/kg every 6 h for 24–48 h.

Table 64.5 Suggested treatment protocol for an MH crisis

1. Discontinue all triggering anesthetic agents.
2. Hyperventilate with 100% oxygen. The circle system and CO_2 absorbent need not be changed.
3. Inform the surgeon: request to expedite and terminate the procedure.
4. Call for help.
5. Have the MH cart brought to the operating room.
6. Designate people to prepare the dantrolene.
7. Administer an initial dose of 2.5 mg/kg of dantrolene as soon as possible. Response to dantrolene should occur within minutes. If not, administer dantrolene as necessary, titrating to heart rate, muscle rigidity and temperature. Average effective dose of dantrolene is 2.5mg/kg but occasionally 10 mg/kg or more may be necessary.
8. Place arterial and central venous catheters and obtain blood gases, electrolyte levels, and clotting studies STAT.
9. Institute electronic temperature monitoring.
10. Treat arrhythmias with lidocaine or procainamide.
11. Administer sodium bicarbonate guided by arterial blood gas results.
12. Control hyperthermia with surface cooling, infusion of cooled normal saline and body cavity lavage as necessary to maintain core temperature of 38°C.
13. Maintain urine output at a minimum of 2 ml/kg/h with intravenous fluids, furosemide and mannitol.
14. After the MH crisis is controlled, transfer the patient to the ICU and observe for recrudescence of malignant hyperthermia.
15. Follow creatinine phosphokinase, calcium, electrolytes and clotting studies until normalized. Observe for disseminated intravascular coagulation.
16. Obtain ECG and follow post-operatively.

Further dantrolene therapy should be based on clinical and laboratory findings.

Once these life-saving measures have been instituted, appropriate monitoring of the patient should be the next priority. The ECG will already be in use and is a necessary monitor for arrhythmias. Although most arrhythmias will respond to dantrolene therapy, refractory cases can be treated with lidocaine or procainamide 10 mg/kg.

The temperature should be monitored at various sites. A Foley catheter should be inserted to monitor urine output. An arterial catheter for pressure measurement and blood gas analysis as well as a central venous catheter should be placed. Arterial and venous blood gases and serum electrolyte levels should be drawn and sent as STAT. The metabolic acidosis should be corrected with sodium bicarbonate, guided by the results of the arterial blood gas. If arterial blood gas data are not available, an initial dose of 2 meq./kg should be administered. In a fulminant MH crisis, it may be difficult to correct the blood pH above 7.20.

Fever should be controlled using any of a variety of techniques, including surface cooling with ice and hypothermic blanket, intravenous cooling with iced saline (not lactated Ringer's solution), body cavity lavage with iced saline or extracorporeal circulation with heat exchanger. One liter of intravenous iced saline every 10 min for 30 min is effective in lowering the core temperature. In order to avoid hypothermia, cooling should not progress below 38°C but should be restarted if the temperature rises above this level.

Urine output should be closely monitored and maintained at a minimum of 2 ml/kg/h. To achieve this high urine flow, a generous volume of saline, mannitol 12.5 mg and furosemide 50 mg should be given intravenously. The diuretics may be repeated for a total of four doses. In addition, central venous pressure and arterial blood pressure should be maintained at adequate levels to optimize urine output. Experience has shown that with early recognition and prompt institution of treatment, recovery from an MH crisis is likely.

THE MALIGNANT HYPERTHERMIA ASSOCIATION OF THE USA

The Malignant Hyperthermia Association of the USA was organized in 1981. Its primary goals are to educate patients and their families as well as members of the medical community about MH, its diagnosis and treatment. The organization also raises funds to support research into the condition and has established a databank of MH cases. A 24-h emergency number has been established to assist physicians in the management of an MH crisis. The MH Hotline telephone number is (209) 634-4917, request Index Zero, Malignant Hyperthermia Consultant List.

ACKNOWLEDGMENT

I wish to thank Richard B. Schwartz, MD, PhD, for his advice in the preparation of this manuscript.

REFERENCES

1. Deufel T, Golla A, Iles D et al 1992 Evidence for genetic heterogeneity of malignant hyperthermia susceptibility. AM J Hum Genet 50: 1151–1161
2. Gronert GA 1980 Malignant hyperthermia. Anesthesiology 53: 395
3. Rosenberg H 1988 Clinical presentation of malignant hyperthermia. Br J Anaesth 60: 268
4. Brownell A K W 1988 Malignant hyperthermia: relationship to other diseases. Br J Anaesth 60: 303
5. Harrison G G, Morrell D F 1980 Response of MHS swine to I.V. infusion of lignocaine and bupivacaine. Br J Anaesth 52: 385
6. Paasuke R T, Brownell A K W 1986 Amide local anaesthetics and malignant hyperthermia. Can Anaesth Soc J 33: 126
7. Morrison D H 1983 Placental transfer of dantrolene (letter). Anesthesiology 59: 265
8. Glassenberg R, Cohen H 1984 Intravenous dantrolene in a pregnant malignant hyperthermia susceptible patient. Anesthesiology 61A: 404
9. Crawford J S 1972 Hyperpyrexia during pregnancy. Lancet 1: 1244
10. Cupryn J P, Kennedy A, Byrick R J 1984 Malignant hyperthermia in pregnancy. Am J Obstet Gynecol 150: 327
11. Gibbs J M 1984 Unexplained hyperpyrexia during labour. Anaesth Intensive Care 12, 4: 375
12. Lips F J, Newland M, Dutton G 1982 Malignant hyperthermia triggered by cyclopropane during cesarean section. Anesthesiology 56: 144
13. Weingarten A E, Korsh J I, Neuman G C et al 1987 Postpartum uterine atony after intravenous dantrolene. Anesth Analg 66: 269
14. Cunliff M, Lerman J, Britt B A 1987 Is prophylactic dantrolene indicated for MHS patients undergoing elective surgery? Anesth Analg 66: S35
15. Beebe J J, Sessler D 1988 Preparation of anesthesia machines for patients susceptible to malignant hyperthermia. Anesthesiology 69: 395
16. Lennon R L, Olson R A, Gronert G A 1986 Atracurium or vecuronium for rapid sequence endotracheal intubation. Anesthesiology 64: 510
17. Britt B (ed) 1987 Malignant hyperthermia. Martinus Nijhoff Publishing, Boston

65. Septic shock in obstetrics

C. K. Lineberger

Septic shock is a clinical syndrome of hypotension and hypoperfusion induced by an infective agent and mediated by host defense systems. It is the most frequent cause of death in the intensive care unit in the USA and its incidence is increasing, in part because of increased use of immunosuppressive drugs, broad-spectrum antibiotics and invasive monitoring devices.

Obstetric patients seem to have much lower mortality from septic shock than the general population (0–3% versus 40–90%).[1] However, because the overall mortality in parturients is very low, septic shock contributes a significant percentage of the deaths occurring in obstetric patients.

The sources of septic infection in obstetrics are premature rupture of membranes with subsequent chorioamnionitis, endometritis, pyelonephritis, wound infections and septic abortions.[2] Common pathogens in the septic

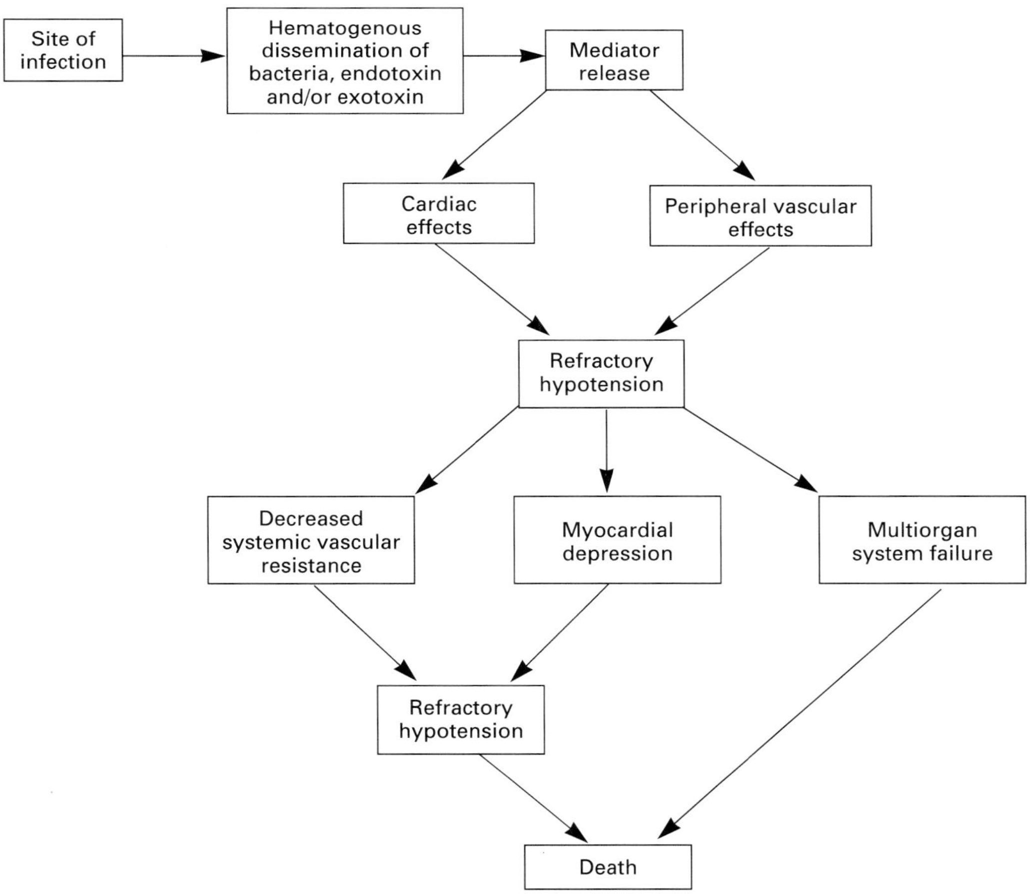

Fig. 65.1 The pathophysiology of septic shock. (Adapted from ref. 4 with permission.)

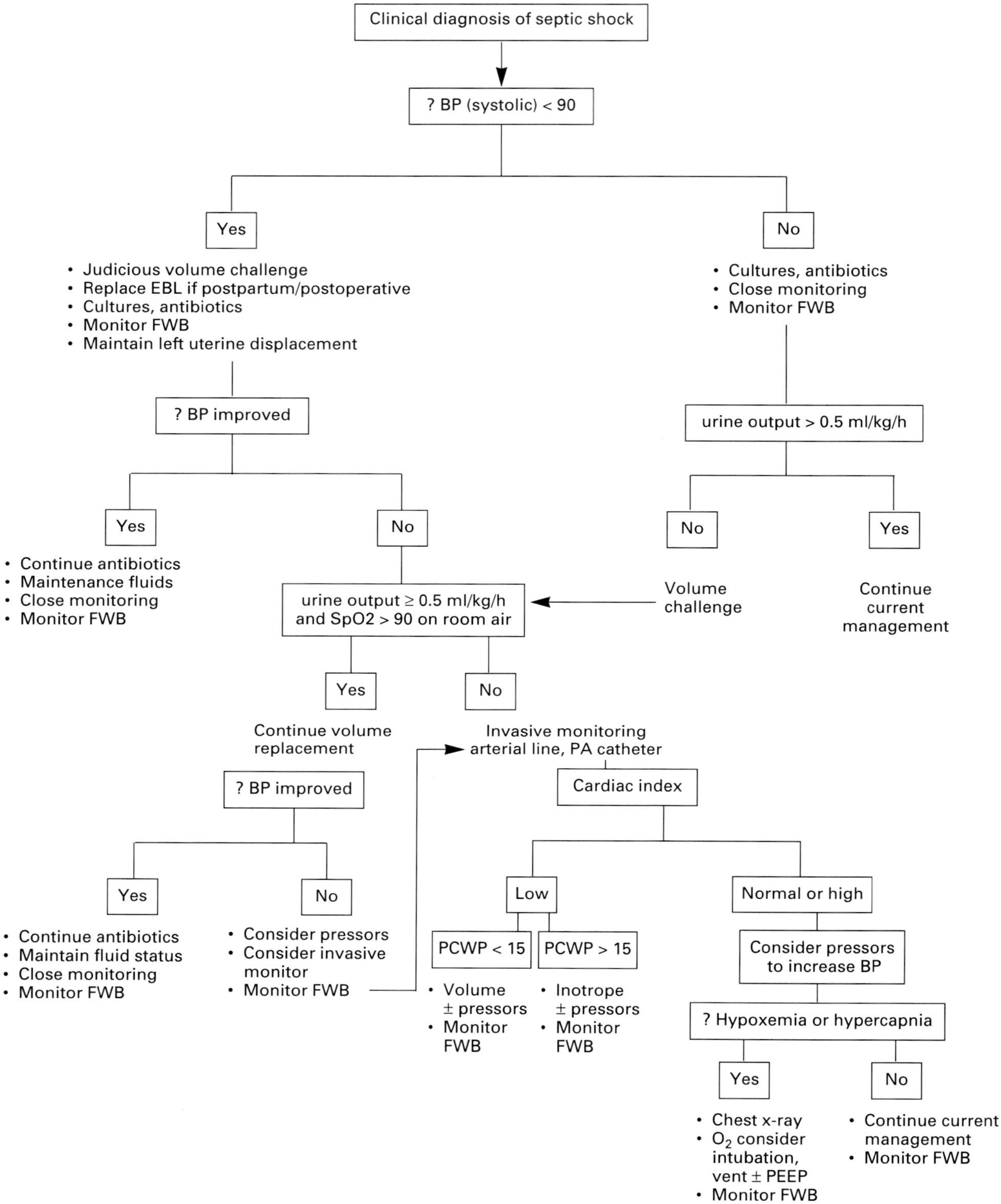

Fig. 65.2 A decision tree for the treatment of the septic obstetric patient. EBL, estimated blood loss; FWB, fetal well-being; BP, blood pressure.

parturient are *Escherichia coli*, *Klebsiella* spp., *Enterobacter* spp., *Proteus* spp., *Pseudomonas* spp., *Streptococcus* spp., and *Bacteroides* spp.[3]

The mainstay of therapy for sepsis and septic shock is eradication of the nidus of infection. In obstetrics, this often equates with delivery, such as in the case of chorioamnionitis, but other problems may involve surgical procedures, such as drainage of abcesses. Appropriate antibiotic therapy is essential but does not replace the need for surgical drainage or debridement if a pus collection can be located.

Concomitant supportive therapy is essential to minimize morbidity or mortality from septic shock. Support of the circulation with volume, vasopressors and inotropes as indicated is crucial (Fig. 65.1), as death is usually the sequela of severe hypoperfusion of vital organs. Careful attention must also be paid to avoiding and/or treating complications such as acute respiratory distress syndrome (ARDS), disseminated intravascular coagulation, acute tubular necrosis and hepatic failure, which occur frequently in this setting. Any treatment of the pregnant patient must include consideration of the effects of therapy on the fetus if the fetus is likely to survive (e.g. the effects of vasopressors on uteroplacental perfusion).

Certain therapies directed toward neutralizing the mediators of septic shock (i.e. naloxone, monoclonal antibodies, prostaglandin inhibitors, etc.) are in experimental stages of development and cannot be uniformly recommended.[4]

Anesthesiologists may be called on to assist in the management of these critically ill patients either pre- or post-partum, to assist in managing delivery of the patient, or often in the post-partum period to anesthetize a patient for a procedure such as dilation and curettage or hysterectomy.

The basic principles of caring for parturients apply to these patients as well. These include prophylaxis against aspiration of gastric contents (nonparticulate antacid, metoclopramide and rapid-sequence induction of general anesthesia utilizing cricoid pressure), prevention of aortocaval compression by left uterine displacement and a thorough understanding of the physiologic changes occurring during pregnancy.

Attention to ventilation and oxygenation is of prime importance because of the additional stress of the hypermetabolic state of sepsis superimposed on that of pregnancy, which is complicated by decreased lung volumes and functional residual capacity. Supplemental oxygen should be provided and oxygen saturation monitored continuously with a pulse oximeter. Arterial catheterization should be considered early in the course of the disease to allow frequent arterial blood gas determinations and close monitoring of blood pressure. The development of ARDS is an ominous complication of sepsis and should be treated with intubation, mechanical ventilation and positive end-expiratory pressure as necessary.

Another primary goal of anesthetic management in these patients is to optimize perfusion and cardiac performance (see Fig. 65.2). Initial attempts should be directed toward ensuring adequate preload. This consists of preventing aortocaval compression and providing volume replacement. Further therapy with inotropes and vasopressors should, in general, be guided by information derived from pulmonary artery catheterization (i.e. cardiac index, stroke volume and systemic vascular resistance).

When choosing an anesthetic technique one must always consider the patient's overall condition. Although recent animal work indicates that prior treatment of septic patients with antibiotics may minimize the risk of epidural or meningeal infection following regional anesthesia,[5] regional anesthesia may be contraindicated in patients with septic shock for one of the following reasons. First, the patient may have developed a coagulopathy, which would prohibit the use of regional anesthesia. Additionally, patients who are hypotensive, volume depleted and with limited myocardial reserve may tolerate a subarachnoid- or epidural-induced sympathectomy very poorly. However, there may be a role for regional anesthesia in select patients who are infected, but less seriously ill, provided that appropriate antibiotic therapy has been instituted.[6]

General anesthesia may be undertaken safely, utilizing a rapid-sequence induction, with ketamine 1–2 mg/kg and succinylcholine 1.5 mg/kg. Alternatively, patients who have had adequate intravascular volume replacement may tolerate small doses of thiopental, although caution must be exercised. Continuous monitoring of fetal heart rate should be employed to help prevent detrimental decreases in uteroplacental perfusion, particularly if vasopressors are utilized.

Post-operatively, provisions must be made to continue the aggressive care and monitoring initiated in the labor suite or operating room. An intensive care setting may be necessary to provide the optimum care for these patients, who are susceptible to developing further complications post-operatively or post-partum. Close monitoring of cardiorespiratory, renal and metabolic function must be provided, with rapid institution of support if necessary. Consultation with subspecialists such as infectious disease, renal and gastroenterology experts may be required if significant improvement does not occur rapidly once the infectious source is eradicated.

REFERENCES

1. Creasy R K, Resnick R (eds) 1989 Maternal and fetal medicine: principles and practice. W B Saunders, Philadelphia, p 457
2. Camann W R, Tuomala R 1991 Infectious disease. In Datta S (ed) 1991 Management of high-risk pregnancy. Mosby-Yearbook Medical Publishers, St Louis, p 536–563
3. Lee W L, Clark S L, Cotton D B et al 1988 Septic shock during pregnancy. Am J Obstet Gynecol 159: 410–416
4. Hoffman W D, Natanson C 1989 Bacterial septic shock. Anesth Clin North Am 7: 845–867
5. Carp H, Bailey S 1992 The association between meningitis and dural puncture in bacteremic rats. Anesthesiology 76: 739–742
6. Chestnut D H 1992 Spinal anesthesia in the febrile patient. Anesthesiology 76: 667–669

66. Trauma and burns in pregnant women

S. Halevy K. J. Freese

INTRODUCTION

There is paucity of information concerning the anesthetic management of pregnant patients who sustain traumatic injuries. This is in spite of the fact that the trauma is the most common nonobstetric cause of death during pregnancy, and accidental trauma is the most common cause of death under 40 years of age.[1–3] Most of the available articles, including those in recent monographs, are essentially a repetition of physiologic changes in pregnancy, teratologic data, and even a discussion of the perimortem indication for cesarean delivery.[1,4,5]

The pathophysiology and management of trauma have been the subject of a number of excellent reviews and recent textbooks. Similarly, the various aspects of the physiology of pregnancy have been reviewed. Here, the authors will only attempt to emphasize common areas of concern to the anesthesiologist and intensive care specialist without repeating details that can be found elsewhere.

The most common injuries to pregnant patients are those of the central nervous system, chest and abdomen. The uterus and urinary tract are also frequently involved. These injuries may be further subdivided into blunt and penetrating trauma. Burns are also classified among traumatic injuries. In addition, some authors include a variety of other injuries which are not always considered traumatic, such as chemical, physical and radiation injuries.

Trauma is an enormously diverse subject. It is also a confusing subject as the intensive care specialist is often unfamiliar with the physiology of the pregnant woman and the obstetrician may know little of the intensive care of trauma patients. There are, however, several important factors that must be considered in the case of the pregnant patient subjected to practically any kind of trauma.

1. The expanded blood volume together with the increase in cardiac output may maintain the blood pressure until the patient has lost a considerable amount of her blood volume. During pregnancy, the blood volume increases, reaching its peak around the 32nd week, and the cardiac output increases by approximately 50% at the time of delivery. This is especially important since the incidence of trauma appears to increase toward the end of pregnancy.
2. Hypoxic damage to the fetus is usually directly proportional to that of the mother because there is no uteroplacental autoregulation. Immediate institution of fetal monitoring after trauma is mandatory. This will determine both the adequacy of placental perfusion as well as fetal well-being. Furthermore, fetomaternal hemorrhage has been recently given particular attention and maternal blood should be routinely analyzed for fetal red blood cells using the Kleihauer–Betke test.[6–9]
3. Placental separation, one of the most common complications of trauma during pregnancy and the leading single cause of fetal death,[10] should be immediately recognized, as its major complication, disseminated intravascular coagulation, is difficult to diagnose and even more difficult to treat, especially when the diagnosis is delayed. For these reasons, cardiotocographic monitoring should be maintained for at least 4 h.[8,11–14]
4. A well-established and clinically demonstrated fact is that pregnant patients develop hypoxia much more rapidly than nonpregnant controls. This is the result of a number of cardiopulmonary changes during pregnancy. The end result is that the oxygen reserves are more rapidly depleted during periods of hypoxia. Furthermore, a classic 5-min limit of maternal hypoxia has been established beyond which fetal resuscitation is considered problematic to impossible without significant brain damage.
5. Delayed gastric emptying is caused by both trauma and pregnancy. Therefore, these patients must be considered as having a full stomach and every measure should be taken to prevent aspiration. Aspiration pneumonitis and respiratory distress syndrome are associated with an extremely high mortality in the pregnant trauma patient.

6. Cardiorespiratory resuscitation of pregnant patients in general and injured pregnant patients in particular is very difficult due to the presence of the enlarged gravid uterus. A series of recommendations have been recently outlined for pregnant women.[15]

BLUNT TRAUMA

Accidental injuries are reported to occur in 6 or 7% of all pregnancies. While trauma caused by accidents is recognized as the third or fourth major cause of death, depending upon the study, the most common causes of death by blunt trauma in pregnant patients are those involving motor vehicles followed a long way behind by falls. Abdominal trauma accounts for nearly 80% of these injuries, while chest trauma is responsible for about 20%.[16,17] In both instances, trauma may be caused by direct and/or indirect forces. Indirect forces include rotational or torquing motion caused by tangential blows and sudden accelerations or decelerations. However, one must remember that about 50% of fatalities by accident are caused by central nervous system injuries. Injuries to the neck and spinal cord, major vessels, long bones and the pelvis require early recognition and treatment. The design of effective seat belts for pregnant women is a matter of continuous concern.[10,18,19]

The evaluation of traumatic injuries of pregnant patients is beyond the scope of this article. However, it must be stressed that the symptoms of these injuries are notoriously unreliable even with today's increasingly sophisticated technology.[20,21] In this respect, the most significant factor associated with abdominal injuries caused by blunt trauma is the fact that they are frequently unrecognized.[20] Repeat physical examinations are essential.[13,22]

The management of trauma in pregnant patients is a simple extrapolation from nonpregnant trauma patient management.[23,25]

Considering the complications of trauma, a recent prospective study found abruptio placentae and fetomaternal transfusion to be the most significant.[24] Interestingly, there were no reliable predictive diagnostic or prognostic signs of either complication. In an earlier but frequently quoted article, the authors reported a high incidence of hemorrhage and shock and stressed again the importance of prompt maternal resuscitation in overall fetal outcome.[26] Most authors agree that peritoneal lavage is an extremely important diagnostic tool which, in many cases, determines the indication for laparotomy.[10, 27] A final observation concerns two rare complications of trauma that are practically unique to pregnancy. Rupture of either the uterus or urinary bladder can occur, the latter in association with pelvic fractures. Both types of organ ruptures are severe and life-threatening and obviously related to the anatomic situation of these organs during pregnancy.

PENETRATING TRAUMA

Penetrating injuries resulting from gunshot and stabbing are the third major category of injuries during pregnancy. They occur much less frequently than blunt trauma. However, gunshot wounds appear to be rapidly increasing in number for the past several years.

It is important to remember, especially in the case of gunshot injuries, that the trajectory is of lesser importance than the kinetic energy dissipated by the penetrating object. Furthermore, in the case of a bullet, the velocity is more important than the size of the bullet. In addition, as in the case of blunt trauma, damage from contrecoup and inertial forces must be considered. In summary, all these factors greatly amplify the effect of the penetrating object.[17] Obviously, as the pregnancy progresses, the uterus is the organ frequently affected by penetrating trauma.

There are two major problems to take into consideration:

1. The exploration of the wound is practically mandatory; and
2. Possible injury to the fetus must be considered when there is an abdominal wound.[10]

In fact, in this type of trauma, the injury to the fetus is also more severe.[23] This is the main reason why the perinatal mortality in penetrating trauma by gunshot to the uterus is exceedingly high. In contrast, maternal mortality is significantly lower because of the protection offered by the pregnant uterus.[23] In general, stab wounds to the abdomen are significantly less dangerous than gunshots because of the aforementioned additional physical forces created by the bullet which result in more damage.[10,17] The same general observations concerning the diagnosis and procedures mentioned in connection with blunt trauma injuries apply to penetrating trauma as well.

BURNS

Burns or thermal injuries sustained during pregnancy are today the object of extensive pathophysiologic and psychosocial studies since the literature on the subject is, at best, scarce. A relatively small number of pregnant patients sustain burn injury (about 4%), since most burn patients (about 80%) are adult men or children. Clearly, there is a striking lack of data in the literature concerning the main therapeutic problem, fluid requirement, in pregnant burn patients. At present, a prospective study in the USA with the participation of 182 burn care resources is designed to collect data and provide guidelines concerning burned pregnant patients. However, one of the anticipated problems with this study is the fact only 0.1% of pregnant burn patients will require hospitalization, and only 4–7% of burn patients are women between 15 and 39 years of age.

Burns represent a very special form of traumatic injury, damaging the skin, the largest organ in the body, with a multitude of consequences. The cardiovascular system suffers from intravascular hypovolemia due to generalized increase in capillary permeability. Cardiac performance is compromised, possibly as a result of some unknown humoral factors released from injured areas. Pulmonary function is affected by upper airway burns, circumferential chest wall involvement, inhalation of noxious gases and carbon monoxide poisoning. The metabolic rates are dramatically elevated. Gastrointestinal bleeding, sepsis and renal failure are life-threatening later complications. There are also a number of other complications related to the nature of the burns. For instance, electrical burns are complicated by myoglobinuria and neurologic damage.

Although burns, including thermal injuries, may be caused by a variety of agents, e.g. flame, explosions, scalding, electricity and chemicals, the pathology and therapy depends on two basic factors, the depth of the burn and the size of the affected area. The significance of burn depth is based on skin capacity for re-epithelialization with formerly third-degree burns, now called full-thickness burns, losing their capacity for regeneration.

It appears that pregnancy does not influence the pathology of burns.[25] Based on the available information, the management of burns in pregnancy differs little from that of nonpregnant patients.[28]

Delivery has been recommended for patients with over 50% burns and those in their second and third trimesters, since it has been hypothesized that the chances of fetal survival will not improve by waiting.[29] This problem has become a matter of heated debate. Preterm labor is known to occur quite frequently during the acute phase of the burn which is associated with, first, high levels of histamine followed by release of many vasoactive substances such as serotonin, bradykinin, prostaglandins and leukotrienes. Later, infection may be responsible for the release of phospholipase A, which, in turn, is responsible for further increases in prostaglandins.[2,25,28,30] The question of tocolytic therapy and its potential side-effects in burn patients is still open. A study of 19 patients at the US Army Institute of Surgical Research concluded that obstetric intervention is not necessary unless the patient is extremely ill.[2,31,32] The conclusion is that, similar to other types of trauma, fetal survival depends on maternal survival and, of course, gestational age.[28,32,33,34]

Aggressive therapy, both fluids and surgical, has been recently recommended for pregnant women with burns over 15%.[24] The main reason for this recommendation is based on uterine hypoperfusion caused by hypotension, fluid loss and shock. Low uterine perfusion is, in turn, responsible for fetal hypoxia and acidosis and even initiation of premature labor.[32,34] Unfortunately, there are insufficient data available to be able to establish a working protocol since most data are empirical. Until more knowledge is accumulated and studies are completed, it is difficult to reach any practical conclusions.

CONCLUSION

Giving first consideration to physiologic alterations caused by pregnancy, the current management of trauma in pregnant patients is very similar to that of nonpregnant patients. Perhaps the most important single factor for anesthesiologists to remember in the resuscitation of the pregnant trauma victim is the same as in the management of any pregnant patient, i.e. the avoidance of the supine position to prevent aortocaval compression and its consequences. The second factor to be taken into consideration is early and prolonged cardiotocographic monitoring. The third element of concern is that the physiologic and anatomic changes of pregnancy make the classic physical findings less reliable and delay the institution of effective treatment. In 1984 the American College of Surgeons Committee on Trauma formalized the life support recommendation for Trauma in Pregnancy. In essence, the guidelines recognize the importance of the knowledge of both the mechanism of trauma and physiologic changes of pregnancy along with the need for fetal assessment, i.e. fetal maturity, and well-being. Teamwork between emergency and trauma specialists, obstetrician, anesthesiologist and pediatrician is essential.

REFERENCES

1. Haycock C E 1985 Burns and other trauma in pregnancy. In: Haycock C E (ed) Trauma and pregnancy. PSG, Littleton, MA pp 57–68
2. Baker D P 1982 Trauma in pregnant patient. Surg Clin North Am 62: 275–289
3. Jackson F C 1979 Accidental injury: the problem and the initiatives. In: Buchsbaum H J (ed) Trauma in pregnancy. W B Saunders, Philadelphia pp 1–21
4. Erian M, Wu W-H 1985 Anesthetic management of the traumatized parturient. In: Haycock C E (ed) Trauma and pregnancy. PSG, Littleton, MA pp 80–92
5. Ramanathan S, Porges R M 1991 Anesthetic care of the injured pregnant patient. In: Capon L M, Miller S M, Turndorf H (eds) Trauma: anesthesia and intensive care. J B Lippincott, Philadelphia pp 599–628
6. Rose P G, Strohm P L, Zuspan F P 1985 Fetomaternal hemorrhage following trauma. Am J Obstet Gynecol 153: 844–847
7. Pearlman M D, Tintinalli J E, Lorenz R P 1990 A prospective study of outcome after trauma during pregnancy. Am J Obstet Gynecol 162: 1502–1510
8. Goodwin T M, Breen M T 1990 Pregnancy outcome and fetomaternal hemorrhage after noncatastrophic trauma. Am J Obstet Gynecol 162: 665–671
9. Farmer D L, Adzick N S, Crombleholme W R, Crombleholme T M, Longaker M T, Harrison M R 1990 Fetal trauma: relation to maternal injury. J Pediat Surg 25: 711–714

10. Crosby W M 1983 Traumatic injuries during pregnancy. Clin Obstet Gynecol 26: 902–912
11. Higgins S D, Garite T J 1984 Late abruptio placenta in trauma patients: implications for monitoring. Obstet Gynecol 63: 10S–12S
12. Kettel L M, Branch D W, Scott J R 1988 Occult placental abruption after maternal trauma. Obstet Gynecol 71: 449–453
13. Esposito T J, Gens D R, Smith L G, Scorpio R 1989 Evaluation of blunt abdominal trauma occurring during pregnancy. J Trauma 29: 1628–1632
14. Lavin J P, Miodovnik M 1981 Delayed abruption after maternal trauma as a result of an automobile accident. J Reprod Med 26: 621–624
15. Lee R V, Rodgers B D, White L M, Harvey R C 1986 Cardiopulmonary resuscitation of pregnant women. Am J Med 81: 311–318
16. Cohen-Addad N 1985 Neonatal aspect of the injured fetus. In: Haycock C E (ed) Trauma and pregnancy. PSG, Littleton, MA pp 103–120
17. Zolli A F, Neville W E 1985 Chest trauma in pregnancy. In: Haycock C E (ed) Trauma and pregnancy. PSG, Littleton, MA pp 120–135
18. Crosby W M 1979 Automobile injuries and blunt abdominal trauma. In: Buchsbaum H J (ed) Trauma in pregnancy. W B Saunders, Philadelphia pp 101–127
19. Lane P L 1989 Traumatic fetal deaths. J Emerg Med 7: 433–435
20. McAnena O J, Moore E E, Marx J A 1990 Initial evaluation of the patient with blunt abdominal trauma. Surg Clin North Am 70: 495–515
21. Drost T F, Rosemurgy A S, Sherman H F, Scott L M, Williams J K 1990 Major trauma in pregnant women: maternal/fetal outcome. J Trauma 30: 574–578
22. Williams J K, McClain L, Rosemurgy A S, Colorado N M 1990 Evaluation of blunt abdominal trauma in the third trimester of pregnancy: maternal and fetal considerations. Obstet Gynecol 75: 33–37
23. Patterson R M 1984 Trauma in pregnancy. Clin Obstet Gynecol 27: 32–38
24. Pearlman M D, Tintinalli J E, Lorenz R P 1990 Blunt trauma during pregnancy. New Engl J Med 323: 1609–1613
25. Gonik B 1989 Intensive care monitoring of the critically ill pregnant patient. In: Creasy R K, Resnik R (eds) Maternal fetal medicine. W B Saunders, Philadelphia pp 845–874
26. Rothenberger D, Quattlebaum F W, Perry J F, Zabel J, Fischer R P 1978 Blunt maternal trauma: a review of 103 cases. J Trauma 18: 173–179
27. Rothenberger D, Quattlebaum F W, Perry J F, Zabel J, Fischer R P 1977 Diagnostic peritoneal lavage for blunt trauma in pregnant women. Am J Obstet Gynecol 129: 479–481
28. Rayburn W, Smith B, Feller I, Varner M, Cruikshank D 1984 Major burns during pregnancy: effects on fetal well-being. Obstet Gynecol 63: 392–395
29. Matthews R N 1982 Obstetric implications of burns in pregnancy. Brit J Obstet Gynaecol 89: 603–609
30. Deitch E A 1990 The management of burns. New Engl J Med 323: 1249–1253
31. Amy B W, McManus W F, Goodwin C W, Mason A, Pruitt B A 1985 Thermal injury in the pregnant patient. Surg Gynecol Obstet 161: 209–212
32. Taylor J W, Plunkett G D, McManus W F, Pruitt B A 1976 Thermal injury during pregnancy. Obstet Gynecol 47: 434–438
33. Deitch E A, Rightmire D A, Clothier J, Blass N 1985 Management of burns in pregnant women. Surg Gynecol Obstet 161: 1–4
34. Bartle E J, Sun J H, Wang X-W 1988 Burns in pregnancy. J Burn Care Rehabil 9: 485–487

67. Acute carbon monoxide poisoning in pregnancy

S. B. Corn

Acute carbon monoxide poisoning is the leading cause of death due to poisoning, and it is estimated that between 1500 and 3500 deaths occur per year.[1–3] As a better understanding of this entity is realized, more accounts of true carbon monoxide poisoning during pregnancy are being reported. It is important that obstetric anesthesiologists have a thorough understanding of this clinical state, so that prompt diagnosis, appropriate monitoring and immediate therapy may be instituted to avoid the deleterious effects of carbon monoxide poisoning on the mother and the developing fetus.

CHEMICAL ASPECTS OF CARBON MONOXIDE

Carbon monoxide poisoning and its mechanisms have been known since Claude Bernard reported in 1857 that this gas causes death by producing hypoxia.[4] Carbon monoxide is a colorless, odorless, tasteless, nonirritating gas produced by the incomplete combustion of carbonaceous material. Almost any fire produces carbon monoxide. Other sources of carbon monoxide include automotive exhaust, thick smoke, gas heaters (not natural gas), home and industrial heating systems, erythrocyte destruction and cigarette smoke.[2] Automotive fumes may produce a carboxyhemoglobin (HbCO) level greater than 20%, erythrocyte destruction usually gives a 1% HbCO level and cigarette smoke may give a HbCO level between 2 and 15%.[5,6]

SIGNS AND SYMPTOMS ASSOCIATED WITH CARBON MONOXIDE EXPOSURE

The signs and symptoms seen with carbon monoxide exposure relate to the percentage of carboxyhemoglobin (Table 67.1). The often-cited cherry-red appearance of the carbon monoxide-poisoned patient is variable in its presentation.

Table 67.1 Carbon monoxide poisoning: signs and symptoms with percentage HbCO

HbCO(%)	Signs and Symptoms
0–10	None
10–20	Tightness across forehead, slight headache, dilation of cutaneous blood vessels
20–30	Throbbing headache
40–50	As above, with possibility of syncope; increased respiration and heart rate
50–60	Syncope, increased respiratory and pulse rates; coma with intermittent convulsions; Cheyne – Stokes respiration
60–70	Coma with intermittent convulsions; depressed cardiovascular and respiratory function, possible death
70–80	Weak pulse, slow respiratory rates; respiratory failure and death

DIAGNOSIS OF CARBON MONOXIDE POISONING

The diagnosis may not be immediately obvious, however the aforementioned signs and symptoms coupled with the history usually lead to the suspicion of carbon monoxide poisoning. The definitive diagnosis is made with the HbCO level determined by multiple band spectrophotometry (see below).

The HbCO level is very important for diagnosis, but the presence of signs, symptoms and history of exposure to carbon monoxide justify the institution of therapy and any delay in administering that therapy is inappropriate.[4]

An HbCO level of greater then 20% is considered to be carbon monoxide poisoning. However, many victims receive supplemental oxygen therapy before blood samples are drawn, thus lowering their HbCO level upon admission. Owing to this possible reduction in HbCO level, the clinician must thoughtfully consider the diagnosis of carbon monoxide poisoning in patients with a history and presentation suggestive of this entity, even if the HbCO level is not markedly elevated. Interestingly, the $P\text{aCO}_2$ may be normal, increased or decreased.

Included in the differential diagnosis are anemic hypoxia, circulatory hypoxia, specific organ hypoxia, and increased oxygen-requiring states (i.e. febrile states and thyrotoxicosis) and improper oxygen utilization states (i.e. cyanide poisoning). Cyanide poisoning may occur concomitantly with carbon monoxide poisoning in burn- and fume-exposed victims. These patients are unable to utilize oxygen because cyanide interferes with the electron transport of the cytochrome oxidase system.

BIOLOGIC CONSIDERATIONS OF CARBON MONOXIDE POISONING

The toxic effects of carbon monoxide are a result of tissue hypoxia. It is known that hemoglobin has an affinity for carbon monoxide that is 200–250 times greater than that for oxygen. Carbon monoxide freely combines with hemoglobin (Hb) to form carboxyhemoglobin (HbCO). Carbon monoxide also interferes with the release of oxygen from hemoglobin. Carbon monoxide has this effect by shifting the hemoglobin curve to the left, thus further reducing the amount of oxygen available to the tissues, and this explains why tissue anoxia occurs at levels of arterial hemoglobin concentrations tolerated by anemic patients. One is better off with a 50% reduction in hemoglobin concentration than a 50% level of HbCO. Carbon monoxide also interferes with cellular oxidative metabolism via the intracellular cytochrome oxidase system.[2]

Van Hoesen et al[2] explained that the effects of carbon monoxide are dramatic for the pregnant patient and that the fetus is even more vulnerable than the mother to the hypoxic effects of carbon monoxide. Fetal HbCO concentrations depend on maternal HbCO concentration, placental diffusing capacity of carbon monoxide, endogenous fetal carbon monoxide production and the relative affinity of maternal and fetal hemoglobin for carbon monoxide and oxygen. Normal human fetal: maternal HbCO concentration is 1.1:1. This demonstrates that the fetal HbCO levels are 10–15% higher than maternal levels at steady state.

The fetal hemoglobin dissociation curve lies to the left of the maternal curve. Since the normal fetal arterial $P\text{O}_2$ is low, the fetal system normally operates on the steep part of the curve, thus a small drop in oxygen tension results in a large drop in oxygen concentration.[2]

Before the fetal HbCO level has risen, there will already have been a fall in the maternal arterial oxygen content, leading to fetal hypoxia. Also, as the fetal HbCO level rises, it will further shift the hemoglobin dissociation curve to the left, making it even more difficult for the fetus to unload oxygen, possibly leading to drastic hypoxia in the fetus[2] (Fig. 67.1).

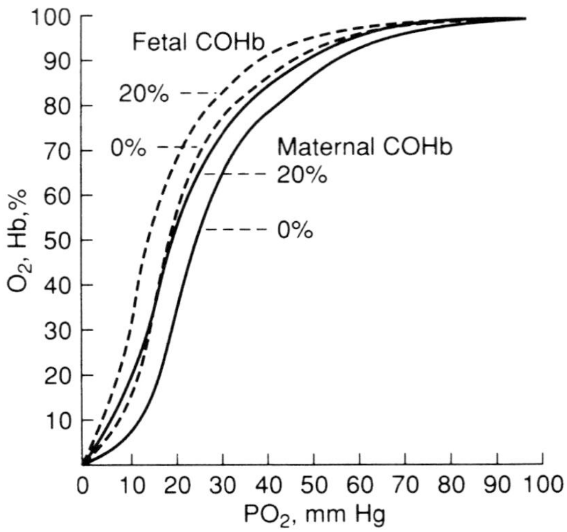

Fig. 67.1. Effect of carboxyhemoglobin on the hemoglobin dissociation curve. (From ref. 2 with permission.)

A mathematical model has been developed[7] that examines the exchange of carbon monoxide between the human fetus and the mother. The findings demonstrated that fetal HbCO levels lag with respect to maternal HbCO levels by several hours. However, during uptake, fetal HbCO levels eventually rise above maternal HbCO levels. The elimination of carbon monoxide from the fetus lags considerably behind the mother. With increased inspired oxygen concentration, the time for elimination of the maternal HbCO is reduced but the time for elimination of the fetal HbCO is not reduced nearly as much as the mother. These physiologic considerations will have important implications for the treatment of the pregnant patient exposed to carbon monoxide.

TREATMENT OF THE PREGNANT PATIENT EXPOSED TO CARBON MONOXIDE

Standard care and monitoring apply to these patients as they would to any patient with a history of smoke inhalation and possible thermal airway injury. Depending on gestational age, fetal monitoring may be appropriate. The limitations of pulse oximetry are discussed below.

The definitive treatment of carbon monoxide poisoning is to facilitate elimination of the gas via the lungs.

1. Remove the victim from the carbon monoxide source.
2. Assess ventilation and the need for intubation.
3. Increase inspired oxygen concentration to 100%.
4. Decrease patient activity to decrease tissue oxygen needs.

Oxygen competes with carbon monoxide for the same site on the Hb molecule, so that increasing the oxygen tension will increase the competition for the sites. Removing the victim from the carbon monoxide source will decrease the alveolar partial pressure of carbon monoxide but, even with the alveolar partial pressure close to zero, there is less than a 2 mmHg gradient from blood to alveoli to remove carbon monoxide from the hemoglobin.[8] An illustration will put this elimination process in perspective: Breathing room air the HbCO half-life is 5 h for the nonpregnant patient; on 100% FiO_2, the half-life decreases to 1 h.

Numerous studies have looked at the use of hyperbaric oxygen therapy (HBO) for the treatment of acute carbon monoxide poisoning. The first systematic studies evaluating the physiologic effects of HBO for the treatment of carbon monoxide poisoning were conducted in the 1950s.[9] HBO increases arterial and tissue oxygen tensions far in excess of that achieved with breathing 100% oxygen. With increasing oxygen partial pressures, the rate of release of carbon monoxide from HBO is increased, thus decreasing the HbCO half-life.[3] It has been proposed that there may be additional mechanisms by which HBO therapy functions.

Carefully conducted clinical studies have not been performed, and some investigators have questioned whether HBO therapy confers a benefit over 100% oxygen in the treatment of acute carbon monoxide poisoning.[8,10,11] Additional concern arises with the use of HBO in the pregnant patient because of the relative lack of information on the risk of high partial pressures of oxygen on the fetus. However, there have been numerous reports that show a decrease in morbidity and mortality in patients with acute carbon monoxide poisoning who have had HBO therapy.[12–14]

It is known that carbon monoxide has toxic effects on the fetus in all stages of pregnancy.[15–17] With this in mind and the knowledge that carbon monoxide elimination from the fetus is much slower than in the mother, it is of considerable interest to try to hasten the carbon monoxide elimination process.

Van Hoesen et al[2] have reviewed numerous studies employing HBO in the pregnant patient. They remark that many of the adverse effects noted in various studies may have been secondary to the excessive hyperbaric pressures and time periods used in treatment. They also reviewed many studies that report improved fetal outcome with HBO use, without detrimental effects to the fetus. Studies in the Soviet Union employing HBO therapy in several hundred pregnant patients during all stages of gestation report improved fetal circulation and reduced perinatal complications and mortality without any evidence of retinopathy or adverse effects secondary to HBO.[18–20] Van Hoesen et al, who have done an extensive review of the literature, believe that the benefits of HBO therapy in the pregnant patient with acute carbon monoxide poisoning far outweigh the risks and state that HBO therapy should be considered in any pregnant patient with acute carbon monoxide poisoning. They recommend the following steps (from Van Hoesen et al[2] with permission):

1. Administer HBO therapy if the maternal HbCO level is above 20% at any time during the exposure.
2. Administer HBO therapy if the patient has suffered or demonstrates signs of any neurologic injury regardless of the HbCO level.
3. Administer HBO therapy if signs of fetal distress are present (i.e. fetal tachycardia, decreased beat-to-beat variability on the fetal monitor or late decelerations) consistent with the HbCO levels and exposure history.
4. If HBO treatment is unavailable, administer 100% oxygen by a tightly fitting mask for five times as long as needed to reduce maternal HbCO to normal (less than 5%).
5. If the patient continues to demonstrate neurologic signs or signs of fetal distress 12 h after initial treatment, additional HBO treatments may be indicated. Multiple HBO treatments have been suggested to be beneficial in severely poisoned and nonresponsive patients exposed to carbon monoxide.

MONITORING AND CARBON MONOXIDE POISONING

Pulse oximetry has been recommended as a standard of care for every general anesthetic and is routinely used in many settings, including the obstetric operating room and recovery room.[21]

Pulse oximetry provides an instantaneous, noninvasive means of determining the arterial oxygenation based on determining light absorption between a light-emitting diode and a nonselective photodetector. The oximeter 'assumes' that there are only two species of hemoglobin present in the blood [i.e. oxyhemoglobin (HbO) and deoxyhemoglobin (Hb)]. To distinguish between these two species, the oximeter emits light at two different wavelengths (i.e. one emits red at 660 nm and the other infrared at 940 nm). The oximeter makes use of the relative absorbance of these wavelengths of light to calculate the arterial oxygen saturation.[22] However, when another species of hemoglobin is present (i.e. HbCO, which absorbs very similarly to oxyhemoglobin at 660 nm), erroneous readings will result. Numerous studies[23–25] have demonstrated that when clinically significant quantities of HbCO are present, substantial differences may be seen between the pulse oximeter oxygen saturation reading and the actual arterial oxygen saturation. Therefore, a normal oximeter saturation reading in a patient exposed to carbon monoxide cannot be regarded as accurate, for the actual arterial saturation may be significantly lower. A 'low' oximeter reading in this carbon monoxide-exposed patient may represent severe hypoxemia.

In the care of patients exposed to carbon monoxide, an arterial blood gas analysis must be immediately performed and the laboratory should be requested to report a measured HbCO level and a measured arterial oxygen saturation employing a multiple band spectrophotometer.

The accuracy of the pulse oximeter for use on the neonate has been questioned, since fetal hemoglobin differs from adult hemoglobin in its amino acid sequence and thus may differ in its absorbance characteristics. However, studies report an insignificant effect on the extinction curves employed by the pulse oximeter, with a negligible effect on the pulse oximeter reading.[22,23,26,27]

REFERENCES

1. Wharton M, Bistowish J M, Hutcheson R H, Schaffner W 1989 Fatal carbon monoxide poisoning at a motel. J Am Med Assoc 261: 1177–1178
2. Van Hoesen K B, Camporesi E M, Moon R E et al 1989 Should hyperbaric oxygen be used to treat the pregnant patient for acute carbon monoxide poisoning? J Am Med Assoc 261: 1039–1043
3. Thom S R 1989 Hyperbaric oxygen therapy. J Intensive Care Med 4: 58–74
4. Winter P M, Miller J N 1976 Carbon monoxide poisoning. J Am Med Assoc 236(13): 1502–1504
5. Wald N J, Idle M, Boreham J, Bailey A 1981 Carbon monoxide in breath in relation to smoking and carboxyhaemoglobin levels. Thorax 36: 366–369
6. Nordenberg D, Yip R, Binkin N J 1990 The effect of cigarette smoking on hemoglobin levels and anemia screening. J Am Med Assoc 264(12): 1556–1559
7. Hill E P, Hill J R, Power G G, Longo L D 1977 Carbon monoxide exchanges between the human fetus and mother: a mathematical model. Am J Physiol 232(3): H311–H323
8. Grim P S, Gottlieb L J, Boddie A, Batson E 1990 Hyperbaric oxygen therapy, J Am Med Assoc 263(16): 2216–2220
9. Pace N, Strajman E, Walker E L 1950 Acceleration of carbon monoxide elimination in man by high pressure oxygen. Science 111: 652–654
10. Kumar S 1984 Hyperbaric oxygen in the treatment of carbon monoxide poisoning (abstract). Br Med J 289: 1315
11. Raphael J C, Elkharrat D, Jars-Guincestre M C et al 1989 Trial of normobaric and hyperbaric oxygen for acute carbon monoxide intoxication. Lancet 2: 414–419
12. Goulon M, Barois A, Rapin M et al 1986 Carbon monoxide poisoning and acute anoxia due to breathing coal gas and hydrocarbons. J Hyperbaric Med 1: 23–41
13. Krantz T, Thisted B, Strom J, Sorenson M B 1988 Acute carbon monoxide poisoning. Acta Anaesthesiol Scand 32: 278–282
14. Norkool D M, Kirkpatrick J N 1985 Treatment of acute carbon monoxide poisoning with hyperbaric oxygen: a review of 115 cases. Ann Emerg Med 14: 1168–1171
15. Astrup P, Olsen H M, Trolle D et al 1972 Effects of moderate carbon monoxide exposure on fetal development. Lancet 2: 1220–1222
16. Ginsberg M D, Myers R E 1976 Fetal brain injury after maternal carbon monoxide intoxication. Neurology 26: 15–23
17. Ginsberg M D, Myers R E 1974 Fetal brain damage following maternal carbon monoxide intoxication: an experimental study. Acta Obstet Gynecol Scand 53: 309–317
18. Proshina I V, Kuzmina N V, Borisenko S S 1983 Hyperbaric oxygenation in the prevention and treatment of pregnancy and placental insufficiency. Akush Ginekol 6: 20–23
19. Aksenova A, Proshina I V, Smirnova L K et al 1979 Methods of prenatal diagnosis of fetal hypoxia and control of the effectiveness of its treatment with hyperbaric oxygen. Akush Ginekol 11: 15–18
20. Molzhaninov E V, Chaika V K, Domanova A I et al 1983 Experience and prospects of using hyperbaric oxygenation in obstetrics. In Proceedings of the Seventh International Congress on Hyperbaric Medicine, Moscow, 1981. Moscow, Nauka, Vol 1, p 139–141
21. Eichorn J H, Cooper J B, Cullen D J et al 1986 Standards for patient monitoring during anesthesia at Harvard Medical School. J Am Med Assoc 256: 1017–1020
22. Alexander C M, Teller L E, Gross J B 1989 Principles of pulse oximetry: theoretical and practical considerations. Anesth Analg 68: 368–376
23. Barker S J, Tremper K K 1987 The effects of carbon monoxide inhalation on pulse oximetry and transcutaneous $P\mathrm{O}_2$. Anesthesiology 66: 677–679
24. Tremper K K, Barker S J 1989 Pulse oximetry. Anesthesiology 70: 98–109
25. Gonzalez A, Gomez-Arnau J, Pensado A 1990 Carboxyhemoglobin and pulse oximetry (letter). Anesthesiology 73: 573
26. Pologe J A, Raley D M 1987 Effects of fetal hemoglobin on pulse oximetry. J Perinatol 7: 324–326
27. Anderson J V 1987 The accuracy of pulse oximetry in neonates: effects of fetal hemoglobin and bilirubin. J Perinatol 7: 323

68. The principles of intensive care in obstetrics

D. Watson E. Yau M. A. Hayes S. A. Macklin

INTRODUCTION

Severe illness may occur coincidentally or as a consequence of pregnancy. Traditionally there appears to have been a reluctance to transfer seriously ill obstetric patients to intensive care unit (ICUs), and many of these patients have been managed in the past on labor suites or postnatal wards in isolated obstetric units. Graham and Luxton[1] report that approximately one ICU admission may be expected for every 1000 obstetric deliveries in Nottingham, England. Our own experience in a newly opened teaching hospital obstetric unit reveals a greater frequency of ICU admission from the labor wards.[2]

During the first four complete years since the opening of the Homerton Hospital, a university hospital affiliated to the Medical College of St. Bartholomew's Hospital, London, there have been 100 obstetric patients admitted to the ICU, and in the same period there were 16 905 deliveries (Table 68.1). This is five times the frequency of ICU admission quoted by the Nottingham group, even though the justification for such admissions were broadly similar. Three of our mothers died. Admission policies and case mix clearly differ from city to city[3] depending on whether the obstetric units have medical or nursing personnel trained in critical care medicine. It is generally accepted, however, that women with complications of pregnancy should be managed as other patients with similar life-threatening conditions.

The Reports on Confidential Enquiries into Maternal Deaths[4] have recorded the changing pattern of ultimately fatal illnesses in the obstetric population since the triennial system of reporting began in 1952. This is shown in Figure 68.1 and summarizes the contents of this chapter, since treatment protocols for many of these medical or surgical problems now regularly involve access to sophisticated monitoring equipment, elective ventilatory support

Table 68.1 Reasons for pregnancy-associated ICU admission. Deaths associated with these admissions are shown in brackets

Cause of ICU admission	1987	1988	1989	1990
Hypertensive diseases of pregnancy	11	10(1)	22(1)	25
Hemorrhage	4	4	2	2
Anesthesia	0	1	0	0
Others				
Amniotic fluid embolism	1	0	0	0
Left ventricular failure	1	0	0	0
Sickle cell disease	1	0	2	2
Pre-existing malignancy	1(1)	0	0	0
Small bowel infarction	1	0	0	0
Abdominal wound abscess	1	0	0	0
Hepatocellular dysfunction	1	0	0	1
Thyrotoxicosis	0	1	0	0
Pneumonia	0	1	1	0
Hyperemesis gravidarum	0	0	1	0
Trauma	0	0	1	0
Malaria	0	0	1	0
Totals	22	17	31	30
Obstetric deliveries	3650	3498	3775	3982

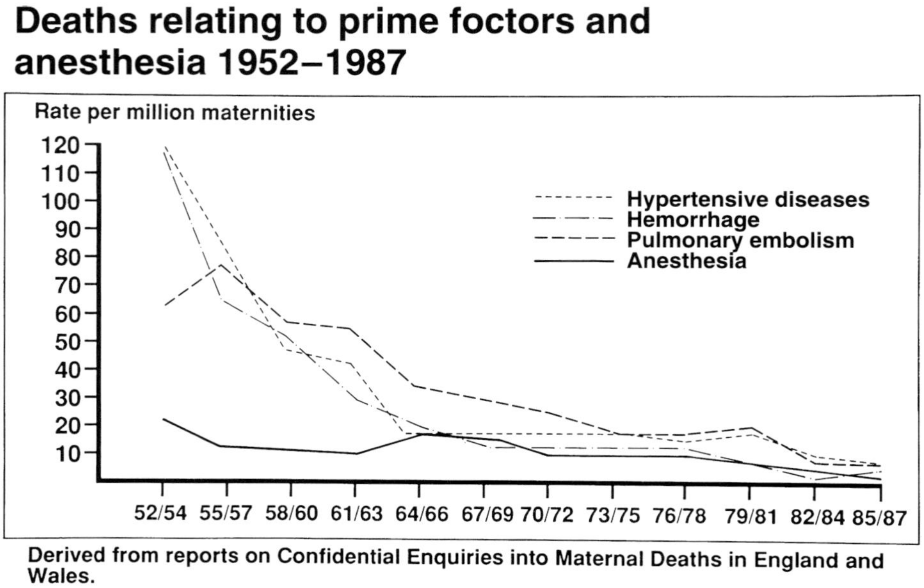

Fig. 68.1 Maternal mortality in England and Wales relating to prime factors, 1952–87

and 1 : 1 trained nurse to patient care. More frequent ICU admissions are warranted therefore for obstetric patients with pregnancy-associated emergencies.

ASPIRATION OF GASTRIC CONTENTS DURING ANESTHESIA

Although multiple-system organ dysfunction syndrome (MSODS) represents the final common pathway of critical illness, its etiology is multifactorial and may be preventable. This has particular relevance to aspiration pneumonitis consequent upon the soiling of the lungs with acidic gastric contents. The severity of aspiration pneumonitis depends on the acidity of the gastric contents aspirated into the lungs as well as their volume. Although in the early Confidential Enquiries the contribution of these anesthetic deaths was only small in comparison with other life-threatening conditions, their contribution remained depressingly constant and represented one of the commonest causes of maternal death in the UK. This was despite the introduction of epidural anesthetic techniques and the widespread administration of antacids to women about the time of delivery.

Various studies have now discredited the particulate antacid, magnesium trisilicate, as effective prophylaxis against acid gastric contents. The pattern of routine prophylaxis has now shifted in the UK to one of H_2-receptor blockade coupled with the administration of nonparticulate antacid. A recent national survey has demonstrated that ranitidine and 0.3 M sodium citrate are the favored combination nationwide.[5] Previously a regimen involving the regular prescription of oral ranitidine together with the administration of 0.3 M sodium citrate before any operative intervention has been shown to be effective in controlling gastric acidity and stomach volumes.[6] Organizational changes prompted by the recommendations of the Confidential Enquires have also meant that unsupervised junior staff no longer undertake anesthesia for cesarean delivery without adequate training and skilled assistance. The importance of correctly applied cricoid pressure and a rehearsed failed intubation drill have been emphasized repeatedly in successive reports.

It should not be forgotten that in Mendelson's original paper[7] women only died from asphyxia and not from the aspiration pneumonia that now carries his name. The increased lethality from the aspiration of acid gastric contents into the lungs may be due to the widespread practice of intermittent positive-pressure ventilation, which serves to blow the acidic juices throughout the lung fields disseminating the inhaled gastric contents and enlarging the acid burn to the capillary endothelium. The free and liberal administration of crystalloid solutions either as an adjunct to epidural analgesia/anesthesia or as a nutritional supplement during labor has also served to exacerbate any capillary leak by providing a 'saline tide' not experienced by Mendelson's patients. The unthinking use of ergometrine or Syntometrine, both of which are pulmonary vasoconstrictors, also contributes to the expulsion of fluid into the pulmonary interstitial space worsening any edema following from acid aspiration. The resulting hypoxia and hypovolemia lead to maldistribution of blood flow in the splanchnic bed and generalized tissue hypoxia, which inevitably progress without aggressive intervention to MSODS. The initiating factor for this sequential organ shutdown appears to be disseminated intravascular inflammation emanating from the damaged bowel mucosal barrier and impaired liver macrophage function.[8] This final common pathway seems to be shared by all the triggering pathologies for MSODS and is well understood by intensive care specialists managing patients suffering from overwhelming sepsis.

THE CAPILLARY LEAK SYNDROME: IMPLICATIONS FOR THERAPY

The human body can be divided into three compartments (Fig. 68.2). The intravascular space is the smallest space, containing some 5 l of fluid. It is sensitively monitored by measurements of heart rate, blood pressure, central venous pressure and pulmonary artery occlusion pressure (PAOP). The intravascular space abuts the extracellular space (14 l) through a semipermeable membrane at the capillary level. The exchange of nutrients to the intracellular metabolic apparatus (23 l) must traverse the extracellular space and is pressure driven, as shown in Figure 68.3. The arteriolar pressure is approximately 35 mmHg. A membrane semipermeable to protein is responsible for the generation of colloid oncotic pressure. In health, fluid rich in oxygen and low in acid is driven from the arteriolar end of the capillary into the extracellular space and toward the cellular membrane. At the venous end of the systemic capillary, the intravascular pressure is approximately 15 mmHg. At the venous end of the capillary, colloid oncotic forces are responsible for drawing in fluid low in oxygen and high in carbon dioxide and acid from the extracellular space. This blood then returns to the heart to pass through the pulmonary circulation to be reoxygenated. This simple schematic of the microcirculation can, therefore, be used to summarize the pathology of several critical events as well as to understand some of the pitfalls of therapy.

If a pregnant patient suffers life-threatening hemorrhage, any resulting hypotension will prejudice tissue oxygen delivery and, since metabolism must continue anerobically, there will be an inevitable worsening of any

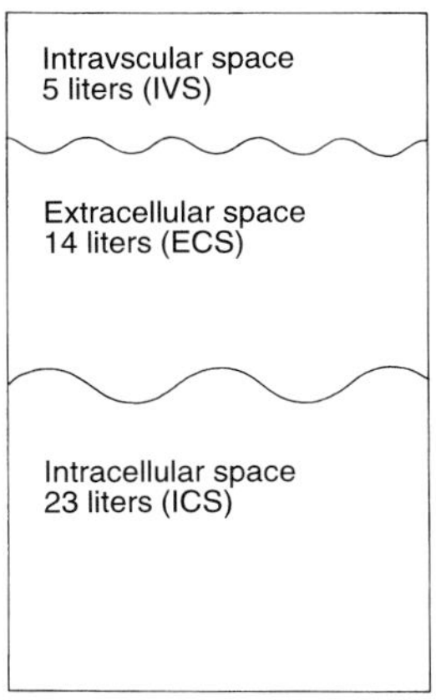

Fig. 68.2 The distribution of body water in an average adult woman.

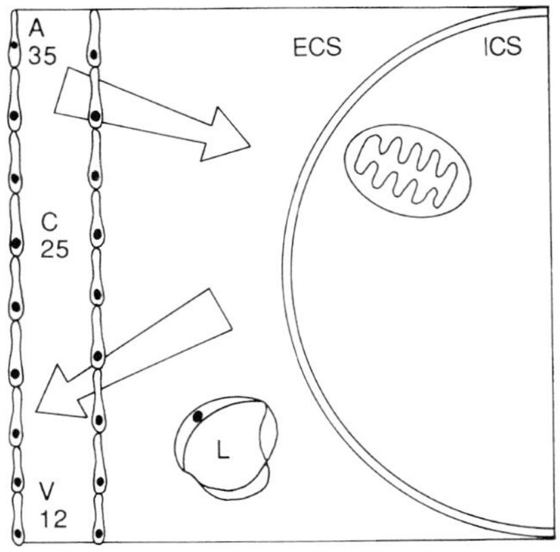

Fig. 68.3 A schematic representation of the microcirculation.

lactic acidosis. Successful restoration of tissue oxygenation is dependent on rapid fluid resuscitation and surgical control of hemorrhage.

If a pregnant patient suffers accidental acid aspiration, the resulting chemical burn to the capillary endothelium or any resulting systemic endotoxemia will inevitably lead to the development of an internal chemical burn. The destruction of the semipermeable membrane locally or body-wide will inevitably lead to a failure of tissue fluid homeostasis with the subsequent development of edema. The volume of fluid exiting the arteriolar end of the capillary will increase through imbalance of forces, and the reabsorption of fluid at the venous end of the capillary will effectively cease. Although lymphatic drainage will endeavor in the short-term to compensate for this imbalance, eventually local tissue water will increase. In the lung this leads to a deterioration in gas exchange with ensuing hypoxemia. In the tissues this leads to a distancing of the cellular apparatus from the capillary membrane exacerbating tissue hypoxia.

If the pregnant woman is allowed to remain supine, the gravid uterus can occlude the intra-abdominal vena cava, thereby preventing forward flow of blood. This will serve to both diminish cardiac output and hinder reabsorption of fluid from the venous end of the capillary as venous pressure rises. When venous end-capillary pressure rises by about 25 mmHg the reabsorption of fluid will have effectively ceased. The supine hypotensive syndrome of pregnancy must be avoided at all costs when resuscitating the critically ill obstetric patient by placing the patient's pelvis into the left lateral position with a wedge or bolster under the right hip.

HEMORRHAGIC SHOCK: THE CRYSTALLOID/COLLOID DEBATE

The pathophysiology of hemorrhage, sepsis and supine hypotension can be influenced deleteriously by injudicious fluid therapy, as outlined in Figure 68.4.[9]

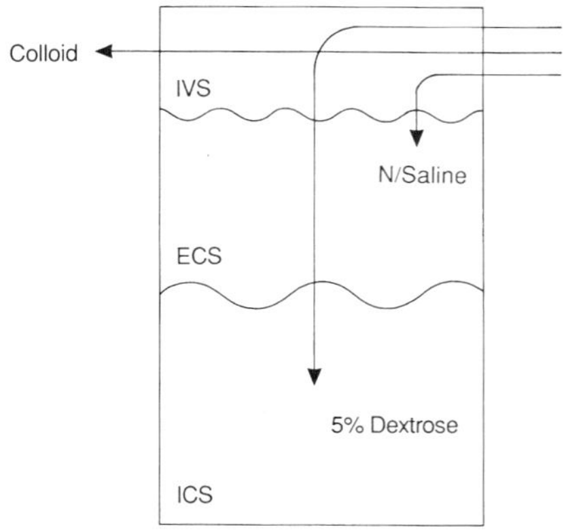

Fig. 68.4 A schematic representation of the effects of crystalloid and colloid resuscitation on various tissue spaces.

If a liter of normal saline is administered intravenously, some minutes after the infusion is complete there will have been a redistribution of this crystalloid solution through the body compartments. About one-tenth of this solution will remain intravascularly as measured by the heart rate, blood pressure, central venous pressure and pulmonary capillary wedge pressure. Nine-tenths will dissipate into the tissues and, since normal saline solution is hypernatremic relative to plasma, it preferentially expands the extracellular space where sodium is the predominant extracellular cation. Normal saline is, therefore, an extracellular expander.

If a liter of dextrose 5% is rapidly infused intravenously then the same redistribution of fluid from the intravascular space occurs, but since dextrose 5% contains only sugar in water the absence of ionic constituents means that it will distribute through the body compartments according to their relative volumes. Since the intracellular space is the largest of the body compartments (23 l) it is preferentially filled by dextrose solutions. Dextrose 5% is, therefore, an intracellular space expander. Unlike the intravascular space, there exist very poor markers for the integrity of the extracellular and intracellular spaces. The presence or absence of tissue edema with an assessment of tissue turgor and thirst are the vague indices of tissue hydration.

By way of contrast, the expansion of the intravascular space by colloidal solutions can be sensitively gauged by repeated measurements of central venous and PAOP. Blood, plasma and plasma substitutes such as Haemaccel and Gelofusin are intravascular expanders. However, administration of the last two solutions is complicated since they are subsequently metabolized to sugar and water with a variable saline content. After approximately 4 h they behave not as colloidal intravascular expanders but resuscitators of the extracellular and intracellular spaces.

THE MAINTENANCE OF TISSUE OXYGENATION DURING OBSTETRIC EMERGENCIES

Treatment priorities for the pregnant patient are the same as for the nonpregnant woman. The best therapy for the fetus is to treat the mother. The goal of resuscitation in critical illness is the maintenance of tissue oxygenation. For the pregnant patient with increased tissue oxygen needs because of the fetoplacental unit, this demands early attention to the airway and respiratory performance together with the restoration of cardiac output. Nevertheless, it must be emphasized that the management of life-threatening bleeding by the administration of supplementary oxygen, the rapid infusion of crystalloid, colloid or type-specific blood and the correction of any accompanying coagulopathy is doomed to fail unless definitive measures include surgical control of the hemorrhage. Furthermore, the simultaneous problems of hypovolemia and hypoxia are frequently misinterpreted during the early progression of aspiration pneumonitis. Similar difficulties are encountered in the patient with preeclamptic toxemia.

PREECLAMPSIA

Preeclampsia and eclampsia are the commonest causes of maternal death in the western world.[4,10] The fundamental disorders in toxemia of pregnancy are increased arterial reactivity with generalized vasoconstriction. Adrenergic hyperactivity may be compensatory as well as aggravatory; intravascular volume reduction results from increased intravascular tone and capillary permeability. Platelet activation and fibrin deposition complicate the microangiopathy with renal, pulmonary and cerebral circulations variably involved. Eclampsia complicates the severe clinical disorder, not necessarily the very high blood pressure, and reflects neuromuscular hyperreactivity. It is usually accompanied by cerebral edema and intracranial hemorrhages.[11]

Intensive care specialists routinely manage patients with cerebral edema following blunt head trauma. Therapy is directed to optimize the cerebral blood volume and control intracranial pressure. Factors that influence cerebral blood flow are shown in Figure 68.5. Most head injury protocols stipulate that unconscious patients who have suffered severe head trauma are electively intubated and hyperventilated to control oxygenation and prevent hypercarbia. The blood pressure is carefully monitored following arterial cannulation. Circulating volume is restored with colloidal solutions while simultaneously attempting to limit tissue edema by restricting crystalloid administration. This approach is facilitated by frequent measurement of central venous pressure or PAOP. Seizures are prevented by the administration of antiepileptic drugs. The patient is managed head up with a dedicated nurse in close attendance.

Such practice runs contrary to the traditional management of the preeclamptic patient who used to be heavily sedated and nursed flat in a darkened room. The preferred sedative in the UK used to be diazepam or heminervin.

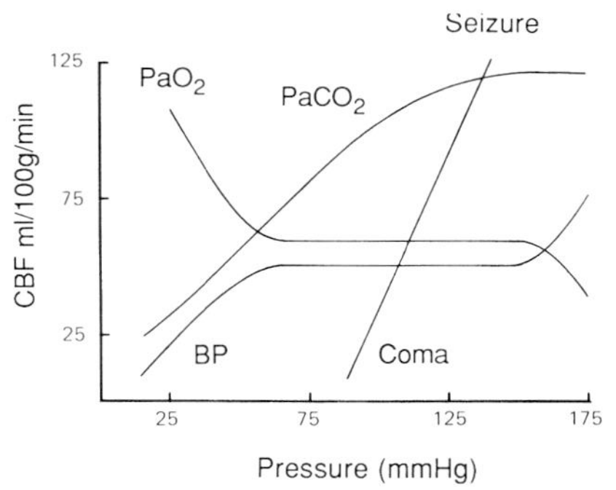

Fig. 68.5 Factors influencing cerebral blood flow.

Although the latter is an excellent antiepileptic, it has to be infused intravenously in a carrier solution of crystalloid solution. Large volumes could, therefore, be unwittingly prescribed to these women, exacerbating cerebral, pulmonary and tissue edema. The control of hypertension in the context of a reduced circulating volume was frequently bolus doses of vasodilators such as hydralazine. Fundamentally, clinicians have remained unable to reliably predict those who may have seizures so that 75% of all eclamptic seizures still occur in hospital in the UK. The mortality from preeclampsia/eclampsia has remained unchanged since 1972 (Fig. 68.1).

In the light of our new understanding of the pathophysiology of preeclampsia and experience with managing other conditions characterized by leaking capillary membranes, diminished intravascular volume and tissue edema, a multidisciplinary approach to the management of preeclamptic patients is rapidly evolving in centers that care for large numbers of such patients. Patients may benefit from admission to high-dependency nursing units if they require intravenous antihypertensive medication monitored with indwelling intra-arterial and central venous pressure lines. Antihypertensive medication should be continuously infused and bolus administration should be avoided. Increasingly, sublingual nifedipine is being prescribed, whereas hitherto clinicians might have administered intravenous hydralazine or labetalol.[12] Relative systolic hypertension is tolerated in the early post-partum hours, as is appropriate oliguria with documented high urinary osmolality. Crystalloid solutions are restricted to 1.2 l/day and repletion of intravascular volume is slowly undertaken with judicious colloid administration until a spontaneous diuresis is observed. Indications for a pulmonary artery flotation catheter are pulmonary edema, profound oliguria (less than 0.5 ml/kg/h) despite fluid challenge and severe uncontrollable hypertension.

Eclamptic patients are electively ventilated post-partum for 24 h or until such time as recovery of consciousness is demonstrated clinically in many centers in the UK. Patients with antenatal hypertension, proteinuria and hyperreflexia currently receive phenytoin 15 mg per kg body weight intravenously as a loading dose at 25 mg/min under ECG monitoring.[13] A second dose of 500 mg is administered orally or intravenously 12 h later and then maintenance therapy with 300 mg daily in divided doses is prescribed together with rantidine 150 mg orally every 6 h by way of prophylaxis against acid aspiration syndrome. Should surgical delivery of the fetus be necessary, then 0.3 M sodium citrate is administered in the anesthetic room together with the implementation of an anesthetic protocol for the operative management of these women. This restricts the use of epidural blockade because of the attendant risks of coagulopathy and raised intracranial pressure.

MISCELLANEOUS

There are numerous medical conditions which carry increased risk for the pregnant woman and her fetus, e.g. cardiopulmonary diseases, diabetes and sickle cell disease. There are emergencies which may involve the pregnant women, e.g. trauma, hemorrhage, cardiopulmonary collapse and pulmonary embolism.[14]

CONCLUSION

There is heated debate regarding the relative merits of some regimens over other protocols, e.g. magnesium sulfate versus phenytoin therapy in pregnancy-induced hypertension; routine prophylaxis against acid aspiration and the crystalloid versus colloid controversy. The aim of intensive care management, nevertheless, is to maintain patients in as near normal physiologic condition as possible until the risk of multiple organ shutdown is diminished and recovery under way. Successive triennial Reports on Confidential Enquiries into Maternal Deaths in England and Wales have sought to highlight recurring shortcomings and unacceptable patterns of care for women with life-threatening complications of pregnancy. ICU admission is just as warranted for the woman with a pregnancy-associated emergency as any other critically ill patient.

REFERENCES

1. Graham S G, Luxton M C 1989 The requirement for intensive care support for the pregnant population. Anesthesia 44: 581–584
2. Yau E H S, Groves P A, Wathen N C, Watson J D 1990 The requirement for intensive care support for the pregnant population. Anesthesia 45: 65–66
3. Hughes R L 1990 The requirement for intensive care support for the pregnant population. Anesthesia 45: 65
4. Department of Health 1991 Report on Confidential Enquiries into Maternal Deaths in the United Kingdom 1985–1987. HMSO, London
5. Tordoff S G, Sweeney B P 1990 Acid aspiration prophylaxis in 288

obstetric anesthetic departments in the United Kingdom. Anesthesia 45: 776–780
6. Gillett G B, Watson J D, Langford R M 1984 Ranitidine and single-dose antacid therapy as prophylaxis against acid aspiration syndrome in obstetric practice. Anesthesia 39: 638–644
7. Mendelson C L 1946 Aspiration of stomach contents into lungs during obstetric anesthesia. Am J Obstet Gynecol 52: 191–205
8. Marshall J 1992 The gut–liver axis in multiple organ failure. In: Lamy M, Thijs L G (eds) Intensive care and emergency medicine, Vol 16. Springer, Berlin, pp 220–238
9. Twigley A J, Hillman K M 1985 The end of the crystalloid era? A new approach to peri-operative fluid administration. Anaesthesia 40: 860–871
10. Kaunitz A M, Hughes J M, Grimes D A, Smith J, Rochat R W, Kafrissen M E 1985 Causes of maternal mortality in the United States. Obstet Gynaecol 65: 605–612
11. Redman C W G 1988 Eclampsia still kills. Br Med J 296: 1209–1210
12. Fenakel K, Fenakel G, Appelman Z, Lurie S, Katz Z, Shotam Z 1991 Nifedipine in the treatment of severe preeclampsia. Obstet Gynecol 77: 331–337
13. Slater R M, Smith W D, Patrick J et al 1987 Phenytoin infusion in severe pre-eclampsia. Lancet 1: 1417–1421
14. Kilpatrick S J, Matthay M A 1992 Obstetric patients requiring critical care. A five year review. Chest 101: 1407–1412

HEMODYNAMIC CHANGES IN THE HELLP SYNDROME – A CASE REPORT

Compiled in the Departments of Anaesthesia and Intensive Care Medicine, St Bartholomew's Hospital at Homerton, London

INTRODUCTION

Preeclamptic toxemia (PET) is a disease of pregnancy characterized by hypertension, proteinuria and edema which may progress to generalized convulsions up to 48 h after delivery of fetus and placenta. Fulminant PET patients may require admission to the intensive care unit for invasive cardiovascular monitoring, intravenous antihypertensive medication, intermittent positive-pressure ventilation and the control of convulsions. We report a case of a patient with severe PET complicated by the syndrome of hemolysis, elevated liver enzymes and low platelet count (HELLP) who required invasive hemodynamic monitoring.

CASE REPORT

A 28-year-old moderately obese Asian woman (G5, P3, height 165 cm, weight 75 kg) presented to the delivery suite at 33 weeks' gestation complaining of severe frontal headache, epigastric pain and vomiting. She was confused and agitated with marked hyperreflexia, peripheral edema, and with a blood pressure of 230/130 mmHg together with a tender epigastrium. Catheterization resulted in the drainage of only 3 ml of urine. Investigations revealed a hemoglobin concentration of 13.3 g/dl, a platelet count of 137×10^6 and a normal coagulation screen. Biochemical analysis showed a serum sodium concentration of 136 mol/l, potassium of 3.5 mmol/l, urea of 6.0 mmol/l and a urate of 0.45 mmol/l. Urinalysis demonstrated +++ proteinuria.

Hydralazine was commenced at 3 mg/h by intravenous infusion and a loading dose of phenytoin (15 mg/kg) was administered by slow intravenous infusion. The fetal heart rate fell to 90 bpm with slow recovery. The decision was taken to perform an emergency cesarean delivery for fetal distress and the patient was premedicated with 150 mg of ranitidine orally and 10 mg of metoclopramide by intramuscular injection. She was transferred to the adjacent anesthetic room lying in the left lateral position, with 4 l/min oxygen administered via a face mask.

The left radial artery was cannulated under local anesthesia in the anesthetic room and 25 ml of 0.3 M sodium citrate was given orally prior to 3 min of acute oxygenation/denitrogenation. Anesthesia was induced by rapid-sequence injection of midazolam 2 mg and thiopental 350 mg followed by succinylcholine 100 mg to facilitate tracheal intubation. It was noted that there was only minimal glottic edema. Anesthesia was maintained with oxygen, nitrous oxide and isoflurane and further neuromuscular relaxation was provided by atracurium. A left internal jugular catheter was inserted with difficulty after failure to identify the right internal jugular vein.

A live female infant was delivered operatively and required intubation and ventilatory support because of persistent bradycardia. Following delivery, maternal anesthesia was maintained by an opioid-relaxant sequence. At the end of surgery the trachea was extubated when the patient awoke and she was then transferred to the intensive therapy unit (ITU).

On admission to the ITU, she was drowsy and hyperreflexic with flexor plantar responses. She was hypertensive despite receiving 3 mg/h hydralazine. She was anuric with a central venous pressure measured at 3 mmHg. The abdomen was tender but the uterus was well contracted following oxytocin administration. A higher dose of hydralazine (10 mg/h) was required to control hypertension; the pulse rate rose to 140 bpm, and this was controlled with intravenous propranolol 2 mg. She remained anuric. 12 h following admission, the hemoglobin concentration and the platelet count had fallen with prolongation of the INR and a rise in the thrombin time. In addition, a dextrose and insulin infusion was required to control a rising serum potassium concentration and calcium resonium was given per rectum. Hematologic advice was sought and her consumptive coagulopathy was treated with blood, fresh-frozen plasma and platelet transfusions.

The patient was by now increasingly restless with a nonproductive cough and the blood pressure had again become increasingly difficult to control. Pulse oximetry showed progressive arterial desaturation despite increasing the inspired oxygen concentration. Coarse crepitations could be heard throughout both lung fields and the chest radiograph confirmed the presence of pulmonary edema. The arterial $Pa\text{O}_2$ was 48 mmHg (6.4 kPa). Intubation and ventilation followed intravenous injection of 100 mg of lidocaine, 1 mg of fentanyl, 20 mg of etomidate and 100 mg of succinylcholine. The glottis was not edematous and intubation, with cricoid pressure, was uncomplicated. After intubation the patient became hypotensive and the hydralazine infusion was discontinued, but this was only a temporary event and subsequent hypertension required reinstitution of hydralazine. A pulmonary artery catheter was inserted via the left internal jugular route and this demonstrated a pulmonary artery occlusion pressure (PAOP) of 14 mmHg, a surprisingly low cardiac index (CI) of 2.2 l/min/m^2 and an initial systemic vascular resistance index (SVRI) of 2683 dynes. sec/cm^5/m^2, which subsequently rose to over 4000 dynes. sec/cm^5/m^2. It was decided to discontinue the hydralazine administration and commence an infusion of sodium nitroprusside. This resulted in an immediate and substantial fall in SVRI and blood pressure and a dramatic rise in CI and left ventricular stroke work index (LVSWI). The changes in blood pressure and SVRI are shown in Figure 68.6. The changes in CI and LVSWI are shown in Figure 68.7.

Despite improved hemodynamics the patient remained oliguric. The serum potassium concentration remained elevated despite dextrose and insulin infusion and ion-exchange resins. Continuous arteriovenous diafiltration was started via an arteriovenous fistula fashioned in the right forearm. The coagulopathy continued to be a source

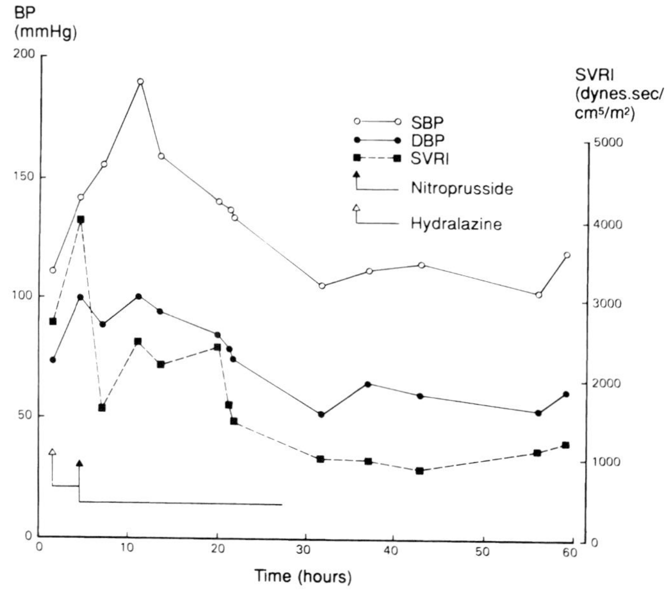

Fig. 68.6 Changes in systolic (SBP) and diastolic (DBP) blood pressure and systemic vascular resistance index (SVRI) in patient and the response to hydralazine and sodium nitroprusside treatment.

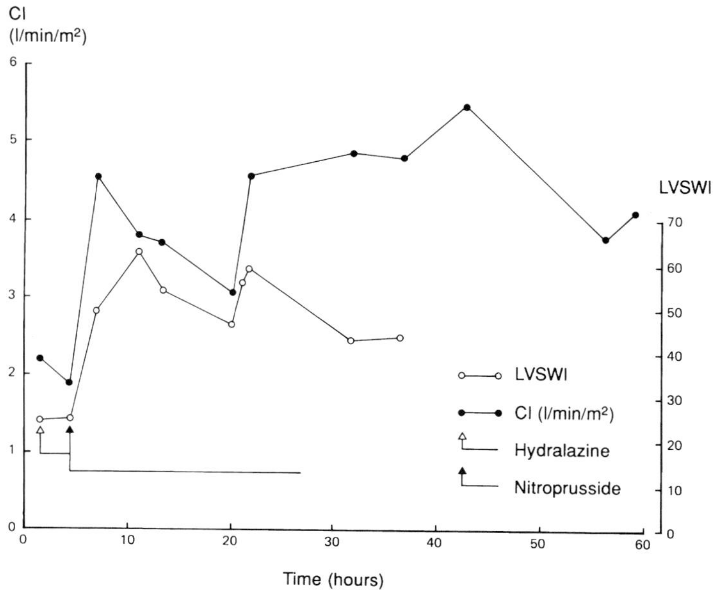

Fig. 68.7 Changes in cardiac index (CI) and left ventricular stroke work index (LVSWI) in patient in response to hydralazine and sodium nitroprusside treatment.

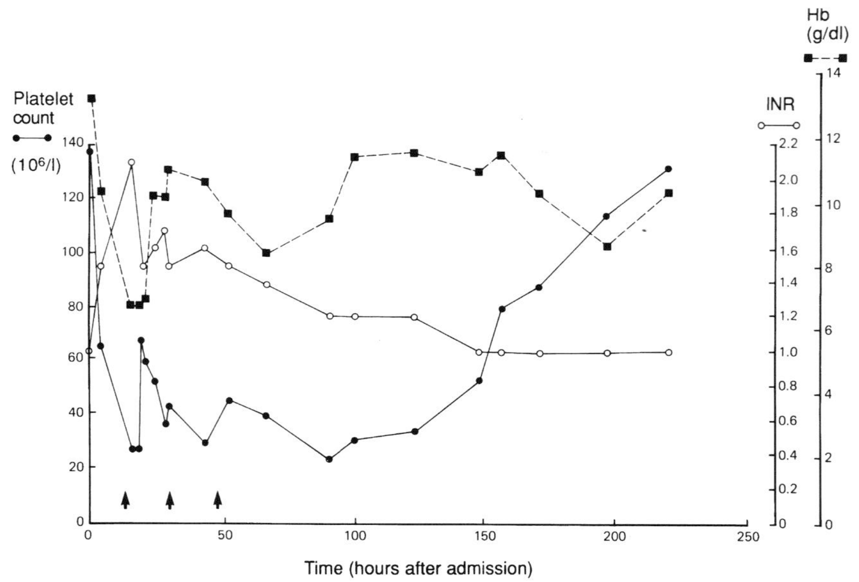

Fig. 68.8 Changes in hemoglobin concentration, coagulation status (INR) and platelet count in patient.

of concern. The changes in her hemoglobin, international normalized ratio and platelet count are shown in Figure 68.8. Analysis of the serum showed the presence of hemolysis and a diagnosis of the HELLP syndrome was made since, although liver function tests were not available, the patient had become clinically jaundiced. The first measured liver function test 50 h after admission demonstrated the serum bilirubin to be 221 μmol/1 and the aspartate aminotransferase (AST) was 1440 IU/C. The changes in her serum AST concentrations can be seen in Figure 68.9. Retrospective analysis of serum from the time of admission showed that the serum AST had been elevated at 435 IU/C but the bilirubin had been normal at the time of presentation to hospital.

During the course of the following week, daily ultrasound scans of the liver failed to demonstrate hepatic congestion or subcapsular hematomata and serum bilirubin and AST levels reached a plateau. Phenytoin was discontinued after 5 days with normal therapeutic levels. She progressed to the polyuric phase of acute renal failure and was weaned from the ventilator.

Fourteen days after admission she was discharged from the ITU to the care of the nephrologists with a residual low creatinine clearance. Subsequent investigations demonstrated a negative anti-neutrophil cytoplasmic antibody but positive anti-Ro antibodies suggestive of systemic lupus erythematosus (SLE). She was also positive for anti-thyroid antibodies. The infant was found to have a congenital tricuspid stenosis, complete heart block and was also positive for anti-Ro antibodies.

In conclusion, clinical protocols should emphasize the importance of a multidisciplinary approach to the management of the preeclamptic patient. This is in line with recommendations following Reports on Confidential Enquiries into Maternal Deaths in England and Wales. We report a patient with HELLP syndrome whose early referral and transfer to a general intensive care unit according to such a protocol enabled prompt institution of invasive cardiovascular monitoring and multiple system support. We believe this contributed to her survival.

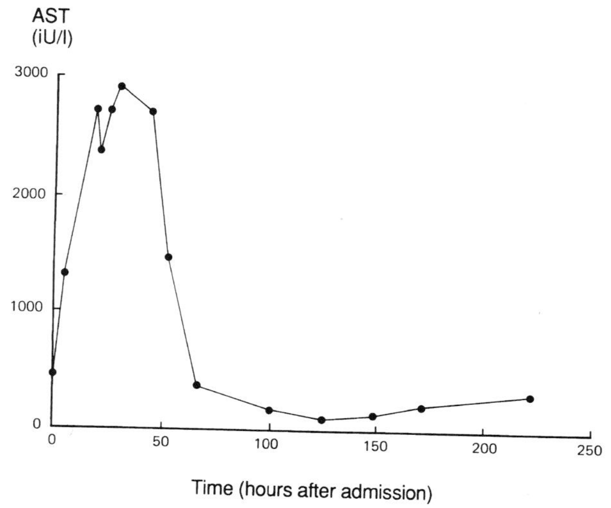

Fig. 68.9 Changes in serum aspartate transaminase concentrations (AST) in patient.

ACKNOWLEDGEMENTS

We would like to thank Mr N Wathen for his permission to present his patient, the King's Liver Unit for their helpful advice and the nursing staff of the Intensive Care Unit at St Bartholomew's at Homerton, London, for their assistance.

69. Regional anesthesia in obstetric patients with previous spinal surgery

L. A. Hortvet

A history of previous major spinal surgery is considered by some anesthesiologists to be a relative contraindication to intraspinal anesthesia because of questions regarding its safety and efficacy. The guidelines are unclear because the available literature concerning the topic is very limited.

In the North American population, the prevalence of scoliosis is approximately 0.4%. Spinal curves of less than 10° are equally common in males and females, whereas curves of greater than 20°, which require treatment are seven times more frequent in females.[1] Idiopathic scoliosis is more common than other causes, which include neurologic diseases (poliomyelitis, neurofibromatosis, cerebral palsy), myopathic disorders (muscular dystrophy, myotonic dystrophy), connective tissue disorders (rheumatoid arthritis, Marfan's syndrome), vertebral anomalies and infection (particularly tuberculosis).[2] Thoracolumbar curves are more common than isolated thoracic or lumbar curvature. The severity of the disease is determined by measuring the degree of spinal curvature. Curves of greater than 60°, if untreated, can lead to cardiopulmonary compromise, progressive deformity, and early death due to cardiorespiratory failure.

In female parturients with untreated scoliosis, pregnancy may exacerbate both the degree of spinal curvature and the extent of cardiopulmonary compromise. Maternal morbidity and mortality correlate well with the severity of functional impairment that existed in the prepregnant state. Patients who have undergone corrective surgery for scoliosis tolerate pregnancy, labor and delivery well, although the incidence of operative delivery in these patients is 2.4 times greater than that for normal parturients.[2]

Treatment for scoliosis is most frequently sought because of symptoms of back pain, but also for curve progression, poor body image and deterioration of pulmonary function.[3] In a skeletally immature patient, spinal curves of less than 40–45° are usually best treated with an orthotic device, whereas curves of greater than 45–50° are usually managed by spinal fusion with internal fixation.[4] The object of spinal fusion is to create a bony fusion of the spinal curve that should include all rotated vertebrae.

In 1947, Paul R. Harrington began to develop his surgical treatment for scoliosis while working with poliomyelitis patients, among whom he saw a high prevalence of spinal deformities and pulmonary compromise. He developed the Harrington instrumentation as a means of halting progression and gaining correction of the spinal deformity. This technique consists of decortication of the laminae and transverse processes followed by removal of the spinous processes together with the interspinous soft tissue. Next, a distraction and compression system is applied. This system comprises a smooth distraction rod with ratchets at its upper end, a threaded compression rod with hooks locked into position by twisting nuts on the threaded rod and a selection of hooks. Afterward, facets are fused in the thoracic area and lateral transverse processes are fused in the lumbar region; then an autogenous iliac bone graft is added. Newer methods of spinal fusion include the Lugue and Cotrel–Dubousset techniques.[4]

Spinal fusion should not be extended caudally to L4, because fusion to L5 is associated with a high incidence of low back pain at long-term follow-up. Harrington fusion to L5 or S1 also produces an unacceptable loss of lumbar lordosis and increases stress on the lower back. Idiopathic scoliosis does not involve L5 or S1, so fusion to these levels is not necessary.[4]

Early surgical correction (prior to adulthood) results in significant increases in lung volume post-operatively and prevents the cardiopulmonary complications. The degree of curvature is reduced by 50%, and 85–90% of back pain is relieved. There may be a long-term increased incidence of degenerative disease due to a reduction in the number of mobile lumbar spinal segments, which leads to increased mechanical stress on those segments below the level of fusion.[2] Other complications are most commonly perioperative, due to anesthetic complications or to cord injury (less than 0.5% of cases), direct trauma, vascular compromise or overdistraction with neurologic impairment. Early post-operative complications include wound infection; pulmonary, gastrointestinal, and urinary problems; and hook dislodgment. Late post-operative problems include failure to produce a solid spinal arthrodesis, which results in increased stress on the rod, metal fatigue and rod breakage and bursitis.[4]

EPIDURAL ANESTHESIA

Epidural anesthesia after major spinal surgery has been considered as relatively contraindicated because of a number of potential complications. The epidural space may be difficult to identify because of surgical and degenerative changes. Insertion of a needle through a midline or lateral approach in the fused region may not be possible because of the presence of scar tissue and bone graft. Ideally, the needle should be inserted below the lowest fused segment, however this area often undergoes retrolisthesis and spondylolisthesis; furthermore, 20% of patients have fusions involving L4–L5.[2] Multiple attempts may be necessary for successful epidural placement. Surgical obliteration of the epidural space may lead to unintentional dural puncture. An epidural blood patch may be difficult to perform if a significant post-dural puncture headache results. Blood vessel trauma may also be more likely to occur. There is a possibility of introducing infection during the procedure, which is of particular concern in these patients because of the presence of a foreign body. There may be unpredictable spread of local anesthetic, resulting in a 'patchy' block. This is attributed to injury to the ligamentum flavum during surgery, which causes adhesions or obliteration of the epidural space in some areas. An increased volume or concentration of local anesthetic may be required to achieve an adequate block.[2] Patients with idiopathic scoliosis or neuromyopathic syndromes that predispose to scoliosis may have an increased incidence of malignant hyperthermia. Significant respiratory compromise may occur if intercostal muscles are paralyzed as a result of a high level of anesthesia. Persistent back pain may exist even after surgical correction of scoliosis, and pregnancy may exacerbate this problem. Coincidental exacerbation of musculoskeletal or neurologic symptoms secondary to the underlying disorder may be attributed to the epidural anesthetic, which may pose a medicolegal issue. Finally, these patients have a high degree of anxiety regarding their backs and they may be reluctant to consent to epidural anesthesia.

The significance of most of these potential complications of epidural anesthesia is *not* supported by the limited literature that exists. In 1985, Hubbert[5] discussed his experience with attempted epidural anesthesia in 17 obstetric patients with Harrington rod spinal fusion. Nine attempts resulted in epidural anesthesia, whereas two resulted in unintentional dural puncture. Numerous 'false' losses of resistance were encountered and 11 patients underwent multiple attempts at various interspaces, using both midline and lateral approaches. In one patient, blood was encountered in each of three attempts. The volume and concentration of local anesthetic required to produce an adequate epidural block did not differ from patients without spinal fusion, and no patients reported post-partum back pain or other complications.

In 1989, Crosby and Halpern[2] reported a retrospective study of 16 patients with previous Harrington rod instrumentation for correction of idiopathic scoliosis who requested epidural anesthesia for labor. Of the nine epidural procedures, four required multiple attempts and two never received adequate anesthesia. Complications included failure to identify the epidural space despite attempts at two interspaces, blood vessel trauma and dural puncture. 38% of their patients required operative delivery.

Daley et al,[6] in 1990, reviewed their experience with 18 patients who had a history of previous major spinal surgery and who requested epidural anesthesia for labor. 15 of 21 attempts produced satisfactory anesthesia; however, four patients required larger than usual doses of local anesthetic. No correlation was seen between the ease of insertion or quality of anesthesia and the surgical level.

Feldstein and Ramanathan,[1] in 1985, reported successful lumbar epidural anesthesia for labor and cesarean delivery in three patients with a history of extensive spinal surgery. They found no difference in onset of action, spread, dose requirement, highest sensory level achieved or duration of action of local anesthetic from that expected for normal parturients.

In 1978, Carlson et al[7] reported a successful epidural anesthetic for cesarean delivery in a 25-year-old woman with severe, uncorrected idiopathic kyphoscoliosis. As they discussed, lesions of the lumbar spine may cause changes in the pelvic architecture severe enough to lead to dystocia. Thoracic spinal lesions may cause disorders of normal cardiac and pulmonary function that are exacerbated as a result of the normal rise in cardiac output during pregnancy and labor as well as the encroachment of the enlarging uterus on the nondistensible thorax, which does not allow the normal increase in maternal alveolar ventilation to occur. Carlson et al suggested several advantages of epidural anesthesia for patients with scoliosis: avoidance of the use of respiratory depressants such as opioids during labor; minimization of the undesirable rise in cardiac output during labor; and a means of providing post-operative analgesia, which attenuates the reduction in vital capacity that normally follows abdominal surgery because of pain-induced limitation of respiratory excursion.[7]

Few large studies involve epidural anesthesia for obstetric patients after major spinal surgery. However, the existing literature fails to show any long-term complications due to the procedure. Despite the potential short-term complications, the available reports indicate that epidural anesthesia is safe and usually effective for these patients.[3,8–11]

An antepartum anesthetic consultation is necessary in order to discuss anesthetic and analgesic options with the patient in a relatively stress-free environment. The patient must be advised of the potential difficulties of epidural needle insertion as well as the lack of evidence for long-term adverse sequelae. Furthermore, the prelabor consultation affords the anesthesiologist an opportunity to obtain a complete history and physical examination, which should include documentation of existing low back pain, or cardiopulmonary or neurologic dysfunction. Spine radiographs and operative reports should be obtained to determine the lowest level of fused vertebrae. If these are not available, the lower extent of spinal surgery must be estimated based on patient history (which is often unreliable) and physical examination. No spinous processes will be palpable in the fused region, and the incisional scar usually extends to one level below the lowest level of the fusion.

Many spinal fusions have the appearance of Swiss cheese on radiographic examination. The midline approach to the epidural space may not be possible with an appliance in place. However, it is a reasonable approach in the patient with a long fusion, particularly in the lower lumbar area, even when no spinous processes are palpable.

Patients with a history of major spinal surgery should *not* be automatically denied epidural anesthesia for labor and delivery. Insertion of the epidural needle and catheter may be attempted, providing that the patient and anesthesiologist are both aware of the increased incidence of short-term complications and of the possibility of failure to obtain satisfactory anesthesia.

SUBARACHNOID ANESTHESIA

Although some anesthesiologists avoid subarachnoid anesthesia in obstetric patients who have undergone previous spinal surgery, the limited available literature suggests that subarachnoid anesthesia is a safe and effective alternative to general anesthesia for these patients. In 1980, Berkowitz and Gold[12] performed 42 successful subarachnoid anesthetics in patients with previous lumbar laminectomies without complications. Interestingly, they pointed out that, while some anesthesiologists are reluctant to perform subarachnoid anesthesia in patients with previous spinal surgery, radiologists routinely perform myelograms in patients with laminectomies or spinal fusions, injecting a radiopaque dye into the subarachnoid space. In Hubbert's 1985 report[13] on epidural anesthesia for patients with spinal fusions, two out of 17 patients received adequate subarachnoid anesthesia (after unintentional dural puncture or unsuccessful epidural placement) without complications.

Subarachnoid anesthesia is a useful alternative for obstetric patients with previous spinal surgery after an unintentional dural puncture occurs or when epidural placement is unsuccessful. Furthermore, subarachnoid blocks may have some advantages over epidural anesthesia. Subarachnoid injection may be technically easier in these patients, due to disruption of the epidural space by surgery or degenerative changes. A subarachnoid anesthetic may also provide a more reliable and complete spread of local anesthetic solution with less likelihood of obtaining a 'patchy' block, as is sometimes seen with epidural anesthesia (thought to be secondary to adhesions and obliteration of areas of the epidural space). In 1990, Moran and Johnson,[14] while administering continuous spinal anesthesia to an obstetric patient with severe kyphoscoliosis and congenital heart disease, found that a distortion of the spinal column may cause an alteration in the normal gravity-directed distribution of hyperbaric local anesthetic solution in the cerebrospinal fluid. They suggested that the local anesthetic layers in the dependent areas of the spinal column caused a unilateral block that they were able to raise by the addition of an isobaric local anesthetic solution. Bozeman and Chandra,[15] in 1980, explained this phenomenon on the basis of Valentino's myelography, which showed a unilateral distribution of contrast in patients with severe scoliosis. They proposed that the dura on the convex side of the spine stretches, which presses the spinal cord against the opposite surface of the spinal canal, squeezing the subarachnoid space between the spinal canal wall and the cord. This would hinder movement of local anesthetic in the subarachnoid space. Discrepancies have also been found in the height of the block that can be achieved with both epidural and subarachnoid anesthesia despite utilization of a number of maneuvers to raise the level of the block.

Subarachnoid and epidural anesthesia carry similar risks of complications, such as blood vessel trauma (possibly less for subarachnoid anesthesia because of the smaller needle size), subdural catheter placement (particularly after multiple attempts or dural puncture),[16] introduction of infection, respiratory compromise due to intercostal muscle paralysis, coincident exacerbation of low back pain during labor and delivery and patient anxiety. An additional disadvantage to subarachnoid anesthesia may be the difficulty in performing an epidural blood patch on these patients should a significant post-dural puncture headache occur. For this reason, the smallest possible spinal needle should be used. Subarachnoid opioids or low-concentration local anesthetic solutions may also be administered via a continuous subarachnoid catheter. Such a catheter may actually reduce the incidence of post-dural puncture headache by creating an inflammatory reaction, which seals the hole in the dura after the catheter is removed, thus preventing cerebrospinal fluid leakage into the epidural space. Because of the greater ease of insertion and more reliable anesthesia, subarachnoid anesthesia may be preferable to epidural anesthesia for cesarean delivery, and may be used for labor (with a subarachnoid catheter and small doses of lipophilic opioid with or wihtout low concentrations of hyperbaric local anesthetic) in obstetric patients with previous major spinal surgery.

REFERENCES

1. Feldstein G, Ramanathan S 1985 Obstetric lumbar epidural anesthesia in patients with previous posterior spinal fusion for kyphoscoliosis. Anesth Analg 64: 83
2. Crosby E T, Halpern S H 1989 Obstetric epidural anesthesia in patients with Harrington instrumentation. Can J Anaesth 36: 693
3. VanDam B E 1988 Operative treatment of adult scoliosis with posterior fusion and instrumentation. Orthop Clin North Am 19: 353
4. Renshaw T S 1988 The role of Harrington instrumentation and posterior spine fusion in the management of adolescent idiopathic scoliosis. Orthop Clin North Am 19: 257
5. Hubbert C H 1985 Epidural anesthesia in patients with spinal fusion. Anesth Analg 64: 843
6. Daley M D, Rolbin S, Hew E, Morningstar B 1990 Continuous epidural anesthesia for obstetrics after major spinal surgery. Can J Anaesth 37: S112
7. Carlson W, Engelman D R, Bart J 1978 Epidural anesthesia for cesarean section in kyphoscoliosis. Anesth Analg 57: 125
8. Crawford J S, James F M, Nolte H et al 1981 Regional analgesia for patients with chronic neurological disease and similar conditions. Anesthesia 36: 821
9. King H A 1988 Selection of fusion levels for posterior instrumentation and fusion in idiopathic scoliosis. Orthop Clin North Am 19: 247
10. Vaagenes P, Fjaerestad I 1981 Epidural block during labour in a patient with spina bifida cystica. Anesthesia 36: 299
11. Walpole J B 1974 Continuous lumbar epidural block in labour in the presence of a Meurig Williams plate from L1–L4. Br J Anaesth 46: 163
12. Berkowitz S, Gold M I 1980 Spinal anesthesia for surgery in patients with previous lumbar laminectomy. Anesth Analg 59: 881
13. Hubbert C H 1985 Epidural anesthesia in patients with spinal fusion. Anesth Analg 64: 843
14. Moran D H, Johnson M D 1990 Continuous spinal anesthesia with combined hyperbaric and isobaric bupivacaine in a patient with scoliosis. Anesth Analg 70: 445
15. Bozeman P M, Chandra P 1980 Unilateral analgesia following epidural and subarachnoid block. Anesthesiology 52: 356
16. Howard R, Anderson W 1990 Subdural catheterization and opiate administration in a patient with Harrington rods. Can J Anaesth 37: 712

70. Kyphoscoliosis and pregnancy

E. Margaria   I. Castelletti   S. Treves

The association of kyphoscoliosis and pregnancy presents potentially serious problems for mother and baby.[1] Kyphoscoliosis causes deformed lungs with a limited capacity to provide proper oxygenation, causing strain and damage to the heart.

According to Chapman,[2] the average life span of patients with scoliosis is 30 years. In Jensen's study[3] of 50 pregnant women with kyphoscoliosis, all of whom died, 26.2% were 29 or under, while 73.8% were 30 or over.

An extremely important factor in the prognosis is vital capacity. Usually[4] it decreases during pregnancy: the rigidity of the thoracic cage limits pulmonary expansion, whilst, at the same time, diaphragmatic flattening results in poor 'abdominal' respiration. Fearl[5] stated that thoracic surgeons consider a vital capacity of 1000–1200 ml to be the lower limit for surgery. Patients with vital capacity lower than this are at increased risk. Dugan[6] presented a case review of a 36-year-old woman with a severe kyphoscoliosis and a vital capacity of 600 ml. She died 5 h after the vaginal delivery of a living

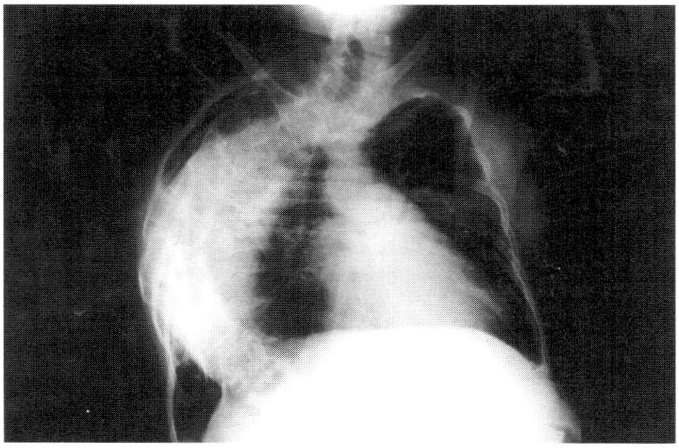

Fig. 70.1 Anteroposterior radiogram of the thorax of the patient.

A: Test - Results Vicatest - 5EU

DAT : 060691   Wt KG : 43
PT NO : 12   HT CM : 147
TEMP : 18   M/F : F
A Y : 32

	Expiration			Inspiration		
PAR.	ACT.	NORM.	%	ACT.	NORM.	%
IVC	-	2.80	-	-	2.80	-
FVC	0.85	2.79	30	0.77	2.79	28
FV0.5	0.57	1.81	31	0.42	-	-
FV1	0.68	2.41	28	0.61	2.20	28
FV3	0.82	2.71	30	0.76	-	-
FV1%	80	75	107	79	-	-
FV1/VC	-	83	-	-	-	-
MVV	20	97	21	-	-	-
PF	2.9	6.0	48	1.0	-	-
MF75%	2.9	5.5	53	0.2	-	-
MF50%	0.8	4.0	20	0.5	-	-
MF25%	0.2	1.9	11	1.0	-	-
MMF	0.5	3.7	14	0.5	-	-
MEF50%/MIF50%			160			

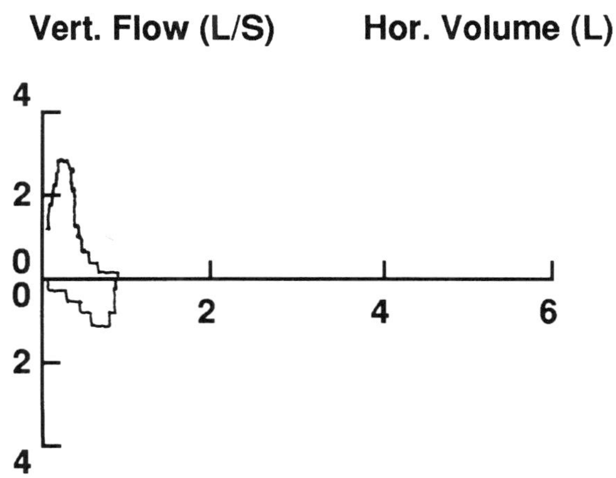

Fig. 70.2 (A) Respiratory values in patient.

B: Test - Results Vicatest - 5EU

DAT : 309091 Wt KG : 50
PT NO : 12 HT CM : 155
TEMP : 22 M/F : F
A Y : 29

PAR.	Expiration ACT.	NORM.	%	Inspiration ACT.	NORM.	%
IVC	-	3.25	-	-	3.25	-
FVC	3.56	3.22	111	3.49	3.22	108
FV0.5	2.50	2.09	120	1.92	-	-
FV1	3.07	2.80	110	3.43	2.61	131
FV3	3.43	3.12	110	3.49	-	-
FV1%	86	80	108	98	-	-
FV1/VC	-	84	-	-	-	-
MVV	92	106	87	-	-	-
PF	7.4	6.5	114	3.9	-	-
MF75%	7.4	5.9	125	3.4	-	-
MF50%	4.2	4.2	100	3.1	-	-
MF25%	1.5	2.0	75	3.9	-	-
MMF	3.7	3.9	95	3.4	-	-
MEF50%/MIF50%			135			

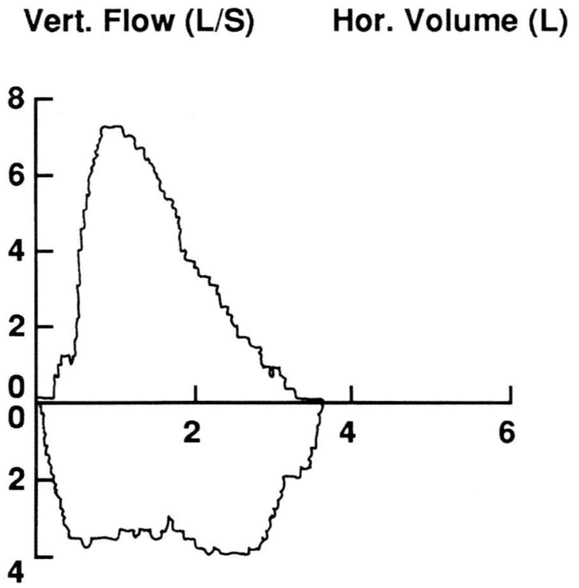

Fig. 70.2 (B) Respiratory values of a normal subject of similar age and weight.

male infant with generalized convulsions and cardiorespiratory failure.

CASE REPORT

A 31-year-old patient came to our attention in the twentieth week of pregnancy. She complained of a very severe kyphoscoliosis (90%) resulting from poliomyelitis when she was 2 years old (Fig. 70.1). In fact, this patient was completely dependent as her upper extremities were atrophic and she was paralytic in her lower extremities. Her vital capacity was about 800 ml and her arterial PO_2 75 mmHg (Fig. 70.2). This pathologic picture was complicated by obstructive lung disease.

The patient and her husband, while knowing the extremely elevated risk for both mother and child resulting from the pregnancy, were determined to proceed with delivery. The mother was hospitalized and her physicians proposed a therapeutic schema based on pulmonary function, respiratory physiotherapy, corticosteroids, heparin and low residue diet to maintain patient's weight at around 40 kg.

The clinical situation becomes critical at the thirty-first week of gestation (Table 70.1): the patient required oxygen by mask to avoid severe respiratory insufficiency and appeared to be extremely distressed. The need for cesarean delivery was discussed and this course was decided upon.

Via an epidural catheter at the level of L1–L2, 10 ml of bupivacaine 0.5% plus 0.05 mg of piperidine were administered. The patient was given 100% oxygen. After 10 min she gave birth to a baby girl weighing 1670 g, who was intubated and transferred to the neonatal intensive care unit, where she required respiratory assistance for 9 days. Following this she was treated for 30 days in the premature babies department.

The mother was observed and administered oxygen for 24 h in the intensive care unit. She left the hospital after 13 days without complications. The clinical and laboratory findings had improved but respiratory values were decreased compared with the prepregnant values.

We look forward to following the neonate's outcome with particular attention to eventual chronic hypoxic damage that could have been developed in utero.

Table 70.1 Respiratory parameters

Date	FVC	FEV_1(L)	PO_2 (mmHg)	PCO_2 (mmHg)	Residual functional capacity (L)
	VN = 2.79	VN = 2.41			
21/6/91	0.89	0.68	70	29	29
1/8/91	0.81	0.54	66.8	28	30
24/8/91	0.72	0.57	63	28.8	35**
5/9/91	0.66	0.49	52.9	36.4	30

**Prepartum respiratory values.
FEV, forced expiratory volume in I S; FVC: forced vital capacity.
VN: normal value

REFERENCES

1. Kopenhager T 1977 A review of 50 pregnant patients with kyphoscoliosis. Br J Obstet Gynaecol 84: 585–587
2. Chapman E M
3. Jensen J
4. Berman A T 1982 The effects of pregnancy on idiopathic scoliosis. Pregnancy and scoliosis 7: 76–77
5. Fearl C S
6. Dugan R J 1957 Kyphoscoliosis and pregnancy. Am J Obstet Gynecol 73: 89–93

SECTION 6

Maternal and neonatal outcome

71. Maternal mortality

Part A UK view *J. H. McClure*
Part B USA view *N. E. Oriol*

PART A
UK VIEW
J. H. McClure

Details of all deaths in pregnancy and deaths within 42 days of delivery or termination of pregnancy irrespective of the duration of pregnancy are published at 3-yearly intervals within the UK in the Reports on Confidential Enquiries into Maternal Deaths (CEMD).[1] Late deaths which occur between 43 days and 1 year after pregnancy are also considered if the death is thought to have resulted from a complication of pregnancy. This is particularly relevant if life has been sustained by intensive therapy, including artificial ventilation.

The CEMD reports were initiated in 1952 in England and Wales, and 1991 saw the publication of the first UK report combining information from the four countries of the UK.[2] Previously England and Wales had published reports 3-yearly, Scotland 5-yearly and Northern Ireland varied between 4 and 10 years. The small numbers of deaths in each of the constituent countries caused difficulty in maintaining confidentiality and, therefore, it was decided to assess the cases from the four countries together to make further use of the information available. The 1985–87 UK report and preceding reports represent the largest running series of continuous clinical audit in the world.

DEFINITIONS

There is international agreement to subdivide causes of obstetric deaths into 'direct' and 'indirect'. ICD-9 (ninth revision of the International Classification of Diseases) defines *direct* obstetric deaths as 'those resulting from obstetric complications of the pregnant state (pregnancy, labor and puerperium), from interventions, omissions, incorrect treatment, or from a chain of events resulting from any of the above'. *Indirect* obstetric deaths are defined as 'those resulting from previous existing disease, or disease that developed during pregnancy and which was not due to direct obstetric causes, but which was aggravated by physiologic effects of pregnancy'. Only those deaths from other causes (fortuitous deaths) which happen to occur in pregnancy or the puerperium are excluded from maternal mortality as internationally defined. The numerator is thus defined, but any comparison of rates must also include a firm definition of a denominator. Great care must be taken in interpreting figures using alternative denominators such as maternities, births or conceptions.

Maternities refer to the numbers of mothers delivered, births include twins and other multiple births, and conceptions include maternities and legal abortions. It is now customary for the Office of Population Censuses and Surveys (OPCS) in the UK to publish annual estimates of conceptions.

TRENDS

The maternal mortality rate (MMR), defined as number of maternal deaths per 1000 births, has been recorded in England and Wales since 1847. Figure 71.1 illustrates a sudden reduction which began in 1937 when the MMR was around 4000 per million.

The fall in 1937 is considered to have been due to the introduction of sulphonamides and a simultaneous reduction in the virulence of the hemolytic streptococcus, reducing maternal death due to sepsis.

Improving maternal health, new antibiotics, increasing hospital confinement and better midwifery and obstetric care have all contributed to the continuing decline in maternal mortality rate. Figure 71.2 expresses the MMR on a logarithmic scale, and it can be seen that the reduction in MMR from 1937 is almost linear and that MMR,

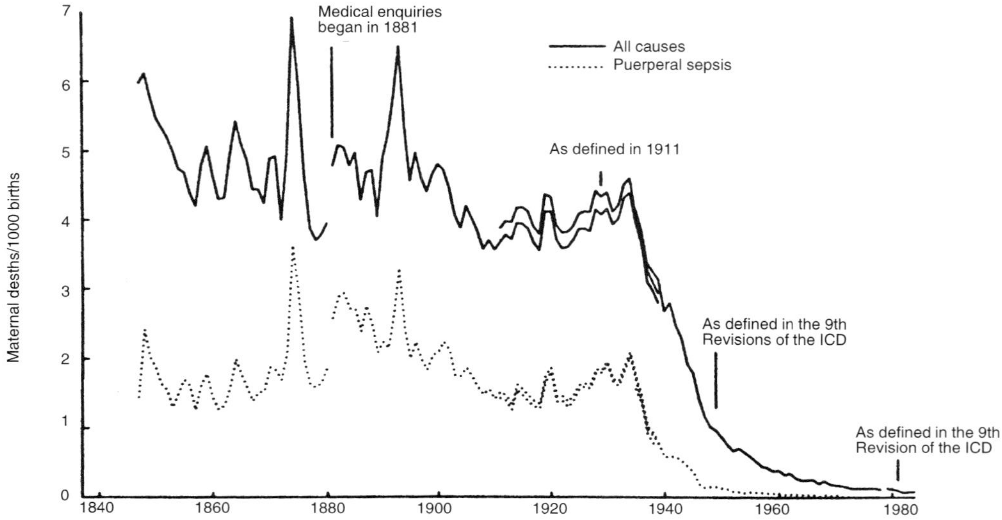

Fig. 71.1 Maternal mortality, England and Wales, 1847–1984.

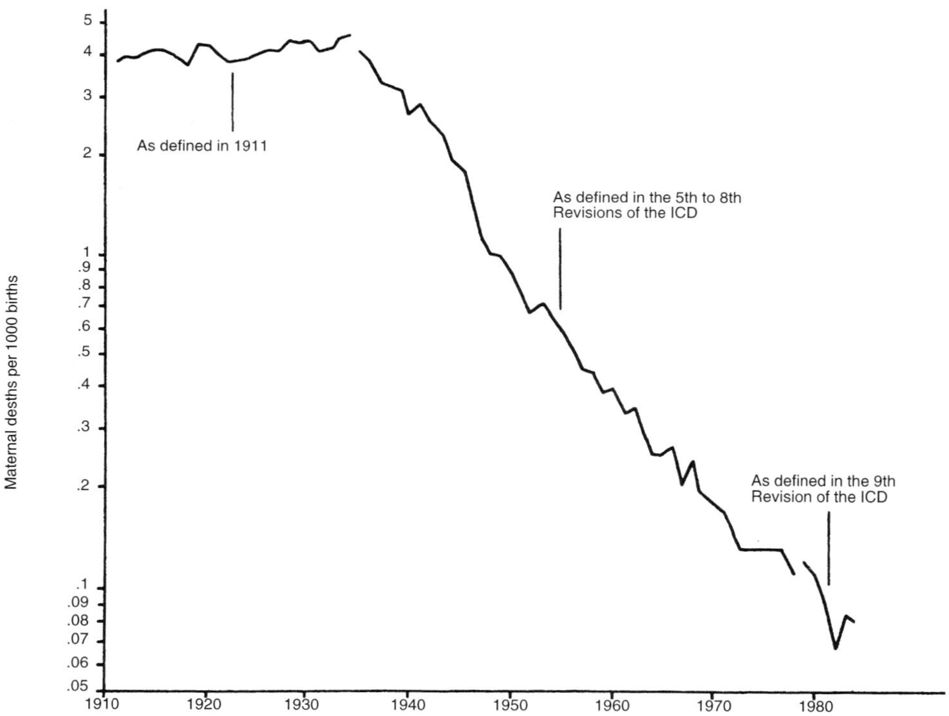

Source: OPCS mortality statistics

Fig. 71.2 Maternal mortality, England and Wales, 1911–84 plotted on logarithmic scale.

in fact, halved every 10 years over the period of the Confidential Enquiries 1952–87.

The Confidential Enquiry includes deaths of women after legal or spontaneous abortion. Some of the reduction in maternal mortality since 1970 reflects the introduction of legal abortion, which was intended to reduce and, in the longer term, eliminate deaths after illegal abortion. Since 1970 there has been a steady decline in deaths from illegal abortion. In 1970–72 there were 37 deaths from illegal abortion and in the 1985–87 report there were none. The legal abortion rate for Great Britain has shown a sustained increase since 1970 (Fig. 71.3).

In the UK the MMR, expressed per 100 000 total births, has fallen from 67.1 in the triennium 1955–57 to 7.6 in the triennium 1985–87. This represents a reduction of approximately 20% per triennium, assuming a constant rate of fall. It has been estimated that maternal deaths per 1000 births are 6.4 in Africa, 4.2 in Asia and 2.7 in Latin America, compared with 0.3 in all developed countries and less than 0.1 in northern and middle Europe. This is consistent with the 1985–87 rate of 0.07 in the UK.

AGE AND PARITY

Maternal mortality is closely related to maternal age and parity. Analysis of the 1976–87 figures reveals that direct maternal death rates follow a 'J'-shaped pattern, being lowest for women aged 20–24 years and then rising with age, particularly for mothers aged 35 years and over. There is a similar pattern of direct maternal mortality with parity, being 'J'-shaped, with lowest rates for women in their second pregnancy.

CAUSES OF DEATH

The first six triennia, 1952–54 to 1967–69, were dominated by deaths from hypertensive diseases of pregnancy, pulmonary embolism, hemorrhage and abortion (Table 71.1).

Deaths from abortion, often associated with criminal interference, showed little real improvement during these two decades, and abortion was the main cause of death between 1958–60 and 1967–69. Between 1961–63 and 1967–69 increasing provision of beds for hospital confinement, expansion of the maternity services and better midwifery and obstetric care contributed to the reduction in deaths from hypertensive diseases, pulmonary embolism and hemorrhage. The introduction in 1962 of a combined preparation of oxytocin and ergometrine for intramuscular use is considered to have contributed to the reduction in deaths from post-partum hemorrhage.

The two major causes of maternal death in England and Wales since the 1970–72 triennium have been pulmonary embolism and hypertensive disorders of pregnancy. The numbers and percentage of direct maternal deaths for the triennia between 1970 and 1987 are shown in Table 71.2.

Table 71.2 shows the most dramatic falls in deaths due to abortion and anesthesia. While the abortion deaths can be related to the introduction of the 1967 Abortion Act, the fall in anesthetic deaths is considered to be due to improved anesthetic services and the increased resource provided to this service within maternity hospitals in the UK.

There were 249 maternal deaths in the triennium 1985–87 in the UK. 139 (56%) were classified as direct, 84 (34%) as indirect and 26 (10%) as fortuitous.

Deaths associated with anesthesia

The number of deaths directly associated with anesthesia, six in 1985–87, has shown a steady decline since figures

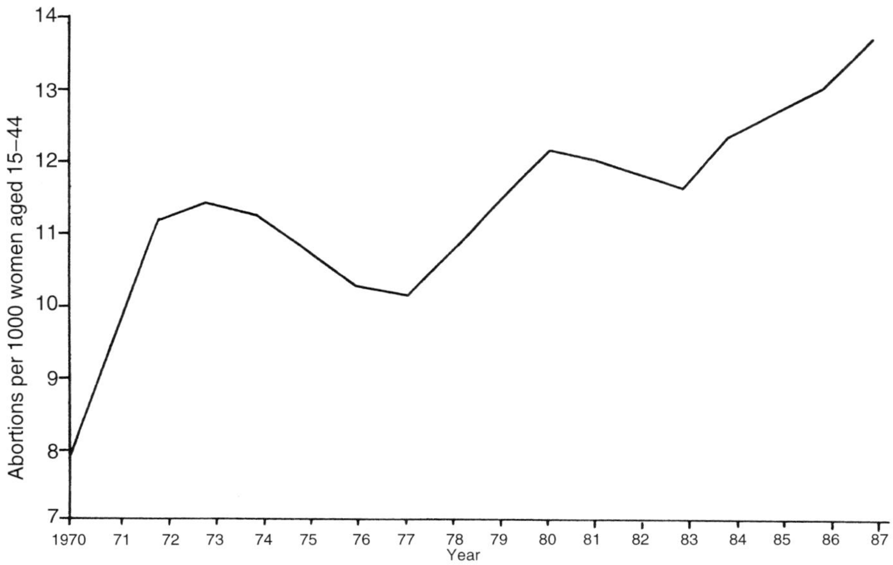

Source: England and Wales, OPCS AB Series data
Scotland, Scottish Health Statistics

Fig. 71.3 Legal abortion rate, Great Britain 1970–87.

Table 71.1 Numbers of direct maternal deaths by cause 1952–54 to 1967–69

Causes	1952–54	1955–57	1958–60	1961–63	1964–66	1967–69
Hypertensive diseases of pregnancy	246	171	118	104	67	53
Pulmonary embolism	138	157	132	129	91	75
Abortion	153	141	135	139	133	117
Hemorrhage	188	130	130	92	68	41

Table 71.2 Cause of direct maternal deaths/numbers and percentages, England and Wales 1970–87, compared with UK, 1985–87

	Triennium		Cause of direct maternal death										
			Pulmonary embolism	Hypertensive disorders of pregnancy	Anesthesia	Amniotic fluid embolism	Abortion	Ectopic pregnancy	Hemorrhage	Sepsis, excluding abortion	Ruptured uterus	Other direct causes	All deaths
England and Wales	1970–72	No.	51	43	37	14	73	34	30	30	11	20	343
		%	14.9	12.5	10.8	4.1	21.3	9.9	8.7	8.7	3.2	5.8	100
	1973–75	No.	33	34	27	14	27	19	21	19	11	22	227
		%	14.5	15.0	11.9	6.2	11.9	8.4	9.3	8.4	4.8	9.7	100
	1976–78	No.	43	29	27	11	14	21	24	15	14	19	217
		%	19.8	13.4	12.4	5.1	6.5	9.7	11.1	6.9	6.5	8.8	100
	1979–81	No.	23	36	22	18	14	20	14	8	4	19	178
		%	12.9	20.2	12.4	10.1	7.9	11.2	7.9	4.5	2.2	10.7	100
	1982–84	No.	25	25	18	14	11	10	9	2	3	21	138
		%	18.1	18.1	13.0	10.1	8.0	7.2	6.5	1.4	2.2	15.2	100
	1985–87	No.	24	25	5	9	6	11	10	6	5	20	121
		%	19.8	20.7	4.1	7.4	5.0	9.1	8.3	5.0	4.1	16.5	100
UK	1985–87	No.	29	27	6	9	6	16	10	6	6	24	139
		%	20.9	19.4	4.3	6.5	4.3	11.5	7.2	4.3	4.3	17.3	100

were accurately attributed to being due to the administration of anesthesia (Table 71.3).

Deaths associated with anesthesia have been due to difficulty with tracheal intubation, inhalation of stomach contents, failure of post-operative care, hemorrhage and other miscellaneous causes. There is commonly a history of inexperienced personnel being presented with an emergency cesarean delivery with little or no experienced help or skilled assistance. In spite of the observed dramatic reduction in deaths associated with anesthesia it is still apparent that 'substandard care' is contributory. The term 'substandard care' takes into account not only failure in clinical care, but also some of the underlying factors that may have produced a low standard of care for the patient. This includes situations produced by the action of the woman herself, or her relatives, which may be outside the control of the clinicians. It also takes into account shortage of resources for staffing facilities and administrative failure in the maternity services and the back-up facilities such as anesthetic, radiologic and pathology services.

Table 71.3. Deaths associated with anesthesia, estimated rate per million pregnancies and percentage of direct maternal deaths England and Wales 1970–87, compared with UK 1985–87

		Number of deaths directly associated with anesthesia	Rate per million pregnancies	Percent of direct maternal deaths
England and Wales	1970–72	37	12.8	10.8
	1973–75	27	10.5	11.9
	1976–78	27	12.1	12.4
	1979–81	22	8.7	12.4
	1982–84	18	7.2	13.0
	1985–87	5	1.9	4.4
UK	1985–87	6	N/A	4.3

The commonest cause of maternal death associated with anesthesia in the triennium 1985–87 was misplacement of the tracheal tube. The typical picture was of an obese woman of short stature presenting for emergency cesarean delivery under general anesthesia. Unrecognized misplacement of the tracheal tube in the esophagus rapidly causes anoxia, leading to death or permanent neurologic damage. Tracheal intubation is more difficult in late pregnancy due to:

1. obesity;
2. anatomic factors;
3. inappropriately applied cricoid pressure;
4. inadequate anesthesia or relaxation;
5. fluid retention;
6. poor assistance.

The extra anesthetic equipment required for a difficult intubation includes:

1. a laryngoscope with a blade in line with the axis of the handle (polio blade);
2. long introducers (gum-elastic, rubber or plastic-coated malleable wire);
3. laryngeal masks;
4. large-bore orogastric tubes;
5. a laryngotomy kit.

The absolute need for a skilled anesthetic assistant cannot be overemphasized, and a failed intubation drill should be agreed to and practiced by all those involved in obstetric anesthesia.

It must be said, however, that the anoxic deaths due to misplaced tubes were not simply due to failure to intubate the trachea but to failure to recognize or admit that the esophagus had been intubated by mistake.

If an anesthesiologist fails to intubate the trachea and cannot maintain a satisfactory airway with continued cricoid pressure, it is now recommended in the UK that priority should be given to the mother's safety and she should be allowed to recover consciousness. Senior help can then be summoned and an alternative strategy, perhaps under spinal anesthesia, employed once help has arrived.

Modern monitoring equipment should ensure that tracheal intubation can be confirmed after each and every placement of a tracheal tube. The presence of a regular alveolar plateau of carbon dioxide in the expired gas is the only certain method of ensuring that the tube is in the trachea. It is now considered essential that a rapid carbon dioxide analyzer should be provided in every location where anesthetics are given so that the position of the tube can be checked immediately after intubation and the adequacy of ventilation monitored throughout the anesthetic.

The prevalence of death due to aspiration pneumonitis or Mendelson's syndrome has declined, presumably due to better antacid prophylaxis or the reduced use of general anesthesia. Most UK centres are using H_2-receptor blockers given early in labor combined with 0.3 M sodium citrate solution and cricoid pressure should general anesthesia be indicated.

Figures are not available to determine the actual increased proportion of operative procedures carried out under epidural or spinal anesthesia, but the decline in deaths due to tracheal tube problems and aspiration pneumonitis may well reflect the decline in use of the hurried general anesthetic in obstetric practice.

Post-operative care

Anesthesiologists in the UK now accept a major responsibility for the patient in the immediate post-operative period. This responsibility includes care of the airway, the respiratory and circulatory systems and provision of pain relief. The anesthetic management was considered to have contributed to deaths in some cases of preeclampsia, hemorrhage and delayed recovery from anesthesia. The anesthesiologist is responsible for the patient until full recovery has occurred but cannot be expected to fulfill this obligation if appropriate facilities are not provided.

It is recommended that every obstetric unit should have a designated recovery area where post-operative patients should remain until they are fully conscious and in a stable cardiorespiratory state. It should be ensured that adequate therapeutic and monitoring equipment is provided and that there are clear lines of responsibility and delegation. Large units dealing with high-risk patients with preeclampsia or other life-threatening conditions require a high dependency area where skilled nursing can be provided on a continual supervision basis.

Hypertensive disorders of pregnancy

This remains a major cause of maternal death, second only to pulmonary embolism in the UK. This is despite recent advances in antenatal care and the control of hypertension and convulsive disease. In 1985–87 there were 27 deaths due to this cause in the UK, 12 patients dying from pulmonary complications, especially adult respiratory distress syndrome (ARDS), and 11 from intracerebral hemorrhage. Anesthesia or sedation was considered to have contributed to three of these deaths as two patients died within the first 2 h after emergency cesarean delivery and the third received excessive sedation when labor was induced at 26 weeks' gestation.

Uncontrolled hypertension is a serious life-threatening condition at any time during pregnancy and in the puerperium. The management of labor, operative delivery and post-partum care in the patient with severe preeclampsia demands a team approach. It is often difficult to identify women who will develop eclampsia, and this makes management difficult. Anesthetic staff should be involved early even if operative delivery is not planned to assist with analgesia, sedation, antihypertensive therapy and monitoring. Epidural anesthesia is commonly used, but it takes time to become established and fails to control blood pressure in women with severe disease. Additional parenteral antihypertensive therapy may be required. Careful fluid therapy under central venous pressure monitoring is advisable as the arterial blood pressure is controlled.

The choice of anesthetic technique for operative delivery in women with severe preeclampsia is influenced by the maternal and fetal condition and the urgency of delivery. The question of the coagulation status of the patient needs to be considered. The hemodynamic status of the eclamptic or preeclamptic mother before, during and after delivery is complex and not fully understood.

It is recommended that anesthesiologists and obstetricians in training should receive formal instruction in this difficult aspect of care. Senior staff should be consulted early and specialized regional teams to assist in the management of these cases should be established as recommended in the last three Triennial Reports.

The emergence of ARDS as the eventual cause of death in cases of preeclampsia or eclampsia is noteworthy. Artificial ventilation in these cases was indicated initially because of ventilatory failure due to eclampsia, heavy sedation or unrecognized aspiration of gastric contents. It was continued because of worsening gas exchange in the lungs due to alveolar membrane dysfunction and pulmonary edema. It is hoped that careful monitoring of arterial pressure and venous filling pressures with restriction of fluid intake may reduce the incidence of ARDS in this type of patient.

Thrombosis and thromboembolism

Pulmonary embolism is now the most common cause of maternal death in the UK (Table 71.2). The deaths appear to be evenly distributed in the antepartum and post-partum period. Post-partum pulmonary emboli are generally seen in mothers who have been restricted to bed for long periods following cesarean delivery. Risk factors include previous thromboembolism, obesity, immobilization, operative delivery and lupus anticoagulant. The role of the anesthesiologist in preventing thromboembolism is crucial, and consideration should be given to the role of regional anesthesia in encouraging lower limb blood flow and early mobilization. Heparin prophylaxis should not be a contraindication to epidural or spinal anesthesia provided common sense is employed in the timing of heparin administration. Full heparin anticoagulation is still considered a contraindication to central neural blockade. Other simple methods such as intermittent calf compression with inflatable leggings and the use of prophylactic antibiotics, particularly in the obese patient having a cesarean delivery, may reduce the risk of wound infection and the increased period of bed rest associated with it.

Indirect deaths – cardiac disease

84 maternal deaths (34% of the total) were classified as indirect, i.e. resulting from previous existing disease, or disease that developed during pregnancy and which was not due to direct obstetric causes, but which were aggravated by the physiologic effects of pregnancy. These deaths were not included in Table 71.2, but constitute a group of great significance to the anesthesiologist. The largest single entity within this classification is death due to cardiac disease, either congenital or acquired. The number of mothers with congenital heart disease proceeding with pregnancy is increasing, often against medical advice. Congenital heart disease, whether surgically corrected or not, presents a significant risk since pregnancy and labor increases the workload of the heart, which may have little reserve functional capacity. Careful maintenance of central venous and arterial pressures is essential and, should anesthesia be indicated, accurate direct hemodynamic monitoring is indicated. The choice of anesthetic technique will depend on the cardiac lesion presenting and the expertise of the individual anesthesiologist. The need for early involvement of the cardiologist and the anesthesiologist with the obstetrician in a team approach is emphasized. Patients with severe disease may require delivery in a specialized cardiac unit.

Ischemic heart disease in women of child-bearing age is increasing in prevalence and should be suspected in women who smoke or have essential hypertension or diabetes. Mothers with ischemic heart disease may be at increased risk of subendocardial ischemia secondary to falls in diastolic arterial pressure during epidural anesthesia, falls in cardiac output due to aortocaval compression or acute rises in arterial pressure seen in light general anesthesia.

There has been a change in perception of the role and responsibilities of anesthesiologists in the management of obstetric cases. They need to be involved from an early stage in the monitoring and management of high-risk patients, such as those with severe preeclampsia or cardiac disease, even if operative delivery is not planned. It is the duty of anesthesiologists to ensure that appropriate facilities are requested, but they cannot be expected to fulfill this obligation if they are not provided.

ACKNOWLEDGEMENTS

The figures and tables in this chapter are reproduced with permission from source material provided by the Office of Population Censuses and Surveys and the Department of Health.

REFERENCES

1. Reports on Confidential Enquiries into Maternal Deaths in England and Wales 1952–84. Eleven Triennial Reports. HMSO, London
2. Report on Confidential Enquiries into Maternal Deaths in the United Kingdom 1985–87 1991. HMSO, London

PART B
USA VIEW

N. E. Oriol

INTRODUCTION

'Maternal mortality study and reporting are less than exciting, but like all epidemiology, they are necessary to more precisely know where our attention must be directed to prevent its occurrence' comments May and Greiss[1] in the discussion following their review of maternal mortality in North Carolina.

Maternal mortality statistics are often used as a yardstick by which to measure such intangibles as health of a community, availability of health care, medical advances, reproductive freedom, poverty and the status of women.[2-7] Yet interestingly, Barker and Osmond[2] demonstrated that the study of maternal mortality can serve as a predictor of the future health risks (i.e. cerebral vascular accidents) of the cohort born to the maternal population measured. Maternal mortality review committees have set the example for the use of outcome statistics and confidential audits to promote continuing medical education, peer review and quality assurance.[8] However, for obstetric anesthesiologists, maternal mortality statistics could also be used to assign a risk index to their patients and, therefore, sharpen awareness of the inherent risk factors in the obstetric patient in much the same way that the cardiovascular anesthesiologist assesses risk factors for coronary artery disease in the cardiovascular patient.

This chapter will present information based on maternal mortality statistics gathered in the USA. We will evaluate recent trends and associations, followed by an in-depth look at issues relevant to anesthetic practice.

The chapter will be divided into seven sections:

1. Definitions and data collection as a means to evaluate from a common base the many disparate epidemiologic studies.
2. Trends over time and across the various geographic regions in the USA.
3. Examination of the current causes of maternal mortality.
4. Associations and confounders (age, weight, race and socioeconomic status).
5. Anesthesia-related maternal mortality.
6. Development of a risk profile for the pregnant patient.
7. Conclusion.

DEFINITIONS AND DATA

In order to summarize and compare the maternal mortality literature, we must understand the common ground from which maternal mortality statistics are derived and analyzed. 'Definitions of maternal deaths vary from one authoritative source to another, authors and data-collecting agencies count differently'.[9] The literature moves between discussions of pregnancy-related, reproduction-related and childbirth-related deaths, leaving the critical reader to calculate the comparisons. Rates and ratios are used interchangeably and the denominators are often unspecified. In an effort to facilitate an interpretation of the maternal mortality literature, this section will present common terminology and methodologic considerations.

Pregnancy to death interval

Most studies have established their own definition of maternal mortality relative to the time interval between the termination of the pregnancy and the maternal death. The resultant profusion of definitions was one reason for the establishment of the National Pregnancy Mortality Surveillance (NPMS). This reporting system was established in 1983 by a collaboration between the Division of Reproductive Health of the Centers of Disease Control (CDC) and the Maternal Mortality Collaborative, a special interest group of the American College of Obstetricians and Gynecologists (ACOG). This national surveillance, under the auspices of the CDC, gathers information from state maternal mortality committees, health departments and private physicians. The collaboration chose the working definition of maternal mortality as 'a woman's death that was caused or contributed to by pregnancy and that occurred *during or within 1 year after the end of pregnancy*'.[10] However, many important studies and most international studies use other time intervals. Therefore, when studying the same population, different reporting sources would find different maternal mortality ratios. Time intervals of 42 days [World Health Organization (WHO)], 72 days[11] and 90 days [American Medical Association (AMA)][10] from the termination of pregnancy are some commonly used limits. In 1987 Bassell and Marx,[12] noting that 16% of deaths occur > 42 days after parturition, suggested that 'extension of the tabulation period past that time should be the aim'. More recently, it has been argued that current life-sustaining capabilities require an extension to 1 year.[1] Of note, anesthesia deaths accounted for 8–10% of the late deaths, i.e. deaths > 42 days after parturition.[13,14]

Mortality classifications

Which outcomes of the pregnancy are included in the maternal mortality ratio varies in each study. Many studies include mortality related to abortion and ectopic pregnancy in their calculations of maternal mortality ratios, while some studies limit themselves only to mortality associated with childbirth. To be accurate, *reproductive mortality* refers to deaths associated with reproduction and its control including birth control, sterilization and, presumably, in vitro fertilization, while *pregnancy-related mortality* refers to deaths associated with any pregnancy regardless of site or duration including ectopic, abortion and parturition. *Maternal mortality* implies death associated with parturition only, but most studies use this term synonymously with pregnancy-related deaths.

Classifications of causal relationship

Traditionally, the broad classifications of the causal relationship between pregnancy and death are: *direct*, caused by pregnancy; *indirect*, caused by a nonobstetric condition, exacerbated by pregnancy; and *nonmaternal*, incidental, not related to pregnancy at all, i.e. trauma, suicide. However, this classification is controversial. It is argued that, for example, suicides resulting from depression due to pregnancy or deaths in accidents caused by inappropriate seat belts are deaths that would not have happened if the patient had not been pregnant and, therefore, are appropriately called maternal deaths.[15] In response to such criticism the NPMS adopted the categories of *pregnancy related* to describe deaths resulting from a complication of pregnancy or from events that aggravate unrelated conditions by the physiologic or pharmacologic effects of pregnancy and *pregnancy associated* to describe deaths from any cause during pregnancy or within 1 year of the termination of pregnancy.[13,16]

Cause of death codes

The International Classification of Diseases (ICD) established by WHO assigns codes for specific causes of morbidity and mortality. Until 1980 anesthesia was not listed as a separate code and therefore all anesthesia-related deaths were listed as indirect and classified as a complication of the particular obstetric procedure, i.e. death from spinal shock during a cesarean delivery was counted as a cesarean death, not an anesthetic death. Since 1980, the ninth revision of the International Classification of Diseases (ICD-9) has listed anesthesia as a separate cause of death under codes 168–169.9, 349 and 349.0 (Table 71.4).[17] This is an improvement over the older codes, but to be truly useful for educational purposes 'These categories are rather broad'; the 'unidimensional codes are inadequate, [giving] insufficient evidence of the sequence of steps to death'. '[We] need to know outcome, immediate cause and underlying condition'.[18] Whatever way the categories are defined, accuracy of assignment depends on the certifying physician's assessment and reporting of the facts.

Assigning cause of death

The problem of inaccurate assessments of the cause of death can be due to several factors: lack of medical history details by the certifying physician, fear of litigation,[19] low autopsy rate or even, after an autopsy, a lack of understanding on the part of the pathologist of the potential relationship of the death to issues of pregnancy.[9,19–23] The problem of inadequate information with which to assign a cause of death is potentially solvable, as has been shown by the United Kingdom Confidential Inquiry Report, by using confidential reporting as the source of information followed by an in-depth review of each case.[24] The many published studies that utilize thorough reviews of medical records to determine the sequence of events that lead up to the maternal death gave the most helpful information.[1,9,11,15,21–23,26–30]

Table 71.4 The International Classification of Diseases 9th revision, clinical modification (ICD-9-CM)

Code	Description
668	Complications of the administration of anesthetic or other sedation in labor and delivery Includes Complications arising from the administration of a general or local anesthetic, analgesic or other sedation in labor and delivery Excludes Reaction to spinal or lumbar puncture (349.0)
668.0	Pulmonary complications Inhalation aspiration of stomach contents or secretions Mendelson's syndrome Pressure collapse of lung following anesthesia or sedation in labor and delivery
668.1	Cardiac complications Cardiac arrest or failure following anesthesia or other sedation in labor and delivery
668.2	Central nervous system complications Cerebral anoxia
668.8	Other complications of anesthesia or other sedation in labor and delivery
668.9	Unspecified complications of anesthesia and other sedation
349	Other and unspecified disorders of the nervous system
349.0	Reaction to spinal or lumbar puncture

Assignment of responsibility

Although most studies classified deaths as preventable or not preventable and tried to assign responsibility, i.e. patient, doctor, hospital, determining whether or not a death is preventable is controversial. Who should make such a determination? One study used information gathered by a review committee for over 30 years. During the early years of this review period the committee defined every anesthetic death as preventable.[28] In this chapter, issues of preventability will not be addressed as the assignments, even by review committees, were often arbitrary and because the notion of preventability is only a reflection of the medical knowledge at one moment in time and is not an intrinsic property of the obstetric process itself. In an effort to address this issue, the NPMS has devised a new classification scheme that allows for multiple factors, distinguishing among immediate and underlying cause of death, associated obstetric conditions and complications and outcomes of pregnancy. This scheme provides enough detail to assess, for prevention purposes, the circumstances and pathophysiology that led up to each maternal death. Such detail is necessary to understand and educate, and to prevent maternal deaths.[10]

Data collection

Identification and statistical analysis of maternal deaths also varies from study to study. The literature of maternal mortality is a morass of statistics, derived from information that is gathered in any one of a number of less-than-perfect ways, imperfections due in part to the nature of the events that are being measured.

One problem is to identify the entire cohort of maternal or, more correctly, pregnancy-related deaths. Most commonly the deaths are culled from a review of the coded cause of death on death certificates using the broad ICD codes. However, death certificates are only as thorough as the questions asked and as accurate as the person who completes the form. A recent pregnancy or an early pregnancy may go unrecognized or simply unrecorded, and many state death certificates do not ask if a recent pregnancy had occurred. The cause of death may be accurately listed, while its relationship to a recent pregnancy may be unspecified. Some studies have employed other, more detailed techniques such as linkage, by mother's name, birth certificates and reproductive age on death certificates. The accuracy of this technique is dependent on the mother using her real name.[11] Studies using multiple sources of information have found that standard vital statistic methods significantly under-report by as much as 112%.[14,23,31,32] Other methods to increase discovery include addition of medical examiner cases, manual death certificate review, the review by ICD coding and hospital-based confidential reporting. The last appears to have the greatest potential for accurate and thorough discovery.[10,11,14,27]

Data analysis

The problem of achieving valid statistical analysis is formidable. It is almost impossible to document case-specific rates except in hospital-based surveys.[23] The number of deaths may be discoverable and the number of live births known, but the total number of pregnancies or specific cases cannot be determined by any current accounting techniques. Therefore, most epidemiologic studies only calculate the maternal mortality *ratio* as opposed to the *rate*. Using the number of live births as the denominator, yields a *ratio*, i.e. the number of maternal deaths per 100 000 *live births*, whereas the *rate* would be the number of maternal deaths per 100 000 *pregnancies*. A ratio includes maternal deaths after both abortive pregnancies and live births in the numerator, but includes only live births in the denominator. Even more difficult to ascertain are *case-specific rates*, such as the number of deaths due to general anesthesia per number of cases of general anesthetics given. At best we must assume how common a given procedure is performed and estimate how likely it is to lead to a bad outcome.

TRENDS OVER TIME AND ACROSS REGIONS

Historical trends

In 1600 the maternal mortality ratio is estimated to have been 2200/100 000. This has greatly improved. The maternal mortality ratio was ≈ 10/100 000 over the past decade.[12,14] In 1915 the USA began mandatory birth registration and started keeping maternal mortality statistics. Since that time there has been a steady reduction in the maternal mortality ratio. In 1915 the maternal mortality ratio was 700/100 000, and in 1930 it was 670/100 000.[33] There was a 90% decline from 1915 until now, with the most significant decrease between 1930 and 1980 and little change since 1980.[12,23,29,34] One study even found a recent increase.[23] This reduction in maternal mortality has occurred in all industrialized nations despite the adoption of very different standards of obstetric care delivery systems. For example: in the USA obstetricians deliver in hospitals; in the Netherlands midwives deliver at home; in New Zealand midwives deliver in hospitals and in the UK midwives and general practitioners deliver at home and in hospitals. Each country used a different system for deploying obstetricians/midwives/general practitioners providing either hospital and/or home deliveries,[34] yet all had a parallel decline in maternal mortality. The obvious explanations for the improvement in mortality are the discovery of antibiotics, the advent of blood banking, the legalization of abortion, better understanding of the physiology of hypertension and the development of safe operative and anesthetic techniques.[15,28,34,35] In an interesting natural experiment that proves the importance of modern medical advances in the improvements in maternal mortality, a study of a religious group in the USA that avoids obstetric care found an estimated maternal mortality ratio of 872/100 000 for the years 1975–82, worse than the maternal mortality ratio of 1915.[36]

Medical trends

During the earlier years the main causes of maternal mortality were the classic triad of bleeding, hypertension and infection (due to septic abortions and puerperal fever).[37] This triad is now replaced by deaths due to embolic events, hypertension and ectopic pregnancy.[12,14,31,38] When comparing large national studies, these trends are found consistently and reflect the major changes in the practice of medicine listed above.[15] However, some smaller studies observe other trends, which may reflect specific local standards of care or the results of local educational efforts based on their individual populations.[9,28,30,39] Also, some of the more detailed studies, with a higher percentage of autopsy data, question the trends claimed by the more general studies.[9,14,20,23,39,40] In particular, the reported increase in embolic events that has been identified in many studies is not borne out in some studies with a higher autopsy rate.

Table 71.5 Cause of maternal death, by outcome of pregnancy, USA,* 1979–86 (Adapted from Koonin et al[13])

	Outcome of pregnancy							
	Live birth		Stillbirth		Ectopic		Abortion†	
Cause of death	No.	%	No.	%	No.	%	No.	%
Pulmonary embolism	370	27.1	47	17.9	10	2.9	24	19.4
Pregnancy-induced hypertension	307	22.5	59	22.4	1	0.3	1	0.8
Hemorrhage	249	18.3	89	33.9	305	88.9	43	34.8
Infection	101	7.4	22	8.4	6	1.7	35	28.2
Anesthesia complications	65	4.8	3	1.1	4	1.2	11	8.9
Cardiomyopathy	53	3.9	4	1.5	0	0.0	1	0.8
Other	218	16.0	39	14.8	17	5.0	9	7.3
Total maternal deaths	1363	100	263	100	343	100	124	100

* Including Puerto Rico.
† Includes spontaneous and induced abortions.

Regional trends

Although the trends over time in the USA as a whole seem to follow in an orderly, steadily improving fashion, closer inspection of each particular region demonstrates inequalities. Specifically, maternal mortality statistics of the four main geographic regions (the north-east, north-central, south and west), showed the medical improvements reaching the north-east first. That advantage was taken away by population shifts and the increasing regionalization of poverty. By 1974–78, the west had the lowest maternal mortality ratio and the south the highest. More recently (1979–86), the north-central has the lowest and the north-east now has the highest. The association between ethnic minorities and poverty appears to explain why the areas with the highest minority population have the highest maternal mortality ratio. These trends may reflect the access to, or quality of, prenatal care afforded the poorer, minority populations.[12,13]

The *Healthy People 2000* objectives issued by the Surgeon General call for a reduction in maternal mortality to no more than 5/100 000[41] for any ethnic group or country. This goal will not be met without a major effort to respond to the information garnered from inquiry into maternal mortality.

CAUSES OF DEATH

The list of the common causes of maternal mortality varies according to the outcome of the pregnancy, i.e. live birth, stillbirth, ectopic or abortion (Table 71.5).[14] However, considering all outcomes combined, most nationwide studies find that the common causes are: pulmonary embolism (combined thrombotic and amniotic); pregnancy-induced hypertension; hemorrhage; infection; and anesthesia.[10,13,14,21] In many statewide studies, the reported incidence of each diagnosis depends on the thoroughness of the surveillance and the percentage of diagnoses established by autopsy.[1,9,11,15,16,22,23,25,27,29–31,42] However, regardless of the survey technique or the outcome of pregnancy, these five causes listed above are always among the most common (joined occasionally by cerebrovascular accidents and cardiomyopathy).[13,43] In addition to these five causes, when ectopic pregnancy is counted as a cause of death and not an outcome, it becomes the first or second most common cause of death. In this section I will discuss four of the leading causes of death and deaths associated with three specific outcomes of pregnancy: ectopic pregnancy, cesarean delivery and abortion. Anesthesia as a cause of death will be discussed in a separate section.

Embolism

Improvements in medical management have caused the classic triad of catastrophes of hemorrhage, infection and toxemia to be replaced by the less treatable catastrophe of pulmonary embolism (combined thrombotic and amniotic). However, in the maternal mortality surveys that have a high percentage of autopsies, it has been found that embolism is overdiagnosed clinically, and many of the cases of 'sudden unexpected death' are in fact caused by pulmonary edema. This discrepancy has led some to speculate that pulmonary embolism, being untreatable, is overdiagnosed in this litiginous society. There is further speculation that pulmonary edema is more common in smaller (obstetric units) due to underutilization of central venous pressure monitoring in acutely ill pregnant patients.[9,23,30,44] Regardless of the actual ranking, most large surveys agree that, as a cause of death, embolism is not decreasing at the same rate as other causes. Although thrombotic and amniotic embolism are combined in many surveys, the mechanism by which they cause death are completely unrelated and deserve separate consideration. Thrombotic pulmonary embolism is the number one cause of death after live birth outcomes, while amniotic embolism is the number three cause of death after stillbirth.[13,14,27,30] Risk factors for amniotic fluid embolism include increased age, multiparity, prolonged labor, forceful contractions and the use of uterine stimulants.[45] The risk factors for thrombotic embolisms are less clear. Prolonged bed rest is considered a risk factor for thrombotic embolism. However, since 1950, with the change in medical management to early ambulation after cesarean delivery, thrombotic embolism has become less common and some report that the incidence of thrombotic embolism is no worse for cesarean than vaginal delivery.[45] In the 1960s, the increased awareness of thrombotic embolism and the increased use of lung scans created an apparent increase in incidence. Several recent studies with a high autopsy rate addressed the question of an overdiagnosis of thrombotic embolism. One study with an 84% autopsy rate found thrombotic embolism was the fourth most common cause of death, accounting for only 17% of the autopsy-verified maternal deaths. An interesting trend has been noted in the relative timing which may help differentiate embolism from edema. This is that pulmonary edema tends to occur within 0–4 days after delivery, whereas thrombotic embolism usually occurs more than 6 days following delivery.[23]

Hypertension

Hypertension as a cause of death has decreased in incidence over the past 30 years.[1,9,13,23] The most dramatic improvement occurred between 1954 and 1960[15, 22] Little improvement has been documented since 1960, although the impact of new therapies such as low-dose aspirin has yet to be measured. Even so, pregnancy-induced hypertension remains one of the five leading causes of death in almost all studies, being the number one cause of death after a live birth and the number two cause of death after a stillbirth.[13]

Much of the improvement in mortality due to pregnancy-induced hypertension is accounted for by a decreased incidence of intracranial hemorrhage, believed to be the result of aggressive management and early diagnosis.[9] In general, maternal mortality secondary to hypertension increases with age, parity and inadequate therapy. Although pregnancy-induced hypertension is more common in primiparas, death due to pregnancy-induced hypertension is more common in multiparas. Currently 40% of the deaths due to pregnancy-induced hypertension are associated with intracranial hemorrhage. The risk factors for intracranial hemorrhage are increased age, increased parity, higher blood pressure and coagulopathy. Seizures do not constitute a risk factor.[15,23,30,46,47] 29% of deaths due to pregnancy-induced hypertension are associated with pulmonary edema. Frequently, the pulmonary edema is not appreciated until after the patient has experienced respiratory distress.[23]

Hemorrhage

Nationally, hemorrhage is the number one cause of death after stillbirth, number four after livebirth and number one after ruptured ectopic pregnancy.[13] The hemorrhage is most often post-partum, followed by hemorrhage associated with abruptio and then placenta previa. 50% of fatal hemorrhages are associated with disseminated intravascular coagulation.[30] An interesting and unfortunately consistent finding is that fatal hemorrhage is often unrecognized and, when recognized, the severity is underappreciated.[1,15,23–25,30] Of patients who die after obstetric hemorrhage unrelated to disseminated intravascular coagulation, 71% are hypovolemic while 27% are hypervolemic. Despite the continuing trend of unappreciated hemorrhage, there has been an overall decline in the incidence of death due to hemorrhage.[15,16,22,30,43] Second to the advent of blood banking, the majority of this decline was due to a decreasing incidence of uterine atony and a decreasing incidence of delayed transfusion.[15] Although one state documented that the most common cause of hemorrhage was uterine rupture after high forceps delivery, this relationship was discovered and corrected with targeted education.[30]

Infection

In 1918 puerperal sepsis caused 40% of maternal mortality. Despite the recognition by the mid-nineteenth century that puerperal sepsis was an infection spread by poor hygiene and aseptic technique, outbreaks continued to occur as late as 1927.[48] After the 1940s, infection other than puerperal sepsis as a major cause of maternal mortality was eliminated first by effective antibiotic therapy and second by legalization of abortion and the elimination of illegal septic abortions.[1] Septic abortions accounted for 22% of the deaths due to infection. 95% of all infection-related deaths occurred before 1973, the year the Roe vs. Wade decision legalized abortion. Currently, infection is the third or fourth cause of death overall[1,30] and continues to be an important cause of death after cesarean delivery.

Infection with human immunodeficiency virus (HIV) is becoming an important consideration in all mortality studies. 80% of the women with HIV are of reproductive age. In New York City HIV is the leading cause of death in women of reproductive age. Originally there was some concern that the decrease in cell-mediated immunity in the second and third trimester of pregnancy would predispose the HIV-infected parturient to experience an acceleration of the disease or hasten the onset of AIDS.[49] This has not been borne out. There is also no evidence that HIV infection increases the incidence of obstetric or anesthetic complications.[50–52]

Ruptured ectopic pregnancy

When considered as a cause of death and not as an outcome, ruptured ectopic pregnancy is the second leading cause of maternal mortality. 1.4% of all pregnancies are ectopic, whereas 13% of maternal deaths are associated with an ectopic pregnancy.[53] The incidence of ectopic pregnancy has increased steadily, while the fatality from ectopic pregnancy has decreased steadily, from a fatality rate of 35.5 per 10 000 in 1970 to 4.9 per 10 000 in 1986.[53] Even though there has been improvement in fatality rate, ruptured ectopic pregnancy is not improving as rapidly as other causes and is considered the first or second leading cause of death overall,[43,53] and it is the leading cause of death in Blacks.[22] The actual mechanism of death is usually hemorrhage[13] belatedly diagnosed.[15]

The risk of having an ectopic pregnancy increases with age, but the fatality is highest for teenagers. Black teenagers have a risk of death four times that of White teenage children. Reasons for this disparity may include the promptness of the response to the patients' complaints, the quality of care available and access to newer diagnostic technologies.[53] A similar disparity in access to care exists for rural White teenagers, in whom ectopic pregnancy remains a persistent preventable cause of death.[30]

Cesarean delivery

Until the late nineteenth century, cesarean delivery had a mortality risk between 75 and 100%. Women delivering through a traumatic hysterotomy caused by a bull's horn stood a better chance of survival than those delivered by a surgeon.[54] By the beginning of the twentieth century cesarean delivery had a 6% chance of mortality. By 1980 it had improved to 0.3%. Current reports cite a maternal mortality ratio of 0–277/100 000 with sepsis, embolism, anesthesia and hemorrhage as the mechanism of death. Anesthesia accounts for between 20 and 25% of the cesarean deaths[23,25,37,55] emergency cesarean deliveries having a greater risk than elective. According to some reviews, both emergency and elective cesarean delivery are associated with greater risk than vaginal delivery.[46,56] However, on closer inspection, the increased risk may be due to coexisting disease and not the surgical procedure itself.[15,27]

Abortion

The component of reproductive mortality due to abortion has decreased to < 0.1%. However, general anesthesia is playing an increasingly important role as the mechanism of abortion-related death.[43] The CDC reviews all cases of abortion-related deaths in the USA. In 1972–75, 7.7% of the abortion deaths were due to anesthesia; 29.4% between 1980 and 85.[57] Most of these deaths were attributed to hypoventilation or loss of the airway. Many deaths occurred in the recovery room. The majority of patients received only a short-acting barbiturate.[57] Obviously, more care needs to be taken with this 'minor procedure'.

ASSOCIATIONS AND CONFOUNDERS (age, weight, race and socioeconomics)

Although there are well-defined common causes of death, they do not affect all women equally. There are specific demographic and personal characteristics associated with increased risk of dying. These associations suggest that factors other than the specific obstetric condition or procedure are important in determining risk. The commonly recognized associations with increased risk include: age greater than 35, obesity, non-White ethnicity and poor socioeconomic status.

Age

Common knowledge suggests that the extremes of reproductive age are a high risk for poor maternal outcomes. The teenage parturient is not at greater risk of death than those in the 20–24 year age group and is at significantly less risk than those over 35 years old.[58] The exception to this is the Afro-American teenager with ectopic pregnancy who is more likely to die of hemorrhage associated with ruptured ectopic pregnancy due to delayed diagnosis.[53]

The specific risks of advanced age are not well defined. Several studies have demonstrated an association between age over 35 and an increased risk of death, especially from pregnancy-induced hypertension and hemorrhage.[47] However, after controlling for parity, this risk is less important. In fact, when age and educational level are considered together, the effect of age vanishes completely. This suggests that the delayed child-bearing of the college-educated woman does not increase her risk as much as the high parity of someone who begins child-bearing early and continues child-bearing into the third decade.[32,47]

Weight

The medical consequences of obesity are well documented, as are the obstetric risks.[59,60] Obesity is also associated with a greater difficulty of diagnosis of the abdominal and pelvic problems of ectopic pregnancy and uterine rupture leading to increased incidence of misdiagnosis. Also, management of the critically ill obese obstetric patient can be extremely difficult. Obesity is associated with a more extreme response to many of the complications of pregnancy. In particular, of the patients dying from hypertension, anesthesia or embolism, 15% are obese, while only 5–9% of patients dying from all other causes are obese.[14,57] Two studies that examined anesthetic-related deaths found that 28–80% of the anesthesia deaths occurred in obese women.[26,28] Even routine anesthetic management of the obese patient is not without increased risk due to greater difficulty with airway management combined with less respiratory reserve. Airway management of the obese patient is hampered by the effect of redundant tissue: visualization of the trachea is more difficult, and anesthesia by mask can be almost impossible, leading to an increased risk of failed intubation with no way to ventilate and making it harder to perform a cricothyroidotomy.

Race

All studies that specify race or ethnicity found a disparity between the mortality rate between White and non-White patients. The differences between Black and White mortality rates was greatest for ectopic pregnancy, abortion and anesthesia.[14] Ectopic pregnancy is the number 1 cause of death for Blacks, pregnancy-induced hypertension for Native Americans and hemorrhage for Whites.[22] The relative risk of death was 3–4 times greater for non-White than for White patients when considering all causes of death,[13,29,42] but, when considering anesthesia-related deaths only, the risk was 30 times higher.[26,57] The nonmedical confounders behind this association are: poverty (1980 United States Bureau of Census, 61% of Blacks are below United States poverty level) and access to high-quality prenatal, obstetric and hospital care. The medical confounders are: sickle cell anemia, hypertension and diabetes mellitus in the Afro-Americans and hypertension in Native Americans. However, deaths from hypovolemia, infection or anoxia are more likely to be due to problems of medical management rather than the confounding effect of coexisting disease.

Given the genetic mix that is represented by the title 'non-White', it is unlikely that there is any genetic predisposition to increased mortality. More likely the differences reflect medical management: inability of some physicians to recognize cyanosis in the non-White patient, less access to excellent medical care as a group or as an individual, and a disproportionate amount of poverty within the group termed non-White. Studies that examine adverse reproductive outcome in college-educated Afro-Americans suggest that the poor outcome is due to some inherent biologic risk in Afro-Americans, since these studies claimed to control socioeconomic and education.[61] However, another interpretation may be that access to equal quality care is still denied these women because of their racial identity rather than educational level or ability to pay.[62] This would seem to be a plausible explanation, at least for anesthesia-related risk, in which anoxia from loss of the airway is the most common problem rather than coexisting disease.

Socioeconomic status

Despite the many advancements in the practices of obstetrics and anesthesiology, maternal mortality remains significantly higher for women of low socioeconomic status. What has been termed the *feminization of poverty* is nowhere clearer than in the direct correlation that can be made between poverty and high-risk factors in maternal deaths.[4] Common health problems arise simply from poor diet and stress. Although some health services are available to women living in poverty, many are inaccessible to the most needy, complicated by lack of health insurance and dwindling resources for programs such as Medicaid, Aid to Families with Dependent Children and other important services. Low-income women are also at greater risk of suffering from untreated sexually transmitted diseases and pelvic inflammatory disease, which can lead to complications such as ectopic pregnancy. Ectopic pregnancies appear especially dangerous for Black women. Black women, who are more than three times as likely as White women to die in childbirth, are overall at greater risk simply because of their disproportionate representation among women living in poverty.[3,4]

The relationship between poverty and family planning services in reducing maternal death is hard to prove, but easy to understand.[63] When women give birth more frequently than optimal, with babies spaced too closely together, and with little access to medical services, the risk to the mother's health is obviously greater and must be taken into account when developing the patient's risk profile.[7] 'Categorical funding' such as prenatal care only, focusing on the fetus rather than the woman, is actually inadequate for the health of both.[3] Comprehensive services including family planning, pre- and antenatal care and parenting education are needed to address both societal needs and the overall health of mother and child.[4]

The relationship between education and maternal mortality is also an important area of concern. Education appears to have a major impact through family planning: the more highly educated, the lower the parity. This relationship begins in high school when there is a direct correlation between how well a young girl is doing in high school and her risk of unplanned pregnancy. Thus, teenage pregnancy and lack of education work together to perpetuate poverty and increase maternal mortality.

ANESTHESIA-RELATED MATERNAL MORTALITY

Anesthesia, as a significant factor among the causes of maternal mortality, was first spotlighted in the 1970 Triennial Report from England and Wales. About that time, the works of Marx, Crawford, Morgan and others highlighted the major risks associated with obstetric anesthesia and led the way to the improved outcomes witnessed over these past two decades. In the largest recent national surveillance, anesthesia as a cause of death was sixth overall, fifth of livebirths and fourth of abortive outcomes.[13] However, most studies under-report anesthesia-related deaths, often not even listing anesthesia as a cause of death but counting the anesthetic deaths under the procedure.[29] Of the studies that count anesthesia separately, a wide range of anesthesia-related maternal mortality rates have been reported: 33% in one hospital in England in 1958–78, 12% in England and Wales in 1979–81, 8% in the USA in 1980–85 and 0% in Sweden in 1973–79.[10,64–66]

In the USA, obstetric anesthesia has improved over the past two decades.[26,28] However, the practice of obstetric anesthesia continues to be plagued by a lack of trained physicians dedicated to the pregnant patient.[67] Anesthesia in the USA has remained one of the most common causes of preventable obstetric deaths. Although the absolute number of deaths due to all causes is declining[13,14,43] anesthesia as a cause is declining less rapidly[1,14,16,23,25,30] and, among some populations, is beginning to take the lead.[1,9,14] Furthermore, if we include the important role the anesthesiologist plays in the resuscitation of the critically ill perioperative patient, initiating central monitoring, managing intravascular volume replacement and directing recovery room care, then the number of deaths that are traceable to anesthetic management becomes even greater.[1,23,30,53,57]

Two papers highlight the role that anesthesia plays in maternal mortality. One paper by Sachs et al[28] looked at the risk associated with the different trends in anesthetic management, techniques and monitoring over the past three decades.

Sachs et al[28] reported on 37 anesthesia-related deaths that occurred in the Commonwealth of Massachusetts between 1954 and 1985. The study used data collected by the Committee on Maternal Welfare which was created in Massachusetts in 1941. Its continuing objective is to improve the safety of childbirth through a detailed review of every maternal death. Because the committee's objective is to educate and not discipline, it receives great cooperation from clinicians and institutions. In fact, legislation prevents its findings from being used in litigation. In the event of a maternal death an investigator reviews the case and reports to the committee. Autopsies are encouraged and the autopsy rate was greater than 70% for all but 2 years of the study period. The committee is composed of obstetricans from teaching hospitals and community hospitals, anesthesiologists, internists, pathologists and a representative from the public health department. They review the findings and assign a primary cause of death and associated events. Of 886 maternal deaths that occurred during the study period, 37 (4.2%) were judged to be due to complications associated with anesthesia (see Table 71.6).

Table 71.6 Deaths directly due to an anesthetic accident (Reproduced with permission from Sachs et al[28])

Year	Number*	Percent death†	Rate ‡
1954–57	4	1.8	0.9
1958–61	10	4.9	2.2
1962–65	5	2.8	1.2
1966–69	9	8.3	2.4
1970–73	6	8.1	2.7
1974–77	0	0	0
1978–81	1	2.8	0.4
1982–85	2	6.7	0.6
Total	37	4.2	1.3

* Death directly related to anesthesia.
† Percent of maternal deaths.
‡ Number of anesthetic-related deaths per 100 000 live births in Massachusetts.

Cause of death

Of the 37 deaths, 16 (43.2%) were due to aspiration and 21 (56.8%) to cardiorespiratory arrest. Of the 16 aspiration deaths, 13 were associated with anesthesia by mask, two with endotracheal intubation and one occurred during a regional anesthetic. Of the 21 cardiorespiratory arrests, 16 were associated with neuraxial blockade and five with general endotracheal anesthesia (Table 71.7).

Anesthetic technique

Of the 37 deaths, 13 deaths were associated with anesthesia by mask and 16 deaths were associated with neuraxial anesthesia (14 spinals and two caudals). Of the 14 deaths associated with spinal anesthesia, 10 were due to cardiovascular collapse and in all but two cases small doses of tetracaine (<8 mg) were used. Eight deaths were associated with general endotracheal anesthesia, three were caused by cardiac arrest associated with hypotension, one by cardiac arrest associated with a nonanesthetic drug reaction and four were directly due to problems of intubation (see Table 71.8).

Training of anesthesia-personnel

During the first decade of the study, anesthetics were given by a variety of health care providers, a circulating nurse, obstetricians, residents, nurse anesthetists and anesthesiologists. During the second decade, anesthesiologists were involved in 12 of the 17 deaths and, in the last

Table 71.7 Anesthetic deaths: cause of death (Reproduced with permission from Sachs et al[28])

Year	Aspiration	Cardiorespiratory
1955–64	11	6
1965–74	5	12
1975–85	0	3
Total	16	21

Table 71.8 Anesthetic deaths: types of anesthesia (Reproduced with permission from Sachs et al[28])

Year	Total	Mask	Regional	General endotracheal anesthesia
1955–64	17	10	6	1
1965–74	17	3	10	4
1975–85	3	0	0	3
Total	37	13	16	8

decade, all three deaths were attended by an anesthesiologist. Of the 20 deaths that occurred during the first two decades and were attended by an anesthesiologist, 10 were associated with either inadequate vigilance or lack of equipment.

Monitoring of vital signs

15 of the 37 patients who died had no monitoring of vital signs; in two cases, all medical personnel left the room after a spinal had been initiated. Of the three deaths in the last decade, two happened despite excellent vigilance, preparation and manpower.

Based on the observations of the events that led up to each of these deaths, Sachs et al[28] concluded with recommendations considered standard in the anesthesia literature, but important to restate given that in the USA approximately 25% of cesarean deliveries and 45% of vaginal deliveries have the anesthetic managed or directed by an obstetrician. The recommendations include:

1. There should be the capability to intubate any parturient receiving a general anesthesia and the person administering any regional anesthetic should be prepared to treat all possible complications such as 'total spinal' and, therefore, be skilled at tracheal intubation.
2. Every intubation in a parturient should be confirmed by capnography.
3. Antacids should be given routinely prior to an anesthetic but oral intake after the start of active labor should be avoided (although this point is now being debated).[68]
4. Vital signs should be monitored continuously following administration of a regional anesthetic.
5. Pulse oximetry should be used, especially in the patient undergoing a regional anesthetic with supplemental sedation for cesarean delivery.[28]

The second paper by Endler et al[26] looked at the demographic and physical characteristics of those patients who died as a direct result of anesthesia. They found specific traits that related to increased risk. Non-White race, obesity and hypertension all correlated with increased anesthesia mortality. Sachs et al[28] found similar trends, and these findings have been echoed in many other studies and reflect areas for improvement in training anesthesiologists and assessing risk.[1,9,14,25]

Endler et al,[26] reviewed anesthesia-related maternal deaths that occurred in Michigan from 1972–1984. 15 deaths were considered to be primarily due to anesthesia and in four deaths anesthesia was a contributory factor. The deaths, identified through a variety of reporting mechanisms, were reported in detail by a regional visiting obstetrician and forwarded to the Sub-Committee on Maternal Mortality of the Michigan State Medical Society Committee on Maternal and Perinatal Health. The 10-member subcommittee, consisting of obstetricians, pathologists and anesthesiologists, reviewed the report and classified the death and identified the contributing factors.

Anesthetic technique

Failure to secure a patent airway was the predominant cause of death in recent years. There were no deaths associated with regional anesthesia since 1980.

Patient characteristics

13 deaths occurred in Black patients and two in White, although the overall population distribution in Michigan is 85% White and 15% nonWhite.

Weight

80% of the patients were obese. The mean age was 24 (range 16–34).

Confounding medical conditions

50% of the patients were hypertensive and 80% of the cases were emergent.[26]

Despite these detailed studies, some sources question the importance of anesthesia as a cause of maternal mortality. This contention is based on the suggestion that anesthesia-related death has reached an irreducible minimum.[1,69,70] However, it is important to remember that maternal mortality studies can only report the trends they uncover, which is a reflection of the instrument used to analyze the data. If deaths are classified by the operative procedure – not the specific cause of death – and if cause of death is determined by superficial inspection rather than in-depth inquiry or autopsy, we will not be able to establish the true incidence of anesthesia-related maternal mortality. Frequently, only deaths directly due to airway problems or regional anesthesia are counted as anesthesia-related deaths. This may seriously underestimate the importance of anesthetic management and encourage, by lack of attention, the current trend whereby anesthesia as a cause of death does not improve at the same rate as other causes.

RISK PROFILE

Death represents only the tip of the iceberg of anesthetic-related harm. Morbidity due to 'near misses', an obvious extension of mortality, has been virtually impossible to document in a systematic, epidemiologic study. Maternal mortality ratios are too crude a statistic. Case-specific mortality rates or a patient registry of adverse outcomes with detailed histories would be very useful. Until these are available we must extract and utilize the only information available to us. Information regarding maternal mortality should lead to something more than statements about the health of society or the position of women or even more than enhanced education. It should be converted into clinically useful information that can direct attention and medical management. We should develop a risk assessment protocol similar to the risk assessment used by the cardiovascular anesthesiologist in determining the need for invasive monitoring and then target high-risk patients for more intensive scrutiny and aggressive management. From a review of the literature it appears that age over 35, especially when combined with lower than average educational level or multiparity, is a significant risk. Non-White racial identity is also a risk factor, as is obesity. The risks associated with these characteristics are confounded by the presence of coexisting medical conditions such as hypertension and infection.

Risk associations are:

1. Age greater than 35 – at risk for ectopic pregnancy, pregnancy-induced hypertension and peripartum hemorrhage.
2. Non-White race – at risk for problems of airway management, misdiagnosed ectopic pregnancy and pregnancy-induced hypertension.
3. Obesity – at risk for airway problems, pregnancy-induced hypertension and embolism.

Specific anesthesia-related risk-reducing protocols include:

1. Invasive monitoring: patients with two or more risk factors should be considered candidates for invasive monitoring when managing peripartum hemorrhage.
2. Afro-Americans: an often cited excuse for the higher rate of anoxic deaths among Afro-Americans is the inability to detect cyanosis in dark-skinned patients. Physicians should be taught to observe the coloration of mucous membranes at least, or preferably make the use of pulse oximetry standard in the obstetric suite. Furthermore, Comroe in the 1960s demonstrated that cyanosis is a late and unreliable sign of hypoxia.[72] Given the increase in anoxic deaths associated with general anesthesia for cesarean delivery and therapeutic abortions, pulse oximetry should be considered standard for all pregnant patients receiving general anesthesia or heavy sedation both during the operative procedure and in the recovery room.[71]
3. Emergency anesthesia in the obese patients: it is often suggested that regional anesthesia is the technique of choice for the obese patient. This author agrees, but recognizes that in inexperienced hands, i.e., the occasional obstetric anesthesiologist, performing an epidural may be technically difficult and both epidural and spinal may give an unpredictable block. Some authors suggest awake intubation for these patients, which is certainly a safe alternative. Another suggestion for the emergency case is a continuous spinal anesthetic utilizing an epidural catheter thus allowing the speed of a spinal and the controllability of an epidural. It should be noted that smaller catheters may not be suited for these patients because of the greater likelihood of kinking the catheter by the redundant skin. Microcatheters are no longer FDA approved at this time (1994).

CONCLUSION

All this begins as a life that enveloped another potential life ends. Accurate maternal mortality statistics depend primarily upon the physician attending the woman at the time of her death. Every effort should be made to salvage something positive from that loss – perhaps the prevention of a similar event.[44]

The study of maternal mortality is a powerful tool to help improve medical management and, if we permit, medical science. Over the past three decades significant changes have been brought about by work of the many maternal mortality committees. However, the work is not yet completed. Not only have we failed to reach the agenda for the year 2000 set forth by the Surgeon General's Office, but we are witnessing an increase in the disparity between the risk of death faced by different populations. Clearly, there are institutional barriers such as a real problem of access. However, there are also problems of physician training and manpower distribution. As our population continues to grow in diversity our knowledge must keep up with the particular requirements of each ethnic group. We must have universally available accurate means of assessing oxygenation status in every delivery, operating and recovery room. If ectopic pregnancy is underdiagnosed in the teen populations, then this deficiency must be made known to the emergency room physicians that care for these young women. As obstetric anesthesiologists we must take responsibility for our role in resuscitation of the sick parturient and make pulmonary edema and fatal hemorrhage even rarer causes of death. Finally, as academic physicians, we must make research and training in this area of women's health as important and as attractive as any other area of health care.

REFERENCES

1. May W J, Greiss Jr F C 1989 Maternal mortality in North Carolina: a forty-year experience. Am J Obstet Gynecol 161: 555–561
2. Barker D J, Osmond C 1987 Death rates from stroke in England and Wales predicted from past maternal mortality. Br Med J 295: 83–86
3. Chavkin W, St. Clair D 1990 Beyond prenatal care: a comprehensive vision of reproductive health. JAMWA 45: 55–57
4. McBarnette L 1987 Women and poverty: the effects on reproductive status. Women Health 12(3–4): 55–81
5. Simkin P 1989 Childbearing in social context. Women Health 15: 5–21
6. Sundstrom-Feigenberg K 1988 Reproductive health and reproductive freedom: maternal health care and family planning in the Swedish health system. Women Health 13(3–4): 35–55
7. Winikoff B, Sullivan M 1987 Assessing the role of family planning in reducing maternal mortality. Studies Fam Plan 18: 128–143
8. Cook R 1989 The role of confidential enquiries in the reduction of maternal mortality and alternatives to this approach. Int. J Gynecol Obstet 30: 41–45
9. Gabel H D 1987 Maternal mortality in South Carolina from 1970 to 1984: an analysis. Obstet Gynecol 69: 307–311
10. Koonin L M, Atrash H K, Rochat R W, Smith J C 1988 Maternal mortality surveillance, United States, 1980–1985. MMWR 37: 19–29
11. Allen M H, Chavkin W, Marinoff J 1991 Ascertainment of maternal deaths in New York City. Am J Public Health 81(3): 380–382
12. Bassell G M, Marx G F 1987 Anesthesia-related maternal mortality. In Shnider S M, Levinson G (eds) Anesthesia for Obstetrics, 2nd edn. Williams & Wilkins, Baltimore, pp 325–333
13. Koonin L M, Atrash H K, Lawson H W, Smith J C 1991 Maternal mortality surveillance, United States, 1979–1986. MMWR 40: 1–13
14. Rochat R W, Koonin L M, Atrash H K, Jewett J F 1988 Maternal mortality in the United States: report from the Maternal Mortality Collaborative. Obstet Gynecol 72: 91–97
15. Sachs B P, Brown D A, Driscoll S G, Schulman E, Acker D, Ransil B J, Jewett J F 1988 Hemorrhage, infection, toxemia, and cardiac disease, 1954–85: causes for their declining role in maternal mortality. Am J Public Health 78: 671–675
16. Rumbolz W L 1991 A report of maternal deaths in Nebraska for the years 1987, 1988 and 1989. Neb Med J 76(2): 31–34
17. Commission on Professional and Hospital Activities 1980 International Classification of Diseases, 9th revision. Clinical modifications, 2nd printing, Edwards Brothers, Ann Arbor
18. Chamblee R F, Evans M D 1982 New dimensions in cause of death statistics. Am J Public Health 72: 1265–1270
19. Wright R F, Smith J C 1990 State level expert review committees – are they protected? Public Health Rep 105: 13–23
20. Dawson I 1988 The confidential enquiry into maternal deaths: its role and importance for pathologists. J Clin Pathol 41: 820–825
21. Kaunitz A M, Hughes J M, Grimes D A, Smith J C, Rochat R W, Kafrissen M E 1985 Causes of maternal mortality in the United States. Obstet Gynecol 65: 605–612
22. Moses V, DePersio S R, Lorenz D, Oberle M W, Rochat R, Fermo A 1987 A thirty-year review of maternal mortality in Oklahoma, 1950–1979. Am J Obstet Gynecol 157: 1189–1194
23. Lehmann D K, Mabie W C, Miller J M, Pernoll M L 1987 The epidemiology and pathology of maternal mortality: Charity Hospital of Louisiana in New Orleans, 1965–1984. Obstet Gynecol 69: 833–840
24. Morgan M 1987 Anaesthetic contribution to maternal mortality. Br J Anaesth 59: 842–855
25. Dorfman S F 1990 Maternal mortality in New York City, 1981–1983. Obstet Gynecol 76: 317–323
26. Endler G C, Mariona F G, Sokol R J, Stevenson L B 1988 Anesthesia-related maternal mortality in Michigan, 1972 to 1984. Am J Obstet Gynecol 159: 187–193
27. Sachs B P, Brown D A J, Driscoll S G, Schulman E, Acker D, Ransil B J, Jewett J F 1987 Maternal mortality in Massachusetts: trends and prevention. New Engl J Med 316: 667–672
28. Sachs B P, Oriol N E, Ostheimer G W, Weiss J B, Driscoll S, Acker D, Brown D A, Jewett J F 1989 Anesthetic-related maternal mortality, 1954 to 1985. J Clin Anesth 1: 333–338
29. Syverson C J, Chavkin W, Atrash H K, Rochat R W, Sharp E S, King G E 1991 Pregnancy-related mortality in New York City, 1980–1984: causes of death and associated risk factors. Am J Obstet Gynecol 164: 603–608
30. Varner M W 1989 Maternal mortality in Iowa from 1952 to 1986. Surg Gynecol Obstet 168: 555–562
31. Benedetti T J, Starzyk P, Frost F 1985 Maternal deaths in Washington state. Obstet Gynecol 66: 99–101
32. Dorfman S F 1985 Pregnancy for older parents. In: Cherry S H, Berkowitz R L, Kase N G (eds) pp 579–583
33. Adair R L 1935 Maternal, fetal and neonatal morbidity and mortality. Am J Obstet Gynecol 29: 384–95
34. Editorial 1989 Lessons from history – maternal and infant mortality. Lancet 2: 140
35. Cunningham F G, MacDonald P C, Gant N F 1989 Obstetrics in broad perspective. In: Williams obstetrics, 18th edn. Appleton & Lange, Norwalk, CT, pp 1–6
36. Kaunitz A M, Spence C, Danielson T S, Rochat R W, Grimes D A 1984 Perinatal and maternal mortality in a religious group avoiding obstetric care. Am J Obstet Gynecol: 150: 826–831
37. Pritchard J A, MacDonald P C, Gant N R 1985 In: Williams' obstetrics. Appleton Century Crofts, Norwalk, CT, pp 3–4
38. Centers for Disease Control 1985 Maternal mortality: pilot surveillance in seven states. MMWR 34: 709–711
39. Antler J, Fox D M 1976 The movement toward a safe maternity: physician accountability in New York City 1915–1940. Bull Hist Med 50: 569–595
40. Birge E A 1970 Autopsy in maternal demise. Wis Med J 69: 78
41. Dept of Health and Human Services. Public Health Service 1991 Healthy people 2000: national health promotion and disease prevention objectives. US Department of Health and Human Services, Public Health Service, DHHS publication No. PHS91–1120, Washington DC
42. New York State Department of Health 1989 Documentation of maternal mortality. N Y State J Med 89(4): 238–239
43. Rosenberg M J, Rosenthal S M 1987 Reproductive mortality in the United Sates: recent trend and methodologic considerations. Am J Public Health 77: 833–836
44. Dorfman S F 1985 Maternal mortality in the United States. In: Cherry S H, Berkowitz R L, Kase N G (eds) Rovinsky and Guttmacher's medical, surgical and gynecologic complications of pregnancy, 3rd edn. Williams & Wilkins, Baltimore pp 590–594
45. Teirsyein A S, Lesser M 1985 Pulmonary function and pulmonary disease in pregnancy. In: Cherry S H, Berkowitz R L, Kase N G (eds), pp 88–108
46. Albright G A, Stevenson D K, Ferguson J E 1986 Anesthetic and obstetric risks. In: Albright G A, Ferguson J E, Joyce T H, Stevenson D K (eds) Anesthesia in obstetrics, maternal, fetal and neonatal aspects, 2nd edn. Butterworths, Boston
47. Fonteyn V J, Isada N B 1988 Nongenetic implications of childbearing after age thirty-five. Obstet Gynecol Surv 43: 709–720
48. King C 1991 The New York Maternal Mortality Study. A conflict of professionalization. Bull Hist Med 65: 476–502
49. Koonin L M, Ellerbrock T V, Atrash H K et al 1989 Pregnancy-associated deaths due to AIDS in the United States. J Am Med Assoc 261: 1306–1309
50. Chu S Y, Buehler J W, Berkelman R L 1990 Impact of the human immunodeficiency virus epidemic on mortality in women of reproductive age, United States. J Am Med Assoc 264: 225–229
51. Nicholas S W, Sondheimer D L, Willoughby A D et al 1989 Human immunodeficiency virus infection in childhood, adolescence and pregnancy: a status report and maternal research agenda. Pediatrics 83: 293–308
52. Selwyn P A, Schoenbaum E E, Davenny K et al 1989 Prospective study of human immunodeficiency virus infection and pregnancy outcomes in intravenous drug users. J Am Med Assoc 261: 1289–1294
53. Lawson H W, Atrash H K, Saftlas A F, Finch E L 1989 Ectopic pregnancy in the United States, 1970–1986. MMWR 38: 1–10
54. Harris R P 1887 Cattle-horn lacerations of the abdomen and uterus in pregnant women. Am J Obstet Gynecol 20: 43

55. Leo J D 1990 Cesarean section and other obstetric operations. In: Scott J R, DiSaia P J, Hammond C B, Spellacy W N (ed) Danforth's obstetrics and Gynecol, 6th edn. J B Lippincott, Philadelphia. p 640
56. Miller Jr J M 1988 maternal and neonatal morbidity and mortality in Cesarean section. Obstet Gynecol Clinics N Am 15: 629–638
57. Atrash H K, Cheek T G, Hogue C J R 1988 Legal abortion mortality and general anesthesia. Am J Obstet Gynecol: 158: 420–424
58. Lee K, Corpuz M 1988 Teenage pregnancy: trend and impact on rates of low birth weight and fetal, maternal, and neonatal mortality in the United States. Clin Perinatol 15: 929–942
59. Fancieullo G, Johnson M D 1992 Morbid obesity. In: Ostheimer G W (ed) Manual of obstetric anesthesia, 2nd edn. Churchill Livingstone, New York pp 322–329
60. Gross T, Sokol R J, King K C 1980 Obesity in pregnancy: risks and outcome. Obstet Gynecol 56: 446–450
61. Schoendorf K C, Hogue C J, Kleinman J C, Rowley D 1992 Mortality among infants of black as compared with white college-educated parents. New Engl J Med 326: 1522–1526
62. Wise P H, Pursley D M 1992 Infant mortality as a social mirror (editorial comment). New Engl J Med 326: 1558–1560
63. Duke R C, Speidel J J 1991 Women's reproductive health: A chronic crisis. J Am Med Assoc: 266: 1846–1847
64. Moldin P, Hokegard K H, Nielsen T F 1984 Cesarean section and maternal mortality in Sweden 1973–1979. Acta Obstet Gynecol Scand 63: 7–11
65. Morgan B M 1980 Maternal death: a review of maternal deaths at one hospital from 1958 to 1978. Anaesthesia: 35: 334–348
66. Turnbull AC, Tindall U R, Robson G, Dawson I M P, Cloake E P, Ashley J S 1986 Report on confidential enquiries into maternal deaths in England and Wales 1979–81. HMSO, London
67. Gibbs C P, Krischer J, Peckham B M, Sharp H, Kirschbaum T H 1986 Obstetric anesthesia: a national survey. Anesthesiology: 65: 298–306
68. Elkington K W 1991 At the water's edge: where obstetrics and anesthesia meet. Obstet Gynecol 77: 304–308
69. Conklin K A 1990 Can anesthetic-related maternal mortality be reduced? Am J Obstet Gynecol: 163: 253–254
70. Taylor 1989 Maternal mortality in North Carolina [see comments]. Am J Obstet Gynecol 161: 560
71. Vandam L D 1990 The senses as monitors. In: Blitt C D (ed) Monitoring in anesthesia and critical care medicine, 2nd edn. Churchill Livingstone, New York pp 19–20

72. Resuscitation of the pregnant woman

S. S. Schwalbe

Pregnancy is most often considered as a benign physiologic process that occurs in young, healthy women. While this may be true for the vast majority of pregnancies, it is, unfortunately, not always the case. For example, Ginz[1] estimated the rate of myocardial infarction to be about 1 per 10 000 deliveries, with an overall mortality rate of 28%. Sullivan and Ramanathan[2] noted that the prevalence of heart disease in pregnancy ranged from 0.4% to 4.1%, and that among gravid women in class III or IV of the New York Heart Association's functional classifications, the maternal mortality was as high as 6.8%.

Causes of cardiac arrest during pregnancy are numerous and include hemorrhage, pulmonary embolism, amniotic fluid embolism, myocardial infarction, pheochromocytoma, laryngeal edema secondary to preeclampsia, local anesthetic toxicity, hypoxia from anesthetic mishap, electrocution from operating room equipment, motor vehicle accidents and other trauma. Such occurrences are far from routine in the delivery suite; nevertheless, the labor team must be conversant with basic resuscitative techniques.

CARDIOPULMONARY RESUSCITATION (CPR)

The first step in resuscitation for a suspected cardiac arrest should always be a check for consciousness. Loss of consciousness ensues 5–11 s following the loss of cerebral blood flow.[3] Therefore, a patient who is even slightly arousable cannot have suffered a cardiac arrest. Once unconsciousness has been confirmed, the next steps are the classic ABCs of resuscitation: airway, breathing and circulation.

A patent airway must be achieved immediately. The goal is to relieve the obstruction that occurs when there is loss of muscle tone. Most often such obstruction in the unconscious patient is caused by the tongue. Two methods of opening the airway have been recommended: the head tilt–jaw thrust maneuver and the head tilt–chin lift maneuver.

After opening the airway, any vomitus or foreign material visible in the oropharynx should be wiped away, and a check made for the presence of spontaneous breathing. Sometimes, in cases of respiratory arrest, merely relieving the obstruction and opening the airway by one of the maneuvers described above may be all that is necessary to restore spontaneous respiration. There should, however, be no unnecessary delay at this point. A pregnant woman, particularly one in labor, has little oxygen reserve.[4] Even brief periods of apnea will not be tolerated well by either mother or fetus. In the presence of apnea, artificial respiration should begin immediately. In the hospital setting, equipment such as a bag–valve–mask device or a pocket mask should be readily available and is the preferred mode of therapy to deliver supplemental oxygen. The jaw thrust maneuver can be used to maintain the patient's airway while using these devices. If mouth-to-mouth ventilation is chosen outside the hospital, it should begin with two full breaths of 1–1.5 s each. This differs from the old technique of four quick initial breaths, which is more likely to force air into the esophagus, leading to regurgitation and pulmonary aspiration.[5]

Aspiration is an ever-present danger in the unconscious parturient. A combination of mechanical and hormonal factors retards gastric emptying in the parturient to the point at which food may be retained for more than 24 h.[6] Therefore, even if ventilation is thought to be adequate by either the mouth-to-mouth or the bag–valve–mask technique, these should be considered only temporary measures. Control of the airway by endotracheal intubation must be accomplished as soon as possible.

Once the airway has been opened and artificial ventilation has begun, the next step is to palpate the carotid artery. If pulsations are absent, the diagnosis of cardiac arrest is confirmed, and external chest compression (closed-chest cardiac compression) should begin.

With the hands over the lower sternum, and not overlying the xiphoid, the sternum should be compressed 1.5–2 in (3.75–5.0 cm) with each effort, at a rate of 80–100 compressions per min. The ratio of compression to ventilation should be 5 to 1, with a 1–1.5 s pause for ventilation.[5]

It had long been thought that these cardiac compressions generate blood flow by a direct compression of the heart between the sternum and spine, the 'cardiac pump' mechanism proposed by Kouwenhoven et al in 1960.[7] There is now growing evidence to suggest that a second mechanism may be of equal or greater importance for maintaining blood flow during CPR.[8,9] This 'thoracic pump' mechanism is based on the observation that external chest compression increases the intrathoracic pressure, which is transmitted equally to all thoracic structures. Since arteries tend to resist collapse, such a pressure increase should be almost fully transmitted to the extrathoracic arteries. Venous collapse and the presence of valves in the venous system prevent full transmission of this pressure increase to extrathoracic veins. A pressure gradient is created between the extrathoracic arteries and veins, causing antegrade flow during compression. During the relaxation phase between compressions, the intrathoracic pressure falls below the extrathoracic venous pressure, resulting in venous return to the right side of the heart.

With this mechanism in mind, it is clear that even minor degrees of aortocaval compression imposed by the gravid uterus may have a profound effect on the success or failure of the resuscitative efforts. Any compression of the inferior vena cava will seriously impede the venous return to the heart. In addition, obstruction of the lower aorta would represent a significant obstacle to flow, hindering the development of an appropriate arteriovenous pressure gradient during chest compressions.

It is therefore imperative that uterine displacement be maintained during CPR. A wedge or sandbag should be placed under the right hip to provide a left lateral tilt to the pelvis of approximately 30°. The position of the torso will not be greatly affected and chest compressions should still be possible without difficulty. If circumstances make this approach cumbersome or impractical, the uterus can be deviated manually by having the patient's abdomen displaced to the left and slightly cephalad. If it is possible to raise the patient's legs, this simple maneuver may also help to improve venous return.

If hemodynamic stability still cannot be achieved despite attempts at uterine displacement, then abdominal delivery of the baby must be performed immediately. It would be a serious mistake to defer cesarean delivery until the mother has 'stabilized' since such stabilization may never occur without delivery and relief of the aortocaval compression. Several cases have occurred in which prompt delivery led to adequate maternal resuscitation and recovery.[10,11] In addition to relief of aortocaval compression, delivery of the child improves the thoracic compliance, which is decreased during pregnancy. This may have a further beneficial effect on chest compressions, as well as improve the ability to ventilate the patient.

A review of agonal and post-mortem cesarean deliveries also demonstrates the importance of this procedure to the infant.[12] Most of the children who survived such emergency cesarean deliveries were delivered within 5 min of the onset of maternal cardiac arrest. As the time to delivery extends beyond 5 min, the chances for survival of the fetus diminish markedly, and the probability of severe neurologic damage increases. This is demonstrated clearly in Table 72.1.

In the first and second trimesters the degree of aortocaval compression exerted by the uterus may be minimal, and an emergency abdominal delivery may offer less in terms of effective resuscitation at this time in pregnancy. If CPR fails to maintain peripheral circulation, emergency thoracotomy with open chest cardiac massage must be considered. In certain clinical situations (e.g. chest trauma, severe emphysema, cardiac tamponade), open chest massage may also be necessary to produce adequate perfusion of the brain and heart.[5]

ACID–BASE BALANCE

The primary mode of therapy for acid–base imbalances during a cardiac arrest is the establishment of adequate alveolar ventilation.[13] To this end, frequent determination of arterial blood gas values can be used to assess the adequacy of ventilation and guide further therapy. In late pregnancy, the $Paco_2$ should normally be between 32 and 34 mmHg.

As a general rule, in the treatment of acidosis, hyperventilation is preferred over the exogenous administration of sodium bicarbonate, which may be counterproductive. However, if the patient remains severely acidotic, sodium bicarbonate may be administered in an initial dose of 1 mEq/kg. Hyperventilation to the point at which the $Paco_2$ falls below 25 mmHg is to be avoided, as is overuse of sodium bicarbonate, since both of these events will have a deleterious effect on placental transfer of oxygen.

Table 72.1 Survival rate of infants according to interval between cardiac arrest and delivery (Reproduced with permission from ref. 12)

Cases	No. of patients	Percent
0–5 min	42 (normal infants)	70
6–10 min	7 (normal infants) 1 (mild neurologic sequelae)	13
Subtotal	8	
11–15 min	6 (normal infants) 1 (severe neurologic sequelae)	12
Subtotal	7	
16–20 min	1 (severe neurologic sequelae)	1.7
21+ min	1 (normal infant) 2 (severe neurologic sequelae)	3.3
Subtotal	3	
Total	61	100

VASOPRESSORS

On the labor floor, anesthesiologists often give ephedrine to counteract the hypotension that may result from a regional blockade. However, during cardiac arrest or severe cardiovascular depression ephedrine may not be a sufficient myocardial stimulant.[14] Epinephrine has been used in these situations primarily for its alpha-adrenergic properties,[15] and the value of its beta-adrenergic effects in this situation is controversial. The recommended intravenous dose of epinephrine (0.5–1.0 mg every 5 min during resuscitation) is more than enough to reduce uterine blood flow and adversely affect an already compromised fetus.[16] As mentioned above, early delivery of the infant gives the child the best chance of survival.

DIRECT CURRENT CARDIOVERSION

Some concern has been raised as to the risk of fetal morbidity during the treatment of maternal arrhythmias with direct current (DC) shock. Few cases of DC cardioversion for supraventricular arrhythmias have been reported during pregnancy, and the experience with ventricular defibrillation is even more limited. However, a review of these cases, which employed energies as high as 300 J, showed no adverse infant outcomes related to the use of this therapy.[17] At present, there appears to be no contraindication to the use of direct current shock.

SPECIFIC THERAPIES

The 1992 National Conference on Cardiopulmonary Resuscitation (CPR) and Emergency Cardiac Care (ECC) established suggested algorithms for the treatment of specific dysrhythmias.[5] The treatment algorithms for ventricular fibrillation, bradycardia, pulseless electrical activity (electromechanical dissociation) and asystole, are presented in Figures 72.1–72.4.

SPECIAL SITUATIONS

The resuscitative regimens for two special syndromes are detailed below. Prompt appropriate management may save the lives of mother and fetus in these unusual, but critical situations.

Amniotic fluid embolism

Amniotic fluid embolism (AFE), an uncommon complication of pregnancy, is nevertheless one of the most dangerous, having a reported maternal mortality rate of 86%.[18] Clinically, the awake patient often presents with

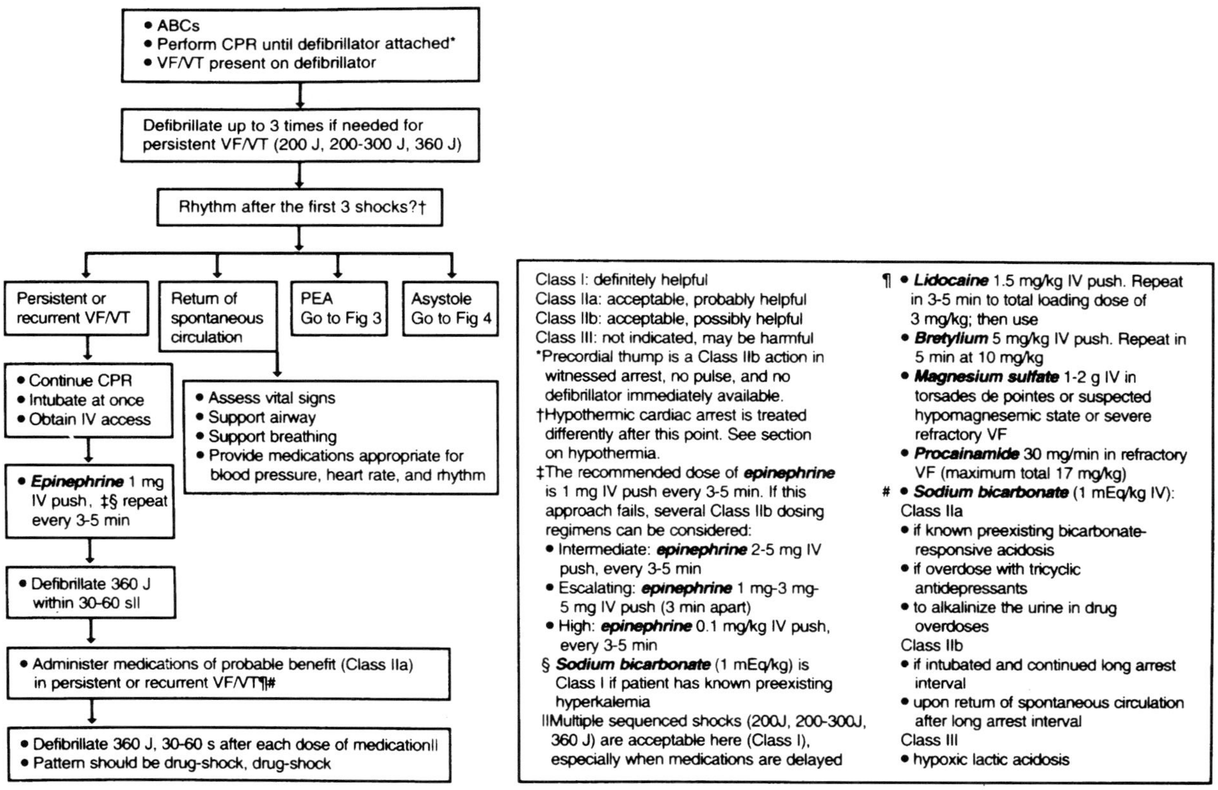

72.1 Algorithm for ventricular fibrillation.

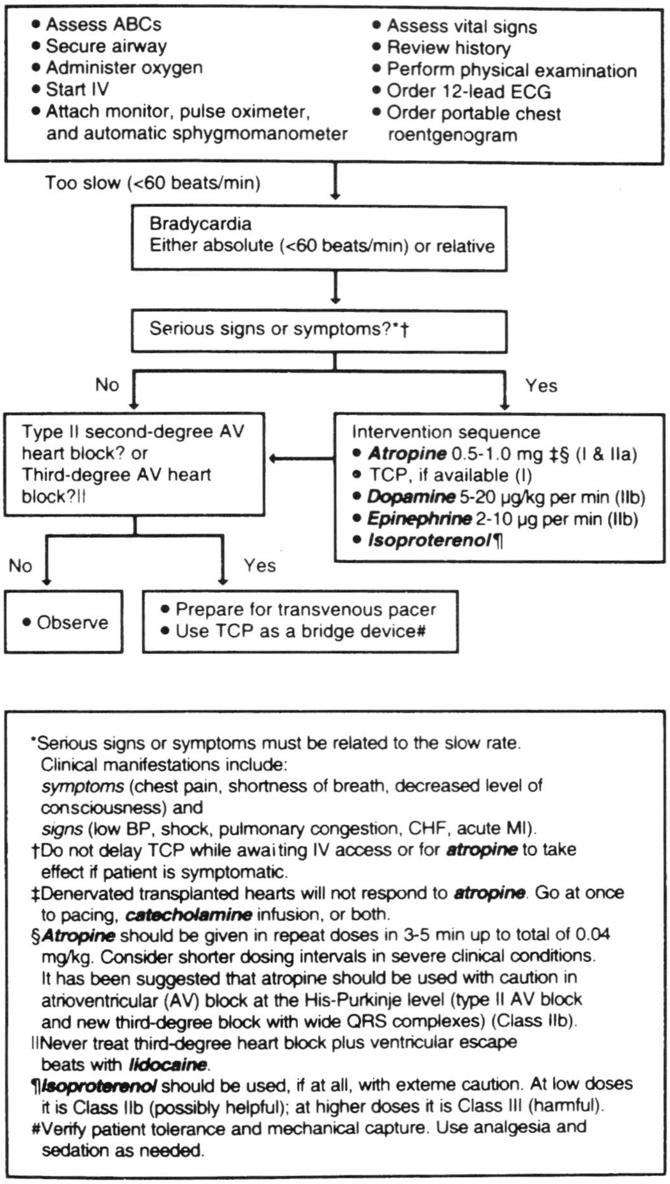

72.2 Algorithm for bradycardia.

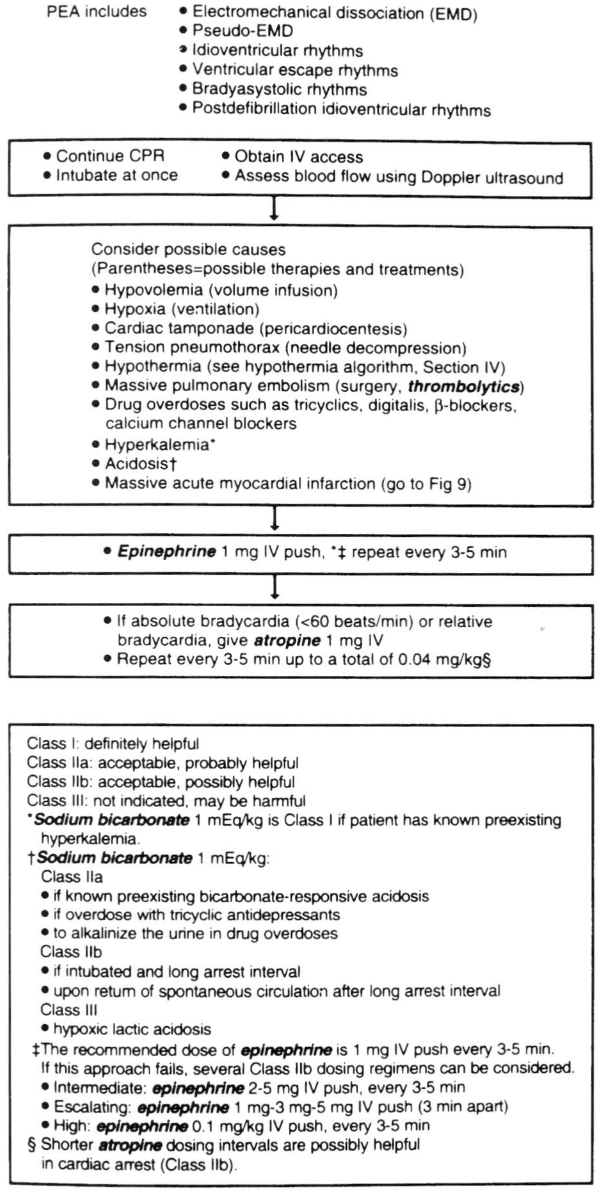

72.3 Algorithm for pulseless electrical activity (PEA) (electromechanical dissociation (EMD)).

anxiety, shivering, coughing and sudden respiratory distress, almost always without chest pain. Besides the mechanical blockage of the pulmonary vessels by amniotic fluid and other fetal debris, an anaphylactoid reaction may also develop, causing bronchospasm and enhancing pulmonary artery constriction. The result is severe hypoxia and an acute pulmonary hypertension which may lead to acute pulmonary edema. 25–50% of AFE patients die in the first hour from this initial insult. Of the patients who do survive this period, most develop a diffuse intravascular coagulopathy. This clotting defect is usually thought of as a late development, but it can be an early event. In Morgan's review of 272 cases, the presenting signs and symptoms were respiratory in 51%, cardiovascular in 27% and hematologic in 12%. Convulsions were the first signs in 10% of the patients.[18]

Diagnosis is often difficult and rests upon a high index of suspicion combined with recovery of fetal squames and other amniotic debris from a central venous catheter inserted into the mother's right atrium.[19] Recent investigations, however, have shown that squames and trophoblastic cells can be recovered from the maternal circulation even in pregnancies where there is not overt clinical evidence of amniotic fluid embolism.[20,21] The question of how much amniotic fluid is necessary to precipitate the clinical picture of embolism has yet to be answered.

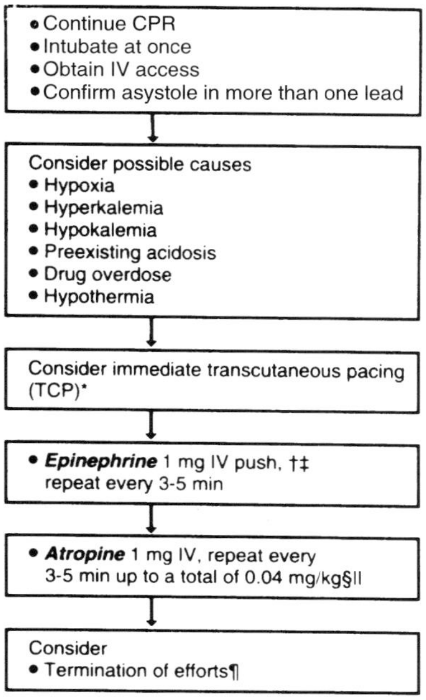

Class I: definitely helpful
Class IIa: acceptable, probably helpful
Class IIb: acceptable, possibly helpful
Class III: not indicated, may be harmful
*TCP is a Class IIb intervention. Lack of success may be due to delays in pacing. To be effective TCP must be performed early, simultaneously with drugs. Evidence does not support routine use of TCP for asystole.
†The recommended dose of ***epinephrine*** is 1 mg IV push every 3-5 min. If this approach fails, several Class IIb dosing regimens can be considered:
- Intermediate: ***epinephrine*** 2-5 mg IV push, every 3-5 min
- Escalating: ***epinephrine*** 1 mg-3 mg-5 mg IV push (3 min apart)
- High: ***epinephrine*** 0.1 mg/kg IV push, every 3-5 min

‡***Sodium bicarbonate*** 1 mEq/kg is Class I if patient has known preexisting hyperkalemia.
§Shorter ***atropine*** dosing intervals are Class IIb in asystolic arrest.
||***Sodium bicarbonate*** 1 mEq/kg:
Class IIa
- if known preexisting bicarbonate-responsive acidosis
- if overdose with tricyclic antidepressants
- to alkalinize the urine in drug overdoses

Class IIb
- if intubated and continued long arrest interval
- upon return of spontaneous circulation after long arrest interval

Class III
- hypoxic lactic acidosis

¶If patient remains in asystole or other agonal rhythms after successful intubation and initial medications and no reversible causes are identified, consider termination of resuscitative efforts by a physician. Consider interval since arrest.

72.4 Algorithm for asystole treatment.

Treatment of AFE must be geared toward (1) improvement of oxygenation, (2) support of the cardiovascular system and (3) treatment of the coagulopathy. Severe ventilation–perfusion inequalities usually develop following entry of amniotic fluid into the pulmonary vasculature, leading to profound hypoxia. Intubation and positive-pressure ventilation with 100% oxygen should be instituted promptly in an effort to enhance oxygenation. Positive end-expiratory pressure (PEEP) is often beneficial. A bronchodilating agent, such as terbutaline, isoproterenol or aminophylline, may aid in relieving bronchospasm.

As mentioned above, a central venous catheter should be inserted to aspirate blood for examination for fetal squames and amniotic debris. Blood should also be obtained for coagulation studies and for cross-match of blood. A pulmonary artery catheter should be placed as soon as is practicable, in order to monitor the patient's hemodynamic status properly. Although historically the teaching has been to watch for acute failure of the right heart secondary to pulmonary hypertension, there may be as much to fear from left-sided heart failure. A review by Clark et al[22] of reported data from AFE patients with pulmonary artery catheters in place revealed a general pattern of left heart failure, even in patients with only mildly elevated pulmonary artery pressure. This suggests that inotropic support may often be necessary, and may be guided by data obtained with the pulmonary artery catheter.

The coagulopathy that develops in these women may be difficult to bring under control. Intravascular volume must be maintained and replacement of clotting factors with cryoprecipitate, fresh-frozen plasma and platelets should continue as necessary.

In addition to the cardiopulmonary and hematologic complications, uterine atony is often a problem in these cases, and should be treated in the standard fashion. The potential adverse consequences of severe hypovolemia in these patients are considerable, and efforts to control uterine bleeding promptly are vital.

Bupivacaine cardiotoxicity

Bupivacaine has become popular in obstetrics owing to its excellent analgesic properties combined with long duration of action. Unfortunately, it also carries the potential for cardiotoxicity when the drug is unintentionally injected intravascularly.[23]

Although high plasma levels of all local anesthetics possess the propensity to cause ventricular arrhythmias, the cardiotoxic effects of bupivacaine are significantly greater than those of other local agents.[24] Several cases of cardiac arrest in pregnant women caused the widespread removal of the 0.75% concentration from the labor suite. However, several healthy parturients died after receiving 0.5% bupivacaine for lumbar epidural block and a few succumbed after single-dose injections of 0.25% bupivacaine into the caudal canal. This indicates that the patient's susceptibility to this complication depends not on the concentration employed but on the actual dose injected. Therefore, strict adherence to the recommended safeguards for epidural blockade, that is, appropriate test dosing, fractionation of the therapeutic dose and ready availability of drugs and equipment for treatment of adverse effects, is imperative for all concentrations of this anesthetic.

Cardiac depression due to bupivacaine has been particularly difficult to reverse, because of a prolonged blockade of cardiac sodium channels. Lidocaine blocks these channels in a fast in–fast out manner, resulting in a rapid recovery from the blockade, while bupivacaine blocks these channels in a fast in–slow out fashion, resulting in delayed recovery during diastole.[25] If tachydysrhythmias should develop during bupivacaine administration, they are probably best treated with bretylium and DC cardioversion, rather than with lidocaine.

Since the cardiac toxicity of bupivacaine is further aggravated by hypoxia and acidemia, resuscitative efforts must begin at the first sign of dysrhythmia. Control of the airway, ventilation with 100% oxygen and correction of acid–base imbalances are of key importance here, as they are with other causes of cardiac arrest. Diazepam or barbiturates may be given parenterally for control of any seizure activity.

As mentioned earlier, the importance of quickly relieving aortocaval compression cannot be overemphasized. Marx[11] reported the fate of five healthy gravidas who received 0.75% bupivacaine during attempted epidural anesthesia for cesarean delivery. All five had a short grand mal seizure followed by disappearance of pulse and blood pressure. All required external cardiac compression for more than 10 min. In three the infant was delivered with no delay and the mother survived intact. In the other two, delivery was postponed for several minutes, and both suffered irreversible brain damage. Kasten and Martin,[26] using a dog model, also demonstrated that relief of aortic and vena caval compression was a necessity for effective resuscitation from a bupivacaine-induced cardiac arrest.

REFERENCES

1. Ginz B 1970 Myocardial infarction in pregnancy. J Obstet Gynaecol Br Cwlth 77: 610–615
2. Sullivan J M, Ramanathan K B 1985 Management of medical problems in pregnancy – severe cardiac disease. New Engl J Med 78: 377–379
3. Rossen R, Kabat H, Anderson J P 1943 Acute arrest of cerebral circulation in man. Arch Neurol Psychiatry 50: 510–528
4. Archer G W, Marx G F 1974 Arterial oxygentension during apnoea in parturient women. Br J Anaesth 46: 358–360
5. Emergency Cardiac Care Committee and Subcommittees, American Heart Association 1992 Guidelines for cardiopulmonary resuscitation and emergency cardiac care. J Am Med Assoc 268: 2175–2295
6. Crawford J S 1956 Some aspects of obstetric anesthesia. Br J Anaesth 28: 201–208
7. Kouwenhoven W B, Jude J R, Knickerbocker G G 1960 Closed chest cardiac massage. J Am Med Assoc 173: 1064–1067
8. Rud M T, Maughan W L, Effron M, Freund P, Weisfeldt M L 1980 Mechanism of blood flow during cardiopulmonary resuscitation. Circulation 61: 345–352
9. Werner J A, Greene H L, Janko C L, Cobb L A 1981 Visualization of cardiac valve motion in man during external chest compression using two-dimensional echocardiography. Implications regarding the mechanism of blood flow. Circulation 63: 1417–1421
10. Depace N L, Betesh J S, Kotler M N 1982 'Postmortem' cesarean section with recovery of both mother and offspring. J Am Med Assoc 248: 971–975
11. Marx G F 1982 Cardiopulmonary resuscitation of late-pregnant women. Anesthesiology 56: 156
12. Katz V L, Dotters D J, Droegmueller W 1986 Perimortem cesarean delivery. Obstet Gynecol 68: 571–576
13. Donegan J H 1981 New concepts in cardiopulmonary resuscitation. Anesth Analg 60: 100–108
14. Caplan R A, Ward R J, Posner K, Cheney F W 1988 Unexpected cardiac arrest during spinal anesthesia: a closed claims analysis of predisposing factors. Anesthesiology 68: 5–11
15. Yakaitis R W, Otto C W, Blitt C D 1979 Relative importance of alpha and beta adrenergic receptors during resuscitation. Crit Care Med 7: 293–296
16. Rossenfeld C R, Barton M D, Meschia G 1976 Effects of epinephrine on distribution of blood flow in the pregnant ewe. Am J Obstet Gynecol 124: 156–163
17. Cullhed I 1983 Cardioversion during pregnancy. Acta Med Scand 214: 169–172
18. Morgan M 1979 Amniotic fluid embolism. Anesthesia 34: 20–32
19. Killam A 1985 Amniotic fluid embolism. Clin Obstet Gynecol 28: 32–36
20. Clark S L, Pavlova Z, Greenspoon J, Horenstein J, Phelan J P 1986 Squamous cells in the maternal pulmonary circulation. Am J Obstet Gynecol 154: 104–106
21. Lee R V, Rodgers B D, White L M, Harvey R C 1986 Cardiopulmonary resuscitation of pregnant women. Am J Obstet Gynecol 81: 311–318
22. Clark S L, Montz F J, Phelan J P 1985 Hemodynamic alterations associated with amniotic fluid embolism: a reappraisal. Am J Obstet Gynecol 151: 617–621
23. Albright G A 1979 Cardiac arrest following regional anesthesia with etidocaine or bupivacaine. Anesthesiology 51: 285–287
24. Kotelko D M, Shnider S M, Dailey P A, Brizgys R V, Levinson G, Shapiro W A, Koike M, Rosen M A 1984 Bupivacaine-induced cardiac arrhythmias in sheep. Anesthesiology 60: 10–18
25. Clarkson C W, Hondeghem L M 1985 Mechanism for bupivacaine depression of cardiac conduction: fast block or sodium channels during the action potential with slow recovery from block during diastole. Anesthesiology 62: 396–405
26. Kasten G W, Martin S T 1986 Resuscitation from bupivacaine-induced cardiovascular toxicity during partial inferior vena cava occlusion. Anesth Analg 65: 341–344

73. Perinatal mortality

E. B. Skerman

OVERVIEW

Natality and mortality statistics are determined from birth and death certificates from each state. These statistics are compiled by the National Center for Health Statistics and provide a variety of useful data such as evaluation of health care systems as well as the health of the population studied. The usefulness of these statistics is limited by differences in defining specific terminology and reporting requirements at the state, national and international levels.[1]

An example of this problem concerns the definition of stillbirth or fetal death (synonomous terms). Some states report a stillbirth according to weight (from 350 to 500 g); others report by gestational age (from 16 to 20 weeks); and some utilize both weight and age.[2]

Uniformity in statistical reporting is essential to correctly evaluate the quality of perinatal health care, to identify a particular area for improvement and to establish criteria to achieve the desired solution.[3]

DEFINITIONS

To attain uniformity in reporting, the World Health Organization[4] recommends: 'National perinatal statistics should include all fetuses and infants delivered weighing at least 500 grams or, when birth weight is unavailable, the corresponding gestational age (22 weeks) or body length (25 cm crown to heel), whether alive or dead.' Further recommendations concerning countries reporting statistics include: 'Countries should present, solely for international comparisons, standard perinatal statistics in which both the numerator and denominator of all rates are restricted to fetuses and infants weighing 1000 grams or more or, when birth weight is unavailable, the corresponding gestational age (28 weeks) or body length (35 cm crown to heel).'

The American Academy of Pediatrics and the American College of Obstetricists and Gynecologists as well as six other prominent national health organizations prepared, reviewed and approved the following definition of fetal death:[5]

> death prior to the complete expulsion or extraction from the mother of a product of human conception, fetus and placenta, irrespective of the duration of pregnancy; death is indicated by the fact that, after such expulsion or extraction, the fetus does not breathe or show any other evidence of life, such as beating of the heart, pulsation of the umbilical cord, or definite movement of voluntary muscles. Heartbeats are to be distinguished from transient cardiac contractions; respirations are to be distinguished from fleeting respiratory efforts or gasps. This definition excludes induced terminations of pregnancy.

Perinatal mortality comprises the total number of stillbirths or fetal deaths and neonatal deaths. Neonatal death is defined as death of an infant within the first 28 days after birth and may be subdivided into early and late neonatal death. Early neonatal death refers to the death of a liveborn infant within the first 7 days of life. Late neonatal death is defined as death of a liveborn infant after the seventh day but not later than the 28th day after birth. The neonatal mortality rate is calculated per 1000 live births. The perinatal mortality rate is determined by the sum of stillbirths and neonatal deaths per 1000 total births.[6]

STATISTICAL INFORMATION

Fetal death or stillbirth amounts to an estimated 15–20% of overall perinatal mortality in clinically diagnosed pregnancies.[2] According to the World Health Organization,[4] the probability of fetal death by gestational age is greatest post conception and drops rapidly until 16 weeks' gestation. Fetal death is said to occur in less than 1% of pregnancies after 20 weeks' gestation.[3,7]

Causes of fetal death vary, however approximately one-third of all stillbirths are unexplained by either fetal or maternal pathologic conditions. This failure is most likely due to not having appropriate studies performed on the fetus and placenta. Most investigators report that chromosomal aberrations are responsible for first-trimester abortions, with the type of abnormality varying according to gestational age, parental age and reproductive history. According to Warburton,[8] 55% of fetal deaths up to 28 weeks' gestation are due to trisomies. Other causes of stillbirth are related to single or multiple anomalies such as heart defects, neural tube defects and urinary tract anomalies.[9] Stillbirth of an infant may occur without warning in an apparently normal pregnancy.

Chronic or acute states of fetal anoxia are most commonly due to placental abruption secondary to a maternal pathologic condition or event and are responsible for about 20% of all stillbirths.[4] The second most common cause of fetal anoxia is cord accident. The most significant maternal conditions adversely affecting fetal oxygenation are diabetes and pregnancy-induced hypertension.

By studying statistical data related to maternal mortality and altering maternal care, the medical community has been able to effect a decrease in the maternal mortality rate. Improvement in maternal mortality has caused the perinatal mortality rate to decline. In support of this statement, Davidson[10] recommends using maternal mortality reviews as a historic model. He proposes a process that will encourage cities and states on a national level and hospitals on a local level to develop specific guidelines for in-depth reviews of fetal and infant mortality and to examine the reasons for each death seriously and comprehensively.

Since the 1950s, the mortality rates for neonates and infants have been gradually decreasing.[7] In 1976, the neonatal mortality rate was 10.9%, and in 1985 the rate had dropped to 7.0%. Within the USA, the District of Columbia has the highest rate (15.9%), followed by Delaware (10.6%). The states reporting the lowest neonatal mortality rates are Montana (5.0%) and Alaska (5.1%).[7]

Analysis of infant mortality rates shows that very low birthweight (less than 1500 g) is the principal predictor of mortality in the neonatal period.[2] Concerns have been raised about variables affecting the collection of these weight data and recognizing the importance of birthweight to infant mortality. Variation in state-reported rates of births of infants weighing less than 500 g does appear. There is a twofold difference between the neonatal mortality rate of Montana, the state with the lowest rate, and Delaware, the state with the highest rate. National statistics were examined in an attempt to estimate the incidence of underreporting.[1] The analyses concluded that there may be approximately 1.1 neonates with weights of less than 500 g who are not reported out of every 1000 live births.

POSSIBLE CAUSES OF UNDERREPORTING

Part of the problem of underreporting may be attributed to the individual state's definition of terms. Other factors that must be considered may be perceptual problems in the clinical setting. For instance, if a baby is declared to weigh more than an arbitrary amount, and thus considered live at the time of birth, the family would then be faced with the expense of a funeral. Monetary reimbursement for medical or hospital care for delivery as opposed to a spontaneous abortion may be another issue to consider in the reporting of live births. How a birth is described may also affect the use of reimbursement codes.

HISTORY OF NEONATAL INTENSIVE CARE

In the 1920s and 1930s, specially designed centers for the care of premature neonates were established in the USA. Many centers trace their origin in part to the work of Dr Julius Hays Hess from Chicago,[11] who became intrigued by the fetal specimens at various stages of gestation that were on exhibition at fairs and expositions in the USA and Europe in the early 1900s. During the 1940s and 1950s, the study of academic neonatology evolved with the establishment of uniform standards of care for the neonate, recognizing their need for isolation, thermal stability, proper nutrition and specialized nursing care.

The establishment of these specialized centers was the forerunner of the neonatal intensive care units, which began to develop in the late 1950s and through the 1960s. It was also during this period that the concept of intensive care for adults and children evolved. During the 1960s, the rapid expansion of neonatal care resulted in more aggressive medical and surgical care of neonates, with the focus primarily on the low-birthweight infant.

With improved knowledge to identify high-risk factors for both the mother and fetus, a new era of obstetric and neonatal care has evolved. Advanced technology has enabled physicians to assess fetal health, including fetal maturation, and diagnose congenital anomalies, and has permitted aggressive management of preterm birth. Utilization of the multidisciplinary approach is essential to assess, intervene and manage the neonate.[12] In substantiation of the effectiveness of the multidisciplinary approach, intrauterine fetal surgery has been undertaken in a few instances, although this treatment is still in experimental stages. Harrison et al[13] successfully performed intrauterine fetal surgery to correct congenital diaphragmatic hernia. Other procedures such as fetal blood exchange for hematologic disease have also been successfully performed. Thus, ongoing research and advancing technology have enabled neonatal practitioners to improve the survivability of the preterm or ill neonate, thereby reducing mortality and long-term morbidity. Immediate aggressive resuscitation is a key factor in decreasing neonatal mortality and morbidity with these infants.[14]

Avery and Mead[15] demonstrated in 1959 that respiratory distress syndrome (RDS) was due to a deficiency in pulmonary surfactant. For over 30 years, researchers have looked for methods to prevent or more successfully treat RDS in premature infants. Artificial surfactant therapy for prevention and treatment of RDS has recently become a reality.

Clinical trials using artificial pulmonary surfactant have shown promising initial results by reducing the duration and severity of RDS and chronic lung disease in the infants affected by RDS at birth. Artificial surfactant therapy can be initiated in the delivery room or in the first few hours of life. The therapy involves the installation of the surfactant preparation directly into the trachea through an endotracheal tube. Positive-pressure ventilation may or may not be utilized in the acute phase of therapy.

FACTORS PREDISPOSING TO PERINATAL MORTALITY

Prevention of preterm birth remains the most important unresolved issue currently confronting obstetricians and neonatologists. Immaturity (weight of less than 1000 g) accounts for up to 50% of all perinatal deaths as well as increases in long-term morbidity.

In a study by Amon et al,[16] maternal diagnoses responsible for preterm birth were found to include the following factors, listed according to their frequency of occurrence:

1. Idiopathic preterm labor;
2. Chorioamnionitis;
3. Premature rupture of membranes;
4. Pregnancy-induced hypertension;
5. Incompetent cervix.

Their study encompassed three variables: maternal diagnosis primarily responsible for delivery, past obstetric outcome, and antepartum and intrapartum factors.

Of interest, their study showed that, of the patients with idiopathic preterm labor, the majority had received no prenatal care. In addition, after their admittance to the hospital, most were in advanced stages of labor with little or no opportunity to try to arrest labor.[16]

METHODS OF DECREASING PERINATAL MORTALITY

Prenatal care must begin early so that those parturients who are at high risk can be identified as soon as possible and effective therapy against preventable maternal factors instituted, thereby prolonging pregnancy. Maternal characteristics that relate to the increased incidence of preterm delivery such as idiopathic preterm labor and incompetent cervix may be identified and managed more aggressively.

Factors responsible for predisposing the fetus to premature delivery or intrauterine growth retardation may be identified and altered through patient education. One of the most devastating problems in the USA today concerns maternal drug abuse, specifically 'crack' cocaine. Not only is maternal health affected, but the fetus is exposed to the barrage of chemical assault each time the mother uses the drug. Intervention for addicted mothers has proven most successful in programs designed to manage all the mother's needs rather than just those relating to her pregnancy.[17] Prevention of perinatal complications through patient and community education is vital in fighting this growing problem as well as other alterable behavioral problems.[18]

Miller and Merritt[19] identified the following behavioral factors that strongly relate to low-birthweight delivery:

1. Low maternal weight for height;
2. Lack of adequate weight gain in pregnancy;
3. No prenatal care;
4. Delivery before age 17 or after age 35;
5. Smoking during pregnancy;
6. Use of alcohol and addicting drugs.

Traditionally, obstetric approaches have been primarily focused on treatment rather than timely identification of those women at risk. Creasy et al, in 1980,[20] modified a risk scoring system initially devised by Papiernik and Kaminski,[21] which identifies women at increased risk for preterm delivery. Included in their criteria are a variety of factors relating to pregnancy, such as socioeconomic status, reproductive history, daily habits and any current complication of pregnancy.

Recommendations to improve the perinatal mortality rate include:

1. Increased availability of prenatal care;
2. Early prenatal care;
3. Identification of those parturients at high risk;
4. Education with the aim of altering behavioral characteristics;
5. Early maternal transport to a tertiary care center if delivery is inevitable;
6. Aggressive resuscitation of the preterm infant;[14]
7. Medical/surgical intervention, if indicated, incorporating a multidisciplinary approach;
8. Uniformity regarding definitions of terms and criteria.

Eisner et al[22] noted that, within the USA, the greatest risk factor for low birthweight is no prenatal care.

In a desire to learn from experiences of countries whose infant mortality rates have decreased more quickly than those of the USA, the National Center for Health Statistics established an International Collaborative Effort on Perinatal and Infant Mortality (ICE). Research has been carried out with scientists from Denmark, the

Federal Republic of Germany, the UK, Israel, Japan, Norway and Sweden. Two symposia have been held, the first in August 1984 and the second in March 1990. Reports at the latter symposium made one point of special interest: in the Scandinavian countries almost every pregnant woman receives high-quality prenatal care early. This is a goal that must be emphasized in the USA, with every effort made to increase the quality and quantity of prenatal care available to all women and thereby more favorably affect perinatal mortality.

REFERENCES

1. Wilson A L, Fenton L J, Munson D P 1986 State reporting of live births of newborns weighing less than 500 grams: impact on neonatal mortality rates. Pediatrics 78: 850–854
2. National Center for Health Statistics 1985 Final mortality statistics, 1983 Advance report: monthly vital statistics report. National Center for Health Statistics, 34(6 suppl 2): Sept 26
3. Block B S 1990 Evaluating the quality of perinatal health care. Am J Perinatol 7: 146–153
4. World Health Organization 1977 Manual of the international statistical classification of diseases, injuries and causes of death. World Health Organization, Geneva, p 763–768
5. Friogoletto F D, Little G A 1988 Guidelines for perinatal care 2nd edn. American Academy of Pediatrics and the American College of Obstetricians and Gynecologists, Elk Grave Village, Illinois
6. Cunningham F G, MacDonald P C, Gant N F 1989 Williams obstetrics, 18th edn. Appleton & Lange, East Norwalk CT, p 1–2
7. Information Science Research Institute 1988 Infant and perinatal mortality rates by age and race, United States, each state and county: 1976–1980, 1981–1985. Maternal and Child Health Studies Project, Information Science Research Institute, Vienna, VA, p 1–19
8. Warburton D 1987 Chromosomal malformations and syndromes associated with stillbirth. Clin Obstet Gynecol 30: 268–277
9. Hall B D 1987 Nonchromosomal malformations and syndromes associated with stillbirth. Clin Obstet Gynecol 30: 278–283
10. Davidson E C 1991 A strategy to reduce infant mortality. Obstet Gynecol 77: 2–5
11. Friogoletto F D, Little G A 1988 Guidelines for perinatal care 2nd edn. American Academy of Pediatries and the American College of Obstetricians and Gynecologists, Elk Grave Village, Illnois
12. Lorenz R P, Kuhn M H 1989 Multidisciplinary team counseling for fetal anomalies. Am J Obstet Gynecol 161: 263–266
13. Harrison M R, Adzick N S, Longaker M T et al 1990 Successful repair in utero of a fetal diaphragmatic hernia after removal of herniated viscera from the left thorax. New Engl J Med 322: 1582–1584
14. Hack M, Fanaroff A A 1986 Special report: changes in the delivery room care of the extremely small infant (< 750 gm). New Engl J Med 314: 660–664
15. Avery M E, Mead J 1959 Surface properties in relation to atelectasis and hyaline membrane disease. Am J Dis Child 97: 517–523
16. Amon E, Anderson G D, Sibai B M et al 1987 Factors responsible for preterm delivery of the immature newborn infant (< 1000 gm). Am J Obstet Gynecol 156: 1143–1148
17. Marsh J C, Miller N A 1985 Female clients in substance abuse treatment. Int J Addict 20: 995–1019
18. Herron M A, Katz M, Creasy R K 1982 Evaluation of a preterm birth prevention program: preliminary report. Obstet Gynecol 59: 452–456
19. Miller H C, Merritt T A 1977 Fetal growth in humans. Year Book Medical Publishers, Chicago
20. Creasy R K, Gummer B A, Liggins G C 1980 System for predicting spontaneous preterm birth. Obstet Gynecol 55: 692–697
21. Papiernik E, Kaminski M 1974 Multifactorial study of the risk of prematurity at 32 weeks of gestation: a study for the frequency of 30 predictive characteristics. J Perinat Med 2: 30–35
22. Eisner V, Brazie J V, Pratt M W et al 1979 The risk of low birthweight. Am J Public Health 69: 887–893

74. Resuscitation and care of the newborn

Part A USA view *G. W. Ostheimer*
Part B European view *I. A. Laing*

PART A
USA VIEW
G. W. Ostheimer

Birth is a time of physiologic stress and change for the fetus. Usually, the asphyxial stress of birth is mild to moderate, and the neonate is able to compensate for it. When the neonate's compensatory ability is decreased or the asphyxial stress is excessive, resuscitative intervention is necessary to assist in the conversion from fetal to neonatal physiology.

Who should assume responsibility for resuscitation of the depressed neonate? Guideline VII of the American Society of Anesthesiologists (ASA) 'Guidelines for Regional Anesthesia in Obstetrics' state:* 'Qualified personnel, *other than the anesthesiologist attending the mother,* should be immediately available to assume responsibility for resuscitation of the depressed newborn.' (The primary responsibility of the anesthesiologist is to provide care to the mother. If the anesthesiologist is also requested to provide brief assistance in the care of the newborn, the benefit to the child must be compared to the risk to the mother.)

The 'Guidelines for Perinatal Care'[1] state:

> The first minutes of life may determine the quality of that life. The need for prompt, organized, and skilled response to immediate neonatal emergencies requires written policies delineating responsibility for immediate newborn care, resuscitation, selection and maintenance of necessary equipment, and training of personnel in proper techniques.

Routine care

The delivering physician or nurse–midwife is responsible for providing immediate postdelivery care of the newborn and for ascertaining that the newborn adaptations to extrauterine life are proceeding normally unless the care has been transferred. The hospital rules and regulations should include protocols for the transfer of medical care of the neonate in both routine and emergency circumstances. Routine care of the healthy newborn may be delegated to appropriately trained nurses, or transferred to a family physician or pediatrician.

Information to be transmitted to the physician caring for the infant after delivery includes both the infant's and the mother's name and medical record number; the mother's blood type, serology result, rubella status, hepatitis B screen result, diabetes screen, exposure to group B streptococci, and record of substance abuse; and the presence of fetal anomalies.

At least one person skilled in initiating resuscitation should be present at every delivery. The skills and responsibilities of that individual should be defined at the institutional level.

Resuscitation

Recognition and immediate resuscitation of a distressed neonate requires an organized plan of action and the immediate availability of qualified personnel and equipment as described in the American Academy of Pediatrics and the American Heart Association *Textbook of Neonatal Resuscitation*. Responsibility for identification and resuscitation of a distressed neonate should be assigned to a qualified individual, who may be a physician or an appropriately trained nurse–midwife, labor and delivery nurse, nurse–anesthetist, nursery nurse, or respiratory therapist. The provision of services and equipment for resuscitation should be planned jointly by the directors of the departments of obstetrics, anesthesia, and pediatrics, with the approval of the medical staff. A physician should be designated to assume primary responsibility for initiating, supervising, and reviewing the plan for management of depressed neonates in the delivery room. The following factors should be considered in this plan:

- A list of maternal and fetal complications that require the presence in the delivery room of someone specifically qualified in all aspects of newborn resuscitation should be developed.
- Individuals qualified to perform neonatal resuscitation should demonstrate the following capabilities:
  - Skills in rapid and accurate evaluation of the newborn condition, including Apgar scoring.
  - Knowledge of the pathogenesis and causes of a low Apgar score (eg, hypoxia, drugs, hypovolemia, trauma, anomalies, infections, and prematurity), as well as specific indications for resuscitation.
  - Skills in airway management (eg, laryngoscopy, endotracheal intubation, suctioning of the airway), artificial ventilation, cardiac massage, emergency administration of drugs and fluids, and maintenance of thermal stability. The

ability to recognize and decompress tension pneumothorax by needle aspiration is also a desirable skill.
- Procedures should be developed to ensure the readiness of equipment and personnel and to provide for intermittent review and evaluation of the effectiveness of the system.
- Contingency plans should be established for multiple births and other unusual circumstances.
- A physician for the neonate need not be present at a delivery provided that no complications are anticipated and another skilled individual is present to care for the neonate.
- The resuscitation steps should be documented in the records.

However, it would seem that these guidelines are not necessarily followed. Gibbs et al[2] found that in small units in the USA, with fewer than 500 deliveries per year, personnel other than an anesthesiologist, nurse anesthetist, pediatrician or obstetrician perform neonatal resuscitation after vaginal delivery almost 50% of the time, and, for cesarean delivery, 25% of the time.

CARDIOVASCULAR PHYSIOLOGY (FETUS TO NEONATE)

The fetal circulation operates in parallel, in contrast to the adult circulation, which operates in series.[3,4] In the fetus, oxygenated blood returns from the placenta via the umbilical vein, largely bypassing the liver through the ductus venosus. Owing to a streaming effect, this blood is preferentially shunted from the right atrium through the foramen ovale to the left atrium and via the left ventricle into the systemic circulation. This streaming of ductus venosus blood to the left side of the circulation enhances the oxygen content of the blood perfusing the organs of highest oxygen consumption – the heart and the brain.

Desaturated blood returns from the upper part of the body via the superior vena cava and streams into the right ventricle. Right ventricular output encounters high pulmonary vascular resistance due to arteriolar vasoconstriction. About 90% of this right-sided output passes through the ductus arteriosus and enters the aorta distal to the branches of the aortic arch; thus less well-oxygenated blood perfuses the lower body, which has a lower oxygen consumption (Fig. 74.1).

At birth, two primary events initiate the conversion from fetal to adult circulatory patterns.[5] First, cessation of umbilical artery flow (by clamping the cord or exposing the cord to air) increases systemic vascular resistance and aortic pressure, and the clamping of the umbilical vein decreases venous return and right atrial pressure. This effects a decrease in the right-to-left shunts both at the foramen ovale from the right atrium to the left and at the ductus arteriosus from the pulmonary artery to the aorta. Second, the expansion of the lungs at birth stimulates pulmonary vasodilation, with resulting falls in pulmonary vascular resistance and pulmonary arterial pressure, which helps to reduce further the right-to-left flow through the

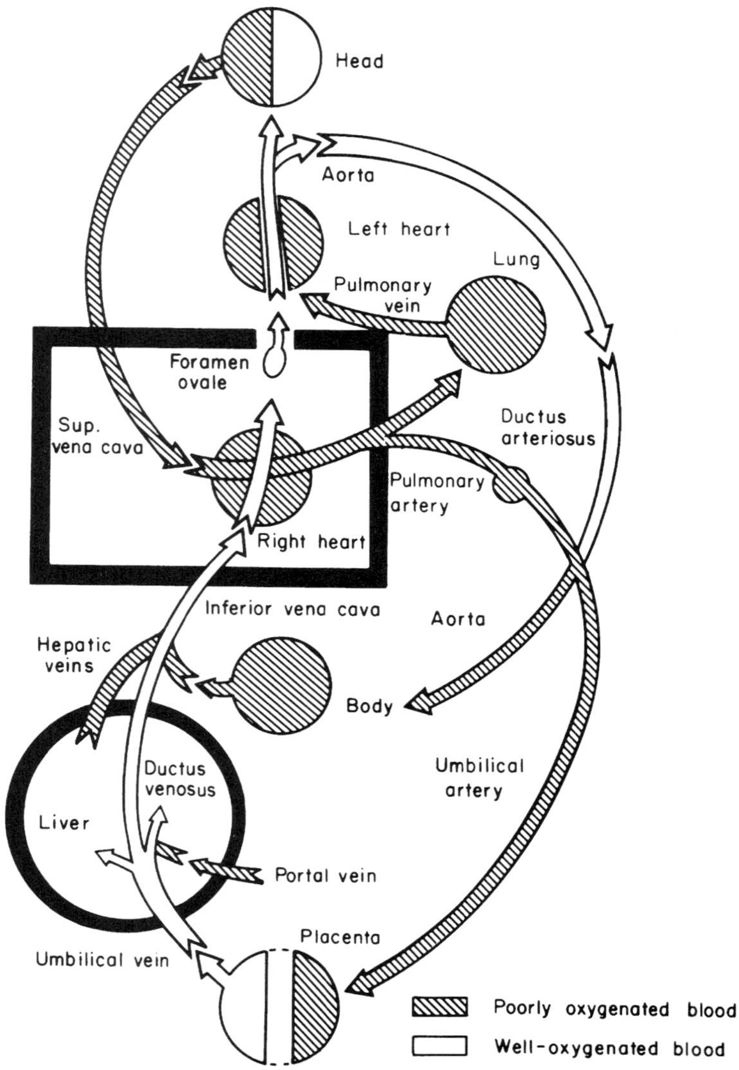

Fig. 74.1 Fetal circulation. (Modified from ref. 29 with permission.)

patent ductus arteriosus. Pulmonary blood flow increases, oxygenation improves and left atrial pressure rises, further decreasing the shunt across the foramen ovale (Figs. 74.2 and 74.3).

The hallmarks of conversion to adult circulation are a rise in systemic arterial pressure, accomplished mainly by cord clamping, and a rise in pulmonary blood flow, accomplished by filling the lungs with air. Therefore, the major effort of resuscitation is usually to assist the neonate with the initiation of ventilation. More severely depressed neonates may require additional forms of intervention.

The adult circulatory pattern is established rapidly in the normal, healthy neonate. However, for the first 2 weeks of life (longer in the premature neonate), the circulation can revert to the fetal pattern when the neonate is subjected to certain stresses such as hypoxemia, acidosis, hypercarbia, hypovolemia, shock and hypothermia.[5]

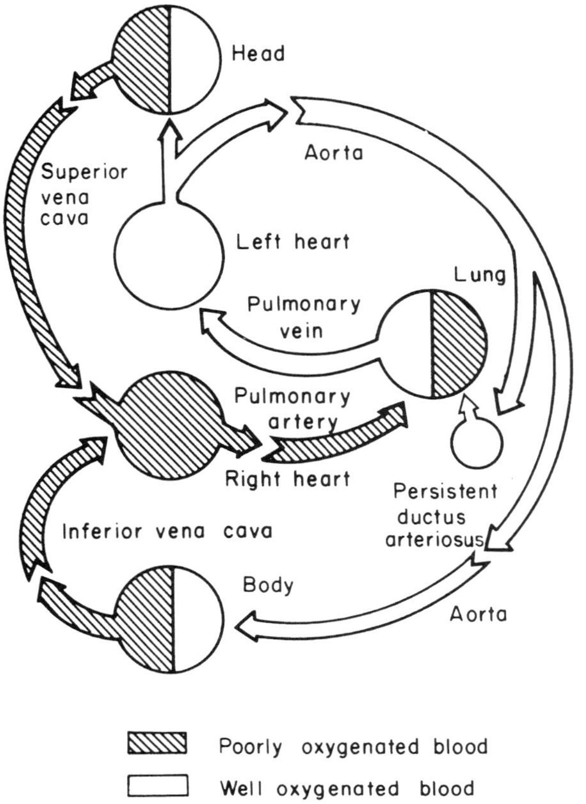

Fig. 74.2 Post-delivery circulation: intermediate phase. (Modified from ref. 29 with permission.)

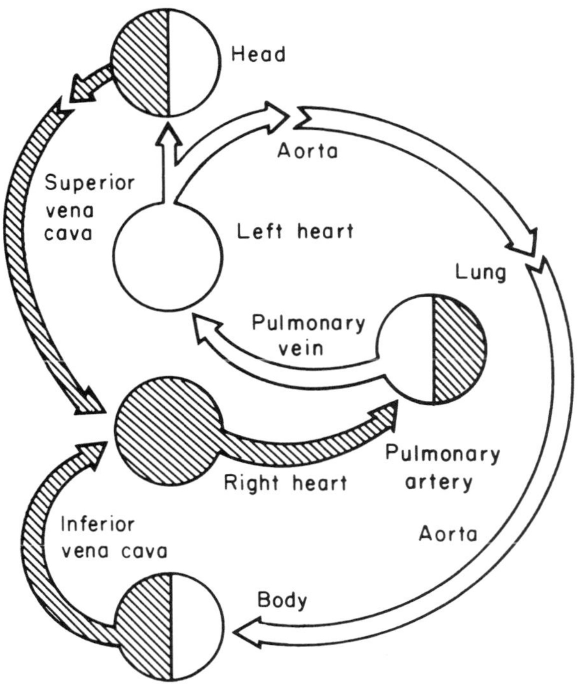

Fig. 74.3 Normal circulation: final phase. (Modified from ref. 29 with permission.)

RESPIRATORY SYSTEM

The fetal lung develops by a budding process from the foregut at approximately 24 days of gestation. By 20 weeks, the airways are lined with epithelium and pulmonary capillaries are developing in the mesenchyme. By 26–28 weeks, the capillaries are close to the developing airways so that oxygen and carbon dioxide exchange could occur, making extrauterine life possible. Surfactant-like material is present in the airway epithelium between 22 and 24 weeks but is not present on the alveolar surface until 26–28 weeks. Steroids administered to the mother facilitate the development of the epithelial cells lining the alveoli and the production of surfactant. The onset of fetal breathing is stimulated by stress (usually hypoxia) and amniotic fluid can be drawn into the lung, as can be demonstrated by meconium aspiration in the stillborn.[6,7]

Normal neonates will begin spontaneous respirations within 30–60 s of birth. Stimuli to breathe include rebound of the thoracic cage after vaginal birth, mild to moderate hypoxia, cord clamping, a cold environment and tactile stimulation. (Note: only gentle stimulation is needed. Vigorous spanking, cold and hot water baths and other excessive stimulation have no therapeutic value and may be harmful.) The volume of the first breath is 20–75 ml. Subsequent tidal volume is 15–20 ml. When rhythmic breathing is established and the lungs are fully expanded, the normal respiratory rate is 30 – 40 breaths/min. In the first few hours of life, during the resorption of residual lung fluid, respiratory rates may be as high as 60–90 breaths/min. Central cyanosis should clear by 5 min after birth. Some peripheral cyanosis may persist because of peripheral vasoconstriction. During vaginal delivery, the baby's chest is compressed with a pressure of 30–250 cmH_2O.[8] This 'squeeze' expresses much of the fluid from the lungs, but the lungs remain collapsed and are not aerated. In order to expand the lungs against the collapsing forces of alveolar tension and elastic pulmonary recoil, the neonate exerts 40 – 80 cmH_2O negative pressure.[9,10] The resuscitator may, therefore, need to use higher than normal pressures when assisting with the initiation of ventilation, so long as the potential for pneumothorax is kept in mind (Fig. 74.4). The neonate will respond to a large rapid inflation of its lungs with a sharp inspiration of its own (Head's paradoxical reflex).

CARDIOVASCULAR SYSTEM

The heart rate may vary from 100 to 200 beats/min (bpm) during the first 30 min of life, but should stabilize at 120 + 50 bpm thereafter. Normal blood pressure varies with birthweight, as shown in Table 74.1.[1] A systolic pressure less than 50 mmHg in a term neonate is abnormally low

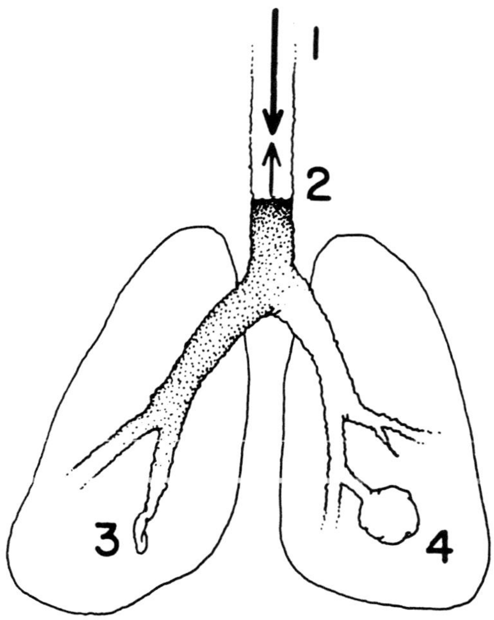

Fig. 74.4 The lung immediately after delivery. Expansion of the collapsed lung requires higher pressures than those needed to move air into the lungs (1) once aerated. Several forces must be overcome: outward flow of fluid in the trachea and bronchi (2); surface tension of the collapsed alveoli (3); and elastic forces of the lung (4). (Modified from ref. 30 with permission.)

and should be treated promptly with intravascular volume expansion. Normal intravascular volume is 85–100 ml/kg in the newborn.

THERMOREGULATION

Humans are homeothermic, that is we increase our heat production when exposed to a cold environment to maintain body temperature. Poikilotherms, such as reptiles, cannot increase their heat production and their body temperature drifts to that of the environment. There are two methods of increasing heat production: a physical method of muscle contraction (shivering), used by children and adults, and a chemical method used by neonates called *nonshivering thermogenesis* (Fig. 74.5). When the neonates are cold stressed, they increase their oxygen consumption and metabolic activity. Large amounts of norepinephrine are released (in contrast to epinephrine in adults), which activates an adipose tissue lipase to break down brown fat (so called because of its rich vascular supply) into triglycerides and nonesterified fatty acids (NEFAs). The NEFAs may pass out of the cell, are oxidized to carbon dioxide and water in the cell – which is an exothermic (heat-producing) reaction – or are re-esterified with glycerol to form triglycerides. Adipose tissue is not able to phosphorylate the glycerol derived from the triglycerides; therefore, re-esterification via the coenzyme A–NEFA complex requires a supply of α-glycerol phosphate derived from glucose that comes from outside the cell. Resynthesis of triglycerides is also an exothermic reaction because of the utilization of adenosine triphosphate (ATP) in the formation of the coenzyme A–NEFA complex.

Table 74.1 Normal neonatal blood pressures

Birthweight (kg)	Pressure (mmHg)	
	Systolic	Diastolic
<1.0	40–60	15–35
1.0–2.0	50–65	20–40
2.0–3.0	50–70	25–45
>3.0	50–80	30–50

Nonshivering thermogenesis occurs mainly in the brown fat of the neonate, which is found in an interscapular mass (the 'hibernating gland'), muscles and blood vessels entering the thoracic inlet and the abdominal viscera, especially around the kidneys and adrenal glands. The venous drainage from the interscapular adipose tissue joins the drainage from the muscles of the back to form the external vertebral plexus, which drains to the rich venous plexus around the spinal cord, which in turn enters the jugular or azygous veins, depending on the level, thus supplying heat to the spinal cord and the heart (Fig. 74.6).

We must strive to maintain a neutral thermal environment (32–34°C for neonates) at which metabolism (as reflected by oxygen consumption) is minimal yet sufficient to maintain body temperature. Minimal oxygen consumption occurs when the difference between skin and the environmental temperature is less than 1.5°C.

The infant, born into the cold environment of the delivery room, suffers an enormous heat loss, initially by evaporation since the neonate is wet from amniotic fluid and has a large surface area. Once the skin is dried, heat loss is mainly by radiation. Dahm and James[12] investigated heat loss in the first 30 minutes after delivery and found that wet infants exposed to room air lost nearly five times more heat than those who were dried and warmed.

In vigorous infants, promptly drying the skin and wrapping the baby in a warm blanket is almost as effective in decreasing heat loss as placing the baby under a radiant heater. However, in depressed or immature infants, who may be more asphyxiated or have reduced energy stores, an overhead radiant heater maintains body temperature while allowing access to the patient during resuscitation.

ROUTINE DELIVERY ROOM CARE OF THE NORMAL NEONATE

The following measures are all that is necessary in 85–90% of deliveries:

1. aspiration of the mouth and nose by bulb syringe;

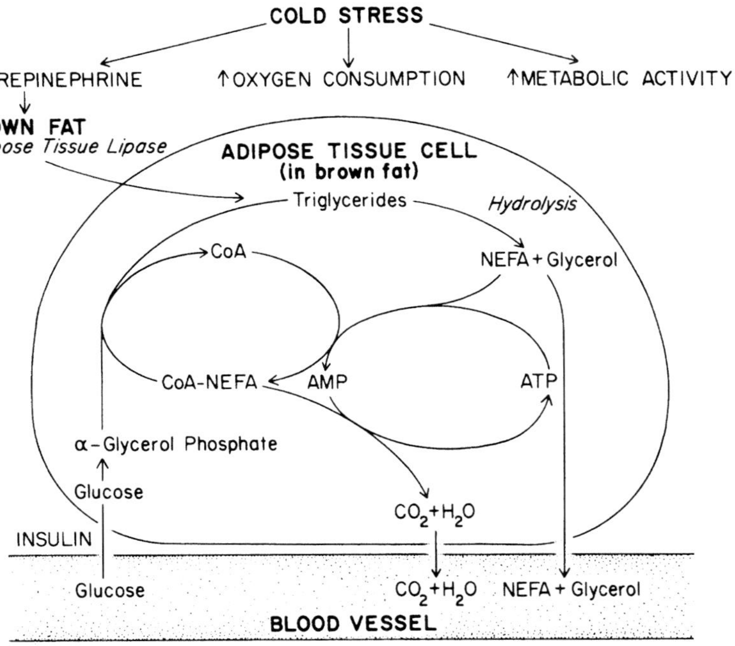

Fig. 74.5 Nonshivering thermogenesis. (From ref. 30 with permission.)

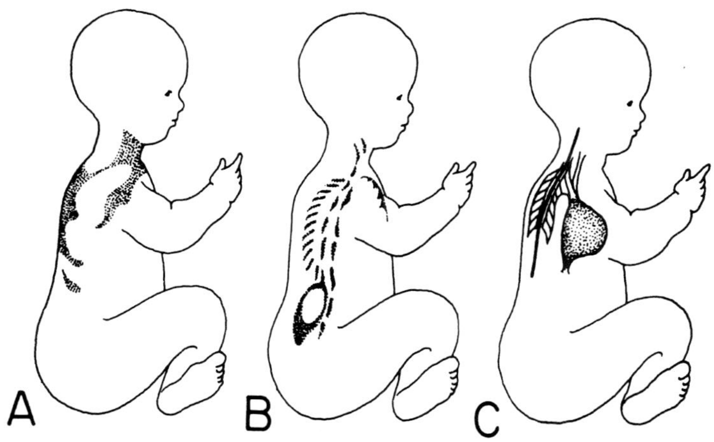

Fig. 74.6 (A and B) Sites of brown fat. (C) Route of venous drainage.

2. drying the skin and maintaining normal newborn temperature;
3. routine identification procedures;
4. ophthalmic prophylaxis (required by law in most states).

In the remainder, in whom neonatal depression has occurred, further measures will be necessary.

PRINCIPLES OF NEWBORN RESUSCITATION

The principles of newborn resuscitation are the same as those for adult resuscitation:

1. airway management;
2. breathing; and
3. circulation or adequate cardiac output to maintain cerebral oxygenation.

After birth of the baby's head, the oropharynx is suctioned with a bulb syringe before the baby's first breath and while the chest is still compressed in the vaginal canal (vaginal squeeze) to prevent aspiration of mucus and debris into the trachea with the onset of respiration (Fig. 74.7). The baby is then delivered; the umbilical cord is clamped and cut and the newborn is transferred by the obstetrician to a warmed bassinet that has been placed in a 20-30° head-down position to facilitate the gravity drainage of liquid material into the oropharynx. A slight

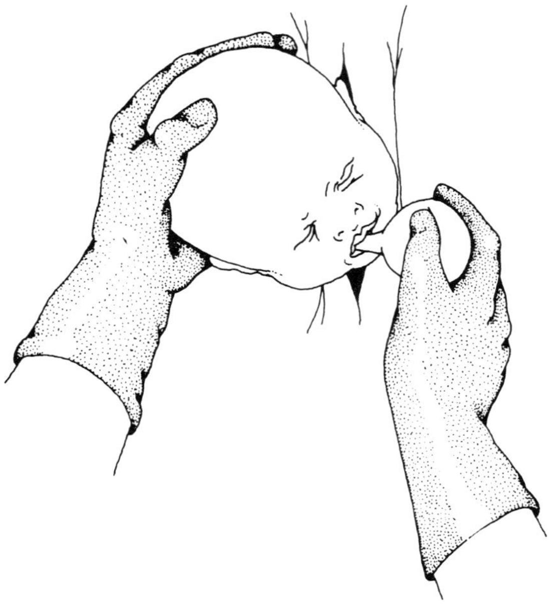

Fig. 74.7 Pharyngeal suction with the baby's head on the perineum. (Modified from ref. 30 with permission.)

lateral tilt of the newborn concentrates the pooling of secretions into one corner of the oropharynx. Management of the airway is accomplished by gentle suction with a bulb syringe – if possible – not a plastic or rubber suction catheter. Cordero and Hon[13] investigated the effect of nasopharyngeal or oropharyngeal stimulation on heart rate and respiration. In 41 infants who received repeated nasopharyngeal suction with a bulb syringe, no decreases in heart rate or respiration were noted. However, in 46 neonates who were suctioned blindly with a catheter through the nose or mouth, seven developed severe cardiac arrhythmias and five became apneic. These undesirable responses resulted from stimulation of afferent vagal fibers in the posterior pharynx of already highly vagotonic newborns.

Gentle slapping of the feet is all the stimulation needed for the healthy newborn. Spanking, cold-water showers, jackknifing, 'milking' the trachea, dilation of the anal sphincter, alternating hot and cold baths, rocking beds and excessive rubbing of the back are *condemned* as having no therapeutic value and are potentially harmful.

RESUSCITATION EQUIPMENT

Every delivery area should have the following equipment readily available for the resuscitation of the newborn:

1. A source of 100% oxygen.
2. A bag and mask for intermittent positive-pressure ventilation (IPPV). A flow-through system that requires positive pressure for oxygen delivery should be used since most neonates will not need positive-pressure ventilation, just oxygen therapy.
3. A bulb syringe for suctioning the nose and oropharynx.
4. A DeLee suction catheter with mucus trap for aspiration of mucus, meconium, blood and other secretions or stomach contents.
5. Laryngoscopes with size 0 and 1 straight blades.
6. Endotracheal tubes (Cole orotracheal tubes or straight endotracheal tubes with stylets in place in sizes 1.5 mm, 2.0 mm, 2.5 mm, 3.0 mm and 3.5 mm). The Cole tubes are more rigid and do not require a stylet. If the neonate requires long-term ventilation, the oral tube should be changed to a straight nasotracheal tube when the infant's condition is stable.
7. Oral airways, size 00 and 0, are rarely needed but should be available.
8. A radiant heater with servomechanisms.

A neonatal 'code cart' should also be available and should contain equipment for vascular access and blood sampling, intravenous infusion, drugs commonly employed in resuscitation and charts showing typical doses and dilutions.

With the increasing concern about body fluid contaminated with hepatitis or human immunodeficiency virus (HIV), personnel participating in newborn resuscitation are using one of several devices that allows aspiration of fluids from the mouth, trachea and stomach of the newborn by vacuum suction (<80 cmH_2O). This approach should eliminate the possibility of inhaling contaminants through a mask or gauze covering while aspirating via the endotracheal tube or DeLee suction apparatus.

EVALUATION AND TREATMENT OF THE DEPRESSED NEONATE

Apgar scoring

It is easy to recognize the vigorous, healthy, normal neonate and the severely depressed neonate needing immediate cardiopulmonary resuscitation. Between these two extremes lie varying degrees of neonatal depression. While the Apgar scoring system was not meant to be used as a guide to resuscitators, it has proven useful as a means of quantifying the degree of depression (Table 74.2). The 1-min score[14] is used here as a guide to the intervention required. However, resuscitation should not be delayed awaiting the 1-min Apgar score. A follow-up score is determined at 5 min of life and will indicate the progress of the neonate. Additionally, 10-, 15- and 20-min scores may be assigned to document the response of the neonate to the resuscitation efforts.

Table 74.2 The Apgar scoring system

Evaluation	Sign	Stimulus	Score 0	Score 1	Score 2
Appearance	Color	Visual assessment	Blue, pale	Body pink, extremities blue	Completely pink
Pulse	Heart rate	Count cord pulse or auscultate heart	Absent	< 100 bpm	> 100 bpm
Grimace	Reflex irritability	Flick sole of foot	No response	Some motion	Cry
Activity	Muscle tone	Manipulate extremity	Limp, flaccid	Some flexion of extremities	Well-flexed
Respiration	Respiratory effort	Visual assessment	Absent	Slow, irregular hypoventilation	Good strong cry

Vigorous, crying infant (Apgar score 7–10)

No therapy is necessary beyond the routine measures mentioned above.

Moderate depression (Apgar 4–6)

1. Administer 100% oxygen by mask (Fig. 74.8).
2. Stimulate by slapping the feet or by drying the skin with a soft cloth towel or blanket.
3. If the heart rate is below 100 bpm and/or respirations are inadequate, begin IPPV by bag and mask and continue it as long as necessary.
4. Monitor the heart rate and spontaneous respiratory efforts. If these deteriorate or fail to improve, treat as a severely depressed neonate.

Severe depression (Apgar score 0–3)

1. Administer 100% oxygen by bag and mask as soon as possible.
2. If there is no response (increased heart rate, increased respiratory effort) within a few minutes, perform laryngoscopy, suction the oropharynx and/or trachea and intubate the trachea to facilitate ventilation (Fig. 74.9).
3. Initiate closed-chest cardiac massage (CCCM) if the heart rate remains below 100 bpm. Place both thumbs over the mid to lower third of the sternum and the fingers behind the chest.[15,16] Compress the chest at a rate of 120 bpm, depressing the sternum two-thirds of the way to the vertebral column (see Fig. 74.8).
4. Monitor the adequacy of cardiopulmonary resuscitation. With proper intubation and ventilation, the chest should expand and breath sounds should be heard in both

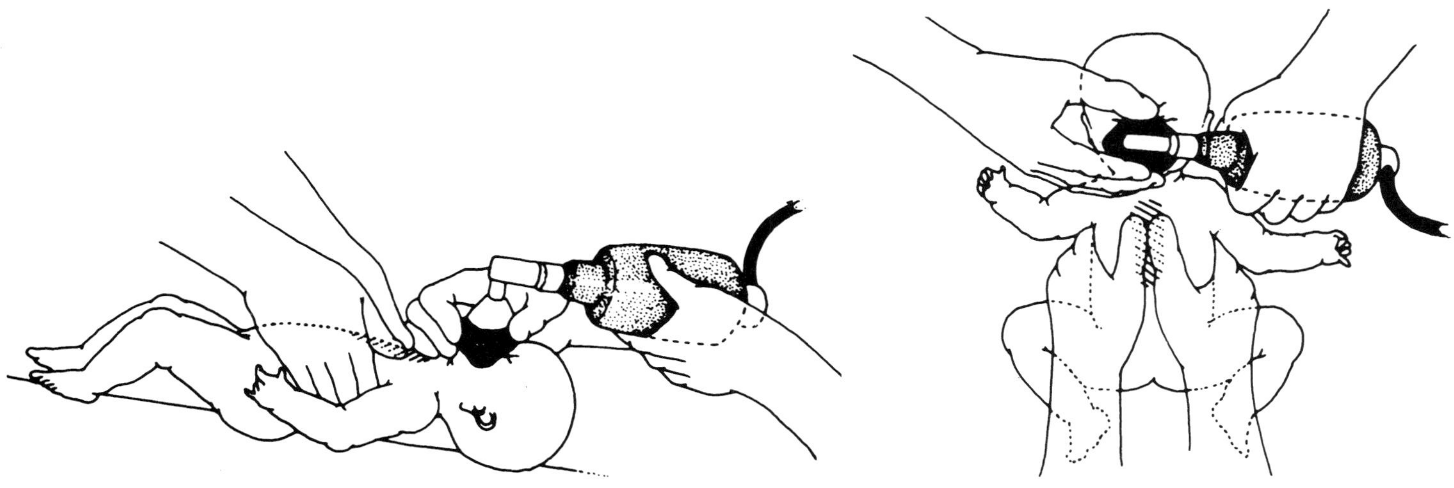

Fig. 74.8 Technique of ventilation and closed-chest cardiac massage. (From ref. 30 with permissions.)

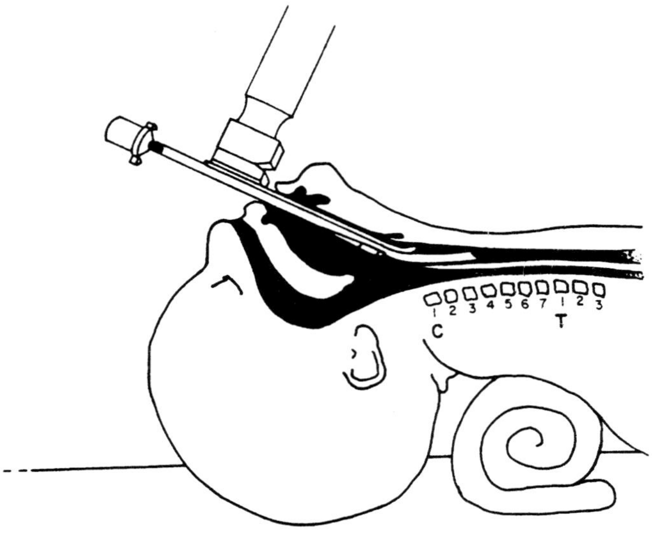

Fig. 74.9 Laryngoscopy and endotracheal intubation with a Cole (shouldered) tube.

axillae (Fig. 74.10). Auscultate over the abdomen to rule out esophageal intubation. If ventilation and/or intubation are difficult, repositioning of the head may be necessary. Because of the relatively large head of the neonate, as well as the edema fluid (caput) that collects over the occiput during labor, the neck may be flexed enough to compress the trachea when the baby is supine. Placing a small roll under the baby's shoulders will alleviate this problem by extending the neck (Fig. 74.11). However, excessive hyperextension may also compress the soft trachea of the neonate.

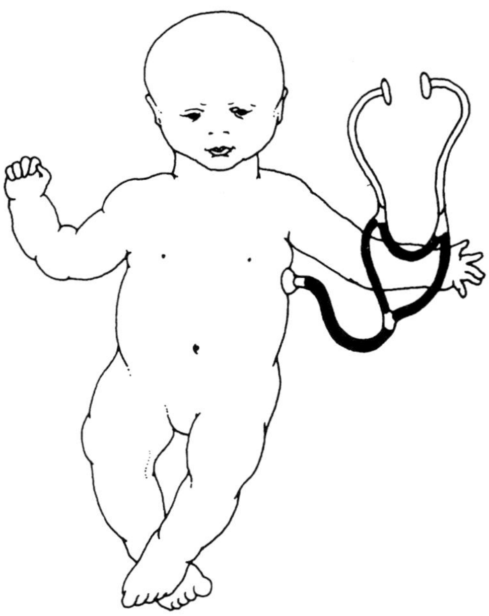

Fig. 74.10 Evaluation of ventilation by auscultation. (Modified from ref. 30 with permission.)

5. Gastric aspiration should not be done in the first few minutes of life in order to avoid causing any arrhythmias from nasopharyngeal or oropharyngeal stimulation – unless there is massive gastric dilation secondary to IPPV with the bag and mask or a tracheoesophageal fistula is suspected. Cordero and Hon[13] suggest that after 5 min of age the neonate has become physiologically more stable and will tolerate passage of a nasogastric tube.

CONTINUED MODERATE TO SEVERE DEPRESSION

The newborn that fails to respond to adequate ventilation with oxygen and circulatory support with CCCM will require further therapy.

Pharmacologic intervention

Drugs commonly used in neonatal resuscitation are administered through an umbilical artery or vein catheter, although epinephrine can be given intratracheally if vascular access has not yet been established. A 5- or 8-French catheter can be threaded into the umbilical artery, although intense vasoconstriction of the artery may necessitate use of the umbilical vein in the immediate resuscitative period. In the latter case, the catheter should be threaded no more than 2 cm into the vein to avoid cannulation of a major hepatic vessel.

Drugs used in pharmacologic resuscitation

Sodium bicarbonate (1–2mEq./kg). The neonate suffering from severe birth asphyxia and not responding well to oxygen and ventilatory support probably has a respiratory and metabolic acidosis. This initial dose of sodium bicarbonate will improve the acidosis, but further doses should be administered only as indicated by the infant's pH. A sample of blood (arterial or venous) should be drawn for blood gas analysis upon insertion of the umbilical artery or vein catheter. Ventilation must be adequate to reverse the respiratory component of the acidosis.

Bicarbonate therapy has several potential complications.[17–20] It is a hyperosmolar solution, and its rapid administration in the acidotic and hypoxic newborn can lead to profound vasodilation and hypotension due to skeletal muscle vasodilation and venous pooling. Because of its lower osmolarity, a 0.22 mmol/ml solution is preferred to the 0.45 mmol/ml solution. It should be given in an intravenous infusion (5–10% dextrose or 0.45% saline) so that the solution can serve as a diluent to decrease the bolus effect of the sodium bicarbonate. Excessive sodium bicarbonate therapy has been shown to cause hypernatremia, which has been implicated in intravascular cerebral hemorrhage in the sick neonate.[20]

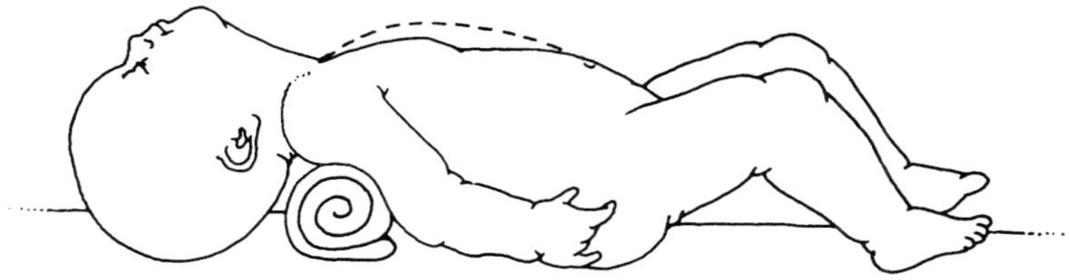

Fig. 74.11 Moderate hyperextension to relieve soft tissue obstruction. (Modified from ref. 30 with permission.)

However, appropriate doses, guided by the infant's pH, appear to be safe in this regard.

Dextrose (2 g/kg i.v. push, then 5–8 mg/kg/min). Severely asphyxiated infants are often hypoglycemic because of their increased catecholamine levels, with initial elevation of glucose and stimulation of insulin secretion in the presence of decreased glycogen reserves and immature gluconeogenetic pathways.[5] Neonates born to diabetic mothers are at risk for hypoglycemia because of prolonged exposure to maternal hyperglycemia, with fetal islet cell hyperplasia and elevated insulin secretion. Those neonates who are small for gestational age or have suffered from uteroplacental insufficiency may also develop hypoglycemia because of depleted glycogen stores. Hypoglycemia in these infants may be of later onset and they will require longer monitoring of blood glucose levels.

Epinephrine (adrenaline) (0.01–0.1 mg/kg) The hypotensive, bradycardic infant who is still acidotic may require this high dose of epinephrine for cardiac stimulation. In the nonacidotic infant, the usual dose of epinephrine is 0.01 mg/kg.

Naloxone (0.1 mg/kg i.v. or 0.2 mg/kg i.m.) Naloxone is used to reverse opioid-related depression only. If the mother has received opioids, the neonate may require naloxone. If this is so, the neonate should be observed for at least 4 h after naloxone administration for evidence of recurrence of opioid depression.

If the mother has received general anesthesia for delivery, the anesthetic can have a depressant effect on the newborn. Usually all the baby needs is oxygen, stimulation, and time to 'wake up'. Naloxone is not necessary in this setting, unless the mother has received opioids as a part of the anesthetic.

Other drugs may be needed in prolonged resuscitation. The indications for and methods of their use are not discussed here in the context of the acute resuscitative effort, and their use is the prerogative of the attending pediatrician.

SPECIFIC NEONATAL PROBLEMS

Meconium staining

Passage of meconium by the fetus is thought to occur in response to hypoxic stress in the ante- or peripartum period.[21] Meconium staining is present in 8–15% of all pregnancies, with a higher incidence in the post-term pregnancy. Over half of infants born through meconium-stained fluid will have meconium in their tracheas, and if left untreated many will develop meconium aspiration syndrome.[22–24] Since the treatment for meconium aspiration syndrome is only supportive and symptomatic, efforts have been concentrated on the prevention of the syndrome through effective airway suctioning at birth.[23–25] Immediately after the delivery of the infant's head, while the chest is still in the birth canal, the oropharynx and nasopharynx should be suctioned thoroughly by the obstetrician, using a bulb syringe or a DeLee apparatus. Immediately after delivery and, if possible, before the infant has taken his first breath, laryngoscopy and tracheal suctioning should be performed by the most experienced person present, regardless of the presence or absence of meconium in the oropharynx and nasopharynx since the obstetrician may have already completely cleared the upper airways of meconium. Tracheal suctioning should be repeated until no further meconium can be aspirated. An assistant should monitor the baby's heart rate during suctioning, since pharyngeal stimulation can cause bradycardia and other arrhythmias through vagal reflexes.[13] If the heart rate slows substantially, oxygen by mask or by clean tracheal tube should be given, with positive pressure ventilation as necessary. Infants who have aspirated meconium should receive chest physical therapy and postural drainage with suctioning, and should be monitored closely for the occurrence of respiratory distress. This sequence of immediate, thorough pharyngeal and tracheal suctioning has been found to be safe, and its implementation has greatly reduced the incidence and severity of meconium aspiration syndrome and its subsequent mortality.[23,24]

How often has the obstetric anesthesiologist heard that if there is thin meconium present in the airway at delivery it is not necessary to aspirate the trachea of the newborn? Chen et al[26] demonstrated that even small amounts of meconium in aspirated amniotic fluid can result in inactivation of surface-active material from the alveolar lining of the lungs. Therefore, it behooves us to be very aggressive in the management of the neonate with meconium in the amniotic fluid. However, the occurrence of in utero

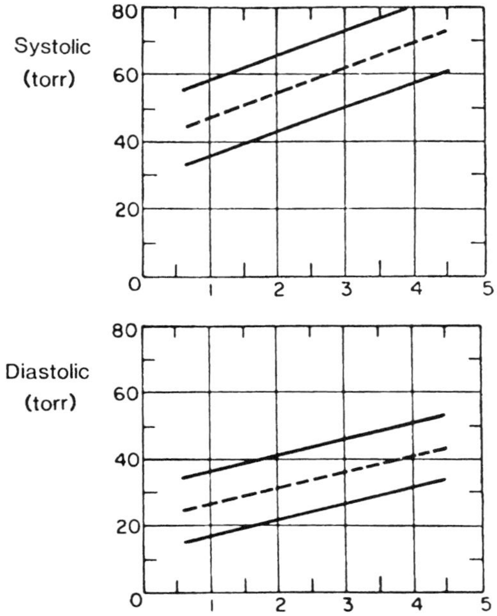

Fig. 74.12 Neonatal systolic and diastolic aortic blood pressure (From ref.11 with permission.)

meconium aspiration is still a devastating problem. If we could eliminate this potentially disastrous occurrence during the later stages of pregnancy or during labor, we would virtually eliminate the meconium aspiration syndrome.

Neonatal shock

Serious hypovolemia with secondary hypoperfusion and tissue hypoxia can occur as a result of numerous factors. Sequestration of blood in the placenta because of elevation of the infant above the mother at the time of cord clamping, prolapsed umbilical cord, placental abruption, placenta previa and rupture of the umbilical cord can significantly decrease the neonate's circulating blood volume. Low-birthweight infants may have decreased total protein concentrations, with a resultant shift of fluid out of the intravascular space because of low intravascular oncotic pressure. Also, maternal sepsis transmitted to the fetus may present as neonatal shock.

A decreasing blood pressure, tachycardia, pallor, decreased urine output, decreasing hematocrit and metabolic acidemia all indicate that volume expansion may be needed. The preferred therapy is 20 ml/kg of fresh, uncontaminated heparinized fetal whole blood obtained from the placenta, which may be difficult to obtain.[27,28] If this is unavailable, fresh whole adult blood or packed red blood cells and fresh-frozen plasma in the same quantity may be used. 5% albumin (1 g/kg) can also serve as a volume expander. Finally, if no blood products are available, lactated Ringer's solution or 0.45% normal saline may be used. The neonate's blood pressure, pulse, respiration and temperature should be monitored carefully to detect any deterioration before such a change becomes a crisis.

Constant monitoring of the hypotensive neonate is vital to proper management. Measurement of the infant's blood pressure should become a routine part of the physiologic evaluation at birth if a problem exists and all infants should have a screening blood pressure measured on admission to the nursery (Fig. 74.12). The neonate is 'recovering' from the asphyxia of delivery and should have the same evaluation as a patient 'recovering' from anesthesia and surgery.

SUMMARY

The simple mnemonic ABCDE summarizes the five key principles of neonatal resuscitation:

1. *A*irway;
2. *B*reathing;
3. *C*irculation;
4. *D*rugs;
5. *E*valuation of concurrent and causative problems and maintenance of a neutral thermal *E*nvironment.

REFERENCES

1. Freeman R K, Poland R L 1992 Guidelines for perinatal care 3rd edn. American Academy of Pediatrics and the American College of Obstetricians and Gynecologists, Elk Grove Village, Illinois
2. Gibbs C P, Krischer J, Peckham BM et al 1986 Obstetric anesthesia: a national survey. Anesthesiology 65: 298–306
3. Behrman R E, Lees M H, Peterson E N et al 1970 Distribution of the circulation in the normal and asphyxiated fetal primate. Am J Obstet Gynecol 108: 956–969
4. Rudolph A M, Heymann M A 1974 Fetal and neonatal circulation and respiration. Ann Rev Physiol 36: 187–207
5. Bowen F W 1982 Resuscitation and stabilization of the neonate. In Bolognese R J (ed) Perinatal medicine: management of the high risk fetus and neonate. Williams & Wilkins, Baltimore, p. 445–453
6. Brown B L, Gleicher N 1981 Intrauterine meconium aspiration. Obstet Gynecol 57: 26–29
7. Turbeville D F, McCaffress MA, Block M F et al 1979 In utero distal pulmonary meconium aspiration. South Med J 72: 535–536
8. Karlberg P 1960 The adaptive changes in the immediate post-natal period, with particular reference to respiration. J Pediatr 56: 585–604
9. Vyas H, Milner A D, Hopkin I E 1981 Intrathoracic pressure and volume changes during the spontaneous onset of respiration in babies born by cesarean section and by vaginal delivery. J Pediatr 99: 787–791
10. Milner A D, Vyas H 1982 Lung expansion at birth. J Pediatr 101: 879–886
11. Versmold H T, Ketterman J A, Phibbs R H et al 1981 Aortic blood pressure during the first 12 hours of life in infants with birth weight 610–4220 grams. Pediatrics 67: 607–613
12. Dahm L S, James L S 1972 Newborn temperature and calculated heat loss in the delivery room. Pediatrics 49: 504–513
13. Cordero L, Hon E H 1971 Neonatal bradycardia following nasopharyngeal stimulation. J Pediatr 78: 441–447
14. Apgar V 1953 A proposal for a new method of evaluation of the newborn infant. Curr Res Anesth Analg 32: 260–267

15. Todres I D, Rogers M C 1975 Methods of external cardiac massage in the newborn infant. J Pediatr 86: 781–782
16. Fiholt D A, Kettrick R G, Wagner H R, Swedlow D B 1986 The heart is under the lower third of the sternum. Am J Dis Child 140: 646–649
17. Simmons M A, Adcock E W, Bard H et al 1974 Hypernatremia and intracranial hemorrhage in neonates. New Engl J Med 291: 6–10
18. Volpe J 1974 Neonatal intracranial hemorrhage–iatrogenic etiology (editorial). New Engl J Med 291: 43–45
19. Cote C J, Greenhow D E, Marshall B E 1979 The hypotensive response to rapid intravenous administration of hypertonic solutions in man and in the rabbit. Anesthesiology 50: 30–35
20. Wheeler A S, Sadri S, Gutsche B B et al 1979 Intracranial hemorrhage following intravenous administration of sodium bicarbonate or saline solution in the newborn lamb asphyxiated in utero. Anesthesiology 51: 517–521
21. Walker J 1953 Fetal anoxia. J Obstet Gynecol Br Cwlth 60: 162–180
22. Gregory G A, Gooding C A, Phibbs R H et al 1974 Meconium aspiration in infants: prospective study. J Pediatr 85: 848–852
23. Ting P, Brady JP 1975 Tracheal suction in meconium aspiration. Am J Obstet Gynecol 122: 767–771
24. Carson B S, Losey R W, Bowes W A, Simmons M A 1976 Combined obstetric and pediatric approach to prevent meconium aspiration syndrome. Am J Obstet Gynecol 126: 712–715
25. Frantz I D, Wang N S, Thach B T 1975 Experimental meconium aspiration: effects of glucocorticoid treatment. J Pediatr 86: 438–441
26. Chen C T, Toung T J K, Rogers M C 1983 Effect of intra-alveolar meconium on pulmonary surface tension properties. Crit Care Med 13: 233
27. Paxson C L 1979 Collection and use of autologous fetal blood. Am J Obstet Gynecol 134: 708–710
28. Golden S M, O'Brien W F, Metz SA 1982 Anticoagulation of autologous cord blood for neonatal resuscitation. Am J Obstet Gynecol 144: 103–104
29. Ostheimer G W 1980 Resuscitating the depressed neonate. Contemp Obstet Gynecol 15: 27
30. Ostheimer G W 1978 Newborn resuscitation. Weekly Anesthesiology Update, Princeton, N J.

PART B
EUROPEAN VIEW

I. A. Laing

INTRODUCTION

All institutions in which infants are delivered should have an identified member of staff whose responsibility it is to carry out assessment and resuscitation of the newborn. The responsible individual must be immediately available, on site and kept in regular practice. The quality of emergency resuscitation carried out in a tertiary referral center (level 3 facility) is expected to be different from that in a 'cottage hospital' (level 1 facility).

Antenatal identification of the 'at-risk' fetus (Table 74.3) should help to make this disparity acceptable by having the compromised infant transferred in utero to an appropriate referral center and delivered into the hands of a neonatologist. Nevertheless, general practitioners, midwives and other paramedical staff should be able to improve the condition of the distressed newborn. The following recommendations for basic and advanced resuscitation are as it should be practiced in the UK.[1]

NEED FOR RESUSCITATION

The minutes immediately before and after birth are times of acute stress for the fetus and newborn. Normally the fetus can tolerate brief asphyxial stress, and the newborn can adapt to the changes imposed by post-natal life. When, however, stress on the fetus is excessive or the neonate can compensate only partially, resuscitation becomes necessary to allow complete adaptation from the fetal to the post-natal state. The physiologic changes which occur at this time have been reviewed by McKlveen and Ostheimer.[2]

EQUIPMENT FOR NEONATAL RESUSCITATION

Table 74.4 shows essential equipment for basic resuscitation of the newborn. Most units in Europe carry out resuscitations using a trolley such as the Vickers Resuscitaire

Table 74.3 Risk factors predictive for possible resuscitation

Maternal	Fetal	Labor/delivery
Fever	Multiple	Fetal distress
Heavy sedation	Preterm	Forceps delivery
Acute illness	Post-term	Abnormal presentation
Diabetes	Anomaly	Antepartum hemorrhage
Hypertension	Growth retardation	Prolonged labor
Drug abuse	Isoimmunization	Prolapsed cord
Prolonged rupture of membranes		Cesarean delivery for the above

Model 165, which includes a radiant heater, overhead lighting, adjustable tilting surface, suction, oxygen outlet with variable pressure relief valve (10–30 cmH_2O), stop-clock and auxiliary oxygen mounts. Self-inflating bags such as the Cardiff, Ambu or Laerdal are available for gas insufflation. The infant Laerdal system is suitable for children under 7 kg and has a 240-ml bag and a 600-ml reservoir. With the reservoir connected, high oxygen concentrations may be delivered either passively to the spontaneously breathing infant or actively via a face mask with adequate seal, or directly to an endotracheal tube. The Laerdal system also incorporates a pressure relief valve, which blows off at approximately 45 cmH_2O and can be easily overridden if necessary.

BASIC RESUSCITATION

The objectives of resuscitation of the newborn are:

1. to expand the lungs and establish alveolar ventilation;
2. to increase arterial oxygen to safe levels;
3. to support cardiac output;
4. to minimize heat loss.

Table 74.4 Equipment for neonatal resuscitation

Designated surface
Radiant heater with thermostatic control
Dry warm towels and a heat source for such
Stethoscope
Oxygen source with flowmeter
Ventilation system with pressure regulator and gauge
Suction apparatus with pressure regulator and gauge
Suction catheters, gauge 8 and 10
Bag and mask with reservoir
Stop-clock
Syringes 2,5 and 10 ml
Needles 21 and 23 gauge
Drugs (see Table 74.5)

Preparing for resuscitation

1. Check equipment (Table 74.4).
2. Check drugs which may be required (Table 74.5).
3. Obtain details of maternal history.
4. Establish team of care givers and their roles.
5. If time allows, meet the family and discuss the anticipated course.

At birth the stop-clock is activated to time subsequent events of the resuscitation, including all assessments (e.g. the Apgar score, Table 74.6) and interventions (e.g. endotracheal intubation).

Some units carry out acute care of the newborn in the mother's delivery room, while others have a designated draught-free room where resuscitation is carried out. In hospital, resuscitation of the newborn should take place in a room whose ambient temperature is 24–26°. Thermoregulatory processes may be impaired by a difficult birth, perhaps as a result of impaired blood supply to the stores of brown fat.[3] With practice and meticulous technique the care team should nevertheless be able to keep the smallest and most compromised infant warm. Immediately after birth the infant is thoroughly dried, including the trunk, limbs, groins, head and neck. The child is then wrapped in a second warm towel, also covering the scalp area, from which a large heat loss may otherwise occur. The infant is

Table 74.6 The Apgar score

	0	1	2
Heart rate	Absent	Less than 100	Greater than 100
Respiratory	Absent	Shallow, irregular	Strong cry
Muscle tone	Limp	Some flexion	Active, well flexed
Reflex/ irritability	Absent	Grimace	Cry/sneeze
Color	Pale or deep blue	Peripherally blue	Pink

Table 74.5 Drugs used in neonatal resuscitation

Drug	Dosage/route	Indications	Comments
Dextrose 10%	2 ml/kg i.v.	Hypoglycemia	Give over 2 min
Sodium bicarbonate 0.45 mEq./ml (2mEq.)/Kg	4 ml/kg i.v.	Metabolic acidosis	Give over 2 min
Vitamin K	1 mg i.m. if over 2 kg 0.5 mg i.m. if less than 2kg	All infants, to prevent hemorrhagic disease	Give in midline of anterior thigh
Naloxone (0.02 mg/ml)	2 ml if over 2 kg 1 ml if less than 2 kg	Reverse opioid	Follow i.v. dosage with 1 ml i.m.
Calcium gluconate 10%	1 ml/kg i.v.	Improve low cardiac output	Give over 10 min. Do not mix with sodium bicarbonate
Epinephrine (adrenaline) 1:10000	0.5 ml/kg i.v. or e.t.	Correct asystole or profound bradycardia	May cause tachyarrhythmias
Atropine	0.01 mg/kg i.v.	Correct vagal bradycardia	May cause tachycardia
Fresh-frozen plasma	10 ml/kg i.v.	Correct acute hypovolemia	May repeat dosage over half an hour
0 negative blood	10 ml/kg i.v.	Correct acute hypovolemia, especially after fetal blood loss	May repeat dosage over half an hour or more

then placed supine on the designated resuscitation surface underneath the radiant heat warmer. The trolley surface may be horizontal but with a 10° slope at the head end allowing gentle extension of the neck. Alternatively it may help to place a small towel behind the infant's shoulders, thus promoting neck extension, which facilitates airway opening and visualization.

Tactile stimulation may be all that is necessary to initiate adequate respiration in the newborn: if this is so, drying the child's skin or gentle flicking of the soles of the feet will be sufficient. There is no place for inflicting painful stimuli. Mechanical suction of the anterior nares and anterior oropharynx may be beneficial if there is a large volume of mucus. Because of the hazards of ingesting infectious secretions, it is unacceptable for a member of staff to use mouth suctioning for any reason in the delivery room.[4] If the child is blue but breathing spontaneously, oxygen by funnel or face mask may be directed to the infant's nose, while being careful to ensure that no seal of the funnel or mask occurs on the infant's face. NB: Only a bag and mask system which delivers oxygen at all times *irrespective of whether or not the bag is compressed* should be used for this purpose. Traditionally the degree of oxygenation of a newborn has been assessed visually, but the pulse oximeter may now have an important part to play during resuscitation,[5] particularly when caring for the extreme preterm infant in whom retinopathy of prematurity must be prevented if possible.

If the infant's breathing is absent or irregular or persistently shallow, resulting in bradycardia or cyanosis, artificial ventilation with bag and mask will be required. A circular mask which provides a good seal around the infant's mouth and nose should be chosen. The mask, when tightly sealed around the infant's airway, should not extend below the chin, nor should it press on eyeballs. The infant's airway is opened by gentle extension of the neck, holding the mandible forward with the tips of the fourth and fifth fingers of the left hand. When the mask is firmly applied, the seal is achieved using pressure from the thumb and index fingers of the left hand. Intermittent breaths are given by squeezing the resuscitation bag with the right hand, listening to ensure there is no leak of air at the face seal, and watching that the chest wall rises with each insufflation. Compression of the bag is with fingertips, and must not be too forceful, since unintentional high pressures may be achieved even when there is a functioning relief valve. Oxygen flow should be 4–6 l/min, and the insufflation rate may be 30–40/min. If chest wall movement is poor, check (a) the flow rate, (b) that the reservoir and bag fill adequately, (c) that the infant is positioned with the neck gently extended and (d) that there is no leak of oxygen around the mask.

If the infant fails to improve with the above measures, immediate endotracheal intubation is indicated.

The Apgar score

Some clinicians use the Apgar score (Table 74.6) as a guide to management of the infant during resuscitation. It has the advantage of being a widely used assessment, and undoubtedly has an important role in describing the infant's condition, especially for retrospective analysis. It is true that, in general, infants with an Apgar score of 8–10 need no resuscitation, those with totals 5–7 will respond to stimulation and 'blow-by' oxygen, those with scores of 3–4 may be helped by bag and mask ventilation, while those who achieve totals of only 0–2 need immediate endotracheal intubation. However, heart rate and respiratory effort are the most important clinical features measured, and the experienced clinician can guide a resuscitation efficiently based largely on these two parameters.

External closed chest cardiac massage

Even during a basic resuscitation unexpected asystole or profound bradycardia may occur, and so all neonatal care givers should be familiar with this technique. The priority during any resuscitation is to achieve good bilateral lung expansion and ventilation. External cardiac compression is indicated if the newborn's heart rate remains consistently below 60 bpm despite adequate ventilation. Repeated firm pressure on the sternum compresses the heart against the spinal column, and transmits blood from the ventricles into the main arteries. This is best done by standing to the side of the child, and facing the infant's head. The lower chest is firmly grasped with both hands, the fingertips being as close to the spine as possible, and the thumbs applying rhythmic compressions on the sternum at approximately 100–120 bpm.[6] Some neonatologists coordinate ventilation and cardiac compression, e.g. three beats of compression followed by a single inflation of the chest. It may be at least as effective to allow the compressor and inflator to continue independently of each other. A clinician should listen and feel briefly for spontaneous cardiac output every 30–60 s, and reassess the value of continuing the resuscitation.

Unexpected meconium during a basic resuscitation

If meconium is noted to be present immediately prior to delivery, the oropharynx and nasopharynx should be aspirated prior to delivery of the infant's trunk. Suction should be carried out using a mechanical device, or by a spontaneously inflating bulb, or by oral suction with a fail-safe fluid trap or filter. Ideally someone skilled in neonatal intubation should be summoned, and meanwhile 'blow-by' oxygen is directed to the infant's face until there is no evidence of cyanosis. Positive-pressure ventilation should be avoided prior to inspection of the vocal cords, unless the infant is persistently apneic and bradycardic despite tactile stimulation.

ADVANCED RESUSCITATION

Additional skills are required when the sick newborn needs acute intensive care at the time of birth. Someone responsible for providing this high degree of care must be available within every tertiary referral center (level 3) at all times, and should be rapidly available at centers where any 'at risk' infants are delivered (see Table 74.3). The additional equipment required for this more complex level of resuscitation is shown in Table 74.7.

Endotracheal intubation

Prior to endotracheal intubation, if time allows, all equipment should be checked, ensuring that the laryngoscope is fully functioning and that the gas flow is at appropriate pressure and volume. Although some practitioners will by choice insert a nasotracheal tube when it is clear that the infant will be ventilated long term, most prefer to use the orotracheal route initially, and may change to a nasotracheal method of ventilation subsequently. Some pediatricians prefer a shouldered endotracheal tube for orotracheal intubation, while others choose a straight tube. The intubator should be thoroughly familiar with the chosen tube beforehand: introducers (stylets) to stiffen the tube are rarely necessary if the practitioner's technique is adequate. The size of endotracheal tube is selected on the basis of anticipated birthweight of the infant (Table 74.8).

The infant is placed as before on the surface under the radiant heater, with neck gently extended. The laryngoscope is held in the left hand. The fingers of the practitioner's right hand open the infant's mouth and allow the laryngoscope blade to slide behind the tongue, lifting it gently up. Some prefer to keep the blade in the midline, but it may be an advantage to slip the blade along the right half of the tongue and then lift it up and to the left, thus allowing maximal space for the endotracheal tube (in the right hand) to approach from the angle of the mouth. If this technique is used, it allows visualization of the vocal cords even after insertion of the tip of the tube into the larynx. Whether the midline or right-side technique is employed, the tip of the laryngoscope blade should reach the epiglottis, which is then lifted gently anterior to display the larynx. If the laryngoscope has been advanced too far, the esophagus will be seen. The blade is then slowly withdrawn until the larynx or epiglottis is visualized, and the intubation is carried out as before. Occasionally it is necessary to ask an assistant to provide downward pressure on the thyroid cartilage, which may help an anteverted larynx to come more easily into view.

Table 74.7 Additional equipment required for advanced resuscitation

Two laryngoscopes with straight blades sizes 0 and 1
Spare bulb and batteries
Endotracheal tubes, sizes 2.0, 2.5, 3.0 and 3.5 mm internal diameter
Adhesive tape 1 cm
Endotracheal tube fixation method, e.g. holder and stockinette hat
Suture forceps and strong silk suture
Suction catheters, gauge 4, 6 and 8
Umbilical venous catheters, gauges 3.5 and 5
Three-way stopcocks with Luer lock fittings
Butterfly needles, gauge 21 and 23
Intravenous catheters, gauges 22, 24 and 26
Trocars and catheters, gauges 10 and 12
Heimlich valve for pleural drainage
Blood culture bottles, universal containers, tubes for blood tests, including capillary tubes for blood gas analysis
Sterile umbilical venous catheter tray

Table 74.8 Appropriate endotracheal tube size for birthweight

Birthweight (kg)	Endotracheal tube (internal diameter in mm)
Less than 0.8	2.0
0.8 to 2.0	2.5
2.0 to 3.5	3.0
Greater than 3.5	3.5

Common errors

1. Tube in too far: this should not occur if the shouldered tube is advanced gently only until the shoulder sits on the vocal cords, or if the straight tube is advanced only as far as the mark (approximately 2 cm from the tip).
2. Tube becomes dislodged after intubation: this should not occur if the well-placed tube is held firmly between index finger and thumb of the left hand *which are resting immediately on the infant's mandible and maxilla respectively*.
3. Intubation of the esophagus: this should not occur if the infant is well positioned, the pharynx is suctioned free of mucus and the tube tip is seen to enter the larynx as described above.
4. Unsuccessful intubation attempted for too long: if the tube is not passed successfully in 30 s, it should be withdrawn and bag and mask insufflation used instead.

Inflating the lungs via the endotracheal tube

Oxygen should be delivered at 4–6 l/min. The system should allow peak inflation pressures of 20–30 cmH_2O. Infants who have already cried effectively can usually be ventilated with lower peak pressures, and infants who are of very low birthweight should be ventilated if possible with initial peak pressures of around 20 cmH_2O. Infants who have not cried and have not inflated their lungs spontaneously will need higher pressures and prolonged inspiratory times of 2–3 s for the first few inflations. The practitioner should look at the infant's chest movement and listen with the stethoscope to insure that there is satisfactory bilateral air entry.

Poor bilateral air entry may be due to an esophageal intubation, inadequate inflation pressures or (less likely) pulmonary hypoplasia, a laryngeal web or laryngeal agenesis. Poor air entry on one side is usually due to intubation of a main bronchus, almost always the right side. The tube can be slowly withdrawn while listening for improved air entry on the side which was previously poorly inflated. A pneumothorax or a diaphragmatic hernia (usually on the left side) can also result in asymmetrical breath sounds.

Vascular access

Although it is occasionally possible to insert an effective peripheral intravenous catheter, usually the infant who is in need of acute resuscitation is poorly perfused. Some authors then recommend cannulation of the umbilical artery,[2] which has the advantage of providing arterial gas samples for assessment: others continue to worry about injecting drugs into the arterial system with the possible hazards of vasospasm and perhaps even necrotizing enterocolitis. Because of its rapidity, simplicity and perhaps safety, umbilical venous catheterization may be the method of choice to allow reliable administration of fluids and drugs. Insertion of any umbilical catheter is strictly a sterile procedure.

Technique

A 10-cm syringe is filled with 5% dextrose and attached to an umbilical catheter (gauge 5 for a term infant, 3.5 for a preterm infant). The catheter is carefully filled with dextrose solution and checked to make sure that no air bubbles persist. A ribbon ligature is tied loosely round the base of the umbilicus, and the cord is cleaned with chlorhexidine. Artery forceps are clipped on to the side of the cord, 3–4 cm from the base. The cord is transected above the forceps, and the umbilical catheter with syringe attached is threaded into the largest (and thinnest walled) of the three vessels seen. The ribbon ligature is used to control hemorrhage. The catheter is inserted to a depth of approximately 4 cm, when venous blood can then be freely aspirated into the 10-ml syringe. The ligature is then pulled firmly to fix the catheter. A check is made to insure that the blood column in the catheter does not pulsate. The catheter can subsequently be sutured firmly to the umbilical cord.

SPECIAL PROBLEMS

Meconium aspiration

There is a great deal of individual variation in the management of meconium aspiration, but the following principles are important.

1. The oropharynx and nasopharynx should be aspirated thoroughly by the obstetrician, ideally before delivery of the infant's trunk.
2. If meconium is present in the posterior oropharynx then the infant should be intubated and the laryngotracheal fluid aspirated.
3. The largest possible suction catheter should be used so that copious, viscous meconium can be removed: this can be achieved by passing the largest gauge of catheter down the endotracheal tube, or by attaching mechanical suction to the endotracheal tube itself.
4. A blocked endotracheal tube should be replaced as rapidly as possible.
5. Positive-pressure ventilation should be delayed if the infant's condition is stable and meconium continues to be aspirated, but if the infant is sick, cyanosed, bradycardic or deteriorating, oxygen should be urgently given by positive-pressure ventilation.
6. The inexperienced intubator may be confronted with an energetic infant who 'refuses' to be intubated. It is probably safest to allow the child to clear the meconium spontaneously, rather than risk the complications of a traumatic, asphyxiating intubation. Oral suction and 'blow-by' oxygen are recommended.
7. The stomach can be emptied of meconium via a gauge 8–10 catheter passed via *the mouth* into the stomach.
8. There is little evidence that saline lavage of the trachea improves the prognosis during acute resuscitation of the infant with meconium aspiration syndrome.[7]

Diaphragmatic hernia

This condition may have been diagnosed antenatally but still frequently presents unexpectedly at birth. A combination of persisting cyanosis, respiratory distress and a displaced apex beat (usually towards the right side of the chest) should alert the clinician to the diagnosis. The abdomen may be scaphoid. Occasionally bowel sounds may be heard in the chest, most frequently on the left side.

Bag and mask resuscitation is contraindicated because this will cause gastric and intestinal gaseous distension, thus aggravating the condition. If necessary the infant should be intubated and given intermittent positive-pressure ventilation. A large-bore orogastric tube is passed, and put on free drainage or continuous suction. An urgent chest radiograph is arranged and the infant is transferred to a neonatal intensive care unit for further acute care. Some children are extremely difficult to ventilate because of pulmonary hypoplasia, and high pressures may be required. Some infants may show persistent pulmonary hypertension of the newborn, and so hypoxia must be avoided if possible.

Pharmacologic muscle relaxation may be required to achieve satisfactory ventilation. There is continued controversy as to whether infants with congenital diaphragmatic hernia should be transferred urgently to an operating room for emergency surgery, or whether the prognosis is improved by a day or two of intensive medical care. In Europe few centers are as yet carrying out extracorporeal membrane oxygenation (ECMO). However, in the United Kingdom, a multicentered, randomized, controlled trial of ECMO versus maximal, conventional intensive care is being performed.

Pneumothorax

Pneumothorax may occur spontaneously or during resuscitation. The diagnosis is suspected when cyanosis and respiratory distress are accompanied by asymmetrical air entry. If the pneumothorax is on the left side, the cardiac apex is displaced to the right (as in diaphragmatic hernia, see above). A left-sided pneumothorax may displace the spleen downwards, and similarly a right-sided pneumothorax may cause downward displacement of the infant's liver.

Initial management should be with an exploratory needle. This may be done best using a 23-gauge butterfly catheter attached to a three-way stopcock on the end of a 10-ml syringe. The catheter should be inserted in the second intercostal space anteriorly in the mid-clavicular line, or else in the fifth intercostal space in the anterior axillary line. If a pneumothorax is present, then gentle suction brings gas into the syringe, which can then be expelled via the stopcock and the suction repeated. A definitive catheter can then be inserted and connected to a Heimlich valve.

TRAINING OTHERS

Although the current author has put forward the view that many aspects of resuscitation, including endotracheal intubation, can be expertly handled by those other than pediatricians, it is a mistake for any institution to teach too many members of staff these techniques: this serves merely to dilute the experience of each. A guide to resuscitation, such as this chapter, can convey principles only: the importance of regular practice has already been emphasized. Although a plastic mannikin is very helpful in providing the novice with practice in endotracheal intubation, frequently the artificial textures mislead the student. With parental permission, and with the acquiescence of other care givers, a senior member of staff should teach intubation on any infant recently dead. Best of all, however, is the experience gained in the delivery room, where the novice learns all the resuscitation techniques in the immediate presence of an experienced teacher.

ETHICAL DECISIONS

Labor ward is seldom the best place for ethical decisions to be made. Problems regarding the wisdom of proceeding with a resuscitation arise most frequently with the extremely low-birthweight infant, the very asphyxiated infant and the child with multiple severe congenital abnormalities. Recent advances in antenatal diagnosis now often allow parents to have detailed discussions with their advisors prior to delivery of the malformed infant: armed with accurate diagnosis and prognosis it is frequently possible to formulate a plan which may specify the degree of appropriate intervention by the pediatrician. In the absence of such prior information however, it is usually wise for the team to embark on full resuscitation, transferring the infant to the neonatal unit after preliminary stabilization. Thereafter an informed consensus may be reached as to how to proceed in the interests of the child and family. It is important for the entire care-giving team to recognize that major technological advances in neonatology create new questions about the wisdom of aggressive intervention.[8] The answers are elusive but must be found, otherwise for a small number of children one may regret that the neonatal resuscitation was so expert.

REFERENCES

1. Working Party of the British Paediatric Association, College of Anaesthetics, Royal College of Midwives, and Royal College of Obstetricians and Gynaecologists 1990 Resuscitation of the Newborn. Chameleon Press, London
2. McKlveen R E, Ostheimer G W 1987 Resuscitation of the Newborn. Clin Obstet Gynecol 30: 611–620
3. Schubring C 1986 Temperature regulation in healthy and resuscitated newborns immediately after birth. J Perinat Med 14: 27–33
4. Ballard J L, Musial M J, Myers M G 1986 Hazards of delivery room resuscitation using oral methods of endotracheal suctioning. Pediatr Infect Dis 5: 198–200
5. Sendak M J, Harris A P, Donham R T 1986 Use of pulse oximetry to assess arterial oxygen saturation during newborn resuscitation. Crit Care Med 14: 739–740
6. David R 1988 Closed chest cardiac massage in the newborn infant. Pediatrics 81: 552–554
7. Rosegger H, Engele H, Haas J 1987 Tracheobronchial lavage – a supplementary measure in the initial management of meconium aspiration syndrome. Wiener Klinische Wochenschrist 99: 843–847
8. Young E W D, Stevenson D K 1990 Limiting treatment for extremely premature, low-birth-weight infants (500 to 750 g). Am J Dis Child 144: 459–552

75. Anesthetic management of the pregnant surgical patient

A. M. Malinow

Anesthetic management of the pregnant surgical patient must address the well-being of both the mother and fetus. The patient's surgical condition, pregnancy-induced physiologic changes and possible adverse effects (both direct and indirect) of anesthesia all have a bearing on anesthetic management. Attention must be paid to the duration of the planned surgical procedure, possible sequelae from anesthesia and surgical intervention, the condition of the pregnancy and the gestational age and viability of the fetus.

Nonobstetric surgery is required in about 1% of pregnancies.[1–4] Surgery may be directly related to pregnancy (e.g. cerclage procedures), associated with pregnancy (e.g. torsion of an ovarian pedicle) or incidental to pregnancy (e.g. trauma or appendicitis).[5] The consultant anesthesiologist must be patient and understanding in answering difficult questions from both the patient and surgeon about 'what is best'. Decreasing the psychological stress of the patient and surgeon will help optimize operating room conditions.

FETAL CONSIDERATIONS

Teratogenicity

Teratogenic susceptibility/resistance differs among species, making any correlation between animal data and humans difficult. Retrospective epidemiologic studies of anesthetic exposure provide the only human data available; direct control of the experimental conditions has been lost. For a teratogenic effect to occur, a fetus must be exposed to a teratogenic dose of drug for a particular duration and during a susceptible period of embryonal development. In humans, the susceptible period of organogenesis is days 14–56. Development of the central nervous system and peripheral nervous system continues into the neonatal period. Results of multiple surveys reveal that *there is no increase in the incidence* of congenital abnormalities in pregnant patients who have undergone surgery during this period.[1–4,6,7] These thoughts must be tempered with the fact that the number of anesthetic exposures during pregnancy reported in the world literature is insufficient to detect possible human teratogenesis. Matching of gestational age, duration of anesthetic exposure, dose of drug and surgical stress can best be accomplished in animal models. The only controlled experimental data are all from animal studies.

Inhalation agents

Halothane, isoflurane, enflurane and nitrous oxide have not been shown to be associated with congenital malformations in rats repeatedly exposed to anesthetic concentrations of inhaled agent.[8]

Nitrous oxide controversies

The use of nitrous oxide during early pregnancy presents a difficult problem. Nitrous oxide inhibits methionine synthetase activity through the inactivation of vitamin B_{12}, interfering with thymidine and, therefore, DNA synthesis.[9] 24-h exposure of pregnant rats to 50% or greater inspired nitrous oxide concentrations will produce teratogenic effects.[10]

In humans, only significant exposures (approximately 2 h or more) to nitrous oxide have resulted in altered enzyme activity.[9] Additionally, epidemiologic studies have presented evidence, albeit weak, that early nitrous oxide exposure in clinically administered anesthetic concentrations does not produce teratogenic effects.[11] Some animal data report a degree of protection conferred by supplemental (intramuscular) folinic acid,[12] although this is controversial.[10] Administration of supplemental folinic acid to pregnant surgical patients is routinely practiced at some major obstetric anesthesia centers.[13]

Effect on gestational viability

Surgery and/or anesthesia in early pregnancy lead to an increased risk of spontaneous abortion.[6] Traditionally, surgical procedures anatomically distant to the pregnant, and therefore irritable, uterus were thought to carry a lower risk of premature labor and possible pregnancy loss. However, recent large epidemiologic surveys present conflicting evidence.[6,7] Pregnancy loss is increased particularly when associated with gynecologic procedures[2,6] and general anesthesia for nonabdominal procedures.[6] More low-birthweight infants (due to both prematurity and intrauterine growth retardation) are born to mothers who have had surgery and anesthesia during pregnancy.[7] This increased incidence is not associated with a specific type of anesthesia or surgery. While the results of these studies are statistically significant, the authors admit that the causative factors are still unknown.[6,7] Nitrous oxide has been associated with increased reproductive loss in the pregnant rat model.[8,10] Interestingly, the use of low-concentration isoflurane in combination with 50% nitrous oxide has adverse reproductive effects similar to those in nonexposed rats.[14]

Indirect effects

Volatile inhaled agents in concentrations of greater than 0.5 MAC (minimum alveolar concentration) will decrease uterine tone. Up to 1 MAC, inhaled agents will produce uterine artery vasodilation and increased blood flow; above 1 MAC the decrease in maternal cardiac output will offset this vasodilation, decreasing uterine artery flow.[15]

Direct and indirect effects of other agents

The maternal administration of 100% *oxygen* will not raise the fetal oxygen much above 60 mmHg[16] and will not predispose the fetus to the adverse effects of hyperoxia. Maternal hyperventilation may decrease fetal oxygen levels because of effects on uterine blood flow[17] and a left shift of the maternal oxyhemoglobin dissociation curve.

Certain *opioids* (morphine, meperidine and hydromorphone) have been associated with animal fetal abnormalities,[18] although never in humans. Fentanyl, alfentanil and sufentanil have been shown not to be teratogenic.[19] Fentanyl has shown no deleterious effects on uterine blood flow.

Barbiturates in a single dose have not been shown to be teratogenic. However, barbiturates may further decrease uterine blood flow in an already hypoperfused placenta.

Diazepam has been associated with different fetal abnormalities, notably cleft lip,[20] although this relationship is controversial.[21] The fetal half-life of diazepam is about 30 h, which might cause delayed neurobehavioral effects in the fetus if premature delivery is necessary.

Antisialagogues seem to have little, if any, effect on the fetus.

Muscle relaxants do not readily cross the placenta, yet can be measured in the fetal circulation after very large maternal doses. This may necessitate the need for ventilatory support in infants delivered in the perioperative period.

Ketamine in doses greater than 1.5 mg/kg will increase uterine tone and, therefore, decrease uterine blood flow. This tonic effect is seen throughout the second and third trimesters of pregnancy.[22]

Vasopressors have predominantly indirect fetal effects, affecting uterine blood flow. Predominantly β-adrenergic agonists are preferred,[23] yet there may be a place for α-adrenergic agents in *severely hypotensive patients*.[24]

Drugs used for prophylaxis against acid aspiration [e.g., histamine-2 (H_2) antagonists] have not been shown to have significant fetal effect in the dosage regimens commonly employed.

Local anesthetics have well-known indirect effects on the fetus. Although presumably cytotoxic, they have not been shown to be teratogenic.[25] The effects of local anesthetics on neurobehavioral scores has been discussed.

Sodium nitroprusside (SNP) has caused fetal cyanide toxicity in laboratory animals when doses far exceeding safe clinical anesthetic practice have been administered.[26] SNP has been used without harm for induced hypotension.[27,28]

Nitroglycerin and *trimethaphan* are used often during the management of preeclampsia and have proven human safety records.

Mannitol will cause bulk flow of water from the fetus across the placenta, but has been used without apparent harm in low doses.[29]

Chronic administration of β-*adrenergic blocking agents* has been associated with intrauterine growth retardation as well as expected fetal β-adrenergic blockade. Acute intravenous administration of labetalol in the gravid ewe model has produced insignificant fetal β-adrenergic blockade.[30] Clinical observation of infants born to mothers chronically treated with oral labetalol did not demonstrate significant β-adrenergic blockade.[31] Acute intravenous administration of esmolol in nonhypertensive gravid ewes has produced fetal hypoxemia.[32]

MATERNAL CONSIDERATIONS

Safeguarding the pregnant patient during surgery requires knowledge of the anesthetic implications of the altered physiology of pregnancy.

Hematologic system

Hematocrit values less than 35% are considered abnormal, although many pregnant women with a lower hematocrit carry to term and deliver without adverse outcome. Intraoperative blood loss should be replaced keeping this level in mind. Pregnancy is a hypercoagulable state. Early ambulation or the use of minidose heparin should be considered when appropriate in patients who are confined to bed for extended periods of recovery.

Cardiovascular system

Cardiac output is 40% above prepregnant values by the early third trimester. Increased plasma volume, venous capacitance and cardiac output keep systemic arterial and central venous pressures at essentially nonpregnant values. Aortocaval compression will decrease cardiac output or uterine blood flow or both. Uterine displacement is required at all times during the second half of pregnancy.

Respiratory system

Renal excretion of bicarbonate offsets the respiratory alkalosis produced by normal maternal hyperventilation ($Pa\text{CO}_2$ = 32 mmHg). Pregnancy-associated increase in minute ventilation as well as decrease in dead space significantly decrease the arterial-to-alveolar carbon dioxide gradient toward zero.[33] End-tidal capnography is, therefore, additionally helpful in intraoperative monitoring. Pulse oximetry is invaluable. Increased oxygen demand, increased cardiac output and decreased functional residual capacity lower apneic blood oxygen tensions faster in the pregnant woman. Denitrogenation before induction along with facile laryngoscopy and intubation of the trachea are obligatory. The possible anatomically difficult airway in the pregnant patient requires extra attention to be given to preinduction positioning of the patient. Immediate availability of endotracheal tubes in a wide selection of internal diameters as well as a short-handled laryngoscope is prudent. Vascular, friable nasopharyngeal muscosa may make passage of gastric tubes a bloody mess. Gentle insertion of well-lubricated gastric tubes is necessary. If the gastric tube is used only during the operative procedure, oral placement is an easier and safer choice. Finally, mucosal vasoconstrictors may have negative effects on uterine blood flow.[34]

Renal system

Blood urea nitrogen and serum creatinine are decreased to 5–10 mg/dl and 0.5 mg/dl respectively. These values should be considered when interpreting laboratory data. The possibility of urinary stasis due to ureteral compression by the gravid uterus makes meticulous fluid management necessary in an attempt to minimize the need for bladder catheterization.

Gastrointestinal system

Pharmacologic means to alter gastric acidity and volume should be an integral part of acid aspiration prophylaxis. When appropriate, regional anesthesia with intact airway reflexes is preferable to general anesthesia. If general anesthesia is selected, rapid-sequence induction of general anesthesia is routinely advised. If the surgical condition warrants a more deliberate induction of general anesthesia (e.g. severely increased intracranial pressure), experienced personnel should be available to maintain cricoid pressure and otherwise assist the anesthesiologist from induction of anesthesia through endotracheal intubation.

Central nervous system

The MAC of inhaled agents decreases during pregnancy.[35] This is especially important if inhalation analgesia is contemplated. Loss of protective airway reflexes in a possibly anesthetized patient demands careful titration of agent to effect, and then only in the most experienced hands. A fasting pregnant patient presenting electively for surgery in the first trimester would possibly (but rarely) be a candidate for inhalation analgesia. The gravida presenting for surgery in the second trimester and beyond should be treated with the same precautions as the nonfasting patient presenting emergently for surgery. Neural sensitivity to local anesthetics increases during pregnancy.[36] The induction of surgical epidural or subarachnoid anesthesia will require less anesthetic in the pregnant patient. Use of continuous epidural or subarachnoid catheters allows the anesthesiologist to titrate the dose of local anesthetic to desired effect.

GENERAL RECOMMENDATIONS

First trimester

Possible teratogenic effects should be kept in mind but there is no reason to avoid general anesthesia if appropriate for the planned surgical procedure or if requested by the patient. The use of nitrous oxide in the first trimester as well as in the entire pregnancy is controversial. Maintenance of general anesthesia can easily be accomplished while avoiding the use of nitrous oxide.

Second and third trimester

Support of uteroplacental perfusion is of prime importance. Uterine displacement is essential in the supine pregnant patient, especially after 20 weeks' gestation. Intermittent comparison of brachial blood pressure to blood pressure distal to the uterus (e.g. popliteal area) is helpful in detecting occult supine hypotension. Fetal heart rate should be monitored throughout the perioperative period by personnel familiar with its interpretation in all pregnancies that are thought to be viable. Obstetric consultation should be readily available to evaluate fetal well-being before, during and after the procedure as well as to treat obstetric complications such as premature labor. Gastrointestinal changes demand acid aspiration prophylaxis. Rapid-sequence induction of general anesthesia is indicated.

Remember: **Meticulous care of the mother will help ensure fetal well-being.**

REFERENCES

1. Smith B E 1963 Fetal prognosis after anesthesia during gestation. Anesth Analg 42: 521
2. Shnider S M, Webster G M 1965 Maternal and fetal hazards of surgery during pregnancy. Am J Obstet Gynecol 92: 891
3. Brodsky J B, Cohen E N, Brown B W et al 1980 Surgery during pregnancy and fetal outcome. Am J Obstet Gynecol 138: 1165
4. Konieczko K M, Chapk J C, Nunn J F 1987 Fetotoxic potential of general anesthesia in relation to pregnancy. Br J Anaesth 59: 449
5. Weingold A B (ed) 1983 Surgical diseases in pregnancy. Clin Obstet Gynecol 24(4): 793
6. Duncan P G, Pope W D B, Cohen M M et al 1986 Fetal risk of anesthesia and surgery during pregnancy. Anesthesiology 64: 790
7. Mazze R I, Kallen B 1989 Reproductive outcome after anesthesia and operation during pregnancy: a registry study of 5405 cases. Am J Obstet Gynecol 161: 1178
8. Mazze R I, Fujinaga M, Rice S A et al 1986 Reproductive and teratogenic effects of nitrous oxide, halothane, isoflurane and enflurane in Sprague–Dawley rats. Anesthesiology 64: 339
9. Nunn J F 1987 Clinical aspects of the interaction between nitrous oxide and vitamin B12. Br J Anaesth 59: 3
10. Fujinaga M, Mazze R I, Baden J M 1988 Reconsiderations of the mechanisms of nitrous oxide teratogenicity. Anesthesiology 69: A658
11. Crawford J S, Lewis M 1986 Nitrous oxide in early human pregnancy. Anesthesia 41: 900
12. Keeling P A, Rocke D A, Nunn J F et al 1986 Folinic acid as protection against nitrous oxide teratogenicity in the rat. Br J Anaesth 58: 528
13. Marx G F 1985 The N_2O dilemma. Obstet Anesth Dig 5: 126
14. Fujinaga M, Baden J M, Yhap E O et al 1987 Reproductive and teratogenic effects of nitrous oxide, isoflurane, and their combination in Sprague–Dawley rats. Anesthesiology 67: 960
15. Biehl D R, Yarnell R, Wide J G et al 1983 The uptake of isoflurane by the foetal lamb in utero: effect on regional blood flow. Can Anaesth Soc J 30: 581
16. Baraka A 1972 Correlation between maternal and foetal pO2 and pCO2 during cesarean delivery. Br J Anaesth 42: 434
17. Levinsohn G L, Shnider S M, deLorimier A A et al 1974 Effects of maternal hyperventilation on uterine blood flow and fetal oxygenation and acid–base status. Anesthesiology 40: 340
18. Geber W F, Schramm L C 1975 Congenital malformations of the central nervous system produced by narcotic analgesics in the hamster. Am J Obstet Gynecol 123: 705
19. Fujinaga M, Mazze R I, Jackson E C et al 1988 Reproductive and teratogenic effects of sufentanil and alfentanil in Sprague-Dawley rats. Anesthesiology 67: 166
20. Safra M J, Oakley G P 1975 Association between cleft lip with and without cleft palate and prenatal exposure to diazepam. Lancet 2: 478
21. Rosenberg L, Mitchell A A, Parsells J L et al 1983 Lack of relation of oral clefts to diazepam use during pregnancy. New Engl J Med 309: 1282
22. Galloon S 1976 Ketamine for obstetric delivery. Anesthesiology 44: 522
23. Ralston D H, Shnider S M, deLorimier A A 1974 Effects of equipotent metaraminol, mephenteramine and methoxamine on uterine blood flow in the pregnant ewe. Anesthesiology 40: 354
24. Ramanathan S, Friedman S, Moss P et al 1984 Phenylephrine for the treatment of maternal hypotension due to epidural anesthesia. Anesth Analg 63: 262
25. Fujinaga M, Mazze R I 1986 Reproductive and teratogenic effects of lidocaine in Sprague-Dawley rats. Anesthesiology 65: 626
26. Naulty J S, Cefalo R C, Lewis P E 1981 Fetal toxicity of nitroprusside in the pregnant ewe. Am J Obstet Gynecol 139: 708
27. Kofke W A, Wuest H P, McGinnis C A 1984 Cesarean section following ruptured cerebral aneurysm and neuroresuscitation. Anesthesiology 60: 242
28. Rigg D, McDonogh A 1981 Use of sodium nitroprusside for deliberate hypotension during pregnancy. Br J Anaesth 53: 985
29. Neuman B, Lam A M 1986 Induced hypotension for clipping of a cerebral aneurysm during pregnancy: a case report and brief review. Anesth Analg 65: 675
30. Eisenach J C 1989 Maternally administered labetalol produces less adrenergic blockade in fetus than in mother. Anesthesiology 71: A915
31. MacPherson M, Broughton Pipkin F, Rutter N 1986 The effect of maternal labetalol in the newborn infant. Br J Obstet Gynecol 93: 539
32. Eisenach J C, Castro M I 1989 Maternally administered esmolol produces fetal beta adrenergic blockade and hypoxemia. Anesthesiology 71: 718
33. Shankar K B, Moseley H, Kumar Y et al 1986 Arterial to end-tidal carbon dioxide tension difference during cesarean section. Anesthesia 41: 698
34. Woods J R, Plessinger M A, Clark K E 1987 Effect of cocaine on uterine blood flow and fetal oxygenation. J Am Med Assoc 257: 957
35. Palahniuk R J, Shnider S M, Eger II E I 1987 Pregnancy decreases the requirements of inhaled anesthetic agents. Anesthesiology 41: 82
36. Datta S, Lambert D H, Gregus J et al 1983 Differential sensitivity of mammalian nerve fibers during pregnancy. Anesth Analg 62: 1070

76. Anesthesia for fetal surgery

C. A. Burchman

Anesthesia for fetal surgery is a provocative possibility. In the most basic sense, it is the merging of the management of two distinct, yet joined, organisms. The most fundamental principles of obstetric anesthetic care must apply. In addition, perinatal (actually *antenatal*) considerations apply.

Fetal intervention was first described by Liley in 1963[1] for treatment of infants with erythroblastosis fetalis. Until recently, few therapeutic options existed when serious fetal anomalies were present. If pregnancy was not medically terminated, many of these infants would die in utero or shortly after birth.

In the subsequent 25 years, the potential for fetal surgery improved dramatically. Today, surgical intervention early in fetal development (for conditions such as diaphragmatic hernia, hydronephrosis and obstructive hydrocephalus) is a viable option because of improvements of intrauterine diagnostic capabilities and new surgical techniques.[2–4]

Anesthesia can have a profound effects on both the mother and fetus. Minimal clinical data are available upon which to base decisions regarding the management of anesthesia for fetal surgery.[1–4]

PHYSIOLOGIC CHANGES OF PREGNANCY

The physiologic changes of pregnancy influence the conduct of anesthesia. Aortocaval compression can become clinically important as early as the 10th week of gestation. At term, the maternal cardiac output has increased by 25%, the plasma volume by 50% and the red cell mass by 30% (resulting in the physiologic anemia of pregnancy).[5] Pregnancy is associated with alterations in the levels of several coagulation factors (plasma fibrinogen is increased by 50%; factors VIII and XII are increased, whereas factors XI and XIII are usually decreased). The fibrinolytic system may be depressed, especially plasminogen activator and antithrombin III. Venous stasis in the lower extremities, due to the enlarged gravid uterus and compression of the inferior vena cava, may be associated with an increased risk of thrombophlebitis. As the uterus increases in size, maternal oxygen consumption and minute alveolar ventilation increase and the functional residual capacity declines. The pregnant patient compensates for the increases in minute ventilation by renal excretion of bicarbonate to maintain a normal acid–base balance. Thus, with reduced cardiopulmonary reserve, the pregnant patient rapidly becomes hypoxic when apneic. She has less ability to buffer the acidotic state.

PHARMACOKINETIC CONSIDERATIONS

Uptake, distribution, metabolism and excretion of anesthetic agents are altered in pregnancy.[6] These alterations are secondary to an increased cardiac output, increased volume of distribution, altered plasma protein levels and enzyme activity, increased glomerular filtration rate, altered hepatic function and increased minute ventilation. Pregnant patients are more sensitive to the effects of general and local anesthetic agents. Thus, the mean alveolar concentration of volatile agents needs to be reduced by approximately 25–50% and the dosage of local anesthetics diminished by about one-third. This reduction in anesthetic requirement may be due in part to an altered hormonal state, particularly increased levels of progesterone.[7]

Pregnant patients are at increased risk for aspiration of gastric contents. Nonparticulate antacids, metoclopramide and cimetidine may be given preanesthetically.[8] Induction of general anesthesia should be performed in a 'rapid-sequence' fashion with cricoid pressure (Sellick's maneuver).

Considerations in maintenance of uteroplacental perfusion include avoidance of aortocaval compression and maintenance of adequate maternal blood pressure and cardiac output with intravenous volume expansion and ephedrine. Pure α-agonists should be avoided because of the reported deleterious effect of these agents on placental perfusion.[9] Supplemental oxygen should be administered. Pure oxygen administration to the mother for extended periods does not cause retinopathy of prematurity in the fetus unless hyperbaric pressures are used.[10] Maternal $P\text{aco}_2$ should be kept in the normal range. Maternal stress and drugs that increase uterine tone (ketamine in doses greater than 1 mg/kg and neostigmine) should be avoided.

REGIONAL VERSUS GENERAL ANESTHESIA

For surgical procedures on the fetus, regional anesthesia is intuitively appealing because it may limit the amount of fetal drug exposure, thereby reducing the risk of exposure to possible toxic or teratogenic effects of anesthetic agents. Regional approaches may also reduce the risk of maternal aspiration associated with general anesthesia.[11] However, regional anesthesia does not completely prevent the maternal stress response to anxiety, nor does it provide fetal anesthesia or block the response of the fetus to surgery-induced stress. Anand et al[12] demonstrated that preterm infants undergoing surgery had a substantial hormonal response indicative of stress if not given adequate anesthesia. Regional anesthesia cannot provide uterine relaxation or fetal neuromuscular block. Fetal movement may occur and disrupt the operative field. In such situations, intramuscular injections of muscle relaxants into the fetus have been reported to maintain a motionless surgical field.[13] Therefore, general anesthesia offers several advantages for fetal surgery.[14]

In a recent case report of fetal surgery, the author and his associates chose general anesthesia for several reasons. With general anesthesia, there is maternal skeletal muscle relaxation, uterine smooth muscle relaxation, fetal immobility, fetal anesthesia, maintenance of normal uteroplacental perfusion and a block of maternal awareness.[15–18] To minimize toxic drug effects on the fetus, agents with minimal biodegradation and long safety records in pregnant humans should be used. The reduction of the maternal stress response and the maintenance of placental perfusion are of equal importance. Isoflurane has some merits that may make it the volatile anesthetic of choice. It undergoes the least biodegradation, has an excellent safety record in obstetric anesthesia and provides good uterine and skeletal muscle relaxation.

Nitrous oxide should be avoided because of its inhibitory effect on the activity of vitamin B_{12}-dependent enzymes (methionine synthetase and thymidylate synthetase).[19] Methionine synthetase catalyzes the conversion of homocystine to methionine, a precursor of myelin. Interference with either of these enzymatic processes could theoretically compromise normal fetal development. Vanucci and Wolf [20] observed that nitrous oxide in conjunction with muscle relaxation led to profound metabolic alterations in fetal rat brains, suggestive of inhibition of aerobic metabolism. The combination of mild hypoxia and nitrous oxide produced more anomalies than hypoxia alone.[21] Nitrous oxide, when given to rats for 1 or 2 days, caused a high incidence of fetal death and malformations.[22] For these reasons, many authors recommend avoiding fetal exposure to nitrous oxide during the first and second trimesters. Theoretically, intravenous alfentanil may be a useful adjunct for general anesthesia in fetal surgery. Its rapid redistribution and metabolism allow it to be used as a continuous intravenous infusion. Alfentanil can be used to maintain a profound maternal opioid effect that will rapidly dissipate when discontinued. It does tend to accumulate on the fetal side of the placenta, and this accumulation may provide a prolonged level of stress reduction in the fetus after surgery. Alfentanil has not been correlated with any teratogenic effects to date.

NEUROMUSCULAR BLOCKADE

Succinylcholine, because of its highly ionized state at normal body pH, minimizes fetal exposure and is rapidly metabolized by maternal and fetal plasma cholinesterase. Although the levels and activity of fetal cholinesterase at 20 weeks' gestation are not well documented, succinylcholine has been reported to be rapidly metabolized by premature infants.[23] Nondepolarizing agents such as pancuronium and d-tubocurarine are highly ionized compounds that are slow to cross the placenta.[24,25] The amount of these drugs that reaches the fetus after maternal administration is small. Adequate fetal skeletal muscle relaxation cannot be ensured when conventional doses are administered only to the mother. Direct fetal intramuscular injections of 3mg/kg d-tubocurarine to immobilize the fetus during surgery have been reported.[13] Fetal cardiac output is heart rate dependent. Pancuronium may be preferred over d-tubocurarine for intrauterine fetal surgery because it has been shown to maintain a higher fetal heart rate and mean arterial pressure.[26–28] Fetal movement did not occur in a case when 1.5% isoflurane in oxygen was used, and no additional fetal muscle relaxants were required.[15]

The use of a sterile neonatal pulse oximeter for monitoring of the fetus is a consideration. However, a technical problem may be encountered. The pulse oximeter probe is attached to the fetus with an adhesive band. The risk of denuding the immature dermal layers with this adhesive is of concern, since the manipulation of the fetus by surgeons caused a noticeable sloughing of the dermis in one case.[15] A sterile probe without adhesive would be advantageous. Seeds et al[26] have used fetal heart rate monitoring, utilizing the standard scalp electrode, with a reference electrode on the maternal abdomen.

A QUESTION OF ETHICS

The question arises as to what could be done therapeutically in the event that the monitors suggest fetal compromise. Ensuring stable maternal hemodynamics and ventilation and the avoidance of aortocaval compression is the fundamental doctrine for preservation of fetal homeostasis.

Although fetal surgery is at its inception, it is clear that as technology improves, these procedures will become more widely used. Early animal and human studies indicate that these surgical procedures can correct what would otherwise be fatal abnormalities. As technology becomes more sophisticated, ethical conflicts become unavoidable. Most fetal malformations do not pose a threat to maternal health, whereas general anesthesia and laparotomy do. Ethical guidelines need to be developed for fetal surgery.

REFERENCES

1. Liley A W 1963 Intrauterine transfusion of foetus in haemolytic disease. Br Med J 2: 1107
2. Frigoletto F D, Birholz J C, Greene M F 1982 Antenatal treatment of hydrocephalus by ventriculoamniotic shunting. J Am Med Assoc 248: 2496
3. Golbus M S, Harrison M R, Filly R A et al 1982 *In utero* treatment of urinary tract obstruction. Am J Obstet Gynecol 142: 383
4. Berkowitz R I, Glickman M G, Smith G W et al 1982 Fetal urinary tract obstruction: what is the role of surgical intervention *in utero*? Am J Obstet Gynecol 144: 367
5. Bonica J J 1980 Obstetric analgesia and anesthesia. World Federation of Societies of Anesthesiologists, p 2
6. Davis A G, Moir D D 1986 Anaesthesia during pregnancy. Clin Anaesthesiol 4: 233
7. Flanagan J L, Datta S, Lambert D et al 1987 Effect of pregnancy on bupivacaine-induced conduction blockade in the isolated rabbit vagus nerve. Anesth Analg 66: 123
8. Solanki D R, Suresh M, Ethridge H C 1984 The effects of intravenous cimetidine and metoclopramide on gastric volume and pH. Anesth Analg 63: 599
9. Shnider S M, Levinson G 1987 Anesthesia for obstetrics, 2d edn. Williams & Wilkins, Baltimore, p. 32.
10. Ricci B, Calagero G 1988 Oxygen induced retinopathy in newborn rats: effects of prolonged normobaric and hyperbaric oxygen supplementation. Pediatrics 83: 193
11. Spielman F J, Seeds J W, Corke B C 1984 Anesthesia for fetal surgery. Anesthesia 39: 756
12. Anand K J S, Sippel W G, Green A 1987 A randomized trial of fentanyl anesthesia in preterm babies undergoing surgery. Lancet 1: 243
13. De Crespigny L C, Robinson H P, Ross A W, Quinn M Curarization of fetus for intrauterine procedures. Lancet 1: 1164
14. Levine M D, McNeil D E, Kabuck M M et al 1974 Second trimester fetoscopy and fetal blood sampling: current limitations and problems. Am J Obstet Gynecol 120: 937
15. Johnson M J, Birnbach D J, Burchman C A et al 1989 Fetal surgery and general anesthesia: a case report and review. J Clin Anesth 1: 363
16. Delany A G 1983 Anesthesia in the pregnant women. Clin Obstet Gynecol 20: 795
17. Duncan P G, Pope W D, Cohen M M, Greer N 1986 Fetal risk of anesthesia and surgery during pregnancy. Anesthesiology 20: 795
18. Warren T W, Datta S, Ostheimer G W et al 1983 Comparison of the maternal and neonatal effects of halothane, enflurane, and isoflurane for cesarean deliveries. Anesth Analg 62: 516
19. Nunn J F, Chanarin I 1985 Nitrous oxide inactivates methionine synthetase. In Eger EI (ed) Nitrous oxide. Elsevier, New York p 211
20. Vanucci R C, Wolf J W 1978 Oxidative metabolism in fetal rat brain during maternal anesthesia. Anesthesiology 48: 238
21. Smith B E, Gaub M I, Moya F 1965 Teratogenic effects of anesthetic agents. Anesth Analg 44: 726
22. Fink B R, Shepard T H, Blendau R J 1967 Teratogenic activity of nitrous oxide. Nature 214: 146
23. Escobichon P J, Stephens D S 1973 Perinatal development of human esterases. Clin Pharmacol Ther 14: 41
24. Abouleish E, Wingard L B, de la Vega S, Uy N 1980 Pancuronium in cesarean section and its placental transfer. Br J Anesth 52: 531
25. Kivalo I, Saarikoski S 1972 Placental transmission and foetal uptake of 14C-dimethyl-tubocurarine. Br J Anaesth 44: 557
26. Seeds J W, Corke B C, Spielman F J 1986 Prevention of fetal movement during invasive procedure with pancuronium bromide. Am J Obstet Gynecol 155: 818
27. Chestnut D H, Weiner C P, Thompson C S, McLaughlin G L 1988 Intravenous administration of D-tubocuraine and pancuronium in fetal lambs (abstract). Anesthesiology 69: A652
28. Harrison M R, Anderson J, Rosen MA et al 1982 Fetal surgery in the primate. Anesthetic, surgical and tocolytic management to maximize fetal-neonatal survival. J Pediatr Surg 17: 115

77. Anesthesia for post-partum surgery

Part A UK view *G. O'Sullivan*
Part B USA view *B. L. Koffel*

PART A
UK VIEW
G. O'Sullivan

The international definition of maternal death includes all deaths occurring during pregnancy or before 42 days post-partum. The latest Report on Confidential Enquiries into Maternal Deaths in the United Kingdom (1985–87) shows that many of these deaths occur post-partum.[1] Since delivery is the definitive treatment for pre-eclampsia/eclampsia it is perhaps not surprising that in this latest report 26 of the 27 deaths due to hypertensive disorders of pregnancy occurred post-partum. Pulmonary complications were the immediate cause of death in 12 of the patients, while anesthesia or excessive sedation contributed to three of the deaths. Six of the 10 deaths from maternal hemorrhage occurred post-partum, as did 14 of the 29 deaths attributed to thromboembolic disease. Therefore the role of the obstetric anesthesiologist in the risk management of the pregnant patient must include pre-, intra- and post-partum care.

Surgery in the post-partum period will be required for indications both related and unrelated to the pregnancy and delivery. In the UK tubal ligation is very rarely performed in the early post-partum period, it most usually being carried out at the time of cesarean delivery or alternatively delayed until several months post-partum. One of the factors that separates surgery in the post-partum period from any other surgery in essentially fit young women is the persistence of the physiologic changes of pregnancy. The timing and speed of return of the physiologic parameters to the nonpregnant physiologic baseline state cannot always be identified precisely. Serial physiologic measurements during pregnancy and in the early post-partum period are often limited by ethical and safety considerations and by patient compliance. Thus comparison of experimental results which have been made using many different methodologies must be carefully interpreted, particularly when they might influence anesthetic technique.

GASTRIC FUNCTION DURING PREGNANCY AND THE PUERPERIUM

Gastroesophageal reflux is one of the risk factors associated with aspiration pneumonitis. Symptoms of reflux occur in approximately 75% of pregnant women at term,[2] while in other women in the third trimester of pregnancy lower esophageal pH monitoring indicates that gastroesophageal reflux can be asymptomatic.[3] Measurements of gastroesophageal reflux by lower esophageal pH monitoring made prior to delivery and 36 h post-partum have shown that there is a statistically significant decrease in gastroesophageal reflux by the second day after delivery.[4] Intragastric pressure is considerably increased and the position of the stomach itself is distorted during pregnancy. In many women the increase in intragastric pressure is not matched by a similar increase in the gastroesophageal pressure gradient,[5] thereby increasing the potential for passive regurgitation of gastric contents into the pharynx. Although no serial measurements have been made, it can be postulated that intragastric pressure will rapidly fall as the uterus involutes post-partum.

Results of studies on gastric acid secretion during pregnancy and the puerperium are summarized in Table 77.1. Studies during the 1920s and 1930s indicated that gastric acid secretion was significantly decreased during pregnancy, with the greatest decrease occurring in mid-pregnancy.[6–10] One of these studies[7] advocated the use of dilute hydrochloric acid as prophylaxis against nausea and vomiting during pregnancy, while another[9] suggested that the anemia seen in pregnancy was due to a deficiency of a 'gastric factor' absent as a result of the fall in gastric acidity throughout pregnancy. In 1953 an

Table 77.1 Summary of studies evaluating gastric acidity during pregnancy and the puerperium

Reference	Method of assessment	Time of assessment	Gastric acidity
6	Test meal	Early and late pregnancy	Decreased, especially in early pregnancy
7	Test meal	Early and late pregnancy	Decreased, especially in early pregnancy
8	50 ml 7% alcohol 0.3 mg histamine	Throughout pregnancy Post-partum	Decreased, maximum in months 3–6
9	Test meal	Throughout pregnancy Post-partum	Progressive decrease during pregnancy
10	300 ml 7% alcohol 0.3 mg histamine	Third trimester	Minimal decrease
12	Basal secretion 0.1 mg/10 kg histamine	Throughout pregnancy	Decreased in the first and second trimesters
13	0.5 mg histamine	Throughout pregnancy Post-partum	No significant change
14	X-ray	Labor (10 subjects)	Delayed in two subjects
15	X-ray	Labor (12 subjects)	Delayed in one subject
16	X-ray	Pregnancy and labor	Pregnancy, no delay Labor, slight delay Labor + narcotics, marked delay
17	Double sampling test meal	Pregnancy and labor	Pregnancy, delayed? Labor, delayed
19	Paracetamol absorption	Labor	Labor, slight delay Labor + narcotics, marked delay
22	Paracetamol absorption	Pregnancy First 2 h post-partum 18–36 h post-partum	Pregnancy, no delay First 2 h post-partum, delayed 18–36 h post-partum, no delay

improvement in ulcer symptoms was noted in 90% of 334 pregnancies in 118 women, however by the sixth month post-partum ulcer symptoms had recurred in over 75% of the women.[11] In perhaps the most comprehensive study[12] of gastric secretion during pregnancy basal and histamine-augmented (0.4 mg of histamine acid phosphate per 10 kg body weight) gastric secretion were measured in 10 nonpregnant women and 30 pregnant women equally distributed throughout the three trimesters of pregnancy. There was no significant difference in the rates of basal secretion between the pregnant and nonpregnant females; however, when the subjects were divided into groups according to the stage of gestation, the mean basal secretion in the middle trimester was decreased (though not significantly) relative to the first and third trimesters. The response to histamine acid phosphate (0.4 mg/10 kg) was significantly depressed in the first and second trimester compared with the response seen in the third-trimester mothers.

The overall conclusion to be drawn from the studies on gastric acid secretion during pregnancy (most of which show a wide inter-subject variation) must be that gastric secretion is decreased in early pregnancy and returns to normal levels in the last trimester (Table 77.1). In those studies in which mothers were assessed post-partum, no significant difference was shown between them and the antepartum controls.[8,9,13]

Another factor influencing acid reflux and regurgitation from the stomach will be the size of the residual gastric volume, itself determined by the rate of gastric secretion and emptying. The emptying of the gastric contents from the stomach to the duodenum is the result of highly complex interrelationships between hormonal, muscular and electrical influences, and therefore any technique that simply measures the rate of transfer of liquids or solids from the stomach to the duodenum will not necessarily detect subtle changes in motility or the pattern of emptying. Improvements in the assay techniques for gastrointestinal peptides, neurotransmitters and prostaglandins and the elucidation of the factors influencing such events as the migrating myoelectric complex further highlight the complexity of gastrointestinal motility. It is, therefore, not surprising to find that gastric emptying studies, including studies performed during pregnancy and labor, have produced varying results.

Although X-ray studies of gastric emptying during

pregnancy and labor would be ethically unacceptable today, several such studies have been performed in the past. Hirscheimer et al[14] gave 10 fasting primigravidas in early labor a thin barium mixture. Radiographs were then taken at hourly intervals during labor with the subjects in the standing position; no food, fluid or medication was allowed during the study. Two of the 10 patients showed delayed and the remainder normal gastric emptying. In a similar study, Crawford[15] administered barium to 12 women in the first stage of labor, only one of whom demonstrated a delay in gastric emptying. In another radiologic study evaluating gastric emptying in pregnancy and labor, a barium meal was administered to 42 pregnant women on three separate occasions: (a) late in the third trimester of pregnancy, (b) late in the third trimester but following an intramuscular injection of meperidine 100 mg and scopolamine 0.4 mg and (c) in active labor following meperidine 100 mg and scopolamine 0.4 mg.[16] An upright film was taken 3 h after the meal and at 2 hourly intervals thereafter, and the percentage of barium retained in the stomach at these times was measured. Pregnancy had no effect on gastric emptying, and 5 h after the test meal all the barium had been evacuated from the stomach. Meperidine given during the third trimester of pregnancy caused approximately 7.5% retention of the barium at 5 h, but the combination of labor plus meperidine caused the greatest delay in the evacuation of the barium, with up to 20% retention at 5 h.

In 1970 Davison et al[17] used a double sampling technique to measure gastric emptying in 11 nonpregnant female controls, 11 females in the third trimester of pregnancy and eight women in established labor. The mean ± S E M total emptying time was significantly longer in the pregnant patients, being 119.5 ± 17.2 min compared with a mean time of 74.8 ± 8.5 min in the nonpregnant women; the half-life of gastric emptying was not significantly different in the two groups. Labor was shown to cause all the measured parameters to be prolonged, and the pattern of emptying was no longer exponential.

An alternative and noninvasive approach to the measurement of gastric emptying is to estimate it indirectly from the absorption kinetics of orally administered paracetamol.[18] This technique of estimating gastric emptying was applied to 56 women during labor and the puerperium; of the 28 patients given meperidine or diamorphine during labor, 12 had achieved maximum paracetamol concentration before the opioid was administered and these 12 subjects plus 10 post-partum patients acted as controls.[19] Established labor caused some delay in gastric emptying, but this delay was minimal compared with the effect of opioids. Gastric emptying in those receiving epidural analgesia was similar to that seen in the patients who had received no analgesia. The concomitant use of metoclopramide did not reverse the delay in gastric emptying caused by opioids.

Thus evidence to date suggests that pregnancy does not significantly alter gastric emptying but that established labor causes a slight delay in gastric emptying that is very markedly potentiated by the use of opioid analgesia. This is further substantiated by a study which showed that the largest residual gastric volumes in patients undergoing cesarean delivery were found in those women who had received meperidine during labor.[20]

In a survey on aspiration prophylaxis in the post-partum period it was found that 50% of the 225 obstetric anesthesiologists questioned administer preoperative antacids for 3 days post-partum, while 5% still give preoperative antacid 6 weeks after delivery. It was also found that 50% of the anesthesiologists employ a rapid-sequence induction during the first two post-partum days, while 5% still persist with this practice for more than 4 weeks after delivery.[21]

The question which must be answered is: what happens to emptying in the early post-partum period? In a recent study the paracetamol absorption technique was used to measure gastric emptying (a) during pregnancy, (b) during the first 2 h post-partum and (c) between 18 and 36 h post-partum. Gastric emptying was found to be delayed in those mothers investigated in the first 2 h after a normal vaginal delivery. The gastric emptying times measured 18–36 h after delivery were not significantly different from the emptying times achieved in the same women during their third trimester of pregnancy; in addition these times were similar to those seen in the nonpregnant control group.[22]

When gastric volume and pH were measured in post-partum patients undergoing tubal ligation more than 8 h after delivery, it was shown that the pH and volume were not significantly different from nonpregnant female controls.[23] Similarly, James et al[24] were unable to demonstrate that two of the frequently defined parameters for aspiration (pH < 2.5, volume > 25 ml) were any different between women early (1–8 h) and late (9–25 h) in the post-partum period and elective surgical controls. The fact that gastric emptying has been shown to be delayed in the first 2 h post-partum confirms that exactly the same precautions against acid aspiration should be provided to newly delivered mothers requiring anesthesia. However, by 24 h after delivery, gastric emptying will have returned to the prepartum baseline in normal post-partum mothers.

The pattern of emptying *during* the first day post-partum has not been elucidated and awaits further study. One question must however be considered: would situations such as the retention of the products of conception delay the return of gastric emptying to normal and thereby in these patients extend the period for which full precautions against aspiration would be required? The appropriate preventive and prophylactic measures against pulmonary aspiration of gastric contents aim at producing a high intragastric pH with a low intragastric volume.

Mendelson in his original paper proposed the withholding of solid food during labor and the administration of warm antacid prior to surgery. The advent of the H_2-antagonists[25] and more recently omeprazole[26] has further improved the safety profile, and where necessary these agents should be administered, in the same regimens as those used for cesarean delivery, in women requiring surgery in the hours immediately following delivery.

CARDIOVASCULAR AND HEMATOLOGIC SYSTEMS

Cardiac output increases gradually until early in the third trimester, and this increase is maintained until delivery, an effect mediated by an increase in both stroke volume and heart rate. In the third trimester cardiac output is significantly influenced by maternal position: if the mother lies in the supine position the inferior vena cava will be compressed and consequently venous return and cardiac output will decrease.[27] Pain and uterine contractions increase cardiac output during labor, while placental autotransfusion further increases cardiac output immediately post-partum. Depending on the volume of blood loss at delivery, cardiac output probably returns to prepartum levels during the first 2 weeks post-partum. Regional distribution of blood flow is altered during pregnancy, there being a large increase in flow to the skin, kidneys and uterus. Again, pain and uterine contractions will increase blood pressure during labor, but it probably rapidly returns to prepartum levels shortly after delivery.[28] Pregnancy causes little change in systolic pressure, but a fall in peripheral vascular resistance results in a decline in diastolic pressure, which produces an increase in pulse pressure.

Blood volume increases by between 35 and 40% during pregnancy, and the relatively greater increase in plasma volume results in a fall in hemoglobin, hematocrit and red cell count.[29] Blood loss at delivery will vary between 250 and 1000 ml depending on the mode of delivery; this loss at delivery is compensated for by autotransfusion from the placental bed and the increase in peripheral vascular resistance. Blood volume returns to normal prepartum levels on approximately the third day post-partum, although obviously the blood loss at delivery will influence these changes.[30] Thus in the healthy mother the cardiovascular and hematologic changes of pregnancy should not significantly influence surgery in either the early or late post-partum period, while venocaval occlusion by the gravid uterus, which can have major cardiovascular effects in late pregnancy, is obviously no longer a factor in the immediate post-partum period.

Unfortunately, it would appear that obstetricians, midwives and anesthesiologists frequently underestimate the volume of blood loss at delivery and in the early post-partum period. The maternal mortality report for 1985–87[1] shows that, of the 10 deaths from hemorrhage, four were caused by placental abruption and six by post-partum hemorrhage, of which four were associated with cesarean delivery. This suggests that failure to appreciate both intra- and post-operative blood loss and to quickly and adequately replace this loss with colloid and, where necessary, blood exposes some mothers to unnecessary life-threatening situations. The routine post-partum use of an oxytocin infusion (20 units in 500 ml of crystalloid solution) following cesarean or vaginal delivery in a mother at risk from post-partum hemorrhage might reduce post-partum blood loss. All delivery units should provide protocols and guidelines for the management of severe obstetric hemorrhage and should be capable of providing facilities for intensive care and immediate blood and blood products transfusion. Adequate venous access should be established and central venous pressure should be used to monitor fluid loss and replacement. Pressurized infusion pumps should be available. A urinary catheter must be inserted and urine output closely monitored, while in severe cases intra-arterial blood pressure monitoring will be helpful.

When disorders of coagulation are responsible for severe prepartum hemorrhage, specialist advice should be sought from a hematologist. Pregnancy results in an increase in plasma fibrinogen and factors VII, VIII and X. The platelet count decreases slightly during pregnancy but platelet function remains unchanged. Plasma fibrinolytic activity is decreased during pregnancy but returns to normal shortly after placental separation.[28] This alteration in coagulation and fibrinolytic factors provides protection against peripartum hemorrhage but, unfortunately, is probably the cause of the greater incidence of thromboembolic disease during pregnancy and the puerperium.

Although venous thromboembolism remains one of the commonest causes of maternal death, it would appear from the latest maternal mortality report that the diagnosis is not always considered, particularly in the antepartum patients.[1] Since the post-partum deaths from thromboembolic disease are most frequently associated with cesarean delivery, the anesthesiologist must remain vigilant to this complication particularly in the obese, the older parturient and those who have been immobilized. If the post-partum patient complains of leg pain, chest pain or dyspnea, a venogram and lung scan should be performed and, if necessary, full anticoagulant therapy should be commenced.

RESPIRATORY SYSTEM

Functional residual capacity, residual volume and expiratory reserve volume progressively decrease during pregnancy. Tidal volume increases to about 40% above the nonpregnant level, while there is only a minor increase in respiratory rate. The rise in serum progesterone probably stimulates this increase in ventilation and consequently arterial $P\text{CO}_2$ is decreased. Oxygen consumption increases during pregnancy, but the greatest increase will be seen during labor, when it may reach 100% above prelabor values. In addition, hyperventilation during uterine contractions results in hypoventilation and a fall in oxygen saturation between contractions. Following delivery, functional residual capacity, residual volume and closing volume rapidly return to normal, and thus apnea should not result in the rapid fall in $P\text{aO}_2$ seen in the apneic pregnant patient at term.[31] Airway resistance and chest wall compliance are decreased during pregnancy; the latter, however, returns to normal immediately after delivery, which suggests that this change is mechanically rather than hormonally induced. Failed intubation during general anesthesia for cesarean delivery remains a common cause of anesthetic-related maternal mortality.[1] Some of the factors associated with difficult intubation in the obstetric patient, such as the need to apply cricoid pressure with the patient lying in the tilted position, should no longer be of major importance if general anesthesia is required post-partum. However, in the first hours post-partum when gastric residual volume may be increased as a result of the delaying effect of labor and opioids on gastric emptying, all measures to prevent regurgitation and pulmonary aspiration of gastric contents must be taken if general anesthesia is required; these should include the administration of antacid, H_2-antagonists and a rapid-sequence induction of anesthesia.

Total body water increases continuously during pregnancy, and although there are wide interindividual variations the increase at term will vary between 7 and 10 l. During the last trimester of pregnancy any increased fluid load is excreted slowly, and water intoxication has been described in women receiving oxytocin-containing solutions for the treatment of post-partum hemorrhage.[32] Thus, intravenous fluids and oxytocin must be carefully prescribed and monitoring is necessary both during labor and in the hours following delivery. While lung water has not been measured during pregnancy, post-partum radiologic measurements of lung water have shown that in some women interstitial lung water is increased, and it has been speculated that this factor might increase the severity of Mendelson's syndrome.[33] Although a diuresis occurs in the first 4–5 days post-partum it is possible that the lungs might still be more susceptible to aspiration. Maternal deaths from acid pulmonary aspiration most commonly occur at the time of induction of emergency general anesthesia, however aspiration has occurred in the post-partum period in women who were excessively sedated either following anesthesia for cesarean delivery or in an attempt to control the symptoms of preeclamptic toxemia. While these deaths actually represent a failure of care in the semiconscious patient, the potential for pulmonary aspiration of gastric contents immediately post-partum cannot be ignored.

SURGERY DURING THE FIRST 24 HOURS POST-PARTUM

Surgery during the first 24 h post-partum will be required, in most instances, because of events relating to the preceding labor and delivery, e.g. evacuation of the retained products of conception, perineal resuturing and control of post-partum hemorrhage. Ideally, all delivery units should have at least two fully equipped operating theaters in which surgery, both elective and emergency, can be speedily and efficiently performed. Anesthetic facilities must include an electrocardiograph, a pulse oximeter, automatic blood pressure monitoring, an end-tidal capnograph, a warming blanket and a blood warmer. Facilities and equipment must also be available for the rapid transfusion of blood. Uncertainty regarding the gastric residual volume immediately post-partum means that *all mothers must be considered to have a full stomach*. Thus, regardless of the surgical procedure (which is often of short duration and minimally invasive) anesthetic technique in this situation must aim to minimize the hazard of acid pulmonary aspiration with prophylactic administration of antacids and H_2 antagonists and, if general anesthesia is chosen, protection of the airway with the insertion of a cuffed endotracheal tube is mandatory. Although regional anesthesia circumvents the problems associated with general anesthesia in the obstetric patient, it should not be initiated post-partum without first assessing the circulatory status of the patient. Blood loss should be measured, and when necessary cross-matched blood should be available. If blood loss has been controlled and vital signs are stable, then the careful establishment of a regional block is probably not contraindicated. However, if blood loss is continuous and/or the mother has developed a bleeding diathesis, then general anesthesia becomes the method of choice. In a busy obstetric unit with an active epidural service it is likely that between 25 and 40% of patients will have an epidural in situ following its use for pain relief during labor and delivery. In almost all instances, but not in the mother with severe post-partum bleeding, it would seem judicious to extend the epidural block with either lidocaine or bupivacaine and where necessary to use epidural opioids to provide effective post-operative analgesia. In those patients who have not received a regional anesthetic during labor the options for post-partum surgery include epidural, spinal or general anesthesia.

Epidural anesthesia

Surgery in the early post-partum period is often of short duration, and thus epidural anesthesia offers no great advantage over spinal anesthesia, and it may even take longer to achieve effective anesthesia than to perform the surgery. Obviously, if there is already an epidural catheter in situ this should be used to provide effective anesthesia. The block should be extended to a level compatible with the proposed surgery. Evacuation of the uterus will require anesthesia to T7–8, but should the surgery necessitate a higher block then the hazards of the associated sympathetic block must be considered. Vital signs must be monitored and colloids and vasopressors may be required to treat hypotension. Epidural opioids (fentanyl 100 µg or diamorphine 2.5 mg) can be used both to improve the quality of the local anesthetic block and to provide post-operative analgesia. However, should blood loss become severe and accompanied by signs of circulatory shock, it may, on some occasions, be necessary to convert to general anesthesia.

Spinal anesthesia

The advantages of spinal anesthesia for post-partum surgery include the speed of onset and the excellent quality of anesthesia, the small dose of local anesthetic used and the rapid and smooth recovery. The objection to spinal anesthesia for post-partum patients has always been the morbidity associated with a post-dural puncture headache. However, the advent of the pencil-point needles such as the Sprotte and Whitacre has significantly reduced this complication, and this is reflected in the increased use of spinal anesthesia for cesarean delivery.[34] When a headache does occur it is usually mild to moderate, responds well to simple analgesics and only rarely requires an epidural blood patch. Prior to establishing spinal anesthesia, an intravenous catheter should be inserted and the mother should receive acute intravascular volume expansion with 500–1000 ml of crystalloid; in addition, a vasopressor such as ephedrine should be available to treat hypotension. Hyperbaric bupivacaine 0.5% in 8% glucose is the only local anesthetic currently licensed in the UK for subarachnoid use. A larger dose of local anesthetic will be required than for cesarean delivery as it has been demonstrated that approximately 30% more bupivacaine will be needed in the post-partum patient to achieve the same height of block as the patient requiring a cesarean delivery.[35] The final level of block and, therefore, the dose of local anesthetic required will obviously be dictated by the nature and extent of the surgery. Overall, spinal anesthesia is probably the most appropriate technique for those surgical procedures which are most commonly encountered in the first 24 h post-partum.

General anesthesia

In those women who did not have an epidural catheter inserted during labor it may be prudent in some circumstances to perform surgery in the first 24 h post-partum under general anesthesia. Severe and life-threatening post-partum hemorrhage can complicate many post-partum obstetric emergencies, and this dangerous situation should not be compounded by the sympathetic block associated with regional anesthesia. Thus, in surgical procedures in which bleeding is likely to be both prolonged and difficult to control or there is a coagulation defect, regional anesthesia is contraindicated and general anesthesia would then become the method of choice. General anesthesia may also be required if there are other contraindications to regional anesthesia or if the patient refuses a regional block. In rare complications such as acute inversion of the uterus, if the inversion cannot be rapidly replaced, then the mother should receive a general anesthetic and the uterus should be replaced either manually or by using a hydraulic technique. Theoretically, the uterine relaxation associated with general anesthesia should allow for easier replacement of the uterus – an oxytocin infusion should then be used to prevent uterine relaxation and reinversion of the uterus.

The delay in gastric emptying caused by labor may have been exacerbated if opioids were administered to relieve pain, and thus gastric residual volume is likely to be large. Intravenous ranitidine 50 mg should be given as soon as it is apparent that surgery is necessary and 30 ml of 0.3 M sodium citrate should be administered orally immediately prior to induction of anesthesia. The mother should lie in the supine position for the induction of anesthesia, thus eliminating one of the causes of difficult intubation seen in the obstetric patient, that is distortion of the larynx caused by the misapplication of cricoid pressure in the patient lying in a tilted position. The lithotomy position should also be avoided as this raises intragastric pressure and may reduce the signs of significant hypovolemia. Adequate acute oxygenation/denitrogenation should be carried out prior to a rapid-sequence induction of anesthesia. In the event of hemorrhage, the induction dose of thiopental should be reduced or, alternatively, ketamine (1–2 mg/kg) can be used. Serum cholinesterase activity, which is reduced during pregnancy, remains depressed post-partum. While succinylcholine has a similar duration of action in nonpregnant and term pregnant patients, its action has been demonstrated to be significantly prolonged post-partum, which difference has been attributed to the greater volume of distribution in the term patient.[36] However, this minimal prolongation of the action of succinylcholine in the post-partum patient does not mean that the intubating dose of succinylcholine should be reduced, as this could result in inadequate muscle relaxation and consequent difficulties with intubation. Anesthesia should be maintained using a balanced anesthetic technique to include nitrous oxide, oxygen, intravenous opioid and a concentration of volatile agent which is appropriate to the surgery being performed. The loss of uterine tone associated with higher concentrations of volatile agents might be advantagous in certain circumstances, e.g. evacuation of a retained placenta, but can also increase bleeding and the incidence of uterine perforation. Post-operatively an infusion of oxytocin (20 units of oxytocin in 500 ml of crystalloid) will be required to maintain uterine tone. The mother should be extubated awake in the left lateral position and should be carefully observed in the recovery/high-dependency area until it is appropriate for her to be transferred with her baby to the post-natal ward.

SURGERY LATER THAN 24 HOURS POST-PARTUM

Choice of anesthesia during this time should be governed by the nature of the surgical procedure and the same principles used in a nonpregnant woman of the same age should be applied. The commonest obstetric indication for surgery more than 24 h after delivery will be a secondary post-partum hemorrhage. Retained placental products can precipitate severe hemorrhage, and if the patient is pyrexial as a result of superimposed uterine infection then the uterus may easily be perforated during a dilation and curettage. Again, where necessary, hypovolemia should be corrected and blood and blood products should be available. If blood loss is not severe or is under control then the anesthesiologist can choose between spinal, epidural or general anesthesia. In the normal post-partum mother, gastric emptying at this time will be similar to that seen in nonpregnant females, and thus full prophylaxis against Mendelson's syndrome (acid aspiration) is not strictly necessary. Should emergency surgery under general anesthesia be required then it would be prudent to administer antacids and H_2 antagonists and to perform a rapid-sequence induction with cricoid pressure.

REFERENCES

1. Report on Confidential Enquiries into Maternal Deaths in England and Wales, 1985–1987. 1991 London: HMSO
2. Bainbridge E T, Temple J G, Nicholas S P, Newton J R, Boeiah V 1983 Symptomatic gastro-oesophageal reflux in pregnancy. A comparative study of white Europeans and Asians in Birmingham. Br Clin Pract 37: 53–57
3. Hey V M F, Cowley D J, Ganguli P C, Skinner L D, Ostock D G, Sharp D S 1977 Gastro-oeosphageal reflux in late pregnancy. Anaesthesia 32: 372–377
4. Vanner R G, Goodman N W 1989 Gastro-oesophageal reflux in pregnancy at term and after delivery. Anaesthesia 44: 808–811
5. Lind F J, Smith A, McFuer D K, Coopland A T, Crispin J S 1968 Heartburn in pregnancy – a manometric study. Can Med Assoc J 98: 571–574
6. Nakai T 1925 On the gastric juice of the pregnant woman. J Biochem (Tokyo) 5: 465–477
7. Arzt F 1926 On the gastric juice during pregnancy. Am J Obst Gynecol 12: 879–883
8. Strauss M B, Castle W B 1932 Studies of anemia in pregnancy. Gastric secretion in pregnancy and the puerperium. Am J Med Sci 184: 655–662
9. Goodall J R, Gottlieb R 1936 The association of pregnancy, hypochromic anaemia and achlorhydria. Can Med Assoc J 35: 50–33
10. Labate J S 1939 The effect of pregnancy on gastric secretion. Am J Obstet Gynecol 38: 650–653
11. Clark D H 1953 Peptic ulcer in women. Br Med J 1: 1254–1257
12. Murray F A, Erskine J P, Fielding J 1957 Gastric secretion in pregnancy. Br J Obstet Gynaecol 64: 373–381
13. Clark D H, Tankel H I 1954 Gastric acid and plasma histaminase during pregnancy. Lancet 2: 886–887
14. Hirscheimer A, January D A, Daversa J J 1938 An X-ray study of gastric function during labor. Am J Obstet Gynecol 36: 671–673
15. Crawford J S 1956 Some aspects of obstetric anaesthesia. Br J Anaesth 28: 201–208
16. La Salvia L A, Steffen E A 1950 Delayed gastric emptying time in labor. Am J Obstet Gynecol 50: 1075–1081
17. Davison J S, Davison M C, Hay D M 1970 Gastric emptying line in late pregnancy and labour. Br J Obstet Gynecol 77: 37–41
18. Heading R C, Nimmo W S, Prescott L F, Tothill P 1973 The dependence of paracetamol absorption on the rate of gastric emptying. Br J Pharmacol 47: 415–421
19. Nimmo W S, Wilson J, Prescott L F 1975 Narcotic analgesics and delayed gastric emptying during labour. Lancet 1: 890–893
20. Holdsworth J D 1978 Relationship between stomach contents and analgesia in labour. Br J Anaesth 50: 1145–1148
21. Herrema I 1990 Aspiration prophylaxis policies in early pregnancy and post-partum. Obstet Anaesth Association Meeting, The London Hospital, March 1990
22. Whitehead E M, O'Sullivan G, Smith M, Dean Y 1993 An evaluation of gastric emptying times in pregnancy and the puerperium. Anaesth 48: 53–57
23. Blouw R, Scatliff J, Craig D B, Palahniuk R J 1976 Gastric volume and pH in postpartum patients. Anesthesiology 45: 456–457
24. James C F, Gibbs C P, Banner T 1984 Postpartum perioperative risk of aspiration pneumonia. Anesthesiology 61: 756–759
25. O'Sullivan G, Sear J W, Bullingham R E S, Carrie L E S 1984 The effect of magnesium trisilicate mixture, metoclopramide and ranitidine on gastric pH, volume and serum gastrin. Anaesthesia 39: 973–978
26. Ewart M C, Jan G, Gin T, Kotur C F, Oh T E 1990 A comparison of the effects of omeprazole and ranitidine on gastric secretion in women undergoing elective Caesarean section. Anaesthesia 45: 527–530
27. Ueland K, Novy M J, Peterson E N, Metcalfe J 1969 Maternal cardiovascular dynamics. IV. The influence of gestational age on the maternal cardiovascular response to posture and exercise. Am J Obstet Gynecol 104: 856–864
28. Hytten F, Chamberlain G 1991 Clinical physiology in obstetrics, 2nd edn. Blackwell Scientific Publications, Oxford
29. Chesley L C 1972 Plasma and red cell volumes during pregnancy. Am J Obstet Gynecol 112: 440–449
30. Ueland K 1976 Maternal cardiovascular dynamics. VII. Intrapartum blood volume changes. Am J Obstet Gynecol 126: 671–677
31. Archer G W, Marx G F 1974 Arterial oxygen tension during apnoea in parturient women. Br J Anaesth 46: 358–359
32. Bilek W, Dorr P 1970 Water intoxication and grand mal seizures due to oxytocin. Can Med Assoc J 103: 379–382
33. Maclennan F M, Macdonald A F, Campbell D M 1987 Lung water during the puerperium. Anaesthesia 42: 141–147
34. Cesarini M, Torrielli F, Lalaye F, Mene J M, Caliro C 1990 Sprotte needle for intrathecal anaesthesia for Cesarean Section: incidence of postdural puncture headache. Anaesthesia 45: 656–658
35. Abouleish E I 1986 Postpartum tubal ligation requires more bupivacaine for spinal anesthesia than does Cesarean section. Anesth Analg 65: 897–900
36. Leighton B L, Cheek T G, Gross J B , Apfelbaum J L, Shantz B B, Gutsche B B, Rosenberg H 1986 Succinylcholine pharmacodynamics in peripartum patients. Anesthesiology 64: 202–205

PART B
USA VIEW

B. L. Koffel

Surgery in the post-partum period may be required for a variety of elective or emergent conditions. Elective post-partum sterilization procedures are relatively benign when compared with an emergency obstetric hysterectomy in a patient with a coagulopathy. A brief review of the physiologic changes of the post-partum period precedes a discussion of obstetric situations that may require surgical intervention and their anesthetic management.

PHYSIOLOGY OF THE PUERPERIUM

The maternal physiology as altered by pregnancy does not immediately revert to the nonpregnant state at delivery. The exact time course of reversal is unknown. Some changes are exaggerated in the immediate post-partum period; others gradually reverse, while some do so dramatically. The highest level of cardiac output occurs immediately after delivery, which is attributed to the autotransfusion and increased venous return associated with uterine involution.[1] The increased blood volume returns to prepregnant levels within several days. This conservation of red cells allows the mother to tolerate the blood loss of delivery with minimal decrease in hemoglobin or hematocrit.[2]

While the mechanical reasons for the increased gastric volume in pregnancy are at least partially mitigated after delivery, hormonal and pharmacologic reasons for delayed gastric emptying may persist for days. Labor itself and the use of opioids during labor can also delay emptying.[3] In the post-partum patient, the volume and pH of gastric contents have been reported to be independent of the length of time from delivery.[4] In one study, patients more than 9 h and less than 23 h after delivery had the smallest gastric volumes. Nonetheless, a significant number of patients (40–73%) were still considered ‘at risk’ for aspiration pneumonitis.[5] Another study confirms that a high percentage of post-partum patients (33%) are ‘at risk’ for aspiration.[6] A small study of eight women does suggest that gastric emptying (measured by paracetamol absorption) does not change between the first and third post-partum days.[7] Nevertheless, post-partum patients should be considered at high risk for aspiration pneumonitis and, in this regard, should be managed as if the patient were still pregnant. The increased sensitivity to anesthetic agents may rapidly dissipate after delivery. The requirements for local anesthetics are higher 8–24 h post-partum than in the parturient.[8]

Pseudocholinesterase activity is decreased for 2–3 days post-partum. However, the action of succinylcholine in a 1 mg/kg dose is only prolonged by 3 min in the post-partum patient.[9]

ELECTIVE POST-PARTUM SURGERY

The only elective procedure routinely performed in the post-partum period is sterilization.

Timing of surgery

The Committee on Obstetrics: Maternal and Fetal Medicine of the American College of Obstetricians and Gynecologists (ACOG) has stated:[10]

> The decision as to when to proceed with anesthesia and surgery should be based on the anesthesiologist’s assessment of the patient and judgment of the relative risks and benefits for that patient.

The anesthesiologist must be aware of the risks and benefits of various choices in timing. Technically, the surgery is a simple procedure when the uterine fundus is near the umbilicus. The fundus remains so for at least 2 days post-partum, allowing ample time to perform the procedure.

Certain elements of maternal risk may decrease with a delay of 8–24 h. Post-partum hemorrhage, which occurs in about 5% of parturients, can occur without warning and be life-threatening even after an apparently uneventful vaginal delivery.[11] The incidence decreases dramatically after 10 h in multiparous women.[12] Post-partum hemorrhage presenting during a tubal ligation might be difficult to diagnose initially and would clearly increase maternal risk during post-partum sterilization.

The prognosis of any infant can better be predicted several hours rather than minutes after delivery. Immediate post-partum tubal ligation carries the risk of sterilization prior to a full evaluation of the neonate. However, immediate post-partum tubal ligation may avoid the need for an additional anesthetic in a patient who already has anesthesia for labor and/or delivery. Continuous epidural or spinal techniques can easily be extended to provide surgical anesthesia for a tubal ligation. Therefore, the patient with a continuous technique may incur the least additional risk if an immediate sterilization is performed. Exceptions should be made when there have been complications of the labor and/or delivery, for example: major blood loss or cardiac compromise.

In contrast, a patient who delivers without anesthesia is probably best served by a tubal ligation 8–24 h later. That is, women delivering before midnight would have their procedure the next day and those delivering after midnight the next day after that. With the demands of decreasing hospital stay, spinal anesthesia can be used for immediate post-partum sterilization. We believe general anesthesia should not be induced in the immediate post-partum period solely for a tubal ligation.

These guidelines assume that patient load and staffing can accommodate what is fundamentally an elective procedure. Other activities in the labor and delivery suite should not be compromised.

Anesthetic management

The considerations of acid aspiration prophylaxis, difficult intubation and fluid requirements to avoid hypotension are the same for post-partum surgery as for cesarean delivery. Recent and/or ongoing blood loss may modify the choice of anesthetic technique and raise the question of postponement to 6 weeks post-partum.

An in situ continuous lumbar epidural (or subarachnoid) catheter may be used to provide anesthesia for an immediate post-partum tubal ligation. If immediate surgery is not to be done, the catheter should be removed. Catheter tip migration (and subsequent inadequate surgical anesthesia) is common in ambulatory patients. Local anesthetic agents may be chosen, as in Table 77.2. Subarachnoid anesthesia is most frequently used for the tubal ligation in the post-partum period and is preferable to epidural anesthesia because of its speed of onset and reliability of block. Drug dosage may need to be increased by the second day after delivery. Epidural anesthesia induced only for tubal ligation is more time-consuming and is not usually considered unless specifically indicated for other reasons.

The decreased likelihood of problems with intubation and/or aspiration makes regional anesthesia preferable to general anesthesia. General anesthesia may be used for surgery the next day after delivery at the patient's request. A rapid-sequence induction should be followed by endotracheal intubation. Routinely, intravenous thiamylal 5 mg/kg or thiopental 4 mg/kg and succinylcholine 1–1.5 mg/kg is used to induce anesthesia. Anesthesia is maintained with 70% nitrous oxide in oxygen and intravenous opioid supplementation while using a succinylcholine infusion for muscle relaxation. Volatile anesthetic agents are usually avoided, as the risk of uterine relaxation may still exist.

EMERGENCY POST-PARTUM SURGERY

Obstetric considerations

Post-partum hemorrhage is the most frequent reason for emergency surgery in the immediate post-partum period.

Causes of post-partum hemorrhage include:

Table 77.2 Recommended anesthetic agents for post-partum sterilization

Regional anesthesia
Epidural
Lidocaine 2% with 1 : 200 000 epinephrine
Chloroprocaine 3%
Subarachnoid *
Hyperbaric lidocaine 5%⁺
Hyperbaric bupivacaine 0.75%⁺

* More dilute solutions may be used with a continuous subarachnoid technique.
⁺ Epinephrine may be added, if desired.

1. Uterine atony (failure of the uterus to contract and adequately compress vessels at the placental implantation site). Predisposing factors include:
   a. An overdistended uterus prior to delivery (multiple gestations, polyhydramnios, macrosomia):
   b. Prolonged labor;
   c. Rapid labor;
   d. Vigorous use of oxytocin stimulation during labor;
   e. Multiparity;
   f. Hypotension;
   g. Uterine infection;
   h. Amniotic fluid embolism.
2. Laceration/injury to the perineum, vagina, cervix, or uterus. Predisposing events include:
   a. Delivery of a large infant;
   b. Mid-forceps delivery;
   c. Forceps rotation;
   d. Delivery through an incompletely dilated cervix;
   e. Intrauterine manipulation;
   f. Vaginal birth after cesarean delivery;
   g. Dührssen's incisions.
3. Retained placental tissue, which may be due to an abnormally adherent placenta (placenta accreta, increta or percreta) or a normal placenta incompletely removed.
4. Uterine inversion, which is a rare cause of hemorrhage that should be immediately recognized in order to prevent life-threatening consequences. Blood loss in this situation is frequently underestimated.

Anesthetic considerations

Hypovolemia is a major risk factor in emergency post-partum surgery. Estimating blood loss is notoriously unreliable in determining blood loss.[2] Cardiovascular changes of hypovolemia should be evaluated in every patient. The presence of hypotension, tachycardia or orthostatic changes may be the first clues of hypovolemia. Its presence should directly affect the choice of anesthetic technique.

Anesthetic management

If a regional anesthetic is preferred, subarachnoid anesthesia is frequently chosen for its speed of onset and reliability. The spinal anesthetic technique is similar to that for vaginal delivery. Intravenous hydration is extremely important because of the possibility of unrecognized hypovolemia. Regional anesthesia with its sympathetic blockade often exaggerates hypotension, possibly increasing maternal morbidity and mortality. Therefore, general anesthesia is usually used in the hypovolemic patient.

For emergency post-partum surgery, optimal care would include:

1. Availability of compatible blood products;
2. Determination of maternal hemoglobin/hematocrit;

3. Placement of large intravenous catheters (two catheters required for major hemorrhage);
4. Use of a blood and fluid warmer;
5. Colloid or blood infusion;
6. Capacity to directly measure maternal systemic blood pressure and central venous pressures.

After premedication and denitrogenation, general anesthesia is induced, in a rapid-sequence fashion, with thiamylal or thiopental (up to 4 mg/kg), ketamine (up to 1 mg/kg) or etomidate (up to 0.2 mg/kg), depending on the degree of hypovolemia. Endotracheal intubation is facilitated with succinylcholine (1–1.5 mg/kg). Muscle relaxation is maintained with a succinylcholine infusion or a nondepolarizing relaxant, depending on the anticipated duration of the procedure. Volatile agents are avoided unless they are specifically indicated for their uterine relaxant properties (e.g. in the initial management of uterine inversion). Nitrous oxide, opioids and/or benzodiazepines are used to maintain anesthesia as tolerated.

Blood replacement

A post-partum patient hemorrhaging in the delivery room encompasses all the indications for a potential disaster. Obstetric hemorrhage is still one of the major causes of maternal mortality.[13] Seemingly minor hemorrhage can progress to major blood loss within minutes. Transfusion will not be necessary in all patients. In fact, hemorrhage is rare enough that autologous blood donation is not encouraged for pregnant patients not at high risk for complications (e.g. placenta previa).[14] Yet, every patient having emergency surgery for post-partum hemorrhage should have compatible blood products available. The risks of transfusion warrant an initial attempt to correct hypovolemia with crystalloid or colloid, although packed red cells, platelets and fresh-frozen plasma may be necessary in certain patients. Uncross-matched O negative blood or, preferably, type-specific blood can be used in the emergency situation. Dilutional coagulopathy and thrombocytopenia are common and should be treated when they occur. Early determination of platelet count may be helpful.

Massive hemorrhage and transfusion can lead to disseminated intravascular coagulation (DIC). Additionally, DIC is associated with the following obstetric conditions:

1. Placental abruption;
2. Fetal death;
3. Severe preeclampsia/eclampsia;
4. Amniotic fluid embolism;
5. Saline abortion;
6. Septicemia and intravascular hemolysis.

Table 77.3 Laboratory findings in DIC

Early
Decreased fibrinogen
Decreased platelet count
Increased fibrin degradation products
Abnormal red cell morphology
Late
Prolongation of prothrombin time
Prolongation of partial thromboplastin time
Prolongation of thrombin time

Diagnosis of acute DIC does not generally require laboratory evaluation. Hemorrhage associated with any of the above conditions with supporting laboratory abnormalities (Table 77.3) should be considered DIC.

The management of DIC focuses on treatment of the underlying disease (i.e. removal of the source of thromboplastin or bacterial endotoxin) as soon as possible. Administration of procoagulant factors and/or platelets is frequently necessary. The use of heparin is controversial and not recommended.

REFERENCES

1. Hansen J M, Ueland K 1966 The influence of caudal analgesia on cardiovascular dynamics during normal labor and delivery. Acta Anaesthesiol Scand Suppl 23: 449–452
2. Pritchard J A 1965 Changes in the blood volume during pregnancy and delivery. Anesthesiology 26: 395–399
3. O'Sullivan G M, Sutton A J, Thompson S A et al 1987 Noninvasive measurement of gastric emptying in obstetric patients. Anesth Analg 66: 505–511
4. Rennie A L, Richard J A, Milne M K et al 1979 Post-partum sterilisation – an anaesthetic hazard? Anaesthesia 34: 267–269
5. James C F, Gibbs C P, Banner T 1984 Postpartum perioperative risk of aspiration pneumonia. Anesthesiology 61: 756–759
6. Blouw R, Scatliff J, Craig D B et al 1976 Gastric volume and pH in postpartum patients. Anesthesiology 45: 456
7. Gin T, Cho A M W, Lew J K L, Lau G S N, Yuen P M, Critchley J A J H, Oh Te 1991. Gastric emptying in the postpartum period. Anaesth Intensive Care 19: 521
8. Abouleish E I 1986 Postpartum tubal ligation requires more bupivacaine for spinal anesthesia than does cesarean section. Anesth Analg 65: 897
9. Leighton B L, Cheek T G, Gross J B et al 1986 Succinylcholine pharmacodynamics in peripartum patients. Anesthesiology 64: 202–205
10. Committee on Obstetrics 1987 Maternal and Fetal Medicine: Postpartum tubal sterilization: Appropriate timing of surgery after vaginal delivery. ACOG Committee Opinion No. 50
11. Lewis J M, Fontrier T 1988 Near misses in anesthesia: lessons learned. Butterworths, Boston
12. Pritchard J A, MacDonald P C, Gant N F 1985 Williams obstetrics, 17th edn. Appleton-Century-Crofts, East Norwalk, CT
13. Rochat R W, Koonin L M, Atrash H K et al 1988 Maternal mortality in the United States: report from the maternal mortality collaborative. Obstet Gynecol 72: 91–97
14. The National Blood Resource Education Program Expert Panel 1990 The use of autologous blood. J Am Med Assoc 263: 414–417

78. Transplantation

W. R. Camann

The transplantation of organs for various disease states has become commonplace. Replacement of kidneys, hearts and livers are now routinely performed with excellent survival rates. Many of these procedures are performed in women of child-bearing age, thus the obstetric anesthesiologist may, on occasion, encounter patients with transplanted organs presenting for anesthetic care during labor and delivery. Anesthetic implications include alterations in organ function, physiology and pharmacology, as well as the effects of immunosuppression.

RENAL TRANSPLANTATION

Renal transplantation is now considered routine therapy for those afflicted with end-stage renal disease (ESRD). Five-year survival rates of 80% and 40% are observed in patients receiving living, related donor and cadaveric kidneys respectively.[1] These survival rates are expected to rise as advances are made in immunosuppressive therapy and treatment of rejection episodes. Although patients with ESRD maintained on dialysis therapy are often anovulatory, a return to normal menstruation is common following a successful renal allograft. Approximately 1 in 50 women of child-bearing age with a functioning renal transplant becomes pregnant.[2]

In general, pregnancy outcome in this patient population is good.[3] Approximately 10% of patients will experience a rejection episode during gestation; however, this rate is equal to that seen in the nonpregnant population. Permanent deterioration of allograft function during pregnancy occurs in approximately 10%, but this also does not differ from the rate seen in the general nonpregnant renal transplant population.[3] Nevertheless, numerous factors contribute to the classification of these patients as 'high risk' during pregnancy.

Infectious complications are of particular concern because of the state of immunosuppression.[1] The most common bacterial infection is in the urinary tract. Viral infections, such as herpes simplex or cytomegalovirus, are more common in renal transplant recipients and pose special problems for the pregnant patient. A general rule is that these patients often manifest infections with uncommon pathogens. Thus, appropriate cultures and aggressive therapy are mandatory whenever infection is suspected.

Premature labor and premature rupture of membranes are significantly increased in this patient population.[4,5] The reasons for this are unclear, although marginal renal function and chronic steroid therapy may be contributory. Pregnancy-induced hypertension is also more common in these patients and may account for some of the instances of premature delivery.[5] The diagnosis of preeclampsia may be difficult, as chronic hypertension, proteinuria and edema are common in these patients.

All renal transplant recipients receive some degree of immunosuppressive therapy. The most common regimen is a combination of cyclosporin A (CsA), azathioprine (Imuran) and a corticosteroid, usually prednisone. Side-effects of these agents may be of significance to the anesthesiologist. CsA is commonly associated with systemic hypertension, and most patients ultimately require antihypertensive medication. The mechanism for this effect is CsA-induced activation of the sympathetic nervous system.[6] Azathioprine may be associated with thrombocytopenia and abnormalities of liver function. Chronic steroid therapy results in a host of systemic manifestations. Glucose intolerance, avascular neurosis of bone, hypertension, poor wound healing, peptic ulcer disease and obesity (with possible airway distortion) are all commonly seen and all have well-known implications for anesthetic care. Thin, fragile skin warrants caution with application of tape and automated blood pressure cuffs should be used with caution since high inflation pressures can result in skin abrasions. In addition, bolus ('stress') doses of parenteral steroids are recommended during labor and delivery – whether vaginal or cesarean.

Anesthetic considerations

Renal transplant recipients with good renal function can receive virtually any type of anesthesia. The preanesthetic evaluation should include attention to current medical therapy and possible side-effects. Laboratory evaluation should include white cell count, hematocrit and renal and liver function, along with a coagulation profile. Careful assessment of bony abnormalities, joint dysfunction and airway anatomy is important. Epidural anesthesia for labor is well tolerated, although care should be exercised with positioning after institution of the block and with taping to secure the epidural catheter. Cesarean delivery should be performed for obstetric indications and either epidural or subarachnoid anesthesia may be used. However, epidural anesthesia may be preferable, as less rapid and profound hemodynamic effects allow for more judicious fluid management, which may be an important factor if renal function is marginal or preeclampsia is a concern. In addition, prolonged operative time (owing to previous abdominal surgery) may also favor continuous epidural or subarachnoid anesthesia.

CARDIAC TRANSPLANTATION

Cardiac transplantation has become an accepted mode of treatment for end-stage cardiomyopathy. The most common indication for cardiac transplantation in young patients is viral cardiomyopathy, although congenital heart disease, valvular dysfunction and peripartum cardiomyopathy may be the etiology in a small percentage of patients. (Liberalization of recipient criteria has allowed ischemic cardiomyopathy owing to coronary artery disease to become a major indication for transplantation. However, this group of patients is generally older and unlikely, although not impossible,[7] to be of concern to the obstetric anesthesiologist.) Current survival rates after cardiac transplantation average 80–90% at 1 year and 60–70% at 5 years.[8] Most patients with nonrejecting cardiac allografts are able to resume normal lifestyles, including reproductive endeavors. Childbirth, both vaginally[9] and by cesarean delivery,[10] has been reported, with a minimum of complications.

Anesthetic considerations

The preanesthetic evaluations should include careful assessment of exercise tolerance, especially any changes noted by the patient during pregnancy. The time interval since the transplant is important, as the incidence of rejection decreases as this time interval increases. However, cardiac transplant recipients undergo accelerated coronary artery atherosclerosis such that allograft coronary artery disease is detected in up to 40% of patients by 3–5 years after transplantation.[11] The current pharmacologic and immunosuppressive regimen should be noted.

Physiology and pharmacology

The physiologic hallmark of the heart transplant recipient is the fact that the donor allograft is void of any efferent or afferent autonomic or somatic innervation.[12] The denervated state results in several anesthetic implications.

1. Any maneuver acting via reflex vagal activity (i.e. carotid sinus massage or oculocardiac reflex) will not be effective in these patients.
2. Pharmacologic agents acting via vagal pathways (e.g. atropine and neostigmine) will be free of cardiac effects. However, peripheral actions on vascular tone and peripheral cholinergic receptors will still be intact.
3. Only direct-acting vasoactive agents will reliably produce inotropic or chronotropic effects.
4. Baseline tachycardia is common, owing to absence of vagal tone.
5. Chronic denervation results in 'up-regulation' of cardiac β-adrenergic receptors. Thus, extreme sensitivity to β-agonist drugs is seen.[13] (Even small amounts of epinephrine in local anesthetic solutions may have profound chronotropic effects).[10]
6. A chronotropic response to stress (such as hypovolemia or vasodilation) is delayed, thus adequate cardiac output is dependent on maintenance of adequate preload (the Starling mechanism). Increasing preload is useful prior to anesthetic maneuvers that are likely to result in vasodilation.
7. Afferent denervation implies that myocardial ischemia will not be felt as chest pain or angina. Thus, these patients usually undergo yearly cardiac catheterization to assess the allograft for the development of coronary artery disease.

Effects of immunosuppression

The concerns in cardiac transplantation are similar to those encountered in the renal transplant recipient. Cardiac transplant recipients are similarly likely to develop hypertension owing to chronic cyclosporine use and usually require antihypertensive therapy. To date, no fetal compromise has been noted to the offspring of cardiac transplant recipients, although only a few such cases have been reported.

Management during labor

Successful vaginal deliveries have been accomplished both with[14] and without[9] epidural anesthesia. Primary concern should be directed toward maintenance of adequate intravascular volume as labor itself may be associated with marked degrees of dehydration. In addition to adequate hydration, careful avoidance of aortocaval compression is essential, as decreased venous return and subsequent inadequate cardiac filling will be poorly tolerated by the patient with a transplanted heart. In light of these concerns, one may argue that invasive monitoring of central venous pressures during labor is warranted. However, the nonrejecting donor allograft with documented preserved ventricular function should tolerate volume changes quite well. Moreover, a major cause of morbidity in these immunocompromised patients is infection, thus the risk of catheter-induced sepsis probably outweighs the information that would be obtained from such monitoring.

Epidural anesthesia is well tolerated during labor. Low concentrations of local anesthetic with opioid will aid in minimizing the degree of sympathectomy. If hypotension should occur, the first course of management should include uterine displacement to relieve aortocaval compression and increased fluid infusion. If vasopressors are necessary, either ephedrine or phenylephrine may be used. However, ephedrine has both direct and indirect mechanisms of action, and may thus be slightly less effective than expected. If a chronotropic agent is required, then isoproterenol (not atropine) should be utilized.

Management of cesarean delivery

Epidural anesthesia is the technique of choice for cesarean delivery as the sensory level can be slowly raised, allowing time for adequate intravascular volume expansion to compensate for the ensuing sympathetic blockade. Subarachnoid anesthesia may, in theory, not be as well tolerated owing to the rapidity of the sympathetic blockade. However, both intraspinal and general anesthesia have been successfully used for a wide variety of nonobstetric surgical procedures in heart transplant recipients.[15] If general anesthesia should be required, one might consider using ketamine rather than thiopental as an induction agent so as to preserve some degree of sympathetic tone.

As with renal transplant patients, appropriate attention to aseptic technique should be employed, and 'stress' steroid coverage is usually required.

OTHER TRANSPLANTS

Successful pregnancies and deliveries have been reported after both bone marrow[16] and hepatic transplantation.[17] Experience in these areas, as for other organs (such as lung, pancreas and combined heart–lung) is extremely limited and anesthetic care must be individualized to the clinical status of the patient at the time of delivery.

REFERENCES

1. Graybar G B, Tarpey M 1987 Kidney transplantation. In Gelman S (ed) Anesthesia and organ transplantation. WB Saunders, Philadelphia, p 61–110
2. Penn I, Makowski E L, Harris P 1980 Parenthood following renal transplantation. Kidney Int 18: 221–223
3. Lau R J, Scott J 1985 Pregnancy following renal transplantation. Clin Obstet Gynecol 28: 339–350
4. Davison J M, Lindheimer M D 1982 Pregnancy in renal transplantation recipients. J Reprod Med 27: 613–617
5. Fine R N 1982 Pregnancy in renal allograft recipients. Am J Nephrol 2: 117–122
6. Scherrer U, Vissing S F, Morgan B J et al 1990 Cyclosporine-induced sympathetic activation and hypertension after heart transplantation. New Engl J Med 323: 693–699
7. Curiel P, Spinelli G, Petrella A et al 1990 Postpartum coronary artery dissection followed by heart transplantation. Am J Obstet Gynecol 163: 538–539
8. Fragomen L S, Kaye M P 1988 The registry of the International Society for Heart Transplantation: Fifth official report. J Heart Trans 7: 249–253
9. Lowenstein B R, Vain N W, Perrone S V et al 1988 Successful pregnancy and vaginal delivery after heart transplantation. Am J Obstet Gynecol 158: 589–590
10. Camann W R, Goldman G A, Johnson M D et al 1989 Cesarean delivery in a patient with a transplanted heart. Anesthesiology 71: 618–620
11. Renlund D G, Bristow M R, Lee H R, O'Connell J B 1988 Medical aspects of cardiac transplantation. J Cardiothorac Anesth 2: 500–511
12. Kent K M, Cooper T 1974 The denervated heart – a model for studying autonomic control of the heart. New Engl J Med 291: 1017–1021
13. Yusef S, Theodoropoulos S, Mathias C J 1987 Increased sensitivity of the denervated transplanted human heart to isoprenaline both before and after β-adrenergic blockade. Circulation 75: 696–704
14. Camann W R, Jarcho J A, Mintz K J, Greene M F 1991 Uncomplicated vaginal delivery fourteen months after cardiac transplantation. Am Heart J 121: 939–941
15. Bailey P L, Stanley T H 1990 Anesthesia for patients with a prior cardiac transplant. J Cardiothroac Anesth 4 (suppl 1): 38–47
16. Deeg H J, Kennedy M S, Sanders J E et al 1983 Successful pregnancy after marrow transplantation for severe aplastic anemia and immunosuppression with cyclosporine. J Am Med Assoc 250: 647
17. Newton E R, Turskoy N, Kaplan M, Reinhold R 1988 Pregnancy and liver transplantation. Obstet Gynecol 71: 499–500

79. Anesthesia for in vitro fertilization procedures

M. J. Segal   M. D. Johnson

The first live birth produced by an externally fertilized human egg was reported in England in 1978.

In vitro fertilization (IVF) involves four steps:

1. exogenous hormonal stimulation of multiple ovarian follicles;
2. collection of the oocytes;
3. fertilization of the oocyte and growth of the embryo outside the body; and
4. replacement of the embryo back into the uterus.

On day 3 of the menstrual cycle, menotropins (a combination of luteinizing hormones and follicle-stimulating hormones) are administered to promote ovarian follicular growth and maturation. Follicular growth is monitored with ultrasonography and serial estrogen levels. When the follicles reach an average diameter of 1.5 cm, human chorionic gonadotropin is administered to stimulate ovulation. Oocytes are aspirated from the follicles 34–36 h later, transferred to culture medium, incubated and then fertilized. The oocytes are collected either by transabdominal laparoscopy or by transvaginal ultrasound-directed needle aspiration. A transvesical approach, in which the needle is guided transurethrally through the posterior wall of the bladder to the ovarian follicle, may also be used. After fertilization, the embryo is transferred to the uterus via a fine catheter inserted through the cervix. The harvest of oocytes requires some form of analgesia or anesthesia, whereas the replacement of the embryo is a relatively painless procedure.

A newer technique, gamete intrafallopian transfer (GIFT), allows fertilization to take place in the fallopian tube rather than in culture medium. As the name implies, oocytes and sperm are injected directly into the fallopian tubes and fertilization and implantation of the embryo in the uterine wall occurs naturally. The GIFT procedure is usually performed by laparoscopy or minilaparotomy.

PREANESTHETIC EVALUATION

The IVF patient population can be very challenging from an anesthetic standpoint. These patients are generally older than most obstetric patients, and frustrated from months to years of unsuccessful attempts at pregnancy. Hormonal therapy prescribed to hasten oocyte maturation may contribute to emotional lability. Anxiety can increase gastric acidity and decrease gastric emptying, thus the incidence of nausea and risk of aspiration is increased. To offset the increased risk of aspiration, the 'full stomach' protocol used in obstetric patients should be the standard approach to these patients. This is a completely elective, but urgent, procedure. Very real time constraints exist because the oocytes must be harvested within a small window of time.

ANESTHETIC OPTIONS

An optimal anesthetic for IVF will provide safety and comfort with a brief recovery period, as this is an ambulatory patient population. Benzodiazepines are useful as premedicants. Midazolam is preferable to diazepam because of its shorter half-life. Also, because midazolam is water soluble, it is not associated with the venous irritation often produced by diazepam. In early pregnancy, diazepam is considered to be teratogenic. This is a potential but unproven risk with midazolam. However, oocyte harvest occurs before conception, so this problem should not be an issue. Sodium citrate (0.3mol/l) should be routinely considered as a premedicant along with metoclopramide and histamine-2(H_2) receptor antagonists.

General anesthesia is commonly administered for laparoscopy. The use of the Trendelenburg position and the insufflation of the abdomen with carbon dioxide may lead to difficulties with spontaneous respiration plus nausea and vomiting when major regional anesthesia is used. The anesthetic options for transvaginal or transvesical ultrasound needle aspiration include local, general and regional (subarachnoid, epidural, continuous spinal) anesthesia.

ANESTHETIC TECHNIQUES

Local/monitored anesthesia care

The nature of this procedure is one of multiple exposures to brief, but intense stimulation. Most of the discomfort is generally from passage of the needle through the posterior vaginal wall and peritoneum. Local anesthesia is frequently inadequate and patients typically require heavy sedation, which increases recovery room stay.

General anesthesia

General anesthesia has its drawbacks, which include post-operative somnolence and long recovery room stays. In addition to the inherent risk of aspiration with general anesthesia, volatile agents, nitrous oxide and opioids all may increase the incidence of nausea and vomiting in the post-operative period.

Subarachnoid anesthesia

Subarachnoid anesthesia is frequently used because the onset time is rapid and the duration of the procedure is usually predictable (1–1.5 h). These benefits must be weighed against the possibility of a post-dural puncture headache, which is 1–5% with a 26-gauge, Quincke point, spinal needle. The use of 27-gauge or conical-point spinal needles may decrease further the risk of post-dural puncture headache. The sedation requirements are significantly reduced as compared with monitored anesthetic care. This is helpful in decreasing the incidence of post-operative nausea and vomiting. In addition to anxiety and opioids, nausea may be due to peritoneal traction and bleeding. At least a T6 level is necessary with subarachnoid anesthesia to minimize discomfort from peritoneal traction. Nausea can also occur from either hypotension or the addition of epidural or subarachnoid opioids. The addition of fentanyl improves the quality of a subarachnoid block and relieves some discomfort from peritoneal manipulation as well as providing 2–3 h of post-operative analgesia.[1] We commonly add fentanyl 10–25 μg to 10–15 mg of 0.75% hyperbaric bupivacaine or 50–75 mg of 5% hyperbaric lidocaine for this procedure.

Continuous spinal anesthesia

Small-gauge catheters for continuous spinal anesthesia are presently under investigation for use in IVF. These 24- to 32-gauge microcatheters offer the advantages of a titratable level with reduced local anesthetic requirements. Using various concentrations of lidocaine, including the 5% hyperbaric formulation, these microcatheters allow rapid onset with a controllable duration and level of anesthesia; this reduces recovery room stay, which is important in these ambulatory patients. Unfortunately, at present, these microcatheters are technically more difficult to use and multiple attempts at placement may be necessary until one is successfully inserted. This increases cost as well as preparation time. (Editors' note: at present, catheters <28 gauge have been removed from the USA market by the FDA). In preliminary reports, the incidence of post-dural puncture headache is similar to that seen with 26-gauge needles, as these microcatheters are placed through a 26-gauge spinal needle. As facility with continuous subarachnoid catheters increases, this technique may play an important role in anesthesia for IVF.

Epidural anesthesia

Epidural anesthesia offers the advantage of decreased risk of post-dural puncture headache as compared with subarachnoid anesthesia. An epidural anesthetic may be preferable when the duration of the case is expected to take longer such as with aspiration of many follicles. A T6 level is desirable to minimize peritoneal discomfort. The disadvantages of epidural anesthesia are the increased doses of local anesthetic required, the longer onset time compared with subarachnoid anesthesia and the higher failure rate.

Despite adequate levels of anesthesia, some patients still experience uncomfortable peritoneal symptoms. Epidural (and subarachnoid) fentanyl has been shown to relieve intraoperative discomfort due to intra-abdominal manipulations.[2] Usually epidural administration of 2% lidocaine 10–15 ml is sufficient to achieve a T6 level and adding fentanyl 50 μg will improve the quality of the block as well as provide 2–3 h of post-operative analgesia.[2]

Diluting the fentanyl in at least 10 ml of preservative-free normal saline or local anesthetic has been shown to shorten the onset time and increase the duration of analgesia as compared with use of less diluent.[3]

Fentanyl is most commonly used, because although morphine gives longer analgesia (12–24 h) the risk of respiratory depression, while low, is still present. Highly lipid-soluble opioids such as fentanyl may produce a more segmental block and have not been associated with respiratory depression. The side-effects of epidural (or subarachnoid) fentanyl are nausea, vomiting, pruritus and urinary retention. These symptoms are usually transient and mild, and do not require treatment. Small doses of naloxone or diphenhydramine may be useful in treating these side-effects.

REFERENCES

1. Hunt C O et al 1989 Perioperative analgesia with subarachnoid fentanyl-bupivacaine for cesarean delivery. Anesthesiology 71: 535–540
2. Naulty S J, Datta S, Ostheimer G W et al 1985 Epidural fentanyl for postcesarean delivery pain management. Anesthesiology 63: 694–698
3. Birnbach D J, Johnson M D et al 1989 Effect of diluent volume on analgesia produced by epidural fentanyl. Anesth Analg 68: 808–810

SECTION 7

Structure and function

80. Education in obstetric anesthesia

M. A. Hauch

INSTRUCTIONAL OBJECTIVES

The foundation upon which education in obstetric anesthesia rests is a core of knowledge essential to the field. The full scope of maternal physiologic alterations attendant to pregnancy and principles of perinatal pharmacology need to be understood. Management of parturition, techniques of inducing regional and general anesthesia in the parturient and the management of their complications are basic to the practice of safe obstetric anesthesia. The fundamentals of operative delivery, management and considerations of the high-risk obstetric patient and the anesthetic nuances for nonobstetric surgery during pregnancy and post-partum surgery need to be accentuated.

In addition to maternal, fetal and neonatal physiologic considerations, the dynamics of the change from intra- to extrauterine life must be taught in the education program. Pre- and intrapartum assessment, effects of maternally administered drugs on the fetus and neonate and the principles of neonatal resuscitation are particular areas for emphasis.

An understanding of the pharmacokinetics and pharmacodynamics of local anesthetics, as well as the use of epidural and subarachnoid opioids, should be incorporated into the teaching curriculum. Drug interactions with commonly used oxytocics and tocolytics deserve review.

Although drug administration is fundamental to the practice of obstetric anesthesia, a knowledge base in nonpharmacologic analgesia is as essential. Any busy obstetric anesthesiologist will confirm the fact that the patient educated in prepared childbirth classes is frequently more cooperative.[1]

With the exposure of a CA-3 and CA-4 resident to an active labor and delivery service, the value of the knowledge gained in understanding the logistics of such a service will pay handsome dividends. This trainee may some day be given the task of organizing anesthetic services in a new facility. Determining what considerations should go into the creation of the physical side of an obstetric anesthesia service cannot be taught from a textbook.

TECHNICAL OBJECTIVES

Regional anesthesia techniques play a major role in the management of the obstetric patient. Trainees in this field must have facility in the placement of epidural and subarachnoid blocks. Exposure to a large clinical service is advisable as these procedures are mastered with practice.

The administration of general anesthesia is much less common today than in the past. However, the skills necessary to induce and maintain a parturient with a general anesthetic are vital for cesarean and, infrequently, vaginal deliveries.

The knowledge of invasive monitoring, specifically intra-arterial and central venous monitoring, is a further technical objective in the indoctrination of trainees in obstetric anesthesia.

ADMINISTRATIVE OBJECTIVES

It is the philosophy of the Section of Obstetric Anesthesia at the Brigham and Women's Hospital that CA-3 and CA-4 residents receive some training in the administration of the service itself. Residents acquire expertise in the role of sound clinician, strategist and diplomat when dealt the responsibility of 'acting' director. Operating rooms for cesarean and vaginal deliveries, obstetric surgical emergencies, and in vitro fertilization all fall under the observant attention of the 'fellow'. Furthermore, the management of the labor suite for the coordination of consultations and epidural catheter placement, as well as supervision and teaching of less experienced residents, are other administrative tasks.

METHODS OF INSTRUCTION

An effective teaching program blends many sources of instruction: teaching in the labor and delivery suites, didactic programs by residents and staff, audiovisual materials, computer-assisted learning programs and, of course, independent study.

To quote Osler, 'The art of the practice of medicine is to be learned only by experience; 'tis not an inheritance; it cannot be revealed.'[2] As imparted in the beginning of this chapter, even the 'modest country doctor' may furnish the resident with a vital link in the education chain.[2] With stated instructional and technical objectives in mind, the resident and teacher may discuss their case in advance and apply what has been learned to the present situation.

The didactic program should consist of formal lectures given by both the attending and resident staff. Clinical case discussions and morbidity and mortality issues should be incorporated into the agenda. The capacity to discuss successes and errors of fellow trainees in such a forum is useful.

Independent study is the basis of self-education. The use of a departmental library with relevant journals, major reference texts, monographs and books dealing with specific topics is vital to the acquisition of knowledge. Resources such as audiovisual aids, photocopying machines, and computer-assisted literature searches are invaluable.

METHODS OF EVALUATION

Cognitive skills may objectively be assessed by written examination. The ABA/ASA (American Board of Anesthesiology/American Society of Anesthesiologists) In-Training Examination attempts to accomplish this goal. A subset of questions, related to the practice of obstetric anesthesia, may audit the residents' knowledge base. Direct observation by the clinical staff may also gauge resident proficiency on the technical aspects of obstetric anesthesia care.

The judgment and attitude of the resident are values not easily measured. Evaluations of these characteristics are by definition subjective, and thus are open to bias. Periodic self-assessment, with peer and staff review, may lend objectivity.

CONTINUING MEDICAL EDUCATION

The foundation for scholarship in continuing medical education remains motivation for self-education and the maintenance of an active, alert interest in important advances in the field. If spurred by the ideal combination of curiosity and proper training, the candidate will mature into a clinical scholar.

REFERENCES

1. Bonica J J 1980 Obstetric Analgesia and Anesthesia. World Federation of Societies of Anesthesiologists, Amsterdam
2. Osler W 1919 Johns Hopkins Hosp Bull 30: 198–202

Academic and clinical goals in obstetric anesthesia

One of the basic goals of the Department of Anesthesia at the Brigham and Women's Hospital has been to develop a solid set of concepts and skills relating to obstetric anesthesia to serve as a knowledge base for our trainees. To aid in this endeavor, we have created a set of clinical and academic goals that, when mastered, will allow our residents to practice obstetric anesthesia with skill and expertise.

ACADEMIC GOALS

From the texts recommended at the end of this section, a resident should acquire a basic fund of knowledge in the following areas by the end of the rotation:

1. Maternal physiologic changes during pregnancy
   a. Cardiovascular system
   b. Respiratory system
   c. Acid–base balance
   d. Gastrointestinal system
   e. Hepatic system
   f. Neurologic system
   g. Renal system
   h. Hematologic system.
2. Uterine blood flow
   a. Changes during pregnancy
   b. Effects of local/general anesthesia
   c. Effects of vasopressors/antihypertensives.
3. Maternal uptake/distribution, placental drug transport, and perinatal effects (including neurobehavioral effects and transfer of drugs into breast milk) of:
   a. Volatile anesthetics, barbiturates, ketamine, muscle relaxants, opioids, sedatives, tranquilizers, and scopolamine and their effects depending on the *route* of administration (i.e., intravenous, intramuscular, etc.)
   b. Local anesthetics
   c. Antihypertensives
   d. Anticoagulants
   e. Tocolytics
   f. Hypoglycemics/glucose administration.
4. Physiology of labor
   a. Stages of labor
   b. Effects of analgesia and anesthesia on labor
   c. Suppression of preterm labor. Be able to describe mechanism(s) of action and the anesthetic considerations of:
      (i) β-sympathomimetics
      (ii) magnesium channel blockers
      (iii) calcium channel blockers
      (iv) prostaglandin synthesis inhibitors
      (v) ethanol
      (vi) progestational agents

- d. Dystocia
  - (i) fetal
  - (ii) maternal
  - (iii) diagnosis/management
- e. Induction/augmentation of labor
  - (i) amniotomy and its anesthetic considerations
  - (ii) oxytocin and its anesthetic considerations
  - (iii) prostaglandins and their anesthetic considerations
  - (iv) ergot derivatives and their anesthetic considerations.

5. Local anesthetics
   - a. basic structure, properties, and mode of action of
     - (i) lidocaine with/without epinephrine
     - (ii) bupivacaine
     - (iii) mepivacaine
     - (iv) chloroprocaine
     - (v) tetracaine

     In addition, be able to discuss factors that affect toxic reactions to local anesthetics, the classification of reactions to local anesthetics, and reactions to vasopressor (epinephrine) in the local anesthetic
   - b. maternal absorption and placental transfer, including prevention and treatment of central nervous and cardiovascular system toxicities.
6. Inhaled anesthetics and ketamine
   - a. Uptake and distribution during pregnancy
   - b. Inhalation analgesia and its maternal and perinatal effects
   - c. Inhalation anesthesia and its maternal/perinatal effects
   - d. Ketamine maternal/perinatal effects.
7. Use of paracervical, pudendal, and perineal infiltrative blocks
   - a. Anatomic landmarks
   - b. Drugs commonly used
   - c. Associated maternal and fetal complications.
8. Basic concepts of major regional anesthesia in obstetrics
   - a. Vertebral column anatomy
   - b. Regional block
     - (i) cardiovascular effects
     - (ii) respiratory effects
     - (iii) spinal dermatomes
     - (iv) pain pathways
   - c. Indications and contraindications, including:
     - (i) coagulopathy
     - (ii) neurologic diseases
     - (iii) hypovolemia
     - (iv) drug allergy
     - (v) fever
     - (vi) backache
     - (vii) scoliosis

     Be able to discuss *why* the above may be considered absolute/relative contraindications.
   - d. Complications due to regional anesthesia. Be able to discuss the incidence(s), depending on the technique chosen (i.e. spinal versus epidural), and be able to formulate a treatment plan for each of the following:
     - (i) cardiovascular
     - (ii) headache
     - (iii) backache
     - (iv) bladder dysfunction
     - (v) neurologic sequelae
     - (vi) infection.
9. Subarachnoid anesthesia
   - a. Techniques (preparations, landmarks and procedures)
   - b. Local anesthetics used and their administration
   - c. Subarachnoid opioids: mechanism of action, drugs used, systemic effects and associated complications.
10. Lumbar epidural anesthesia
    - a. Techniques (preparations, landmarks and procedures)
    - b. Local anesthetics used and their administration
    - c. Epidural opioids: mechanism of action, drugs used, systemic effects and associated complications
    - d. Use of continuous epidural infusions, including patient-controlled epidural anesthesia.
11. Caudal anesthesia
    - a. Techniques (preparations, landmarks and procedures)
    - b. Local anesthetics used and their administration
    - c. Complications.
12. Cesarean delivery
    - a. Indications for cesarean delivery, including:
      - (i) failure to progress
      - (ii) breech presentation
      - (iii) cephalopelvic disproportion
      - (iv) previous cesarean delivery
      - (v) fetal distress
    - b. Selection of anesthetic. Be able to discuss why certain techniques are chosen over others
    - c. General anesthesia
      - (i) management of induction, intraoperative anesthesia, and emergence
      - (ii) significance of delivery intervals and concentrations of volatile agents
      - (iii) pros and cons of nitrous oxide
      - (iv) complications of general anesthesia, including diagnosis and management of aspiration and failed intubation
    - d. Regional anesthesia
      - (i) significance of delivery intervals

- (ii) maternal/neonatal effects of anesthetic induced hypotension.

13. Emergency delivery
    a. Vaginal delivery
    b. Cesarean delivery
    Be able to discuss why certain anesthetic techniques are chosen over others.
14. The high-risk parturient
    Be able to discuss (1) why the following maternal health complications pose problems for an obstetric anesthesiologist and (2) the anesthetic management of these patients during labor and delivery.
    a. Cardiac disease, including:
        (i) congenital heart disease
        (ii) valvular lesions
        (iii) associated pulmonary hypertension
        (iv) cardiomyopathy: restrictive
    b. Respiratory disease
        (i) restrictive
        (ii) obstructive
    c. Diabetes
        (i) classifications
        (ii) management
        (iii) associated maternal/neonatal complications
    d. Morbid obesity
    e. Airway abnormality
    f. Miscellaneous, including thyroid disease, malignant hyperthermia, coagulopathy, and neuromuscular disease.
15. Obstetric complications
    Be able to discuss the diagnosis, obstetric management and anesthetic considerations/management for each of the following:
    a. abnormal presentations
        (i) Breech, face, brow, and compound presentations
        (ii) Transverse lie
        (iii) Prolapsed cord
        (iv) Multiple gestation
    b. Pregnancy-induced hypertension
        (i) Classification
        (ii) Diagnosis
    c. Premature rupture of membranes
    d. Hemorrhage
        (i) Placenta previa
        (ii) Placental abruption
        (iii) Uterine rupture
        (iv) Post-partum hemorrhage (uterine atony, retained placenta, birth trauma, uterine inversion, placenta accreta, disseminated intravascular coagulation)
    e. Embolism: amniotic fluid, air and thrombus.
16. Anesthesia for nondelivery surgery during pregnancy
    a. General surgery
        (i) preoperative evaluation and management
        (ii) intraoperative management
        (iii) use of tocolytics
        (iv) perioperative fetal monitoring
        (v) anesthetic considerations including teratogenic effects and other problems
    b. Cerclage placement
        (i) anesthetic management
    c. Post-partum tubal ligation
        (i) Anesthetic management.
17. The fetus and the neonate
    a. Physiology of fetus and newborn
    b. Antepartum fetal assessment
        (i) electronic fetal heart rate monitoring
        (ii) fetal pH monitoring
        (iii) nonstress testing
        (iv) oxytocin challenge testing
        (v) biophysical profile
        (vi) fetal lung maturity testing
    c. Diagnosis and management of peripartum fetal asphyxia
    d. Evaluation of the neonate
    e. Resuscitation of the neonate
    f. Specific neonatal disorders and their management
        (i) meconium aspiration
        (ii) diaphragmatic hernia
        (iii) tracheoesophageal fistula
        (iv) sepsis
        (v) respiratory distress syndromes.

CLINICAL GOALS

1. Be able to set up an operating room to administer anesthesia for an obstetric case (vaginal or cesarean delivery).

2. Become proficient at the placement and management of an epidural anesthetic for delivery. Aim for *at least* 40–50 epidural catheter placements in a month-long rotation.

3. Become proficient in the performance and management of spinal anesthesia for vaginal and cesarean delivery.

4. Be able to administer safely general anesthesia for emergent and nonemergent vaginal and cesarean deliveries.

5. Be able to evaluate preoperatively and design a safe plan for the anesthetic management of:

a. a healthy parturient presenting for vaginal delivery with/without the use of forceps;

b. a healthy parturient presenting for elective cesarean delivery;

c. a healthy parturient presenting for emergency cesarean delivery;

d. a parturient with preeclampsia/eclampsia (pregnancy-induced hypertension);

e. a parturient with antepartum/intrapartum/post-partum hemorrhage.

6. Become familiar with the diagnosis and management of a neonate in distress.

7. Be able to discuss at length the questions following the case histories below. Brief answers are provided to guide you.

Case 1

A 35-year-old parturient with a 38-week gestation has mild pregnancy-induced hypertension (BP 150/90). She fails to progress after 4 h of labor at station + 1 with cervical dilation 4 cm. She received butorphanol 2 mg i.m. × 2 with little relief. The obstetrician starts an oxytocin infusion, which improves the progress of labor, but the patient becomes very uncomfortable. There are intermittent type I decelerations on the fetal monitor strip. The obstetrician anticipates a vaginal delivery and requests your assistance for pain relief.

Questions

1. Why doesn't the obstetrician do a paracervical block (PCB)?

   Answer. *The* main drawback to a PCB is the possible production of fetal bradycardia. This is thought to be due to fetal hypoxia/acidosis resulting from uterine artery vasoconstriction from local anesthetic applied in close location to the artery, which causes decreased uteroplacental perfusion. Second, the block is only effective during the first stage of labor because the perineal sensory fibers are not blocked with this technique.

2. What are the advantages/disadvantages of a lumbar epidural block in this patient?

   Answer. An epidural block is able to block pain pathways extending from T10 to S5, thus providing total pain relief during all stages of labor. Because of its continuous technique, it is especially useful in cases of prolonged labor. In the patient with pregnancy-induced hypertension, its vasodilating action and ability to lower catecholamine levels usually result in an improvement in uteroplacental perfusion and a lowering of maternal blood pressure.

   In the inadequately hydrated patient, however, it may precipitate sudden maternal hypotension, resulting in decreased uteroplacental perfusion and fetal distress.

3. What are the advantages/disadvantages of magnesium therapy in patients with pregnancy-induced hypertension?

   Answer. Magnesium sulfate, by its effects on the peripheral neuromuscular junction, acts as an anticonvulsant and also reduces hyperreflexia. It also is a mild vasodilator and improves uterine blood flow by reducing uterine hyperactivity.

   High doses can produce maternal muscle weakness, hypotension and even cardiac/respiratory failure. Magnesium sulfate potentiates neuromuscular block.

Case 2

A 26-year-old primigravida at 38 weeks' gestation presents in active labor with a fetus in the breech position. The obstetrician asks you to provide help with pain relief.

Questions

1. How would you proceed at this point?

   Answer: The decision to deliver this baby by vaginal or cesarean delivery should be made promptly by the obstetrician. Vaginal delivery of a breech infant may result in umbilical cord compression or prolapse and/or a traumatic delivery for both mother and fetus.

   If the obstetrician believes the infant can be delivered vaginally, perineal anesthesia can be supplied with a pudendal, spinal or epidural block. On occasion, general anesthesia (following a rapid-sequence induction) may be required (rarely), using a volatile agent to relax the uterus and allow manipulation and delivery of the head.

   If obstetric indications mandate a cesarean delivery, anesthesia can be accomplished with regional or general anesthesia depending on the urgency of the situation.

2. The obstetrician specifically ask you to administer a caudal block for this patient. What are its drawbacks?

   Answer: Because of their close proximity, the caudal needle may pierce the patient's rectum or the presenting fetal part. This may result in a toxic administration of local anesthetic to the fetus. Because a large volume of local anesthetic is required to produce analgesia using this technique, unintentional injection into the subarachnoid space would produce a high or total spinal block. In addition, unintentional intravascular injection would produce central nervous system excitation or convulsions. Most anesthesiologists believe that caudal block is technically more difficult to perform than a spinal or epidural block.

3. After some length, vaginal delivery was accomplished

but the infant is born with an initial Apgar score of 3. The mother is fine but only you and the obstetrician are in the room. What should you do?

Answer: This score indicates severe cardiorespiratory depression. While you are calling for additional help, intermittent positive-pressure ventilation with 100% oxygen should be administered by bag and mask. If there is not an immediate response, intubation and closed-chest cardiac massage should be instituted. Drug therapy with sodium bicarbonate, epinephrine and dextrose should be considered if resuscitation is prolonged.

REFERENCES

1. Shnider S M, Levinson G 1987 Anesthesia for obstetrics, 2nd edn. Williams & Wilkins, Baltimore
2. Datta S, Ostheimer G W 1987 Common problems in obstetric anesthesia. Year Book Medical Publishers, Chicago
3. Albright G A, Ferguson J E, Joyce T H, Stevenson D K 1986 Anesthesia in obstetrics: maternal, fetal, and neonatal aspects, 2nd edn. Butterworths, Boston
4. James F J, Wheeler A S, Dewan D M 1988 Obstetric anesthesia: the complicated patient, 2nd edn. F A Davis, Philadelphia
5. Crawford J S 1984 Principle and practice of obstetric anaesthesia, 5th edn. Blackwell Scientific Publications, Oxford
6. Beard R W, Nathaniels P W 1984 Fetal physiology and medicine. The basis of perinatology, 2nd ed. Marcel Dekker, New York

81. Organization of an anesthetic service for obstetrics

PART A
AUSTRALIA

P. Brownridge M. J. Cousins

As in other developed countries, the delivery of anesthetic services to obstetric patients in Australia has gradually improved during the last two decades. These improvements reflect an increase in the number of specialist anesthesiologists within the community; an increased demand for proficiently administered anesthesia and analgesia in modern obstetric practice; and recognition of the need for higher professional training in obstetric anesthesia.* Maternal mortality related to anesthesia has decreased over the years despite an undoubted increase in the number of anesthetics administered to obstetric patients. Examination of the Triennial Reports on Maternal Deaths in Australia also reveals that there has been a marked decline in the number of deaths in which the anesthetic was administered by a general practitioner or nonspecialist – although, unfortunately, the status of the anesthesiologist has not been specified in recent reports (Table 81.1). This trend reflects the growth of anesthesia as a specialty in Australia in the last three decades.

However, despite improvements in the overall quality of anesthetic service available for obstetric patients in Australia, there remain considerable differences between individual units in the standard of anesthetic care that is available. As elsewhere, these differences are related to factors such as the size and category of maternity unit (e.g. free-standing or contained within a general hospital; teaching or nonteaching; private or public); local consumer demand; financial constraints; and professional attitudes within each unit towards the role of the anesthesiologist in obstetric pain management.

The annual birth rate in Australia during the past 25 years has ranged between 222 000 and 264 000. The majority of births occur in a hospital environment – home deliveries accounting for only 0.5% of births. Unfortunately, information regarding the distribution of births by size of hospital is very limited. Although each of the six states and two territories publish annual maternal and

*The Australian and New Zealand college of Anaesthetists

Table 81.1 Maternal deaths associated with anesthesia in the Commonwealth of Australia, 1964–84*

Status of the anaesthesiologist	1964–66	1967–69	1970–72	1973–75	1976–78	1979–81	1982–1984
Consultant/registrar	3	4	3	NS	NS	NS	NS
Resident medical officer/other	3	3	NS	NS	NS	NS	NS
General practitioner	12	7	NS	NS	NS	NS	NS
Total	18	14	13	4	6	6	3

* Taken from the Triennial Reports on Maternal Deaths in Australia (published by the National Health and Medical Research Council of Australia, Canberra).
NS, not stated.

perinatal reports, the data are not sufficiently consistent to present an overall picture of the standard of obstetric anesthesia service in Australia, or to permit a comparison to be made between different geographic regions. There are even inconsistencies in the definition of terms. For example, obstetric units in New South Wales are classified (according to the facilities that are available) into five different levels, whereas in Victoria there are only three levels of classification. Some of the other states simply classify the place of confinement into metropolitan, teaching, private and country hospitals – but do not specify the distribution of births according to hospital size. It is not possible, therefore, to estimate the entire range of anesthetic services available to obstetric patients in Australia.

The constraints that small obstetric units impose on standards of anesthetic care in the UK have already been described.[1] From the limited data available, it is likely that the position in Australia is similar – if not worse – than that which exists in Britain. For example, in the State of Victoria more than 170 maternity units exist for the delivery of approximately 60 000 births a year, of which 44% occur in units with fewer than 1000 deliveries a year (including 4.6% in hospitals with fewer than 100 births a year).[2] In South Australia fewer than 20 000 deliveries a year take place in 91 maternity units; 27.2% occur in units with fewer than 500 births a year (including 8.6% in units with fewer than 100 births a year).[3]

These data – from only two Australian states – imply that anesthetic services must be less than ideal in some places. In all states there are many small, geographically isolated, maternity units which are remote from specialist anesthetic care. In rural areas and in many large country towns anesthesia is provided by general practitioners. While general practitioners who practice anesthesia must be accredited by the hospital board, they obviously cannot be expected to have the same experience as a specialist.

In the metropolitan areas most anesthetic procedures carried out in private maternity units are performed by registered specialists. However, although most privately run units have access to a specialist anesthesiologist, they do not generally have resident medical staff. The ability of such units to respond adequately to an obstetric emergency is therefore questionable.

The relatively small proportion of deliveries occurring in teaching hospitals in Australia also presents difficulties for undergraduate and postgraduate training. In Adelaide, for example, fewer than 10 000 deliveries a year occur within the five teaching hospitals that have maternity beds. Quite apart from organizational difficulties, this relatively small number of deliveries limits teaching and clinical exposure of trainees in obstetric anesthesia. A similar state of affairs probably exists in other capital cities. In Western Australia, for instance, only 46% (or approximately 11 500) of deliveries occur in the metropolitan teaching and public hospitals.[4]

As has been described in other countries, the smaller the obstetric unit, the more difficult it is to provide a safe, efficient and cost-effective anesthetic service.[1,5,6] Bromage has reasoned that for a self-contained obstetric unit to provide a viable 24-h anesthesia coverage a throughput of at least 3000 deliveries (and preferably 5000) a year is required.[7] Yet, as elsewhere, small units remain popular in the community and there has been little attempt to reduce their number in Australia. Factors such as public pressure, vested interests and political inertia all influence the national delivery of obstetric health care and these factors are unlikely to change significantly in Australia within the foreseeable future.

There has not yet been a nationwide survey of obstetric anesthetic services in Australia. Most metropolitan public hospital maternity units, however, would have a full-time consultant anesthesiologist (or director) who is responsible for the overall organization of the service. Outside the capital cities the position is less certain because many hospitals with public maternity beds do not have ready access to a specialist anesthesiologist.

The situation in the private sector is even more conjectural. In many metropolitan private hospitals an accredited visiting anesthetic specialist is appointed to act as a liaison officer, one of whose functions is to discuss anesthesia-related problems with colleagues and determine anesthetic policies. Most private obstetric units have a roster of anesthetic specialists available for the unit – although it is not always clear whether the 'on-call' anesthesiologist is in close proximity and free from other commitments. As noted previously, the vast majority of private maternity units in Australia do not have resident medical staff.

ORGANIZATION OF OBSTETRIC ANESTHESIA AT FLINDERS MEDICAL CENTRE

Flinders Medical Centre is a general teaching hospital within the The Flinders University of South Australia, and has foundation chairs in both anesthesia and intensive care and in obstetrics and gynecology. The obstetric anesthetic service was established when the hospital was first commissioned in 1975. The labor and delivery suite currently delivers approximately 2800 babies a year and is adjacent to the neonatal unit, operating theatres and the adult intensive care unit. The cesarean delivery rate is approximately 20% (of which 85% are performed utilizing the regional anesthesia) and epidural rate during labor is currently 52%. The unit attracts complicated deliveries from the southern region of South Australia and has a retrieval service (including retrieval by air) for both neonates and adults. It is the only obstetric centre in South Australia that has both adult and neonatal intensive care facilities.

Staffing

A full-time director of obstetric anesthesia is responsible for the provision and organization of anesthetic services to the maternity unit. During normal hours (i.e. 0800–1800h, Monday to Friday) anesthesia and analgesia within the labor and delivery suite are generally administered by a consultant anesthesiologist – usually, the director. Apart from providing a stable clinical service there are other benefits associated with units which are administered by someone who has a special interest in obstetric anesthesia. For example, activities such as consultation and daily follow-up of patients, clinical audit and quality assurance, formulation of policies and guidelines, teaching and antenatal education, clinical research and communication with other disciplines (including nursing staff) can all be achieved more readily when someone is made responsible for administration of the anesthetic service. Obstetric anesthesia has become a recognized subspecialty during the last two decades in most developed countries and advances in this field have invariably emanated from centers that have appointed an anesthesiologist with a special interest in obstetrics to supervise and develop the service.

Outside normal hours, anesthesia is provided by one of two anesthetic registrars or the consultant 'on call'. If these staff are all occupied a second rostered consultant is available. Only registrars who have had at least 1 year of experience in anesthesia are rostered to the obstetric unit. These staffing arrangements ensure that an experienced anesthesiologist is available to the obstetric unit at all times. Our adult intensive care unit is also close by so that resuscitation can be implemented immediately in an emergency.

Despite our obstetric unit having somewhat less than the ideal number of deliveries (i.e. more than 3000) per year, anesthetic cover is adequate and cost-effective. This has been made possible by virtue of the obstetric unit being within a general surgical hospital.

A trained midwife is in attendance with each patient throughout labor on a one-to-one basis. Apart from pudendal block, obstetricians do not perform anesthetic procedures in our unit; and nursing staff do not administer anesthesia at all in Australia except for perineal infiltration and epidural top-ups in some hospitals.

Facilities and equipment

The maternity and delivery suite has 10 delivery rooms, two side rooms and a recovery area. Each room is equipped with suction, oxygen, nitrous oxide (Midogas), a tipping delivery bed, a lateral tilt wedge and a range of intravenous apparatus, regional anesthesia trolleys, infusion pumps and blood warmers. Extra monitoring equipment is readily available from the adjacent operating theaters if required.

There is no dedicated obstetric operating theater in our maternity unit: patients requiring cesarean delivery must be transferred to one of the nearby general theaters. While this arrangement is very cost-effective, it can interrupt surgical schedules and there exists a potential for delay if all of the theaters are occupied. Having to move hurriedly to a strange and alien area, surrounded with unfamiliar faces, also represents an added source of anxiety for the patient and her partner. A dedicated, en suite obstetric theater is a more pleasant and less-threatening environment for the patient. It is also much easier to organize a properly supervised trainee rotation in obstetric anesthesia when the obstetric unit has its own theater.

Policies, protocols and guidelines

Policies related to obstetric anesthesia and analgesia are determined after discussion within the Department of Anesthesia and Intensive Care and, when necessary, with other departments in the hospital. Policies are reviewed from time to time and modified in the light of new knowledge or changing circumstances. Whenever possible they are determined by mutual agreement. For example, the following policies apply in our own unit:

1. analgesia in labor is principally determined by patient choice;
2. all patients must receive oral sodium citrate prior to cesarean delivery;
3. an anesthetic assistant proficient in the application of cricoid pressure must be present before the induction of general anesthesia;
4. epidural meperidine is prescribed for post-operative analgesia following cesarean delivery performed under epidural blockade.

Protocols and instructions for nursing staff are contained in a Nursing Procedure Manual. There are protocols for the preparation of patients for general and regional anesthesia; the administration of epidural drugs; the removal of epidural catheters; the treatment of hypotension; and management of patients following an unintentional dural puncture. The authors are not in favor of written instructions for medical staff concerning practical procedures or matters of clinical judgment: consequently there are no formal protocols for the attention of anesthetic staff in the maternity unit. There are, however, *guidelines* for the management of complications such as failed intubation; systemic local anesthetic toxicity; high spinal block; and unintentional dural puncture. These guidelines are not clinical directives, as such, but are there for the assistance of staff in the event of a complication.

Finally, there are guidelines outlining our approach to pain management during labor. These are designed to acquaint newly appointed staff with the way pain relief has developed in our unit and so promote a consistent source of information for patients seeking guidance about analgesia. Epidural analgesia, for example, is managed by midwives who are permitted to determine – as well as administer – top-up doses according to the needs and circumstances of each individual patient. We believe that this practice confers considerably more flexibility in obstetric epidural pain management than can be achieved with other regimens.

Communication with other disciplines

Modern obstetric care involves staff from several disciplines – including obstetricians, midwives, perinatologists, anesthesiologists, antenatal educators and physiotherapists – each with different backgrounds and areas of expertise. A cooperative and harmonious atmosphere can exist only if there is regular communication between these professional groups. It is important, therefore, that the members of each specialty have the opportunity to listen to each other and to exchange ideas.

There are various ways in which channels of communication can be established or improved. All staff are encouraged to attend clinical meetings, 'grand rounds', audits and other educational activities that are of mutual interest; and each discipline has the opportunity to periodically present reviews of recent developments or research in their field. A weekly presentation of obstetric cases is another valuable forum for informal education and discussion between staff of different disciplines.

Business meetings – at which matters of policy, funding and organization can be discussed – are convened on a regular basis with senior representatives from the various departments. It is important that matters that have been discussed are then conveyed to other members of the department. The most effective communication often occurs informally – during morning coffee, lunch or afternoon tea. Proper communication ultimately means the free exchange of opinions among colleagues who respect each other's points of view and who have established an atmosphere of trust and understanding. Without these qualities communication exists in name only.

Teaching and training

An essential feature of any obstetric unit, irrespective of size, is to ensure that all staff are adequately trained and able to deal with obstetric emergencies or complications. This implies a regular review of the standard of training in patient resuscitation and in the management of complications. In our own unit, nursing staff are trained and examined each year in resuscitation with the aid of a mannikin. In addition to the educational outlets described in the previous section, the nursing division also has weekly 'in-service' lectures including topics related to obstetric anesthesia.

As with other clinical specialties, teaching in obstetric anesthesia is most effective when carried out informally at the bedside. A clinical round each morning of patients in labor and in the post-natal wards is an excellent opportunity for teaching trainees in anesthesia, undergraduates in their obstetric term and trainee midwives. Unfortunately, for logistical reasons, it has not been feasible to have a formal rotation in obstetric anesthesia for our own trainees. Departmental service requirements have had to take priority over training needs. As noted previously, this shortcoming in training is largely a consequence of the relatively small size of our maternity unit (2800 deliveries a year) and the absence of a dedicated operating theater. However, all registrars receive training and experience in obstetric anesthesia and analgesia.

Audit and quality assurance

Obstetric analgesia and anesthesia are topics well suited for clinical auditing. Concurrent audit of epidural analgesia during labor, for example, allows us to evaluate our service; to compare it with other centers; and to determine any deficiencies or shortcomings.[8] Once the latter have been identified, it is then possible to modify clinical practices or introduce changes in procedure. A concurrent obstetric analgesia audit has been partly responsible for initiating changes in epidural pain management within our own unit. Finally, a detailed audit also provides a resource for continuing education and a database for further studies.

When a complication occurs only infrequently, a different type of audit is required. In this case, it is preferable that someone who has an interest in the complication is notified so that detailed records can be maintained. This allows one individual in a department to become experienced in the presentation, symptomatology, treatment and outcome of an otherwise uncommon complication. The management of unintentional dural puncture is an example of this type of audit.[9]

The anesthesiologist and antenatal education

Obstetric patients should know what choices of pain relief are available to them long before they go into labor. Accordingly, antenatal preparation classes in our unit includes a session on obstetric analgesia. This session is conducted informally by someone well experienced in discussing the topic. The class is kept sufficiently small to remain intimate and the participants encouraged to share their opinion and experiences. In this way, a successful class promotes patient confidence as well as providing reliable and authoritative information about obstetric pain relief and anesthesia. Antenatal classes are also educational for the anesthesiologist: he becomes more familiar with matters that are of concern to the child-bearing public and learns how to handle questions sympathetically yet honestly.

A booklet entitled *Soothing the Pain of Childbirth* has been written for patients attending our maternity unit. This booklet describes and illustrates the methods of analgesia that are available to them. It is written in simple English and is easily understood. The booklet complements information that is presented at the antenatal class and is an additional source of reference for the patient.

There are also two educational video programs which have been produced for the benefit of patients attending our unit. The first, entitled 'Precious Moments', shows a cesarean delivery performed under epidural anesthesia. The other shows various methods of analgesia being used in childbirth (transcutaneous nerve stimulation, intramuscular opioid, nitrous oxide inhalation and an epidural block). These videos provide insight for the patient who has not experienced labor or a cesarean delivery before. They are shown at regular intervals on the antenatal ward and are available for private viewing at any time.

The obstetric anesthesiologist can make a valuable contribution, therefore, in preparing women for childbirth. These activities are time-consuming but well worthwhile in helping to make patients feel more confident.

SUMMARY AND CONCLUSIONS

The organization of anesthetic services in obstetrics is dependent upon several factors, including financial resources, manpower, public demand and the way in which health care is provided. Australia enjoys a high standard of obstetric care and a relatively high ratio of specialist anesthesiologists per unit of population; but there are many small maternity units in remote areas – and even in capital cities – without properly organized anesthetic services. The extent of deficiencies in the provision of obstetric anesthetic services is unknown because there are only very limited data available.

The anesthetic organization of a medium-sized obstetric unit in an Australian teaching hospital is described. Our experience suggests that the appointment of a full-time director of obstetric anesthesia can improve the standard of clinical service, encourage better teaching and promote research. The relatively small number of deliveries in our unit, however, and the absence of a dedicated obstetric theater has limited the amount of supervision, teaching and clinical exposure of trainees in obstetric analgesia and anesthesia.

REFERENCES

1. Report 1987 Anaesthetic services for obstetrics – a plan for the future. The Association of Anaesthetists of Great Britain and Ireland, London
2. Report 1990 Having a baby in Victoria – final report of the ministerial review of birthing services in Victoria. Department of Health, Melbourne
3. Report 1989 Pregnancy outcome in South Australia 1988. South Australian Health Commission, Adelaide
4. Report 1990 Perinatal statistics in Western Australia 1988. Health Department of Western Australia, Perth
5. Reynolds F 1986 Obstetric anaesthetic services. Br Med J 293: 403–404
6. Gibbs C P, Krischer J, Peckham B M, Sharp H, Krischbaum T H 1986 Obstetric anesthesia: a national survey. Anesthesiology 65: 298–306
7. Bromage P R 1980 Epidural analgesia: demand and supply. In: Doughty A (ed) Epidural analgesia in obstetrics: a second symposium. Lloyd-Luke, London
8. Brownridge P 1990 Concurrent audit of midwife-managed epidural analgesia during labor. Pain suppl 5: 401
9. Brownridge P 1983 The management of headache following accidental dural puncture in obstetric patients: case series and review. Anaesth Intens Care 11: 4–15

PART B
ARGENTINA

P. J. Kelly

Very few obstetric units have formally designated obstetric anesthetic services in Argentina. This is because hospitals either deal exclusively with obstetrics and gynecology (of which there are fewer than 20 in the whole country) or have a large obstetrics department.

Public hospitals (either national, provincial or county owned), university hospitals and large private hospitals have an anesthesia department responsible for all anesthetics given, no matter what the surgical specialty. Within such departments two circumstances have to be considered:

1. The total number of procedures performed is relatively small and thus the same anesthesiologists administer obstetric anesthetics and all other anesthetic procedures.
2. The total number of deliveries is large enough to merit a separate obstetric anesthetic service or an 'on-call team' dedicated exclusively to obstetrics.

In the latter situation, the special 'obstetrics on-call team' is composed of some of the regular members of the anesthesia department who work 24 h days exclusively in obstetrics. Currently the delivery rooms are separate from the operating theaters, but cesarean deliveries and dilation and curettage are done in the surgical area with very few exceptions. In this instance the anesthetic procedure started for a normal delivery is continued by the same anesthesiologist in the operating theater. Post-operative analgesia is administered either by the surgeon (most frequently), or by the anesthesiologist. Obviously, the total number of anesthesiologists depends on the average delivery rate. In small private hospitals or clinics, groups of anesthesiologists take care of obstetric anesthesia as a whole. Most of them are organized as 'on-call teams', but many deliveries are done by the same anesthesiologists who perform every type of anesthesia when 'on call'.

PART C
UK

M. Harmer

The provision of obstetric care in the UK is predominantly hospital based, but the size of each individual unit may vary widely throughout a region or the country as a whole, depending upon geographic and demographic factors. The size of a unit may vary from one delivering fewer than 500 mothers to one delivering in excess of 4000 mothers per annum. While there are still a large number of the smaller units in the UK, they probably account for only about 1% of all deliveries, and those units delivering more than 4000 mothers per annum account for about 20% of all deliveries. Over 50% of all deliveries are carried out in units undertaking between 2000 and 4000 deliveries per annum. It is obvious that with such diversity of unit size the organization of an obstetric anesthesia service must differ accordingly.

STAFFING

The actual organization and provision of an optimum, safe obstetric anesthesia service is the responsibility of each health district, and such responsibility is further devolved on the hospital in which the unit is sited. In the past, the provision of staff for an obstetric anesthesia service has been organized by the Division of Anesthesia (a medico-managerial subcommittee) for that particular hospital. More recently though, with the introduction of management changes brought about by the restructuring of the National Health Service, the responsibility lies with the clinical director of anesthetic services for the hospital. Whilst this clinical director is responsible for the allocation of staff, the other aspects of the provision of a service, such as equipment, drugs, nonmedical assistance, etc., may partly or wholly rest with the clinical director of obstetric services.

The day-to-day management of the obstetric anesthesia service is the responsibility of a named consultant anesthesiologist. This consultant will, with the help of his/her colleagues, organize and be accountable for all aspects of teaching, training and maintenance of equipment and ensuring appropriate standards of practice. In addition, he/she will also be a member of the district maternity services liaison committee, which acts to provide a link between the hospital services and the community.

The provision of an obstetric anesthesia service should aim to ensure that an anesthesiologist who is skilled and experienced in obstetric anesthesia and analgesia is immediately available at all times for elective operative deliveries, emergencies and for the provision of pain relief in labor. The Obstetric Anaesthetists' Association recommends that trainee anesthesiologists should have at least 1 year's experience before working on the obstetric unit. In larger units (those delivering more than 3000 mothers per annum) there is usually sufficient workload to justify the allocation of a dedicated anesthesiologist, but in smaller units such an allocation of staff may represent uneconomical use of manpower and some arrangement of shared cover with another anesthetic subspecialty might have to be considered.

The majority of obstetric units in the UK that provide a 24-h anesthetic service (generally those mentioned above) do so by the use of trainee anesthesiologists, particularly for 'out-of-hours' cover. These trainees are supported and supervised by more senior staff – usually consultants. These senior staff provide 24 h on-call cover for the trainee and will, in addition, have a number of fixed daytime sessions allocated to the obstetric unit during which time elective operative procedures can be performed. The number of consultants and their sessional commitments varies from unit to unit, but the organization of the service should ensure that these are sufficient to provide adequate coverage for the unit. While the actual allocation of senior staff to obstetric sessions may vary around the regions in the UK, hospitals are encouraged to provide consultant staff in accordance with the recommendations of the Obstetric Anaesthetists' Association. These recommendations state that there should be at least one consultant anesthesiologist session (half-day) per week for each 500 deliveries with full-time consultant cover (10 sessions) being provided if a unit has more than 3000 deliveries per year. It is most unusual for a hospital to have a consultant anesthesiologist who works solely in obstetrics; the majority of hospitals have a group of three or four so that on-call rotations are not too onerous and periods of leave are possible.

If a hospital fails to provide a proper obstetric anesthesia service, the department of anesthetics may have its recognition for training withdrawn. Such an eventuality would follow one of the regular visits from representatives of the Royal College of Anaesthetists, part of whose role is to ensure adequate support for staff being trained.

FACILITIES

Most larger obstetric units are attached to general hospitals, but around the UK there are still a number of isolated, often small, units. Obviously the facilities that are immediately available in these two types of hospitals will vary and, indeed, even the larger obstetric unit on a general hospital site may be largely self-contained with very little link with the main hospital. In particular, the obstetric unit may have its own operating suite. However, certain standards must always be met and include the provision of a full complement of anesthetics, monitoring and resuscitation equipment. There must also be skilled nonmedical assistance readily available and a designated area for mothers recovering from anesthesia or in need of careful observation. The larger units may also have their own high-dependency units. In general, the facilities available in the obstetric unit should be similar to those in the hospital's main operating suite.

PROVISION OF ANESTHETIC COVER FOR SMALL UNITS

If a unit delivers fewer than 2000 mothers per annum, it will be difficult to provide, or indeed justify, continuous anesthetic cover. If one assumes that approximately one-third of mothers will at some time during labor and delivery need the attention of an anesthesiologist, it would follow that in an average 24 h period there would be two anesthetic interventions. With such demand it would be uneconomical to provide a dedicated anesthesiologist and some joint cover may be the only answer, but such arrangements may endanger the immediate response time desirable in obstetric anesthesia practice. The most common joint arrangement in such units is to combine the obstetric cover with that of the intensive care unit.

The very small obstetric unit (fewer than 500 deliveries per annum) is often sited distant from a large hospital and is unlikely to have resident anesthetic cover. In such circumstances, there is little possibility of providing comprehensive anesthetic cover, and mothers likely to require intervention should either not be admitted to that unit or, if problems arise later, should be transferred to a larger unit. The most logical solution to the problem would be the closure of such units, but this is often not easy as local public pressure to keep such units open may be intense.

OBSTETRIC FLYING SQUAD

In addition to providing 'in-house' obstetric care for the local population, all health districts in the UK have a responsibility to provide facilities to treat major problems occurring outside the hospital. Such problems may include ante- and post-partum hemorrhage, prolapsed cord, retained placenta or the need for neonatal resuscitation. Most districts provide this service by the use of an obstetric flying squad. The need for such a facility will depend upon the number of home confinements and the geographic distribution of mothers in the district. Traditionally the obstetric flying squad consists of an obstetrician, an anesthesiologist, a pediatrician and a midwife. This team is transported by ambulance, with their equipment, to the scene of the problem, where necessary care can be given. More recently, a paramedic-based service has been introduced in Cardiff and may become the model for other districts.

SUMMARY

While the provision of an obstetric anesthesia service in the UK is the responsibility of each District Health Authority, the actual organization is executed by the hospital's department of anesthetics (or, more recently, the clinical director of anesthetic services). The day-to-day running of the service is further devolved to a designated consultant anesthesiologist. The cover of a medium-sized obstetric unit (the most common in the UK) is usually achieved by trainees providing the 'frontline' care with consultants providing a 24 h senior back-up. However, small units often have to develop compromise solutions to maintain cover, or, if such cover is unavailable, face closure.

PART D
SWEDEN

L. Irestedt P. Belfrage

INTRODUCTION

The development of a generally available obstetric anesthesia service in Sweden started in the early 1970s. 10 years later the majority of Swedish delivery units could provide women in labor with an effective pain relief service (including the administration of epidural anesthetics) on a 24 h basis. During the 1980s the responsibility of the anesthetic departments in hospitals with delivery units to provide an effective obstetric anesthesia service has been established. Until the late 1960s the routine obstetric management of women in labor was provided by midwives, and with rather little interest from the responsible obstetrician unless complications leading to surgical intervention occurred. The obstetric management was conservative and essentially unchanged for decades. The relief of obstetric pain was restricted to the use of nitrous oxide, meperidine or sedatives such as chlorpromazine. Nitrous oxide was often used intermittently in concentrations up to 100%, and open-mask anesthesia with chloroform during the actual delivery was used frequently. Until that time obstetricians and anesthesiologists paid little attention to pain in obstetrics. During the late 1960s the generally conservative management of laboring women changed towards a more active approach. This modern obstetric era also included a rapidly increasing interest in obstetric pain relief.

In 1950 Risholm[1] published a paper regarding conduction anesthesia in obstetrics, but this early paper remained very isolated in Scandinavia in spite of the positive results with epidural anesthesia for obstetric pain relief reported from the USA and Canada.[2,3] Several Scandinavian studies did underline the need for more effective obstetric pain relief. In a retrospective Norwegian study published in 1970, Lind[4] showed that 50% of 500 recently delivered women regarded their delivery as being very painful. 17% judged the pain as being unbearable. The study also documented that a third of the patients judged the given analgesia (meperidine and nitrous oxide) as being without effect. In 1970, Hollmén[5] in Oulu published his experiences with lumbar epidural anesthesia as a method of obstetric pain relief. At about the same time, Belfrage[6] and Raabe[7] started a series of investigations regarding obstetric pain relief with bupivacaine at the Karolinska Hospital in Stockholm, and Zador[8] correspondingly studied lidocaine in Uppsala. The demonstration of the evident need for effective obstetric pain relief in at least one-third of all parturients and the scientific investigations showing that obstetric pain relief can be accomplished without harmful maternal or neonatal effects were the two main factors that created a very rapidly increasing demand for an effective obstetric anesthetic service during the 1970s in Scandinavia.

A political debate regarding a woman's right to be given adequate pain relief during labor started in the beginning of the 1970s, and representatives from various women's organizations were very active in arguing for expanding resources for the management of pain during labor. The issue became politically important and, in 1975, the Swedish parliament decided that every women in labor had the right to receive adequate alleviation of pain. This decision was, in a sense, rather premature since the resources required for obstetric analgesia on a 24 h basis were not available in the majority of the Swedish hospitals at that time. Since then, however, staffing, education and other resources have been improved and, as shown in Table 81.2, the various forms of analgesia during delivery reached their maximal incidence around 1985. Since then the use of obstetric pain relief has decreased rather significantly, reflecting a strong current public opinion that delivery and pregnancy are normal processes which should not be interfered with by various obstetric interventions such as obstetric analgesia. Table 81.2, which is derived from a database generated at the Swedish National Board of Health and Welfare, shows that in 1989 around 17% of all women undergoing vaginal delivery received epidural or paracervical block, while 25% received a pudendal block at the end of delivery. Opioids (mainly meperidine) were used in around one-third of all deliveries, while nitrous oxide was used in 60% of all deliveries.

ROLE OF MIDWIVES

Most of the routine obstetric analgesia will be given by midwives. The midwife can, at her own discretion, give 100–200 mg of meperidine during an uncomplicated labor. She can also give nitrous oxide in normal labor. For delivery, a midwife can decide to administer a bilateral pudendal block, which will also be used for the suturing of a perineal rupture or a perineotomy (episiotomy).

A Swedish midwife will have the following formal and practical training. All are initially registered nurses, which requires 2 years of training. To become a midwife requires one further year of training. During this last year there will be 8 h of theoretical training in anesthesia, after which 2 weeks will be spent in a department of anesthesia under the supervision of a nurse anesthetist or an anesthesiologist. Most of the training will concentrate on obstetric analgesia, epidural block, anesthesia for cesarean delivery, etc. The trainee midwife will also spend about 20 weeks working practically in an obstetric department. During this time period, the trainee will deliver, under supervision, about 50 patients and will also, if needed, give these patients analgesia with meperidine, nitrous oxide and pudendal block.

ROLE OF OBSTETRICIAN

The overall responsibility for analgesia (policy-making, etc.) rests with the obstetricians, and the midwives will work under this directive. The obstetrician will be directly responsible for providing analgesia in complicated or pathologic cases. It will also be the responsibility of the obstetrician to order the administration of major regional anesthesia. Epidural block is given by the anesthesiologist after consultation with the obstetrician. Paracervical block will be be given by the obstetrician.

The training of the obstetrician follows the following format. All doctors receive 2 months of training in obstetrics and gynecology, during which they attend one or two theoretical lectures on obstetric anesthesia, and between 1 and 2 weeks will be spent in an obstetrics department as practical training. Later on, during specialized training in obstetrics and gynecology, additional training in obstetric anesthesia will be more advanced. There is a basic requirement of 3 years training in an accredited department of obstetrics and gynecology and 1 year of training in an accredited surgical department for an obstetrician/gynecologist. There will be 1 week of intensive theoretical training in perinatal medicine, which is followed by an examination. The specialist in obstetrics and gynecology will also spend 6 months training in an anesthetic department. During this period there will be ample training in obstetric anesthesia, from both a theoretical and a practical point of view.

PARACERVICAL BLOCK

Paracervical block has played a rather important role in obstetric pain alleviation in both Sweden and in Finland. Because of its easy administration it quickly increased in popularity, especially in certain Swedish hospitals. As is seen from Table 81.2 the maximum incidence of paracervical block was recorded around 1985, after which it has decreased in popularity. The well-known side-effect of fetal bradycardia, which occurs in about 5–15% of deliveries and which can occasionally lead to fetal damage or death, contributed to a decrease in its use. During the years 1985–88 there was on average one case of severe fetal damage or fetal death annually reported to the Swedish Board of Health and Welfare. Since around 6000–8000 paracervical blocks were annually performed in Sweden during the same time period the frequency of severe fetal damage or death was thus 1 per 5000–10 000 blocks. It is doubtful whether this represents an acceptable risk limit, and the decreasing number of paracervical blocks performed in Sweden during the last few years reflects increasing support for this opinion.

Table 81.2 Frequency of various methods for obstetric pain relief in Sweden 1975–89 (in percent of the total number of vaginal deliveries per year) (Source: National Birth database, Swedish Medical Board of Health and Welfare)

	1975	1980	1985	1987	1988	1989
Opioids (mainly meperidine)	Uncertain data	Uncertain data	49	45	41	33
Nitrous oxide	64	52	52	54	56	57
Paracervical block	4	9	12	9	8	6
Pudendal block	53	70	62	49	39	24
Epidural block	2	10	16	13	12	11

ANTENATAL CARE

An effective and well-organized antenatal care system in Sweden is an important major factor in the provision of adequate pain relief. At the regular antenatal visits mothers are informed by midwives about the available pain relief methods and usually also visit the delivery unit where they are going to be delivered to become familiar with the delivery room and the nitrous oxide apparatus. Through the antenatal care system, high-risk deliveries will also be identified and the handling of the delivery will be planned and discussed by obstetricians, neonatologists and anesthesiologists.

REFERENCES

1. Risholm L 1950 Conduction anesthesia in obstetrics. Acta Soc Med Upsal 55: 323
2. Bonica J J, Backup C E, Anderson D et al 1957 Peridural block, analysis of 3637 cases and a review. Anesthesiology 18: 723
3. Hellman K 1965 Epidural anesthesia in obstetrics: a second look at 26127 cases. Canad Anaesth Soc J 12: 398
4. Lind B 1970 Obstetrical anesthesia in Norway. Acta Anaesthesiol Scand Suppl 37 186
5. Hollmén A 1970 Lumbar epidural analgesia as an obstetric analgesic method. Acta Anaesthesiol Scand Suppl 37: 251
6. Belfrage P 1975 Lumbar epidural blockade with bupivacaine. A pharmacological and clinical study. Academic dissertation. Karolinska Institute
7. Raabe N 1976 Lumbar epidural analgesia for vaginal delivery. Academic dissertation. Karolinska Institute
8. Zador G 1974 Continuous lumbar peridural analgesia and pudendal block for vaginal delivery. Effects on the mother, fetus and uterine activity using lidocaine in different dosage forms. Academic dissertation. Uppsala University

PART E
ITALY

E. Margaria E. Gollo

The most recent guidelines regarding health care provision in Italy are contained in a ministerial decree of 13 September 1988. Hospital organization should conform to a model in which distinct specialties are allocated a fixed number of beds.

Allocation of resources to regions is based on 6.5 beds for every 1000 inhabitants, assuming an average bed occupancy of not less than 70–75%. Obstetric and gynecologic specialties must have a minimum number of staff, below which the management of the department becomes uneconomic.

Obstetric and gynecologic units defined by the ministerial decree as those serving a large population must be organized as model-type unit of 32 beds. Each unit, which has an average of at least 600 deliveries per year (and in any case no fewer than 300), is provided with five physicians, 17 nurses and three–six midwives, depending on workload. There is no distinction between obstetric and gynecologic units. Anesthetic services should be organized by the medical and administrative heads because this service does not conform to the organizational model.

Anomalies are to be found in the organization of schools specializing in anesthesiology. For example, a doctor can administer anesthesia, as long as he is not the head of his department, even without a special qualification. To achieve such a qualification requires 4 years' study, not necessarily including a course in obstetric anesthesia: such a course is included in the curriculum of anesthesiology schools, but each school director can choose whether or not to include it.

A problem with analyzing the organization of the obstetric service in Italy is that administratively there is no functional difference between beds in obstetric units and those in gynecologic units, and this makes it difficult to gather statistical information. To find out how many beds are used for obstetrics or gynecology the information must be obtained directly from each hospital. From information we have gathered from many hospitals in the country we have calculated that about 40% of the total number of beds in obstetric and gynecologic units are used for obstetrics. Based on this indirect but reasonable approximation we corrected the information obtained from the Ministry of Health.

It is also necessary to consider differences in the quality of health care in the hospitals we studied. Only in large cities are there major specialized centers as well as university departments. Much more common are provincial hospitals catering to all medical and surgical specialties. Recently, many obstetric departments in these small

Table 81.3 Structure of obstetric and gynecologic care in the Italian regions (Source: Ministry of Health, 1988)

Region	Number of units	Patients	Hospital beds	Average stay (days)	Rate of utilization (%)
Piedmont	56	90 071	2206	5.4	60.0
Aosta Valley	1	2404	60	6.3	69.0
Lombardy	110	203 445	4938	5.8	63.1
Trentino	15	20 109	542	6.0	64.2
Venetia	57	90 904	2705	6.5	59.6
Friuli	17	29 792	756	5.1	55.2
Liguria	25	37 351	1039	5.6	55.5
Emilia-Romagna	47	73 000	2040	5.6	55.1
Tuscany	49	80 162	1833	6.0	54.8
Umbria	17	18 948	572	7.2	58.3
Marche	27	27 411	867	6.5	56.4
Latium	62	87 741	2126	5.9	66.5
Abruzzo	20	27 258	925	6.8	54.8
Molise	6	9047	239	7.5	77.9
Campania	51	75 127	1955	5.9	62.9
Apulia	63	104 029	2866	6.1	60.8
Basilicata	11	12 654	363	6.9	66.2
Calabria	35	43 327	1397	5.8	49.0
Sicily	72	96 173	2602	5.2	53.4
Sardinia	18	29 814	840	6.6	54.4

hospitals have closed because of the declining birth rate. It is not cost-effective to maintain an obstetric unit undertaking fewer than 300 deliveries a year.

Table 81.3 shows that there are no regional differences between the length of stay in obstetric and gynecologic units and that underutilization of existing hospital facilities is common. In order to obtain more accurate figures it was necessary to amend the aggregate ministerial data to take into account responses to direct questioning of hospitals.

Table 81.4 shows a comparison of the female population (15–44 years) and live newborns with the number of obstetric and gynecologic beds by region. It can be seen that hospital facilities are equally distributed throughout the major Italian regions but that such facilities are used more in the central and northern regions of Italy, probably for cultural and social reasons.

Perinatal mortality in Italy is higher than in the rest of Europe (Fig. 81.1), although the rate has fallen from 31.2 per thousand in 1970 to 13.2 per thousand in 1988. Again there is a regional imbalance, with the perinatal mortality rate being higher in the south of Italy than in the north and center (Table 81.5 and Fig. 81.2). Perinatal mortality is a very important indicator of the quality of obstetric services.

The safety and efficiency of delivery must be guaranteed in both small hospitals and large specialized centers.

Table 81.4 Comparison of obstetric and gynecologic beds and female resident population (A) and live newborns (B) (%) (Source: Elaboration of Istat data)

	(A)	(B)
Italy	0.9	21.37
Center and north	0.99	25.92
South	0.91	16.43

Regional and general anesthesia must only be administered in the presence of highly trained medical and paramedical staff, and apparatus for immediate maternal and neonatal resuscitation must be on hand. The availability of an anesthesiologist and obstetrician and neonatologist in the obstetric unit not only ensures optimum obstetric care and pain relief but also provides a greater margin of safety in the recognition and prompt treatment of complications.

Ideally, units undertaking more than 1000 deliveries per year should have the following facilities:

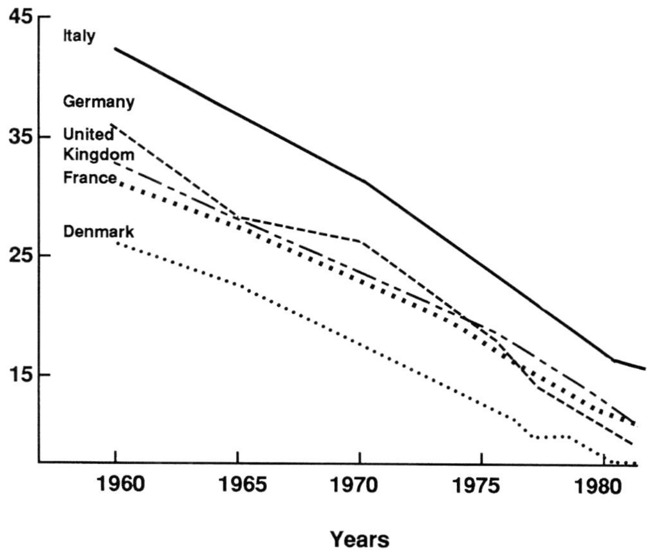

Fig. 81.1 Perinatal mortality in Europe from 1960 to 1980. (From ref. 1)

Table 81.5 Perinatal mortality in Italy, 1988 (Source: Istat data)

	Age less than 1 day	Age 1–6 days	Total	Rate*
Italy	1782	1663	3445	12.4
Center and north	830	661	1491	10.6
South	952	1002	1954	14.5

* Deaths before 1 week per 1000 newborns.

1. An anesthetic induction room containing two beds that can be used to perform regional anesthesia for vaginal delivery. The room must contain equipment to monitor cardiovascular and respiratory function and cardiotocographs to monitor the fetus and uterine activity at regular, frequent intervals.

2. Delivery boxes containing all the equipment required for administering general anesthesia and for maternal and neonatal resuscitation including:

a. equipment for the placement of intravenous catheters (peripheral or central venous);

b. drugs for intravenous administration: parasympathetic antagonists, sympathomimetic agents, sympathomimetic amines, barbiturates, opioid analgesics, steroids, uterine stimulants, neuromuscular blocking agents, premedication drugs, sedatives and neuroleptics, intravenous induction agents, volatile anesthetics, cardiovascular drugs, electrolytes and infusion fluids;

c. equipment necessary for maintaining the airway: aspirators, nasogastric and oral and nasal tracheal tubes of various sizes and possibly a fiber-optic bronchoscope for difficult intubation;

d. anesthesia respirators and monitors, which must be checked every day and before every anesthetic procedure.

3. In every room there must be a neonatal unit including an infrared heating unit for the primary resuscitation of the newborn. An intravenous set for the umbilical vein must be available, and an incubator in case of transfer to another department.

4. An operating theater for elective or emergency cesarean delivery.

5. Hematologic laboratory facilities available 24 h a day.

6. A blood transfusion center with the capacity to undertake autologous or homologous transfusions.

The personnel in the obstetric unit must be highly specialized: for every 8-h shift there must be one anesthesiologist, one obstetrician, one neonatologist, one nurse anesthetist, one midwife, one surgical nurse, three general

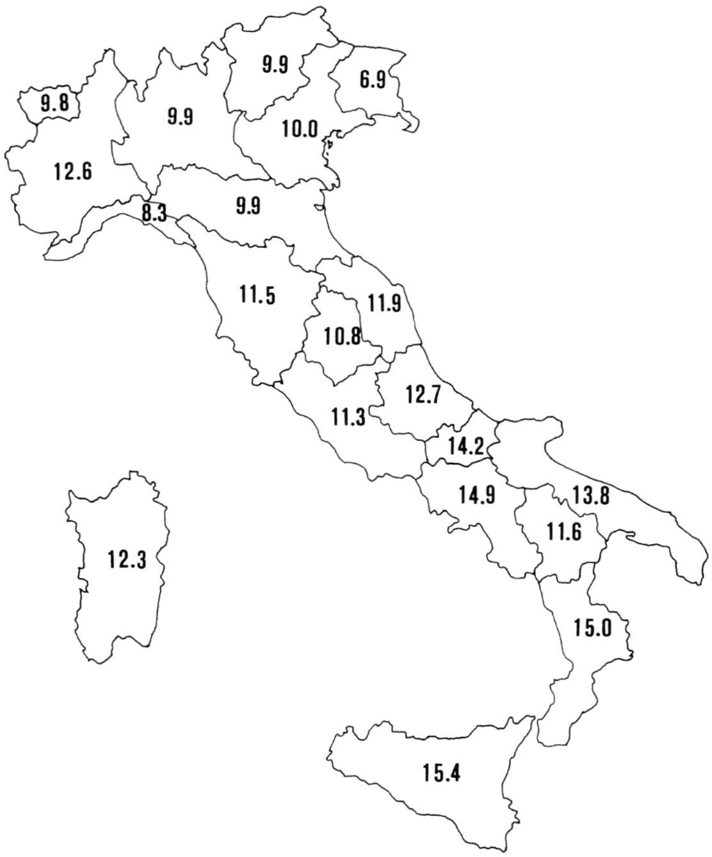

Fig. 81.2 Perinatal mortality in Italy, 1987. (Source: Istat data, 1989.)

nurses, one laboratory physician and one laboratory technician. With three shifts a day and taking into account rest periods and holidays each of the numbers above should be multiplied by 8.

To provide an adequate obstetric anesthetic service we suggest that the following measures should be adopted:

• Training of physicians. The medical curriculum should include a course on obstetric anesthesia, as should specialist post-graduate courses on obstetrics and gynecology.

• Antenatal education. During preparatory classes mothers must be informed by an anesthesiologist of the anesthetic possibilities and their advantages and disadvantages.

• There should in every hospital be a consulting room in which pregnant patients can receive check-ups and further information to help them decide if they wish to receive regional or general anesthesia. The patient should receive two visits from the anesthesiologist. At the first visit, about week 15–20 of pregnancy, basic blood investigations are performed and others requested if necessary. This first meeting is important to determine whether there are any physical problems masked by the usual changes in pregnancy. The second meeting should take place between weeks 30 and 35. On this occasion, as well as checking the patient's physical condition, the topic of analgesia during labor can be introduced.

• During the delivery an anesthesiologist should be with the patient at all times and do all that is possible for the comfort of the mother and newborn.

REFERENCES

1. Pachi A, Astrei G 1985 Tutela della salute della gestante e del concepito. Acta Medica, Rome
2. Istat 1989 Annvario Statistico Italiano

PART F
FRANCE

D. Benhamou B. O'Kelly

The organization of an obstetric anesthetic unit is of major importance since parturients are usually healthy young patients for whom delivery is generally a happy event and, if complications occur, they may have tragic consequences. In this context, the medical team has to find the proper balance between an excessive medical and technologic presence and a 'patient-friendly' environment. At first glance, the main aim of a well-organized obstetric unit is to improve conditions of safety for parturients. This implies that risks have been defined and can be managed. The management of obstetric risks cannot be based solely on personnel and technical facilities but requires the existence of an organizational structure in order to create and maintain links between the different elements of the structure (Fig. 81.3). Unfortunately, in France, as in most other occidental countries, the situation is far from optimum.

THE MATERNITY AND THE MEDICAL TEAM

In the ideal maternity unit here there should be a certain number of deliveries per year, since below a critical number the medical and nursing staff will inevitably be less experienced, fewer in number and also less often present if their commitment to the unit is on a part-time basis. Moreover, it is usual that the larger the obstetric unit, the greater the technical means available to reduce maternal and neonatal mortality. Also, the presence in the maternity unit 24 h a day of obstetricians, pediatricians and anesthesiologists seems mandatory (especially when high-risks pregnancies are managed) and more readily achieved in larger units. Grenom and Lacore[1] in a recent survey of all French maternity units, have shown that a senior obstetrician was in the maternity unit around the clock only in 1 out of 2 university teaching hospitals, in 47% of private medical centers and in 19% of general hospitals. Very similar percentages were obtained when the authors looked at the anesthetic coverage for obstetric anesthesia.

Another necessary component of the ideal maternity unit is a recovery room organized to accept pregnant patients as well as post-operative or post-delivery patients 24 h a day.[2] No specific data relating to the recovery period of obstetric patients in France are available but the general French survey performed from 1978 to 1981[3] as well as the Enquiry in England and Wales[4] both confirm the importance of the recovery period.

A less than ideal situation can be found by looking at the inappropriate geographic 'mismatching' of maternity units

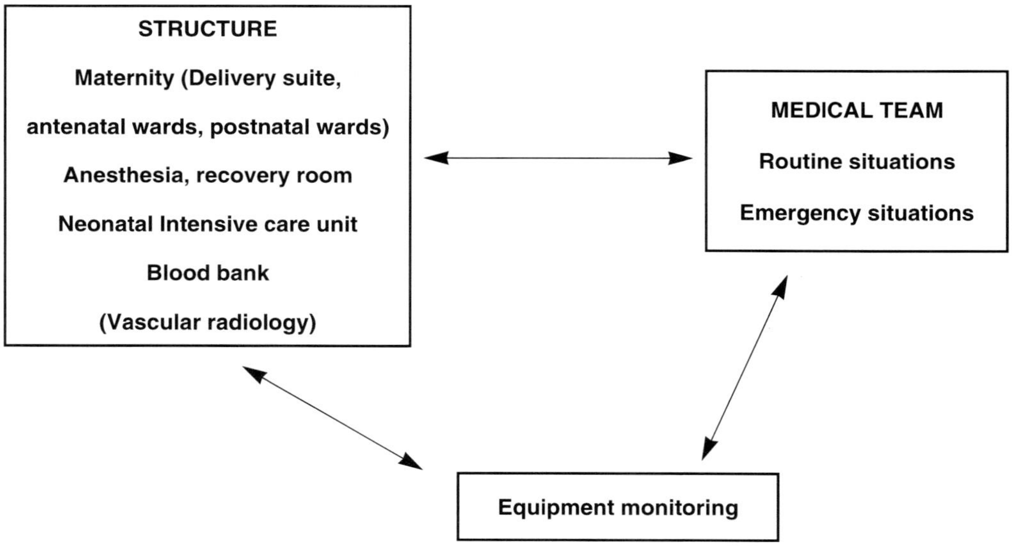

Fig. 81.3 Conditions of safety.

caring for high-risk pregnancies and neonatal intensive care units. In Paris, for example, only 3 out of the 12 maternity units that have more than 2000 deliveries per year are located in a medical center containing a neonatal intensive care unit.

Finally, when considering the organization of an ideal maternity unit, the presence of an efficient blood bank (hemorrhage remains one of the leading causes of maternal death) and of a vascular radiologist who is able to perform hypogastric artery embolization at all times is recommended.[5]

ORGANIZATION AND MEDICAL ACTIVITIES OF THE MEDICAL TEAM

The permanent presence of anesthesiologists in the maternity unit offers many advantages. By regular discussions with obstetricians and pediatricians, a better standard of care will be obtained. By increasing the number of preanesthetic visits during pregnancy, better information and an improved care will be offered at the time of labor and delivery, especially when dealing with anxiety and doubts concerning epidural anesthesia. French anesthesiologists working in obstetric anesthesia often consider that a ratio of one anesthesiologist for 500 deliveries would be optimal. This has not been substantiated by any study, but calculations indicate that this ratio can be considered as a reasonable goal to reach. Finally, the presence of experienced anesthesiologists will give them time to teach residents, with special emphasis being placed on anticipating and treating different serious obstetric emergencies. In a recent national survey, a questionnaire was sent to all French anesthesiologists to investigate the efficacy of procedures used in the prophylaxis against aspiration of gastric contents.[6] Of the 297 obstetric anesthesiologists who responded, only 40% were able to describe adequately the technique of applying cricoid pressure. This percentage was not different between university teaching hospitals and smaller units and was surprisingly similar between physicians using the technique routinely and those not, suggesting that a major place remains for teaching.[7]

Finally, improved monitoring of patients during cesarean deliveries remains a legitimate goal which must be reached without delay. Like many other societies, the French Society of Anesthesia and Intensive Care has recently published its own recommendations for monitoring during operations.[8] These recommendations are very similar to those of the other countries.[9] Specific recommendations for monitoring during labor or during major conduction anesthesia have recently been made available.[10]

In conclusion, with our increasing participation in obstetric activities, greater means (human and technical) are required. These new needs should be rapidly recognized by the French government in order to place obstetric anesthesia where it should be, i.e. as an interesting and important medical activity caring for young healthy patients in order to minimize maternal and neonatal morbidity and mortality and provide adequate pain relief during labor.

REFERENCES

1. Grenom A, Lacore V 1987 Conclusion: résultats de l'enquête prospective sur les conditions de l'analgésie obstétricale en 1985. In: Arnette (ed) Médecine périnatale. Lyon, pp 55–62
2. Harris AP 1990 The obstetric recovery room. Postanesthesia care unit problems. Anesthesiol Clin N Am 8: 311–322
3. Hatton F, Tiret L, Maujol L, N' Doye P, Vourc'h G, Desmonts J M, Otteni J C, Scherpereel P 1983 Enquête épidémiologique sur les anesthésies. Premiers résultats. Annales Françaises d'Anesthésie et de Réanimation 2: 333–385
4. Department of Health Report 1989 on Confidential Enquiries into maternal deaths in England and Wales 1982–1984. HMSO London
5. Henk H J, Scattenkerk M E, De Vries J E et al 1987 Non-surgical treatment of pelvic hemorrhage in obstetric and gynecologic patients. Crit Care Med 15: 534–535
6. Benhamou D 1993 French obstetric anaesthetists and acid aspiration prophylaxis. Eur J Anaesthesiol 10: 27–32
7. Wraight W J, Chamney A R, Howells T H 1983 The determination of an effective cricoid pressure. Anaesthesia 38: 461–466
8. Société Française d'Anesthésie et de Réanimation 1989 Recommandations concernant la surveillance des patients en cours d'anesthésie
9. Winter A, Spence A A 1990 An International consensus on monitoring. Br J Anaesth 64: 263–266
10. Société Française d'Anesthésie et de Réanimation 1992 Recommandations concernant la pratique de l'analgésie Obstetricale

PART G
USA

G. W. Ostheimer

QUALITY OF CARE

The regionalization of perinatal care has produced an increased demand on the anesthesiologist to participate actively in obstetric care. Fewer new facilities are constructed because they have to receive approval from a board granting a certificate of need; as a result, existing facilities are either closed or combined and upgraded to provide care for the uncomplicated to the most complex high-risk pregnancy. Regardless of the level of obstetric care, the quality of anesthetic practice in the delivery suite must be the same as that provided in the operating suite of the same institution. There cannot be two levels of anesthetic care in the same institution. The parturient and her fetus, soon to be a neonate, need and demand the highest quality of anesthetic care available to any patient in that particular institution.

Location

The anesthesiologist responsible for the organization of the anesthetic services in a new hospital or facility should help coordinate the location of the delivery suite in an easily accessible area of the institution close to the admitting and laboratory facilities and equally accessible to the operating suite; ideally, it should be on the same floor. The availability of anesthesiologists is often dependent on the accessibility of the delivery rooms. The transitional nursery should be immediately adjacent to the obstetric suite with easy access to the neonatal intensive care unit. Depending on the construction of the hospital, it would be expedient to have the regular nursery and the post-partum unit on the same floor; however, in many institutions, this may be impossible. The prepartum fetomaternal intensive care unit should be part of or immediately adjacent to the obstetric suite. A schematic approach to the logistic problem is shown in Figure 81.4.

DETERMINING MATERNITY BED NEED

The overall number of beds in a maternity unit cannot be determined by a simple formula. The number of adult beds must include those in the fetomaternal intensive care unit, labor area and post-partum units. The neonatal beds include those in the transitional, regular and neonatal intensive care units. Each hospital must have its bed capacity calculated according to the size and geographic location of the institution, population served, accessibility,

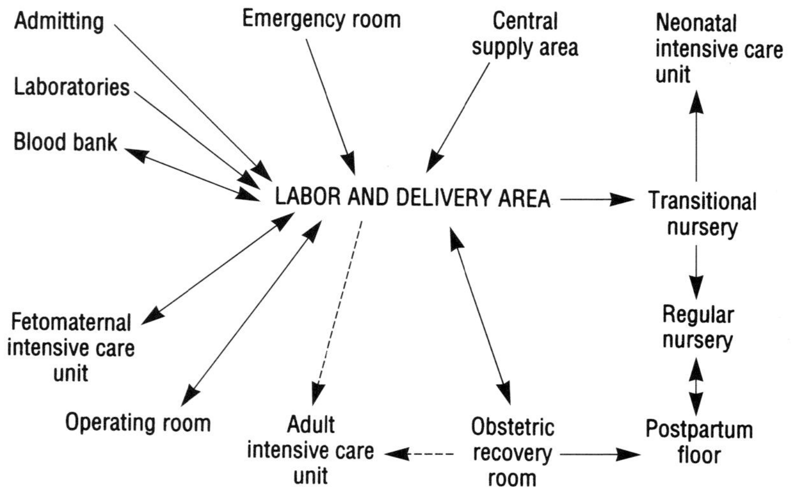

Fig. 81.4

average length of stay, population projections, economic factors and regionalization requirements.

As one might expect, each state has its own formula for determining bed need. One of the early approaches was based on a set number of beds per thousand population, adjusted for the density of the particular population. Later improvements focused on future populations and suggested minimum utilization standards based on an 80% overall occupancy. This plan attempted to calculate total bed need for the future on a current demand basis and did not take into account the need by service.

Service-specific formulas have been recently developed. The Public Health Service formula[1] calculates an average daily census for a maternity unit by dividing the projected census days by 365. This average daily census is then divided by the expected occupancy rate to obtain the number of beds needed. This formula can only be applied when patient turnover is extremely regular and the patients do not require urgent treatment so that their admissions can be scheduled. Neither of these conditions can be applied to maternity services, in which patients' arrivals are unpredictable and unscheduled. Therefore, this approach is being replaced by another formula based on the principle that patients should have equal access to beds regardless of a facility's size.

This translates into providing each unit with sufficient beds that the probability (determined by the Poisson distribution) of all beds being filled simultaneously is kept below an acceptable threshold. For larger units, the Poisson distribution can be approximated by the more convenient computer-adapted normal distribution. Thus, the number of beds required to ensure a specific probability of immediate patient access is taken from a simple formula using only the average daily census and a constant derived from the normal probability distribution. Unfortunately, maternity services do not satisfy the assumptions about length of stay that lead to a Poisson-distributed bed census and the normal distribution is not accurate for smaller services.

Fortunately, mathematical models developed by statistical theorists can be used instead for maternity services analysis. The 'finite-state, birth–death' queuing model has been used to plan emergency services and applies directly to maternity services. It assumes simply that patient arrivals are unpredictable and unscheduled; it imposes no restrictions on the distribution of length of stay and it assumes that the number of beds is fixed. From information on average patient arrival rates, average lengths of stay and number of beds, the queuing model will predict occupancy, or service, levels. The bed-need predictions of the complicated queuing model for specific service levels can be accurately approximated by a simple formula involving two constants, K_1 and K_2 (which depend on the service level), and the average daily census presented by the maternity unit. The higher the service level, the greater the cost and need for beds. The constants for the 99% service level are $K_1 = 0.91$ and $K_2 = 2.6$; and for 95% service level $K_1 = 0.84$, $K_2 = 2.1$.

Sample calculations using the queuing formula for a 100-patient average daily census (ADC) are as follows:

Beds needed for a 99% service level:

$$= K_1 \times \text{ADC} + K_2 \times \sqrt{\text{ADC}}$$
$$= 0.91 \times 100 + 2.6 \times \sqrt{100}$$
$$= 0.91 \times 100 + 2.6 \times 10$$
$$= 91 + 26$$
$$= 117 \text{ beds}$$

Beds needed for a 95% service level:

$$= \text{K}_1 \times \text{ADC} + K_2 \times \sqrt{\text{ADC}}$$

$$= 0.84 \times 100 + 2.1 \times \sqrt{100}$$
$$= 0.84 \times 100 + 2.1 \times 10$$
$$= 84 + 21$$
$$= 105 \text{ beds}$$

The use of the queuing system for establishing maternity bed need will result in nearly equal service levels for all sizes of maternity units and considerable cost savings, especially with larger maternity units, because utilization will be more accurately predicted.[1]

INNOVATIONS

It is not my purpose to suggest architectural arrangements for the construction of the labor and delivery area; common sense dictates that the delivery rooms should be immediately adjacent to the labor rooms. In new facilities, several of the labor rooms should be convertible to delivery rooms with the inclusion of the appropriate beds that can function as delivery tables. This innovation will help foster the concept of family-oriented maternity care in which all the facilities of the institution, such as blood banks, laboratories and intensive care units, are immediately available but the parturient can deliver in a home-like environment, which may be more conducive to parent – infant bonding. Some or all of the delivery rooms should be convertible to major operating rooms for cesarean deliveries and post-partum surgical procedures. A minor operating room may be included for obstetric-related gynecologic procedures such as dilation and curettage. Regardless of the details of the arrangement of the delivery suite, one fact is clear: every full anesthetizing location must have the equipment necessary to provide complete anesthetic care from simple monitoring functions to full-scale anesthesia with the appropriate physiologic monitors for any obstetric emergency.

LABOR ROOM

What considerations should be made for anesthesia in a labor room? The amount of equipment needed depends on whether anesthesia will be inducted in a combination labor–cesarean delivery room or in a room used only for labor and vaginal delivery. In the latter situation, wall outlets must accommodate oxygen, suction, sphygmomanometer, emergency call system and adequate lighting. I personally would like to see non-invasive arterial blood pressure monitors, pulse oximeters and ECG apparatus in every labor room. Hangers for intravenous bottles can be part of the labor room or attached to the labor bed. The labor bed must be capable of being placed in a head-up or head-down position. Suction catheters and oxygen delivery systems must be in each labor room and ready for immediate use.

If the labor room is also to function as a cesarean delivery room, and therefore as a surgical location, the usual equipment found in a regular operating delivery room must be available. Compact anesthesia machines and wall-mounted cabinets can provide the essential equipment, while their presence can be unobtrusive to the occupants of the labor room. Although an electrocardiograph is not mandatory for each labor–vaginal delivery room, an emergency cart must be immediately available in the labor area that will contain the standard drugs and equipment for emergency care. It should also contain an electrocardiograph, intra-arterial transducer, central venous pressure equipment, a defibrillator and a cardiac resuscitation board. Uterine displacement equipment is mandatory in each labor and delivery room. If regional blocks are initiated in the labor room, essential anesthetic and resuscitative equipment must be on a cart brought into the room before the block is performed.

In my opinion, the obstetric service should provide an electronic fetal monitor for each patient in labor. Electronic fetal heart rate monitoring provides essential information not available via auscultation, because few labor attendants – physicians, midwives or nurses – ever listen to the entire contraction cycle. One cannot be aware of variations in fetal heart rate unless one listens from the beginning of one contraction to the beginning of the next contraction. Auscultation of the fetal heart rate between contractions will miss late decelerations and variable decelerations; it will identify only the very ominous prolonged late decelerations that demand immediate intervention, and perhaps cesarean delivery, unless vaginal delivery is imminent. Although 'full-cycle' auscultation has been shown to be adequate monitoring in comparative studies, its use necessitates 'one-on-one' nursing, which is a luxury few hospitals can afford. Therefore, I do not see a return to auscultation in place of continuous electronic fetal heart rate monitoring.

For maternal monitoring during regional anesthesia in a labor-delivery room, I would like to see the development of a noninvasive blood pressure finger cuff to be worn on one finger accompanied by a pulse oximeter worn on another finger of the same hand. Designs attempted to date by various companies have been cumbersome and unreliable.

DELIVERY ROOM

The delivery room must be equipped to provide appropriate anesthesia for vaginal or abdominal (cesarean) delivery, post-partum tubal ligation and any emergency obstetric surgery. The same quality of anesthetic equipment available in the general operating suite must be available in the delivery room.

Modern delivery rooms should have piped-in nitrous oxide and oxygen provided through an overhead unit to prevent personnel from becoming entangled in coils of tubing. Suction is most efficient if aided by gravity and led to floor bottles. There is no need to provide explosive gases in the delivery area since all procedures can be done with a variety of nonexplosive agents. The expense of conductive flooring and appropriate grounding is excessive and not justified for new or refurbished areas; most important, delivery room personnel today are unfamiliar with the precautions necessary when explosive agents are in use.

An automated noninvasive blood pressure monitor, pulse oximeter, capnograph or mass spectrometer, temperature probe, electrocardiograph and ventilator should be mounted on the anesthetic machine, which should be equipped with fail-safe devices, an oxygen analyzer and precision vaporizers. The availability of central venous pressure, arterial blood pressure and pulmonary arterial blood pressure transducers would be useful. A fetal heart rate monitor must be available. The immediate availability of all necessary fluids, infusion apparatus, nerve stimulator and other standard anesthetic equipment is essential. Scavenging devices are necessary in all anesthetizing locations to minimize the contamination of the environment by trace gases. Endotracheal intubation utilizing rapid induction and cricoid pressure is mandatory if general anesthesia is administered for vaginal or cesarean delivery. Depending on the individual needs of the institution, disposable or reusable inhalation equipment may be selected. Disposable regional anesthesia trays are recommended since aseptic meningitis appears to be related to turnover of the hospital personnel preparing the kits, because inexperienced workers may deviate from appropriate cleaning technique.

An anesthetic supply area should be easily accessible and should contain additional equipment including blood warmers and a refrigerator to keep perishable medications and cold intravenous solutions to administer during a hyperthermic crisis. This area should also have a designated shelf for specialized equipment boxes that will contain appropriate equipment and drugs to deal with difficult intubation (including fiber-optic endoscopy equipment, materials for transtracheal jet ventilation and cricothyroidotomy/tracheotomy kits), malignant hyperthermia and cardiac arrest (thoracotomy kit).

PROCEDURE ROOM

It would be to the advantage of the anesthesia team if a large room (minimum 400 square feet) were included in the design of the delivery suite. This area would allow the administration of multiple epidural anesthetics simultaneously, particularly in preparation for cesarean delivery. This procedure room should be fully stocked with the appropriate anesthesia equipment, including an anesthetic machine with appropriate monitoring equipment, intravenous fluids and administration sets, block trays, wall outlets for oxygen and suction and electric fetal monitors.

An efficient labor and delivery unit demands the services of the anesthetic care team coupled with skilled obstetric nursing care. Often, the labor and delivery nurses are the first to observe hypotension and fetal heart rate changes and should initiate appropriate therapy at once. This may include increasing the rate of intravenous fluid administration, giving oxygen by mask, placing the parturient in the lateral position, discontinuing the oxytocin infusion, correlating the monitoring of the uterine contractions and the fetal heart rate and notifying the obstetric and anesthetic care team about the problem.

TRANSITIONAL NURSERY

The labor and delivery suite should be on the same floor and physically connected to the neonatal intensive care unit and the regular nurseries by a transitional nursery. This area would contain bassinets to observe neonates with potential problems and incubators to facilitate transfer to the specialized acute care area. This area would provide acute intensive care from the moment the neonate arrives (minutes after delivery) until he or she has stabilized sufficiently to allow transfer to an acute care area. A small number of intensive care beds should be available at all times in the transitional nursery. Radiant heaters are essential since one of the major problems after delivery is the loss of temperature in the neonate. This factor alone can precipitate the continuation or recurrence of acidosis and hypoxia and lead to persistent fetal circulation.

RECOVERY AREA

A recovery room or area in the labor and delivery suite is essential in order to allow close observation of the mother for the first few hours after delivery. It should be immediately adjacent to the delivery and obstetric operating rooms. Ideally, there should be a separate nursing station for the recovery area, which should be as fully equipped as the post-anesthetic and surgical recovery area. Accessibility to the adult intensive care areas is desirable (see Fig. 81.3). Minimal facilities include wall-mounted oxygen and suction outlets, direct and indirect lighting, sphygmomanometers, pulse oximeters, curtains to divide the room into individual private areas, routine and emergency drugs, cardiopulmonary resuscitation cart, and cardiac monitor with defibrillator. A large pleasant room is preferable to small cramped cubicles. Curtains will give the parturient, father and neonate a chance to interact in a private area without diminishing the effectiveness of the nursing care by making observation difficult. The number of recovery room beds should equal one-third of the number of labor beds in a busy service.

Family-oriented obstetric care may allow post-partum recovery in the combination labor – delivery room or labor room if nursing coverage is sufficient. Recovery area personnel should be qualified to provide the intensive care that may be necessary in routine or emergency situations. Continuous teaching and monitoring by the obstetric anesthesia service is necessary to maintain a high standard of care.

ADMINISTRATION

The obstetric anesthesia section should have office facilities adjacent to the labor and delivery area. A conference room with teaching facilities and audiovisual equipment should be available and can be shared with the departments of obstetrics and neonatology. On-call rooms must be adjacent to the obstetric suite so that there can be an immediate response to an emergency call.

PERSONNEL

Determining need

The requirements for anesthetic personnel in the labor and delivery area are difficult to ascertain. Coverage may range from the 'on-call' situation, in which the anesthesiologist responds to the needs of the service from the surgical suite, to anesthetic personnel who are in attendance in the labor and delivery suite 24 h a day. It would be very difficult to contrast our situation at the Brigham and Women's Hospital with any other hospital. At present, we have approximately 10 000 deliveries a year. We are an academic department of anesthesia that trains fellows and residents in obstetric anesthesia.

Anesthesia care team

Although the number of available anesthesiologists is increasing throughout the USA, I do not believe there are adequate numbers at this time to provide 24 h-a-day coverage in the labor and delivery areas throughout the level III hospitals in the USA, let alone the level II or I hospitals. (A level III hospital is able to handle any obstetric or neonatal problem and has the appropriate personnel available 24 h a day; level II hospitals can offer advanced but not all encompassing perinatal care and level I hospitals offer routine obstetric and neonatal care.) Therefore, our initial premise in providing obstetric anesthesia care is the appropriate utilization of the anesthesia care team. Depending on the institution, the anesthesia care team may involve anesthesiologists only up to and including anesthesiologists and residents and/or nurse anesthetists. At the Brigham and Women's Hospital, the anesthesia care teams include staff anesthesiologists, fellows in obstetric anesthesia, residents on their obstetric anesthesia rotation, and, on occasion, certified nurse anesthetists. All types of obstetric pain relief are available, with the exception of inhalation analgesia, which has not been used in our institution in more than 25 years. We do not see any need to utilize an archaic form of pain relief while jeopardizing the mother's health if she has had parenteral sedatives and opioids that in combination with inhaled analgesics may lead to a general anesthetic state, with the possibility of regurgitation and aspiration into the unprotected airway. Paracervical block is an excellent technique that is utilized for gynecologic procedures; however, it has not been used on our obstetric service for pain relief in more than 15 years.

Coverage in the labor and delivery area is provided by a minimum of one staff anesthesiologist 24 h a day, supplemented with a combination of fellows, residents and nurse anesthetists. Obviously, this is reasonable both for patient care and on a financial basis since we are administering anesthesia to approximately 70% of our total number of deliveries.

Is it possible to provide adequate anesthesia care in the smaller units throughout the country? I believe that adequate obstetric anesthesia care can be provided on an 'on-call' basis in which the anesthesiologist is in reasonable proximity to the labor and delivery suite. The level of care provided should include major regional anesthesia and general endotracheal anesthesia for vaginal and cesarean delivery. Depending on the particular circumstances in each institution, this may not provide for the provision of continuous epidural anesthesia on a 24 h-a-day basis.

A member of the anesthesia care team often must assist in the resuscitation of the neonate if a pediatrician or pediatric nurse trained in neonatal resuscitation is not available. Such expertise may not be available in many of the 5000 hospitals in the USA that provide obstetric care. It must be kept in mind that 'qualified personnel, *other* than the anesthesiologist attending the mother, should be immediately available to assume responsibility for resuscitation of the newborn Guideline (VII of Guidelines for Regional Anesthesia in Obstetrics). It is the responsibility of the hospital overall to make sure that qualified personnel are available. The attending anesthesiologist acts as a 'Good Samaritan' if he or she assists in the resuscitation since the primary responsibility is to the parturient.

When is it possible to provide continuous obstetric coverage other than in an academic institution? I believe that approximately 2000 deliveries a year could be considered borderline for full-time coverage of an obstetric service by a designated anesthesiologist given:

1. A cesarean delivery rate of 20% (2000 × 20% = 400 cesarean deliveries).
2. 50% of the vaginal deliveries would require only parenteral medication: opioids and/or tranquilizers and local infiltration or pudendal block (1600 × 50% = 800 vaginal deliveries).

3. 2000 – 400 = 1600 vaginal deliveries – 800 requiring no major anesthetic = 800 deliveries that would require a major anesthetic (spinal or epidural).

We are discussing the administration of anesthesia to 1200 parturients a year. An average of 3–4 deliveries a day requiring anesthesia provides enough work for the anesthesia care team.

REFERENCES

1. Department of Public Health 1977 Commonwealth of Massachusetts: Regionalization of maternity and newborn care in Massachusetts, Final Report, August 1, 1974– September 30, 1976, Boston

PART H
SPAIN

J. De Andrés

OBSTETRIC ANESTHESIA: ORGANIZATIONAL CONSIDERATIONS

Health care is a fundamental public right in Spain. Care is free for the vast majority of the population. The country's political system comprises 19 autonomous areas and the central government has delegated organizational aspects of the National Healthcare System (NHS) to these regional authorities. However, throughout the country the cost of health care is equal and is paid for by direct income deductions imposed upon all Spanish citizens. All health care is free, with the exception of a proportion of drug prescriptions outside of the hospital setting. To this fundamental funding system, a number of additional, minor contributions are made by public entities such as local governments etc., or foundations that specifically collaborate with health centers.

Since the creation of the Spanish Society of Anesthesiology, Critical Care and Pain Therapy (Sociedad Española de Anestesiología Reanimación y Terapéutica del Dolor, SEDAR) in 1952, considerable interest has centered on development within the speciality of obstetric anesthesia. In 1976, the Section of Obstetric – Gynecologic Anesthesia was formed, in addition to other specific areas of subspeciality interest. The National Commission on Medical Specialities, which is dependent upon the Ministry of Universities for its training program for specialities in anesthesiology, considered a number of general and specific areas in which knowledge is essential to achieve an adequate professional level in this particular field. Teaching activities, however, are the specific competence of each hospital, through the mediation of teaching commissions and regulation by the head of the department of anesthesia; in the case of level III centers, this function corresponds to the head of the service of obstetric and gynecologic anesthesia. Activities include theoretical training and a rotation system through emergency areas, delivery wards and operating theaters.

With these basic concepts in place, the effective provision of coverage for anesthesia in obstetrics will directly depend upon the level of the hospital involved (i.e. I, II or III), whether, for example, it is a university or nonuniversity center, and the internal organization of the hospital. In addition, consideration should be given to the pressure exerted by the birth rate, which has decreased drastically in Spain in recent years and now reflects a regression in population growth: in my city (Valencia), the number of births varies between 9600 and 1900 births/year, depending on the hospital involved. Cesarean deliveries are performed in 17.9–20% of cases. The cesarean delivery rate has progressively increased in recent years as a result of legal considerations.

At present, the obstetric anesthesia team in a level III hospital is contained within the possesses a Service of Obstetric–Gynecologic Anesthesia that is physically separated from the rest of the hospital in a mother–infant pavilion. In lower level centers (I and II), the Service of Obstetric–Gynecologic Anesthesia forms part of the central service of anesthesia, with no dedicated staff or administration. Obstetric care is provided by at least one staff anesthesiologist on call for 24 h; a second specialist may be placed on duty if necessary, together with a resident in training after his or her second year. Work is organized on an 'on-call' basis, and involves the management of systemic pathology in pregnancy and preventive measures in the initial stages of disease development. The midwife administers sedation intramuscularly during early labor, while the anesthesiologist intervenes in 20–70% of deliveries, depending on the type of hospital and service. The anesthesiologist is usually assisted by a nonspecialized nurse attached to the surgical team or delivery ward. No specialist nursing staff is contemplated at this time in Spanish health care legislation.

The techniques utilized include general and regional anesthesia. The proportions involved depend on the prevailing tendencies in anesthetic practice. General anesthesia is preferentially employed in 95% of cases, with the exception of those areas in which epidural anesthesia is traditionally performed, usually cesarean and elective deliveries. Other forms of regional anesthesia, such as pudendal anesthesia for expulsion, the induction of paracervical block or subarachnoid techniques, are little used. The increased presence of the anesthesiologist in obstetric areas – especially in level III centers and universities – has led to an increase in the application of regional anesthetic techniques, particularly continuous epidural anesthesia in early-stage dilation and in certain cases for the control of post-delivery pain. Clearly, in other types of hospitals, the need for 'on-call' anesthesiologists to deal simultaneously with obstetric care and general emergency medical and surgical situations leads to the restriction of obstetric anesthesia except in emergency settings.

Neonatal critical care is the responsibility of the pediatrician, who decides the type of therapy and the measures to be adopted in each specific case. In the absence of a pediatrician, the anesthesiologist is responsible for immediate resuscitation until the pediatrician arrives. If no specialist with adequate training is available (as may occur in level I and II centers), the anesthesiologist is in charge of the mother and newborn until full stabilization of both is achieved.

Finally, in private practice there exist dedicated obstetric–gynecologic hospitals with high-quality anesthesia services, and with an internal organization similar to that of the National Healthcare System. However, general practice centers on the liberal professional; the patient chooses her obstetrician, but only rarely indicates preferences as regards the anesthesiologist or anesthetic technique to be performed. Nevertheless, the demand for epidural anesthesia is increasing – even though it is still regarded as a 'special service'. Acute neonatal resuscitation is usually the responsibility of the anesthesiologist.

PART I
CHILE

J. Riquelme H. Lacassie

In Chile, obstetric anesthesia is practiced in two different situations:

1. practice in state funded hospitals;
2. private practice.

In the hospitals that belong to the National Health Care System, obstetric anesthesia services are provided by the anesthesia department, which covers in the mornings (1) labor and delivery rooms, (2) obstetric operating rooms and (3) gynecologic operating rooms. During the afternoons and at night, there is only one anesthesiologist in attendance to cover the various procedures.

The anesthetic coverage last year in one of the State Hospitals in Santiago, Chile, was as follows.

Total deliveries	11 154	100.00%
Anesthetics administered		
Regional anesthesia		
(Epidural and spinal)	5360	48.05%
Local		
(perineal infiltration)	4379	39.25%
General	80	0.71%
Total anesthetics	9819	88.03%
Without anesthesia	1335	11.96%

Anesthesia by perineal infiltration for delivery only was administered by the obstetrician or the midwife.

Private patients have an obstetric team formed by an obstetrician, a midwife, a neonatologist and an anesthesiologist.

Considering the total number of deliveries in this situation, 90% have a continuous epidural anesthesia for labor, vaginal or cesarean delivery, 9.5% receive spinal anesthesia for vaginal or cesarean delivery and only 0.5% receive a general anesthetic for cesarean delivery.

70% of the anesthetic costs are paid by the national health system called FONASA (Fondo Nacional de Salud), 25% by private health care systems and the rest by charity.

During a continuous epidural anesthetic in the National Health Care system or private practice, we use the intermittent top-up procedure instead of the continuous-infusion pump, because the latter is very expensive in our country. The top-up doses are administered by the anesthesiologist in charge.

82. Standards for obstetric anesthesia

G. W. Ostheimer

JOINT STATEMENT ON THE OPTIMAL GOALS FOR ANESTHESIA CARE IN OBSTETRICS

After several attempts at creating standards or guidelines for the conduct of obstetric anesthesia by various groups and committees, this 'Joint Statement on the Optimal Goals for Anesthesia Care in Obstetrics' was approved by the American Society of Anesthesiologists (ASA) House of Delegates on 21 October 1986, and by the American College of Obstetricians and Gynecologists (ACOG) Board of Directors on 5 March 1988. It is printed here in its entirety.

The joint statement from the ASA and the ACOG has been designed to address issues of concern to both specialties. Good obstetric care requires the availability of qualified personnel and equipment to administer general or regional anesthesia on either an elective or emergent basis. The extent and degree to which anesthesia services are available varies widely among hospitals. However, for any hospital providing obstetric care, certain optimal anesthesia goals should be sought. These include:

1. Availability of a person qualified to administer an appropriate anesthetic whenever necessary. For many women, regional anesthesia (spinal or epidural) will be the most appropriate anesthetic.
2. Availability of a person qualified to maintain support of vital functions in any obstetric emergency.
3. Availability of anesthesia and surgical personnel such that emergency cesarean deliveries can be started within 30 min of recognition of the need.
4. Appointment of a qualified anesthesiologist to be responsible for all anesthetics administered. In many obstetric units, obstetricians or obstetrician-supervised nurse anesthetists administer the anesthetics. The administration of general or regional anesthesia requires numerous medical judgements and technical skills. Nurse anesthetists are not trained as physicians and cannot be expected to make medical decisions. Obstetricians seldom have sufficient training or experience in anesthesia to allow them to properly supervise nurse anesthetists.

Persons administering or supervising obstetric anesthesia should be qualified to manage the infrequent but occasionally life-threatening complications of major regional anesthesia such as respiratory and cardiovascular failure, toxic local anesthetic convulsions or vomiting and aspiration. Mastering and retaining the skills and knowledge necessary to manage these complications requires adequate training and frequent application.

To ensure the safest and most effective anesthesia for obstetric patients, the director of anesthesia services with the approval of the medical staff must develop and enforce written policies regarding provision of obstetric anesthesia. It is the responsibility of the director of anesthesia services and the medical staff to review each individual's qualifications and competence and to determine which agents and techniques may be used.

5. Availability of a qualified obstetrician during administration of anesthesia. Major conduction anesthesia (epidural, caudal of spinal) and/or general anesthesia should not be administered until the patient has been examined, and the fetal status and progress of labor evaluated by a qualified physician who is readily available to supervise the labor and to deal with any obstetric complications that may arise.
6. Availability of equipment, facilities and support personnel equal to that provided in the surgical suite. This should include the availability of a properly equipped and staffed recovery room capable of receiving and caring for all patients recovering from major regional or general anesthesia. Birthing facilities, when used for anesthesia, must be appropriately equipped to provide safe anesthetic care during labor and delivery, or post-anesthesia recovery care.
7. Personnel other than the surgical team should be immediately available to assume responsibility for resuscitation of the depressed neonate. The surgeon and anesthesiologist are responsible for the mother and may not be able to leave her to care for the neonate even when a regional anesthetic is functioning adequately. Individuals qualified to perform neonatal resuscitation should demonstrate:

a. Skills in rapid and accurate evaluation of the neonatal condition, including Apgar scoring.

b. Knowledge of the pathogenesis and causes of a low Apgar score (asphyxia, drugs, hypovolemia, trauma, anomalies and infection), as well as specific indications for resuscitation.

c. Skills in airway management, laryngoscopy, endotracheal intubation, suctioning of the airway, artificial ventilation, cardiac massage and maintenance of thermal stability.

In larger maternity units and those functioning as high-risk centers, 24 h in-house anesthesia, obstetric and neonatal specialists are usually necessary. Preferably, the obstetric anesthesia service should be directed by an anesthesiologist with special training or experience in obstetric anesthesia. These units will also frequently require the availability of more sophisticated monitoring equipment and specially trained nursing staff.

A recent survey jointly sponsored by the ASA and ACOG found that many hospitals in the USA have not yet achieved the above goals. Deficiencies were most evident in smaller delivery units. Some small delivery units are necessary because of geographic considerations. Currently, 54% of hospitals providing obstetric care have fewer than 500 deliveries per year. Providing comprehensive care for obstetric patients in these small units is extremely inefficient, not cost-effective and frequently impossible. Thus, the following recommendations would seem appropriate:

1. Whenever possible, small units should consolidate.[1]
2. When geographic factors require the existence of smaller units, these units should be part of a well-established perinatal regionalization system.

The availability of the appropriate staff to assist in the management of a variety of obstetric problems is a necessary feature of good obstetric care. The presence of a pediatrician at a high-risk cesarean delivery or an anesthesiologist at a breech delivery are examples. Frequently, these professionals spend a considerable amount of time but may eventually not be required to perform the tasks for which they are present. Reasonable compensation for these standby services is justifiable and necessary.

A variety of other mechanisms has been suggested to increase the availability and quality of anesthesia services in obstetrics. Improved hospital design to place labor and delivery suites closer to the operating room would allow for more efficient supervision of nurse anesthetists. Anesthesia equipment in the labor and delivery area must be similar to that in the operating room.

Finally, interpersonal relations between obstetricians and anesthesiologists could be improved. Joint meetings between the two departments should be encouraged. Anesthesiologists should recognize the special needs and concerns of the obstetricians and obstetricians should recognize the anesthesiologist as a consultant in the management of pain and life-support measures. Both should recognize the need to provide high-quality care for all patients.

GUIDELINES FOR REGIONAL ANESTHESIA IN OBSTETRICS

(approved by House of Delegates on October 12, 1988 and last amended on October 30, 1991)

These guidelines apply to the use of regional anesthesia or analgesia in which local anesthetics are administered to the parturient during labor and delivery. They are intended to encourage quality patient care but cannot guarantee any specific patient outcome. Because the availability of anesthesia resources may vary, members are responsible for interpreting and establishing the guidelines for their own institutions and practices. These guidelines are subject to revision from time to time as warranted by the evolution of technology and practice.

Guideline I

Regional anesthesia should be initiated and maintained only in locations in which appropriate resuscitation equipment and drugs are immediately available to manage procedurally related problems.

Resuscitation equipment should include, but is not limited to: sources of oxygen and suction, equipment to maintain an airway and perform endotracheal intubation, a means to provide positive pressure ventilation, and drugs and equipment for cardiopulmonary resuscitation.

Guideline II

Regional anesthesia should be initiated by a physician with appropriate privileges and maintained by or under the medical direction of such an individual.

Physicians should be approved through the institutional credentialing process to initiate and direct the maintenance of obstetric anesthesia and to manage procedurally related complications.

Guideline III

Regional anesthesia should not be administered until: (1) the patient has been examined by a qualified individual; and (2) the maternal and fetal status and progress of labor have been evaluated by a physician with privileges in obstetrics who is readily available to supervise the labor and manage any obstetric complications that may arise.

Under circumstances defined by department protocol,

qualified personnel may perform the initial pelvic examination. The physician responsible for the patient's obstetrical care should be informed of her status so that a decision can be made regarding present risk and further management.

Guideline IV

An intravenous infusion should be established before the initiation of regional anesthesia and maintained throughout the duration of the regional anesthetic.

Guideline V

Regional anesthesia for labor and/or vaginal delivery requires that the parturient's vital signs and the fetal heart rate be monitored and documented by a qualified individual. Additional monitoring appropriate to the clinical condition of the parturient and the fetus should be employed when indicated. When extensive regional blockade is administered for complicated vaginal delivery, the standards for basic anesthetic monitoring should be applied.

Guideline VI

Regional anesthesia for cesarean delivery requires that the standards for basic anesthetic monitoring be applied and that a physician with privileges in obstetrics be immediately available.

Guideline VII

Qualified personnel, other than the anesthesiologist attending the mother, should be immediately available to assume responsibility for resuscitation of the newborn.

The primary responsibility of the anesthesiologist is to provide care to the mother. If the anesthesiologist is also requested to provide brief assistance in the care of the newborn, the benefit to the child must be compared to the risk to the mother.

Guideline VIII

A physician with appropriate privileges should remain readily available during the regional anesthetic to manage anesthetic complications until the patient's postanesthesia condition is satisfactory and stable.

Guideline IX

All patients recovering from regional anesthesia should receive appropriate postanesthesia care. Following cesarean delivery and/or extensive regional blockade, the standards for postanesthesia care should be applied.

1. A Postanesthesia Care Unit (PACU) should be available to receive patients. The design, equipment and staffing should meet requirements of the facility's accrediting and licensing bodies.
2. When a site other than the PACU is used, equivalent postanesthesia care should be provided.

Guideline X

There should be a policy to assure the availability in the facility of a physician to manage complications and to provide cardiopulmonary resuscitation for patients receiving postanesthesia care.

In addition, the 1990 House of Delegates voted not to require the use of pulse oximetry during the recovery of the obstetric patient in whom regional anesthesia was used for labor and vaginal delivery.

Further developments in this area will undoubtedly occur in the future. For clarification of any issue, please refer to the ASA Home Office for the latest information.

REFERENCES

1. Committee on Perinatal Health 1977 Toward improving the Outcome of Pregnancy – Recommendations for the Regional Development of Maternal and Perinatal Health Services, The National Foundation-March of Dimes, New York.

83. Financial considerations

Part A Australia *S. P. Gatt*
Part B USA *G. W. Ostheimer*
Part C UK *M. Harmer*
Part D Belgium *A. Van Steenberge*
Part E Canada *D. Writer*
Part F France *D. Benhamou B. O'Kelly*
Part G Italy *E. Margaria*
Part H Argentina *P. J. Kelly*
Part I Spain *J. De Andrés*

PART A
AUSTRALIA
S. Gatt

INTRODUCTION

Australia is approximately the same size as North America and has a population of about 17.5 million. With the exception of the indigenous Aborigines, most of the population is concentrated in a handful of large cities distributed along a relatively narrow coastal strip. The majority of the large urban areas are along the eastern seaboard.

Financial arrangements in obstetric anesthesia are similar throughout the Australian Federation of six states and two territories. Each of the state capitals has at least one level III unit dedicated to maternity services. This is usually a free-standing, university-affiliated, tertiary referral women's health center providing obstetrics, gynecology, neonatology, breast screening and surgery, urology and infertility/reproductive endocrinologic technologies. These obstetric-gynecologic university teaching centers offer a full range of support services including obstetric and neonatal intensive care units. There has been an attempt to reduce the number of free-standing maternity units and to amalgamate them with the larger teaching hospitals to create 'mega-campuses' providing the entire gamut of health services.

While there are some minor variations from state to state with regard to relative proportions of insured versus uninsured ('private') patients, private practice costs, salary scales for specialist and junior anesthetic staff and rates of remuneration for visiting medical staff (see below), health care funding is the same for all states and territories.

WHO IS RESPONSIBLE FOR THE BILL FOR OBSTETRIC ANESTHESIA SERVICES?

All Australian citizens, except those who are disadvantaged and below the 'safety net' level, pay a levy on their income tax of 1.4% to cover the costs of Medicare.

Obstetric patients can opt for three combinations of obstetric service:

1. private – obstetrician of choice; private room
2. private shared - doctor of choice; shared hospital accommodation
3. public hospital – hospital doctor; shared accommodation in a public hospital

and several styles of obstetric management:

a. hospital care;
b. doctor- or midwife-supervised birthing center delivery;
c. obstetrician-, general practitioner- or midwife-supervised home birth with hospital care for privately insured mothers available in both the public and private hospital sectors.

Australia spends 8.1% of its gross domestic product (GDP) on health. This is higher than the percentage in the UK (6.1%) but lower than Canada (8.6%) and the US (11.2%) (see Fig. 83.1). This translates into an annual health expenditure of A$1415 (almost US$1000) per annum for every Australian. The total expenditure on health of $23.4 billion comes from: federal government (35.8%), state government (33.4%) and the private sector, mainly health insurance funds (30.67%) (see Fig. 83.2). Each state contributes a different proportion of

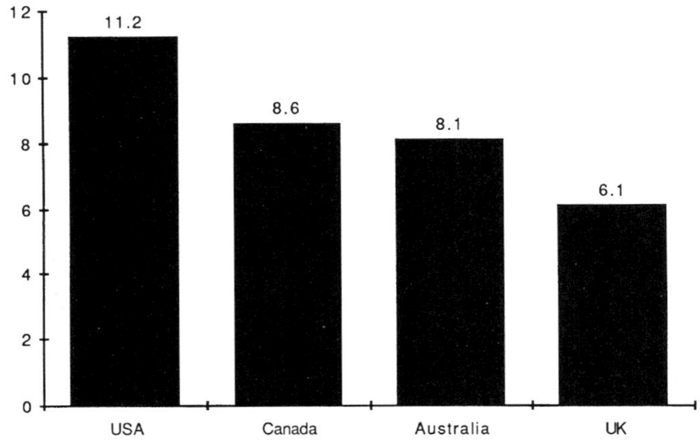

Fig. 83.1 Comparison of health spending as a percentage of gross domestic product. (Modified with permission from Schieber G J, Poullier J P 1989 Overview of international comparisons of health care expenditures, Health Care Financing Review, Department of Health and Human Services, Baltimore, USA.)

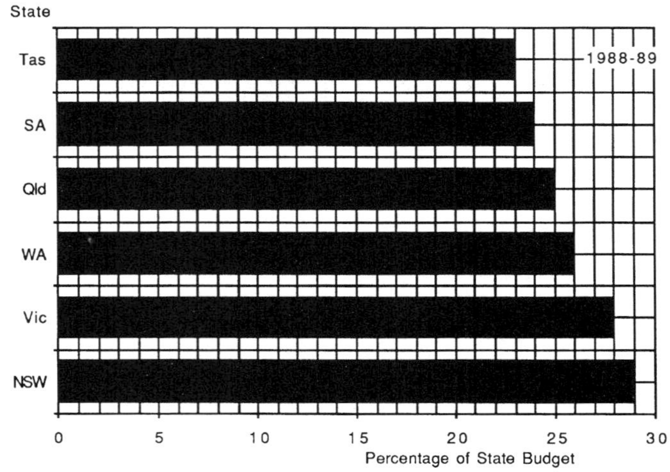

Fig. 83.3 Percentage of state budget that each state spends on government hospitals. From state government figures for 1989.

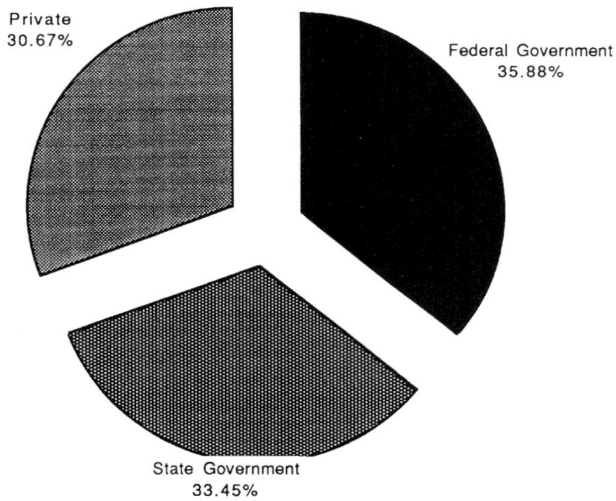

Fig. 83.2 Source of funds showing the percentage of health expenditure derived from federal and state governments and 'private' sources. The last group includes health insurance funds, accident compensation, employer-funded schemes and individuals' co-payments. (Modified with permission from Macklin J 1990 Setting the agenda for change. The National Health Strategy Canberra, p. 13.)

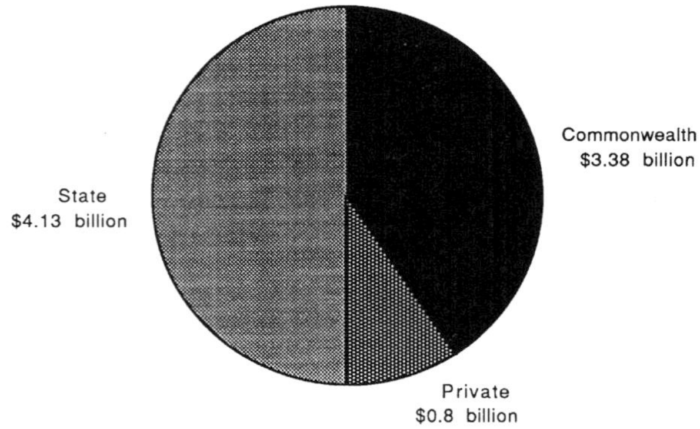

Fig. 83.4 Expenditure on public hospitals in Australia in billions of A$. Source: Official figures, Commonwealth Department of Community Services and Health, 1989–90.

its state budget to hospital services. New South Wales contributes the greatest proportion of its total budget (29%) to hospital services (see Fig. 83.3).

The public hospitals are funded from the three separate sources:

a. the Commonwealth Government (about 40%);
b. the State Health Department (about 48%);
c. other sources, predominantly patient fees (about 12%) (see Fig. 83.4)

In 1993, the proportion of the Australian population with private insurance is 40.7%. This is considerably less than in June 1982, when 67.9% were privately insured. A significant proportion of privately insured mothers are cared for in public hospitals.

HOW ARE FEES FOR OBSTETRIC ANESTHESIA DETERMINED?

The number of *full-time* obstetric anesthesiologists in Australia is very small – no more than one or two in each large city. The bulk of obstetric anesthesia is provided by 'generalists', who often work in more than one hospital and who are required to provide obstetric services as a component of their contract.

These anesthesiologists are hospital-based, full-time or part-time, state or federal salaried staff, salaried clinical academics or visiting medical officers (VMOs). The public patients are cared for either by the salaried staff or by the visiting staff. The VMOs are paid on a fee-for-service, honorary or sessional basis. While wide variations in salary

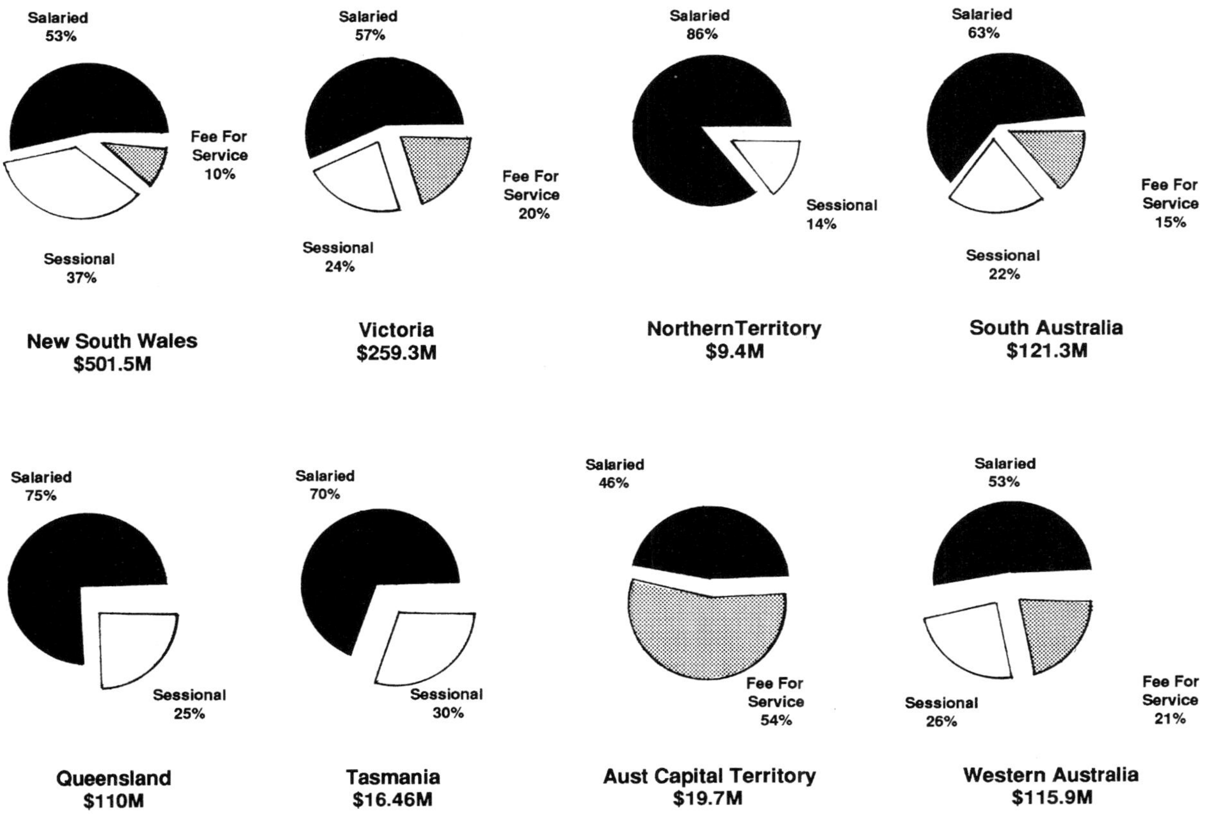

Fig. 83.5 State comparisons showing medical remuneration as a percentage of medical expenditure for public patients in public hospitals. (Reproduced with permission from Hospital Services in Australia, Access and Financing, 1991 National Health Strategy, Canberra, p. 89.)

do not exist from state to state for salaried staff, there are wide variations in sessional payments to VMOs and in the relative proportions of sessional vs. fee-for-service vs. salaried work that is available (Fig. 83.5). For example, the sessional rate per hour for a senior obstetric VMO anesthesiologist in New South Wales is A$135/h (almost US$100/h), while across the state border in Victoria it is A$54/h (almost US$40/h).

Private patients are billed using three recognized fee schedules:

- the Commonwealth Government Medicare Benefits Schedule of Fees and Rebates;
- the Australian Medical Association List of Medical Services and Fees, and;
- the Relative Value Guide of the Australian Society of Anesthetists.

Of the Australian Society of Anesthetists' members, about one-third are staff specialists and two-thirds are VMOs. In billing private patients, most obstetric anesthesiologists use the Relative Value Guide (RVG) of the Australian Society of Anesthetists (ASA) or the Australian Medical Association (AMA) recommended fee, which is based on the ASA RVG. The Commonwealth Government (Medicare) Schedule is used mainly to determine the level of rebate that the patient will receive from Medicare. There is essentially only one difference between the ASA's RVG and the AMA's RVG. While the AMA recommends a unit value of A$28.00 (US$20.00), the ASA suggests a range of A$21.50 to A$36.00 (US$15 to US$25) per unit. In the USA, the same RVG units attract A$40 to A$100 (US$28 to US$70) for different states of the US.

RATES OF REMUNERATION: SALARIED STAFF SPECIALISTS AND VISITING MEDICAL OFFICERS

Salaried obstetric anesthesia specialists in NSW in 1993 are paid from $A76 322 (US$55 000) for a first year specialist rising to $A94 181 (US$68 000) for a fifth and subsequent year specialist to treat patients in public hospitals. On June 30 each year, they can elect to charge between three schemes:

- scheme A, in which they get a 20% salary supplement on base salary but are not allowed to charge private patients;

• scheme B, in which the anesthesiologist is allowed to charge private patients up to a maximum of 25% of salary;
• scheme C, in which the physician takes a drop in base salary but is allowed to draw a maximum of 100% of base salary as private practice supplement.

Visiting medical officers (VMOs) in NSW are paid A$153.13 per hour (specialists) or A$163.13 per hour (senior specialists) for treating public patients and charge private patients directly in both public and private hospitals.

IS THE MEDICARE REBATE ADEQUATE?

In recent years, the Medicare rebate has not kept pace with either the consumer price index (CPI) or the average weekly earnings (AWE). The co-payment that the patient or her guarantor has to pay has become progressively larger (see Fig. 83.6).

The co-payment (portion of the doctor's account which the patient has to meet) change has been largest in those physician groups with the smallest increase in numbers. Between 1985 and 1990, the number of anesthesiologists increased by about 7% and co-payments actually decreased by almost 1%. In contrast, there was no increase in the number of obstetricians practicing but the co-payments increased by over 15% (Fig. 83.7).

Overall, in NSW, anesthesiologists charge about 19% above[6] 'the schedule' (Medicare rebate) fee. In other states, the 'gap' ranges from about 17% to 21%.

IS THE REBATE ANESTHESIOLOGISTS RECEIVE FAIR?

The rebates anesthesiologists receive for their services in Australia are dramatically less than those received by other specialists. The rebate per anaesthesiologist is 28% of the rebate received by an ophthalmologist and 33% of the rebate received by an ENT surgeon.

Between 1984 and 1991, anesthesia rebates rose by only 29% as compared with a total benefits rise of 86% and the anesthesia share of Medicare benefits fell from 2.9% to 2%.

The situation is particularly poor in obstetric anesthesia, where the rebate for an epidural block for analgesia in labor is A$64.00 (US$45) as compared with A$450.00 (US$315; £180) in the UK. To add insult to injury, little provision has been made in the rebate schedule for the newer methods of analgesia for labor and delivery (e.g.

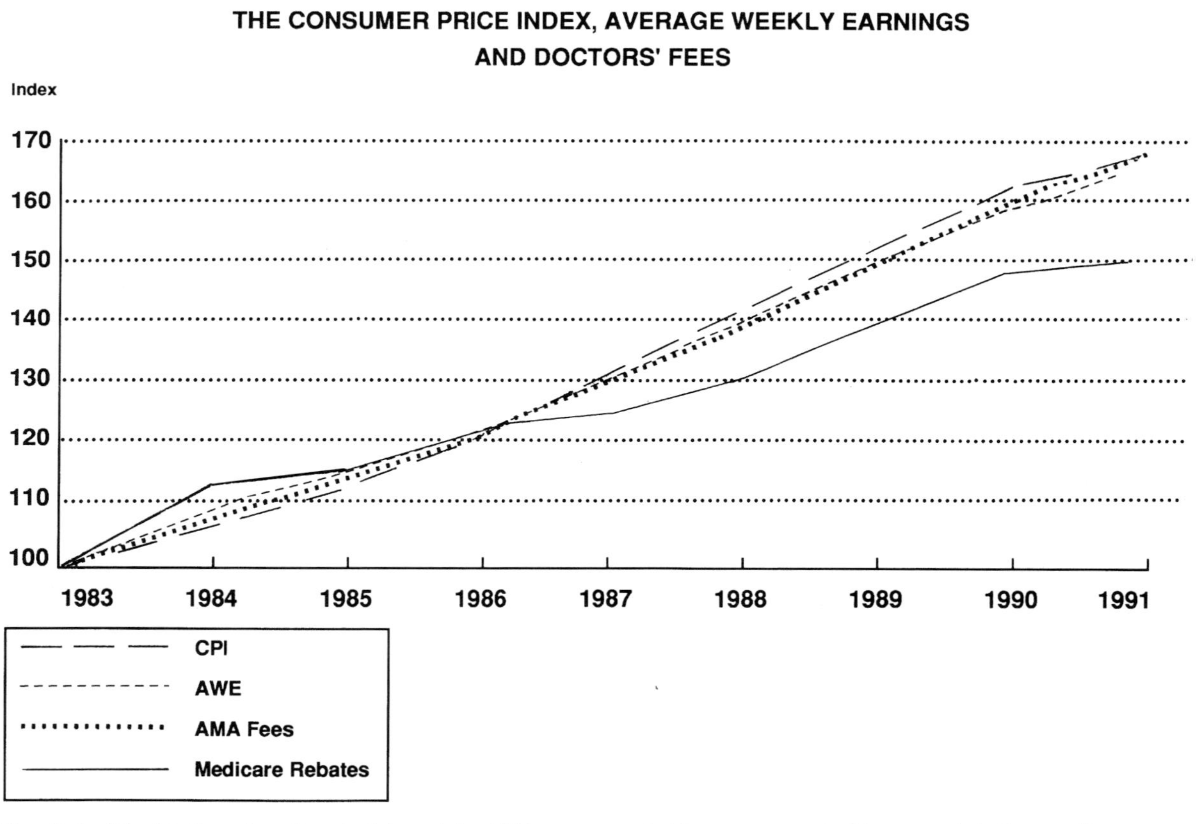

Fig. 83.6 The Medicare benefits schedule and the AMA recommended fee as compared with economic indicators (the consumer price index, CPI, and average weekly earnings, AWE) of Australians, 1983–1991. (Reproduced with permission from Arnold P 1992 NSW Doctor, 5B.)

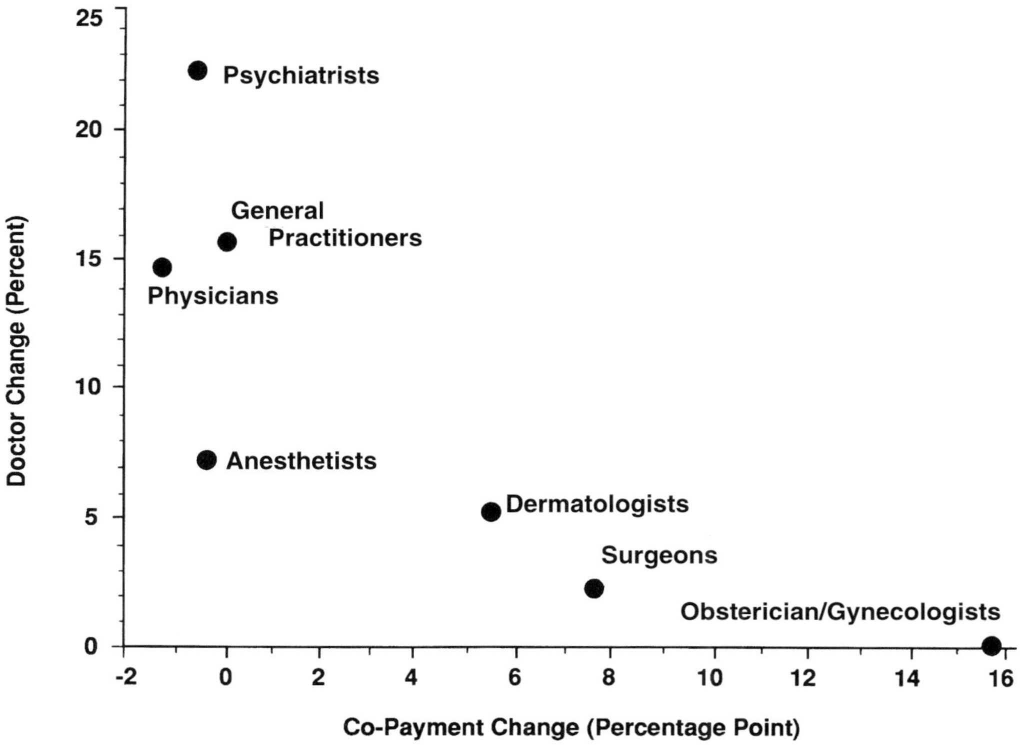

Fig. 83.7 Comparison of change in co-payment and change in doctor numbers from 1985 to 1990 to show that the doctor groups that grew fastest were also the ones with the smallest growth in co-payments. (After Richardson J 1991 The effects of consumer copayments in medical care. National Health Strategy, Canberra, with permission.)

epidural patient-controlled analgesia; epidural infusion; combined spinal–epidural techniques) or for the additional expertise and time required for the rapidly increasing use of regional anesthesia for cesarean delivery.

Post-operative pain relief attracts a very poor Medicare rebate. Techniques such as intravenous patient-controlled analgesia, continuous subarachnoid catheter analgesia, ambulatory continuous infusion and intermittent epidurals, multiple agent epidurals and continuous epidural infusion with stepwise volume decrement either do not draw a benefit or have such low rebate value as to make them financially unattractive methods of pain relief even though they may be clinically superior.

While the need for tighter monitoring, better informed consent, greater involvement of 'support partners' in both vaginal and cesarean delivery is recognized and the use of better, but potentially more hazardous, techniques of anesthesia and analgesia in labor and delivery continues to rise, the rebate attracted for this work is, at worst, non-existent and, at best, static at pre-1985 rates (Fig. 83.8).

The situation in obstetric intensive care is even worse. It was not until very recently that some provision has been made in the Medicare rebate schedule for obstetric anesthesiologists/intensive care specialists who delivered prolonged care to mothers in obstetric high-dependency or intensive care units.

CONCLUSION

While some of the discrepancy between what a service is worth and what is paid for it has, in part, been addressed by the introduction of the ASA and AMA Relative Value Guides, this has only been achieved by the patient or her guarantor having to pay the 'unfunded gap' between what

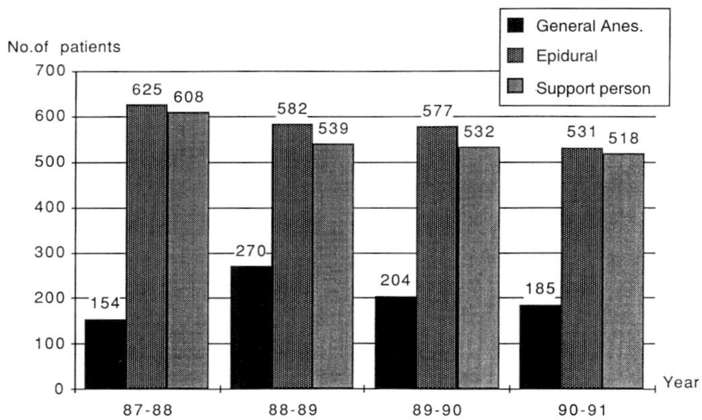

Fig. 83.8 Number of patients undergoing cesarean delivery at the Royal Hospital for Women, Paddington, Sydney, Australia, between 1987 and 1991. Of 3128 mothers having Cesarean delivery, 2197 (70.2%) had a supporting partner in the operating suite during the operation.

has been charged for the service and what Medicare and the private health funds are prepared to pay for the service. Besides, this method of billing private patients is not universally available to all anesthesiologists.

The Australian system of obstetric anesthesiologist remuneration is also flawed in that two methods of payment operate simultaneously in parallel within the same hospital. For identical services to a privately insured mother within the same institution, two doctors of equal seniority, competence and expertise are paid at different rates. To a large degree, Australian anesthesiologists have been able to stave off unnecessary government interference in fee setting but find themselves having to live within a nonuniform system in which an additional amount of time and effort put into the carrying out of duties does not necessarily increase the level of financial remuneration.

By and large, the nonindigenous Australian public, irrespective of financial or social status, has access to a wide choice of high-quality obstetric anesthesia. However, on the basis of risk involved, quality and duration of care, length of training and expertise and effort devoted to the task, the Australian obstetric anesthesiologist remains poorly compensated both in comparison with his/her anesthesiologist peers and in relation to other physicians and surgeons.

PART B
USA
G. W. Ostheimer

The issue of reimbursement for obstetric anesthesia services is as complex in the USA as in any country in the world. There are a myriad of third-party payers that can be charged for obstetric anesthesia services. Third-party payers denote a payer other then the patient directly and can include private 'commercial' insurance companies, health care maintenance organizations, the federal government, the state government and, in many cases, the hospital where the care is provided. 'Free care' for the mother and her infant is a major portion of the free care provided by private and public hospitals in the USA. In addition, several cities and states have special programs to insure adequate perinatal care for the women and neonatal care for children. However, the level of reimbursement varies from state to state and often within a state. Reimbursement for obstetric anesthetic care for a patient with private 'commercial' insurance can vary from literally full pay from the moment of induction until the delivery, an appropriate dollar cap or may be a fixed amount ranging from adequate to absurd. In many parts of the USA, anesthesiologists request a deposit be made prior to admission for labor and delivery in order to guarantee some remuneration for their services.

Using the above as a base for our discussion, let us assume that 50% of a population being served by the obstetric anesthesia team will pay their bill in some fashion. Collections for obstetric services rarely exceed 60% of the bill that is rendered. Therefore, without a reasonable number of deliveries and reasonable compensation for anesthetic services, it is not difficult to understand why anesthesiologists are not interested in providing obstetric anesthetic care in the USA. When third-party payers, the federal government and the state government decide to provide appropriate reimbursement for services rendered, anesthesiologists will become more interested in providing their services in the labor and delivery suite.

However, let us assume that the anesthesia department in a particular hospital has decided to provide obstetric anesthesia care using an anesthesia care team. Using the figure of 2000 as the minimal number of deliveries to make it financially feasible, we assume that at least 60% of the total number of women delivering must receive a major anesthetic in some form to even come close to providing satisfactory reimbursement. If the level of reimbursement is inadequate or the services are not adequately utilized and the hospital demands 24-h-a-day coverage by the anesthesia care team, I believe it is the responsibility of the hospital to make up the difference so that the anesthesia department can break even financially given the compensation received for services provided. Only by putting the appropriate financial squeeze on the administration of the hospital will the administrators and physicians realize that perhaps regionalization of certain aspects of medical care may be more financially feasible in the long run. Obviously, hospitals in rural areas must provide level I or routine obstetric services to their population. However, level II or III units should have adequate populations to provide more sophisticated perinatal services. It is absurd for 8 out of 10 hospitals in a metropolitan area to provide obstetric anesthesia services and not perform more than 1500 deliveries each.

Regionalization into level II or III hospitals would provide an extremely high level of maternal–fetal–neonatal care and meet all the needs of the metropolitan area. State Departments of Public Health should help (force?) hospitals to consolidate their services and provide open staffing for more efficient delivery of perinatal health care. Hospital administrations must realize that they cannot provide all the services from 'birth to death'; they must provide those services that they can most efficiently. Therefore, while one hospital is the cardiac regional center, another hospital could be the perinatal center and have a sufficient number of deliveries to provide continuous obstetric, anesthetic and neonatal intensive care services.

It took personnel interested in perinatal medicine many years to convince obstetricians that the uterus is the best transport incubator for the fetus. How many years will it take us to convince state and hospital administrators that the amount of money available for medical care is finite and that hard-nosed decisions must be made in order to provide the best possible medical care for the citizens of a particular area?

In summary, approximately 2000 deliveries are required to make 24-h-a-day obstetric anesthesia 'in-house' relatively feasible, assuming that 60% of these patients receive a major anesthetic. Otherwise, obstetric anesthesia services should be on a consultative or per-case basis, which takes into account what other demands are being made on the anesthetic services of the hospital. If the hospital administration sees 24-h-a-day obstetric anesthesia coverage as a selling point for their hospital over other hospitals with maternity services in the area and the number of deliveries does not come up to the rate mentioned, hospitals must supplement the income of the anesthesia department to come close to a 'break even' basis. The anesthesia department cannot be in a deficit position for providing services. Obviously, 24-h-a-day coverage of obstetric anesthesia services must be made economically feasible by direct or third-party payments.

One does not like to forecast the future, but it would appear that we are adequately training enough physicians in obstetric anesthesia to be comfortable with providing that service. However, with the exception of the level III perinatal centers, anesthesia care for obstetrics remains the function of the anesthesiologist who is a 'generalist' – trained to provide obstetric anesthesia on a 'case-by-case' or consultative basis, primarily because of manpower and financial constraints.

PART C
UK
M. Harmer

In the past, financial considerations for the provision of an obstetric anesthesia service did not weigh heavily on the anesthesiologist's mind; the National Health Service in the UK provides free obstetric care to all patients and the clinician's role was to identify to the District Health Authority areas that needed additional funding. However, the recent introduction in British hospitals of self-governing trusts and the appointment of clinical directors responsible for budgets has meant that all clinicians are becoming more financially aware of their environment.

FUNDING OF THE OBSTETRIC SERVICE IN THE UK

Traditionally it has been the responsibility of the District Health Authority to provide adequate obstetric care for the community; this included the provision of an obstetric anesthesia service. The level of the anesthetic staffing varied from district to district and depended on numerous factors including the influence of local clinicians. In providing staff and facilities, the District Health Authority would take into account many factors, such as unit workload, type of workload (simple or complex obstetric care), development of additional services and past performance. They would then allocate funds from their budget or perhaps seek financial support from the Department of Health.

In the new climate of trust hospitals, the same level of staff and facilities is expected but the funding on this occasion must be generated in a different way. Instead of the District Health Authority funding the obstetric service at a particular hospital, it is the responsibility of that hospital to negotiate contracts with the District Health Authority (and possibly surrounding Health Authorities) for the provision of care. By necessity this has to be done on an average cost-per-patient basis. Once the contract for care of a specific number of patients has been agreed, the hospital involved must balance its own budget and any changes in staff or facilities must be funded internally. This is the basis of the purchaser–provider agreement. However, many large, tertiary referral obstetric units may experience difficulty in keeping within budget as the contracted fee per patient may be adequate for 'normal' deliveries but more complex problems incur additional costs.

Funding the tertiary referral center has always been a problem because of cross-boundary flow. In the past, a District Health Authority with a large, referral obstetric unit would fund that unit for all the work carried out in it. Any patient referred from another health district for specialist care (either of the mother or the neonate) would be readily treated and then the Health Authority in the area which the patient was resident would be billed for the service. However, the costs involved were always averaged out and the 'tertiary referral' district was rarely fully reimbursed. Such cross-boundary referrals and billing continues in the new arrangements but on a more formal, contractual basis.

At present, within each hospital the budget is devolved to clinical directors. As far as the provision of an obstetric anesthetic service is concerned, the budget for medical staff rests with the clinical director of anesthetic services, while the budget for facilities, drugs and nonmedical staff (anesthetic assistants) rests with the clinical director of obstetric services. Equipment is often funded on a shared basis. This division of funding can lead to areas of conflict when medical staff are made available but the facilities are inadequate, or vice versa. At the end of the financial year, each clinical directorate is expected to be within budget. Any 'profit' on the year can be used to improve patient services (by employing more staff or by the purchase of new equipment). However, there is no financial benefit to the staff for staying within budget (except that regular overspending may lead to a reduction in staff numbers). Occasionally, additional money may be made available from central funds for particular developments or for the implementation of centrally-commissioned reports.

FINANCIAL REMUNERATION

The National Health Service works on a salaried basis with no item of service arrangement with staff undertaking whatever work is generated. This means that it is not necessary to carry out procedures in order to ensure continuing income and so is ideally suited to the unpredictable workload associated with obstetric anesthetic practice. Staff-in-training are paid at an hourly rate for the work that they undertake (though the rates vary according to whether it is day or night work), while consultants are given a fixed salary for the provision of a number of half-days of work and a commitment to provide out-of-hours emergency cover. The fact that salaries are the same for staff working in busy referral units as in smaller, 'simple obstetrics' units puts greater pressure on managers of smaller units to consider carefully the cost benefits of having full anesthetic cover for their obstetric unit and perhaps attempt some lesser degree of provision.

While staff are becoming less financially naive with regard to funding of the obstetric services (including obstetric anesthesia), there can be little doubt that the simple concept of the purchaser–provider contract has definite problems. Contracts for a hospital to undertake a certain number of a certain type of operation can be regulated. Such regulation is very difficult in the obstetric population, and some flexibility in funding allocation must be introduced in the obstetric field to allow for the changing customer population.

MONITORING OF SERVICE COSTS

In order to be able to balance the budgets each year, one element of the change to clinical directorates was to include the provision of adequate information technology and equipment. Because of the nonnecessity of providing itemized bills in the past the whole area of information technology has been largely overlooked and the development of such systems has been very slow. Until such systems are in place it is difficult to see how accurate budgeting, particularly for drugs and disposable items, can be achieved. In the meantime the budgets depend upon 'gross' itemization and estimates. Once more accurate figures are available it will be easier to look at the cost-effectiveness of certain techniques or staffing employed in the obstetric unit.

While pressure is placed on greater cost awareness, overall financial considerations still tend to come low on the list of priorities for most obstetric anesthesiologists.

PART D
BELGIUM
A. Van Steenberge

CONSIDERATIONS

The financial aspect of pain relief in obstetrics influences the practice of obstetrics in Belgium. Since 1984, epidural analgesia for labor and delivery has been paid for by compulsory health insurance. This has substantially increased the practice of regional analgesia and anesthesia in obstetrics. There is however a wide variety in this practice depending on the kind of payment the anesthesiologist receives.

Doctors paid on a salary basis receive no direct income from providing obstetric analgesia or anesthesia. It is part of their professional duties. Anesthesia for cesarean delivery is provided by the anesthesiologist on duty if urgent or on the weekend, whereas elective cesarean deliveries are included in the surgical schedule. Pain relief for vaginal delivery is dependent on the number of staff members as the law forbids paramedics to inject drugs into an epidural catheter.

The outcome is that often in small units (fewer than 1000 deliveries per year) which account for over 40% of the country's total births, the salaried anesthesiologist provides epidural analgesia for vaginal delivery only during daytime hours from 0800 h till circa 1800 h from Monday until Friday.

This restricted coverage for epidural analgesia increases the induction rate to more than 50% in some of these maternity hospitals.

Anesthesiologists who are paid on a fee-for-service basis receive a specific amount for providing epidural analgesia for vaginal delivery. This is a fixed sum reviewed yearly by a commission made up of doctors and representatives of the mutual funds. This amount is charged to – and paid by – the social security system via the mutual funds (Table 83.1). The patient is not directly involved. Membership of one of the five mutual funds is compulsory for anyone living in Belgium. In private practice, the anesthesiologist is entitled to double this amount for

Table 83.1 Reimbursement of social security via mutual funds

Epidural analgesia	$US*	ECU*
Labor–vaginal delivery	175	144
Cesarean delivery +	195	161
Cesarean delivery – weekend ‡/night-time	384	317

* $US1 = 33 Belgian francs; I ECU = 40 Belgian francs.
+ For epidural analgesia for labor followed by cesarean delivery only the cesarean delivery component is reimbursed.
‡ Weekends are from 0800 h Saturday to 0800 h Monday. Night-time is from 2100 h to 0800 h.

patients staying, for nonmedical reasons, in a single room. This supplement has to be charged to and paid by the patient. Some patients benefit from a complementary insurance, covering this health expense. Complementary insurance paid for by employers as a fringe benefit for employees is quite common in Belgium.

ACTUAL STATUS

In small units with a small staff and in which doctors are paid on a fee-for-service base the practice works as follows: a staff member or a senior assistant well versed in regional anesthesia and obstetric problems places the epidural catheter and administers the test dose, which happens to be the therapeutic dose (bupivacaine 12.5 mg, epinephrine 12.5 μg and sufentanil 10 μg in a 10-ml bolus). He or she observes closely the outcome for at least 20 min. When uneventful analgesia occurs within less than 15 min, the staff member instructs the parturient about the use of a patient-controlled and time-locked epidural analgesia pump which will deliver the same amount of drug. The parturient does her own top-ups under the close surveillance of an experienced midwife, who checks blood pressure, fetal heart rate, etc. before the top-up and thereafter. The anesthesiologist is present continuously when there is a maternal and/or fetal pathology or distress, when fetopelvic disproportion exists and also when three or more laboring women are receiving epidural analgesia.

In those small units with a poor financial income from the obstetric workload, a pool of income and expenses of the anesthesia department provides compensation. Interestingly, those small units often have a very close relationship and understanding of the entire team. This is an absolute prerequisite for safe and efficient practice.

In large maternity units (> 1500 deliveries per year) in which fee-for-service is applied, the financial income permits the organization of a permanent obstetric analgesia service, with an experienced anesthesiologist present at all times.

In training centers, the senior assistants usually rotate and are present at all times and a staff member is on call.

PART E
CANADA
D. Writer

INTRODUCTION

Canada, a federal state, consists of 10 provinces and two national territories (the Yukon and the Northwest Territories). Its population is approximately 26 million, three-quarters of whom live in urban areas concentrated in the southern part, in variable proximity to the border with the USA.

HEALTH CARE IN CANADA

The federal government and provinces share responsibility for health care. While the federal government oversees health promotion and protection and health services for Canada's indigenous populations, the provinces run the hospital services, through hospital insurance programs.

The Medical Care Act of 1966 established Canadian Medicare as it exists today, when the federal and provincial governments introduced a universal health program, financed within provinces mainly by taxation (plus supplements from general revenues) and cost shared by contributions from the federal government. In 1977, the Established Programs Fiscal Arrangements Act came into being, by which the federal government initiated a system of block funding, instead of cost sharing, allowing provinces to use federal funds in any area of their health program, according to need.

PHYSICIANS' REMUNERATION

Under Medicare, most physicians receive remuneration on a fee-for-service basis. The value of their services is determined by the provincial medical societies or associations, which represent the physicians' interest in economic negotiations with provincial governments. The resultant fee schedule lists the mutually agreed fees, but provinces deduct a percentage (generally 10%) for 'administrative' costs. Before 1984, physicians had the right to 'extra bill' for their services, and hospitals could levy user charges. However, the Canada Health Act of 1984 put an end to these practices, and reaffirmed and clarified some essential principles of Medicare: universality – all residents of Canada must be entitled to health services; comprehensiveness – all medically necessary services must be covered ('insured services'); accessibility – services must be provided on uniform terms and conditions and reasonable access not impeded. Thus private medicine (except in some very specialized areas) does not exist in Canada.

The Act also provided for the federal government to levy financial penalties against provinces and territories that failed to comply with these principles. Under these penalties provincial governments lose $1 of Medicare cash grants for every $1 collected from patients in user fees and extra billing. Extra billing by physicians and hospitals has virtually disappeared, but, to contain costs, some provinces have redefined services which are 'medically necessary' (e.g. tubal ligation may not be universally insured.)

OBSTETRIC ANESTHESIA SERVICES IN CANADA

Canada has only two dedicated maternity hospitals – the Grace Hospital in Vancouver, British Columbia, and its 'sister' institution in Halifax, Nova Scotia. Elsewhere across the country obstetric anesthesia is provided in maternity units attached to general hospitals. In the larger busy institutions, such as the Grace Hospitals, anesthesiologists remain in-house, on a 24-h basis. However, in the majority of maternity units within teaching, regional or community hospitals, it is rarely financially feasible to provide 24-h, in-house anesthesia. Larger hospitals may offer dedicated daytime coverage, but night-time and weekend coverage is usually provided by anesthesiologists on call (or in-house) for the general surgical operating rooms.

METHODS OF FUNDING OBSTETRIC ANESTHESIA IN CANADA

Fee-for-service physician remuneration

Most anesthesiologists offering obstetric anesthesia services receive payment on a fee-for-service basis, according to the provincial fee schedule. Fees differ between provinces, and two kinds exist: procedural fees (a predetermined fee, unrelated to the duration of the procedure), and a 'relative value' system, which values each procedure in units of anesthetic work. Most provinces use this latter system. Relative value scales should enable similar rewards for different anesthetic services, but obstetric anesthesia is the 'Cinderella' of anesthetic subspecialties, with an unfavorable fee schedule. In general, a procedure has a number of basic units, plus additional units paid on a time basis (e.g. 1 unit/15 min). The number of basic units usually relates to the anesthetic complexity of the procedure.

Advantages of fee-for-service remuneration include:

a. the system rewards the anesthesiologist's willingness to work;
b. scheduled fees frequently generate 'premiums' for after-hours, weekend and holiday work.

Disadvantages include:

a. unpredictable health-care funding;
b. potential conflict between fee-for-service remuneration and academic goals and productivity;
c. the temptation to 'overservice' patients;
d. the system (generally) does not reward 'in-house' anesthetic coverage; and
e. work disruptions or stoppages diminish the anesthesiologist's income.

Global/block funding

Some Canadian institutions have developed this system because the demand for obstetric anesthesia services varies considerably over a 24-h period, and the fee-for-service system may not provide a 'competitive' income, if much of the 24-h period is spent 'standing by'.

The advantages of this method are:

a. predictable health-care budgeting;
b. consistent physician remuneration, irrespective of workload.

The disadvantages are:

a. governments consider the funding comprehensive, and the system allows no flexibility for increased workload;
b. physician dissatisfaction may result if workload increases;
c. funding does not differentiate between elective and emergency work.

Sessional fees

In some institutions, sessional fees, over and above the provincial fee schedule, enable anesthesiologists to provide in-house availability. The advantage of this method is that the economic incentive recognizes the frequently considerable demands of obstetric anesthesia. The disadvantage is that governments (and hospitals) may be vulnerable to curtailment of services, if sessional fees become inadequate.

Salary

This is usually considered the least attractive of the payment options. It has the advantage of predictable health-care budgeting but the disadvantages that:

a. the system rarely compensates for changes in workload, evening or weekend cover;
b. patient care may suffer, since salaried individuals lack incentives to provide 'inessential' services, such as labor analgesia.

EXAMPLES OF PAYMENT FOR OBSTETRIC ANESTHESIA

The two Grace Hospitals present an interesting contrast in funding anesthesia services. The Grace Hospital,

Vancouver, has approximately 8000 deliveries per year, and anesthesiologists rotate to provide 24-h in-house anesthesia, with at least one additional anesthesiologist during the daytime for the elective 'surgical' list (e.g. cesarean delivery). Weekend and night-time coverage ensures one in-house anesthesiologist, plus a second on call-back, in the event of an excessive workload. The province remunerates the hospital via block funding, which precludes any billing for physician services (approximate 1990 cost C$1.8 million).

The Grace Maternity Hospital, Halifax, undertakes approximately 6000 deliveries annually. A team of six anesthesiologists provides 24-h in-house coverage, and each is remunerated on a fee-for-service basis. The physician cost of anesthesia services approximates C$700 000.

The following are examples of frequently billed procedures:

1. *Epidural analgesia for labor*:
   - Insertion: 7 base units + 1 additional unit for each 15 min of anesthetic time;
   - Maintenance: 1 unit/30 min, to maximum of 6 units (i.e. 3 h);
   - Final delivery time: 1 unit/15 min anesthetic time.

   Thus, an epidural block that takes approximately 30 min to establish (including preoperative assessment, performance of the procedure and the necessary documentation), that is maintained for some 4 – 5 h and that requires the anesthesiologist's attendance at the delivery for 30 min will generate 17 units. In 1991, the value of a unit was C$13.06; by 1993 this had fallen to C$11.11. One inherent disadvantage of this system is that it fails to compensate anesthesiologists adequately for protracted 'epidurals' that make frequent demands on their time. Further, in Nova Scotia and some other provinces, epidural analgesia for labor does not attract 'premium' fees. In Ontario, on the other hand, premium fees apply to all obstetric anesthesia services.
2. *Anesthesia for cesarean delivery:*
   - Basic units: 7;
   - Time units: 1 unit per 15 min anesthetic time.

Thus, a cesarean delivery under epidural anesthesia, which takes 1 h 30 min from initial establishment of the i.v. catheter to return of the patient to the recovery room, will generate 13 units (approximately C$170). Anesthesia for cesarean delivery and other obstetric 'surgical' procedures (e.g. retained placenta) carries a premium of approximately 35% in Nova Scotia during evening/night hours and on weekends. In some provinces (e.g. Ontario) the premium fee increases to 50% overnight and on weekends, while in others premium fees may not apply to any anesthetic procedures.

The two systems exemplified above emphasize the previously noted advantages and disadvantages of each. Global budgeting compensates the anesthesiologist irrespective of workload, and quiet or busy days are equally remunerated. However, when workload becomes excessive, or at weekends when 'confined' in-house, anesthesiologists may question whether they are fairly remunerated by the system. In contrast, fee-for-service remuneration compensates the anesthesiologist for an excessive workload, especially when the procedure involves the additional payment of a premium fee; however, there is no financial return for 'stand-by' hours, when the level of clinical activity is low, but the anesthesiologist stays in-house for considerations of safety.

FISCAL CONSIDERATIONS *vs.* PRACTICE STANDARDS

The Canadian Anesthetists' Society, which represents the vast majority of anesthesiologists across Canada, publishes 'Guidelines to the Practice of Anesthesia', which are updated annually.[1] With respect to obstetric anesthesia, these guidelines state 'In an obstetrical unit, it is acceptable to supervise more than one patient receiving regional analgesia for labour. Due care must be taken to ensure that each patient is adequately observed by a suitably trained person following an established protocol.' This statement is not intended to encourage simultaneous anesthesia for concurrent operative procedures, which the Society considers unacceptable, but the guideline allows anesthesiologists ethically to bill for concurrent patients having labor analgesia.

THE FUTURE

Health care in Canada, and most western countries, faces a funding crisis, as escalating costs account for an increasing percentage of gross national product (GNP). Physician staffing and remuneration has come under close scrutiny, and a recent report commissioned by provincial health ministers noted:[2]

> Although there is no single 'best' way to pay physicians in all circumstances, too little use is made of alternatives to fee-for-service as a payment method in Canada.

The report suggested the elimination of fee-based payment in academic institutions; global funding contracts for highly specialized, but relatively uncommon services (e.g. obstetric anesthesia); and sessional payments or salaries, instead of fee-for-service, in certain situations (e.g. the emergency department).

The authors felt that a strong case could be made for limiting health care expenditure (especially medical care expenses) to that necessary to account for general inflation, population growth and changes in the population's need. I therefore believe that medical manpower and physician remuneration in Canada will undergo review as a matter of some urgency. Obstetric anesthesia services will almost certainly become subject to global funding contracts, and the Barer–Stoddart report presages an end to fee-for-service remuneration.

In the end, the method and magnitude of funding will depend upon 'social choice'. Global budgeting probably represents the best way in which to fund obstetric anesthesia, but anesthesiologists must work to ensure that the sums allotted compare favorably with those in other areas of anesthetic and medical practice. For them to do otherwise might signal an end to the present high level of service. Obstetric anesthesiologists must proclaim, loud and clear, the message that pregnant women and their unborn children deserve only the highest standards of anesthesia care, and this must be appropriately funded.

REFERENCES

1. Guidelines to the Practice of Anesthesia as recommended by the Canadian Anesthetists Society. 1991 Can J Anesth, 38 (8) (Suppl): 1–15
2. Barer M L, Stoddart G L 1991 Toward integrated medical policies for Canada. Report prepared for the Federal/Provincial/Territorial Conference of Deputy Ministers of Health. Health and Welfare Canada, Ottawa

PART F
FRANCE

D. Benhamou B. O'Kelly

In order to understand the French system of health care and particularly the financial aspects of obstetric anesthesia, one needs to describe (1) the system of financing general medical expenditure and the tariff system of medical costs and (2) the relationship between medical needs and economic considerations.

The health care of the very large majority of the French population is provided by a system called 'Social Security'. This principle is theoretically a simple one: financial contributions ('input') deducted automatically from every French salary serves to cover the medical expenditure ('output'). Individual contributions are calculated as a ratio of the salary until a certain maximal level of salary is reached, above which contributions do not increase. The cost of each procedure is calculated by a schedule of charges defined by the 'Social Security'. The unitary cost of every medical procedure is the basis of funding.

As will be described later, some practitioners working in private practice charge fees for a given medical procedure which are higher than the unitary predefined values. A patient choosing such a practitioner will be personally responsible for a larger part of the payment. When one looks at the specific problem of obstetrics, the French schedule of charges defines two simple situations (normal delivery and twin delivery), which form the basis for funding. To these two basic contractual payments can be added many additional contractual payments arising from specific obstetric situations. The need for epidural anesthesia represents one of these additional costs. However, there is no agreement between the Social Security and physicians concerning the indications for its provision. For example, epidural analgesia/anesthesia will be funded only if there is an 'obstetric indication'. In other words, this theoretically excludes provision of epidural analgesia 'only' for pain relief during a normal delivery. The reality is different for many reasons and particularly because the definition of an 'obstetric indication' is, of course, very large and this term can be interpreted very differently by different physicians and by different funding organizations.

The French health care system is a two-tier system consisting of a public system, on the one hand, and a private system on the other, the only similarity being their final aim of improving the health of the population. In all other respects they are fundamentally different. Financial resources of private and public hospitals differ markedly.

Public hospitals meet their expenditures with money from different sources (Fig. 83.9), the most important of which is an endowment from the Social Security. This

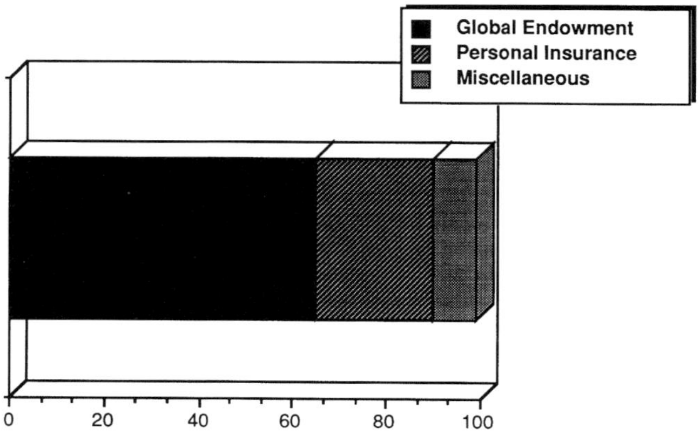

Fig. 83.9 How public hospitals meet their expenditure.

global endowment is given to cover routine expenditure and is not intended to pay for capital spending. This endowment is increased annually, taking into account the rate of inflation. In contrast, the majority of private medical centers work on a fee-for-service system, i.e. payment of a charge per item of health care received. For example, to the basic charge of a day in hospital, the private medical center adds further charges in respect of every additional item of care, e.g. charges for operating room or delivery room stay, charges for catheterization, endoscopy, etc.

Having described the organization of the French health care system, the question that now arises is how the increasing need for obstetric anesthesia can be financed within this system. This problem is common to most developed countries in which expenditure on obstetric anesthesia has always been low. The need for an improved service requiring increased funding is obvious to both patients (parturients) and anesthesiologists. However, the French Ministry of Health seems unwilling, probably for economic reasons, to admit the need to increase funding. If patients are to be provided with an epidural service of good quality day and night, proof that the presence of an anesthesiologist in the maternity unit 24 h a day reduces maternal mortality must be produced. Intuitively this would seem to be logical, although some anesthesiologists disagree.[1] Moreover, the current awareness in France of the need for the provision of better obstetric anesthesia care is counterbalanced by the fact that the national schedule of charges is not sufficiently profitable for anesthesiologists. They believe that a 12-h labor beginning during the night and requiring the permanent presence of an anesthesiologist near the delivery room deserves a much higher remuneration than that received at present. The logical consequence of this situation is a much less enthusiastic use of epidural anesthesia for pain relief during labor, and this typically leads to a situation of less than optimal care.

REFERENCES

1. Singer M M 1987 No evidence that anesthesiologists enhance care of the parturient. Anesthesiology 67: 152

PART G
ITALY
E. Margaria E. Gollo

In the Italian National Public Health Service, medical practice is governed by laws and decrees, and financial regulations and rules are issued by every region of the country.

The latest National Contract (1988–91) provides many controls regarding medical practice, including anesthetic practice. There is no mention of anesthetic specializations (obstetrics, pediatrics, etc.).

Physicians may work full time (38 h/week) or part time (28–30 h/week); 4 h/week must be reserved for refresher activity. The total amount of overtime in 1 year cannot exceed 50 h. Gross annual salaries are as follows:

(Art. 108 DPR 384 28/XI/90)
- Medical assistant: full time, L18 071 000; part time, L13 553 000.
- Assistant to head of department: full time, L25 211 000; part time, L18 908 000.
- Head of department: full time, L35 593 000; part time, L25 195 000.

These values increase by 6% every 2 years (on an eight-point scale); after this the increase is 2.5% of the eighth scale every 2 years. To these amounts must be added, with the same progressive increments applied to the base salary, some annual additions for:

- Full time: Assistant: L13 300 000;
  Assistant to head of department:
  16 520 000:
  Head of department: L19 780 000.
- Specialization Assistant:
  part time L1 238 000;
  full time L1 650 000.
  Assistant to head of department:
  part time L1 620 000:
  full time L2 160 000.
  Head of department: part time
  L2 520 000;
  full time L3 360 000.
- Medical management (head of department): L1 2000 000.
- Home availability: L80 000/24 h.
- Exposure to X-rays, gases: L50 000/month).

Extra payments are also available for night duty and attendance during holidays.

Moreover, incentive payments are available to medical staff to improve the service to the public. Doctors can choose to do this outside their normal duty hours ('plus orario') but more than 7 and 5 h per week respectively for full-time and part-time staff. Every 6 months these hours are checked and money received by the hospital for supplying services (clinics, laboratory, radiology, outpatients, etc.), is divided:

- 45% to the medical team who provided the service;
- 55% to all staff (medical and administrative staff).

For example, anesthesiologists at the S. Anna Hospital in Turin can almost double their salary with the 'plus orario' on top of the basic salary.

Doctors are allowed to practice privately within the public system during duty hours if patients are hospitalized in private rooms. Outside duty hours, private practice can be undertaken in consulting rooms or by visiting patients. Patients pay the doctor, who reserves a percentage for the hospital.

When a full-time doctor works in private clinics, the patient pays for the service in the doctor's hospital. The administration department of the hospital keeps 5% of the fee plus taxes (30–45%) and returns the remainder to the doctor with his salary. A doctor working part-time in a hospital may freely carry on private medical practice without telling or paying the hospital. All doctors have 30 holidays per year, but anesthesiologists have 8 more days and radiologists 15 more days.

PART H
ARGENTINA
J. Kelly

In Argentina the proportion of parturients receiving anesthesia for vaginal delivery is quite different depending on where the delivery takes place. In public hospitals other than those specializing in obstetrics, very few women receive an epidural anesthetic for normal delivery. Anesthesia is requested only for difficult cases, mainly because of a shortage of anesthesiologists resulting from insufficient funds. The contrary is true in private and community hospitals, where the anesthesiologist is paid on a fee-for-service basis for almost every case. This was the result of a 'union-type' request to the insurance companies by the anesthesiology societies and of a long campaign in the non-medical press by women's organizations more than two decades ago.

The fee for an epidural anesthetic for a normal delivery is exactly the same as for a cesarean delivery. The total fee varies slightly depending on the time of day (day or night) and the insurance involved (from US$90 to US$300).

Most purely private and insured patients also receive anesthesia, because the possibility is suggested to them early in their pregnancy by the obstetrician or the midwife in charge of teaching breathing exercises prior to delivery. Sometimes, the anesthesiologist is asked to have a special session with a small number of patients to explain to them what can be done for their pain relief and how it works, in both the mother and the fetus.

PART I
SPAIN
J. De Andrés

At present, most working doctors are associated with the National Healthcare System (NHS). In the last 5 years, labor contracts have been exclusive in character, i.e. private practice in free time is prohibited for those physicians under contract to the NHS. As a result, only those specialists contracted before this time are presently able to choose between exclusive public service or a combination with private practice. In this sense, few physicians are exclusively dedicated to the private practice of their professions.

Specialists working at different levels (I, II or III) receive a fixed monthly salary from the National Healthcare System that is independent of the number of interventions involved and varies between 280 000 Spanish pesetas for a staff specialist and 397 000 pesetas for a Head of Service (US$2200–3200). In addition to this basic salary, supplements are paid for 24 h duty coverage, with variable compensations for duties on holidays, etc. This amounts to an average of 20 000 pesetas (US$127) per duty. Other supplements may stem from university teaching activities, the amount being highly variable and dependent on the number of lecture hours and professional status.

Improvements in equipment are funded by the economic and administrative management of each hospital on a yearly basis, from resources assigned by the National Healthcare System. This is done following an analysis of the needs defined by the service of anesthesiology in order to maintain the standards of care, and is based on an annual memorandum or report of the activities of the service, with consideration of the advances afforded by new technologies in obstetric anesthesia.

In private practice, an obstetric patient may receive care through the coverage afforded by private insurance companies, or choose her physician herself. In this sense, two options exist in this country:

1. *Closed entities* correspond to hospitals with their own staff provisions. The staff members may be under contract to the hospital or constitute active society members. In either case, the physician receives a fixed monthly salary from the hospital depending on the contract, or participates in the benefits of the institution according to an agreed percentage.
2. *Open entities* place their hospitals at the disposal of 'freelance' professionals. These may, in turn, be organized independently into teams to afford 24-h coverage to obstetric patients through an 'on call' system; alternatively, there may simply be an agreement between the

anesthesiologist and obstetrician to provide coverage. In both cases, charge rates are established directly between the anesthesiologist and patient – mean cost being 30 000 pesetas for a cesarean delivery (US$240), 20 000 pesetas (US$160) for a vaginal delivery under general anesthesia, 30 000 pesetas (US$240) when performed with epidural anesthesia and 20 000 pesetas (US$160) for an obstetric currettage. These rates may vary according to the ASA risk involved or particular circumstances, such as surgery on holidays, etc. The material employed in performing anesthesia belongs to the clinic and is charged by the clinic on top of the anesthesiologists's fees.

The anesthesiologist is rarely selected by the obstetric patient, and is usually accepted as an integral part of the obstetric team which, in effect, is actively chosen by the patient. However, delivery under epidural anesthesia is becoming more widely accepted as a 'special service' provided by the anesthesiologist and regarded as a 'luxury' on the part of the patient. Hence, the expense involved is seen as being greater.

84. Socioeconomic considerations

Part A General *J. Gardiner*
Part B USA view *E. B. Skerman* *J. H. Skerman*

PART A
GENERAL
J. Gardiner

Poverty is very good in poems, but is very bad in a house. It is very good in maxims and in sermons, but is very bad in practical life.

Henry Ward Beecher, Proverbs from Plymouth Pulpit, 1887

In developed countries health care can cost up to 10% of the total national income. The working anesthesiologist has only recently had to think in economic terms. Fluctuating economies and changing attitudes to the concept of the 'bottomless pit' for health care have challenged doctors' moral attitude that medical attention be provided to all regardless of how it is financed.

In less developed countries governments are often unable to provide the minimum requirements for a doctor let alone a patient.

GLOBAL PICTURE

Maternal mortality rates in developing countries 10–100 times higher than in UK or USA point to a serious health problem for these societies.[1] What is needed is improved literacy and general health awareness; a change in attitude toward entering hospital plus improved nutrition. In this context improved obstetric and anesthetic factors has only a miniscule benefit. However, medical professionals have always operated at a personal level. Teaching programs sponsored by developed countries in Central Africa and India have been most beneficial. Spinal anesthesia has a major role. Dextrose can be added to lidocaine in local pharmacies and thus provides a means of anesthesia that can be safely taught to local health workers. Regional anesthesia, although popular in certain centers, is still poorly accepted as a reliable economic means for providing operative anesthesia.[2] An unreliable availability of anesthetic cylinders and equipment, back-up services, together with medical and electrical supplies is still a reality.

In a hospital in Central Africa the only induction agent available to an anesthesiologist was diazepam 10 mg. In a life-threatening situation and with only time-expired succinylcholine, laryngeal spasm followed attempted intubation and resulted in death following hypoxia and aspiration (D. Riordan, personal communication). This incident occurred in 1989, and the economic reality was the scarcity of agents for regional or general anesthesia. This is an extreme example of shortages. In most developing countries, general anesthesia is available for mothers, but analgesia in childbirth receives very little attention – the busy Kuala Lumpur General Hospital has one Entonox cylinder to six delivery cubicles.[3]

In developed countries, intranational differences can highlight disadvantaged groups. For instance, minorities such as immigrants in Amsterdam[4] or American non-whites, have maternal loss that is still 3–4 times the rate of loss among white mothers.[5] With one or two notable exceptions, in all Western countries, unequal economic redistribution allows those in the lowest socioeconomic categories to receive a shrinking share of an often expanding economic pie.

TREND IN DEVELOPED SOCIETIES

It has become customary in Western societies to attribute the dramatic decrease in maternal and neonatal mortality to confinement in the hospital, with the availability of qualified doctors, nurses and physiotherapists and laboratory and pharmaceutical back-up. Western industrial societies attribute the decrease in maternal mortality to improved obstetric medical care rather than improved socioeconomic status of mothers.[6] The most recent UNICEF report identifies Ireland as having the lowest maternal mortality rate in the world, despite its low level of expenditure on health care. Both Canada and the USA invest more than twice as much as Ireland on health care as percent of GDP, yet record rates of maternal mortality per 100 000 births of 5 and 8 (Tables 84.1 and 84.2).[7,8] However increased interest in alternative birthing options is leading to modifications in existing practice, permitting labor in less formal, home-like settings, such as a hospital room with some of the conveniences of the home. This approach can accommodate the desire for a choice of analgesia/anesthesia available in conventional centers.

Since the 1970s, in the developed countries, the family unit has become smaller, with a greater investment by both partners in each delivery and with the expectation of 100% success with each confinement. There is enormous pressure on the services to provide care in keeping with these elevated aspirations.

Table 84.1 Maternal mortality rate by country. UNICEF evaluated maternal mortality figures in all member countries over the 1980s and took average figures for deaths directly related to childbirth. It is illuminating that countries with freely available abortion have higher maternal mortality rates and Ireland, with no abortion, has the world's lowest. Those who died giving birth could not necessarily have been saved by abortion. The maternal deaths in the industrialized countries (with the lowest mortality rates) were as follows:

Rank	Country	Maternal deaths per 100 000 births
1	Ireland	2
2	Australia, Belgium, Denmark, Israel, Norway	3
7	Italy	4
8	Canada, Germany, Greece, Spain, Sweden, Switzerland	5
14	Austria, USA, UK	8
17	Bulgaria, France	9
19	Czechoslovakia, Holland, Portugal	10
22	Finland, Japan, Poland	11
25	New Zealand	13

Group average: 13 maternal deaths per 100 000 births (Source: The Progress of Nations 1993 and The State of the World's Children 1994, UNICEF reports).

Table 84.2 Maternal mortality and health spending in $US by country

	1987	1980s
	GDP per capita on healthcare	Maternal mortality per 100 000 births
1. Ireland	7541	2
2. Belgium	11 802	3
3. Holland	12 252	10
4. Italy	12 254	4
5. UK	12 340	8
6. Australia	12 612	3
7. France	12 803	9
8. Japan	13 182	11
9. Germany	13 323	5
10. Denmark	13 329	3
11. Canada	17 211	5
12. USA	18 338	8

The implication, in the event of complications, is the relegation of fault to the negligence of the medical team. This has brought with it its own socioeconomic side-effects for both the hospital and the anesthesiologist, e.g. inflated premiums to defray the costs of the subsequent medical protection insurance, which itself is a measure of the high awards and settlements disposed by the courts. The clinical 'knock-on' effect is the increased tendency to perform cesarean delivery at any hint of potential abnormality in neonatal or maternal behavior during labor. It is argued that this represents the emergence of 'defensive' medical practice which is becoming acceptable in an increasingly litigious society.

STAFFING AND THE ECONOMY

There is a worldwide crisis in health care which is only partly economic. It is inevitable that as a country becomes more prosperous the state invests more on health care programs. However, costs of health systems have been escalating relative to national income. Health care systems are seeking to hold down health spending. Many countries are remaking their systems, while others are introducing new initiatives. The medical profession must learn to be accountable for their share of the health budget. Directives relating to prescribing practices, as well as research budgets, while economically imperative, are perceived as encroaching on medical autonomy and greeted with dismay.

Budgetary constraints are mainly reflected in reduced levels of staffing and restricted medical facilities for patients. The recommendations of the European Commission to further reduce the working hours of non-consultant hospital doctors to 39 h per week mean that more personnel must be employed in order to maintain the same service, or that existing staff be paid more by way of overtime, further straining hospital budgets.

In Britain, the market approach to the funding of health care is as yet having a mixed reaction. The concept of competition for the provision of services is not appealing to doctors. While there will be more consultants to treat illness, the teaching aspect of their work is of little interest to lay managers. The perception is that a service rationalized by accountants and administrators might not be in the best interests of the patient.

Other countries, such as The Netherlands, Sweden and Germany, have embarked on cost-containment or pro competitiveness laws. None of these reforms is popular with the doctors.

In Japan, with similar medical standards to the UK and more obstetric and neonatal staff but noticeably fewer anesthesiologists, the maternal mortality rate is twice that in the UK. While it is impossible at the moment to determine the reasons for this, the lack of trained anesthesiologists must be a contributory factor.[9]

CLINICAL PRACTICE

Patients in lower socioeconomic groups may be unsure of their eligibility for benefits or treatment.[10] While superficially they may appear to enjoy normal health, there may be latent health hazards, such as poor nutrition or short stature associated with heavy smoking, excessive drinking or a drug habit.[11] This is exacerbated by depressed levels of health education awareness.

In the hospital situation, these factors can increase apprehension and fear to an unacceptable level. The patient may often mask anxiety by aggressive and uncooperative behavior. Such groups would include mothers in special categories such as single adolescents, female prisoners, AIDS carriers and the traveling community. Many patients in these groups will have left the formal education system at an early age and be partly or totally illiterate.[12]

An American study[13] identified a correlation between lower cesarean delivery rate and lower socioeconomic status.

Puerperal depression does not seem to be associated with a single factor, but may very well be affected by psychosocial stress disturbances, or nonobservance of sociocultural rituals.[14–16] It is tempting to theorize that optimal standards for analgesia/anesthesia during labor would reduce the incidence of puerperal depression. This, however, has not been confirmed by research findings. Contrary to accepted opinion, few are resigned to the pain of childbirth. Extroversion of the pain, which is associated with certain sociocultural values, does not appear to increase the pain threshold.[17]

The presence of a partner at the birth can be reassuring for the patient but has implications for the health care providers.[18] In the performance of a specific procedure, the presence of an emotionally involved observer can place extra stress on the anesthesiologist. The rightful privilege of allowing or prohibiting such presence must always rest with the specialist in this situation.

Childbirth educators have a major role in preparing mothers for what to expect, and for what is available to them by way of analgesia and anesthesia during the delivery. Unfortunately, those most in need of this knowledge are the ones who either do not receive it or neglect to avail themselves of it. Providing analgesia for someone who is entirely lacking in both knowledge and awareness of the complexities of birthing, accompanied by an elevated level of fear and apprehension, can prove a distracting and dangerous mix for the obstetric anesthesiologist.

While health budgets are not limitless, much more money and resources will have to be allocated to improve the standard care of disadvantaged people. Anesthesiologists must lobby for the necessary finances which they believe will allow them to improve the quality of treatment they provide for their patients. A positive European approach to the situation in developing countries would be for an international body such as the European Academy of Anesthesia or the World Federation of Societies of Anesthesiologists, or the newly formed European Society of Anesthetists to give specialist recognition to a candidate for time spent on a primary health care team and thus make it attractive for young doctors to add this item to their curriculum vitae. There should be special emphasis on a teaching program for local providers.

There is no substitute for treating mothers at any level of the social spectrum with the utmost dignity and consideration. In the delivery suite, anesthesiologists, by their special position and function, can maintain a high level of morale, for both patients and staff, in striving for the highest standards of care. It is thus in the interests of all parties in the obstetric experience to ensure the maintenance of these standards.

REFERENCE

1. Zahr C A, Royston R 1991 Maternal mortality – a global factbook. WHO, Geneva
2. Greene N M 1993 The role of spinal anaesthesia in developing countries. In: Update in anaesthesia. World Federation of Societies of Anaesthesiologists. Great Britain p 1–2
3. Saunders J 1986 Clinics in Anaesthesiology
4. Rozendaal G 1989 The immigrant mother. Conference on maternal and neonatal care, Bruges
5. Rypens Medical Licensure Examinations. Lippincott p 749 et seq
6. Loudon I 1986 Obstetric care, social class, and maternal mortality. Br Med J 293: 606–608
7. UNICEF 1993 The Progress of Nations
8. UNICEF 1994 The State of the World's Children
9. Rosen M, Fujimuri M 1985 Maternal mortality and manpower. Anesthesia 2: 892 – 895
10. Muller C 1998 Medicaid: the lower tier of health care for women. Women Health 14: 81–102
11. Kappel B et al 1987 Short stature in Scandinavian women. An obstetrical risk factor. Acta Obstet Gynaecol Scand 66: 153 –158
12. Clinical Report 1989 Rotunda Hospital, Dublin p 39
13. Gould J B et al 1989 Socio-economic differences in rates of cesarean section. New Engl J Med 321: 233–239
14. Cox J L 1988 Childbirth as a life event: socio-cultural aspects of postnatal depression. Acta Psychiatr Scand (suppl) 344: 75–83
15. Kennerley H, Gath D 1986 Maternity blues reassessed. Psychiatry 4: 1–17
16. Kennerley H, Gath D 1989 Maternity blues. III. Association with obstetric psychological and psychiatric factors. Br J Psychiatr 155: 367–373
17. Wiesenberg M, Caspi Z 1989 Cultural and educational influences on pain in childbirth. J Pain Symptom Manage 1989 4: 13–19
18. Palkovitz R 1987 Fathers' motives for birth attendance. Maternal Child Nurs J 16: 123 –129

PART B
USA VIEW

E. B. Skerman J. H. Skerman

INTRODUCTION

Obstetric anesthesia presents a unique challenge to the anesthesiologist. Two patients (sometimes more with multiple births) are being treated, thereby demanding experienced care. During this past decade, the advances made in obstetrics and fetal/newborn medicine have been astounding. Along with these breakthroughs made in obstetrics, the practice of obstetric anesthesia has been greatly enhanced through knowledge gained by researchers concerning neural pain pathways and pharmacokinetics of neuraxial opioids. With all this new knowledge, obstetricians, perinatologists and neonatologists have begun to realize the importance of the multidisciplinary approach to patient care, which includes the active participation of an obstetric anesthesiologist. Coincidentally, obstetricians' and parturients' expectations demand a high level of safety as well as comfort, which has expanded the role of the obstetric anesthesiologist.

Despite the aforementioned advances in obstetric anesthesia, there are problems which have persisted and continue to perplex the practice. The purpose of this chapter is to discuss the concerns confronting the practice of obstetric anesthesia in the USA. Lack of anesthesia coverage in obstetric suites is the most consistent on-going problem; however, other problems which have developed as a result of inadequate anesthetic coverage for obstetrics will also be discussed.

Two major studies have been published on problems associated with obstetric anesthesia practice.[1,2] Though the surveys were almost 25 years apart, both identified anesthesia coverage for obstetrics as a current problem. Gibbs et al[1] documented the lack of full-time anesthesiologists, who were available in only 21% of all hospitals responding, and this figure dropped to 15% on nights and weekends. While the percentage of anesthesiologists involved in cesarean delivery increased from 40% in the 1962 study by Phillips and Frazier[2] to 70% in the latest study by Gibbs et al in 1986,[1] this percentage has not changed appreciably since 1970, when the American College of Obstetricians and Gynecologists (ACOG) reported their results from a survey conducted on all maternity units in the USA.[3] All three surveys concluded that an anesthesiologist was available on a 24-h basis in only a very small percentage of those hospitals responding, and the greatest lack of obstetric anesthesia coverage was noted in the smaller hospitals (<500 births/year). The reasons for this include the fact that labor and delivery suites historically have not been thought of as a priority area when compared with the operating room. Demands on the anesthesia staff from other areas of the hospital; i.e., surgery, recovery room, intensive care, teaching and research, are often prioritized ahead of obstetrics.[4] One might suppose this may be due to the antiquated idea that labor and delivery is a natural process without need of medical intervention. For some few parturients this may be acceptable, but most women anticipate the availability of some form of pain relief should it be desired or become necessary. Unfortunately, according to Gibbs et al,[1] 32% of all hospitals in their survey offered no form of anesthetic support, not even the availability of parenteral medications, to patients in labor. The authors further documented that 15% of those same hospitals provide no anesthesia for delivery and, interestingly, these hospitals also deliver 500 or fewer infants on an annual basis. Often when an institution has an anesthesia staff that is unable to provide adequate coverage to the obstetric unit, two levels of care result. The quality of anesthetic practice in the labor and delivery suite *must be the same* as that provided in the operating room. There cannot be two levels of anesthetic care within the same institution: one that applies to the surgical suite and another for the delivery suite.[5] In a recent survey conducted by Minnich and Minnich[6] for the purpose of determining common monitoring standards of anesthetic practice for patients in labor and delivery, varying standards for patients in the operating suites versus patients in the labor and delivery suites were unintentionally demonstrated. Their survey revealed that 98% of the respondents offered a labor epidural service and 85% of the respondents provided 24-h 'in-house' anesthesia coverage for parturients. The noninvasive blood pressure monitor was used most often as the only monitoring device – during epidural catheter placement 52%, during maintenance 73% and during delivery 53%. 2% of the respondents used no monitors during placement, 3% used none during maintenance and 3% used none during delivery. In this survey, 6% of the respondents were from Canadian hospitals and 91% were from institutions in the USA. The resultant comparison of the USA and Canadian monitoring practices reveals a difference in the percentage of respondents using no monitoring equipment – during placement of epidural catheters USA 1.7%, Canada 10.0% ($P < 0.01$); during maintenance USA 2.8%, Canada 20.0% ($P < 0.001$); and during delivery USA 3.2%, Canada 30.0% ($P < 0.001$). Though the number of Canadian respondents is small, the data clearly demonstrate some significant differences in the monitoring practices of parturients, while the monitoring standards for patients receiving regional anesthesia in the operating room are shown to be very different. The parturient and her fetus, soon to be a newborn, demand and need the highest quality of anesthetic care available. Should a maternal or fetal emergency occur, it is crucial that a skilled anesthesiologist be available to select, administer and manage his/her anesthetic care.

Each anesthetic area must maintain properly functioning equipment necessary to provide anesthetic care, ranging from usual and customary monitoring to complete anesthetic care of the parturient receiving general anesthesia, with all appropriate additional hemodynamic monitoring for any possible obstetric emergency. This shortcoming has also been documented by Gibbs et al:[1] 43% of the anesthesiologists and 47% of the obstetricians agreed that anesthesia equipment in the maternity units is inferior to that in the operating rooms. We must strive to ensure that the following statement agreed upon independently by JCAHO,[7] ASA[8] and ACOG[9] is instituted and maintained: 'The anesthesia personnel and equipment in the maternity unit shall be equivalent to that provided the emergency patient in the operating room suites.'[7–9] Barnes[10] noted the irony of a situation that can frequently occur in hospitals in the USA:

> The removal of a brain tumor in a 70 year old patient usually calls for a team of seven people, including an anesthesiologist and one assistant, who will work six to eight hours, whereas the birth of the baby at four A.M. is often attended by one physician, one nurse and inadequate or haphazard anesthesia coverage. At best, the life expectancy of the tumor patient is 18 months; that of the baby and the mother a combined total of over 120 years.

In many hospitals in the USA, this same situation exists today as it did in 1963, when Barnes first made this statement. Furthermore, it validates the fact of an ongoing problem concerning the lack of anesthesia coverage and the double standards of anesthetic care for parturients versus surgical patients.

With the exception of very isolated, small hospitals and/or remote clinics, it has been hoped that the above surveys would eventually cause hospitals delivering 500 or less babies per year to consolidate to regional maternity centers and to strongly discourage the development of small obstetric services.[11] When geographic factors require the existence of smaller units, these units should be part of a well-established regional perinatal system.[4] These measures would be a great step forward in solving the perpetual problem of lack of qualified obstetric anesthesia coverage. Unfortunately, only two states, Michigan and Massachusetts, seem to have adopted this policy to date. The most recent trend has been in the exact opposite direction, with many smaller hospitals attempting to attract the business of health maintenance organizations (HMOs) by offering obstetric services as part of a 'full service' hospital.[12] It is hoped that all members of the anesthesia care team in these situations will begin to monitor their obstetric patients during all phases of regional or local anesthesia, as it is known that anesthesia is not without risks, particularly in the labor and delivery suite.

In order to prevent an untoward outcome resulting from an anesthetic procedure, strict adherence to safety monitoring standards must be followed. This enables the anesthesiologist to sometimes anticipate problems early, and also to take appropriate interventive action to prevent possible injury to either the parturient or fetus. Two other sources of long-standing contention among anesthesiologists trying to provide coverage for obstetrics concern the location and unpredictability of the obstetric service. Labor and delivery is often isolated from the operating suite; this fact, coupled with the unpredictability of the service, causes difficulties in scheduling and management of the two areas using a limited anesthesia staff.[1,5]

The consolidation of smaller obstetric services into one larger regional center would again cure these problems. This clearly is no help to those currently affected, but appears to be the only solution short of providing more anesthesiologists or personnel for the anesthesia care team and/or remodeling the institution. Since many small hospitals cannot justify a larger staff, or specifically the hiring of an obstetric anesthesiologist, it is necessary to have an anesthesiologist who accepts obstetrics as part of his/her practice responsibility.[13] Though the smaller institutions may not be able to afford an obstetric anesthesiologist, this is not an acceptable reason to deny obstetric patients the services of an anesthesia staff. In this day and age of litigation, it would seem that to fail to offer parturients anesthesia for labor and delivery could be considered grounds for a malpractice suit. With the variety and acute nature of perinatal complications, which could and all too often do occur, many of which are life-threatening and usually unpredictable, the need for 'around the clock' competent anesthesia coverage available to the labor suite is entirely justified.

Another source of controversy identified relates to the changing relationships between patients and medical staff. At present in the USA, many patients 'shop around' to find a physician and hospital whose practices conform to the patients' ideas or desires. This is particularly true in obstetrics and, unfortunately, the price paid for attracting patients into a practice or hospital is often less than optimal care for the patient. Obstetricians have preceded other physicians in their acceptance of this attitude of consumerism along with some private hospitals in the marketing competition with other hospitals.

Currently, there is conflict between obstetricians and obstetric anesthesiologists as to the prudence of allowing patients to eat during labor.[12–15] Proponents of the more liberal intake policy feel that the parturient will be less stressed, less likely to require an intravenous infusion and less likely to require medical intervention. One obstetrician writes 'from our patients' perspective, the ability to satisfy basic needs such as hunger and thirst is important.'[16] There are no statistics on maternal mortality or morbidity caused by parturients *not* eating while in labor. Though many physicians do allow ice chips, water and/or clear liquids for the laboring patient as long as there is no maternal or fetal contraindication, Abouleish and Merriman[17] feel that there may still be an unnecessary additional risk owing to the acidity of some of the clear liquids. Chestnut and Cohen[18] recently stated a well-known fact that some healthy parturients unexpectedly require general anesthesia for emergency situations. In the land of litigation and expensive malpractice insurance premiums, it is an unnecessary risk to ignore established safety standards for parturients, which have been based on knowledge gained from years of research and statistical study. The concern of anesthesiologists, as stated by Campbell,[12] is that 'it underscores our failure to educate both obstetricians and patients adequately about the risks of pulmonary aspiration of gastric contents'.

Perhaps the need for obstetric anesthesia has not been realized or appreciated by some patients, physicians or hospital administrators. Many women do not realize the dangers of childbirth; this is shown in the USA by the increasing trend for women (who obviously think they and their unborn infant are immune to obstetric complications) to choose to deliver at home. Many women also do not realize the need for obstetric analgesia during labor until they desire or require pain relief and none is immediately available. There is no other circumstance in medical practice that allows patients to suffer severe pain, amenable to safe intervention, while under a physician's care.[19] It is the primary responsibility of obstetricians to demand from hospital administrators that their patients have available the same anesthetic coverage that is provided for emergency surgery patients.

Insufficient remuneration from insurance carriers is another area of concern among obstetric anesthesiologists and a disincentive to anesthesiologists to provide coverage for obstetrics.[1] In some states, third-party insurance companies want to pay the anesthesiologist only for placement of the epidural catheter, even if another member of the anesthesia care team administers or monitors continuous infusions.[12] What these third-party insurance companies do not understand is that patient responsibility and management of care is not over for the anesthesiologist when the last piece of tape secures an epidural catheter to the parturient's back. Since the anesthesiologist can safely monitor more than one laboring patient at a time, this helps to compensate for the disparity between the amount of anesthesia time spent covering the labor unit versus what is actually paid for by the insurance companies. These third-party companies should be challenged for their lack of knowledge. Similarly, the American Society of Anesthesiologists (ASA) and the American College of Obstetricians and Gynecologists (ACOG) have received reports that some third-party insurance companies have denied reimbursement for labor epidurals, unless a physician has documented the presence of a 'medical indication' for epidural anesthesia.[19] In the ACOG committee's opinion, a maternal request is sufficient justification for pain relief during labor and, therefore, third-party companies should not deny reimbursement.[19]

According to Ostheimer,[5] collections in obstetric anesthesia rarely exceed 60% of the total bill. Therefore, it is not difficult to understand why some anesthesiologists are reluctant to provide obstetric anesthesia care when unreasonable compensation as well as insufficient numbers of deliveries are the order. Ostheimer further states 'when third party payers and the government decide to provide appropriate reimbursement for service rendered, anesthesiologists will be more interested in providing their services for the labor and delivery area.'[15] Regionalization of maternity care would increase both numbers of deliveries and, hopefully, remuneration. If reimbursement is not adequate, it is recommended that hospital administration make up the difference, as departments of anesthesiology cannot provide services if operating in a position of financial deficit.

In Canada and the USA, many residency or training programs offer the specialty of obstetric anesthesia, and many obstetricians are now required to include a study of anesthesia for obstetrics in their postgraduate curriculum. This can be of great benefit for the two specialties in that it fosters greater understanding, thereby improving interpersonal relationships between the two specialties. This appreciation is clearly needed, as reflected in the survey by Gibbs et al:[1] 22% of the anesthesiologists and 46% of the obstetrician respondents stated that anesthesiologists are not sufficiently trained in obstetric anesthesia. It was also stated that 73% of the anesthesiologists and 59% of the obstetricians feel that obstetricians lack sufficient background in anesthesia. Despite this fact, 84% of the obstetricians agree they tend to dictate the type and timing of anesthesia provided to maternity patients.[1,20]

It is to be hoped that with obstetricians' realizing the benefits of good anesthesia practice by an anesthesiologist who not only enjoys obstetrics, but is attuned to the unique needs of the obstetric patient, obstetric anesthesiologists will gain the respect they deserve from obstetricians who have previously been resistant to other practitioners being involved in the care of their patient.

FACTORS RESPONSIBLE FOR CHANGING ATTITUDES ABOUT OBSTETRIC ANESTHESIA

The recent advances in obstetric anesthesia have been brought about by an increased interest and greater appreciation of the value of good anesthesia practice by parturients, obstetricians, neonatologists, pediatricians and anesthesiologists. Currently, patients are more informed of the benefits of anesthesia through articles in newspapers, and magazines, radio and television programs, conversations with friends or even being with a friend or family member during her labor. Many parturients accept they will have anesthesia for childbirth and additionally they expect the best methods to be available to them.[10] This new interest in obstetric anesthesia occurred first in the USA,[21] then Canada,[22] Great Britain[23] and later in Finland,[24] Sweden[25] and Norway.[26] As a result of this, the Committee on Obstetric Anesthesia of the World Federation of Societies of Anesthesiologists (WFSA) developed the text of *Obstetric Analgesia–Anesthesia*, which has been translated and distributed to anesthesiologists and obstetricians worldwide. There has also been more active participation by many young couples to become more educated in the physiologic changes associated with pregnancy, labor and delivery.[27] These enlightened young couples have shown a great interest in becoming active participants in the process of childbirth, including acquiring knowledge of the types of anesthesia available for the expectant mother and baby.[10]

The development of obstetric anesthesia has also been influenced by the obstetricians' appreciation of their obligation to provide their patients with the best and safest anesthetic care. The archaic misconception that obstetric anesthesia is simple and requires no specialized expertise has been replaced with the knowledge that its administration and particular management is often complex and certainly a very specialized entity of obstetric practice. No longer is it acceptable to sedate the patient to unconsciousness, or offer only encouragement to relieve the pain of labor and delivery.

In the USA, obstetric anesthesia has also gained acceptance and status among anesthesiologists as reflected by the number of abstracts, articles, journals and books being published on this subject. Acceptance is also reflected by the establishment of organizations such as the Society for Obstetric Anesthesia and Perinatology (SOAP), the Obstetric Anesthetists Association, and many meetings and symposia such as the Gertie Marx Symposium.

Recommendations to alleviate the problems associated with inadequate coverage in the practice of obstetric anesthesia in the USA consistently are to consolidate or regionalize smaller obstetric services into a larger perinatal center. The geographically remote hospitals or clinics and the small rural hospitals should affiliate with a regional center. Not only would the economics of obstetric anesthesia benefit by providing sufficient numbers of deliveries, but, even more important, the standards of patient care would be very high and research possibilities would be outstanding because of the expanded knowledge base gained from each individual's clinical teaching and experiences pooled into one institution.

There is yet much uncertainty as to the policies the US government will make involving health care. It is hoped more regionalization of services will develop and, if so, one area should definitely be obstetric care. Regulation of physicians' fees should not be dictated by attorneys or insurance companies, or the government; instead, physicians should be allowed to establish their own standards for fees.

The first anesthetized childbirth for an American woman occurred on April 7, 1847, when Henry Wadsworth Longfellow administered ether to his wife Fanny, for the delivery of their third child. They both declared it to be 'a gift from God'.[28]

Since the dawn of recorded time women have been in search of a remedy to help ease the sufferings of the travail of labor. The 'roots' of obstetric anesthesia came from these times, and thankfully medicine has come a long way since then.

REFERENCES

1. Gibbs C P, Krischer J, Peckhan B M et al 1986 Obstetric anesthesia: a national survey. Anesthesiology 65: 298–306
2. Phillips O C, Frazier T M 1962 Obstetric anesthetic care in the United States. Obstet Gynecol 19: 796–802
3. American College of Obstetrics and Gynecologists 1970 A report on the committee on maternal health. National study of maternity care, survey of obstetric practice and associated services in the hospitals in the United States. Chicago, American College of Obstetricians and Gynecologists
4. Heyman H J 1990 Systemic analgesia in labor: still a viable option? In: Reisner L S (ed) Anesthesiology clinics of North America, Vol 8, WB Saunders Company, Philadelphia, pp 43–54
5. Ostheimer G W 1992 The labor and delivery suite. In: Ostheimer G W (ed) Manual of obstetric anesthesia, 2nd edn. Churchill Livingstone, New York, pp 443–449
6. Minnich M E, Minnich S J 1992 Monitoring practices for epidural analgesia in obstetrics. SOAP Abstracts, Charleston S C, p 36
7. Joint Commission on Accreditation of Healthcare Organizations 1989 Surgical and anesthesia services. In: Accreditation manual for hospitals. JCAHO, Chicago, pp 269–279
8. American Society of Anesthesiologists, House of Delegates 1985 Guidelines for patient care in anesthesiology. Park Ridge, IL, American Society of Anesthesiologists, October 16
9. American Academy of Pediatrics and American College of Obstetricians and Gynecologists 1992 Personnel for perinatal care services. In: Guidelines for perinatal care, 3rd edn. Elk Grove Village, IL p 74
10. Barnes A C 1963 Quoted in Medical Tribune 4: 24
11. Levinson G, Schnider S M 1986 Obstetric anesthesia coverage – a continuing problem. Anesthesiology 65: 245–246
12. Campbell C 1993 Clinical dilemmas in obstetrics. In: Stoelting R K (ed) Advances in anesthesia, Vol 10. Mosby-Year Book, St Louis, pp 195–218
13. Campbell C 1993 Challenges in obstetrical anesthesia. In: Barash P G, Cullen B F, Stoelting R K (eds) Clinical anesthesia updates, Vol 4. J B Lippincott, Philadelphia, pp 1–10
14. Douglas M J 1988 Commentary: the case against a more liberal food and fluid policy in labor. Birth 15: 93–94
15. McKay S, Mahan C 1988 How can aspiration of vomitus in obstetrics best be prevented? Birth 15: 222–229
16. Elkington K W 1991 At the water's edge: Where obstetrics and anesthesia meet. Obstet Gynecol 77: 304–308
17. Abouleish E, Merriman T 1991 In obstetrics: keep the water colorless and clear. Anesth Analg 73: 674
18. Chestnut D H, Cohen S E 1991 At the water's edge: Where obstetrics and anesthesia meet. Obstet Gynecol 77: 965–966

19. The American College of Obstetricians and Gynecologists 1993 Pain relief during labor. ACOG Committee Opinion No. 118. Washington, DC
20. Charles-Rawlins J, Stein D J, Grunebaum A et al 1993 Anesthesiology rotations for OB/GYN residents. A survey of obstetric anesthesiology education. SOAP Abstracts, Indians Wells, CA, p 8
21. Marx G F, Orkin L R 1969 Physiology of obstetric anesthesia Charles C Thomas, Springfield, IL
22. Eisen S M, Rosen N, Winesanker H et al 1960 The routine use of lumbar epidural anesthesia in obstetrics: Clinical review of 9,532 cases. Can Anaesth Soc J 7: 280–286
23. Crawford J S 1977 Obstetric analgesia and anesthesia. Br J Anaesth 49: 19–23
24. Hollmen A, Jarvinen P A 1970 Conduction analgesia in obstetrical practice. Ann Chir Gynaecol Scand 59: 61–65
25. Cullhed S, Lofstrom B 1961 Obstetric analgesia with pethidine and scopolamine. Lancet 1: 75–77
26. Lind B 1970 Obstetric analgesia in Norway. Acta Anaesth Scand Suppl 37: 186–188
27. Watson-Lubric R, Ernst E K M 1975 Psychological analgesia (natural childbirth and psychoprophylaxis). In Bonica J J (ed) Clinics in obstetrics and gynaecology. Obstetric analgesia and anesthesia, recent advances and current status, Vol 2. W B Saunders, London
28. Knight N 1983 Pain and its relief, catalog of an exhibition at the National Museum of American History, Smithsonian Institution, Washington, DC, p 52

85. Obstetric anesthesia in developing countries

Part A Guatemala *I. Guasp L. M. Padilla*
Part B The Philippines *R. R. Joco*

PART A
GUATEMALA
I. Guasp L. M. Padilla

There is a vast difference between the standard of care in underdeveloped areas of Central America and that of more industrialized and commercially oriented countries. In Guatemala in 1989, 77% of births took place at home and only 20% in a hospital setting. This is a reflection of the type of medical assistance available: only 20.8% of births were attended by a physician and 30% by a midwife. Of the rest, 37% received 'empiric assistance' from a lay person knowledgeable and familiar with the birthing process, while 12% of parturients had no outside help at all.

The maternal mortality rate in Guatemala was 1.04 per 1000 live births. This is in a country in which the birth rate is 36 per 1000 habitants compared with a world birth rate of 9.7 per 1000. On a national level, 56% of the maternal deaths occurred due to complications originating at the time of parturition, 14% due to complications arising earlier in gestation, 12.5% due to puerperal sepsis, 11.5% due to abortion, and 6% due to 'miscellaneous' causes (L. Moreles Padilla, unpublished observation).[1] The three most common etiologies of maternal death in hospitalized parturients in two major hospitals in Guatemala City were as follows:

Hospital General S. Juan de Dios	*Hospital Roosevelt*
1. Hemorrhage	1. Sepsis
2. Eclampsia	2. Eclampsia
3. Sepsis	3. Hemorrhage

The cesarean delivery rate for the parturients in these two hospitals has ranged from 15% to 17%. This prevalence is considerably higher than the national rate, since only about 20% of all births are in a hospital. Approximately 70% of the parturients in the two hospitals received epidural anesthesia, 30% received general anesthesia but only 1–2% received spinal anesthesia.

The most popular local anesthetic drug used in Guatemala is lidocaine, the 2% solution – with or without added epinephrine – for epidural anesthesia and the 5% hyperbaric solution for spinal anesthesia. This pertains to both the national and the poorer private hospitals. In the financially more secure private hospitals, however, 0.5% bupivacaine has become the agent of choice for epidural anesthesia in cesarean deliveries.

General anesthesia for cesarean delivery is conducted using a neuroleptic technique following acute denitrogenation, rapid sequence induction with thiopental 5 mg/kg and endotracheal intubation with the aid of succinylcholine-induced relaxation. Fentanyl 50–100 µg is the preferred opioid. In the last 5 years, the prevalence of failed intubation was zero and there was only one case of pulmonary inhalation of gastric contents.[2]

An estimate of the percentage of parturients, overall or hospitalized, who receive some form of pain relief for labor and non-operative vaginal delivery is difficult to obtain. It is reported, however, that all hospitalized primigravidas are treated with local infiltration for performance and repair of an episiotomy. Whether a regional block is ever offered to these select few remains unclear.

Perinatal mortality is high. In 1990, the four leading causes of fetal deaths were: congenital anomalies, placental complications, rhesus incompatibility and maternal eclampsia. The most frequent etiologies of mortality in the post-natal period are outlined below (number of perinatal deaths per 10 000 live births):

- Miscellaneous and poorly defined perinatal afflictions 99.54
- Intrauterine hypoxia and asphyxia at birth 37.40
- Perinatal infections and sepsis 21.50

- Deaths related to premature birth and/or intrauterine growth retardation 19.46
- Other 16.41

After even a cursory review of the demographics of Guatemala's birth practices and its maternal and perinatal mortality, it becomes evident that limited access to obstetric care presents a major problem to pregnant and birthing women. In this country with approximately 8.5 million inhabitants, there are only 40 anesthesiologists. Undoubtedly, greater availability of qualified care would result in a more favorable pregnancy outcome.

REFERENCES:

1. "Guatemala a Cifras de Salud, 1987 y 1988": Direccion General de Servicios de Salud, Guatemala y datos no publicados de la Seccion de Informatica de la Direccion General de Servicios de Salud del Ministerio de Salud Publica Y Asistencia Social
2. Review of monthly statistics of the Departamento de Anestesia de los Hospitales Nacionales, communiques Dr Morales Padilla

PART B
THE PHILIPPINES
R. R. Joco

Maternal and child health in the Philippines reflects the vast economic differences between the opposite ends of the social scale. Since health insurance is virtually nonexistent, patients have to provide for their own health care. With unemployment and underemployment approaching 70%, this leads to a significant disparity in access to meaningful pre-, intra- and post-partum care. While modern medical facilities are available in metropolitan Manila, the mostly rural population relies on a mixture of superstitions, local 'hilots' or traditional birth attendants, midwives and poorly equipped rural, provincial or regional hospitals.

In this small country with 60 million inhabitants, separated by more than 7000 islands, the 1988 birth rate was 27.6 per 1000 population, the maternal mortality rate was 1.1 per 1000 live births and the neonatal death rate was 9.8 per 1000 live births.

The techniques used for obstetric anesthesia in the Philippines are basically similar to those employed in the USA. Monitoring, however, is limited by a lack of equipment. Mass spectrometry, capnography, pulse oximetry, electrocardiography and neuromuscular block monitoring are not available for routine use. Intraoperative controlled ventilation and blood pressure measurements are achieved manually. Electrocardiography is utilized only for very sick patients and those with cardiac problems. Invasive monitoring is limited to radial arterial lines and central venous pressure measurements through a median basilic vein cutdown.

Most modern anesthetic agents and drugs are available. Because of the high cost of isoflurane, enflurane and halothane are preferred as inhalation agents. Succinylcholine, pancuronium bromide, atracurium and vecuronium are utilized for muscular relaxation. Sodium thiopental is commonly employed for induction of general anesthesia and diazepam or midazolam for sedation. Local anesthetic drugs such as lidocaine, bupivacaine and tetracaine are available.

At the University of the Philippines-Philippine General Hospital, a well-known government hospital, the majority of vaginal deliveries are performed with local perineal infiltration or with a pudendal block administered by the obstetrician. Only a small percentage of women receive either continuous lumbar epidural block with 0.25% bupivacaine or inhalational analgesia with 50% nitrous oxide–oxygen with or without low concentrations of a volatile anesthetic. Spinal (saddle) block with tetracaine or lidocaine is favored for forceps deliveries. In 1990, at this institution, 74% of parturients undergoing cesarean delivery received spinal anesthesia, 16% received general anesthesia and 10% received epidural block. General anesthesia was mainly reserved for emergency cesarean deliveries undertaken for massive third-trimester bleeding, prolapsed umbilical cord or severe fetal distress. For nonemergency cases, spinal anesthesia was the preferred technique because of the ease of administration, rapid and reliable anesthesia and minimal effect on the neonate.

Needless to state, the conduct of obstetric anesthesia in the Philippines remains a challenge to the anesthesiologist's skills.

ACKNOWLEDGEMENTS

The author thanks Dr Nestor do Lacruz, Far Eastern University, and Dr Sylvia Acusta, University of the Philippines, for valuable information and advice.

86. Liability

Part A UK view *T. A. Thomas* *T. H. Taylor*
Part B USA view *R. M. Knapp*

PART A
UK VIEW
T. A. Thomas *T. H. Taylor*

Liability: the condition of being answerable, bound or obliged by law or equity.

Shorter Oxford English Dictionary

INTRODUCTION

When liability is discussed in the context of medical practice, it is usually assumed to refer to the legal accountability defined above. The word does have other connotations, however, particularly those of duty, responsibility and probability. These shades of meaning are important. If an anesthesiologist is aware of the probability of risk to his patient and subsequently discharges his responsibility to that individual by avoiding the risks, the practitioner will have nothing to answer for in English Common Law. An important part of that duty is the advice given to the patient of the most suitable method of treatment and the information given about risks and possible limitations of that treatment. Risk management techniques should be employed as part of the decision-making process, and their proper use will either prevent or limit any future allegations of negligence that may be made.

This approach is of particular importance in the practice of obstetric anesthesia because of two unusual features. In the first instance the mother-to-be and her family correctly regard pregnancy as a physiologic event and thus expect that no ill effect will ensue. Secondly, the presence of the fetus adds the burden of care of a second patient to the anesthesiologist's duty, and this care of the second patient may conflict with the duty owed to the first. There is also an expectation of a perfection of outcome which is not seen anywhere else in anesthetic practice. This very understandable view is held by members of the public because they are not informed of, and have little understanding of, the inherent risks of pregnancy, operative delivery or analgesia/anesthesia during labor.

LIABILITY AND THE BRITISH LEGAL SYSTEM

One, probably definitive, view of liability is contained in Kennedy and Grubb.[1]

> Legal liability for medical accidents can take a number of forms. Doctors can be held strictly liable for all the adverse consequences resulting from medical treatment, or only for adverse consequences resulting from their negligence. Those held liable can be either individual practitioners or groups of individuals acting collectively.

They go on to detail individual types of liability.

> *Strict liability* exists when individual doctors are held responsible to the patient for all the adverse outcomes of medical treatment.
>
> *No-fault liability* imposes liability on doctors as a group. The group might be the whole profession or only those doctors involved in the treatment which gave rise to the adverse outcome.
>
> *Negligence liability* is the current rule. Under this rule, only those doctors whose standard of care is deemed inadequate by the courts are held liable for the adverse consequences of their actions.

The object of establishing this type of liability for a medical mishap is twofold: first to compensate the victim of the accident, in so far as it is possible to do so, with money; and second to deter individuals or groups from acting negligently. In the UK the determination of liability is through Tort Law. This system is basically adversarial and, therefore, lengthy and expensive lawsuits are needed to establish fault. Some such suits fail to establish negligence and are, therefore, unsuccessful in obtaining compensation, irrespective of the needs of the claimant. Patients are rarely given freely a full explanation of the medical accident because of the antagonism inherent to the system and are even less likely to receive an apology from the hospital or doctor concerned. Ironically, this refusal to explain or apologize probably causes more patients to pursue claims into the courts than would otherwise be the case. Failure to explain and apologize is a practice to be deprecated for it is unmannerly, inconsiderate, unwise and poor risk management. In the UK at least, an expression of sympathy and explanation of events is often all that a patient is seeking when making the initial complaint.

The deterrent effect of this system on erring doctors is minimal and only derives from the small proportion of cases that reach the courts and, therefore, the public domain. Furthermore, the medical defense organizations only take to the courts those cases in which there seems to be a good defense in that the treatment given was correct and normal. The doctors who have to appear in court are therefore likely to be those who carried out correct treatment, in a proper way, to which the patient has taken exception, or in which a genuine accident has occurred. The obviously negligent practitioner is most unlikely to suffer the embarrassment of a court appearance because these cases are settled out of court by negotiation. The inevitable consequence of this system is that, from time to time, the courts will find in favor of a plaintiff even though an apparently correct treatment has been given. Medical practitioners react to the risk of litigation by building more and more defensive practices into their routine treatment of patients. There is already some evidence to show that this is now occurring in the UK.[2]

The number of claims has risen in the last decade, as has the value of each claim (Tables 86.1 and 86.2).

Naturally the cost of 'insuring' against such claims has risen commensurately (Table 86.3). The escalation of cost comes from a group of 'high-risk' specialties. Obstetrics accounted for most of the increase shown in Table 86.2 because of the rising number and great value of the claims for babies alleged to have suffered brain damage at birth as a result of negligence of their attendants (Table 86.1). The financial peril of the defendants is enhanced in these cases because there is no time limit for the initiation of claims on behalf of a minor. Since individuals with mental impairment never reach the age of majority in law their claims are never statute barred. Other specialities are less expensive and in an approximate descending order include: orthopedic surgery, accident and emergency surgery, pediatrics and general surgery. It was also found that the rate of claim against younger doctors in their training years, who were paying lower 'privilege' premiums, was higher than against established practitioners. The high-risk practitioners were clearly being subsidized by low-risk doctors; e.g., general practitioners and laboratory doctors. Interestingly, the number of claims in relation to anesthesia has fallen in the UK, as it has in the USA and Australia, for a number of reasons, not least of which is the proper use of risk management and critical incident analysis techniques. The excessive rise in the cost of identifiable 'high-risk' specialties as opposed to the more modest increases in 'low-risk' specialties led the Medical Protection Society in 1988 to institute 'differential' rates according to the perceived risk of each specialty. The concept of mutuality in general, which had been pursued satisfactorily for many years, was thus abandoned in favor of mutuality between equivalent groups of doctors. This system has been operating elsewhere for some time and is especially successful in Canada. The result of this entirely logical approach would be to place a very heavy financial burden on the individual members of high-risk specialty groups. In this context the phrase 'high risk' indicates a high actuarial risk of incurring cost, not a high incidence of medical accidents. The high cost to the individual in the high-risk specialty groups, if not reimbursed by the employer either directly or through higher salaries, would almost certainly distort recruitment to those specialties. This consequence has already been experienced in the

Table 86.1 Claims and costs in obstetrics (Source: Sir Donald Acheson, Chief Medical Officer, speaking at the Royal College of Midwives, 6 December 1990)

	Cerebral palsy claims per year	Average cost (excluding legal costs) per claim settled (per case) (pound sterling)
1983	50	250 000
1989	200	700 000
1990	600 (estimated)	1 000 000 plus

Table 86. 2 Annual costs of negligence claims (MPS only)

Year	Cost (pounds sterling)
1985	10 million
1986	13 million
1987	17.7 million
1988	22 million (up to October)
1990	NHS Indemnity for Hospital and Community Services

Table 86.3 Annual subscriptions

Year	Cost (pounds sterling)
1978	40
1979	70
1980	95
1981	120
1982	135
1983	195
1984	264
1985	288
1986	336
1987	576
1988	1080
1989*	1350 (MDU) MPS differentials

* Medical insurance in the UK changed to NHS vicarious indemnity at this point

USA and was seen in the UK to be of such detriment to the community that government intervention became inevitable.

In the UK, the National Health Service has always assumed vicarious liability for most of its employees. Kennedy and Grubb[1] point out that 'under this liability rule the fault of an individual employee renders the employer liable for the adverse consequences resulting from the employee's actions'. On 1 January 1990, the British government introduced 'National Health Service Indemnity'. Under this arrangement, liability is assumed by employing authorities for all claims against hospital and community health practitioners provided that the claim arises from work undertaken during treatment of National Health Service patients on health authority premises. The employing authorities also become responsible for the legal costs entailed in such cases and, therefore, it is they who decide how to conduct the case. Individual practitioners will have no influence over this decision, and the only gesture made so far by the NHS Indemnity provisions is that:

> In deciding how a case should be handled, and in particular whether to resist a claim or seek an out-of-court settlement, health authorities and those advising them should pay particular attention to any potentially damaging effect on the professional reputation of the practitioner(s) concerned. They should also have clear regard to:
> (i) any point of principle or of a wider application raised by the case; and
> (ii) the costs involved.
>
> It is open to the practitioner concerned to employ at his or her expense an expert adviser, but the practitioner can be represented separately in court only with the agreement of the Court. The plaintiff and the health authority may agree to separate representation for the practitioner, but under normal circumstances the health authority should not do so if it considers that this would lead to additional costs or damages falling on the health authority.

Under the agreement, subsequently signed by all parties, the individual health authorities take over all previous and future known, and unknown liability, the so-called 'tail'. The negotiations with the government actuary led to a sum being set aside from the reserve of each of the UK defense societies and placed in an 'NHS Indemnity' fund. This is to be used to assist the funding of existing claims and is expected to be exhausted in 3 years.

General practice and private medicine are excluded from these arrangements. Both of these categories involve less risk, the first by the nature of the work and the second because the incidence of claims arising from private practice seems to be lower than from NHS practice in the same specialty, probably because medical care in the private sector is undertaken personally by fully trained specialists. The defense organizations continue to offer full cover both for these groups and also offer an advisory service for those engaged in full-time NHS work. Bearing in mind the slight influence that practitioners will have over employers' decisions in the future, the importance of retaining advisory cover with a medical defense organization cannot be too strongly emphasized. Their advice is also valuable when facing the many quasijudicial proceedings that occur in the NHS, and in providing evidence for Coroner's courts and less commonly in criminal proceedings. All these activities are outside the scope of NHS indemnity.

CLAIMS, CAUSATION AND RISK MANAGEMENT

It is important to realize that many claims do in fact begin with a simple complaint from a patient or patient's relative. The complaint is often based more on a wish to understand what has occurred and why than a desire to punish the doctor or hospital concerned. Appropriate sympathetic and honest communication at this stage will frequently satisfy the complainant and will certainly show the individual or hospital to be caring and considerate if matters proceed to a civil suit. To pursue their complaint through the courts the plaintiff must be able to show that an individual, group or authority has been negligent in the discharge of its duty of care.

Under UK law a number of criteria must be met before a plaintiff can establish a claim for negligence. In the first instance it is quite clear that the doctor or health authority concerned must, at the material time, have owed the patient a duty of care and that this duty of care has not been fulfilled. Next the patient must also show that he or she has in fact been harmed. These two factors, acceptance of a duty of care and proof of harm, must be linked by causation; that is, the breach of duty must be clearly shown to be the cause of the damage. The difficulty in establishing the link can lead to the failure of claims. Unfortunately, a patient who has clearly suffered harm often attracts the attention of the media, and even if the doctor is not blamed the publicity can cause great damage to the practitioner's reputation. This occurs because it is easy to imply, in media reports, that harm has been done to the plaintiff, but more difficult to see, in the absence of full scientific scrutiny, that the damage was not caused by the actions alleged against the doctor or the drugs used. If a 'no fault' scheme was instituted causation would still need to be established to make a claim justifiable.

The duty of care that is owed to a patient is established by the contemporary standards of care of the day. To escape blame an anesthesiologist must be shown to have practiced to a standard that matched the contemporary state of knowledge and in a way that was consistent with the practice of other anesthesiologists of good standing. To make any comparison the courts must have available evidence from experts to be called by both sides. It is regrettable that practicing doctors are often not available for lengthy court proceedings, and this is becoming an area which retired practitioners occupy. The standards current at the time of the incident are sometimes difficult to identify, but will include the use of appropriate techniques and the awareness of potential risks. The standards of monitoring employed and the degree of supervision afforded to doctors in training are also factors that are likely to be taken into consideration. It is also important that, as far as is possible, sufficient information about the procedures, techniques and risks has been given to patients prior to treatment to allow them to give consent to the procedure on a reasonably informed basis. However, it must be stated that the criteria applied in this respect in the UK are perhaps not so stringent as elsewhere in the world.[3]

The identification and appropriate communication of risk is a necessary part of any discussion of liability. Good risk management depends on three factors: identification of risk, assessment of risk and response to risk. All three should form part of good contemporary obstetric anesthetic management. The principal areas of risk, and therefore potential liability, associated with mortality and morbidity in pregnant patients include:

1. failed intubation;
2. aspiration of gastric contents;
3. hypotension;
4. awareness;
5. neurologic sequelae following regional anesthesia;
6. pain or discomfort during regional anesthesia;
7. anaphylaxis.

Clear evidence that a practitioner has appreciated the risks, communicated them to the patient and responded appropriately to events which may cause harm to the patient will be considered by the courts and may indeed reduce a practitioner's liability.

Individual departments can assist defense of claims by instituting protocols outlining appropriate preparations and safe techniques for the conduct of anesthesia.

THE BRITISH COURT – SOME CURRENT ATTITUDES

Some of the most publicized anesthesia-related claims appearing in British courts in the last decade have involved awareness, inadequate regional anesthesia and maternal hypoxic brain damage. Some of the cases will be used to illustrate the judge's attitude to the problems.

Awareness during cesarean delivery under general anesthesia

In 1985 Mr Justice Russel awarded Mrs Margaret Ackers £13 775 plus costs against the Wigan Health Authority because she was aware during cesarean delivery. This was, for the UK, a high award in an area in which claims were previously not common. The publicity entailed led to many further claims, mostly funded by Legal Aid. However, in 1989 and again in 1990 the Medical Protection Society successfully defended two anesthesiologists against similar claims in two separate actions. It was shown to the courts in both instances (Ludlow v Swindon Health Authority and Taylor v Worcester and District Health Authority) that, although it was possible that the plaintiff may have been aware at some stage of the operation, no negligence occurred. In each case the anesthesiologist had employed a standard technique of general anesthesia for cesarean delivery that was accepted practice nationally and was also approved in the protocols laid down by the hospital departments concerned. The technique at the time included the use of antacid prophylaxis to reduce the acidity of gastric contents, acute oxygenation to prevent hypoxia during endotracheal intubation and application of cricoid pressure to prevent regurgitation. Induction was carried out with thiopental and endotracheal intubation facilitated by succinylcholine. A longer acting relaxant was given to allow intermittent positive-pressure ventilation with nitrous oxide in 50 : 50 mixture with oxygen to which 0.5% halothane had been added until delivery. Following delivery an intravenous opioid, 20 mg of papaveretum, was administered and the volatile agent discontinued. This technique, which was considered appropriate at the time, has since been shown to be associated with awareness in some 9 of 2500 (0.35%) of patients. In both cases the anesthesiologists, both doctors in training, had followed the method and produced a good anesthetic record of their technique. Neither anesthesiologist was negligent since both correctly and properly used the standard technique approved at the time (1983 and 1985) albeit the patient suffered a known complication. Both cases were dismissed and no damages were awarded to the plaintiff. The techniques employed were acceptable at that time as good contemporary practice and contemporary standards were clearly used to judge the quality of care. Subsequently practices have changed and currently, for cesarean delivery under general anesthesia, higher equivalent concentrations of volatile agent, preferably isoflurane, would be used. Anyone using the earlier method in present (1990) or future practice might expect a less sympathetic hearing in the courts should a claim for awareness be launched against him/her.

Inadequate regional anesthesia

A considerable number of claims have arisen implying negligence in the conduct of regional anesthesia. The claims are based on the fact that patients suffered discomfort or pain during operative delivery under regional epidural anesthesia. The increasing use of regional anesthesia for cesarean delivery and for pain relief during labor has undoubtedly brought this liability to prominence. Some of the cases are genuine failures of the technique, combined with a reluctance on the part of the anesthesiologist to convert to a general anesthetic. The majority, however, arise because patients are not warned sufficiently clearly that regional techniques for obstetric patients are fallible, having a failure rate of up to 5%. The patient's expectation of a labor or cesarean delivery free of all discomfort cannot always be achieved. When it is not they will be disappointed. To avoid this disappointment it is vitally important to inform patients of the limitations of regional analgesia/anesthesia and warn them that some sensation will remain and that there is a possibility of some discomfort or pain occurring. This information should be given during preanesthetic visits. The patient's response to the warning will assist the anesthesiologist in assessing the patient's suitability for delivery under regional analgesia/ anesthesia. Those patients who are judged to be unsuitable for a regional technique should be advised clearly, and the fact recorded in the notes by the visiting anesthesiologist.

Maternal hypoxia

Maternal deaths in the UK are the subject of the Reports on Confidential Enquiries into Maternal Deaths. However, tragedies occur, especially from accidental hypoxia during anesthesia, which do not kill the patient, but cause brain and other damage. Failed intubation, disconnections of anesthetic breathing systems, inhalation of stomach contents and anaphylactoid responses are among the causes. The first two are clearly not defensible and should now be preventable with proper clinical observation, the use of failed intubation protocols and adequate monitoring. In this context advisory standards for monitoring during anesthesia and recovery have been issued by The Association of Anaesthetists of Great Britain and Ireland in 1988, in addition to those available in the USA and Australia. These standards are likely to become the standards accepted by the courts as being reasonable normal practice, and hence departure from them may be construed as negligent.

Regurgitation and aspiration of gastric contents can cause marked hypoxia with the possibility of hypoxic brain damage.[4] In 1989 it was held by Mr Justice MacDermott that an anesthesiologist was not negligent when there was aspiration of acid gastric content during a difficult intubation preceding a hysterectomy in a nonpregnant patient. Severe chest complications resulted, which led to a hospital stay of 1 month (Chambers V Southern Health and Social Services Board). However, preinduction therapy to control the acidity and volume of gastric contents and the use of cricoid pressure until intubation is achieved are now standard techniques in obstetric cases. Omission of either in a case of damage from aspiration would lead to liability in any resulting claim.

Hypotension

Severe hypotension still occurs in obstetric anesthesia despite its recognition by anesthesiologists as a risk factor. It can occur during general anesthesia but is more common during regional anesthesia. It occurs more frequently in pregnant than nonpregnant patients because of aortocaval compression, and without early recognition and treatment is potentially harmful to both mother and fetus. Good practice dictates the use of lateral uterine deviation, acute hydration with intravenous fluid and ephedrine to prevent or limit the fall in blood pressure. Mothers receiving epidural or subarachnoid anesthesia should be warned of the possibility of hypotension. The signs and symptoms of hypotension are easily explained and readily recognized by the patient herself. She is likely to give the earliest warning of the change in blood pressure, allowing rapid effective treatment to be instituted. Appropriate monitoring of pulse and blood pressure in obstetric patients receiving anesthesia is now an accepted standard. It will identify changes and the effect of treatment and will help prevent maternal and fetal harm. It is now essential to show conclusively that appropriate monitoring has been employed in all obstetric cases. Falling short of the accepted standards will attract such opprobrium and cost in lawsuits that neither medical staff nor their employing authority or trust can afford the risk.

Anaphylaxis

This rare but dangerous reaction to many of the commonly used intravenous anesthetic drugs is well known. In some circumstances the results can be devastating, and lead to death or brain damage of the patient. Although damage may not be prevented, it is reasonable to expect that proper treatment was carried out by the anesthesiologist, including the use of epinephrine, and that the diagnosis be confirmed by the analysis of suitable serial samples of blood for complement C3 and C4 and immunoglobulin IgE. Confirmation of the diagnosis is of some importance because the signs of anaphylaxis may be almost indistinguishable from the signs of an esophageal intubation. The former is an isolated event and is a complication of anesthesia. Harm arising from it cannot be held to be due to negligence, provided the correct treatment is instituted at the outset. Harm arising from failure to diagnose and treat an esophageal intubation is a different matter.

CONCLUSIONS

Anesthesiologists should remember that obstetric patients probably have higher expectations of their care and its results than any other patient group. Giving birth is an emotional event with the potential for great joy or great sadness. The possibility of disappointment with one or other element of care during the intrapartum period is commensurately great. Inadequacy of pain relief or anesthesia is particularly keenly felt. Careful antenatal anesthetic advice will prevent much misunderstanding and should be available for all patients. Antenatal preparations and discussion of analgesia and anesthesia that are well documented are particularly helpful later, for instance, during labor when patients are in distress and often unable to communicate and plan clearly. A clear note that a form of treatment has been discussed and agreed on will be particularly helpful.

The recent changes in UK indemnity arrangements have yet to make their full impact on health care and the conduct of claims against doctors and health authorities. There are already signs that the current 'NHS Indemnity' arrangements will be a stopgap measure. The Chief Medical Officer in the Department of Health has already shown that there are worries that funds for patient care may be seriously depleted by meeting the costs of both successful and unsuccessful negligence claims by patients.

One benefit of this may be an attempt to impose a higher standard of care, for example by making compulsory the standards of monitoring during anesthesia promulgated by both the Association and College of Anesthetists, which are similar to those already adopted elsewhere in the world. Establishing with more reliability the true cause of mortality and morbidity, especially of the fetus, is also becoming a priority. For instance, there are signs that more resources will be diverted to establishing that predelivery events are the principal cause of cerebral palsy and some stillbirths. Finally one is left to speculate that in the UK at least the door may be opening to a 'no fault' system of liability.

REFERENCES

1. Kennedy I, Grubb A 1989 Medical law: text and materials. Section 5, Medical malpractice, Butterworths, London, p 475
2. Jones M, Morris A 1989 Law lecturers at Liverpool University. J Med Defence Union, Summer edition
3. Siddaway versus the Board of Governors of the Bethlem Royal Hospital and Maudsley Hospital Health Authority and others 1985 House of Lords Times Law Reports 22
4. Department of Health 1989 Report on Health and Social Subjects, 34. Report on Confidential Enquiries into Maternal Deaths in England and Wales 1982–84, HMSO, London

PART B
USA VIEW
R. M. Knapp

The overlap between clinical and legal issues in obstetric anesthesia is more extensive than most anesthesiologists realize. A variety of legal questions besides those of malpractice and informed consent can have an impact on obstetric anesthetic practice.

For most anesthesiologists, however, malpractice is the major legal issue of obstetric anesthesia – and with good reason. A recent study found that among anesthetic malpractice claims, those relating to obstetric anesthesia cost almost three times as much to settle as the non-obstetric claims.[1]

Therefore, it is reasonable that the topic of negligence should begin the legal discussion concerning obstetric anesthesia.

NEGLIGENCE

Negligence is the legal theory that supports almost all claims against anesthesiologists. Under the theory of negligence, a court will award damages if certain conditions can be demonstrated. First, there must be some actual and measurable damage. Merely feeling wronged, or even suffering a provable wrongdoing but not suffering a loss, will not entitle a person to an award. Second, the anesthesiologist must have been under a duty to act in the interest of the injured patient. Third, the duty to the patient must not have been fully met. Fourth, the failure of the anesthesiologist to meet the duty must have caused the injury at issue. To prevail in court, the attorney for the plaintiff must show that all four of these conditions occurred, whereas the defendant's attorney need only show that one did not.

Evidence

The expert witness

Most cases revolve around the issue of whether or not the anesthesiologist fulfilled his duty to the patient. This is another way of saying that the issue is whether anesthesiology was correctly practiced. Since few laws, if any, dictate how anesthesiology must be practiced, the courts must ask other anesthesiologists to answer this question.

The answers of 'expert' anesthesiologists are often the best evidence a court has on which to make its decision. The importance of these answers is seen in the latitude of expression granted by courts to medical experts. It is underscored by the high regard in which courts hold the expert physician's opinion.

As a rule, expert opinions on anesthetic care are given by physicians – but not always anesthesiologists! This is partly a matter of witness credibility and partly a matter of who the court is likely to recognize as an expert. For example, in one case a court was asked to decide whether an epidural catheter should have been left in a parturient for several days following a cesarean delivery. The testimony of a registered nurse concerning the propriety of this act was given no standing by the court, which noted that the nurse's opinion pertained to '... the exercise of medical judgment or involves decisions and treatment exclusively within the scope of a physician.'[2] Since nothing indicated that the nurse was qualified to express an expert opinion on anesthesiology, the court concluded that the testimony of the physicians would stand unrebutted on that issue.

Another sign of the court's regard for the expert physician is the fact that an expert need not agree with all, most, or even many other experts in his field. In fact, his opinion may be a minority view or it may simply be a theory that he happens to hold (unfortunately)!

An example of this was demonstrated in a case involving the possibly cardiotoxic nature of bupivacaine. Two obstetric anesthesiologists were allowed to testify to the existence of this property (of cardiotoxicity) even though their theories were not widely accepted.[3] In allowing their views into evidence, the court pointed out that peer acceptance affected only how much weight the injury might give to their theory. The degree of peer acceptance should not determine whether a jury should hear the theory in the first place, particularly when the theory was contradicted by other testimony.

Given the deference and the latitude accorded to the expert anesthesiologist by the court, it is essential that the expert shows a corresponding respect for the court's needs. A witness should be familiar with, and should truthfully describe, current practice and opinion in his area of expertise. He should be ready to substantiate his opinion when he agrees with a widely held practice and to distinguish it when he does not. In short, an expert anesthesiologist should, when asked, ably represent both his own opinions and those of his peers. Neither justice nor the profession is served when these principles are disregarded.

Standards

In recent years the American Society of Anesthesiologists (ASA) and other organizations have supported practice guidelines and standards that address issues in obstetric anesthesia.[4] Standards may serve several purposes but, from a liability standpoint, they seem to provide irrefutable evidence of what constitutes acceptable care. In fact, to the anesthesiologist, standards may appear to dictate the *legally* acceptable response to a given clinical situation. It turns out, however, that the courts have quite a different view.

Several courts have been asked to rule on the admissibility of standards to answer questions about specific episodes of anesthetic care. Each court found that the standards could be properly admitted, but only as *evidence*. The different courts variously described standards as evidence of accepted practice, guides for measuring care and a substitute for expert testimony; but each court refused them any more deference than would be shown a human witness. This gives standards the weight of expert testimony but it also gives the jury the freedom to disregard any standard it finds unhelpful.

The specific point which was emphasized by each court is that standards are not conclusive in determining negligence. In other words, a standard cannot by itself *dictate* the applicable standard of care to which a physician should be held.

This position reflects the court's understanding that standards are generally based on what is customary to an industry or profession. Custom is by definition rooted in the past and so the custom of a profession or an industry may well lag in the adoption of new practices. For this reason, the courts reserve to themselves the right to determine negligence based on all the currently available evidence.[5]

This is a philosophy that anesthesiologists should encourage. Even where a standard may appear to reflect the correct response to a clinical situation, all the relevant evidence should be examined before a judgment is made. The label of 'negligent' is too stigmatizing and too emotionally devastating to apply solely on the basis of some single, though simple, rule.

Duty

Good Samaritan statutes and the newborn infant

Establishing the anesthesiologist's duty to the parturient is seldom difficult. Duty will arise out of either an explicit or implicit agreement to provide coverage for obstetric anesthesia and it will be confirmed by the act of providing care.

The newborn infant, however, can raise an entirely separate question of duty. This is because the anesthesiologist's commitment to the mother does not imply an equal commitment to the infant after delivery occurs. At delivery, the infant becomes a second patient, separate from its mother.

At some time after delivery, an infant usually becomes the patient of a pediatrician, who then owes a duty of care to the infant. At the moment of delivery, however, the pediatrician is often absent. This leaves the obstetrician, the anesthesiologist and the nurse to jointly decide how to manage, and who has responsibility for, any complications concerning the infant. In the absence of a pediatrician, the anesthesiologist is frequently *assumed* to have that responsibility.

In law, there is no reason to assume that a patient – physician relationship exists between the newborn infant and the anesthesiologist. In fact, several states have statutes that have been used to deny both the relationship and duty that goes with it. These statutes are often called 'Good Samaritan' statutes, because they protect people who voluntarily render emergency assistance to an injured person.

As a rule, a Good Samaritan statute prevents a person from being liable for negligent acts or omissions committed while *voluntarily* providing emergency care. Such a statute may even relieve a physician of the duty to take reasonable care when volunteering assistance in a medical emergency.

In consideration of this principle, an appellate court was asked to determine if a Good Samaritan statute provided immunity to an anesthesiologist asked to resuscitate an infant.[6] The court found that in general there is *no* immunity for the anesthesiologist where either he has an employment *duty* to aid the infant or there is a pre-existing doctor–patient relationship with the infant. However, if a duty to the infant does not exist prior to the delivery, then it is not suddenly created simply because an anesthesiologist works at a hospital, is in a delivery room and has a doctor–patient relationship with the infant's *mother*.

According to the court, the question of the anesthesiologist's immunity with regard to the newborn infant turns on the issue of the *duty*. Where there is a duty there can be no immunity, and vice versa.

Duty, in turn, is largely determined by the basis on which an anesthesiologist assists in neonatal resuscitation. If a jury finds that he assists by chance and on an irregular basis, then no duty will be found. On the other hand, if it finds that he assists because he is either expressly or customarily required to resuscitate, then a duty to the infant will likely be found.

The message of the appellate court to the anesthesiologist is that his duty to a particular infant is a question of fact and of individual practice, and of institutional practice rather than of law. His practice with regard to infant resuscitation *in general* will largely determine his duty to a particular infant.

Breach of duty

Consent

Most questions about an anesthesiologist's performance are concerned with medical issues. However, the anesthesiologist's failure to obtain the patient's informed consent for an anesthetic may also be seen as actionable. The requirements of informed consent can present a confusing issue for the anesthesiologist because the standard is derived from judicial rather than medical practice. Furthermore, the stress and pain of labor have led many anesthesiologists to question whether any obstetric consent is truly 'informed'. Fortunately, it turns out that this issue is much easier to resolve than it first appears.

Informed consent

In those cases addressing the adequacy of anesthetic consent during labor, the courts have not made the subjective claims of the parturient the focus of their inquiry.[7] Instead, they have noted these three common factors that *together* support a finding of informed consent: the information given to the parturient, the absence of the parturient's objection to the proposed anesthetic and the parturient's cooperation while the procedure is performed.

This analysis favors the anesthesiologist, since two of the three factors are satisfied at the outset. It is unlikely that an anesthetic will be given over the objection of the parturient or without her cooperation.

The final factor, the information given to the parturient, also favors the anesthesiologist. This is because the courts did not base their findings exclusively on the parturient's opinion nor did they seek a specific kind of documentation. Instead, they looked mainly for assurance that reasonable information was given. Their view of reasonable information included a brief description of the anesthetic and its effects and a general acknowledgment of serious risks with the approximate chance of their occurrence. The courts also take note that an opportunity was provided for the parturient to ask questions. Once this exchange takes place, a brief notation on the chart will suffice to show that consent for an anesthetic was appropriately obtained.

Jehovah's Witnesses

People of certain religious beliefs will not consent to the administration of blood or blood products even when they are necessary to preserve life. Most physicians do not share these beliefs. Also, most physicians will, if forced to choose, prefer to preserve life rather than allow it to slip away for want of a blood transfusion.

The rights claimed here by the patient, self-determination and freedom of religious expression, are among the most important in American law. On the other hand, the state also has very compelling interests in preserving life, preventing suicide, protecting the interests of innocent third parties and maintaining the ethical integrity of the medical profession.[8] The conflict between these interests can become sharp in the obstetric setting, particularly when the parties in conflict are the mother on one hand and her infant and her physician on the other.

One particular philosophy has guided the resolution of

this conflict in recent decades. It is best quoted, 'Parents may be free to become martyrs themselves. But it does not follow they are free, in identical circumstances, to make martyrs of their children before they have reached the age of full and legal discretion when they can make that choice for themselves.'[9] In the obstetric setting this has been interpreted to mean that a mother may not refuse the benefit of transfusion where the result would be a dependent child deprived of parental support.[10]

The case that underscores the importance of the dependent child involved a father of two children. He was allowed to refuse a transfusion, but only because his family was able to demonstrate that the children could be adequately provided for by a close extended family and with the assets of a family business.[11] It should be noted, however, that these conditions required a judicial hearing to affirm. In the emergency situation, the anesthesiologist and the obstetrician may not have the benefit of extensive fact-finding or judicial direction. In this case, the sole guidance available may be the knowledge that judicial deference has traditionally been given to the needs of dependent children.

Minors

There is no uniform guideline for obtaining a minor's consent for an anesthetic. In several states, a pregnant minor is considered completely emancipated and her consent is the same as that of an adult. There are also several states with statutes that provide a specific age at which a minor is allowed to consent to general medical treatment.

When deciding how best to handle the issue of minor consent, these considerations may be of help. First, it is most helpful to get the advice of a professional who is familiar with the issue. Local attorneys who work in hospital risk management are likely to have a practical answer from their own experience. It is also important to keep in mind that, while consent is an important part of patient care, it is usually not the element of negligence that controls a claim. This is another way of saying that in any clinical situation there are usually several important aspects that must all be kept in perspective. The issue of age, and its affect on consent, has its place; and so do all the other considerations that affect an obstetric patient.

Finally, the realities of society and current practice are recognized by the courts. As one attorney recently put it:[12]

> Even in the absence of statute, there have been no cases reported within the past 30 years in which a parent successfully sued a physician for nonnegligent care of an adolescent without the parent's knowledge . . . In effect, the legal principle now applied is that if a young person (aged 14 or 15 years or older) understands the nature of proposed treatment and its risks, if the physician understands the nature of proposed treatment and its risks, if the physician believes that the patient can give the same degree of informed consent as an adult patient, and if the treatment does not involve very serious risks, the young person may validly consent to receiving it.

LAWS AND REGULATIONS

Not every legal issue in obstetric anesthesia is based on negligence, and not every one is resolved in a malpractice trial. Issues not involved with negligence may be decided in several contexts. The most common are case law, statutory law and the regulatory process.

Case Law

Case law is law made by judges on the bench, one case at a time. These decisions are based on the application of legal principles to a question not answered by statute or regulation, or on the application of a statutory principle to a specific question that was not considered by the legislature. This latter is especially likely to happen when the courts are asked to adapt the existing law to a changing society.

There is one societal change that is especially familiar to obstetric anesthesiologists. As social custom has changed, the person who is expected or who may expect to be present at a delivery has also changed. This has lead to conflicts between parturients and hospitals. One of these conflicts involved a hospital whose policy allowed 'immediate family' only in the delivery room. The dispute ultimately came before an appellate court for resolution.[13]

In this case the mother wanted the child's unmarried father to be present at the delivery. The hospital staff had some difficulty with this request and refused it on the grounds that hospital policy restricted the delivery room to 'immediate family' only. Since the father did not technically qualify, he was refused permission to attend the delivery even though he otherwise satisfied all the hospital's requirements. The court that ultimately heard this case decided that the civil rights of the parents were at issue. The court cited a civil rights statute that forbade discrimination on the basis of marital status in places of public accommodation, and it concluded that the hospital's policy was 'impermissibly discriminatory'. The result was that the father could not be excluded from the delivery room solely for lack of a marriage relationship with the mother, particularly where the hospital routinely allowed other nonmedical support persons at deliveries.

Interestingly, the court decided the issue even though the delivery had already taken place at a hospital that did not contest the father's presence. The court felt a decision was needed because the civil rights issue was both publicly significant and likely to recur.

Statutory law

State statutes can directly affect the practice of obstetric anesthesia. In California, for example, the scope of practice of nurse anesthetists is defined in the Nurse Anesthetist Act. This Act excludes nurse anesthetists from the practice of medicine or surgery. To some people, this also excluded them from performing regional anesthesia and, thus, obstetric anesthesia.

This apparent exclusion, however, merely set the stage for a statutory conflict over regional anesthesia. The reason was that a second statute, the Nursing Practice Act, allowed nurses to perform 'standardized procedures'. Where the first statute seemed to foreclose regional anesthesia to nurses as the practice of medicine, the second statute appeared to allow nurses to perform regional procedures if the procedures were properly defined. Not surprisingly, soon after the Nurse Anesthetist Act took effect, the following question was put to California's Attorney General: May a certified Registered Nurse Anesthetist lawfully administer regional anesthetics pursuant to a 'standardized procedure?'

The Attorney General reconciled the two statutes in an opinion that cited extensively from statutes, legislative history, court cases, and a legal nursing text. The final conclusion was that a nurse anesthetist could, indeed, '. . . lawfully administer a regional anesthetic when ordered by and within the scope of licensure of a physician, dentist, or podiatrist . . . but not pursuant to a "standardized procedure."'[14]

The primary impact of this opinion was to clarify statutory intent with regard to nurse anesthetists and regional anesthesia. The opinion clearly determined that the legislature intended to allow nurse anesthetists to administer regional anesthesia in California. In fact, the scope of permissible regional procedures for the nurse appeared to encompass whatever was permitted a medical practitioner.

There is another side to this opinion, though. In considering the statutory breadth of nursing practice, the opinion also affirms the domain of medical practice. In anesthesia, the practice of medicine encompasses the decision to induce or to withhold anesthesia. This decision may not be part of a 'standardized procedure', and it must be made by a medical practitioner. Only after the decision is made may the anesthetic procedure be delegated to a nurse anesthetist.

As a legal point, then, the line where anesthesia becomes the practice of medicine in California is where a medical judgment is required, rather than where a procedure occurs. As a matter of statute, the nurse anesthetist may legally perform regional anesthesia, but only based on the judgment, the initiative and the responsibility of a medical practitioner (but not necessarily an anesthesiologist).

Regulation

The Food and Drug Administration (FDA) is one of the most influential regulatory agencies in obstetric anesthesia, primarily through its drug approval process. Unfortunately, the purpose and significance of this process is widely misunderstood, sometimes to the detriment of both anesthesiologists and their patients. For example, during the 1980s, the clinical use of epidural and subarachnoid opioids expanded enormously, particularly in obstetric anesthesia. Despite the profession's acceptance of these techniques, many individual anesthesiologists encountered resistance to them in their own institutions. A rationale frequently cited was the lack of FDA 'approval' of most opioids for epidural or subarachnoid use. The impression given was that a lack of 'approval' meant the practice was either illegal or negligent. However, neither of these implications was true, according to both the FDA and the federal courts.

FDA approval is actually *labeling* approval and not physician *usage* approval. The approval process defines what may go into a drug's labeling, and approved labeling is required before a drug may lawfully enter the marketplace.

Individual physician use is not a concern that the FDA's approval process is intended to address. The specific intent of Congress, as recorded in the legislative history of both the original Food, Drug, and Cosmetic Act and its 1962 amendments, is that the FDA *cannot* interfere in medical practice. In fact, the FDA itself has pointed out that that passage of the act in 1983 was predicated on the explicit understanding that the act would not regulate the practice of medicine between physician and patient.[15]

Practically speaking, this means that once a physician has legally obtained any lawfully available medication, he does not need the approval of the FDA to vary the conditions of use from those found on the package insert. The courts have consistently upheld this right of physicians, ruling that the physician's use of legally obtained medications is the practice of medicine. As one court explained, prescribing beyond the directions in the package insert implies neither illegal nor unethical behavior. Congress did not intend the FDA to interfere with medical practice by limiting the physician's ability to prescribe according to his best judgment.[16]

With regard to obstetric anesthesia, it is clear that the careful and conscientious use of epidural and subarachnoid opioids is not illegal, unethical or negligent.

CONCLUSION

It is obvious that a significant number of legal issues may arise out of obstetric anesthetic practice. Taken together, they illustrate this point: Even though an anesthesiologist hardly needs to be a lawyer to practice good obstetric anesthesia, knowing certain legal principles will help a good anesthesiologist practice with that much more certainty.

REFERENCES

1. Chadwick H S et al 1989 A review of obstetric anesthesia malpractice claims. SOAP Abstracts, Seattle, p 64
2. *Fountain v. Cobb General Hospital*, 306 S.E. 2d 37 (Ga.App. 1983)
3. *Douglas v. Lombardino*, 693 P. 2d 1138 (Kan. 1985)
4. Palmer S K, Gibbs C P 1989 Risk management in obstetric anesthesia. Int Anesthesiol Clin 27(3): 188
5. *Darling v. Charleston Community Memorial Hospital*, 211 N.E. 2d 253 (1965)
6. *Clayton v. Kelly*, 357 S.E 2d 865 (Ga.App. 1987)
7. Knapp R M 1990 Legal view of informed consent for anesthesia during labor. Anesthesiology 72: 211
8. *Superintendent of Belchertown v. Saikewicz*, 370 N.E. 2d 417, 425 (1977)
9. *Prince v. Massachusetts*, 321 U.S. 158 (1944)
10. *Application of President & Directors of Georgetown College*, 331 F.2d 1000 (1964)
11. *In re Osborne*, 294 A. 2d 372 (1972)
12. Holder A R 1987 Minors' rights to consent to medical care. J Am Med Assoc 257: 3400
13. *Whitman v. Mercy-Memorial Hospital*, 339 N.W. 2d 730 (Mich. App. 1983)
14. 67 Op. Atty. Gen. Cal. 122, 4–5–84
15. *Legal Status of Approved Labeling for Prescription Drugs; Prescribing for Uses Unapproved by the Food and Drug Administration*, 37 Fed Reg 16503 (1972)
16. *United States v. Evers*, 453 F. Supp. 1141, 1150 (1978)

87. The labor and delivery suite

G. W. Ostheimer

QUALITY OF CARE

The regionalization of perinatal care has produced an increased demand on the anesthesiologist to participate actively in obstetric care. Fewer new facilities are constructed because they have to receive approval from a board granting a certificate of need; as a result, existing facilities are either closed or combined and upgraded to provide care for the uncomplicated to the most complex high-risk pregnancy. Regardless of the level of obstetric care, the quality of anesthetic practice in the delivery suite must be the same as that provided in the operating suite of the same institution. There cannot be two levels of anesthetic care in the same institution. The parturient and her fetus, soon to be a neonate, need and demand the highest quality of anesthetic care available to any patient in that particular institution.

LOCATION

The anesthesiologist responsible for the organization of the anesthetic services in a new hospital or facility should help coordinate the location of the delivery suite in an easily accessible area of the institution close to the admitting and laboratory facilities and equally accessible to the operating suite; ideally, it should be on the same floor. The availability of anesthesiologists is often dependent on the accessibility of the delivery rooms. The transitional nursery should be immediately adjacent to the obstetric suite with easy access to the neonatal intensive care unit. Depending on the construction of the hospital, it would be expedient to have the regular nursery and the post-partum unit on the same floor; however, in many institutions, this may be impossible. The prepartum fetomaternal intensive care unit should be part of or immediately adjacent to the obstetric suite. A schematic approach to the logistic problem is shown in Figure 87.1.

DETERMINING MATERNITY BED NEED

The overall number of beds in a maternity unit cannot be

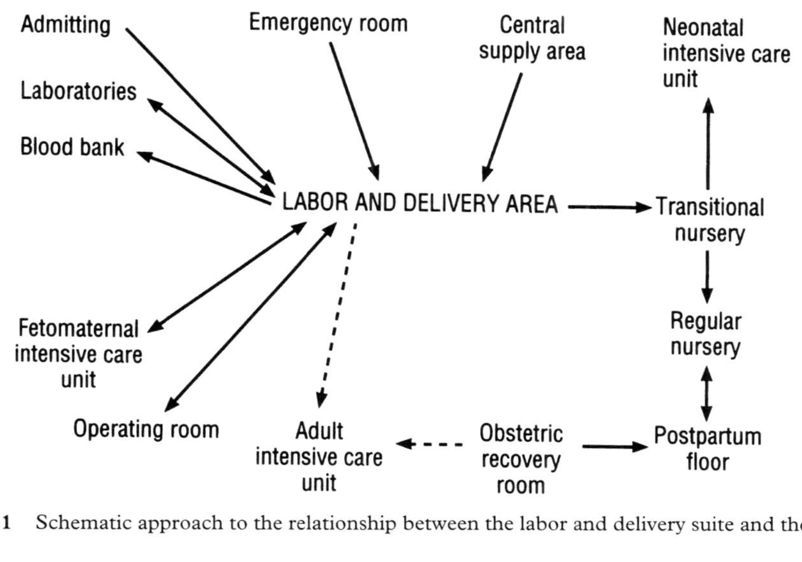

Fig. 87.1 Schematic approach to the relationship between the labor and delivery suite and the hospital.

determined by a simple formula. The number of adult beds must include those in the fetomaternal intensive care unit, labor area, and post-partum units. The neonatal beds include those in the transitional, regular, and neonatal intensive care units. Each hospital must have its bed capacity calculated according to the size and geographic location of the institution, population served, accessibility, average length of stay, projections, economic factors, and regionalization requirements.

As one might expect, each state has its own formula for determining bed need. One of the early approaches was based on a set number of beds per thousand population, adjusted for the density of the particular population. Later improvements focused on future populations and suggested minimal utilization standards based on an 80% overall occupancy. This plan attempted to calculate total bed need for the future on a current demand basis and did not take into account the need by service.

Service-specific formulas have been recently developed. The Public Health Service formula[1] calculates an average daily census for a maternity unit by dividing the projected census days by 365. This average daily census is then divided by the expected occupancy rate to obtain the number of beds needed. This formula can only be applied when patient turnover is extremely regular and the patients do not require urgent treatment so that their admissions can be scheduled. Neither of these conditions can be applied to maternity services, in which patients' arrivals are unpredictable and unscheduled. Therefore, this approach is being replaced by another formula based on the principle that patients should have equal access to beds regardless of a facility's size.

This translates into providing each unit with sufficient beds so that the probability (determined by the Poisson distribution) of all beds being filled simultaneously is kept below an acceptable threshold. For larger units, the Poisson distribution can be approximated by the more convenient computer-adapted normal distribution. Thus, the number of beds required to ensure a specific probability of immediate patient access is taken from a simple formula using only the average daily census and a constant derived from the normal probability distribution. Unfortunately, maternity services do not satisfy the assumptions about length of stay that lead to a Poisson-distributed bed census and the normal distribution is not accurate for smaller services. Fortunately, mathematical models developed by statistical theorists can be used instead for maternity services analysis. The 'finite-state, birth–death' queuing model has been used to plan emergency services and applies directly to maternity services. It assumes simply that patient arrivals are unpredictable and unscheduled; it imposes no restrictions on the distribution of length of stay and it assumes that the number of beds is fixed. From information on average patient arrival rates, average lengths of stay and number of beds, the queuing model will predict occupancy, or service, levels. The bed-need predictions of the complicated queuing model for specific service levels can be accurately approximated by a simple formula involving two constants, K_1 and K_2 (which depend on the service level), and the average daily census presented by the maternity unit. The higher the service level, the greater the cost and need for beds. The constants for the 99% and the 95% levels are 99% service level: $K_1 = 0.91$, $K_2 = 2.6$; 95% service level: $K_1 = 0.84$, $K_2 = 2.1$.

Sample calculations using the queuing formular for a 100-patient average daily census (ADC) are as follows:

Beds needed for a 99% service level:

$$\begin{aligned} &= K_1 \times \text{ADC} + K_2 \times \sqrt{\text{ADC}} \\ &= 0.91 \times 100 + 2.6 \times \sqrt{100} \\ &= 0.91 \times 100 + 2.6 \times 10 \\ &= 91 + 26 \\ &= 117 \text{ beds} \end{aligned}$$

Beds needed for a 95% service level:

$$\begin{aligned} &= K_1 \times \text{ADC} + K_2 \times \sqrt{\text{ADC}} \\ &= 0.84 \times 100 + 2.1 \times \sqrt{100} \\ &= 0.84 \times 100 + 2.1 \times 10 \\ &= 84 + 21 \\ &= 105 \text{ beds} \end{aligned}$$

The use of the queuing system for establishing maternity bed need will result in nearly equal service levels for all sizes of maternity units and considerable cost savings, especially with larger maternity units, because utilization will be more accurately predicted.[1]

INNOVATIONS

It is not my purpose to suggest architectural arrangements for the construction of the labor and delivery area; common sense dictates that the delivery rooms should be immediately adjacent to the labor rooms. In new facilities, some of the labor rooms should be convertible to delivery rooms with the inclusion of the appropriate beds that can function as delivery tables. This innovation will help foster the concept of family-oriented maternity care in which all the facilities of the institution such as blood banks, laboratories and intensive care units are immediately available but the parturient can deliver in a homelike environment, which may be more conducive to parent–infant bonding. Some or all of the delivery rooms should be convertible to major operating rooms for cesarean deliveries and post-partum surgical procedures. A minor operating room may be included for obstetric-related gynecologic procedures such as dilation and curettage. Regardless of the details of the arrangement of the delivery suite, one fact is clear: every full anesthetizing location must have the equipment necessary to provide complete anesthetic care from simple monitoring functions to full-scale anesthesia with the appropriate physiologic monitors for any obstetric emergency.

LABOR ROOM

What considerations should be made for anesthesia in a labor room? The amount of equipment needed depends on whether anesthesia will be inducted in a combination labor–cesarean delivery room or in a room used only for labor and vaginal delivery. In the latter situation, wall outlets must accommodate oxygen, suction, sphygmomanometer, emergency call system, and adequate lighting. Hangers for intravenous bottles can be part of the labor room or attached to the labor bed. The labor bed must be capable of being placed in a head-up or head-down position. Suction catheters and oxygen delivery systems must be in each labor room and ready for immediate use.

If the labor room is also to function as a cesarean delivery room, and therefore as a surgical location, the usual equipment found in a regular operating delivery room must be available. Compact anesthesia machines and wall-mounted cabinets can provide the essential equipment while their presence can be unobtrusive to the occupants of the labor room. Although an electro-cardiograph is not mandatory for each labor–vaginal delivery room, an emergency cart must be immediately available in the labor area that will contain the standard drugs and equipment for emergency care. It should also contain a combination electrocardiographic and arterial monitor, central venous pressure equipment, a defibrillator, and a cardiac resuscitation board. Uterine displacement equipment is mandatory in each labor and delivery room. If regional blocks are initiated in the labor room, essential anesthetic and resuscitative equipment must be on a cart brought into the room before the block is performed.

In my opinion, the obstetric service should provide an electronic fetal monitor for each patient in labor. Electronic fetal heart rate monitoring provides essential information not available via auscultation, because few labor attendants – physicians, midwives, or nurses – ever listen to the entire contraction cycle. One cannot be aware of variations in fetal heart rate unless one listens from the beginning of one contraction to the beginning of the next contraction. Auscultation of the fetal heart rate between contractions will miss late decelerations and variable decelerations; it will identify only the very ominous prolonged late decelerations that demand immediate intervention, and perhaps cesarean delivery, unless vaginal delivery is imminent. Although 'full-cycle' auscultation has been shown to be adequate monitoring in comparative studies, its use mandates 'one-on-one' nursing, which is a luxury few hospitals can afford. Therefore, I do not see a return to auscultation in place of continuous electronic fetal heart rate monitoring.

For maternal monitoring during regional anesthesia in a labor-delivery room, I would like to see the development of a noninvasive blood pressure finger cuff to be worn on one finger accompanied by a pulse oximeter worn on another finger of the same hand. Designs attempted to date by various companies have been cumbersome and unreliable.

DELIVERY ROOM

The delivery room must be equipped to provide appropriate anesthesia for vaginal or abdominal delivery, postpartum tubal ligation, and any emergency obstetric surgery. The same quality of anesthetic equipment available in the general operating suite must be available in the delivery room.

Modern delivery rooms should have piped-in nitrous oxide and oxygen provided through an overhead unit to prevent personnel from becoming entangled in coils of tubing. Suction is most efficient if aided by gravity and led to floor bottles. There is no need to provide explosive gases in the delivery area since all procedures can be done with a variety of nonexplosive agents. The expense of conductive flooring and appropriate grounding is excessive and not justified for new or refurbished areas; most important, delivery room personnel today are unfamiliar with the precautions necessary when explosive agents are in use.

An automated noninvasive blood pressure monitor, pulse oximeter, capnograph or mass spectrometer, temperature probe, electrocardiograph, and ventilator should be mounted on the anesthetic machine, which should be equipped with fail-safe devices, an oxygen analyzer, and precision vaporizers. The availability of central venous pressure, arterial blood pressure, and pulmonary arterial blood pressure transducers would be useful. A fetal heart rate monitor must be available. The immediate availability of all necessary fluids, infusion apparatus, nerve stimulator, and other standard anesthetic equipment is essential. Scavenging devices are necessary in all anesthetizing locations to minimize the contamination of the environment by trace gases. Endotracheal intubation utilizing rapid induction and cricoid pressure is mandatory if general anesthesia is administered for vaginal or cesarean delivery. Depending on the individual needs of the institution, disposable or reusable inhalational equipment may be selected. Disposable regional anesthesia trays are recommended since aseptic meningitis appears to be related to turnover of the hospital personnel preparing the kits, because inexperienced workers may deviate from appropriate technique.

An anesthetic supply area should be easily accessible and should contain additional equipment including blood warmers and a refrigerator to keep perishable medications and cold intravenous solutions to administer during a hyperthermic crisis. This area should also have a designated shelf for specialized equipment boxes that will contain appropriate equipment and drugs to deal with difficult intubation (including fiberoptic endoscopy equipment, materials for transtracheal jet ventilation, and cricothyroidotomy/tracheotomy kits), malignant hyperthermia, and cardiac arrest. Equipment for the routine care and resuscitation on the neonate is listed in Chapter 74.

PROCEDURE ROOM

It would be to the advantage of the anesthesia team if a large room (minimum size, 400 square feet) were included in the design of the delivery suite. This area would allow the administration of multiple epidural anesthetics simultaneously, particularly in preparation for cesarean delivery. This procedure room should be fully stocked with the appropriate anesthesia equipment, including an anesthetic machine with appropriate monitoring equipment, intravenous fluids and administration sets, block trays, wall outlets for oxygen and suction and electric fetal monitors.

An efficient labor and delivery unit demands the services of the anesthetic care team coupled with skilled obstetric nursing care. Often, the labor and delivery nurses are the first to observe hypotension and fetal heart rate changes and should initiate appropriate therapy at once. This may include increasing the rate of intravenous fluid administration, giving oxygen by mask, placing the parturient in the lateral position, discontinuing the oxytocin infusion, correlating the monitoring of the uterine contractions and the fetal heart rate, and notifying the anesthetic care team about the problem.

TRANSITIONAL NURSERY

The labor and delivery suite should be on the same floor and physically connected to the neonatal intensive care unit and the regular nurseries by a transitional nursery. This area would contain bassinets to observe neonates with potential problems and incubators to facilitate transfer to the specialized acute care area. This area would provide acute intensive care from the moment the neonate arrives (minutes after delivery) until he or she has stabilized sufficiently to allow transfer to an acute care area. A small number of intensive care beds should be available at all times in the transitional nursery. Radiant heaters are essential since one of the major problems after delivery is the loss of temperature in the neonate. This factor alone can precipitate the continuation or recurrence of acidosis and hypoxia and lead to persistent fetal circulation.

RECOVERY AREA

A recovery room or area in the labor and delivery suite is essential in order to allow close observation of the mother for the first few hours after delivery. It should be immediately adjacent to the delivery and obstetric operating rooms. Ideally, there should be a separate nursing station for the recovery area, which should be as fully equipped as the postanesthetic and surgical recovery area. Accessibility to the adult intensive care areas is desirable (Fig. 81.1). Minimal facilities include wall-mounted oxygen and suction outlets, direct and indirect lighting, sphygmomanometers, pulse oximeters, curtains to divide the room into individual private areas, routine and emergency drugs, cardiopulmonary resuscitation cart, and cardiac monitor with defibrillator. A large pleasant room is preferable to small cramped cubicles. Curtains will give the parturient, father, and neonate a chance to interact in a private area without diminishing the effectiveness of the nursing care by making observation difficult. The number of recovery room beds should equal one-third of the number of labor beds in a busy service.

Family-oriented obstetric care may allow post-partum recovery in the combination labor–delivery room or labor room if nursing coverage is sufficient. Recovery area personnel should be qualified to provide the intensive care that may be necessary in routine or emergency situations. Continuous teaching and monitoring by the obstetric anesthesia service is necessary to maintain a high quality standard of care.

ADMINISTRATION

The obstetric anesthesia section should have office facilities adjacent to the labor and delivery area. A conference room with teaching facilities and audiovisual equipment should be available and can be shared with the departments of obstetrics and neonatology. On-call rooms must be adjacent to the obstetric suite so that there can be an immediate response to an emergency call.

PERSONNEL

Determining need

The requirements for anesthetic personnel in the labor and delivery area are difficult to ascertain. Coverage may range from 'on-call' situation, in which the anesthesiologist responds to the needs of the service from the surgical suite, to anesthetic personnel who are in attendance in the labor and delivery suite 24 h a day. It would be very difficult to contrast our situation at Brigham and Women's Hospital with any other hospital. At present, we are approaching 11 000 deliveries a year. We are an academic department of anesthesia that trains fellows and residents in obstetric anesthesia.

Anesthesia care team

Although the number of available anesthesiologists is increasing throughout the United States, I do not believe there are adequate numbers at this time to provide 24 h-a-day coverage in the labor and delivery areas throughout the Level III hospitals in the United States, let alone the Level II or I hospitals. (A Level III hospital is able to handle any obstetric or neonatal problem and has the appropriate personnel available 24 h a day; Level II hospitals can offer advanced but not all encompassing perinatal care and Level I hospitals offer routine obstetric and neonatal care.) Therefore, our initial premise in providing obstetric anesthesia care is the appropriate utilization of the anesthesia care team. Depending on the institution, the anesthesia care team may involve anesthesiologists only up to and including anesthesiologists and residents and/or nurse anesthetists. At Brigham and Women's Hospital, the anesthesia care teams include staff anesthesiologists, fellows in obstetric anesthesia, residents on their obstetric anesthesia rotation, and, on occasion, certified nurse anesthetists. All types of obstetric pain relief are available, with the exception of inhalation analgesia, which has not been used in our institution in more than 25 years. We do not see any need to utilize an archaic form of pain relief while jeopardizing the mother's health if she has had parenteral sedatives and narcotics that in combination with inhaled analgesics may lead to a general anesthetic state, with the possibility of regurgitation and aspiration into the unprotected airway. Paracervical block is an excellent technique that is utilized as previously presented in Chapter 30 for gynecologic procedures; however, it has not been used on our obstetric service for pain relief in more than 15 years.

Coverage in the labor and delivery area is provided by a minimum of one staff anesthesiologist 24 h a day, supplemented with a combination of fellows, residents, and nurse–anesthetists. Obviously, this is reasonable both for patient care and on a financial basis since we are administering anesthesia to approximately 70% of our total number of deliveries.

Is it possible to provide adequate anesthesia care in the smaller units throughout the country? I believe adequate obstetric anesthesia care can be provided on an 'on-call' basis in which the anesthesiologist is in reasonable proximity to the labor and delivery suite. The level of care provided should include major regional anesthesia and general endotracheal anesthesia for vaginal and cesarean delivery. Depending on the particular circumstances in each institution, this may not provide for the provision of continuous epidural anesthesia on a 24 h-a-day basis.

A member of the anesthesia care team often must assist in the resuscitation of the neonate if a pediatrician or pediatric nurse trained in neonatal resuscitation is not available. Such expertise may not be available in many of the 5000 hospitals in the United States that provide obstetric care. It must be kept in mind that qualified personnel, *other* than the anesthesiologist attending the mother, should be immediately available to assume responsibility for resuscitation of the depressed neonate (Standard VI of 'Standards/Guidelines for Conduction Anesthesia in Obstetrics'). It is the responsibility of the hospital overall to make sure that qualified personnel are available. The attending anesthesiologist acts as a 'Good Samaritan' if he or she assists in the resuscitation since the primary responsibility is to the parturient.

When is it possible to provide continuous obstetric coverage other than in an academic institution? I believe that approximately 2000 deliveries a year could be considered borderline for full-time coverage of an obstetric service by a designated anesthesiologist given:

1. A cesarean delivery rate of 20% (2000 × 20 % = 400 cesarean deliveries).
2. 50% of the vaginal deliveries would require only parenteral medication: narcotics and/or tranquilizers and local infiltration or pudendal block (1,600 × 50% = 800 vaginal deliveries).
3. 2000–400 = 1600 vaginal deliveries −800 requiring no major anesthetic = 800 deliveries that would require a major anesthetic (spinal or epidural).

We are discussing the administration of anesthesia to 1200 parturients a year. An average of three to four deliveries a day requiring anesthesia provides enough work for the anesthesia care team.

Reimbursement

The one problem with the above calculation is that it does not take into account the reimbursement where these deliveries are taking place. Inherent to the above calculation is the factor that at least 50% of the population being served by obstetric anesthesia will completely pay their bill. This is presumptuous in many states.

Collections for obstetric anesthesia rarely exceed 60% of the total bill. Therefore, without a reasonable number of deliveries and reasonable compensation for anesthetic services, it is not difficult to understand why anesthesiologists are not that interested in providing obstetric anesthesia care. When the third-party payers and the government decide to provide appropriate reimbursement for services rendered, anesthesiologists will be more interested in providing their services forth labor and delivery area.

However, let us assume that the anesthesia department in the particular hospital has decided to provide obstetric anesthesia care using an anesthesia care team. Using the figure of 2000 as the minimal number of deliveries to make it financially feasible, we assume that at least 60% of the total number of women delivering must receive a major anesthetic in some form to even come close to providing satisfactory reimbursement. If the level of reimbursement is inadequate or the services are not adequately utilized and the hospital demands 24 h-a-day coverage by the anesthesia care team, I believe it is the responsibility of the hospital to make up the difference so that the anesthesia department can break even financially given the compensation received for services provided. Only by putting the appropriate financial squeeze on the administration of the hospital will the administrators and physicians realize that perhaps regionalization of certain aspects of medical care may be more financially feasible in the long run. Obviously, hospitals in rural areas must provide Level I or routine obstetric services to their population. However, Level II or III units should have adequate populations to provide more sophisticated perinatal services. It is absurd for 8 out of 10 hospitals in a metropolitan area to provide obstetric anesthesia services and not perform more than 1500 deliveries each.

Regionalization into Level II or III hospitals would provide an extremely high level of maternal–fetal–neonatal care and meet all the needs of the metropolitan area. State Departments of Public Health should help (force?) hospitals to consolidate their services and provide open staffing for more efficient delivery of perinatal health care. Hospital administrations must realize that they cannot provide all the services from 'birth to death'; they must provide those services that they can most efficiently. Therefore, while one hospital is the cardiac regional center, another hospital could be the perinatal center and have a sufficient number of deliveries to provide continuous obstetric, anesthetic, and neonatal intensive care services.

It took personnel interested in perinatal medicine many years to convince obstetricians that the uterus is the best transport incubator for the fetus. How many years will it take us to convince state and hospital administrators that the amount of money available for medical care is finite and that hard-nosed decisions must be made in order to provide the best possible medical care for the citizens of a particular area?

In summary, approximately 2000 deliveries are required to make 24 h-a-day obstetric anesthesia 'in-house' relatively feasible, assuming that 60% of these patients receive a major anesthetic. Otherwise, obstetric anesthesia services should be on a consultative or per-case basis, which takes into account what other demands are being made on the anesthetic services of the hospital. If the hospital administration sees 24 h-a-day obstetric anesthesia coverage as a selling point for their hospital over other hospitals with maternity services in the area and the number of deliveries do not come up to the rate mentioned, hospitals must supplement the income of the anesthesia department to come close to a 'break even' basis. The anesthesia department cannot be in a deficit position for providing services. Obviously, 24 h-a-day coverage of obstetric anesthesia services must be made economically feasible by direct or third-party payments.

One does not like to forecast the future, but it would appear that we are adequately training enough physicians in obstetric anesthesia to be comfortable with providing that service. However, with the exception of the Level III perinatal centers, anesthesia care for obstetrics remains the function of the anesthesiologist who is a 'generalist' – trained to provide obstetric anesthesia on a 'case-by-case' or consultative basis, primarily due to manpower and financial constraints.

REFERENCES

1. Department of Public Health, Commonwealth of Massachusetts: Regionalization of maternity and newborn care in Massachusetts, Final Report, August 1, 1974–September 30, 1976, Boston, 1977

SECTION 7

Controversies

88. Is epidural analgesia the best method of pain relief in the world today?

Part A Anesthesiologists' view *D. R. Gambling G. H. McMorland*
Part B Obstetrician's view *J. F. Pearson*
Part C Mothers' view of childbirth *B. M. Morgan*

PART A
ANESTHESIOLOGISTS' VIEW
D. R. Gambling G. H. McMorland

This chapter will address the issue of pain relief in labor, although many statements will also apply to analgesia or anesthesia for operative delivery. Epidural analgesia will be compared with other methods of relieving labor pain, bearing in mind the various needs and facilities throughout the world.

Melzack et al[1] have shown that, even after careful prenatal preparation for controlled childbirth, most women do experience significant pain during labor. Pain, associated with a long, exhausting labor, is an acute stress, associated with progressive increase in endogenous catecholamine release.[2] This, in turn, may lead to decreased uterine activity and longer labors,[3] as well as a reduction in uterine blood flow that may cause acute fetal asphyxia.[4,5]

The specifications for the ideal labor analgesic would include:

1. universally available and acceptable;
2. affordable;
3. adequate analgesia throughout labor;
4. no adverse effect on progress or outcome of labor;
5. no adverse effect on fetus or neonate;
6. no maternal side-effects;
7. noninvasive, with rapid onset and offset times;
8. controllable;
9. no need for monitoring, special equipment, vigilance, expertise or training.

Unfortunately, this ideal analgesic is unlikely to ever exist. The pharmacologic agents now in use do not fit all of these criteria and regional blocks fall far short. Psychoprophylaxis provides some benefit in certain communities, but frequently requires some additional form of analgesia. Hypnosis and psychotherapy have their proponents, but require trained therapists and are time-consuming.

Epidural analgesia is regarded as the standard by which other analgesic techniques are measured. A multitude of clinical trials have been done over the past two decades to assess epidural analgesia during labor and a comprehensive analysis of these trials is summarized in a book chapter by Dickersin[6] which is recommended reading. It will reduce maternal plasma epinephrine levels, during labor, by 56% and also block the expected rise in plasma catecholamine levels at the height of each contraction.[7] Administered via an indwelling catheter, epidural analgesia is a versatile technique. It provides good to excellent pain relief, which can be adjusted to serve the strength and frequency of uterine contraction at each stage of labor. Associated morbidity is minimal and complications are few in number. While intermittent 'top-up' doses, given by anesthesiologist or midwife, are effective, continuous epidural infusions[8,9] and patient-controlled epidural analgesia[10–16] are becoming increasingly popular around the world.

A survey in Sweden, in 1982, reported an epidural rate of 13.4% during labor, while continuous infusions were used in 50% of the reporting institutions.[8] It was felt that the continuous infusion technique provided safe, stable analgesia and was a valuable aid in organizing a 24-h obstetric analgesia service, without increasing the staff requirements. In our view, patient-controlled epidural analgesia (PCEA) is a safe, perhaps optimal, method of providing analgesia during labor. Bupivacaine consumption is low, and thus toxic drug levels or significant motor block are unlikely. The self-administered increments are small and the consequent risk of complications, related to subarachnoid or intravascular injection, is low. The parturient retains control over a critical part of her labor experience and patient satisfaction is high. If the concentration of bupivacaine is no higher than 0.125%, with addition of 1:800 000 epinephrine, maternal plasma drug levels are low and analgesia is usually associated with little or no motor block.[17] The use of epidural opioids in this setting has allowed the anesthesiologist to reduce the concentration of local anesthetic necessary to produce adequate analgesia.[18]

Other advantages of epidural analgesia relate to the lack of maternal sedation. The mother is fully alert and able to participate in labor and birth. Systemic local anesthetic or opioid levels are low and immediate breastfeeding is safe and encouraged. The risk of pulmonary aspiration of regurgitated gastric contents is reduced to almost zero.

Epidural analgesia is frequently associated with an increased rate of forceps delivery.[19] Whether this is due to the effect of the epidural block or to an increased demand for epidural analgesia by women experiencing difficult labor is subject to debate. In the authors' institution the overall rate of forceps delivery, in primigravidas without epidural analgesia, is about 10%, while it rises to 30–40% in those who receive epidural block during labor. However, examination of the labor records shows that frequently the epidural block is commenced just before the forceps delivery; and in many of the other cases the epidural is requested because of abnormal labor due to malposition, or other obstetric complications, when the labor is more painful and prolonged. Chestnut et al[20] reported that continuous infusion of a dilute solution of bupivacaine and fentanyl, through the second stage of labor, did not increase the forceps delivery rate compared with a saline control. Epidural analgesia inhibits endogenous oxytocin secretion from the pituitary gland.[21] Infusion of a dilute oxytocin solution during labor will improve contractions and reduce the forceps delivery rate.[22]

The other disadvantages of lumbar epidural analgesia include the need for trained anesthesiologists to initiate and maintain the block. An intravenous infusion of crystalloid solution is necessary to reduce the risk of hypotension associated with peripheral vasodilatation secondary to sympathetic blockade. Risks associated with needle and catheter placement include blood vessel perforation, dural puncture, paresthesias and infection. Continuous monitoring of mother and fetus is essential and this, in turn, requires attendance of trained staff. Other reported disadvantages of this technique include motor block if stronger solutions of local anesthetic are used; asymmetric sensory block, due to misplaced catheter, fibrous bands and septae; and neurologic complications, usually temporary.

GEOGRAPHIC CONSIDERATIONS

The availability and safety of epidural analgesia services in obstetric units have been the subjects of reviews and surveys from many countries, including Canada,[23–26] the UK,[27–29] the USA,[30] New Zealand,[31] Sweden,[8] Japan[32] Norway.[33] and Australia.[34,35]

McMorland et al[23] recommended the definition of minimum standards for training in obstetric anesthesia. Scott and Aitken[27] in their Scottish survey, noted that medium-sized hospitals should be expected to achieve a standard that is equal to that expected of large hospitals. They also stated that some special arrangements are necessary for smaller hospitals. Frank et al[29] observed that, while 16 out of 22 units reported the continuous presence of an anesthesiologist, there was no uniform pattern of instruction to midwives regarding 'top-ups' and subsequent care. He recommended the establishment of standards for midwife training, particularly in dealing with emergencies associated with epidural analgesia. Gibbs et al[30] reported a similar variation in procedures and availability of personnel in the USA. The Japanese study[32] noted that, although the Japanese have a less negative attitude to anesthesia and analgesia during labor than patients in some other countries, epidural analgesia is not as frequently employed. This is related to a shortage of Japanese anesthesiologists practicing obstetric anesthesia. Lind and Hoel[33] compared the provision of labor analgesia in Norway in 1969 and 1985 (Table 88.1).

The establishment of universal standards, based on the resources available in urban teaching hospitals, would effectively prohibit the provision of epidural analgesia in smaller institutions. The authors agree with Scott and Aitken's recommendation[27] that smaller hospitals require special arrangements that are compatible with their resources. Whether this service should even be offered in small, isolated hospitals is controversial. Physicians, in these circumstances, may feel that they lose their technical skills and have higher complication rates.[25] National standards committees may stipulate manpower requirements that make provision of an obstetric anesthesia service difficult in mid-sized hospitals. In some large city hospitals the workload may be too great for the available staff to provide a full, 'on demand', obstetric anesthesia service.

On the other hand, there are those countries and states that are unable to provide, or afford, an obstetric anesthesia service. This may be the result of political, social, economic or geographic realities.[36] A discussion of whether epidural analgesia is the best method of pain relief

Table 88.1 Labor pain relief in Norway (percent of patients)

	1969	1985
Mothers left unattended	69	17
Husbands present	6	86
Analgesic given (epidural)	31 (0)	75 (14)
Mothers satisfied with care	80	80
Dissatisfied because of lack of analgesia	17	15

becomes academic and irrelevant in these circumstances. In other countries, traditional remedies, religious beliefs, local customs and the expectations of the parturients and their attendants all influence the management of labor analgesia.

Even in the so-called 'developed' countries, the provision of an obstetric epidural service for parturients is not consistent. Cultural and social influences significantly affect demand for analgesia during labor. It has been suggested that Dutch parturients, for example, expect less analgesia than their American counterparts. This is probably due less to difference in pain thresholds than to differences in societal and cultural influences that determine expectations.[36] Consumerism has played a role in increasing epidural rates in some communities.[37]

Table 88.2 Epidural drugs used during labor

Anesthesiologists surveyed from	Local anesthetic for labor			Epidural opioids–frequency of use in labor
	Type	Percent	Volume	
Australia	B	0.375–0.5	12–24	Seldom
Austria	B	0.25–0.375	8–12	Sometimes
Denmark	B	0.25	6–10	Never
Finland	B	0.5	4–5	Never
France	B	0.25	6–12	Usually
Hungary	B	0.25–0.5	8	Seldom
Iceland	B	0.25	6–8	Never
Israel	B	0.375–0.5	10–12	Seldom
New Zealand	B	0.5	10–25	Usually
Singapore	B	0.125–0.5	6–8	Sometimes
Spain	B	0.375	6–10	Sometimes
Sweden	B	0.25	3–6	Never
UK	B	0.125–0.5	6–16	Sometimes
Zimbabwe	M/L	0.25–0.5/1–2	10–15	Seldom

B, bupivacaine; M, mepivacaine; L, lidocaine.

ALTERNATIVES TO EPIDURAL ANALGESIA

Hypnosis, acupuncture and transcutaneous electrical nerve stimulation (TENS) are all relatively safe, cheap and nonpharmacologic means of providing some analgesia in early labor.[38] None is as effective as epidural analgesia. In China, where acupuncture is an old, traditional form of analgesia, an epidural service is provided in some of the larger hospitals.[39] In many of the more remote parts of the country, acupuncture is still a useful and effective form of therapy. However, Scott[40] feels that acupunture is used less as an anesthetic technique in China, especially in large city hospitals, than we have been led to believe. TENS provides some pain relief in early labor, allows for continued ambulation and may reduce opioid requirements.[41] However, it may interfere with the function of the electronic fetal heart rate monitor.

Parenteral opioids have been the mainstay of labor analgesia for decades and are still widely regarded as the best alternative therapy when epidural analgesia is not available. Philipsen and Jensen[42] however, reported, that parturients preferred low-dose epidural analgesia over parenteral meperidine, particularly in regard to pain relief and incidence of side-effects. Opioids appear to be most effective during labor when given intravenously as patient-controlled analgesia.[43,44]

Inhalation analgesics, with the exception of nitrous oxide, are no longer widely used during labor. A report from Nigeria[45] stated that 87% of women received satisfactory pain relief from inhalation of 50% nitrous oxide (Entonox). In spite of the effect of nitrous oxide on vitamin B_{12} metabolism, and its potential for long-term environmental damage,[46] it is still likely to be used for labor analgesia, around the world, into the foreseeable future. It has a rapid onset of action, has negligible respiratory or cardiovascular depression, is nonirritant and is inexpensive.

Paracervical blocks have fallen from favor because of reported fetal bradycardia (and even death) and maternal systemic drug toxicity. However, they are still used in many places because of the ease of administration and effective analgesia during the first stage of labor.[47] *Caudal analgesia* is now seldom used because it requires larger

Table 88.3 Rates for epidural catheterization in labor and cesarean delivery rates

Anesthesiologists surveyed from	Epidural rate (%)	Epidural catheter	Cesarean delivery rate (%)
Australia	10–35	Usually	10–20
Austria	10–35	Always	10–20
Denmark	<10	Always	10–20
Finland	<10	Always	10–20
France	35–50	Always	10–20
Hungary	35–50	Usually	20–30
Iceland	10–35	Always	10–20
Israel	10–35	Always	10–20
New Zealand	10–35	Always	10–20
Singapore	10–35	Always	12
Spain	50–75	Always	10–20
Sweden	10–35	Always	10–20
UK	10–26	Usually	10–30
Zimbabwe	<10	Usually	>30

volumes of local anesthetic solution than lumbar epidural analgesia, blocks the sacral segments during first-stage labor and carries a high risk of fetal injury.

Continuous subarachnoid analgesia, using microcatheters inserted through small-gauge needles, may become more widely used as an alternative to epidural analgesia.[48,49] However, there have been reported complications and side-effects and it is too early to determine the value of this technique in parturients. Single dose subarachnoid opioids have been used in laboring women but have a brief duration of action and are associated with pruritus, nausea and sedation.[50,51]

PRESENT WORLDWIDE PRACTICE

Anesthesiologists from around the world were recently informally surveyed. Letters were sent to the members of the WFSA (World Federation of Societies of Anesthesiologists) Committee on Obstetric Anesthesia and Analgesia; and one of the authors (DG) interviewed registrants at an international anesthesia meeting. The survey included 26 anesthesiologists, representing 20 countries. 17 of these countries reported provision of an obstetric epidural analgesia service. Most of the respondents claimed that their replies were reasonably representative of practice in their country. The responses are summarized in Tables 88.2 and 88.3.

Although the survey indicated some regional differences in use of epidural analgesia for obstetrics, it also demonstrated many similarities in the epidural and cesarean delivery rates among the various countries. Data from Cyprus, Jamaica, Japan and Kenya are not included in the tables. Representatives from these countries reported little, or no, use of epidural analgesia during labor. The reasons given were financial restraints, as well as lack of dedicated obstetric anesthesiologists and trained nurses. Egypt was also included in the survey and reported an increase in the epidural rate, during labor, over the last 10 years, as a result of an increase in the number of trained anesthesiologists in that country. Our contact in Egypt also stated that epidural analgesia for obstetrics is generally available in other Middle East countries, notably Saudi Arabia, Jordan and Syria.

SUMMARY

Ideally epidural analgesia should be universally available for those women who request it. Politico–economic realties do not always allow for this provision. For many women throughout the world, in 1993, nitrous oxide and parenteral opioids would be considered a luxury. For them, quality of care is not the prime consideration, survival is. Alternatives to epidural analgesia are available and may be more suitable in those countries without trained staff and appropriate facilities. In countries with comprehensive epidural services many anesthesiologists use continuous epidural infusions with low dose bupivacaine and an opioid such as fentanyl or meperidine. This has in all likelihoods made epidural services safer and therefore more attractive to community hospitals with fewer staff. In this age of consumerism, throughout the developed world, patient-controlled epidural analgesia offers the parturient participation in her own pain relief. She can titrate epidural analgesia to a level which is satisfactory, with minimal potential for adverse effects. In the future though, continuous subarachnoid analgesia may prove to be a superior technique, but suitable catheters are not currently available and considerable clinical research will be required to prove any advantage.

REFERENCES

1. Melzack R, Taenzer P, Feldman P, Kinch R A 1981 Labour is still painful after prepared childbirth training. Can Med Assoc J 125: 357–363
2. Lederman R P, McCann D S, Work B A et al 1977 Endogenous plasma epinephrine and norepinephrine in last-trimester pregnancy and labor. Am J Obstet Gynecol 129: 5–8
3. Lederman R P, Lederman E, Work B A, McCann D S 1978 The relationship of maternal anxiety, plasma catecholamines and plasma cortisol to progress in labor. Am J Obstet Gynecol 132: 495–500
4. Morishima H O, Yeh M N, James L S 1979 Reduced uterine blood flow and fetal hypoxemia with acute maternal stress: experimental observation in the pregnant baboon. Am J Obstet Gynecol 134: 270–275
5. Shnider S M, Wright R G, Levison G et al 1979 Uterine blood flow and plasma norepinephrine changes during maternal stress in the pregnant ewe. Anesthesiology 50: 524–527
6. Dickersin K 1991 Pharmacological control of pain during labour. In: Chalmers I, Enkin M, Keirse M J N C (eds). Effective Care in Pregnancy and Childbirth, Vol. 2. Oxford University Press, Oxford
7. Shnider S M, Abboud T K, Artal R et al 1983 Maternal catecholamines decrease during labor after lumbar epidural anesthesia. Am J Obstet Gynecol 147: 13–15
8. Hanson B, Matouskova-Hanson A 1985 Continuous epidural analgesia for vaginal delivery in Sweden. Report of a nationwide inquiry. Acta Anaesthesiol Scand 29: 712–715
9. Taylor H 1983 Clinical experience with continuous epidural infusion of bupivacaine at 6 ml per hour in obstetrics. Can Anaesth Soc J 30: 278–286
10. Gambling D R, Yu P, Cole C et al 1988 A comparative study of patient-controlled epidural analgesia (PCEA) and continuous infusion epidural analgesia (CIEA) during labour. Can J Anaesth 35: 249–254
11. Lysak S Z, Eisenach J C, Dobson C E 1990 Patient-controlled epidural analgesia during labor: a comparison of three solutions with a continuous infusion control. Anesthesiology 72: 44–49
12. Gambling D R, McMorland G H, Yu P, Lazo C 1990 Comparison of patient-controlled epidural analgesia and conventional intermittent 'top-up' injections during labor. Anesth Analg 70: 256–261
13. Ferrante F M, Lu L, Jamison S B, Datta S 1991 Patient-controlled epidural analgesia: demand dosing. Anesth Analg 73: 547–552
14. Paech M J 1992 Patient-controlled epidural analgesia in labour–is a continuous infusion of benefit? Anaesth Intensive Care 20: 15–20
15. Purdie J, Reid J, Thorburn J, Asbury A J 1992 Continuous epidural analgesia: Comparison of midwife top-ups, continuous infusions and patient-controlled epidural administration. Br J Anaesth 68: 580–584
16. Gambling D R, Huber C J, Berkowitz J et al 1993 Patient-

controlled epidural analgesia in labour: varying bolus dose and lockout interval. Can J Anaesth 40: 211–27

17. van Zundert A, Burm A, van Kleef J et al 1987 Plasma concentrations of epidural bupivacaine in mother and newborn: 0.125% v 0.375%. Anesth Analg 66: 435–441
18. Westmore M D 1990 Epidural opioids in obstetrics–a review. Anaesth Intens Care 18: 292–300
19. Chestnut D H 1991 Epidural anesthesia and instrumental vaginal delivery (editorial). Anesthesiology 74: 805–808
20. Chestnut D H, Laszewski L J, Pollack K L et al 1990 Continuous epidural infusion of 0.625% bupivacaine/0.0002% fentanyl during the second stage of labor. Anesthesiology 72: 613–618
21. Goodfellow C F, Hull M G R, Swaab D F et al 1983 Oxytocin deficiency at delivery with epidural analgesia. Br J Obstet Gynaecol 90: 214–216
22. Saunders N J S, Spiby H, Gilbert L et al 1989 Oxytocin infusion during second stage of labour in primiparous women using epidural analgesia: a randomised double-blind, placebo-controlled trial. Br Med J 299: 1423–1426
23. McMorland G H, Jenkins L C, Douglas M J 1986 A survey of obstetric anaesthesia practice in British Columbia. Can Anaesth Soc J 33: 185–194
24. Palahniuk R J 1988 Obstetric epidural anaesthesia in remote hospitals (editorial). Can J Anaesth 35: 448–450
25. Orser B 1988 Obstetrical epidural anaesthesia in a Canadian outpost hospital. Can J Anaesth 35: 503–506
26. Webb R J, Kantor G S A 1992 Obstetrical epidural anaesthesia in a rural Canadian hospital. Can J Anaesth 39: 390–393
27. Scott D B, Aitken R E 1986 Obstetric anaesthetic services in Scotland in 1982. Anaesthesia 41: 370–374
28. Frank M, Heywood A, MacLeod D M 1988 Survey of the practice of epidural analgesia in a sample of regional obstetric units. Anaesthesia 43: 54–58
29. Rosen M 1988 Anaesthetic services in obstetrics (letter). Br Med J 296: 790
30. Gibbs C P, Krischer J, Peckham B M 1986 Obstetric anesthesia: a national survey. Anesthesiology 65: 298–306
31. Richardson T 1988 Epidural anaesthesia for obstetrics: where are we? NZ Med J 101: 657–658
32. Arai M, Nishijima M, Tatsumi H 1989 Analgesia and anesthesia during labor in Japan and developed countries. Asia Oceania J Obstet Gynaecol 15: 213–221
33. Lind B, Hoel T M 1989 Alleviation of labor pain in Norway. An interview investigation in 1969 and 1986. Acta Obstet Gynecol Scand 68: 125–129
34. Watts R W 1992 Obstetric epidural services in rural South Australia. Anaesth Intens Care 20: 345–353
35. Watts R W 1992 A five-year prospective analysis of the efficacy, safety and morbidity of epidural anaesthesia performed by a general practitioner anaesthetist in an isolated rural hospital. Anaesth Intens Care 20: 348–353
36. Senden I P M, v. d. Wetering M D, Eskes T K A B et al 1988 Labor pain: a comparison of parturients in a Dutch and an American teaching hospital. Obstet Gynecol 71: 541
37. de Haven Pitcock C, Clark R B 1992 From Fanny to Fernand: the development of consumerism in pain control during the birth process. Am J Obstet Gynecol 167: 531–587
38. Douglas M J 1991 Alternatives to epidural analgesia during labour (editorial). Can J Anaesth 38: 421–424
39. Huang S T, Peng C H, Chuah E C et al 1988 Obstetric epidural service in Keelung Chang Gung Memorial Hospital (a review of 288 cases in the past 33 months). Mz Tsui Hsueh Tsa Chi 26: 395–398
40. Scott D B 1989 Travels in China (editorial). Reg Anesth 14: 53–54
41. Hughes S C, Dailey P A, Partridge C 1987 Transcutaneous electrical nerve stimulation for labour analgesia (abstract). Anesth Analg 67: S99
42. Philipsen T, Jensen N H 1990 Maternal opinion about analgesia in labour and delivery. A comparison of epidural blockade and IM pethidine. Eur J Obstet Gynaecol Reprod Biol 34: 205–210
43. Robinson J O, Rosen M, Evans J M et al 1980 Self-administered intravenous and intramuscular pethidine. A controlled trial in labour. Anaesthesia 35: 763–770
44. Rosaeg O P, Kitts J B, Koren G, Byford L J 1992 Maternal and fetal effects of intravenous patient-controlled fentanyl analgesia during labour in a thrombocytopenic parturient. Can J Anaesth 39: 277–281
45. Soyannwo O A 1985 Self-administered entonox in labour: a report of experience in Ibadan. Afr J Med Sci 14: 95–98
46. Logan M, Farmer J G 1989 Anaesthesia and the ozone layer (editorial). Br J Anaesth 63: 645–647
47. Day T W 1989 Community use of paracervical block in labor. J Fam Pract 28: 545–550
48. McHale S, Mitchell V, Howsam S, Carli F 1992 Continuous subarachnoid infusion of 0.125% bupivacaine for analgesia during labour. Br J Anaesth 69: 634–636
49. Kestin I G, Madden A P, Mulvein J T, Goodman N W 1992 Analgesia for labour and delivery using incremental diamorphine and bupivacaine via a 32-gauge intrathecal catheter. Br J Anaesth 68: 244–247
50. Honet J E, Arkoosh V A, Norris M C et al 1992 Comparison among intrathecal fentanyl, meperidine and sufentanil for labor analgesia. Anesth Analg 75: 734–739
51. Boreen S, Leighton B L, Kent H, Norris M C 1992 Intrathecal meperidine for labor analgesia: preliminary communication. Int J Obstet Anesth 1: 149–152

PART B
OBSTETRICIAN'S VIEW
J. F. Pearson

It's nice work if you can get it and you can get it if you try.

(Popular song)

The answer to the question as to whether epidural analgesia (EA) is the best method of pain relief in the world today has to be 'it all depends'. It all depends on where you are and who you are. The vast majority of women in the world today do not have access to this mode of analgesia. Much depends also on the cultural background. Women in some Mediterranean cultures firmly believe that screaming loudly during contractions is necessary for the baby to be born healthy and thus might not take kindly to having their labor pains obtunded, while other cultures encourage a state of stoical silence. The expectations of the patient differ greatly. What might be considered satisfactory pain relief in one cultural setting may be considered to be unsatisfactory and even undesirable in another. For instance, a Swedish study has shown that women wishing to deliver their babies at their local hospital consider that the absence of an epidural is more than made up for by the sense of security that she feels in more familiar surroundings.[1] Kloosterman[2] was of the opinion that 80–90% of women are capable of normal delivery without medical intervention. His views were reflective of those common in Holland in the 1960s and have been used to support the anti-interventionist views of the natural childbirth movement.[3]

In the UK during the 1930s most births took place at home. By 1958, 49% of all births took place in hospital. By 1970 this had risen to 66% and by 1981 to 95%. This last increase was consequent upon the recommendations of the Peel Committee[4] that all births should take place in hospital for reasons of maternal and fetal safety.

During the late 1960s and early 1970s EA became increasingly used in the UK because of 'consumer demand'. Its effectiveness and relative safety for the woman and her baby, especially when compared with general anesthesia, were widely appreciated. Indeed, the availability and usage of EA is sometimes quoted as an index of the quality of an obstetric anesthetic service. A report of the National Medical Consultative Committee for Scotland in 1975 stated 'An optimum obstetric anaesthesia and analgesia service is one which provides all forms of anaesthesia and analgesia for all women who wish or require such a service at all times. Without the availability of epidural analgesia for labor and for all types of operative delivery, including Cesarean section, modern obstetric practice is incomplete'.[5] The Social Services Committee of 1980 recommended that there should be an epidural service in all consultant-led units.[6] A recent review on the availability of EA was performed on all obstetric units recognized by the Royal College of Obstetricians and Gynaecologists for training purposes. It showed that between the years 1982 and 1986, when 3.4 million deliveries occurred, EA was not regularly available to all who would want it or in whom it might have been recommended on medical grounds. This survey demonstrated a wide variation in the use of epidural analgesia/anesthesia, with nearly fivefold differences between the rates in the highest and lowest geographic regions. These findings gave rise to concern in the Health Service which has, as an objective, equality of availability of health services for all. It clearly emphasized that whether or not a woman gets an epidural depends on where she lives.[7] Such a patchy distribution of services may well be characteristic of most of the developed world.

Most of this textbook contains detailed discussion by expert obstetric anesthesiologists regarding virtually all aspects of this important subject. Obstetricians tend to have more limited concerns and, by and large, when faced with the need to deliver women presenting with unusual medical or surgical problems, will see themselves as just one member of a team. So when dealing with a severe maternal cardiac disorder such as Eisenmenger's syndrome, the obstetrician would be expected to recognize the importance of referral to a regional center where cardiologist, anesthesiologist and obstetrician can plan optimum peripartum care. The same goes for a multitude of hematologic, respiratory, neurologic and endocrinologic diseases, all of which may present the obstetrician and anesthesiologist with special problems. These self-evident considerations aside, the main concerns of the obstetrician with respect to the use of EA lie with its effect on labor, especially on instrumental delivery and its use in certain obstetric situations, particularly in severe preeclampsia. The remainder of this chapter will therefore consider these two controversial aspects of care in some detail.

EPIDURAL ANALGESIA AND THE FIRST STAGE OF LABOR

When continuous epidural analgesia was first introduced into obstetric practice within the UK, assessment of labor had traditionally consisted of intermittent vaginal examinations, often at intervals of 4 h or less frequently (to reduce the risk of infection). The most common indication for vaginal examination was to assess progress in order to determine the most appropriate analgesic for the patient. For instance, it was generally considered that if the woman was close to full cervical dilation, narcotic analgesia was best avoided for fear of its depressant effect upon the child. With epidural block and pain-free labor came the realization that it was very important to be able to predict the onset of the second stage of labor. It was fortunate, therefore, that Friedman's[8] method of graphically charting cervical dilation and descent of the presenting part was at that time entering European clinical practice, and somewhat later the composite partogram was devised by Philpott and Castle[9] in Rhodesia and was being introduced into British obstetrics. This graphic evaluation of progress revolutionized the understanding of the mechanisms of labor.

Much work was done to assess the effect of EA on the progress of labor. The effect of EA on the latent phase of labor is difficult to assess, largely because the onset of the latent phase is nebulous and has no easily definable endpoint, but the consensus view is that there is some slowing if EA is used prior to the active phase.[10] Once active-phase labor is established, most clinical studies are in agreement that labor is not impeded in any major way by EA.[11] But there may be transient inhibition of contractions immediately following EA for periods of up to 30 min.[12]

EPIDURAL ANALGESIA AND THE SECOND STAGE OF LABOR

Studies of the effect of EA on the duration of the second stage of labor and its bearing upon the condition of the newborn infant have focused on two important possibilities:

1. that prolongation of the second stage of labor might aggravate or cause fetal asphyxia;
2. that prolongation of the second stage of labor may result in an increased risk of potentially traumatic delivery.

Fetal asphyxia

A study of fetal acid–base variables in parturients by Wood et al[13] indicated that a degree of progressive fetal asphyxia was inherent in the second stage of labor and that the degree of fetal acidosis was time dependent. They subsequently[14] performed a prospective controlled study which showed that reducing the duration of the second stage, by forceps if necessary, diminished fetal metabolic acidosis. Pearson and Davies[15] found that it was possible to abolish the maternal metabolic acidosis which occurs in the second stage of labor by fully depressing the bearing-down reflex using EA and by ensuring that the mother did not push. This did not, however, prevent the fetal metabolic acidosis. They concluded that a degree of progressive fetal asphyxia was intrinsic to the normal second stage of labor and was possibly the result of placental site retraction.

While these studies were carefully performed, the conclusions of both groups of workers have since partially been discounted, the reason being that both studies were performed on women in whom the second stage of labor was conducted in the supine position, and we now know that aortocaval compression may result in a degree of fetal asphyxia even in the absence of hypotension and that the use of left lateral tilt[16] will usually prevent this development. Maresh et al[17] performed a prospective randomized study of the second stage of labor conducted with EA and showed that, provided lateral tilt was used, the fetus tended not to develop the incremental acidosis observed by earlier workers. They suggested that, given these precautions, there need be no arbitrary limit to the second stage of labor on the grounds that such prolongation of itself causes fetal asphyxia.

Recently, using the pulse pressure measured in the toe, Kinsella et al[18] showed that the usually recommended 15° left lateral tilt was not always sufficient to abolish aortic compression in the first stage of labor. They demonstrated that aortic compression was often relieved by the head becoming engaged within the pelvic cavity, that is below the level of the aortic bifurcation. Unfortunately, values were not given for full cervical dilatation and the second stage of labor.

Fetal trauma

'The position, stated simply, is that extradural anesthesia introduces an increased risk of trauma which affects both the mother and the child, and trauma, it scarcely needs to be argued, is one risk of childbirth which can no longer be tolerated'. This powerful and unequivocal condemnation of EA was written by O'Driscoll in 1975.[19] His thesis was argued as follows: (a) extradural anesthesia causes a sharp increase in forceps deliveries; (b) tentorial tears with subarachnoid hemorrhage for the fetus and genital laceration with hemorrhage for the mother are caused by forceps; (c) it therefore follows that, because EA is associated with increased instrumental delivery, it also causes tentorial tears. In support of this contention the author stated that, in the previous 10 years, 20 000 primigravidas had been delivered in his hospital, and all 20 babies dying from tentorial tears had been delivered by forceps. It seems that a good case was being made against the misuse of forceps rather than the use of EA and that any other conclusion could not be justified.

PROGNOSTIC SIGNIFICANCE OF ABNORMAL ACTIVE-PHASE DILATION PATTERNS

The later part of the active phase of labor (the deceleration phase) reflects cephalopelvic relationships. At this stage, retraction of the cervix occurs together with the descent of the presenting part, which continues into the second stage. The duration of this phase of labor is increased in cephalopelvic disproportion and in persistent occipitoposterior positions and Friedman[8] suggested that deceleration phases greater than 3 h in nulliparas and 1 h in multiparas should be considered abnormal. In clinical practice the duration of the 7–10 cm cervical dilation interval has been shown to be a good guide to the mother's subsequent performance during the second stage of labor. Short 7–10 intervals are associated with a high likelihood of spontaneous delivery, but longer 7–10 intervals are associated with an increased incidence of forceps delivery.[20]

A prolonged deceleration phase has been shown to be associated with a 10-fold increase in both cesarean delivery and forceps delivery rates over that expected in the normal parturient population, for both nulliparous and multiparous women. The vast majority of cesarean deliveries are for cephalopelvic disproportion and include a significant proportion of failed forceps. Not surprisingly, such labors have a very high incidence of other forms of active-phase dystocia occurring concurrently. Protraction disorders predominate (63% in nulliparas and 36% in multiparas), and, furthermore, as might be expected, fetal macrosomia is a potent contributory factor.[10]

These serious abnormalities of the active phase of labor are frequently managed by EA so they also reflect the very sort of mechanical disorder which, if unrecognized or managed inappropriately, will sometimes lead to traumatic damage to the fetus, for which EA is sometimes unfairly blamed.

MANAGEMENT IMPLICATIONS FOR THE SECOND STAGE OF LABOR

For the parturient with an averaged-sized infant in normal progressive labor who chooses EA, the second stage of labor may be prolonged not because of poor uterine performance but because sensory blockade of roots S2, 3 and 4 obtunds the bearing-down reflex, and this considerably reduces the power of her expulsive efforts. In the absence of hypotension, prolongation of the second stage of labor is unlikely of itself to be injurious to either mother or fetus provided aortocaval occlusion is avoided. The current trend is to allow the second stage to continue until delivery can be conducted either spontaneously or with outlet forceps. This technique is certainly preferable to the earlier one of automatic delivery frequently from mid-cavity after some arbitrary interval (usually 1 h) following full cervical dilatation and has led to a marked reduction in forceps delivery rates for uncomplicated 'failure to progress'.

Chestnut et al[21] evaluated the analgesic efficacy and the influence of continuing an epidural infusion of 0.125% bupivacaine beyond 8 cm dilation in a well-designed double-blind trial. The second stage of labor was prolonged and there was an increased frequency of instrumental delivery. Importantly, and in contrast to earlier non-blinded studies, the maintenance of EA did not result in an increased incidence of abnormal positions of the vertex or the more frequent performance of cesarean delivery. Furthermore, there were no significant differences between the groups in either Apgar scores or umbilical cord blood acid–base values.

The need or justification for delivering by forceps is almost entirely within the purview of the attending obstetrician, and there are no properly validated objective criteria by which one can judge the effect of an intervention designed to reduce forceps usage. Nevertheless certain management strategies have been evaluated.

The effect of allowing the epidural to wear off was assessed by Phillips and Thomas,[22] who found no differences in second-stage duration. The pain scores, incidence of malposition and forceps rate were actually all higher in patients in whom the block was allowed to wear off.

In a small number of parturients, oxytocin release during the second stage of labor was shown to be diminished.[23] This has led to the suggestion that the need for forceps could be reduced by oxytocin augmentation of uterine activity. As yet no satisfactory double-blind prospective randomized controlled trial of this treatment modality has been performed.

Dosage of bupivacaine may be very important. Turner et al[24] reported a trial of 517 women which showed that low-dose, low-volume bupivacaine resulted in a lower incidence of forceps delivery. Marcoux et al[25] performed a randomized controlled trial of 371 women receiving a single dose of bupivacaine 20 ml of 0.375% or 15 ml of 0.5%. The lower dosage resulted in 22% mid forceps vs. 43% in the high-dose group, and rotational forceps occurred three times more frequently in the high-dosage group.

The already high maternal satisfaction from conventional epidural analgesia can be enhanced by the addition of a lipid-soluble opioid (e.g., fentanyl). This combination allows smaller quantities of bupivacaine to be used without compromising analgesic effect and without depressant effects on the neonate.[26] Because the site of action of opioids is the spinal cord itself rather than the spinal nerves, it has been found possible to achieve satisfactory perineal anesthesia without incurring the side-effects incumbent on allowing caudal spread of the local anesthetic agent.[27] The most striking finding of a recent study was that women receiving bupivacaine and fentanyl were twice as likely to deliver spontaneously than those treated with bupivacaine alone.[28] The disadvantage of this technique is that it is very labor intensive for the anesthetic staff and the search for less demanding regimens continues. This approach, if perfected, would avoid the distress to the patient of allowing the block to 'wear off' and the potential dangers of hyperstimulation inherent in the use of oxytocin and as such is the most attractive currently available option to the obstetrician.

EPIDURAL ANALGESIA AND PREECLAMPSIA

This continues to be a controversial topic. Proponents of

EA extoll the lack of need for drugs that may depress both mother and neonate; the provision of ideal pelvic floor relaxation for vaginal delivery especially important in the premature infant; and excellent analgesia for forceps or ventouse delivery. A further bonus is that the block can be quickly extended for cesarean delivery if indicated.

Pain-induced hyperventilation during contractions is abolished and maternal lactate accumulation and metabolic acidosis is minimized.[29,30] Circulating levels of catecholamines are increased in preeclampsia, thus possibly interfering with placental perfusion. Epidural analgesia/anesthesia decreases catecholamine levels, which is advantageous,[31] may improve both uteroplacental and renal blood flow and might even possibly prevent the development of eclampsia.[32] The stabilization of maternal blood pressure diminishes the likelihood of acute hypertensive crises which can precipitate intracranial hemorrhage.[33] The relatively alert patient is also less likely to aspirate gastric contents.[34] However, reservations have been expressed on the grounds that marked post-epidural hypotension may cause fetal asphyxia and that there may be the possibility that local anesthetic agents may predispose to convulsions. There is little evidence to support this latter contention and, indeed, local anesthetic agents have been used successfully to treat status epilepticus.[35]

By 1980, there was a large body of opinion supported by clinical studies to the effect that properly managed lumbar epidural block was the method of choice in severe preeclampsia provided that hypertension was controlled and that coagulopathy was excluded. Following the work of Joyce et al[36] acute hydration of the patient with severe preeclampsia to a central venous pressure (CVP) of 4–6 cmH_2O was advocated, the usual regimen being 2 l of crystalloid together with salt-free albumin with the caution that, in some cases, an increase of only 2–3 cmH_2O may occur.[34] It was found that the higher the diastolic pressure the more acute hydration was required to raise the CVP, and with diastolic pressures greater than 100 mmHg, colloid (as 5–25% albumin) is necessary to raise the CVP.[37] The early work using this method demonstrated that acute hydration improved urinary output and decreased diastolic blood pressure and the institution of EA was also free from the risk of hypotension.

The subsequent experience of 'acute loading' severely preeclamptic patients has indicated that this procedure is by no means devoid of risk.

Simultaneous measurements of CVP and pulmonary capillary wedge pressure (PCWP) have been shown to be poorly correlated.[38] Central venous pressure measurements are usually low in severe preeclampsia, but in a disturbingly high proportion of severe preeclamptics PCWP may be increased.[39] The relatively high PCWP has been thought to be the result of a cardiovascular hyperdynamic state, but the present consensus leans towards the view that the raised PCWP is more likely to be the result of peripheral vasoconstriction.[40] Severe preeclamptic women may also have low serum albumin and low plasma colloid osmotic pressure plus elevated PCWP due to increased cardiac afterload and are thus in great danger of pulmonary edema, which can sometimes be precipitated by acute loading these patients to the levels of CVP previously advocated. Owing to this hazard, we have abandoned this practice in Cardiff. Other times of increased liability to pulmonary edema are (a) when EA diminishes and (b) 18–26 h later.

In severely preeclamptic women managed with EA, measurements of mean arterial pressure (MAP) and systemic vascular resistance (SVR) rose to pre-epidural values 2 h following delivery when the epidural block wore off.[41] If blood pressure is poorly controlled this may result in increased afterload with an increase in hydrostatic pressure within the alveolar capillaries. The increased antidiuretic hormone (ADH) secretion immediately following childbirth or, especially, following cesarean delivery impairs satisfactory elimination of the fluid overload. After delivery in severe preeclampsia the colloid osmotic pressure, already low, continues to fall due to the mobilization of the water in the extravascular space, which dilutes the intravascular colloid and in the absence of a diuresis further increases the intravascular volume, thus further increasing the danger of pulmonary edema.

A case history presented by Newsome et al[41] illustrates this relationship:

> A pregnant pre-eclamptic woman was admitted with pulmonary edema, epidural analgesia was initiated and pulmonary edema improved (MAP and SVR was diminished) only to recur in the post-partum period with elevated PCWP, low cardiac output and elevated SVR. The institution of afterload reduction therapy with hydralazine reduced the pulmonary edema with a return of cardiac output towards normal levels and a decrease in SVR.

Clinical strategies to minimize the hazard of pulmonary edema need to be directed towards the lowering of PCWP and increasing plasma colloid osmotic pressure. In Cardiff we have found that this may be readily achieved by limiting the volume of parenteral fluid to 1.5 l in the first 24 h post delivery, by treating hypertension using a vasodilator such as hydralazine and by the early use of furosemide to induce an early diuresis (J F Pearson, G Foat, S Bailey, unpublished observations). Furosemide, by removing water from the intravascular space, also tends to increase colloid osmotic pressure, which inhibits filtration from the pulmonary capillary bed into the alveoli. Furosemide also lowers PCWP in two other ways, firstly by a direct action on venous capacitance vessels and, secondly, by a diuretic-induced fall in intravascular volume and pressure.[42]

If attention is carefully directed towards the normalization of maternal hemodynamic and osmotic equilibrium, there is no reason why epidural analgesia should not be freely used in severe preeclampsia but, as most of the more severe cases are managed by cesarean delivery rather than induction of labor in our unit, our preference tends towards the use of general rather than regional anesthesia.

SUMMARY

EA remains probably the best method of obstetric analgesia in the world today. Availability even in the most developed countries remains limited for political and financial reasons. Women given the choice prefer to stay close to home rather than travel some distance in order to receive an epidural anesthetic.

There is little doubt that EA and its consequences require a higher level of supervision from both anesthetic and midwifery staff than more traditional methods, and because of this EA is often only available in the larger hospitals. Second-stage delay with increased forceps delivery rates do not necessarily incur other penalties for the mother and her child but are held by some groups of consumers as examples of unnecessary and 'unjustifiable' medical intervention in a 'natural' process. The advent of new techniques such as low-dose bupivacaine enhanced by opioids promises to answer such objections.

It is feasible and possibly advantageous to use EA as an adjunct in the management of severe preeclampsia, but in this area it should not be used without 'state-of-the art' maternal hemodynamic monitoring.

REFERENCES

1. Fallman M L, Kebbon M, Nilson B A, Zador G 1974 Pain and analgesia in childbirth (in Swedish). Lakartidningen 71: 1407–1411
2. Kloosterman G L 1975 Quoted in Suzanne Arms. Immaculate deception. Houghton Mifflin
3. Claxton R 1986 Natural birth in hospital: how to avoid interference. In: Claxton R (ed) Birth matters, issues and alternatives in childbirth. Unwin Paperbacks, London p 133
4. Peel Committee Report 1970 Standing Maternity and Midwifery Advisory Committee. HMSO, London
5. National Medical Consultative Committee 1985 Obstetric Anaesthesia and Analgesia in Scotland. Report to the Scottish Home and Health Department. SHHD, Edinburgh
6. Social Services Committee 1980 Second Report 1979–1980 Perinatal and Neonatal Mortality (Chairman Mrs Renee Short). HMSO, London
7. Hibbard B M, Scott D B 1990 The availability of epidural anaesthesia and analgesia in obstetrics. Br J Obstet Gynaecol 97: 402–405
8. Friedman E A 1965 The graphic analysis of labor. Am J Obstet Gynaecol 68: 1568–1571
9. Philpott R H, Castle W M 1972 Cervicographs in the management of the primigravida. 1. The alert line for detecting abnormal labour. J Obstet Gynaecol Br Cwlth 79: 592–598
10. Friedman E A 1978 Labor, clinical evaluation and management, 2nd edn. Appleton Century Crofts, New York
11. Studd J W W, Crawford J S, Duignan N M, Rowbotham C H F, Hughes A O 1980 The effect of lumbar epidural analgesia on the rate of cervical dilatation and the outcome of labour of spontaneous onset. Br J Obstet Gynaecol 87: 1015–1021
12. Lowensohn R I 1974 Intra-partum epidural anaesthesia: an evaluation of effects of uterine activity. Obstet Gynecol 41: 388
13. Wood C, Ng K H, Hounslow D, Benning H 1973 The influence of differences of birth times upon fetal condition in normal deliveries. J Obstet Gynaecol Br Cwlth 80: 289–294
14. Wood C, Ng K H, Hounslow D, Benning H 1973 Time – an important variable in normal delivery. J Obstet Gynaecol Br Cwlth 80: 295–300
15. Pearson J F, Davies P 1974 The effect of continuous lumbar epidural analgesia upon fetal acid–base status during the second stage of labour. J Obstet Gynaecol Br Cwlth 81: 975–979
16. Eckstein K L, Marx G F 1974 Aorto-caval compression and uterine displacement. Anesthesiology 40: 92–96
17. Maresh M, Choong K H, Beared R W 1983 Delayed pushing with lumbar epidural analgesia in labour. Br J Obstet Gynaecol 90: 623–627
18. Kinsella S M, Whitwam J G, Spencer J A D 1990 Aortic compression by the uterus: identification with the Finapres digital arterial pressure instrument. Br J Obstet Gynaecol 97: 700–705
19. O'Driscoll K 1975 An obstetrician's view of pain. Br J Anaesth 47: 1053–1059
20. Davidson A C, Weaver J B, Davies P, Pearson J F 1976 The relation between ease of forceps delivery and speed of cervical dilatation. Br J Obstet Gynaecol 83: 279–283
21. Chestnut D H, Vandewalker G E, Owen C L et al 1987 The influence of continuous epidural bupivacaine analgesia on the second stage of labor and method of delivery in nulliparous women. Anesthesiology 66: 774–780
22. Phillips K C, Thomas T A 1983 Second stage of labour with or without extradural analgesia. Anaesthesia 38: 972–976
23. Goodfellow C F, Hull H G R, Swaab D F 1983 Oxytocin deficiency at delivery with epidural analgesia. Br J Obstet Gynaecol 90: 214–219
24. Turner M J, Silk J, Gordon H 1987 Bupivacaine concentration and mode of delivery. Lancet 1: 1496–1497
25. Marcoux S, Mailloux J, Fontaine J Y, Le Clerk M 1987 Bupivacaine concentration and obstetric delivery. Lancet 2: 330–331
26. Chestnut D H, Owen C L, Bates J N 1988 Continuous infusion epidural analgesia during labor: a randomized double-blind comparison of 0.0625% bupivacaine/0.0002% fentanyl versus 0.125% bupivacaine. Anesthesiology 68: 754–759
27. Reynolds F, O'Sullivan G 1989 Epidural fentanyl and perineal pain in labour. Anaesthesia 44: 341–344
28. Murphy J D, Henderson K, Bowden M I, Lewis M, Cooper G M 1991 Bupivacaine versus bupivacaine plus fentanyl for epidural analgesia: effect on maternal satisfaction. Br Med J 302: 563–567
29. Pearson J F, Davies P 1973 The effect of continuous lumbar epidural analgesia on the acid–base status of maternal arterial blood during the first stage of labour. J Obstet Gynaecol Br Cwlth 80: 218–224
30. Pearson J F, Davies P 1973 The effect of continuous lumbar epidural analgesia on maternal acid–base balance and arterial lactate, concentration during the second stage of labour. J Obstet Gynaecol Br Cwlth 80: 225–229
31. Abboud T, Artal R, Sarkis F, Henriksen E H, Kammula R K 1982 Sympathoadrenal activity, maternal, fetal and neonatal responses after epidural anesthesia in the preeclamptic patient. Obstet Gynecology 114: 915–918
32. Jouppila P, Jouppila R, Hollmen A, Koivula A 1982 Lumbar epidural analgesia to improve intervillous blood flow during labor in severe preeclampsia. Obstet Gynecol 59: 158–161
33. Hodgkinson R, Husain F J, Hayashi R H 1980 Systemic and pulmonary blood pressure during caesarean section in parturients with gestational hypertension. Can Anaesth Soc J 27: 389–394
34. Gutsche B B, Cheeck T G 1987 Anesthetic considerations in preeclampsia-eclampsia. In: Snider S H, Levinson G (eds) Anesthesia in obstetrics, 2nd edn. Williams & Wilkins, Baltimore p 225–242
35. Ritchie J M, Greene N M 1980 Local anesthetics. In: Gilman A G, Goodman L S, Gilman A (eds) The pharmacological basis of therapeutics, 6th edn. MacMillan, New York p 307
36. Joyce III T H, Debnath K S, Baker E A 1979 Preeclampsia – relationship of CVP and epidural analgesia. Anesthesiology 51: S297
37. Joyce III T H, Loon M 1981 Preeclampsia: effect of albumin 25% infusion. Anesthesiology 55: A313

38. Benedetti T J, Cotton D B, Read J C, Miller F C 1980 Hemodynamic observations in severe pre-eclampsia with a flow directed pulmonary artery catheter. Am J Obstet Gynecol 136: 465–470
39. Rafferty T D, Berkowitz R L 1980 Hemodynamics in patients with severe toxaemia during labor and delivery. Am J Obstet Gynecol 138: 263–270
40. Zemel M B, Zemel P C, Berry S et al 1990 Altered platelet calcium metabolism as an early predictor of increased peripheral vascular resistance and preeclampsia in urban black woman. New Engl J Med 323: 434–438
41. Newsome L R, Bramwell R S, Curling P E 1986 Severe preeclampsia: hemodynamic effects of lumbar epidural anesthesia. Anesth Analg 65: 31–36
42. Dikshit K, Vyden J K, Forrester J S 1973 Renal and extra-renal hemodynamic effects of furosemide in congestive heart failure after acute myocardial infarction. New Engl J Med 288: 1087–1090

PART C
MOTHERS' VIEWS OF CHILDBIRTH
B. M. Morgan

The quality of maternity services, as measured by maternal and perinatal mortality rates, is an indication of the standard of health care in a community. But the quality of health care must also be judged by the consumer's satisfaction.

The mother's experience of childbirth is seen, from a sociological point of view, as more important than the experience of the same woman receiving other forms of health care. The reason is believed to be long-term effect of the mother's experience on the entire family, its interpersonal relationships and the consequences to the developing child.[1,2]

A satisfying experience of childbirth leads mothers to greater self-esteem and more self-control and independence.[3] Women who are allowed an active participating role in childbirth are reported as having a more satisfying experience than those who rely on others.[4] Childbirth is a 'major life event with intense personal significance'.[5] Women believe that a satisfactory experience is related to positive mental health and confidence, and these qualities are beneficial in a mother. An unsatisfactory experience produces increased rates of depression and thus a less satisfactory development of family relationships.[2] Maternal depression leads to relative lack of awareness of and response to the child's emotional needs.[6]

What constitutes a satisfactory experience? Certainly the outcome of a healthy mother and baby must be part of it, but it is not the only factor. Mothers believe that 'increased safety has been bought at the expense of women's dignity, fulfillment and autonomy'.[7] This is the basis of the controversy between women and the medical profession. The conflict is about 'who has the right to dictate what the birth experience will be'.[8] Women believe that the mother is central to the birth process.[9] They believe that obstetricians concentrate wholly on the fetus and the birth of a healthy baby, and the obstetricians' fear that it may be jeopardized has resulted in the dehumanizing of childbirth.[10] Women want to have responsibility for their own childbirth experience and outcome, and not have their bodies taken over and controlled by the obstetrician.[1] It may be that this controversy will fade away as more obstetricians become unwilling to take the entire responsibility for the outcome of the baby and are eager, where possible, to hand this back to the mother. The mother is concerned with much more than just the birth. In the present climate the obstetrician may face the medicolegal costs of a damaged child but the mother, even though obedient to the obstetrician, often has to face the emotional, social and family consequences of caring for the disabled child for life. Her claim that the responsibility for the birth process is hers is therefore very strong.

It is impossible to divorce childbirth from pain. Its control forms an essential part of the mother's experience. Her ability to deal with the pain of labor with emotional and social support forms a central core of antenatal teaching. The consequences of systemic or regional analgesia are a common cause of an unsatisfactory childbirth experience.

Epidural analgesia is seen as not only interventionist but leading to a 'cascade of intervention' in childbirth.[11] Mothers believe that epidural pain relief in labor is bought at the price of longer labors, obstetric interventions, postpartum perineal pain and bladder and back problems.[12,13] Studies have shown that painless labor does not automatically equate to a satisfactory experience of childbirth, especially in primiparas with instrumental deliveries.[14,15] Other studies have shown no difference in the mothers' self-esteem whatever the analgesia, but a less positive feeling about the childbirth experience in those with epidural analgesia.[16] However, in Kitzinger's study,[17] 50% of women found childbirth a completely positive experience with epidural analgesia and only 18% regretted it, and that usually because of inadequate blocks or forceps delivery. For most women, being allowed to choose their analgesia, or avoid it, seems more important than the type of analgesia they receive.

Most mothers accept that when the pregnancy or labor is abnormal or the fetus is at risk then all necessary interventions must be used. However, it is possible that the psychological impact of this technological childbirth may be similar to the psychological side-effects of high-technology treatment for other very sick patients.[18] These women may require greater emotional support and counselling post partum than those having easier births. It is helpful if the mother has been informed antenatally about all forms of treatment she may encounter and if the reasons for them are discussed with her at the time.

A satisfying experience of childbirth is as various as the range of women who produce children. For many, an unmedicated labor with a normal vaginal delivery and the emotional support of a sympathetic person offers a chance to mobilize inner resources and take responsibility for the progress and outcome of the birth.[19–21] This constitutes for the woman the most satisfactory experience, and any other form of delivery is likely to make her feel inadequate, and dependent on others rather than being self-reliant.

For other women a painless labor with epidural analgesia provides a means of taking control of themselves during the labor and birth.[17] A passive compliance rather than active participation[22] is their preferred experience. To subject these women to childbirth without regional analgesia is likely to provide them with a harrowing experience, which may be seen as anything but fulfilling or satisfactory.

An increasing number of women express the view that elective cesarean delivery is their preferred experience of childbirth. They regard labor and vaginal delivery as unpleasant, undesirable and possibly unsafe. These women consider elective cesarean delivery on request to be a feminist issue.

Deciding what to do with their own bodies and exercising an informed choice is essential for all women. What is important is that the woman feels she is allowed an active participating role in her experience of birth rather than having to submit to a labor ward routine[23] over which she has no control.

Huttle et al[4] have described the idea of 'the mastery of childbirth': mobilizing inner resources, self-reliance, independence and self-control. This key to the success of the experience is a sense of personal control. Some mothers have what is described as an 'internal locus of control', i.e. the woman believes in her ability to control her life rather than be controlled by others. She believes that her experience of pregnancy will be determined by her own ability to cope. This view is contrasted by women with an 'external locus of control', that is those who believe that their experience will be controlled by doctors or midwives (the so-called 'powerful others'). Other women again believe that luck or fate determines whether they have a satisfactory experience of childbirth ('chance locus of control').

It is impossible for birth attendants, midwives and doctors to perceive the mother's experience of labor. Midwives view the experience of labor as more pleasant than do mothers.[24] There are also large differences between mothers' views of obstetric interventions and what obstetricians believe mothers' views to be.[25] This is also obviously true for many obstetric anesthesiologists, who frequently regard the experience of childbirth without regional anesthesia with horror, and the women who select this as incomprehensible, or even masochistic. Mothers believe that avoiding the treatment for pain often results in nonintervention in labor.[19,20] Being physically active by walking around during labor and adopting the upright position in the second stage has been shown in some studies to be beneficial in encouraging a normal outcome of labor,[26,28] others have found no benefit.[29,30] But many mothers feel that this active participation in childbirth is the crux of a satisfying experience.

Women who wish to have and succeeded in having normal labors with no intervention and supportive social circumstances usually find the experience satisfying.[21] However, women who wish to have a 'natural childbirth' and fail to achieve this may require treatment for depression for some months post partum.[31,32] Obviously, mothers must be encouraged to have aims that are realistic, but obstetric staff must also be encouraged to keep the mother's wishes in mind and help her whenever possible to achieve her desires within the bounds of safety.

This particularly applies to the use of analgesia in labor. Personal support by a sympathetic person has been shown to reduce the occurrence of complications in labor[33] and is believed by many mothers to be more important than any analgesia.[34]

Irrespective of the mother's attitude to the experience of the birth itself, she also needs to negotiate the greater reality of childbirth. 'Childbirth is a life event with considerable loss and uncertain gain'.[1] Oakley[1] suggests that in the 'transition to motherhood the gap that exists between expectations and reality of the whole birth process contradicts the mother's too romantic expectations'. An effort to bridge the gap that exists between expectations and reality is the basis for antenatal education classes. Information regarding the birthing process is believed to be important in increasing the number of mothers who have a positive experience of childbirth. Imparting knowledge, instilling confidence and providing a forum for dealing with childbirth-related fears are the crucial aspects of prenatal classes.[35] Crowe and Von Baeyer[35] suggest that women with a high level of confidence expect to exercise a significant role in their own pain management, and this is likely to increase their satisfaction and allow them a more positive experience of childbirth. The psychological determinants of a positive childbirth experience – attitudes, expectations and beliefs – are unlikely to be readily influenced.[36] But improving information can lead to the increased sense of security that mothers gain from antenatal education. The aim must be to have more mothers emerging from childbirth as 'exalted rather than demoralized, confident rather than afraid'.[37]

High antenatal levels of maternal anxiety have been reported as being associated with more pain in labor[38] and also with less pain,[35] possibly because very anxious women expect more pain than they experience and those with low levels of anxiety are surprised and shocked by the pain that they have. There is a correlation between an unfavorable birth experience and birth not being as the mother expected it to be, leaving the impression that 'the reality of birth, the pain, the unpredictability and the stress may not be accurately conveyed to primiparous women in antenatal classes'.[39]

One of the professed goals of childbirth education has been the use of psychological methods for the avoidance of pain in labor.[40] Psychoprophylaxis based on Pavlov's concept of conditioned reflexes is known as the Lamaze method. Its aim is to reduce the perception of pain by focusing attention on things other than pain awareness.[41] Pain, however, has been shown not to be minimized by antenatal education preparation,[42] but acceptance of the pain, and plans and strategies to overcome it, are developed, often increasing the woman's satisfaction. Reduced use of analgesia has been used as a measure of the effectiveness of antenatal psychoprophylactic education.[43–45]

This view that antenatal education will reduce the requirements for analgesia is regarded now as of less significance than the view that pain must be accepted by the mother. During antenatal classes she must develop coping techniques which allow her to feel in control of herself. Pain in labor is seen as 'a side-effect of a task willingly undertaken or pain with a purpose'.[46] Increased enjoyment of childbirth has been shown not to be dependent on a reduction of the pain experienced[47,48] but on the mother's being in control.

The wishes and desires of the mother or parents should be discussed antenatally and detailed in a 'birth plan'.[49] This can result in some labor ward procedures being avoided where possible. It reduces not only antagonism between parents and staff but also the sense of failure that the mother feels when her unrealistic and inflexible targets cannot be met and she has to decide on a different course of action. It is important that the woman is allowed to detail her wishes regarding epidural analgesia on her 'birth plan', and these should be upheld whenever possible. A 'birth plan' allows the mother to feel that she has some control over her childbirth experience. It also increases the awareness of obstetricians and midwives of the mother's wishes and needs. It may be an important tool in making the professionals more consumer oriented.

The vocal wishes of various women's consumer groups for home deliveries has induced many obstetric units to provide a more friendly environment for childbirth, with birthing rooms or birthing centers rather than surgical or intensive care-like suites. However, many women feel that, although this is welcome, it does not address the problem of attitude. That is, professionals view childbirth as dangerous rather than as a physiological event that occasionally becomes pathological. The result of this attitude is 'interference' in labor. In a study of low-risk primigravidas, those delivered in a general practitioner unit had less analgesia, augmentation or electronic monitoring than those delivered in a consultant unit. In spite of this there were fewer neonates with low Apgar scores and fewer needing intubation in the general practitioner unit.[50] Klein et al[50] suggest that there is a strong case to be made that the care of low-risk women should be primarily supportive care by midwives. It must, however, be emphasized that the more 'at risk' the mother or fetus, the greater the supportive role of the midwife must be to minimize the mother's emotional trauma by the need for technological intervention in childbirth. Home births are favored because of greater maternal emotional fulfillment. Women delivered at home are more likely to be satisfied with their analgesia and report their attendants as very helpful than those delivered in hospital.[51]

CESAREAN DELIVERY

The ambivalence about epidural analgesia and the consequences on the progress and outcome of the labor are not applicable to anesthesia for cesarean delivery. The conscious mother can have some experience of childbirth, but the unconscious woman has none. Mothers have reported cesarean delivery utilizing regional block as almost as good as a natural birth and a positive experience.[52] There have been no studies comparing general and regional anesthesia as regards maternal views of her childbirth experience.

Even so, it may be that the most important contribution that the obstetric anesthesiologist can make to the mother–child relationship is regional anesthesia for cesarean delivery. Identifying and claiming the infant are important factors in the maternal attachment process.[53] When the mother is unaware of the actual delivery, her identification with the child appears to require more conscious effort.

The existence of the maternal sensitive period has been shown to occur during the first hours of the newborn's life. Studies have shown that mothers having contact within the first 12 h of life as compared with those who do not exhibit an increased maternal interaction with more fondling, kissing, eye-to-eye contact and increased tendency to hold the infant.[54–56]

These effects are likely to be more important among mothers already at special risk of child abuse, that is the young primiparas with some emotional disturbance, often in need of the attention of the social worker and infant admission to the special care baby unit.[57] Cesarean delivery was twice as common among at-risk women who abused their children than among a similiar group who did not.

Mothers delivered by emergency cesarean delivery with a period of amnesia after the delivery had less eye-to-eye contact with the infant at 1 month and felt that the baby did not become a person until later than a similar group having a vaginal delivery.[58] In this study even mothers at low risk of child abuse delivered by cesarean delivery seemed to be more likely to have difficulty in establishing a relationship with their child than those having a vaginal delivery. But another study on the parental adjustment to cesarean delivery, without mentioning the type of anesthetic, found no differences in mother–infant behavior when compared with a vaginal delivery group.[59] Poor inner-city women exhibited little disappointment at emergency cesarean delivery whether under general or regional anesthesia.[60]

Emergency cesarean delivery is perceived as the most negative birth experience but can be mitigated by the use of regional anesthesia, being able to hold the baby immediately and have the father present throughout.[53,61] The impact of these forms of childbirth on the mother can also be reduced by intensive post-partum nursing and emotional support.[62,63]

The presence of the father at the birth has become an 'essential emotional support to the mother'. Shearer[64] has declared that, although there is no proof that his presence is beneficial, there is also no proof that it is beneficial to exclude him. There has not been a lot of work done on the effect of the birth experience on the father himself,[65] nor has there been any evidence of a paternal sensitive period or an improved father–child relationship.[66,67]

It is obviously important to expand our understanding of the mother's view of her childbirth experience. However, 'opinions or reactions' must be viewed with caution. The use of words and feelings or 'soft outcomes' must be regarded with a certain measure of cynicism. Many of the studies have defects in methodology[68] with small numbers and lack of controls. Many studies have a middle-class bias and lack the broader view of other social classes and ethnic groups. Most serious of all criticisms is the tendency to generalize the results and reinforce the strongly held opinions of the investigators. There cannot be any childbirth experience that will be satisfactory to all women even if the process is normal, much less when things go wrong.

The work of obstetric anesthesiologists consists largely of attempting to improve the mother's experience of childbirth, by giving her pain relief. Life saving is a less frequent but obviously important part of their duties. Therefore, the obstetric anesthesiologist must be sensitive to the mother's views of her experience and must be prepared to be taught by mothers how this experience can be improved. Sensitivity to maternal reactions is needed rather than trying to impose our own views or experiences on women. The obstetric anesthesiologist may be in the unique position to improve the mother's reactions to her child by having her conscious during cesarean delivery with regional anesthesia. Several studies have shown improvements in the outcome of labor, maternal–child bonding and successful breastfeeding when sympathetic nonprofessional companions stay with the laboring woman to provide her with reassurance and praise.[33,69–73] No studies have shown an improvement in the outcome of labor or better parenting with the use of regional analgesia and painless labor. It may be that a supportive sympathetic companion in labor will also provide an acceptable level of pain relief.

REFERENCES

1. Oakley A 1980 Women confined: towards a sociology of childbirth. Martin Robertson, Oxford
2. Plotsky H, Sherenshefsky P 1973 Psychological meaning of labour delivery experience. In: Yarrow L, Sherenshefsky P (eds) Psychological aspects of a first pregnancy and early postnatal adaptation. Raven Press, New York
3. Humenick J S 1981 Mastery: the key to childbirth satisfaction. A review. Birth 6: 79–83
4. Huttle F A, Mitchell-Fisher M Z, Meyer A E 1972 A quantitative evaluation of psychoprophylaxis in childbirth. J Psychosomatic Res 16: 81–85
5. Kitzinger S 1980 The complete book of pregnancy and birth. A A Knopf, New York
6. Lee M C, Gotlib I H 1989 Maternal depression and child adjustment: a longitudinal analysis. J Abnorm Psychol 98: 78–85

7. Simkin P, Enkin M 1989 Antenatal classes. In: Chalmers I, Enkin M, Keirse M (eds) Effective care in pregnancy and childbirth, Vol 1. Oxford University Press, Oxford, pp 318–334
8. Varney Burst H 1983 The influence of consumers in the birthing movement. Topics Clin Nurs 5: 42–54
9. Editorial 1982 New dimensions in obstetric audit (leading article). Lancet 2: 857–858
10. Macintyre S 1977 The management of childbirth: a review of sociological research issues. Soc Sci Med 11: 477–484
11. Avard D M, Nimrod C M 1985 Risks and benefits of obstetric epidural analgesia. A review. Birth 12: 215–225
12. William S, Hepburn M, McTwain G 1985 Consumers' view of epidural anaesthesia. Midwifery 1: 32–36
13. Newson K 1984 Care during labour. Br J Obstet Gynaecol 91: 609–610
14. Billevicz-Driemel A M, Milne M D 1976 Long-term assessment of extradural analgesia for relief of pain in labour. II. Sense of deprivation after extradural analgesia in labour: relevant or not? Br J Anaesth 48: 139–144
15. Morgan B M, Bulpitt C J, Clifton P, Lewis P J 1982 Analgesia and satisfaction in childbirth. Lancet 2: 808–810
16. Slavazza K, Mercer R T, Marut J S 1985 Anaesthesia and analgesia for vaginal childbirth: differences in maternal perception. J Obstet, Gynecol Neonatal Nurs 14: 321–329
17. Kitzinger S 1987 Some women's experience of epidurals – a descriptive study. National Childbirth Trust, London
18. Oakley A 1983 Social consequences of obstetric technology: the importance of measuring 'soft' outcomes. Birth 10: 96–108
19. Jennings B 1982 Childbirth choices: are there safe options? Nurse Pract 7: 26–37
20. Milner I 1986 Choosing a natural or an active childbirth. Nursing 3: 39–45
21. Crafter H R 1987 Study of a couple's planned labour. Midwives Chron Nurs Notes 100: 302–303
22. Poore M, Cameron Foster J 1989 Epidural and no epidural anaesthesia: differences between mothers and their experience of birth. Birth 12: 205–213
23. Gillespie S A 1981 Childbirth in the 1980s: what are the options? Issues in Health Care of Women 3: 101–128
24. Bradley C, Brewin C R, Duncan S L B 1983 Perceptions of labour: discrepancies between midwives and patients ratings. Br J Obstet Gynecol 90: 1176–1179
25. Cartwright A 1979 The dignity of labour: a study of childbearing and induction. Tavistock, London
26. Stewart P, Spiby H 1989 Posture in labour. Br J Obstet Gynaecol 66: 1258–1260
27. Mendez-Bauer C, Arroyo J, Garcia Ramos A et al 1975 Effect of standing position on spontaneous uterine contractility and other aspects of labour. J Perinat Med 3: 39–100
28. Flynn M, Kelly J, Hollins G, Lynch P F 1978 Ambulation in labour. Br Med J 2: 591–593
29. McManus T J, Calder A A 1978 Upright posture and the efficiency of labour. Lancet 1: 72–74
30. Gardosi J, Sylvester S, Lynch C B 1989 Alternative positions in the second stage of labour: a randomised controlled trial. Br J Obstet Gynecol 66: 1290–1296
31. Sandelowski M 1984 Expectations for childbirth versus actual experiences: the gap widens. Maternity Child Nurs J 9: 237–239
32. Stewart D E 1982 Psychiatric symptoms following attempted natural childbirth. Can Med Assoc J 127: 713–716
33. Sosa R, Kennell J, Klaus M, Robertson S, Urrutia J 1980 The effect of a supportive companion on parental problems, length of labour and mother–infant interaction. New Eng J Med 309: 597–600
34. Morgan B M, Bulpitt C J, Clifton P, Lewis P J 1984 The consumers attitude to obstetric care. Br J Obstet Gynaecol 90: 624–628
35. Crowe K, Von Baeyer C 1989 Predictors of a positive childbirth experience. Birth 16: 2: 59–63
36. Genest M 1981 Preparation for childbirth – evidence for efficacy. A review. J Obstet Gynecol Neonatal Nurs 10: 82–85
37. Morris N 1960 Human relations in obstetric practice. Lancet 1: 913–915
38. Klusman L E 1975 Reducing pain in childbirth by the alleviation of anxiety in pregnancy. J Consult Clin Psychol 43: 162–165
39. Knight R G, Thirkettle J A 1987 The relationship between expectations of pregnancy and birth, and transient depression in the immediate postpartum period. J Psychosomatic Res 31: 351–357
40. Beck N C, Siegel L J 1980 Preparation for childbirth and contemporary research on pain, anxiety and stress reduction. A review. J Psychosomatic Med 42: 429–447
41. Lamaze F 1984 Painless childbirth. The Lamaze method. Contemporary books, Chicago
42. Melzack R, Taenzer P, Feldman P, Kinch R A 1981 Labour is still painful after prepared childbirth training. Can Med Assoc J 125: 357–363
43. Doering S G, Gutwhistle 1975 Preparation during pregnancy and ability to cope with labor and delivery. Am J Orthopsychiatr 45: 825–837
44. Zax M, Sameroff A J, Farnum J E 1975 Childbirth education, maternal attitudes and delivery. Am J Obstet Gynecol 123: 185–190
45. Scott J R, Rose N B 1976 Effects of psychoprophylaxis (Lamaze preparation) on labor and delivery in primiparas. New Engl J Med 294: 1205–1207
46. Kitzinger S 1978 Pain in childbirth. J Med Ethics 4: 119–121
47. Norr K L, Block C R, Charles A, Meyering S, Meyers E 1977 Explaining pain and enjoyment in childbirth. J Health Soc Behav 18: 260–275
48. Willmuth R, Weaver L, Borenstein J 1978 Satisfaction with prepared childbirth and locus of control. J Obstet Gynaecol Neonatal Nurs 3: 33–37
49. Ekeocha G E O, Jackson P 1985 1985 The 'birthplan' experience. Br J Obstet Gynaecol 92: 97–101
50. Klein M, Lloyd I, Redman C et al 1983 A comparison of low-risk women booked for delivery in two systems of care. Br J Obstet Gynaecol 90: 118–122
51. O'Brien M 1978 Home and hospital: a comparison of the experiences of mothers having home and hospital confinements. J Royal Coll Gen Pract 28: 460–466
52. Hardwick M 1983 Caesarean section under epidural. A personal account. Br Med J 287: 35–36
53. Marut J, Mercer R 1979 Comparison of primiparas' perception of vaginal and caesarean births. Nurs Res 28: 260–266
54. Klaus M H, Jerrauld R, Kleger N C et al 1972 Maternal attachment – importance of the first postpartum days. New Engl J Med 286: 460–463
55. McClennan M, Cabiaca W 1980 Effects of early mother–infant contact following caesarean birth. Obstet Gynecol 56: 52–55
56. Hales D J, Lozoff B, Soso P et al 1977 Defining the limits of the maternal sensitive period. Dev Med Child Neurol 19: 454–456
57. Lynch M A, Roberts J 1977 Predicting child abuse. Signs of bonding failure in the maternity hospital. Br Med J 1: 624–626
58. Trowell J 1982 Possible effects of emergency cesarean section on the mother–child relationship. Early Hum Dev 7: 41–51
59. Culp R E, Osofsky H J 1989 Effects of Cesarean Delivery on parental depression, marital adjustment and mother–infant interaction. Birth 16: 53–57
60. Sandelowski M, Bustamante R 1986 Cesarean births outside the natural childbirth culture. Res Nurs Hlth 9: 84–88
61. Cranley M S, Hedahl K J, Pegg S H 1983 Women's perceptions of vaginal and caesarean deliveries. Nurs Res 32: 10–15
62. Bradley C F, Ross S E, Warnyca J 1983 A prospective study of mothers' attitudes and feelings following caesarean and vaginal births. Birth 10: 79–83
63. Cohen M 1977 Minimizing emotional sequelae of Caesarean birth. Birth 4: 114–119
64. Shearer E C 1984 Some limits on small studies of fathers' attendance at Caesarean birth. Birth 11: 15
65. Richman J 1982 Men's experiences of pregnancy and childbirth. In: McKee L, O'Brien M (eds) The father figure. Tavistock, London
66. Palkovitz R 1985 Fathers' birth attendance, early contact and extended contact with the newborn: a critical review. Child Dev 56: 392–406
67. Rodholm M 1981 Effects of father–infant postpartum contact on their interaction 3 months after birth. Early Hum Dev 5: 79–85

68. Reid M 1983 A feminist sociological imagination? A review article. Soc Health Illness 5: 83–94
69. Berteh T D, Nagashima-Whalen L, Dykeman S, Kennell J H, McGarth S 1990 Labour support by first-time fathers: direct observations with a comparison to experienced doulas. J Psychosomatic Obstet Gynecol 11: 251–260
70. Oakley A 1989 Can social support influence pregnancy outcome? Br J Obstet Gynaecol 96: 260–262
71. Klaus M H, Kennel J H, Robertson S S, Sosa R 1986 Effects of social support during parturition on maternal and infant morbidity. Br Med J 293: 585–587
72. Kennell J, Klaus M, McGroth S, Robertson S, Hinkley C 1988 Medical intervention: the effect of social support during labour. Pediatr Res 23: 211A
73. Hofmeyr G J, Nikodem V C, Wolman W L, Chalmers B E, Kramer T 1991 Companionship to modify the clinical birth environment: effects on progress and perceptions of labour and breastfeeding. Br J Obstet Gynaecol 98: 756–764

89. Intravenous hydration

Part A A positive view *G. F. Marx*
Part B A critical view *D. B. Scott*
Part C Acute hydration before cesarean delivery *S. D. Belzarena*

PART A
A POSITIVE VIEW
G. F. Marx

Intravenous hydration is beneficial during labor, advantageous before general anesthesia, and required before institution of major regional anesthesia for labor analgesia and cesarean delivery.

LABOR

Labor is an energy-consuming process comparable to moderate to severe muscular exercise: oxygen consumption increases, aerobic and anaerobic carbohydrate metabolism rise, and electrolytes are lost by sweating.[1,2] Prolonged or complicated labor may readily lead to 'exhaustion' with arterial and central venous hypotension as a result of dehydration and metabolic acidosis.[3] Prevention consists of the intravenous infusion of a balanced electrolyte solution containing 5% dextrose. Use of a salt solution provides needed electrolytes and additionally avoids the occurrence of water retention when oxytocin is administered. The antidiuretic effect of oxytocin can induce water intoxication with convulsions and cerebral edema in parturients receiving intravenously high doses of oxytocin together with large amounts of electrolyte-free solutions.[4] Dextrose not only supplies energy substrate but also prevents the development of maternal – and consequent fetal – hypoglycemia. Gravid women become clinically hypoglycemic at blood glucose levels of less than 3.3 mmol/l (60 mg/dl), whereas in nonpregnant individuals signs of hypoglycemia do not appear until the level has declined to 2.2–2.8 mmol/l (40–50 mg/dl).[5] Furthermore, gravidas live in a state of 'accelerated starvation', characterized by a tendency toward fasting hypoglycemia.[6] First, the fuel demands of the fetus are met primarily by the consumption of glucose and, second, secretion of insulin in response to glucose is augmented. In the fetus, hypoglycemia is defined as a glucose level below 2.2 mmol/l (40 mg/dl); since its concentration is always 1.1–1.7 mmol/l (20–30 mg/dl) lower than that of the mother,[7] the fetus of a hypoglycemic mother invariably becomes hypoglycemic too. In nondiabetic gravidas, clinical signs of hypoglycemia, such as diaphoresis, jitteriness or drowsiness, rarely develop. In contrast, the fetus-in-utero responds to maternal fasting with decreased breathing movements, decreased low-voltage electrocortical activity and, at times, heart rate abnormalities.[8,9]

Oral intake by the woman in labor – except for ice chips or small sips of clear fluid – increases her risk of pulmonary aspiration of gastric contents should anesthesia become necessary. Therefore, adequate intravenous hydration with a balanced electrolyte solution containing dextrose is indicated for maternal and fetal reasons. However, the dextrose load should not exceed 20 g/h in order to avoid the development of fetal hyperglycemia which, in turn, may lead to reactive hypoglycemia after birth.[10] The value of giving laboring women receiving epidural analgesia both electrolytes and dextrose was confirmed in a well-controlled study in which 25 parturients received Hartmann's solution and 25 others were given dextrose in half-normal saline.[11] The volume required for prevention of hypotension during the course of labor was significantly less in the dextrose–saline group (1.80 ± 0.96 l) than in the Hartmann's solution group (2.96 ± 1.16 l). Maternal and cord plasma sodium concentrations at delivery were lower in the dextrose–saline group, while β-hydroxybutyrate levels were markedly increased in women receiving Hartmann's solution. Glucose concentrations were substantially higher in the saline–dextrose group but no value was at the level of hyperglycemia. Thus, expansion of the intravascular blood volume necessary prior to induction of epidural analgesia can be achieved with minimal biochemical disturbances using dextrose in an electrolyte solution.

ANALGESIA AND ANESTHESIA

For inhalation analgesia and general anesthesia, maintenance of adequate hydration is usually sufficient. Blood and plasma losses at delivery must, however, be considered. After vaginal delivery of a term infant, the average blood loss amounts to 400–500 ml and, after abdominal delivery, to 900–1000 ml. The decline in total blood volume is approximately twice that of measured blood loss, apparently as a result of translocation of plasma into traumatized tissues.[12] Confirmation of normoglycemia prior to induction is beneficial as hypoglycemia can cause serious problems in anesthetized patients because of blockade by anesthesia of the usual compensatory mechanism.[13] In general, hypoglycemia stimulates the release of epinephrine from the adrenal medulla; this induces the breakdown of glycogen to glucose in liver and muscles and simultaneously leads to increases in systolic pressure and heart rate. However, the output of epinephrine is decreased during deep general anesthesia as well as during major regional anesthesia.

For major regional block, acute (forced) intravenous hydration, also called preload, is required to prevent the hypotension from major regional block. The specific cardiovascular responses associated with sympathetic blockade of spinal or epidural anesthesia are exaggerated in the pregnant woman. There are three reasons. First, neurogenic vasoconstrictor tone is increased; i.e., vascular tone is more dependent upon sympathetic control.[14] Second, the effect of blood trapping in the peripheral vascular bed of the anesthetized part is aggravated by the large amount of blood contained in the uterus. And third, the sympathetic blockade and pooling of blood in the splanchnic area may potentiate the effects of aortocaval compression. Thus, central venous and arterial hypotension tend to develop at levels of sympathetic blockade that would not affect maintenance of normal blood pressure in the nonpregnant woman.

Maternal hypotension is associated with a proportionate decrease in uterine blood flow.[15] Therefore, significant falls in blood pressure must be prevented or, if they occur, immediately and vigorously treated. Apart from avoidance of aortocaval compression, prevention consists primarily of an increase in effective circulating blood volume by the intravenous infusion of an electrolyte-containing solution; for additional treatment, the intravenous injection of a small dose of vasopressor with predominantly central action may be indicated.

The advantage of intravenous fluid load over the sole use of vasopressors was demonstrated in term pregnant ewes.[15] When a peripheral vasopressor was administered for treatment of hypotension from spinal block, maternal pressure was restored to normal but uterine blood flow did not improve, indicating that the drug induced both peripheral and uterine vasoconstriction. In contrast, when intravenous dextran or dextrose in water was infused rapidly, both maternal pressure and uterine blood flow improved simultaneously. Based on this report, the use of acute hydration for prevention of hypotension from major regional block was evaluated in healthy parturients. As a preliminary measure, the safety of infusing 1 l of Ringer's lactate solution within 20–30 min was examined in 10 healthy women, five in active labor and five awaiting elective cesarean delivery. Arterial and central venous pressures (CVP) were measured while 1000 ml of Ringer's lactate with dexrose was infused within 20–30 min. The average rise in CVP amounted to 1 cm H_2O and the maximum rise to no more than 2 cm H_2O in both groups. Thereafter, fluid preloading with 1 l of Ringer's lactate solution was used in 14 women undergoing scheduled cesarean delivery under spinal block and the results were compared with those of five similar parturients who had received less than 100 ml of the same solution. After spinal block to sensory levels of T2–T6, but before delivery, CVP fell significantly in both groups ($P < 0.01$); in the acutely hydrated women, post-block CVP was in the range of magnitude experienced by the controls before the anesthetic and, consequently, arterial pressure declined only slightly. In contrast, in the controls, both CVP and arterial pressure decreased significantly ($P < 0.01$) (Fig. 89.1).[16] Adequate uterine displacement is an obvious prerequisite to the effectiveness of acute hydration so that the increased circulating blood volume can return to the heart without impediment. A subsequent investigation [17] involving 60 gravidas revealed that in the absence of acute intravenous hydration, ephedrine – even in large doses – was not uniformly successful in circumventing post-block hypotension. However, in conjuction with fluid loading, the drug proved to be a safe and dependable adjunct, both prophylactically and therapeutically.

The efficacy of fluid loading prior to regional block in parturients has been confirmed with consistency. In one study,[18] maternal blood pressure and fetal heart rate were recorded in 104 parturients in whom lumbar epidural block was initiated during labor. All women were lying on their left side, but only 51 received an intravenous infusion of 1 l of an electrolyte-containing solution immediately before the extradural injection. This fluid load decreased the prevalence of maternal hypotension from 28% to 2% ($P < 0.005$) and of fetal heart rate abnormality from 34% to 12% ($P < 0.025$). In another assessment,[19] the effect of lumbar epidural block on placental intervillous blood flow was studied in 38 healthy gravidas scheduled for elective cesarean delivery by means of the intravenous Xenon-133 method. Of the 24 women who received extradural anes-

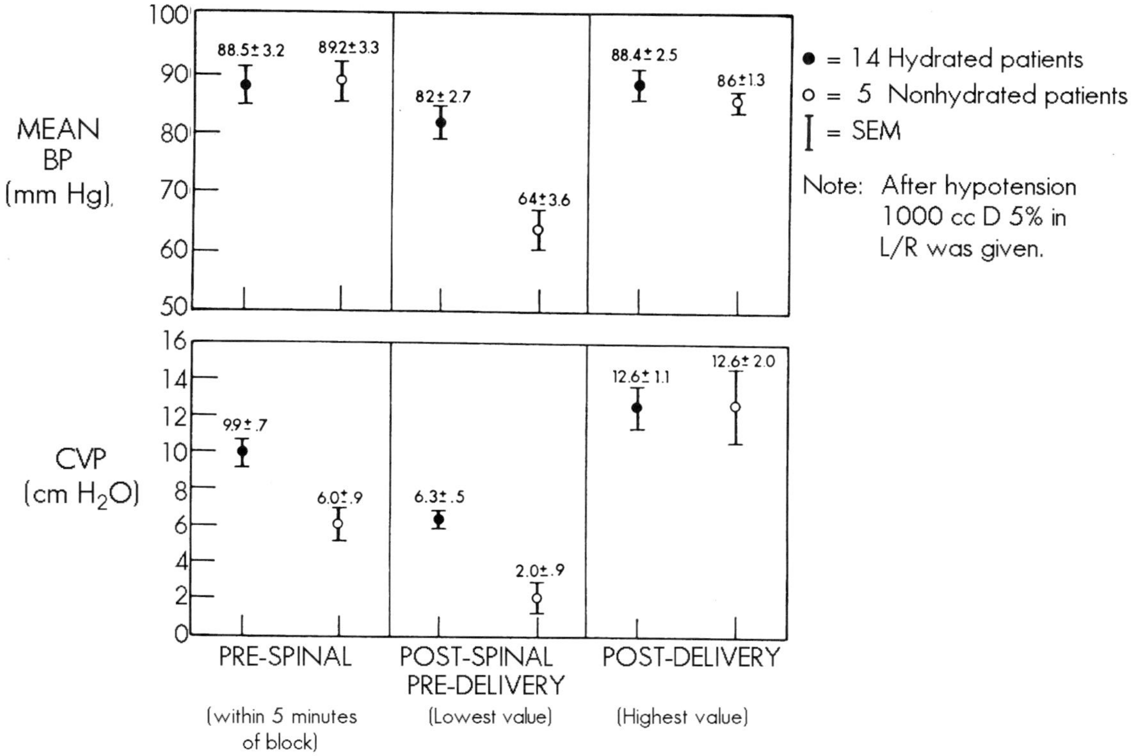

Fig. 89.1 Central venous and mean arterial pressures compared in hydrated and nonhydrated cesarean section patients (sensory level T2 – T6).

thesia 11 were infused with a plasma expander (Haemaccel), 10 ml/kg, while 13 were not given any preloading treatment. The remaining 14 women who served as controls were delivered under general anesthesia after termination of the blood flow measurements. When no preloading infusion had been administered, maternal mean arterial pressure as well as intervillous blood flow declined significantly following institution of the block ($P < 0.05$ and 0.01 respectively). In contrast, the intervillous blood flow of the acutely hydrated group was not different from that of the control patients. Finally, the effects on maternal and neonatal whole-blood lactate, pyruvate, excess lactate, lactate–pyruvate ratio, and base excess of a preload of 1200 ml of four different intravenous solutions before epidural anesthesia for elective cesarean delivery were determined in four equal groups of 22 parturients.[20] The intravenous solutions were as follows: normal saline 1200 ml, Ringer's lactate 1200 ml, Ringer's lactate 800 ml + 5% dextrose in saline 400 ml, and Plasma-Lyte A solution 1200 ml. All four fluids, despite differences in their effects on lactate and pyruvate concentrations, produced clinically satisfactory maternal and neonatal conditions and outcome. Umbilical vein blood glucose was significantly greater in the dextrose–saline group than in the other groups, but there was no significant difference in the umbilical artery blood glucose concentration among the four groups, and there was no case of neonatal hypoglycemia. Administration of up to 20 g of glucose to a fasting mother was recommended as this may improve the neonatal condition (secondary to increased fetal breathing movements and increased electrocortical activity) without adversely affecting neonatal blood excess lactate, lactate–pyruvate ratio, or blood glucose concentration. This is reassuring since maternal hypoglycemia is most hazardous during regional anesthesia – as needed for cesarean delivery because of the marked decrease in epinephrine output. In fact, cases have been reported of healthy parturients undergoing elective cesarean delivery whose post-block hypotension was difficult to reverse until their low blood glucose concentration had been normalized.[20] It is important to realize that pregnant women scheduled for morning surgery tend to be hypoglycemic since they are advised to forego snacks after dinner. In a group of 50 healthy gravidas who had been fasting since 1900 h the evening before, fasting blood glucose at 0800 h measured below 3.3 mmol/l (60 mg/dl) in 32 women (64%) and below 2.2 mmol/l (40 mg/dl) in 15 women (30%); thus, only three of the gravidas were not hypoglycemic on arrival to the obstetric operating room.[21]

Depending on the gravida's size, acute hydration with 1200–1500 ml of a balanced electrolyte solution is used most frequency before institution of regional anesthesia for elective cesarean delivery. Administration of a preload of 2000 ml is associated with a high incidence of electrographic changes suggestive of myocardial ischemia, possibly due to circulatory overload.[22,23] In parturients in labor requiring emergency cesarean delivery, a lesser amount of prehydration suffices because of the redistribution of blood volume following each uterine contraction.[24] With the low levels of blockade needed for labor and vaginal delivery, acute hydration with only about 500 ml is adequate in the healthy gravida.

In conclusion, although the judicious use of ephedrine or phenylephrine does not appear to impair the fetus-in-utero, appropriate acute hydration before regional anesthesia obviates the use of vasopressor therapy in most healthy parturients.

REFERENCES

1. Sampson J J, Rose E M, Quinn R 1945 Estimation of the work of obstetric labor and its significance in heart disease. Am J Obstet Gynecol 49: 719–734
2. Marx G F, Greene N M 1964 Maternal lactate, pyruvate, and excess lactate production during labor and delivery. Am J Obstet Gynecol 90: 786–793
3. Marx G F, Desai P K, Habib N S 1980 Detection and differentiation of metabolic acidosis in parturients. Anesth Analg 59: 929–931
4. Storch A S 1971 Acute water intoxication associated with continuous slow infusion of oxytocin; a case report. Obstet Gynecol 37: 109–110
5. Bergman M, Seaton T B, Auerhahn C C et al 1986 The incidence of gestational hypoglycemia in insulin-dependent and non-insulin-dependent women. NY State J Med 86: 174 –177
6. Freinkel N, Dooley S L, Metzger B E 1985 Care of the pregnant woman with insulin-dependent diabetes mellitus. New Engl J Med 313: 96–101
7. Phillips L, Lumley J, Paterson P et al 1968 Fetal hypoglycemia. Am J Obstet Gynecol 102: 371–377
8. Richardson B, Hohimer A R, Mueggler P et al 1982 Effects of glucose concentration on fetal breathing movements and electrocortical activity in fetal lambs. Am J Obstet Gynecol 142: 678–683
9. Langer O, Cohen W R 1984 Persistent fetal bradycardia during maternal hypoglycemia. Am J Obstet Gynecol 149: 688–690
10. Mendiola J, Grylack L J, Scanlon J W 1982 Effects of intrapartum glucose infusion on the normal fetus and neonate. Anesth Analg 61: 32–35
11. Evans S E, Crawford J S, Stevens I D et al 1986 Fluid therapy for induced labor under epidural analgesia: biochemical consequences for mother and infant. Br J Obstet Gynaecol 93: 329–333
12. Pritchard J A, Baldwin R M, Dickey J C et al 1962 Blood volume changes in pregnancy and the puerperium. II. Red blood cell loss and changes in apparent blood volume during and following vaginal delivery, cesarean section, and cesarean section plus total hysterectomy. Am J Obstet Gynecol 84: 1271–1281
13. Engquist A, Brandt M R, Fernandez A et al 1977 The blocking effect of epidural analgesia on the adrenocortical and hyperglycaemic responses to surgery. Acta Anaesthesiol Scand 21: 330–335
14. Assali N S, Prystowsky H 1950 Studies on autonomic blockade. I. Comparison between the effects of tetraethylammonium chloride (TEAC) and high selective spinal anesthesia on the blood pressure of normal and toxemic pregnancy. J Clin Invest 29: 1354–1366
15. Greiss F C, Crandell D L 1965 Therapy of hypotension induced by spinal anesthesia during pregnancy. Observations on gravid ewes. J Am Med Assoc 191: 793–796
16. Wollman S B, Marx G F 1968 Acute hydration for prevention of hypotension of spinal anesthesia in parturients. Anesthesiology 29: 374–380
17. Marx G F, Cosmi E V, Wollman S B 1969 Biochemical status and clinical condition of mother and infant at cesarean section. Anesth Analg 48: 986–993
18. Collins K M, Bevan D R, Beard R W 1978 Fluid loading to reduce abnormalities of fetal heart rate and maternal hypotension during epidural analgesia in labor. Br Med J 2: 1460–1461
19. Huovinen K, Lehtovirta P, Forrs M et al 1979 Changes in placental intervillous blood flow measured by the Xenon^{133} method lumbar epidural block for elective cesarean section. Acta Anaesthesiol Scand 23: 529–533
20. Ramanathan S, Masih A K, Ashok U et al 1984 Concentrations of lactate and pyruvate in maternal and neonatal blood with different intravenous fluids used for prehydration before epidural anesthesia. Anesth Analg 63: 69–74
21. Marx G F, Domurat M F, Costin M 1987 Potential hazards of hypoglycaemia in the parturient. Can J Anaesth 34: 400–402
22. Palmer C M, Norris M C, Giudici M C et al 1990 Incidence of electrocardiographic changes during cesarean delivery under regional anesthesia. Anesth Analg 70: 36–43
23. Elstein I D, Marx G F 1990 Electrocardiographic changes during cesarean section under regional anesthesia. Anesth Analg 71: 103
24. Clark R B, Thompson D S, Thompson C H 1976 Prevention of spinal hypotension associated with cesarean section. Anesthesiology 45: 670–674

PART B
A CRITICAL VIEW

D. B. Scott

The use of intravenous fluids to prevent or treat hypotension following epidural or spinal anesthesia is widely practiced in Europe and in North America.

RATIONALE

The use of 'preloading' (for preinduction fluid loading) with fluid is based on the concept that increasing the blood volume will increase cardiac output, which in turn will increase arterial pressure or at least prevent it from decreasing. In addition, preloading will correct any minor degree of dehydration. The term 'preloading' will be used in this chapter but acute intravascular hydration and volume expansion are used elsewhere.

Though the practice varies widely in regard to the amount infused, and whether the fluid is a colloid or an electrolyte, the same beneficial results are claimed. This fact is, in itself, suspicious because if the above rationale is correct, the volume and nature of the infusion would be of prime importance. Most of the papers on the subject suffer from serious methodological problems which include:

1. No controls *not* receiving preloading were used. The almost total acceptance of preloading ensures that many would now consider the use of such controls as unethical.
2. The mechanism itself; i.e., the purported increase in cardiac output, is hardly ever confirmed by actual measurement. Where this has been done (see below) the results do not uphold the theory.
3. The other or alternative mechanism; i.e., correction of dehydration, has received even less scientific enquiry. Nevertheless, the idea that a patient who has had no oral fluids overnight can have serious and even 'life-threatening' hypovolemia is commonplace but unsubstantiated.
4. The criterion of success in most studies has been the incidence of or lack of hypotension in a series of cases. If hypotension did not occur in a mother, preloading was proclaimed a success. If the arterial pressure did fall, it was not considered that the preloading had failed. In these types of study there have been wide variations in the definition of hypotension, and little regard has been paid to the multiplicity of causative factors in the development of hypotension. These include vasodilation, inferior vena caval (IVC) occlusion (which is *not* always relieved by a pelvic wedge), vasovagal fainting and hemorrhage. While the vasodilation resulting from the sympathetic block acts as the 'trigger' in most cases, it is uncommon for even high blocks to cause hypotension in young healthy patients who are not pregnant.

While epidural anesthesia is used for both cesarean delivery and for relief of pain in labor, only the first of these will be considered in detail here. For pain relief, the anesthetic is not extensive and the fully lateral position, with total relief of IVC occlusion, can (and should) be used. Hypotension, therefore, is seldom a problem and preloading is even less appropriate than for cesarean delivery.

CIRCULATORY CHANGES DURING CESAREAN DELIVERY PERFORMED UNDER EPIDURAL OR SPINAL ANESTHESIA

During pregnancy there are considerable changes in the circulation relevant to the anesthesia. There is an increase in blood volume and cardiac output. The gravid uterus at term takes a substantial proportion of the cardiac output, and this is abruptly stopped at delivery. The IVC is occluded in most mothers when lying supine and the adequacy of the venous return depends upon the collateral venous drainage via the paravertebral and azygos veins.[1] In a substantial number of mothers (perhaps as many as 50%), this collateral venous return is not adequate to ensure a normal cardiac output.[2] In these circumstances, the sympathetic system is activated to increase peripheral resistance and increase venous tone in the capacitance vessels, thus keeping the arterial pressure within normal limits. A very few mothers (1–2%) react to this increased sympathetic activity by developing a sudden vasovagal attack which causes profound hypotension – the so-called 'supine hypotensive syndrome.'[2] Excluding this small group, it is not possible to say which mothers have a normal cardiac output and which have compensation in response to a reduced output when lying supine. If the epidural/spinal anesthetic removes the compensatory vasoconstriction, the arterial pressure will decrease and the IVC occlusion will be 'revealed'.[3] Mothers anesthetized in this way are very susceptible to the development of hypotension if IVC occlusion is present. The incidence of hypotension in patients receiving a general anesthetic is much lower, although it may still occur and the supine position should be avoided.

While tilting the patient (usually to the left) into a semilateral position can relieve the IVC occlusion, and is widely used in cesarean delivery, such relief is not guaranteed in all patients. The full lateral position is to be preferred during the onset of epidural/ spinal anesthesia and the patient is turned to the tilted/wedged position only when the surgical team is ready to operate.

Partial occlusion of the aorta can also occur in the supine position.[4] This can reduce the uterine blood flow, but is seldom life-threatening to the mother. Indeed, the arterial pressure above the occlusion is likely to rise.

If the spinal or epidural anesthetic extends into the upper thoracic segments, then bradycardia and a decrease in inotropy of the myocardium can occur. However, the sudden development of bradycardia is much more commonly the result of a vasovagal attack (as happens in the supine hypotensive syndrome). The rapid changes in sympathetic/parasympathetic balance, not to mention the psychosomatic effects of having an abdominal operation while fully conscious, are the probable causes of vagal overactivity. That the vagus is involved is further confirmed by the appearance of other signs and symptoms, such as nausea and vomiting along with pallor and profuse sweating. Moreover, the administration of a sympathomimetic vasopressor rapidly relieves these symptoms and signs, as well as the hypotension.

CIRCULATORY EFFECTS OF FLUIDS

A rapid infusion of fluid to a normally hydrated subject will increase blood volume, but it is doubtful if this increase is sustained long enough to be of clinical importance. Electrolyte solution rapidly leaves the vascular compartment, while colloid will displace plasma electrolytes and fluids into the extracellular space. While there is some evidence that in hypovolemic patients in shock, electrolyte solutions are of clinical value, this is more the result of increasing the extracellular fluid volume than of increasing the blood volume.[5,6]

In the context of cesarean delivery, Robson et al[7] report the effects of a fluid load given before and during the onset of epidural anesthesia. After preloading with 600–1000 ml of Hartmann's solution, followed by 500 ml every 15 min (total volume of fluid 1600–2200 ml), cardiac output increased initially by 10%, but had returned to control values by the time the block was effective (30 min). 25% of the mothers were excluded from the analysis because, despite the fluid, they became hypotensive and required ephedrine! Whatever effect intravenous (i.v.) fluids may have, they do not reverse the primary trigger to hypotension, namely the vasodilation.

EFFICACY OF FLUID LOADING IN PREVENTING HYPOTENSION

The vast majority of papers presenting evidence for the value of preloading have used the incidence of hypotension in a series of cesarean deliveries. Interpreting these studies is not made easy by the wide variations in the volume of fluid infused, the use of colloid or crystalloid, variations in the definition of hypotension and the lack of controls not being preloaded.

Even taken at face value, the efficacy of preloading is very poor, the prevalence of hypotension being 7–63% in published papers.[8] In a fairly large recent study of 60 patients, colloid was compared with crystalloid, and hypotension occurred in 63% of patients with colloid and 25% with crystalloid.[8] This high prevalence of failure can hardly be described as a therapeutic triumph.

SAFETY OF INTRAVENOUS FLUIDS

While large quantities of i.v. fluid are well-tolerated by young healthy mothers, this is not necessarily the case in those with heart disease or those with problems of renal function and fluid balance; e.g., in preeclamptic toxemia.

A death has been reported in a patient who had aortic incompetence and who collapsed soon after an epidural anesthetic was established. Including the preloading, a total volume of 6 l of fluid was given, without the benefit of central venous pressure measurements.[9] This is an example of the misplaced enthusiasm for large amounts of intravenous fluids.

CONCLUSION

Hypotension is to be avoided during cesarean delivery and there is no substitute for frequent measurements of blood pressure and vigilance on the part of the anesthesiologist. This applies regardless of any precautions instituted to avoid hypotension.

The possible causes of hypotension are many, but the precipitating factor is almost always vasodilation. This is not reversed by fluid loading. Fluid depletion and dehydration are very uncommon conditions in late pregnancy.

When vasodilation is the underlying cause, then hypotension can be rapidly reversed with a vasopressor, much more rapidly than the infusion of a large fluid volume, which in any case is frequently ineffective. Using an appropriate vasopressor, a reduced uterine blood flow is not to be expected.[10,11] Once the baby has been delivered, hypotension is most unusual.

Cesarean delivery performed under epidural/spinal anesthesia has an excellent safety record in regard to both fetal morbidity and maternal mortality.[12] Fluid loading has fortunately not materially affected this record, but it remains both illogical and ineffective. Critical comparative studies on the appropriate use of fluids and vasopressors are eagerly awaited.

REFERENCES

1. Kerr M G, Scott D B, Samuel E 1964 Studies of the inferior vena cava in late pregnancy. Br Med J 1: 532–533
2. Lees M M, Kerr M G, Scott D B et al 1967 Circulatory effects of the supine posture in late pregnancy. Clin Sci 32: 453–465
3. Crawford J S 1984 Principles and practice of obstetric anaesthesia. Blackwell Scientific Publications, Oxford, pp 13–14
4. Bieniarz J, Maqueda R, Caldeyro-Barcia R 1966 Compression of the aorta by the uterus in late human pregnancy. I. Variations between femoral and brachial artery pressure with changes from hypertension to hypotension. Am J Obstet Gynecol 1966: 95: 795–808
5. Shires G T, Coln D, Carrico C J et al 1964 Fluid therapy in haemorrhage shock. Arch Surg Lond 88: 688
6 Moore F D, Dagher F J, Boyden C M et al 1966 Haemorrhage in normal man. Ann Surg 163: 485
7. Robson S, Hunter S, Boys R et al 1989 Changes in cardiac output

during epidural anesthesia for cesarean section. Anaesthesia 44: 475–479
8. Murray A M, Morgan M, Whitwan J G 1989 Crystalloid versus colloid for circulatory preload for cesarean section. Anaesthesia 44: 463–466
9. Alderson J D 1987 Cardiovascular collapse following epidural anesthesia for cesarean section in a patient with aortic incompetence. Anaesthesia 42: 643–645
10. Hollmen A I, Jouppila R, Albright G A et al 1984 Intervillous blood flow during cesarean section with prophylactic ephedrine and epidural anaesthesia. Acta Anaesthesiol Scand 28: 396–400
11. Shnider S M, de Lorimer A A, Hall J W 1970 Vasopressors in obstetrics. II. Fetal hazards of methoxamine administration during obstetric spinal anesthesia. Am J Obstet Gynaecol 106: 680–686
12. Confidential Enquiry into Maternal Deaths in England Wales, 1982–84. HMSO, London, p 95

PART C
ACUTE HYDRATION BEFORE CESAREAN DELIVERY

S. D. Belzarena

The decrease in maternal arterial pressure before delivery may be deleterious for the neonate. Hypotension may adversely affect the Apgar score, neurobehavioral assessment and measured values from umbilical blood gases, demonstrating some fetal stress. Since avoiding this complication is paramount for maternal and fetal well-being, certain procedures should be followed. Acute hydration of the parturient before induction of anesthesia is one of the important steps prior to induction.

Acute administration of Ringer's lactate to prevent maternal hypotension was first recommended in 1968.[1] Since then, a number of studies have proposed many ways to avoid hypotension during abdominal delivery. Nevertheless, everyone has employed his/her own (different) criteria for maternal hypotension, and for this reason it must be remembered that changes in the definition of hypotension from one study to another may affect the results and, sometimes, these changes are not so subtle. The most frequent criteria used for hypotension are shown in Table 89.1.

Reading the methodology section of 79 papers published between 1989 and 1992 related to anesthesia for cesarean delivery, all authors state that patients were acutely hydrated and most of them received Ringer's lactate solution, the volume of which varied between 1 and 2 l. Is this practice then effective and safe? Effectiveness will be achieved by avoiding maternal hypotension, while safety will be demonstrated by the absence of adverse effects derived from rapid infusion of fluids on the mother and the neonate.

Arterial pressure values in pregnant patients acutely hydrated before cesarean delivery may be affected by different factors (Table 89.2). First of all, the selected technique of regional anesthesia can alter the percentage of patients developing hypotension. Many believe that epidural anesthesia produces less hypotension than spinal anesthesia, as a result of faster sympathetic blockade after spinal anesthesia. However, data from many authors[2–6] demonstrate that there are no significant differences in maternal hypotension after epidural or spinal anesthesia. Moreover, incremental doses of epidurally administered

Table 89.1 What is maternal hypotension? Usual criteria used in studies of hypotension during cesarean delivery

20% decrease in systolic blood pressure
30% decrease in systolic blood pressure
Systolic blood pressure below 100 mmHg
Systolic blood pressure below 90 mmHg

Table 89.2 Factors that may influence maternal hypotension during cesarean delivery

1. Selected regional anesthesia
   - Epidural
   - Spinal
2. Fluids
   - Speed of infusion
   - Volume of infusion
   - Type of fluid
     - Colloid
     - Crystalloid
3. Patient in labor or not
4. Left uterine displacement

local anesthetics cause the same degree of hypotension as single-shot epidural anesthesia.[3,4] Addition of epinephrine to the local anesthetic increases the number of hypotensive patients because of its vasodilating beta effects.[2]

Type of fluid administered (crystalloid or colloid), volume of infusion and speed of infusion may have some influence on the incidence of maternal hypotension. It is controversial whether crystalloid or colloid solution is better for acute loading before abdominal delivery. However, the former is more frequently employed, mainly because of its low cost. In one study, published in 1989, there was no difference between crystalloids and colloids, and patients who had received hydroxyethylstarch presented more decrease in systolic arterial pressure than those that had received Ringer's lactate (63% vs. 40%).[7] Volume appears to be the more important issue, as was demonstrated by Lewis et al in 1983.[8] They increased the preload volume from 1 to 2 l and significantly decreased the number of patients with hypotension. On the other hand, doubling the speed of volume infusion from 20 to 10 min had no influence on hypotension.[9]

Other measures are also important. Left uterine displacement diminishes aortocaval compression. Wrapping of the legs may be useful, although this technique is not commonly used.[10] Vasopressors, administered before or at the same time as acute hydration may help to avoid hypotension. Nevertheless, while some say that prophylactic ephedrine is useful,[11] others do not confirm this fact.[12,13] Finally, and beyond our control, whether the patient is actually in labor or not affects the incidence of hypotension. As early as 1976 it was demonstrated that laboring patients have significantly less hypotension during subsequent delivery,[6] and these results have been confirmed.[12]

What are the consequences of the acute infusion of fluid on the mother and the neonate? Acute administration of a large volume of liquid causes acute hemodilution, which intensifies the pre-existing gestational hemodilution. It also produces an acute increase in blood volume that may increase myocardial work. In the lung, increases in water content may lead to post-operative morbidity.

Carvalho et al[14] studied the consequences of hemodilution, showing that plasma volume presents the highest increase when infusion begins and that as the volume infused increases it is feasible to have hemoglobin values below 10 g dl. In fact, in their first study,[14] 50% of patients demonstrated lower than normal hemoglobin levels. Their second study pointed out that cord blood gas values from neonates were normal but had a statistically significant trend toward metabolic acidosis.[15]

Wennberg et al[16] infused a very large volume of fluid into their pregnant patients (30 ml/kg of Ringer's acutate or 15 ml/kg of dextran 70), making cardiovascular measurements and evaluating the intrathoracic content of water. They demonstrated that this large amount of fluid posed no burden for the cardiovascular system, but that after crystalloid fluid loading there was a significant increase of water in the lungs. This fact, caused by the reduction in plasma oncotic pressure, may lead to post-operative pulmonary morbidity, and was specifically assessed by Ramanathan et al[4] using only crystalloid or a combination of crystalloid and colloid. They found with every solution low values of plasma proteins, confirming plasma dilution, and without post-operative lung morbidity. Both studies showed normal Apgar scores and neonatal cord blood gas analysis.

Blood gas measurements, Apgar score and neurobehavioral assessments (ENNS) of neonates were performed by Corke et al[17] after acutely loading their patients with 1 or 1.5 l of Ringer's lactate with 5% glucose. Their results demonstrated no changes related to acute hydration, although neonates from hypotensive patients presented a slight but significantly higher value for hydrogen concentration.

In conclusion, acute hydration of pregnant patients will be effective in preventing maternal hypotension during regional anesthesia for cesarean delivery depending on the actual volume infused (about 2 l of crystalloids, mainly Ringer–lactate), concomitant left uterine displacement and whether the patient is laboring or not. This kind of acute fluid loading appears to cause no harm to mother or neonate who do not have complications. There are no studies evaluating its consequences on mothers with hematologic, cardiovascular or respiratory diseases or those with fetal distress of any origin.

REFERENCES

1. Wollman S B, Marx G 1968 Acute hydration for prevention of hypotension of spinal anesthesia in paturients. Anesthesiology 29: 374–380
2. Wilson C M, Moore J, Ghaly R G, Flynn R, McClean E, Dundee J W 1988 Plasma concentrations of bupivacaine during extradural anesthesia for cesarean section. The effect of adrenalin. Anesthesia 43: 12–15
3. Laishley R S, Morgan B M 1988 A single dose epidural technique for cesarean section. A comparison between 0.5% bupivacaine plain and 0.5% bupivacaine with adrenaline. Anesthesia 43: 100–103
4. Ramanathan S, Masih A, Rock I, Chalon J, Turndorf H 1983

Maternal and fetal effects of prophylactic hydration with crystalloids or colloids before epidural anesthesia. Anesth Analg 62: 673–678
5. Mathru M, Rao T L K, Kartha R K, Shanmugham M, Jacobs H K 1980 Intravenous albumin administration for prevention of spinal hypotension during cesarean section. Anesth Analg 59: 655–658
6. Clark R B, Thompson D S, Thompson C H 1976 Prevention of spinal hypotension associated with cesarean section. Anesthesiology 45: 670–674
7. Murray A M, Morgan M, Whitwam J G 1989 Crystalloid versus colloid for circulatory preload for epidural cesarean section. Anesthesia 44: 463–466
8. Lewis M, Thomas P, Wilkes R G 1983 Hypotension during epidural analgesia for cesarean section. Anesthesia 38: 250–253
9. Rout C C, Akoojee S S, Rocks A D, Gouws E 1992 Rapid administration of crystalloid preload does not decrease the incidence of hypotension after spinal anesthesia for elective cesarean section. Br J Anaesth 68: 394–397
10. Bhagwanjee S, Rocke D A, Rout C C, Koovarjee R V, Brijball R 1990 Prevention of hypotension following spinal anesthesia for elective cesarean section by wrapping of the legs. Br J Anaesth 65: 819–822
11. Gutsche B B 1976 Prophylactic ephedrine preceding spinal anesthesia for cesarean section. Anesthesiology 45: 462–465
12. Rolbin S H, Cole A F D, Hew E M, Pollard A, Virgint S 1982 Prophylactic intramuscular ephedrine before epidural anesthesia for cesarean section: Efficacy and actions on the foetus and newborn. Can J Anaesth 29: 148–153
13. Brizgis R V, Dailey P A, Shnider S M, Kotelko D M, Levinson G 1987 The incidence and neonatal effects of maternal hypotension during epidural anesthesia for Cesarean section. Anesthesiology 67: 782–786
14. Carvalho J C A, Mathias R S, Senra W G et al 1990 Avaliaçâo da expansão volémica durante anestesia peridural para cesarea através da concentraçâo de hemoglobina (abstract). Rev Bras Anesth CBA: 137
15. Carvalho J C A, Mathias R S, Senra W G et al 1991 Expansâo volémica materna durante anestesia peridural para cesarea e suas repercussões sobre o recém nascido (abstract). Rev Bras Anest CBA: 72
16. Wennberg E, Frid I, Haljamäe H, Wennergren M, Kjellmer I. 1990 Comparison of Ringer's acetate with 3% dextran 70 for volume loading before extradural cesarean section. Br J Anaesth 65: 654–660
17. Corke B C, Datta S, Ostheimer G W, Weiss J B, Alper M H Spinal anesthesia for cesarean section. 1982 Anesthesia 37: 658–662

90. Who does top-ups?

Part A Australia *P. Brownridge*
Part B UK *M. Harmer*
Part C USA *T. H. Joyce N. H. Blass*
Part D Belgium *A. Van Steenberge*
Part E Sweden *L. Irestedt P. Belfrage*
Part F Argentina *P. J. Kelly*

PART A
AUSTRALIA
P. Brownridge

Responsibility for the ongoing administration of epidural medication within the Commonwealth of Australia is subject to guidelines determined by the Faculty of Anaesthetists of the Royal Australasian College of Surgeons* and by the professional bodies that regulate nursing practice within each of the six states and two territories of Australia.

Faculty Guidelines for the Conduct of Epidural Analgesia in Obstetrics (1987) include the following statements:[1]

Once epidural analgesia has been established, and the response of the patient to the agent has been tested, further doses to maintain analgesia may be administered by other members of the medical or nursing staff, provided that:

1. The dose has been prescribed by the anesthetist.
2. The anesthetist delegating the 'top-up' procedure is satisfied that the person who will carry out the task is competent to do so.
3. The person carrying out the task is satisfied that he or she is competent to do so.
4. In the event of complication or adverse reaction, a person expert in the management of such problems is readily available.

The guidelines also include a statement on the administration of epidural opioids:

Evidence is accumulating that safe analgesia can be provided by intermittent or continuous injection of narcotics into the epidural space and the Faculty believes that similar principles should apply in these techniques.

The guidelines stipulate that patients 'must be nursed in an area staffed in a manner which will ensure frequent observation by persons competent to recognise untoward effects, and able to judge the necessity for further doses', and conclude with the statement: 'At all times the ultimate responsibility for the patient's care remains that of the anaesthetist.'

Nursing Board guidelines differ somewhat between the states and territories of Australia, but only the Australian Capital Territory (ACT) specifically prohibits nursing staff from administering epidural medication. The Nursing Board of Western Australia and the Nursing Council of Victoria both demand that nurses are 'certified competent in epidural top-up procedure' – although the actual requirements for certification are not specified. Nursing guidelines for the remaining states and for the Northern Territory are broadly similar and compatible with the Faculty guidelines.

Apart from the ACT, therefore, professional bodies within Australia approve the administration of drugs (local anesthetics and/or opioids) via the epidural route by nurses – provided that the above guidelines are met. Individual obstetric units are ultimately responsible for interpreting professional guidelines and formulating policies concerning the degree of nurse involvement in the management of epidural analgesia. There are no data currently available, however, to establish the extent to which top-up doses are administered by obstetric nurses (midwives) in Australia.

LIMITATIONS ASSOCIATED WITH TOP-UPS ADMINISTERED BY PHYSICIANS

Many obstetric units in Australia demand that all epidural medication must be administered by medically qualified practitioners. While such restrictions may be entirely appropriate, top-up doses administered solely by physicians do have limitations. Even in well-staffed units, for example, it is not always feasible to provide top-up doses as and when required. The parturient must then put up with unpredictable intervals of unnecessary pain. Furthermore, if the patient is already distressed when the physician eventually arrives, she is more likely to receive a top-up dose that will produce the most immediate and prolonged effect. In these circumstances it is not surprising that local anesthetics are commonly administered in dosages greater than are strictly necessary or desirable.

Various attempts have been made to overcome some of the logistic difficulties associated with physician-administered epidural top-ups. Epidural management via a continuous, or patient-controlled, infusion device has become popular in some centers. There are still limitations, however, associated with such devices: the infusion is limited to a single, predetermined preparation; the preset delivery rate (in the case of constant flow rate devices) may be greater than is really necessary; patient mobility is restricted; and the apparatus may be inconvenient or unpopular with the parturient. The relative merits of various epidural regimens used in labor are discussed more fully elsewhere.[2]

An alternative approach is to permit top-up doses to be given by the attending nurse or midwife. In Australia, a qualified midwife is constantly present throughout labor; the midwife is well placed, therefore, to administer further analgesia as soon, and as often, as it is required. Moreover, by developing a close rapport and empathy with the patient, the midwife is able to determine individual needs and requirements. As discussed in the next section, the midwife can confer a more responsive and adaptable quality to epidural pain management than can be achieved by other means.

In addition to the labor and delivery ward, the postnatal area is also usually staffed in Australia by midwives who are experienced in epidural management. Furthermore, in comparison with other surgical wards, the postnatal ward enjoys a relatively generous ratio of nurse-to-patient in Australia. A properly staffed obstetric unit presents an opportunity, therefore, to extend epidural analgesia into the post-operative period.

EPIDURAL 'TOP-UP' DOSES DETERMINED AND ADMINISTERED BY MIDWIVES: THE FLINDERS EXPERIENCE

At Flinders Medical Centre, Adelaide, epidural analgesia managed by midwives during labor was approved in 1976; and following surgery in 1983. Approximately 1200 patients receive epidural analgesia during labor each year in our unit. We believe that this number provides sufficient clinical experience for midwives to become competent and confident in epidural management. Only experienced midwives are permitted to administer top-up doses (or supervise its conduct) according to our protocol. Facilities for resuscitation are readily available at all times in our unit. Our experience with this practice can be summarized as follows.

During childbirth

At first in our unit, the epidural drug of choice throughout labor was the local anesthetic, bupivacaine 50 mg. Provided the anesthesiologist was satisfied with the patient's response to the initial dose, subsequent top-ups were administered by the midwife on a patient-demand basis and according to a simple protocol. It became apparent, however, that the resulting profound degree of analgesia was unnecessary, and that the associated side-effects of dense neural blockade were frequently a source of patient criticism and complaint.

Dose-related side-effects of epidural analgesia include diminished patient awareness of uterine contractions and of giving birth; sensations of weakness, numbness and paresthesia of the lower limbs; reduced mobility; bladder distension; shivering; and symptoms related to postural hypotension. Impaired sensory and motor function may also – directly or indirectly – lead to a greater need for obstetric intervention (e.g. urinary catheterization, instrumental delivery and episiotomy).

As with other sources of acute pain, analgesia requirements during childbirth are peculiar to each individual, are usually unpredictable and frequently alter as labor progresses. Women requesting epidural analgesia do not, strictly speaking, desire or demand 'analgesia' (i.e. *absence* of pain); rather, they seek sufficient relief to render painful contractions *tolerable* again. This distinction becomes particularly relevant once it is appreciated that the incidence and severity of side-effects are largely determined by the density of neural blockade.

In an attempt to overcome some of these disadvantages of epidural analgesia and to allow greater flexibility in management, we introduced the practice of permitting midwives to determine – as well as administer – epidural medication in 1983. When several agents are prescribed, then the density of analgesia can be adjusted by the midwife according to patient preference or clinical circumstances. In our experience, during the past 10 years, the introduction of this simple modification in epidural management has proved safe, efficacious and practical. Our practice may be summarized as follows.

Providing the patient's response to the initial epidural dose has been satisfactory, subsequent doses are administered by the attending midwife according to a protocol (summarized later in the chapter) on a patient-demand basis. Unless a contraindication exists, the following premixed preparations (contained in volumes of 10 ml) are prescribed: bupivacaine 12.5 mg + meperidine (pethidine) 25.0 mg; bupivacaine 25.0 mg; and bupivacaine 50.0 mg. When further analgesia is requested, the midwife determines and administers whichever preparation seems most appropriate. (A smaller dose than that which has been prescribed may be given at the midwife's discretion.)

Each top-up dose is administered slowly, via an epidural filter, with the patient in a lateral recumbent position. Prior aspiration of the catheter is not performed unless so instructed by the anesthesiologist. In the case of bupivacaine 0.5%, the injection is divided into two 5-ml increments (separated by at least 5 min), and the height of block assessed before giving the second increment. (We have not found it feasible to delineate the dermatomal spread of neural blockade when using the low-dose bupivacaine/meperidine mixture, and accordingly have not introduced the practice of routinely assessing the upper sensory level of block after each top-up – as has been recently recommended[3].) Blood pressure is monitored every 5 min for 20 min after each top-up. (Epidural analgesia is not regarded as an indication per se for continuous fetal monitoring in our unit.)

Our experience with this regimen during the last 3 years may be illustrated by referring to data obtained from a concurrent audit of patients who have received epidural analgesia in our unit.

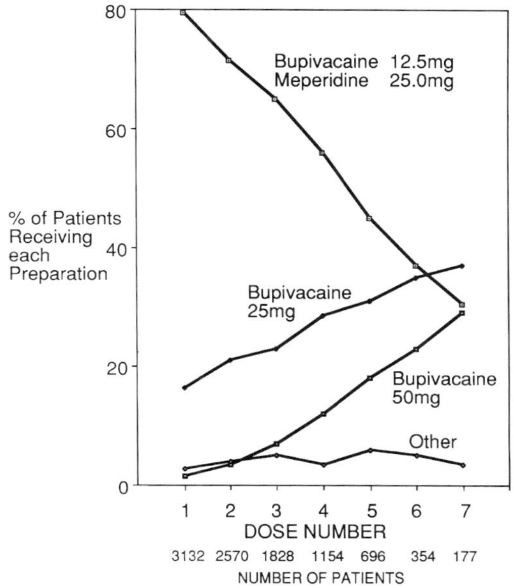

Fig. 90.1 Diagram showing epidural agents administered during labor at Flinders Medical Centre in the 3-year period 1987–89 (Other = lidocaine and miscellaneous preparations used in a clinical trial). Note that the low-dose bupivacaine – meperidine mixture was most commonly used initially but that more potent analgesia was required as the duration of labor increased. (Reproduced with permission from ref. 4.)

Epidural medication administered during labor

The low-dose bupivacaine – meperidine mixture has been the most commonly used preparation, although there is a tendency for stronger doses of bupivacaine to be used with increasing duration of labor (Fig. 90.1).

As reported previously, the bupivacaine–meperidine mixture usually provides satisfactory analgesia for contraction pain but is not always adequate during the transitional stage and at delivery.[5] This clinical impression is in accordance with other studies which have demonstrated that a drug combination of opioid and local anesthetic appears to behave synergistically. The addition of fentanyl 80 µg, for example, to a relatively small dose of bupivacaine (e.g., 12.5 mg) produces analgesia that is consistently more rapid in onset, more complete and of longer duration than that provided by bupivacaine alone.[6]

Complications

During the 3-year audit period no serious complication has occurred as a consequence of a midwife-administered top-up (e.g., a high spinal block or convulsion). Overall experience gained during the past 18 years in the author's unit supports the proposition that midwife-managed epidural analgesia is a safe practice provided that recommended procedures are strictly observed.[2,7]

Side-effects

Side-effects which may be related to a top-up dose have included nausea or vomiting (12%); shivering (7%); pruritus (6%); and significant hypotension (3%). Shivering is invariably associated with local anesthetic agents, but is very rarely witnessed following the meperidine-containing preparation. This protective effect of meperidine against local anesthetic-induced shivering has been demonstrated previously.[8] Pruritus has been associated solely with the meperidine-containing mixture, but has only been severe in one patient. This low incidence of distressing pruritus – when compared with many other epidural opioids – seems to be a feature peculiar to meperidine.

Weight-bearing/ambulation during labor

Provided there are no medical contraindications, symptoms of postural hypotension or significant leg weakness, patients receiving the low-dose bupivacaine – meperidine mixture are permitted to ambulate. In this way, more than a third of patients have been sufficiently mobile to be able to walk around during labor. Only 10% of those who wished to weight-bear were unable to do so because of leg weakness or symptoms of hypotension. The remaining patients were either prohibited from walking for some medical or obstetric reason or were simply disinclined. Previously, restricted mobility associated with epidural analgesia was a major source of discontent among patients and staff. Being able to move easily allows the patient to feel more 'in control' and reduces the burden upon nursing staff.

Urge to bear down at delivery/urinary catheterization

90% of patients having a vaginal delivery during the last 3 years in our unit have retained the urge to bear down. Those requiring an instrumental delivery usually received more potent analgesia and so the urge to bear down was obtunded deliberately.

Spontaneous micturition occurred in at least 45% of patients. A urinary catheter was required in 26% – usually in association with an instrumental or cesarean delivery. In the remainder, the records were not sufficiently complete to determine whether a catheter was required after delivery or not. Urinary catheterization, therefore, need not be an inevitable accompaniment of epidural analgesia.

Obstetric outcome and method of delivery

The introduction of midwife-managed epidural analgesia in 1983 was accompanied by a dramatic reduction in obstetric intervention. The *overall* instrumental delivery rate associated with epidural analgesia has more than halved (from 65% to 28%), and there has been an even larger decline in the number of rotation deliveries (from 18% to 4.5%). While the relationship between epidural analgesia and obstetric intervention is complex and controversial, there can be little doubt that spontaneous delivery is more likely to occur when the parturient remains aware of fetal descent and is able to bear down effectively and naturally. We believe that the higher spontaneous delivery rate witnessed in recent years is primarily attributable to the lesser degrees of neural blockade that can be achieved when top-up doses are determined by midwives.

Consumer evaluation following delivery

Overall patient satisfaction in our unit compares favorably with that reported from centers using more traditional, denser, degrees of epidural blockade. 83% of patients rated their satisfaction with pain relief between 7 and 9 (on a 1–9 visual analog scale ranging from 'completely dissatisfied' to 'fully satisfied').

Other favorable comments recorded by patients in our audit include: 'feeling relaxed' (68%); 'feeling aware' (62%); 'feeling in control' (53%), and 'able to move easily' (40%).

Apart from 'feeling numb' (20%) and 'feeling drowsy' (14%), the only tangible disadvantage associated with our practice has been 'severe pain at delivery' reported in 17% of cases. In some cases this was aggravated by the need for an urgent instrumental delivery before the block could be made denser; in others, a top-up dose may have been deliberately withheld at the request of the obstetrician or the patient. As reported previously, however, pain experienced at delivery is not necessarily a source of consumer dissatisfaction.[3] This suggests that delivery pain is acceptable to many women if accompanied by spontaneous birth.

Our audit, therefore, supports the notion that properly trained and experienced midwives can manage epidural analgesia safely, simply and effectively. Furthermore, by adjusting dosage to meet individual needs, the midwife can confer considerable flexibility and subtlety to epidural pain management. Childbirth pain is rarely perceived by the parturient in isolation and, in practice, most mothers will 'weigh' the pain relief provided by epidural analgesia against the side-effects. We contend, therefore, that obstetric patients feel more satisfied when they can exercise some control over the strength and quality of epidural analgesia.

It is unlikely that any single epidural preparation will be entirely satisfactory throughout labor for all patients. Epidural management based upon a single drug preparation and upon a rigid delivery system cannot be expected, therefore, to satisfy individual needs.

When midwives are permitted to determine top-up doses, they initially choose the preparation containing the smallest dose of bupivacaine. We believe this to be intrinsically safer, since it is unlikely that a life-threatening outcome would occur if a patient accidentally received, say, 12.5 mg of bupivacaine intravenously, or even subarachnoid.

A confidential survey of midwives in our unit has confirmed unanimous endorsement of the concept of midwife-managed epidural analgesia (unpublished observations). Quite apart from benefits to the patient it has become apparent that professional satisfaction can also be enhanced when the midwife is able to exercise judgment and responsibility in the management of obstetric pain.

The influence of our practice upon the newborn is currently under study. Preliminary results of a clinical trial suggest that there are negligible effects on neonatal neurobehavior – as might be anticipated from the relatively small cumulative dosage of local anesthetics and of meperidine that is usually employed.

Following surgery

The presence of a surgical wound poses an extra burden for the nursing mother: a burden which does not apply to other kinds of abdominal surgery. It is difficult for the mother to breastfeed and care for her baby when she is troubled with post-operative pain and fatigue. There are good reasons, therefore, for trying to make the post-operative period as comfortable as possible. An epidural catheter is a very convenient route for providing ongoing analgesia after cesarean delivery or other sources of pain following delivery (e.g., trauma to the lower birth canal or perineum, hemorrhoids and uterine 'after pains').

For epidural drugs to be administered safely in a post-natal ward, the top-up procedure must be foolproof and patient supervision satisfactory. These constraints have prohibited the use of post-operative epidural analgesia in many units. There is also controversy about which drug is most appropriate for epidural use and about the best means of administration (intermittent top-ups, continuous infusion or patient-controlled epidural analgesia).

Local anesthetics are not really suitable for post cesarean delivery pain (except possibly in very low dosage and combined with an opioid). Any significant degree of neural blockade in the post-operative period interferes with patient mobility and spontaneous micturition; postural hypotension may be a nuisance and there is a potential for the development of skin pressure areas. Tachyphylaxis develops after a time with all local anesthetics and there is always a risk that a high spinal block might suddenly occur. Extensive neural blockade also presents a considerable workload for nursing staff.

Epidural opioids are free from the above problems but have their own disadvantages. Pruritus is a nuisance with some opioids (and in some cases may be protracted and severe); excessive sedation may interfere with maternal – infant interaction; and central effects can lead to respiratory depression. With some opioids (notably morphine), respiratory depression can occur several hours later – when patient surveillance tends to be more relaxed. The potential risk for the development of undetected, life-threatening central depression has been the major disincentive to the introduction of epidural opioids in post-operative pain management.

Epidural meperidine has been used in the management of post-operative pain by the author since 1980. The following protocol is observed:

1. The initial dose of meperidine must be administered by an anesthesiologist. Subsequent top-up doses may be delegated to nursing staff only if the anesthesiologist is satisfied with patient response to this initial dose.
2. Epidural meperidine may be administered by a registered nurse competent in epidural procedures, provided that the dose and frequency of injection are properly prescribed.
3. Epidural meperidine (50 mg in 10 ml of preservative-free saline) is drawn up into a 10 ml syringe and double-checked. The dose is then administered via an epidural filter over the course of 3–5 min.
4. The patient is closely observed over the following 15 min. If excessive drowsiness, or a respiratory rate below 8/min occurs, the resuscitation team is notified and naloxone 0.4 mg administered intravenously.

Provided that the epidural catheter is still in situ, analgesia is usually achieved within 10 min, and lasts for approximately 3–4 h. A double-blind within-patient trial has demonstrated that epidural meperidine 50 mg compares favorably with other treatments (intramuscular meperidine 100 mg, epidural bupivacaine 25 mg) and is preferred by most subjects.[9]

Epidural meperidine is usually maintained for up to 48 h after cesarean delivery in our unit, although the epidural catheter sometimes becomes displaced before then. Once neural blockade has regressed patients are encouraged to become mobile and the urinary catheter is removed. There has never been any suggestion that the incidence of urinary retention is increased by epidural meperidine following cesarean delivery. As noted previously, epidural meperidine seems to be associated with a very low incidence of pruritus.

It has been our experience that epidural meperidine administered by nursing staff on a patient-demand basis is only marginally more labor intensive than giving intramuscular injections. In our view, close monitoring of the patient's clinical response (outlined in our protocol) for 15 min after each injection by a trained nurse is adequate. We consider it unnecessary to monitor blood pressure after a top-up dose any more frequently than following an intramuscular opioid.

During the last 10 years in our own unit and at the Queen Victoria Hospital, Adelaide, approximately 11 000 obstetric patients have received over 100 000 doses of epidural meperidine postoperatively (J. Crowhurst, personal communication). During this period there has been one potentially serious complication following a nurse-administered top-up – when a patient became unresponsive and peripherally cyanosed 5 min after receiving her second dose of meperidine.[10] The patient's condition rapidly improved following oxygen and intravenous naloxone, and she made a complete recovery. Subsequent radiologic investigation confirmed that the epidural catheter was sited subarachnoid. This incident remains the only occasion that patient resuscitation has been required following a nurse-administered epidural top-up in these two centers.[9]

CONCLUSIONS

Except in the ACT, epidural top-ups (local anesthetics and opioids) may be administered by nursing staff in Australia provided that guidelines issued by the relevant professional bodies are met. The extent to which nursing staff are permitted to manage epidural analgesia in Australian obstetric units is currently unknown. Many smaller units are presumably unable to meet the guidelines, while others may have decided to exclude nurse-administered top-ups as a matter of policy.

Our experience supports the notion that, in ideal circumstances, epidural analgesia can be managed safely and effectively by nursing staff. The midwifery-trained nurse in Australia is usually proficient in epidural management and the nurse-to-patient ratio is such that proper patient supervision can generally be provided both during labor and post-natally.

Several epidural opioids have been reported as providing excellent analgesia after cesarean delivery. The different physicochemical properties of opioid drugs, however, have a profound influence on clinical response – particularly the onset time and duration of analgesia and the interval for the potential development of central nervous system (CNS) depression. These properties have important clinical implications when choosing an opioid for intermittent injection. It is important that any significant CNS depression caused by the drug is revealed quickly and during the patient surveillance period. After a decade of experience in our obstetric unit, we believe that meperidine 50 mg satisfies this requirement and that any CNS depression will become apparent within the 15-min observation period. It is our contention, therefore, that epidural meperidine is suitable for administration on a patient-demand basis by nurses observing a simple protocol in the post-natal ward. Other opioids may prove to be equally suitable but there have been no comparative studies as yet to confirm this. (In Australia, diamorphine is unfortunately not available for medical use.)

During labor, there is considerable variation in epidural analgesia requirements both between, and within, individuals. In an attempt to meet these different requirements, and to provide more flexibility in pain management, we permit midwives to determine – as well as administer – prescribed epidural medication. Thus, analgesia can be adjusted to meet individual need. A low-dose preprepared mixture of bupivacaine and meperidine has proved to be extremely popular in our unit.

Introduction of this simple modification in epidural management has been associated with a dramatic increase in patient mobility (including ambulation) during labor and in the spontaneous delivery rate; a marked reduction in shivering and catheterization of the bladder; and fewer episodes of hypotension. Undoubtedly, the greater responsibility for epidural management accorded to our midwives has also enhanced their professional satisfaction.

REFERENCES

1. Faculty of Anaesthetists 1987 Guidelines for the conduct of epidural analgesia in obsterics (P14). Policy document. Royal Australasian College of Surgeons, Melbourne.
2. Brownridge P 1990 Epidural medication after the initial dose: reflections on current methods of administration during labour. Anaesth Intens Care 18: 300–308
3. Jones M J T, Bogod D G, Rees G A D, Rosen M 1988 Midwives' assessment of the upper sensory level after epidural blockade. Anaesthesia 43: 557–559
4. Brownridge P 1991 Epidural analgesia in the first stage of labour. Current Anaesth Crit Care 2: 92–100
5. Brownridge P 1988 Epidural bupivacaine-pethidine mixture: clinical experience using a low-dose combination in labor. Aust NZ J Obstet Gynaecol 28: 17–24
6. Justins D M, Francis D, Houlton P G, Reynolds F 1982 A controlled trial of extradural fentanyl in labour. Br J Anaesth 54: 409–414
7. Crawford J S 1985 Some maternal complications of epidural analgesia for labour. Anaesthesia 40: 1219–1225
8. Brownridge P 1986 Shivering related to epidural blockade with bupivacaine in labour, and the influence of epidural pethidine. Anaesth Intens Care 14: 412–417
9. Brownridge P, Frewin D B 1985 A comparative study of techniques of postoperative analgesia following caesarean section and lower abdominal surgery. Anaesth Intens Care 13: 123–130
10. Brownridge P, Wrobel J, Watt-Smith J 1983 Respiratory depression following accidental subarachnoid pethidine. Anaesth Intens Care 11: 237–240

PART B
UK
M. Harmer

The past decade has seen a rapid increase in the number of units using continuous epidural infusions during labor. These have gained in popularity for a number of reasons: they allow a more even level of analgesia to be attained; they tend to be associated with less motor weakness; and they can diminish the frequency of, or even the need for, intermittent top-ups. However, unless a fast infusion rate of a relatively high concentration of local anesthetic is used, top-ups are unlikely to be totally eliminated. The person responsible for topping up epidurals varies in units throughout the UK. One can consider the options as: anesthesiologists; nonanesthetic medical staff; midwives; patients. Many factors will influence the choice of staff who will undertake this duty; sadly, all too often tradition and lack of staff may be more influential in this choice than patient safety.

ANESTHESIOLOGISTS

There are no independently-practicing nurse anesthetists in the UK, and all anesthesiologists, staff-in-training or consultants, are medically qualified. The likelihood of anesthesiologists carrying out top-ups will be largely dictated by their availability – it is obviously not possible in units which do not have a dedicated obstetric anesthesiologist.

However, even in units with full anesthetic cover, the task of topping up may be delegated to other staff.

While virtually all epidurals for labor in the UK will be inserted by an anesthesiologist who will initiate the block, there is no universal agreement over who is best placed to carry out the subsequent top-ups. The arguments in favor of the anesthesiologist are based predominantly on safety and teaching grounds. The pregnant mother at term presents particular problems with regard to resuscitation should the local anesthetic solution be unintentionally injected subarachnoid producing a 'total spinal'. An anesthesiologist with knowledge of airway management and cardiovascular resuscitation would seem to be the ideal person to have available if such a situation should occur. However, does the anesthesiologist need to give the drug?; It is probably sufficient for the anesthesiologist to be readily available should a problem occur. The argument that topping up is a good training exercise probably carries greater strength. It is surprising to most anesthesiologists just how varied an epidural block can be, with partial block being a not uncommon problem. By ensuring that the anesthesiologist does the top-ups it is possible to teach, in a hands-on fashion, the options available to ameliorate anything less than a satisfactory block. Many staff-in-training will initially object to this chore until they appreciate the benefits that they can gain from this process. On an organizational and financial basis it might be more viable to have a dedicated obstetric anesthesiologist at all times if it can be seen that his or her time is more fully occupied.

The main argument against anesthesiologists topping up the epidural is that it is a waste of their time, particularly so if it occurs at night and the alternative would be a period of sleep. If top-ups are to be done by anesthesiologists, many would question the logic of disturbing someone's sleep only for them to wearily inject a dose of local anesthetic before returning to bed. In this sleepy condition, is an unintentional subarachnoid injection more or less likely?

The debate over anesthesiologists performing top-ups continues and, while it is unusual in the UK for this to happen, many would consider it the ideal method of providing top-ups. Gradually, its advocates on the grounds of safety and training seem to be convincing other centers. However, the anesthesiologist top-up still remains very rare.

NONANESTHETIC MEDICAL STAFF

The rarity of an epidural being inserted by nonanesthetic medical staff has largely led to a situation of such staff distancing themselves from the process of epidural aftercare. There are, in some centers, enthusiastic obstetricians who may be closely involved in the provision of analgesia and may on occasion be involved in the topping up of epidurals, but such a situation is extremely rare. Occasionally, in units where the anesthesiologist is responsible for performing top-ups, other medical staff may be expected to perform a top-up if the anesthesiologist is already occupied elsewhere. With limited understanding of epidurals and limited experience in cardiopulmonary resuscitation, this could be considered inappropriate. Generally speaking, nonanesthetic medical staff will seldom be involved in topping up epidurals and, if they are, it tends to be on an occasional basis.

MIDWIVES

The majority of units in the UK use a system of topping up for epidurals by midwives. In most units this originally arose out of necessity owing to the unavailability of a dedicated, full-time obstetric anesthesiologist. Originally midwife topping up was taught and protocols agreed on an informal basis. However, currently such top-up regimens are controlled by the criteria laid down by the United Kingdom Central Council for Nursing, Midwifery and Health Visiting. These criteria are:

1. that the ultimate responsibility for such a technique should be clearly stated to rest with the doctor;
2. that written instructions regarding the dose are provided;
3. that in all cases the dose given by a midwife should be checked by one other person;
4. that the initial dose through the catheter should be given by the doctor;
5. that the instructions should be given by the doctor as to the posture of the patient at the time of injection, observation of blood pressure and measures to be taken in the event of any side-effects;
6. that the midwife should be thoroughly instructed in the technique so that the doctor concerned is satisfied as to the midwife's ability.

In addition to fulfilling these criteria, the anesthesiologist should be in the hospital whenever an epidural anesthetic is in use, and a person capable of resuscitating the mother must also be present in the delivery suite. What is worrying is that, while the anesthesiologist may be in the hospital when an epidural is in use, there is no requirement for him/her to be on the delivery suite; should a problem arise with an unintentional subarachnoid injection and the development of a 'total spinal', the anesthesiologist is probably the only person able to cope adequately with the problem.

It is clear from the widespread use of midwives to top-up epidurals that they are able to provide a safe, effective service. However, some might argue that by placing restrictions on dose of drug and patient position, the midwife will never be able to attain the same perfection of block that can be achieved by the anesthesiologist. On grounds of safety, over the years there have been a few cases of death in the UK following midwife top-ups, but this is probably no more common than with other staff (including anesthesiologists) performing the task. The very large number of uneventful top-ups performed by midwives would attest to the safety of the technique.

PATIENT-CONTROLLED TOP-UPS

The traditional top-up dose given by the anesthesiologist or the midwife has been of a reasonably large volume (about 10 ml) and has often been given as a single injection with no preliminary checking of catheter position. Such large single doses are potentially hazardous and great emphasis over the years has been placed on the importance of fractionating the dose (giving smaller volumes more often). While it is often hard to control human nature and try to ensure that small doses only are given with a safe interval between, the introduction over the last decade of patient-controlled analgesia pumps allows exact criteria to be set and adhered to.

In recent years, there has been a great deal of interest in the use of patient-controlled pumps to carry out top-ups, but their use in the UK for this purpose is still very much in its infancy. By ensuring that only a small dose can be given each time with a known interval between, it is difficult to see how excessively high blocks could develop. The main problem is in deciding on the concentration of local anesthetic to be used and the size of the incremental dose. In addition, the ability of this type of top-up to cope with patchy or unilateral blocks is very uncertain.

CONCLUSION

The position in the UK is that the majority of units use a midwife-based system for topping up epidural blocks. Several units believe that the best person to administer the top up is the anesthesiologist and, while this may represent a gold standard, it is not without its problems. It may well be that patient-controlled top-ups will continue to expand and may eventually become the standard method of topping up.

PART C
USA

T. H. Joyce *N. H. Blass*

In 1970 the American College of Obstetricians and Gynecologists completed a survey which found that in more than 80% of vaginal deliveries patients were attended by nonphysicians for anesthetic coverage.

In 1974, in a survey of the state of Ohio, Nicholson and Joyce found a similar distribution, with 10% of patients being attended by a nonmedical person and general anesthesia being used in more than 50% of all vaginal deliveries (T. Joyce, unpublished results). Over the past 16 years the number of physician anesthesiologists and nurse anesthetists has increased to the point that 80% of women undergoing vaginal delivery have fully trained anesthesia personnel available to attend them. During this time, epidural analgesia for labor and vaginal delivery has become increasingly popular as the '*Cadillac*' of labor analgesic techniques. Thus, the following question naturally arises. Who does the 'top-ups' when labor outlasts the initial dose of local anesthetic?

Anesthesiologists, nurse anesthetists, obstetricians, labor nurses and midwives have all been assigned the responsibility for 'top-ups'. The guidelines for obstetric anesthesia issued by the American Society of Anesthesiologists state that regional anesthesia should be initiated by a physician with appropriate privileges and maintained by/or under the medical direction of such an individual.[1] At this time the majority of 'top-ups' are done by a member of the anesthesia health care team. However, the policies of the anesthesia department must designate which individuals may give 'top-ups' and what training is required to qualify for 'epidural privileges' since one must be deemed competent to manage those anesthetic complications that can arise from this form of anesthesia.

Repeated injections of local anesthetic of local anesthetic–opioid combinations can be done on a time schedule when the sensory level begins to recede or when the patient complains of pain. The advent of continuous-infusion epidural analgesia has modified the older technique of repeat boluses. When boluses are used the admonition for fractionated injection applies. The refill of an empty syringe on a pump requires the same check of vital signs, sensory level, review of obstetric progress and any interaction with the epidural anesthetic by mother and/or fetus, and appropriate charting of this check and the syringe refill. Recently, the use of *patient*-controlled epidural catheter injection has clouded the issues of responsibilities for the management of labor analgesia.

At Baylor University Department of Anesthesia (Houston) and at the Department of Anesthesiology at the Medical College of Virginia the 'anesthesia care team' concept is operant.[2,3] Physicians, residents, nurse anesthetists and student nurse anesthetists all place and inject epidural catheters under the direction of a faculty physician. In this mode of practice, all treatment is supervised by the assigned responsible anesthesiologist. Generally, epidural anesthetics are begun with 8–10 ml of 0.25% bupivacaine injected in 3–5 ml increments every 2–3 min. Once a satisfactory T10 level is reached, a continuous-infusion syringe pump (currently Baxter autosyringe or Harvard pump) is attached to inject 0.125 % bupivacaine at 10–12 ml/h. Lidocaine or 2-chloroprocaine can also be used. If an opioid is to be used to intensify the analgesia, fentanyl 50 µg in a bolus is most commonly used, although sufentanil, alfentanyl, meperidine, butorphanol, and clonidine have all been used. Fentanyl can then be added to the infusion in a concentration of 1–2 µg/ml of local anesthetic if deemed desirable.

The most frequent problem faced by the management team is that of the occasional unblocked dermatome or 'hotspot'. Commonly, the patient is placed on the side with the unblocked segment down and 5–6 ml of 0.25% bupivacaine is fractionally injected. If more than one segment is not blocked or bilateral segments are unblocked, the epidural catheter is repositioned or replaced. If unblocked or delayed block of segments continues, the diagnosis of subdural catheter migration must be considered. 'Hotspots' have also been successfully treated by the injection of fentanyl 50 µg in 5–6 ml of sterile preservative-free saline provided an opioid has not been used in the initial injection.

The use of continuous infusion of local anesthetic agents for 2 h or more generally produces perineal anesthesia in 80% of patients for vaginal delivery, with or without outlet forceps. When using a low concentration of local anesthetic in the infusion, an additional dose for perineal muscular block is required for a trial of mid-forceps. In this situation we commonly administer an adequate additional local anesthetic in a concentration and volume to produce relaxation of the pelvic musculature. 10–12 ml of 2% lidocaine or 3% chloroprocaine can produce the appropriate block.

If changes in the fetal heart rate or pattern lead the obstetrician to elect urgent or emergent cesarean delivery, the anesthetic must be evaluated for a surgical level in view of the urgency of the surgery. A change to 3% 2-chloroprocaine (18–25 ml) will generally produce solid surgical anesthesia in 5–6 min; 2%-lidocaine will generally produce similar surgical anesthesia in 8–10 min. Alkanization of 2% lidocaine will produce surgical anesthesia in approximately the same time frame as 3% 2-chloroprocaine. Our patients receive 30 ml of 0.3 M sodium citrate by mouth from the nursing staff as soon as surgery is contemplated. Metaclopropramide 10 mg i.v. and an H_2-blocker (ranitidine or cimetidine) intravenously may be given, (time permitting) if desired.

Epidural catheters are removed either in the delivery room or in the recovery room by a member of the anesthesia health care team who is responsible for appropriate completion of the anesthesia record.

In summary, each institution should have a policy delineating the requirements for accrediting individuals for the insertion, injection and management of epidural anesthesia/analgesia in the obstetric patient. When the 'anesthesia health care team' concept is used, special care must be given to delineate the decision-making roles of all nonphysicians and trainees.

REFERENCES

1. Guidelines for Regional Anesthesia in Obstetrics 1991. American Society of Anesthesiologists, Park Ridge, Illinois
2. Policies and Procedures, Department of Anesthesia, Baylor College of Medicine, Houston, Texas
3. Policies and Procedures, Department of Anesthesia, Medical College of Virginia, Richmond, Virginia

PART D
BELGIUM

A. Van Steenberge

A dedicated midwife is entitled to inject or reinject the epidural catheter provided she is properly trained and supervised by an experienced anesthesiologist. The usual standard precautions are to be taken: a functioning i.v. catheter (>16 gauge), oxygen and a suitable mask should be immediately available; the bed should be able to be placed in the Trendelenburg position; the left lateral position is the rule; and ephedrine 5 mg/ml must be at hand.

The syringe containing the local anesthetic solution must be prepared by the anesthesiologist. The name of the parturient, the content per milliliter and the volume to be given must be labeled on the syringe as well as ordered on the chart.

The first so-called test dose, equal to the therapeutic dose, is to be administered by the anesthesiologist. Each therapeutic dose being a test dose, the subsequent doses should be identical to the first dose.

The established method is to inject bupivacaine 10–12.5 mg, epinephrine 10–12.5 μg with sufentanil 8 μg in a 10-ml bolus. The total dose of sufentanil should not exceed 30 μg. This mixture, even if injected intravenously or subarachnoid, will not cause a disaster. Intravenous injection will give clear warning signals within less than 1 min lasting no longer than 90 s. No analgesia will ensue. If injected into the cerebrospinal fluid, anesthesia will spread to dermatome T2–3 within 5–10 min. This situation can be controlled by simple, standard precautions which are within the realm of any experienced midwife. No harm to the mother or the fetus will result.

Maternal and fetal pathology as well as fetopelvic disproportion or the confinement of three or more parturients at one time entail the constant care of the anesthesiologist. Further presence of the anesthesiologist is requested during each injection in the epidural space and the subsequent 20 min if there have been problems with the placement of the needle or catheter or perforation of dura or a vessel wall. The same rule applies when the first dose has not resulted in at least a substantial relief of pain.

Skill and experience of the midwife gained during the injection into the epidural catheter and the observation and care related to it will contribute to the safety and comfort of the mother and the fetus.

In addition, the presence of a qualified physician to supervise labor and to deal with any obstetric complication that may arise is essential.

Keen attention by the midwife will help to discover

minor problems before any incident or accident becomes manifest. These problems will be easy to correct when managed at once.

An instructed and interested midwife becomes a positive asset in the obstetric team through active participation in the provision of epidural analgesia/anesthesia.

PART E
SWEDEN

L. Irestedt   P. Belfrage

While the administration of nitrous oxide, opioids and pudendal block in the noncomplicated delivery is left to the midwives and the administration of paracervical block to the obstetrician, epidural block for obstetric analgesia is performed by an anesthesiologist after being contacted by the responsible obstetrician. The anesthesiologist will perform the epidural block usually through an indwelling epidural catheter. The anesthesiologist will document his procedures in the anesthetic record, check the analgesic response and prescribe top-up doses and top-up intervals or infusion rates if a continuous infusion is being used. In the routine case, the midwife will then independently handle the infusion of the local anesthetic agent or the top-up dosage under the direction of the anesthesiologist and the obstetrician. The most frequently used local anesthetic solution for obstetric pain relief is bupivacaine 0.25% with or without epinephrine 5 μg/ml. There is a tendency to decrease the bupivacaine concentration to 0.125% and add small doses of sufentanil (10–30 μg) in order to decrease motor blockade of the legs. The majority of delivery units use a continuous-infusion technique, but several major hospitals in Sweden still prefer an intermittent technique. Today, the majority of delivery units in Sweden are staffed and organized in a way that allows the possibility of effective pain relief during delivery including the administration of epidural anesthesia on a 24-h basis. In the large county hospitals and in the university hospitals the anesthesia service is mostly divided into various anesthetic sections. Obstetric anesthesia is usually organized within the section of obstetric and gynecologic anesthesia under the supervision of a senior consultant. It must be emphasized that there are no private delivery units in Sweden, implying that the frequency of epidural anesthetics for obstetric pain relief is not influenced by any economic incentive for the anesthesiologist. The specialist training in Sweden includes a 1-week full-time course in obstetric anesthesia and analgesia followed by examination including the knowledge of one major textbook in obstetric anesthesia and analgesia.

PART F
ARGENTINA

P. J. Kelly

Anesthesiologists are responsible for all anesthetics given, including 'top-ups'. Midwives or obstetricians cannot give top-ups. In places far from cities, some surgeons give some epidural anesthetics themselves although this situation is avoided because of the increasing medicolegal problems in the country.

91. Vaginal birth after cesarean delivery

Part A USA view *N. E. Oriol C. Johnson*
Part B European view *Y. Darbois D. Sfoggia M. Henry D. Vauthier J. Seebacher*

PART A
USA VIEW

N. E. Oriol C. Johnson

In October 1988, the American College of Obstetricians and Gynecologists (ACOG) decided that vaginal birth after a previous cesarean delivery, or the trial of labor (TOL), was an acceptable alternative to elective repeat cesarean delivery.[1] The guidelines established by ACOG have not adequately addressed the risks of epidural anesthesia for the relief of labor pain during a TOL; however, reports in the obstetric literature have suggested that it is safe. The purpose of this section is to review the literature on trial of labor and examine the role of epidural anesthesia.

CESAREAN DELIVERY

Between 1970 and 1984, the cesarean delivery rate increased from 5.5% to 18% in the USA.[2] In 1985, cesarean delivery was the most frequently performed major operation in America, exceeding the combined total of all tonsillectomies, appendectomies and mastectomies.[3] The most common reason for performing a cesarean delivery in this country is a history of a prior cesarean delivery. The origin of the elective repeat cesarean delivery came from the belief that the risk of uterine rupture in a laboring 'scarred' uterus outweighed the maternal and neonatal risks of an elective repeat cesarean delivery.[4] It was determined that the type of uterine incision played a significant role in the severity of uterine rupture during labor after cesarean delivery.[5,6] A uterine incision on the upper segment of the uterus (classical incision) is more likely to rupture without warning. The classical incision is 10 times more likely to rupture than the low transverse uterine incision, resulting in excessive hemorrhaging and extrusion of the fetus into the abdomen.[5,6] Ruptured incisions of the lower uterine segment form a dehiscence or window that is relatively avascular; these incisions rarely result in abdominal extrusion of the fetus and rarely interfere with the birthing process.[5,6]

TRIAL OF LABOR

In 1981, the National Institutes of Health decided that vaginal birth after cesarean delivery in patients with a lower segment uterine scar should be considered the reasonable alternative to elective repeat cesarean delivery.[7] Since that time, numerous retrospective and prospective studies have been performed examining the last 30 years of obstetrics in the USA. The results of such studies have shown that a TOL can be safely tolerated by patients with low transverse uterine incisions, by patients with more than one prior low transverse cesarean delivery, and by those with oxytocic induction or augmentation of labor.[8–12] The overall success rate for a TOL is 60–80% and increases to 90% when the indication for the previous cesarean delivery was a breech presentation. When the indication for the previous cesarean delivery was fetopelvic disproportion or failure to progress, the success rate is 55–65%.[8-13] The rationale for attempting a TOL is the decreased maternal and fetal morbidity and mortality from vaginal delivery when compared with the elective repeat cesarean delivery.[1,8,9,14] The increase in maternal morbidity associated with cesarean delivery is due to a 0.31% prevalence of bladder laceration, a 0.09% prevalence of ureteral injury, a 30–50% increase in blood loss, increased chance of wound infection, increased hospital stay (from 2.5 to 4.5 days), increased risk of post-operative thrombophlebitis (from 0.25–0.1% with vaginal delivery to 2–10% with cesarean delivery) and longer post-operative recovery period compared with a successful TOL.[1,5,8,9,14]

In this era of cost containment, economic factors need

to be considered. In a 1984 study performed by Flamm et al,[13] the total cost for a vaginal delivery after cesarean delivery was $2087, compared with $5101 for elective repeat cesarean delivery.

Cesarean delivery may not be a benign event for the fetus or neonate. Poorly timed elective cesarean delivery can result in iatrogenic prematurity, which causes fetal morbidity or death. Elective cesarean delivery has been associated with persistent fetal circulation in term infants, which can be a fatal condition.[15–18] However, with the use of amniocentesis and biochemical evaluation of amniotic fluid to determine fetal lung maturity, the occurrence of iatrogenic prematurity should be a rare event.

There are two types of uterine separation associated with a TOL: incomplete rupture and complete rupture. Incomplete rupture is a relatively benign event and is not associated with increased maternal or fetal morbidity or mortality. It is usually an incidental finding, detected by vaginal palpation of the uterine scar after a vaginal delivery or noted during direct visualization at cesarean delivery. The prevalence of incomplete rupture with a TOL is 0.5–3.0%.[8,19–33] Complete uterine rupture is associated with significant maternal morbidity and fetal morbidity or mortality.[34] The prevalence of complete rupture is 0.3–0.5% with a TOL, compared with 1 per 800 to 1 per 3000 (0.125–0.3%) for spontaneous rupture of unscarred uteri.[8,9,35–38] In our review of 10 967 patients, presented in 14 studies from 1980 to 1989, there were no maternal deaths related to the TOL. There were a total of nine fetal deaths secondary to scar rupture during the TOL. This gives a perinatal mortality rate (PMR) of less than 1 per 1000 births. In a study by Meehan and Magani,[23] the PMR in 1498 patients with one or more cesarean delivery scars delivered between 1972 and 1982 was analyzed. Repeat elective cesarean delivery was performed in 654 of the patients, and the PMR was 4.5 per 1000 births. TOL was attempted in 844 patients, and the PMR dropped from 40 per 1000 births to 20 per 1000 births by the end of the study. In view of the improvement in the PMR and the added risk to the mother with elective cesarean delivery, obstetricians advocate a policy of TOL with informed consent in selected cases.[23]

Analysis of the Meehan and Magani study looking at PMR secondary to complete uterine rupture reveals a PMR of only 4.7 per 1000 births. Combination of the present study with the Meehan and Magani study yields a PMR resulting from complete uterine rupture of 1 per 1000 to 4.7 per 1000 births, which is equal to the PMR for elective cesarean delivery. Thus, complete uterine rupture is not a significant contributor to the PMR resulting from a TOL.

THE USE OF EPIDURAL ANESTHESIA

The American College of Obstetricians and Gynecologists[1] have adopted the following guidelines for trial of labor.

> A woman with a low transverse uterine incision in the absence of a contraindication (classical incision) should be encouraged to attempt a trial of labor. There are insufficient data to assess the safety or danger of labor for women with a previous low vertical incision. Likewise, the effects of labor on patients with more than one fetus, a breech presentation or an estimated fetal weight greater than 4000 g have not been substantiated. Continuous electronic fetal monitoring and 24-h blood banking capabilities could be available. Anesthesia coverage and an obstetrician capable of evaluating labor and performing an emergency cesarean delivery should be in house.

Although the 'classic' signs and symptoms of rupture are abdominal pain between contractions or a severe tearing sensation followed by cessation of uterine contractions, the majority of ruptures usually present with signs of fetal distress diagnosed by continuous fetal heart rate (FHR) monitoring.[34] FHR patterns heralding complete rupture are severe variable decelerations or a prolonged

Table 91.1 Trial of labor data from 14 studies

Reference	Year	No. of patients	With epidural	Without epidural	Complete rupture	Rupture frequency (%)
29	1980	119	77	42	2	1.7
19	1982	92	41	51	2	2.2
21	1982	207	19	188	0	0
32	1983	717	98	619	3	0.42
31	1983	222	71	151	4	1.8
28	1984	115	115	0	1	0.87
13	1984	230	73	157	0	0
27	1985	732	0	732	2	0.27
10	1987	272	153	119	1	0.37
33	1987	1781	85	1696	8	0.45
9	1987	1796	178	1618	5	0.28
8	1988	1776	131	1595	3	0.17
25	1989	1498	187	1311	4	0.27
23	1989	1350	345	1005	6	0.44
Total		10967	1623	9344	41	
Overall rupture incidence						0.37

deceleration. Associated with the FHR changes can be loss of pressure tracing on the internal uterine pressure monitor.[8–11,24] In Tables 91.1 and 91.2 data are presented from 14 TOL studies between 1980 and 1989. There were 10 967 patients who attempted a vaginal birth after a cesarean delivery. A total of 41 complete uterine ruptures occurred, giving a rupture frequency of 0.37%. Of the 10 967 patients undergoing a TOL, 1623 had epidural catheters placed for relief of labor pain (Table 91.1). The presentation of 37 of the 41 ruptures is shown in Table 91.2. The Meehan et al[25] study failed to mention the presenting signs and symptoms of their four ruptures and none of them had epidural anesthesia.

The prevalence of uterine rupture in patients with epidural anesthesia (14 of 1623) was 0.86%. The prevalence of uterine rupture in patients without epidural anesthesia (23 of 9344) was 0.25%. The prevalence of rupture in the epidural group is three times greater than that in the nonepidural group. However, because of the small sample size of uterine ruptures, the increased prevalence of ruptures in the epidural group is not clinically significant. Three of the 14 ruptures presented with 'classic' abdominal pain alone, seven with fetal distress alone and two with both fetal distress and abdominal pain; one was an incidental finding at cesarean delivery, and one presented with post-partum bleeding.

It is interesting that five of 14 (35%) complete ruptures in the epidural group presented with abdominal pain, compared with four of 23 (17%) in the nonepidural group (Table 91.2). Two of the five ruptures in the epidural group presented with abdominal pain associated with monitored fetal distress. All of the studies alluded to the fact that satisfactory epidural anesthesia was obtained. However, none gave specific levels of epidural sensory or motor block at the time of uterine rupture. Overall, abdominal pain alone or in association with monitored fetal distress was present in only nine of the 41 (22%) uterine ruptures (Table 91.2). Fetal distress alone was the presenting sign of rupture 50% of the time in the epidural group and 61% of the time in the nonepidural group. Overall, uterine rupture presented with signs or symptoms other than abdominal pain 76% of the time, with fetal distress presenting by itself 52% of the time (Table 91.2). Thus, the single most reliable sign of uterine rupture is fetal distress rather than abdominal pain. Of note, however, is the fact that if abdominal pain is going to occur with complete uterine rupture there will be the development of 'breakthrough pain' despite the presence of epidural anesthesia. Crawford[26] referred to this phenomenon as the 'epidural sieve.'

The presentation of uterine rupture as it relates to the presence or absence of epidural anesthesia, oxytocin, and prostaglandin administration is shown in Table 91.3. 23 of the 41 (56%) ruptures occurred in patients without epidural anesthesia, compared with only 18 of 41 (44%) ruptures in patients with epidural anesthesia. This suggests that there is no increased incidence of uterine rupture in patients with epidural anesthesia. 19 of the 41 (46%) ruptures occurred in patients who did not receive any agent for induction or augmentation of labor (oxytocin or prostaglandin). 22 of 41 (54%) patients developing ruptures received either intravenous oxytocin or vaginal prostaglandin, which does not represent a significant clinical difference from the nonoxytocin group.

Table 91.2 Presenting signs of uterine rupture*

Presenting signs of rupture	Number of patients who ruptured	With epidural (n = 1623)	Without epidural (n = 9344)
Abdominal pain	4	3	1
Fetal distress	21	7	14
Incidental finding at cesarean delivery	3	1	2
Fetal distress and abdominal pain	5	2	3
Post-partum bleeding	4	1	3
Total	37	14	23
Rupture incidence		0 .86%	0 .25%

* Data from Table 91.1. The four ruptures from Meehan et al[25] are not included because their presentation is not mentioned in the study.

Table 91.3 Rupture presentation related to epidural anesthesia, oxytocin and prostaglandin use

Presentation	Epidural	Epi + Oxy	Oxy	PG	Nothing	Epi + PG
Abdominal pain alone	0	3	0	1	0	1
Abdominal pain and fetal distress	1	1	2	0	1	0
Fetal distress alone	7	3	5	0	5	0
Incidental finding at cesarean delivery	1	0	2	0	0	0
Post-partum bleeding	0	1	0	0	3	0
Presentation not given*	0	0	3	0	1	0
Total	9	8	12	1	10	1

Epi, epidural; oxy, oxytocin; PG, prostaglandin.
* Meehan et al.[25]

Horenstein and Phelan[27] studied the risks and benefits of oxytocin usage in 732 patients who underwent a TOL. In their study, 40% of the patients received oxytocin for either induction or augmentation of labor and 60% did not receive oxytocin. The prevalence of incomplete rupture in the oxytocin and nonoxytocin groups was 3% and 2%, which is not clinically significant. There were only two complete ruptures, one with oxytocin and one without oxytocin. Flamm et al[8] performed a similar study and found no increased incidence of incomplete rupture with oxytocin usage in a TOL. There were three complete ruptures in their study, one with oxytocin and two without oxytocin.

The present review of the literature confirms the obstetric clinical impression that complete uterine rupture is not significantly increased with oxytocin use for induction/augmentation of labor. Nine of the 41 (22%) ruptures occurred in patients who received epidural anesthesia and induction/augmentation of labor, compared with 10 of 41 (24%) ruptures in patients who received no epidural anesthesia and no induction/augmentation of labor. There appears to be no increased risk of complete uterine rupture with the combination of epidural anesthesia and oxytocin.

Studies have shown that epidural anesthesia does not have a negative effect on the success rate of vaginal delivery with trial of labor. Phelan et al[9] studied 1796 women undergoing a TOL. Epidural anesthesia was administered to 178 patients, all of whom also received oxytocin for augmentation of labor. When the cesarean delivery rate for the combination of epidural anesthesia and oxytocin was compared with that for patients who received oxytocin alone, there was no significant difference (approximately a 31% incidence of cesarean delivery for both groups). Flamm et al[8] had similar results. Among 1776 patients who underwent a TOL, 181 patients received epidural anesthesia for relief of labor pain; 134 (74%) delivered vaginally. The success rate in this group did not differ from those who did not have epidural anesthesia (1180 of 1595, or 74%).

CLINICAL RECOMMENDATIONS

We recommend that sensory analgesia with intraspinal opioids or sensory anesthesia with local anesthetics with or without opioids rather than complete anesthesia be the goal for relief of labor pain. The lowest possible local anesthetic concentration and dose – with or without opioids – should be considered. We prefer continuous epidural anesthesia using bupivacaine 0.0625–0.125% with fentanyl 1–2 μg/ml. This mixture is administered at a rate of 8–12 ml/h after the establishment of the anesthetic using a variety of drugs. It is our conclusion from the literature and our practice that epidural anesthesia is safe during a TOL provided appropriate fetal heart rate and uterine contraction monitoring are used.

REFERENCES

1. Committee on Obstetrics 1988 Maternal and fetal medicine: guidelines for vaginal delivery after a previous Cesarean birth. American College of Obstetricians and Gynecologists Newsletter No. 64
2. Notzon F C, Placek P J, Taffel S M 1987 Comparison of national Cesarean-section rates. New Engl J Med 316: 386–389
3. Nation Center for Health Statistics Monthly Vital Statistics Report 1985 Advance Report of Final Natality Statistics. Vol. 34. US Government Printing Office, Washington, DC, p 6
4. Cragin E B 1916 Conservatism in obstetrics. NY State J Med 104: 1
5. Hibbard L 1986 Cesarean section and other surgical procedures. In Gabbe S G, Neibyl J R, Simpson J L (eds) Obstetrics: normal and problem pregnancies. Churchill Livingstone, New York, p 517
6. Pritchard J A, MacDonald P C 1980 Williams obstetrics, 16th edn. Appleton & Lange, East Norwalk, CT, p 861
7. National Institutes of Health 1981 Cesarean Childbirth. NIH Publication No. 82–2067. Bethesda, MD
8. Flamm B L, Lim O W, Jones C et al 1988 Vaginal birth after Cesarean Section: results of a multicenter study. Am J Obstet Gynecol 158: 1079–1084
9. Phelan J P, Clark S T, Diaz F, Paul R H 1987 Vaginal birth after Cesarean. Am J Obstet Gynecol 157: 1510–1515
10. Stovall T G, Shaver D C, Solomon S K, Anderson G D 1987 Trial of labor in previous Cesarean section patients, excluding classical Cesarean sections. Obstet Gynecol 70: 713–717
11. Pruett K M, Kirshon B, Cotton D B, Poindexter AN 1988 Is vaginal birth after two or more Cesarean sections safe? Obstet Gynecol 72: 163–165
12. Anon 1978 Induction of labor. Technical Bulletin No. 49. American College of Obstetricians and Gynecologists, Washington, DC
13. Flamm B L, Dunnett C, Fischermann E, Quilligan E J 1984 Vaginal delivery following Cesarean section: use of oxytocin augmentation and epidural anesthesia with internal tocodynamic and internal fetal monitoring. Am J Obstet Gynecol 148: 759–763
14. Eisenkop S M, Richman R, Platt L D, Paul R H 1982 Urinary tract injury during Cesarean section. Obstet Gynecol 60: 591–596
15. Chervenk F A, Herslinger R, Freedman R, Lamastra P 1986 Current perspectives on iatrogenic neonatal respiratory distress syndrome. J Reprod Med 31: 53–57
16. Heritage C K, Cunningham M D 1985 Association of elective repeat Cesarean delivery and persistent pulmonary hypertension of the newborn. Am J Obstet Gynecol 152: 627–629
17. Hjalmarson O, Krantz B, Jacobsson B et al 1982 The importance of neonatal asphyxia and Cesarean section as risk factors for neonatal respiratory disorders in an unselected population. Acta Paediatr Scand 71: 403–408
18. Evrard J R, Gold E M 1978 Cesarean section: risk/benefit. Perinatal Care 2: 4
19. Demianczuk N N, Hunter D J, Taylor D W 1982 Trial of labor after previous Cesarean section: prognostic indicators of outcome. Am J Obstet Gynecol 142: 640–642
20. Gibbs C E 1980 Planned vaginal delivery following Cesarean section. Clin Obstet Gynecol 23: 507–515
21. Merrill B S, Gibbs C E 1978 Planned vaginal delivery following Cesarean section. Obstet Gynecol 52: 50–52
22. Case B D, Corcoran R, Jeffcoate N, Randle G H 1971 Cesarean section and its place in modern obstetric practice. J Obstet Gynecol Br Commonw 78: 203–214
23. Meehan F P, Magani I M 1989 True rupture of the Cesarean scar (a 15-year review. 1972–1987). Eur J Obstet Gynecol Reprod Biol 30: 129–135
24. Uppington J 1983 Epidural analgesia and previous Cesarean section. Anaesthesia 38: 336–341
25. Meehan F P, Burke G, Casey C, Sheil J G 1989 Delivery following Cesarean section and perinatal mortality. Am J Perinatol 6(1): 90–94
26. Crawford J S 1976 The epidural sieve and MBC (minimal blocking concentration): a hypothesis. Anaesthesia 31: 1277–1280
27. Horenstein J M, Phelan J P 1985 Previous Cesarean section: the

risks and benefits of oxytocin usage in a trial of labor. Am J Obstet Gynecol 151: 564–569
28. Rudick V, Niv D, Hetman-Peri M et al 1984 Epidural analgesia for planned vaginal delivery following previous Cesarean section. Obstet Gynecol 64: 621–623
29. Carlsson C, Nybell-Lindahl G, Ingemarsson I 1980 Extradural block in patients who have previously undergone Cesarean section. Br J Anaesth 52: 827–830
30. Eckstein K L, Oberlander S G, Marx G F 1973 Uterine rupture during extradural blockade. Can J Anaesth J 20: 566–568
31. Martin J N, Harris B A, Huddleston J F et al 1983 Vaginal delivery following previous Cesarean birth. Am J Obstet Gynecol 146: 255–263
32. Meier P R, Porreco R P 1982 Trial of labor following Cesarean section: a two-year experience. Am J Obstet Gynecol 144: 671–678
33. Molloy B G, Sheil O, Duigan N M 1987 Delivery after Cesarean section: review of 2,176 consecutive cases. Br Med J 294: 1645–1647
34. Eden R D, Parker R T, Gall S A 1986 Rupture of the pregnant uterus: a 53-year review. Obstet Gynecol 68: 671–674
35. Brudenell M, Chakravarti S 1975 Uterine rupture in labor. Br Med J 2: 122–123
36. Smith A M 1975 (letter) Uterine rupture in labor. Br Med J 2: 446
37. Schrinsky D C, Benson R C 1978 Rupture of the pregnant uterus: a review. Obstet Gynecol Surv 33: 217–232
38. Caggiano A P, Breen J L 1968 Uterine rupture: an analysis of 27 patients. Int Surg 50: 368–376

PART B
EUROPEAN VIEW

Y. Darbois D. Sfoggia M. Henry D. Vauthier J. Seebacher

SCARRED UTERI

Cesarean delivery is one of the most common surgical procedures performed in France, and more than half of these are repeat cesarean deliveries. However, in the past 10 years, the attitude of obstetricians has changed and vaginal delivery may now be considered, despite a scarred uterus, under certain conditions. This change in attitude is the result principally of an increase in the number of patients requesting vaginal birth after a cesarean delivery, but also of a reduction in maternal morbidity and in fetal morbidity.

The most important risk associated with vaginal delivery following a previous cesarean delivery is uterine rupture. There are three types of rupture:

- *Complete rupture* involving the muscle and serosa with opening of the amniotic cavity and expulsion of the fetus into the peritoneal cavity: this is extremely rare.
- *Incomplete sub serous rupture*, with occasional protrusion of the amniotic sac.
- *Dehiscence* or significant thinning of the muscularis mucosa.

Only complete rupture carries an immediate risk for the fetus and mother. Uterine rupture is uncommon (1%), irrespective of the type of delivery, i.e. whether by cesarean or vaginally. Maternal mortality is now reduced and fetal mortality is not higher in vaginal delivery.[1] Such prognostic arguments are in favor of 'testing the scar'.

ANTENATAL MANAGEMENT

Before saying 'yes' to a request for a vaginal delivery after cesarean delivery, it is essential to look for favorable or unfavorable criteria by history and examination.[2–5]

There are two types of scars:

1. *Gynecologic scars.*[2] Myomectomies with or without opening of the uterine cavity and hysteroplasties yield good-quality scars, albeit corporeal. Tubouterine reinsertions or resections of the interstitial portion of the fallopian tube are more fragile. Uterine ruptures following gynecologic surgery are exceptional and often dehiscence is confused with protrusion of the membranes.
2. *Obstetric scars.* In this case the prognosis depends on the location. Cesarean scars in the body of the uterus are usually of poor quality, with a major risk of rupture. Low-segment cervical cesarean delivery leaves a much more solid scar, whether it is transverse or vertical. Vertical,

segmental hysterotomy may sometimes be ascending or in the body with the same prognosis as corporeal cesarean delivery.

Examination to assess the quality of the scar must be considered, with some reservations. Hysterography long after a cesarean delivery is only a contraindication for vaginal delivery if there is a deformation or a fistula greater than 6 mm.[2,3] Ultrasound examination during pregnancy measures the lower segment but does not take into account the status at the end of pregnancy.[4–6] Lastly, during labor, it has been suggested that the uterine scar should be evaluated by pelvic examination, as the fingers reach up to the lower segment. The ideal situation is to have the surgical report, the test labor report, the indication for the cesarean delivery, and the report of the post-partum period (infection). At the end of pregnancy, after 37 weeks, examinations should include a fetopelvic comparison with conventional pelvimetry [2–7] or computed tomography and fetal ultrasound to determine the presentation and placental insertion and to estimate fetal weight. The contraindications for 'testing the scar' will be determined after reviewing these data, leading to a routine prophylactic cesarean delivery (Table 91.4).

The rate of repeat prophylactic cesarean delivery is 30–40%. Dehiscence of the uterine scar is only found in 2 or 3 % of cases, confirming that uterine rupture is uncommon.

'TESTING THE SCAR' FOLLOWING CESAREAN DELIVERY

This may be considered in 60% of patients having undergone previous cesarean delivery, and vaginal delivery is possible in two-thirds of these patients. This trial of labor must take place in the labor room with an obstetrician and an anesthetic team present. In addition, there must be an operating theater available at all times. Attempted vaginal delivery requires the routine recording of uterine dynamics and fetal heart as soon as labor begins. In addition to the usual criteria, monitoring includes careful examination for signs of prerupture, which are unfortunately often not obvious.[8–13]

Table 91.4 Indications and contraindications for trial of labor

	Vaginal birth after prior cesarean delivery (Trial of labor)	Prophylactic cesarean delivery
Scar	Segmental cesarean Gynecologic surgery	Corporeal cesarean Segmental-corporeal
Indication for the first cesarean delivery	Fetal distress	Fetopelvic disproportion
Time between the two births	Two years	One year
Follow-up hysterography	No anomaly	Leakage of contrast media
Current pregnancy	Normal course	Breech; low placental insertion Abnormal pelvis or fetopelvic disproportion

Pain is inconsistently present and nonspecific. *Mctromenorrhagia* is rare, whereas bleeding during normal labor is common; maternal hemodynamic shock is uncommon because hemorrhaging is low grade. *Stagnation of dilatation* is undoubtedly the best sign: the absence of mechanical dystocia suggests ineffective contractility and raises the possibility of dehiscence. *Unexpected uterine hypertonia* has the same significance. *Anomalies of fetal cardiac rhythm* are inconsistent and late. The signs are relatively nonspecific (pain, bloody fluid), and not very sensitive. Normal progression of labor is the differentiating criterion; dilatation must progress evenly without faltering. Any anomaly warrants a cesarean delivery, especially uterine hypertonia. This raises the problem of the use of oxytocin.[5–14]

The use of oxytocin is acceptable if mechanical conditions are ideal, i.e. non-fetopelvic disproportion (weight lower than 4000 g) with good fetal accommodation if there is documented hypokinesis and **if** there are no signs of fetal distress. The insertion of an internal pressure monitor to obtain accurate intrauterine pressure measurements is proposed if hypokinesis is suspected but doubtful. It allows the adjustment of the flow rate of oxytocin according to the intensity of uterine contractions. Under these circumstances oxytocin increases the probability of vaginal delivery without exposure to the risk of uterine rupture or fetal distress and associated epidural analgesia does not increase the risk of uterine rupture.[15–20] For reasons of effectiveness and safety, induction of labor may be considered in patients with a scarred uterus when cervical conditions are favorable (Bishop score).[17–21]

Should instrumental delivery be routine? If this is the first vaginal delivery, it is mandatory. For subsequent deliveries, the answer depends on the estimated fetal weight and progression of the presentation, bearing in mind that a previous delivery is certainly a favorable factor but that the scar may have become more vulnerable. Expulsive efforts must, therefore, be kept to a minimum.

Manual exploration of the uterus is justified if it is important to detect uterine rupture or dehiscence so that it may be sutured or to decide on cesarean delivery for future pregnancies. One may then base the decision on a follow-up hysterography. Palpation during manual verification of the uterus may make the scar more vulnerable and should therefore be gentle. Abdominal compression and uterine massage after delivery should be prohibited because this entails the risk of segmental rupture.

EPIDURAL ANALGESIA[14–19, 20]

Epidural analgesia was discredited in the past because it was thought to mask a potential uterine rupture; it is now used increasingly. All authors now agree that pain associated with rupture is not relieved by epidural analgesia. This pain is due to intraperitoneal hemorrhaging following uterine rupture causing peritoneal irritation. The peritoneum is supplied by sensitive fibers that course to T4. Only analgesia that ascends to T4 can be responsible for delayed diagnosis of uterine rupture (large diffusion, excessive concentrations of local anesthetics, combination with opioid derivatives).

In practice, epidural anesthesia must not go above T9. The concentration of local anesthetics must remain at or below 0.25% bupivacaine (continuous or intermittent doses). In our team, we contraindicate the opioids since the association with bupivacaine delays the diagnosis of the rupture (three cases). Temporary hypokinesis caused by the epidural is readily corrected by oxytocin and compensated by the cervical relaxation at induction. Such analgesia enables instrumental extractions and manual exploration of the uterus without requiring general anesthesia.

SPECIAL CASES

In order to further reduce the number of cesarean deliveries, one may sometimes decide to test the uterine scar on a twice-operated uterus, in the event of breech presentation or a macrosomic fetus. This must be specifically requested by the patient and requires a perfect cephalopelvic comparison with a large pelvis (promonto-retropubic diameter + useful transverse > 24 cm) and perfect dynamics with close monitoring.

CONCLUSIONS

Vaginal delivery with scarred uterus is often accepted with the patient agreement, because maternal and fetal morbidity has improved.

The use of oxytocin does not increase the risk of uterine rupture. The use of epidural analgesia is now accepted by numerous teams without deleterious effects.

REFERENCES

1. Palaric J C, Berger O, Giraud J R 1989 Conduite obstétricale en présence d'un utérus cicatriciel. In: Puech (ed) 19e journées nationales de médecine périnatale. Arnette, Paris, p 167–174
2. Boulanger J C H 1984 Utérus cicatricle et accouchement. In: Tournaire (ed) Mises à jour en gynécologie obstétrique. Vigot, Paris p 203–235
3. Delarue T, Pele P 1981 Prévention des ruptures et pré-ruptures des utérus antérieurement césarisés. J Gyn Obstet Biol Rep 10: 259–267
4. Boisselier P H, Maghioracos P, Marpeau L 1987 Evolution dans les indications de césariennes de 1977 à 1983 à propos de 18.605 accouchements. J Gynécol Obstet Biol Reprod 16: 251–260
5. Barrat J, Maria B 1985 Les utérus cicatriciels In: Vokaer R (ed) Traité d'Obstétrique Tome II Masson, Paris, p 275–285
6. Michaels W H 1988 Ultrasound diagnosis of defects in the scarred lower uterine segment during pregnancy. Obstet Gynecol 72: 144–146
7. Delarue T, Maheo A, Souplet J P 1988 Indications et contre-indications de l'anesthésie péridurale en obstétrique. Rev Fr Gynecol Obstet 83: 427–437
8. Picaud A, Nlomenze A R, Ogowet N 1990 L'accouchement des utérus cicatriciels. A propos de 606 cas pour 62193 accouchements. Rev Fr Gynécol Obstet 85: 387–392
9. Picaud A, Nlomenze A R, Ogowet N 1989 Les ruptures utérines. A propos de 31 cas observés au Centre Hospitalier de Libreville. Rev Fr Gynécol Obstet 84: 411–416
10. Mintz P, Herlicoviez M, Tilliard J P 1987 Utérus cicatriciel et déhiscence utérine. A propos de 20 observations. Rev Fr Gynécol Obstet 87: 97–105
11. Pruett K, Kirshan B, Cotton D B 1988 Unknown uterine scar and trial of labor. Am J Obstet Gynecol 159: 807–810
12. Silver R, Gibbs R 1987 Predictors of vaginal delivery in patients with a previous cesarean section who require oxytocin. Am J Obstet Gynecol 156: 57–60
13. Laot T, Leung BF 1987 Rupture of the gravid uterus. Eur J Obstet Gynecol Reprod Biol 25: 175–180
14. Rudigoz R C, Chardon C 1990 Césariennes en 1988. Problémes obstétricaux posés par les utérus cicatriciels. Rev Fr Gynécol Obstet 85: 105–108
15. Flamm B L, Funett C, Fishermann E 1984 Vaginal delivery following Cesarean section: use of oxytocin augmentation and epidural anesthesia with internal tocodynamic and internal fetal monitoring. Am J Obstet Gynecol 48: 759–763
16. Camus M, Ropert J F, Planchais O Déclenchement du travail sur uterus cicatriciel. J Gynecol Obstet Biol Reprod 21: 89–102
17. Canis M, Schoeffler P, Monteillard C 1985 Accouchement après césarienne. Utilisation de l'anesthésie péridurale et des ocytociques. A propos de 87 cas. Rev Fr Gynecol Obstet 80: 49–53
18. Stovall T, Shaver D C, Facog 1987 Trial of labor in previous cesarean section patients, excluding classical Cesarean section. Obstet Gynecol 70: 713–717
19. Flamm B, Newman L, Thomas S 1990 Vaginal birth after Cesarean delivery: results of a 5 year multicenter collaborative study. Obstet Gynecol 76: 750–754
20. Camus M, Lefebvre G, Scebacher J 1989 Utérus cicatriciel. Accouchement par voie basse sous analgésie péridurale. J Gynecol Obstet Biol Reprod 18: 379–387
21. Crawford J S 1976 The epidural sieve and minimal blocking concentration, a hypothesis. Anaesthesia 31: 1278–1285
22. Rosen M G, Dickinson J C 1990 Vaginal birth after Cesarean. An analysis of indicators for success. Obstet Gynecol 76: 865–869

The text and tables of this section are reproduced with modification from Regional Anesthesia 15: 304, 1990, with permission.

92. Anesthetic considerations for parturients with herpes simplex and chorioamnionitis

B. L. Loferski

HERPES SIMPLEX VIRUS TYPE II

Over the past decade, the incidence and prevalence of infection with genital herpes simplex virus (HSV) has dramatically increased, especially in the reproductive age group.[1] The herpes simplex virus causes a chronically recurring disease process that is characterized by asymptomatic periods interspersed with episodes of viral reactivation from its latent phase in sensory ganglia and post-ganglionic nerve fibers. Approximately 1% of obstetric patients have a history of HSV infection. Many controversies and concerns surround the anesthetic care of the parturient with HSV.

The virus

The herpesviruses are double-stranded DNA viruses and include cytomegalovirus, Epstein–Barr virus, varicella-zoster virus and the herpes simplex virus. Two different subtypes of viruses, HSV-I and HSV-II, are responsible for genital herpes infection. The HSV-II subtype leads to 93% of primary infection and 98% of recurrent infections. The remainder of the infections are caused by HSV-I.

The disease

Primary maternal HSV infections are associated with viremia, and symptoms include fever, headache and lymphadenopathy. Approximately 8% of these patients have aseptic meningitis.[2] During the first 20 weeks of gestation, there is an associated increase in frequency of stillbirths, spontaneous abortions and congenital malformations.[3] Transplacental transmission may occur during the primary infection.

Recurrent episodes, on the other hand, are manifested by localized outbreaks and, since viremia is absent, the occurrence of systemic symptoms and meningitis is rare. Viral shedding in the birth canal, however, can occur for up to 2 weeks after healing of the lesion. Asymptomatic shedding can also occur.[4] Of women with a confirmed history of recurrent infection, 1.4% will have virus in the lower genital tract at the time of labor.[5]

Neonatal infection

The incidence of HSV infection in the neonate is estimated to be between 1 : 2500 and 1 : 10 000 deliveries per year.[3] The consequences of this infection can be heartbreaking. The virus is usually transmitted to the neonate during delivery by passage through an infected maternal genital tract. Ascending infection, especially with prolonged rupture of membranes, or transplacental virus transmission can occur.

Clinical evidence of infection is usually present between 5 and 17 days of life. It can be limited to the skin, eyes and mouth, or it can affect the central nervous system and visceral organs to cause hepatitis, pneumonitis, disseminated intravascular coagulopathy and encephalitis.[6] Death can occur in up to 50% of infants with disseminated disease, even with antiviral therapy.

Women with active genital lesions or positive cultures at term are advised to avoid neonatal exposure by undergoing cesarean delivery.

Anesthesia

The use of regional anesthesia in obstetric patients with HSV infections is a controversial topic. Two major issues arise. The first issue centers around the possibility of introducing the virus into the central nervous system during the placement of a subarachnoid or epidural anesthetic, resulting in meninigitis or encephalitis, especially during the primary infection when viremia is present. Second, if post-operative headache or neurologic sequelae occur, it may be difficult to exclude the regional anesthetic from the differential diagnosis in a patient with HSV infection.

The literature on this topic has been limited to date. Ravindran et al, in 1982,[7] reported a study in which 30 patients with HSV infection who received epidural anesthesia had no complications related to anesthesia.[7] The authors, however, did not indicate if any patient had a primary infection.

In 1986, Ramanathan et al[8] reported a retrospective series of patients with recurrent genital herpes infection who underwent cesarean delivery. None of the patients who received general (28 patients) or epidural (48 patients) anesthesia developed any neurologic or anesthetic complications. Indeed, 75% of patients who received epidural anesthesia had lesions at the time of delivery. Crosby et al,[9] in 1989, presented the results of a 6-year retrospective analysis of 89 patients with active recurrent HSV infections who received epidural anesthesia and had no septic or neurologic complications related to anesthesia.

Most recently, Bader et al[10] performed a 6-year retrospective study of the anesthetics of 169 patients who underwent cesarean delivery because of both primary and recurrent HSV infection (awaiting publication). None of the 164 patients with recurrent infection had anesthetic-related complications with either subarachnoid or epidural anesthesia. Of the five patients with no previous history of HSV infection, three received spinal anesthesia and two received general anesthesia. The only post-operative complication was a transient leg weakness, which spontaneously resolved in a patient with the diagnosis of primary HSV infection who received a spinal anesthetic.

These studies demonstrate that both subarachnoid and epidural anesthetics are safe choices for a parturient with recurrent HSV infection. The safety of regional anesthesia for parturients with primary infection remains unclear.

CHORIOAMNIONITIS

Chorioamnionitis is present in approximately 1% of all parturients and is one of the most common infectious processes to occur in the pregnant woman.[11] It is usually accompanied by fever, chills, elevated white cell count and fetal tachycardia, and is a frequent cause of both maternal and fetal sepsis as well as congenital pneumonia. Both aerobic and anaerobic bacteria found in the lower genital tract may be responsible for chorioamnionitis. The most common organisms are group B streptococci and *Escherichia coli*.[12]

The complex mechanism of this process includes direct placental transport of maternal blood-borne infectious agents to the fetus and amniotic fluid as well as ascending infection through ruptured membranes into the intrauterine cavity. Amniotic fluid generally protects against infection with specific antibacterial substances, including lysozymes and immunoglobulins. Rupture of the amniotic membrane has a potential to lead to infection, especially with prolonged duration. Delivery of the fetus is the only definitive cure.

Anesthesia

Although epidural anesthesia is desired by many pregnant women, it may be denied by the anesthesiologist to the febrile patient for fear of seeding bacteria into the epidural or subarachnoid space. To date, no clear relationship has been demonstrated between the febrile parturient and the possibility of bacteremia. Blanco et al, in 1981[11], reported the frequency of bacteremia in febrile pregnant women as 9%. Therefore, approximately 90% of these patients had negative cultures. In another study, these investigators reported that there is an 8% prevalence of bacteremia in chorioamnionitis and that approximately half of these patients with positive blood cultures were not febrile.[13] Absence of fever does not mean absence of bacteremia.

There have been no reports of epidural abscess or meningitis following regional anesthesia in patients with chorioamnionitis. A recent retrospective study by Vaddadi et al[14] assessed the use of epidural anesthesia in parturients with chorioamnionitis. Of the 115 patients who received regional anesthesia, none developed signs or symptoms of epidural abscess or meningitis. The authors did not include blood cultures in their study, so the incidence of actual bacteremia was not available.

Recently, Carp and Bailey[15] attempted to further delineate the relationship between bacteremia and the risk of developing meningitis after dural puncture. 40 chronically bacteremic rats were studied 24 h after undergoing cisternal puncture. Bacteremic rats after cisternal puncture showed evidence of central nervous system infection, whereas bacteremic animals not having cisternal puncture had sterile spinal fluid. In addition, in the absence of bacteremia, the cisternal puncture did not result in infection. While this study suggests the possibility that bacteremia is a risk factor in developing meningitis, the extrapolation to humans undergoing intraspinal anesthesia is not clear.

REFERENCES

1. Brown Z A, Berry S, Vontver L A 1986 Genital herpes simplex virus infections complicating pregnancy. J Reprod Med 31: 440
2. Corey L, Adams H G, Brown Z A et al 1983 Genital herpes simplex virus infections: clinical manifestations, course and complications. Ann Intern Med 98: 958
3. Stagno S, Whitley R J 1985 Herpes virus infections in pregnancy. New Engl J Med 313: 1327
4. Brock B, Selke S, Benedetti J et al 1990 Frequency of asymptomatic shedding of herpes simplex virus in women with genital herpes. J Am Med Assoc 203: 418
5. Arvin A, Hensleigh P A, Prober C G et al 1986 Failure of antepartum maternal cultures to predict the infants risk of exposure to herpes simplex virus at delivery. New Engl J Med 315: 796
6. Kibrick S 1980 Herpes simplex infection at term. What to do with mother, newborn, and nursery personnel. J Am Med Assoc 243: 157

7. Ravindran R S, Gupta C D, Stoops C A 1982 Epidural analgesia in the presence of patients with herpes simplex virus (type 2) infection. Anesth Analg 62: 714
8. Ramanathan S, Sheth R, Turndorf H 1986 Anesthesia for cesarean section in patients with genital herpes infection: a retrospective study. Anesthesiology 64: 807
9. Crosby E T, Halpern S H, Rolbin S H 1989 Epidural anesthesia for cesarean section in patients with active recurrent genital herpes simplex infections: a retrospective review. Can J Anesth 36: 701
10. Bader A M, Camann W R, Datta S 1990 Anesthesia for cesarean section in patients with herpes simplex virus type 2 infections. Reg Anesth 15: 261
11. Blanco J D, Gibbs R S, Castaneda Y S 1981 Bacteremia in obstetrics: Clinical course. Obstet Gynecol 58: 621
12. Schnider S, Levinson G 1987 Anesthesia for obstetrics, 2nd edn. Williams & Wilkins, Baltimore
13. Gibbs R S, Castillo M S, Rodgers P J 1980 Management of acute chorioamnionitis. Am J Obstet Gynecol 136: 709
14. Vaddadi A, Ramanathan J, Angel J et al 1989 Epidural anesthesia in women with chorioamnionitis (a retrospective study). Anesthesiology 71 (suppl): A 863
15. Carp H, Bailey S 1989 Meningitis after dural puncture in bacteremic rats. Anesthesiology 71 (suppl): A 862

93. Effect of lumbar epidural anesthesia on the progress of labor and the incidence of operative deliveries

R. C. Chantigian   P. D. M. Chantigian

Epidural anesthesia is currently a common technique of pain relief used during labor. In 1981, Gibbs et al[1] surveyed approximately 1200 US hospitals about the type of analgesia used in obstetrics and found that 16% of women received epidural anesthesia during labor. The frequency of epidural anesthesia use depended on the size of the obstetric service. In hospitals reporting over 1500 births, the epidural rate was 22%; in hospitals with 500–1499 deliveries, the epidural rate was 13%; in hospitals with fewer than 500 deliveries, the rate was 9%. In 21% of the hospitals surveyed, epidural anesthesia for labor was not available.

In hospitals where epidural anesthesia is available, the frequency of epidural anesthesia administration is commonly between 20 and 80%. At the Mayo Clinic from 1986 to 1988, the epidural rate for all women who delivered (vaginal and cesarean) was 47% and for women who delivered vaginally was 43%.

With its widespread use, concern has been raised as to whether epidural anesthesia may lead to an increase in maternal and/or fetal morbidity or mortality. Several aspects must be considered in order to address this concern. Do the pharmacologic (direct drug effect) or physiologic effects (maternal blood pressure and uterine blood flow) of epidural anesthesia adversely affect the mother or fetus? Does the epidural anesthetic affect the mechanism of labor? Does the use of epidural anesthesia lead to more operative deliveries? If epidural anesthesia does affect labor or the mode of delivery, does this lead to an adverse maternal or fetal outcome?

This section reviews the available data as they relate to the effects of epidural anesthesia on the progress of labor and the incidence of operative deliveries. (Epidural anesthesia refers to epidural sensory analgesia provided by local anesthetics with or without opioids as well as sensory and motor anesthesia. Instrumental deliveries refer to vaginal deliveries in which obstetric forceps or vacuum extraction is employed, whereas operative deliveries include instrumental as well as cesarean deliveries.)

EFFECT OF LUMBAR EPIDURAL ANESTHESIA ON THE PROGRESS OF LABOR

The progress of labor is affected by several factors, including the frequency and strength of the uterine contractions, the size and position of the fetus, and the size and shape of the pelvis. Commonly, these are referred to as the 'three P's': power, passenger, and pelvis. *If* epidural (peridural) anesthesia has an effect, perhaps one could refer to the four P's: power, passenger, pelvis, and peridural.

Forces in labor

Two forces are involved in the progress of labor and both must be evaluated. The primary force is produced by the uterine muscle (involuntary) and the secondary force is produced by an increase in intra-abdominal pressure (voluntary).

The uterus is composed of smooth muscle and, like all smooth muscle, has the intrinsic capacity to contract and relax. This intrinsic activity may be modified by many factors. Estrogen, oxytocin, α-adrenergic drugs, prostaglandins and mechanical manipulation of the cervix (e.g. by digitally stripping the membranes from the lower uterine segment or by the insertion of internal fetal monitors) stimulate uterine contractions. Progesterone, magnesium sulfate, calcium channel blockers (e.g. nifedipine), prostaglandin synthetase inhibitors (e.g. indomethacin), alcohol, aminophylline and β-adrenergic drugs inhibit uterine contractions. In addition, a decrease in uterine blood flow that may occur with hypotension can decrease uterine contractions. This primary force is important in both the first and second stages of labor.

Intra-abdominal pressure can be increased by two sets of muscles, the abdominal wall muscles and the diaphragm. This secondary force is important during the second stage of labor.

First stage of labor

Effects of epidural anesthesia on uterine contractions

In 1961, Vasicka and Kretchmer[2] looked at the effects of regional anesthesia (23 subarachnoid anesthetics and 12 lidocaine epidural anesthetics) on uterine contractions. In the absence of hypotension, regional anesthesia did not interfere with uterine contractions. In some patients, the intensity of the contractions decreased about 10–20 mmHg for up to 30 min, then the intensity of the contractions resumed to preanesthetic levels. One patient developed hypotension, which was associated with a marked drop in uterine activity. They noted no inhibition of the effects of exogenously administered oxytocin. Whether this temporary inhibition of uterine contractility was an effect of the epidural anesthesia or the effect of the fluid bolus given at the start of epidural anesthesia is unclear.

In 1970, Sala et al[3] saw no changes in spontaneous uterine contractions (Montevideo units) in five women in spontaneous labor when epidural anesthesia (lidocaine without epinephrine) was started. These women had previously received meperidine, promazine and promethazine intravenously for analgesia. In addition, they did not see any changes in uterine contractions in the same women when artificial cervical dilation was performed after the epidural anesthesia had been established.

In 1976, Raabe and Belfrage[4] noted a decrease in uterine contraction pressure but not frequency after the administration of epidural anesthesia using bupivacaine with epinephrine. The depression in pressures lasted about 30 min, and then the pressures resumed to preanesthetic levels.

Also in 1976, Matadial and Cibils[5] noted no significant changes in uterine activity when 1.0–1.5% lidocaine without epinephrine was administered epidurally (activity increased in 14 cases, decreased in 16 cases). However, when 1.0–1.5% lidocaine with epinephrine was used, a decrease in uterine activity was noted (activity increased in 12 cases, decreased in 39 cases). The decrease in activity was a decrease in pressure generated with no decrease in the frequency of the contractions.

In 1977, Schellenberg[6] failed to show a decrease in uterine activity with epidural 0.25–0.5% bupivacaine without epinephrine. He stressed the avoidance of aortocaval compression during labor when evaluating the effect of an epidural anesthetic on uterine activity; this was not consistently done in previous studies.

In 1977, Jouppila et al[7] saw a mild increase in uterine activity when 0.5% bupivacaine was administered; when 0.5% bupivacaine with 1 : 200 000 epinephrine was administered, a mild fall in uterine activity was seen. All patients had left uterine displacement to avoid aortocaval compression. Although these changes were not significant when comparing the uterine activity before and after epidural administration within each group, the change in uterine activity between the two groups (bupivacaine without and bupivacaine with epinephrine) was significant. Clinically, this was reflected in longer induction-to-delivery times in the epinephrine group. They recommended avoiding the addition of epinephrine to the local anesthetic solutions used for epidural anesthesia during labor since it decreases uterine activity.

In several studies, Abboud et al[8–10] failed to see any significant changes in uterine activity after establishing epidural anesthesia with bupivacaine, lidocaine or chloroprocaine without epinephrine,[8] lidocaine with epinephrine[9] or bupivacaine with epinephrine.[10]

Clinical studies on the duration of the first stage of labor (see Table 93.1)

In 1972, Crawford[11] reported shorter first stages of labor in multiparous women compared with primiparous women. This observation held true when spontaneous labors were compared with induced labors. He also

Table 93.1 Mean duration of the first stage of labor (hours)

	Primipara		Multipara	
	Epidural	No epidural	Epidural	No epidural
Crawford[11]				
Spontaneous labor	8.7	8.9	6.4	5.7
Induced labor	10.3	12.1	7.1	6.5
Joupilla et al[12]				
Entire first stage	9.6	7.8	5.3	5.0
IDI*	3.5	3.7	2.1	2.3
Robinson et al[13]	8.2	8.3	6.0	6.4
Studd et al[14]				
Spontaneous labor	8.4	5.7	5.2	3.5
Augmented labor	12.4	11.9	9.2	10.0

* The IDI is the time interval from the induction of epidural anesthesia to delivery. For women without epidural anesthesia, an equivalent time from similar cervical dilation was used.

demonstrated slightly shorter duration of the first stage of labor in primiparous women and a slightly longer duration of the first stage of labor in the multiparous women who received epidural anesthesia compared with those who did not. The local anesthetic was bupivacaine.

In 1979, Jouppila et al[12] reported poor progress of labor prior to establishing epidural anesthesia in women who elected to have epidural anesthesia when compared with a control group. After the block was established, the subsequent course of labor was similar. This suggests that women with longer latent phases of labor are more likely to receive epidural anesthesia.

In 1980, Robinson et al[13] reported similar durations of the first stage of labor for primiparous and multiparous women in their epidural group when compared respectively with primiparous and multiparous women in the control group. Women in the control group received meperidine and perphenazine intramuscularly and/or inhalation analgesia (50% nitrous oxide or 0.35% methoxyflurane in oxygen).

In 1980, Studd et al[14] noted that epidural anesthesia did not affect the rate of cervical dilation in women with spontaneous labors or with labors augmented with oxytocin. However, the overall duration of the first stage of labor was longer in women who received epidural anesthesia compared with the control group. This may be explained by the fact that women who later received epidural anesthesia had less cervical dilation on admission (2.7 cm for primiparas and 3.3 cm for multiparas) than women in the control group (3.8 cm for primiparas and 4.6 cm for multiparas). In women with augmented labors, the duration of labor was similar in the epidural and control groups.

Second stage of labor

Effects of epidural anesthesia on voluntary expulsive forces

In 1972, Johnson et al[15] looked at the effects of regional anesthesia on the intrauterine pressure developed during the second stage of labor. They found an increase in voluntary or 'pushing' effort (pressure produced above the peak of a uterine contraction) as the second stage of labor progressed in women with no or local anesthesia. Women who received pudendal nerve blocks pushed better after the block was established. With epidural anesthesia (1% lidocaine), a slight decrease in voluntary effort was noted overall (46 mmHg produced after the block compared with 55 mmHg before the block). A closer look demonstrated that one-third of patients pushed better after the epidural was started, and two-thirds pushed less effectively. When looking at the voluntary effort and the level of anesthesia produced, two-thirds of patients with an anesthetic level of T10 or lower pushed better, whereas all patients pushed less effectively when the level was T9 or higher.

Clinical studies on the duration of the second stage of labor (see Table 93.2)

In 1972, Crawford[11] reported longer durations of the second stage in primiparous women compared with multiparous women, and in women who received epidural anesthesia (0.25 and/or 0.5% bupivacaine) compared with those who did not. Because of the longer second stage of labor seen with epidural anesthesia, more instrumental deliveries were performed for a diagnosis of failure to progress or prolonged second stage.

In 1979, Bleyaert et al[16] achieved short second stages with 0.125% bupivacaine with 1 : 800 000 epinephrine in 3000 women (1496 primiparas and 1504 multiparas). The second stage lasted 21 min for primiparous and 14 min for multiparous women. Note that 61% of the primiparous and 27% of the multiparous women had instrumental deliveries.

In 1979, Jouppila et al[12] looked at the duration of the second stage in women with or without epidural anesthesia in a prospective, nonrandomized study of 200 women (77 primiparas and 23 multiparas in the epidural group, and 77 primiparas and 23 multiparas in the control group). They used a low-dose epidural technique

Table 93.2 Mean duration of the second stage of labor (min)

	Primiparas		Multiparas	
	Epidural	No epidural	Epidural	No epidural
Crawford[11]				
Spontaneous labor	58	46	39	19
Induced labor	59	47	37	20
Bleyaert et al[16]	21		14	
Joupilla et al[12]	17	15	7	8
Robinson et al[13]	54	42	30	18
Studd et[14]				
Spontaneous labor	64	44	46	18
Augmented labor	58	46	33	20

consisting of 4 ml of 0.5% bupivacaine per dose repeated as needed. In the control group, meperidine (50–150 mg) was administered intramuscularly for first-stage analgesia in 58% of the primiparous and in 30% of the multiparous women. They did not find a significant difference in the duration of the second stage in women with or without epidural anesthesia.

In 1980, Robinson et al[13] found a significant increase in the duration of the second stage of labor in patients receiving epidural anesthesia (0.5% bupivacaine) compared with their control group (meperidine with perphenazine and/or inhalation analgesia consisting of nitrous oxide or methoxyflurane).

In 1980, Studd et al[14] also found a significant increase in the duration of the second stage of labor in women who had epidural anesthesia compared to those without. They observed this in women with spontaneous labors as well as in women whose labors were augmented with oxytocin.

Clinical studies on the duration of the second stage of labor

How long should the second stage be? The first time limit placed on the duration of the second stage was made in 1817 by Denman.[17] 'The use of forceps is not indicated until the second stage of labor has lasted six hours and all other means of delivery have been tried.' In 1861, Hamilton recommended a shorter duration of the second stage: 2 h.[17]

In 1952, Hellman and Prystowsky[17] looked at 13 377 deliveries performed for the years 1937–49. For primiparous women, 40% delivered spontaneously and 60% by forceps. For multiparous women 80% delivered spontaneously and 20% by forceps. Overall, 77% delivered within 1 h and 92% delivered within 2 h. An increase in fetal mortality was noted when the second stage of labor was greater than 150 min. They also noted an increase in maternal post-partum hemorrhage and puerperal febrile reactions when the second stage of labor was longer than 150 min.

In 1974, Pearson and Davies,[18] looked at fetal acid–base values during the second stage of labor in a control group of 13 patients who received meperidine and/or promazine, and in two epidural groups, one group of eight women who pushed and a group of seven women who did not push during the second stage. They noted progressive fetal acidosis in all three groups. The fall in pH was fastest in the control group, less in the epidural group who pushed and the least in the epidural group whose mothers did not push. All women labored in the supine position.

In 1977, Cohen[19] looked at 4403 nulliparous women to determine the effects of the duration of the second stage of labor on neonatal outcome and maternal morbidity. He noted no increase in perinatal mortality or poor 5-min Apgar scores with a progressive lengthening of the second stage. A significant increase in post-partum hemorrhage was noted after a second stage of 3 h. This was thought to be related to the increase in mid-forceps and cesarean deliveries that were performed. If only normal spontaneous vaginal deliveries and low forceps were reviewed, no increase in hemorrhage was seen. He concluded: 'It would thus appear that the elective termination of labor simply because an arbitrary period of time has elapsed in the second stage is clearly not warranted.'

In 1983, Maresh and Choong[20] compared women who pushed early in the second stage with women who pushed late in the second stage. (A top-up dose of local anesthetic was administered if they had the urge to push early in the second stage.) The top-up dose delayed the start of pushing by a mean of 96 min. In both groups, the women pushed for an average of 50 min. In the early pushing group, the spontaneous delivery rate was 35%, whereas in the late pushing group the spontaneous delivery rate was 50%. There was no increase in abnormal fetal heart rate abnormalities and there was no decrease in umbilical cord pH or Apgar scores.

In 1990, Moon et al[21] noted that neonates born after a prolonged second stage (at least 2 h) did not have an increase in newborn acidosis (umbilical artery pH less than 7.20) or low 5-min Apgar scores (< 7), nor did they need neonatal intensive care unit admission more often when compared with neonates born after a normal second stage (less than 2 h).

The American College of Obstetrics and Gynecology (ACOG)[22] recently revised the guideline for the approximate duration of the second stage of labor. For the nulliparous woman, the diagnosis of a prolonged second stage is made when more than 3 h with a regional anesthetic or more than 2 h without a regional anesthetic has elapsed. For the parous women, more than 2 h with a regional anesthetic or more than 1 h without a regional anesthetic is considered a prolonged second stage.

Although a time limit can be a helpful guideline, it remains that: a guideline. With the current technology available for monitoring the fetus and the mother, assessment on a case-by-case basis can allow continuation of the second stage unless intervention is indicated.

Conclusions

There is a wide variation in the reported duration of the first and second stages of labor. The optimal duration of the second stage of labor is still controversial. However, in most of the studies describing the duration of the second stage, neonates have been delivered well within the current ACOG guidelines.

In the very early stages of labor (latent phase), any analgesic may slow labor; confounding conclusions could be drawn regarding the length of the first stage if studies include patients who have received epidural anesthesia in the latent phase. Most recent studies reviewing the effects of epidural anesthesia on the duration of the first stage of labor or the rate of cervical dilation look primarily at the active phase of the first stage of labor.

Epidural anesthesia appears to have little effect on the rate of cervical dilation or the duration of the first stage of labor (active phase). If hypotension is avoided, epidural anesthesia has minimal effect on uterine contractions. In several studies, a short-term (< 30 to 60 min) and probably insignificant depression in uterine intensity develops mainly when epinephrine-containing local anesthetics are used. Perhaps a slight β-adrenergic effect of absorbed epinephrine causes this observed decrease. After 30 min, uterine activity returns to normal.

The second stage of labor may be prolonged in women who have epidural anesthesia compared with women who do not receive epidural anesthesia. Several reasons for the longer second stage of labor in women who receive epidural anesthesia have been suggested, including loss of the bearing-down reflex (urge to push) and the generation of lower intra-abdominal pressures with expulsive efforts (too weak to push, too exhausted from a long labor to push). How the patient is managed may have an effect on the duration of the second stage. The level and density of anesthesia can be adjusted to allow more sensation and better expulsive efforts. Appropriate coaching on the timing, direction and duration of the 'pushing' efforts is important.

EFFECT ON THE INCIDENCE OF OPERATIVE DELIVERIES

Controversy abounds regarding the question 'Does epidural anesthesia given during labor have an effect on the incidence of operative deliveries (forceps deliveries, vacuum extractions or cesarean deliveries)?'

This section reviews the concerns surrounding the performance of operative deliveries, the studies that look at the association of epidural anesthesia with the frequency of operative deliveries, observations that support as well as observations that oppose the view that epidural anesthesia increases the incidence of operative deliveries, factors associated with the performance of operative deliveries and ways to achieve a low incidence of operative deliveries.

Concerns about operative deliveries

Cesarean delivery

Cesarean delivery has been associated with a two- to fourfold increase in maternal mortality when compared with vaginal deliveries.[23–25] The incidence of maternal mortality for women undergoing cesarean delivery ranges from 1 per 2500[26] to none reported in 10 231 consecutive deliveries.[27] Approximately half of the maternal deaths associated with cesarean delivery are attributed to the operative procedure and the rest attributed to the obstetric complications leading to the cesarean delivery.[23]

Cesarean delivery has a greater frequency of maternal morbidity than vaginal delivery. The incidence ranges from 10 to 80%! In 1981, Amirikia et al[28] reviewed 9718 patients who underwent cesarean delivery. They reported a maternal morbidity of 28% with endometritis, urinary tract infection, anemia, wound infections and fever being the five most common etiologies. In 1976, Jones[29] reported an overall maternal morbidity of 49%, with significant morbidity in 12% of 2563 patients undergoing cesarean delivery.

Though infrequent, neonatal complications due to cesarean delivery can occur. These include traumatic delivery, blood loss (e.g. cutting through the placenta) and iatrogenic prematurity.[23]

Instrumental deliveries

Over the course of the past several decades, the trends and theories behind the use of forceps, and later vacuum extractors, have varied. Initially, they were instruments of last resort, used to achieve delivery when all other means had been exhausted. Later, maternal exhaustion and a prolonged second stage (⩾ 2 h) became indications for intervention.

In 1920, DeLee[30] promoted the concept of 'prophylactic forceps operations' to shorten painful labors, to help preserve the integrity of the birth canal and to decrease the stress of labor and delivery on the fetus. Since that time, concerns about the safety of forceps deliveries have led to several conflicting reports.[31–36]

In 1973, Niswander and Gordon[34] reviewed the neonatal outcome in a collaborative project of nearly 30 000 neonates. They looked at several neonatal factors, including the neonatal death rate, 1- and 5-min Apgar scores, Bayley Scales of Mental and Motor Development at 8 months of age and the Stanford–Binet Intelligence Quotient at 4 years of age. They found the 'prophylactic forceps operation' to be a safe method of delivery. It did not increase the chance of neonatal death or neurologic impairment of the neonate: 'Whether the operation is 'protective' to the infant is less certain, although the data suggest this possibility.'[34]

In 1983, Richardson et al[36] did an extensive review of the literature concerning the safety of mid-forceps delivery. They believed that 'the bulk of evidence suggests that it [mid-forceps] can be a useful and safe tool in the armamentarium of the obstetrician, *when properly indicated and skillfully applied.*'

In 1984, Friedman et al[32] looked at the effects of mid-forceps and low-forceps deliveries on 7-year intelligence quotient data (Stanford–Binet Intelligence Scale) with matched controls. Outcome for low-forceps cases was similar to that for the controls. However, mid-forceps delivery cases were associated with nearly a six-point reduction in scores compared with the control cases. They concluded, 'unless one can provide justification in the form of documentable benefit on a case-by-case basis to counterbalance the potential risk, midforceps procedures should no longer be done.'

In 1984, Gilstrap et al[33] studied 704 women who underwent forceps delivery compared with 303 spontaneous vaginal deliveries and 111 cesarean deliveries. No significant differences in acidosis were seen in infants delivered by low forceps, mid-forceps or cesarean delivery when performed for similar reasons. Significantly more neonates delivered by cesarean delivery had Apgar scores ≤6 at 1 and 5 min. Infants delivered spontaneously compared with those delivered by low forceps had no significant difference in acidosis or low Apgar scores. Vaginal wall lacerations and lower post-delivery hematocrits were more common with mid-forceps than low-forceps delivery.

In 1986, Dierker et al[31] compared neurologic outcome of 110 infants delivered by mid-forceps with a matched group of 110 infants delivered by cesarean delivery at 2 years of age or older unless death occurred earlier. Their match included the indication for operative delivery (dystocia or fetal distress), something not consistently done in previous studies, as well as birthweight, gestational age, sex and race. They found no difference in abnormal neurologic outcomes between the two groups.

Even in the absence of physical morbidity to the mother or neonate, emotional and psychological trauma in the mother can occur. As stated by Morgan et al[37], 'The mother's satisfaction with her experience of childbirth is lessened in forceps delivery even when it is not traumatic'.

Outlet and low-forceps deliveries as well as vacuum deliveries are considered by most to be relatively safe modes of delivery. Although the safety of mid-forceps deliveries is controversial, most studies[31,33,36] support the judicious use of mid-forceps deliveries in select circumstances by skilled operators.

Epidural anesthesia and operative deliveries

When one looks at studies (Tables 93.3 and 93.4) that report the incidence of operative deliveries in women with and without epidural anesthesia, three trends are noted.

First, there is a large difference between studies in the incidence of operative deliveries in women who have received epidural anesthesia (6–93%).

Second, in most studies, women who received epidural anesthesia have about a 2–10 times greater frequency of

Table 93.3 Frequency of operative deliveries (%): retrospective and prospective nonrandomized studies

	Primipara		Multipara		All	
Reference	Epidural	No epidural	Epidural	No epidural	Epidural	No epidural
			Vaginal and cesarean deliveries			
38					93	
39					91	
40					90	
41	75		40		70	
42					68	
43					65	
44					58	14
45	70		27		55	
14	64	23	32	7	53	14
46	48		16		44	
47					33	
8					31	
48					19	15
49					19	
50	22		7		17	
51	15		6		12	
7					11	
			Vaginal deliveries only			
52					65	
53	71	22	42	6	58	11
54	52	23	43	7	50	20
37	55		35		47	
16	61		27		44	
55	52	14	26	2	43	6
56	51	42	17	16	33	26
57	18				18	
12	8	3	0	0	6	2

Table 93.4 Frequency of operative deliveries (%): prospective randomized studies

Reference	Primipara		Multipara		All	
	Epidural	No epidural	Epidural	No epidural	Epidural	No epidural
			Vaginal and cesarean deliveries			
13	61	27	30	6	49	19
58					42	37
59					31	9

operative deliveries than women who deliver without epidural anesthesia.

Third, primiparous women have a higher frequency of operative deliveries than multiparous women in both the epidural groups and in the control groups. This is important since more primiparous women receive epidural anesthesia than multiparous women, making studies that do not differentiate the primiparous from the multiparous patients more difficult to interpret.

Does epidural anesthesia directly cause an increase in operative deliveries? Are there other factors that result in operative deliveries that are also associated with an increased use of epidural anesthesia? If so, this may lead to the erroneous conclusion that it is the epidural anesthetic causing the increased rate of operative delivery.

Observations supporting the view that epidural anesthesia increases the incidence of operative deliveries

Many women who have epidural anesthesia do not push effectively. This may be due to the inability to feel the contractions, the loss of the urge to 'push' or the bearing-down reflex, or not knowing when, how long or in what direction to focus the 'pushing efforts'. Some women are too weak to push (muscle weakness from the local anesthetic) or are too exhausted to push. These factors can lead to a prolonged second stage, which may be considered an indication for an instrumental or operative delivery.

Patients with epidural anesthesia are comfortable and have better perineal and pelvic relaxation; they will tolerate an operative delivery better than patients without such anesthesia. Instrumental deliveries are then easier to perform or to teach, and may increase the likelihood of an instrumental delivery.

Epidural anesthesia may increase the frequency of fetal malpresentations (e.g. occiput posterior) because of relaxation of the muscles of the pelvic sling.

Hoult et al[53] in a prospective nonrandomized study reported a more than threefold increase in fetal malpresentations in women who received mainly 0.5% bupivacaine epidural anesthesia (21%) compared with a control group (6%). The incidence of malpresentations was not affected by the timing of induction of anesthesia (less than or greater than 4 cm cervical dilation).

Kaminski et al[54] reported a 27% incidence of occiput posterior (OP) presentation in the epidural group and 8 % in the control group. Raabe et al[46] reported a 9% incidence of OP presentation in the epidural group. Their control group had a 3% incidence of OP presentations. Both groups of investigators thought that the increase in OP presentations in the epidural group could be related to either (1) pelvic floor relaxation or (2) selection bias (e.g. more patients with OP presentations request epidural anesthesia because of more painful and longer labors).

Studd et al[14] reported a 20-fold increase in rotational forceps deliveries, but no increase in cesarean delivery in women who received epidural anesthesia compared with their control group.

This increase in malpresentation was not seen in the studies by Jouppila et al[12] or by Maltau and Anderson[50] and Matouskova et al[48] who advocated the use of lower doses of local anesthetics.

Some prospective randomized studies seem to indicate an increase in the incidence of instrumental deliveries in patients with epidural anesthesia.

In 1971, Noble et al[59] looked at the incidence of instrumental deliveries in women with and without epidural anesthesia. They initially had 245 patients in the study but deleted 43 patients (18%). Most of the deleted patients in the epidural group delivered before the epidural anesthetic could be performed, whereas most of the patients in the nonepidural group were deleted because inadequate analgesia was obtained, leading to the request for epidural anesthesia. In the remaining 202 patients (100 with epidurals, 102 controls), 30 forceps deliveries occurred in the epidural group and only six in the control group. There was also one cesarean delivery in the epidural group and three in the control group. Although they showed a higher incidence of operative deliveries in the epidural group, they noted better neonatal outcome in the epidural group as noted by the Apgar scores and the umbilical cord artery blood pH.

In 1980, Robinson et al[13] noted an increase in instrumental deliveries in their epidural group compared with their control group (meperidine and inhalation analgesia). This was significant only for the primiparous patients, in which the epidural group had twice the number of instrumental deliveries. They deleted a large number of patients because they did not complete the interview process, the clinical considerations dictated a deviation in analgesic plan or labor was too advanced when they were admitted.

Observations opposing the view that epidural anesthesia increases the incidence of operative deliveries

Some women experience severe pelvic and perineal pain and cannot push effectively. Establishing epidural anesthesia can allow the patient to push more effectively and shorten the second stage of labor.

The likelihood may be greater when an epidural anesthetic is placed in women who are having an abnormally prolonged and painful labor than in those who are experiencing a normal labor. In these cases, the epidural anesthetic will allow the mother to rest free of pain, allowing time for further progression of labor and culminating in a vaginal delivery. In these cases, an instrumental delivery may be implemented to end the long and exhausting labor, not because of a direct effect of the epidural anesthetic.[60–62]

Epidural anesthesia may be placed more often in women who are destined to have an operative delivery as a result of other factors, whether or not an epidural anesthetic is used. This theory may be looked at indirectly in two ways.

In 1969, Doughty[56] reported a decrease in the incidence of operative deliveries over a timespan of 13 years as the frequency of epidural anesthesia increased. They suspected that epidurals were initially placed in patients with difficult or abnormal labors, but as time continued epidurals were being placed in more women with normal labors. Note the trend of decreasing instrumental deliveries (100 to 24%) as the frequency of epidural anesthesia increased from 2 to 82% over the three time periods (1957 to 1962; 1963 to 1965; 1966 to 1969) (see Table 93.5).

In 1983, Bailey and Howard[63] looked at the effect of starting an epidural service on the incidence of operative deliveries. The first 2 years of their study were before epidural anesthesia was available and served as their control. The following 3 years were after epidural anesthesia was introduced. They reported a very small increase in the incidence of instrumental deliveries (14 to 15%) and cesarean deliveries (7 to 9%) despite a dramatic increase in the incidence of epidural anesthesia performed (0 to 43%) (see Table 93.6).

In 1983, Rudick et al[47] did a similar study over a 2-year period. They noted a slight increase in instrumental deliveries (9 to 11%) when the epidural anesthesia rate rose from 0.1 to 37%.

A prospective randomized study suggests no effect of epidural anesthesia on the incidence of instrumental deliveries.

In 1989, Philipsen and Jensen[58] compared epidural anesthesia with meperidine analgesia during labor. They found no significant difference between the groups with respect to the duration of the first stage or second stage of labor or the incidence of instrumental deliveries. Epidural analgesia did provide better pain relief than meperidine.

Table 93.5 Frequency of operative vaginal deliveries under epidural anesthesia over several years (From ref. 56 with permission)

	Instrumental deliveries (%)			
Years	Epidural*	Primiparas	Multiparas	All
1957–62	2	100	100	100
1963–65	37	87	56	75
1966–69	82	42	11	24
All years (1957–69)	52	51	17	33

* Percentage of all vaginal deliveries under epidural anesthesia.

Factors associated with the selection of operative deliveries

As mentioned previously, the trends in the use of forceps have varied over the past decades. In 1968, in a study by Duthie et al[38] the instrumental rate was 93% for vaginal deliveries; it would have been 100% but a few women requested delivery without forceps. As cesarean delivery has become safer, as the use of 'prophylactic forceps' has fallen out of favor and with the development of the silastic vacuum cup, forceps deliveries are currently performed less often.

In 1990, Notzon[35] looked at the rate of operative cesarean deliveries (21 countries) and operative vaginal deliveries (14 countries) for the years 1975–86. The cesarean deliveries varied from 7 to 32% and for operative vaginal deliveries, from 2 to 16%. For most countries that

Table 93.6 Frequency of obstetric deliveries (%) for 2 years before and 3 years after an epidural anesthesia service became established (From ref. 63 with permission)

	Before		After		
	1976	1977	1978	1979	1980
All patients					
NSVD	74	74	69	71	71
Instrumental	14	14	17	15	15
Cesarean	8	7	9	9	9
Epidural rate	—	—	27	37	43
Primiparas					
NSVD	63	63	54	56	58
Instrumental	24	24	29	28	27
Cesarean	7	8	11	9	10
Epidural rate	—	—	49	67	72
Multiparas					
NSVD	81	81	77	78	79
Instrumental	8	8	10	8	9
Cesarean	8	7	8	9	7
Epidural rate	—	—	14	21	26

NSVD, normal spontaneous vaginal delivery.
Note: Breech and twin deliveries were excluded.

reported both cesarean and operative vaginal rates, cesarean delivery rates rose as operative vaginal delivery rates fell.

Thus, studies done on the incidence of instrumental deliveries may be affected by the 'trend of the times'.

Some physicians tend to perform instrumental deliveries more often than others.[64] At the Mayo Clinic for the years 1987 and 1988, the incidence of instrumental vaginal deliveries was 15% for all deliveries. When uncomplicated primiparous patients who delivered vaginally at the Mayo Clinic were reviewed, the incidence of instrumental deliveries for women was 21% for the family physicians and 33% for the obstetricians. Furthermore, the incidence of instrumental deliveries for the obstetricians ranged from 20 to 74%! The training and skill of the individual may influence the frequency with which instruments will be used.

Unresolved fetal distress is an indication for prompt delivery. If the second stage of labor has been achieved and the fetal presentation is favorable, an instrumental vaginal delivery may be attempted.

In women with a prolonged second stage, ie ineffective pushing or 'maternal exhaustion' an instrumental delivery can end the long labor.

Although not commonly admitted, an instrumental delivery may be performed as a matter of convenience to shorten the stay of the physician at the obstetric suite.

Academic programs usually involve resident training. It is easier to teach proper instrument placement and maintain patient satisfaction when patients are comfortable (i.e. have epidural anesthesia).

Achieving a lower incidence of operative deliveries

1. Use operative deliveries only when obstetrically indicated and not when obstetrically convenient or for teaching purposes.
2. Allow the second stage to be longer. In many of the studies in this chapter a short second stage was decreased further by use of instruments. The ACOG guidelines[22] reflect a view allowing the second stage to be longer. (See the section on duration of the second stage.)
3. Adjust the epidural block to allow a greater chance for a spontaneous delivery.
   a. Decrease the density of the epidural block (by using a lower concentration and/or smaller volumes of local anesthetic) to allow mild sensation of contractions or perineal pressure. This may allow the parturient to retain the urge to push and may increase the efficacy of the expulsive efforts.

Crawford[11] noted that about 50% of patients who delivered spontaneously under epidural anesthesia lost the urge to push, whereas about 70% of patients who had instrumental deliveries lost the urge to push. He also noted that the concentration of bupivacaine made a difference. When 0.25% bupivacaine was used, 50% of women lost the urge to push, whereas 75% of women lost the urge to push when 0.5% bupivacaine was used.[45]

Thorburn and Moir[44] compared 0.5% bupivacaine (group A, 6–8 ml/dose) with 0.25% bupivacaine (group B, 10–14 ml/dose; group C, 6–8 ml/dose). They noted a higher frequency of spontaneous deliveries when a lower concentration or smaller volume was used; group A had 32%, group B had 39%, and group C had 53% spontaneous deliveries. They also noted less motor block and less sensory anesthesia in group C.

Some investigators use a low concentration of local anesthetics to retain the urge to push in the parturient, whereas others use a low volume of a high concentration (i.e. 0.5% bupivacaine), producing a more segmental block.[12,51]

Although the concentration of local anesthetic may be important, other factors such as total dose may also be important. Jouppila et al[12] achieved a 6% instrumental rate with 0.5% bupivacaine (4 ml/dose), whereas Bleyaert et al[16] had a 44% instrumental rate with 0.125% bupivacaine (10 ml/dose).

It has been suggested the epidural anesthetic should be turned off during the second stage so that the parturient can push better. Theoretically this is because the parturient is either too weak to push or too comfortable (and thus not motivated) to push. However, the data in Table 93.7 does not consistently support this approach.

A better approach would be to individualize the epidural block. If the patient is comfortable and pushing well, maintain the epidural block at its current level. Some women, if it hurts to push, will not push effectively. Thus, anesthesia should be maintained. For others, mild sensation will increase

Table 93.7 Letting the epidural wear off: frequency of instrumental deliveries (%)

Drug	Epidural wear off	Epidural continued	Significance
Bupivacaine, intermittent[65]	43	25	NS
0.75% Lidocaine, continuous[66]	35	31	NS
0.125% Bupivacaine, continous[67]	28	53	$P < 0.05$
0.0625% Bupivacaine + 0.002% fentanyl, continuous[57]	15	21	NS

NS, not significant.

Table 93.8 Continuous-infusion epidural anesthesia: three different local anesthetics (From ref. 8 with permission)

	Group I Bupivacaine (23 Pts)	Group II Chloroprocaine (19 Pts)	Group III Lidocaine (19 Pts)
First stage	286 min	301 min	390 min
Second stage	171 min	113 min	67 min
NSVD	10 (43%)	16 (84%)	16 (84%)
Forceps and vacuum delivery*	6 (26%)	1 (5%)	2 (11%)
Cesarean	7 (30%)	2 (11%)	1 (5%)

* Only one of the cesarean deliveries was for fetal distress.

the effectiveness of their expulsive efforts, in which case the epidural block may be adjusted to allow some return of sensation.

b. High concentrations and large volumes of some local anesthetics may cause muscle weakness. If this is the problem, a local anesthetic with a good differential blockade such as bupivacaine at a low concentration (0.125% or less) may be tried. If pain relief is not sufficient, the addition of an epidural opioid, such as fentanyl, may help as this produces no motor blockade.

c. Consider using a lower concentration of local anesthetic (such as 0.25% bupivacaine or 1% lidocaine or lower concentrations) for sensory anesthesia during the first stage of labor. This may decrease the incidence of abnormal fetal presentations.[48,50]

If the fetus is in the OP position, consider the use of epidural anesthesia with a higher concentration of local anesthetic (such as 0.5% bupivacaine or 2% lidocaine); this may relax the pelvic floor and allow spontaneous rotation during the first stage or can enable the physician to more easily turn the fetus to an occiput anterior position in the second stage of labor. Less trauma may result to the mother and the fetus.[39,52] The approach of making the block more dense should be fully discussed with the obstetrician or family physician prior to its use.

d. Perhaps the choice of local anesthetic makes a difference. Abboud et al[8] reported a higher rate of instrumental deliveries with bupivacaine compared with lidocaine and chloroprocaine (see Table 93.8). Further work in this area is needed.

e. Over the past few years, the continuous infusion of local anesthetic into the epidural space has become widely used. The level of anesthesia is better maintained than with the bolus-injection technique. Once the level of anesthesia is established, fine tuning of the epidural block is possible during the entire labor.

4. In some cases, the patient is exhausted from her long labor. Permitting her to rest before pushing may be helpful.

5. The assistance of a good labor coach can overcome the parturient's lack of sensation by directing the timing and direction of the expulsive efforts.[52]

Conclusions

There is a wide variation in the operative delivery rates cited in the literature for women receiving epidural anesthesia. This may be a reflection of the wide variation in their obstetric and anesthetic management. Other differences between studies include the patient populations (e.g. primiparous or multiparous women versus combined), the stage at which the epidural is initiated, the concentration and amounts of drugs used, the length of the second stage and, perhaps more importantly, the views of the obstetrician or family physician and the patient regarding the use of operative obstetrics.

The administration of epidural anesthesia during labor is associated with a higher incidence of operative deliveries. Whether the epidural 'caused' the operative delivery or whether other factors leading to operative delivery are also associated with an increased use of epidural anesthesia is unclear. For some labors, a different management plan may decrease the likelihood of operative deliveries.

This chapter looks at the effects of epidural anesthesia on the course of labor and the incidence of operative deliveries. Regardless of the findings, the benefit of providing analgesia may far outweigh any perceived problem with the use of an epidural anesthesic during labor, especially for the woman who is experiencing the pain!

REFERENCES

1. Gibbs C P, Krischer J, Peckham B M et al 1986 Obstetric anesthesia – a national survey. Anesthesiology 65: 298–306
2. Vasicka A, Kretchmer H 1961 Effect of conduction and inhalation anesthesia on uterine contractions. Experimental study of the influence of anesthesia on intra-amniotic pressures. Am J Obstet Gynecol 82: 600–611
3. Sala N L, Schwarcz Jr R L, Althabe Jr O et al 1970 Effect of epidural anesthesia upon uterine contracility induced by artificial

cervical dilatation in human pregnancy. Am J Obstet Gynecol 106: 26–29
4. Raabe N, Belfrage P 1976 Epidural analgesia in labour. IV. Influence on uterine activity and fetal heart rate. Acta Obstet Gynecol Scand 55: 305–310
5. Matadial L, Cibils L A 1976 The effect of epidural anesthesia on uterine activity and blood pressure. Am J Obstet Gynecol 125: 846–854
6. Schellenberg J C 1977 Uterine activity during lumbar epidural analgesia with bupivacaine. Am J Obstet Gynecol 127: 26–31
7. Jouppila P, Jouppila R, Kaar K, Merila M 1977 Fetal heart rate patterns and uterine activity after segmental epidural analgesia. Br J Obstet Gynaecol 84: 481–486
8. Abboud T K, Afrasiabi A, Sarkis F et al 1984 Continuous infusion epidural analgesia in parturients receiving bupivacaine, chloroprocaine, or lidocaine – maternal, fetal, and neonatal effects. Anesth Analg 63: 421–428
9. Abboud T K, David S, Nagappala S et al 1984 Maternal, fetal, and neonatal effects of lidocaine with and without epinephrine for epidural anesthesia in obstetrics. Anesth Analg 63: 973–979
10. Abboud T K, Sheik-ol-Eslam A, Yanagi T et al 1985 Safety and efficacy of epinephrine added to bupivacaine for lumbar epidural analgesia in obstetrics. Anesth Analg 64: 585–591
11. Crawford J S 1972 The second thousand epidural blocks in an obstetric hospital practice. Br J Anaesth 44: 1277–1286
12. Jouppila R, Jouppila P, Karinen J M, Hollmen A 1979 Segmental epidural analgesia in labour – related to the progress of labour, fetal malposition and instrumental delivery. Acta Obstet Gynecol Scand 58: 135–139
13. Robinson J O, Rosen M, Evans J M et al 1980 Maternal opinion about analgesia for labour – a controlled trial between epidural block and intramuscular pethidine combined with inhalation. Anaesthesia 35: 1173–1181
14. Studd J W W, Crawford J S, Duignan N M et al 1980 The effect of lumbar epidural analgesia on the rate of cervical dilatation and the outcome of labour of spontaneous onset. Br J Obstet Gynaecol 87: 1015–1021
15. Johnson W L, Winter W W, Eng M et al 1972 Effect of pudendal, spinal, and peridural block anesthesia on the second stage of labor. Am J Obstet Gynecol 113: 166–175
16. Bleyaert A, Soetens M, Vaes L et al 1979 Bupivacaine, 0.125%, in obstetric epidural analgesia – experience in three thousand cases. Anesthesiology 51: 435–438
17. Hellman L M, Prystowsky H 1952 The duration of the second stage of labor. Am J Obstet Gynecol 63: 1223–1233
18. Pearson J F, Davies P 1974 The effect of continuous lumbar epidural analgesia upon fetal acid-base status during the second stage of labour. J Obstet Gynaecol Br Cwlth 81: 975–979
19. Cohen W R 1977 Influence of the duration of second stage labor on perinatal outcome and puerperal morbidity. Obstet Gynecol 49: 266–269
20. Maresh M, Choong K H 1983 Delayed pushing with lumbar epidural analgesia in labour. Br J Obstet Gynaecol 90: 623–627
21. Moon J M, Smith C V, Rayburn W F 1990 Perinatal outcome after a prolonged second stage of labor. J Reprod Med 35: 229–231
22. American College Obstetricians Gynecologists Committee 1989 Opinion: Obstetric forceps. No. 71: 1–2
23. Hibbard L T 1986 Cesarean section and other surgical procedures. In Gabbe S G, Niebyl J R, Simpson J L (eds) Obstetrics: normal and problem pregnancies. Churchill Livingstone, New York, p 517–546
24. NIH 1981 The cesarean birth task force: NIH consensus development statement on cesarean childbirth. Obstet Gynecol 57: 537–545
25. Zuspan F P, Quilligan E J 1988 Cesarean childbirth. In Zuspan F P, Quilligan E J (eds): Douglas–Stromme operative obstetrics 5th edn. Appleton & Lange, East Norwalk, CT, p 473–515
26. Sachs B J, Brown D A J, Driscoll S G et al 1987 Maternal mortality in Massachusetts: trends and prevention. New Engl J Med 316: 667–672
27. Frigoletto Jr F D, Ryan K J, Phillippe M 1986 Maternal mortality rate associated with cesarean section: an appraisal. Am J Obstet Gynecol 136: 969–970
28. Amirikia H, Zarewych B, Evans T N 1981 Cesarean section: a 15-year review of changing incidence, indications and risks. Am J Obstet Gynecol 140: 81–90
29. Jones O H 1976 Cesarean section in present-day obstetrics: presidential address. Am J Obstet Gynecol 521–530
30. DeLee J B 1920 The prophylactic forceps operation. Am J Obstet Gynecol 1: 34–44
31. Dierker Jr L J, Rosen M G, Thompson K, Lynn P 1986 Midforceps deliveries: long-term outcome of infants. Am J Obstet Gynecol 154: 764–768
32. Friedman E A, Sachtleben-Murray M R, Dahrouge D, Neff R K 1984 Long-term effects of labor and delivery on offspring: a matched-pair analysis. Am J Obstet Gynecol 150: 941–945
33. Gilstrap III L C, Hauth J C, Schiano S, Connor K D 1984 Neonatal acidosis and method of delivery. Obstet Gynecol 63: 681–685
34. Niswander K R, Gordon M 1973 Safety of the low-forceps operation. Am J Obstet Gynecol 117: 619–630
35. Notzon F C 1990 International differences in the use of obstetric interventions. J Am Med Assoc 263: 3286–3291
36. Richardson D A, Evans M I, Cibils L A 1983 Midforceps delivery – a critical review. Am J Obstet Gynecol 145: 621–632
37. Morgan B M, Rehor S, Lewis P J 1980 Epidural analgesia for uneventful labour. Anaesthesia 35: 57–60
38. Duthie A M, Wyman J B, Lewis G A 1968 Bupivacaine in labour – its use in lumbar extradural analgesia. Anaesthesia 23: 20–26
39. DeVere R D 1969 Epidural analgesia. Proc R Soc Med 62: 186–188
40. Browne R A, Catton D V 1971 The use of bupivacaine in labour. Can Anaesth Soc J 18: 23–32
41. Brown S E, Vass A C R 1977 An extradural service in a district general hospital. Br J Anaesth 49: 243–246
42. Graffagnino P, Seyler L W 1938 Epidural anesthesia in obstetrics. Am J Obstet Gynecol 35: 597–602
43. Brownridge P 1982 A three year survey of an obstetric epidural service with top-up doses administered by midwives. Anaesth Intensive Care 10: 298–308
44. Thorburn J, Moir D D 1981 Extradural analgesia – the influence of volume and concentration of bupivacaine on the mode of delivery, analgesic efficacy and motor block. Br J Anaesth 53: 933–939
45. Crawford J S 1972 Lumbar epidural block in labour – a clinical analysis. Br J Anaesth 44: 66–74
46. Raabe N, Belfrage P 1976 Lumbar epidural analgesia in labour – a clinical analysis. Acta Obstet Gynecol Scand 55: 125–129
47. Rudick V, Niv D, Golan A et al 1983 Epidural analgesia during labor in 1,200 monitored parturients. Isr J Med Sci 19: 20–24
48. Matouskova A, Dottori O, Forssman L, Victorin L 1975 An improved method of epidural analgesia with reduced instrumental delivery rate. Acta Obstet Gynecol Scand 54: 231–235
49. Hanson A L, Hanson B 1985 Continuous mini-infusion of bupivacaine into the epidural space during labor – experience from 1000 deliveries. Reg Anesth 10: 139–144
50. Maltau J M, Andersen H T 1975 Continuous epidural anesthesia with a low frequency of instrumental deliveries. Acta Obstet Gynecol Scand 54: 401–406
51. Hollmen A, Jouppila R, Pihlajaniemi R et al 1977 Selective lumbar epidural block in labour. A clinical analysis. Acta Anaesth Scand 21: 174–181
52. Mastroianni Jr L, Kelly J V, Lavietes S, Carbone P 1956 The use of continuous epidural combined with continuous caudal anesthesia for labor and delivery. Am J Obstet Gynecol 71: 300–303
53. Hoult I J, MacLennan A H, Carrie L E S 1977 Lumbar epidural analgesia in labour–relation to fetal malposition and instrumental delivery. Br Med J 1: 14–16
54. Kaminski H M, Stafl A, Aiman J 1987 The effect of epidural analgesia on the frequency of instrumental obstetric delivery. Obstet Gynecol 69: 770–773
55. Walton P, Reynolds F 1984 Epidural analgesia and instrumental delivery. Anaesthesia 39: 218–223
56. Doughty A 1969 Selective epidural analgesia and the forceps rate. Br J Anaesth 41: 1058–1062
57. Chestnut D H, Laszewski L J, Pollack K L et al 1990 Continuous

epidural infusion of 0.0625% bupivacaine – 0.0002% fentanyl during the second stage of labor. Anesthesiology 72: 613–618

58. Philipsen T, Jensen N-H 1989 Epidural block or parenteral pethidine as analgesic in labour; a randomized study concerning progress in labour and instrumental deliveries. Eur J Obstet Gynecol Reprod Biol 30: 27–33
59. Noble A D, Craft I L, Bootes J A H et al 1971 Continuous lumbar epidural analgesia using bupivacaine – a study of the fetus and newborn child. J Obstet Gynaecol Br Cwlth 78: 559–563
60. Climie C R 1964 The place of continuous lumbar epidural analgesia in the management of abnormally prolonged labour. Med J Austral 2: 447–450
61. Maltau J M, Andersen H T 1975 Epidural anesthesia as an alternative to cesarean section in the treatment of prolonged, exhaustive labour. Acta Anaesth Scand 19: 349–354
62. Moir D D, Willocks J 1967 Management of incoordinate uterine action under continuous epidural analgesia. Br Med J 111: 396–400
63. Bailey P W, Howard F A 1983 Epidural analgesia and forceps delivery – laying a bogey. Anaesthesia 38: 282–285
64. Doughty A 1978 Epidural analgesia in labour – the past, the present and the future. J R Soc Med 71: 879–884
65. Phillips K C, Thomas T A 1983 Second stage of labour with or without extradural analgesia. Anaesthesia 38: 972–976
66. Chestnut D H, Bates J N, Choi W W 1987 Continuous infusion epidural analgesia with lidocaine: efficacy and influence during the second stage of labor. Obstet Gynecol 69: 323–327
67. Chestnut D H, Vandewalker G E, Owen C L, Bates J N, Choi W W 1987 The influence of continuous epidural bupivacaine analgesia on the second stage of labor and method of delivery in nulliparous women. Anesthesiology 66: 774–780

94. Should obstetricians give major regional anesthesia?

Part A European view *J. F. Pearson*
Part B USA view *D. M. Sherline*

PART A
EUROPEAN VIEW
J. F. Pearson

Much early European experience of regional anesthesia in obstetrics was gained by obstetricians who, discerning the hazards to the mother of general anesthesia, sought local techniques such as perineal infiltration and pudendal block to provide adequate anesthesia for operative vaginal delivery. In an effort to improve first-stage analgesia, techniques such as caudal epidural block were introduced into obstetric practice in the USA. It was during World War II that the special flexible needles for the performance of caudal epidural block were smuggled to Oxford in a 'Bundles for Britain' parcel. The Oxford school then began the tradition of the obstetrician providing caudal epidural block. Later, obstetricians began to use intermittent paracervical block and attempts were made to develop it as a continuous technique using catheters implanted in the paracervical tissues. Why then did obstetricians persist for so long?

The emerging answer is by no means simple but, in essence, the availability of suitably trained anesthetic staff depends on cost-effective resource allocation, which in turn relates to the size and site of maternity units.

The size of the anesthetic staffing problem was illustrated by the UK National Birthday Trust Survey of 1982.[1] This survey demonstrated that 30% of confinements occurred in units delivering fewer than 2000 babies per year. These units constituted 70% of the 524 units investigated. In the 222 units delivering fewer than 500 babies per year, there was no anesthesiologist on the premises, and in the 148 units delivering 501–2000 babies per year, 26% of deliveries occurred in the absence of an anesthesiologist.

With respect to the availability of epidural anesthesia within the UK, the most recent survey for the years 1982–86 inclusive covered 271 units and represented about 3.4 million deliveries and 565 000 epidural blocks.[2] The overall epidural rate for the 5-year period was 17%, with national rates varying from 21% in Scotland to 6% in Northern Ireland. In England there were also significant regional variations, from 26% in the Trent region to 10% in the NE Thames region. Epidural rates were also considered in relation to unit size, classifying those with over 3000 deliveries as 'large', 1500–3000 as 'intermediate' and fewer than 1500 deliveries as 'small'. In general, epidural rates tended to be higher in large units, but there were considerable variations, with a rate as low as 0.2% in one large unit and as high as 35% in one small unit. Few units had staffing up to the levels recommended by the Association of Anaesthetists (1987).[3]

In Sweden, a national survey of obstetric anesthesia between 1983 and 1986 showed a mean epidural rate of 16%, which is similar to the UK experience but, in contrast, the paracervical block rate was 12%.[4] This study echoed the UK study in that it revealed that epidural block was given more frequently in the larger regional hospitals, but was more frequently provided during daylight hours. The simpler forms of analgesia such as parenteral opioids and pudendal block were usually administered in Sweden by midwives on their own initiative. Paracervical block was usually administered by the obstetrician in charge of the case, but continuous lumbar epidural block was normally given by a specialist anesthesiologist. It seems that both the UK and Swedish services are acting under similar constraints, and both surveys highlighted the same sort of problems. In the UK much progress has been made in rationalizing services by reducing the number of babies born in small units. (In 1983 only 1% of babies were born in units delivering fewer than 500 per year.[1])

In smaller units, which are required to exist for geographical reasons, current UK recommendations are that the managerial and medical staff must endeavor to ensure that all 'facilities' are made available at the place of birth.[5] The forward planning document *Anaesthetic Services for Obstetrics* (1987) stated 'Mothers should be given information if the range of anaesthetic services available in a unit is restricted. Admission to a unit with a comprehensive service should be offered as an alternative'.[3] This, however, would not compensate for those occasions when epidural anesthesia becomes indicated during the course of labor in circumstances when patient transfer is an unsafe option. It is of more than passing interest to note that in Sweden women considered the geographical proximity of the local maternity hospital to be more important than the prospect of travelling 50–100 km to be able to obtain an epidural anesthetic.[5]

The reluctance of Swedish women to travel for an epidural block must also be viewed within the context of a system in which 12% of women are provided with obstetrician-administered paracervical block – a form of anesthesia that has long been unfashionable in the UK. Introduced several decades ago in France and Germany, it enjoyed a considerable vogue in North America in the 1960s. The technique is relatively simple. Its demise in the UK followed documentation of a 30% prevalence of fetal heart rate changes and a significant incidence of neonatal respiratory depression.[6] Its continued popularity in Sweden probably indicates that the degree of fetal risk is not so high as to prohibit its use.

In 1987, a Melbourne general practitioner attempted to provide a caudal epidural block in a patient in the second stage of labor. The anesthetic agent was unintentionally injected into the fetal brain and the baby was stillborn. A Coroner's inquest resulted. The matter was referred to in a publication from the Medical Defence Association of Victoria, concluding with the advice that 'if Doctors are still using caudal blocks in obstetrics, they should cease to do so; the next time it happens, the Coroner may be expected to deal harshly with the Doctor concerned'.[7]

Despite the above, because many labor wards in Australia – even in central Melbourne – are not provided with adequate anesthetic services, obstetricians remain the main providers of regional anesthesia. Dennerstein[8] recently (1990) reported a personal series of 670 consecutive caudal blocks. There was no morbidity attributable to the technique and satisfactory pain relief was achieved in 88% of women. The author suggested that caudal epidural anesthesia should be taught to obstetricians, particularly as we seem so far away from achieving the ideal of total anesthetic coverage on every labor ward. The editorial comment on this paper was: 'Not many obstetricians in Australia perform their own caudal blocks in patients requiring forceps delivery or manual removal of the placenta. This paper indicates that the practice is safe when training is appropriate and expertise is maintained by regular use of the technique.'

Serious but non-fatal complications associated with epidural block do occur, the frequency of which has been assessed as occurring only once in every 4–5000 epidural anesthetics in the UK.[9]

It is not surprising that an obstetrician with appropriate training should have a series of 670 consecutive caudal blocks in 20 years without serious maternal morbidity.

Whether one sides with the Melbourne Coroner or the Melbourne obstetrician, there is little doubt that in most of the world skilled specialist obstetric anesthetic services on a round-the-clock basis at immediate readiness is an unrealistic goal. While organizational and logistic debates continue, it is important to search for other equally effective and safe analgesic/anesthetic methods which demand less in the way of resources and perhaps to modify regional techniques to reduce the level of skilled supervision presently essential for the achievement of safety.

Therefore, obstetricians will continue to provide their patients with regional anesthesia until anesthetic staffing levels in European hospitals will be able to provide a round-the-clock obstetric anesthetic coverage.

REFERENCES

1. Morgan B 1987 Anaesthetic facilities In: Chamberlain G V P, Gunn P (eds) Birthplace. Report of the confidential enquiry into the facilities available at the place of birth. John Wiley, London, p 167–202
2. Hibbard B M, Scott D B 1990 Availability of epidurals in obstetrics. Br J Obstet Gynaecol 97: 402–405
3. Association of Anaesthetists of Great Britain and Ireland 1987 Anaesthetic services for obstetrics – a plan for the future. Association of Anaesthetists, London
4. Gerdin E, Cnattingius 1990 Obstetric analgesia in Sweden. Br J Obstet Gynaecol 97: 789–796
5. Fallman M-L, Kebbon M, Nilson B A, Zador G 1974 Pain and analgesia in childbirth (Swedish). Lakart idningen 97: 789–796
6. Schnider S M, Asling J H, Holl J W, Margolis A J 1970 Paracervical block anesthesia in obstetrics. I. Am J Obstet Gynecol 107: 619–625
7. Defence Update 1989 1: 42
8. Dennerstein G 1990 Caudal Analgesia by the Obstetrician. Aust New Zealand J Obstet Gynaecol 30: 203–205
9. Scott D B, Hibbard B M 1990 Serious non-fatal complications: association with extradural block in obstetric practice. Br J Anaesth 64: 537–541

PART B
USA VIEW
D. M. Sherline

The question of whether or not obstetricians should administer anesthesia to their patients is certainly not a new one, but a question that does require reconsideration. In 1993, the answer to that question is the same as it has been for years: yes and no.

First, there are certain criteria that must be met before there can be a resolution of this question:

The obstetrician must be:

1. Competent to administer the regional anesthetic.
2. Competent to deal with the immediate complications associated with the placement of the block. This should include, but not be limited to, airway problems, blood pressure alterations and management of complications associated with the anesthetic agents used.
3. Competent to assure knowledgeable maternal and fetal monitoring of the patient during initiation and maintenance of the anesthetic.
4. Able to maintain a positive working relationship with the department of anesthesia should back-up be necessary in case of an obstetric or anesthetic complication.

The department of anesthesia must:

1. Recognize the professional competence of the obstetrician.
2. Respond to requests for assistance when needed.
3. Recognize the right of *all* obstetric patients to adequate pain relief when requested.
4. Be knowledgeable regarding obstetric anesthesia and the placement and management of regional anesthetics.

Given that these criteria are met, then the local situation can vary from that of an academic health center with a full staff of obstetricians, family practitioners, anesthesiologists and nurse anesthetists, to that of a small institution where there may be unavailability of fully trained anesthesiologists, nurse anesthetists, or obstetricians. Availability may vary from 24-h in-hospital call to call-back for all personnel when needed. In some institutions, adequate numbers of willing personnel may be available to administer anesthesia for cesarean delivery but not for vaginal deliveries. In rare situations, the obstetrician wishing to utilize regional block for cesarean delivery may need to initiate the block and have a nurse anesthetist monitor the patient and, if necessary, provide general analgesia or anesthesia support.

The obstetrician must avoid being placed in a situation where there is less than adequate monitoring of the mother and the fetus. Statistically, the chance is small that there will be both an obstetric and anesthetic complication at the same time, but it must be considered and one must be prepared.

Initiating the block may be the easiest part of regional anesthesia. Adequate monitoring of the anesthetic, maintenance and management of complications, should they occur, all require extra skills and time and may be more difficult than initiation of the anesthetic.

Although it seems to contradict my earlier statement regarding the right of all laboring patients for adequate pain relief, obstetricians and anesthesiologists must remember that if they cannot insure adequate knowledgeable management and monitoring after the initiation of the anesthetic then the block itself should not be initiated. It is unrealistic, and unprofessional, for anesthesiologists to refuse to offer regional anesthesia to all laboring patients and to then refuse to aid obstetricians competent and willing to offer this service to their patients. The primary concern must be patient safety and comfort, not who does the anesthetic.

In summary, then, yes, obstetricians who are trained in the initiation and management of regional anesthesia, appropriate maternal and fetal monitoring and management of immediate anesthetic complications, *and* who have the willing cooperation of their anesthesiologist colleagues, should be able to initiate their own regional anesthetics.

Suggested anesthetic curriculum for obstetricians:

1. Historical perspective
   a. Simpson
   b. Channing
   c. Meigs
   d. Others
      (i) Hingson, continuous caudal
      (ii) Bonica, physiologic basis of obstetric anesthesia
2. Obstetric physiology
   a. Maternal pain pathways
   b. Placental physiology
      (i) Placental transfer
         Gases
         Drugs
      (ii) Metabolism
         Drugs
   c. Fetal Physiology
      (i) Enzyme induction
         Premature infant
      (ii) Blood flow
      (iii) Fetal blood/tissue levels
      (iv) Doppler studies
   d. Obstetric considerations
      (i) Patient-oriented practice
3. Anesthetic considerations
   a. Techniques

(i) General
(ii) Regional
  Lumbar epidural
  • Techniques
    – Continuous
    – Infusion
  • Drugs
    – Local anesthetic agents
      Bupivacaine
      • Concentration
      2-chloroprocaine
      Lidocaine
    – Opioids
      Agents
      Complications
      • Ventilation
      • Other
      • Side-effects
  Caudal (historical)
  Spinal
(iii) Local
  Paracervical
  Pudendal
  Local infiltration
(iv) Hypnosis
(v) Psychoprophylaxis, natural childbirth

b. Personnel problems
  (i) Anesthesiologist
    Joint ACOG/ASA statement
    Time commitment
    Monitoring
    • Equipment
    • Personnel
      – Self
      – CRNA (Certified registered nurse anesthetist)
      – Ob RN (Obstetric nurse)
      – Other
  (ii) Certified registered nurse anesthetist
  (iii) Obstetrician
    Training
    Time
    Professional liability
  (iv) Family medicine specialist
    ACOG/ASA statement
    Obstetric/gynecologic consultation
  (v) Cost

4. Summary and conclusions
  a. Major problems
    (i) Cost
    (ii) Personnel
5. Possible Solutions
  a. Alternative non-drug analgesic techniques
    (i) TENS
    (ii) Hypnosis
    (iii) Acupuncture
  b. New drugs/systems
    (i) Patient-controlled analgesia
    (ii) Paracervical block revisited?
  c. Increasing funding
    (i) Reimbursement levels
    (ii) Indigent care
  d. Alternative professionals (anesthesiologists with increasing responsibilities or, with trauma and major cases, critical care consultants, postoperative patient-controlled analgesia services).

95. Should neonatologists do all newborn resuscitations?

Part A USA view *J. W. Scanlon*
Part B European view *I. A. Laing*

PART A
USA VIEW
John W. Scanlon

The answer to the question posed in the chapter title is an enthusiastic and unequivocal 'no', and 'yes'.

Certainly a critically ill newborn does not care who performs the resuscitation, only that it is appropriate, skilled, swift and available. With proper training, and practice, physicians from each of the natal disciplines (obstetrics, anesthesia and pediatrics) can satisfactorily carry out most acute delivery room care. Certainly, specifically trained nurses (midwives, nurse anesthetist, delivery room and NICU nursing specialists) and respiratory therapists can also resuscitate the newborn.[1] Even lay resuscitators have been trained for this task, and special equipment has been designed specifically for their use in developing nations.[2] In fact, Blundell described the basic tenets of neonatal resuscitation, including endotracheal intubation, more than 150 years ago.[3] You do not need 6 years of post-graduate medical education to resuscitate a newborn!

However, the resuscitator must be immediately available when needed and must devote all attention and thinking to that one baby's problems. Responsibility for both mother and baby means that one or the other receives less than full attention. It is my belief that everyone involved in the birthing process *must* be trained in newborn resuscitation and its several components must be regularly reviewed at frequent intervals. Courses offered by the American Heart Association and the American Academy of Pediatrics are particularly useful. Each hospital has a direct responsibility to ensure a competent resuscitator's prompt availability if obstetric services are offered.

What then is the role of the neonatologist in newborn resuscitation? There are a few special circumstances which require the additional training and experience gained during the three post-pediatric residency years of a Neonatal–Perinatal Medicine Fellowship. Managing an extremely premature, very low-birthweight newborn in the delivery room is an excellent example. Technical skills, including intubating via a tiny larynx, catheterizing minute umbilical vessels, surfactant insufflation, drug dosage computations and recognizing incipient thermal stress, are more familiar to the neonatologist and to the NICU team. Another example is gathering pertinent historical information about perinatal and intrapartum events and assessing their potential impact on the fetus, soon-to-be newborn. Prepartum consultation regarding very high-risk perinatal circumstances requires the extensive training necessary to become a neonatologist. One final example: because concerns about viability and attendant ethical considerations regarding selective nontreatment decisions are regularly explored in the NICU, sensitivity and experience about this issue can be profitably applied during acute delivery room situations.[4,5]

The neonatologist has another, even more important role, which is organizing and supervising the hospital's neonatal resuscitation services. Therefore a 'yes' response to the chapter title query is also in order. Delivery room resuscitation is a team event and should not be an 'Oh, my gosh, what do I do now?' chaotic experience.

Essential components of all neonatal resuscitations are anticipation and preparedness. Communication is a third. Recognizing which fetuses may be compromised, or at risk for compromise*, falls to the obstetrician/perinatologist. The anesthesiologist has acute responsibility for maternal pain management and cardiorespiratory stability during parturition.

Neonatologists should help train members of the resuscitation team as well as collect and analyze information about delivery room events in a timely fashion. They should also be involved in establishing policy about which categories of babies need to be triaged to the NICU, and who should care for them (pediatrician or neonatologist). Certainly, the neonatologist should review their subsequent care. This includes monitoring outcomes (morbidity and mortality) for quality assurance and improvement. The neonatologist should also liaise with referral hospitals, hospital administrators, and others involved in providing acute newborn services. This newborn resuscitation coordinator/neonatologist must also be able to provide direct care when necessary as part of the institution's program for newborn resuscitation.

Individual hospitals meet their particular obligation for neonatal resuscitation in various ways which depend on immediately available direct care personnel, level of neonatal intensive care on site, the hospital's avowed mission and the personalities of participating newborn specialists. At the Columbia Hospital for Women, a physician in neonatal medicine and NICU nurse are available around the clock to attend any high-risk delivery when requested. There is a STAT paging system linking the NICU and delivery room (and well-baby nurseries) for unanticipated emergencies. There is a 'hands-off' communication system between each delivery room and the NICU, as well as a hotline telephone between NICU and the labor area. Help, and more help, can be summoned promptly, information exchanged and required equipment properly deployed using these systems. Special data sheets are used to document pertinent care descriptors at 1-min intervals.[6] The Section of Neonatology provides direct care, oversight, and, with our NICU nursing staff, education and documentation about the newborn resuscitation system in a planned and organized fashion.

Therefore, there should be participation by neonatologists in each neonatal life-saving event, at least from an organizational perspective. Institutional responsibility from the hospital's perspective can be specifically delegated, but the overall responsibility for newborn resuscitation should never become a political issue.

*Another euphemism for asphyxia, such as 'stress' and 'distress'.

REFERENCES

1. Moore J, Andrews L, Henderson C, Zuspan K J, Hertz R H 1989 Neonatal resuscitation in community hospitals. Am J Obstet Gynecol 161: 849–854
2. Milner A D, Upton C J, Green J, Stokes G M 1990 A device for domiciliary neonatal resuscitation. Lancet 1: 273–277
3. Dunn P 1989 Dr. James Blundell and neonatal resuscitation. Arch Dis Child 64: 494–495
4. Berseth C L, Kenny T D, Durand R 1988 Longitudinal development in pediatric residents of attitudes toward neonatal resuscitation. Am J Dis Child 140: 91–95
5. Lantos J D, Miles S H, Silverstein M D, Stocking C B 1988 Survival after cardiopulmonary resuscitation in babies of very low birthweight. New Engl J Med 318: 91–95
6. Daze A M, Scanlon J W 1981 Code pink, a system for neonatal resuscitation. University Park Press, Baltimore, MD p 86, Figure 1

FURTHER READING

Daze A M, Scanlon J W 1981 Code pink: a system for neonatal resuscitation. University Park Press, Baltimore, M D

Jacobs M M, Phibbs R H 1989 Prevention, recognition and treatment of perinatal asphyxia. In: Hageman T R (ed) Clin Perinatol 16: 785–808

Kimberlin L V, Kucera V S, Lawrence P B, Newkirk A, Stenske J S 1989 The role of the neonatal intensive care nurse in the delivery room. In: Hageman J R (ed) Clin Perinatol 16: 1021–1028

PART B
EUROPEAN VIEW
I. A. Laing

The title 'neonatologist' does not automatically confer on the individual the ability to carry out resuscitations better than any of his/her colleagues. Neither is it possible that a neonatologist can be present whenever a newborn infant requires resuscitation. Nevertheless, the abilities which have tempted a doctor into a career in neonatology (as with anesthesiology) may include a facility with hand and eye, a degree of calm under stress and the ability to communicate clearly with other members of the care-giving team. The physician who best takes charge of a resuscitation will have these qualities. But at least as important as possession of such attributes is the opportunity to use them frequently. The consultant (attending physician) who intubates an infant once a year may show less skill than the neonatal nurse who performs laryngoscopy and inserts endotracheal tubes several times per week.

Before deciding who should resuscitate infants, a number of questions must be addressed. In a given region where are infants delivered? Who delivers them? What level of expertise is thought to be required? What if this prediction is wrong?

WHERE ARE THE INFANTS DELIVERED?

In the UK a small but increasing number of infants are delivered at home. Occasionally they are born on the way to hospital. However, most infants in Europe are born either in a 'cottage hospital', offering simple nursery facilities (level 1), or in a 'district general hospital' with special care facilities (level 2) or in a 'tertiary referral center', which can provide full intensive care (level 3) for sick infants.

WHO DELIVERS THEM?

It is a legal requirement in the UK that a home delivery should be supervised by a registered midwife, or else that the parents have made adequate efforts to summon midwifery help. Most mothers delivering *at home* should be parous, have had an uneventful previous pregnancy and have received antenatal care which has failed to identify any risk factors to mother or fetus. If such a mother then delivers at term there is only a small risk that newborn resuscitation will be required. In the *cottage hospital*, delivery may be carried out by a trained midwife or by a general practitioner who has (often due to geographical necessity) maintained his/her obstetric skills. In the *district general hospital* a team of experienced midwives, supported by obstetricians, will supervise the labors, monitoring closely, and with facilities for 'on-site' cesarean delivery if required: there may be a resident junior anesthetist (anesthesiologist) and pediatrician in attendance. A special care unit will be available to provide thermoregulatory care, supplementary oxygenation, monitoring, gastric feeding and intravenous drug therapy. In the *tertiary referral center*, most deliveries are carried out by midwives, but if high-risk pregnancies have been appropriately referred to the institution, supervision and intervention by obstetricians will be common. In all tertiary referral centers, a neonatal unit must be readily available with facilities for full intensive care, as well as to provide enough special care and routine nursery care. The neonatal unit will be run by a team of neonatologists and pediatricians, who train junior pediatricians in the resuscitation and care of the newborn. Pediatricians and anesthesiologists should be present in the referral center at all times.

WHAT LEVEL OF EXPERTISE IS THOUGHT TO BE REQUIRED?

The midwife undertaking a *home* delivery should be competent in the clearing of a newborn's airway, the intramuscular injection of vitamin K and naloxone, delivery of oxygen by face mask, and positive-pressure ventilation by bag and mask, and should have the knowledge and skills to keep a newborn child warm. In the delivery room and nursery of a *cottage hospital*, the midwife and general practitioner must also have these skills, and must be able safely to apply mechanical suction to the nasal passages and oropharynx. The pediatricians and anesthesiologists working in a *district general hospital* must have all the above skills, but also they must be able to intubate the neonate's trachea with ease, carry out short-term assisted ventilation, set up intravenous infusions, administer drugs appropriately, and provide all the short-term care necessary for a 24-week gestation neonate weighing 600 g, or a 42-week gestation infant with meconium aspiration syndrome. The *tertiary referral center* should have the additional abilities to provide long-term intensive care, with full investigational and therapeutic facilities. This level 3 facility should also be able to provide an experienced team for transferring the sickest of infants speedily and safely from one hospital to another.

WHAT IF THE PREDICTION IS WRONG?

The community midwife is at lowest risk of being required to resuscitate a neonate, but is most vulnerable if called upon to do so and must know how to contact immediately an emergency team that can transfer the infant rapidly to a district general or tertiary referral center. The level 1 or level 2 hospitals must have an arrangement with the tertiary referral center such that any sick infant may be found an intensive care bed as soon as possible. The referral center should take responsibility for the transfer of all sick infants within the area, and must travel with full resuscitative and monitoring facilities, including a portable incubator and ventilator (with air and oxygen mix), all necessary drugs, pulse oximeter and equipment for suction and intravenous infusions. In Europe, because of the even distribution of large cities, it is rarely necessary to provide an air ambulance service, although, in some remote areas, helicopter and fixed-wing flights may occasionally be required.

CONCLUSIONS

It is logical that the choice of care-giver responsible for resuscitating infants should depend on the institution, the availability of expertise and the complexity of problem anticipated. There is no reason why a competent nurse or midwife should not be trained to intubate infants in a tertiary referral center, or why a skilled neonatal nurse should not resuscitate a compromised infant in an intensive care unit. The abilities to recognize a problem, formulate an appropriate plan and carry out life-saving treatment are products of training and practice, rather than the result of being dubbed neonatologist or anesthesiologist. In most tertiary referral centers in the UK the ultimate responsibility for infant resuscitation lies with the neonatologist, but many a junior resident has reason to be glad that an anesthesiologist was on the labor ward when a crisis occurred.

96. Nutrition during pregnancy: implications for mother and fetus

R. Martin

The nutritional status of a woman during pregnancy is of particular concern to an obstetrician. In general, maternal weight gain correlates well with both fetal weight gain and outcome. Maternal protein–calorie malnutrition (PCM) is related directly or indirectly to several complications of pregnancy, including intrauterine growth retardation (IUGR) and preeclampsia. Because of the implications for labor and delivery, (i.e. growth retarded fetuses might tolerate poorly labor or abrupt alterations in utero-placental flow which can result in emergent deliveries) anesthesiologists should have an appreciation of maternal nutrition.

The maternal and fetal circulations are separated by the placenta, which maintains a concentration gradient between them. Placental growth is important to ensure continued blood flow and nutrient supply for the fetus. This is of particular importance in pregnancies complicated by primary PCM.

This chapter will review the nutritional interrelationship between mother and fetus in normal gestation as well as the adaptive mechanisms which accompany maternal PCM.

NUTRITIONAL REQUIREMENTS IN PREGNANCY

During pregnancy, an increase in energy substrates is necessary because of the metabolic demands of the fetus and placenta. In addition, maternal metabolic work is increased as a result of the various alterations in physiology necessary to sustain the pregnancy. The average total extra energy necessary to meet all these functions during pregnancy is 80 000 kcal, or about 300 kcal/day in addition to basal needs (Table 96.1).[1] The rate of energy expenditure rises asymptomatically, reaching its maximum near the end of the first trimester and remaining at that level until term. Maternal factors, such as expanded blood volume, fat accumulation and growth of the uterus and breasts account for the second-trimester increase in energy expenditure, whereas the third-trimester burden is mainly due to growth of the fetus and placenta.

The increased dietary or energy intake is also reflected in weight gain. At term, the average weight gain in US women is 11 kg or 24 lb. Weight gain begins at the end of the first trimester and increases linearly (Fig. 96.1). Based on experiments in the rat, the shifts in maternal stores during gestation have been divided into an anabolic and a catabolic phase, which correlate well with human gestation. The former period corresponds to the first two trimesters, during which protein stores are accumulated. Fat stores are also accumulated owing to an increased conversion of glucose to fatty acids (lipogenesis) and a decrease in free fatty acid release from adipose tissue (lipolysis) in response to a relative hyperinsulinemia. Other contributing factors are the increased serum levels of progesterone and a secondary reduction in the secretion of free cortisol.

During the catabolic phase or third trimester, fetal demands increase more rapidly and are met by mobilizing maternal muscle protein stores. Triglyceride formation from fatty acids in adipose tissue declines as maternal lipolysis leads to net mobilization of free fatty acids. This is reflected in decreased tissue responsiveness to insulin as gestation progresses. Concentrations of estrogen increase, as well as the synthesis of corticosteroids by the maternal adrenal gland, mediated by ACTH secretion. Cortico-

Table 96.1 Recommended energy and protein intake for women

Age (years)	Energy needs (Kcal/day)	Protein needs (g/day)
19–24	2200	46
25–50	2200	50
Pregnancy		
First trimester	0	+ 10
Second trimester	+ 300	+ 10
Third trimester	+ 300	+ 10
Post-partum		
Lactation	+ 500	+ 15

Adapted for Recommended Dietary Allowances, 10th Rev. ed. 1989, Nutritional Research Council National Academy of Sciences.

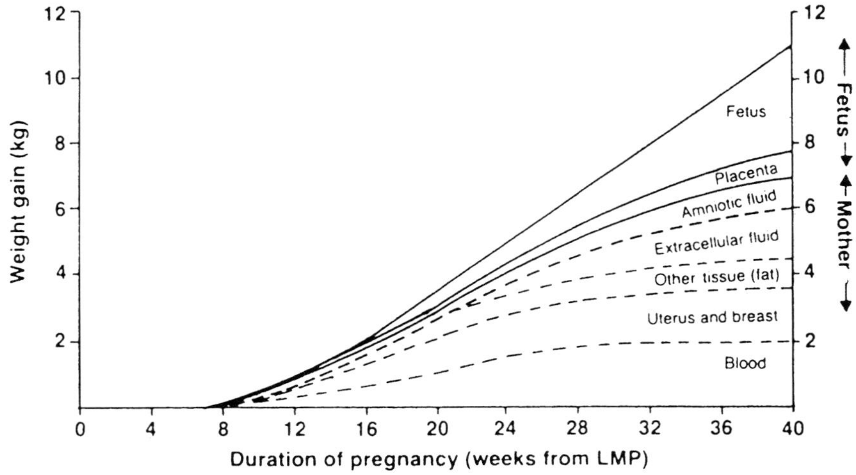

Fig. 96.1 Pattern and components of maternal weight gain during pregnancy. Adapted from Pitkin, RM: Obstetrics and gynecology. In Anderson, CE, Coursin, DB and Schneider, HA, Eds.: Nutritional Support of Medical Practice. Harper and Row, Hagerstown, Md., 1977.

steroids foster catabolism of maternal muscle protein to maintain amino acid pools for fetal uptake.

The composition of maternal weight gain as either protein or fat has been approximated by indirect means. Total body potassium determinations in pregnant teenage girls demonstrate an accumulation of potassium that is greater than the estimations for lean tissue gain from fetus, placenta and accessory tissues.[2] A similar study in older pregnant women (24–34 years old) also demonstrated excess potassium retention; however, the difference was not as large as in the younger group. These findings support the belief that maternal lean body mass increases during pregnancy. Results from nitrogen balance studies have led to similar conclusions.[3] An estimate of the protein need of obstetric patients has been made by calculating the amounts of nitrogen added during pregnancy in the known sites of protein storage: blood, breast, uterus, fetus, placenta and amniotic fluid. The result corresponds to approximately 1 kg of protein. Spread out over the duration of pregnancy, this means that an accretion of 4 g/day of protein is necessary in order to achieve optimal levels. In order to achieve this positive protein balance, an approximate intake of 1.3 g protein/kg/day is recommended (calculated from the recommended dietary allowance for the nonpregnant woman with the addition of 30 g each day for pregnancy). The remainder of maternal weight gain is fat tissue.

NUTRITIONAL SUPPORT OF THE PLACENTA

The pivotal organ in maternal–fetal nutrient transfer is the placenta. The placenta has a variety of functions, including endocrine support of the pregnancy and transport of nutrients and respiratory gases to the fetus against a concentration gradient. It produces several protein hormones, including human chorionic gonadotropin (HCG), human placental lactogen (HPL) and possibly human chorionic corticotropin (HCC). Both HCG and HPL are secreted primarily into the maternal circulation. HCG reaches its maximum level at day 70 of gestation, then declines gradually,[4] but HPL rises slowly throughout gestation and disappears rapidly after delivery. HPL has a diabetogenic, glucose-sparing effect and also stimulates maternal lipolysis, causing an increase in maternal serum free fatty acid levels.[5] Since the mother can then utilize larger amounts of free fatty acids as fuel, this frees maternal stores of glucose and amino acids for use by the fetus. HCG stimulates the corpus luteum to produce progesterone during the first trimester, and may possibly direct steroid production by the fetal gonads[6] while increasing the catabolism of glycogen.[7] This may have a glucose-sparing effect in the placenta and make more glucose available for the fetus.

The progesterone produced by the placenta also has a diabetogenic, glucose-sparing effect in the mother. The primary role of estrogen is in stimulating uterine growth by increasing local DNA and protein synthesis. Another estrogen effect is to increase placental and uterine blood flow, thus increasing the transport of nutrients to the fetus.

Table 96.2 lists substances that cross the placenta as well as currently accepted transport mechanisms. In the case of glucose, both placental metabolism and facilitated diffusion contributed to the differences in concentration between maternal and fetal circulation.[8]

An active transport of amino acids is suggested by the fourfold higher concentration of amino acids in the fetal circulation when compared to that of the mother.[9] In addition, amino acid concentrations in umbilical venous blood exceed those in umbilical arterial blood. Large proteins and polypeptides cross the placenta very slowly, probably by pinocytosis or through breaks in the membranes.[10] Free fatty acids exchange readily, although not

Table 96.2 Substances that cross the placenta and currently accepted mechanism of transport

Transport mechanism	Substances transported
Passive diffusion	Oxygen
	Carbon dioxide
	Fatty acids
	Steroids
	Nucleosides
	Electrolytes
	Fat-soluble vitamins
Facilitated diffusion	Sugars
Active diffusion	Amino acids
	Some cations
	Water-soluble vitamins
Solvent drag	Electrolytes
Pinocytosis, breaks in membrane	Proteins

as quickly as oxygen and carbon dioxide.[11] The diffusion of cholesterol and steroids is relatively slow and depends upon their molecular configuration.

Water-soluble vitamins are found in higher concentrations in the fetal blood than in the maternal blood.[12] Although they are probably actively transported, their protein binding in the fetal blood is also increased and might account for the large gradient. Fat-soluble vitamins readily cross the placenta by passive diffusion.

The concentration of water in both circulations is affected by both hydrostatic and osmotic pressure differences. Changes in the concentration of any of the above-mentioned substances can affect the osmotic pressure gradient across the placenta and thereby influence water exchange. The osmotic water flux is also influenced by water shifts, due to carbon dioxide exchange, between erythrocytes and plasma, which can then affect the plasma concentration of numerous solutes.

FETAL AND PLACENTAL GROWTH

Fetal growth, as measured by changes in fetal body weight, increases gradually throughout pregnancy. Biochemical analyses of various organs have shown that fetal growth is proliferative up to the 25th week of gestation but becomes both hyperplastic and hypertrophic thereafter.[13] This pattern is similar to the growth pattern of the placenta. In early gestation, the placenta is larger than the fetus and probably has greater growth requirements. In later gestation, the rate of fetal growth exceeds that of the placenta. This is reflected by an increase in the ratio of fetal/placental weight. Because of this shift, the placenta must increase the amount of substrate per gram of placental tissue which is transferred into the fetal circulation to meet fetal growth needs.[14] This osmotic gain in turn affects fetal blood volume, venous return, cardiac output and delivery of nutrients to fetal tissues.

There are several recently recognized growth factors that may also play a role in fetal growth. The fetal blood concentration of somatomedin A has been correlated with birth weight. Somatomedin A has binding sites in the placenta and there is indirect evidence that it is synthesized there. Somatomedin C, found in fetal erythrocytes, also has placental binding sites. It is found in increasing concentrations in the fetal pig placenta as gestation advances while at the same time insulin binding is decreasing. This suggests a possible role for somatomedin in placental growth.[15] Human placental lactogen (HPL) has been shown to increase somatomedin production, which suggests that HPL may regulate placental growth through this mechanism.[16] In addition to the somatomedins, there are insulin-like growth factors (IgF1 and IgF2) about which little is known.

SUBSTRATES

Carbohydrates

During pregnancy, fasting plasma glucose concentrations are somewhat lower than in the nonpregnant state, and they do not change significantly as pregnancy progresses. Fasting plasma insulin concentrations, however, rise slightly during pregnancy. In response to a standard glucose load, there is a rise in serum glucose during the first hour, with a return to fasting levels by $2-2\frac{1}{2}$ h. There is, though, a wide range in serum glucose values. In some patients there is only a small rise in serum glucose, whereas in others there is a secondary increase after the first peak. The resulting response for the former is probably rapid, causing an increase in diffusion from plasma to the extracellular space, as well as increased uptake by tissue. For the latter response, there is a corresponding secondary rise in plasma insulin. As pregnancy progresses, the time necessary to reach maximum glucose concentration increases. By 38 weeks of gestation, the mean time to peak plasma glucose is 55 min, compared with 34 minutes in the nonpregnant state. Return to fasting level, however, is still attained in $2-2\frac{1}{2}$ h.[17] The insulin response is characterized by a gradually increasing peak value throughout gestation as well as a delay in reaching this peak. By 2 h, the insulin level is still above the fasting concentration.

The glomerular filtration rate (GFR) rises in pregnancy to about 50% above the prepregnancy level.[17] With the rise in postprandial glucose levels, this means an increase in the filtered load presented to the renal tubules. It has been shown that with elevated plasma glucose levels, tubular reabsorption increases, but with decreasing efficiency, which leads to glycosuria. In a study of urinary glucose excretion in 30 healthy pregnant women, it was found that 10 women excreted glucose in the normal, nonpregnant range of less than 100 mg/24 h.[18] The rest excreted more that 100 mg/24 h on some days. Of the latter group, 10 women excreted as much as 1000 mg/24 h. All patients had normal oral glucose tolerance tests. Evaluation of possible influencing variables (relationship to meals, time of day, etc.) showed no significant relationship. In addition to the glucose loss from glycosuria during pregnancy, there is also increased excretion of water-soluble vitamins as well as amino acids. In well-nourished women during pregnancy, this loss does not affect maternal–fetal nutritional balance. In the presence of PCM, however, intermittent glycosuria could be another potentially significant source of nutritional loss.

Intravenous glucose tolerance tests (IGTT) have been used in infants and neonates to calculate the rate of disappearance of glucose (Kg). In healthy full term infants, the mean Kg starts at 1%/min and increases to 2%/min by 6 months (similar to the adult level). Infants of diabetic mothers have higher Kg values within the first 24 h after birth, as do infants who are small for gestational age (SGA) or those with significant hypoglycemia. The Kg values for premature infants that were appropriate for gestational age (AGA) were less than those of full-term infants for the first 24 h; however, there was a rapid increase in the Kg. In SGA infants, after the first 24 h, the Kg decreased to a pattern similar to that of the AGA infants.[19]

Amino acids

As mentioned previously, the placenta has an active transport mechanism for amino acids, specifically the L-amino acids. Studies in rhesus monkeys, looking at the ratio of amino acid levels in cord and maternal blood (C/M), demonstrated that the cord blood levels were greater than those of the mother for all amino acids.[20] For lysine, taurine and 3-methyl-histidine, the elevated C/M is secondary to an increase in free amino acids in the fetus as well as reduced maternal levels. For the other amino acids, the elevated ratio is due entirely to a reduction in maternal serum levels. Taurine, alanine, lysine and 3-methyl-histidine levels were elevated in full-term monkey fetuses as compared with 1-year-old animals. The serum levels of the other amino acids were either unchanged or decreased.

Ghadimi and Pecora[21] studied free amino acid levels at delivery in simultaneously drawn cord and maternal serum in humans during the second and third trimesters of pregnancy. As in the monkey, cord blood has a higher concentration of amino acids than maternal blood. The fetal/maternal ratios all favored the fetus, most showing a twofold greater concentration in the fetus. When maternal blood was analyzed 6–8 weeks postpartum, all amino acid concentrations were found to have increased from maternal levels at delivery. When the fetuses were stratified for gestational age (immature, < 30 weeks; premature, 30–37 weeks; and full term, > 37 weeks) the differences in C/M ratios were larger in the immature deliveries. Three diabetic mothers and their full-term infants were also included. Their C/M ratios did not differ from those of nondiabetic women with full-term deliveries. The amino acids in the Krebs-ornithine cycle, i.e. aspartic acid, glutamic acid and ornithine, have higher ratios in the immature group than in the full-term group. This suggests an immaturity of the Krebs-ornithine cycle in early pregnancy, resulting in increased fetal concentrations of these amino acids.

These data indicate that the placenta concentrates amino acids in the fetal circulation. This system is probably best suited for periods of maternal nutritional deprivation.

Fatty acid and ketone metabolism

The fetus needs fatty acids for structure (i.e. phospholipids) and storage. Although the fetus can synthesize some fatty acids, it cannot make essential fatty acids. Linoleic acid accounts for approximately 2.5% of fetal adipose tissue stores.[22] This indicates that fatty acids cross the placenta in sizable amounts. Studies in perfused human placentas have demonstrated fatty acid transfer and suggest that the flow to the fetus is determined by the free fatty acid concentration in the maternal serum. Elphick et al[23] infused 200 ml of a fat emulsion (10% Intralipid) over 1 h into 6 pregnant women at 1–2 h prior to delivery. The umbilical vein levels of all triglyceride fatty acids were higher than those in the umbilical artery, indicating placental transfer secondary to the establishment of a large maternal–fetal gradient of oleic and linoleic acids. There was a similar increase for free fatty acids. Maternal phospholipid levels were only slightly affected, with no significant umbilical venous–arterial difference. The profile of the venous–arterial cord levels for both free fatty acids and triglycerides reflects the imprint of the infused fat emulsion.

During periods of maternal fasting, there is a reduction in both maternal and fetal serum glucose levels. The resulting maternal lipolysis and free fatty acid mobilization lead to increased ketone body formation. Because the fetus has limited ability to mobilize hepatic glycogen stores, increase gluconeogenesis, or extract free fatty acids from maternal serum, its serum ketone concentration also increases. This is the result of both placental transfer and endogenous production in the fetus. Under normal conditions in the human, measurements of arterial–venous differences show that the fetal brain extracts glucose, ketone bodies and oxygen. This utilization is particular for the fetus. When one compares fractional extraction rates of ketone bodies by brain in the neonate, infant and adult, there is a gradual decrease with increasing age. This would explain why neonates are able to tolerate periods of hypoglycemia better than older infants.

Vitamins

Vitamin deficiency is a concern during pregnancy and is seen commonly in women with PCM. Baker et al analyzed vitamin profiles of 174 women and their newborn infants at term.[24] 133 of these women reported having taken supplemental vitamins during their pregnancy. There was a 1:2 to 1:5 ratio of serum vitamin levels between the mother and the neonate for all the women and infants studied. The exceptions were vitamins A, B6, E and beta-carotene. Of the mothers found to be hypovitaminemic, serum levels of folate, thiamine and vitamins B12, C and A were the most depressed. In women not taking supplemental vitamins, the levels of nicotinate and vitamin B6 were also depressed. In this latter group, the incidence of low serum folate and thiamine levels was 71% and 53%, respectively. The hypovitaminosis was also seen in the neonate. Based on these results, it is evident that most vitamins cross the placenta and accumulate in the fetus against a concentration gradient. The fat-soluble vitamins are the exception.

Baker et al[25] studied placental transfer in two groups of women (hypovitaminemic and normovitaminemic) who took no supplemental vitamins throughout gestation. In the hypovitaminemic group, the vitamin depletion in both maternal and fetal serum was the same as in the above-mentioned study, however, the placentas of these women had depressed levels of only B12 and folate when compared with placentas of normovitaminemic women. This suggests that the placenta not only is selective in the transport of vitamins but as a growing organ has its own vitamin requirements.

Trace elements and minerals

The need for iron supplementation during pregnancy is well established and has been reviewed.[26] Deficiency states of minerals and trace elements are rare. Dawson et al[27] measured maternal plasma levels in 244 pregnant adolescents. These women had not had any mineral supplements. The samples were drawn serially from the 10th week of pregnancy to term. Their serum concentrations of calcium, magnesium, iron and zinc decreased progressively throughout pregnancy. Plasma copper levels rose slightly. All pregnancies in this series were uncomplicated. The role of the placenta in the maternal–fetal exchange of minerals and trace elements is still not clearly defined.

THE EFFECTS OF MATERNAL NUTRITIONAL DEPRIVATION ON THE FETUS AND PLACENTA

Studies in pregnant rats pair-fed 50% of the food normally consumed by nonpregnant controls showed no change in body composition of the mother. However, fetal mean body weights were significantly reduced.[28] When pregnant rats were restricted to 75% or their ad libitum intake, the mothers gained 9 g of net body weight while the mean fetal weight remained within control values. With a decrease in the restriction to 50% of normal intake, the mothers lost 8% of the initial weight, with a decrease in mean fetal weight of 12%. At a 25% intake restriction, there was a 32–36% loss of initial body weight, with a 45–56% decrease in mean fetal weight. This was also associated with a 64–92% embryonic death rate.[29] These data suggest that there is no apparent effect on fetal growth in food-restricted rats unless the restriction is so severe that the mother cannot gain weight.

If nutrients are available and the mother increases her intake above normal, a portion of the excess goes to the fetus. When food intake is severely limited, however, the fetus is not favored over the mother. The maternal preference for nutrients is continued with refeeding. In pregnant guinea pigs, a low protein diet resulted in a 10–12% reduction of maternal weight, a 50% fetal mortality and a 22–38% reduction in fetal birth weight.[30] Pigs fed a low-protein diet during pregnancy lost 17% of initial body weight, while the fetuses were 33% below control weight.[31] The same has been found in rhesus monkeys.[32,33] When rats were restricted to 24% of normal intake for the first 5 days of pregnancy and then allowed to eat ad libitum for the remainder of the pregnancy, maternal and fetal weights were similar to those of controls. If refeeding was not permitted until the last 12 days of pregnancy, however, maternal net body weight increased 23% while fetal body weight decreased 7% when compared with controls. When refeeding was begun during the last 10 days of gestation, maternal body weight increased by 21% and fetal body weight decreased by 12%.[34] This demonstrates that the mother is favored over the fetus when nutrients are available. These results also support the concept that nutrients go preferentially to the mother rather than the fetus during periods of starvation.

The Dutch famine during the winter of 1944–45 demonstrated the effects of starvation on maternal weight gain. It has been estimated that the average daily intake during this time was approximately 1200 calories. When this occurred during the second and third trimesters, there was a 250 g decrease in mean fetal body weight (10% reduction). Rosso has estimated that the mean loss of weight for the mother was 1.5 kg of initial body weight or less than 3%.[35] This is consistent with the experimental animal data described previously and suggests that with semistarvation, the mother maintains her own body stores rather than adapting to maintain fetal growth. If there are extra body stores, then she can maintain normal fetal growth even with inadequate food intake. If the stores are small, however, the amount of food intake becomes the critical factor in the maintenance of fetal growth.

The metabolic changes that the mother undergoes during starvation are still largely unknown. In pregnant rats that have been protein-restricted, the rate of urea synthesis and the levels of hepatic enzymes involved in amino acid catabolism are reduced.[36,37] Women on low protein diets have reduced urea excretion, which suggests

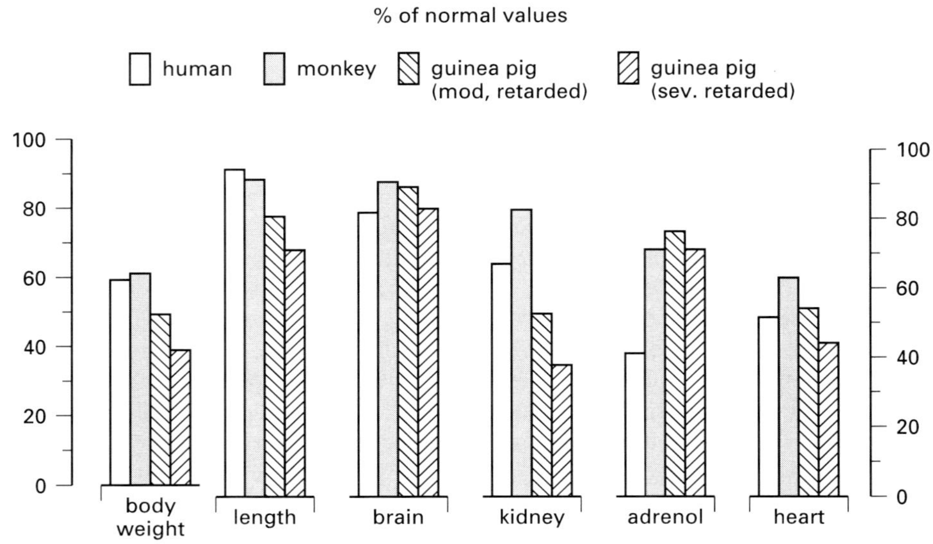

Fig. 96.2 Comparative organ size in growth retarded fetuses of man, monkey and guinea pig. From Leafeber, HN, Jones, CT and Rolph, TP: Some of the consequences of intrauterine growth retardation. p. 47. In Visser, HKA, Ed.: Nutrition and metabolism of the fetus and infant. Martinus Nijhoff, The Hague, p 47 1979.

a similar mechanism to reduce amino acid catabolism,[38] although the reason for this is not clear. In humans as well as in experimental animal models, protein restriction beginning just after conception causes a significant reduction in the expected expansion of plasma volume.[39,40] If blood volume is inadequate, uterine blood flow may be decreased, with subsequent compromise of fetal development. It has been shown that the volume of maternal plasma correlates with infant birth weight.[41]

The lack of normal plasma volume expansion and its consequent reduction in uterine blood may adversely influence nutrient transfer across the placenta. In addition, changes in placental morphology may reduce the size of the effective exchange area and thereby the rate of transfer for substances moved by simple or facilitated diffusion. A reduction in the metabolic activity of the trophoblast would influence active transport. Measurements of maternal cardiac output and regional blood flow have shown less expansion in cardiac output and placental blood flow for malnourished pregnant rats compared with controls, although the percentage of cardiac output distributed to the uterus was the same for both groups.[42] It was the lack of plasma volume expansion that accounted for the decreased placental blood flow and decreased nutrient supply.

The primary cause for the lack of weight gain in the nutritionally growth-retarded fetus is decreased placental transport. This is suggested by the frequent occurrence of hypoglycemia seen in nutritionally growth-retarded guinea pig fetuses. Plasma-free fatty acids in these fetuses are also depressed as is the arterial oxygen saturation.[43] In both guinea pig and human fetuses that suffer from nutritional IUGR, venous alanine concentrations are elevated owing to increased protein catabolism. Fetal serum ammonia levels are high because of inadequate clearing by the placenta, as well as a poorly developed fetal urea cycle. Fetal hepatic glycogen is reduced in the rat,[44] but not in the monkey[45] or guinea pig.[43] Triglyceride stores are also reduced with nutritional IUGR. Both glycogen and triglycerides are rapidly mobilizable energy stores for the neonate. Decreased glycogen storage probably accounts for the hypoglycemia that occurs frequently in human newborns who have experienced PCM during gestation.

Our understanding of fetal changes in response to maternal malnutrition is largely based on animal studies. A consistent feature seen with nutritional IUGR in both animal models and humans is an asymmetric effect on organ growth.[43] Length is not affected as much as the decrease in body weight. When compared with the reduction in total body weight, the decrease in brain weight is proportionally less and the decrease in lung, heart and kidney weight is the same (Fig. 96.2).

In addition to a decrease in organ weight, there are also changes in morphology. The liver shows less cytosol, fewer mitochondria, and less endoplasmic reticulum. Hepatic enzyme function is also altered. Low levels of phosphoenolpyruvate carboxykinase suggest impairment of gluconeogenesis. Decreased activity of aminotransferase is consistent with reduced rates of peripheral amino acid metabolism.[43]

In the brain, the decrease in mass is associated with a fall in DNA, RNA and protein content. In humans, most neurogenesis and some myelination have occurred by 26 weeks of gestation. If growth restriction starts after that time, brain mass at birth is reduced, but if postnatal nutrition is adequate, 'catch-up' growth will compensate to produce a normal size brain.[46] Growth restriction before 26 weeks, however, leads to permanent stunting of brain growth and measurable neurologic damage.[47]

The skeletal system is affected by nutritional IUGR. In guinea pigs, there is delayed ossification, probably secondary to a decrease in factors that cause sulfate to be incorporated into cartilage.[43] These changes are caused primarily by decreased nutrient supply, although secondary changes in circulating levels of insulin have an effect as well.

There is clearly a relationship between maternal weight gain, fetal weight gain and fetal outcome. A question yet to be answered is whether one can quantitate the relationship between the degree of maternal weight loss and the severity of fetal outcome. It is, of course, important to know what populations are at increased risk for weight loss.

SUMMARY

Because maternal and fetal well-being correlate with maternal weight gain, nutrition during pregnancy is a major concern. With an underweight parturient (prepregnancy weight 10% or more below ideal body weight, or a woman with inadequate weight gain (<1 kg per month during the second or third trimesters), there is an increased risk of nutritional deficiency. These women encompass a spectrum of problems:

1. adolescents
2. women with low incomes, for whom food purchase is an economic hardship
3. women with a history of frequent conceptions
4. women with a history of infants with low birth weights
5. diseases that influence nutritional status: diabetes, inflammatory bowel disease, mental depression
6. drug addiction and/or alcoholism.

These problems are well known to obstetric anesthesiologists because of the greater incidence of fetal decompensation during labor and delivery, requiring emergent delivery. In addition, several of the above problems are predisposing factors for pregnancy-induced-hypertension or preeclampsia.

Although there is little known about metabolic changes during labor and delivery, with even less known about resuscitative measures for nutritionally compromised parturients and their fetuses, recognition of the problem is an important first step. Anesthesiologists who are involved in the care of obstetric patients should have an appreciation of maternal–fetal nutrition and its implication for certain diseases and the potential impact during labor and delivery.

REFERENCES

1. Recommended dietary allowances 10th Rev 1989 National Academy of Sciences, Washington DC, p 33
2. King J C, Calloway D H, Margen S 1973 Nitrogen retention, total body 40K and weight gain in teenage pregnant girls. J Nutr 103: 772
3. Calloway D H 1974 Nitrogen balance during pregnancy. In: Winick M (ed) Nutrition and fetal development. John Wiley, New York, p 79
4. Grumbach M M, Kaplan S L, Sciarra J J et al 1968 Chorionic growth hormone-prolactin (CGP): secretion, disposition, biological activity in man and postulated function as 'growth hormone' of the second half of pregnancy. Ann NY Acad Sci 148: 501
5. Kalikhoff R K, Kisselbah A H, Kim H K 1978 Carbohydrate and lipid metabolism during normal pregnancy: relationship to gestational hormone action. Semin Perinatol 2: 291
6. Abramovich R, Baker T G, Neal P 1974 Effect of human chorionic gonadotropin on testosterone secretion by the fetal human testis in organ culture. J Endocrinol 60: 179
7. Gabbe S G, Demers L M, Greep R O et al 1972 The effects of hypoxia on placental glycogen metabolism. Am J Obstet Gynecol 114: 540
8. Widdas W F 1952 Inability of diffusion to account for placental glucose transfer in the sheep and consideration of the kinetics of a possible carrier transfer. J Physiol (London) 118: 23
9. Young M, Prenton M A 1969 Maternal and fetal plasma amino acid concentrations during gestation and in retarded fetal growth. J Obstet Gynaecol Br Commonw 76: 333
10. Brambell F W R 1954 Transport of proteins across the fetal membrane. Cold Spring Harbor Symposium. Quant Biol 19: 71
11. Robertson A F, Sprecher H 1968 A review of human placental lipid metabolism and transport. Acta Paedoatr Scand 57: (suppl) 183: 1
12. Snelling C E, Jackson S H 1977 Blood Studies of vitamin C during pregnancy, birth and early infancy. J Pediatr 14: 447
13. Widdowson E M, Grabb D E, Milveer R D G 1972 Cellular development of some human organs before birth. Arch Dis Child 47: 652
14. Rosso P 1975 Changes in transfer of nutrients across the placenta during normal gestation in the rat. Am J Obstet Gynecol 122: 2761
15. D'Ercole A J, Foushee D B, Underwood L E 1976 Somatamedin-C receptor ontogeny and levels in porcine fetal and human cord serum. J Clin Endocrin Metabol 43: 1069
16. Takano K T, Hizuka N, Shizuma N 1977 The effects of growth hormone and fasting on the serum levels of somatomedin in rats and man determined by radioreceptor assay. Acta Endocrinol (Copenh) 85: 189
17. Davison J M 1974 Changes in renal function and other aspects of homeostasis in early pregnancy. J Obstet Gynaecol Br Commonw 81: 1003
18. Lind T, Hytten F E 1972 The excretion of glucose during normal pregnancy. J Obstet Gynaecol Br Commonw 79: 961
19. Isles T E, Dickson M, Farquhar J W 1968 Glucose tolerance and plasma insulin in newborn infants of normal and diabetic mothers. Pediatr Res 2: 198
20. Kerr G R, Waisman H A 1967 Transplacental ratio of serum amino acids during pregnancy in Rhesus monkey. In: Nyhan W L (ed) Amino acids metabolism and genetic variation. McGraw Hill, New York p 429
21. Ghadimi H, Pecora P 1964 Free amino acids of cord plasma as compared with maternal plasma during pregnancy. Pediatrics 30: 500
22. Widdowson E M, Southgate D A T, Hey E N 1979 Body composition of the fetus and infant. In: Visser H K A (ed) Nutrition and metabolism of the fetus and infant. Martinus Nijhoff, The Hague p 169
23. Elphick M C 1978 The passage of fat emulsion across the human placenta. Br J Obstet Gynaecol 85: 610
24. Baker H 1975 Vitamin profile of 174 mothers and newborns at parturition. Am J Clin Nutr 28: 56
25. Baker H 1981 Role of placenta in maternal–fetal vitamin transfer in humans. Am J Obstet Gynecol 141: 792

26. Pritchard J A 1970 Anemias complicating pregnancy and the puerperium. In: Maternal nutrition and the course of pregnancy. National Academy of Sciences, Washington DC
27. Dawson E B 1969 Plasma vitamins and trace metal changes during teenage pregnancy. Am J Obstet Gynecol 104: 953
28. Child C M 1920 Some considerations concerning the nature and origin of physiological gradients. Biol Bull 39: 147
29. Eastman N J, Jackson J 1968 Weight relationships in pregnancy. 1. The bearing of maternal weight gain and pre-pregnancy weight on birth weight in full term pregnancies. Obstet Gynecol Surv 23: 1003
30. Young M, Widdowson E 1975 The influence of diets deficient in energy or in protein in conceptus weight and the placental transfer of non-metabolizable amino acid in the guinea pig. Biol Neonate 27: 184
31. Pond W G, Stracham D N, Sinha Y N et al 1969 Effect of protein deprivation of the swine during all or part of gestation on birth weight, postnatal growth rate and nucleic acid content of the brain and muscle of progeny. J Nutr 99: 61
32. Riopelle A J, Hill C W, Li S C 1975 Protein deprivation in primates v. fetal mortality and neonatal status of infant monkeys born of deprived mothers. Am J Clin Nutr 28: 989
33. Riopelle A J 1975 Weight gain of non-pregnant and pregnant monkeys fed low protein diets. Am J Clin Nutr 28: 802
34. Berg B N 1965 Dietary restriction and reproduction in the rat. J Nutr 87: 344
35. Rosso P 1981 Nutrition and maternal–fetal exchange. Am J Clin Nutr 34: 744
36. Beaton G H, Beare J, Ryu M H et al 1954 Protein metabolism in the pregnant rat. J Nutr 54: 291
37. Naismith D J 1973 Adaptations in the metabolism of protein during pregnancy and their nutritional implications. Nutr Rep Int 7: 383
38. Beydoun S N, Cuenca V G, Evans L P 1972 Maternal nutrition. 1. The urinary urea nitrogen/total nitrogen as an index of protein nutrition. Am J Obstet Gynecol 114: 198
39. Blechner J N, Stenger V G, Prystowsky H 1974 Uterine blood flow in women at term. Am J Obstet Gynecol 129: 633
40. Bruce N W 1976 The distribution of blood flow to the reproductive organs of the rat near term. J Reprod Fertil 45: 359
41. Croall J, Sheriff S, Matthews J 1978 Non-pregnant maternal plasma volume and fetal growth retardation. Br J Obstet Gynaecol 85
42. Kava R, Rosso P 1979 Mechanisms for fetal growth retardation in undernourished pregnant rats. Fed Proc 38: 871
43. LaFever H N, Jones C T, Rolph T P 1979 Some of the consequences of intrauterine growth retardation. In: Visser H K A (ed) Nutrition and metabolism of the fetus and infant. Martinus Nihjoff, The Hague, p 43
44. Hehenauer L, Oh W 1969 Body composition in experimental intrauterine growth retardation in the rat. J Nutr 99: 23
45. Myers R G, Hill D E, Holt A B et al 1971 Fetal growth retardation produced by experimental placental insufficiency in the Rhesus monkey 11. Chemical composition of the brain, liver, muscle and carcass. Biol Neonate 18: 379
46. Dobbing J 1964 The influence of early nutrition on the development of myelination of the brain. Proc R Soc Lond (Biol) 159: 503
47. Fancourt R, Harvey D R, Norman A P et al 1976 Follow-up study of small for dates babies. Br Med J 1: 1435

97. Use of hyperbaric oxygen

E. M. Camporesi

Carbon monoxide poisoning is the leading cause of fatal poisoning in the USA, accounting for over 3500 deaths per year.[1] Carbon monoxide is a colorless, odorless gas produced by the incomplete combustion of hydrocarbons. The most frequent sources of exposure are from automobile exhaust, faulty heating systems and smoke inhalation from fires. Although uncommon, carbon monoxide poisoning does occur during pregnancy, thus raising concern not only for the mother at risk, but for the developing fetus as well. The deleterious fetal effects of carbon monoxide exposure during pregnancy have been extensively described.[2,3] Management and treatment of the intoxicated pregnant patient is inconsistent. Hyperbaric oxygen (HBO) therapy is used routinely as the preferred treatment for severe carbon monoxide poisoning in the nonpregnant patient; however, its use during pregnancy is controversial because of possible adverse fetal effects of oxygen at high partial pressures. Review of the literature indicates that the clinical use of HBO during pregnancy and the risks of treatment of the fetus have never been thoroughly examined, although one case has been reported[4] and others have suggested its use.[5,6] The safest and most effective therapy needs to be established to ensure proper treatment of these patients. The most complete study of carbon monoxide poisoning during pregnancy and successful treatment with HBO was presented by van Hoesen et al,[6] with a discussion of the pathophysiology of maternal and fetal carbon monoxide poisoning, a critical review of the experimental and clinical use of HBO therapy during pregnancy and recommendations regarding the use of HBO for acute carbon monoxide poisoning in the pregnant patient.

CARBON MONOXIDE PATHOPHYSIOLOGY

The affinity of hemoglobin for carbon monoxide is over 200 times greater than for oxygen. Carbon monoxide competes with oxygen for the same binding site on the hemoglobin molecule, thus blocking the uptake of oxygen. As HbCO levels rise, the oxygen-carrying capacity of the blood decreases. The initial binding of carbon monoxide onto the hemoglobin molecule changes its structure, which increases its affinity for the remaining oxygen molecules. This produces the characteristic 'left shift' of the oxyhemoglobin dissociation curve (ODC), therefore a lower tissue $P\text{O}_2$ is required to unload oxygen to the tissues. Additionally, carbon monoxide interacts with cytochrome oxidase at the cellular level, producing a direct cellular toxicity by disrupting intracellular respiration.[7]

In addition to external sources, carbon monoxide is produced endogenously by the breakdown of heme pigments. During pregnancy, endogenous maternal carbon monoxide production is increased as a result of increased red cell turnover and the endogenous production by the fetus.[3] Fetal HbCO concentration depends upon maternal HbCO concentration, placental diffusing capacity of carbon monoxide, endogenous fetal carbon monoxide production and the relative affinities of maternal and fetal hemoglobin for carbon monoxide and oxygen. During normal steady-state production, the human fetal–maternal HbCO concentrations ratio is 1.1 to 1. Hence, fetal HbCO levels are 10–15% higher at steady state than maternal HbCO levels.[3]

Extensive experimental work on carbon monoxide poisoning during pregnancy was conducted by Longo and Hill[8] utilizing pregnant sheep. They demonstrated a lag time in the uptake of carbon monoxide by the fetus relative to the mother. Maternal HbCO concentration rose rapidly during the first 2 h and then reached a steady-state at 7–8 h. Fetal HbCO concentration rose more slowly, equaling maternal levels at 5 h and then surpassing them later before reaching a steady state. The reverse was also true for carbon monoxide elimination; the half-life of elimination for maternal carbon monoxide was 4 h, whereas the half-life for fetal carbon monoxide elimination was 7.5 h. These experimental data are in agreement with a mathematical model proposed by Hill et al[9] describing the relationship between maternal and fetal carboxyhemoglobin.

The fetus is more vulnerable than the mother to the hypoxic effects induced by carbon monoxide. The fetal ODC normally lies to the left of the maternal curve. Normal fetal arterial Po_2 is low, at about 20 mmHg with an oxygen content of 12 ml/100 ml. The fetal system normally operates on the steep part of the ODC, thus a small drop in oxygen tension can dangerously lower the fetal arterial oxygen concentration. In acute carbon monoxide exposure, there is a reduction in oxygen content. Even before the fetal HbCO concentration has risen, the fall in the maternal oxygen content in the uterine artery will cause a significant decrease in fetal oxygen content, leading to fetal hypoxia. As the fetal HbCO level begins to rise, the fetal ODC will shift further to the left, exaggerating the effect and resulting in dramatic hypoxia in the fetus.

Numerous experimental models have demonstrated the widespread toxic effects of carbon monoxide on the fetus exposed during all stages of gestation. These include teratogenicity, neurologic dysfunction, decreased birthweight and increased risk of fetal death. Reports in humans of carbon monoxide intoxication during pregnancy have been summarized;[3,6] there are eight reported cases of fetal demise from maternal carbon monoxide poisoning in which the mother survived and 11 cases in which both the mother and fetus died. Of more interest are those cases in which both the mother and fetus survived but the fetal outcome was poor. Many of the surviving infants subsequently developed somatic and neurologic sequelae including malformation of limbs, hypotonia and areflexia, persistent seizures, mental and motor disabilities and microcephaly. Autopsies of infants who died at a later time showed brain damage consisting of injury to the basal ganglia, abnormalities of the cerebellum and neuronal loss in the cortex resembling injuries seen in anoxic encephalopathy. In summary, the degree of fetal carbon monoxide saturation and effects of hypoxia on the fetus depend on the duration of exposure, the amount of carbon monoxide to which the fetus is exposed and the stage of fetal development. The fetus is more susceptible to carbon monoxide poisoning than its mother for two reasons: first, fetal carbon monoxide levels at equilibrium are higher and elimination time is longer than for maternal carbon monoxide levels and, second, the fetal ODC is shifted to the left and the Po_2 is normally low, thus a small decrease in maternal and fetal oxygen tension and a relatively low level of fetal HbCO can result in significant fetal tissue hypoxia or anoxia.

Experimental use of hyperbaric oxygen during pregnancy

The use of HBO for the treatment of carbon monoxide poisoning was first suggested by Pace et al in 1950.[10] HBO is effective as a treatment for carbon monoxide intoxication because it quickly increases arterial oxygen content with oxygen dissolved in the plasma; the high oxygen tension rapidly reduces the carbon monoxide level in the blood, and HBO hastens carbon monoxide removal from intracellular cytochromes.[7] Breathing fresh air, the half-life of HbCO is 5 h 20 min. Administration of 100% oxygen by a tight-fitting mask decreases this half-life to approximately 80 min. HBO with 100% oxygen at 3 ATA reduces the HbCO half-life to 23 min.[11]

The use of HBO during pregnancy is controversial because of possible adverse fetal effects induced by high oxygen partial pressures.[12] It is important to note, however, that the pressure and duration of exposure in these experiments exceeded those routinely used for therapeutic treatment of carbon monoxide poisoning in humans. In addition, some experimental data have shown that HBO can be used safely during pregnancy.[12]

CLINICAL USE OF HYPERBARIC OXYGEN DURING PREGNANCY

The most extensive trials of HBO and pregnancy have been reported from the Soviet Union,[13] where more than 700 pregnant women have been treated with HBO during all stages of gestation for hypoxemia of various etiologies, including congenital heart defects, toxemia, placental insufficiency, miscarriages, anemia and diabetes. According to these reports, HBO significantly improves various conditions of mother and fetus and reduces perinatal complications and mortality.[3] In the case reported by van Hoesen et al,[6] the patient presented with a dangerously high HbCO level of 47.2% on admission to the emergency room with obvious neurologic involvement and presumed fetal hypoxia. One 90-min treatment at 2.4 ATA reduced the maternal HbCO level to 2.4%. The initial fetal heart rate of 170 bpm with possible late decelerations was highly suggestive of fetal hypoxia. The rapid decrease of FHR to normal after only a few minutes of HBO indicates that HBO was probably extremely beneficial in this case. Cesarean delivery would be an alternative to HBO in this situation, however the potential reversibility of carbon monoxide intoxication by HBO makes cesarean delivery a less attractive option.

RECOMMENDATIONS FOR HBO DURING PREGNANCY

Guidelines for treatment of carbon monoxide intoxication with HBO[14] suggest that patients with HbCO level greater or equal to 25% be treated regardless of symptoms. Patients with HbCO levels less than 25% should be given HBO if neurologic findings are present. Although no guidelines have been set for the pregnant patient, it has been suggested that HBO treatment should be more liberal in pregnant patients because of enhanced fetal vulnerability to carbon monoxide and hypoxia.[8] This suggestion is based upon the higher steady-state levels and the longer elimination half-time in the fetus as compared with the mother.

As previously noted, blood carboxyhemoglobin levels do not necessarily reflect the clinical status of the patient.[8] This becomes particularly important in the case of the pregnant patient. One cannot estimate the fetal HbCO concentration only on the basis of a maternal blood sample. The fetal HbCO level depends on the exposure pattern and equilibration with maternal HbCO. We recommend HBO therapy if signs of fetal distress are present, i.e. fetal tachycardia, decreased beat-to-beat variability on fetal monitor or late decelerations, consistent with the HbCO levels and exposure history.

If HBO is unavailable, 100% oxygen should be administered by a tight-fitting mask for five times as long as needed to reduce maternal HbCO to normal (< 5%). If the patient continues to demonstrate neurologic signs or signs of fetal distress 12 h after initial treatment, additional HBO treatments may be indicated. Multiple HBO treatments have been suggested to be beneficial in severely poisoned and nonresponsive carbon monoxide exposed patients.[14]

REFERENCES

1. Winter P M, Miller J N 1976 Carbon monoxide poisoning. J Am Med Assoc 236: 1520–1504
2. Astrup P, Olsen H M, Trolle D, Kjeldsen K 1972 Effect of moderate carbon monoxide exposure on fetal development. Lancet 2: 1220–1222
3. Longo L D 1977 The biological effects of carbon monoxide on the pregnant woman, fetus and newborn infant. Am J Obstet Gynecol 129: 69–103
4. Hollander D I, Nagey D A, Welch R, Pupkin M 1987 Hyperbaric oxygen therapy for the treatment of acute carbon monoxide poisoning in pregnancy. J Reprod Med 32: 615–617
5. Jennings R T 1987 Women and the hazardous environment: when the pregnant patient requires hyperbaric oxygen therapy. Aviat Space Environ Med 58: 370–374
6. Van Hoesen K B, Camporesi E M, Moon R E, Hage M L, Piantadosi C A 1989 Should hyperbaric O_2 be used to treat the pregnant patient for acute carbon monoxide poisoning? A case report and literature review. J Am Med Assoc 261: 1039–1043
7. Piantadosi C A 1982 Carbon monoxide, oxygen transport and oxygen metabolism. J Hyperb Med 2: 27–44
8. Longo L D, Hill E P 1977 Carbon monoxide uptake and elimination in fetal and maternal sheep. Am J Physiol 232: H323–H330
9. Hill E P, Hill J R, Power G G, Longo L D 1977 Carbon monoxide exchanges between the human fetus and mother: a mathematical model. Am J Physiol 232: H311–H323
10. Pace N, Strajman E, Walker E L 1950 Acceleration of carbon monoxide elimination in man by high pressure oxygen. Science 111: 652–654
11. Peterson J E, Steward R D 1970 Absorption and elimination of carbon monoxide by inactive young men. Arch Environ Health 21: 165–171
12. Ferm V H Teratogenic effects of hyperbaric oxygen. Proc Soc Exp Biol Med 116: 975–976
13. Molzhaninov E V, Chaika V K, Domanova A I, Belousov G V, Zolotukhin N S, Akimova I K 1983 Experience and prospects of using hyperbaric oxygenation in obstetrics. In: Proceedings of the 7th International Congress on Hyperbaric Medicine, Moscow, 1981, Vol 1. Nauka, Moscow, pp 139–141
14. Hyperbaric oxygen therapy: a committee report. Bethesda M D, Undersea and Hyperbaric Medical Society, Bethesda M D, 1986 pp 33–36

98. Computers and fetal monitoring

N. E. Oriol   D. P. Landry   F. M. Bennett

INTRODUCTION

Electronic fetal heart rate (FHR) monitoring was introduced by Hon in 1963.[1] Today, fetal heart rate monitoring is considered a labor management standard for high-risk pregnancy.[2–6] However, no study has proven a consistent relationship between continuous electronic monitoring and improved fetal outcome. Indeed, several recent studies[7,8] have even suggested that electronic monitoring is associated with an increased instrumental or operative delivery rate and is not predictive of positive neurologic outcome.[9] Despite the lack of epidemiologic evidence of the utility of FHR monitoring, there is a considerable body of data relating various fetal states and particular patterns of the FHR trace.[10–15] With the advent of relatively inexpensive, powerful computers it has become possible to examine the fetal ECG (FECG) in much more detail. In this chapter we will examine the monitoring of fetal heart rate variability (FHRV) as a tool in assessing the physiologic state of the fetus during labor and delivery.

A typical FECG recorded from a scalp electrode is shown in Figure 98.1. As can be clearly seen, the heart rate is not constant but varies about a mean value. The variability in heart rate observed between contractions is referred to as baseline variability and may provide information concerning the overall state of the fetus.[11,15,16–19] In addition, heart rate will change in response to a contraction. The timing of these heart rate changes relative to the onset of uterine contraction reflects the ability of the fetus to respond to the stress of changes in uteroplacental blood flow or fetal blood flow and thus provides additional information concerning the physiologic state of the fetus.[20–22]

In this chapter we first briefly review the history and current practice of FHRV monitoring relating some of the observations which have motivated its use. We then briefly examine arguments regarding the physiologic basis of heart rate variability (HRV). Finally, we discuss the current state and potential future applications of FHRV monitoring by reviewing some recent advances in adult cardiology, including monitoring of adult heart rate variability in both health and disease by spectral analysis and nonlinear dynamic techniques and the implications these developments may have for FHRV monitoring. Current techniques of FHRV monitoring are relatively superficial.[23–29] The application of more sophisticated methods based on spectral and nonlinear dynamic (e.g. chaos theory) analysis techniques to determine the structure of heart rate variability in greater detail may provide a more sensitive method of assessing the state of the fetus.

FETAL HEART RATE MONITORING

The aim of fetal heart rate monitoring is to identify fetuses at risk for intrapartum asphyxia and to intervene to avoid a poor outcome. Several investigators have shown that preterm infants are at risk of poor intellectual development,[30,31] and survivors of respiratory distress syndrome have lower average IQs.[30] In 1958, Hon first suggested that the practice of averaging fetal heart rate masked information about the fetal state and that the variability between the individual beats was important. The first

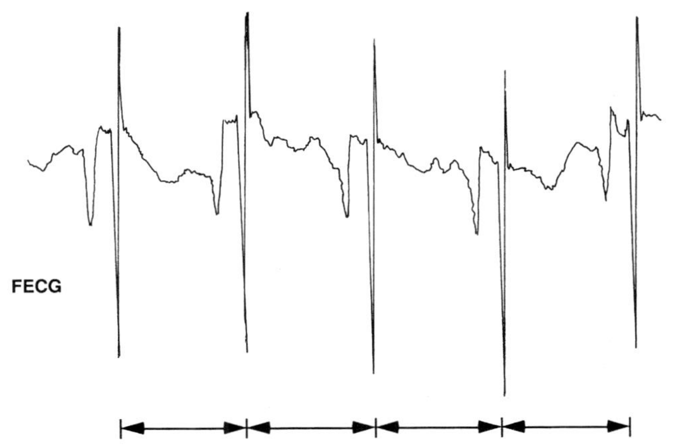

Fig. 98.1A

application of continuous fetal heart rate variability monitoring as a predictor of neonatal outcome was by Hon and Lee[1] in 1963. They documented the absence of variability in a dying fetus. Hammacher et al[11] in 1968 were the first to correlate decreased baseline variability and poor outcome in a large series of patients. Decreased FHRV has subsequently been reported to be predictive of intrauterine deaths[32] and has been associated with low Apgar scores[18] and fetal acidosis.[18,19] The degree of association has varied between studies. This might be because of methodologic differences in experimental design as well as in classifying FHRV.[25,33,34]

In addition, changes in FHRV have been associated with specific pathologic states. Anencephalic fetuses (and adults with severe brain damage) have virtually no HRV unless both the hypothalamus and medulla are intact.[33,35] Infants with respiratory distress syndrome[34,36] and infants at risk for cardiovascular collapse[37] have diminished HRV. In order to better understand how changes in HRV can relate to different fetal conditions it is helpful to examine the current thinking about the underlying physiologic processes responsible for normal HRV.

PHYSIOLOGIC BASIS FOR HEART RATE VARIABILITY

Variability of the beat-to-beat heart rate is a feature of the adult as well as the fetal and neonatal cardiovascular systems.[38] As clinicians, we are usually only aware of averaged vital signs. We take a pulse for 30 s, double it, and record the result as the 'true' heart rate. Even ECG monitors average the heart rate over several beats, thereby smoothing out the instantaneous fluctuations. It has become clear in recent years that these variations are not necessarily due to random noise but result from both interactions between the various components of the cardiovascular control system and the nonlinear nature of the cardiovascular system.[38-43] Thus, one would expect that perturbations to the cardiovascular system should produce changes in the variability of beat-to-beat heart rate.

Heart rate variability is thought to be caused by an interplay of a number of different factors.[40,44,45] These include:

1. inputs to the cardiovascular controller from peripheral baroreceptors and chemoreceptors which form negative feedback loops as well as inputs concerned with thermoregulatory processes;[46]
2. nonlinear interactions of the parasympathetic and sympathetic nervous systems and their effects upon the electrical conduction system of the heart;
3. intrinsic time delays in the responses of the sympathetic and parasympathetic nerves to changes in baroreceptor input[45,47,48] and
4. intrinsic factors in the sinoatrial node.

The human fetus shows an increase in HRV with decreasing heart rate, increasing gestational age, increasing post-natal age, fetal breathing, fetal movement and active sleep.[49-54] Vagal blockade results in an increase in fetal heart rate and a decrease in HRV,[43,45] suggesting that the parasympathetic cardiac inhibitor system plays an important role in the HRV of the human fetus. The sympathetic nervous system appears to have a much smaller effect on FHRV.[56] Changes in FHRV in the absence of a change in the mean heart rate (HR) is very common,[33] but the mechanisms for this effect are unclear. Similar effects have also been reported in the neonatal lamb.[44,57] Other factors described below can also affect FHRV.

Hypoxia decreases human FHRV and increases baseline heart rate,[58-61] but reports in humans[14] as well as animals[58-61] have demonstrated an increased FHRV and decreased heart rate with early hypoxia. These seemingly contradictory data may reflect differential effects of acute versus chronic hypoxia.[33,62] However, it appears unlikely that the changes in HRV during hypoxia are due primarily to changes in pH. In fetal lambs, decreases in pH to 6.9 produce little or no change in FHRV.[15] In addition, the metabolic and blood buffering systems of the fetal lamb appear to withstand up to an hour of hypoxia with little change in pH.

Most anesthetic agents decrease FHRV,[62,63,64] but this does not appear to be to the detriment of the fetus. Parasympatholytics will decrease FHRV, but β-agonists will decrease variability only if the fetal heart rate goes above 160 beats/min.[60]

Early data have shown that heart rate *decreases* progressively after birth as a function of post-natal age but that HRV *increases* as a function of gestational age.[27,58] As neonates grow to adolescence there is a general trend of decreases in both sympathetic and parasympathetic activity. Sympathetic activity stabilizes at approximately age 12, whereas parasympathetic activity continues a slow decline throughout adulthood. Changes in HRV concomitant with uterine contractions during labor have also been studied[65] and may be of particular diagnostic value.

HEART RATE VARIABILITY DURING LABOR

There are two types of fetal heart rate variability which are classified according to whether they are linked to a contraction. Baseline variability refers to HRV that is observed between contractions.[66,67] Transient HRV refers to changes in heart rate that may occur in association with a contraction.[65] Typically, there is a transient decrease in heart rate during a contraction. These transient changes in heart rate are further classified as early, late or variable depending on the timing of the onset of the cardiac deceleration relative to the onset of a uterine contraction. The timing of these decelerations may provide some information as to the status of the fetus.[13,68,69]

Early decelerations are generally thought to be secondary to increases in fetal intracranial pressure and do not indicate fetal distress.[65] However, late decelerations may indicate fetal distress. They are thought to represent utero-placental insufficiency and are a sign of reduced fetal reserve.[13] Variable decelerations (variable onset time and/or variable shape of deceleration) are often a sign of umbilical cord compression[40,70] and can frequently be alleviated by maternal position changes. There is evidence that late or variable decelerations in combination with decreased baseline variability may indicate fetal acidosis.[33]

QUANTIFICATION OF HEART RATE VARIABILITY

Powerful portable computers have enabled more complex analysis of heart rate variability. As in standard fetal heart rate monitors, these advanced techniques treat heart rate as a time series, i.e. a sequence of instantaneous heart rate values (Fig. 98.1B), each value corresponding to a single cardiac cycle. Instantaneous heart rate is typically calculated by identifying the time interval between R-waves on successive beats. The instantaneous heart rate is then calculated as 60/R–R interval(s). For example, an R–R interval of 0.5 s corresponds to an instantaneous heart rate of 120 beats/min. The heart rate time series may then be analyzed to provide clinically important information concerning the status of the cardiovascular system in particular and the state of the patient in general.

Two of the common indices of FHRV are instantaneous (beat-to-beat) variability and long-term variability. Instantaneous variability may be defined as the value of the absolute difference in heart rate between successive beats. Long-term variability may be calculated as the standard deviation of the instantaneous heart rate. This is calculated over a predefined interval. A major limitation of such indices is that they contain no information concerning the temporal dependence of the variations in heart rate. To understand this concept better, consider the following example. Two simulated heart rate tracings are shown in Figure 98.2. In Figure 98.2A, it is assumed that heart rate varies in a sinusoidal fashion, whereas in Figure 98.2B heart rate is random, i.e. the heart rate of any beat is independent of the heart rate of any other beat. Over any

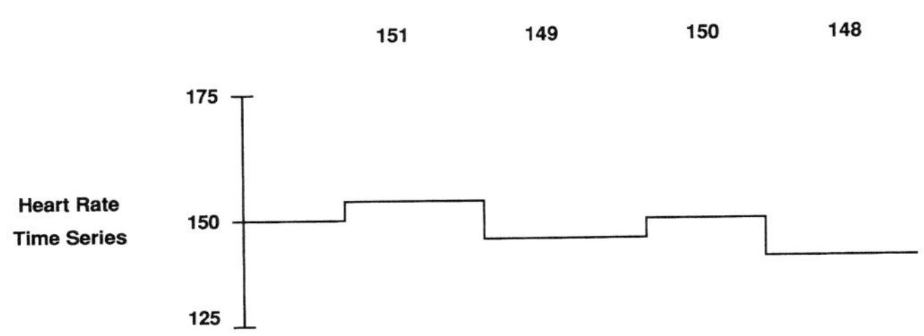

Fig. 98.1B

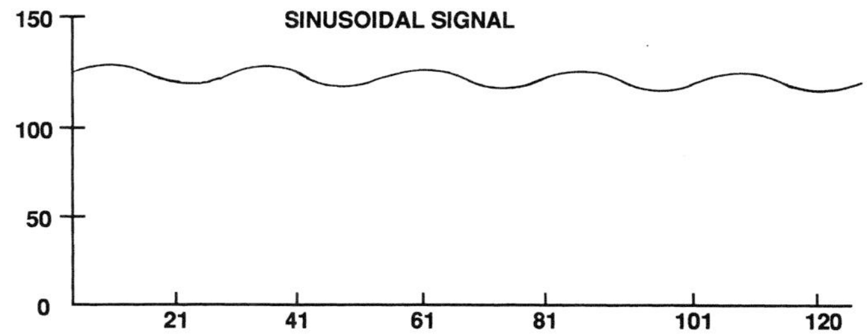

Fig. 98.2A

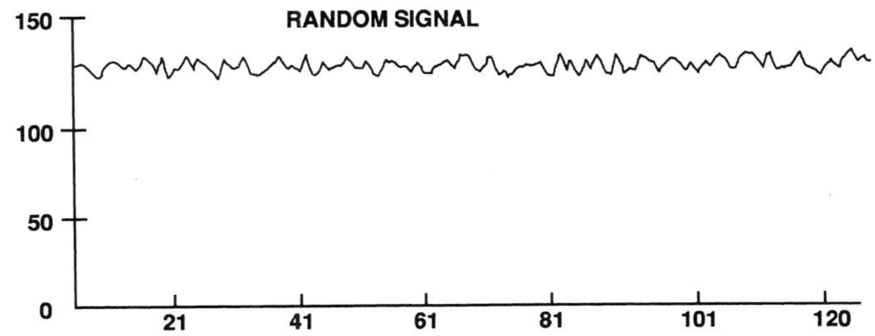

Fig. 98.2B

given interval, the long-term variability calculated as described above could be the same for both signals, even though the dynamic mechanisms of the signals are different. It would be reasonable to expect that the state of the underlying physiologic processes that generated these two curves would be vastly different. An increasing number of data show that the healthy heart rate variability of adults at rest is neither periodic nor random but instead has a complex pattern reminiscent of nonlinear chaos.[41] While chaotic time series may appear random on first inspection, their dynamics have in fact a very complex deterministic structure.[41]

Spectral analysis is a powerful technique for characterizing time series and has been widely applied to the study of cardiovascular control, particularly in the adult.[38] Any time series, such as beat-by-beat heart rate, may be represented as a finite sum of sinusoids, each having a distinct frequency, amplitude and phase. These sinusoids may be displayed as a plot of amplitude versus frequency, which allows an assessment of the relative contributions of various frequency components to the heart rate signal. If heart rate varied with time as a single sinusoid with fixed frequency (Fig. 98.2A), the amplitude of the spectral plot would consist of a single spike at that particular frequency (Fig. 98.3A). If, on the other hand, the variability in heart rate was completely random (Fig. 98.2B), the spectrum would consist of a single value of the amplitude across all frequencies (Fig. 98.3B). If the heart rate dynamics was chaotic, the spectral plot would follow a $1/x$ form, i.e. amplitude would decrease logarithmically with increases in frequency (Fig. 98.3C).

Akselrod et al and others[38,42] have shown that the power

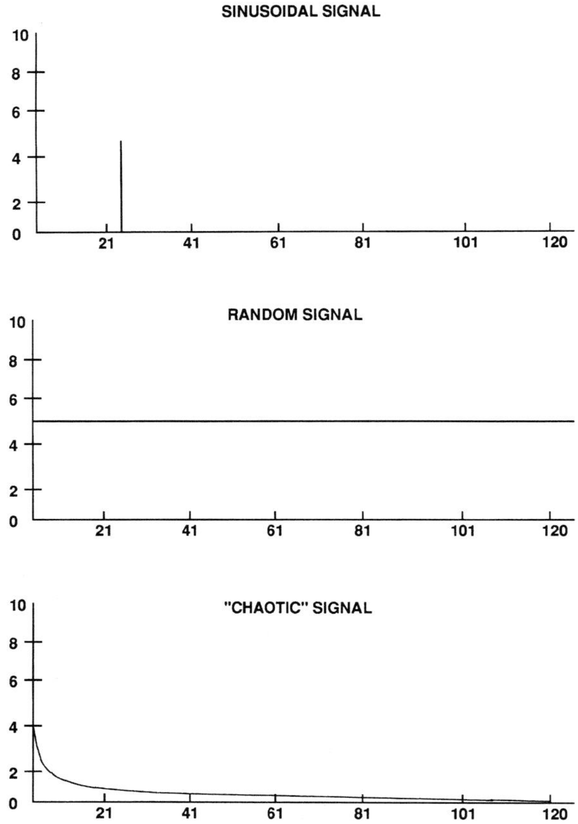

Fig. 98.3

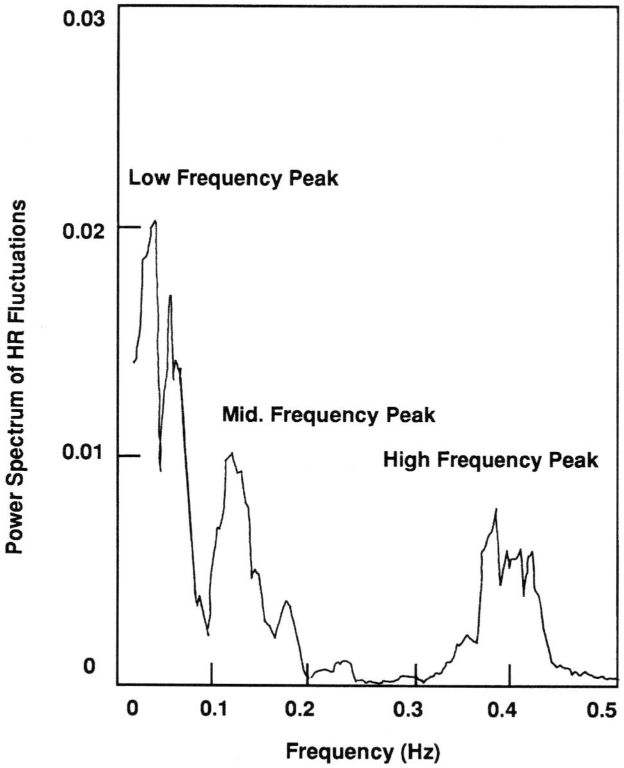

Fig. 98.4

spectral density (PSD) of heart rate in the normal, healthy adult has three major components:

1. a low-frequency peak below 0.1 Hz mediated by both sympathetic and parasympathetic nervous systems;
2. a mid-frequency peak between 0.1 and 0.3 Hz reflecting primarily parasympathetic activity; and
3. a high-frequency peak occurring at greater than 0.3 Hz that corresponds to respiratory effects on heart rate (Fig. 98.4).

The PSD is a plot of power (which is proportional to the square of the amplitude) versus frequency. An oscillation having a greater amplitude would have a greater power. Changes in the PSD may be indicative of disease that produces alterations in the cardiovascular control system. For example, reduced PSDs are seen in patients after transplantation, and further changes in the PSD may be used to identify rejection.[71] A decreased heart rate PSD is also seen in patients following myocardial infarction and correlates with an increased mortality.[72,73] Changes in heart rate PSD have also been observed in patients with congestive heart failure,[74] hypertension[75] and diabetes.[76] Thus, monitoring heart rate variability by spectral analysis in the adult may provide a means of assessing the health of the cardiovascular system. Some evidence suggests this may also be true in the neonate.

Gordon et al[37] observed a 10-fold decrease in the ratio of low-frequency spectral peaks to high-frequency peaks in children who died following cardiac surgery. Changes in the heart rate PSD has been noted in asphyxiated term infants,[77] and in children who subsequently died of sudden infant death syndrome (SIDS).[78,79] The application of spectral analysis techniques in the newborn is made somewhat more complex by the observations that (1) maturational effects may alter the heart rate PSD,[80] (2) the effect of arousal state on HRV may be particularly powerful in the newborn,[48,81] and (3) the physiologic understanding of the origin of the spectral peaks in newborns is less well understood than in adults.[44,75–76,82]

The recent emergence of theories for nonlinear dynamics, such as chaos theory, and their application to the study of the cardiovascular system, has provided a potentially powerful set of tools for studying and monitoring the dynamics of the cardiovascular system.[83–86] 'Chaos' or other nonlinear dynamic analysis can be used to describe erratic time varying changes in cardiovascular variables. Such dynamics are not random, but possess a complex structure which may reflect the nature of the cardiovascular system. Thus, a random time series and a chaotic or other nonlinear time series could have the same mean and variance but the detailed structure of the variability would be substantially different. Recent evidence suggests that changes in the complexity of the heart rate dynamics may be associated with changes in the state or health of the cardiovascular system and some reports suggest that normal sinus rhythm may, in fact, be chaotic.[39,41] A decrease in the complexity of the signal dynamics may foreshadow an impending cardiovascular emergency. For example, it has been observed that the complex dynamics of sinus rhythm can be altered to states in which there is either a marked reduction in variability or the heart rate varies in a periodic, sometimes almost sinusoidal, pattern in heart failure.[74] Also, there is a decrease in complexity of heart rate dynamics with aging.[87,88] Thus, quantitation and monitoring of the loss of physiologic chaos and/or complexity may provide an important method for both predicting the onset of arrhythmias as well as assessing the overall stability of the cardiovascular system and for quantifying the effects of maturation and aging. These nonlinear dynamic analysis techniques are just beginning to be applied to fetal heart monitoring.[89,90] It is important to re-emphasize that fetal hypoxia is often accompanied by a substantial decrease in variability and, most likely, complexity. This may be similar to the loss in heart rate complexity of adults prior to the onset of fatal arrhythmias.[73]

As noted earlier, the analysis of fetal heart rate during contractions has been primarily restricted to determining the magnitude and timing of the deceleration. Other indices such as the deceleration area[91,92] include an element of the response dynamics, not just the delay. Only preliminary attempts at examining HRV during the contraction have been made. The effect of uterine contractions on instantaneous and long-term variabilities of HR have been examined in normal fetuses by calculating these indices over the first and second half of the contraction. Both long-term and instantaneous variability increase during the first half of the contraction but return to precontraction levels in the second half. To describe more completely the HR dynamics during a contraction it will be necessary to be able to determine:

1. the magnitude of the deceleration;
2. the time delay between the onset of a contraction and the deceleration;
3. the dynamics of the deceleration (i.e. how fast does HR decrease?); and
4. how the beat-to-beat variability is affected.

SUMMARY

Current techniques for assessing FHRV are relatively limited because they do not adequately quantify complex dynamics. When compared with the techniques currently being applied to the study of adult HRV, the methods of assessing FHRV are primitive. The application of new techniques, including spectral and nonlinear dynamic analysis, to the study of FHRV may provide more reliable tests of fetal well-being and developmental state and give rise to improved monitoring tools. In addition, it would also be desirable to develop better and more complete techniques of describing the transient changes in heart rate which occur during uterine contractions. Finally, in order for fetal heart rate monitoring to reach its ultimate potential as a diagnostic and monitoring tool it will be necessary to understand the basic mechanisms whereby changes in fetal physiology affect the complex structure of heart rate dynamics underlying these complex physiologic fluctuations.

REFERENCES

1. Hon E H, Lee S T 1963 The electronic evaluation of the fetal heart. VII. Patterns preceding fetal death: further observations. Am J Obstet Gynecol 87: 814
2. American College of Obstetricians and Gynecologists 1988 Statement on fetal heart rate monitoring. ACOG Newsletter 32(11): 5
3. Rooth G et al 1987 Guidelines for the use of fetal monitoring. Int J Gynaecol Obstet 25: 159–167
4. Van den Berg P, Schmidt S, Gesche J, Saling E 1987 Fetal distress and the condition of the newborn using cardiotocography and fetal blood gas analysis during labour. Br J Obstet Gynaecol 96: 72–75
5. Sykes G S, Molloy P M, Johnson P, Stirrat G M, Turnbull A C 1983 Fetal distress and the condition of newborn infants. Br Med J 287: 93–94
6. Zuspan F P, Quilligan E J, Lams J D, Van Geijn H P 1979 Predictors of intrapartum fetal distress: the role of electronic fetal monitoring. Am J Obstet Gynecol 135: 287–291
7. Hess O W 1980 Impact of electronic fetal monitoring on obstetric management. J Am Med Assoc 244: 682–686
8. Banta H D, Thacker S B 1979 Assessing the costs and benefits of electronic fetal monitoring. Obstet Gynecol Surv 34: 627–642
9. Shy K K, Lutht D A, Bennett et al 1990 Effects of electronic monitoring, as compared with periodic auscultation, on the neurologic development of premature infants. New Engl J Med 322: 588–593
10. Murphy K W, Johnson P, Moorcraft J, Pattinson R, Russell V, Turnbull A C 1990 Birth asphyxia and the intrapartum cardiotocograph. Br J Obstet Gynaecol 97: 470–479
11. Hammacher K, Huter K A, Bokelmann J, Werners P H 1968 Foetal heart frequency and perinatal condition of the foetus and newborn. Gynaecologia 166: 3449–3460
12. Van Geijn H P 1985 The value and interpretation of fetal heart rate patterns. In: Clinch J, Matthews T (eds) Perinatal Medicine. MPT Press, Lancaster pp 71–78
13. Rosen K G, Kjellmer 1975 Changes in fetal heart rate and ECG during hypoxia. Acta Physiol Scand 93: 59–166
14. Thaler L, Timor-Tritsch I E, Blumenfeld Z 1985 Effect of acute hypoxia on human fetal heart rate – the significance of increased heart rate variability. Acta Obstet Gynecol Scand 64: 47–50
15. Dalton K J, Dawes G S, Patrick J E 1977 Diurnal, respiratory and other rhythms of fetal heart rate in lambs. Am J Obstet Gynecol 127: 414–424
16. Smith J H, Anand K J S, Cotes P M et al 1988 Antenatal fetal heart rate variation in relation to the respiratory and metabolic status of the compromised human fetus. Br J Obstet Gynaecol 95: 980–989
17. Visser G H A, Sadovsky G, Nicolaides K H 1990 Antepartum fetal

heart rate patterns in small for gestational age third trimester fetuses: Correlations with blood gases obtained at cordocentesis. Am J Obstet Gynecol 182: 698–703
18. Beard R W, Simons E G 1971 Diagnosis of foetal asphyxia in labour. Br J Anaesthes 43: 874–885
19. Zanini B, Paul R H, Huey J R 1980 Intra-partum fetal heart rate; correlation with scalp pH in the preterm fetus. Am J Obstet Gynecol 136: 43–47
20. Melchoir J, Bernard N 1985 Incidence and pattern of fetal heart rate alterations during labor. In: Kunzel W (ed) Fetal heart rate monitoring. Springer-Verlag Berlin pp 73–81
21. Itskovitz J, Goetzman B W, Rudolph A M 1978 The mechanisms of late decelerations of the heart rate and its relationship to oxygenation in normoxemic and chronically hypoxemic fetal lambs. Am J Obstet Gynecol 141: 66–73
22. Kunzel W 1985 Fetal heart rate alterations in partial and total cord occlusion. In: Kunzel W (ed) Fetal heart rate monitoring. Springer-Verlag, Berlin
23. Pello L C, Rosevear S K, Dawes G S, Moulden D M, Redman C W G 1991 Computerized fetal heart rate analysis in labor. Obstet Gynecol 78: 602–610
24. Freeman R 1990 Intrapartum fetal monitoring – a disappointing story. New Engl J Med 322: 624–626
25. Trimbos J B, Keirse M J N C 1978 Observed variability in the assessment of antepartum cardiotocograms. Br J Obstet Gynaecol 85: 900–906
26. Flynn A M, Kelley J, Matthews K 1982 Predictive value of and observer variability in several ways of reporting antepartum cardiotocograms. Br J Obstet Gynaecol 89: 434–440
27. Lotgering F K, Wallenberg H C S, Schouten H J A 1982 Interobserver and intraobserver variation in the assessment of antepartum cardiotocograms. Am J Obstet Gynecol 144: 701–705
28. Nielsen P V, Stigsby B, Nickerson C, Nim J 1987 Intra- and inter-observer variability in the assessment of intrapartum cardiotocograms. Acta Obstet Gynecol Scand 66: 421–424
29. Borgotta I, Shrout P E, Divon M Y 1988 Reliability and reproducibility of non-stress test readings. Am J Obstet Gynecol; 159: 554–558
30. Field T M, Sostek A, Goldberg S, Shuman H (eds) Infants born at risk. Spectrum Press, New York
31. Drillen D M 1964 The growth and development of the prematurely born infant. Williams & Wilkins, Baltimore
32. Tushuizen P B, Soot J E, Ubachs J M 1974 Fetal heart rate monitoring of the dying fetus. Am J Obstet Gynecol 120: 922–931
33. Martin C B 1982 Physiology and clinical use of fetal heart rate variability. Clin Perinat 9: 339–352
34. Kero P 1974 Heart rate variation in infants with respiratory distress syndrome. Acta Paediat Scand 250 (suppl): 1
35. Lowensohn R I, Weiss M, Hon E H 1977 Heart rate variability in brain damaged adults. Lancet 1: 626–628
36. Aarimaa T, Oja R, Antila K, Valimaki I 1988 Interaction of heart rate and respiration in newborn babies. Pediat Res 24: 745–750
37. Gordon D, Herrera V L, McAlpine L et al 1988 Heart rate spectral analysis: a noninvasive probe of cardiovascular regulation in critically ill children with heart disease. Pediat Cardiol 9: 69–77
38. Akselrod S, Gordon D, Ubel F A, Shannon D C, Barger A C, Cohen R J 1981 Power spectrum analysis of heart rate fluctuation: a quantitative probe of beat-to-beat cardiovascular control. Science 213: 220–222
39. Saul J P, Kaplan D T, Kitney R I 1989 Nonlinear interactions between respirations and heart rate: classical physiology or entrained nonlinear oscillators. Inst Electr Electron Eng 299–303
40. Kitney R I, Rompelman O (eds) 1980 The study of heart rate variability. Oxford University Press, New York
41. Goldberger A L 1991 Is the normal heartbeat chaotic or homeostatic. News in Physiol Sci 6: 87–91
42. Pomeranz B, Macaulay R J B, Caudill M A et al 1985 Assessment of autonomic function in humans by heart rate spectral analysis. Am J Physiol 248: H151–153
43. Raeder E A, Berger R, Kenet R, Kiely J P 1987 Assessment of autonomic cardiac control by power spectrum of heart rate fluctuations. J Appl Cardiol 2: 283–300
44. Siimes A S I, Valimaki I A T, Antila K J et al 1990 Regulation of heart rate variation by the autonomic nervous system in neonatal lamb. Pediat Res 27: 383–391
45. Giddens D P, Kitney R I 1985 Neonatal heart rate variability and its relation to respiration. J Theor Biol 113: 759–780
46. Kitney R I 1975 An analysis of the nonlinear behaviour of the human thermal vasomotor control system. J Theor Biol 52: 231–248
47. Koizumi K, Terui N, Kollai M 1985 Effect of cardiac vagal and sympathetic nerve activity on heart rate and rhythmic fluctuations. J Auton Nerv Syst 12: 251–259
48. Warner H R, Russell R O 1969 Effect of combined sympathetic and vagal stimulation on heart rate in the dog. Circ Res 24: 567–573
49. Katona P G, Frasz A, Egbert J 1980 Maturation of cardiac control in full-term and pre-term infants during sleep. Early Human Dev 4: 145–159
50. Siass B, Hodgman J E, Cabal L, Hon E H 1979 Cardiac and respiratory activity in relation to gestation and sleep states in newborn infants. Pediat Res 13: 1163–1166
51. Valimaki I A, Rautahurju P M, Roy S B, Scott K E 1974 Heart rate patterns in healthy term and premature infants and in respiratory distress syndrome. Eur J Cardiol 1: 411–419
52. Wheeler T, Cooke E, Murrils A 1979 Computer analysis of fetal heart rate variation during normal pregnancy. Br J Obstet Gynaecol 86: 186–197
53. Siimes A S I, Valimaki I A T, Sarajas H S S, Sakone K, Oja R T 1984 Heart rate variation in relation to age and sleep state in neonatal lambs. Acta Physiol Scand 537 (suppl): 7–15
54. Divon M Y, Zimmer E Z, Platt L D, Paldi E 1985 Human fetal breathing: associated changes in heart rate and beat-to-beat variability. Am J Obstet Gynecol 151: 403–406
55. Hon E H, Bradfield A H, Hess O W 1961 The electronic evaluation of the fetal heart rate. V. The vagal factor in fetal bradycardia. Am J Obstet Gynecol 82: 291
56. Warner H R, Cox A 1962 A mathematical model of heart rate control by sympathetic and vagus efferent information. J Appl Physiol 17: 349
57. Gronlund J U, Antila K J, Siimes A S I 1989 Beta-adrenergic control and inter-relationships between heart rate and blood pressure in neonatal lambs. Med Biol Eng Comput 27: 163–170
58. Korner P I 1971 Integrative neural cardiovascular control. Physiol Rev 51: 312–367
59. Ikenouse T, Martin C B, Murata Y et al 1981 Effect of acute hypoxia and respiratory acidosis on the fetal heart rate in monkeys. Am J Obstet Gynecol 141: 797–806
60. Martin C B, Van der Wildt B, Jongsma H W et al 1979 Mechanisms of late decelerations in the fetal heart rate. A study with autonomic blocking agents in fetal lambs. Eur J Obstet Gynecol Reprod Biol 9: 361–373
61. Martin C R 1978 Regulation of the fetal heart rate and genesis of FHR patterns. Semin Perinatol Med 2: 131–146
62. Field D R, Parer J T, Auslender R, Baker W B et al 1991 Fetal heart rate variability and cerebral oxygen consumption in fetal sheep during asphyxia. Eur J Obstet Gynecol Reprod Biol 42: 145–153
63. Hon E H 1975 An introduction to fetal heart rate monitoring, 2nd edn. Harty, New Haven
64. Yeh S Y, Paul R H, Cordero L et al 1974 A study of diazepam during labor. Obstet Gynecol 43: 363–373
65. Thaler I, Timor I E, Goldberg I 1988 Interpretation of the fetal ECG during labor: the effect of uterine contractions. J Perinat Med 16: 373–379
66. Kariniemi V, Katila T, Laine H, Ammala P 1980 On-line quantification of fetal heart rate variability. J Perinat Med 8: 213–216
67. Kariniemi V, Ammala P 1981 Short-term variability of fetal heart rate during pregnancies with normal and insufficient placental function. Am J Obstet Gynecol 139: 33–37
68. Saito J, Okamura K, Akagi K et al 1988 Alteration of FHR pattern associated with progressively advanced fetal acidemia caused by cord compression. Nippon Sanka Fujinka Gakkai Zasshi 40: 775–780
69. Akagi K, Okamura K, Endo C H et al 1988 The slope of the fetal heart rate deceleration is predictive of fetal condition during repeated umbilical cord compression in sheep. Am J Obstet Gynecol 159: 516–522
70. Tortosa M N, Acien P 1990 Evaluation of variable decelerations of

fetal heart rate with the deceleration index: Influence of associated abnormal parameters and their relation to the state and evolution of the newborn. Eur J Obstet Gynecol Reprod Biol 34: 235–245
71. Sands K E F, Appel M L, Lilly L S, Schoen F J, Mudge G H, Cohen R J 1989 Power spectrum analysis of heart rate variability in human cardiac transplant recipients. Circulation 79: 76–82
72. Kleiger R E, Miller J P, Bigger J T, Moss A J 1987 Decreased heart rate variability and its association with increased mortality after acute myocardial infarction. Am J Cardiol 59: 256–262
73. Myers G A, Martin G J, Magid N M et al 1986 Power spectral analysis of heart rate variability in sudden cardiac death: comparison to other methods. Inst Electr Electron Eng Trans Biomed Eng 33: 1149–1156
74. Saul J P, Arai Y, Berger R D, Lilly L S, Colucci W S, Cohen R J 1988 Assessment of autonomic regulation in chronic congestive heart failure by heart rate spectral analysis. Am J Cardiol 61: 1292–1299
75. Mancia G, Ferrari A, Gregorini L et al 1983 Blood pressure and heart rate variabilities in normotensive and hypertensive human beings. Circ Res 53: 96–104
76. Ewing D J, Campbell I W, Clarke B 1980 Assessment of cardiovascular effects in diabetic autonomic neuropathy and prognostic implications. Ann Intern Med 92: 308–311
77. Divon M Y, Winkler H, Yeh S Y, Platt L D, Langer O, Merkatz I R 1986 Diminished respiratory sinus arrhythmia in asphyxiated term infants. Am J Obstet Gynecol 155: 1263–1266
78. Gordon D, Southall D P, Kelly D H et al 1986 Analysis of heart rate and respiratory patterns in sudden infant death syndrome victims and control infants. Pediat Res 20: 680–684
79. Kluge K A, Harper R M, Schechtman V L, Wilson A J, Hoffman H J, Southall D P 1988 Spectral analysis assessment of respiratory sinus arrhythmia in normal infants and infants who subsequently died of sudden infant death syndrome. Pediat Res 24: 677–682
80. Baldzer K, Dykes F D, Jones S A, Brogan M, Carrigan T A, Giddens D P 1989 Heart rate variability analysis in full-term infants: Spectral indices for study of neonatal cardiorespiratory control. Pediat Res 26: 188–195
81. Griffin R L, Caron F J M, van Geijn H P 1985 Behavioral states in the human fetus during labor. Am J Obstet Gynecol 152: 828–833
82. Hathorn M K S 1989 Respiratory modulation of heart rate in newborn infants. Early Human Dev 20: 81–99
83. Ruelle D 1980 Strange attractors. Mathematical Intell 2: 126
84. Smith J M, Cohen R J 1984 Simple finite element model accounts for wide range of cardiac dysrhythmias. Proc Nat Acad Sci USA 81: 233–237
85. Kelso J A S, Mandell A J, Shlesinger M F (eds) 1988 Dynamic patterns in complex systems. World Scientific, Teaneck, N J
86. Goldberger A L, Rigney D R Nonlinear dynamics at the bedside. In: Glass L, Humter P (eds) Theory of heart. Springer, Berlin
87. Kaplan D T, Furman M I, Pincus S M, Ryan S M et al 1991 Ageing and the complexity of cardiovascular dynamics. Bio Phys J 59: 945–949
88. Lipsitz L A, Mietus J, Moody G B, Goldberger A L 1990 Spectral characteristics of heart rate variability before and during postural tilt relation to ageing and risk of syncope. Circulation 81: 1803–1810
89. Karin J, Hirsch M, Akselrod S 1993 An estimate of fetal autonomic state by spectral analysis of fetal heart rate fluctuations. Pediatr Res 34: 134–138
90. Chaffin D G, Goldberg C E, Reed K L 1991 The dimension of chaos in the fetal heart rate. Am J Obstet Gynecol 165(5): 1425–1429
91. Tournaire M, Yeh S Y, Forsythe A, Hon E H 1973 A study of fetal heart rate deceleration areas: I. Preliminary exploration. Obstet Gynecol 42: 711–717
92. Beguin F, Yeh S Y, Forsythe A, Hon E H 1975 A study of fetal heart rate deceleration areas: II. Correlation between deceleration areas and fetal pH during labor. Obstet Gynecol 45(3): 292–298

99. Is continuous fetal heart rate monitoring necessary with epidural anesthesia?

R. Martin

The issue of fetal heart rate (FHR) monitoring during normal labor and delivery has been addressed by the American College of Obstetrics and Gynecology (ACOG) and the specific recommendations are:[1]

1. The fetal heart rate tracing should be examined before an epidural block is initiated.
2. Once the mother is positioned for the block, the FHR should be rechecked.
3. If placement of the epidural block takes more than 5–10 min, the FHR should be rechecked.
4. When an adequate level of epidural analgesia is established, the FHR should be checked every 15 min during active labor and at least every 5 min during the second stage of labor.

The American Society of Anesthesiologists (ASA) has established Guidelines for Conduction Anesthesia in Obstetrics. The guidelines of importance to our discussion include:[2]

Guideline I

Major conduction anesthesia (lumbar or caudal epidural, subarachnoid or bilateral lumbar sympathetic block) shall be initiated and maintained only in locations in which appropriate resuscitation equipment and drugs are immediately available to manage procedurally related problems (e.g. hypotension, respiratory depression, convulsions and myocardial depression).

Resuscitation equipment shall include: sources of oxygen and suction, equipment to maintain an airway and perform endotracheal intubation and a means to provide positive-pressure ventilation. Drugs and equipment for cardiopulmonary resuscitation shall be immediately available.

Guideline II

Major conduction blocks in obstetrics shall be initiated and maintained by or under the direction of a physician with appropriate privileges.

Physicians must be approved through the institutional credentialing process to administer or supervise the administration of obstetric anesthesia and must be qualified to manage procedurally related complications.

Guideline III

Major conduction anesthesia should not be administered until the patient has been examined, and the fetal status and progress of labor evaluated by a qualified physician who is readily available to supervise the labor and to deal with any obstetric complications that may arise.

The ACOG recommendations provide a definite answer to the question posed for this chapter. The recommendations by the ASA do not dictate obstetric management but are meant to answer the 'What if. . . ?' questions that relate to the inherent dangers, however small, of the use of an anesthetic technique.

Whether continuous electronic FHR monitoring offers advantages over intermittent auscultation has been the focus of a number of ongoing studies.

Probably more important in the decision as to how the mother and fetus are monitored is the availability of adequate nursing staff to provide 'one-on-one' coverage; that is, the ability to have one nurse take care of one parturient at a time. At a busy obstetric service, particularly a tertiary referral center, this might not be possible except for the sick or problem parturient. As a result, electronic FHR monitoring, either external or internal, is a necessary adjunct to an overstretched nursing staff.

THE ISSUES BEHIND THE ANSWER

Monitoring the fetus throughout parturition has evolved considerably because of biochemical and technical advances that result in a more knowledgeable assessment of the fetus. During labor and delivery, the fetus can be monitored directly with FHR monitoring, either externally or internally, as well as by fetal scalp blood sampling. Monitoring techniques are used not only for diagnostic purposes, thereby serving a preventive role, but are also necessary for treatment, should the fetus be stressed.

In this chapter stress to the fetus will be defined as either hypoxia or asphyxia, because the supply of oxygen to the fetus is crucial. Any diminution or cessation of oxygenation results in an immediate change in the biochemical status of the fetus that affects all organs, particularly the heart and the brain. There are compensatory responses by the fetus, but the fetal reserve capacity is limited. Therefore, it is important to recognize the fetal response to stress, identify the cause and treat it as quickly as possible.

Anesthesia and analgesia, as an integral part of obstetric delivery, can affect the outcome of labor and delivery, depending on the status of the fetus. In a small number of cases, the effect can be detrimental. For this reason, it is important to have an understanding of the potential impact of epidural anesthesia on the mother and fetus.

In an attempt to delineate the issues that the above question raises, this chapter will point out the effects of local anesthetics in the epidural space. This will be considered in some detail because of the possible consequences to the mother and fetus. Particular diseases in obstetrics in which there is a greater likelihood of fetal asphyxia and/or hypoxia, will be mentioned because of the need to monitor the fetus closely. Finally, two case reports will be presented to illustrate some of the points made.

EFFECTS OF EPIDURAL ANESTHESIA ON THE PARTURIENT AND THE FETUS

An epidural anesthetic, when administered to a parturient, may affect the fetus in one of two ways:

1. through effects of local anesthetics on the fetus through fetal uptake (i.e. directly);
2. indirectly through changes in maternal uterine blood flow and/or oxygenation that secondarily affect the fetus.

As these changes may alter FHR, which reflects fetal well-being, the effects of regional anesthesia must be considered before attempting to answer the original question.

Direct effects of local anesthetics on the fetus

Several factors contribute to the direct effects of local anesthetics on the fetus:

- placental transfer;
- fetal uptake and distribution;
- fetal biotransformation and excretion; and
- toxicity in the fetus.

It is worth considering each of these issues in some detail.

Placental transfer of local anesthetics

Table 99.1 is a compilation of current data on the maternal and fetal blood concentrations of local anesthetics after maternal epidural administration. This demonstrates that local anesthetics cross the placenta from the maternal to the fetal blood and appear in measurable quantities in the fetal circulation. Although local anesthetics cross the placenta by passive diffusion,[14,15] other factors influence the amount transported: drug binding[14] and metabolism by maternal proteins and the placenta itself;[14,16] changes in maternal blood flow;[14,15] active transport across the placenta; and a number of disease states (diabetes mellitus, preeclampsia, pregnancy-induced hypertension) that could alter placental permeability to local anesthetics.[14–16]

The pK_a of the individual local anesthetic can also influence the amount that crosses the placenta. Local anesthetics are weak bases with pK_as between 7.6 and 8.7 so that it is the unionized form that crosses the placenta. Thus, at a given pH, the higher the pK_a, the less local anesthetic that is in the unionized form and, therefore, available to cross the placenta. As an example, the proportion of 2-chloroprocaine, with a pK_a of 8.7, in the unionized form at pH 7.4 is 4.8%, compared with 24% for lidocaine (pK_a 7.9) and 17% for bupivacaine (pK_a 8.1).[17,18] At similar maternal blood levels, more lidocaine would cross the placenta than bupivacaine and 2-chloroprocaine.

Of the two structural groups of local anesthetics, amides and esters, the amides are metabolized principally in the

Table 99.1 Concentrations of commonly used local anesthetics (LA) in maternal and neonatal blood after maternal epidural administration

LA	*n*	Maternal dose (mg)	Maternal blood (µg/ml)	Fetal blood (µg/ml)	Reference
Bupivacaine	18	37.3	0.77	0.16	3
	70	47.7	0.54	0.01	4
	21	56.7	0.22	0.08	5
	32	96.7	0.24	0.08	5
Lidocaine	9	266	2.8	1.6	6
	6	398	2.8	1.7	7
	6	423	2.3	1.2	8
	46	502	2.6	1.8	9
Etidocaine	81	250	1.33	0.38	10
Mepivacaine	25	374	2.9	1.8	8
	26	341	1.8	0.8	11
	30	776	3.5	2.6	11
Chloroprocaine	34	838	3.9	3.0	12
	17	852	2.7	6.6	13

liver. Because the volume of distribution of the amide local anesthetics is large, the liver is able to metabolize a fraction of an injected or absorbed dose. This leads to relatively long half-lives (i.e. 90 min for lidocaine in a non-pregnant human)[19] and slow decline in plasma concentrations. When large doses of an amide local anesthetic are given frequently over a long period of time, fetal levels begin to rise, indicating systemic accumulation.[20,21]

Ester local anesthetics are hydrolyzed by either plasma or liver esterases.[19,22] Although the placenta has an esterase, there is no indication that it contributes significantly to the hydrolysis of ester-linked local anesthetics.[23,24] The hydrolysis occurs quickly, such that for procaine maternal intravenous doses of 4 mg/kg result in no placental transfer.[25] With larger doses, up to 10 mg/kg, umbilical concentrations of procaine are 8.5 μg/ml and are not associated with any detrimental effect on the fetus.[26]

Uptake and distribution by the fetus

The pattern of venous return and then the distribution of cardiac output directly determines the concentration of local anesthetics in fetal tissues.[25,27] The bulk of umbilical artery blood is channeled through the liver.[28] Whether the fetal liver, like the adult, can remove a substantial amount of lidocaine during a single passage, preventing high drug levels, is not known. The next organs to receive a large amount of local anesthetic (although less than in the umbilical artery) are the heart and the brain. In the guinea pig, the fetal myocardium contains high concentrations of local anesthetics after maternal administration.[29] Because the blood–brain barrier is poorly developed, concentrations of local anesthetics after maternal administration are first measured within minutes, then peak at 20–30 min, with a decline similar to that in plasma.[30,31]

Because hypoxia and asphyxia can cause systemic acidosis, this shift in pH can have several effects on the distribution of local anesthetics. Acidosis increases the fetal to maternal lidocaine ratio because of trapping the ionized form of lidocaine in the fetal circulation, resulting in increased lidocaine concentrations.[32] Fetal catecholamine production is increased, resulting in greater flow through the ductus venosus, which shunts a larger portion of umbilical artery blood flow to the heart and brain.[33] In addition, a rising fetal $P\text{CO}_2$ will also increase cerebral blood flow.[33] The above compensatory changes in the circulation increase the concentration of local anesthetics in these organs. Cerebral vascular permeability is also increased, thus enhancing local anesthetic diffusion across the blood–brain barrier.[34] It is possible that acidosis could also decrease protein binding of local anesthetics (as has been demonstrated with bilirubin–albumin)[35] to increase the amount of free drug available to cross the blood–brain barrier.

Biotransformation and excretion by the fetus

As mentioned above, for amide local anesthetics, the liver is the primary site of local anesthetic metabolism.[19] Although fetal hepatic enzymatic activity is less than in adults, Shnider and Way[36] found similar decay curves for maternal and fetal plasma lidocaine concentrations, after administering 3 mg/kg to the mother. Brown et al[37] followed neonatal plasma levels for lidocaine, mepivacaine and bupivacaine for up to 24 h after delivery with epidural anesthesia. The half-life for these local anesthetics were: 9 h for mepivacaine, 3 h for lidocaine and slightly less than 2 h for bupivacaine.

Amniotic fluid[38] and neonatal urine[6] contain measurable quantities of local anesthetics and their metabolites after maternal administration. One study found increasing quantities of lidocaine metabolites in neonatal urine with time after maternal epidural anesthesia,[6] so that, unlike the adult, where the kidney plays a minor role in excreting local anesthetics, fetal and neonatal renal excretion is probably significant.

Toxicity in the fetus

Although lumbar epidural blood with local anesthetics rarely results in toxic fetal blood levels, there are several situations in which fetal toxicity can develop:

1. unintentional intravenous injection of local anesthetic;
2. epidural injection of large doses over a brief period of time;
3. prolonged infusion of local anesthetics;
4. direct fetal injection (usually seen with a paracervical block).

The organ systems first affected are the central nervous and cardiovascular systems because of blood flow distribution. In addition, the fetus might be more sensitive to local anesthetics than an adult because the fetal capacity for binding local anesthetics to plasma proteins is 50–60% of that of an adult.[39] This results in more free form of the drug being available in the fetus.

With CNS toxicity, the most common findings are tremors, twitching and convulsions, associated with neonatal depression.[40] Subtle neurobehavioral changes have been described by Scanlon et al[41] in the absence of neonatal depression, 2–8 h after the use of epidural lidocaine and mepivacaine for an uncomplicated labor and delivery. A subsequent study found no neurobehavioral effect after the use of bupivacaine and 2-chloroprocaine.[42] Long-range studies demonstrate that any changes noted, as with lidocaine, are transient and short-lived.[43]

Unlike adults, in whom the response of the cardiovascular system to toxic doses of local anesthetics is peripheral vasodilation, decreased myocardial contractility, bradycardia and hypotension,[17,44] the fetal response is variable.

Studies in fetal lamb preparations have demonstrated bradycardia with large doses of mepivacaine[45] and lidocaine.[46] Tachycardia and acidosis have also been described with large doses of lidocaine. The changes noted were also related to gestational age, with fetuses less than 120 days responding minimally compared with older fetuses.[47]

Indirect effects of local anesthetics on the fetus

Epidural blockade can cause changes in uterine blood flow because of maternal hypotension.[48] The loss of sympathetic tone results in venous pooling. The fact that approximately one-sixth of maternal blood volume is in the uterus and that both the aorta and the inferior vena cava can be partially or completely occluded makes the parturient at term susceptible to hypotension.[49] The decrease in blood pressure can be minimized by acute hydration with crystalloid, just prior to the administration of the block, rapid treatment of a downward trend in blood pressure with ephedrine and crystalloid and left uterine displacement.[45]

The treatment of maternal hypotension with vasopressors can result in constriction of uterine vessels leading to a decrease in uterine blood flow.[50,51] Vasopressors with predominant α-adrenergic activity, such as methoxamine, phenylephrine or norepinephrine decrease uterine blood flow, causing fetal asphyxia.[52,53] Metaraminol, which has both α- and β-adrenergic activity, also decreases uterine blood flow.[53] Ephedrine and mephentermine have predominant β-activity and are effective at increasing maternal blood pressure without causing uterine artery vasoconstriction.[53,54] It is thought that the mechanism of action is by central stimulation, resulting in positive inotropic and chronotropic activity, with little effect on uterine blood flow.

Local anesthetics can cause uterine artery vasoconstriction through direct action on the vascular wall in vitro.[55,56] However, concentrations well above those seen in clinical use are required to demonstrate a decrease in uterine blood flow.

Because the uterine muscle has both α- and β–adrenergic receptors, it can respond with hypertonus to a wide number of catecholamines. In addition, local anesthetics can cause uterine hypertonus and tetanus.[57] Predominant α-adrenergic drugs, such as methoxamine, result in uterine hypertonus and a decrease in uterine blood flow.[58] The α-effects of epinephrine predominate at high levels and can also cause myometrial tetany. The β-effects are at the other extreme and cause smooth muscle relaxation and uterine hypotonus. The transient uterine relaxation that is seen after establishment of an epidural block is due to the low levels of circulating local anesthetic following absorption from the epidural space.[58] With high levels of local anesthetics found after unintentional intravenous injection, uterine hypertonus results.[57]

Fetal consequences of decreased uterine blood flow

The effects of maternal hypotension on the fetus relate directly to the etiology, depth and duration of the hypotension as well as the basal fetal state. An episode of hypotension can increase risk to the fetus when uterine blood flow is further reduced by either uterine artery vasoconstriction or uteroplacental insufficiency. When uterine blood flow is decreased for a prolonged period of time, fetal asphyxia results.

The fetal organ systems first affected by severe hypotension are the central nervous system, the heart and the lungs. In monkeys, maternal blood pressure of 40 mmHg or less causes fetal asphyxia with a reduction in fetal Po_2 from 31 mmHg to 15 mmHg. With mild asphyxia (pH 7.10) there is no permanent organ system damage, but when severe asphyxia (pH 7.00) lasts several hours fetal death from cardiovascular failure results.[59,60] When the stress is intermediate, permanent brain damage with lesions similar to those of human cerebral palsy occurs.[60,61] Hypoxia and acidosis may be causative factors in adult respiratory distress syndrome because pulmonary hypoperfusion may lead to depletion of pulmonary surfactant.[62,63]

In humans, there are few studies that can examine this issue in a systematic manner because of the limited ability to monitor the fetus and measure maternal uterine blood flow. However, it has been shown that after the onset of an epidural block late decelerations in the FHR tracing can develop when the maternal systolic blood pressure drops below 100 mmHg for 5–7 min.[64] This is quickly corrected with oxygen and conventional measures to increase blood pressure (left uterine displacement, increased intravenous fluid administration and ephedrine). Transient decreases in maternal blood pressure do not adversely affect the FHR tracing.[65]

Maternal hypoxia

Maternal hypoxia, while a rare complication of epidural anesthesia, can be due to maternal convulsions from toxic blood levels of a local anesthetic or from an unintentional total spinal block. The prevalence of convulsions can be as high as 0.5% in large series of epidural anesthetics.[66] Total spinal anesthesia occurs in approximately 0.03% of patients receiving lumbar epidural anesthesia and may quickly result in profound hypotension, unconsciousness and cardiac arrest.[66] For both convulsions and a 'total spinal', the primary treatment is to maintain the maternal airway and provide adequate oxygenation. Then treatment of seizures with a benzodiazepine or support of maternal circulation with vasopressors and intravenous fluids must be undertaken.[67]

Fetal reaction to stress

During labor and delivery, the main causes of stress for the fetus are hypoxia and asphyxia. Fetal hypoxia is due to the mother breathing a hypoxic mixture of gases and results in decreased oxygen tension presenting to the uteroplacental unit. Fetal asphyxia is secondary to a reduction of at least 50% in uterine blood flow. In addition to decreased oxygen tension, there is also increased carbon dioxide tension, producing both metabolic and respiratory acidosis. With prolonged asphyxia, the fetus switches to anerobic metabolism and there is a build-up of lactic acid. Metabolic acidosis subsequently develops.

The fetal responses to hypoxia or asphyxia are:

1. bradycardia (due to increased vagal activity) with hypertension;
2. slight decrease in ventricular output;
3. redistribution of blood from the splanchnic bed to the heart, brain, placenta and adrenal glands[68]
4. decrease in fetal breathing movements (from 39% to 7% of the time);
5. terminal gasping movements (with asphyxia);
6. increased α-adrenergic activity.

In chronically instrumented sheep, fetal oxygen consumption decreases as much as 60% from control values with hypoxia.[69] This is accompanied by fetal bradycardia, increase in fetal blood pressure and progressive metabolic acidosis. The fetal sheep can tolerate this state for approximately 1 h. These changes are rapidly reversed with restoration of oxygenation.[70] Fetal cerebral[71] and myocardial[72] oxygen consumption have been shown to remain constant. When hypoxia is prolonged or proceeds to asphyxia, these compensatory mechanisms are lost.

The ability to reverse the effects of hypoxia or asphyxia depends on the recognition of signs and symptoms. This is where fetal monitoring is crucial.

OBSTETRIC CONSIDERATIONS

Aside from normal labor and delivery in healthy parturients, there are a number of conditions or diseases in obstetrics in which the fetus is at increased risk of a sudden alteration in oxygenation. In these cases, where possible, the mother and fetus should receive close, careful monitoring not only during labor and delivery but during the course of pregnancy as well. These conditions generally reflect vascular compromise that results in decreased uteroplacental perfusion and a compromised fetus. Because these conditions can occur either acutely or chronically, the fetus can deteriorate very quickly or slowly accordingly. Epidural anesthesia may play an integral part in the management of some of these diseases.

Antepartum hemorrhage leads to an acute decrease or cessation of uteroplacental perfusion, placing the fetus at immediate risk of death. The most common causes are:

1. abruptio placentae;
2. placenta previa;
3. uterine rupture.

In these cases, epidural or regional anesthesia is relatively contraindicated because of the possible exacerbation of hypotension with the vasodilation produced by the sympathetic block, potential associated clotting abnormalities and the emergent need for delivery. Fetal monitoring is imperative to follow the condition of the fetus.

More likely to include epidural anesthesia as a part of the management in labor and delivery are a number of diseases with a chronic decrease in uteroplacental perfusion and/or oxygen supply:

1. Hypertensive disorders of pregnancy, including preeclampsia and eclampsia, are characterized by an underlying vasoconstriction that results in marginal placental function. The vasodilating effects of the sympathetic blockade from epidural anesthesia during labor has been shown to improve uteroplacental blood flow.[73]
2. Diabetes in pregnancy covers a wide range of symptoms and treatment, but placental abnormalities have been found with even mild, well-controlled gestational diabetes.[74] A 35–45% decrease in placental blood flow, compared with healthy parturients, means decreased oxygen transport and buffering capacity.[75] Concomitant problems are major congenital anomalies, respiratory distress syndrome, macrosomia and neonatal hypoglycemia, all of which mean a significant risk for fetal morbidity and mortality.
3. Acute exacerbations of asthma, as can occur in 25–40% of parturients with underlying asthma, are associated with an increased incidence of preterm delivery, low-birthweight infants and perinatal death.[76]
4. Obesity is associated with an increased risk of hypertensive diseases of pregnancy, diabetes, malpresentation (especially breech presentation) and high-birthweight infants.[77,78]

These disease states occur in many of the people who undergo careful monitoring during pregnancy and, as a result, they may require an elective induction of labor for a positive oxytocin challenge test, post-dates gestation, worsening symptoms or have a compromised fetus that is intrauterine growth retarded.

Deviations from the labor curve (protracted active phase, prolonged descent) place both the mother and fetus at increased risk of morbidity and mortality. With prolonged labor, particularly with ruptured membranes, there is an increased incidence of chorioamnionitis.[79] When the disorder becomes an arrest due to cephalopelvic disproportion, a cesarean delivery is essential.

Multiple gestations present several stresses to the mother, fetuses and health care providers:

1. Premature labor occurs 6–10 times more frequently than in single gestations.[80,81] This accounts for the significant morbidity and mortality.
2. Preeclampsia and eclampsia.
3. Prolonged labor, possibly due to ineffective uterine contractions from the distended uterine myometrium.
4. Maternal anemia, despite the increase in blood volume (occurs 40% more frequently than with single gestations).
5. Antepartum and post-partum hemorrhage. Uterine distension contributes to this and results in a uterus that does not contract after the delivery of the placenta. Blood loss with delivery is twice that occurring with a single fetus. Manual extraction of the placenta is required twice as often as for a single gestation.
6. Supine hypotension is more severe and frequent because of the large uterus compressing the aorta and inferior vena cava.
7. Increased incidence of malpresentation.

Substance abuse is a broad term that covers a wide range of drugs that can have several effects, but is increasingly seen over a wide socioeconomic range. In general, parturients who are substance abusers are treated as high-risk pregnancies, not only because they present late in their pregnancy for prenatal care or frequently have no prenatal care, but also because of other associated problems: preterm labor, placental abruption, intrauterine growth retardation and preeclampsia. While fetal monitoring during labor and delivery is imperative, the use of epidural anesthesia depends on the level of patient cooperation. In some instances, general anesthesia might be necessary to effect a controlled cesarean delivery.

CASE REPORTS

A.B. is a 28-year-old G3P2 woman who presented to the labor and delivery unit in premature labor with ruptured membranes at 36 weeks' gestation. She had a prior history of intravenous drug abuse but denied any drug use during this pregnancy. On vaginal examination, the cervix was dilated 4 cm. TDx of the amniotic fluid was 112 (mature). The obstetrician decided to let labor progress. A fetal scalp electrode was placed and the FHR tracing was reactive. The patient requested epidural anesthesia. Accordingly, an epidural catheter was placed uneventfully in the L3–4 interspace. After an initial dose of 12 ml 0.25% bupivacaine, a bilateral T10 level was obtained and a continuous infusion of 0.125% bupivacaine with 2 μg/ml fentanyl was started. The patient was comfortable. Over the next 4 h, her cervix fully dilated (to 10 cm.) During the second stage of labor, the FHR demonstrated progressively deeper variable decelerations with each contraction and pushing. Because the obstetrician felt that the patient was not pushing effectively, she requested that the rate of the epidural infusion be decreased. After a total of 3 h of pushing and because of deep variable decelerations, the obstetrician elected to perform a low forceps vaginal delivery. In the delivery room, with her legs in stirrups, the patient complained of perineal discomfort. A top-up dose of 10 ml 2% lidocaine was administered. Within 1 min, the patient's eyes rolled back, she complained of difficulty breathing, her fingers twitched and she quickly became unresponsive with no frank seizure activity. The FHR decreased to 50 beats/min. Forceps were then used to deliver a liveborn female infant with Apgars of 2 and 8. The mother continued to breathe spontaneously throughout the episode of unresponsiveness. Her oxygen saturation was 98–100% and her pulse was 70–80. She was treated with supplemental oxygen and observation. She quickly regained consciousness and was alert throughout the episiotomy repair, so that she could complain of pain from the suturing. Rather than use the epidural catheter again, the obstetrician injected lidocaine locally. After the repair and just prior to removing the epidural catheter, an attempt to aspirate fluid was negative.

C.D. is a 19-year-old G1P0 woman with a 38-week gestation who was admitted to labor and delivery with worsening preeclampsia. She had been on the high-risk obstetric service as an inpatient for bed rest for the past week. On admission to labor and delivery unit, her blood pressure was 170/105 and was associated with bilateral pitting ankle edema, two beats of clonus and proteinuria. Intravenous magnesium sulfate was begun and a Foley catheter was placed in her bladder. Over a 3 h period her blood pressure fell to 150/90. The obstetricians decided to induce labor with intravenous oxytocin. A consultant anesthesiologist was called because of the patient's preeclampsia and weight (260 lb). During 5 h of oxytocin stimulation, the cervix dilated to 3 cm and the blood pressure remained 150/95. The amniotic membranes were ruptured and a fetal scalp electrode was placed. Because the patient complained of painful uterine contractions, an epidural catheter was placed after checking the patient's clotting parameters (prothrombin time, partial thromboplastin time, platelet count and fibrinogen), which were normal. A T9 level was achieved with 10 ml 0.25% bupivacaine. A continuous infusion of 0.125% bupivacaine with 2 μg/ml fentanyl was begun. The patient's blood pressure fell to 130/80 and remained at that level over the next 6 h as the cervix dilated to 8 cm. During this time, the patient developed a fever of

100.2°F (°C) and fetal tachycardia was noted. She was begun on antibiotics. After another hour, with adequate contractions induced by the maximal dose of oxytocin, the cervix was still 8 cm. An arrest of dilation due to cephalopelvic disproportion was diagnosed and a decision for cesarean delivery was made. The epidural infusion was stopped and 0.5% bupivacaine was used to raise the level of anesthesia to T4. This was done over a 30-min period and 30 ml of bupivacaine was used. There was no change in the fetal tachycardia during this time. A cesarean delivery was performed and a liveborn, female infant with Apgar scores of 7 and 8 was delivered. Post-operatively, the epidural catheter was left in place and a continuous infusion of 0.25% bupivacaine with 2 μg/ml fentanyl was used for a period of 8 h for analgesia while the magnesium sulfate was gradually reduced. After the epidural infusion was completed the patient was started on patient-controlled morphine. Her blood pressure was observed for 2 h while motor and sensory function returned. She was transferred to her room with a blood pressure of 130/85.

These two cases illustrate several points about the impact of epidural anesthesia on the mother and fetus. In the first case, a possible intravascular injection resulted in fetal bradycardia and transient maternal unresponsiveness. While the latter was obvious, the former was diagnosed by continuous fetal heart rate monitoring and led to rapid forceps delivery. The initial Apgar score of 2 could have reflected the brief period of hypoxia from the bradycardia, possible uterine artery vasoconstriction by high maternal levels of lidocaine and fetal systemic effects of lidocaine 'trapped' within the fetal circulation. The neonate quickly recovered, as evidenced by the Apgar score of 8 at 5 min.

In the second case, the epidural served as part of the treatment of the elevated blood pressure during and after labor and delivery. The vasodilation and relief of pain by the lumbar sympathectomy produced by the epidural anesthetic was achieved slowly to prevent rapid changes in blood pressure. Similarly, when the decision for cesarean delivery was made, bupivacaine was used to slowly raise the level of the block to T2. Although this took 30 min and 30 ml of 0.5% bupivacaine, there was no maternal hypotension to further stress the fetus.

SUMMARY

As discussed at the beginning of this chapter, the ACOG recommendations answer the question as to whether fetal heart rate monitoring is necessary during epidural anesthesia. The answer of 'yes' leaves open the issue of whether continuous electronic monitoring, as opposed to intermittent auscultation of the FHR, is desirable. This issue, in most hospitals, is solved by the availability or lack of adequate nursing coverage.

Epidural anesthesia, while safe and effective during labor and delivery, does have potential complications that can quickly place both the mother and fetus at risk of hypoxia or asphyxia. This can occur rapidly and requires prompt recognition to treat and reverse the cause before there is significant damage. This is where continuous FHR monitoring, in addition to monitoring the mother, is important in both diagnosis and treatment.

There are a number of diseases and conditions particular to obstetrics that place an infant at increased risk of stress during labor and delivery. Given the association of epidural anesthesia with some of these conditions, it is important to monitor both the mother and fetus closely.

REFERENCES

1. ACOG 1988 Statement on Fetal Heart Rate Monitoring. ACOG Newsletter 32: 5
2. ASA 1991 Guidelines for conduction of anesthesia in obstetrics. ASA
3. Reynolds F, Taylor G 1971 Plasma concentrations of bupivacaine during continuous epidural analgesia in labor. Br J Anaesth 43: 436–440
4. Reynolds F, Hargrove R I, Wyman J B 1973 Maternal and fetal plasma concentrations of bupivacaine after epidural block. Br J Anaesth 45: 1049–1053
5. Hyman M D, Shnider S M 1971 Maternal and neonatal blood concentrations of bupivacaine associated with obstetrical conduction anesthesia. Anesthesiology 34: 81–86
6. Shnider S M, Way E L 1968 Plasma levels of lidocaine (Xylocaine) in mother and newborn following obstetrical conduction anesthesia: clinical applications. Anesthesiology 29: 951–958
7. Blankenbaker W L, DiFazio C A, Berry F A 1975 Lidocaine and its metabolites in the newborn. Anesthesiology 42: 325–330
8. Brown W U, Bell G C, Lurie A O et al 1975 Newborn blood levels of lidocaine and mepivacaine in the first postnatal day following maternal epidural anesthesia. Anesthesiology 42: 698–707
9. Epstein B S, Banerjee S G, Coakley C S 1968 Passage of lidocaine and prilocaine across the placenta. Anesth Analg 47: 223–227
10. Lund P C, Cwik J C, Gannon R T et al 1977 Etidocaine for caesarean section – effects on mother and baby. Br J Anaesth 49: 457–460
11. Cowles G T 1965 Experience with lumbar epidural block. Obstet Gynecol 26: 734–739
12. Philipson E H, Kuhnert B R, Syracuse C D 1985 Fetal acidosis, 2-chloroprocaine and epidural anesthesia for Cesarean section. Am J Obstet Gynecol 151: 322–324
13. Aboud T K, Afrasiabi A, Saskis F et al 1984 Continuous epidural analgesia in parturients receiving bupicaine, chloroprocaine or lidocaine – maternal, fetal and neonatal effects. Anesth Analg 63: 421–428
14. Mirkin B L 1975 Perinatal pharmacology: placental transfer, fetal localization and neonatal disposition of drugs. Anesthesiology 43: 156–170
15. Moya F, Smith B 1965 Uptake, distribution and placental transport of drugs and anesthetics. Anesthesiology 26: 465–476
16. Yaffe S J, Juchau M R 1974 Perinatal pharmacology. Ann Rev Pharmacol 14: 219–238
17. Moya F, Thorndike V 1963 The effects of drugs used in labor on the fetus and newborn. Clin Pharmacol Ther 4: 628–653
18. Covino B G, Vassallo H G 1976 Local anesthetics: mechanisms of action and clinical use. Grune & Stratton, New York p 104

19. Levinson G, Shnider S M 1973 Placental transfer of local anesthetics, clinical implications. In: Marx G F (ed) Parturition and perinatology. Williams & Wilkins, Philadelphia pp 173–185
20. Rowland M 1974 Local anesthetic absorption, distribution and elimination. In: Eger E I (ed) Anesthetic uptake and action. Williams & Wilkins, Baltimore pp 332–360
21. Gordon H R 1968 Fetal bradycardia after paracervical block: correlation with fetal and maternal blood levels of local anesthetic (Mepivacaine). New Engl J Med 279: 910–914
22. Moore D C, Bridenbaugh L D, Bagdi P A et al 1968 Accumulation of mepivacaine hydrochloride during caudal block. Anesthesiology 29: 585–588
23. deJong R H 1970 Physiology and pharmacology of local anesthetics. Charles C Thomas, Springfield, IL pp 176–204
24. Hingson R A, Cull W A, Benziner M 1961 Continuous caudal analgesia in obstetrics. Anesth Analg 40: 119–129
25. Holmes F 1960 The supine hypotensive syndrome: its importance to the anesthetist. Anaesthesia 15: 298–306
26. Usubiaga J E, LaTuppa M, Moya F et al 1968 Passage of procaine hydrochloride and para-amino benzoic acid across the human placenta. Am J Obstet Gynecol 100: 918–923
27. Rudolph A M 1974 Congenital diseases of the heart. Year Book Medical Publishers, Chicago pp 1–28
28. Rudolph A M, Heymann M A 1968 The circulation of the fetus in utero. Circ Res 21: 163–184
29. Stave U W 1970 Physiology of the perinatal period. Appleton Century Crofts, New York p 147
30. Finster M, Morishima H O, Boyes R N et al 1972 The placental transfer of lidocaine and its uptake by fetal tissues. Anesthesiology 36: 159–163
31. Wilkinson G R, Lund P D 1970 Bupivacaine levels in plasma and cerebrospinal fluid following peridural administration. Anesthesiology 33: 482–486
32. Biehl D, Callender K, Shnider S M et al 1976 The effect of fetal acidosis on lidocaine blood levels. Abstracts of Scientific Papers. American Society of Anesthesiologists Annual Meeting, San Francisco p 535
33. Cohn H E, Sacks E J, Heymann M A et al 1974 Cardiovascular responses to hypoxemia and acidemia in fetal lambs. Am J Obstet Gynecol 120: 817–824
34. Lending M, Slobody L B, Mestern J 1961 Effect of hyperoxia, hypercapnia and hypoxia on blood–cerebrospinal fluid barrier. Am J Physiol 200: 959–962
35. Odell G B 1959 Studies in kernicterus. 1. The protein binding of bilirubin. J Clin Invest 38: 823–833
36. Shnider S M, Way E L 1968 The kinetics of transfer of lidocaine (Xylocaine) across the human placenta. Anesthesiology 29: 951–958
37. Brown W U, Bell G C, Alper M H 1976 Acidosis, local anesthetics and the newborn. Obstet Gynecol 48: 27–30
38. Brown W U, Bell G C, Weiss J B et al 1977 Mepivacaine in amniotic fluid following maternal epidural anesthesia. Anesthesiology 47: 384–386
39. Mather L E, Long G J, Thomas J 1971 The binding of bupivacaine to maternal and foetal plasma proteins. J Pharm Pharmacol 23: 359–364
40. Teramo K, Benowitz N, Heymann M A et al 1974 Effects of lidocaine on heart rate, blood pressure and electrocardiogram in fetal sheep. Am J Obstet Gynecol 118: 935–949
41. Scanlon J W, Brown W U, Weiss J B et al 1974 Neurobehavioral responses of newborn infants after maternal epidural anesthesia. Anesthesiology 40: 121–128
42. Scanlon J W, Ostheimer G W, Lurie A O et al 1976 Neurobehavioral responses and drug concentrations in newborns after maternal epidural anesthesia with bupivacaine. Anesthesiology 45: 400–405
43. Tronick E, Wise S, Als H et al 1976 Regional obstetric anesthesia and newborn behavior: effect over the first ten days of life. Pediatrics 58: 94–100
44. deJong R H 1970 Physiology and pharmacology of local anesthetics. Charles C Thomas, Springfield, IL pp 63–84
45. Rosen M A, Thigpen J W, Shnider S M et al 1985 Bupivacaine-induced cardiotoxicity in hypoxia and acidotic sheep. Anesth Analg 64: 1089–1096
46. Morishima H O, Heymann M A, Rudolph A M et al 1972 Toxicity of lidocaine in the fetal and newborn lamb and its relationship to asphyxia. Am J Obstet Gynecol 112: 72–79
47. Teramo K, Benowitz N, Heymann M A et al 1976 Gestational differences in lidocaine toxicity in the fetal lamb. Anesthesiology 44: 125–130
48. Greiss Jr F C 1966 Pressure–flow relationship in the gravid uterine vascular bed. Am J Obstet Gynecol 96: 41–47
49. Adamson K, Mueller-Heubach E, Myers R E 1971 Production of fetal asphyxia in the rhesus monkey by administration of catecholamines to the mother. Am J Obstet Gynecol 153: 870–877
50. Greiss Jr F C, Gobble Jr F L 1967 Effect of sympathetic nerve stimulation on the uterine vascular bed. Am J Obstet Gynecol 97: 962–967
51. Nimwegan D V, Dyer D C 1974 The action of vasopressors on isolated uterine arteries. Am J Obstet Gynecol 118: 1099–1103
52. Eng M, Berges P U, Ueland K et al 1971 The effects of methoxamine and ephedrine in normotensive pregnant primates. Anesthesiology 35: 354–360
53. James F M, Greiss Jr F C, Kemp R A 1970 An evaluation of vasopressor therapy for maternal hypotension during spinal anesthesia. Anesthesiology 33: 25–34
54. Shnider S M, deLorimier A A, Holl J W et al 1968 Vasopressors in obstetrics. 1. Correction of fetal acidosis with ephedrine during spinal anesthesia. Am J Obstet Gynecol 102: 911–919
55. Gibbs C P, Noel S C 1976 Human uterine artery responses to lidocaine. Am J Obstet Gynecol 126: 313–315
56. Gibbs C P, Noel S C 1977 Responses of arterial segments from gravid human uterus to multiple concentrations of lignocaine. Br J Anaesth 49: 409–411
57. Belitzky R, Deland L G, Novick L M 1970 Oxytocic effect of intramyometrial injection of procaine in a pregnant woman. Am J Obstet Gynecol 107: 973–975
58. Smith N T, Corbascio A N 1970 The use and misuse of pressor agents. Anesthesiology 33: 58–101
59. Myers R E, Mueller-Heubach E, Adamson K 1973 Predictability of the state of fetal oxygenation from a quantitative analysis of the component of late deceleration. Am J Obstet Gynecol 115: 1083–1094
60. Myers R E 1972 Two patterns of perinatal brain damage and their conditions of occurrence. Am J Obstet Gynecol 112: 246–276
61. Brann A W, Myers F D 1977 The effects of intrauterine asphyxia on the full term neonate. Clin Perinatol 4: 149–161
62. James L S 1959 Physiology of respiration in newborn infants and in the respiratory distress syndrome. Pediatrics 24: 1069–1101
63. Chu J, Clements J A, Cotton E K 1967 Neonatal pulmonary ischemia. 1. Clinical and physiological studies. Pediatrics 40: 709–782
64. Hon E H, Reid B L, Hehre F W 1960 The electronic evaluation of the fetal heart rate. II. Changes with maternal hypotension. Am J Obstet Gynecol 70: 209–215
65. Elmer H, Barcohana J, Bartoshok A K 1960 The influence of postspinal hypotension on the fetal electrocardiogram. Am J Obstet Gynecol 80: 569–572
66. Kandel P F, Spoerel W E, Kinch R A H 1966 Continuous epidural analgesia for labor and delivery: review of 1000 cases. Can Med Assoc J 95: 947–953
67. Norris S, Harris L J, Eisen S M 1960 Epidural anesthesia in obstetrics and gynecology. Obstet Gynecol 16: 15–20
68. Cohn H E, Piesecki G J, Jackson B T 1974 Cardiovascular responses to hypoxemia and acidemia in fetal lambs. Am J Obstet Gynecol 129: 817–824
69. Parer J T 1980 The effect of acute maternal hypoxia on fetal oxygenation and the umbilical circulation in the sheep. Eur J Obstet Gynecol Reprod Biol 10: 125–136
70. Mann L I 1970 Effects in sheep of hypoxia on levels of lactate, pyruvate and glucose in blood of mothers and fetus. Pediatr Res 4: 46–54
71. Jones M D, Sheldon R E, Peeters L I et al 1977 Fetal cerebral oxygen consumption at different levels of oxygenation. J Appl Physiol 43: 1080–1084
72. Fisher D J, Heymann M A, Rudolph A M 1982 Fetal myocardial

oxygen and carbohydrate consumption during acutely induced hypoxemia. Am J Physiol 242: H657–661

73. Jouppila P, Jouppila R, Hollman A, Koivula A 1982 Lumbar epidural analgesia to improve intervillous blood flow during labor in severe pre-eclampsia. Obstet Gynecol 59: 158–161
74. Jones C J P, Fox H 1976 Placental changes in gestational diabetes. An ultrastructural study. Obstet Gynecol 48: 274–280
75. Nylund L, Lunell N-O, Lewander R, Persson B, Sarby B 1982 Uteroplacental blood flow in diabetic pregnancy: Measurements with indium 113 m and a computer-linked gamma camera. Am J Obstet Gynecol 114: 298–302
76. Bahna S L, Bjerkdal T 1972 The course and outcome of pregnancy in women with bronchial asthma. Acta Allergy 27: 397–406
77. Tracy T A, Miller G L 1969 Obstetric problems of the massively obese. Obstet Gynecol 33: 204–208
78. Maeder E C, Barno A, Mecklenburg F 1975 Obesity: a maternal high-risk factor. Obstet Gynecol 45: 669–671
79. Duff P, Sanders R, Gibbs R S 1983 The course of labor in term patients with chorioamnionitis. Am J Obstet Gynecol 147: 391–395
80. Friedman E A, Sachtleben M 1964 The effect of uterine overdistension on labor. 1. Multiple pregnancy. Obstet Gynecol 23: 164–172
81. Little W A, Friedman E A 1958 The twin delivery: factors influencing second twin mortality. A review. Obstet Gynecol Surv 13: 611–623

100. Neurologic complications of regional anesthesia in obstetrics

P. R. Bromage

Neurologic sequelae to regional anesthesia for childbirth present unique problems of etiology and diagnosis because there are two potential sources of neural injury, and due to poor reporting practices the precise incidence of each is still unknown at the present time. Pregnancy and parturition exact their own intrinsic tolls of neurologic deficits, most of which are transient and recoverable, but a very few may result in permanent paraplegia. No formal prospective study of the incidence of this intrinsic type of injury has ever been carried out. A few small-sample surveys were done several decades ago before the liberal practice of pre-emptive abdominal delivery became commonplace. Those figures suggested that the incidence of intrinsic maternal palsy lay somewhere between 1:2100 and 1:6400 during the third and fourth decades of the twentieth century.[1–4]

The incidence of post-partum neurologic sequelae directly attributable to regional anesthesia is also unknown, with widely varying estimates based on incomplete retrospective surveys. The overall etiologic picture is further confused by the creation of a third etiologic source from the interplay of the other two. Here there is a more complex situation where post-anesthetic neural sequelae may have arisen from pre-existing, occult neural pathology that is triggered by the stresses of pregnancy, childbirth and obstetric surgery, and where major regional anesthesia is a possible but unproven contributory factor.

The margins of these three categories are indistinct and it is often difficult, or impossible, to categorize the precise cause of injury with more than a moderate degree of probability. Nevertheless, improved reporting practices and advances in diagnostic technology during the past decade have brought the overall picture into increasingly clear focus, and a three-class categorization provides a useful working approach to etiology and diagnosis.

In any instance of post-partum neurologic injury there are clearly important medical and medico-legal reasons to distinguish between the unavoidable intrinsic maternal causes and the extrinsic iatrogenic components of the injury. This distinction is necessary, not only for appropriate management of the unfortunate individual involved, but also for the attainment of an objective vision of the interventional risks and benefits of regional anesthesia when set against the background balance of risks inherent in natural childbirth. The following examples of the three major categories outlined above will illustrate the diagnostic issues to be resolved, and the directions in which future developments may evolve to improve the safety and appropriate use of spinal and epidural anesthesia in obstetric pain management.

CATEGORY 1. POST-ANESTHETIC NEUROLOGIC SEQUELAE SOLELY ATTRIBUTABLE TO NON-ANESTHETIC CAUSES

Anecdotal case reports and small retrospective surveys of intrinsic obstetric paralysis extend from 1838 to the present time,[1–6] but no large scale prospective studies have been performed because of the formidable practical problems involved. Such a study would require carefully documented pre-delivery and post-delivery neurologic examinations in every mother enrolled in the survey, whether they delivered by natural childbirth or by anesthesia-assisted delivery, in order to distinguish between pre-existing neurologic conditions and injuries arising de novo from labor and delivery alone, and those that might be attributable to regional anesthesia.

At the University of Manitoba, Ong and his colleagues have performed one of the most thorough surveys of neurologic deficits.[7] They evaluated neurologic outcome after 25 827 deliveries in the eight-year period between 1975 and 1983, and they made several interesting observations:

1. No permanent sequelae developed: all the neurologic sequelae were transient and none lasted longer than 3 days.
2. Only 10 of the 45 cases of neurologic deficits had been recorded in the *hospital* record – an indication that retrospective studies of hospital records are not reliable sources of accurate statistics.

3. The incidences of transient neurologic sequelae in the epidural and general anesthesia groups were similar and 5–14 times greater than after delivery with inhalation analgesia, or with no analgesia at all. However, both of these anesthetic groups of patients were likely to include a larger proportion of women who would have developed more serious neurologic injury if they had been allowed to undergo prolonged and difficult forceps delivery.
4. Although the size of the study population was substantial, it was still too small to uncover the incidence of rare, catastrophic cases of neurologic injury attributable to pre-existing disease. Estimates from other studies suggest that a population sample approximately 40 times larger would be required to compare the respective incidences of permanent neurologic sequelae due to intrinsic obstetric causes and anesthesia related events.

One preliminary large scale postal survey, prepared on behalf of the Royal College of Obstetrics and Gynaecologists and the College of Anaesthetists of England was published in 1990.[8] The purpose of this retrospective survey was solely to establish the magnitude of the problem, and it focused on serious non-fatal complications associated with extradural block in obstetric practice, in a sample of 505 000 women from a survey population of 2 580 000 deliveries in the five-year period between 1982 and 1986 inclusive. 108 adverse events were reported from this 19.6% sample of women who had received epidural blocks. Of these 108 events, 29 cases were non-neurologic (e.g. acute toxicity, anaphylaxis, high spinal), making an incidence of 79 out of 505 000 or 1:6400. Pre-delivery neurologic status was not recorded in this preliminary study and so it is impossible to draw any conclusions regarding the contribution of intrinsic maternal palsy to the aggregate number of reported neurologic sequelae. However, 38 of the 108 adverse events were reported as neuropathy of a single nerve. This lower motor neuron type of injury is commonly associated with purely obstetric causes, and so if these 38 cases are excluded, the incidence of anesthesia-related injury would be approximately 1:12 000 cases and close to a generally held estimate of 1:11 000 for anesthesia related injuries,[9] while intrinsic obstetric related injuries would be approximately 1:13 000. These two ratios are very close to one another and they do indicate the need for a very large, very carefully designed and very expensive study, if this matter of intrinsic versus extrinsic obstetric palsy is ever to be settled to any reasonable degree of probability.

Compression nerve trauma

Transient post-partum maternal paralysis most often arises from some degree of cephalopelvic disproportion. The fetal head may compress the lumbosacral trunk as it descends in front of the ala of the sacrum, producing partial injury of the sciatic nerve and classic foot drop.[5] Branches of the lumbar plexus (e.g. lateral femoral cutaneous nerve of thigh – L2, L3; obturator nerve, L2, L3, L4) may be compressed as they course through the pelvis. The femoral nerve, as it passes through the inguinal ligament, is at risk for kinking and ischemic damage from energetic and prolonged flexion of the thighs during a difficult second stage of labor.[15] The resulting injury of a weakened quadriceps and hypoesthesia in the saphenous distribution is largely preventable by ensuring that the mother extends the thighs and relaxes hip flexion between second stage contractions.[10]

Improperly padded lithotomy supports are a peripheral cause of foot drop unrelated to anesthesia or the process of childbirth. Pressure of the metal supports may cause trauma to the common peroneal nerve as it winds around the neck of the fibula just below the knee and care should be taken to cushion this area during forceps deliveries in the lithotomy position.[11]

The severity of compression nerve trauma may range from mild and transient ischemic neuropraxia to complete physical interruption of the axonal elements (axonotmesis). Both extremes of injury usually recover but in different time scales. Mild ischemic neuropraxia may occur in 2–6 days. Since complete axonotmesis heals by axonal regeneration at rates of 0.25–2.00 mm per day, full recovery of long nerves from the lumbosacral trunk may take as long as 2–3 years.[12]

Ischemic injury to the spinal cord

The spinal cord, in common with the brain, can suffer permanent ischemic injury of 'spinal stroke' from inadequate blood flow due to vascular disease or severe arterial hypotension. Conditions that lower arterial inflow pressures, or raise venous outflow pressures, may jeopardize net capillary blood flow and lead to spinal cord infarction. This simple principle of vascular dynamics has become increasingly well-recognized as an underlying mechanism in some previously little-understood but catastrophic forms of post-partum paralysis that may have seemed attributable to regional anesthetic injury.

Obstruction of arteries to the spinal cord

Prior to 1960 it was thought that maternal paralyses, following long labors with cephalopelvic disproportion, were almost entirely explicable by mechanical pressure of fetal parts on nerves of the lumbosacral plexus. By the mid 1960s evidence had become available that interruption of blood flow in ascending branches of the internal iliac arteries was an alternative and more sinister explanation in a significant number of cases.

Between 1962 and 1966 Lazorthes and his colleagues at Toulouse demonstrated a dual and reciprocal blood supply to the termination of the spinal cord. They demonstrated that the primary source descends from the artery of Adamkiewicz (arteria magna) which usually arises from the lower thoracic and lumbar segments between T9 and L2. A secondary and more tenuous supply ascends through the iliolumbar and lateral sacral branches of the internal iliac arteries. These two arterial sources, both ultimately dependent on the integrity of the aorta, anastamose in a small circulus surrounding the tip of the conus medullaris. The relative contributions of these two sources are unequal but reciprocal.[13,14] In 85% of the population the main supply to the conus is from above, via the arteria magna, and the iliac contribution is proportionately tenuous and possibly expendable. In the remaining 15% of the population the arteria magna arises from the upper half of the descending aorta in the neighborhood of T5, and then the ascending iliac branches, lying on the ala of the sacrum, assume a greater contribution to the tip of the conus and the cauda equina. It is these ascending arteries and their territory that are vulnerable to obstruction and injury during protracted labor and instrumental delivery.

Lazorthes' anatomical statistics received clinical confirmation 14 years later in a report of obstetric maternal paralysis from Nigeria. Between 1966 and 1976, 34 cases of maternal palsy were studied at the University of Ibadan. Of these 34 mothers 29 (85%) made a partial or complete recovery. The remaining five mothers (15%) did not recover but remained permanently paraparetic.[6] Subsequent correspondence revealed that none of these five women had received regional anesthesia – a point of great potential medico-legal interest.[15]

Further confirmation of the vulnerability of the iliac arterial supply to the lumbar enlargement comes from reports of sudden paraplegia following intragluteal injections of antibiotics. The anatomic basis for this injury is thought to be accidental injection into the superior gluteal artery and then by direct passage through the rich anastomoses between the superior gluteal artery and the iliolumbar and lateral sacral arteries supplying the cauda equina and the tip of the conus medullaris. Retrograde flow into these arteries has also been postulated, but direct anastomotic flow appears to be a more likely route. Eight cases of this injury have been reported since 1966. One such recent case showed marked atrophy of the thoracolumbar cord on magnetic resonance imaging (MRI), consistent with the late effects of a vascular lesion.[16] Misplaced suspicion is likely to fall on any coincidental spinal or epidural anesthesia if injuries such as these are inflicted during the perioperative period.

A variety of rare diseases and 'natural' causes entirely unrelated to type of anesthesia or anesthetic technique may arise in the peripartum period, and some of these may overlap with precipitating factors to be described later in this chapter. The random nature of these associated but unrelated temporal events is illustrated by scattered reports of paralysis following well-conducted general anesthesia, without any form of supplementary regional anesthesia.[17–21] In every case of neurologic deficit, an independent and urgent neurologic consultation should be sought. But, before doing so it is incumbent on the anesthetist to perform his own neurologic examination and to arrive at his own working diagnosis, based on the classic differential categories of trauma, congenital abnormalities, infection, vascular accidents, degenerative disease and new growth that must be considered in every case where a neurologic deficit arises after anesthesia.

Paralysis due to infection may be viral,[19,21] bacterial[17] or parasitic in origin.[22] Transverse myelitis is most commonly due to para-infectious involvement of the cord or to multiple sclerosis.[23] Hemangiomas of the spinal column are common congenital vascular anomalies and these tend to enlarge during the late stages of pregnancy causing a wide spectrum of local vascular changes and neurologic symptoms. Physical expansion of the hemangioma may cause local compression of the spinal cord and progressive leg weakness, sometimes without disturbing sphincter control.[24] Vascular catastrophes of the spinal cord may arise from an arteriovenous malformation (AVM) causing venous hypertension and reduced capillary flow within the cord,[25,26] or rarely, from rupture of an AVM,[27,18] or from a spinal embolus due to air,[28] or cartilage fragments from a peripheral operative site.[29] Intraspinal neoplasms may be primary or metastatic in origin and may become manifest for the first time following vascular changes associated with regional or general anesthesia.[20] Congenital or acquired intraspinal cysts are extremely rare causes of paralysis that should be included in the long list of differential diagnoses.[30–34]

Regional anesthesia is a very visible *potential* cause of post-anesthetic paralysis and a most plausible target for medico-legal action when any neurologic deficit arises, regardless of whether it is likely to fall in this *category of unrelated injury* or not. For this reason many anesthetists have developed strong reservations about using regional anesthesia unless driven to it by indisputable clinical indications. One 12-month sample of three cases of major paralysis from a single North American institution provides a retrospective glimpse of how close to the brink of medico-legal jeopardy the liberal use of regional anesthesia can bring practitioners of the art.[35]

This sample included one case of permanent paraplegia from an epidural abscess, one bilateral femoral neuropathy and one patient with acute postoperative quadriplegia who recovered after urgent cervical laminectomy performed within a few hours of her primary operation. All three of these neurologic sequelae followed careful general anesthesia without regional anesthesia. During the preoperative informed consent process, each of these patients had been offered and had agreed to either regional or general anesthesia as appropriate alternatives, but on the day of operation, for reasons of convenience, general anesthesia was administered to all three patients.[35] Anesthesia was not incriminated in any of these three cases but it is almost certain that it would have been blamed if spinal or epidural blockade had been used as the primary or supplementary anesthetic, as originally planned in each case.

CATEGORY 2. POST-ANESTHETIC NEUROLOGIC SEQUELAE ATTRIBUTABLE TO REGIONAL ANESTHESIA

Accidental wrongful injections

Wrong drug

Accidental wrongful injections will always remain an inherent, but hopefully remote hazard of invasive regional anesthesia. Wrongful injections are not the sole prerogative of habitually careless or stupid individuals. They are usually due to preoccupation with several simultaneous technical problems or to inattention induced by sleep deprivation or extreme physical fatigue.[36] Wrongful injections can happen in anyone's hands and most of us have been guilty of such a seemingly inexcusable accident at some point in our careers. This writer was the recipient of one of these events in 1947 during an experiment into the respiratory effects of norepinephrine. The operator, who went on to develop a most distinguished career in medicine, mistakenly administered an undiluted intravenous bolus of one milligram norepinephrine instead of an intended injection of one milligram of atropine. The sequence of events was instructive. First, deep-seated upper abdominal ache developed followed closely by headache, suggesting that splanchnic vasoconstriction precedes peripheral vasoconstriction. Shortly afterwards, violent intolerable orthopnea erupted as the systolic pressure rose to 300 mmHg and then gradually subsided without sequelae. All syringes had been labeled with large labels by the experimental subject but the single operator was busy with equipment adjustments and recording apparatus and simply had not noticed the label on the syringe. It was fortunate that the offending syringe contained norepinephrine and not epinephrine, for a one milligram intravenous bolus of epinephrine is generally considered to be a fatal dose and ventricular fibrillation might have been added to the problems of acute left ventricular failure.

Since that incident the writer has always favored low-dose norepinephrine instead of epinephrine as the safer agent for restoration of blood pressure in acute hypotensive emergencies, or for prolonged catecholamine replacement in operations performed under total sympathetic blockade.

The catalog of accidental wrongful injections into the epidural space is long and varied. Once an epidural catheter is in place the patient is at the mercy of human error and the possibility of chemical injury and permanent paralysis. Some extraordinarily bizarre epidural injections that led to permanent paralysis have been reported including collodion.[9] One case of epidural paraldehyde during labor seems almost unbelievable because one would imagine that sense of smell alone would warn the perpetrator. That case resulted in permanent, painful quadriplegia and was awarded the largest monetary damages in Britain to that date.[37]

The outcome of most injurious chemical injections is dose- and concentration-dependent. Some relatively common wrongful injections such as epidural barbiturates seem comparatively innocuous and published accounts relate that the patient became sleepy from vascular absorption of the barbiturate but no lasting paralysis occurred.[38–41] Potassium is less forgiving; published accounts reflect a dose-dependent severity of injury ranging from intense but recoverable motor block and painful depolarizing muscle spasms from the high extracellular potassium, to permanent paralysis.[42–45] Recent reports of wrongful epidural injections include cephazolin[46] and ranitidine in a phenol-containing solution;[47] fortunately, neither of these two cases suffered permanent damage.

These types of accident can only be avoided by constant awareness of their lurking danger. All those in attendance must exercise sustained informed vigilance, with scrupulous attention to clear, accurate labeling of all syringes and infusions, and strict segregation of intraspinal medications from all other routes of administration.

Wrong site

Wrong access site. Patients with multiple venous access sites and under surveillance in busy intensive care facilities are candidates for accidental wrongful epidural connections. Two published accounts of parenteral nutriiton via epidural catheters illustrate this potential danger. One patient who had undergone esophagectomy received 160 ml of hyperosmolar TPN (2000 m.osmol/kg) via his epidural catheter before the error was detected.[48] The other patient had undergone total colectomy. He received 300 ml intralipid TPN 'piggy backed' into a brightly labeled epidural catheter over a period of more than 8 h.[49] Neither case suffered any apparent neurologic damage and it is interesting to note that both patients remained pain free for 24 h after their polypharmic epidural adventure. Perhaps this remarkable analgesic effect may reflect partial but reversible neurologic damage from the very highly osmotic parenteral solutions.

Occult epidural catheter misplacement. To understand the ability of epidural and subarachnoid catheters to migrate to unintended places and the hazards that such migrations entail, it is necessary to consider some basic mechanical properties of the meninges and the catheters themselves. First, the dura mater is tough, resilient and highly resistant to penetration by flexible plastic catheters.[50] Second, the flimsy arachnoid membrane is an important pharmacologic barrier but a very poor mechanical barrier.[51] In many places the arachnoid is very loosely attached to the dural tube and these two membranes are easily separated to reveal the subdural space between them.[52] Third, indwelling epidural catheters have been shown to move outwards or inwards for distances of up to 3 cm.[53] While inward catheter movements (either during insertion or afterwards) cannot penetrate normal intact dura, passage into the underlying subdural space becomes easy if a small cut is made in the dura by rotating the epidural needle.[54,55] In fact, Mehta and Maher recommended just such needle trauma as a precise technical maneuver for intentional cannulation of the subdural space in the management of intractable malignant pain.[56]

Subdural block is characterized by a loculated but extensive pattern of anesthetic spread.[57] As long as the catheter remains in the subdural space, small incremental injections may do no harm,[58,59] but there is the constant danger of further penetration through the delicate arachnoid into the subarachnoid space, and sudden, massive subarachnoid block accompanied by acute arterial hypotension and respiratory arrest if the migration is not detected.[60]

Two contemporary clinical studies from separate institutions (summarized in Table 100.1) provide estimates of accidental subdural and subarachnoid puncture during attempted epidural cannulation in a combined sample of 5682 patients.[57,61] The incidences of both sites of accidental cannulation are very similar and sufficiently common to indicate the need for a high degree of vigilance during continuous epidural infusions. Monitoring should include regular observations of the upper segmental level of analgesia and the intensity of motor block in the lower limbs to give warning of unexpected extensive anesthetic spread, or the remote possibility that some unsuspected neurologic complication may be developing.

Spinal cord injection. Direct injury to the spinal cord may occur during attempted epidural or subarachnoid punctures above the termination of the cord. In conscious patients puncture of the spinal cord is signalled by intense lancinating pain, but this warning sign is absent in anesthetized patients and then permanent paralysis may follow undetected injury to the cord. Subsequent magnetic resonance imaging (MRI) or CT scan may reveal intracord air bubbles as direct anatomical evidence of injury in such cases.[62] Controversy still exists over the propriety of performing thoracic epidural cannulation in anesthetized patients. Some maintain that the risk is small enough to justify the practice in skilled hands[63] while others hold that although the risk may be numerically small, it is potentially catastrophic and only to be undertaken in extraordinary circumstances.[64]

Table 100.1 Epidural catheters: indirect evidence of subdural and subarachnoid migration

Reference		Subdural	Subarachnoid	
	n		Immediate	Delayed
57	2181	0.82%		
61	3500		0.4%	0.2%

Backache

Backache after epidural or subarachnoid anesthesia may arise from a variety of causes. Most are due to needle trauma during induction and are benign and self-limiting. Severe backache is more likely to be due to other causes, some of which are directly related to the anesthetic. Non-anesthetic causes that may be temporarily associated with anesthesia but only indirectly related to it are less frequent and these will be considered separately.

Chemical backache

In the 1980s sporadic reports of arachnoiditis following epidural analgesia with 3% chloroprocaine led to extensive laboratory investigations. The cause was eventually traced to sodium bisulphite, an antioxidant included in the formulation.[65–70] In 1987 the manufacturers replaced sodium bisulphite with the chelating agent disodium ethylene diamine tetraacetic acid (EDTA) and since that time no further cases of 'chloroprocaine arachnoiditis' were reported

However, trouble did not stop there. Shortly after the new formulation became available, reports began to appear of severe post-epidural backache. The back pain was described as very severe, centered deep to the site of epidural injection and lasting approximately 12 h in patients who had received total doses of 23–40 ml epidural chloroprocaine.[71] Two studies in human volunteers indicated that the backache was dose-dependent, without adverse sequelae and probably attributable to the EDTA in the new formulation. Moreover, backache was unlikely to arise if the total epidural dosage was limited to 20 ml or less of 3% chloroprocaine.[72,73]

Postpartum backache

Prolonged backache lasting for more than 3–6 weeks is rare in surgical patients and is almost entirely confined to obstetric patients. Two reports from Birmingham, England suggest that this difference may be due to a combination of anesthetic and obstetrical factors. In a series of 11 701 deliveries during the 8-year period from 1978–1985 the same incidence of prolonged backache (10.5%) was found in women who had delivered by natural childbirth without epidural analgesia, as in those who had cesarean delivery under general or epidural anesthesia, without prior trial of labor. This background incidence of 10.5% rose significantly to 18.7% in women who had received epidural analgesia for labor and delivery, or for trial of labor before cesarean delivery.[74,75]

To understand this apparently profound and deleterious effect of epidural analgesia, one has to appreciate the historical and pharmacological setting in which the series was collected. At that time many British anesthetists were employing surgical concentrations of bupivacaine in the range of 0.375–0.5% for relief of pain in labor when their counterparts in North America were using analgesic concentrations of 0.25% bupivacaine[76] or the more appropriate 0.125% solution favored in Belgium.[77]

Surgical concentrations of local anesthetics, such as those used for relief of pain in labor in the Birmingham study, cause two undesirable effects. First, partial motor block of the muscles of the pelvic floor relaxes the pelvic gutter and removes the normal muscular resistance required to maintain flexion and rotation of the fetal head during its descent through the pelvis, so that a high incidence of malrotation results and duration of the second stage of labor becomes unduly prolonged.[78,79] Second, intense analgesia masks the pain of severe joint strain and permits the mother to adopt and maintain postures during the second stage of labor that may place excessive strain on vertebral and sacroiliac joints, possible prolapse of intervertebral discs, and result in prolonged backache and post-partum disability. Recent trends toward more selective epidural deafferentation, with very low concentrations of local anesthetics mixed with potent lipid-soluble opioids, permit an improved functional compromise between adequate pain relief and preservation of motor tone that is likely to safeguard the natural forces of labor while protecting the integrity of maternal structures from excessive joint strain.[89]

In spite of the high prevalence of post-partum backache, complaints of persistent back pain cannot be ignored and careful search must be made to exclude non-anesthetic causes that may require timely intervention to prevent progression to permanent disability.[81]

CATEGORY 3. POST-ANESTHETIC SEQUELAE ATTRIBUTABLE TO PREDISPOSING PATHOLOGY WHERE MAJOR REGIONAL ANESTHESIA MAY BE A CONTRIBUTORY FACTOR

This is the most complicated of the three broad etiologic categories because it embraces combinations of the other two main categories, and each of these contains its own subset of variables, any one of which may become the basis for an adverse neurologic outcome.

Vascular complications

Classically, 'spinal stroke' or the anterior spinal artery syndrome, is caused by obstruction to part of the arterial inflow to the spinal cord as in the cases of permanent postpartum paralysis cited under *Category 1*. Pure arterial ischemia affects the anterior two-thirds of the cord with loss of motor power and pain and temperature sensation but with sparing of the posterior columns carrying vibration sense and position sense from joint capsules. Infarction arising from obstruction to venous outflow may be less clear-cut with some sparing of motor and pain sensation.[82]

Figure 100.1 outlines the basic physical determinants of spinal cord capillary flow that are common to tissues within any body compartment, whether it be a skull, a limb fascial compartment or the spinal canal. In very rare instances a severe alteration of one of the three pressures in Figure 100.1 may be sufficient to halt capillary flow and cause a localized area of infarction in the cord, but more commonly two, and sometimes all three of the pressures have been affected adversely by a combination of circumstances. Vascular causes of neurologic deficits are conveniently categorized under the three pressures P1, P2 and P3 shown in Figure 100.1.

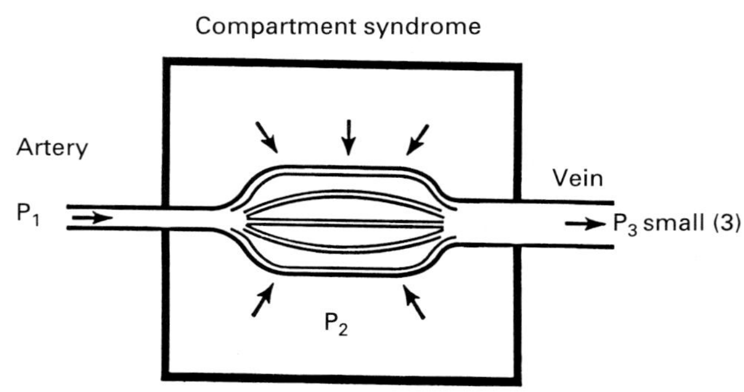

Tissue flow $\alpha \frac{\Delta P_1 - P_3}{P_2}$

$P_1 - P_3 > P_2$ = Health

$P_1 - P_3 \leq P_2$ = Sickness

in

- Skull and spine
- Heart
- Lungs
- Limbs
- Gravid uterus

etc

Fig. 100.1 Conceptual relationships of arterial (P1) tissue (P2) and venous (P3) pressures to capillary blood flow and outcome in closed compartments. P_1–$P_3 > P_2$ = health, P_1–$P_3 \leq P_2$ = sickness in skull and spine, heart, lungs, limbs, gravid uterus, etcetera.

Inadequate perfusion pressure (P1)

Prolonged reduction of arterial pressure (P1 in Fig. 100.1) is an extremely rare cause of anterior spinal artery syndrome after childbirth.[82] Reports of paraplegia following arterial hypotension in non-pregnant patients have usually been associated with prolonged periods of low systolic pressure of 55–65 mmHg lasting more than one hour.[83,84,85] Severe and prolonged hypotension in childbirth is most unusual unless associated with torrential hemorrhage, as in placenta accreta, and followed by coagulopathy and prolonged bleeding.

Adrenaline-containing solutions are sometimes mistakenly cited as a putative cause of spinal cord ischemia in cases of postoperative paralysis where ample alternative causes existed.[83,85,86,87] Three major animal studies of spinal cord blood flow, two with radioactive microspheres and one with the hydrogen clearance technique have all failed to show a reduction of flow with adrenaline, and at the time of writing there is no objective evidence to support the notion that epidural adrenaline has any deleterious effect on spinal cord blood flow.[88,89,90]

Spinal cord tissue pressure (P2)

Changes of epidural pressure are transmitted directly to the spinal and intracranial subarachnoid space, and from thence to the tissues of the spinal cord (P2 in Fig. 100.1).[70] Measurements of epidural and subarachnoid pressures in dogs reflect a simple hydraulic relationship between epidural and subarachnoid pressure, arterial inflow pressure and spinal cord function. Abrupt cord dysfunction occurs when the net spinal perfusion pressure falls below levels in the region of 30–35 mmHg.[70] During childbirth both epidural injections and the natural forces of labor increase epidural pressures and contribute to the overall resistance that must be overcome to maintain viable capillary flow within the cord. The part played by epidural injections is usually small in normal patients of childbearing age, with 10 ml bolus injections increasing epidural pressures by approximately 8 mmHg for 30 s or so.[91] During the first stage of labor each uterine contraction causes a very similar pressure change,[92] but during active expulsive efforts of the second stage, the Valsalva-like efforts raise epidural pressures to 50 mmHg or more, with a correspondingly severe effect on capillary flow within the cord and exacerbation of any underlying impairment of flow due to pre-existing pathology such as spinal stenosis, sclerederma or arteriovenous malformation.[93,94]

These experimental and clinical data illustrate two practical aspects of the occasional association between epidural analgesia and an adverse neurologic sequel. First, complications may be attributable, not to epidural blockade itself but, to the manner of its induction if surges of high intraspinal pressure are generated by hasty injection of large epidural volumes. Second, epidural analgesia should be induced very cautiously and the blood pressure maintained at normotensive levels in patients who display signs of disease or anomalies that may impair epidural compliance and spinal cord blood flow.

Space-occupying lesions such as epidural or subdural hematomas and epidural abscesses that may cause pressure on the cord are discussed in their appropriate chapters on hematologic and infective conditions.

Venous outflow pressures (P3)

Venous infarction of the spinal cord is caused by anything that raises venous outflow pressure to a point where capillary flow is halted for a period of 5 min. High venous pressures in the cord may be due to a generalized rise of venous pressure or to local pathology causing venous hypertension in a limited area of the cord.

Venous hypertension

Generalized venous hypertension from right-sided heart failure or raised intrapulmonary pressure sufficient to cause a neurologic deficit is unlikely to be encountered in childbirth. However, pressure within the azygos venous system and hence in the spinal canal may be raised to high levels if occlusion of the inferior vena cava is allowed to occur.[95] The supine hypotensive syndrome from caval occlusion is now well recognized and avoided by prevention of the supine position during labor. But even today, many patients are still placed in the lithotomy position during the second stage of labor without the precaution of left pelvic tilt. In the presence of severe lordosis this oversight may be sufficient to cause appreciable kinking of the inferior vena cava and raised pressure in the spinal veins draining into the azygos system.

Localized venous hypertension: spinal arteriovenous malformations

Vertebral angiomas are found in approximately 10% of the population, with a 2:1 female predominance.[96,97] These vascular anomalies are remnants of the complex vascular rearrangements in the azygos venous compartment that accompany closure of the embryonic neural tube and its surrounding mesodermal structures during fetal development. Most of these vascular anomalies are harmless but a small minority occur as arteriovenous malformations (AVMs) in the meninges or spinal cord itself, and these anomalies are of great interest to the practicing anesthesiologist because of their potential to cause venous infarction of the cord under the vascular stresses of childbirth and anesthesia.

The hemodynamic properties of spinal AVMs have become increasingly well recognized since the introduction of selective spinal arteriography in the 1970s[98] and more recently following rapid advances in magnetic resonance imaging (MRI) in the 1980s.[99] Intraspinal AVMs have the following characteristics:

1. Approximately 25–30% of spinal AVMs are associated with a cutaneous angioma or nevus in the same metamere.[100] Central venous pressures are transmitted directly to these nevi by valveless veins and so a cough or Valsalva maneuver will distend them and assist in their detection on physical examination.
2. The majority of spinal AVMs arise in the thoracic area but the resulting neural impairment is usually confined to the caudal parts of the neuraxis in the conus medullaris and the cauda equina.[101] One or more small branches of an intercostal artery send feeders to a nidus of neighboring venous networks draining into one or more tortuous longitudinal epidural veins spanning several vertebral segments, and sometimes the entire length of the spinal canal.[98,99]
3. Arterial inflow pressure to the AVM is transmitted through the valveless spinal veins resulting in high venous outflow pressures in the affected segments of the cord.
4. AVMs tend to enlarge in response to the hormonal changes of pregnancy, and symptoms of sensory and motor loss in the legs may emerge in the third trimester or shortly after delivery.[25]

The clinical implications of these vascular anomalies follow logically from their physical characteristics. First, detection of a cutaneous nevus on the trunk or limbs should arouse suspicion that it is likely to be accompanied by a spinal AVM in the same metamere, with engorged epidural veins extending cranially or caudally over several segments, presenting a target for trauma from epidural or spinal needles and catheters, and necessitating extreme technical caution. Any additional history of sensory or motor changes in the legs should be taken as a sign that pathologic changes are already in progress and that spinal or epidural blockade should be avoided altogether. Second, efforts should be made to maintain arterial pressure at normal levels throughout the perioperative period if suspicion of an intraspinal AVM has been aroused by the presence of a cutaneous nevus. Acute hypertension may rupture a dilated epidural vein causing fulminant epidural hematoma formation and acute paraplegia,[102] while arterial hypotension may precipitate venous infarction of the cord from inadequate capillary blood flow.[94]

In the light of contemporary evidence it is probable that a significant proportion of unexplained paraplegias and cauda equina syndromes following spinal puncture or general anesthesia were precipitated by changes of hemodynamic and intraspinal pressures superimposed upon a localized area of impaired capillary flow within the substance of the spinal cord and within the vascular territory of an unrecognized and unsuspected AVM.[102,103,104,105,106,107]

Spinal hematoma

Bleeding into the epidural, subdural or subarachnoid space may give rise to hematoma formation and compression of the spinal cord. Recent advances in coagulation problems are discussed in Chapter 55. Little progress has been made in the development of tests to predict the danger of intraspinal hematoma formation from spinal puncture in conditions where coagulation processes may be compromised.

There is general agreement that the platelet count is a good predictor and that low counts below 100×10^9 l are associated with prolonged bleeding times. Counts below $50–60 \times 10^9$/l should be considered as a contraindication to spinal or epidural anesthesia.[108] Thromboelastography appears to be a useful diagnostic advance but it is still under evaluation and it is an expensive and time-consuming test.[109]

It is the opinion of this author and others that the modified Ivy bleeding time remains the best clinical test available to anesthetists for rapid bedside prediction of the danger of intraspinal hematoma formation.[110,111] In spite of recent criticism that the Ivy bleeding time is insensitive and unreliable in the hands of non-hematologists,[112,113] it does provide repeatable results *in trained hands*, and anesthetists can readily acquire the requisite technical skill using the disposable Simplate II device. The test is particularly useful while on night duty in a busy obstetric unit when results are needed in a hurry and when laboratory response times are likely to be slow. Modified Ivy bleeding times of 10 min or less can be accepted with assurance that abnormal intraspinal bleeding is unlikely to occur. Nevertheless, the anesthetist is still responsible to exercise due vigilance in the post-partum period to ensure that full motor and sensory function has returned after a subarachnoid or epidural block and that spinal cord compression is not developing.

Infection

Difficult decisions must be made when epidural and subarachnoid anesthesia are indicated in patients who show evidence of infectious pathology that may place them in *Category 1* of the three classes of neurologic risk but who will enter *Category 3* once a central block is performed. Example of such dilemmas include patients with chorioamnionitis who would be likely to benefit from regional anesthesia for vaginal or abdominal delivery, those with acute herpes simplex infection[114] or individuals known to be HIV-positive. Three basic safety conditions are required to address the associated but usually unrelated risk of regional anesthesia in these cases.[115]

1. A fully informed consent process where the risks and the benefits of the proposed anesthetic plan are disclosed and accepted.
2. Exercise of prudent precautions to avoid bacterial infection of the spinal canal. This may include administration of appropriate antibiotics before induction of central neural blockade.[116,117]
3. Possession and exercise of necessary skills and vigilance to recognize early signs of impending neurological complications and to institute appropriate diagnostic and therapeutic steps in a timely fashion. Urgent spinal decompression remains the cardinal factor in neurologic recovery from an acute epidural abscess.[118,119,120,121]

SUMMARY

The background risk of obstetric neurologic injury from 'natural' causes is small and imprecisely known. The evolution of interventional pain management has brought its own rare and imprecisely known share of side-effects and neurologic risk. When these two categories of risk are superimposed it is often difficult or impossible to identify the role played by each in the final picture. To contain the iatrogenic risks and avoid potential complications requires educated vigilance. That vigilance must be sustained from the time the patient is seen until the remote effects of the analgesic procedure have completely dissipated.

Next in importance to vigilance is speed of appropriate therapeutic response, since the period of grace to save a compromised spinal cord is in the range of 6–12 h. Magnetic resonance imaging (MRI) with gadolinium enhancement has virtually replaced ionized radiography as the premier imaging technique and it has supplanted CT scan and myelography except in cases where MRI is unavailable or contraindicated.[122,123,124] While MRI is expensive, economy achieved by eliminating former diagnostic imaging procedures has made it both a safe and cost-effective instrument, well suited to the current societal needs of careful cost-containment.[125]

REFERENCES

1. Tillman A J B 1935 Traumatic neuritis in the puerperium. Am J Obstet Gynecol 29: 660–666
2. Chalmers J A 1949 Traumatic neuritis of the puerperium. J Obstet Gynaecol Brit Emp 56: 205–216
3. Hill E C 1962 Maternal obstetric paralysis. Am J Obstet Gynecol 83: 1452–1460
4. Murray R R 1964 Maternal obstetric paralysis. Am J Obstet Gynecol 88: 399–403
5. Beatty T E 1838 Second report of the new Lying-in-Hospital, Dublin. Dublin J Med Sci 12: 273–313
6. Bademosi O, Osuntokun B O, Van der Werd H J, Bademosi A K 1980 Obstetric neuropraxia in the Nigerian African. Int J Gynaecol Obstet 17: 611–614
7. Ong B Y, Cohen M M, Esmail A, Cumming M, Kozody R, Palahniuk R J 1987 Paresthesia and motor dysfunction after labor and delivery. Anesth Analg 66: 18–22
8. Scott D B, Hibbard B M 1990 Serious nonfatal complications associated with extradural block in obstetric practice. Br J Anaesth 64: 537–541
9 Usubiaga J E 1975 Neurological complications following epidural anesthesia. International Anesthesiology Clinics, Little Brown, Boston, p 19
10. Redick L F 1992 Maternal perinatal nerve palsies. Postgard Obstet Gynecol 12: 1–6
11. Goldstein P J 1978 The lithotomy position. In: Martin J T Positioning in anesthesia and surgery. W B Saunders, Philadelphia p 142–150
12. Brain R W, Walton J N 1969 Brain's diseases of the nervous system, 7th edn. Oxford University Press, Oxford, p 9–12; 756–759
13. Lazorthes G, Poulhes J, Bastide G, Chancolle A R, Zadeh O 1962 La vascularization de la moelle epiniere (etude) anatomique et physiologique. Rev Neurol 106: 535–557
14. Lazorthes G, Gouaze A, Bastide G, Soutoul J H, Zadeh O, Santini J J 1966 La vascularization arterielle du renflement lombaire: études des variations et des suppleances. Rev Neurol 114: 109–122
15. Bademosi O 1984 Personal communication
16. Tesio L, Bassi L, Strada L 1992 Spinal cord lesion after penicillin gluteal injection. Paraplegia 30: 442–444
17. Male C G, Martin R 1973 Puerperal spinal epidural abscess. Lancet i: 608–609
18. Guy M J, Zahra M, Sengupta R P 1979 Spontaneous spinal subdural haematoma during general anaesthesia. Surg Neurol 11: 199–200
19. Neumark J, Feichtinger W, Gassner A 1980 Epidural block in obstetrics followed by aseptic meningoencephalitis. Anesthesiology 52: 518–519
20. Martin H B, Gibbons J J, Bucholz R D 1992 An unusual presentation of spinal cord tumor after epidural anesthesia. Anesth Analg 75: 844–846
21. Gutowski N J, Davies A O 1993 Transverse myelitis following general anesthesia. Anaesthesia 48: 44–45
22. Rizzi I 1935 Su un rara caso di rammollimento ischemico del midollo spinale di natura parassitaria. Contributo allo studio delle mieliti degenerative. Revista di Pathologia Nervosa e Mentale 45: 397–422
23. Jeffery D R, Mandler R N, Davis L E 1993 Transverse myelitis: retrospective analysis of 33 cases, with differentiation of cases associated with multiple sclerosis and parainfectious events. Archiv Neurol 50: 532–535
24. Redekop G J, Del Maestro R F 1992 Vertebral hemangioma causing spinal cord compression during pregnancy. Surg Neurol 38: 210–215
25. Symon L, Kuyama H, Kendall B 1984 Dural arteriovenous malformations of the spine: clinical features and surgical results in 55 cases. J Neurosurg 60: 238–247
26. Liu C L, Yang D J 1988 Paraplegia due to vertebral hemangioma during pregnancy: a case report. Spine 13: 107–108
27. Newbery J M 1977 Paraplegia following general anaesthesia. Anaesthesia 32: 78–79
28. Wikler A, Marmor J, Hurst A 1937 Air embolism to the spinal cord following attempted pneumothorax. J Am Med Assoc 109: 430–431
29. Moorhouse D F, Burke M, Keohane C, Farrell M A 1992 Spinal cord infarction caused by cartilage embolus to the anterior spinal artery. Surg Neurol 37: 448–452
30. Hyndman O R, Gerber W F 1946 Spinal extradural cysts, congenital and acquired. J Neurosurg 3: 474–486
31. Gindre-Barrucand T, Charleux F, Turjman F, Jouvet A, Confavreux A, Deruty R, Froment J C 1991 Magnetic resonance imaging contribution to the diagnosis of spinal cord compression by a subdural arachnoid cyst. Neuroradiology 33: 87–89
32. Manno N J, Uihlein A, Kernohan J W 1965 Intraspinal epidermoids. J Neurosurg 19: 754–765

33. Pear B L 1969 Iatrogenic intraspinal epidermoid sequestration cysts. Radiology 92: 251–254
34. Halcrow S J, Crawford P J, Craft A W 1985 Epidermoid spinal cord tumour after lumbar puncture. Arch Dis Child 60: 578–579
35. Schreiner E J, Lipson S F, Bromage P R, Camporesi E M 1983 Neurological complications following general anaesthesia. Three cases of major paralysis. Anaesthesia 38: 226–229
36. Moore-Ede M 1993 The twenty-four society. Addison-Wesley Reading, Massachusetts
37. Brahams D 1982 Record award for personal injuries sustained as a result of negligent administration of epidural anaesthetic. Lancet 1: 159
38. Forestner J E, Raj P P 1975 Inadvertent epidural injection of thiopental. A case report. Anesth Analg 54: 406–407
39. Wells D, Davies G, Wagner D 1987 Accidental injection of epidural methohexital. Anesthesiology 67: 846–848
40. Aghdami A, Keenan R L, Boyan C P 1979 Inadvertent caudal injection of thiopental. Anesthesiology Review 6: 38–39
41. Cay D L 1984 Accidental epidural thiopentone. Anaesth Int Care 12: 61–63
42. Bromage P R 1978 Epidural analgesia. W B Saunders, Philadelphia, p. 662–663
43. Lin D, Becker K, Shapiro H M 1986 Neurologic changes following epidural injection of potassium chloride and diazepam: a case report with laboratory correlations. Anesthesiology 65: 210–212
44. Tessler M J, White I, Naugler-Colville M A, Biehl D R 1988 Inadvertent administration of potassium chloride. A case report. Can J Anaesth 35: 631–633
45. Shanker K B, Palkar N V, Nishkala R 1985 Paraplegia following epidural potassium chloride. Anaesthesia 40: 45–47
46. Kopacz D J, Slover R B 1990 Accidental cephazolin injection: safeguards from patient-controlled analgesia. Anesthesiology 72: 944–947
47. McGuinness J P, Cantees K K 1990 Epidural injection of phenol-containing ranitidine preparation. Anesthesiology 73: 553–555
48. Patel P C, Sharif A M Y, Farnando P U E 1984 Accidental infusion of total parenteral nutrition solution through an epidural catheter. Anaesthesia 39: 383–384
49. Bickler P, Spears R, McKay W 1990 Intralipid solution mistakenly infused into epidural space. Anesth Analg 71: 712–713
50. Hardy P A J 1986 Can epidural catheters penetrate dura mater? An anatomical study. Anaesthesia 41: 1146–1147
51. Bernards C, Hill H F 1990 Morphine and alfentanil permeability through the spinal dura, arachnoid and pia mater of dogs and monkeys. Anesthesiology 73: 1214–1219
52. Blomberg R G 1987 The lumbar subdural extraarachnoid space of humans: an anatomical study using spinaloscopy in autopsy cases. Anesth Analg 66: 177–180
53. Phillips D C, Macdonald R 1987 Epidural catheter migration during labour. Anaesthesia 42: 661–663
54. Meiklejohn B H 1987 The effect of rotation of an epidural needle: an in vitro study. Anaesthesia 42: 1180–1182
55. Woerth S D, Bullard J R, Calpert C C 1977 Total spinal anesthesia, a late complication of epidural anesthesia. Anesthesiology 47: 380–381
56. Mehta M, Maher R 1977 Injection into the extra-arachnoid subdural space. Anaesthesia 32: 760–766
57. Lubenow T, Keh-Wong E, Kristof K, Ivankovich O, Ivankovich A D 1988 Inadvertent subdural injection: a complication of an epidural block. Anesth Analg 67: 175–179
58. Brown G, Atkinson G L, Standiford S B 1989 Subdural administration of opioids. Anesthesiology 71: 611–613
59. Collier G B, Gatt S P, Lockley S M 1993 A continuous subdural block. Br J Anaesth 70: 462–465
60. Reynolds F, Speedy H M 1990 The subdural space: the third place to go astray. Anaesthesia 45: 120–123
61. Okell R W, Sprigge J S 1987 Unintentional dural puncture. A survey of recognition and management. Anaesthesia 42: 1110–1113
62. Oswalt K 1989 Medical/legal issues in regional anesthesia. Amer Soc Reg Anesth News November, p 4
63. Gough J D, Williams A B, Vaughan R S, Khalil J F, Butchart E G 1988 The control of post-thoracotomy pain. A comparative evaluation of thoracic epidural fentanyl infusions and cryo-analgesia. Anaesthesia 43: 780–783
64. Bromage P R 1989 The control of post-thoracotomy pain. Anaesthesia 44: 445
65. Ravindran R S, Bond B K, Tasch M D, Gupta C D, Luerssen T G 1980 Prolonged neural blockade following regional analgesia with 2-chloroprocaine. Anesth Analg 59: 447–451
66. Covino B G, Marx G F, Finster M, Zsigmond E K 1980 Prolonged sensory/motor deficits following inadvertent spinal anesthesia. Anesth Analg 59: 399–400
67. Reisner L S, Hocjman B N, Plummer M H 1980 Persistent neurologic deficit and adhesive arachnoiditis following intrathecal 2-chloroprocaine injection. Anesth Analg 59: 452–454
68. Barsa J, Batra M, Fink B R, Sumi S M 1982 A comparative in vivo study of local neurotoxicity of lidocaine, bupivacaine, 2-chloroprocaine and a mixture of 2-chloroprocaine and bupivacaine. Anesth Analg 61: 561–567
69. Gissen A J, Datta S, Lambert D 1984 The chloroprocaine controversy. II. Is chloroprocaine neurotoxic? Reg Anesth 9: 135–145
70. Gissen A J, Datta S, Lambert D 1984 The chloroprocaine controversy. I. A hypothesis to explain the neural complications of chloroprocaine epidural. Reg Anesth 9: 124–134
71. Fibuch E F, Opper S E 1989 Back pain following epidurally administered Nesacaine-MPF. Anesth Analg 69: 113–115
72. Hynson J M, Sessler D I, Glosten B 1991 Back pain in volunteers after epidural anesthesia with chloroprocaine. Anesth Analg 72: 253–256
73. Stevens R A, Chester W L, Artuso J D, Bray J G, Nellestein J A 1991 Back pain after epidural anesthesia with 2-chloroprocaine in volunteers. Reg Anesth 16: 199–203
74. MacArthur C, Lewis M, Knox E G, Crawford J S 1990 Epidural anaesthesia and long term backache after childbirth. Br Med J 301: 9–12
75. MacArthur C, Lewis M, Knox E G 1992 Investigation of long term problems after obstetric epidural anaesthesia. Br Med J 304: 1279–1282
76. Bromage P R 1969 An evaluation of bupivacaine for epidural analgesia in obstetrics. Can J Anaesth 16: 46–56
77. Vanderick G, Geerinckx K, Van Steenberge A, De Muylder E 1974 Bupivacaine 0.125% in epidural block analgesia during childbirth: clinical evaluation. Br J Anaesth 46: 838–844
78. Johnson W L, Winter W W, Eng M, Bonica J J, Hunter C A 1972 Effect of pudendal, spinal, and peridural block anesthesia on the second stage of labor. Am J Obstet Gynecol 113: 166–175
79. Walton P, Reynolds F 1984 Epidural analgesia and instrumental delivery. Anaesthesia 39: 218–223
80. Vertommen J D, Vandermeulen E, Van Aken H, Vaes L, Soetens M, Van Steenberge A, Mourisse P, Willaert J, Noorduim H, Devlieger H, Van Assche A F 1991 The effects of the addition of sufentanil to 0.125% bupivacaine on the quality of analgesia during labor and on the incidence of instrumental deliveries. Anesthesiology 74: 809–814
81. Simon J N, Mokriski B, Gillies B S, Martz D G, Keene C L, Malinow A M 1989 Spinal cord compression following labor and delivery with epidural analgesia. Reg Anesth 14: 256–258
82. Foo D, Rozier A B 1983 Anterior spinal artery syndrome and its natural history. Paraplegia 21: 1–10
83. Urquhart-Hay D 1969 Paraplegia following epidural analgesia. Anaesthesia 24: 461–470
84. Urquhart-Hay D, Teague C A 1974 Spinal thrombophlebitis after prostatectomy with hypotensive anaesthesia. Case report. New Zealand Med J 79: 654–656
85. Harrison P 1975 Paraplegia following epidural analgesia. Anaesthesia 30: 778–782
86. Bromage P R 1974 Spinal thrombophlebitis after hypotensive anaesthesia. New Zealand Med J 80: 519 (C)
87. Bromage P R 1976 Paraplegia following epidural analgesia: a misnomer. Anaesthesia 31: 947–949
88. Kozody R, Palahniuk R J, Wade J G, Cumming M 1984 The effect of subarachnoid epinephrine and phenylephrine on spinal cord blood flow. Can J Anaesth 31: 503–508
89. Porter S S, Albin M S, Watson W A, Bunegin L, Patoja G 1985

Spinal cord and cerebral blood flow responses to subarachnoid injection of local anesthetics with and without epinephrine. Acta Anaesth Scand 29: 330–338
90. Dohi S, Takeshima R, Naito H 1987 Spinal cord blood flow during spinal anesthesia in dogs: The effects of tetracaine, epinephrine, acute blood loss and hypercapnia. Anesth Analg 66: 599–606
91. Usubiaga J E, Wikinski J A, Usubiaga L E 1967 Epidural pressure and its relation to spread of anesthetic solutions in the epidural space. Anesth Analg 46: 440–446
92. Bromage P R 1961 Continuous lumbar epidural analgesia for obstetrics. Can J Anaesth 85: 1136–1140
93. Eastwood D W 1991 Anterior spinal artery syndrome after epidural anesthesia in a pregnant diabetic patient with scleredema. Anesth Analg 73: 90–91
94. Woodall N, Huggins N J, Jewkes D A 1990 Postoperative paraplegia in a patient with an unsuspected arteriovenous-malformation. Br J Anaesth 64: 638–641
95. Galbert M W, Marx G F 1974 Extradural pressures in the parturient patient. Anesthesiology 40: 499–502
96. Junghanns H 1932 Uber die Haufigkeit gutartiger Geschwulste in den Wirbelkorpern (Angiome, Lipome, Osteome) Arch fur Klinische Chirurgie 169: 204–212
97. Ross J S, Masaryk T J, Madis M T et al 1987 Vertebral hemangiomas: MR imaging. Radiology 165: 165–169
98. Kendall B E, Logue V 1977 Spinal epidural angiomatous malformations draining into intrathecal veins. Neuroradiology 13: 181–189
99. Hirsch N P, Child C S, Wijetilleka S A 1985 Paraplegia caused by spinal angioma–possible association with epidural analgesia. Anesth Analg 64: 937–940
100. Doppman J L, Wirth F P, Di Chiro G, Ommaya A K 1969 Value of cutaneous angiomas in the arteriographic localization of spinal-cord arteriovenous malformations. New Eng J Med 281: 1440–1444
101. Mourier K L, Gelbert F, Rey A et al 1989 Spinal dural arteriovenous malformations with perimedullary drainage: indications and results of surgery in 30 cases. Acta Neurochirurgica (Wien) 100: 136–141
102. Eastwood D W 1991 Hematoma after epidural anesthesia: relationship of skin and spinal angiomas. Anesth Analg 73: 352–354
103. Dunn D W, Ellison J 1981 Anterior spinal artery syndrome during the postpartum period. Arch Neurol 38: 263
104. Warner D O, Danielson D R, Restall C J 1987 Temporary paraplegia following spinal anesthesia in a patient with a spinal cord arteriovenous malformation. Anesthesiology 66: 236–237
105. Sghirlanzoni A, Gemma M, Pareyson D, Cimino C, Boiardi A 1989 Spinal arteriovenous fistula: a possible cause of paraparesis after epidural anaesthesia. Anaesthesia 44: 831–833
106. Awad I A, Barnett G H 1990 Neurological deterioration in a patient with spinal arteriovenous malformation following lumbar puncture. J Neurosurg 72: 650–653
107. Metzger G, Singbartl G 1991 Spinal epidural hematoma following epidural anesthesia versus spontaneous spinal subdural hematoma. Two case reports. Acta Anaesth Scand 35: 105–107
108. Ramanathan J, Sibai B M, Vu T, Chauhan D 1989 Correlation between bleeding times and platelet counts in women with preeclampsia undergoing cesarean section. Anesthesiology 71: 188–191
109. Tuman K J, McCarthy R J, March R J et al 1991 Effects of epidural anesthesia and analgesia on coagulation and outcome after major vascular surgery. Anesth Analg 73: 689–704
110. MacDonald R 1991 Editorial. Aspirin and extradural blocks. Br J Anaesth 66: 1–3
111. Bromage P R 1992 Epidural anesthesia in the anticoagulated patient. Anesthesiology Review 19: 22–24
112. Rodgers R P C, Levin J 1990 A critical reappraisal of the bleeding time. Seminars in Thrombosis and Hemostasis 16: 1–20
113. Editorial 1991 The bleeding time. Lancet 337: 1447–1448
114. Bader A M, Camann W R, Datta S 1990 Anesthesia for cesarean delivery in patients with herpes simplex virus type-2 infections. Regional Anesthesia 15: 261–263
115. Davies J M, Thistlewood J M, Rolbin S H, Douglas M J 1988 Panel summary. Infections and the parturient: anaesthetic considerations. Can J Anaesth 35: 270–277
116. Yoder P R, Gibbs R S, Blanco J D, Castaneda Y S, St Clair P J 1983 A prospective, controlled study of maternal and perinatal outcome after intra-amniotic infection at term. Am J Obstet Gynecol 145: 695–701
117. Carp H, Bailey S 1990 Meningitis after dural puncture in bacteremic rats. Anesthesiology 73: A 862
118. Hancock D O 1973 A study of 49 patients with acute spinal extradural abscess. Paraplegia 10: 285–288
119. Baker A S, Ojemann R G, Swartz M N, Richardson E P 1975 Spinal epidural abscess. New Engl J Med 293: 463–468
120. Russell N A, Vaughan R, Morley T P 1979 Spinal epidural infection. Canad J Neurol Sci 6: 325–328
121. Danner R L, Hartman B J 1987 Update of spinal epidural abscess: 35 cases and review of the literature. Rev Infect Dis 9: 265–274
122. Sze G, Bravo S, Krol G 1989 Spinal lesions: quantitative and qualitative temporal evolution of gadopentate dimeglumine enhancement in MR imaging. Radiology 170: 849–856
123. Byrne T N 1992 Spinal cord compression from epidural metastases. New Engl J Med 327: 614–619
124. Arlien-Soborg P, Kjaer L, Praestholm J 1993 Myelography, CT, and MRI of the spinal canal in patients with myelopathy: a prospective study. Acta Neurol Scand 87: 95–102
125. du Boulay G H, Hawkes S, Lee C C, Teather B A, Teather D 1990 Comparing the cost of spinal MR with conventional myelography and radiculography. Neuroradiol 32: 124–136

101. Ethical problems: Jehovah's Witness

V. Manica

Caring for a patient who is a Jehovah's Witness can pose ethical, moral, and legal problems for the anesthesiologist. In the operating room, the anesthesiologist oversees the administration of blood and blood products. A conflict can develop as a result of the refusal of Jehovah's Witness patients to accept blood or blood products, including whole blood, packed erythrocytes, plasma and platelets. Some, but only a small minority, will accept albumin, antihemophilic products (cryoprecipitate) or immune serum globulin.

RELIGIOUS BACKGROUND

Their refusal of blood (whole blood, packed erythrocytes, plasma and platelets) tranfusion is based on a literal interpretation of certain passages from the Bible:

> . . . every moving thing that liveth shall be meat for you; even as the green have I given you all things. But flesh with the life thereof, which is the blood thereof, shall ye not eat. (Genesis, 9: 3, 4)

> . . . therefore I said unto the children of Israel, ye shall eat the blood of no manner of flesh: for the life of all flesh is the blood thereof: whosoever eateth it shall be cut off (Leviticus, 17:14)

> . . . wherefore my sentence is: that they abstain from meats offered to idols, and from fornication, and from things strangled, and from blood.' (Acts, 15:19, 20)

ETHICAL CONSIDERATIONS

Physicians are ethically bound by the oath of Hippocrates or Maimonides to preserve life, and this may require the use of blood transfusion. Conversely, physicians have a moral obligation to respect their patients' wishes, including their religious beliefs. However, the physicians can be placed in a precarious ethical and legal position when patients endanger their lives by refusing certain medical treatments (e.g. blood transfusion).

LEGAL CONSIDERATIONS

In many situations, these decisions are made by another party, on behalf of the patient. Examples include the parent deciding for a minor child, or a patient's family stating that the patient should not receive a blood transfusion. Because of these controversies, the issue of blood transfusion for these patients has been addressed by different courts of law. Unfortunately, the law has been very ambiguous, with decisions varying from case to case and from state to state. To minimize these potential problems, each hospital should develop specific protocols to guide the management of such patients who refuse blood transfusions on religious beliefs. These protocols should address both elective and emergency situations.

Pregnant Jehovah's Witnesses pose a special problem, because the mother's management also directly involves the unborn fetus. The courts seem to favor, at least at this point, the viable fetus in late gestation. The rights of the fetus early in gestation, however, have not been completely addressed, since this issue involves determining when a fetus becomes viable, as well as the rights of termination of gestation in early pregnancy.

For example, a pregnant Jehovah's Witness patient who may or may not have minor dependent children at home cannot endanger her life by refusal of blood transfusion because of religious beliefs, because she has a responsibility to the community to care for her minor, born or unborn, children. Several states have this case law. As a result, she could be forced by a court order to receive the undesired, but necessary, treatment. The interest of the unborn fetus in late pregnancy will supersede the mother's rights or wishes and the state's interests will prevail.

When admitting these pregnant patients, it should be made clear that, if the situation requires, blood will be transfused to save the life of the fetus. This issue should be addressed during the pregnancy by the obstetric care team and the position of the physician and the hospital explained to the patient. In the event that a pregnant patient refuses blood therapy, but an emergency situation ensues, a court order must be sought in order to proceed with the blood transfusion.

MEDICAL CONSIDERATIONS

The anesthesiologist should always discuss all alternatives with the patient and her family and also conduct a detailed interview to find out to what specific blood product transfusion the patient has an objection. However, it is the responsibility of the primary care physician to have already discussed the subject with the patient. For nonobstetric surgery in the pregnant patient, where the prospect of transfusion is high and the patient agrees to autotransfusion, autologous blood should be made available, if this is unacceptable to the patient, then a cell saver technique may be used during the procedure, provided there is a continuous circuit and the blood does not leave this circuit. The use of the cell saver may not be feasible at operative delivery because of contamination of the blood with amniotic fluid, fetal cells, meconium and adipose tissue.

Plasma substitutes are another alternative that has been used to replenish blood volume; these include both crystalline and colloid solutions. Administration of crystalloids (normal saline and lactated Ringer's) can lower the hematocrit by hemodilution, but is followed by marked intraoperative edema. Conversely, colloid administration can result in prolonged anemia and hypervolemia postoperatively, with difficulty in removing the colloid solutions by diuresis. Hetastarch (Hespan) solutions have been used successfully as plasma expanders, but they increase the risk of coagulopathy if administered in large volumes. Some of the most recent studies have concluded that a total amount of 1.5 per/kg of normal body weight of Hespan will avoid possible complications. Desmopressin (DDAVP), a synthetic vasopressin, has also been used in cases where coagulation times were prolonged, so it could have some place in the management of Jehovah's Witness patients preoperatively. Fluosol DA, a synthetic oxygen-carrying compound, has been used in certain circumstances, but it requires either general anesthesia and endotracheal intubation or a hyperbaric chamber in order to obtain $P\text{aO}_2$ over 300 mmHg. It has been effective in the treatment of short-term anemia, but it is not yet approved by the Food and Drug Administration for this use, because of reported anaphylactic reactions. Epsilon-aminocaproic acid (EACA), a synthetic lysine analog, is an antifibrinolytic agent that inhibits plasmin formation by binding plasminogen to fibrin. It has been used to control severe bleeding in post-partum hemorrhage, however an increased incidence of pulmonary edema precludes its use. Recombinant human erythropoietin, immune serum globulin, danazol, conjugated estrogens and polymerized stroma-free hemoglobin are some of the other products investigated as alternative choices for the management of nonpregnant Jehovah's Witness patients when blood transfusions are refused and emergency situations arise.

REFERENCES

1. Benson K T 1989 The Jehovah's Witness patient: considerations for the anesthesiologist. Anesth Analg 69: 647
2. Samuels J 1989 Preanesthetic assessment: the patient who is a Jehovah's Witness. Anesthesiol News 21
3. Wong D H, Jenkins L C 1989 Surgery in Jehovah's Witnesses Can J Anesth 36(5): 578
4. Gibbs R F 1988 Blood transfusion for Jehovah's Witnesses. In Legal Medicine. American Society of Legal Medicine, CV Mosby, St. Louis, p 365
5. *Raleigh-Fitkin-Paul Morgan Memorial Hospital v. Anderson* 1964, 42 N. J. 421, 201 A.2d 537
6. *Jefferson v. Griffin Spalding County Hospital Authority* 1981, 274 S.E. 2d. 457
7. *Roe v. Wade*, 410 US 113, 93 S Ct 705 (1973)
8. *Application of the President and Directors of Georgetown College* 1964, 331 F 2d. 1000
9. Bragg L E 1990 Management strategies in the Jehovah's Witness patient. Contemp Surg 36: 45
10. Stone D J 1988 DDAVP to reduce blood loss in Jehovah's Witnesses. Anesthesiology 69(6): 1028
11. Howell P J, Bamber P A 1987 Severe acute anaemia in a Jehovah's Witness. Survival without blood transfusion. Anaesthesia 42: 44
12. Sacks D A, Koppes R H 1986 Blood transfusion and Jehovah's Witness: medical and legal issues in obstetrics and gynecology. Am J Obstet Gynecol 154(3): 483
13. Brigham and Women's Hospital 1983 Hospital policy for administering blood to Jehovah's Witnesses. Brigham and Women's Hospital, Boston
14. Bonakdar M I, Ecknous A W 1982 Major gynecologic and obstetric surgery in Jehovah's Witnesses. Obstet Gynecol 60: 587
15. Tremper K K, Levine E 1981 The perioperative treatment of severely anemic patients with a perfluorochemical blood substitute, Fluosol D A-20%. Anesthesiology 55(3): A9
16. Dixon J L 1981 Jehovah's Witness. The surgical/ethical challenge. J Am Med Assoc 246: 2471
17. Dornette W H 1972 Jehovah's Witnesses and blood transfusion: the horns of a dilemma. Anesth Analg 52: 272
18. Jehovah's Witnesses and the Question of Blood 1977. Watchtower and Bible Tract Society, New York, p1

Index